BIRTH DEFECTS
❖ ENCYCLOPEDIA ❖

The Comprehensive, Systematic, Illustrated Reference Source for the Diagnosis, Delineation, Etiology, Biodynamics, Occurrence, Prevention, and Treatment of Human Anomalies of Clinical Relevance

VOLUME II
I – Z

Mary Louise Buyse, M.D.

Editor-in-Chief

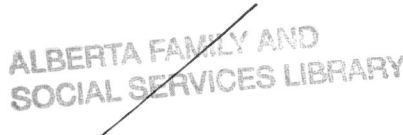

CENTER FOR BIRTH DEFECTS INFORMATION SERVICES, INC.

Dover Medical Building   30 Springdale Avenue   Box 1776   Dover, MA 02030   U.S.A.

Tel. (508) 785-2525   **BDFax** (508) 785-BDIS   Fax. (508) 785-2526

The **BIRTH DEFECTS ENCYCLOPEDIA**
is a service of the
Center for Birth Defects Information Services, Inc.

Dover Medical Building
30 Springdale Avenue   Box 1776
Dover, MA   02030   U.S.A.

Published in association with
Blackwell Scientific Publications

238 Main Street,
  Cambridge, Massachusetts 02142, USA
Osney Mead, Oxford OX2 0EL, England
25 John Street, London, WC1N 2BL, England
23 Ainslie Place, Edinburgh, EH3 6AJ, Scotland
54 University Street, Carlton, Victoria 3053, Australia

Other editorial offices:

Arnette SA, 1 rue de Lille, 75007 Paris, France
Blackwell-Wissenschaft, Düsseldorfer Str. 38, D-10707, Berlin,
  Germany
Blackwell MZV, Feldgasse 13, A-1238 Vienna, Austria

Distributors:

USA
  Blackwell Scientific Publications
  238 Main Street
  Cambridge, Massachusetts 02142
  (Telephone orders: 800-759-6102 or 617-225-0401)

Canada
  Times Mirror Professional Publishing
  130 Flaska Drive
  Markham, Ontario L6G 1B8
  (Telephone orders: 800-268-4178 or 905-470-6739)

Australia
  Blackwell Scientific Publications (Australia) Pty Ltd
  54 University Street
  Carlton, Victoria 3053
  (Telephone orders: 03-347-0300)

Outside North America and Australia
  Blackwell Scientific Publications, Ltd.
  c/o Marston Book Services, Ltd.
  P.O. Box 87
  Oxford   OX2 0DT
  England
  (Telephone orders: 44-865-791155)

Typeset by The William Byrd Press
Printed and bound by Arcata/Halliday

Blackwell Scientific Publications, Inc.
©1990 by The Center for Birth Defects Information Services, Inc.
Printed in the United States of America
94 5 4 3

The opinions expressed in this Encyclopedia are those of the
individual authors and editors and are not official statements of the
institutions or Government agencies with which authors and editors
may be affiliated.

All rights reserved. No part of this book may be reproduced in any
form or by any electronic or mechanical means, including
information storage and retrieval systems, without permission in
writing from the publisher, except by a reviewer who may quote
brief passages in a review.

Articles prepared by officers or employees of the United States
Government fit the description in the U.S. Copyright Act of a
"United States Government work" and are subject to the free use
and copyright provisions of the Act.

Library of Congress Cataloging in Publication Data

Birth defects encyclopedia : the comprehensive, systematic,
  illustrated reference source for the diagnosis, delineation,
  etiology, biodynamics, occurrence, prevention, and treatment of
  human anomalies of clinical relevance / Mary Louise Buyse,
  editor-in-chief.
      p.   cm.
  Includes index.
  ISBN 0-86542-228-1
    1. Abnormalities, Human—Dictionaries. I. Buyse, Mary Louise.
    [DNLM: 1. Abnormalities—encyclopedias.   QS 13 B619]
QM690.B57   1990
616'.043–dc20
DNLM/DLC
for Library of Congress
                                                        90-522
                                                        CIP

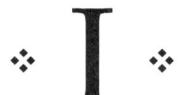

ICHTHYOSIFORM ERYTHROKERATODERMA, ATYPICAL WITH DEAFNESS   2861

Includes:
Burns syndrome
Cornification, disorder of (one form)
Deafness-ichthyosiform erythroderma
Ichthyosiform erythroderma-corneal involvement-deafness
Keratitis-Ichthyosis-Deafness (KID) syndrome
Senter syndrome

Excludes:
Phytanic acid storage disease (0810)
Skin, erythrokeratodermia, variable (0361)
Skin, keratosis follicularis spinulosa decalvans (2867)
Storage disease, neutral lipid type (2859)

Major Diagnostic Criteria: A generalized disorder of cornification characterized by follicular hyperkeratosis and perioral furrowed plaques in conjunction with neurosensory deafness. Progressive neovascularizing keratitis develops in most patients.

Clinical Findings: The disorder of cornification in these patients is quite unique, and is characterized by 1) fixed keratotic plaques; 2) diffuse palmoplantar keratoderma; and 3) a generalized hyperkeratosis with prominent, follicular keratoses elsewhere on the body. The dermatosis presents at birth as erythematous, diffusely thickened skin that desquamates in the first week of life. Fixed, keratotic plaques, often with an erythematous base, are most common on the extremities and face, producing an aged or leonine appearance. Whereas most patients display generalized hyperkeratosis, skin thickening, and follicular prominence, in others, involvement may be limited to the face and extremities. Follicular hyperkeratosis may result in significant alopecia. The nails are hypoplastic or dystrophic, and teeth may be small and carious. The histopathology of the skin is characteristic but not diagnostic, demonstrating "basket-weave" hyperkeratosis.

Neurosensory deafness is nonprogressive and may be severe. Ocular involvement is characterized by keratoconjunctivitis, which progresses to neovascularization and pannus formation. Although keratitis commonly begins in infancy, the onset may be delayed until the second decade. Some patients develop recurrent skin infections, including multiple abscesses, atypical, granulomatous fungal infections, and recurrent deep tissue infections, e.g., pneumonia, otitis, and urinary tract infections. However, an immunologic basis for these lesions has not been established. Squamous cell carcinoma of the tongue has been reported.

Complications: Visual impairment due to progressive keratitis with scarring. The coexistence of deafness, which although nonprogressive may be severe, can add to the sensory handicap. Recurrent skin infections may lead to discomfort and disability. Recurrent pneumonia, otitis, and urinary tract infections may produce morbidity in some patients with this syndrome.

Associated Findings: Tight heel cords, 17%; impaired sweating, 13%. Other reported findings in single patients include cryptorchidism, hepatomegaly, pes cavus, **Hernia, inguinal**, neuropathy, and growth retardation.

Etiology: Most cases have been sporadic. A family with two affected sibs has been reported, suggesting possible autosomal recessive inheritance.

Pathogenesis: Unknown. Elevated serum steroid disulfate levels were reported in one patient.

MIM No.: 24215

POS No.: 3528

CDC No.: 757.197

Sex Ratio: F12:M10 (observed).

Occurrence: A recent literature review identified 23 cases from North America, Europe, and Vietnam.

Risk of Recurrence for Patient's Sib:
See Part I, *Mendelian Inheritance.*

Risk of Recurrence for Patient's Child:
See Part I, *Mendelian Inheritance.*

Age of Detectability: The skin is usually abnormal at birth, but the distinctive cutaneous phenotype may not become apparent until late in infancy. Deafness is congenital and nonprogressive. Keratitis usually begins in infancy, but onset may be delayed until adolescence.

Gene Mapping and Linkage: Unknown.

Prevention: None known. Genetic counseling indicated.

Treatment: Effective therapies for progressive keratitis are unknown. Cutaneous infections should be cultured and treated appropriately. Oral synthetic retinoids are considered experimental because of their toxicity.

Prognosis: Probably normal for life span. Intelligence is normal.

Detection of Carrier: Unknown.

Support Groups: San Francisco; Foundation for Ichthyosis and Related Skin Types (FIRST)

References:
Skinner BA, et al.: The keratitis, ichthyosis and deafness (KID) syndrome. Arch Dermatol 1981; 117:285–289. * †
Legrand J, et al.: Un syndrome rare oculo-auriculo-cutane (syndrome de Burns). J Fr Ophthalmol 1982; 5:441–445. †
Harms M, et al.: KID syndrome (keratitis, ichthyosis, and deafness) and chronic mucocutaneous candidiasis: case report and review of the literature. Pediatr Dermatol 1984; 2:1–7. *
Frieden IJ, Esterly NB: Selected genodermatoses in infants and children. Clin Dermatol 1985; 2:14–32. * †

WI013   **Mary L. Williams**

Ichthyosiform erythryoderma, unilateral-ipsilateral malformations
See LIMB REDUCTION-ICHTHYOSIS

ICHTHYOSIFORM HYPERKERATOSIS, BULLOUS CONGENITAL   2852

Includes:

Bullous congenital ichthyosiform erythroderma
Bullous erythroderma ichthyosiformis congenita of Brocq
Bullous ichthyosis
Cornification, disorder of, bullous type (DOC 3)
Epidermolytic hyperkeratosis
Ichthyosis, bullous type
Ichthyosis congenita, wet type

Excludes:

Ichthyosiform erythroderma, non-bullous congenital
Ichthyosis congenita, dry type
Ichthyosis hystrix, Curth-Macklin type (2857)
Nevus, epidermal nevus syndrome (0593)

Major Diagnostic Criteria: Affected infants are born with widespread areas of blistered or denuded skin. After the newborn period, a severe, generalized hyperkeratosis ensues, that may be accentuated on palms and soles and around joints. Skin biopsy showing histological features of epidermolytic hyperkeratosis is required for the diagnosis, and excludes all other generalized disorders of cornification.

Clinical Findings: The newborn presents with widespread areas of denuded skin, resembling the infant with one of the severe mechano-bullous disorders (**Epidermolysis bullosum**). On careful examination, however, areas of hyperkeratosis may be present. After the neonatal period, as hyperkeratosis becomes prominent, the mechano-bullous component recedes; but focal blistering may continue, and bullae are most often induced by secondary infection rather than trauma. The scales are usually dark and warty, forming a ridged pattern which is particularly evident in the flexures. Verrucous hyperkeratoses in occluded areas become macerated and secondarily colonized by bacteria, producing a foul body odor. Scales may be shed in thick clumps of nearly full-thickness stratum corneum, leaving behind a pink, denuded, and often tender base. An underlying erythroderma is usually evident. Palmoplantar keratoderma is always present but varies in severity. Facial involvement may occur but without ectropion. Although the hair shaft itself is spared, severe scalp involvement results in "nit-like encasements" of hair shafts. Secondary nail dystrophy due to periungual inflammation is common.

Many patients have demonstrated limited and/or localized disease; in this cases, flexural involvement with the formation of spiney ridges is an important diagnostic sign. A wide range in the severity of disease expression occurs in this disorder, but most of this variability apparently is interfamilial rather than intrafamilial.

The skin biopsy distinguishes this disorder from any other generalized disorder of cornification. The epidermis is acanthotic, and the cells of the upper spinous and granular cell layers exhibit intracellular vacuolization; dense clumps of granular material that appear to be enlarged keratohyalin granules but in fact represent clumped keratin filaments; and dense, massive, hyperkeratosis. These features have been termed *epidermolytic hyperkeratosis*.

The histopathologic features of epidermolytic hyperkeratosis are not unique to this generalized disorder of cornification, but occur in such diverse settings as solitary acanthomas, epidermis overlying dermatofibromas, within epidermoid cyst walls, and as an incidental finding on oral mucosa. Furthermore, some kindreds with palmoplantar keratoderma exhibit the histology of epidermolytic hyperkeratosis, but are not at risk for this generalized disease. While epidermolytic hyperkeratosis observed in these other settings does not appear to be part of the phenotypic expression of bullous congenital ichthyosiform hyperkeratosis, there is still some uncertainty as to the relationship of epidermal nevi exhibiting this histopathologic feature and the present disorder.

Complications: The thick, macerated scales in intertriginous areas become heavily colonized with microorganisms resulting in foul body odor. Recurrent blisters on hands and feet may interfere with physical activities, as may thick keratoderma in these areas. Newborns with widespread areas of denuded skin are at high risk for sepsis and fluid/electrolyte imbalance.

Associated Findings: None known.

Etiology: Autosomal dominant inheritance with variability in expression, probably largely interfamilial. At least 50% of the cases reported in literature were sporadic, suggesting new mutations. The rare instances of more than one affected sibling of unaffected parents may represent instances of incomplete penetrance of a dominant trait; or of a phenotypically similar, recessively-inherited trait.

Pathogenesis: The underlying metabolic abnormality is undetermined. The epidermis is hyperproliferative. On electron microscopy, keratin filaments are clumped in lower epidermal cell layers and form ring-like perinuclear shells in upper spinous and granular cell layers. Intraepidermal vesiculation and clefting occurs as a result of loss of desmosomal attachment. Abnormal keratin profiles have been reported by two different groups, but the specific abnormality reported in each case was different, and these changes may represent a secondary disturbance of keratin synthesis consequent to epidermal hyperproliferation. Deficiency of lysosomal α-mannosidase in one patient with this disorder has been observed, but this finding awaits confirmation.

MIM No.: *11380, 14680

CDC No.: 757.190

Sex Ratio: Presumably M1:F1.

Occurrence: First recognized by Nikolsky in the late nineteenth century, numerous cases have been reported worldwide.

Risk of Recurrence for Patient's Sib:
See Part I, *Mendelian Inheritance*. Rare instances of more than two affected siblings with unaffected parents, suggest risk may be increased above general population in this setting.

Risk of Recurrence for Patient's Child:
See Part I, *Mendelian Inheritance*.

Age of Detectability: May be diagnosed *in utero* by fetal skin biopsy because the abnormal clumping of keratin filaments is expressed early in gestation (at least by 20 weeks). Because some amniotic fluid cells exhibit a similar clumped keratin pattern, it may be possible to diagnose this disorder by amniocentesis and examination of the sediment for abnormally cornified cells.

Gene Mapping and Linkage: Unknown.

Prevention: None known; genetic counseling is indicated.

Treatment: Careful attention to fluid and electrolyte balance in affected newborn and surveillance for sepsis. Topical keratolytic agents may be employed to remove thick scales, but are often poorly tolerated because of the blistering tendency of the skin. Systemic toxicity from absorption of these agents, especially corticosteroids and salicylates may occur. Blisters should be cultured and systemic antibiotic administered, because after the neonatal period these are often induced by bacterial infection, particulary *Staphylococcus aureus*. Use of antibacterial soap may improve body odor due to heavy bacterial colonization. Use of oral synthetic retinoids is controversial because of the significant toxicity of these agents, as well as their teratogenecity (see **Fetal retinoid syndrome**). Also, skin fragility with blisters may be exacerbated by retinoids.

Prognosis: Increased morbidity/mortality in neonatal period. Thereafter normal life span. Social adaptation may be impaired by severity of skin involvement. Intelligence is normal.

Detection of Carrier: By clinical examination.

Special Considerations: The term *epidermolytic hyperkeratosis* is in widespread use, because it emphasizes the distinctive skin histopathology in this generalized disorder of cornification, and permits distinction from all other such disorders. However, this histopathology may be seen in other clinical contexts, some of which are genetically transmitted (e.g. an autosomal dominant form of palmoplantar hyperkeratosis) and some of which are not (e.g. normal oral mucosa or over benign skin fibromas). With the exception of epidermal nevi with this histopathology, these other instances do not appear to be part of the phenotypic spectrum of this disorder.

Two reported instances of a father with an epidermal nevus that exhibited the histopathology of epidermolytic hyperkeratosis having an offspring with the generalized disorder of cornification may represent variable expression of the disorder or unrelated, chance occurrence. No instances are reported of the reverse; i.e., a parent with the generalized disorder of cornification with a child with partial expression (i.e., an epidermal nevus). Moreover, monozygotic twins have been discordant for epidermal nevi with epidermolytic hyperkeratosis.

While the histopathology is diagnostic, all features may not be equally well-developed in the fetus and neonate. Careful evaluation by electron microscopy is required looking for clumped keratin filaments, because the abnormal light microscopic features may not be well developed.

Support Groups: Raleigh, NC; Foundation for Ichthyosis and Related Skin Types (FIRST)

References:

Simpson JR: Congenital ichthyosiform erythroderma. Trans St Johns Hosp Derm Soc 1964; 50(New Series):53–104. *

Goldsmith LA: The ichthyosis. Prog Med Genet 1967; 1:185–240.

Holbrook KA, et al.: Epidermolytic hyperkeratosis: ultrastructure and biochemistry of skin and amniotic fluid cells from two affected fetuses and a newborn infant. J Invest Dermatol 1983; 80:222–227.

Lookingbill DP, et al.: Generalized epidermolytic hyperkeratosis in the child of a parent with nevus comedones. Arch Dermatol 1984; 120:223–226.

Eady RAJ, et al.: Prenatal diagnosis of bullous ichthyosiform erythroderma. J Med Genet 1986; 23:46–51.

Williams ML, Elias PM: Genetically transmitted, generalized disorders of cornification: the ichthyosis. Dermatologic Clinics 1987; 5:155–178. * †

WI013   **Mary L. Williams**

ICHTHYOSIS   1511

Includes:

> Collodian baby
> Lamellar exfoliation of the newborn
> Palmo-plantar keratodermas

The ichthyoses encompass a number of unrelated acquired and inherited disorders having in common the accumulation of visible scale on the skin surface. Ideally, the term *ichthyosis* should be replaced because of its derogatory connotations. The ichthyoses may be considered disorders of cornification, where cornification represents those processes leading to the production and maintenance of a normal stratum corneum. Scaling may result either from epidermal hyperproliferation resulting in excessive production of stratum corneum, often with features of incomplete cornification, or from abnormal retention of stratum corneum (i.e., failure to desquamate). The causes of acquired ichthyoses

and the number of genetically transmitted disorders are numerous. At present little is known about their pathogenesis; however, several of the genetic forms are known to be due to inborn errors of lipid metabolism, and among the causes of acquired ichthyosis are some cholesterol-lowering drugs and essential fatty acid deficiency. Because lipids are segregated to the intercellular spaces in stratum corneum, they are in a position to mediate cohesion and desquamation (for review, see Williams and Elias, 1986).

The genetic forms constitute a heterogeneous group exhibiting a wide range of severity of skin involvement, ranging from relatively mild, focal seasonal scaling to severe constrictive horny plates incompatible with life, as well as exhibiting a spectrum of organ system involvement, ranging from skin alone to severe multisystem disease (Goldsmith, 1976; Rand and Baden, 1983; Williams and Elias, 1987).

The clinical features of the individual inherited forms of ichthyosis are described elsewhere in individual articles. Most of the severe forms are evident at birth, and the milder forms usually become evident within the first year of life. However, age of onset is not invariably a reliable indicator of acquired vs. genetic causes; i.e., some genetic forms (e.g., **Phytanic acid storage disease**) may have delayed onset, and, conversely, neonates may be at particular risk for some of the acquired causes (e.g., essential fatty acid deficiency). Evaluation should include a detailed family history, including examination of family members, complete history and physical examination, and, in most instances, a skin biopsy. Usually the biopsy should be obtained from a well-developed area of scaling. Specific laboratory studies, such as examination of a peripheral blood smear, serum lipoprotein electrophoresis, and determination of serum phytanic acid level, may be required to establish or exclude a specific form of ichthyosis.

The appearance at birth of taut, shiny, inelastic, thickened skin with ectropion, eclabion, and fissures; the so-called *collodian baby*, because of the likeness to a film of dried collodian, is not specific to a single genetic disease but may occur in several disorders (Larreque et al, 1976). Most of these infants eventually can be classified as classic **Ichthyosis, lamellar**, congenital ichthyosiform erythroderma, or, in rare instances, another genetic form. However, in many instances, the disorder may resolve. This has been termed *lamellar exfoliation of the newborn* (Reed et al, 1972). Occurrence in sibs suggests that this may also be a genetic entity. The outcome of a collodian baby cannot be predicted, and a precise diagnosis may not be possible until the complete phenotype has developed.

The causes of acquired ichthyosis include xerosis (environmental dry skin), metabolic disorders such as renal insufficiency and hypothyroidism, nutritional deficiency due to malabsorption or essential fatty acid deficiency, and several drugs. In adults it is essential to rule out malignancy as the cause, particularly **Cancer, Hodgkin disease** and bronchogenic carcinoma (Polisky and Bronson, 1986).

Finally, the differential diagnosis of a given patient may include focal disorders of cornification, such as those primarily involving the palms and soles (*palmar-plantar keratodermas*), as well as other genetically determined scaling disorders such as **Darier disease** and **Skin, psoriasis vulgaris**, nongenetic disorders such as pityriasis rubra pilaris, unusual presentations of tinea infections or scabies infestations, and immunologic disorders such as graft vs. host disease.

References:

Reed WB, et al.: Lamellar ichthyosis of the newborn: a distinct clinical entity: its comparison to the other ichthyosiform erythrodermas. Arch Dermatol 1972; 105:394–399.

Goldsmith LA: The ichthyoses. Prog Med Genet 1976; 1:185–240.

Larregue M, et al.: Le bebe collodion evolution a propos de 29 cas. Ann Dermatol Syphiligr 1976; 103:31–54.

Rand RE, Baden HP: The ichthyoses: a review. J Am Acad Dermatol 1983; 8:285–305.

Polisky RB, Bronson DM: Acquired ichthyosis in a patient with adenocarcinoma of the breast. Cutis 1986; 38:359–360.

Williams ML, Elias PM: The ichthyoses. In: Theirs BH, Dobson RL,

eds: Pathogenesis of skin disease. New York: Churchill Livingstone, 1986:519–552.
Williams ML, Elias PM: Genetically transmitted, generalized disorders of cornification. The ichthyoses. Dermatol Clin 1987; 5:155–178.

WI013   **Mary L. Williams**

Ichthyosis congenita (some)
See ICHTHYOSIS, LAMELLAR RECESSIVE
Ichthyosis congenita fetalis
See ICHTHYOSIS, HARLEQUIN FETUS
Ichthyosis congenita gravis
See ICHTHYOSIS, HARLEQUIN FETUS
Ichthyosis congenita, wet type
See ICHTHYOSIFORM HYPERKERATOSIS, BULLOUS CONGENITAL
Ichthyosis follicularis
See SKIN, KERATOSIS FOLLICULARIS SPINULOSA DECALVANS
Ichthyosis hystrix gravior
See NEVUS, EPIDERMAL NEVUS SYNDROME

ICHTHYOSIS HYSTRIX, CURTH-MACKLIN TYPE   2857

Includes: Curth-Macklin syndrome

Excludes:
> **Ichthyosis** (other)
> **Nevus, epidermal nevus syndrome** (0593)

Major Diagnostic Criteria: Generalized or localized disorder of cornification with characteristic skin histopathology of keratin filaments amassed with perinuclear shells and with numerous binucleate keratinocytes.

Clinical Findings: In a large kindred reported by Curth and Macklin (1954), expression varied from palmoplantar hyperkeratosis and focal hyperkeratotic plaques on elbows, knees, and/or ankles, and in severely affected patients, dark, warty hyperkeratoses covering most of the body surface with an underlying erythroderma. Some family members exhibit a milder, generalized hyperkeratosis, clinically resembling **Ichthyosis vulgaris**, while others have had focal hyperkeratosis. Blisters do not occur. This disorder can be distinguished on light microscopy by the presence of numerous (10–30% of total) binucleate keratinocytes and on electron microscopy by the presence of continuous perinuclear shells of keratin filaments within spinous and granular cell layers. In contrast, in bullous congenital ichthyosiform hyperkeratosis, binucleate corneocytes are absent, intraepidermal vesiculation is prominent, and tonofilament clumps are evident ultrastructurally.

Complications: Severe palmoplantar hyperkeratosis may lead to functional impairment and formation of contractures.

Associated Findings: None known.

Etiology: Autosomal dominant inheritance with markedly variable expression.

Pathogenesis: Unknown.

MIM No.: *14659

CDC No.: 757.190

Sex Ratio: M1:F1

Occurrence: In addition to the large kindred from New York City reported by Curth and Macklin (1954), two sporadic cases from the United States and Finland have also been reported.

Risk of Recurrence for Patient's Sib:
See Part I, *Mendelian Inheritance*.

Risk of Recurrence for Patient's Child:
See Part I, *Mendelian Inheritance*.

Age of Detectability: At birth, for severely affected individuals.

Gene Mapping and Linkage: Unknown.

Prevention: None known. Genetic counseling indicated.

Treatment: Topical keratolytic agents (e.g., 5–10% lactic or glycolic acid in petrolatum) are the first line of therapy. Severely affected patients may respond to oral synthetic retinoids. However, in view of the known toxicity of these drugs, treatment should be considered on an individual basis.

Prognosis: Disease is persistent. Normal life span and intelligence.

Detection of Carrier: Clinical examination of the skin for elbow, knee, and palmoplantar hyperkeratoses.

Special Considerations: The term *ichthyosis hystrix* is subject to much confusion in the medical literature. Without the addition of an eponym, it is commonly used to indicate a bilaterally distributed epidermal nevus (i.e., focal warty hyperkeratoses distributed along the lines of cutaneous morphogenesis [the lines of Blashko]), often exhibiting the histopathology of epidermolytic hyperkeratoses. The genetic nature of these nevi is uncertain; identical twins may be discordant for these nevi, but two instances of transmission of bullous congenital ichthyosiform hyperkeratosis to offspring has been reported. These observations are suggestive of a somatic mutation that may on occasion affect the germ cell lines. These nevi can be distinguished from the Curth-Macklin type by the characteristic histopathology and ultrastructure. The dominant, ichthyosis hystrix gravior (porcupine man of Lambert; see **Nevus, epidermal nevus syndrome**) may be the same entity as the Curth-Macklin type; unfortunately, histopathology is unavailable to resolve this question.

Support Groups: San Francisco; Foundation for Ichthyosis and Related Skin Types (FIRST)

References:
Curth HO, Macklin MT: The genetic basis of various types of ichthyosis in a family group. Am J Hum Genet 1954; 6:371–381.
Pinkus H, Nagao S: A case of biphasic ichthyosiform dermatosis: light and electron microscopic study. Arch Klin Exp Dermatol 1970; 237:727–748.
Ollendorff-Curth H, et al.: Follow-up of a family group suffering from ichthyosis hystrix type Curth-Macklin. Humangenetik 1972; 17:37–48.
Kanerva L, et al.: Ichthyosis hystrix (Curth-Macklin): light and electron microscopic studies performed before and after etretinate treatment. Arch Dermatol 1984; 120:1218–1223.

WI013   **Mary L. Williams**

Ichthyosis nigricans
See ICHTHYOSIS, X-LINKED WITH STEROID SULFATASE DEFICIENCY
Ichthyosis simplex
See ICHTHYOSIS VULGARIS

ICHTHYOSIS VULGARIS   2534

Includes:
> Ichthyosis, autosomal dominant
> Ichthyosis simplex

Excludes:
> **Ichthyosis, lamellar dominant** (2854)
> **Ichthyosis, X-linked with steroid sulfatase deficiency** (2532)
> **Ichthyosis** (other)

Major Diagnostic Criteria: Widespread scaly skin, i.e., visible cracking of the stratum corneum. Histologically the stratum corneum is thickened, and, of diagnostic significance, the stratum granulosum is thin to absent. Steroid sulfatase activity and cholesterol sulfate levels in blood and scale are normal, thus excluding **Ichthyosis, X-linked with steroid sulfatase deficiency**.

Clinical Findings: Scaling usually is absent at birth but clinically apparent by age six months. The severity of scaling tends to diminish with ''maturation'' and aging. The scales tend to be fine, white, and adherent. Unlike patients with hyperkeratoses associated with hyperproliferation of the epidermis (e.g., **Skin, psoriasis vulgaris**, **Ichthyosis, lamellar**), patients with ichthyosis vulgaris do not leave a ''trail'' of scales around them. Scaling may lessen in the summer and worsen in the winter, but the seasonal variation is less prominent than it is in **Ichthyosis, X-linked with steroid sulfatase deficiency**. Scaling is more prominent at the calves, spares the neck, and may be associated with palmar hyperkeratosis. Palmar hyperlinearity may be prominent, but it is uncertain whether such hyperlinearity is specific for ichthyosis vulgaris or whether it is more a feature of the often-associated atopic dermatitis.

Although more severe cases of ichthyosis vulgaris are clincally obvious, and may even be confused with X-linked or even lamellar ichthyosis, milder cases may be difficult to differentiate from nonichthyotic "dry skin" present, for example, in patients with atopic dermatitis. The generally quoted incidence of 1:250 persons likely includes such milder cases. The incidence of scaling as severe as that in patients with X-linked ichthyosis doubtless is much lower-perhaps tenfold less-and one large survey of patients with ichthyosis (using clinical and pedigree data) noted an incidence of ichthyosis vulgaris twofold greater than that in X-linked ichthyosis, the latter being approximately 1:6,000 males. Reduction to absence of keratohyaline granules (in the epidermal stratum granulosum) is noted by light microscopy, but some have advocated the more rigorous diagnostic criterion of keratohyaline granule absence by electron microscopy. Reduced keratohyaline granules correlates with reduced amounts of the protein filaggrin and its precursor profilaggrin, but it is not known whether the reduction of that protein causes the scaling and whether the "genetic" abnormality is related directly to that protein (or to other components of the keratohyaline granule or to yet unknown gene products). The phenotype of reduced profilaggrin is maintained in keratinocyte culture.

Complications: Unknown.

Associated Findings: None known.

Etiology: Autosomal dominant inheritance.

Pathogenesis: Unknown.

MIM No.: *14670

CDC No.: 757.195

Sex Ratio: M1:F1

Occurrence: About 1:250, depending on the diagnostic criteria used.

Risk of Recurrence for Patient's Sib:
See Part I, *Mendelian Inheritance.*

Risk of Recurrence for Patient's Child:
See Part I, *Mendelian Inheritance.*

Age of Detectability: Usually clinically evident by age six months.

Gene Mapping and Linkage: Unknown.

Prevention: None known. Genetic counseling indicated.

Treatment: "Keratolytics" to reduce stratum corneum thickness and brittleness, e.g., topical agents containing salicylic acid, lactic acid, urea, or propylene glycol. Avoidance of soap.

Prognosis: Normal life span. Scaling tends to become less severe with maturation and aging.

Detection of Carrier: Clinical examination.

Special Considerations: Clinical heterogeneity probably exists. Some patients have mild "dry skin," and some have considerably more severe scaling. Probably the latter have more complete keratohyaline granule loss, but this finding may wane following successful topical treatment. Diagnostic criteria, especially for those with milder scaling, are now imprecise.

Support Groups: San Francisco; Foundation for Ichthyosis and Related Skin Types (FIRST)

References:
Wells RS, Kerr CB: Clinical features of autosomal dominant and sex-linked ichthyosis in an English population. Br Med J 1966; 1:97–950.
Fartasch M, et al.: Ultrastructural study of the occurrence of autosomal dominant ichthyosis vulgaris in atopic eczema. Arch Dermatol Res 1987; 279:270–272.
Fleckman P, et al.: Keratinocytes cultured from subjects with ichthyosis vulgaris are phenotypically abnormal. J Invest Dermatol 1987; 88:640–645.

EP005   **Ervin H. Epstein, Jr.**

Ichthyosis, autosomal dominant
See ICHTHYOSIS VULGARIS
Ichthyosis, bullous type
See ICHTHYOSIFORM HYPERKERATOSIS, BULLOUS CONGENITAL

ICHTHYOSIS, CONGENITAL ERYTHRODERMIC   2855

Includes:
Collodion baby (some)
Cornification, disorder of, congenital erythrodermic type (DOC 5)
Ichthyosiform erythroderma, non-bullous congenital
Lamellar exfoliation of the newborn

Excludes:
Ichthyosis, harlequin fetus (2856)
Ichthyosis, lamellar dominant (2854)
Ichthyosis, lamellar recessive (2853)
Ichthyosis, linearis circumflexa (2858)
Ichthyosis vulgaris (2534)
Ichthyosis, X-linked with steroid sulfatase deficiency (2532)
Storage disease, neutral lipid type (2859)

Major Diagnostic Criteria: Generalized disorder of cornification affecting entire body surface, often with prominent erythroderma and fine white scales, and compatible histopathology. At birth, infants have collodion baby phenotype.

Clinical Findings: Affected infants are born with a taut, shiny encasement ("collodion membrane"). As this membrane is shed postnatally, an underlying erythroderma and generalized ichthyosis becomes apparent. As in **Ichthyosis, lamellar recessive,** generalized involvement is characteristic, including the face, palms/soles, and all of the flexures. Whereas scales on the trunk, face and scalp are fine and whitish in color, scales on the extensor surfaces of the lower legs may be large, plate-like and dark in color. Severely affected patients exhibit an intense erythroderma and ectropion. Cicatricial alopecia may develop. Secondary nail dystrophies with thickening of the nail plate and ridging are common. The histopathology displays acanthosis, moderate hyperkeratosis, and usually focal or complete parakeratosis. Stratum corneum membrane regions stain with periodic acid-Schiff reagent.

Complications: Although there are no primary systemic manifestations, collodion babies have an increased incidence of premature birth with its attendant perinatal morbidity and mortality. Moreover, collodion babies are at risk for both sepsis and fluid and electrolyte imbalance, particularly hypernatremia, because of their abnormal skin barrier. In severely affected patients, skin tautness may not only produce ectropion and eclabion, and may also compromise the development of nasal and auricular cartilages. Patients may exhibit symptoms of heat intolerance, secondary to eccrine duct obstruction. Although most patients exhibit normal growth and development, mild growth retardation may occur in some severely erythrodermic patients.

Associated Findings: None known.

Etiology: Autosomal recessive inheritance with interfamilial and intrafamilial variability in disease expression.

Pathogenesis: Although the underlying cause is unknown, epidermal cell turnover rates are markedly increased, as in **Skin, psoriasis vulgaris.** Evidence for a primary abnormality in lipid metabolism derives from the observation of a marked increase in hydrocarbon (alkane) content in scales from these patients, which distinguishes this disorder from normals and **Ichthyosis, lamellar recessive.** However, the finding of elevated scale hydrocarbons is not entirely disease-specific, since they occur occasionally in patients with other disorders of cornification. Furthermore, the source of these hydrocarbons in epidermis is not known. Topically applied alkanes induce the hyperproliferative epidermis, suggesting a role in the pathogenesis of this disease.

MIM No.: *24210, *24230

CDC No.: 757.190

Sex Ratio: M1:F1

Occurrence: On the order of 1:180,000. Cases are reported worldwide, without known ethnic predilection.

Risk of Recurrence for Patient's Sib:
See Part I, *Mendelian Inheritance.*

Risk of Recurrence for Patient's Child:
See Part I, *Mendelian Inheritance.*

Age of Detectability: At birth, as collodion baby.

Gene Mapping and Linkage: IC1 (ichthyosis 1, (autosomal recessive); congenital ichthyosiform erythroderma) is unassigned.

Prevention: None known. Genetic counseling indicated.

Treatment: Topical keratolytics (e.g. lactic or glycolic acids) are useful in removing scales but require continual applications. Topical retinoic acid cream may also be effective but is difficult to use. If topical salicylates are used, patients must be observed for signs of salicylism. Oral synthetic retinoids are effective but should be employed only after careful consideration of their long-term toxicity as well as teratogenicity (see **Fetal retinoid syndrome**).

Prognosis: Normal life span for those who survive the neonatal period. Some patients report improvement around puberty. Intelligence is normal.

Detection of Carrier: Unknown.

Special Considerations: *Collodion baby* should not be considered a disease entity, but a descriptive term for an infant born encased in a membranous-like covering, a phenotype that may be common to several disorders of cornification. In most patients (i.e. 2/3 or more), however, congenital erythrodermic ichthyosis is the underlying disorder. Some collodion babies progress to normal skin; they are diagnosed as *lamellar exfoliation of the newborn* in retrospect, which may represent a distinct, autosomal recessive disorder.

Support Groups: Raleigh, NC; Foundation for Ichthyosis and Related Skin Types (FIRST)

References:
Frost P, Van Scott EJ: Ichthyosiform dermatoses: classification based on anatomic and biometric observations. Arch Dermatol 1966; 94:113–126.
Reed WB, et al: Lamellar ichthyosis of the newborn, a distinct clinical entity: its comparison to the other ichthyosiform erythrodermas. Arch Dermatol 1972; 105:394–399.
Larregue M, et al: Le bebe collodion evolution a porpos de 29 cas. Ann Derm Syph (Paris) 1976; 103:31–54.
Williams ML, Elias PM: Elevated n-alkanes in congenital ichthyosiform erythroderma: phenotypic differentiation of two types of autosomal recessive ichthyosis. J Clin Invest 1984; 74:269–300.
Hazell M, Marks R: Clinical, histologic and cell kinetic discriminants between lamellar ichthyosis and non-bullous congenital ichthyosiform erythroderma. Arch Dermatol 1985; 121:489–493.
Williams ML, Elias PM: Heterogeneity in autosomal recessive ichthyosis: clinical and biochemical differentiation of lamellar ichthyosis and non-bullous congenital ichthyosiform erythroderma. Arch Dermatol 1985; 121:477–488. * †
Bernhardt M, Baden HP: Report of a family with an unusual expression of recessive ichthyosis: review of 42 cases. Arch Dermatol 1986; 122:420–433.

WI013   **Mary L. Williams**

Includes:
    Cornification, disorder of, harlequin type (DOC 6)
    Harlequin fetus ichthyosis
    Ichthyosis congenita fetalis
    Ichthyosis congenita gravis

Excludes:
    Ichthyosis, congenital erythrodermic (2855)
    Ichthyosis, lamellar dominant (2854)
    Ichthyosis, lamellar recessive (2853)

Major Diagnostic Criteria: Congenital onset of a severe generalized disorder of cornification composed of massive hyperkeratotic plates and resulting in severe eclabion, ectropion, and underdevelopment of cartilages and digits. Rare survivors from the perinatal period exhibit phenotype of severe generalized ichthyosiform erythroderma.

Clinical Findings: Affected infants are born with massive hyperkeratotic plates that produce grotesque facial features, with severe eclabion and ectropion and often deformities of other body parts, particularly the ears, hands, and feet. There are deep fissures between the hyperkeratotic plates. Many affected fetuses are stillborn, and most of the remaining do not survive more than a few days due to severe constriction of the chest and abdomen, resulting in compromised respiration and feeding. In the few instances in which patients have survived past the perinatal period, a severe generalized scaling disorder with erythroderma has occurred. Eclabion and ectropion improve, and further development of cartilaginous structures such as ears and nose takes place.

    Skin biopsy material demonstrates massive orthohyperkeratosis, but diagnosis rests on the clinical phenotype in the newborn. Premature and excessive cornification occurs by at least 20 weeks *in utero*, and has been used successfully as a guide in prenatal diagnosis.

Complications: A high perinatal mortality is usually due to interference with vital functions produced by severe restrictive skin disease. Fissures between keratotic plates provide a portal of entry for microorganisms, placing newborns at high risk for sepsis. As in collodion babies, problems with fluid and electrolyte imbalance are likely. Deformities of hands and feet, such as mitten-like enclosures due to severe restrictive skin *in utero*, may require surgical correction in survivors. Casting for orthopedic procedures may result in reversion to restrictive skin plates, similar to those present at birth. Development of nose and ear cartilages may proceed in survivors, and ectropion and eclabion improves. However, symptomatic ectropion may require surgical correction.

Associated Findings: None known.

Etiology: Autosomal recessive inheritance.

Pathogenesis: Unknown. No consistent abnormalities in epidermal keratin or lipid composition have been recognized.

MIM No.: *24250

CDC No.: 757.100

Sex Ratio: M1:F1

Occurrence: On the order of 1:300,000. Established literature with no ethnic predilection.

Risk of Recurrence for Patient's Sib:
See Part I, *Mendelian Inheritance.*

Risk of Recurrence for Patient's Child:
See Part I, *Mendelian Inheritance.*

Age of Detectability: Prenatal diagnosis by fetoscopy or fetal skin biopsy has been successful after 20 weeks gestation. Electron microscopy of fetal skin demonstrates premature and excessive cornification.

Gene Mapping and Linkage: Unknown.

Prevention: None known. Genetic counseling indicated.

Treatment: Use of oral synthetic retinoids, e.g., etretinate, may be beneficial in liveborn infants to facilitate shedding of restrictive cornified plates. Use of these retinoids in older survivors is controversial because of long-term toxicity.

Prognosis: Until recently, this disorder was believed to be universally fatal in the perinatal period. One recent survivor suffered an unexpected crib death at age eight months. Other long-term survivors appear to have normal intelligence and life span.

Detection of Carrier: Unknown.

Special Considerations: Some authorities have included this disorder as part of the phenotypic spectrum of lamellar ichthyoses. However, the failure to observe overlapping phenotypes within kindreds suggests that these are genetically distinct disorders. An early report of an abnormal keratin pattern (cross β configuration) has not been confirmed in subsequent studies. Abnormal keratin polypeptides have also been reported in two patients, but the specific abnormalities were not consistent. One patient with harlequin ichthyosis was suspected of having an abnormality in lipid metabolism, with prominent lipid vacuoles histologically and increased sterol ester content. It is possible that the harlequin ichthyosis phenotype may result from several different primary abnormalities of epidermal cornification.

Support Groups: Raleigh, NC; Foundation for Ichthyosis and Related Skin Types (FIRST)

References:

Goldsmith LA: The ichthyoses. Prog Med Genet 1976; 1:185–210. *
Buxman MM, et al.: Harlequin ichthyosis with epidermal lipid abnormality. Arch Dermatol 1979; 115:189–193.
Baden HP, et al.: Keratinization in the harlequin fetus. Arch Dermatol 1982; 118:14–18.
Lawler F, Peiris S: Harlequin fetus successfully treated with etretinate. Br J Dermatol 1985; 112:585–590. †
Williams ML, Elias PM: Genetically transmitted, generalized disorders of cornification: the ichthyoses. Dermatol Clin 1987; 5:165–178. * †

WI013   **Mary L. Williams**

ICHTHYOSIS, LAMELLAR DOMINANT   2854

Includes:

Collodion baby (some)
Cornification, disorder of, lamellar dominant (DOC 6)
Ichthyosiform erythroderma, nonbullous, dominant form
Lamellar ichthyosis, autosomal dominant form
Lamellar ichthyosis, nonbullous congenital

Excludes:

Ichthyosis, congenital erythrodermic (2855)
Ichthyosis, lamellar recessive (2853)

Major Diagnostic Criteria: A generalized disorder of cornification with dominant pedigree and characteristic histopathology.

Clinical Findings: A kindred with a generalized disorder of cornification that phenotypically resembled **Ichthyosis, lamellar recessive** has been documented. Vertical transmission was documented over three generations, and consanguinity was absent. Skin involvement was evident at birth, with encasement in a collodion-like membrane. Thereafter, the entire body surface was involved with a large scale pattern, not as severe as is typical for **Ichthyosis, lamellar recessive.** Erythroderma was absent, as is common in **Ichthyosis, congenital erythrodermic.** Palmoplantar keratoderma was disproportionately severe in these patients, and may provide a useful phenotypic marker for this disorder. Ultrastructural histopathology may be diagnostic, because a prominent transitional zone is seen in the stratum corneum just overlying the stratum granulosum.

Complications: Unknown.

Associated Findings: None known.

Etiology: Presumably autosomal dominant inheritance.

Pathogenesis: Unknown.

MIM No.: 14675

CDC No.: 757.190

Sex Ratio: Presumably M1:F1; M1:F2 observed.

Occurrence: At least one kindred, with an affected grandfather, mother and daughter, has been reported in the literature.

Risk of Recurrence for Patient's Sib:
See Part I, *Mendelian Inheritance.*

Risk of Recurrence for Patient's Child:
See Part I, *Mendelian Inheritance.*

Age of Detectability: Clinically evident at birth as collodion baby.

Gene Mapping and Linkage: Unknown.

Prevention: None known. Genetic counseling indicated.

Treatment: Topical keratolytic agents to remove scale may improve appearance. Use of oral synthetic retinoids in generalized disorders of cornification is controversial because of long-term toxicity and teratogenecity (see **Fetal retinoid syndrome**).

Prognosis: Presumably normal life span and intelligence.

Detection of Carrier: By clinical examination.

Support Groups: San Francisco; Foundation for Ichthyosis and Related Skin Types (FIRST)

References:

Traupe H, et al.: Autosomal dominant lamellar ichthyosis: a new skin disorder. Clin Genet 1984; 26:457–461.
Kolde G, et al.: Autosomal-dominant lamellar ichthyosis: ultrastructural characteristics of a new type of congenital ichthyosis. Arch Dermatol Res 1985; 278:1–5.
Williams ML, Elias PM: Ichthyosis: genetic heterogeneity, genodermatoses, and genetic counseling. (Editorial) Arch Derm 1986; 122: 529–531.

WI013   **Mary L. Williams**

ICHTHYOSIS, LAMELLAR RECESSIVE   2853

Includes:

Collodion fetus (some)
Cornification, disorders of, lamellar recessive (DOC 4)
Desquamation of the newborn
Ichthyosiform erythroderma, Brocq nonbullous form
Ichthyosis congenita (some)
Lamellar exfoliation of the newborn
Lamellar ichthyosis, classical

Excludes:

Ichthyosiform erythroderma, non-bullous congenital
Ichthyosis, congenital erythrodermic (2855)
Ichthyosis, erythrodermic, congenital
Ichthyosis, harlequin fetus (2856)
Ichthyosis, lamellar dominant (2854)
Ichthyosis vulgaris (2534)
Ichthyosis (other)

Major Diagnostic Criteria: Severe, life-long, generalized disorder of cornification with large dark plate-like scales and an underlying erythroderma, affecting the entire skin surface and producing facial tautness with ectropion, in association with compatible histopathology.

Clinical Findings: Generalized hyperkeratosis is evident from birth. The most striking clinical feature is that of large, dark, plate-like ("lamellar") scales. Most patients have an underlying erythroderma of variable intensity. Facial involvement results in significant ectropion. The scalp is involved, but hairs themselves are spared and alopecia does not occur. All flexures are involved as are palms and soles. The disorder is unremitting. Histopathology demonstrates massive orthohyperkeratosis with some acanthosis and papillomatosis; parakeratosis and features of epidermolytic hyperkeratosis are absent; the granular cell layers are well-developed.

Complications: Ectropion may result in corneal injury if uncorrected. Palmoplantar keratoderma may be severe enough to present some functional disability. Generally, the disorder is disfiguring but not physically disabling.

Associated Findings: None known.

Etiology: Autosomal recessive inheritance.

Pathogenesis: Unknown. Scale lipids are composed of an increased proportion of ceramides and free sterols, a pattern reminiscent of palmo-plantar stratum corneum. The epidermis is normoproliferative or only modestly hyperproliferative; excessive stratum corneum may be attributed primarily to stratum corneum retention.

MIM No.: *24210, *24230

CDC No.: 757.190

Sex Ratio: Presumably M1:F1.

Occurrence: On the order of <1:300,000. Cases of **Ichthyosis, congenital erythrodermic** are more common than this phenotype. The two disorders are separated by clinical, histological, histometric and biochemical differences. There appears to be little intrafamilial variability. No ethnic predilections are known.

Risk of Recurrence for Patient's Sib:
See Part I, *Mendelian Inheritance.*

Risk of Recurrence for Patient's Child:
See Part I, *Mendelian Inheritance.*

Age of Detectability: At birth. Prenatal diagnosis may be possible through fetoscopy and fetal skin biopsy with fetal skin showing excessive and premature cornification.

Gene Mapping and Linkage: IC1 (ichthyosis 1, (autosomal recessive); congenital ichthyosiform erythroderma) is unassigned.

Prevention: None known. Genetic counseling indicated.

Treatment: Topical keratolytics (e.g. lactic or glycolic acids) are useful in removing scales but require continual applications. Topical retinoic acid cream may also be effective but are difficult to use. If topical salicylates are used, patients must be observed for signs of salicylism. Oral synthetic retinoids are effective but should be employed only after careful consideration of their long-term toxicity as well as teratogenicity (see **Fetal retinoid syndrome**).

Prognosis: Normal life span. The skin disorder is unremitting and presents a significant cosmetic handicap which may impair psychosocial adaptation. Intelligence is normal.

Detection of Carrier: Unknown.

Special Considerations: For the first half of the 20th Century this disorder was commonly lumped together with **Ichthyosiform hyperkeratosis, bullous congenital** as *ichthyosis congenita*, dry and wet types, respectively, until the characteristic histopathology of epidermolytic hyperkeratosis and dominant inheritance pattern of **Ichthyosiform hyperkeratosis, bullous congenital** were generally appreciated.

Support Groups: Raleigh, NC; Foundation for Ichthyosis and Related Skin Types (FIRST)

References:
Frost P, Van Scott EJ: Ichthyosiform dermatoses. Classification based on anatomic and biometric observations. Arch Dermatol 1966; 94:113–126.

Williams ML, Elias PM: Elevated n-alkanes in congenital ichthyosiform erythrodermal: phenotypic differentiation of two types of autosomal recessive ichthyosis. J Clin Invest 1984; 74:269–300.

Hazell M, Marks R: Clinical, histologic and cell kinetic discriminants between lamellar ichthyosis and non-bullous congenital ichthyosiform erythroderma. Arch Dermatol 1985; 121:489–493. †

Williams ML, Elias PM: Heterogeneity in autosomal recessive ichthyosis: clinical and biochemical differentiation of lamellar ichthyosis and non-bullous congenital ichthyosiform erythroderma. Arch Dermatol 1985; 121:477–488. * †

Sybert VP, Holbrook KA: Prenatal diagnosis and screening. Dermatologic Clinics 1987; 5:17–41.

WI013   **Mary L. Williams**

ICHTHYOSIS, LINEARIS CIRCUMFLEXA   2858

Includes:
> Bamboo hair
> Cornification, disorder of, Netherton type (DOC 9)
> Hair, "bamboo"
> Netherton syndrome

Excludes:
> **Ichthyosis, lamellar recessive** (2853)
> **Trichothiodystrophy** (2559)

Major Diagnostic Criteria: Affected individuals exhibit a distinctive disorder of cornification characterized by circinate lesions formed on either side by a free edge of scale ("double-edged" scale). Some patients may have a generalized hyperkeratosis resembling congenital erythrodermic ichthyosis. Scalp hairs are short and fragile due to structural defects of the hair shaft. Trichorrhexis invaginata, a ball-and-socket intussusception of the hair shaft, is diagnostic of this syndrome.

Clinical Findings: This disorder is characterized by the triad of 1) ichthyosis linearis circumflexa; 2) structural anomalies of the hair shaft, particularly trichorrhexis invaginata; and 3) an atopic diathesis. Ichthyosis linearis circumflexa refers to a generalized hyperkeratosis that, with desquamation, results in a circinate erythematous base with the pathognomonic "double-edged" scale along the margins. At birth, a generalized erythroderma or a collodion baby phenotype may be present. Later, the characteristic migratory, circinate plaques develop. Pruritis is variable but may be severe. Lichenification of the flexural surfaces may be present as a manifestation of the associated atopic dermatitis. The face, scalp, and eyebrows are often affected by dermatitis. Instead of the circinate pattern of ichthyosis linearis circumflexa, some patients phenotypically resemble **Ichthyosis, congenital erythrodermic**. Histopathologic examination is nondiagnostic, revealing features of both psoriasis and atopic dermatitis.

The characteristic hair shaft anomaly of Netherton syndrome is trichorrhexis invaginata, or bamboo hairs. Pili tori and trichorrhexis nodosa may also occur. These hair shaft anomalies result in fragile hairs that usually break off within a few inches of the scalp.

Complications: Pruritis may be severe, related to the atopic status. Anaphylactic reactions to foods may occur.

Associated Findings: The atopic diathesis in these patients manifests as either atopic dermatitis or asthma (see **Skin, atopy, familial**). Anaphylactic reactions to foods have been frequently observed, and marked elevation of serum IgE levels may be present. Other reported findings include a generalized aminoaciduria in up to one-half of patients, mild-to-severe mental retardation, and impaired cellular immunity.

Etiology: Autosomal recessive inheritance. The literature reflects a predominance of females, but well-documented cases in males and reports of consanguinity are most consistent with autosomal recessive inheritance.

Pathogenesis: Unknown. Bamboo hairs represent a ball-and-socket intussusception of the distal hair shaft into the proximal portion resulting from a defect in cornification of the internal root sheath.

MIM No.: *25650

CDC No.: 757.190

Sex Ratio: Presumably M1:F1; observed, M1:F2.

Occurrence: A few dozen cases have been documented.

Risk of Recurrence for Patient's Sib:
See Part I, *Mendelian Inheritance.*

Risk of Recurrence for Patient's Child:
See Part I, *Mendelian Inheritance.*

Age of Detectability: Usually at birth.

Gene Mapping and Linkage: Unknown.

Prevention: None known. Genetic counseling indicated.

Treatment: Avoidance of food allergens. Usual management for atopic dermatitis, if present. Some patients may respond to PUVA (psoralen plus UVA light). Retinoids and antimetabolites should be considered experimental.

Prognosis: Probably normal for life span.

Detection of Carrier: Unknown.

Support Groups: San Francisco; Foundation for Ichthyosis and Related Skin Types (FIRST)

References:

Altman J, Stroud J: Netherton's syndrome and ichthyosis linearis circumflexa: psoriasiform ichthyosis. Arch Dermatol 1969; 100:550–558. *

Hurwitz S, et al.: Reevaluation of ichthyosis and hair shaft abnormalities. Arch Dermatol 1971; 103:266–271. * †

Krafchik BR, Toole JWP: What is Netherton's syndrome? Int J Dermatol 1983; 22:459–462.

Caputo R, et al.: Netherton's syndrome in two adult brothers. Arch Dermatol 1984; 120:220–222.

WI013   **Mary L. Williams**

ICHTHYOSIS, X-LINKED WITH STEROID SULFATASE DEFICIENCY   2532

Includes:

Ichthyosis nigricans
Placental steroid sulfatase deficiency
Steroid sulfatase deficiency disease (SSDD)

Excludes:

Ichthyosis vulgaris (2534)
Ichthyosis (other)

Major Diagnostic Criteria: Widespread scaly skin, i.e., visible thickening and cracking of stratum corneum in a patient with a family history compatible with X-linked recessive inheritance. The diagnosis is confirmed by detecting an absence of steroid sulfatase activity with or without elevated quantities of its substrate cholesterol sulfate.

Clinical Findings: Scaling of skin usually becomes evident by age six months. The scales tend to be dark, adherent, and especially prominent on the lateral calves and (of diagnostic significance when prominent) on the sides of the neck: the typical appearance of a little boy with a dirty neck that soap cannot clean. The scaling is greatly reduced in the summer so that patients almost "moult" in the spring. In some sunny, moist climates (e.g., Southeast Asia, Central America) scaling may be nearly inapparent clinically all year long. Scaling tends to spare the palms and involve the cubital fossae, unlike that in ichthyosis vulgaris, in which the palms are often hyperkeratotic and the cubital fossae are spared. Scaling tends not to improve with advancing age. Even with careful attention to these clinical criteria, differentiation from ichthyosis vulgaris is often difficult, because scales sometimes may be rather lighter in color and less broadly distributed.

The stratum corneum is thickened and granular cells are present in normal numbers (cf. few to no granular cells in ichthyosis vulgaris) in skin biopsy material. Approximately 50% of patients and a smaller percentage of carriers have clinically inapparent corneal opacities detectable only by careful slit-lamp examinations. There is an increased incidence of delayed parturition, but the exact incidence is uncertain. Increased incidences of cryptorchidism and testicular carcinoma have been suggested.

Steroid sulfatase activity can be measured in scale, whole skin or epidermis, leukocytes, cultured fibroblasts, keratinocytes, and amniocytes. Elevated cholesterol sulfate can be measured in stratum corneum and blood. In blood, the cholesterol sulfate is "carried" on low-density lipoproteins (LDL). The sulfates impart an enhanced electronegativity to the LDLs that can be detected by enhanced LDL electromobility on serum lipoprotein electrophoresis.

Complications: Psychologic impairment due to embarassment at visible abnormality and fear of social ostracism.

Associated Findings: None known.

Etiology: X-linked recessive inheritance.

Pathogenesis: Approximately 90% of patients so far studied have deletions of most or all of the steroid sulfatase gene. The absence of steroid sulfatase catalytic activity at the periphery of the cells of the stratum corneum prevents the normal predesquamative desulfation of cholesterol sulfate to cholesterol. The intercellular cholesterol sulfate appears to act as a glue and prevents stratum corneum desquamation, leading to thickening and "cracking" of that layer.

MIM No.: *30810

Sex Ratio: M1:F0. However, one inbred family has been described in which three affected daughters were born to an affected male and a female who most likely was a carrier of the disease.

Occurrence: 1:4,000–6,000 males. Patients have been reported in all major ethnic groups.

Risk of Recurrence for Patient's Sib:
See Part I, *Mendelian Inheritance.*

Risk of Recurrence for Patient's Child:
See Part I, *Mendelian Inheritance.*

Age of Detectability: Clinically evident by age six months, although usually not at birth. Prenatal diagnosis can be made in the first trimester by detecting absence of steroid sulfatase enzyme activity in cultured amniocytes, elevated levels of the enzyme substrate dehydroepiandrosterone in amniotic fluid, or late in pregnancy by detection of abnormally low maternal urinary estriol. Gene deletion is likely to be detectable in chorionic villi.

Gene Mapping and Linkage: STS (steroid sulfatase (microsomal)) has been mapped to Xp22.32.

Prevention: None known. Genetic counseling indicated.

Treatment: "Keratolytics" to reduce stratum corneum thickness, e.g., topical agents containing salicylic acid, lactic acid, urea, or proplyene glycol. Avoidance of soap.

Prognosis: Normal life span.

Detection of Carrier: Peripheral blood leukocyte steroid sulfatase activity is lower in carriers than in normal women. In the 90% of families in which there are gene deletions, detection of a 50% reduction of steroid sulfatase gene sequences should be possible.

Special Considerations: The gene for steroid sulfatase is of particular interest in that it partially escapes X-inactivation (lyonization) and in that it is located in humans just proximal to the pseudoautosomal region (in mice it is located within the pseudoautosomal region). This location near the site of obligate crossing over between the X and Y chromosomes during male meiosis may be related to the very high incidence of gross deletions causing the enzyme deficiency. Rarely do patients have yet larger deletions and associated clinical abnormalities, including chondrodysplasia punctata. It is unclear whether the variably reported associated findings such as corneal opacities, cryptorchidism, and delayed onset of labor, are consequences of absent steroid sulfatase enzyme activity or are due to genomic deletions extending beyond the steroid sulfatase gene into adjacent regions of the X chromosome.

In the very rare multiple sulfatase deficiency, ichthyosis and increased cholesterol sulfate are associated with steroid sulfatase deficiency, but the enzymatic activity of many other sulfatases (e.g., arylsulfatases A and B) is also absent, and death occurs at an early age.

Support Groups: San Francisco; Foundation for Ichthyosis and Related Skin Types (FIRST)

References:

Wells RS, Kerr CB: Clinical features of autosomal dominant and sex-linked ichthyosis in an English population. Br Med J 1966; 1:947–950.

Shapiro LJ, et al.: X-linked ichthyosis due to steroid-sulphatase deficiency. Lancet 1978; I:70–72.

Shapiro LJ, et al.: Non-activation of a X-chromosome locus in man. Science 1979; 204:1224–1226.

Epstein EH Jr., et al.: X-linked ichthyosis: increased blood cholesterol sulfate and electrophoretic mobility of low-density lipoprotein. Science 1981; 214:659–660.

Williams ML, Elias PM: Stratum corneum lipids in disorders of cornification. J Clin Invest 1981; 68:1404–1410.

Bonifas JM, et al.: Cloning of a cDNA for steroid sulfatase. Frequent occurrence of gene deletions in patients with recessive X-chromosome-linked ichthyosis. Proc Natl Acad Sci USA 1987; 84:9248–9251.

Yen PH, et al.: Cloning and expression of steroid sulfatase cDNA and the frequent occurrence of deletions in STS deficiency: implications for X-Y interchange. Cell 1987; 49:443–454.

EP005   **Ervin H. Epstein, Jr.**

Ichthyosis-cataract
See CATARACT-ICHTHYOSIS

ICHTHYOSIS-CHEEK-EYEBROW SYNDROME   3010

Includes:
>   Cheek-eyebrow-ichthyosis syndrome
>   Eyebrow-cheek-ichthyosis syndrome

Excludes: Ichthyosis (other)

Major Diagnostic Criteria: Ichthyosis vulgaris, prominent full cheeks until puberty, sparse lateral eyebrows, and other craniofacial and musculoskeletal anomalies.

Clinical Findings: *Craniofacial:* dysplastic ears (folded helices) (4/4), flat occiput (4/4), full cheeks until puberty (4/4), high-arched palate (4/4), prominent nose (4/4), sparse lateral eyebrows (4/4).
   Musculoskeletal: chest asymmetry (4/4), genu valgum (1/4), kyphoscoliosis (3/4), long fingers and toes (4/4), **Pectus carinatum** (1/4), **Pectus excavatum** (3/4), pes planus (4/4).
   Skin: **Ichthyosis vulgaris** (4/4), widely spaced nipples (3/4).

Complications: Unknown.

Associated Findings: None known.

Etiology: Autosomal dominant inheritance.

Pathogenesis: Unknown. The prominent full cheeks most probably represent excess adipose tissue in the buccal fat pad, which begins to diminish with the onset of puberty.

MIM No.:   14672

POS No.:   4277

Sex Ratio: Presumably M1:F1.

Occurrence: Reported in four generations of a Jewish Sephardic family from Israel.

Risk of Recurrence for Patient's Sib:
   See Part I, *Mendelian Inheritance.*

Risk of Recurrence for Patient's Child:
   See Part I, *Mendelian Inheritance.*

Age of Detectability: During infancy.

Gene Mapping and Linkage: Unknown.

Prevention: None known. Genetic counseling indicated.

Treatment: Supportive. Affected females may find the prominent cheeks disturbing during childhood and early teens, as they may be teased and accused of having the mumps.

Prognosis: Normal life span.

Detection of Carrier: Appears to be fully penetrant in the heterozygous state.

Special Considerations: The acronym *ICE*, sometimes used to describe this condition, has long been used as a descriptor for another distinct disorder; *Iridocorneal endothelial syndrome* (Yanoff, 1979). Use of acronyms, and this acronym in particular, is discouraged in favor of more complete terminology.

Support Groups: San Francisco; Foundation for Ichthyosis and Related Skin Types (FIRST)

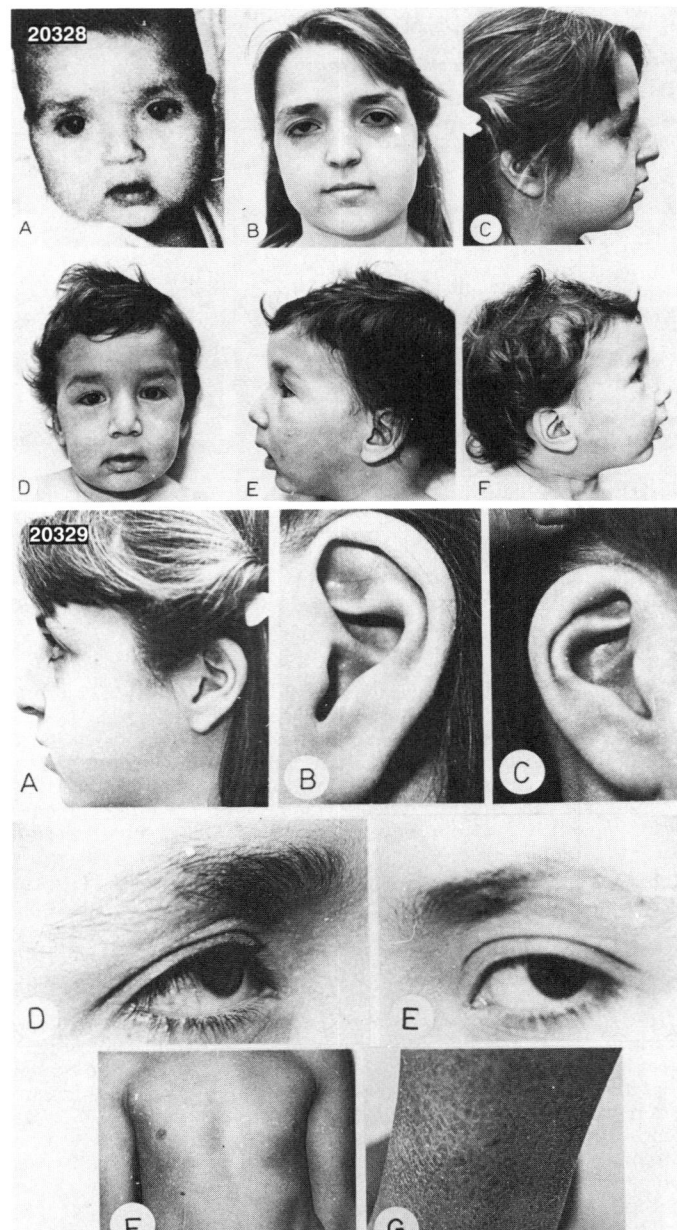

3010-20328:   A–C) The prominent and full cheeks of the proband at the time of infancy and at age 11 years. D–F) The proband's affected brother at age 1 year and 8 months also with full cheeks and sparse lateral eyebrows. **20329:**   Full cheek (A), folded helices (B,C), sparse lateral eyebrows (D,E), chest asymmetry with mild pectus excavatum (F), and icthyosis vulgaris involving the lower extremity (G) in the proband.

References:

Yanoff M: Iridocorneal endothelial syndrome: unification of a disease spectrum. Surv Ophthal 1979; 24:1–2.

Sidransky E, et al.: Ichthyosis-cheek-eyebrow (ICE) syndrome: a new autosomal dominant disorder. Clin Genet 1987; 31:137–142.

G0026   **Richard M. Goodman**

ICHTHYOSIS-COLOBOMA-HEART DEFECT-DEAFNESS-MENTAL RETARDATION 3214

Includes:
 CHIME syndrome
 Ichythyosiform dermatosis-neurologic/ophthalmologic
  abnormalities

Excludes:
 Charge association (2124)
 Gingival fibromatosis-depigmentation-microphthalmia (0413)
 Ichthyosiform erythrokeratoderma, atypical with deafness (2861)
 Ichthyosis, linearis circumflexa (2858)
 Intrauterine exposure to aflatoxin B(1)
 Limb reduction-ichthyosis (2019)
 Phytanic acid storage disease (0810)
 Seizures-ichthyosis-mental retardation (0741)
 Sjogren-Larsson syndrome (2030)
 Skin, erythrokeratodermia, variable (0361)
 Trichothiodystrophy (2559)

Major Diagnostic Criteria: Bilateral retinal coloboma, migratory ichthyosiform dermatosis, normal to small "C" shaped ears with rolled helices, severe developmental delay, and congenital heart defect.

Clinical Findings: At birth, the children appear unusual with brachycephaly; one child had small head circumference and micrognathia. Length and weight are variable ranging from normal to less than the 3rd percentile. Retinal colobomas are usually readily apparent. True or apparent hypertelorism may be noted with epicanthal folds. Muscle tone is usually normal, but, in one child severe hypotonia occurred. Further investigation reveals congenital heart defects: **Heart, tetralogy of Fallot, Heart, transposition of great vessels**, and peripheral pulmonic stenosis. Respiratory distress may occur secondary to congestive heart failure. The

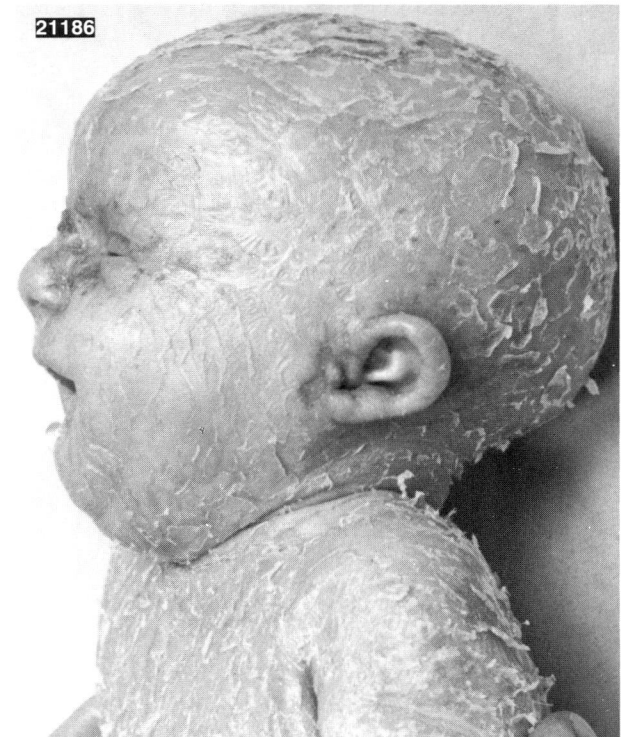

3214B-21186: Micrognathia, "C"-shaped ears with rolled helices, and the scaling of the transitory ichthyosiform rash.

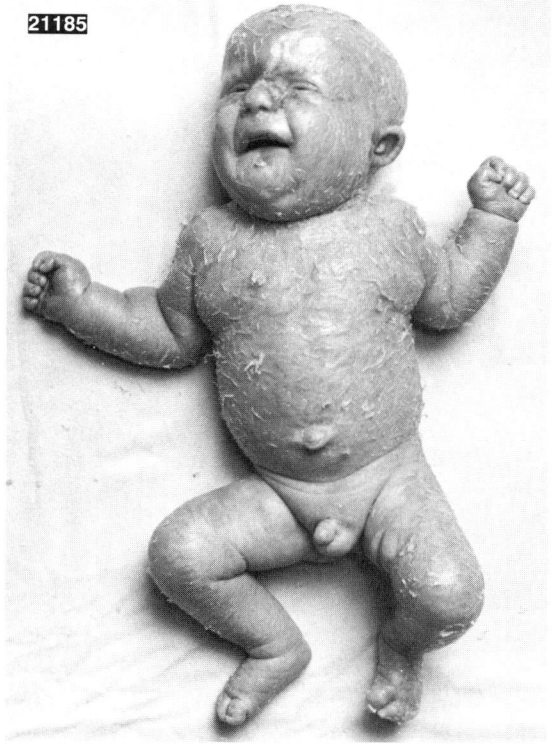

3214A-21185: Generalized distribution of the transient ichthyosiform dermatosis.

diagnosis may remain in doubt until the migratory ichthyosiform rash develops, usually by one week, but it may not appear until 4–6 weeks of life; persisting into late childhood. Developmental delay, hearing deficit and visual impairment are apparent from the outset. Seizures occur in early infancy. Dermatoglyphs show high percent of digital arches.
 Chromosome analyses have been normal. No defects in immunoglobulin levels or cellular immunity have been detected.

Complications: Recurrent respiratory infections; otitis media; cutaneous infections and abscesses, contractures of digits and large joints, and failure to thrive with gastrointestinal reflux in one child.

Associated Findings: Dental anomalies; cleft palate (submucous cleft with bifid uvula); conductive hearing loss; bilateral inguinal hernias, undescended testes and umbilical hernias occurred in one neonate; one child had a large lipoma on the back and one had large bilateral lipomas in the pectoral-axillary areas.

Etiology: Presumably autosomal recessive inheritance.

Pathogenesis: Unknown.

Sex Ratio: M3:F1

Occurrence: Only four children (three reported and one by personal communication) are known in three unrelated families.

Risk of Recurrence for Patient's Sib:
 See Part I, *Mendelian Inheritance.*

Risk of Recurrence for Patient's Child:
 See Part I, *Mendelian Inheritance.*

Age of Detectability: Retinal coloboma, heart defect and ear anomalies are detected at birth or within a few days of life. Scaly skin changes may appear during the first week to month of life.

Gene Mapping and Linkage: Unknown.

Prevention: None known. Genetic counseling indicated.

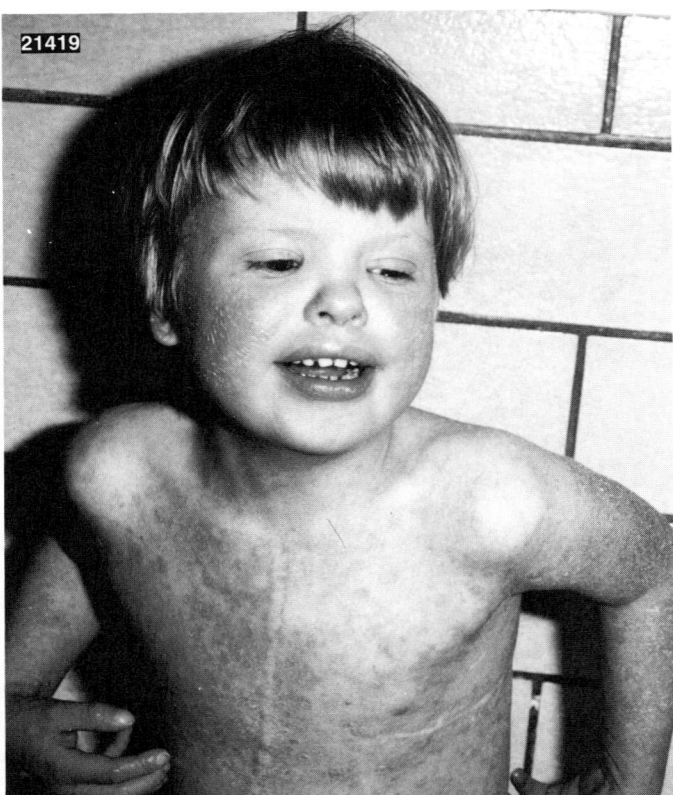

3214C-21419: Note unusual facies, generalized dermatitis and scar from heart surgery.

Treatment: Skin care is the major day-to-day problem. Warm baths followed by total body moisturizing preparations usually controls the scaling and erythroderma. Daily application of a topical steroid was highly effective in the most severely affected child. Keratolytic agents, uric acid and lactic acid preparations, are effective in removing scales and may be required daily. Gastroesophageal reflux may require Nissan fundoplication and gastrostomy tube placement.

Prognosis: Mental retardation is severe. Two children at 4 and 6.5 years chronological age functioned at the 12 and 18 months levels respectively. Two other children at one year have shown little progress beyond 1–2 months level. Ichthyosis persists through childhood.

Detection of Carrier: Unknown.

Special Considerations: The acronym C.H.I.M.E. was drawn from "Coloboma, heart defect, ichthyosiform dermatosis, mental retardation, and ear anomalies" (CHIME).

References:
Zunich J, Kaye CI: New syndrome of congenital ichthyosis with neurologic abnormalities. Am J Med Genetics 1983; 15:331–333.
Zunich J, Kaye CI: Additional case report of new neuroectodermal syndrome (letter). Am J Med Genetics 1984; 17:707–710.
Zunich J, et al.: Congenital migratory ichthyosiform dermatosis with neurologic and ophthalmologic abnormalities. Arch Dermatol 1985; 121:1149–1156.
Zunich J, Kaye CI: Autosomal recessive transmission of new neuroectodermal syndrome. Pediatr Res 1988; 23:271A.

LA007
ZU000

Roger L. Ladda
Janice Zunich

IMINOGLYCINURIA   0520

Includes:
  DeVries hyperglycinuria
  Glycinuria with or without oxalate urolithiasis
  Iminoglycinuria type II
  Renal iminoglycinuria

Excludes:
  Hyperprolinemia (0502)
  Iminoglycinuria of normal newborn

Major Diagnostic Criteria: The homozygotes have normal plasma concentration of proline, hydroxyproline (both imino acids), and glycine, as well as large amounts of imino acids and glycine in urine after 6 months of age. Heterozygotes have glycinuria exceeding 160 μmole/g total urinary nitrogen, or renal clearance exceeding 8.6 ml/min/1.73 M² in one type of heterozygote; the other (silent) type has normal glycine excretion.

Clinical Findings: No proven disease occurs with the trait that affects the common renal tubular reabsorptive mechanism for glycine, proline, and hydroxyproline. Its occasional association with seizures or mental retardation is probably fortuitous. Numerous healthy children and adults have now been recognized with selective impairment of cellular transport of proline, hydroxyproline, and glycine. Plasma levels of affected amino acids are normal. In homozygotes, net renal tubular reabsorption of proline, hydroxyproline, and glycine is about 80%, 80%, and 60%, respectively, of the normal amount. An intestinal transport defect restricted to the iminoglycine group of amino acids has also been identified in some, but not in all, pedigrees. Most heterozygotes have abnormal endogenous glycine reabsorption. Evidence for "silent" heterozygotes exists. On this basis, and on apparent evidence for heteroallelic homozygotes in some pedigrees, it is assumed that more than one mutant genotype determines the renal iminoglycinuric trait.

Complications: Unknown.

Associated Findings: None known.

Etiology: *Iminoglycinuria type I:* autosomal recessive inheritance.
Iminoglycinuria type II (with or without oxalate urolithiasis): autosomal dominant inheritance.

Pathogenesis: Presumed deficiency of high-capacity, low-affinity, group-specific membrane transport system (protein or permease), in brush border membrane common to proline, hydroxyproline, and glycine.

MIM No.: 13850, *24260

Sex Ratio: M1:F1

Occurrence: About 1:17,000 live births for homozygous trait. *All* newborns have *normal* transient neonatal iminoglycinuria of a different mechanism.

Risk of Recurrence for Patient's Sib:
See Part I, *Mendelian Inheritance.*

Risk of Recurrence for Patient's Child:
See Part I, *Mendelian Inheritance.*

Age of Detectability: At birth.

Gene Mapping and Linkage: Unknown.

Prevention: None known. Genetic counseling indicated.

Treatment: Care for associated illnesses (if any).

Prognosis: Normal life span.

Detection of Carrier: Hyperglycinuria in one type of heterozygote.

Special Considerations: Renal iminoglycinuria is normally present in the newborn, reflecting ontogeny of independent transport systems for imino acids and for glycine and not controlled by the iminoglycinuria marker locus (Lasley and Scriver, 1979). Renal tubular conservation of imino acids and glycine approaches adult values by the 6th month of life in normal infants.

Evidence for more than one mutant genotype rests in the different forms of heterozygosity, the demonstration of an intestinal transport defect in some homozygotes, the failure to identify this feature in other homozygotes, and Mendelian evidence for genetic compounds.

References:
Rosenberg LE, et al.: Familial iminoglycinuria: an inborn error of renal tubular transport. New Engl J Med 1968; 278:1407–1413.
Scriver CR: Renal tubular transport of proline, hydroxyproline and glycine. III. Genetic basis for more than one mode of transport in human kidney. J Clin Invest 1968; 47:823–835.
Lasley L, Scriver CR: Ontogeny of amino acid reabsorption in human kidney: evidence from the homozygous infant with familial renal iminoglycinuria for multiple proline and glycine systems. Pediatr Res 1979; 13:65.
Scriver CR: Familial renal iminoglycinuria. In: Scriver CR, et al., eds: Metabolic basis of inherited disease, ed 6. New York: McGraw-Hill, 1989:2529–2538.

SC050   **Charles R. Scriver**

Iminoglycinuria type II
See IMINOGLYCINURIA

Immotile cilia syndrome
See DEXTROCARDIA-BRONCHIECTASIS-SINUSITIS SYNDROME
Immune interferon deficiency
See INTERFERON DEFICIENCY

IMMUNODEFICIENCIES   1508

Recent advances in immunology and molecular biology have been translated into improved understanding of the etiology and management of many disorders of the immune system. Immunodeficiencies constitute a wide spectrum of diseases with a diversity of underlying mechanisms of pathogenesis, ranging from arrest of development to infection with immunosuppressive etiologic agents. While it may be perceived that there has been a steady rise in the number of patients with a diagnosis of primary immune deficiency, it is unlikely that this reflects any change in the incidence of disease. More likely this is due to an increased awareness by the medical community of the possibility of immunodeficiency as well as improved methods of diagnosis.

What are some of the indications of underlying immunodeficiency disease? Recurrent infections, often due to opportunistic organisms, may be an early sign. It is difficult, however, to give specific examples of just what frequency may be cause for concern. Evidently what is needed is sufficient experience with a normal population to recognize the tremendous range of individual variability with regard to susceptibility to routine infections.

Familial clustering of immunodeficiencies may also assist in their diagnosis. Thus it is not uncommon to see families with several symptomatic members. While a single disease entity such as **Immunodeficiency, agammaglobulinemia, X-linked, infantile** may be scattered throughtout a family, patterns of multiple, different syndromes are also not uncommon. It is prudent to consider a more extensive family evaluation when an index case is identified. Further, when a patient has been shown to express one immunodeficiency disorder, it is also recommended to look for other immunologic dysfunctions within that individual as several different immunodefiency syndromes may occur simultaneously or sequentially. One example of this is the increased incidence of atopy associated with immunodeficiencies. Another indication of immune deficiency is a familial tendency to fetal wastage or deaths in early childhood. These should indeed be specifically noted on taking the history. So-called cancer families or families with several members with malignant disease may also be associated with underlying immunodeficiency.

Several significant physical findings are often indicative of immunodeficiency disease. Many such patients have a paucity of peripheral lymphoid tissues including the absence of adenoids and/or tonsils. Occasionally immunodeficient patients may show evidence of growth retardation which may present initially as failure to thrive. This is not to be confused with dwarfism which may also be associated with immunodeficiency diseases. In response to frequent bouts of infection, patients may manifest hepatosplenomegaly. Certain immunodeficiencies may also be associated with specific dysmorphism such as the unique facies noted among patients with **Immunodeficiency, thymic agenesis,** or the bony abnormalities of the ribs found in **Immunodeficiency, severe combined** due to adenosine deaminase deficiency.

Treatment of immunodeficiencies has progressed remarkably. Numerous technical advancements have significantly reduced thier morbidity and mortality. Bone marrow transplantation has emerged as a recognized treatment modality. While at one time it was specifically restricted to closely related, major histocompatibility complex matched, donor-recipient pairs, successful transplantation across this barrier is now a reality. Elimination of mature, post-thymic T-lymphocytes from the donor marrow can significantly reduce the likelihood of serious graft-versus-host disease. Bone marrow transplantation has been successfully used to treat primary immunodeficiencies, a wide variety of hematologic and oncologic disorders, and some inborn errors of metabolism; additional applications are under consideration. Cellular engineering, as exemplified by bone marrow transplantation, may soon be complemented by the transfer of individual genes to replace defective ones in selected recipients. Recent preclinical studies have indicated that definitive treatment of severe combined immunodeficiency with adenosine deaminase deficiency may be achieved by the transfer of functional adenosine deaminase genes to the deficient recipient. We may soon bear witness to the first successful correction of a congenital defect by gene transplantation.

During the last several years a new class of immunotherapeutic agents have been identified, biological modifier substances. As their name implies these drugs are capable of modulating various biologic activities including immunologic functions. Several of these substances were first recognized to be the secretory products of various cells and were called cytokines; the secretory products of lymphocytes have been designated lymphokines. Included among these substances are interferons, interleukins, tumor necrosis factor, B-cell growth factor, supressor and helper factors, etc. The genes for many of these agents have been isolated and cloned and sufficient quantities of these substances have been produced by recombinant DNA technology for pharmacologic application. Biologic modifier substances are finding increasing application in the treatment of immunodeficiency and malignant disorders.

A mainstay in the treatment of humoral immunodeficiency diseases has been replacement therapy with intramuscular (IM) gamma globulin, resulting in significant improvements in morbidity and mortality among patients with humoral immunodeficiencies. Until recently gamma globulin replacement therapy has been limited by how much could be administered at any one time by the IM route. Many patients were thus inadequately treated. The recent development of gamma globulin preparations for intravenous administration have overcome the volume or dosage hurdle, resulting in improved patient management. Moreover this new form of gamma globulin has prompted exploration of its indications in other disease states such as the immune cytopenias and autoimmune syndromes.

Autoimmune diseases also constitute a large class of disorders due to dysfunction of immunoregulatory mechanisms and may occur together with immunodeficiency syndromes. The scientific advances described above have also impacted positively on the diagnosis and management of autoimmune conditions. Several laboratories have demonstrated that **Lupus erythematosus, systemic** is associated with a deficiency of suppressor T-cell functions. Attempts to treat this disorder by the administration of immunosuppressive lymphokines are currently under investigation. **Diabetes mellitus, insulin dependent type** is now thought to be an autoimmune disease. The development of a new generation of immunosuppressive drugs, such as cyclosporin A, has shown some promise in the treatment of this form of diabetes. While cyclosporin A is recognized to cause some serious adverse reactions, such as nephrotoxicity, newer related drugs with diminished side effects are currently under development. It is further likely that a seemingly unrelated array of disorders, including epilepsy, immune cytopenias, hemolytic anemia, myasthenia gravis, multiple sclerosis, pemphigoid, etc. may be responsive to immunomodulatory therapy. Reports of clinical trials are appearing regularly.

The acquired immunodeficiency syndrome (AIDS) is posing a major contemporary challenge to the health sciences. While the etiologic agent, the human immunodeficiency virus, has been characterized, a treatment for this devastating disease remains elusive. Many of the recent and forthcoming gains in our understanding and therapy of other immunologic diseases may have direct application to the AIDS epidemic. Thus it is hoped that the enthusiasm and successes of the disciplines of immunology and molecular biology achieved over the past several decades will also provide unique new treatments for some present day scurges.

SC039

Stanley A. Schwartz

Immunodeficiency 5
See IMMUNODEFICIENCY, X-LINKED LYMPHOPROLIFERATIVE DISEASE

IMMUNODEFICIENCY WITH CENTROMERIC INSTABILITY   2520

Includes:
> Centromeric instability-immunodeficiency
> Chromosome 1, centromeric instability-immunodeficiency
> Chromosome 9, centromeric instability-immunodeficiency
> Chromosome 16, centromeric instability-immunodeficiency
> Immunodeficiency-centromeric instability-facial anomalies (ICF)
> Immunoglobulin deficiency-centromere instability

Excludes:
> **Ataxia-telangiectasia** (0094)
> **Bloom syndrome** (0112)
> Chromosomal breakage syndromes, classical
> **Chromosome instability, Nijmegen type** (2551)

Major Diagnostic Criteria: 1) Severe immunodeficiency including pronounced immunodeficiency and evidence for deficient cell-mediated deficiency; 2) developmental delay and facial abnormalities; and 3) instability of the centromeric regions of chromosomes 1, 9 and 16 resulting in multibranched configurations.

Clinical Findings: In the six patients reported; a series of variable immunodeficiencies, mild developmental delay, facial abnormalities including epicanthic folds, intestinal malabsorption, and severe failure to thrive was present in all.

All patients suffer from severe immunodeficiency associated with instability of the centromeric regions of chromosomes 1, 9 and 16, which results in multi-branched configurations.

Complications: Unknown.

Associated Findings: Pierre-Robin anomaly (micrognathia, cleft palate) in one patient. Internal malformations are poorly documented in the absence of autopsy data.

Etiology: Unknown.

Pathogenesis: None known.

MIM No.: 24286

POS No.: 4375

Sex Ratio: M3:F2

Occurrence: Six families have been reported, with affected sibs in two of the families.

Risk of Recurrence for Patient's Sib: Unknown.

Risk of Recurrence for Patient's Child: Unknown. Affected individuals are not expected to survive to reproduce.

Age of Detectability: First months of life by the finding of immunodeficiency, failure to thrive, developmental delay and the specific multibranched chromosomes 1, 9 and 16. In principle, prenatal diagnosis is feasible on fetal lymphocytes and amniocytes.

Gene Mapping and Linkage: See *Gene Map*.

Prevention: None known. Genetic counseling indicated.

Treatment: Symptomatic. Gammaglobulin replacement therapy and antibiotic treatment may reduce infections.

Prognosis: Long-term prognosis is poor. Three patients were last examined at five years of age and suffered from failure to

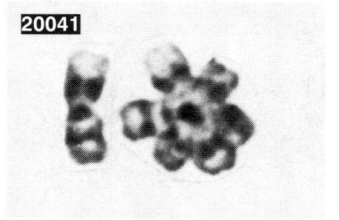 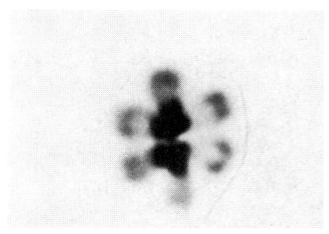

2520-20041: G- and C-banding of centromeric instability.

thrive and recurrent infections. A fourth patient died at the age of 18 months.

Detection of Carrier: Unknown. Extensive chromosomal investigations of the parents of one child were normal.

References:

Hulten M: Selective somatic pairing and fragility at 1q12 in a boy with common variable immunodeficiency. Clin Genet 1978; 14:294 only.

Tiepolo L, et al.: Multibranched chromosomes 1, 9, and 16 in a patient with combined IgA and IgE deficiency. Hum Genet 1979; 51:127–137.

Fryns JP, et al.: Centromeric instability of chromosomes 1, 9, and 16 associated with combined immunodeficiency. Hum Genet 1981; 57:108–110. *

Howard PJ, et al.: Centromeric instability of chromosomes 1 and 16 with variable immune deficiency: a new syndrome. Clin Genet 1985; 27:501–505.

Valkova G, et al.: Centromeric instability of chromosomes 1, 9 and 16 with variable immune deficiency: support of a new syndrome. Clin Genet 1987; 31:119–124.

Turleau C, et al.: Multibranched chromosomes in the ICF syndrome: immunodeficiency, centromeric instability, and facial anomalies. Am J Med Genet 1989; 32:420–424. †

FR030   **Jean-Pierre Fryns**

IMMUNODEFICIENCY, ADENOSINE DEAMINASE DEFICIENCY   2196

Includes:
    ADA deficiency
    Adenosine aminohydrolase deficiency (ADA)
    Adenosine deaminase
    Severe combined immunodeficiency with ADA

Excludes: Nucleoside deaminase deficiencies, other

Major Diagnostic Criteria: Complete absence of adenosine deaminase (ADA) enzymatic activity in the appropriate assay. Lysed erythrocyte ADA activity may be tested in nontransfused patients, with confirmation by testing peripheral blood mononuclear cells, cultured fibroblasts or B-lymphocyte lines. Heterozygous carriers typically have enzyme activity detected at greater than two SD below normal. The gel method is often used for screening, but is not 100% sensitive. Assays that determine the conversion of adenosine to inosine (or to uric acid with addition of xanthine oxidase) are preferred.

Clinical Findings: Patients present with severe combined immunodeficiency (SCID), the prominent features of which are recurrent and severe infections, failure to thrive, and intestinal malabsorption. Of all SCID cases, approximately 20-30% have ADA deficiency as the underlying etiology. This subgroup may be identified clinically by the association of SCID with chondroosseous dysplasia, which is characterized on X-ray by prominent growth arrest lines, paucity of trabeculae, platyspondyly of the vertebral bodies, vertically shortened pelvis with squared ilia, and cupping of the anterior ends of the ribs. Growth plate histopathologic findings are diagnostic and include absence of transition from proliferating to hypertrophic cells, lack of organized columns of hypertrophic cells, and uninterrupted calcified cartilage formation. However, the ADA assay is both necessary and sufficient to confirm the diagnosis. Patients often show signs and symptoms in the first several months of life, but not until ages 4–12 months in 10–15%. The spectrum of severity may relate to small residual amounts of enzyme activity noted in peripheral blood mononuclear cells of those who manifest the disease at the later ages.

Complications: In addition to the complications of SCID, neurologic abnormalities may occur in 10% of patients. Resolution of neurologic manifestations is seen after therapeutic intervention that lowers circulating levels of adenosine and deoxyadenosine. Renal mesangial sclerosis and adrenal cortical fibrosis have also been reported.

Associated Findings: Bony abnormalities.

Etiology: Autosomal recessive inheritance.

Pathogenesis: ADA is a 35–42 kd polypeptide encoded by a single 32 kb locus on the long arm of chromosome 20. It also exists as a higher molecular weight form (280 kd) composed of two ADA molecules joined by a dimeric ADA complexing protein. Electrophoretic studies reveal a series of codominant allelic variants. Analysis of ADA-deficient cells with cDNA probes reveals intact mRNA, and in vitro translation of hybrid-selected mRNA leads to elaboration of appropriate molecular weight proteins that are only weakly immunoprecipitable and exhibit no enzymatic activity. Single point mutations, confirmed by restriction fragment length polymorphism, lead to single amino acid substitutions which appear to render the enzyme inactive and more susceptible to proteolytic degradation. ADA catalyzes the irreversible deamination of adenosine and 2'deoxyadenosine to inosine and 2' deoxyinosine, respectively. In the absence of ADA, phosphorylation to the respective ribo- and deoxyribonucleotides occurs. The accumulation of metabolites has various effects. Deoxyadenosine 5'triphosphate (dATP) appears to block DNA synthesis in mature B-cells by inhibiting ribonucleotide reductase. Deoxyadenosine (dAR) affects immature T-cells in the G0/Gl phase of the cell cycle and inhibits the expression of interleukin-2 receptors. T-cells appear to be very sensitive to dAR accumulation, becoming nonviable before significant phosphorylation to dATP has occurred. Immature murine B-cells are less sensitive in vitro to dAR than activated, complement receptor-bearing B-cells. Inactivation of S-adenosyl homocysteine hydrolase by dAR, depletion of phosphoribosylpyrophosphate, pyrimidine starvation, and depletion of NAD pools may all play a role in the cytotoxic events. Broadly speaking, these findings are consistent with the clinical presentation of profound T-cell but variable B-cell dysfunction.

MIM No.: *10270

Sex Ratio: M1:F1

Occurrence: Accounts for 20–30% of all patients with SCID, and half of the cases of autosomal recessive SCID. More than 20 cases have been documented. Noted in Blacks, West Indian and Mediterranean families.

Risk of Recurrence for Patient's Sib:
    See Part I, *Mendelian Inheritance.*

Risk of Recurrence for Patient's Child:
    See Part I, *Mendelian Inheritance.*

Age of Detectability: Prenatally by determination of ADA activity in cultured amniotic cells.

Gene Mapping and Linkage: ADA (adenosine deaminase) has been mapped to 20q13.11 or 20q13.2-qter.

Prevention: None known. Genetic counseling indicated.

Treatment: Repeated partial exchange transfusions with frozen irradiated RBCs every 2–4 weeks has been shown to ameliorate symptoms. However, immunologic function generally continues to deteriorate. Current therapy is haplo-identical or haplo-mismatched bone marrow transplantation. Retrovirus-mediated transfer of cloned human cDNA has been shown to correct ADA deficiency in vitro in cultured human T- and B-cell lines. ADA deficiency is considered to be the first candidate for attempting in vivo gene replacement therapy. Clinical and biochemical improvement has recently been demonstrated with intramuscular injections of polyethylene glycol-modified bovine adenosine deaminase.

Prognosis: Untreated patients rarely survive beyond age two years except in cases of partial ADA deficiency. With successful bone marrow transplantation, the prognosis is excellent.

Detection of Carrier: Heterozygotes can be detected with 90% accuracy using quantitative assays. Phenotypic studies of ADA showing lack of the expected genetic polymorphism consistent with inheritance of a "null" allele confirms that a family is at risk.

Special Considerations: Partial ADA deficiency has been described. Studies indicate that some may result from genetic compounds at the ADA locus. Similar clinical findings may also be found in **Immunodeficiency, nucleoside-phosphorylase deficiency,** and cytidine deaminase (CDA; cytidine aminohydrolase) deficiency has been described in association with immunologic deficiency.

References:
Simmonds HA, et al.: Correlations between purine levels, clinical and immunological status in ADA deficiency. Adv Exp Med Biol 1985; 195(ptA):93.
Wortmann RL, et al.: Adenosine deaminase deficiency and chondroosseous dysplasia. Adv Exp Med Biol 1985; 195(ptA):81.
Hirschhorn R: Inherited enzyme deficiencies and immunodeficiency: adenosine deaminase (ADA) and purine nucleoside phosphorylase (PNP) deficiencies. Clin Immunol Immunopathol 1986; 40:157.
Kantoff PW, et al.: Correction of adenosine deaminase deficiency in cultured human T and B cells by retrovirus-mediated gene transfer. Proc Natl Acad Sci USA 1986; 83:6563.
Hirschhorn R, Ellenbogen A: Genetic heterogeneity in adenosine deaminase (ADA) deficiency: five different mutations in five new patients with partial ADA deficiency. Am J Hum Genet 1986; 38:13–25.
Hershfield MS, et al.: Treatment of adenosine deaminase deficiency with polyethylene glycol-modified adenosine deaminase. New Engl J Med 1987; 316:589–596.

SL002   Herbert B. Slade

IMMUNODEFICIENCY, AGAMMAGLOBULINEMIA, X-LINKED, INFANTILE   0027

Includes:
Agammaglobulinemia, X-linked, infantile
Bruton agammaglobulinemia
Hypogammaglobulinemia, X-linked

Excludes:
Agammaglobulinemia-thymoma syndrome (0944)
Immunoglobulin G subclass deficiencies
Immunodeficiency, common variable type (0521)
Immunodeficiency, X-linked severe combined (0524)

Major Diagnostic Criteria: Males with absent or severely diminished peripheral and intestinal lymphoid tissue, as demonstrable, for instance, by near absence of tonsils and adenoids. Histologically, plasma cells and germinal centers of lymphoid tissue are absent with or without antigenic stimulation. B-lymphocytes are absent. Absent or very diminished Ig and antibody response to administered antigens. The frequency and severity of bacterial infections increase starting toward the end of the first half-year of life, involving respiratory tract, sinuses, GI tract, and skin.

Clinical Findings: Age of onset of manifestations is usually between 3 and 6 months in males; with repeated bouts of purulent conjunctivitis, otitis media, recurrent upper respiratory infections, bronchitis, and skin infections. Early sinusitis is frequent, and pneumonias begin during the first year of life, often leading to bronchiectasis. Recurrent episodes of septicemia may occur, and meningitis attacks may be seen repeatedly. There is a propensity to contract infectious hepatitis, which, not infrequently, becomes a fatal disease in these patients. Infections with echoviruses, especially those of the high-numbered types, can be devastating. Paralytic poliomyelitis, often associated with live vaccine administration, is unusually frequent. Varicella is another viral disease known to be more severe in these children both by recurrence and may be complicated by occasional accompanying pneumonia. Tonsillar and adenoid tissues are grosely deficient. X-rays reveal clouding of the sinuses with evident infection, obliteration, and destruction of the mastoid air cells, minimal hilar shadows, pulmonary infiltrates, segmental atelectasis, and areas of bronchiectasis, wasting of the tissues, and gaseous distention of the abdomen.

Laboratory findings reveal less than 100 mg% immunoglobulins (Ig), IgM and IgA are absent. IgG is normal at birth but drops to less than 100 mg% in the first 6 months. Peripheral blood is normal, but sometimes there is periodic neutropenia, transient eosinophilia, or monocytosis. B-lymphocytes are absent from the blood and lymphoid tissues. Bone marrow shows absence or severe paucity of plasma cells, but pre-B-lymphocytes recognized by appropriate surface markers and by cytoplasmic but not by surface Ig, are present in normal or near-normal numbers. Bacteriologic investigation of infections demonstrates recurrent diplococcus pneumonias, *Haemophilus influenzae,* meningococcus, streptococcus, and, after antibiotic therapy, usually *Pseudomonas.* ASOT remains negative in spite of documented streptococcal infections. Isoagglutinins are absent, and there is failure to respond to injected antigens such as DPT immunization with production of antibodies. Antibodies to pneumococcal antigens and *H. influenzae* are usually not found.

Complications: Poor growth, clubbing of fingers and toes, erythema nodosum, potbelly, septicemias, bronchiectasis, pulmonary fibrosis and cor pulmonale, cholesteatoma, conductive hearing loss, anemia, diarrhea, hypocalcemia, protein-losing enteropathy, ulcerative colitis, regional enteritis.

Associated Findings: Arthritis of the rheumatoid type in 20–40%, later a dermatomyositis-like illness, agranulocytosis, thrombocytopenia, autoimmune disease, malabsorption, amyloidosis. Persistent echovirus infection may lead to destructive CNS disease. These persistent virus infections may be accompanied by the dermatomyositis syndrome.

Etiology: X-linked recessive inheritance.

Pathogenesis: Pre-B cells fail to develop into B-lymphocytes. The inability to muster a humoral antibody response to pyogenic organisms, which surround the infant, leads to severe infections as soon as the maternal complement or immunoglobulins to the newborn are exhausted. Pneumococcus, *H. influenzae,* meningococcus, streptococcus, and *Pseudomonas aeruginosa* are the most successful invaders under these conditions, spreading from the natural portals of entry inward without effective host resistance. Thus recurrent and later chronic sinopulmonary disease is the outstanding clinical event, together with pyoderma, purulent conjunctivitis, and purulent otitis media. Further uncontrolled spread and dissemination are manifested by septicemias, meningitis, deep abscesses, osteomyelitis, and other parenchymatous pyogenic involvement. Progressive pulmonary impairment with bronchiectasis, fibrosis, and eventual right heart overload from increasing pulmonary vascular resistance are later sequelae. Intestinal involvement with diarrhea, protein-losing enteropathy, and development of regional enteritis and ulcerative colitis are probably consequences of the absence of plasma cells and lymphoid tissue aggregates normally responsible for host resistance in this area. The susceptibility to severe infectious hepatitis and recurrent varicella indicates that B-cell function or antibodies are involved in defense against these organisms. Long-range effects of the chronic infectious processes are physical underdevelopment, amyloidosis, and possible CNS damage. Survival beyond early childhood with the underlying deficiency makes the patient susceptible to rheumatoid arthritis, dermatomyositis-like illness, and autoimmune disease. The pathogenesis of these complications is not understood, but their occurrence in this pure antibody deficiency state indicates that cell-mediated immunity attributed to T-lymphocytes can be responsible for some of the manifestations of autoimmune disease. It has now been established that B-lymphocyte differentiation in these patients is arrested at the level of the pre-B-cell to B-cell differentiation step. Pre-B-cells are present in the marrow, but B-lymphocytes develop poorly or not at all and are not present in the blood.

MIM No.: *30030

Sex Ratio: M1:F0

Occurrence: 1:50,000 live births.

Risk of Recurrence for Patient's Sib:
See Part I, *Mendelian Inheritance.* See Lau et al (1988).

Risk of Recurrence for Patient's Child:
See Part I, *Mendelian Inheritance.* Affected individuals are not expected to survive to reproduce.

Age of Detectability: Neonatal period by study of blood lymphocytes, bone marrow, or lymph node cells.

Gene Mapping and Linkage: AGMX1 (agammaglobulinemia, X-linked 1 (Bruton)) has been mapped to Xq21.33-q22.

Prevention: None known. Genetic counseling indicated.

Treatment: IM immunoglobulin by injection, 0.6 cc/kg/month or 0.3 cc/kg/2 weeks, or plasma from hepatitis-free donors. Any of several preparations of gammaglobulin for intravenous administration given in doses suitable to maintaining the circulating gammaglobulin levels within the normal range of 700–1,300 mg/dl. Avoidance of exposure to infections; regular follow-up. Vigorous antibiotic therapy at earliest signs of infection.

Prognosis: Progressive sinopulmonary disease is occasionally a major problem. Untreated patients rarely survive infancy or early childhood. With good medical attention and preventive immunoglobulin therapy, outlook is much improved. Long-range survivors have now reached adulthood.

Detection of Carrier: RFLP markers have been used to identify carrier state and in early diagnosis (Schuurman et at, 1988).

Special Considerations: This defect has many clinical and laboratory features in common with **Immunodeficiency, common variable type.** However, the absence of B-cells in blood and the clear-cut defect in the humoral antibody-producing capacity without any thymic-mediated involvement makes it possible to distinguish clinically with the help of laboratory evidence. Lymphoreticular malignancy may be increased, although carcinoma and sarcoma are not known to be increased. This is an important prognostic consideration. Recent studies suggest that there may be two distinct and separate forms of X-linked infantile agammaglobulinemia.

References:

Good RA, et al.: Consideration of some questions asked by patients with an attempt at classification. In: BD:OAS 1968; IV(1):17.
Rosen FS, Janeway CA: Diagnosis and treatment of antibody deficiency syndromes. Postgrad Med 1968; 43:188.
Wollheim FA: Primary "acquired" hypogammaglobulinemia: genetic defect or acquired disease? In: 1968; IV(1):311.
Report of a WHO Scientific Group. Primary immunodeficiency diseases. In: 1983; XIX(3):345–360.
Report of a WHO Scientific Group. Primary immunodeficiency diseases 1. Introduction. In: Eibl MM, Rosen FS, eds: Primary immunodeficiency diseases. Amsterdam: Excerpta Medica, 1986:341–375.
Mensick, EJBM, et al.: Immunoglobulin heavy chain gene rearrangements in X-linked agammaglobulinemia. Eur J Immunol 1986; 110:963–967.
Schuurman RKB, et al.: Early diagnosis in X-linked agammaglobulinemia. Europ J Pediat 1988; 147:93–95.
Lau YL, et al.: Genetic prediction in X-linked agammaglobulinaemia. Am J Med Genet 1988; 31:437–448.
World Health Organization. Primary immunodeficiency diseases. Immunodeficiency Reviews 1989; 1:173–205.

G0023   **Robert A. Good**

IMMUNODEFICIENCY, AGRANULOCYTOSIS, INFANTILE KOSTMANN TYPE   2197

Includes:

    Agranulocytosis, infantile Kostmann type
    Kostmann syndrome
    Neutrophil differentiation factor

Excludes:

    Autoimmune neutropenia
    Neutropenia, benign familial (2215)
    Neutropenia, cyclic (0714)

Major Diagnostic Criteria: Persistent severe granulocytopenia, with an absolute neutrophil count less than 500 and often less than 200, is the hallmark of the disorder.

Clinical Findings: Affected infants appear normal, but they are either severely neutropenic at birth or become so in the neonatal period.

During the first few months of life these infants have severe infections. Initially, the infections usually involve the skin and mucosal surfaces, but all organ systems can be involved, with lymphadenitis, pneumonia, peritonitis, liver abscesses, and sep-

ticemia especially common. Infants who survive invariably develop subsequent serious infections. The prompt administration of broad-spectrum antibiotics has prolonged the survival of affected individuals, with survival to adolescence occasionally reported. Although recurrent bacterial infections begin during the first year of life, the other hematopoietic cell lines are not affected, and thus the total white count may be in the normal range because of lymphocytosis and monocytosis. Platelets are not affected, and although there may be an accompanying anemia of chronic illness, the red cell line is unaffected. Examination of the bone marrow shows markedly decreased numbers of mature granulocytes, with a predominance of vacuolated myelocytes and promyelocytes. There may be increased numbers of monocytes, eosinophils, plasma cells, and histiocytes.

Complications: One patient developed acute myelocytic leukemia at 14 years of age, which may indicate an increased susceptibility to neoplasia.

Associated Findings: None known.

Etiology: Autosomal recessive inheritance.

Pathogenesis: Unknown. Evidence obtained from bone marrow culture and from the results of bone marrow transplantation suggests that the cause is a defective stem cell. There are normal or even increased numbers of myeloid colony-forming cells in the marrow, but the maturation of the granulocytes is abnormal. These dysplastic cells either autolyze or are phagocytized by the macrophages in the marrow. Antineutrophil antibodies have not been implicated.

MIM No.: *20270

Sex Ratio: M1:F1

Occurrence: About 75 cases have been reported.

Risk of Recurrence for Patient's Sib:
    See Part I, *Mendelian Inheritance.*

Risk of Recurrence for Patient's Child:
    See Part I, *Mendelian Inheritance.*

Age of Detectability: Always within the first few months of life, but some have been neutropenic at birth.

Gene Mapping and Linkage: Unknown.

Prevention: None known. Genetic counseling indicated.

Treatment: Prompt administration of antibiotics at the first sign of infection has markedly prolonged the survival of affected individuals. For apparently localized infections, oral antibiotics can be tried, but if response is not prompt, parenteral broad-spectrum antibiotics (covering *Staphyloccocus aureus* and gram-negative enteritis) should be started. Prophylactic antibiotics, such as trimethoprim-sulfamethoxazole, have been advocated, but their efficacy has not been documented.

A more permanent therapeutic option is a bone marrow transplant from a compatible sib. With appropriate preconditioning with total body irradiation and cytotoxic drugs, engraftment has been accomplished with the establishment of normal granulocyte maturation. Granulocyte differentiation and subsequent development of circulating granulocytes has occurred following the subcutaneous administration of granulocyte-colony stimulating factor. The use of granulocytic colony stimulating factor should comprise the initial therapy.

Prognosis: In most of the early reports, the affected individuals died in infancy or early childhood. More recently, improvements in supportive care have led to survival into adolescence. The availability of a compatible sib offers the potential for cure by bone marrow transplant, although this procedure is certainly not without risk. A slight number of patients have developed acute leukemia. Amelioration of clinical infections has occurred in response to use of granulocyte-colony stimulating factor.

Detection of Carrier: Unknown.

References:

Kostmann R: Infantile genetic agranulocytosis: a review with presentation of ten new cases. Acta Paediatr Scand 1975; 64:362–368. *

Parmley RT, et al.: Congenital dysgranulocytopoietic neutropenia. Blood 1980; 56:465–475. *

Rappaport JM, et al.: Correction of infantile agranulocytosis by allogeneic bone marrow transplantation. Am J Med 1980; 68:605–609.

Lin CY, et al.: Infantile genetic agranulocytosis in three siblings. Med J Osaka Univ 1981; 31:111–116.

AX001
B0048

Richard Axtell
Laurence A. Boxer

Immunodeficiency, C1r/C1s deficiency
See COMPLEMENT COMPONENT 1, DEFICIENCY OF
Immunodeficiency, cartilage-hair hypoplasia
See METAPHYSEAL CHONDRODYSPLASIA, TYPE McKUSICK

IMMUNODEFICIENCY, COMMON VARIABLE TYPE   0521

Includes:
    Agammaglobulinemia, acquired
    Agammaglobulinemia, adult
    Agammaglobulinemia, late-onset
    Hypogammaglobulinemia, familial
    Immunodeficiency, common varied
    Immunoglobulin deficiencies
    Late-onset immunoglobulin deficiency

Excludes:
    Agammaglobulinemia-thymoma syndrome (0944)
    IgA deficiency, selective
    Immunodeficiency, agammaglobulinemia, X-linked, infantile (0027)
    Immunodeficiency, common variable type (0521)
    Immunodeficiency, X-linked severe combined (0524)
    Immunodeficiency, X-linked with hyper IgM (2524)
    Serum allotypes, human (0476)
    Transcobalamin II deficiency (2624)
    Transient hypogammaglobulinemia of infancy

Major Diagnostic Criteria: Decreased concentration of all or some of the major immunoglobulins (IgG, IgA, IgM) in serum with nearly normal T-cell numbers and function. Conditions secondarily resulting in low serum immunoglobulins must be excluded; i.e. protein loss, drugs, malignancy, infection and **Transcobalamin II deficiency**.

Clinical Findings: Clinical symptoms and infective agents are very similar to those in **Immunodeficiency, agammaglobulinemia, X-linked, infantile**, but somewhat milder. Onset is usually after two years of age, most frequently in the second or third decade. Although occasional patients suffer remarkably few infections, recurrent or persistent sinopulmonary infeciton is the dominant clinical problem occurring in almost 90%. Patients suffer from pulmonary airway, parenchymal and pleural disease with 30–40% going on to develop serious pulmonary impairment (chronic bronchitis, bronchiectasis, interstitial fibrosis and panlobular emphysema). Chronic otitis media is frequent (30%). Gastrointestinal manifestations are found in up to 60% of patients and include chronic diarrhea, malabsorption or protein-losing enteropathy. Giardia lamblia infections occur in 35–65% and Clostridium difficile in 24%. There are decreased small bowel brush border enzyme activities and patchy histological abnormalities of the partial villous atrophy type.

It is likely that some changes are secondary to occult or proven infection. As many as 40% of patients will be anemic with pernicious anemia in approximately five percent. Cancer develops with a markedly increased incidence (5 to 13-fold) in the fifth and sixth decades of life. Stomach cancer is increased 50-fold and lymphoma 30-fold with an undue proportion of lymphomas occurring in female patients. The most common pathogens are high grade encapsulated bacteria but Mycoplasma and Ureaplasma have been identified as significant infectious agents. Echovirus meningoencephalitis and dermatomyositis occur infrequently compared with **Immunodeficiency, agammaglobulinemia, X-linked, infantile**. Patients are also at risk for developing vaccine-associated poliomyelitis.

There is considerable heterogeneity in laboratory findings with variability in numbers of circulating B-cells from nearly normal to very low. These B-cells do not differentiate into immunoglobulin producing plasma cells *in vivo* or *in vitro*. There is diversity with respect to the expression of surface membrane immunoglobulins, B-cell antigens and B-lymphocyte ecto-5′-nucleotidase activity. There are varying degrees of lymphopenia, T-cell subset imbalances and depression of blastogenic responses to mitogens. Laboratory findings may also vary with time in individual patients.

Careful study of family members is indicated and may reveal other antibody deficiency syndromes (especially IgA deficiency and immunoglobulin deficiency with increased IgM), autoimmune diseases and malignancies. This suggests wide intrafamilial variability in expression of a common defect.

Complications: Bronchiectasis, arthritis (7%), gastric carcinoma, lymphoreticular malignancy, cholelithiasis, lymphoid interstitial pneumonia, pseudolymphoma, amyloidosis, transfusion reactions, noncaseating granulomas of lungs, spleen, skin and liver. Echovirus and viral hepatitis infections are particularly troublesome.

Associated Findings: Intestinal nodular lymphoid hyperplasia, splenomegaly, thymoma, alopecia areata, autoimmune hemolytic anemia, neutropenia, sprue-like syndrome, gastric atrophy, achlorhydria, pernicious anemia, thyroid disease, and **Lupus erythematosus, systemic** occur.

Etiology: Autosomal recessive or dominant inheritance.

Pathogenesis: Progressive loss of humoral immune function due to a genetically determined abnormality of B-cell maturation into immunoglobulin-synthesizing and -secreting plasma cells. blocks occur at pre-B, B-cell, and plasma cell levels. Excessive T suppression of B-cell differentiation may be both primary and secondary and is potentially clinically significant if present. Failure of helper T-cell activity and enhanced suppressor activity of monocytes have been described. Autoantibodies to T- or B-cells may be present.

MIM No.: *24050, 14683, *14690, *14691, *14700, *14701, *14702, *14707, *14710, *14711, *14712, *14713, *14716, *14717, *14718, 14720

Sex Ratio: Presumably M1:F1, but some series report a male preponderance.

Occurrence: Sporadic and familial forms occur. True incidence is not known as detection is related to clinical index of suspicion but is less common than IgA deficiency.

Risk of Recurrence for Patient's Sib:
See Part I, *Mendelian Inheritance.*

Risk of Recurrence for Patient's Child:
See Part I, *Mendelian Inheritance.*

Age of Detectability: Onset is at any age but especially after the second decade.

Gene Mapping and Linkage: IGHA1 (immunoglobulin alpha 1) has been mapped to 14q32.33.

IGHA2 (immunoglobulin alpha 2 (A2M marker)) has been mapped to 14q32.33.

IGHJ (immunoglobulin heavy polypeptide, joining region) has been mapped to 14q32.3.

IGHM (immunoglobulin mu) has been mapped to 14q32.33.

IGHV (immunoglobulin heavy polypeptide, variable region (many genes)) has been mapped to 14q32.33.

IGHG1 (immunoglobulin gamma 1 (Gm marker)) has been mapped to 14q32.33.

IGHG2 (immunoglobulin gamma 2 (Gm marker)) has been mapped to 14q32.33.

IGHG3 (immunoglobulin gamma 3 (Gm marker)) has been mapped to 14q32.33.

IGHG4 (immunoglobulin gamma 4 (Gm marker)) has been mapped to 14q32.33.

IGHEP1 (immunoglobulin epsilon pseudogene 1) has been mapped to 14q32.33.

IGHD (immunoglobulin delta) has been mapped to 14q32.33.

IGHE (immunoglobulin epsilon) has been mapped to 14q32.33.

IGKC (immunoglobulin kappa constant region) has been mapped to 2p12.

It is possible that the primary abnormalities may occur in genes which regulate immunoglobulin synthesis.

Prevention: None known. Genetic counseling indicated.

Treatment: Therapy involves replacement of IgG with intravenous immunoglobulin, 0.1–0.6 g/kg/month, with the total dose tailored to individual needs. The higher dose permits achievement of normal serum IgG levels and, in patients with significant sinopulmonary disease, it results in resolution of sinusitis, reduction in cough and improvement in pulmonary function tests. It is the treatment of choice for echovirus-caused meningoencephalitis and dermatomyositis. Adverse reactions to the administration of intravenous immunoglobulin can be prevented by prior administration of hydrocortisone. Specific infections should be treated aggressively with antimicrobial agents. Continous broad-spectrum antibiotics are often necessary. Cimetidine may reverse T suppressor activity, effecting increased serum IgG level and improved clinical status in some patients.

Prognosis: Guarded. There is increased mortality from all causes, but especially from late malignancies.

Detection of Carrier: Unknown.

References:

Wollheim FA: Inherited "acquired" hypogammaglobulinaemia. Lancet 1961; I:316–317.

Waldman TA, et al: Role of suppressor T cells in the pathogenesis of common variable hypogammaglobulinemia. Lancet 1974; II:609–613.

Hermans PE, et al: Idiopathic late-onset immunoglobulin deficiency. Am J Med 1976; 61:221–237.

Kinlen LJ, et al: Prospective study of cancer in patients with hypogammaglobulinaemia. Lancet 1985; I:263–266.

Roifman CM, et al: Benefit of intravenous IgG replacement in hypogammaglobulinemic patients with chronic sinopulmonary disease. Am J Med 1985; 79:171–174.

White WB, Ballow M: Modulation of suppressor-cell activity by cimetidine in patients with common variable hypogammaglobulinemia. New Engl J Med 1985; 312:198–202.

Watts WJ, et al: Respiratory dysfunction in patients with common variable hypogammaglobulinemia. Am Rev Respir Dis 1986; 134:699–703.

RE030   **Elena R. Reece**

Immunodeficiency, common varied
  See *IMMUNODEFICIENCY, COMMON VARIABLE TYPE*
Immunodeficiency, complement component 3
  See *COMPLEMENT COMPONENT 3, DEFICIENCY OF*
Immunodeficiency, erythrophagocytic lymphohistiocytosis
  See *LYMPHOHISTIOCYTOSIS, FAMILIAL ERYTHROPHAGOCYTIC*
Immunodeficiency, functional C1q deficiency
  See *COMPLEMENT COMPONENT 1, DEFICIENCY OF*
Immunodeficiency, granulocyte glycoprotein deficiency
  See *GRANULOCYTE GLYCOPROTEIN CD11/CD18 DEFICIENCY*

IMMUNODEFICIENCY, HYPER IGE TYPE   2211

Includes:
  HIE syndrome
  Hyper IgE, recurrent infection syndrome
  Hyperimmunoglobulin E-recurrent infection syndrome
  Job syndrome

Excludes: Skin, atopy, familial (3150)

Major Diagnostic Criteria: Severe and recurrent staphylococcal infections of the skin and lower respiratory tract from infancy. The diagnosis is confirmed by a history of recurrent furunculosis, staphylococcal pneumonia, and pneumatoceles. Affected individuals have a history of, or current, chronic pruritic dermatitis, with a rash that is not typical atopic eczema. Markedly elevated polyclonal serum IgE, and pronounced eosinophilia of blood and sputum, is found in all affected individuals.

Clinical Findings: Abscesses of the skin and/or lungs have occurred as early as the first day of life, but always begin during infancy and recur throughout life. The condition affects both males and females; members of successive generations within families have been afflicted. It has been reported in Blacks and Whites. In early life there is a predilection for furuncles to localize about the scalp, neck, and face: particularly around the eyes, where hordeolums and even lacrimal gland abscesses occur. Recurrent staphylococcal pneumonia, with resultant persistent pneumatoceles, is typically the major presenting problem. Pneumatocele formation is not seen to this extent in any other clinical condition, including **Granulomatous disease, chronic** (CGD) and **Cystic fibrosis**, where staphylococcal lung infections are common.

Surgical removal of lung cysts that persist for more than six months is usually necessary to prevent superinfection with *Haemophilus* influenzae or other gram-negative organisms or aspergilloma formation. Most have also had chronic or recurrent infections of the ears, sinuses, eyes, and oral mucosa. Fewer have had infections of joints, viscera, and blood. Sites that have usually been spared include the gastrointestinal and urinary tracts, the meninges, and the bones. Exceptions include two patients with cryptococcal meningitis and a rare patient with osteomyelitis. Infrequency of the latter in this condition contrasts with the high frequency of bone infections in CGD. *Staphylococcus aureus*, coagulase positive, has caused infections in all patients. *Candida albicans*, *Haemophilus* influenzae, pneumococci, and Group A streptococci have infected from one-fourth to one-half of patients. Miscellaneous gram-negative rods, *Aspergillus* and *Trichophyton* species, and other fungi, have been pathogens in some cases.

Serum IgE has been noted to rise rapidly during early infancy and is always significantly above the normal 95% confidence interval even when no dermatitis is present. Nevertheless, affected individuals have few or no respiratory allergic symptoms, and the pruritic rash often resembles seborrheic rather that atopic dermatitis in character as well as distribution. Skin testing for IgE-mediated hypersensitivity usually reveals multiple positive reactions to inhalant, food, and pollen allergens and to antigens from infectious agents. High titers of IgE antibodies to staphylococcal and candidal organisms have been detected by radioimmunoassay.

Serum concentrations of immunoglobulins other than IgE are usually normal, although IgD may also be elevated. However, patients usually have impaired anamnestic antibody responses to vaccine antigens, and responses to neoantigens are poor. Cell-mediated immune responses to ubiquitous antigens *in vivo* have been depressed in roughly one-half of patients studied. *In vitro* lymphocyte responses to mitogens have most often been normal, but are usually low to absent following specific antigen stimulation. In addition, responses to mononuclear cells from genetically different members of the patient's family are often low or nondetectable. Percentages and absolute numbers of B- and T-lymphocytes and subpopulations are usually normal, with no increase in IgE-bearing B-lymphocytes. Complement activity and levels of complement components are normal. Polymorphonuclear cell phagocytic and bactericidal functions are normal, as are chemiluminescence and nitroblue tetrazolium dye reduction following phagocytosis. Inconstant chemotactic abnormalities have been reported, but most often both polymorphonuclear and monocyte chemotaxis has been normal. The abscesses are filled with numerous polymorphonuclear cells, and the walls of lung cysts as well as the tissues are heavily infiltrated with eosinophils.

Complications: Superinfected persistent lung cysts are the most common complications, with eventual loss of lobes or of entire lungs if appropriate antibiotic and surgical treatments are not rendered. The second most common complication is cutaneous and other fungal infection. High dose multiple antibiotic therapy is required on a continuing basis. Aspergilloma formation in infected persistent pneumatoceles can lead to fatal hemoptysis. Cryptococcal meningitis and lymphomas have also been reported.

Associated Findings: Osteopenia is present in most patients, with no obvious defect of calcium or phosphorus metabolism, and is seemingly unrelated to the state of activity of the patient. Fractures of bones of the extremities or of the vertebral bodies are common. Coarse facial features are present in a majority, although the basis of this is undetermined. Craniosynostosis has also been reported (Hoger et al, 1985)

Etiology: Familial patterns have suggested autosomal dominant inheritance with incomplete penetrance. Autosomal recessive inheritance of the Job syndrome "variant" has been reported.

Pathogenesis: Disordered IgE regulation and defects in specific immunologic responsiveness are prominent abnormalities; neither is likely to be the primary biologic error.

MIM No.: 14706, *24370

Sex Ratio: M2:F1 is suggested by available data.

Occurrence: Undetermined. 23 cases were seen at one major United States referral center over a 15 year period.

Risk of Recurrence for Patient's Sib:
See Part I, *Mendelian Inheritance.*

Risk of Recurrence for Patient's Child:
See Part I, *Mendelian Inheritance.*

Age of Detectability: In early infancy.

Gene Mapping and Linkage: Unknown.

Prevention: None known. Genetic counseling indicated. Staphylococcal infections can be prevented by continuous prophylaxis with oral antistaphylococcal penicillins or cephalosporins, which should be initiated at time of diagnosis of the hyper-IgE syndrome.

Treatment: In addition to chronic antistaphylococcal antibiotic prophylaxis or therapy, thoracic surgery for persistent pneumatoceles is of utmost importance. Judicious use of other antibiotics or antifungals is indicated for superinfections. Incision and drainage of abscesses is frequently required if antistaphylococcal prophylaxis has not been employed.

Prognosis: If staphylococcal infections are prevented by prophylaxis with antistaphylococcal drugs from an early age, the prognosis is excellent. Many patients reach adulthood. If staphylococcal lung infections lead to persistent pneumatoceles, which become superinfected, death from extensive lung disease can occur at an early age. Extensive fungal superinfection also connotes a poor prognosis.

Detection of Carrier: Unknown.

Special Considerations: Some authors equate this condition with *Job Syndrome* (after "Satan...smote Job with sore boils from the sole of his foot unto his crown. Job 2:7). However, the latter condition was described in 1966 (a year before IgE was discovered) as one in which two red-haired, fair-skinned, nonallergic females with hyperextensible joints had "cold" abscesses. Few patients in the extensive series of hyper-IgE syndrome patients evaluated since 1966 have had red hair or hyperextensible joints. The limited published immunologic data on the two original "Job" patients (who reportedly were found several years later to have elevated serum IgE), and two others, makes it impossible to know whether there is any overlap between the Job and hyper-IgE syndromes. Chemotactic defects were suggested by a few investigators as a prominent feature of the hyper-IgE syndrome. However, numerous subsequent studies have shown this to be a rare and inconsistent defect, ruling out a primary role for chemotactic abnormalities in these patients' infection-susceptibility. Finally, a report from one laboratory stated that such patients have a deficiency in CD8+ T cells (T8+ or suppressor/cytotoxic subset). However, this has not be confirmed.

References:
Buckley RH, et al.: Extreme hyperimmunoglobulinemia E and undue susceptibility to infection. Pediatrics 1972; 49:59–70.
Merten DF, et al.: The hyperimmunoglobulinemia E syndrome: radiographic observations. Radiology 1979; 132:71–78.
Buckley RH, Sampson HA: The hyperimmunoglobulinemia E syndrome. In: Clinical immunology update. New York: Elsevier North-Holland, 1981.
Donabedian H, Gallin JI: The hyperimmunoglobulin E recurrent-infection (Job's) syndrome: a review of the NIH experience and the literature. Medicine 1983; 62:195–208.
Buckley RH: The hyper IgE Syndrome. In: Current therapy in allergy and immunology. Philadelphia: B.C. Decker (Mosby), 1984.
Hoger PH, et al.: Craniosynostosis in hyper-IgE-syndrome. Europ J Pediatr 1985; 144:414–417.

BU042

Rebecca H. Buckley

IMMUNODEFICIENCY, IGG SUBCLASS DEFICIENCIES 2947

Includes:
Antibody deficiencies, partial
IgG heavy chain locus
Immunoglobulin Gm-1
Immunoglobulin Gm-2
Immunoglobulin Gm-3
Immunoglobulin Gm-4

Excludes:
Immunodeficiency, agammaglobulinemia, X-linked, infantile (0027)
Immunodeficiency, combined variable hypogammaglobulinemia (3105)
Immunodeficiency, common variable type (0521)
Immunodeficiency with increased IgM
Immunoglobulin A deficiency (0525)
Selective IgA deficiency
Selective IgM deficiency
Serum allotypes, human (0476)
Transient hypogammaglobulinemia of infancy

Major Diagnostic Criteria: Serum levels of one, two, or three IgG subclasses <2 SD below the mean for age. Clinical use of the designation is usually reserved for the finding of an inability to make expected antibody responses in a patient who is experiencing recurrent or chronic respiratory infections.

Clinical Findings: Clinical symptoms may begin at any age, although onset in infancy or early childhood is common. Patients reported to date have had symptoms localized to the respiratory tract. They most often experience recurrent pneumonia, sinusitis, and otitis media. Recurrent bronchitis and purulent rhinitis have also been reported in these patients. It is likely that IgG subclass deficiency can result in chronic respiratory tract symptoms as well.

Clinical variability is common. It is not clear why some patients with a given IgG subclass or antibody level experience severe symptoms while others with equivalent levels have mild symptoms. It has been suggested that in some patients there may be compensation through other host defense mechanisms.

In many children, IgG subclass deficiency may represent a maturational lag in development of immune function which will disappear with time. In other children and in adults, it may be a permanent, stable deficiency or it may be the precursor to the development of common variable immunodeficiency.

By definition, serum levels of one, two, or three IgG subclasses are <2 SD below mean for age. Patients with deficiency of IgG1 may have difficulty making antibody responses to protein antigens, while those with deficiency of IgG2 may have difficulty with certain polysaccharide antigens. Deficiencies of IgG2 and IgG4 often occur together. IgG2 and IgG2-IgG4 deficiencies have been associated with an IgA deficiency and may explain clinical symptoms in some patients previously thought to have only selective IgA deficiency. Total serum IgG is low usually only if IgG1 is low. A low IgG subclass level is usually associated with an abnormal antibody response in that or another IgG subclass. The latter finding and the documentation of other immune abnormalities in IgG subclass-deficient patients suggest that the low IgG subclass level is a marker of a more global immune abnormality. It should be noted that healthy individuals with a complete absence of one or more IgG subclasses have been reported.

Complications: Chronic otitis media, with hearing loss; chronic sinusitis; chronic bronchitis; reactive airway disease. Bronchiectasis occurs commonly in those patients who experience recurrent or chronic lower respiratory tract infections.

Associated Findings: Possibly defects in other arms of immunity.

Etiology: Possibly autosomal dominant inheritance.

Pathogenesis: Possibly related to inability to make certain V-D-J gene segment rearrangements or to make appropriate class switches to a particular C gene, limiting the antibody repertoire. This might occur because of gene deletion or for other as yet undefined reasons.

MIM No.: *14710, *14711, *14712, *14713

Sex Ratio: Presumably M1:F1.

Occurrence: Undetermined, but studies to date suggest that these may be the most common immunodeficiencies.

Risk of Recurrence for Patient's Sib: Unknown. Multiple affected sibs within a family have been reported.

Risk of Recurrence for Patient's Child: Unknown.

Age of Detectability: After clearance of the majority of maternal transplacentally acquired IgG, i.e., after ages 6–9 months.

Gene Mapping and Linkage: IGHG1 (immunoglobulin gamma 1 (Gm marker)) has been mapped to 14q32.33.

IGHG2 (immunoglobulin gamma 2 (Gm marker)) has been mapped to 14q32.33.

IGHG3 (immunoglobulin gamma 3 (Gm marker)) has been mapped to 14q32.33.

IGHG4 (immunoglobulin gamma 4 (Gm marker)) has been mapped to 14q32.33.

Prevention: None known. Genetic counseling indicated.

Treatment: Some patients may require only antibiotic therapy for acute infections; others, in addition, may benefit from prophylactic antibiotic coverage. Intramuscular gamma globulin has been administered to some patients with benefit, although incomplete resolution of symptoms may be seen because of limitations in dosage. Intravenous gamma globulin has appeared to be useful in eliminating symptoms. Although the optimum dosage has not been determined, it is likely that 300 mg/kg or more must be given about every three weeks. Regression of bronchiectasis has been seen after prolonged therapy with intravenous gamma globulin in high dosage.

Prognosis: Normal life span unless significant pulmonary compromise occurs because of recurrent or chronic lower respiratory tract infections.

Detection of Carrier: Unknown.

Special Considerations: The designation *IgG subclass deficiency* has inherent difficulties. Two and one-half percent of normal people will have a level of any given IgG subclass <2 SD below the mean for age. Also, the serum level of an IgG subclass is a poor predictor of IgG class antibody responses, especially in children. Thus, finding a low level of a subclass in a symptomatic patient does not necessarily indicate that this is the cause of the symptoms. Abnormal subclass-specific antibody responses have been demonstrated in patients who have normal serum levels of IgG subclasses yet experience symptoms identical to those with IgG subclass deficiencies.

It may be that finding a low level of an IgG subclass in an appropriate patient suggests the possibility of an immunodeficiency that may be limited to specific antibody responses or that may include other immune abnormalities. It is clear that finding normal levels of IgG or IgG subclasses does not rule out this possibility. On the other hand, finding a complete absence of one or more IgG subclasses may reflect a gene deletion that has no clinical significance.

In any event, diagnosis of immunodeficiency should rest on demonstration of lack of immune function. For IgG subclass deficiency, this currently should include lack of appropriate antibody responses. Thus, *partial antibody deficiency* may be a preferable term to describe this syndrome.

References:

Schur PH, et al.: Selective gamma-G globulin deficiencies in patients with recurrent pyogenic infections. New Engl J Med 1970; 283:631–634.

Oxelius V-A: Immunoglobulin G (IgG) subclasses and human disease. Am J Med (Suppl) 1984; 76:7–18.

Bjorkander J, et al.: Impaired lung function in patients with IgA deficiency and low levels of IgG2 or IgG3. New Engl J Med 1985; 313:7620–724.

Hanson LA, Oxelius V-A, eds: Proceedings of the First International Symposium on IgG Subclasses. Monogr Allergy, 1986; 20.

Smith TF: Immunodeficiency in chronic pediatric respiratory illness. Hosp Pract 1986; 21:143–158.

Heiner DC: Recognition and management of IgG subclass deficiencies. Pediatr Infect Dis J 1987; 6:235–238.

SM021   **Thomas F. Smith**

IMMUNODEFICIENCY, MYELOPEROXIDASE DEFICIENCY TYPE   2214

Includes: Myeloperoxidase deficiency

Excludes: Granulomatous disease, chronic x-linked (0443)

Major Diagnostic Criteria: The partial or total absence of myeloperoxidase from the azurophilic granules of neutrophils and monocytes. These phagocytes appear normal when stained with Wright's stain, but with a peroxidase stain, the normally strongly positive granules are either markedly decreased or totally absent. Eosinophils and basophils appear normal with Wright's stain and have normal amounts of peroxidase.

Clinical Findings: The disorder is usually discovered serendipitously by the new automated differential counters, which rely on peroxidase positivity to identify neutrophils. The patients are identified as being profoundly neutropenic by automated count, but they have normal numbers of neutrophils on standard Wright's stain. Those with either partial or complete myeloperoxidase deficiency generally have a very benign course, rarely displaying any increased susceptibility to infection. A few people with complete myeloperoxidase deficiency have exhibited increased susceptibility to candidal infections, but they have usually had an additional factor, such as diabetes mellitus, impairing their anticandidal defenses.

Complications: Unknown.

Associated Findings: None known.

Etiology: Originally thought to be straightforward autosomal recessive inheritance, but the recent identification of individuals with varying degrees of myeloperoxidase deficiency suggests that this is a recessive trait with variable expressivity.

Pathogenesis: Neutrophils of affected individuals have normal chemotaxis, normal phagocytosis, a normal respiratory burst, and normal degranulation, but bacterial killing is slower than normal, and candidal killing is markedly impaired. The degree of impairment is directly proportional to the quantitative deficiency of myeloperoxidase in the affected individual's neutrophils. Myeloperoxidase catalyzes the production of the hypochlorous ion, which is an important microbicidal agent.

The normal series of events following the engulfment of a pathogen begins with the occurrence of a respiratory burst, which results in the generation of superoxide by the following reaction: $NADPH + 2O_2 \rightarrow 2O_2- + NADP^+ + H^+$. This superoxide then reacts with the hydronium ion in a reaction catalyzed by superoxide dismutase to form hydrogen peroxide.

$2O_2- + 2H^+ \rightarrow H_2O_2 + O_2$ This hydrogen peroxide usually then reacts with a halide ion (such as chloride), and in the presence of myeloperoxidase a hypohalous anion (one of the principal microbicidal oxidants of phagocytes) is produced.

$H_2O_2 + Cl- \rightarrow$/myeloperoxidase $OCl- + H_2O$

Without myeloperoxidase, hypochlorous acid cannot be generated in significant quantities. Superoxide and hydrogen peroxide are only slightly microbicidal, and thus it is surprising that even individuals with complete myeloperoxidase deficiency have so few infections. Evidently, microbicial oxidants other than OCl- are generated by the respiratory burst because the bacteria are killed, and the respiratory burst is, if anything, prolonged in these individuals. The killing of phagocytized *Candida* is negligible (6%

of normal) in totally deficient individuals and moderately impaired in partially deficient individuals.

The low incidence of invasive candidal infections in these people reflects the presence of independent, probably cell-mediated mechanisms for destroying this pathogen.

MIM No.: *25460

Sex Ratio: M1:F1

Occurrence: Partial deficiency, 1:2,000; total deficiency, 1:4,000.

Risk of Recurrence for Patient's Sib:
See Part I, *Mendelian Inheritance.* Approximately 25% chance of being either partially or completely deficient.

Risk of Recurrence for Patient's Child:
See Part I, *Mendelian Inheritance.* Each child is at risk for being a carrier, but the uncertainty surrounding the mode of inheritance of this disorder makes such an estimation highly speculative.

Age of Detectability: From birth.

Gene Mapping and Linkage: MPO (myeloperoxidase) has been mapped to 17q21.3-q23.

Prevention: None known. Genetic counseling indicated.

Treatment: Parenteral antibiotics for serious infections. Early consideration of empiric antifungal therapy in clinically infected, myeloperoxidase-deficient individuals who fail to respond promptly to antibacterials; especially in the presence of **Diabetes mellitus.**

Prognosis: Vast majority of afflicted individuals appear to live full, unimpaired lives.

Detection of Carrier: Partially affected individuals can be detected by quantitatively assaying neutrophils for myeloperoxidase. The accuracy of such screening is hampered by the variable expressivity of the trait.

References:
Cech P, et al.: Hereditary myeloperoxidase deficiency. Blood 1979; 53:403–411.
Parry MF, et al.: Myeloperoxidase deficiency: prevalence and clinical significance. Ann Intern Med 1981; 95:293–301.
Larrocha C, et al.: Hereditary myeloperoxidase deficiency: study of 12 cases. Scand J Haematol 1982; 29:389–397.
Ross DW, Kaplow LS: Myeloperoxidase deficiency: increased sensitivity for immunocytochemical compared to cytochemical detection of enzyme. Arch Path Lab Med 1985; 109:1005–1006.
Murao S-I, et al.: Myeloperoxidase: a myeloid cell nuclear antigen with DNA-binding properties. Proc Nat Acad Sci 1988; 85:1232–1236.
Forehand JR, et al.: Inherited disorders of phagocyte killing. In: Scriver CR, et al, eds: The metabolic basis of inherited disease, 6th ed. New York: McGraw-Hill, 1989:2779–2801.

AX001   **Richard Axtell**
B0048   **Laurence A. Boxer**

IMMUNODEFICIENCY, NEZELOF TYPE   2216

Includes:
Alymphocytosis, pure
Combined immunodeficiency with immunoglobulins
Nezelof syndrome
Severe combined immunodeficiency, Nezelof type
Severe combined immunodeficiency, variant type
T-lymphocyte deficiency
Thymic aplasia
Thymic dysplasia with normal immunoglobulins

Excludes:
Immunodeficiency, adenosine deaminase deficiency (2196)
Immunodeficiency, agammaglobulinemia, X-linked, infantile (0027)
Immunodeficiency, thymic agenesis (0943)
Immunodeficiency, Wiskott-Aldrich type (0523)
Metaphyseal chondrodysplasia, type Mckusick (0653)

Major Diagnostic Criteria: Severe lymphopenia, diminished lymphoid tissue, and abnormal structure of the thymus are major

findings in patients with Nezelof syndrome, as well as in patients with other forms of severe combined immunodeficiency syndromes (SCIDS). However, Nezelof syndrome can be differentiated from the other SCID subtypes by normal or increased levels of one or more of the major immunoglobulin classes. Antibody formation can be present, but it is often variable. Furthermore, plasma cells are present in the lymphoid tissue and gastrointestinal tract. In contrast to patients with Swiss-type agammaglobulinemia and other SCIDS such as ADA deficiency, the onset of symptoms can be delayed beyond six months of age, with a gradual course and survival beyond 4 years of age.

Clinical Findings: Nezelof syndrome is part of a spectrum of disorders that constitute SCIDS. As with all the clinical subtypes with severe combined immunodeficiency, patients with Nezelof syndrome have recurrent infections and failure to thrive, which often leads to early death. In Nezelof patients the onset of illness usually occurs at about six months of age. It is characterized by failure to thrive, chronic diarrhea, oral candidiasis, recurrent pulmonary infections, and recurrent skin infections. Of the infections, characteristic organisms include measles and varicella, gram-negative bacteria, and opportunistic organisms like *Pneumocystis carinii.* Patients may respond poorly or slowly to antibiotic therapy and other supportive measures. On physical examination, the failure to thrive may be a prominent sign. There is diminished lymphoid tissue such as the tonsils and peripheral lymph nodes, but there may also be hepatosplenomegaly. Aside from pyoderma, some patients may have an eczematoid-type rash.

On the chest X-ray there is usually absence of the thymic shadow. Recurrent or persistent lymphopenia (total lymphocyte count less than 2,000/mm³) is present, and delayed skin hypersensitivity reactions to common antigens such as candida, tetanus, and mumps, are negative.

Serum levels of IgG, IgM, and IgA are normal or elevated. Occasionally there may be a partial deficiency of one of the immunoglobulin isotypes. In addition, patients may have markedly elevated levels of IgD, IgE, or both. Antibody responses are quite variable, but usually deficient. Some patients have preexisting natural antibodies, such as isohemagglutinins, which are naturally occurring antibodies to the ABO blood group antigens. Often patients have deficient antibody formation upon immunization with specific antigens. Autoantibodies have been reported in some patients. In vitro lymphocyte proliferative responses to mitogens are usually reduced or absent. However, lymphocyte proliferative responses in mixed lymphocyte culture in response to allogeneic cells can occur.

Pathologic findings are similar to those of other subtypes of SCIDS. There is diminished lymphoid tissue with abnormal architecture characterized by the absence of follicles and germinal centers. The thymus shows evidence of dysplasia, with predominantly epithelioid cells, rare lymphocytes, and absence of Hassall corpuscles. There is poor architectural demarcation between cortex and medulla. However, in contrast with the other SCID subtypes, plasma cells are present in lymph nodes, bone marrow, and the rectal mucosa.

Complications: As with other patients with severe deficiencies of cellular immunity, Nezelof patients are at risk for graft-vs.-host disease following the administration of viable allogeneic leukocytes by blood transfusion or by intrauterine maternal passage of lymphocytes through the placenta. Thus all blood products, including plasma, should be irradiated. Similarly, these patients are at risk for severe infection following immunization with live vaccines such as polio, bacillus Calmette-Guérin (BCG) or vaccinia. Therefore it is recommended that Nezelof patients, like patients with immunodeficiency disease, not receive any of the live viral or bacterial vaccines for immunizations.

Associated Findings: None known.

Etiology: Both autosomal recessive and X-linked recessive inheritance have been reported. There is a slight preponderance of affected males with Nezelof syndrome. In reviewing 34 cases of Nezelof syndrome, Lawlor et al (1974) found a suggestive or definitive family history either in sibs or a near relative in 55% of families.

Pathogenesis: Possibly a defect in lymphoid stem cell development and differentiation. However, the normal levels of immunoglobulins and plasma cells in the tissues suggest that there may have been some preexisting immunity, with attrition of immunologic function. Thus far, a biochemical or molecular abnormality has not been defined.

MIM No.: *24270

Sex Ratio: M1:F<1

Occurrence: About 50 cases have been described in the literature.

Risk of Recurrence for Patient's Sib:
See Part I, *Mendelian Inheritance.*

Risk of Recurrence for Patient's Child:
See Part I, *Mendelian Inheritance.*

Age of Detectability: In infancy.

Gene Mapping and Linkage: Unknown.

Prevention: None known. Genetic counseling indicated.

Treatment: Prompt, symptomatic treatment of infections is indicated. Bone marrow transplantation from a tissue-matched, compatible donor may be required.

Prognosis: Poor, unless a compatible donor is available for bone marrow transplantation.

Detection of Carrier: Unknown.

References:

Breton A, et al.: Lymphocytophisia avec dysgammaglobulinemie chez un nourrisson. Arch Fr Pediatr 1963; 20:131–139.

Nezelof C, et al.: L'hypoplasie héréditaire du thymus: sa place et sa responsabilité dans une observation d'aplasie lymphocytaire, normoplasmocytaire et normoglobulinemique du nourrisson. Arch Fr Pediatr 1964; 21:897–920.

Rothberg RM, ten Bensel RW: Thymic alymphoplasia with immunoglobulin synthesis. Am J Dis Child 1967; 113:639–648.

Nezelof C: Thymic dysplasia with normal immunoglobulins and immunologic deficiency: pure alymphocytosis. In: Good RA, ed: Immunologic deficiency diseases. New York: March of Dimes Birth Defects Foundation, 1968:104–112.

Lawlor GJ, Jr, et al.: The syndrome of cellular immunodeficiency with immunoglobulins. J Pediatr 1974; 84:183–192.

Rezza E, et al.: Familial lymphopenia with T lymphocyte defect. J Pediatr 1974; 84:178–182.

BA057   **Mark Ballow**

IMMUNODEFICIENCY, NUCLEOSIDE-PHOSPHORYLASE DEFICIENCY   0729

Includes:
Nucleoside-phosphorylase deficiency
Purine-nucleoside: orthophosphate ribosyltransferase

Excludes: Immunodeficiency, adenosine deaminase deficiency (2196)

Major Diagnostic Criteria: Absent to severely reduced red blood cell, lymphocyte, and fibroblast nucleoside-phosphorylase activity; defective cell-mediated immunity, with normal antibody-mediated immunity; and a history of recurrent infections consistent with immunodeficiency disease.

Clinical Findings: Patients may be asymptomatic for periods of several years. Initial manifestations usually include recurrent infection. Fatal varicella infection and progressive vaccinia following smallpox immunization have been reported. A fatal graft-versus-host reaction has been observed. Severe hemolytic anemia has been described in several patients. The oldest identified patient is over age 12 years, and continues to have recurrent infection. Immunologic studies have demonstrated normal B-cell immunity, with absent to severely depressed T-cell immunity. Although enzyme activity is absent at birth, immunologic function

may be normal, and it subsequently declines with age. Measurement of purine nucleosides in the urine and blood reveals increased amounts of inosine, deoxyinosine, guanosine, deoxyguanosine, and decreased amounts of uric acid. Orotic aciduria has been found in some patients. Treatment has included transfer factor, thymus transplantation, thymosin, deoxycytidine, and uridine given orally. In some patients partial reconstitution has been achieved. Infusions of radiated red blood cells as a possible source of enzyme has partially restored immunity in some patients. Patients should not be immunized with attenuated live viral vaccines or receive unirradiated blood products. Autoantibody and autoimmune disease has been described in several patients.

Complications: Unknown.

Associated Findings: Related to underlying immunodeficiency disease.

Etiology: Autosomal recessive inheritance.

Pathogenesis: Undetermined. Because a similar disorder, adenosine deaminase deficiency, also is associated with immunodeficiency disease, it is postulated that the purine salvage pathway is involved in some way in immunodeficiency disease. However, the mechanism whereby a deficiency of enzymes in this pathway results in immunodeficiency is unknown. Pyrimidine "starvation" secondary to the accumulation of adenine nucleotides or to elevated levels of cyclic nucleotides or deoxynucleotides might impair lymphocyte function. Alternatively, increased deoxynucleotides may also impair lymphocyte function by inhibiting ribonucleotide reductase. Inhibition of protein methylation may also occur.

MIM No.: *16405

Sex Ratio: Presumably M1:F1

Occurrence: Undetermined. Established literature.

Risk of Recurrence for Patient's Sib:
See Part I, *Mendelian Inheritance.*

Risk of Recurrence for Patient's Child:
See Part I, *Mendelian Inheritance.* All offspring are obligate carriers, but they are unlikely to manifest the disease as the frequency of the mutant gene appears to be low in the population.

Age of Detectability: At birth. Nucleoside-phosphorylase activity may be quantitated in fibroblasts; therefore the diagnosis can be made in utero.

Gene Mapping and Linkage: NP (nucleoside phosphorylase) has been mapped to 14q11.2.

Prevention: None known. Genetic counseling indicated.

Treatment: At present, nucleoside-phosphorylase cannot be replaced in the patient, either directly or by transfusion. Appropriate immunologic reconstitution for the defined immunodeficiency disease may modify or prevent recurrent infections. Bone marrow transplantation from an appropriate donor should correct the enzyme deficiency.

Prognosis: Guarded due to possible auto-antibody and autoimmune processes.

Detection of Carrier: By analysis of red blood cells for nucleoside-phosphorylase concentration; a carrier has approximately 50% normal concentration.

References:

Giblett ER, et al.: Nucleoside-phosphorylase deficiency in a child with severely defective T-cell immunity and normal B-cell immunity. Lancet 1975; I:1010–1013.

Cohen A, et al.: Abnormal purine metabolism and purine overproduction in a patient deficient in purine nucleoside phosphorylase. New Engl J Med 1976; 295:1449–1454.

Hirschhorn R: Defects of purine metabolism in immunodeficiency diseases. Prog Clin Immunol 1977; 3:67.

Ammann AJ: Immunological abnormalities in purine nucleoside phosphorylase deficiencies in enzyme defects and immune dysfunction. Ciba Found Symp 1979; 55.

Cowan MJ, et al.: Immunodeficiency syndromes associated with inherited metabolic disorders. Clin Haematol 1981; 10:139.

Capapella De Luca E, et al.: Prenatal exclusion of purine nucleoside phosphorylase deficiency. Eur J Pediatr 1986; 145:51–53.

Williams SR, et al.: A human purine nucleoside phosphorylase deficiency caused by a single base change. J Biol Chem 1987; 262:2332–2338.

WA022

AM003

Diane W. Wara

Arthur J. Ammann

IMMUNODEFICIENCY, PLASMA-ASSOCIATED DEFECT OF PHAGOCYTOSIS 0812

Includes:

Complement C5 dysfunction

Leiners disease

Neonatal seborrheic dermatitis

Phagocytosis, plasma-related defect in

Excludes: Complement deficiency, other

Major Diagnostic Criteria: Demonstration in vitro of defective phagocytosis of yeast particles by normal polymorphonuclear leukocytes in the presence of serum or plasma from the patient. Correction of the opsonic defect by the addition of purified human C5 or mouse serum containing C5 ($D_{10}B_2$ old line) which also has C5 ($B_{10}D_2$). Commercial preparations of baker's yeast originally used for this assay have been substantially altered by manufacturers. Currently available preparations are closer to zymosan in cell surface, thereby making their opsonic dependency upon C5 less absolute than previously. The best preparations for the assay are from sources which have been maintained in long-term culture, rather than from retail outlets. Levels of complement components, including C5, are within normal limits.

Clinical Findings: Severe infections recur shortly after birth accompanied by generalized seborrheic dermatitis with a marked inflammatory component, persistent diarrhea (usually associated with bacterial infection) that is resistant to antibiotic and dietary management, and an emaciated appearance.

It is of particular significance that the culture material shows almost exclusively gram-negative bacteria. *Staphylococcus aureus* is the only gram-positive organism seen with any frequency. Patients are likely to be markedly cachectic and show a generalized failure to thrive.

Common laboratory findings include neutrophilia, diffuse hyperglobulinemia, and elevated sedimentation rate. Despite treatment with systemic antibiotics, patients show little change in their clinical state.

Complications: Disability, marked weakness, and death resulting from uncontrolled infection, usually by gram-negative bacteria.

Associated Findings: None known.

Etiology: Possibly autosomal recessive inheritance, although a dominant pattern has been reported in at least one family. In Leiner's (1908) series, twins contracted the disorder at six weeks of age, and both recovered after two months. In another family, two consecutive infants contracted the condition at age six weeks and died after several weeks. Leiner noted that the illness was limited almost exclusively to breast-fed infants.

Pathogenesis: Dysfunction of the 5th component of complement (C5). The ability of patient's serum to enhance phagocytosis of yeast particles can be restored to normal by the addition of highly purified C5.

MIM No.: 17110

Sex Ratio: M1:F1

Occurrence: Some 57 cases were reported between 1902 and 1911. One kinship was reported in the 1960s.

Risk of Recurrence for Patient's Sib:

See Part I, *Mendelian Inheritance.*

Risk of Recurrence for Patient's Child:

See Part I, *Mendelian Inheritance.*

Age of Detectability: At birth, by phagocytosis test.

Gene Mapping and Linkage: Unknown.

Prevention: None known. Genetic counseling indicated.

Treatment: The only effective way to treat this disorder is by the infusion of fresh plasma or blood that contains adequate amounts of C5. Such therapy proved life-saving to two severely afflicted infants. The usual blood bank is not a satisfactory source of active C5; hence the requirement for fresh blood or plasma. Specific antibiotic therapy should be administered.

Prognosis: Based on the experience of Leiner and subsequent families, the mortality rate is approximately 40%. Onset was generally under the age of one month, and duration of the illness varied from several weeks to several months. Fifteen of the original series of 43 infants (1902–1907), and three of the 14 infants in a later series (1907–1911) died. The use of plasma as a source of active C5 may be life-saving, and enable patients to eventually enjoy normal life expectancy. After two years of age, symptoms markedly decreased, hence the importance of early diagnosis and treatment.

Detection of Carrier: The carrier state has been identified by phagocytic assay of yeast particles. However, these values have shown the carrier to be as low as the patient. Hence, the patient and clinically normal members of the family sharing the defect cannot be differentiated.

Special Considerations: Although only a few children have been shown to have this defect, the implications of a humoral deficiency state causing impaired cellular function (such as phagocytosis) are important in understanding normal inflammation.

References:

Leiner C: Über erythrodermia desquamativa, eine eigenartige universelle Dermatose der Brustkinder. Arch Dermatol Syph 1908; 89:163–190.

Miller ME, et al.: A familial, plasma-associated defect of phagocytosis: a new cause of recurrent bacterial infections. Lancet 1968; II:60–63. *

Miller ME, Nilsson UR: A familial deficiency of the phagocytosis-enhancing activity of serum related to a dysfunction of the fifth component of complement (C5). New Engl J Med 1970; 282:354–358. *

Miller ME, Nilson UR: A major role of the fifth component of complement (C5) in the opsonization of yeast particles: partial dichotomy of function and immunochemical measurement. Clin Immunol and Immunopath 1974; 2:246–255.

Nilsson UR, et al.: A functional abnormality of the fifth component of complement (C5) from human serum of individuals with a familial opsonic defect. J Immunol 1974; 112:1164.

Miller ME, Ganges RG: Serum complement-like opsonic activities in human, animal, vegetable, and proprietary milks. Science 1977; 196:1115.

MI014

Michael E. Miller

IMMUNODEFICIENCY, RETICULOENDOTHELIOSIS WITH EOSINOPHILIA 2688

Includes:

Cancer, reticulosis, familial histiocytic, Omenn type

Hemophagocytic reticulosis

Histiocytosis, proliferative

Immunodeficiency, severe combined, Omenn type

Omenn syndrome

Reticulosis, familial histiocytic

Excludes:

Graft-versus-host reaction

Histiocytic storage disorders

Histiocytosis, familial lipochromic

Immunodeficiency, nucleoside-phosphorylase deficiency (0729)

Immunodeficiency, severe combined (0522)

Immunodeficiency, Wiskott-Aldrich type (0523)

Langerhans cell histiocytosis

Letterer-Siwe disease (2181)

Lymphohistiocytosis, familial erythrophagocytic (2946)

Metaphyseal chondrodysplasia with thymolymphopenia (0655)
Viral-associated hemophagocytic syndromes

Major Diagnostic Criteria: Seborrhea-like dermatitis, desquamative erythroderma, eosinophilia, histiocytic lymphadenopathy, and hepatosplenomegaly arising in the early weeks of life and becoming fatal, without immunoreconstitution, within 4–6 months. Exclusion of infections and other histiocytic disorders. Affected sibs and parental consanguinity are commonly noted.

Clinical Findings: The first symptoms may appear within four weeks of birth and are predominantly cutaneous. Dry, reddened skin may have been present from birth, in retrospect, and progressive erythroderma and desquamation occur. Diarrhea, recurrent fevers, failure to thrive, lymphadenopathy, and progressive hepatosplenomegaly follow. Infections and inanition lead to a fatal outcome within 4–6 months if untreated and within 15 months even with aggressive therapy with cytotoxic agents, corticosteroids, and hyperalimentation. Use of matched allogeneic bone marrow transplantation has been reported from Texas Children's Hospital to normalize T-cell subsets, mitogen response, antigen response, and IgE, with freedom from serious infections for two years.

The distinctive hematologic abnormalities are eosinophilia, which may be quite marked, and combined immunodeficiency, with primary involvement of T-lymphocyte subsets. Immature T-cells appear in the peripheral blood, there is functional T-cell suppression of immunoglobulin production and reduction of B-cell populations, 5'-nucleotidase may be markedly deficient, and the T4:T8 ratio is decreased due to a decrease in T4 and an increase in T8. Cutaneous and lymph node biopsies show proliferative infiltration with histiocytes, immature T-cells, and eosinophils. Histologic examination of thymus at postmortem reveals severe atrophy with no Hassall corpuscles. Anemia is common. The clinical features and terminal lymphocyte depletion are suggestive of graft-versus-host disease, possibly intrauterine, in an immunocompromised patient; however, no evidence of cellular chimerism has been detected. Hyperlipidemia and hypofibrinogenemia may be found.

Complications: Life-threatening infections; chronic measles infection from vaccination with measles live virus vaccine; and terminal lymphoma, possibly related to treatments with transfer factor.

Associated Findings: None known.

Etiology: Autosomal recessive inheritance.

Pathogenesis: It is likely that the severe combined immunodeficiency is the underlying mechanism, but its cause is unknown. The autosomal recessive inheritance may be a clue to a primary enzyme deficiency, analogous to ADA and NP deficiencies, but none has been discovered. The deregulation and deficiency of T-cell suppressor subsets account for most of the immunologic abnormalities (including deficiency of B-cell-related 5'-nucleotidase and infectious complications. However, the eosinophilia and the histiocytic proliferation, hallmarks of the clinical disorder, are unexplained, and the prominent cutaneous involvement is unusual. A French child born in germ-free conditions and maintained in a sterile isolator developed skin involvement at day two and successively developed all expected clinical manifestations except that diarrhea appeared only after bacterial contamination.

MIM No.: *26770

Sex Ratio: M1:F1

Occurrence: One highly inbred Roman Catholic Irish-American kindred has accounted for at least 20 homozygotes, seen in more than a dozen medical centers in as many states. (Surnames were mostly Carroll, McDonald, Daley, Donahue, and Gregg.) However, it is clear that unrelated individual cases and multiple cases in unrelated families have occurred in the United States and other countries. Several authors suggest that the disorder is underdiagnosed, partly due to early death and largely due to nosologic confusion. An estimated 150 cases of familial erythrophagocytic lymphohistiocytosis, which may be different and/or heterogeneous, have been reported since 1952.

Risk of Recurrence for Patient's Sib:
See Part I, *Mendelian Inheritance.*

Risk of Recurrence for Patient's Child:
See Part I, *Mendelian Inheritance.* Affected individuals are not expected to survive to reproduce.

Age of Detectability: Clinically evident within 1–2 months after birth. Immunologic tests may be suggestive at birth or even *in utero.*

Gene Mapping and Linkage: Unknown.

Prevention: None known. Genetic counseling indicated.

Treatment: Appeared hopeless for many years. Now aggressive immunoreconstitution therapy, including bone marrow transplantation, may be effective, with nutritional support. Early diagnosis and treatment may be important to the outcome.

Prognosis: Uniformly fatal within six months without treatment; extension to at least 18 months with hyperalimentation and treatment of infections. Possibly curable with allogeneic bone marrow transplantation.

Detection of Carrier: Immunologic tests appear promising. Abnormal distribution of T4+ and T8+ cells in obligatory heterozygotes in a large kindred of affected persons suggests a phenotypic lymphocyte marker.

Special Considerations: Because of its recurrence risk and prospects for carrier detection and prenatal diagnosis, it is clinically important that this disorder be distinguished from other proliferative histiocytoses.

Support Groups: Atlanta; American Cancer Society

References:
Omenn GS: Familial reticuloendotheliosis with eosinophilia. New Engl J Med 1965; 273:427–432.
Ladisch S, et al.: Immunologic and clinical effects of repeated blood exchange in familial erythrophagocytic lympho-histiocytosis. Blood 1982; 60:814–821.
Fischer A, et al.: Heterogeneity of immunologic and enzymatic deficiencies in the familial reticuloendotheliosis syndrome. BD:OAS IXX. New York: March of Dimes Birth Defects Foundation, 1983: 317–319.
Karol RA, et al.: Imbalances of subsets of T lymphocytes in an inbred pedigree with Omenn's syndrome. Clin Immunol Immunopathol 1983; 27:412–427.
Gelfand EW, et al.: Absence of lymphocyte ecto-5'-nucleotidase in infants with reticuloendotheliosis and eosinophilia (Omenn's syndrome). Blood 1984; 63:1475–1480.
Hong R, et al.: Omenn disease: termination in lymphoma. Pediatr Pathol 1985; 3:143–154. †
Nemoto K, Ohnishi Y: Familial hemophagocytic reticulosis: clinicopathologic findings, and cytochemical, immunohistochemical and electron microscopic studies. Acta Path Jpn 1987; 37:1811–1812.
Junker AK, et al.: Clinical and immune recovery from Omenn syndrome after bone marrow transplantation. J Pediatr 1989; 114:596–600.

OM000   **Gilbert S. Omenn**

IMMUNODEFICIENCY, SEVERE COMBINED   **0522**

Includes:
   Bare lymphocyte syndrome
   Agammaglobulinemia, alymphocytotic type
   Agammaglobulinemia, Swiss type
   Aleukia, congenital
   De Vaal disease
   Gitlin syndrome
   Hematopoietic hypoplasia, generalized
   Immunodeficiency, severe dual system
   Nonplasmatic thymic alymphoplasia or alymphocytosis
   Reticular dysgenesis
   Severe combined immunodeficiency (SCID) with
      leukopenia

Severe combined immunodeficiency-lack of HLA on lymphocytes

Excludes:
    Agammaglobulinemia-thymoma syndrome (0944)
    Immunodeficiency, adenosine deaminase deficiency (2196)
    Immunodeficiency, agammaglobulinemia, X-linked, infantile (0027)
    Immunodeficiency, reticuloendotheliosis with eosinophilia (2688)
    Immunodeficiency, thymic agenesis (0943)
    Immunodeficiency, X-linked severe combined (0524)

Major Diagnostic Criteria: In addition to the X-linked type of severe combined immunodeficieny (SCID), there are several autosomal recessive forms of this relatively heterogeneous class of SCID.

In the basic or *Swiss* type, lymphopenia (<1,000 lymphocytes per ml) is usually seen, as well as low numbers of mature T-lymphocytes. Levels of all immunoglobulin classes are low or absent, and no antibody formation is seen upon immunization. T- and B-lymphocyte functions are invariably low. In the *Bare lymphocyte* type, this is combined with a lack of expression of HLA antigens on some cells of hematopoietic origin. In the *Reticular dysgenesis* type, SCID is combined with leukopenia.

Growth and development of infants with severe combined immunodeficiency are generally normal for the first few months of life. Then, length and weight gain cease, and failure to thrive is seen. Intractable diarrhea and chronic or recurrent infections are common.

Clinical Findings: Laboratory findings include lymphopenia and low numbers of T-lymphocytes in circulation. The majority of circulating T-lymphocytes are usually not mature cells, but rather early or late thymocytes (often T10 positive). Mature T-lymphocytes in circulation are usually of maternal origin. Although most patients have low numbers of T- and B-lymphocytes, B-lymphocyte levels may be normal or elevated. The T4:T8 (T-helper to T-suppressor) cell ratio is generally normal. The lymphoproliferative response to mitogens or allogenic cells is decreased. Eosinophilia may be present in certain varieties of SCID. Delayed cutaneous anergy is seen.

All immunoglobulin levels are low. No antibody formation is seen following immunization.

The thymus gland, which may be normal in the X-linked form, is very small (≤2 g) and usually does not undergo normal descenaus. The thymus consists primarily of endodermal cells that have not become lymphoid. Hassall corpuscles are absent, as is corticomedullary distinction.

Depletion is seen in follicular and parafollicular areas of lymph nodes. The tonsils, adenoids, and Peyer patches are underdeveloped or absent.

In the *Bare lymphocyte* type, the failure of HLA expression leads to immunodeficiency affecting both cellular and humoral response to antigens. In the *Reticular dysgenesis*, or De Vaal type, the clinical and laboratory pictures are very similar to those of the more common Swiss type, plus the near absence of granulocytes. Bone marrow aspiration shows hypocellularity with very few lymphoid and granulocytic elements; the main cell type present is the erythroblast. Bone marrow promyelocytes are present, but few mature granulocytes are seen. However, normal erythropoietic and thrombopoietic cells, as well as macrophages in normal or elevated frequency, are present.

Complications: Infants may suffer from graft versus host disease (GVHD) due to maternal lymphocytes, resulting in the appearance of a morbilliform rash in the first few days of life. HLA-identical bone marrow transplantation (BMT) has been reported to result in donor lymphocytes cytotoxic for the maternal lymphocytes and in cessation of GVHD symptomology.

A similar GVHD may also result from the administration of nonirradiated blood or blood products. To prevent this GVHD, all blood and blood products should be irradiated at 3,000 to 6,000 R before transfusion to destroy any lymphocytes present.

Persistent oral thrush may be present throughout the neonatal period, with accompanying moniliasis of the larynx and skin.

Pneumonia is also commonly present, with tachypnea and hyperinflation of the lungs. The pneumonia is often interstitial, due to *Pneumocystis carinii*. Another common and potentially fatal cause of persistent pneumonia is parainfluenza virus, especially type III. Rous sarcoma virus pneumonia has also been reported in SCID patients.

Other common problems include intractable diarrhea; cutaneous bacterial infections, especially by *Pseudomonas aeruginosa*; and severe viral infections, including varicella, herpes group, vaccinia, measles, papovavirus, and enterovirus. Unusual viral infections, such as adenovirus hepatitis and necrotizing bronchitis, and parainfluenza type III pancreatitis have been reported. Vaccinations with live vaccines, such as bacille Calmette Guérin or polio, are often fatal.

Associated Findings: Patients may present with skin eruptions resembling **Letterer-Siwe disease**. Malignant reticuloendotheliosis (see **Lymphohistiocytosis, familial erythrophagocytic**) and noma, a necrotizing gingivostomatitis, have also been reported.

Etiology: Autosomal recessive inheritance.

Pathogenesis: The defect(s) involved may be in T-lymphocytes, stem cells, or the thymus. Thymic defect(s) may be intrathymic or due to abnormal embryogenesis of the thymic epithelium.

Bare lymphocyte syndrome has been interpreted as a pretranslational regulatory defect of expression in two genes (Sullivan et al, 1985).

Reticular dysgenesis probably is not in the multipotent hematopoietic stem cell, but in development of the myelomonocytic and lymphoid cells.

MIM No.: *20250, *20292, *26750

CDC No.: 279.200

Sex Ratio: M1:F1

Occurrence: About 1:500,000 live births in the general population, and 1:10,000 in first cousin matings.

Risk of Recurrence for Patient's Sib:
    See Part I, *Mendelian Inheritance.*

Risk of Recurrence for Patient's Child:
    See Part I, *Mendelian Inheritance.*

Age of Detectability: Prenatal diagnosis is possible. This diagnosis is usually performed in the mid-to-late second trimester (18–22 weeks gestation) using a microsample of pure fetal blood obtained at fetoscopy. Diagnostic criteria include lymphocyte count, total T-lymphocytes, T-lymphocyte subsets, and T-lymphocyte function. The latter is measured by response to mitogens such as phytohemagglutinin. Cell-mediated lympholysis with fetal lymphocytes is unreliable. B-lymphocyte levels may be normal or elevated. A source of error in these diagnoses is the presence of maternal lymphocytes, which may increase or normalize test results. Laboratory findings associated with SCID are present at birth, although complications do not generally begin to appear until the third month of life.

Gene Mapping and Linkage: Unknown.

Prevention: None known. Genetic counseling indicated.

Treatment: Successful treatment of SCID has been achieved predominantly with bone marrow transplantation (BMT). When HLA-identical marrow is not available, successful transplants may be performed using parental haploidentical marrow. In a 15-year retrospective study, HLA-matched BMT in SCID patients resulted in 68% disease-free survival, while T-lymphocyte-depleted HLA-mismatched BMT resulted in 57% disease-free survival. Although no preparative immunosuppression is needed in SCID patients prior to BMT, transplants may be impeded by nonimmune resistance. Also, SCID patients are highly susceptible to GVHD following HLA-mismatched BMT.

Other treatments that have been at least partially successful include fetal liver cell transplants, fetal thymus implants, and implants of fetal thymus epithelium. None of these treatments, however, have been as satisfactory as BMT. Treatment with thymic hormones has not proved beneficial.

The severe parainfluenza virus and RSV infections that are a common complication of SCID have been reported to be successfully treated with ribavirin.

Prognosis: Before the advent of BMT, prognosis was invariably poor, with death occurring in the first year of life. With BMT, prognosis is quite good.

Reticular dysgenesis is invariably fatal if untreated, with the longest survivor living 119 days. BMT is probably the treatment of choice.

Detection of Carrier: Unknown.

Special Considerations: An additional non-X-linked SCID is seen in **Immunodeficiency, reticuloendotheliosis with eosinophilia**, also known as Omenn syndrome.

References:

Buckley RH: Immunodeficiency. J Allergy Clin Immunol 1983; 72:627–641.

Rosen FS, et al.: The primary immunodeficiencies. New Engl J Med 1984; 311:300–310.

Roper M, et al.: Severe congenital leukopenia (reticular dysgenesis). Immunologic and morphologic characterizations of leukocytes. Am J Dis Child 1985; 139:832–835.

Sullivan KE, et al.: Molecular analysis of the bare lymphocyte syndrome. J Clin Invest 1985; 76:75–79.

Fisher A, et al.: Bone-marrow transplantation for immunodeficiencies and osteopetrosis: European survey, 1968–1985. Lancet 1986; II: 1080–1084.

Borzy MS: Prenatal diagnosis of immunodeficiency diseases. Curr Probl Dermatol 1987; 16:185–196.

Durandy A, et al.: Prenatal diagnosis of severe combined immunodeficiency with defective synthesis of HLA molecules. Prenatal Diag 1987; 7:27–34.

HA081   **Michael T. Halpern**
SC039   **Stanley A. Schwartz**

Immunodeficiency, severe combined, Omenn type
  See IMMUNODEFICIENCY, RETICULOENDOTHELIOSIS WITH EOSINOPHILIA
Immunodeficiency, severe dual system
  See IMMUNODEFICIENCY, SEVERE COMBINED

IMMUNODEFICIENCY, THYMIC AGENESIS   0943

Includes:
  DiGeorge anomaly
  DiGeorge syndrome
  Harrington syndrome
  Pharyngeal pouch syndrome
  Third and fourth pharyngeal pouch syndrome
  Thymic aplasia
  Thymic agenesis
  Thymus and parathyroids, congenital absence of the

Excludes:
  Chromosome 10, monosomy 10p (2457)
  Immunodeficiency, agammaglobulinemia, X-linked, infantile (0027)
  Immunodeficiency, Nezelof type (2216)
  Immunodeficiency, severe combined (0522)
  Reticular dysgenesis

Major Diagnostic Criteria: Congenital hypoparathyroidism, dysmorphic facies, absence of thymic shadow on X-ray, evidence of impaired cell-mediated immunity with decreased numbers of T-cells. Lymph nodes showing depletion in deep cortical areas with normal germinal centers.

Clinical Findings: Neonatal hypocalcemic tetany; dysmorphic facial features: hypertelorism, downward slant of eyes, shortened philtrum, low-set ears with notched pinnae and micrognathia; cardiac malformations mainly conotruncal and aortic arch anomalies. Shortened trachea with reduced number of cartilage rings has been described. There is an increased susceptibility to infection manifested by chronic rhinitis, recurrent pneumonia, abscesses and septicemia. Oral candidiasis and recurrent nonspecific diarrhea are common. Patients are weak, fail to thrive and prone

to sudden death. Less common features include bifid uvula, esophageal atresia, hypothyroidism, urinary tract infections and nephrocalcinosis.

Laboratory findings: Hypocalcemia and hyperphosphatemia are usually present, with decreased levels of parathyroid hormone. However, this may be subclinical and may be detected by EDTA challenge. Hypocalcemia may also resolve with age. Immunologic evaluation reveals depressed cell-mediated immunity, as manifested by the following: failure to develop delayed hypersensitivity, absent or delayed homograft rejection, decreased numbers of lymphocytes, and impaired proliferative responses to mitogens, antigens and allogeneic cells. However, there have been instances when one or more of the above functions have been normal. Functions which are initially normal may later get depressed, and vice-versa. Depressed immunity on rare occasions can spontaneously recover. Lymphopenia may or may not be present. B-cell numbers (immunoglobulin bearing cells) are usually increased. Humoral immunity is intact, with normal levels of immunoglobulins and usually normal antibody response. The quality of antibodies may be poor. Complement components are normal. Lymph nodes show paucity of cells in deep cortical areas and well-developed germinal centers and plasma cells. Chest X-rays may show absence of thymic shadow.

Complications: Convulsions, recurrent infections, nephrocalcinosis.

Associated Findings: Anomalies of the great vessels of the heart, including **Heart, truncus arteriosus**.

Etiology: Thymic agenesis, as part of the DiGeorge anomaly, has multiple etiologies. There have been multiple reports of chromosome abnormalities, espically **Chromosome 10, monosomy 10p** and **Chromosome 22, monosomy 22q**, in association with DiGeorge anomaly. About 15% of patients will have chromosome abnormalities. Teratogenic exposures, especially alcohol (see **Fetal alcohol syndrome**) and retinoic acid (isotretinoin) or other vitamin A derivatives (see **Fetal retinoid syndrome**), have been reported to produce DiGeorge anomaly in humans. DiGeorge anomaly has also been reported in association with **Cerebro-hepato-renal syndrome**. In some families, DiGeorge anomaly appears to be inherited as an autosomal recessive or as an autosomal dominant condition without an obvious chromosome abnormality.

Pathogenesis: The absence of thymus and parathyroid glands has been attributed to a failure of embryonic differentiation of structures derived from the 3rd and 4th pharyngeal pouch endoderm and branchial cleft ectoderm.

Abnormal blood supply to the region of the third and fourth pharyngeal arches may play a role in the pathogenesis of DiGeorge anomaly. Experimentally DiGeorge anomaly may be produced in rodents by restriction of zinc intake to the dam during the crucial period of formation of the aortic arches, pharyngeal pouches, thymus and parathyroids. The syndrome also has been produced with all of its concomitants by administering a zinc chelating antibiotic to the mothers of developing rats at the critical time of formation of the aortic arches, pharyngeal pouches, parathyroid analgen and thymus analgen.

A study of the teratogenic effects of Fertilysin, bis(dichloroacety1)diamine, on hamster embryos was undertaken for a comparison of Fertilysin induced malformations with the DiGeorge anomaly of human patients. In treated hamsters, malformations of the aortic arches were consistently produced. DiGeorge anomaly in humans has also been linked to alcohol; a major basis for zinc deficiency in humans.

DiGeorge anomaly has also been reported in association with retinoic acid (isotretinoin) teratogenicity. Vitamin A derivatives have been known to produce related defects in animals, and recently the teratogenic effect of retinoic acid has been shown experimentally to interfere with neural crest migration into the branchial arches.

MIM No.: 18840

Sex Ratio: Presumably M1:F1.

Occurrence: The birth prevalence of DiGeorge anomaly, including complete and partial cases, is estimated to be 1:20,000 births.

Specific risk factors, other then known teratogens such as alcohol or vitamin A derivatives, are undetermined.

Risk of Recurrence for Patient's Sib: Estimated at 2–4%.

Risk of Recurrence for Patient's Child: Unknown. May be as high as 50%.

Age of Detectability: In infancy. Prenatal chromosomal diagnosis for cases due to chromosome abnormality. Fetal echocardiography may detect associated congenital heart defects.

Gene Mapping and Linkage: DGCR (DiGeorge syndrome chromosome region) has been mapped to 22q11.21-q11.23.

Other genes important for branchial arch development appear to be located in the regions of chromosome 10p13 and chromosome 17p13.

Prevention: Avoidance of alcohol, retinoic acid, and vitamin A derivatives during pregnancy.

Treatment: *For hypoparathyroidism*: substitute function with parathyroid hormone, administer calcium, vitamin D. *For absent thymus*: transplant fetal thymus. Fetal thymus transplantation has completely or partially corrected the immunologic abnormality in the majority of the patients where this approach has been used. The recovery of immunological function was rapid in majority of the patients (from few hours to three weeks, to as long as four to five months). In one patient defect of precursor T-cells was found, along with absence of thymic tissue. Transplantation of two fetal thymuses failed to reconstitute the immune function in this patient with the DiGeorge anomaly.

Goldsobel et al (1987) have described an infant girl with DiGeorge anomaly who underwent successful bone marrow transplantation (BMT) at age 28 1/2 weeks. *In-vitro* incubation of this patient's peripheral blood lymphocytes with thymosin alpha-1 showed no increase in the number of T-cells on two occasions. A fetal thymus for transplantation was not available. The patient was given a bone marrow transplantation using a histocompatible brother as donor. The patient has had a good clinical and immunologic response to bone marrow transplant, with evidence of T-cell engraftment, improved B-cell function, and increased levels of serum, thymic hormone, and thymulin.

Prognosis: Usually failure to grow and develop normally. Neurologic impairment may result from neonatal seizures. Early death by infection is common. Cardiac anomalies, when severe, are a major cause of death. Survivors may be mentally retarded, especially if associated with an unbalanced chromosome abnormality. Long term survival may be complicated by Graves disease.

Detection of Carrier: Chromosome translocation may be detected in cases associated with a chromosome abnormality. Otherwise, undetermined.

Special Considerations: The defect of the thymus is often incomplete, and the clinical findings in the DiGeorge anomaly can be very variable. Normal function of thymic-dependent lymphocytes can be present at birth, but can deteriorate progressively. Circulating T-cells, however, are almost always decreased in number. Thymic dependent lymphoid function can rarely recover. The heterogeneity of the syndrome warrants individualization of each case. In the classic DiGeorge anomaly, the success of thymus grafts is unquestionable: six out of seven cases thus treated are living, whereas only 11 of 35 cases not transplanted are alive. Those surviving have been patients with only partial defects, often minimal, of thymus-dependent function. Chromosome analysis should be performed on all patients. Suspected patients should only be transfused with irradiated blood cells to prevent graft versus host disease.

References:
DiGeorge AM: Congenital absence of the thymus and its immunologic consequences: concurrence with congenital hypoparathyroidism. BD:OAS IV(1). White Plains: The National Foundation-March of Dimes, 1969:116–123.
Lischner HW: DiGeorge syndrome. J Pediatr 1972; 81:1042 only.
Conley ME, et al.: The Spectrum of DiGeorge syndrome. J Pediatr 1979; 94:883–890.
Pahwa S, et al.: Failure of immunologic reconstitution in a patient with
DiGeorge syndrome after fetal thymus transplantation. Clin Immunol Immunopathol 1979; 14:96–106.
Lammer EJ, Opitz JM: The DiGeorge Anomaly as a developmental field defect. Am J Med Genet 1986; 2(suppl.):113–127.
Goldsober AB, et al.: Bone marrow transplantation in DiGeorge syndrome. J Pediatr 1987; 111:40–44.
Pahwa R, Good RA: Immunologic deficiencies. In: Immunology essentials of surgical practice. Toledo-Rereyra L, ed: Littleton, MA: PSG Publishing, 1987:270.
Gidding SS, et al.: Unmasking of hypoparathyroidism in familial DiGeorge syndrome by challenge with disodium edetate. New Engl J Med 1988; 319:1589–1591.
Greenberg F, et al.: Cytogenetic findings in a prospective series of patients with DiGeorge anomaly. Am J Hum Genet 1988; 43:605–611.

PA046
PA005
GR011

Rajendra N. Pahwa
Savita Pahwa
Frank Greenberg

Immunodeficiency, thymic agenesis from exposure to D-penicillamine
See FETAL D-PENICILLAMINE SYNDROME
Immunodeficiency, total C1q deficiency
See COMPLEMENT COMPONENT 1, DEFICIENCY OF

IMMUNODEFICIENCY, TUFTSIN DEFICIENCY TYPE 2217

Includes: Tuftsin deficiency

Excludes: Immunodeficiency (other)

Major Diagnostic Criteria: Patients with congenital tuftsin deficiency have repeated severe infections in childhood and repeated less severe infections in adulthood. These recurrent infections respond quite remarkably to injections of γ-globulin which carry sufficient quantity of tuftsin.

Clinical Findings: The biologic activity of the phagocytosis-stimulating tetrapeptide (Thr-Lys-Pro-Arg) tuftsin is highly specific. It stimulates the phagocytic activity of the blood polymorphonuclear leukocytes, as well as macrophages. A unique familial deficiency of the tetrapeptide has been detected. In such patients, infections occur with high frequency. These are most pronounced in childhood. Biochemical and symptomatic evidence can readily be obtained in one or more children. At least one parent of either sex shows clinical signs or laboratory evidence of defective phagocytosis. Recurring infections respond only temporarily to antibiotics. These include tonsillitis, pharyngitis, bronchitis, broncheolitis, pneumonitis, extensive skin infections, furunculosis (frequent in adults), extensive seborrheic dermatitis in children, lymph node infections that are purulent and draining, and occasionally septicemia.

Laboratory findings include absent tuftsin stimulation of phagocytosis, peptide extracts from patients are inhibitory to normal tuftsin activity, reduction on nitroblue tetrazolium tests below normal values, IgA, IgG_{1-4} and IgM levels within normal limits, complement component C5 is normal quantitatively and functionally, complement component C3 is sometimes diminished (not unduly), polymorphonuclear leukocyte level not diagnostic (it can be low, normal, or increased), plasma opsonic activity to yeast particles normal, response to γ-globulin injection results in dramatically alleviated infection.

In every case of tuftsin deficiency that has been studied, an inhibitory peptide was readily demonstrable. In one patient, the peptide was isolated. Its structure is Thr-Glu-Pro-Arg, representing a replacement of lysine by glutamic acid residue. This was synthesized and proved to be an antagonist to tuftsin Thr-Lys-Pro-Arg.

Complications: The most severe complication in children is pneumococcus and staphylococcus pneumonia, infected eczematous skin, and purulent and draining lymph nodes.

Associated Findings: None known.

Etiology: Autosomal dominant inheritance.

Pathogenesis: A congenital mutation of tuftsin, where the triplets AAA or AAG that code for lysine are mutated to yield GAA or

GAG coding for glutamic acid residue. In the presence of the tuftsin mutant, the rate of phagocytosis remains very low and limits the defensive mechanism, particularly in early childhood.

MIM No.: 19115

Sex Ratio: Presumably M1:F1.

Occurrence: Unknown. Established literature. One New England study identified 20 cases.

Risk of Recurrence for Patient's Sib:
See Part I, *Mendelian Inheritance.*

Risk of Recurrence for Patient's Child:
See Part I, *Mendelian Inheritance.*

Age of Detectability: Early in infancy and childhood. May manifest itself during the first year of life.

Gene Mapping and Linkage: Unknown.

Prevention: None known. Genetic counseling indicated.

Treatment: Antibiotics along with γ-globulin.

Prognosis: Normal life span if treated early and survives childhood.

Detection of Carrier: Clinical history and laboratory examination show the presence in serum trypsin digest of inhibitory peptides to tuftsin activity. Radioimmunoassay shows false high values for tuftsin in serum. This is because the inhibitory peptides are tuftsin mutants that have a strong avidity for tuftsin receptor, about four times that of tuftsin. These false high values are diagnostic of the disease.

References:
Constantopoulos A, et al.: Tuftsin deficiency: a new syndrome with defective phagocytosis. J Pediatr 1972; 80:564–572.
Constantopoulos A, Najjar VA: Tuftsin deficiency syndrome. Acta Paediatr Scand 1973; 62:645–648.
Najjr VA: Tuftsin (Thr-Lsy-Pro-Arg): a natural activator of phagocytic cells with antibacterial and antineoplastic activity. In: Torrence PF, ed: Biological response modifiers. New York: Academic Press, 1985:141–169. *
Bump NJ, et al.: Isolation and subunit composition of tuftsin receptor. Proc Nat Acad Sci 1986; 83:7187–7191.

NA012   **Victor Najjar**

IMMUNODEFICIENCY, WISKOTT-ALDRICH TYPE   0523

Includes:
Aldrich syndrome
Eczema-thrombocytopenia-diarrhea-infection syndrome
Wiskott-Aldrich syndrome

Excludes:
Immunodeficiency, X-linked severe combined (0524)
Thrombocytopenia-absent radius (0941)

Major Diagnostic Criteria: Wiskott-Aldrich syndrome (WAS) is characterized by the triad of eczema, megakaryocytic thrombocytopenia, and recurrent infections. Levels of IgA and IgE are elevated, IgM is low to absent, and IgG level is variable.

Clinical Findings: Accompanying the abnormal immunoglobulin levels is an increase in the fractional catabolic rate for all immunoglobulin classes and for albumin, which is attributed to reticuloendothelial hyperplasia. All four IgG subclasses are generally within normal limits. Patients exhibit an early lack of response to polysaccharide antigens, resulting in the absence of isohemagglutinins. Paraproteins or monoclonal IgG, as well as restricted heterogeneity of immunoglobulins, may be present.

The ability to form specific antibody to antigen progressively declines, and anamnestic responses become decreased or absent.

T-lymphocyte number and function are usually normal at birth and show a progressive decline with age. Both the mixed lymphocyte reaction (MLR) and mitogen response normally become depressed. Lymphopenia is usually not evident until about age six years. T4 and T8 levels are both low, but the T4:T8 ratio is normal. Monocyte chemotactic defects may be present due to a lympho-

cyte product, which has been shown to render monocytes unresponsive to chemotactic stimuli *in vitro*.

There is a progressive loss of lymphoid elements normally in the thymus and in T-dependent areas of lymph nodes, spleen, and other peripheral lymphoid organs.

Microplatelets and thrombocytopenia are evident from birth. Platelets are approximately one-half the normal size and are rapidly catabolized. Megakaryocytes appear normal, although thrombopoiesis is depressed.

Complications: Due to variable thrombocytopenia, bleeding from the circumcision site or bloody diarrhea is often seen in the infant patient. Hemorrhagic syndromes may follow viral infections.

Recurrent infections are seen in the first year of life, often due to encapsulated bacteria, including pneumococcus. Common infections include otitis media, pneumonia, meningitis, and sepsis. As the patient grows older, infections due to *Pneumocystis carinii* and herpes-group viruses become more common. Hematemesis, melena, and chronic diarrhea are often seen.

Infants may have difficulty tolerating standard formulas made with intact protein, potentially resulting in malabsorption syndromes, but often tolerate elemental formulas. Difficulty in tolerating intact protein may persist beyond infancy.

Skin manifestations include thrombopenic purpura, petechiae, pyoderma, chronic viral warts, and intractable eczema.

Associated Findings: Increased incidence of malignant reticuloendotheliosis and lymphomas is seen in older patients, especially frequent are malignancies, particularly lymphomas that involve the CNS. Lymphomatoid granulomatosis has also been reported.

Etiology: X-linked recessive inheritance.

Pathogenesis: Patients appear to lack the 115 kD glycoprotein sialophorin on lymphocyte surface membranes and glycoprotein Ib on platelet surface membranes. This apparent absence may be due to an error in glycosylation, particularly of sialadation. Sialophorin is normally found on all thymocytes, CD4+ and CD8+ lymphocytes, and on a subpopulation of bone marrow cells and peripheral blood B-lymphocytes. Functional studies have suggested that sialophorin may play a role in activation of T-lymphocytes. Lymphocytes from WAS patients have also been reported to have fewer surface microvilli than did lymphocytes from normal individuals.

MIM No.: *30100

Sex Ratio: M1:F0

Occurrence: 1:250,000 male births.

Risk of Recurrence for Patient's Sib:
See Part I, *Mendelian Inheritance.*

Risk of Recurrence for Patient's Child:
See Part I, *Mendelian Inheritance.*

Age of Detectability: Fetal blood may be assessed for platelet number and size. Direct measurement of sialophorin may be possible. Phenotyping of fetal lymphocytes is not useful, because affected fetuses and infants initially have normal numbers of T- and B-lymphocytes. Recurrent infections and inability to produce antibody to polysaccharide antigens become evident within the first few years of life.

Gene Mapping and Linkage: WAS (Wiskott-Aldrich syndrome) has been mapped to Xp11.4-p11.21.

Prevention: None known. Genetic counseling indicated.

Treatment: The predominant treatment is bone marrow transplantation (BMT) following ablation of the recipient's marrow with busulfan or total body irradiation. In patients with advanced lymphoid depletion, BMT may be preformed without prior ablation. BMT is apparently curative for all symptoms with the exception of thrombocytopenia, which persists after transplantation. Cell-mediated lympholysis may also remain lower than normal following BMT. Treatment with transfer factor has not been proven to be beneficial.

Splenectomy may be useful in treating the thrombocytopenia. Synthetic steroids should not be used for eczema or thrombocytopenia, as they may further inhibit the patient's immune function. Topical corticosteroids may be administered.

Prognosis: Without appropriate treatment, survival beyond the teens is rare. The major cause of death is bleeding or infection, but malignancies account for 12% of deaths. With BMT, prognosis is good and even the complicating malignancies may be prevented.

Detection of Carrier: Obligate female carriers have an apparent preferential inactivation of the affected X chromosome in certain cell types. Detection is possible through metabolic stress of platelets.

Special Considerations: Immunodeficiencies in CBA/N mice are similar to those in WAS patients. Both exhibit X-linked inheritance and inability to produce antibody to polysaccharide antigens.

References:

Buckley RH: Immunodeficiency. J Allergy Clin Immunol 1983; 72:627–641.
Rosen FS, et al.: The primary immunodeficiencies. New Engl J Med 1984; 311:300–310. *
Saurat JH, et al.: Cutaneous symptoms in primary immunodeficiency. Curr Probl Dermatol 1985; 13:50–91.
Nahm MH, et al.: Patients with Wiskott-Aldrich syndrome have normal IgG$_2$ levels. J Immunol 1986; 137:3484–3487.
Borzy MS: Prenatal diagnosis of immunodeficiency diseases. Curr Probl Dermatol 1987; 16:185–296.
Mentzer SJ, et al.: Sialophorin, a surface sialoglycoprotein defective in the Wiskott-Aldrich syndrome, is involved in human T lymphocyte proliferation. J Exp Med 1987; 165:1383–1392.
Shapiro RS, et al.: Wiskott-Aldrich syndrome: detection of carrier state by metabolic stress of platelets. Lancet 1987; I:121–123.

HA081
SC039

Michael T. Halpern
Stanley A. Schwartz

IMMUNODEFICIENCY, X-LINKED LYMPHOPROLIFERATIVE DISEASE 2210

Includes:
> Duncan disease
> Epstein-Barr virus-induced lymphoproliferative disease in males
> Immunodeficiency 5
> Infectious mononucleosis, susceptibility to
> Lymphoproliferative disease, X-linked
> Purtilo syndrome

Excludes:
> **Granulomatous disease, chronic X-linked** (0443)
> **Immunodeficiency, agammaglobulinemia, X-linked, infantile** (0027)
> **Immunodeficiency, common variable type** (0521)
> **Immunodeficiency, severe combined** (0522)
> **Immunodeficiency, Wiskott-Aldrich type** (0523)
> **Immunodeficiency, X-linked with hyper IgM** (2524)

Major Diagnostic Criteria: Following infection with Epstein-Barr virus (EBV), males with the X-linked lymphoproliferative syndrome (XLP) experience fatal infectious mononucleosis (two-thirds), acquire hypogammaglobulinemia (one-fifth), or malignant B-cell lymphoma (one-fifth). Maternally-related males show one or more of the three major phenotypes. The diagnosis is confirmed by demonstrating EBV genome in tissues and a failure to mount antibodies to EBV-specific antigens, especially EB nuclear antigen (EBNA).

Clinical Findings: Following infection with EBV, males with XLP most frequently develop life-threatening infectious mononucleosis. Approximately 50% of the males will succumb to infectious mononucleosis by ten years of age. Males surviving the primary EBV infection exhibit acquired hypogammaglobulinemia and/or malignant B-cell lymphoma, generally involving extranodal sites such as the ileocecal region. Young males with the infectious mononucleosis phenotype will show fever, lymphadenomegaly, hepatosplenomegaly, and evidence of liver or bone marrow damage. The peripheral blood shows atypical lymphocytosis,

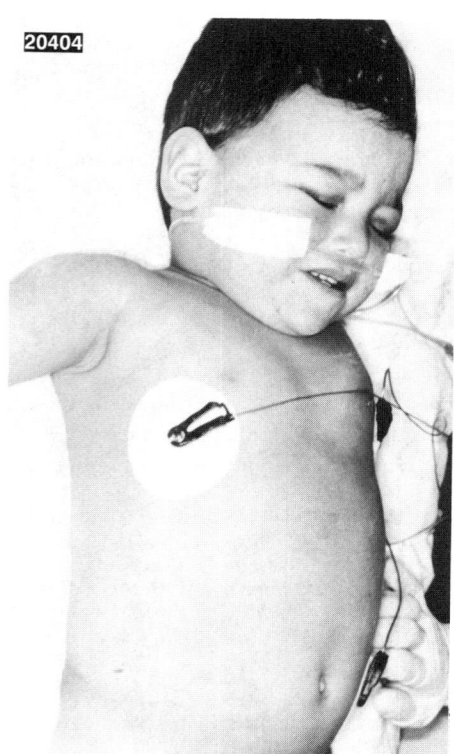

2210A-20404: Fulminant infectious mononucleosis in a 20-month old male. A rash, edema, lymphadenopathy, icterus and hepatosplenomegaly are evident.

especially plasmacytoid forms. Elevated transaminase enzymes and a polyclonal increase in immunoglobulin isotypes are found. The affected males fail to mount antibodies to EBV nuclear antigen. Critical to the diagnosis is identification of maternally related males with similar phenotypes.

The phenotypes can change from one type to another with time. This is likely due to defective immunoregulation of B-cell proliferation or alterations in immune function at various times. Invariably, XLP has been fatal by age 40 years.

Phenotypic variability occurs within a patient, among affected male family members, and between unrelated kindreds who are involved by the syndrome. Penetrance is generally complete. Immunologic and virologic examination for the phenotypes of all family members is essential. Thus far, no females have been affected; however, obligate carrier females of the XLP defect have often shown reactivated EBV infection, i.e., elevated antibodies in their sera to early antigen.

Complications: Massive liver failure associated with hemorrhage or hepatic coma. Also, suppression of bone marrow resulting in virus-associated hemophagocytic syndrome can lead to opportunistic infections by pyogenic agents. The thrombocytopenia these patients develop can lead to fatal hemorrhage. The patients acquiring hypogammaglobulinemia are also subject to opportunistic pyogenic infectious diseases unless they are given gamma-globulin replacement and prophylactic antibiotic therapy. Patients with malignant lymphoma show complications chiefly associated with the chemo- or radiotherapy given to these patients, i.e., opportunistic infections or hemorrhage due to depression of bone marrow.

Associated Findings: Congenital heart or central nervous system defects have occurred in a few affected males.

Etiology: X-linked recessive inheritance.

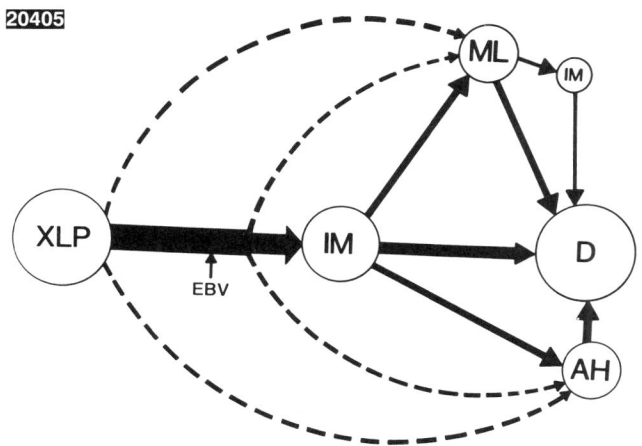

20405

2210B-20405: Natural history of the X-linked lymphoproliferative syndrome (XLP) after infection by Epstein-Barr virus (EBV), shown chronologically. Size of circles indicates relative number of patients thus far showing the various phenotypes, which include life-threatening or fatal infectious mononucleosis (IM) or malignant B cell lymphoma (ML), and acquired hypogammaglobulinemia (AH). Virtually 100% of the patients with XLP will manifest one of the three major phenotypes and the defect eventually leads to death (D). For example, infectious mononucleosis occurs at a median of 2.7 years; malignant lymphoma at 4.9 years; and acquired hypogammaglobulinemia at 6.9 years. Thickness of arrows indicates relative number of patients who subsequently develop various diseases shown. Broken arrows indicate hypothesized rare events that may occur.

Pathogenesis: Current theory postulates an inherited defect in T cells to recognize EBV viral antigens in infected B-cells. T-cells fail to control B-cell proliferation and function following infection by EBV. Tissue damage results from uncontrolled cytoxic cells and cytokines.

MIM No.: *30824

Sex Ratio: M1:F0. Very rare involvement of females is anticipated due to unequal lyonization of the normal X chromosome.

Occurrence: More than 220 patients from 56 kindreds have been registered in the XLP Registry. The affected kindreds have come from the United States, Canada, Great Britain, Scandinavia, France, West Germany, the Middle East, New Zealand and Australia.

Risk of Recurrence for Patient's Sib:
See Part I, *Mendelian Inheritance.*

Risk of Recurrence for Patient's Child:
See Part I, *Mendelian Inheritance.*

Age of Detectability: Usually clinically evident by ten years of age. The affected male is protected by maternally-derived antibodies to EBV for the initial four to six months of life. Defective switching from IgM to IgG antibody production on secondary intravenous challenge with bacteriophage ø0X174 has been detected. Moreover, IgG subclass deficiency prevails in most patients.

Gene Mapping and Linkage: LYP (lymphoproliferative syndrome) has been provisionally mapped to Xq25-q26.

Prevention: None known. Genetic counseling indicated. Early detection of affected males prior to EBV infection by RFLPs linkage analysis permits prophylactic therapy with gammaglobulin containing antibodies to EBV.

Treatment: Testing experimental therapy for the fulminant infectious mononucleosis phenotype is in progress using antiviral agents such as acyclovir and interferon-alpha. High dose intravenous gamma globulin is also recommended. Bone marrow transplantation can potentially reconstitute the immune defect. The individuals with the acquired hypogammaglobulinemia are given replacement immunoglobulin therapy and antibiotics prophylactically. Those developing malignant lymphoma are treated with conventional surgery, radiation therapy and chemotherapy. Care must be taken not to overtreat, as patients with the malignant lymphomas show good prognoses.

Prognosis: Fifty percent of the affected males die by age ten, and 100% by the end of the fourth decade. Approximately 15% of the patients in the Registry are surviving. Patients with hypogammaglobulinemia can maintain relatively normal lives with immunoglobulin replacement therapy. Invariably, patients develop fatal infectious mononucleosis or succumb to infections or hemorrhage.

Detection of Carrier: Pedigree analysis and elevated antibodies to EBV early antigen have been useful but not conclusive in identifying carriers of XLP. Restriction fragment length polymorphism linkage analyses reveals linkage with the DXS42 probe (LOD score 19.4 in seven families).

Special Considerations: The heterogeneity of clinical expression of XLP within an individual and a family must be kept in mind in making the diagnosis. Only a limited number of clinical laboratories are prepared to make the diagnosis.

Physicians are welcome to contact the XLP Registry for consultation in immunodeficiency, EBV detection, and Epstein-Barr virus-induced diseases by calling the University of Nebraska Medical Center, 42nd & Dewey Avenue, Omaha NE 48105, at (402) 559-4244.

References:
Purtilo DT, et al.: X-linked recessive progressive combined variable immunodeficiency (Duncan's disease). Lancet 1975; I:935–941.
Grierson H, Purtilo DT: Epstein-Barr virus infections in males with X-linked lymphoproliferative syndrome. Ann Intern Med 1987; 106: 538–545. *
Harrington DS, et al.: Malignant lymphoma in the X-linked lymphoproliferative syndrome. Cancer 1987; 59:1419–1429.
Skare JC, et al.: Mapping the X-linked lymphoproliferative syndrome. Proc Natl Acad Sci USA 1987; 84:2015–2018.
Purtilo DT, et al.: Detection of X-linked lymphoproliferative disease using molecular and immunovirologic markers. Am J Med 1989; 87:421–424.

PU007   **David T. Purtilo**

IMMUNODEFICIENCY, X-LINKED SEVERE COMBINED   **0524**

Includes:
    Agammaglobulinemia, X-linked recessive lymphopenic type
    Agammaglobulinemia, X-linked Swiss-type
    Alymphocytosis
    Alymphopenic immunologic deficiency, Gitlin form
    Dysplasia, congenital thymic type
    Hypoplasia, X-linked thymic epithelial type
    Immunodeficiency, X-linked severe dual system
    Immunologic deficiency, X-linked lymphopenic type
    Lymphocytophisis
    Lymphopenic hypogammaglobulinemia, X-linked recessive form
    Lymphopenia, X-linked, primary essential type
    Severe combined immunodeficiency, X-linked (SCIDX)
    Thymic alymphoplasia
    Thymic epithelial hypoplasia

Excludes:
    Achondroplasia-agammaglobulinemia
    Agammaglobulinemia-thymoma syndrome (0944)
    Fetal Acquired Immune Deficiency Syndrome (AIDS) infection (2497)
    Immunodeficiency, adenosine deaminase deficiency (2196)

Immunodeficiency, agammaglobulinemia, X-linked, infantile
(0027)
Immunodeficiency, biotin-deficient type
Immunodeficiency, severe combined (0522)
Immunodeficiency, thymic agenesis (0943)
Immunodeficiency, Wiskott-Aldrich type (0523)
Nucleoside phosphorylase deficiency

Major Diagnostic Criteria: Male infant with recurrent severe infections, absent or low isohemagglutinins, absent or low T-cell levels, absent or low immunoglobulins, and positive Schick test following Diphtheria-Pertussis-Tetanus (DPT) immunization. There is no response to skin test antigens and a very low in vitro response to phytohemagglutinin (PHA) stimulation. Lateral X-ray views of oropharynx and retrosternum reveal absence of adenoid and thymic shadows, respectively. B-cell levels are usually elevated. Absence of plasma cells in bone marrow occurs. Without a positive family history of previous male infant deaths, X-linked recessive severe combined immunodeficiency (SCID) may not be distinguishable from autosomal recessive SCID.

Clinical Findings: Recurrent severe infections in a male child, including pneumonia, meningitis, otitis, pyoderma, moniliasis, sepsis, or diarrhea. Eczema, undue susceptibility to common viral diseases (e.g., varicella, morbilli), progressive vaccinia following smallpox vaccination, fatal generalized BCG reactions, absence of lymph nodes, small or absent tonsils, poor growth, furuncles, and a family history of male infant deaths.

Complications: Pneumonitis invariably occurs in these patients. The most common organisms that prove fatal are *Pseudomonas*, enterobacteria, cytomegalovirus, *Pneumocystis carinii*, and *Morbillivirus*. Deaths from varicella pneumonia have also been reported. Other infectious complications include meningitis, sepsis, chronic otitis media, moniliasis, and furunculosis. Chronic diarrhea and malabsorption secondary to fungal or parasitic infections may contribute to marked failure to thrive. Vaccination with any live virus can lead to uncontrollable reactions. Fatal reactions have also been reported following BCG vaccination. Fatal graft-versus-host reactions following fresh whole blood transfusions are among the most common causes of death in these infants who lack the ability to reject histoincompatible lymphocytes. Graft-versus-host disease (GVHD) occurs 7–25 days after transfusion, beginning with a coarse, maculopapular rash over the entire body, followed by diarrhea, hemolytic anemia, hepatosplenomegaly, progressive hepatitis, fever, pancytopenia, and death. A chronic form of GVHD, marked by scaling erythroderma, histiocytic infiltration in the nodes, and chronic diarrhea, may develop secondary to maternal-fetal transfusion or intrauterine transfusion for erythroblastosis fetalis.

Associated Findings: Malabsorption syndrome and lymphoid cancer.

Etiology: X-linked recessive inheritance.

Pathogenesis: Because both thymic-dependent (delayed hypersensitivity) and thymic-independent (circulating antibodies) systems are involved in this disease, an abnormality of the immunologic stem cell line was originally postulated. More recently, elevated B-cell levels and identification of immature non-E-rosetting T-cells (as identified by monoclonal antibodies against T-cells) suggest that other mechanisms may be responsible for the combined immunodeficiency in most patients. Despite these reservations, bone marrow transplantation totally corrects the immunodeficiency. During the first few months of life, these infants are partially protected by placentally transferred circulating antibodies. In the ensuing months, the immunoglobulin levels fall, as no new antibodies are being synthesized and the number of circulating lymphocytes decreases. With the failure of both immunologic systems, recurrent infections follow. On postmortem examination, both gross and microscopic abnormalities are found in the thymus, lymph nodes, spleen, and GI tract. These consist mainly of marked depletion of all lymphoid elements, especially lymphocytes and plasma cells.

MIM No.: *30040

CDC No.: 279.200

Sex Ratio: M1:F0

Occurrence: Less than 1:1,000,000 under one year of age. Seldom seen above two years of age. About 50 cases have been reported in the literature.

Risk of Recurrence for Patient's Sib:
See Part I, *Mendelian Inheritance.*

Risk of Recurrence for Patient's Child:
See Part I, *Mendelian Inheritance.*

Age of Detectability: At birth, by low T-cell levels, elevated B-cell levels, lymph node biopsy, low or absent lymphocyte responses to PHA, inability to reject skin grafts or to form antibody following antigenic stimulation (e.g., typhoid antigen), absent isohemagglutinins, and quantitative low or absent immunoglobulins. A positive family history should increase the index of suspicion.

Gene Mapping and Linkage: SCIDX1 (severe combined immunodeficiency, X-linked 1) has been mapped to Xq13-q21.1.

Prevention: None known. Genetic counseling indicated.

Treatment: Bone marrow transplantation provides an immunologically competent stem cell source from a donor who is histocompatible at the HLA-D/DR locus. If a histocompatible sibling is not available, other approaches can be considered, such as purging the bone marrow of unwanted cells using monoclonal antibodies or using fetal liver as a source of immunologically uncommitted stem cells.

For a number of years, gamma globulin replacement therapy and antibiotics, when necessary, have been used to support these patients. Although this regimen, coupled with good pulmonary hygiene, has probably prolonged the life span of these infants, few have survived beyond the second birthday.

Whenever whole blood transfusion becomes necessary in the treatment of these patients, care must be taken to minimize the number of viable histoincompatible lymphocytes in the transfusate in order to prevent GVHD. This can be accomplished by utilizing buffy-coat-poor blood or frozen red cells after irradiation with 3,000 rads.

Prognosis: Poor, if untreated. Good, if reconstituted by bone marrow transplantation from a histocompatible sib. If a "matched" sibling is not available, newer methods of purging the bone marrow of mature lymphoid cells using monoclonal antibodies have led to moderate success in transplanting bone marrow from a parent. The first recipient of a successful bone marrow transplant has required no further treatment and is completely healthy 20 years later.

Detection of Carrier: Possible through laboratory procedures (Puck et al, 1987)

Special Considerations: Patients with X-linked SCID do not always manifest as severe lymphopenia as do those infants with the autosomal recessive type. Lymphopenia is also occasionally missed when the total lymphocyte count alone is followed. Lymphopenia in these patients refers primarily to decreased numbers of circulating T-cells. B-cell levels are often elevated. The X-linked and autosomal recessive forms may differ on histologic examination of lymphoid tissues, the former group showing generally less severe depletion of lymphoid elements. Occasionally, normal lymphocyte counts are observed in these patients until relatively late in the course of their disease.

References:
Gitlin D, Craig JM: The thymus and other lymphoid tissues in congenital agammaglobulinemia. I. Thymic alymphoplasia and lymphocytic hypoplasia and their relation to infection. Pediatrics 1963; 32:517–530.
Gatti RA, et al.: Immunological reconstitution of sex-linked lymphopenic immunological deficiency. Lancet 1968; II:1366–1369.
Yount WJ, et al.: Immunoglobulin classes, IgG subclasses, Gm genetic markers, and Clq following bone marrow transplantation in X-linked combined immunodeficiency. J Pediatr 1974; 84:193–199.
Buckley RH, et al.: Correction of severe combined immunodeficiency by fetal liver cells. New Engl J Med 1976; 294:1076–1081.
Thomas ED: Current status of bone marrow transplantation. Transpl Proc 1985; 17:428–436.

Puck JM, et al.: Carrier detection in X-linked severe combined immunodeficiency based upon patters of X chromosome inactivation. J Clin Invest 1987; 79:1395–1400.

GA020   **Richard A. Gatti**

Immunodeficiency, X-linked severe dual system
See IMMUNODEFICIENCY, X-LINKED SEVERE COMBINED

IMMUNODEFICIENCY, X-LINKED WITH HYPER IGM   2524

Includes:

Agammaglobulinemia-beta-2 macroglobulinemia
Antibody deficiency-beta-2 macroglobulinemia
Dysgammaglobulinemia antibody deficiency syndrome
Dysgammaglobulinemia, type I
Dysgammaglobulinemia-deficient 7S and elevated 19S
    gammaglobulins
Hyper-IgM syndrome
Immunodeficiency-3

Excludes:

Ataxia-telangiectasia (0094)
Deficiencies of isolated immunoglobulin classes (e.g., IgA)
Fetal rubella syndrome (0384)
Immunodeficiency, agammaglobulinemia, X-linked, infantile
    (0027)
Immunodeficiency, common variable type (0521)
Immunodeficiency, X-linked severe combined (0524)
Immunodeficiency, secondary or acquired
Immunoglobulin A deficiency (0525)
Waldenstrom macroglobulinemia

Major Diagnostic Criteria: Absent or severely diminished IgG, and IgA but IgM levels in excess of 300 mg/100 ml, plus an increased frequency and severity of bacterial infections, with onset during infancy or very early childhood.

Simple paper electrophoresis of serum to measure total gamma-globulins may appear falsely "normal" due to the large amount of IgM produced; therefore quantitative measurement of individual immunoglobulins (IgG, IgA, IgM) is necessary for diagnosis.

Clinical Findings: After age six months, when maternal IgG falls below protective levels, children are noted to have 1) serious persistent or recurrent bacterial infections with unusual frequency, including purulent rhinorrhea, conjunctivitis, otitis media, otitis externa, mastoiditis, sinusitis, facial cellulitis, tonsillitis, stomatitis, gingivitis, lymphadenitis, pneumonia, appendicitis, meningitis and sepsis; and 2) persistent monilial infections of the mouth and skin, and especially the diaper area, may be seen, possibly secondary to broad spectrum antibiotic use.

As early as age three months enlarged tonsils, lymph nodes, liver, and spleen are noted. Associated symptoms and signs may appear: 1) maculopapular rash of the scalp, face, or flexural surfaces; 2) chronic diarrhea/malabsorption; 3) failure to thrive (and possibly secondary developmental delay); 4) oral ulcers; 5) widespread verruca vulgaris; 6) bronchiectasis; 7) barrel chest deformity; 8) digital clubbing; 9) cyclic or persistent neutropenia; and 10) pancytopenia or mild hemolytic anemia possibly secondary to hypersplenism.

Arthritis and nephritis are less commonly reported. *Pneumocystis carinii* has repeatedly been demonstrated on autopsy. Other more commonly cultured organisms include *Haemophilus influenzae*, *Pseudomonas aeruginosa*, *Staphylococcus aureus*, *Streptococcus pneumoniae*, group A β-hemolytic *Streptococcus*, *Escherichia coli*, *Salmonella paratyphi* B, *Neisseria meningitidis*, and *Mycobacterium tuberculosis*.

Biopsied lymphoid tissues histologically demonstrate replacement of normal immunoglobulin-secreting cells with hypertrophied IgM-secreting plasmacytoid cells. Lymph node architecture is variable, ranging from diminished follicular size and number to normal or large follicles. Presence of germinal centers and plasma cells is also variable. Plasmacytoid cells showing specific immunofluorescence with labeled anti-IgM antiserum are described. In cases of malabsorption, small bowel biopsy material shows normal mucosa with lymphocytes, histiocytes, eosinophils, and plasma cells in the lamina propria.

Complications: Arthritis, acute nephritis, B-cell lymphoma of the GI tract especially in males presumed to have the X-linked variety.

Associated Findings: Bronchiectasis, hemolytic anemia, cyclic neutropenia with gingivitis, monilial infections of mucosal surfaces and skin, verruca vulgaris, malabsorption syndrome.

Etiology: X-linked or autosomal recessive inheritance, although in many cases a thorough study of the patient's family has not been reported and no affected relatives are known. Several immunologic defects could be postulated, among these: 1) intrinsic deficiency or absence of certain B-cell subclasses that could differentiate between IgA- and IgG-secreting plasma cells; 2) a block in B-cell differentiation between IgG- and IgA-secreting plasma cells (i.e., failure of the IgM and IgG "switch"); and 3) an additional nonisotype-specific T-cell-mediated suppression of Ig synthesis, in which IgM synthesis is least affected. Such a T-cell abnormality, reported in very few patients, may be inherited in the same way as the B-cell defect or may be a secondary phenomenon due to failure of further B-cell differentiation, causing an imbalance in cellular interactions and thereby leading to increased activity of suppressor T-cells.

Pathogenesis: Cellular immune defects are heterogeneous, with the majority of patients demonstrating an isolated intrinsic B-cell defect, whereas increased activity of T-suppressor cells is uncommon and probably represents assay variability. The phenotypic pattern of surface immunoglobulins on B-lymphocytes shows a large proportion expressing IgM and occasionally IgD. The quantity of IgM secreted by plasma cells is greater than normal. Cell mediated immunity appears intact. Blood group type O, although increased in prevalence in these patients, is not universal, nor is the expression of high levels of isohemagglutinins even in type O subjects. There have even been type O patients described with absence of isohemagglutinins.

MIM No.: *30823

Sex Ratio: M1:<1. Males far outnumber females. X-linked inheritance is believed to be much more common than autosomal recessive inheritance.

Occurrence: More than 25 cases have been reported in the literature.

Risk of Recurrence for Patient's Sib:
See Part I, *Mendelian Inheritance.*

Risk of Recurrence for Patient's Child:
See Part I, *Mendelian Inheritance.*

Age of Detectability: After six months of age.

Gene Mapping and Linkage: HIGM1 (hyper IgM syndrome) has been provisionally mapped to Xq24-q27.

Prevention: None known. Genetic counseling indicated.

Treatment: Therapeutic replacement with pooled gamma globulin, (single donor) plasma, or disaggregated intravenous gamma globulin; avoidance of exposure to infections; and regular medical follow-up. The use of hyperimmune immunoglobulin preparations (e.g., against tetanus, measles, or *Pseudomonas*) may be of value for patients exposed to these infections.

Vigorous antibiotic treatment at the earliest signs of infection, good pulmonary toilet and alternating courses of daily broad spectrum antibiotics in patients with bronchiectasis, nutritional counseling to meet increased metabolic demands of chronic infection, and treatment of malabsorption when present. Breast-fed infants are better protected than are formula-fed infants, particularly against the microbial flora from the intestinal tract of their own mothers. Attempts at permanent correction of the deficient functions by an allograft of immunocompetent tissues carry all the dangers of graft versus host reactions.

Prognosis: Assuming immunoglobulin replacement, appropriate use of antibiotics, and good medical follow-up, most patients survive to lead active, healthy lives; their life span thereafter is directly related to the presence and progression of bronchiectasis.

Detection of Carrier: Unknown.

References:
Kyong, CU, et al.: X-linked immunodeficiency with increased IgM: clinical, ethnic, and immunologic heterogeneity. Pediatr Res 1978; 12:1024–1026.
Brahmi Z, et al.: Immunologic studies of three family members with the immunodeficiency with hyper-IgM syndrome. J. Clin Immunol 1983; 3:127–134.
Levitt D, et al.: Hyper IgM immunodeficiency J Clin Invest 1983; 72:1650–1657.
Pascual-Salcedo D, et al.: Cellular basis of hyper IgM immunodeficiency. J Clin Lab Immunol 1983; 10:29–34.

GA024   **Ellen Garibaldi**

Immunodeficiency-3
See IMMUNODEFICIENCY, X-LINKED WITH HYPER IgM
Immunodeficiency-centromeric instability-facial anomalies (ICF)
See IMMUNODEFICIENCY WITH CENTROMERIC INSTABILITY
Immunodeficiency-microcephaly-malignancy
See CHROMOSOME INSTABILITY, NIJMEGEN TYPE
Immunodeficiency-microencephaly-retardation-skeletal defects
See MICROCEPHALY-RETARDATION-SKELETAL AND IMMUNE DEFECTS
Immunodeficiency-thymoma syndrome
See AGAMMAGLOBULINEMIA-THYMOMA SYNDROME

IMMUNOGLOBULIN A DEFICIENCY   0525

Includes:
Dysgammaglobulinemia type IV
Gamma-A-globulin, selective deficiency of
IgA-Mangel
Isolated IgA deficiency

Excludes:
Ataxia-telangiectasia (0094)
Immunodeficiency, severe combined (0522)
Immunodeficiency, X-linked severe combined (0524)

Major Diagnostic Criteria: IgA in serum more than 3 SD below mean for age. IgA in secretions usually also is low; a few cases with IgA present in secretion.

Clinical Findings: None specific except those of associated defects when these are present. Other laboratory findings: 10% may have anti-IgA antibodies; not all of these can be explained as due to prior plasma or gammaglobulin therapy. Increased IgG, IgM, or more rarely, IgE is found. IgG_2 subclass deficiency may be present in 18% of IgA deficient subjects (see **Immunodeficiency, IgG subclass deficiencies**). These individuals may have more frequent sinopulmonary infections and are candidates for IM or IV gammaglobulin treatment if anti-IgA antibodies are lacking. High levels of antimilk antibodies (hemagglutinating and/or precipitating) are found in 50% and antibovidae antibodies in 40%. Circulating antigen-antibody complexes are found in the sera of 60% and dietary bovine milk antigens are involved in complex formation. Secretory component levels are normal; a rare lack of secretory component has been described, which results in a lack of IgA in secretions. A possible defect in interferon production by lymphocytes after mitogen stimulation has been identified in some patients with selective IgA deficiency. HLA-B8, -DR3, and a particular complotype are found in increased frequency in IgA deficiency.

Complications: Increased susceptibility to respiratory infections, atopic diseases, and GI disease (giardiasis).

Associated Findings: A number of associated defects are present, but whether they are commonly associated epiphenomena or derivative consequences is unknown. The following have been described: **Arthritis, rheumatoid, Lupus erythematosus, systemic,** thyroiditis, pernicious anemia, sprue syndrome, sarcoidosis, hepatic cirrhosis, "lupoid" hepatitis, dermatomyositis, pulmonary hemosiderosis, idiopathic Addison disease, **Sjogren syndrome,** Coombs positive hemolytic anemia, chronic granulomatous disease, scleroderma, regional enteritis, ulcerative colitis,

vitiligo, recurrent parotitis, idiopathic thrombocytopenic purpura, mental retardation, epilepsy (before treatment). Cancers of epithelial origin (gastric or pulmonary) may have an increased incidence. Three instances of IgA deficiency and angio-immunoblastic lymphadenopathy have been reported. A large family with IgA deficiency and correlated early onset chronic obstructive pulmonary disease has been reported. Partial IgA deficiency and circulating immune complexes were found in association with a severe and often fatal respiratory infection in 21/34 infants age four to 24 months.

Etiology: Occurs constantly as a part of congenital agammaglobulinemia syndromes, or unassociated with other immunologic defects. A familial autosomal form has been described. No definite chromosome abnormality has been identified. Since at least some IgA-bearing lymphocytes are present in most if not all cases, this may reflect the presence of an abnormality or suppression of cellular differentiation leading to an inability to secrete IgA, rather than a lack of a gene controlling the constant region of the α chain. This is compatible with the finding that the deficiency has been found to include both IgA_1 and IgA_2 subclasses in studied cases. An immature IgA B-cell (expressing surface IgM, IgD, and IgA) is present in peripheral blood, suggesting that IgA B-cell maturation is arrested at an early stage of differentiation.
Drug-induced IgA deficiency was reported in phenytoin (Dilantin) treated patients with epilepsy, and in a penicillamine treated patient with Wilson disease. The number of IgA-bearing B-lymphocytes was normal in both.

Pathogenesis: Perhaps related to local antibody deficiency, but many people with isolated IgA deficiency seem perfectly normal. Relation to associated diseases is unclear. Hammarstrom et al (1985) reported transferring IgA deficiency from an HLA-matched sib. doner in the course of successful treatment of aplastic anemia by bone marrow transplantation from this doner.

MIM No.: 13710

Sex Ratio: M1:F2

Occurrence: From 1–3:1000 in the normal population; higher in those with collagen diseases, and possibly higher in patients with some cancers.

Risk of Recurrence for Patient's Sib: Unknown.

Risk of Recurrence for Patient's Child: Unknown.

Age of Detectability: At year of age by immunoquantitation.

Gene Mapping and Linkage: Unknown.

Prevention: None known. Genetic counseling indicated.

Treatment: Supportive measures for chronic sinopulmonary infections; avoidance of gluten in **Gluten-sensitive enteropathy,** or lactose in those with lactose intolerance as indicated. Fresh plasma infusions in sprue syndrome and those with chronic respiratory infection may be of benefit, but severe anaphylactic transfusion reactions have occurred in patients lacking IgA and having anti-IgA. If blood transfusions are required, washed and packed cells are indicated.

Prognosis: That of the associated disease; in many cases compatible with normal longevity.

Detection of Carrier: Unknown.

References:
Vjas G, Fudenberg HH: Am(1)₁ the first genetic marker of human immunoglobulin A. Proc Natl Acad Sci USA 1969; 64:1211–1216.
Ammann AJ, Hong R: Selective IgA deficiency: presentation of 30 cases and a review of the literature. Medicine 1971; 50:223–236.
Van Loghem E: Familial occurrence of isolated IgA deficiency associated with antibodies to IgA: evidence against a structural gene defect. Eur J Immunol 1974; 4:57–60.
Koistinen J: Selective IgA deficiency in blood donors. Vox Sang 1975; 29:192–202.
Seager J, et al.: IgA deficiency, epilepsy, and phenytoin treatment. Lancet 1975; II:632–636.
Hjalmarson O, et al.: IgA deficiency during D-penicillamine treatment. Br Med J 1977;1:549.
Cunningham-Rundles C, et al.: Bovine antigens and the formation of circulating immune complexes in selective IgA deficiency. J Clin Invest 1979; 64:272–279.

Cunningham-Rundles C, et al.: Selective IgA and neoplasia. Vox Sang 1980; 38:61–67.

Conley ME, Cooper MD: Immature IgA B cells in IgA deficient patients. New Engl J Med 1981; 305:495–497.

Oxelius VA, et al.: IgG$_2$ subclass deficiency in selective IgA deficiency. New Engl J Med 1981; 304:1476–1477.

Hammarstrom L, Smith CIE: HLA-A, B, C and DR antigens in immunoglobulin A deficiency. Tissue Antigens 1983; 21:75–79.

Hammarstrom L, et al.: Transfer of IgA deficiency to a bone-marrow-grafted patient with aplastic anaemia. Lancet 1985; II:778–781.

G0023
CU006

Robert A. Good
Charlotte Cunningham-Rundles

Immunoglobulin Am2
 See SERUM ALLOTYPES, HUMAN
Immunoglobulin deficiencies
 See IMMUNODEFICIENCY, COMMON VARIABLE TYPE
Immunoglobulin deficiency-centromere instability
 See IMMUNODEFICIENCY WITH CENTROMERIC INSTABILITY
Immunoglobulin Gm-1
 See IMMUNODEFICIENCY, IgG SUBCLASS DEFICIENCIES
 also SERUM ALLOTYPES, HUMAN
Immunoglobulin Gm-2
 See SERUM ALLOTYPES, HUMAN
 also IMMUNODEFICIENCY, IgG SUBCLASS DEFICIENCIES
Immunoglobulin Gm-3
 See IMMUNODEFICIENCY, IgG SUBCLASS DEFICIENCIES
 also SERUM ALLOTYPES, HUMAN
Immunoglobulin Gm-4
 See IMMUNODEFICIENCY, IgG SUBCLASS DEFICIENCIES
Immunoglobulin InV (Km)
 See SERUM ALLOTYPES, HUMAN
Immunologic deficiency, X-linked lymphopenic type
 See IMMUNODEFICIENCY, X-LINKED SEVERE COMBINED
Impacted teeth
 See TEETH, IMPACTED
Imperforate anus, high and low
 See ANORECTAL MALFORMATIONS
Imperforate anus-polydactyly syndrome
 See VATER ASSOCIATION
Imperforate hymen
 See HYMEN, IMPERFORATE
Incarcerated hernia
 See HERNIA, INGUINAL
Incisor, single upper central
 See TEETH, FUSED
Incisors (prominent)-obesity-hypotonia
 See COHEN SYNDROME
Incisors, barrel-shape
 See TEETH, INCISORS, SHOVEL-SHAPED
Incisors, mesiopalatal torsion of central
 See TEETH, MESIOPALATAL TORSION OF CENTRAL INCISORS
Incisors, rotation of upper central
 See TEETH, MESIOPALATAL TORSION OF CENTRAL INCISORS
Incisura mentalis types I, II, III, IV
 See FACE, CHIN FISSURE
Inclusion cysts of the oral mucosa in the newborn
 See MUCOSA, ORAL INCLUSION CYSTS OF THE NEWBORN
Incomplete feminizing testes syndrome
 See ANDROGEN INSENSITIVITY SYNDROME, INCOMPLETE
Incomplete male pseudohermaphroditism, type 1 (Wilson & Goldstein)
 See ANDROGEN INSENSITIVITY SYNDROME, INCOMPLETE
Incomplete testicular feminization syndrome
 See ANDROGEN INSENSITIVITY SYNDROME, INCOMPLETE
Incontinenti Pigmenti Achromians
 See HYPOMELANOSIS OF ITO

INCONTINENTIA PIGMENTI 0526

Includes:
 Bloch-Siemens incontinentia pigmenti
 Bloch-Sulzberger syndrome
 Melanoblastosis cutis linearis
 Pigmented dermatosis, Siemens-Bloch type
Excludes:
 Ectodermal dysplasia, Naegeli type (0703)
 Hypomelanosis of Ito (2264)
Major Diagnostic Criteria: Skin lesions, with or without alopecia, tooth anomalies.

Clinical Findings: Characterized at birth or neonatal period by inflammation and bullae in females. The lesions are arranged in linear fashion and may come and go. They are then replaced by hypertrophic verrucous bands. Then a bizarre pattern of spattered or band-like hyperpigmentation appears mostly on the trunk but also on the scalp and limbs. The hyperpigmentation slowly fades and almost disappears by the third decade. The typical hyperpigmentation is usually preceded by inflammation and blisters. Alopecia of scalp, dental, ocular (vascular abnormalities of the retina and disorders of the retinal pigment epithelium), and osseous anomalies, deformities of ears, small stature, neurologic changes, and occasionally, mental retardation occurs.

Complications: Convulsions, retrolental fibroplasia.

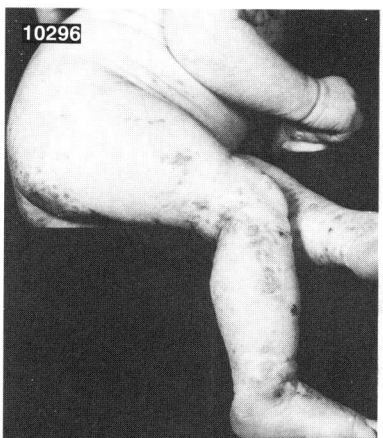
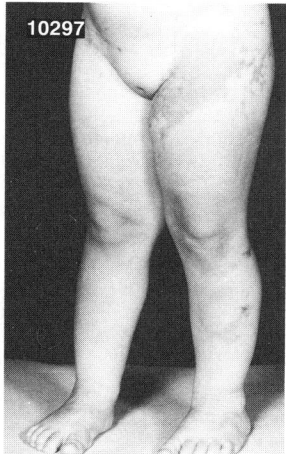
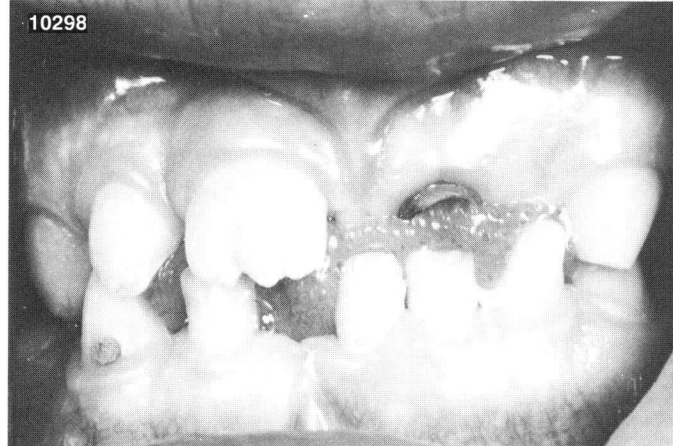

0526-10296: Linear vesicles. **10297:** Spattered hyperpigmentation. **10298:** Dysplastic and conical teeth.

Associated Findings: Supernumerary tragi, chromosomal translocations, **Klinefelter syndrome**, extra ribs, and hemivertebrae.

Etiology: Presumably X-linked dominant inheritance, lethal in males.

Pathogenesis: Unknown.

MIM No.: *30830

POS No.: 3265

CDC No.: 757.350

Sex Ratio: M>0:F1

Occurrence: About 700 cases reported.

Risk of Recurrence for Patient's Sib:
See Part I, *Mendelian Inheritance*.

Risk of Recurrence for Patient's Child:
See Part I, *Mendelian Inheritance*.

Age of Detectability: In childhood.

Gene Mapping and Linkage: IP1 (incontinentia pigmenti 1) has been mapped to Xp11.21-cen.

Prevention: None known. Genetic counseling indicated.

Treatment: Unknown.

Prognosis: Normal life span. Some patients are mentally retarded. Disability may result from neurologic, ocular, osseous and other changes. Reproductive fitness somewhat impaired by major defects.

Detection of Carrier: Unknown.

References:
Carney RG: Incontinentia pigmenti: report of 5 cases and review of literature. Arch Dermatol Syph 1951; 64:126.
Carney RG, Carney RG Jr.: Incontinentia pigmenti. Arch Dermatol 1970; 102:157–162.
Carney RG Jr: Incontinentia pigmenti, a world statistical analysis. Arch Dermatol 1976; 112:535–542.
Wiklund DA, Weston WL: Incontinentia pigmenti: a four generation study. Arch Derm 1980; 116:701–703.
Wieacker P, et al.: X inactivation patterns in two syndromes with probable X-linked dominant, male lethal inheritance. Clin Genet 1985; 28:238–242.
Ormerod AD, et al.: Incontinentia pigmenti in a boy with Klinefelter's syndrome. J Med Genet 1987; 24:439–441.
Spallone A: Incontinentia pigmenti (Bloch-Sulzberger syndrome): seven case reports in one family. Brit J Ophthal 1987; 71:629–634.

CH034   **Philip F. Chance**

Incontinentia pigmenti of Naegeli
See ECTODERMAL DYSPLASIA, NAEGELI TYPE
Index finger polydactyly
See POLYDACTYLY
Indiana type hereditary amyloidosis
See AMYLOIDOSIS, INDIANA TYPE
Indocin△, fetal effects
See FETAL EFFECTS OF NONSTEROIDAL ANTI-INFLAMMATORY DRUGS (NSAIDS)
Indomethacin, fetal effects
See FETAL EFFECTS OF NONSTEROIDAL ANTI-INFLAMMATORY DRUGS (NSAIDS)
Infant of diabetic mother (IDM)
See FETAL EFFECTS FROM MATERNAL DIABETES
Infant of gestational diabetic mother (IGDM)
See FETAL EFFECTS FROM MATERNAL DIABETES
Infantile cerebellar atrophy with retinal degeneration
See OLIVOPONTOCEREBELLAR ATROPHY, DOMINANT WITH RETINAL DEGENERATION
Infantile hemangioendothelioma
See ORBITAL HEMANGIOMA
Infantile malignant osteopetrosis
See OSTEOPETROSIS, MALIGNANT RECESSIVE
Infantile necrotizing encephalomyelopathy
See ENCEPHALOPATHY, NECROTIZING
Infantile paralysis
See POLIO, SUSCEPTIBILITY TO
Infantile phytanic acid storage disease
See PHYTANIC ACID OXIDASE DEFICIENCY, INFANTILE TYPE

Infantile polycystic disease (IPCD)
See KIDNEY, POLYCYSTIC DISEASE, RECESSIVE
Infantile polyposis
See INTESTINAL POLYPOSIS, JUVENILE TYPE
Infantile psychosis
See AUTISM, INFANTILE
Infarction defects in surviving monozygous twins
See FETAL MONOZYGOUS MULTIPLE PREGNANCY DYSPLACENTATION EFFECTS
Infection, Venezuelan equine encephalitis
See FETAL VENEZUELAN EQUINE ENCEPHALITIS INFECTION
Infections, recurrent severe
See GRANULOCYTE GLYCOPROTEIN CD11/CD18 DEFICIENCY
Infectious mononucleosis, susceptibility to
See IMMUNODEFICIENCY, X-LINKED LYMPHOPROLIFERATIVE DISEASE
Inferior vena cava, absent
See VENA CAVA, ABSENT HEPATIC SEGMENT
Inferior vena cava, absent hepatic segment
See VENA CAVA, ABSENT HEPATIC SEGMENT
Inflammation of the brain, skin and joints-infantile relapsing
See INFLAMMATORY DISEASE, NEONATAL BATES-LORBER TYPE

INFLAMMATORY BOWEL DISEASE   **2232**

Includes:
Crohn disease
Granulomatous colitis
Ileocolitis
Intestine, inflammatory bowel diseases
Regional enteritis/ileitis
Ulcerative colitis
Ulcerative proctitis

Excludes:
Colitis due to bacterial, fungal, viral, and protozoal agents
Colitis secondary to systemic disease
Diverticulitis
Drug or irradiation-induced colitis and proctitis
Ileocecal tuberculosis
Irritable bowel syndrome
Ischemic colitis
Pseudomembranous colitis

Major Diagnostic Criteria: The inflammatory bowel diseases (IBD) are chronic diseases characterized by inflammatory lesions of the large and small bowel. The clinical course is extremely variable, with unpredictable remissions and exacerbations and a wide range of local and systemic complications. Diagnosis is based on a combination of clinical, X-ray, and pathologic findings.

Crohn disease: No specific laboratory tests confirm this diagnosis. While classically affecting the small intestine, especially the terminal ileum, large bowel involvement is common as well, and the disease may involve any part of the gastrointestinal tract. Chronic clinical course includes fever, diarrhea, cramping abdominal pain, vomiting, and anemia. Perianal fissure, ulceration, or fistulas may be present at time of diagnosis. On X-ray, distribution of diseased bowel may be segmental. Common findings are strictures, fistulas, abdominal abscesses, and a characteristic "cobblestone" mucosal pattern in affected areas. Sigmoidoscopy findings may be normal, or show lumpy edema or areas of ulceration interspersed with normal areas. On biopsy, most tissue samples show granulomas.

Ulcerative colitis: There are no specific laboratory tests to confirm this diagnosis. The affected area is the large bowel. Common clinical manifestations include bloody rectal discharges, often with recurrent diarrhea, cramping lower abdominal pain, weight loss, and tenesmus. At onset, clinical symptoms may be mild or severe. Constipation may be present. Spontaneous remission and exacerbation of symptoms is characteristic. Diffuse inflammation of the rectal and sigmoid mucosa is seen on proctoscopy in the vast majority of patients. On X-ray, about one-half show involvement of the entire colon.

Clinical Findings: Symptoms at onset, as well as during the course of disease, are highly variable. Each patient's clinical course is characterized by distinct debilitating symptoms and complications. The chronic course will exacerbate and remit in such a variable way that some patients will have minimal social consequences from their disease, while others will require multiple hospitalizations, extensive surgery, and hyperalimentation.

Complications: Complications are numerous, involving virtually all organ systems. Included are skin lesions (aphthous ulcers of the mouth, pyoderma gangrenosum, erythema nodosum); eye lesions (conjunctivitis, iritis, and episcleritis); obstructive hydronephrosis, nephrolithiasis, venous thrombosis, hepatobiliary diseases (pericholangitis, primary sclerosing cholangitis, bile duct carcinoma, cholelithiasis, fatty infiltration of the liver, fibrosis, and cirrhosis of the liver); and musculoskeletal complications (peripheral arthritis, sacroiliitis, and **Ankylosing spondylitis**). Nutritional deficiencies are possible, secondary to decreased intestinal absorption, and growth retardation is seen in some cases with childhood onset. Both Crohn disease and ulcerative colitis patients have an increased risk for carcinomas of the gastrointestinal tract (2–3% of all IBD patients with duration of disease of 20 years or greater). Serious gastrointestinal complications include toxic megacolon, massive gastrointestinal bleeding, and strictures.

Associated Findings: Inflammatory bowel disease is found in increased frequency in two genetic syndromes: **Turner syndrome** and **Albinism, oculocutaneous, Hermansky-Pudlak type**. Four of 135 Turner syndrome patients (3%) in one series developed IBD (two Crohn and two ulcerative colitis). Hermansky-Pudlak syndrome, a tyrosine-positive albinism disorder, has a worldwide distribution. Puerto Rican patients with Hermansky-Pudlak syndrome have a high incidence of granulomatous colitis.

Patients with inflammatory bowel disease and either typical **Ankylosing spondylitis** (approximately 5% of cases) or sacroiliitis show an increased frequency of HLA-B27.

Etiology: Family studies demonstrate an increased family aggregation for both Crohn disease and ulcerative colitis. The etiology(s) appears to be complex, and Mendelian ratios are not observed in families. Crohn disease appears to be more strongly familial than does ulcerative colitis, and a higher monozygotic twin concordance rate has been reported for Crohn disease than for ulcerative colitis. Positive family history for IBD is reported to range from 14% to 30% in Crohn case series; for ulcerative colitis, the proportion of cases with a positive family history ranges from 6% to 8%. Some data suggest that early-onset IBD cases may have an increased incidence of affected second-degree relatives as well (in most series, the increased risk is mainly reported for first-degree relatives). Both Crohn disease and ulcerative colitis appear with increased frequency in relatives of probands with either disease, raising the possibility that these two diseases may be clinical variants of the same underlying disease process.

While environmental factors have been suggested as playing a role in the etiology of both Crohn disease and ulcerative colitis, experimental evidence is unclear at this time. Proposed environmental agents include dietary factors (most notably refined sugars, milk, dietary fiber, carrageenan) and microbial agents (most notably anaerobic bacteria, mycobacteria, and viral agents).

The basic underlying mechanisms in these diseases are unknown. The leading hypotheses are primary immunologic derangements consisting of either autoimmune or immune/toxin interactions.

Pathogenesis: The primary lesion is not yet known for either Crohn disease or ulcerative colitis.

Crohn disease: The early pathologic lesions are scattered superficial ulcers of the bowel. Also found are submucosal edema, lymphatic dilation, and transmural involvement of the bowel wall. Lymphatic involvement suggests a possible role of the immune system in the pathogenesis. Granulomas, found in most but not all Crohn patients, suggest a possible defect in host defenses against environmental agents (either chemical or biologic). Defects in cell-mediated immunity have been found, but these may be secondary to the disease process. Good animal models are not available.

Ulcerative colitis: The diffuse inflammatory reaction seen in the mucosa and submucosa of the colon suggests a possible reaction to cytotoxic agents. Increased plasma cells are found in the colon,

perhaps suggesting an immune reaction. Raised gut bacterial counts, also found in Crohn patients, raise the possibility of a viral or bacterial etiology, although no specific agent is clearly implicated. Other possibilities include an autoimmune etiology or specific immunologic defects originating in the bowel mucosa. It remains difficult to separate primary defects and those secondary to the disease process.

CDC No.: 751.880

Sex Ratio: M1:F0.8–1.6 in Crohn disease (increased in females with older age of onset).

M1:F1 in ulcerative colitis in many populations; slight female preponderance in others (mostly English, English-derived).

Occurrence: *Crohn disease:* 0.27–6.3:100,000 (lowest in Blacks, Asians; highest in northern Europeans, Ashkenazi Jews in Europe, United States).

Ulcerative colitis: 2–7:100,000 (highest in northern Europe).

Since 1950, the incidence of Crohn disease has steadily increased in most populations; this increase appears to be real. No such increase is seen for ulcerative colitis.

Risk of Recurrence for Patient's Sib: *Crohn disease:* 1:25. *Ulcerative colitis:* 1:50. IBD total: Ashkenazi Jew 1:40; non-Jewish 1:100.

Risk of Recurrence for Patient's Child: *Crohn disease:* 1:50. *Ulcerative colitis:* 1:150. IBD total: Ashkenazi Jew 1:40; Non-Jewish 1:100.

The sketchy data suggest that the empiric risk is very much a function of the specific population. All the above data are uncorrected for the age of the relative at risk Actual lifetime risks may be several fold higher, especially among offspring.

Age of Detectability: In infants (less than one year of age) through adulthood. Peak age of detection for Crohn disease is 20–29 years of age; ulcerative colitis at 60–80 years of age.

Gene Mapping and Linkage: A possible association between HLA-DR2 and ulcerative colitis in certain populations have been reported, and between HLA-DR4 and *Crohn disease* in the Japanese. There is also data implicating the involvement of the C3 locus on chromosome 19.

Prevention: None known. Genetic counseling indicated.

Treatment: Medical treatment is primarily symptomatic. Adrenal steroids, ACTH, and immunosuppressive drugs can be useful in controlling active disease in some patients. Sulfasalazine in maintenance doses has been successfully used in preventing relapses in some patients. Use of elemental diet and total parenteral nutrition may play a role in both maintenance and treatment. Surgery may be necessary for severe or debilitating disease in severe acute phases, or for complications.

Prognosis: *Crohn disease:* Even with current treatment, more than 50% of surgically treated, and 90% of medically treated cases, will have recurrent disease. Recurrence soon after resection surgery is a bad prognostic sign, as is extensive involvement of the small bowel.

Ulcerative colitis: Most severe episodes occur during the first year. Modern treatment has greatly improved the death rate due to acute attacks. Childhood and elderly onset have a worse prognosis than adulthood onset (3–5% mortality rate with good care). Risk for gastrointestinal cancer estimated to be increased 10- to 40-fold, with greatest risk to those with onset of colitis before age 30.

Detection of Carrier: Unknown.

Special Considerations: Crohn disease and ulcerative colitis may be the spectrum of one disease, with Crohn disease representing the more severe cases. Equally likely, there may be etiologic and genetic heterogeneity within each disease, with subtypes that may present as either disease.

Support Groups:

New York; National Foundation for Ileitis and Colitis

CANADA: BC; Burnaby; Northwestern Society of Intestinal Research

References:

Arulanantham K, et al.: The association of inflammatory bowel disease and Y chromosomal abnormality. Pediatrics 1980; 66:63–67.

Kirsner JB: Inflammatory bowel disease: clinical, etiologic, and genetic aspects. In: Rotter JI, Samloff IM, Rimoin DL, eds: The genetics and heterogeneity of common gastrointestinal disorders. New York: Academic Press, 1980:261–290.

Mayberry JF, Rhodes J: Epidemiological aspects of Crohn's disease: a review of the literature. Gut 1984; 25:886–899.

Weterman IT, Pena AS: Familial incidence of Crohn's disease in the Netherlands and a review of the literature. Gastroenterology 1984; 86:449–452.

McConnell RB: Genetic aspects of idiopathic inflammatory bowel disease. In: Kirsner JB, Shorter RG, eds: Inflammatory bowel disease, 3rd ed. Philadelphia: Lea & Febiger, 1988:87–95.

Roth M-P, et al.: Familial recurrence risks of inflammatory bowel disease in Ashkenazi Jews. Gastroenterology 1989; 96:1016–1020.

Shohat T, et al.: The genetics of inflammatory bowel disease. In: Gitnick G, ed: Inflammatory bowel disease: a physician's guide. New York: Igukiu-Shoin, 1989.

VA019

Constance M. Vadheim
Jerome I. Rotter

Inflammatory disease, infantile multisystem
See INFLAMMATORY DISEASE, NEONATAL BATES-LORBER TYPE

INFLAMMATORY DISEASE, NEONATAL BATES-LORBER TYPE   2157

Includes:

    Arthropathy-rash-uveitis-mental retardation
    Bates syndrome
    Epiphyseal damage with constitutional symptoms
    Inflammation of the brain, skin and joints-infantile
      relapsing
    Inflammatory disease, infantile multisystem
    Inflammatory disease, neonatal onset multisystem
    Lorber syndrome
    Meningitis-polyarthritis-lymphadenitis-pulmonary
      hemosiderosis

Excludes:

    Arthritis, rheumatoid (2517)
    Infection (rubella, syphilis, toxoplasmosis, etc.)
    Lipogranulomatosis (0598)
    Mucopolysaccharidosis

Major Diagnostic Criteria: Features strongly suggestive of neonatal-onset, multisystem, inflammatory disease include evanescent

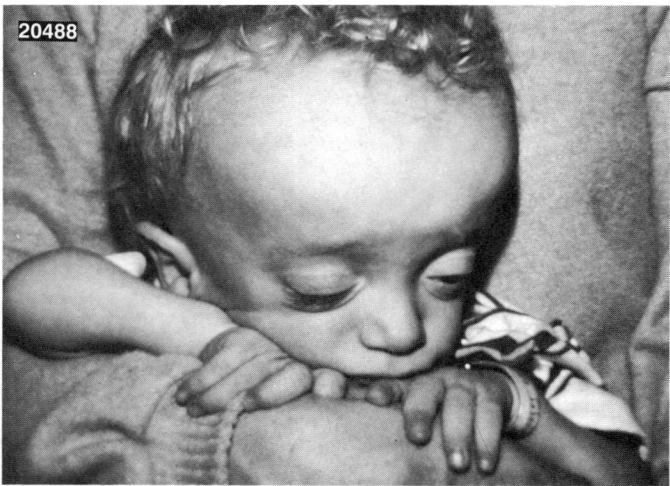

2157A-20488: Inflammatory disease, neonatal Bates-Lorber type; note subject age 18 months with frontal bossing, hydrocephalus, bony enlargement and arthritis of both elbows.

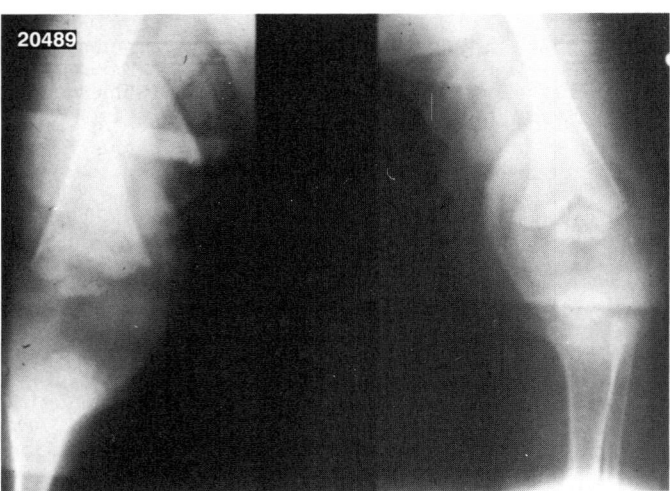

2157B-20489: X-ray of both knees at age 5 months; note soft tissue swelling, epiphyseal erosions of the distal femurs, and periosteal elevations surrounding the femoral metaphyses.

---

rash either similar to the eruption of systemic onset rheumatoid arthritis or to typical urticaria; persistent or intermittent episodes of fever resembling the pattern of systemic onset juvenile rheumatoid arthritis; reticuloendothelial involvement characterized by hepatosplenomegaly or generalized lymphadenopathy; progressive and destructive arthropathy; chronic central nervous system changes, which may include developmental delay, mental retardation, **Hydrocephaly** with persistent open fontanelle, non-bacterial meningitis, cerebral atrophy, and seizures; eye changes such as uveitis, vitreous inflammation, or papilledema. Laboratory changes are nonspecific, but a persistent anemia, leukocytosis, elevated erythrocyte sedimentation rate, and cerebrospinal fluid pleocytosis are usually present. X-ray findings of periosteal elevation, flared metaphyses and abnormal ossification are often seen.

Clinical Findings: The cutaneous findings, fever, lymphadenopathy, and hepatosplenomegaly start characteristically at birth or in the neonatal period. Of 13 patients, nine started at birth, one at two days, one at four months, and in one occurrence the age of onset was not recorded. Destructive arthropathy, then central nervous system and eye involvement usually develop during the first year. Clinical findings in 13 reported children consist of the following: 1. evanescent cutaneous eruption which may be urticarial in appearance or similar to the rash of systemic onset juvenile rheumatoid arthritis (all 13); 2. generalized lymphadenopathy but often very evident in the axillary and inguinal areas (all 13); 3. destructive, particularly bony, and progressive arthropathy involving multiple joints, but most frequently the elbows, wrists, knees, and ankles, and often leading to the formation of severe contractures with a subsequent significant physical disability (all 13); 4. fever suggestive of systemic onset juvenile rheumatoid arthritis persisting in cyclical fashion (12/13); 5. hepatosplenomegaly (9); 6. variable central nervous system abnormalities including persistently open fontanelle (11), hydrocephalus or increased head size (9), delayed developmental milestones (13), and seizures (6); feeding difficulties (4) with subsequent varying degrees of malnutrition, and secondary hearing loss also may be secondary to central nervous involvement; and 7, eye involvement consisting of uveitis (7), sometimes with vitreous inflammatory changes (2), papilledema (7), and optic atrophy (1).

Laboratory findings include a persistent and often severe anemia (usually hypochromic and microcytic) (9/9), an intermittent or persistent leukocytosis (13), and markedly increased sedimentation rate. Immunoglobulin G levels are often elevated (8/10), and antinuclear antibodies negative. Rheumatoid factor may be detected (1/4). Recurrent CSF pleocytosis (mononuclear cells predominantly) is seen (10/10). Low zinc and copper levels are reported in one child with prolonged malnutrition. Profound X-ray changes of periosteal reaction, abnormal epiphyseal ossification centers, and flared metaphyses.

Complications: Marked joint deformities frequently result in gait disturbance and progress to nonambulation.

Inflammatory eye changes may cause visual deficits. There is an apparent susceptibility to infections although measurements of immunologic function in selected cases are normal. One child developed fatal myelomonoblastic leukemia, implying that this may be a premalignant disorder, although this same patient two years previously had been treated with chlorambucil. Almost all patients have experienced some degree of failure to thrive, delayed developmental milestones, and mental retardation as a result of both poor nutrition and chronic inflammatory disease of the CNS (i.e., meningitis).

Associated Findings: Omphalocele, pulmonary hemosiderosis, psoriasis with possibly increased susceptibility to frequent and severe infectious diseases, or development of malignancy.

Etiology: Unknown.

Pathogenesis: Neonatal onset, vitreous inflammation, and early periosteal involvement suggest in utero infection, but a vigorous search to confirm this cause has not been successful. A relationship to psoriasis has been suggested because of biopsy findings in one patient and family history in two patients. Articular manifestations of psoriasis, however, are usually erosive and asymmetric, and chronic CNS inflammatory changes are not seen. The early onset of symptoms, accompanied by developmental delay and variable mental deficiency, is suggestive of progressive organ damage secondary to a metabolic storage disorder. Urinary screening for mucopolysaccharides and oligosaccharides, however, and fibroblast cultures for lysosomal hydrolase and neuroamidase activity in several patients, have yielded normal results; biopsy specimens have also not shown findings consistent with a storage process. Persistent inflammation of the skin and central nervous system suggest an ongoing immune response to sequestered antigens or antigenic fragments, or an inherited deficiency of one of the naturally occurring inhibitors of the inflammatory response.

Sex Ratio: M6:F7

Occurrence: 13 cases have been described in the literature.

Risk of Recurrence for Patient's Sib: Unknown. Two siblings of the opposite sex were affected in one family, but all other cases have been sporadic.

Risk of Recurrence for Patient's Child: There are no reports thus far of any patient having offspring.

Age of Detectability: The presence of maculopapular rash and hepatosplenomegaly at birth should alert the clinician to this disorder. Persistent fever, central nervous system changes, and destructive arthropathy usually follow within the first two to four months of life.

Gene Mapping and Linkage: Unknown.

Prevention: None known. Genetic counseling indicated.

Treatment: In most cases nonsteroidal anti-inflammatory agents or drugs, such as gold or penicillamine, are not very helpful. Corticosteroids are only partially successful in reducing systemic symptoms and improving joint function. Prompt recognition and treatment of infections is needed. A comprehensive program of joint conservation, if started early enough, will lessen the impact of severe joint contractures. Ocular inflammatory disease requires prompt therapy to prevent visual loss, and early audiologic testing is mandatory.

Prognosis: Of 13 patients reported thus far, three have died; causes were haemophilus influenzae pneumonia, necrotizing leukoencephalopathy, and myelomonoblastic leukemia. General clinical outcomes are varied. Severe joint deformities appear to persist, and some degree of mental retardation often occurs.

Detection of Carrier: Unknown.

References:

Lorber J: Syndrome for Diagnosis: dwarfing, persistently open fontanelle, recurrent meningitis, recurrent subdural effusions with temporary alternate-sided hemiplegia, high-tone deafness, visual defect with pseudo-papillaedema, slowing intellectual development, recurrent acute polyarthritis, erythema marginatum, splenomegaly, and iron-resistant hypochronic anemia. Proc R Soc Med 1973; 6:1070–1071.
Ansell BM: Rheumatic disorders in childhood. London, Butterworths, 1980:269–277. †
Prieur A, Griscelli C: Arthropathy with rash, chronic meningitis, eye lesions, and mental retardation. J Pediatr 1981; 99:79–83.
Hassink SG, Goldsmith DP: Neonatal onset multisystem inflammatory disease. Arthritis Rheum 1983; 26:668–673. * †
Goldsmith DP: The right stuff for a new syndrome. J Pediatr 1985; 106:441–443.
Yarom A, et al.: Infantile multisystem disease: a specific syndrome? J Pediatr 1985; 106:390–396. *

G0043   **Donald P. Goldsmith**

INTERFERON DEFICIENCY   3090

Includes:
  Alpha-interferon deficiency
  Antiviral interferon deficiency
  Beta-interferon deficiency
  Fibroblast interferon deficiency
  Gamma-interferon deficiency
  Immune interferon deficiency
  Leukocyte interferon deficiency
  Lymphoblast interferon deficiency

Excludes:
  Antiviral antibody deficiency
  Cell-mediated immunity to viruses

Major Diagnostic Criteria: Decreased levels of one or more types of interferon (IFN) have been described in humans with various disorders, including tumors, leukemia, **Cancer, Hodgkin disease, familial,** chronic hepatitis B infection, the acquired immunodeficiency syndrome (AIDS), recurrent labial herpes, persistent Epstein-Barr virus infection, and congenital cytomegalovirus infection. It is not always possible to determine whether IFN deficiency is primary or secondary in these instances. A deficiency in IFN responsiveness also occurs in malnutrition, corticosteroid therapy, other forms of immunosuppression, and postrenal transplantation, strongly suggesting a secondary defect. Mice subjected to burn injury also have subnormal IFN responses.

IFN is not normally detected in tissue or serum, but is usually detectable during viral infections. Assays for IFN usually measure the inhibition of either virus production or viral cytopathic effect on cultured cell lines.

Clinical Findings: The consequences of IFN deficiency are thought to include 1) decreased resistance to viral infection, possibly due to decreased cellular synthesis of new mRNA and protein (IFN enhances the expression of classes I and II HLA molecules [histocompatibility antigens] on the surface of infected cells, making them more susceptible targets for cytotoxic lymphocytes); 2) decreased natural killer (NK) cell activity; and 3) decreased antibody synthesis.

Few if any of the specific defects in immunity described to date have been proven to be the result of a primary defect in IFN production, although several family studies suggest this may occur. Success in treating certain virus infections and malignancies with IFN suggests that it may play an important role in these disorders.

Alveolar macrophages and peripheral blood monocytes of newborns are more permissive of herpes simplex virus replication than are those of adults. This may be related to an inability of neonatal cells to produce PHA-induced gamma IFN. This inability diminishes until around age six months, when responses are similar to those of adults.

About 30% of patients with recurrent herpes labialis have low levels of IFN. Some children with frequent respiratory syncytial virus (RSV) infections also have low levels of IFN. In both instances, replacement therapy may be beneficial. Therapy with IFN also has been encouraging in some cases of hepatitis B infections and in hairy cell leukemia, Kaposi sarcoma, and renal cell carcinoma. Thus, the possibility of IFN deficiency should be considered in patients with these conditions as well as in persons who have other recurrent or persistent viral infections or as yet unstudied malignancies.

Complications: Interferon deficiency is presumed to cause an unusual susceptibility to infectious diseases and to malignant transformation in a variety of cells.

Associated Findings: IgA deficiency may be associated with IFN deficiency.

Etiology: Possibly autosomal dominant inheritance.

Pathogenesis: There are three major classes of IFN: alpha, beta, and gamma. They have different inducers, cell sources, amino acid sequences, physical properties, antigenicities, and genetic controls. Alpha-IFN is derived predominantly from B-lymphocytes. At least eight different polypeptides may have alpha-IFN activity. Both alpha- and beta-IFN are stable at pH 2.0. Beta-IFN is produced by fibroblasts. It is also comprised of a number of polypeptides that have a significant degree of homology with alpha-IFN molecules. Gamma-IFN (immune IFN) is derived from stimulated T lymphocytes. It may be induced by mitogens, bacterial or viral antigens, or allogeneic cells. It is labile at pH 2.0. A normal newborn infant can produce adequate amounts of alpha-IFN but not gamma IFN.

IFN is a potent regulator of NK activity and an enhancer of IgG antibody production. It also enhances IgE binding to basophils and chemical mediator release from basophils. Deficiency of IFN down-regulates these functions, making the host more susceptible to infections and malignancies.

MIM No.: *14757, *14762, *14764, *14766

Sex Ratio: Presumably M1:F1.

Occurrence: Undetermined despite established literature.

Risk of Recurrence for Patient's Sib:
See Part I, *Mendelian Inheritance.* Single gene defects are likely to cause only partial interferon deficiency. The effects of each defect are not well documented. Several affected patients have been reported to have sibs with low levels of alpha-IFN.

Risk of Recurrence for Patient's Child:
See Part I, *Mendelian Inheritance.* Probably slight.

Age of Detectability: Gamma-IFN deficiency is present in most infants for the first six months of life. Primary deficiency of IFN later in life is uncommon. Deficiency of IFN is often only one aspect of a more widely deranged metabolic state found in a variety of specific diseases.

Gene Mapping and Linkage: IFNA (interferon, alpha (leukocyte)) has been mapped to 9p22-p13.
IFNB1 (interferon, beta 1, fibroblast) has been mapped to 9p22.
IFNB3 (interferon, beta 3, fibroblast) has been mapped to 2p23-qter.
IFNG (interferon, gamma) has been mapped to 12q24.1.
IFNR (interferon production regulator) has been provisionally mapped to 16.
IL6 (interleukin 6) has been mapped to 7p21-p14.

Prevention: None known. Genetic counseling indicated. There is evidence that a nasal spray of alpha-IFN can inhibit rhinovirus infection in a significant number of household contacts.

Treatment: Should be directed toward replacement of the types of IFN that are deficient. Diseases treated to date include the following:
Hairy cell leukemia (HCL): Treatment with alpha-IFN results in decreased hairy cell infiltrates of the bone marrow. Seventy-five percent of HCL patients treated with alpha-IFN achieve sustained improvement in granulocyte, platelet, and hemoglobin levels. Immunity to infections improves, and the need for splenectomy and the mortality rate are reduced.
Kaposi sarcoma in AIDS: IFN has been reported to result in amelioration in approximately 40% of patients. However, there seems to be no augmentation of immunity to opportunistic infection in patients with AIDS.
Non-Hodgkin lymphoma: Treatment with alpha-IFN is frequently effective, especially in the early stages of the disease.
Multiple myeloma, malignant melanoma, renal carcinoma, carcinoma of the bladder, and ovarian cancer: Alpha-IFN is reported to be of benefit in a limited number of patients with these malignancies.

Alpha-IFN has been used prophylactically in organ and tissue transplants to inhibit cytomegalovirus infections. It may inhibit the activation of latent herpes simplex infections. It also may be of value in treating patients with chronic hepatitis B and in interrupting the cycle of recurrent respiratory syncytial virus infection in certain children.
Complication of treatment: A flu-like syndrome occurs in 80–90% of treated patients. It may include fever, chill, fatigue, headache, anorexia, nausea, vomiting, myalgia, arthralgia, low back pain, dry mouth, diarrhea, confusion, depression, hypotonia, skin rashes, hypotension, cardiac arrythmia, and central nervous system toxicity. These symptoms are dose-related and reversible.

Elevated liver enzymes (SGOT and SGPT) may be seen. Hematologic toxicity may result in mild thrombocytopenia and transient granulocytopenia.

Prognosis: Usually depends on the primary or associated disease.

Detection of Carrier: IFN assays on sibs and relatives may provide circumstantial evidence of a carrier state in parents of IFN-deficient children.

Special Considerations: The ramifications of IFN deficiency are not clear. IFN deficiency may be primary or secondary, may contribute to frequent or chronic infections and malignancies, and may play a role in a few autoimmune diseases. Defects in IFN genes and the molecules regulating their expression are poorly understood. Purified natural or recombinant IFN has been used with relative success in treating selected malignancies and viral infections.

References:
Isaacs D, et al.: Deficient production of leucocyte interferon (interferon-alpha) in vitro and in vivo in children with recurrent respiratory tract infections. Lancet 1981; II:950–952.
Naylor S, et al.: Human immune interferon gene is located on chromosome 12. J Exp Med 1983; 57:1020–1027.
Epstein L: Update on interferon. Immunol Allergy Pract 1985; 7:490–497. *

Spiegel R: INTRON A (interferon alfa-2b): clinical overview. Cancer Treat Rev 1985; 12:5–16. *

Taylor-Papadimitriou J: Interferons. Oxford: Oxford University Press, 1985.

Stites D, et al.: Basic and clinical immunology, ed 6. Norwalk, CT: Appleton and Lange, 1987. *

MA079   **Ghodsi Madani**
HE043   **Douglas C. Heiner**

Intermediate (late-onset) cystinosis
  See CYSTINOSIS
Intermediate filament, muscle type
  See MYOPATHY OR CARDIOMYOPATHY DUE TO DESMIN DEFECT
Intermittent branched-chain ketonuria
  See MAPLE SYRUP URINE DISEASE
Internal carotid artery aneurysm of middle ear
  See EAR, ANEURYSM OF INTERNAL CAROTID ARTERY
Internal chondromatosis
  See ENCHONDROMATOSIS
Interphalangeal skin creases, absent distal
  See SKIN CREASES, ABSENT DISTAL INTERPHALANGEAL
Interstitial pyelonephritis, hereditary type
  See NEPHRITIS-DEAFNESS (SENSORINEURAL), HEREDITARY TYPE

INTESTINAL ATRESIA OR STENOSIS   0531

Includes:
  Intestinal polyatresia syndrome, familial
  Jejunoileal atresia and stenosis

Excludes:
  Colon, aganglionosis (0192)
  Colon, atresia or stenosis (0193)
  Duodenum, atresia or stenosis (0300)
  Gastric outlet obstruction, congenital
  Intestinal atresia, multiple (2933)
  Intestinal ileus, isolated meconium ileus (0545)

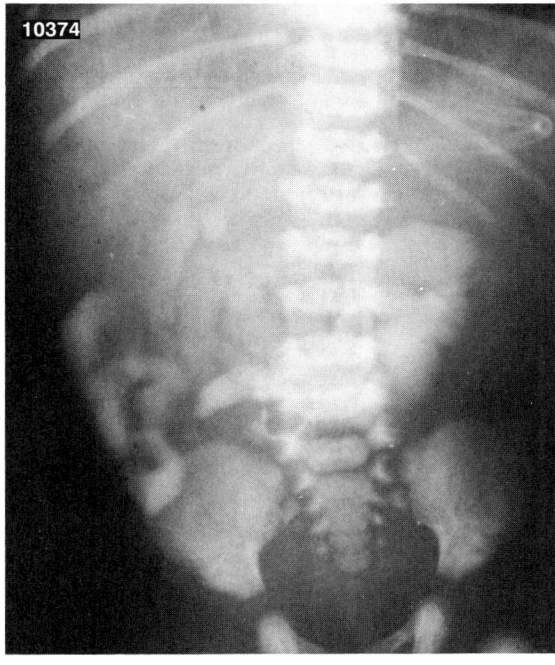

0531-10374: Abdomen in recumbent position. Note Levine tube in stomach; no air distal to stomach; multiple opacities with a calcium density in midabdomen.

Jejunal atresia (2934)
Meconium peritonitis
Pancreas, annular (0062)
Pyloroduodenal atresia, hereditary (2617)
Pyloric stenosis (0848)
Rotational abnormalities of the gastrointestinal tract
Other causes of neonatal intestinal obstruction (bands, hernias)

Major Diagnostic Criteria: Diagnosis of upper intestinal obstruction of the stomach, duodenum, and proximal jejunum rarely requires more than a plain upright X-ray film of the abdomen, demonstrating a double or triple bubble. Obstruction of the distal jejunum, ileum, and colon will require a barium enema following plain X-ray films of the abdomen. The barium study will help to demonstrate a mechanical obstruction or microcolon with proximal intestinal dilation, and will rule out an ileus, gastroenterocolitis of the newborn, or other lesions such as meconium ileus, meconium plug syndrome, or suggestion of Hirschsprung disease not requiring immediate surgery. An upper GI contrast study is necessary in older infants to demonstrate proximal stenosis of the gastrointestinal tract.

Clinical Findings: Vomiting is the most significant clinical finding in all forms of intestinal atresia or stenosis. The vomitus is usually bile stained except in gastric outlet obstruction, when it is clear or coffee-ground in nature. Increasing abdominal distention occurs with the more distal jejunoileal or colonic obstructions. Obstipation is a constant clinical feature; however, the neonate may pass an occasional small, gray, mucoid, pellet-sized stool. Classification of the jejunoileal intestinal atresias is as follows: type I, mucosal atresia with intact bowel and mesentery; type II, blind ends are separated by a fibrous cord; type IIIA, blind ends separated by a V-shaped mesenteric defect; type IIIB, "apple peel" atresia (see **Jejunal atresia**); and type IV, multiple atresias. A nearly similar classification exists for duodenal atresias.
  Small intestine atresias occur in the jejunum (50%), the ileum (43%), and in both the ileum and jejunum, multiple points of atresia occur 7% of the time.

Complications: Dehydration and electrolyte imbalance occur without treatment within 12–48 hours. Aspiration, circulatory collapse, and intestinal perforation with peritonitis and sepsis will follow in a period of hours to several days.

Associated Findings: *Jejunoileal atresia and stenoses*: Low birth weight (30%); rotational abnormalities (10%); meconium peritonitis (12%); meconium ileus (10%); **Cystic fibrosis** (10–20%); multiple atresias (14%); **omphalocele** (5–10%); **gastroschisis** (10–15%).
  Colon atresias and stenoses: Skeletal anomalies such as **Syndactyly, Polydactyly,** absent radius, and club foot are present. Ocular and cardiac anomalies have been noted, as well as abdominal wall defects such as **omphalocele, gastroschisis,** and vesicointestinal fissure.

Etiology: Undetermined, except in **Intestinal atresias, multiple** which is transmitted through autosomal recessive inheritance, and when part of another syndrome sych as **Cystic fibrosis**.

Pathogenesis: Intrauterine vascular accidents during the later gestational period are thought to occur jejunoileal atresia and stenosis, and colonic atresia and stenosis due to volvulus, intussusception, internal hernia, or constriction of the mesentery in a tight gastroschisis or omphalocele defect.

MIM No.: *24315

CDC No.: 751.1

Sex Ratio: M1:F1

Occurrence: Jejunoileal atresia and stenosis occurs in 1:1,000 to 1:5,000 live births throughout the world. It is more often reported in Western countries. Colon atresia and stenosis occurs 1:20,000 live births throughout the world.

Risk of Recurrence for Patient's Sib: Several reports have occurred in the literature with sibs affected; however, incidence is low.

Risk of Recurrence for Patient's Child: Risk of occurrence is low, but has been reported in several families.

Age of Detectability: All atresias and most stenoses present during the newborn period. The remaining 10–20% of stenoses occur before six months of age. Prenatal diagnosis has been performed (Morin et al, 1980).

Gene Mapping and Linkage: Unknown.

Prevention: None known. Genetic counseling indicated.

Treatment: Preoperative treatment includes fluid and electrolyte correction, nasogastric decompression, and temperature control and glucose and hyperbilirubinemia correction in the newborn. Surgical intervention with appropriate gastrointestinal anastomoses and intestinal decompression follows. Rather than performing an extensive intestinal resection in the proximal dilated bowel such as in jejunal atresia, a tapering procedure of the dilated intestine is performed. This conserves length and surface area of bowel for absorption and prevents short gut syndrome. This has resulted in earlier and improved intestinal motility and increased survival. This procedure is usually not necessary in ileal atresia. Usually 20–25 cm of the proximal dilated bowel can be sacrificed safely with a primary anastomosis. Postoperative care includes the necessary neonatal support and surveillance and parenteral and enteral alimentation. Parenteral alimentation may be prolonged in cases of short gut syndrome. Patients with ileal and jejunal atresia must be worked up for cystic fibrosis, since it will occur 10–20% of the time. Other treatment may be necessary for anomalies of other organ systems. The treatment of proximal colon atresia is resection and anastomsis. Distal atreasia: diverting colostomy and at six months to one year, a primary anastomsis.

Prognosis: Excellent except in cases complicated by other complex malformation syndromes, or severe short gut. The distal atresia patients have a better prognosis than is the case in proximal atreasia.

Detection of Carrier: Unknown.

References:
Recomb PP, Karplus M: Familial and hereditary intestinal atresia. Helv Paediatr Acta 1971; 26:561–564.
Melhem RE, et al.: Pyloroduodenal atresia. Pediatr Radiol 1975; 3:1–5.
Morin PR, et al.: Prenatal detection of intestinal obstruction: deficient amniotic fluid disaccharidases in affected fetuses. Clin Genet 1980; 18:217–222.
Blackburn WR, et al.: The familial intestinal poly-atresia syndrome (abstract). Proc Greenwood Genet Center 1983; 2:122–123.
Kirillova IA, et al.: Atresia, stenosis and duplication of the gastrointestinal tract. consideration of their origin. Acta Morphol Acad Sci Hung 1984; 32:9–21.
Grosfeld J: Jejunal atresia and stenosis. In: Welch K, et al.: Pediatric surgery, ed 4. Chicago: Year Book Medical Publishers, 1986, Chapter 85.
Philipport A: Atreasia, stenosis of colon. In: Welch K, et al.: Pediatric surgery, ed 4. Chicago: Year Book Medical Publishers, 1986:984–989.

BE049   **Arthur S. Besser**

INTESTINAL ATRESIAS, MULTIPLE   **2933**

Includes: Intestinal polyatresia syndrome (mucosal or septal variety)

Excludes:
Intestinal atresia or stenosis (0531)
Multiple atresias-foreshortened bowel-prematurity
Pyloroduodenal atresia, hereditary (2617)

Major Diagnostic Criteria: Multiple intestinal atresias that may involve the duodenum, jejunum, ileum, and rectum.

Clinical Findings: The pregnancy may be complicated by hydramnios. The condition is apparent in the neonatal period. The baby has continuous vomiting and usually does not pass meconium. On physical examination the only positive findings are a distended epigastric region, a scaphoid abdomen, and an empty anal canal. X-ray studies of the abdomen reveal a large solitary air bubble in the stomach, with no gas in the intestinal tract. Intraluminal calcifications may be demonstrable.

At laparotomy, the bowel from the duodenum to the rectum has a small caliber, is unused, and has multiple diaphragm-like septa, causing complete discontinuity of the intestinal lumen. In between the septa, there is intestinal lumen.

There is no loss of small bowel loops, no evidence of impairment of the vascular supply in the intact mesentery, and no volvulus, intussusception, internal hernias, or meconium ileus.

Complications: Because of the extensive pathologic lesions, surgery may have complications. With parenteral alimentation some cases may be managed successfully.

Associated Findings: None known.

Etiology: Autosomal recessive inheritance.

Pathogenesis: Unknown.

MIM No.: *24315

CDC No.: 751.100

Sex Ratio: M1:F1

Occurrence: Panethnic. Fewer than 50 patients with the hereditary type have been reported.

Risk of Recurrence for Patient's Sib:
See Part I, *Mendelian Inheritance.*

Risk of Recurrence for Patient's Child:
See Part I, *Mendelian Inheritance.*

Age of Detectability: During the neonatal period. Prenatal detection of intestinal obstruction is possible. The amniotic fluid disaccharidases are deficient when the fetus is affected. Results of low disaccharidase values are best followed by diagnostic ultrasound studies and, when necessary, amniography, for more certain delineation of the defect.

Gene Mapping and Linkage: Unknown.

Prevention: None known. Genetic counseling indicated.

Treatment: Surgical excision of septa with reestablishment of intestinal continuity.

Prognosis: Guarded.

Detection of Carrier: Unknown.

Special Considerations: In all cases of multiple-level intestinal atresia it is very important to keep the possibility of the hereditary type in mind, for proper counseling of the family and for a possible attempt at prenatal diagnosis during future pregnancies.

References:
Mishalany HG, Der Kaloustian VM: Familial multiple-level intestinal atresia: report of two siblings. J Pediatr 1971; 79:124 only.
Guttman FM, et al.: Multiple atresias and a new syndrome of hereditary multiple atresias involving the gastrointestinal tract from stomach to rectum. J Pediatr Surg 1973; 8:633–640.
Dallaire L, Perreault G: Hereditary multiple intestinal atresia: the clinical delineation of birth defects, XVI urinary system and others. Baltimore: Williams & Wilkins, 1974:259–264.
Milunsky A: Diagnosis of fetal abnormalities by ultrasound. In: Milunsky A, ed: Genetic disorders and the fetus, New York: Plenum, 1979:321–330.
Morin PR, et al.: Prenatal detection of intestinal obstruction: deficient amniotic fluid disaccharidases in affected fetuses. Clin Genet 1980; 18:217–222.
Blackburn WR, et al.: The familial intestinal poly-atresia syndrome. Proc Greenwood Genet Center 1983; 2:122–123.
Hauschild R: Familiäere Dunndarmatresie: genetik und humangenetische Beratung. Pediatr Grenzgeb 1983; 22:271–275.

DE030   **Vazken M. Der Kaloustian**
MI039   **Henry G. Mishalany**

INTESTINAL DUPLICATION 0532

Includes:
> Duplication of colon, external genitalia and lower urinary tract
> Enteric cysts
> Enterogenous cysts
> Esophageal duplication (mediastinal cyst of foregut origin)
> Neuroenteric cysts
> Stomach-duodenum-small intestine-rectum, duplication of

Excludes:
> Bronchogenic cysts
> Bronchopulmonary foregut with gastric/esophageal communication
> Esophageal cysts
> Mesenteric or omental cysts
> Other forms of mediastinal cysts of foregut origin

Major Diagnostic Criteria: Demonstration of cystic or communicating duplication of any intestinal structure. X-ray often leads to a presumptive diagnosis. Confirmation is surgical and by histopathology. There are two types of gastrointestinal duplications. One type is the completely enclosed or non-communicating form of duplication or cystic or spherical type. The other type is the communicating or cylindrical type. True duplications must contain gastrointestinal mucosa, but considerable heterotopia occurs.

Clinical Findings: Esophageal duplications present as posterior mediastinal masses which often produce dysphagia, dyspnea and chest pain. They may be seen on plain chest X-ray as a posterior mediastinal mass, often associated with vertebral anomalies. Intra-abdominal duplications most often present as a mass in the right lower quadrant. Abdominal pain, intestinal obstruction, perforation with peritonitis and failure to thrive are other common presentations.

Intra-abdominal duplications may be difficult to diagnose. Barium contrast studies, ultrasound, computerized tomography and nuclear magnetic resonance imaging are useful. Hemorrhage into the gastrointestinal tract may occur with communicating duplications which contain gastric mucosa and become ulcerated.

Complications: Gastrointestinal obstruction, hemorrhage, small bowel contamination syndrome, malabsorbtion, growth failure, meningitis (when communication with the central nervous system exists), torsion with mid-gut volvulus, perforation, and respiratory complications.

Associated Findings: Scoliosis and other vertebral abnormalities.

Etiology: Unknown.

Pathogenesis: There is support for several theories regarding the formation of intestinal duplication. Incomplete fission of the neuroenteric canal in early organogenesis could lead to duplications; a theory particularly applicable when communication between duplications and the central nervous system exists. Defective recanalization of the intestine later in gestation is the most commonly held theory for the pathogenesis of most duplications. Non-communicating diverticulae (intestinal cysts) often enlarge progressively because of secretion by the epithelial lining. Duplications often contain gastric mucosa capable of producing hydrochloric acid, which can produce ulceration of adjacent mucosa.

CDC No.: 751.810

Sex Ratio: M1:F1

Occurrence: 1:40,000–100,000 live births.

Risk of Recurrence for Patient's Sib: Unknown.

Risk of Recurrence for Patient's Child: Unknown.

Age of Detectability: Often in the newborn period or early infancy, but sometimes in older children or adults.

Gene Mapping and Linkage: Unknown.

Prevention: None known. Genetic counseling indicated.

Treatment: Treatment of esophageal duplications is surgical removal by easy separation of the cyst from the esophagus. Treatment of intra-abdominal duplications are divided into 1) simple excision and intestinal anastamosis in the smaller spherical type lesions; 2) simple excision of a rectal duplication; 3) marsupialization or internal drainage of a duodenal lesion; 4) excision of the common wall in the tubular type, especially near the terminal end of the duplication; and 5) mucosal stripping of the duplication when gastric mucosa is present. This latter procedure is preferred in extensive duplications rather than major bowel resections.

Prognosis: With treatment, no reduction of life span or function.

Detection of Carrier: Unknown.

References:
Holder T, Ashcraft K: Pediatric surgery. Philadelphia: W.B. Saunders, 1980.
Welsh K, et al.: Pediatric surgery, 4th ed. Chicago: Yearbook Medical Publishers, 1986.

BE049 **Arthur S. Besser**

INTESTINAL ENTEROKINASE DEFICIENCY 0533

Includes:
> Enterokinase deficiency, primary
> Enteropeptidase deficiency

Excludes:
> Enterokinase deficiency, secondary
> Pancreatic exocrine insufficiency, generalized
> **Trypsinogen deficiency** (0973)

Major Diagnostic Criteria: Diarrhea and failure to thrive begin in early infancy. Normal small bowel histology with decreased enterokinase activity is diagnostic of primary enterokinase deficiency.

Clinical Findings: Patients present from early infancy with diarrhea (100%) and failure to thrive (100%). They will be found to excrete large amounts of fecal nitrogen. As a result of a negative nitrogen balance, hypoproteinemia and edema are usually apparent. Malnutrition may also result in failure of synthesis of pancreatic lipase and amylase, as well as intestinal disaccharidases, leading to generalized malabsorption of all nutrients. Steatorrhea and carbohydrate intolerance are clinically evident in this circumstance.

Complications: Protein malabsorption; malnutrition; failure to thrive (poor weight gain and short stature); hypoproteinemia; generalized pancreatic exocrine dysfunction secondary to malnutrition; intestinal disaccharidase deficiency secondary to malnutrition; and generalized malabsorption.

Associated Findings: Short stature.

Etiology: The finding of this abnormality in sibs, the offspring of unaffected parents, suggests possible autosomal recessive inheritance.

Pathogenesis: The pancreatic peptidases, trypsin, chymotrypsin, carboxypeptidase, and elastase, are secreted as proenzymes that require activation within the intestinal lumen. The peptidopeptidase of intestinal origin that initiates pancreatic propeptidase activation is enterokinase. In the absence of enterokinase, the rate of conversion of trypsinogen to trypsin is subnormal, resulting in concentrations of trypsin that are inadequate for protein hydrolysis, including activation of chymotrypsinogen, procarboxypeptidase, and proelastase. Lipase and amylase are secreted as functional enzymes not requiring activation. They are of normal activity in the patient with enterokinase deficiency.

MIM No.: *22620

CDC No.: 751.880

Sex Ratio: M1:F1

Occurrence: Less than a dozen cases have been reported.

Risk of Recurrence for Patient's Sib: Unknown.

Risk of Recurrence for Patient's Child: Unknown.

Age of Detectability: Early infancy.

Gene Mapping and Linkage: Unknown.

Prevention: None known. Genetic counseling indicated.

Treatment: Orally administered enterokinase or pancreatic extract normalizes intestinal function.

Prognosis: Excellent. Most patients have continued short stature, apparently from early severe malnutrition.

Detection of Carrier: Unknown.

Special Considerations: Study of pancreatic exocrine function is also diagnostic. In baseline and secretin-stimulated samples of duodenal aspirate, trypsinogen levels will be normal, but trypsin will be of low or absent activity. Trypsinogen may be activated to trypsin by incubation with enterokinase or trypsin (16-hour incubation at 4° C results in activation in some patients). The patient's duodenal fluid will have normal tryptic activity after incubation. Enterokinase activity may also be assayed by measuring the hydrolysis of artificial substrates (most recently gly-(Asp)$_4$-Lys-2 naphthylamide) after differentially inhibiting trypsin activity.

Histologic exam should also be performed since some patients with abnormal small bowel mucosa will have low levels of enterokinase activity.

The malnourished patient may have subnormal secretion of all pancreatic enzymes. Therefore, it is necessary to attain a state of adequate nutrition before pancreatic function studies are completed.

References:

Tarlow MJ, et al.: Intestinal enterokinase deficiency: a newly recognized disorder of protein digestion. Arch Dis Child 1970; 45:651–655.

Haworth JC, et al.: Intestinal enterokinase deficiency occurrence in two sibs and age dependency of the clinical expression. Arch Dis Child 1975; 50:277–282.

Follett GF, MacDonald TH: Intestinal enterokinase deficiency. Acta Paediatr Scand 1976; 65:653–656.

Grant DAW, Hermon-Taylor J: Hydrolysis of artificial substrates by enterokinase and trypsin and the development of a sensitive specific assay for enterokinase in serum. Biochim Biophys Acta 1979; 567: 207.

Ghishan FK, et al.: Isolated congenital enterokinase deficiency: recent finding and a review of the literature. Gastroenterology 1983; 85:727–731.

WH007   **Peter F. Whitington**

INTESTINAL HYPOPERISTALSIS, MEGACYSTIS-MICROCOLON TYPE   2317

Includes:

Berdon syndrome
Megacystis-microcolon-intestinal hypoperistalsis syndrome (MMIHS)

Excludes:

Colon, aganglionosis (0192)
Colon, duplication (0194)
Intestinal atresia or stenosis (0531)
Megacystis-megaduodenum syndrome (2316)
Stomach, pyloric atresia (0910)

Major Diagnostic Criteria: Megacystis, dilated small bowel, microcolon, and decreased or absent peristalsis with ganglion cells present.

Clinical Findings: Polyhydramnios occurs in approximately 25% of the cases. Length of gestation is usually term, and birth weight is within normal limits. Notable abdominal distention is present in the neonatal period. Vomiting is frequently encountered and is often with bile. Anatomic (organic) stenosis is absent. Ischemia of the bowel has been reported in a few cases. The proximal small bowel is usually dilated. Microcolon is a consistent finding. It may be malrotated and positioned entirely on the left side. Malfixation of the midgut occurs frequently, but volvulus is rare. Partial or complete absence of intestinal peristalsis, which is largely resis-

tant to treatment, is a constant finding. Reverse peristalsis has been demonstrated in some patients by retrograde passage of contrast medium.

The combined bowel length is frequently shortened to one-third of normal. Intestinal biopsies show mature ganglion cells in dilated and narrow segments of the intestine. Some patients have areas where the ganglion cells are absent or shrunken along with normal ganglion cells. Several patients have increased nerve fibers and mature ganglion cells. X-rays may show dilated air-filled, small intestine loops. The colon and/or rectum may not show gas. A ground glass appearance of the abdomen has been reported. The bladder is enlarged, frequently flaccid with thick walls, and without evidence of obstruction. As much as 700 ml of urine has been recovered by catheterization (usual amount 350–500 ml). Decompression of the bladder may relieve abdominal distention and result in a "prune belly" appearance. One- half of the cases had hydronephrosis. Seventy-five percent had tortuous, dilated ureters. Most did not have vesicoureteral reflux. After bladder drainage, the ureters returned to normal in three patients. Death usually occurs within the first year. There is a report of one person who has survived into adolescence.

Complications: Septicemia has been reported as the cause of death in several infants.

Associated Findings: The abdominal wall musculature in a few patients has been found to be thin and/or flaccid. A small **omphalocele** was present in two female infants. One patient was reported to have mild webbing of the neck. Cytogenetic studies were not mentioned in these reports. Another patient had an intra-abdominal testis, grade III/VI systolic ejection murmur and grade II/VI diastolic murmur of no clinical significance.

Etiology: Almost all cases have been sporadic. Autosomal recessive inheritance has been implied by one report of affected siblings. Another affected female had two healthy siblings and a sibling who died of "intestinal obstruction" at four days of age. An autopsy was not performed. The parents of another affected female were first cousins.

Pathogenesis: Prenatal transient anatomical and/or functional urinary tract obstruction has been considered. A female with a urachal remnant had two healthy brothers and a brother with **Prune-belly syndrome.** This report and intra-abdominal testis in a reported male suggest a common pathogenesis. On the other hand, intestinal hypoperistalsis is a constant feature of this condition and rare in prune belly syndrome. Their different sex ratios also imply that the conditions are different. There are reports inferring that the urinary tract obstruction in this condition is secondary to the intestinal defect. It is not clear whether this is a primary neuropathy or myopathy.

MIM No.: *24921

POS No.: 3830

CDC No.: 751.880

Sex Ratio: M1:F6

Occurrence: A few dozen cases have been reported in the literature. Patients have been reported from the United States, Great Britain, Brazil, the Netherlands, India, Israel, Japan, and Polynesia.

Risk of Recurrence for Patient's Sib:

See Part I, *Mendelian Inheritance.* Most cases of this usually fatal disorder have been sporadic, implying a low risk of recurrence. Two affected siblings and a consanguineous family suggests autosomal recessive inheritance.

Risk of Recurrence for Patient's Child:

See Part I, *Mendelian Inheritance.* No patient is known to have reproduced.

Age of Detectability: May be suspected prenatally by sonographic evidence of cystic abdominal mass in the fetus. Involvement is readily apparent after birth.

Gene Mapping and Linkage: Unknown.

Prevention: None known. Genetic counseling indicated.

Treatment: Palliative surgery. Hyperalimentation is required. Parasympathomimetics, synthetic gastrointestinal stimulants, adrenergic blockers, and multiple gastrointestinal hormones have not been effective in inducing adequate bowel function. A cholinergic drug, bethanechol, did improve the peristalsis in one patient.

Prognosis: Poor; partial function of the urinary tract may appear after bladder drainage. The intestinal dysfunction does not appear to be amenable to treatment.

Detection of Carrier: Unknown.

Special Considerations: Megacystis is usually associated with oligohydramnios. The presence of polyhydramnios in 25% of the pregnancies with an affected fetus is probably due to the intestinal dysfunction. Prenatal volvulus could mimic this condition, while a normal bladder would exclude the diagnosis.

A manometric study of an affected infant documented a marked reduction of the number of total contractions of the stomach and duodenum. The mean amplitude of the contractions was notably diminished when compared to age-matched controls. Rhythmic contractions (type III) showed decreased amplitude and frequency. The findings in the smooth muscle layer are similar to those in **Megacystis-megaduodenum syndrome** (MMS). The gastrointestinal effects usually become evident in late childhood or early adolescence. It may be present neonatally. Megacystis and hydronephrosis may occur in MMS at varying ages. It has been suggested, however, that MMIHS and MMS are part of a spectrum, with the former representing the most severe manifestation.

References:

Berdon WE, et al.: Megacystis-microcolon-intestinal hypoperistalsis syndrome: a new cause of intestinal obstruction in the newborn: report of radiologic findings in five newborn girls. Am J Roentgenol Rad Ther Nucl Med 1976; 126:957–964.

Nelson LH, Reiff RH: Megacystis-microcolon-hypoperistalsis syndrome and anechoic areas in the fetal abdomen. Am J Obstet Gynecol 1982; 144:464–467.

Oliveira G, et al.: Megacystis-microcolon-intestinal hypoperistalsis syndrome in a newborn girl whose brother had prune belly syndrome: common pathogenesis? Pediatr Radiol 1983; 13:294–296.

Puri P, et al.: Megacystis-microcolon-intestinal hypoperistalsis syndrome: a visceral myopathy. J Ped Surg 1983; 18:64–69.

Redman JF, et al.: Megacystis-microcolon-intestinal hypoperistalsis syndrome: case report and review of the literature. J Urol 1984; 131:981–983.

Tomomasa T, et al.: Manometric study on the intestinal motility in a case of megacystis-microcolon-intestinal hypoperistalsis syndrome. J Pediatr Gastroenterol Nutr 1985; 4:307–310.

Winter RM, Knowles SAS: Megacystis-microcolon-intestinal hypoperistalsis syndrome: confirmation of autosomal recessive inheritance. J Med Genet 1986; 23:360–362.

HA069   **James K. Hartsfield, Jr.**

INTESTINAL ILEUS, ISOLATED MECONIUM ILEUS   0545

Includes:
Ileus, isolated meconium
Meconium ileus, isolated

Excludes: Cystic fibrosis (0237)

Major Diagnostic Criteria: Intestinal obstruction in a child with no evidence of cystic fibrosis but with X-rays and operative findings consistent with inspissated meconium.

Clinical Findings: Abdominal distention, bilious vomiting, and failure to pass meconium in neonates. Microcolon and terminal ileum obstructed by inspissated, sticky meconium.

Complications: Intestinal obstruction, perforation and meconium peritonitis.

Associated Findings: Microcolon, **Biliary atresia**, and **Niemann-Pick disease**.

Etiology: Unknown.

Pathogenesis: Presumed to be an abnormal form of meconium.

CDC No.: 759.870

Sex Ratio: M1:F1

Occurrence: Estimated 1:50,000 live births; five percent of all cases of meconium ileus.

Risk of Recurrence for Patient's Sib: Unknown.

Risk of Recurrence for Patient's Child: Unknown.

Age of Detectability: Prenatal ultrasonography shows multiple loops of distended bowel and calcification in fetal abdomen. At birth by X-ray and physical examination.

Gene Mapping and Linkage: Unknown.

Prevention: None known. Genetic counseling indicated.

Treatment: Gastrografin enemas or surgery with normal saline irrigations. Resection of bowel for perforation with some type of exteriorization.

Prognosis: Survival near 100% with appropriate treatment; no long-term consequences anticipated.

Detection of Carrier: Unknown.

References:

Olsen MM, et al.: The spectrum of meconium disease in infancy. J Pediatr Surg 1982; 17:479–481.

Carty H, Brereton RJ: The distended neonate. Clin Radiol 1983; 34:367–380.

Ein SH, et al.: Ileocaecal atresia. J Pediatr Surg 1985; 20:525–528.

Ein SH, et al.: Bowel perforation with nonoperative treatment of meconium ileus. J Pediatr Surg 1987; 22:146–147.

Goldstein RB, et al.; Sonographic diagnosis of meconium ileus in utero. J Ultrasoun Med 1987; 6:663–666.

Zamir O, et al.; Gastrointestinal perforations in the neonatal period. Am J Perinatol 1988; 5:131–133.

SE006   **John H. Seashore**

INTESTINAL LYMPHANGIECTASIA   0534

Includes:
Lymphangiectasia, intestinal
Protein-losing enteropathy with dilated intestinal lymphatics

Excludes:
Lymphedema I (0614)
Lymphedema II (0615)
Mesenteric neoplasms
Protein-losing enteropathy secondary to congestive heart failure

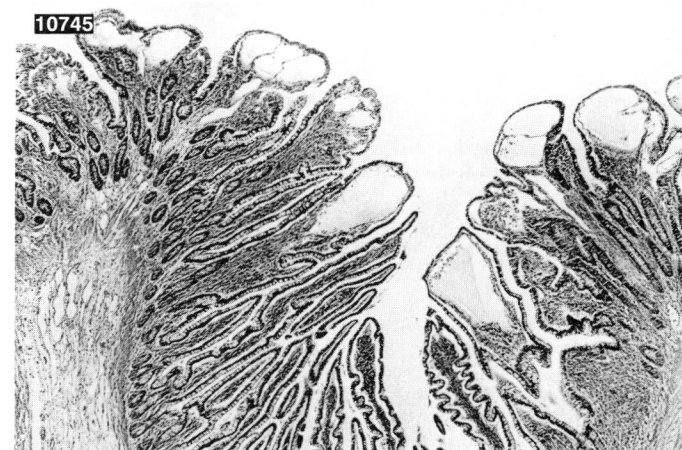

0534-10745: Intestinal biopsy; dilated lymphatic channels are present in mucosa and lamina propria.

Protein-losing enteropathy without dilated lymphatic channels

Whipple syndrome

Major Diagnostic Criteria: Dilated lymphatic channels of the small bowel, as demonstrated by peroral biopsy or laparotomy, is the hallmark morphologic lesion of this disorder and is required for its diagnosis.

The direct demonstration of gastrointestinal (GI) protein loss, hypoalbuminemia, hypogammaglobulinemia, lymphocytopenia, and generalized edema are also important diagnostic features. This syndrome should be differentiated from disorders in which the hypoproteinemia is secondary to decreased protein synthesis, or to accelerated endogenous protein catabolism by direct demonstration of excessive GI protein loss. The diagnosis can be made by determining the intestinal clearance of α1-antitrypsin or by demonstrating increased fecal excretion of intravenously administered radiolabeled macromolecules such as ^{51}Cr labeled serum proteins, ^{59}Fe dextran, ^{95}Nb albumin, or ^{131}I PVP.

Other causes of protein-losing enteropathy with disorders of intestinal lymphatic channels, such as severe congestive heart failure, Whipple syndrome, or mesenteric malignancy, retroperitoneal fibrosis, and inflammatory processes should be ruled out.

Clinical Findings: Patients with intestinal lymphangiectasia have a generalized disorder of development of lymphatic channels with grossly dilated lymphatic vessels in the lamina propria of the small bowel demonstrable in all cases. The patients have edema that may be asymmetric (15%), and that may involve the macula, producing reversible blindness (7%). Chylous effusion is present at the onset or develops during the course of the disease in 45% of the patients. All patients have significant excessive loss of serum proteins into the GI tract through the disordered lymphatic channels. They have hypoalbuminemia (100%) and a marked reduction of IgG (97%). A significant but less marked reduction in the concentration of fibrinogen (30%), transferrin (50%), IgM (40%), and IgA (70%) is noted in many patients.

GI symptoms are usually mild, but may on occasion be entirely absent or severe. Diarrhea and steatorrhea (mild 60%, severe 20%), vomiting (15%), and abdominal pain (15%) are present in these patients. Carbohydrate absorption tests, including glucose, xylose, and lactose tolerance tests, are within normal limits in most of the patients studied. X-rays of the GI tract are completely negative in 20% of the patients. They show mild mucosal edema of the small bowel in 70% of the patients, and show significant segmentation and puddling of the barium in the remaining 10% of the patients. On biopsy of the small bowel, a dilatation of the lymphatic vessels of the lamina propria, the hallmark morphologic lesion of the disease, is revealed. Hypocalcemia and in some cases hypomagnesemia and tetany are present in 12% of the patients and are most common in those patients with steatorrhea. It is thought to be associated with malabsorption or loss of calcium into the GI tract. Lymphocytopenia (mean lymphocyte count 700 compared with 2400 in controls), secondary to the loss of lymphocytes into the bowel, is present in over 90% of the patients. As a consequence of this lymphocytopenia, 83% of the patients show skin anergy and are unable to manifest delayed hypersensitivity responses (tuberculin-type responses), and are unable to reject skin grafts from unrelated donors.

Less frequent findings include anemia and reduction in the serum concentration of fat soluble vitamins and B$_{12}$. Growth retardation (linear growth below 3rd%) is present in the majority of children with onset of edema and diarrhea within the first five years of life. It may be extreme in those patients with associated severe malabsorption.

Complications: Tuberculous infections and reticuloendothelial malignancies develop in 3–5% of the cases, possibly due to the lymphocytopenia and inability to make cellular immune responses. Chronic respiratory diseases (5–10%) associated with the disorder of delayed hypersensitivity and with abnormalities of lymphatics of the lungs. Intestinal obstruction due to adhesions occur especially in those patients with chylous ascites. Deficiency of fat-soluble vitamins, including vitamin K (20%), may cause hypoprothrombinemia.

Associated Findings: Glaucoma, congenital (3 in 75 cases); Peliosis hepatitis (2); Charcot-Marie-Tooth syndrome (2); **Heart, tetralogy of Fallot** (1); **Noonan syndrome** (2); **Hypobetalipoproteinemia** (2); and selective IgA deficiency (see **Immunoglobulin A deficiency**) (1).

Etiology: Possibly autosomal dominant inheritance. The majority of cases (over 75%) are, however, sporadic.

Pathogenesis: The basic defect appears to be a generalized disorder in lymphatic channel development with the most obvious disorder affecting small bowel lymphatics. As a consequence, serum proteins, lymphocytes, as well as lipids, iron, copper, and calcium are lost into the GI lumen. Hypoproteinemia results when the rate of protein loss and catabolism exceeds the body's capacity to synthesize the protein. The edema and effusions are due both to the extreme hypoproteinemia, and the generalized disorder of lymphatic channels. The abnormalities of the *in vivo* cellular (tuberculin-type) responses and the increased incidence in tuberculosis and reticuloendothelial neoplasms appear to be secondary to the lymphocytopenia that results from the loss of lymphocytes into the GI tract.

The hypocalcemia and malabsorption are due to an abnormality of absorption from the bowel, as well as loss of fat and calcium by direct loss of lymph into the bowel.

MIM No.: *15280

CDC No.: 751.880

Sex Ratio: M1:F1.34 (observed).

Occurrence: Approximately 300 cases have been reported; in Black, Oriental and Caucasian races.

Risk of Recurrence for Patient's Sib:
See Part I, *Mendelian Inheritance*. Most cases are sporadic.

Risk of Recurrence for Patient's Child:
See Part I, *Mendelian Inheritance*. Four cases of lymphedema in an offspring or parent of the proband have been reported. Otherwise, there are no reports of an affected individual in two generations. The patients have reproduced, although those patients with chylous ascites, or malabsorption and vitamin deficiency, may have reduced fertility.

Age of Detectability: Generalized edema, chylous effusions, asymmetric edema, diarrhea, or hypocalcemia may be the presenting symptom and is first detected at birth or in the first few weeks of life in 25% of the patients. In the remaining patients, the age of onset ranges to young adult life with, a mean age of onset of 10 years.

Gene Mapping and Linkage: Unknown.

Prevention: None known. Genetic counseling indicated.

Treatment: A very low-fat diet, or a diet in which medium-chain triglycerides are used in lieu of long-chain triglycerides, has been effective in significantly decreasing the hypoproteinemia, GI protein loss, edema, and diarrhea in approximately 50% of the patients. Such therapy has been of value in increasing the growth rate in children. In 5–10% of the cases, resection of a localized area of intestinal lymphangiectasia results in amelioration of the symptoms. There has been a reversal of the protein-losing enteropathy following corticosteroid therapy in some cases.

Diuretics are useful in reducing edema and effusions as well as in reversing blindness in the cases with macular edema. Other therapy, such as surgical relief of intestinal obstruction, or ligation of thoracic duct in patients with isolated chylothorax, may be indicated.

Prognosis: Life expectancy is somewhat shortened. In infancy, death may be related to extreme malabsorption, intestinal obstruction, or infections, especially in debilitated patients. Many cases, especially those with late onset, may be stable over periods from two to more than 40 years. No effect upon intelligence. Approximately 30% of the patients are unable to work because of extreme fatigue and weakness associated with the hypoproteinemia.

Detection of Carrier: Unknown.

Special Considerations: It should be emphasized that the primary features of this disorder, including edema, excessive GI protein loss, lymphocytopenia, and dilated lymphatics of the small intestine, may be seen in patients with Whipple syndrome, mesenteric tumors, or cardiac disorders, especially constrictive pericarditis. Significant care should be taken to rule out congestive failure in all patients with a tentative diagnosis of intestinal lymphangiectasia. The disorders of lymphocyte and protein metabolism are completely reversible in such patients when successful surgical or medical therapy of the cardiac disease is possible. In addition, corticosteroid therapy of patients with intestinal lymphangiectasia secondary to an inflammatory process may lead to remission of the protein losing enteropathy. It should be noted that patients with intestinal lymphangiectasia have skin anergy, and thus skin tests, such as the tuberculin skin test, cannot be used in the diagnosis of such chronic infectious disorders.

References:

Waldmann TA, et al.: The role of the gastrointestinal system in "idiopathic hypoproteinemia." Gastroenterology 1961; 41:197–207.
Jeffries GH, et al.: Low-fat diet in intestinal lymphangiectasia: its effect on albumin metabolism. N Engl J Med 1964; 270:761–766.
Waldmann TA: Protein-losing enteropathy. Gastroenterology 1966; 50:422–443.
Murphy EA: Familial lymphatic dysplasia with intestinal lymphangiectasia. The clinical delineation of birth defects. BDOAS XIII. G.I. tract including liver and pancreas. Baltimore: Williams & Wilkins, 1972:180–181.
Weiden PL, et al.: Impaired lymphocyte transformation in intestinal lymphangiectasia: evidence for at least two functionally distinct lymphocyte populations in man. J Clin Invest 1972; 51:1319–1325.
Waldman TA: Protein-losing gastroenteropathies. In: Berk J, ed: Gastroenterology, vol. 3. Philadelphia: W.B. Saunders, 1985:1814–1834. *

WA007   **Thomas A. Waldmann**

Intestinal monosaccharide intolerance
See GLUCOSE-GALACTOSE MALABSORPTION
Intestinal neurofibromatosis
See NEUROFIBROMATOSIS
Intestinal polyatresia syndrome (mucosal or septal variety)
See INTESTINAL ATRESIAS, MULTIPLE
Intestinal polyatresia syndrome, familial
See INTESTINAL ATRESIA OR STENOSIS

INTESTINAL POLYPOSIS, JUVENILE TYPE   2259

Includes:
  Cystic polyps
  Hamartomatous polyps
  Infantile polyposis
  Inflammatory polyps
  Polyposis coli, juvenile type
  Polyposis, juvenile

Excludes:
  Common juvenile retention polyps
  Intestinal polyposis (all)

Major Diagnostic Criteria: The presence of any polyps of the histologic type described in patients with a family history, or the occurrence of multiple such cystic polyps in any individual.

Clinical Findings: The most common presenting findings are rectal bleeding (75%), prolapse of a polyp (15%), abdominal pain (15%), and diarrhea (9%). The majority of cases present in childhood, although adults are reported. The polyps are fragile and may be passed in the stool. Barium studies or colonoscopy usually reveals multiple pedunculated polyps up to 1cm in diameter in familial cases. Sporadic cases, without a family history of intestinal polyps, are without the associated risks for malignant degeneration and usually have solitary polyps.

The polyps have a smooth, round contour and are not fissured or lobulated, as are adenomatous polyps. On cut section, the polyps have multiple cystic spaces filled with mucin. The predominant histologic feature is increased supporting connective tissue, which contains cystically dilated tubules lined by normal epithelium. No muscularis mucosa is involved in the polyp stalk. Numerous inflammatory cells may be present. In some patients,

juvenile polyps with areas of focal adenomatous changes or carcinoma in situ have been identified.

The polyps may be distributed throughout the stomach, small intestine, and colon, although they are most frequently colonic.

Complications: Thirteen of the 17 families reported through 1985 had some incidence of gastrointestinal, usually but not exclusively, colonic carcinoma. In nine families, the diagnosis of colonic cancer was made before 40 years of age. Thus, the risk for gastrointestinal malignancy is extremely great, approaching that of **Intestinal polyposis, type I.** This has been underestimated in the past, since the index cases are identified in childhood, and the malignancy usually occurs in adulthood. Intussusception, severe blood loss, intestinal obstruction, and malabsorption have been reported in children.

Associated Findings: Failure to thrive, anemia, hypoproteinemia, and hypokalemia. Three families have been identified with cosegregation of pulmonary and CNS arteriovenous malformations, indicating a distinct subtype. **Megalencephaly** has been reported in at least two infants.

Etiology: Autosomal dominant inheritance.

Pathogenesis: Some polyps have developed atypical adenomatous features. These may show areas of malignant degeneration. Separate but coexisting adenomas are also reported in older children and adults. Transformation of juvenile polyps into adenomatous polyps has been suggested.

MIM No.: *17490

CDC No.: 751.880

Sex Ratio: M1:F1

Occurrence: Seventeen families had been documented in the literature as of 1985.

Risk of Recurrence for Patient's Sib:
  See Part I, *Mendelian Inheritance.*

Risk of Recurrence for Patient's Child:
  See Part I, *Mendelian Inheritance.*

Age of Detectability: Varies from nine months to adulthood.

Gene Mapping and Linkage: Unknown.

Prevention: None known. Genetic counseling indicated. Periodic colonic, and possibly gastric, examination is suggested for at-risk family members.

Treatment: Excision biopsy of accessible lesions. Partial colectomy has been required for current bleeding or malignant degeneration. May require an early colectomy in infancy. Strong consideration should be given to prophylactic colectomy in early adulthood.

Prognosis: Good, if bleeding is limited and malignant lesions do not develop. If untreated, the condition can be lethal. Polyps may persist into adulthood.

Detection of Carrier: Air contrast barium enema in late childhood is recommended for at-risk family members.

Special Considerations: Children without a family history of intestinal polyposis or intestinal cancer may frequently have solitary juvenile colonic polyps. These sporadic cases appear to lack the significant potential for GI malignancy that is present in familial cases or in individuals with many (>10) juvenile polyps.

Support Groups: OH; Cleveland; Familial Polyposis Registry

References:

McColl I, et al.: Juvenile polyposis coli. Proc R Soc Med 1974; 57:896–897.
Cox KL, et al.: Hereditary generalized juvenile polyposis associated with pulmonary arteriovenous malformations. Gastroenterology 1980; 78:1566–1570.
Conte WJ, et al.: Juvenile gastrointestinal polyposis and arteriovenous malformations: heterogeneity within juvenile polyposis syndrome and a reassessment of cancer risk. Am J Hum Genet 1982; 34:69A.
Grotsky HW, et al.: Familial juvenile polyposis coli. Gastroenterology 1982; 82:494–501.
Jarvinen H, et al.: Familial juvenile polyposis coli: increased risk of colorectal cancer. Gut 1984; 25:792–800.

Ramaswamy G, et al.: Juvenile polyposis of the colon with atypical adenomatous change and carcinoma in situ. Dis Colon Rectum 1984; 27:393–398.

Grosfeld JL, West KW: Generalized juvenile polyposis coli: clinical management based on long-term observations. Arch Surg 1986; 121:530–534.

C0074
R0036

William J. Conte
Jerome I. Rotter

INTESTINAL POLYPOSIS, TYPE I 0535

Includes:

Colon, familial polyposis
Adenomatous polyposis coli
Adenomatous polyposis, familial
Cancer, intestinal polyposis I
Polyposis, familial

Excludes:

Chromosome 5, monosomy 5q interstitial (2544)
Gingival multiple hamartoma syndrome (0412)
Intestinal polyposis, juvenile type (2259)
Intestinal polyposis, type II (2344)
Intestinal polyposis, type III (0536)

Major Diagnostic Criteria: The presence of 100 or more adenomatous colorectal polyps is diagnostic of familial polyposis coli. Fewer polyps or extraintestinal growths, together with a family history, is highly suggestive.

Clinical Findings: The great majority of individuals with familial polyposis coli are asymptomatic until colorectal cancer occurs. Adenomatous colorectal polyps begin to appear after age 10 years, with an average age of occurrence of 24.5 years. Although a small number of polyps may be seen early in the disease course, hundreds to many thousands of polyps (average approximately 1,000) are evident by the third or fourth decade. The colonic polyps are usually small (less than 0.5 cm), sessile, or early

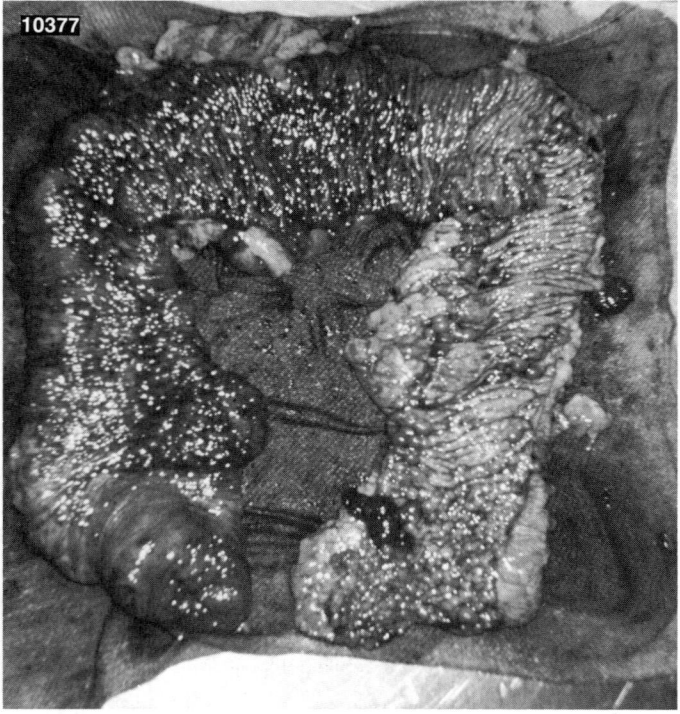

0535-10377: Multiple adenomatous polyps in colon specimen.

pedunculated tubular adenomas that "carpet" the colon. Villous histology is occasionally seen in polyps, and a pattern of fewer (scores to hundreds), larger, more pedunculated polyps has been described in many pedigrees.

Symptoms, including rectal bleeding, diarrhea, abdominal pain, and mucous discharge, begin at an average age of 33 years and are often indicative of colorectal cancer. The average age of cancer diagnosis is 39 years. All untreated individuals will eventually develop colorectal cancer.

Recent studies indicate that upper gastrointestinal polyps occur in **Intestinal polyposis, type I** as often as they are found in **Intestinal polyposis, type II**.

Complications: Colorectal cancer develops in 100% of untreated patients.

Associated Findings: Both desmoids and mesenteric fibromatosis have been reported in patients with familial polyposis coli.

Etiology: Autosomal dominant inheritance with complete penetrance.

Pathogenesis: Unknown.

MIM No.: *17510

Sex Ratio: M1:F1

Occurrence: 1:8300 births.

Risk of Recurrence for Patient's Sib:
See Part I, *Mendelian Inheritance.*

Risk of Recurrence for Patient's Child:
See Part I, *Mendelian Inheritance.*

Age of Detectability: Variable. Colonic polyposis may be seen in the second half of the first decade, and is often present in the second decade. DNA markers are now sufficiently accurate that highly probable diagnoses can be made at birth.

Gene Mapping and Linkage: APC (adenomatosis polyposis coli) has been mapped to 5q21-q22.

There is suggestive evidence that the APC locus regulates *c-myc* expression.

Prevention: None known. Genetic counseling indicated.

Treatment: Effective treatment depends on identification of affected individuals before cancer develops. Screening fiberoptic endoscopy of the colon should be done yearly, beginning at age 10 years, in all individuals at risk. Because polyps are equally distributed throughout the colon, flexible proctosigmoidoscopy is sufficient for screening. In occasional pedigrees where an excess of proximal colonic polyps and cancer is observed, yearly full colonoscopy may be necessary. Once polyps are detected, full colonoscopy should be performed every 6–12 months. Elective colectomy should be planned at the patient's earliest convienience once colonic polyposis is present. Numerous polyps, larger polyps, or villous histology make surgery more urgent. DNA markers may soon obviate the need for screening any but those with the mutant allele.

The optimal surgery is debated. Total colectomy with ileostomy or "ileoanal pull-through" eliminates the risk of colorectal cancer. Many centers have successfully used subtotal colectomy with careful follow-up for coagulation and removal of recurrent rectal polyps.

Screening intervals and treatment guidelines for upper gastrointestinal polyps are presently being developed. Initial upper GI endoscopy should be done once colonic polyps are detected. This should be repeated every 2–3 years until duodenal adenomatous polyps are found. One to two year examinations should then be done. The occurrence of large polyps or polyps with villous or moderately dysplastic histology should prompt consideration of endoscopic or surgical polyp removal.

Treatment of desmoids and mesenteric fibromatosis is a particular problem, since surgical dissection may stimulate their growth.

Prognosis: Good if colorectal cancer is prevented. Survival is somewhat decreased by duodenal cancer, abdominal desmoids and fibromatosis, but complete data are not available.

Detection of Carrier: There is no true "carrier" state, as all individuals with the mutant allele will eventually express the phenotype. DNA markers are now sufficiently accurate that highly probable diagnoses can be made at birth.

Special Considerations: The distinction from Gardner syndrome (see **Intestinal polyposis, type III**) is unclear. Hypotheses regarding the etiology of the two syndromes have included: 1) different mutations or deletions at the same chromosomal location, 2) variable expression of an identical gene defect, and 3) modifying genes separate from the APC locus.

Support Groups: OH; Cleveland; Familial Polyposis Registry

References:

Bussey HJR: Familial polyposis coli. Baltimore, Johns Hopkins Univ, Press, 1975. * †

Luk GD, Baylin SB: Ornithine decarboxylase as a biological marker in familial colonic polyposis. New Engl J Med 1984; 311:80–83.

Haggitt RC, Reid BJ: Hereditary gastrointestinal polyposis syndromes. Am J Surg Pathol 1986; 10:871–887. *

Klemmer S, et al.: Occurrence of desmoids in patients with familial adenomatous polyposis of the colon. Am J Med Genet 1987; 28:385–392.

Leppert M, et al.: The gene for familial polyposis coli maps to the long arm of chromosome 5. Science 1987; 238:1411–1413.

Quirke P, et al.: DNA aneuploidy and cell proliferation in familial adenomatous polyposis. Gut 1988; 29:603–607.

Erisman MD, et al.: Evidence that the familial adenomatous polyposis gene involved in a subset of colon cancers with a complementable defect in c-myc regulation. Proc Natl Acad Sci 1989; 86:4264–4268.

Tops CMJ, et al.: Presymptomatic diagnosis of familial adenomatous polyposis by bridging DNA markers. Lancet 1989; II:1361–1363.

BU036 **Randall W. Burt**

INTESTINAL POLYPOSIS, TYPE II **2344**

Includes:
> Peutz-Jeghers syndrome
> Polyposis, intestinal, II

Excludes:
> **Gastrocutaneous syndrome** (2981)
> **Gingival fibromatosis-depigmentation-microphthalmia** (0413)
> **Gingival multiple hamartoma syndrome** (0412)
> **Intestinal polyposis, juvenile type** (2259)
> **Intestinal polyposis, type I** (0535)
> **Intestinal polyposis, type III** (0536)

Major Diagnostic Criteria: The presence of numerous pigmented spots on the lips and buccal mucosa, together with multiple gastrointestinal hamartomatous polyps, is diagnostic. The histopathology of the polyps is distinctive.

Clinical Findings: Abnormal mucocutaneous pigmentation occurs in infancy or childhood. It is described as multiple 1–5 mm melanotic macules which look like dark freckles but are unusual because of their location. They are most frequently seen on the lips and buccal mucosa but also occur on the face, forearms, palms, soles, digits, perianal area, and, rarely, on the intestinal mucosa. The pigmentation on the lips fades with age, making buccal mucosal pigmentation a more reliable finding in adults. Abnormal pigmentation is present in greater than 95% of affected individuals.

The clinically important feature of the disease is the occurrence of multiple hamartomatous polyps throughout the gastrointestinal tract. The polyps are histologically distinctive and vary in size from 1 mm to 4 cm. They occur in the ileum and jejunum in almost all patients, but they are also found in the rectum, colon, stomach, and duodenum. Polyps are rarely found in the nose, bronchi, renal pelvis, ureters, or bladder. Intestinal polyps usually become symptomatic from complications early in the third decade, although these may occur at a younger age. The average age of diagnosis is 22.5 years.

Complications: The most frequent complications arise secondary to larger polyps and include intestinal obstruction and intussus-

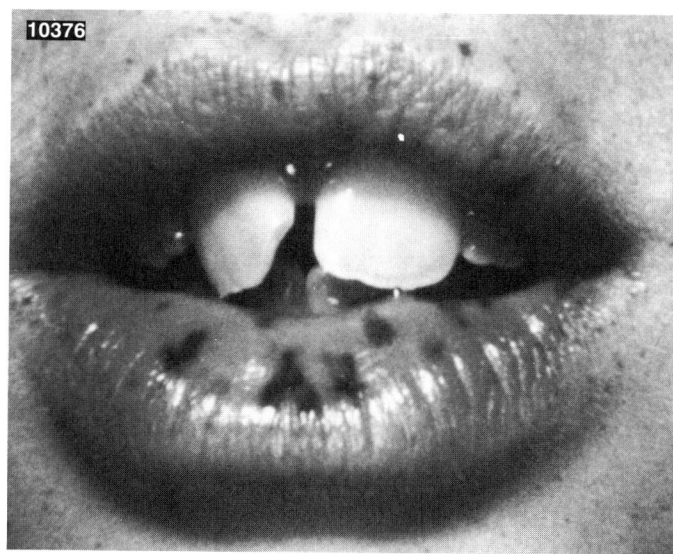

2344-10376: Lip pigmentation in intestinal polyposis II.

---

ception. These complications are heralded by the patient's complaining of severe recurrent colicky abdominal pain. Large polyps also commonly ulcerate and infarct, which results in gastrointestinal blood loss and anemia. Hematemesis may occur from gastric and duodenal polyps.

Recent evidence suggests a 2–13% risk of gastrointestinal cancer. The majority of cancers reported have been present in the stomach or duodenum of patients under the age of 40 years. Cancers also have been reported in the ileum, jejunum, and colon. Concomitant colonic adenomas were seen in the patients with colonic cancer, suggesting the malignancies arose from these lesions. However, adenomatous change in the epithelium of the hamartomatous polyps has been observed. The estimated frequency of neoplastic change in polyps is 3–6%.

Associated Findings: Several extra-intestinal benign and malignant tumors, including breast carcinoma (often bilateral), cervical adenocarcinoma, and benign and malignant ovarian tumors occur. The benign ovarian tumors are "sex cord tumors with annular tubules." These are now considered a phenotypic characteristic of the disease, as they are present in almost all affected females. There is an association with testicular malignancy in males, and pancreatic cancer in both sexes. The overall occurrence of malignancy (gastrointestinal or extra-gastrointestinal) approaches 50%.

Etiology: Autosomal dominant inheritance with high penetrance.

Pathogenesis: Unknown.

MIM No.: *17520

POS No.: 3638

CDC No.: 759.600

Sex Ratio: M1:F1

Occurrence: Estimated at 1:120,000 births.

Risk of Recurrence for Patient's Sib:
> See Part I, *Mendelian Inheritance.*

Risk of Recurrence for Patient's Child:
> See Part I, *Mendelian Inheritance.*

Age of Detectability: Varies from early infancy if pigment spots are present in an individual at risk, to adulthood if melanin spots are absent or family history is not known.

Gene Mapping and Linkage: Unknown.

Prevention: None known. Genetic counseling indicated. It would be prudent to perform yearly occult stool testing, and flexible proctosigmoidoscopy every 3–5 years, beginning in the second decade, in at-risk individuals who have not developed symptoms. Regular breast and gynecologic screening should also be performed in affected individuals.

Treatment: Upper and lower gastrointestinal endoscopy with polypectomy and small bowel X-ray should be performed when any gastrointestinal symptoms develop in an individual who is at risk or who has typical orocutaneous pigmentation. Surgery is indicated for removal of symptomatic small bowel polyps or small bowel polyps larger than 1.5 cm. Intra-operative small bowel endoscopy should be performed when laparotomy becomes necessary, to remove all possible polyps. Upper and lower gastrointestinal endoscopy and small bowel X-ray should be repeated every 2–3 years once the diagnosis is made.

Prognosis: One study reported an actuarial survival identical to the general population (Linos et al, 1981), while another found it to be substantially decreased (Utsunomiya et al, 1975). In the latter study, 43% of deaths which occurred prior to age 30 resulted from complications of the polyposis, while 60% of deaths after that age were due to malignancy.

Detection of Carrier: Unknown.

Support Groups: OH; Cleveland; Familial Polyposis Registry

References:

Utsunomiya J, et al.: Peutz-Jeghers syndrome: its natural course and management. Johns Hopkins Med J 1975; 136:71–82. * †
Linos DH, et al.: Does Purtz-Jeghers syndrome predispose to gastrointestinal malignancy? Arch Surg 1981; 116:1182–1184.
Chen KTK: Female genital tract tumors in Peutz-Jeghers syndrome. Hum Pathol 1986; 17:858–861.
van Coevorden F, et al.: Combined endoscopic and surgical treatment in Peutz-Jeghers syndrome. Surg Gynecol Obstet 1986; 162:426–428.
Giardiello FM, et al.: Increased risk of cancer in the Peutz-Jeghers syndrome. New Engl J Med 1987; 316:1511–1514. *
Konishi F, et al.: Peutz-Jeghers polyposis associated with carcinoma of the digestive organs. Dis Colon Rectum 1987; 30:790–799.
Narita T, et al.: Peutz-Jeghers syndrome with adenomas and adenocarcinomas in colonic polyps. Am J Surg Path 1987; 11:76–81.
Foley TR, et al.: Peutz-Jeghers syndrome: a clinicopathologic survey of the "Harrisburg Family" with a 49-year follow-up. Gastroenterology 1988; 95:1535–1540. *

BU036 **Randall W. Burt**

INTESTINAL POLYPOSIS, TYPE III 0536

Includes:
Gardner syndrome
Hallerman-Streiff syndrome
Oldfield syndrome
Polyposis, Gardner type

Excludes:
Cancer, sebaceous gland tumor-mulitple visceral carcinoma (2743)
Gastrocutaneous syndrome (2981)
Gingival fibromatosis-depigmentation-microphthalmia (0413)
Intestinal polyposis, juvenile type (2259)
Intestinal polyposis, type I (0535)
Intestinal polyposis, type II (2344)
Turcot syndrome (2739)

Major Diagnostic Criteria: One hundred or more adenomatous colorectal polyps with extra-intestinal growths described below is diagnostic of Gardner syndrome. Fewer polyps or extraintestinal growths, together with a family history, is highly suggestive.

Clinical Findings: The colorectal polyposis and cancer occurrence in this disease is virtually identical to that in **Intestinal polyposis, type I**, except for a possible colonic pattern of fewer and larger polyps. The pattern of colonic polyp growth tends to be similar in individuals from the same pedigree.

In addition to colonic polyposis and cancer, individuals with this syndrome exhibit numerous benign extraintestinal growths.

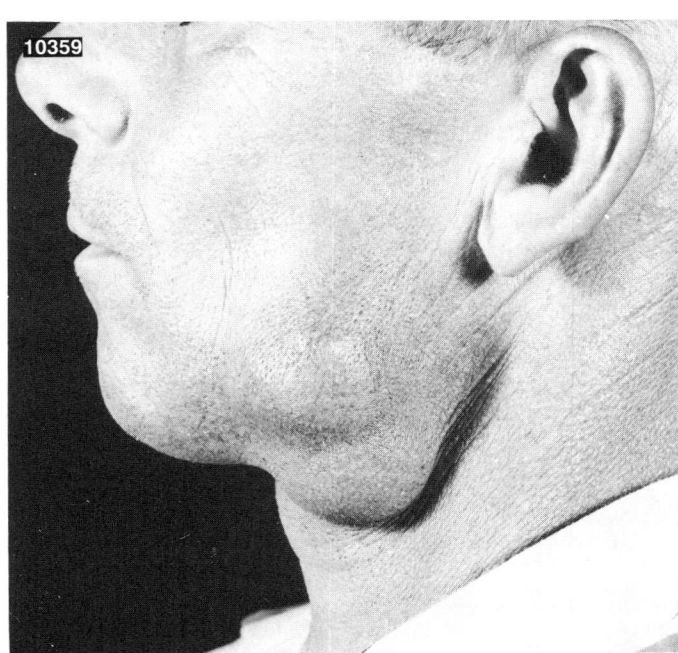

0536A-10359: Osteoma of mandible.

These include osteomas, soft tissue tumors, and dental abnormalities. Osteomas are more commonly observed on the mandible and skull, but may occur on any bone. Soft tissue tumors include epidermoid cysts, sebaceous cysts, fibromas, and lipomas. Supernumerary teeth, unerupted teeth, and odontomas are the most common dental growth defects. The frequency of these benign growths is extremely variable, but usually consistent within a given pedigree. Members of some pedigrees exhibit most or all of

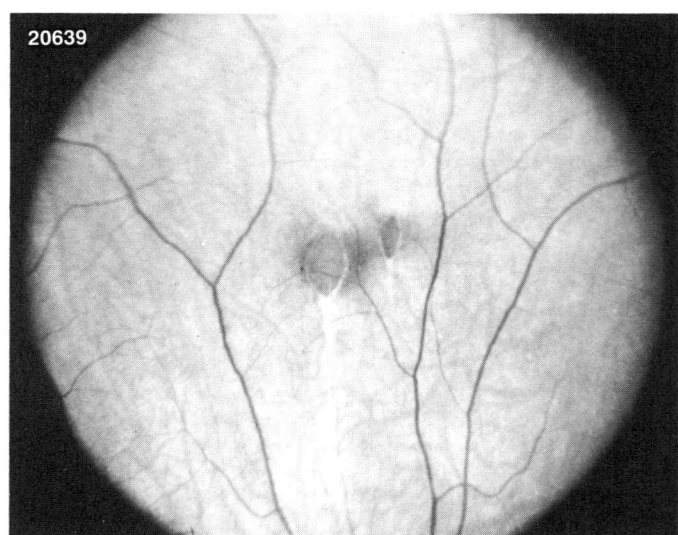

0536B-20639: Intestinal polyposis, Gardner type. Two of a number of brown-black patches of congenital hypertrophy of the retinal pigment epithelium occurring in both eyes of a young male with Gardner Syndrome. The "snow shoe" or "comet-tail" points towards the posterior pole of the eye.

the growths, while only occasional benign lesions are observed in members of other pedigrees. The extraintestinal growths may occur years before colonic polyps are apparent.

Ocular features, particularly of the retina (see **Retina, congenital hypertrophy of retinal pigment epithelium** (CHRPE)) are very helpful in making this diagnosis. CHRPE is pedigree-specific, but is found in virtually all affected individuals in pedigrees in which it is present.

Dermoid tumors and mesenteric fibromatosis are frequent problems (up to 50% of the individuals in some pedigrees). Desmoids often occur postsurgically in the anterior abdominal wall, but may b_ seen prior to surgery and may occur in musculoaponeurotic structures throughout the body.

Gastric, duodenal, and small bowel polyps are a frequent finding. Gastric polyps are numerous small (1–5 mm) sessile hyperplastic polyps of the proximal stomach. They have little or no malignant potential, and occur in up to 50% of cases. Duodenal polyps are seen as numerous 1–5 mm adenomatous polyps and occur in up to 90% of patients. These appear to have some malignant potential, since duodenal cancer occurs in 3–12% of cases. Adenomatous polyps occasionally occur elsewhere in the small bowel, especially the terminal ileum, although cancer is rare outside of the duodenum. Upper gastrointestinal polyps seldom cause symptoms.

Complications: Colorectal cancer develops in all untreated patients at a relatively young age. Problems with extraintestinal manifestations are mainly cosmetic. Although desmoid tumors and mesenteric fibromatosis are benign, they may cause intestinal obstruction, and obstruction or compression of any adjacent structure.

Associated Findings: Cancers of many sites have been reported. The associations are probably coincidental, except for duodenal cancer, central nervous system cancer (see **Turcot syndrome**), and thyroid carcinoma.

Etiology: Autosomal dominant inheritance with virtually 100% penetrance. The frequency of extraintestinal manifestations is variable, but usually consistent within a pedigree.

Pathogenesis: Unknown.

MIM No.: *17530

POS No.: 3766

CDC No.: 759.630

Sex Ratio: M1:F1

Occurrence: 1:14,025 births.

Risk of Recurrence for Patient's Sib:
See Part I, *Mendelian Inheritance.*

Risk of Recurrence for Patient's Child:
See Part I, *Mendelian Inheritance.*

Age of Detectability: Colonic polyposis may be seen in the second half of the first decade, and is often present in the second decade. Extraintestinal manifestations are sometimes observed in the first few years of life. DNA markers are now sufficiently accurate that highly probable diagnoses can be made at birth.

Gene Mapping and Linkage: APC (adenomatosis polyposis coli) has been mapped to 5q21-q22.
Gardner syndrome shares the APC locus.

Prevention: None known. Genetic counseling indicated.

Treatment: Effective treatment depends upon identification of affected individuals before cancer develops. Screening fiberoptic endoscopy of the colon should be done yearly, beginning at ten years of age, in all individuals at risk. Because polyps are equally distributed throughout the colon, yearly flexible proctosigmoidoscopy is sufficient. In occasional pedigrees, where an excess of proximal colonic polyps and cancer is observed, yearly colonoscopy may be necessary. Once polyps are detected, full colonoscopy should be performed every 6–12 months. Elective colectomy should be planned at the patient's earliest convenience once colonic polyposis is present. Numerous polyps, larger polyps, or villous histology make surgery more urgent. DNA markers may soon obviate the need for screening any but those with the mutant allele.

The optimal surgery is debated. Total colectomy with ileostomy or "ileoanal pull-through" eliminates the risk of colorectal cancer. Many centers have successfully used subtotal colectomy with careful follow-up for coagulation and removal of recurrent rectal polyps.

Screening intervals and treatment guidelines for upper gastrointestinal polyps are presently being developed. Initial upper GI endoscopy should be done once colonic polyps are detected. This should be repeated every 2–3 years until duodenal adenomatous polyps are found. One to two year examinations should then be done. The occurrance of large polyps or polyps with villous or moderately dysplastic histology should prompt consideration of endoscopic or surgical polyp removal.

Treatment of extraintestinal growths is cosmetic and symptomatic. Desmoids and mesenteric fibromatosis are particular problems, since surgical dissection may stimulate their growth.

Prognosis: Good if colorectal cancer is prevented. Survival is somewhat decreased by duodenal cancer, abdominal desmoids and fibromatosis, but complete data are not available.

Detection of Carrier: Carriers may exhibit congenital hypertrophy of the retinal pigment epithelium (CHRPE) (see **Retina, congenital hypertrophy of retinal pigment epithelium**) or other extracolonic manifestations before colonic polyposis develops. However, absence of these other manifestations does not exclude the gene (nonpenetrance in an obligate carrier). Ophthalmic examinations, as well as physical examination and regular proctoscopy, are recommended for at-risk individuals. DNA markers are now sufficiently accurate that highly probable diagnoses can be made at birth.

Special Considerations: The distinction from **Intestinal polyposis, type I** is unclear. Hypotheses regarding the etiology of these two syndromes have included: 1) different mutations or deletions at the same chromosomal location, 2) variable expression of an identical gene defect, and 3) modifying agents separate from the APC locus.

Several families have been described which exhibit adenomatous colonic polyposis and brain tumors. This has been termed **Turcot syndrome**. Predominant sebaceous cysts and polyposis coli have been referred to as *Oldfield syndrome*, which may be a variant of Gardner syndrome. Multiple cutaneous sebaceous neoplasms with or without keratoacanthomas in association with adenocarcinomas of the gastrointestinal tract is referred to as *Muir-Torre syndrome* (see **Cancer, sebaceous gland tumor-mulitple visceral carcinoma**). A case of Muir-Torre syndrome has been described in which multiple polyps of the colon were present.

Support Groups: OH; Cleveland; Familial Polyposis Registry

References:
Gardner EJ, et al.: Gastrointestinal polyposis: syndromes and genetic mechanisms. West J Med 1980; 132:488–499. †
Haggitt RC, Reid BJ: Hereditary gastrointestinal polyposis syndromes. Am J Surg Pathol 1986; 10:871–887. *
Burt RW, et al.: Villous adenoma of the duodenal papilla presenting as necrotizing pancreatitis in a patient with Gardner's syndrome. Gastroenterology 1987; 92:532–535. †
Sarre RG, et al.: Gastric and duodenal polyps in familial adenomatous polyposis: a prospective study of the nature and prevalence of upper gastrointestinal polyps. Gut 1987; 28:306–314.
Traboulsi EI, et al.: Prevalence and importance of pigmented ocular fundus lesions in Gardner's syndrome. New Engl J Med 1987; 316:661–667. †
Itoh H, et al.: Treatment of desmoid tumors in Gardner's syndrome: report of a case. Dis Colon Rectum 1988; 31:459–461.
Nakamura Y, et al.: Localization of the genetic defect in familial adenomatous polyposis within a region of chromosome 5. Am J Hum Genet 1988; 43:638–644.

BU036   **Randall W. Burt**

Intestinal polyposis-pigmentary changes of genitalia-megalencephaly
See OVERGROWTH, RUVALCABA-MYHRE-SMITH TYPE

Intestinal pseudo-obstruction-external ophthalmoplegia
See MUSCULAR DYSTROPHY, OCULO-GASTROINTESTINAL

INTESTINAL PSEUDO-OBSTRUCTION SYNDROMES 2330

Includes:
Argyrophil myenteric plexus, deficiency of
Gastric emptying disorders, idiopathic
Megacolon, idiopathic
Megacystis, idiopathic
Megaduodenum, idiopathic
Myopathy, visceral
Pseudo-obstruction, chronic idiopathic intestinal, neuronal
  type
Visceral neuropathy

Excludes:
Colon, aganglionosis (0192)
Endocrine disorders
Gluten-sensitive enteropathy (0423)
Intestinal pseudo-obstruction secondary to amyloidosis
Intestinal pseudo-obstruction secondary to pharmacologic
  causes
Muscle disease, primary
Neurological disease, primary

Major Diagnostic Criteria: Signs and symptoms of chronic intestinal obstruction; no evidence of mechanical obstruction; no evidence of systemic etiologies; histologic evidence for involvement of smooth muscle or enteric nerves.

Clinical Findings: The clinical syndrome is characterized by chronically recurrent attacks suggestive of intestinal obstruction (defined clinically and by X-ray) in the absence of mechanical obstruction (established by appropriate X-ray, endoscopic, or surgical investigations) and in the absence of other recognized etiologies. This is a heterogeneous group of disorders.

In adults, a longstanding history of nonspecific symptoms suggestive of a gastrointestinal motility disorder (dysphagia, early satiety, constipation/diarrhea), or the presence of extraintestinal manifestations (megacystis, ophthalmoplegia), preceding the onset of acute symptoms is characteristic. In contrast, in neonates and infants, severe postprandial abdominal distension and obstruction are often the first manifestations of the disease. The most common symptoms in adults, despite different underlying pathologic lesions (visceral neuropathy, visceral myopathy), are abdominal pain and distension, early satiety, and diarrhea.

Positive findings on esophageal manometry (aperistalsis, incomplete relaxation of lower esophageal sphincter, gastric emptying studies (delayed for solids, variable for liquids), gastrointestinal manometry (usually a hypomotile pattern), and full-thickness biopsy with special silver stains of specimen are not mandatory for the diagnosis of intestinal pseudo-obstruction but allow the classification into visceral neuropathy or visceral myopathy; a more rational approach to management, including surgery; and the detection of asymptomatic but genetically affected relatives.

Complications: The presence and severity of complications depends on the age of the patient (infant vs. adult), primary site of involvement (proximal, distal, or entire GI tract), and degree of functional impairment. Malnutrition is common and can result from decreased food intake (operant conditioning to postprandial pain), maldigestion (impaired gastric dispersion of food), or malabsorption (bacterial overgrowth, sprue-like intestinal lesion, functional or surgical loss of absorptive capacity). In infants, failure to thrive or electrolyte and fluid imbalances are usually secondary to postprandial vomiting and diarrhea. Whereas gastroesophageal reflux appears to be rare in adults, reflux esophagitis and aspiration pneumonia occur in infants secondary to impaired gastroesophageal motility. Narcotic dependence may further compromise GI motility in adults with longstanding symptomatic disease.

Associated Findings: In visceral myopathy: megacystis, vesicoureteral reflux, ophthalmoplegia, ptosis, and small intestine diverticulosis. In visceral neuropathy: autonomic nervous system insufficiency, neurologic abnormalities (ataxia, dysarthria, abnormal pupillary reflexes, abnormal tendon reflexes, mental retardation), and basal ganglia calcification.

Etiology: Intestinal pseudo-obstruction is clearly due to a number of distinct genetic disorders, as both dominant, recessive, and sporadic families have been well described. In addition, different clinical associations have been noted, e.g., a specific pedigree with mental retardation and basal ganglia calcification. Finally, different pathology has been delineated in different pedigrees.

Pathogenesis: In kindreds with visceral myopathies, degenerative changes, and thinning of intestinal smooth muscle, preferentially of the longitudinal layers, have been described. Intestinal neurons were found to be normal. In kindreds with visceral neuropathies, special histologic techniques have revealed degenerative changes of myenteric plexus neurons, including pathognomonic intranuclear inclusions in one family. The intestinal smooth muscle was found to be normal.

MIM No.: *15531, *24318

CDC No.: 751.880

Sex Ratio: M1:F1

Occurrence: Several dozen kinships with inherited patterns have been documented.

Risk of Recurrence for Patient's Sib:
See Part I, *Mendelian Inheritance*.

Risk of Recurrence for Patient's Child:
See Part I, *Mendelian Inheritance*.

Age of Detectability: Clinical detectability is highly variable; usually in the second to fourth decade. Some sporadic cases are detectable in the neonatal period.

Gene Mapping and Linkage: Unknown.

Prevention: None known. Genetic counseling indicated.

Treatment: In mildly symptomatic cases, small frequent feedings and intake of prokinetic agents (metoclopramide, cisapride) may be useful. In severely affected cases, medical therapy is usually ineffective. Surgical interventions (gastrostomy tube, gastrointestinal resections) are useful only in selected cases resistant to conservative management. Long-term total parenteral nutrition is sometimes the only therapy.

Prognosis: Highly variable. Poor in patients with onset in infancy or with diffuse GI involvement.

Detection of Carrier: Gastric emptying studies and esophageal and gastrointestinal manometry may detect subclinically affected individuals.

References:
Byrne WJ, et al.: Chronic idiopathic intestinal pseudo-obstruction syndrome in children: clinical characteristics and prognosis. J Pediatr 1977; 90:585–589.
Schuffler MD, et al.: Chronic idiopathic intestinal pseudo-obstruction. a surgical approach. Ann Surg 1980; 192:752–761.
Schuffler MD, et al.: Chronic intestinal pseudo-obstruction: a report of 27 cases and review of the literature. Medicine 1981; 60:173–196.
Anuras S, et al.: A familial visceral myopathy with external ophthalmoplegia and autosomal recessive transmission. Gastroenterology 1983; 84:346–353.
Mayer EA, et al.: A familial visceral neuropathy with autosomal dominant transmission. Gastroenterology 1986; 91:1528–1536.
Faber J, et al.: Familial intestinal pseudoobstruction dominated by a progressive neurologic disease at a young age. Gastroenterology 1987; 92:786–790.
Mayer EA, et al.: Gastric emptying of a mixed solid-liquid meal in patients with chronic intestinal pseudo-obstruction. Diag Dis Sci 1987; 33:10–18.
Steiner I, et al.: Familial progressive neuronal disease and chronic idiopathic intestinal pseuoobstruction. Neurology 1987; 37:1046–1050.

Hyman PE, et al.: Antroduodenal motility in children with chronic intestinal pseudo-obstruction. J Pediatr 1988; 112:899–905.

MA081
R0036

Emeran A. Mayer
Jerome I. Rotter

Intestinal pseudo-obstruction, idiopathic
See MEGACYSTIS-MEGADUODENUM SYNDROME

INTESTINAL ROTATION, INCOMPLETE   0537

Includes:
> Malrotation
> Malrotation of midgut
> Nonrotation of midgut
> Volvulus of midgut

Excludes:
> **Duodenum, atresia or stenosis** (0300)
> **Intestinal atresia or stenosis** (0531)

Major Diagnostic Criteria: X-ray demonstration of the anatomic abnormality, i.e., the cecum is not in the right lower quadrant, the small bowel is on the right side of the abdomen, and the colon tends to be on the left side of the abdomen. If the patient has undergone midgut volvulus, the duodenum may show complete obstruction and by barium enema the transverse colon may be obstructed.

Clinical Findings: Bile-stained emesis is the most frequent presenting symptom, indicating obstruction distal to the ampulla of Vater. The patient may have cyclic or recurrent vomiting, malabsorption of fat, and recurrent abdominal pain.

Any neonate who has the sudden onset of bile-stained emesis should have appropriate X-ray studies performed on an emergency basis because of the possibility of volvulus of the midgut, which may result in necrosis.

Malrotation is inherently associated with abdominal wall defects such as omphalocele and gastroschisis and with diaphragmatic hernia. The anomaly is evident at the time of surgical correction of these congenital anomalies.

If the patient has an anterior abdominal wall defect, the bowel has not gone through the normal phases of rotation. If the patient has a diaphragmatic hernia, the bowel resides in the thoracic cavity and therefore has not progressed through the normal stages of rotation. In the other patients who have neither an anterior abdominal wall defect nor a diaphragmatic hernia, the rotation of the bowel simply does not occur and there is no known rationale for the lack of rotation.

Complications: Midgut volvulus is the most serious complication. Other complications are malnutrition due to recurrent vomiting and the inability to absorb fats due to obstruction of the mesenteric lymphatics.

Associated Findings: Duodenal stenosis is rarely associated, and should be excluded at the time of surgical correction of the malrotation.

Etiology: Autosomal dominant inheritance has been demonstrated in two families. Most cases appear to be sporadic.

Pathogenesis: During embryonic development, the intestine grows at a more rapid rate than the celomic cavity. Part of the intestine develops in the base of the umbilical cord and in the normal sequence of events returns to the celomic cavity and simultaneously rotates in a counterclockwise direction around the superior mesenteric pedicle. Eventually the cecum and right colon are fixed to the posterior parietes. If the rotation does not proceed to completion, fixation of the right colon does not occur and the entire intestine is on a narrowed pedicle.

MIM No.: *19325

CDC No.: 751.490

Sex Ratio: Presumably M1:F1 (M2:F1 observed in one series).

Occurrence: Of asymptomatic patients having barium enemas, 0–2% have malrotation. One hundred fourteen patients operated on at the Children's Hospital of Los Angeles between 1937 and 1977 and 320 patient operated on at the Boston Children's Hospital through 1967 had malrotation.

Risk of Recurrence for Patient's Sib: Unknown.

Risk of Recurrence for Patient's Child: Unknown.

Age of Detectability: The majority of patients are diagnosed and treated in the first month of life.

Gene Mapping and Linkage: Unknown.

Prevention: None known. Genetic counseling indicated.

Treatment: The only effective therapy for this anomaly is surgical correction of the abnormally narrow mesenteric base by lysis of bands which traverse from the distal small bowel mesentery to the right posterior abdominal wall lateral to the duodenum. If volvulus is present, detorsion is performed prior to lysis of bands.

Prognosis: If the patient is operated on prior to vascular compromise of the small bowel, the prognosis is excellent. If the patient has progressed to necrosis of the entire small bowel and secondary shock, the prognosis is guarded.

Detection of Carrier: Unknown.

Special Considerations: If an infant feeds well during the early hours or days of life and has sudden onset of bile-stained emesis, midgut volvulus secondary to malrotation should be ruled out on an emergency basis. Observation with appropriate X-ray studies may allow the infant to progress to complete bowel necrosis before therapy is instituted.

References:
Stewart DR, et al.: Malrotation of the bowel in infants and children: a 15 year review. Surgery 1976; 79:716–720.
Andrassy RJ, Mahour GH: Malrotation of the midgut in infants and children: a 25-year review. Arch Surg 1981; 116:158–160.
Carmi R, et al.: Familial midgut anomalies: a spectrum of defects due to a single cause? Am J Med Genet 1981; 8:443–446.
Smith EI: Malrotation of the intestine. In: Welch K, et al., eds: Pediatric Surgery, ed 4, Vol 2. Chicago: Yearbook Medical, 1986: 882–895.

W0013

Morton M. Woolley

Intestine, inflammatory bowel diseases
See INFLAMMATORY BOWEL DISEASE
Intimal fibrosis with fibromuscular dysplasia
See ARTERY, RENAL FIBROMUSCULAR DYSPLASIA
Intraadenoidal cysts
See NASOPHARYNGEAL CYSTS
Intraepithelial dyskeratosis
See MUCOSA (ORAL/EYE), INTRAEPITHELIAL DYSKERATOSIS, BENIGN

INTRAHEPATIC CHOLESTASIS OF PREGNANCY (ICP)   3278

Includes:
> Cholestasis associated with oral contraceptive therapy
> Cholestasis, intrahepatic, of pregnancy
> Intrahepatic jaundice of pregnancy, recurrent
> Obstetric hepatosis
> Pregnancy-related cholestasis
> Pruritus gravidarum
> Recurrent intrahepatic cholestasis of pregnancy (RICP)

Excludes:
> **Cholestasis, intrahepatic, recurrent, benign** (3276)
> **Jaundice, intrahepatic cholestatic, Byler type** (2371)
> Liver, acute fatty, of pregnancy
> Preeclampsia/eclampsia associated liver dysfunction

Major Diagnostic Criteria: Jaundice or pruritus associated with elevated serum bile salts during pregnancy or with use of estrogen-containing oral contraceptives, and in the absence of biliary colic, fever or other manifestations of gallstone disease.

Clinical Findings: Patients usually present in the third trimester, but may become symptomatic as early as the second or third month of gestation. Pruritus is the most common initial complaint and can become intolerably severe in some. Fluctuating jaundice may also develop. Patients with a prior history of jaundice not associated with pregnancy or estrogen therapy are excluded from diagnosis. The disease usually recurs in multiparous women, but lack of symptoms during prior pregnancies does not preclude the diagnosis.

The liver may be enlarged and slightly tender. Hepatic histology is notable only for mild hepatocellular cholestasis. The gallbladder may appear distended by ultrasound, but there should be no evidence of biliary obstruction. There is a moderate increase in fasting serum bile acids, cholesterol, alkaline phosphatase, 5' nucleotidase and lipoprotein X. Serum gamma-glutamyl transpeptidase has been reported to be normal. Symptoms and biochemical abnormalities resolve within days after delivery.

Complications: Patients may develop vitamin K deficiency secondary to steatorrhea. The nutritional status of the mother and fetus may also be compromised by fat malabsorption. The incidence of stillbirths, premature deliveries and fetal distress among the offspring of affected mothers appears to be increased as compared to uncomplicated gestations.

Associated Findings: None known.

Etiology: Possibly an autosomal dominant trait that can be transmitted by phenotypically normal males.

Pathogenesis: ICP is speculated to be secondary to reduced inactivation of cholestatic steroid hormones, particularly estrogen. Exaggerated impairment of intravenous sulfobromophthalein clearance after low dose ethinyl estradiol administration has been demonstrated in males with a positive family history of this disorder.

MIM No.: 14748

Sex Ratio: M0:F1 (symptomatic patients are female by definition).

Occurrence: 1:1000–10,000 deliveries overall, 10 to 20 times higher prevalence in Scandinavian countries and Poland, highest incidence in Araucanian Indians of Chile where prevalence approaches 1:10 deliveries.

Risk of Recurrence for Patient's Sib:
See Part I, *Mendelian Inheritance.*

Risk of Recurrence for Patient's Child:
See Part I, *Mendelian Inheritance.*

Age of Detectability: Presumably after puberty.

Gene Mapping and Linkage: Unknown.

Prevention: None known. Genetic counseling indicated.

Treatment: Patients may show improvement in symptoms when treated with phenobarbital or cholestyramine. Cholestyramine does tend to aggravate fat malabsorption. Patients should also receive supplemental fat soluble vitamins, especially vitamin K.

Prognosis: Variable. The condition tends to recur in subsequent pregnancies. No associated residual liver dysfunction has been reported after the post-partum period.

Detection of Carrier: Male carriers may have impaired sulfobromophthalein clearance.

References:
Reyes H, et al.: Sulfobromophthalein clearance tests before and after ethinyl estradiol administration in women and men with familial history of intrahepatic cholestasis of pregnancy. Gastroenterology 1981; 81:226–231.
Reyes H: The enigma of intrahepatic cholestasis of pregnancy: lessons from Chile. Hepatology 1982; 2:87–96.
Holzbach RT, et al.: Familial recurrent intrahepatic cholestasis of pregnancy: a genetic study providing evidence for transmission of a sex-linked, dominant trait. Gastroenterology 1983; 85:175–179.
Riely CA: The liver in pregnancy. In: Schiff L, Schiff ER, eds: Diseases of the liver. Philadelphia: J.B. Lippincott, 1987:1059–1073.

AL037
FI035

Estella M. Alonso
Mark Fishbein

Intrahepatic jaundice of pregnancy, recurrent
See INTRAHEPATIC CHOLESTASIS OF PREGNANCY (ICP)

ISAACS-MERTENS SYNDROME 3271

Includes:

Continuous muscle fiber activity, hereditary
Neuromyotonia

Excludes:

Hyperekplexia (3260)
Jumping Frenchman of Maine (3270)
Myotonia congenita (0701)

Major Diagnostic Criteria: Myokymia (continuous, wormlike contractions of skeletal muscle), pseudomyotonia (difficulty relaxing after forceful grasp as in myotonia, but differing electrophysiologically), and persistent or intermittent abnormal postures of the hands and feet. Hyperhidrosis may also be present.

Clinical Findings: The disorder is quite variable clinically, but the term "Isaacs-Mertens syndrome" is often used in a strict sense to refer to patients who display isolated stiffness and myokymia, the electrophysiologic origin of which appears to be the terminal motor axon or its sprouts (as evidenced by abolition of the continuous motor unit activity by curare but not by peripheral nerve block or sleep). According to this definition, related syndromes with additional clinical features, such as peripheral neuropathy, muscle wasting, episodic titubation, and periodic ataxia, are excluded, as are disorders in which the myokymia is abolished by peripheral nerve block. Isaacs-Mertens syndrome in this narrow sense is usually sporadic, although apparent autosomal dominant inheritance has been described. The disorder is not typically accompanied by an abnormal startle response as in **Hyperekplexia**, and true myotonia is not present. Most reported patients have responded dramatically, although often not completely, to phenytoin or carbamazepine, but not to benzodiazepines (unlike **Hyperekplexia**). Calcium and phosphorus metabolism are normal, despite the presence of ischemia-induced carpopedal spasm (Trousseau's sign) in some patients.

Complications: Cyanosis from respiratory muscle stiffness, and fixed joint contractures, have been reported in severe cases.

Associated Findings: None known.

Etiology: Usually sporadic, although instances of apparent autosomal dominant inheritance have been described.

Pathogenesis: A defect in the terminal motor axonal membrane has been proposed but not proven.

MIM No.: 12102

Sex Ratio: M1:F1

Occurrence: The disorder has been reported in a variety of ethnic groups.

Risk of Recurrence for Patient's Sib:
See Part I, *Mendelian Inheritance.*

Risk of Recurrence for Patient's Child:
See Part I, *Mendelian Inheritance.*

Age of Detectability: Sometimes obvious at birth or in the first few months of life. However, signs and symptoms are often first apparent in the fourth or fifth decades.

Gene Mapping and Linkage: Unknown.

Prevention: None known. Genetic counseling indicated.

Treatment: Phenytoin and carbamazepine have both proven remarkably effective in most patients.

Prognosis: The clinical course is variable; some patients experience complete or partial remission, while others require lifelong treatment.

Detection of Carrier: A thorough family history and examination of first-degree relatives, possibly including electromyography, may occasionally identify mildly affected individuals.

References:

Isaacs H: A syndrome of continuous muscle fiber activity. J Neurol Neurosurg Psychiat 1961; 24:319–325.
Hanson PA, et al.: Contractures, continuous muscle discharges, and titubation. Ann Neurol 1977; 1:120–124.
Ashizawa T, et al.: A dominantly inherited syndrome with continuous motor neuron discharges. Ann Neurol 1983; 13:285–290.
McGuire SA, et al.: Hereditary continuous muscle fiber activity. Arch Neurol 1984; 41:395–396.
Rowland LP: Cramps, spasms and muscle stiffness. Rev Neurol 1985; 141:261–273.

RY001   **Stephen G. Ryan**

Ischiopagus
See TWINS, CONJOINED
Isoimmune hemolytic disease of the newborn
See ERYTHROBLASTOSIS FETALIS
Isolated IgA deficiency
See IMMUNOGLOBULIN A DEFICIENCY
Isolated trypsinogen deficiency
See TRYPSINOGEN DEFICIENCY
Isolated TSH deficiency
See THYROTROPIN DEFICIENCY, ISOLATED
Isoleucine 33 amyloidosis
See AMYLOIDOSIS, ASHKENAZI TYPE
Isomaltase insufficiency
See SUCRASE-ISOMALTASE DEFICIENCY
Isomaltase-sucrase deficiency
See SUCRASE-ISOMALTASE DEFICIENCY
Isoniazid inactivation
See NEUROPATHY, HERITABLE ISONIAZIDE TYPE (INH)
also ACETYLATOR POLYMORPHISM
Isoniazid neuropathy
See NEUROPATHY, HERITABLE ISONIAZIDE TYPE (INH)
Isotretinoin, fetal effects of
See FETAL RETINOID SYNDROME
Isovaleric acid CoA dehydrogenase deficiency
See ACIDEMIA, ISOVALERIC
Isovaleric acidemia
See ACIDEMIA, ISOVALERIC
Israeli hereditary amyloidosis
See AMYLOIDOSIS, ASHKENAZI TYPE
Isthmic spondylolisthesis and spondylolysis
See SPINE, SPONDYLOLISTHESIS AND SPONDYLOLYSIS
Itching, hereditary localized
See PRURITUS, HEREDITARY LOCALIZED
Ito hypomelanosis
See HYPOMELANOSIS OF ITO
IVD deficiency
See ACIDEMIA, ISOVALERIC
Ivemark syndrome
See ASPLENIA SYNDROME

IVIC SYNDROME 3043

Includes:

Deafness-radial hypoplasia-ophthalmoplegia-
thrombocytopenia
Oculo-oto-radial syndrome
Radial hypoplasia-deafness-ophthalmoplegia-
thrombocytopenia

Excludes:

Aase-Smith syndrome (3029)
Heart-hand syndrome (0455)
Lacrimo-auriculo-dento-digital syndrome (2180)
Pancytopenia syndrome, Fanconi type (2029)
Radial-renal-ocular syndrome (2643)
Thrombocytopenia-absent radius (0941)

Major Diagnostic Criteria: The combination of radial ray defects, congenital mixed-type hearing loss, and strabismus should distinguish this condition from other radial anomaly syndromes.

Clinical Findings: All affected individuals have some degree of upper limb anomaly affecting the radial ray, with thumb hypoplasia, triphalangism, or distal placement being the most common. The upper limb hypoplasia can also affect the forearm. Although lower limbs appear normal, retarded growth of the femora and spine occurs, leading to relatively short stature. X-ray evaluation demonstrates an abnormal first metacarpal (absent, short, or long); hypoplastic and sometimes fused carpal bones are also seen in at least one-half of the affected individuals. Proximal fusion of radius and ulna was also present in 4/22 individuals.

Extraocular muscle weakness is present in most affected individuals, with the medial and lateral recti being the most frequently and severely affected. Congenital mixed-type hearing loss is also almost always present, with greater loss in the higher frequencies (above 4,000 cps). Seven affected individuals had mild, incomplete bundle branch block of the heart. Thrombocytopenia and leukocytosis also occurred in some affected individuals. In addition, 3/25 had imperforate anus.

Complications: Strabismus secondary to extraocular muscle weakness.

Associated Findings: Present in one or two individuals were hypoplastic lateral incisors; ocular lens opacities; and unilateral ectopic kidney.

Etiology: Autosomal dominant inheritance.

Pathogenesis: Unknown. A defect in mesenchyme has been postulated.

MIM No.: *14775

POS No.: 3849

Sex Ratio: M1:F1

Occurrence: At least three families have been reported; one each from Venezuela, Italy, and Hungary.

Risk of Recurrence for Patient's Sib:
See Part I, *Mendelian Inheritance.*

Risk of Recurrence for Patient's Child:
See Part I, *Mendelian Inheritance.*

Age of Detectability: Prenatally if major limb defects are present, otherwise at birth.

Gene Mapping and Linkage: Unknown.

Prevention: None known. Genetic counseling indicated.

Treatment: Supportive; surgery for imperforate anus if indicated.

Prognosis: Intellectual development and growth are not impaired; life span is generally normal, with the oldest individual dying at age 110 years, although one affected individual died suddenly at age 3 1/2 years.

Detection of Carrier: Unknown.

Special Considerations: The acronym IVIC stands for Instituto Venezolano de Investigaciones Científicas where Arias conducted his research.

References:

Arias S, et al.: The IVIC syndrome: a new autosomal dominant complex pleiotropic syndrome with radial ray hypoplasia, hearing impairment, internal ophthalmoplegia, and thrombocytopenia. Am J Med Genet 1980; 6:25–29. * †

Sammito V, et al.: IVIC syndrome: report of a second family. Am J Med Genet 1988; 29:875–881. †

Czeizel A, et al.: IVIC syndrome: report of a third family. (Letter) Am J Med Genet 1989; 33:282–283. †

T0007   **Helga V. Toriello**

Ivory exostoses of ear canal
See EAR, EXOSTOSES

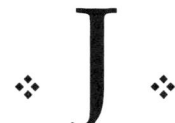 ❖ J ❖

J. Chain
See *LEUKEMIA, ACUTE LYMPHOCYTIC, FAMILIAL*
Jabs syndrome
See *GRANULOMATOSIS-POLYSYNOVITIS, FAMILIAL SYSTEMIC*
Jackson-Weiss craniosynostosis
See *CRANIOSYNOSTOSIS-FOOT DEFECTS, JACKSON-WEISS TYPE*
Jacobs syndrome
See *SYNOVITIS, FAMILIAL HYPERTROPHIC*
Jacobsen syndrome
See *ECTODERMAL DYSPLASIA, HIDROTIC*
also *CHROMOSOME 11, MONOSOMY 11q*
Jadassohn linear nevus sebaceous syndrome
See *NEVUS, EPIDERMAL NEVUS SYNDROME*
Jadassohn-Lewandowsky syndrome
See *NAILS, PACHYONYCHIA CONGENITA*
Jaffe-Lichtenstein disease
See *FIBROUS DYSPLASIA, MONOSTOTIC*
Jansen metaphyseal dysostosis
See *METAPHYSEAL CHONDRODYSPLASIA, TYPE JANSEN*
Jansky-Bielchowsky disease (late infantile NCL or LINCL)
See *NEURONAL CEROID-LIPOFUSCINOSES (NCL)*
Jansky-Bielchowsky-Hagberg disease (late infantile variant of NCL)
See *NEURONAL CEROID-LIPOFUSCINOSES (NCL)*
Janz syndrome
See *SEIZURES, MYOCLONIC, JUVENILE JANZ TYPE*
Japanese-type hereditary amyloidosis
See *AMYLOIDOSIS, TRANSTHYRETIN METHIONINE-30 TYPE*
Jarcho-Levin syndrome
See *SPONDYLOTHORACIC DYSPLASIA*
Jaundice without bilirubin glucuronide in bile
See *UDP-GLUCURONOSYLTRANSFERASE, SEVERE DEFICIENCY TYPE I*
Jaundice, chronic benign
See *HYPERBILIRUBINEMIA, UNCONJUGATED*

JAUNDICE, INTRAHEPATIC CHOLESTATIC, BYLER TYPE   2371

Includes:
Byler disease (Amish kindred)
Cholestasis, progressive idiopathic
Fatal intrahepatic cholestasis
Progressive familial cholestasis

Excludes:
Acidemia, Trihydroxycoprostanic (3275)
Bile ducts, interlobular, nonsyndromic paucity (3277)
Cholestasis, intrahepatic, recurrent, benign (3276)
Hepatitis, neonatal, giant-cell type, nonprogressive
Intrahepatic cholestasis of Pregnancy (ICP) (3278)
Intrahepatic cholestasis, all other recognizable causes of
chronic

Major Diagnostic Criteria: Chronic, progressive cholestasis (as evidenced by jaundice, conjugated hyperbilirubinemia, pruritus, elevated serum bile salt concentration, hypercholesterolemia, and related signs and symptoms) without anatomic obstruction of extrahepatic biliary tract and without other recognizable causes.

Clinical Findings: The cholestasis is unremitting, although it may wax and wane in severity, and leads to progressive biliary cirrhosis. The onset of cholestasis is in the first year, usually in the first month, of life. Death due to hepatic failure or hepatocellular carcinoma occurs in the first or second decades. Usually hepatomegaly and often splenomegaly are present. Pruritus varies in severity; some affected patients exhibit cutaneous mutilation secondary to scratching. Serum bilirubin levels range from 3 to 10 mg/dl early in the course to over 30 mg/dl in the cirrhotic phase. Total serum bile salt concentration is usually between 100 and 200 μM (normal, <10). Hypercholesterolemia is usually mild, i.e., 250–400 mg/dl. Transaminases (ALT and AST) are elevated in the range of 150–500 U/liter and alkaline phosphatase in the range of 400–800 U/liter. Recent observations suggest that a low or normal level of gamma-glutamyl transpeptidase (GGTP), as opposed to high levels in most or all other cholestatic diseases, may be an important diagnostic finding in this disease. Liver biopsy material shows cellular and canalicular cholestasis; variable degrees of lobular disarray, giant cell transformation, and hepatocyte necrosis; and normal to moderately expanded portal areas with small or inapparent bile ducts (sometimes leading to misdiagnosis of a primary ductular hypoplasia syndrome). As the disease progresses, a pattern of micronodular biliary cirrhosis with marked pseudoductular proliferation is observed.

Complications: Cholestasis leads to submicellar concentrations of bile salts in bile, which results in a high incidence of cholecystolithiasis, and in the intestinal lumen, which causes malabsorption of fat and fat-soluble vitamins. All patients have moderate-to-severe growth failure, due to a number of factors: calorie malnutrition, vitamin D-deficient osteomalacia, anorexia secondary to abdominal discomfort, and probable effects of chronic cholestasis on metabolism and utilization of nutrients. Fat-soluble vitamin malabsorption can lead to deficiency states: vitamin D leads to osteomalacia, vitamin E to neuropathy, and vitamin K to prothrombin deficiency.

Cirrhosis with its many complications develops usually after 5–10 years. Hepatoma has developed in several patients in the first or second decades, and is a fatal complication.

Associated Findings: None known.

Etiology: Autosomal recessive inheritance.

Pathogenesis: Primary defect in bile formation leads to reduced bile flow (cholestasis) and retention of bile products. Retained bile products, particularly bile salts, cause hepatomegaly, elevated transaminases, hepatic fibrosis, and cirrhosis.

MIM No.: *21160

CDC No.: 751.880

Sex Ratio: M1:F1

Occurrence: About 75 cases have been reported, but the disease is probably underreported due to confusion with other cholestatic diseases and the absence of specific diagnostic criteria. Byler disease has been documented in the Old Order Amish, and in Greenland Eskimos.

Risk of Recurrence for Patient's Sib:
See Part I, *Mendelian Inheritance*.

Risk of Recurrence for Patient's Child:
See Part I, *Mendelian Inheritance*. To date no affected patients have reproduced. However, the advent of liver transplantation presents the possibility of doing so. In that case, the gene frequency and the risk for recurrence for the patient's child are probably very low, assuming absence of consanguinity.

Age of Detectability: Within the first week of life, if serum bile salt concentration is measured. Clinical detection may be delayed up to one year of age.

Gene Mapping and Linkage: Unknown.

Prevention: None known. Genetic counseling indicated.

Treatment: *Medical:* to increase bile flow: phenobarbital, rifampin; to reduce bile salt concentration: cholestyramine resin; to prevent vitamin deficiencies: supplemental vitamins D, E, and K and close monitoring of vitamin levels.
Surgical: liver transplantation.

Prognosis: All affected patients progress to cirrhosis.

Orthotopic homologous hepatic transplantation corrects the primary defect. However, some of the sequelae of chronic cholestasis, particularly bony abnormalities and neurologic deficits, are not reversible. The prevention of irreversible complications and the early detection of hepatoma improve the prognosis after transplantation.

Detection of Carrier: Unknown.

References:
Clayton RJ, et al.: Byler disease: fatal familial intrahepatic cholestasis in an Amish kindred. Am J Dis Child 1969; 117:112–124.
Ugarte N, Gonzales-Cruss F: Hepatoma in siblings with progressive familial cholestatic cirrhosis of childhood. Am J Clin Pathol 1981; 76:172–177.
Nakagawa M, et al.: Familial intrahepatic cholestasis associated with progressive neuromuscular disease and vitamin E deficiency. J Pediatr Gastro Nutr 1984; 3:385–389.
Nielsen I-M, et al.: Fatal familial cholestatic syndrome in Greenland Eskimo children. Acta Paediat Scand 1986; 75:1010–1016.

WH007   **Peter F. Whitington**

Jaundice, prolonged obstructive
See ALPHA(1)-ANTITRYPSIN DEFICIENCY
Jaw excursion, limitation of
See CAMPTODACTYLY-TRISMUS SYNDROME

JAW, NEUROECTODERMAL PIGMENTED TUMOR   0711

Includes:
Heterotropic pigmented retinoblastoma
Melanotic ameloblastoma
Melanotic neuroectodermal tumor of infancy
Melanotic odontoma
Melanotic progonoma
Neuroectodermal pigmented tumor
Pigmented adamantinoma
Pigmented ameloblastoma
Pigmented epulis, congenital
Progonoma
Retinal anlage tumor
Retinal choristoma

Excludes:
Ameloblastoma
Oral melanoma
Oral nevi
Teeth, epulis, congenital (0360)

Major Diagnostic Criteria: Must be differentiated by microscopic examination. Nonencapsulated infiltrating tumor characterized by moderately vascularized fibrous connective tissue stroma, with tumor cells aggregated into alveolar spaces. Cells are cuboidal about alveolar periphery and decrease in size centrally. Nuclei are round, deeply basophilic, and surrounded by scanty cytoplasm. Pigment may be prominent or inconspicuous. Special stains dramatize presence of melanin pigment.

In view of the X-ray appearance of the irregular, ragged lytic lesion of bone and the clinical feature of rapid growth, care must be exercised to prevent an erroneous diagnosis of malignant neoplasm. Histopathologic examination should precede therapy whenever a pigmented neuroectodermal tumor of infancy is included in the differential diagnosis.

Clinical Findings: Nonulcerated, rapidly growing tumor in jaws of infants almost invariably less than one year of age. It locally destroys bone and displaces teeth. Most cases occur in the maxilla (80%), occasionally in the mandible (10%), both exhibiting midline predilection. Occasionally (10%) other sites are involved: including anterior fontanel, shoulder, and epididymis. High levels of urinary vanilmandelic acid excretion, which returned to normal upon removal of the tumor, were reported in two patients.

Complications: The natural history of untreated lesions is not known, however, disfigurement, displacement of associated teeth, and possible problem of impaired sucking, can occur.

Associated Findings: None known.

Etiology: Hypotheses include: *Neuroectodermal*: arises from cells of the neural crest that migrate to the site of tumor origin during embryogenesis. Identification of high urinary excretion of vanilmandelic acid, which falls to normal upon tumor removal, supports this hypothesis. *Odontogenic*: histogenic hypothesis. *Melanocarcinoma*: original concept, now discredited.

Pathogenesis: The tumor is often present at birth, and grows rapidly destroying bone locally, and displacing associated teeth.

Sex Ratio: M1:F1

Occurrence: Undetermined but presumed rare.

Risk of Recurrence for Patient's Sib: No increased risk reported.

Risk of Recurrence for Patient's Child: Unknown.

Age of Detectability: Often present at birth, almost invariably recognized during the first year of life.

Gene Mapping and Linkage: Unknown.

Prevention: None known. Genetic counseling indicated.

Treatment: Surgical removal indicated.

Prognosis: After surgical removal (slightly in excess of 10% have been irradiated as well), recurrence has occurred in 20% of the treated cases. Recurrences have been associated only with maxillary or mandibular examples of the tumor. Except for local surgical disfigurement, prognosis is excellent. A single incidence of malignant transformation has been noted.

Detection of Carrier: Unknown.

References:
Kerr DA, Pullon PA: A study of the pigmented tumors of jaws of infants (melanotic ameloblastoma, retinal anlage tumor, progonoma). Oral Surg 1964; 18:759.
Borello ED, Gorlin RJ: Melanotic neuroectodermal tumor of infancy - a neoplasm of neural crest origin: report of a case associated with high urinary excretion of vanilmandelic acid. Cancer 1966; 19:196.
Brekke JH, Gorlin RJ: Melanotic neuroectodermal tumor of infancy. J Oral Surg 1975; 33:858.
Dehner LP, et al.: Malignant melanotic neuroectodermal tumors of infancy. A clinical pathologic ultrastructural and tissue culture study. Cancer 1979; 43:1389.

R0039   **Nathaniel H. Rowe**
SA029   **John J. Sauk**

JAW-WINKING SYNDROME   0548

Includes:
Eyelid, winking upon movement of jaw
Marcus Gunn phenomenon
Maxillopalpebral synkinesis
Palpebromaxillary synergy, hereditary
Pterygoid-levator synkinesis
Ptosis, synkinetic
Synkinetic ptosis

Excludes:
Marcus-Gunn phenomenon of the pupil
Reversed Marcus Gunn phenomenon
Winking-jaw phenomenon of Wartenberg

Major Diagnostic Criteria: Retraction of the upper eye lid upon movement of the jaw.

Clinical Findings: The classic Marcus Gunn syndrome, which is the most common, consists of unilateral ptosis at rest with elevation of the apparently paretic upper lid to a level higher than that of the other eye upon opening the mouth, or lateral movement of the lower jaw. Usually if the jaw is deviated to the affected side the ptosis increases, but if deviated to the opposite side maximal retraction occurs. Typically the ptosis recurs if the mouth is held open. Affected individuals habitually open the mouth when looking upwards. The phenomenon occurs more frequently on the left than the right. It rarely occurs bilaterally. Multiple variations of the classic syndrome have been described. Examples are retraction only with side-to-side motion of the jaw, or with masseter function, or with inspiration, or with eye movements.

Complications: Basically cosmetic.

Associated Findings: Amblyopia (50–60%), double elevatory palsy (25%), anisometropia (25–30%), and superior rectus muscle palsy (23%).

Etiology: Unknown except for those families in which an irregular autosomal dominant inheritance pattern exists. Multiple occurrences in the sibship of only one generation may represent autosomal recessive inheritance.

Pathogenesis: The pathogenesis has not been definitely established and many theories have been set forth. Anomalous connections or a reflex arc between the nuclei of the external pterygoid muscle (mesencephalic root C_5) and the levator palpebris (C_3) have been postulated. Antidromic nerve impulses and spread of stimulus rather than direct connection between nuclei also have been implicated.

MIM No.: 15460

CDC No.: 742.800

Sex Ratio: M1:F1

Occurrence: At least 200 cases have been documented. It has been estimated as the cause of 2–5% of congenital ptosis.

Risk of Recurrence for Patient's Sib:
See Part I, *Mendelian Inheritance.*

Risk of Recurrence for Patient's Child:
See Part I, *Mendelian Inheritance.*

Age of Detectability: Soon after birth, since the phenomenon is most noticeable during sucking.

Gene Mapping and Linkage: Unknown.

Prevention: None known. Genetic counseling indicated.

Treatment: Usually unwarranted. Some success has been reported with section of the motor root of the trigeminal nerve. More experience is available using the facial sling procedure involving sectioning the levator aponeurosis and using a fasciala sling to the brow musculature to produce voluntary lid control. Frequently, the identical procedure must be performed on the normal lid as well to produce a symmetrical result and acceptable appearance.

Prognosis: The condition usually grows slowly less noticeable with age.

Detection of Carrier: Unknown.

References:
Falls HF, et al.: Three cases of Marcus Gunn phenomenon in two generations. Am J Ophthalmol 1949; 32:53–59.
Duke-Elder S: System of ophthalmology. vol. 3, pt. 2. Congenital deformities. St. Louis: CV Mosby, 1963:900–902.
Kuder GG, Laws HW: Hereditary Marcus Gunn phenomenon. Can J Ophthalmol 1968; 3:97–105.
Bullock JD: Marcus-Gunn jaw-winking ptosis: classification and surgical management. J Pediat Ophthalmol Strab 1980; 17:375–379.
Doucet TW, Crawford JS: The quantification, natural course, and surgical results in 57 eyes with Marcus Gunn (jaw-winking) syndrome. Am J Ophthalmol 1981; 92:702–707.
Pratt SG, et al.: The Marcus Gunn phenomenon: a review of 71 cases. Ophthalmol 1984; 91:27–29.

DE034
BE026

Monte A. Del Monte
Donald R. Bergsma

Jaws, intraosseous fibrous swelling
See CHERUBISM
Jaws/mouth (small or absent)-low set ears
See AGNATHIA-MICROSTOMIA-SYNOTIA

JEJUNAL ATRESIA   2934

Includes:
Apple peel syndrome
Christmas tree syndrome

Excludes:
Jejunal atresia, mucosal
Jejunal atresia, fibrous cord
Jejunal atresia with large, V-shaped defect in mesentery
Pyloroduodenal atresia, hereditary (2617)

Major Diagnostic Criteria: Complete high jejunal occlusion. The jejunum ends blindly in a dilated proximal loop, 3–4 cm beyond the ligament of Treitz.

Clinical Findings: Bilious vomiting, epigastric distention, and absence of stools in the neonatal period. Plain X-rays of the abdomen show a complete high jejunal occlusion. At laparotomy, the jejunum ends blindly in a dilated proximal loop. The bowel is incompletely rotated and is foreshortened, with a large mesenteric gap, precariously supplied in retrograde fashion by anastomotic arcades from a mesenteric artery.

Complications: If not corrected, the patient will die of starvation.

Associated Findings: None known.

Etiology: Autosomal recessive inheritance.

Pathogenesis: Unknown.

MIM No.: *24360

CDC No.: 751.190

Sex Ratio: M1:F1

Occurrence: At least 57 cases have been reported in the English literature.

Risk of Recurrence for Patient's Sib:
See Part I, *Mendelian Inheritance.*

Risk of Recurrence for Patient's Child:
See Part I, *Mendelian Inheritance.*

Age of Detectability: During the neonatal period. Prenatal detection of intestinal obstruction may be possible by testing the amniotic fluid disaccharidases, which are deficient in affected fetuses. Results of low disaccharidase values are best followed by diagnostic ultrasound studies and, when necessary, amniography for more certain delineation of the defect.

Gene Mapping and Linkage: Unknown.

Prevention: None known. Genetic counseling indicated.

Treatment: Surgical treatment is usually successful.

Prognosis: Good, in the majority of cases.

Detection of Carrier: Unknown.

Special Considerations: In all cases of jejunal atresia it is very important to keep the possibility of the hereditary type in mind, for proper counseling of the family. Thus, if a new child is born, the investigations can be done on time for proper and immediate surgical intervention, if necessary. This may be life-saving.

References:
Mishalany HG, Najjar FB: Familial jejunal atresia: three cases in one family. J Pediatr 1968; 73:753–755. *
Blyth HM, Dickson JAS: Apple peel syndrome (congenital intestinal atresia): a family study of seven index patients. J Med Genet 1969; 6:275–277.
Rickham PP, Karplus M: Familial and hereditary intestinal atresia. Helv Paediatr Acta 1971; 26:561–564.
Grosfeld JL: Jejunoileal atresia and stenosis. In: Welch KJ, et al., Pediatric surgery, ed 4. Chicago: Year Book Medical, 1986:838–848.
Seashore JH, et al.: Familial apple peel jejunal atresia: surgical, genetic, and radiographic aspects. Pediatrics 1987; 80:540–544.

DE030
MI039

Vazken M. Der Kaloustian
Henry G. Mishalany

Jejunoileal atresia and stenosis
See INTESTINAL ATRESIA OR STENOSIS
Jervell syndrome
See CARDIO-AUDITORY SYNDROME
Jeune syndrome
See ASPHYXIATING THORACIC DYSPLASIA
Jewish amyloidosis
See AMYLOIDOSIS, ASHKENAZI TYPE
Job syndrome
See IMMUNODEFICIENCY, HYPER IgE TYPE

JOHANSON-BLIZZARD SYNDROME 2026

Includes:
Ectodermal dysplasia-exocrine pancreatic insufficiency
Malabsorption-ectodermal dysplasia-nasal alar hypoplasia
Nasal alar hypoplasia-hypothyroidism-pancreatic achylia-deafness

Excludes:
Cranio-carpo-tarsal dysplasia, whistling face type (0223)
Ectodermal dysplasias, without malabsorption, other
Oculo-dento-osseous dysplasia (0737)
Oculo-mandibulo-facial syndrome (0738)

Major Diagnostic Criteria: Abnormal craniofacies, including hypoplasia of the nasal alae, hypodontia, sparse hair; malabsorption due to exocrine pancreatic deficiency; and growth and psychomotor retardation.

Clinical Findings: The striking craniofacial features include absent or small alae nasi and short nose from base to tip, creating a beak-like appearance; midline scalp defects over the posterior and/or anterior fontanelles; nasolacrimo-cutaneous fistulae; maxillary hypoplasia; and microcephaly. Hypodontia and microdontia are common. Deciduous and permanent teeth that are present are small, conical, and widely spaced. Hair is sparse, coarse, and dry, with abnormal patterning. There is often an upsweep of frontal hair with extension of the hairline onto the sides of the forehead. Alopecia may be present over the vertex and/or occiput at former site of congenital scalp defects. Imperforate anus or anal stenosis is common. Occasional genito-urinary abnormalities include micropenis, large clitoris, double vagina or vulvar fistula, single urogenital orifice, and various grades of hydronephrosis.

During the first year, failure to thrive due to malabsorption is typical. Laboratory studies of stool and duodenal aspirate document a lipolytic, proteolytic, and amylolytic deficiency of the exocrine pancreas.

Hypotonia and neurosensory deafness are common. Bone age is delayed.

Complications: Respiratory infections appear to be common. Although most cases described have been mentally retarded, a few patients have been mentally normal.

Associated Findings: Asplenia; congenital heart defects including **Heart, transposition of great vessels**, **Pulmonary valve, atresia**, anomalous pulmonary venous return, common atrium, and hypothyroidism.

Etiology: Autosomal recessive inheritance. Sibship recurrence and consanguinity have been documented.

Pathogenesis: Karyotype is normal. Glucose tolerance curve is normal, suggesting normal islet cell function. Sweat chloride is also normal. With thorough studies, all exocrine pancreatic function is deficient. Normal amylase levels from duodenal aspirate is probably salivary in origin.

Autopsy has shown a small thyroid filled with colloid, complete replacement of the pancreas with adipose tissue, with few normal islets, and a brain with abnormal gyri formation and cortical neuronal organization, or structurally normal but small.

MIM No.: *24380

POS No.: 3269

Sex Ratio: Presumably M1:F1.

Occurrence: More than two dozen cases have been reported.

Risk of Recurrence for Patient's Sib:
See Part I, *Mendelian Inheritance.*

Risk of Recurrence for Patient's Child:
See Part I, *Mendelian Inheritance.* Possible infertility with delayed menarche was reported in one case.

Age of Detectability: At birth.

Gene Mapping and Linkage: Unknown.

Prevention: None known. Genetic counseling indicated.

Treatment: Replacement of pancreatic exocrine enzymes and thyroxine. Plastic reconstruction of the ala nasi has been described.

The severity of the imperforate anus or anal stenosis is variable, and may require an anoplasty or colostomy.

Medical treatment consists of a protein hydrolysate diet and oral pancreatin. The malabsorption syndrome of hypoproteinemic edema, chronic anemia, and slow weight gain responds to pancreatic enzyme replacement. Fat soluble vitamins should be monitored. However, the severe growth failure persists. The hypothyroidism, if present, may require more than the usual thyroxine dose because of associated poor intestinal absorption.

Prognosis: Shortened life expectancy because of failure to thrive, frequency of infection, and occasional cardiac defects.

Detection of Carrier: Unknown.

References:
Johanson AJ, Blizzard RM: A syndrome of congenital aplasia of the alae nasi, deafness, hypothyroidism, dwarfism, absent permanent teeth, and malabsorption. J Pediat 1971; 79:982–987. * †
Fox JW, et al.: Surgical correction of the absent nasal alae of the Johanson-Blizzard syndrome. Plast Reconstr Surg 1976; 57:484–486. †
Day DW, Israel JN: Johanson-Blizzard syndrome. BD:OAS VI(B). New York: March of Dimes Birth Defects Foundation, 1978:275–287. * †
Mardini MK, et al.: Johanson-Blizzard syndrome in a large inbred kindred with three involved members. Clin Genet 1978; 14:247–250.
Towne P, White M: Identity of two syndromes: proteolytic, lipolytic and amylolytic deficiency of the exocrine pancreas with congenital anomalies. Am J Dis Child 1981; 135:248–250. †
Zerres K, Holtgrave E-A: The Johanson-Blizzard syndrome: report of a new case with special reference to dentition and a review of the literature. Clin Genet 1986; 30:177–183. * †
Moeschler JB, et al.: The Johanson-Blizzard syndrome: a second report of full autopsy findings. Am J Med Genet 1987; 26:133–138.
Gould NS, et al.: Johanson-Blizzard syndrome: clinical and pathological findings in 2 sibs. Am J Med Genet 1989; 33:194–199. * †

J0010

Virginia P. Johnson

Johnson neuroectodermal syndrome
See ALOPECIA-ANOSMIA-DEAFNESS-HYPOGONADISM, JOHNSON TYPE
Joint contractures-cleft palate-Dandy-Walker malformation
See AASE-SMITH SYNDROME

Joint defects with X-linked mental retardation
See X-LINKED MENTAL RETARDATION-SKELETAL DYSPLASIA
Joint dislocations, multiple, lethal, Larsen-like
See LARSEN SYNDROME, LETHAL TYPE
Joint dislocations-unusual facies-skeletal abnormalities
See LARSEN SYNDROME
Joint dislocations-wormian bones-short stature
See SHORT STATURE-WORMIAN BONES-JOINT DISLOCATIONS
Joint hyperextensibility-facial dysmorphia syndrome
*See FACIAL DYSMORPHIA-JOINT HYPEREXTENSIBILITY
SYNDROME*
Joint hypermobility-cutis laxa-retarded development
See CUTIS LAXA-DELAYED DEVELOPMENT-LIGAMENTOUS LAXITY
Joint instability, familial
See ARTICULAR HYPERMOBILITY, FAMILIAL
Joint laxity, Ehlers-Danlos syndrome
See EHLERS-DANLOS SYNDROME
Joint laxity, familial
See ARTICULAR HYPERMOBILITY, FAMILIAL
Joint laxity-retarded development-cutis laxa
See CUTIS LAXA-DELAYED DEVELOPMENT-LIGAMENTOUS LAXITY
Joints, multiple congenital articular rigidities
See ARTHROGRYPOSES

JOINTS, OSTEOCHONDRITIS DISSECANS   0774

Includes:
Aseptic necrosis
Epiphyseal osteochondritides
Freiburg disease (head of second metatarsal)
Juvenile osteochondritides
Keinbock (carpal semilunar)
Kohler disease (navicular)
Legg-Calve-Perthes disease (capital femoral epiphysis)
Osgood-Schlatter disease (tibial tubercle)
Panner disease (capitellum of humerus)
Perthes disease
Scheuermann disease (vertebrae)
Sever disease (os calcis)
Sindig-Larsen-Johansson disease (patella)
Thiemann disease (phalangeal epiphyses)

Excludes:
Juvenile osteochondroses secondary to trauma or systemic
    disease
Epiphyseal dysplasia, multiple (0358)

Major Diagnostic Criteria: Characteristic clinical presentation, anatomical site, and X-ray appearance.

Clinical Findings: May be asymptomatic or have pain, swelling, and/or limitation of motion.

Complications: Unknown.

Associated Findings: None known.

Etiology: Mostly sporadic, of unknown etiology. A few by autosomal dominant inheritance.

Pathogenesis: Unknown.

MIM No.: *16580, 15060, 18144

Sex Ratio: In the capital femoral epiphysis M4:F1; in the second metatarsal M1:F4; in the elbow M8:F1; in familial cases M1:F1.

Occurrence: Incidence of Perthes disease 1:4,750 live births in South Wales. The osteochondritides are undetermined but presumed rare.

Risk of Recurrence for Patient's Sib:
See Part I, *Mendelian Inheritance.* In the absence of a positive family history, empiric recurrence risks are low (under 1% in Perthes disease).

Risk of Recurrence for Patient's Child:
See Part I, *Mendelian Inheritance.* In the absence of a positive family history, empiric recurrence risks are low (about 3% in Perthes disease).

Age of Detectability: Tend to develop after the appearance of the bony epiphyseal nucleus, thus uncommon in infancy or after adolescence.

Gene Mapping and Linkage: Unknown.

Prevention: None known. Genetic counseling indicated.

Treatment: Orthopedic intervention may be necessary.

Prognosis: Normal life span. May leave some residual disability.

Detection of Carrier: Unknown.

Special Considerations: There is nosological overlap between osteochondritis dissecans and the other juvenile osteochondroses. Furthermore, the conditions in these categories are probably separate entities, each with its own specific pathogenesis. Abnormal development of epiphyses, especially the capital femoral epiphysis, which occurs in several skeletal dysplasias, may lead to problems in the differential diagnosis.

References:
Linden B: The incidence of osteochondritis dissecans in the condyles of the femur. Acta Orthop Scand 1976; 47:664–667.
Petrie PWF: Aetiology of osteochondritis dissecans: failure to establish a familial background. J Bone Joint Surg 1977; 59B:366–367.
Halal F, et al.: Dominant inheritance of Scheuermann's juvenile kyphosis. Am J Dis Child 1978; 132:1105–1107.
Andrew TA, et al.: Familial osteochondritis dissecans and dwarfism. Acta Orthop Scand 1981; 52:519–523.
Phillips HO, Grubb SA: Familial multiple osteochondritis dissecans. J Bone Joint Surg 1985; 67A:155–156.
Hall DJ: Genetic aspects of Perthe's disease: a critical review. Clin Orthop 1986; 209:100–114.

C0066   **J. Michael Connor**

Joints, stiff-dwarfism-eye defects
See DWARFISM-STIFF JOINTS
Jones syndrome
See GINGIVAL FIBROMATOSIS-DEAFNESS, JONES TYPES
Jorgenson syndrome
See ECTODERMAL DYSPLASIA, BASAN TYPE
Joseph disease
See MACHADO-JOSEPH DISEASE

JOUBERT SYNDROME   2908

Includes:
Cerebellar parenchymal disorder, type IV
Cerebellar vermis agenesis, familial
Cerebellar vermis agenesis-neurologic abnormalities
Cerebelloparenchymal disorder IV
Chorioretinal coloboma-Joubert syndrome
Hyperpnea, episodic-abnormal eye movement-ataxia-
    retardation
Joubert-Boltshauser syndrome
Kidneys, cystic-retinal aplasia-Joubert syndrome
Polydactyly-Joubert syndrome
Retinal aplasia-cystic kidneys-Joubert syndrome

Excludes:
Cerebellar agenesis (2011)
Hydrocephaly (0481)
Mouth, wide-intermittent over breathing-mental retardation
Oro-palatal-digital syndrome, Varadi type (2368)
Tectocerebellar dysraphism, isolated-occipital encephalocele
Vermis agenesis (2106)

Major Diagnostic Criteria: Partial or complete absence of the cerebellar vermis is seen in all patients. Pneumoencephalography or CT scan shows an enlarged fourth ventricle communicating with a posterior fossa cyst and abnormally high positioning of the tentorium cerebelli. Alternating tachypnea and apnea, opsoclonus-like eye movements, hypotonia, and mental retardation are also important clinical features.

Clinical Findings: Tachypnea, often likened to the "panting of a dog," in excess of 100 respirations/min, alternating with usually brief periods of apnea, is seen soon after birth. Although not usually associated with respiratory distress, cyanosis, bradycardia, and even death have been noted during the apneic phase. The abnormal respiratory pattern (which resembles cluster breathing and does not show the waxing and waning pattern of Cheyne-Stokes respiration) often subsides after several months. Tachypnea and apnea have been noted while both awake and asleep; tachypnea has been noted during both REM and non-REM sleep, but apnea seems to occur only in non-REM sleep. The opsoclonus-like eye movements may likewise subside, or may persist. Strabismus is frequent. Developmental delay and mental retardation tend to be profound, but two cases are described in which development reverted to normal. Truncal ataxia, as well as wide-based gait, dystonia, athetoid movements, and tongue protrusion are common.

Complications: Death associated with apneic episodes. Blindness. Seizures.

Associated Findings: Dysarthria has been noted in two cases. Retinal colobomas have been noted in eight cases (all male). **Retina, amaurosis congenita, Leber type** has occurred in six cases. Occipital neural tube defects, mostly **Meningocele**, were found in 13 cases.

Other CNS defects include agenesis of the corpus callosum, unsegmented midbrain tectum, brainstem dysplasia, heterotopias, polymicrogyria, and hypoplasia of the cerebellar hemispheres. Less common findings are seizures, hemifacial spasms, **Polydactyly, Syndactyly, Camptodactyly**, renal cysts, and club foot. No consistent pattern of facial dysmorphism has been described. A sibship with features of **Smith-Lemli-Opitz syndrome, Meckel syndrome**, and Joubert syndromes has been described (Casamassima et al, 1987).

Etiology: Autosomal recessive inheritance.

Pathogenesis: Abnormal fusion of the cerebellar plates at the tectum of the fourth ventricle has been postulated. As this process proceeds in a rostal to caudal direction, it is the inferoposterior portion of the cerebellar vermis that is absent in cases of partial agenesis. Secondary disruption of this fusion has also been postulated. The abnormal respiratory pattern may be due to lack of inhibition of the reticular activating system or to an accompanying brainstem dysplasia.

MIM No.: *21330

POS No.: 3593

Sex Ratio: M2.5:F1 observed.

Occurrence: More than 45 cases have been described in the literature.

Risk of Recurrence for Patient's Sib:
See Part I, *Mendelian Inheritance.*

Risk of Recurrence for Patient's Child:
See Part I, *Mendelian Inheritance.* No affected individuals are known to have reproduced.

Age of Detectability: During the neonatal period. At least one case of prenatal diagnosis has been accomplished by comparison of fetal cranial ultrasound to affected sibs' CT scans.

Gene Mapping and Linkage: Unknown.

Prevention: None known. Genetic counseling indicated.

Treatment: Symptomatic for apnea and seizures.

Prognosis: Death has occurred from ages less than one month to 4 1/2 years of age. Survivors tend to be profoundly retarded.

Detection of Carrier: Unknown.

Special Considerations: Agenesis of the vermis itself does not account for the clinical features, as isolated agenesis of the vermis is usually asymptomatic. A number of patients have been described who, in addition to the cerebellar defects and typical symptomatology, have other features which would suggest either variable expression in or heterogeniety of this disorder. Eight males with chorioretinal colobomas may represent a distinct, possibly X-linked recessive entity. Also, Joubert syndrome with retinal aplasia and cystic kidneys (King et al, 1984), Joubert syndrome with polydactyly (Egger et al, 1982), and the cases of Casamassima et al (1987), may represent distinct autosomal recessive conditions.

References:
Joubert M, et al.: Familial agenesis of the cerebellar vermis: a syndrome of episodic hyperpnea, abnormal eye movements, ataxia, and retardation. Neurology 1969; 19:813–825. *
Pfeiffer RA, et al.: Nosology of congenital non-progressive cerebellar ataxia. Neuropediatr 1974; 5:91–102.
Boltshauser E, et al.: Joubert syndrome: clinical and polygraphic observations in a further case. Neuropediatrics 1981; 12:181–191.
Egger J, et al.: Joubert-Boltshauser syndrome with polydactyly in siblings. J Neurol Neurosurg Psych 1982; 45: 737–739.
Aicardi J, et al.: Le syndrome de Joubert: a propos de cinq observations. Arch Fr Pediatr 1983; 40:625–629.
Campbell S, et al.: The prenatal diagnosis of Joubert's syndrome of familial agenesis of the cerebellar vermis. Prenatal Diagn 1984; 4:391–395.
King MD, et al.: Joubert's syndrome with retinal dysplasia: neonatal tachypnea as the clue to a genetic brain-eye malformation. Arch Dis Child 1984; 59:709–718. †
Casamassima AC, et al.: A new syndrome with features of the Smith-Lemli-Opitz and Meckel-Gruber syndromes in a sibship with cerebellar defects. Am J Med Genet 1987; 26:321–326.

CA035   **Anthony C. Casamassima**
PF001   **Rudolf A. Pfeiffer**

JUMPING FRENCHMAN OF MAINE   3270

Includes:
Latah
Myriachit
Ragin' Cajun
Startle syndromes

Excludes:
Epilepsy (all forms)
Hyperekplexia (3260)

Major Diagnostic Criteria: Sudden commands to an affected individual cause excessive startling, often accompanied by jumping, swearing, and other complex behavioral phenomena.

Clinical Findings: The syndrome consists of an exaggerated startle response to sudden acoustic and tactile stimuli accompanied by complex behavioral phenomena, including echolalia, echopraxia, and "forced obedience." Echolalia is involuntary repetition of words, echopraxia is involuntary imitation of gestures, and forced obedience is the allegedly involuntary execution of commands. All of these phenomena are reported in "jumpers" when the stimulus (phrase, command, or gesture) is presented suddenly and forcefully.

Jumping Frenchman of Maine differs from **Hyperekplexia** in that neonatal rigidity is lacking and the startle response consists of jumping and running about excitedly rather than stiffness and unchecked falling.

Complications: Unknown.

Associated Findings: Shyness and ticklishness are described in some patients.

Etiology: Unknown.

Pathogenesis: It is speculated that "jumpers" may have a genetically determined exaggerated startle response, but that the complex behavioral phenomena are culturally or psychiatrically determined.

The condition may be psychiatric in origin. It displays apparently non-Mendelian familial clustering, and has been reported primarily in individuals from the Moosehead Lake region of Maine.

MIM No.: 24410

Sex Ratio: M1:F<1 (significantly more common in males).

Occurrence: Reported primarily in French-Canadian Lumberjacks from the Moosehead Lake region of Maine, although the reported "Ragin' Cajun" Frenchman of Louisiana (McFarling, 1988) is probably related. It has been argued that the disorder is also identical to *latah* and *myriachit* which are complex startle/behavioral syndromes seen in Malaysia and Siberia, respectively.

Risk of Recurrence for Patient's Sib: Unknown.

Risk of Recurrence for Patient's Child: Unknown.

Age of Detectability: Usually but not always apparent by late adolescence.

Gene Mapping and Linkage: Unknown.

Prevention: None known. Genetic counseling indicated.

Treatment: Sedative-hypnotic agents have not been effective. Change of occupation has been beneficial in some cases.

Prognosis: Symptoms generally diminish with age after the second or third decade.

Detection of Carrier: Unknown.

References:

Beard GM: Remarks upon jumpers or jumping Frenchman. J Nerv Ment Dis 1878; 5:526 only.

Stevens HF: Jumping Frenchmen of Maine. Arch Neurology 1966; 12:311–314.

Hardison JE: Are the Jumping Frenchmen of Maine goosey? J Amer Med Ass 1980; 244:70.

Sainte-Hilaire MH, et al.: Jumping Frenchmen of Maine. Neurology 1986; 36:1269–1271.

McFarling DA: "Ragin' Cajuns": the jumping Frenchman of Louisiana. Neurology 1988; 38(Suppl 1):361 only.

RY001   **Stephen G. Ryan**

Junctional epidermolysis bullosa
  See EPIDERMOLYSIS BULLOSUM, TYPE II
Juvenile diabetes mellitus, mild
  See DIABETES MELLITUS, MATURITY ONSET OF THE YOUNG (MODY)
Juvenile diabetes mellitus-optic atrophy-deafness
  See DIABETES (INSIPIDUS/MELLITUS)-OPTIC ATROPHY-DEAFNESS
Juvenile epithelial corneal dystrophy
  See CORNEAL DYSTROPHY, JUVENILE EPITHELIAL, MEESMANN TYPE
Juvenile macular degeneration, hereditary
  See RETINA, FUNDUS FLAVIMACULATUS
Juvenile myoclonic epilepsy (JME), Janz type
  See SEIZURES, MYOCLONIC, JUVENILE JANZ TYPE
Juvenile or adolescent cystinosis
  See CYSTINOSIS
Juvenile osteochondritides
  See JOINTS, OSTEOCHONDRITIS DISSECANS
Juvenile osteoporosis
  See OSTEOPOROSIS, JUVENILE IDIOPATHIC
Juvenile retinoschisis, X-linked
  See RETINOSCHISIS

❖ K ❖

KABUKI MAKE-UP SYNDROME   2355

Includes:

Niikawa-Kuroki syndrome
Short stature-facial and skeletal defects-mental retardation
Skeletal and facial defects-short stature-mental retardation

Excludes:

Aarskog syndrome (0001)
Coffin-Lowry syndrome (0190)
KBG syndrome (0554)
Robinow syndrome (0876)
Tricho-rhino-phalangeal syndrome, type II (0967)
Weaver syndrome (2036)

Major Diagnostic Criteria: The combination of unusual facial appearance (consisting of long palpebral fissures with eversion of lower palpebrae, highly arched, abnormal eyebrows; long, thick eyelashes; large ears; and depressed nasal tip) skeletal anomalies; abnormal dermatoglyphics, short stature and mental retardation.

Clinical Findings: Long palpebral fissures (100%) and eversion of the lateral one-third of the lower palpebra (98%) are the most characteristic features, being remniscent of the actor's make-up of Kabuki (a Japanese traditional play). Other craniofacial anomalies include sparse, arched eyebrows at their lateral half (88%), prominent, large and malformed ears (85%), depressed nasal tip (79%), short nasal septum (93%), high-arched or cleft palate (63%) and malocclusion of teeth (78%). The fifth fingers are short and incurved (89%). Thoraco-lumbar scoliosis (49%) with or without midline defects of the vertebral body such as sagittal clefts is not

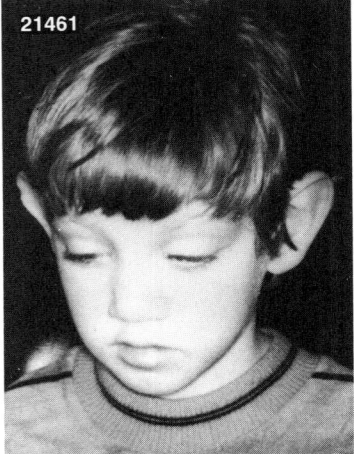

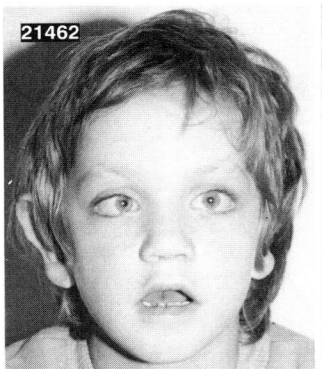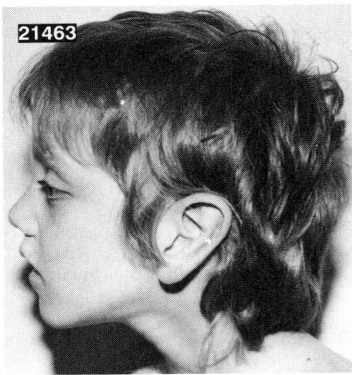

2355B-21461–63: Note large dysmorphic ears, prominent eyes, large nasal bridge, and broad nasal tip.

uncommon. Growth deficiency (73%) usually appears postnatally. Average birth-length is 48.3 cm (49.1 cm after excluding the premature infants) and average birth-weight is 2,868 g (3,153 g and 2,943 g for male and female patients, respectively, excluding the premature). Short stature is evident by 1 year of age, most being at less than two SD below the mean. All patients are mildly to severely mentally retarded. Three-fourths of patients have the fingertip pad which is another characteristic feature. Dermato-glyphic findings include increasing ulnar loop patterns on the fingertip (63%), the absence of the digital triradius c or d (48%), and the presence of the interdigital triradius bc or cd and of hypothenar loops (70%).

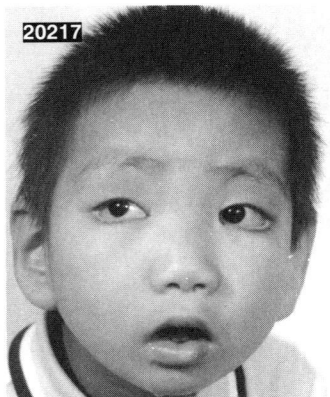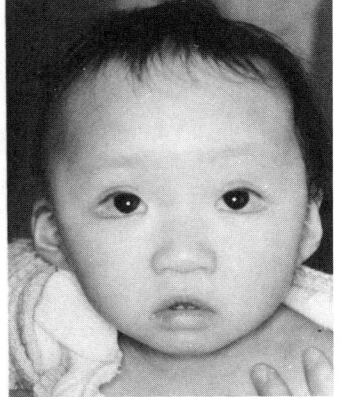

2355A-20217: Note the long palpebral fissures and everted lateral third of the lower eyelid reminiscent of the Kabuki actor's makeup.

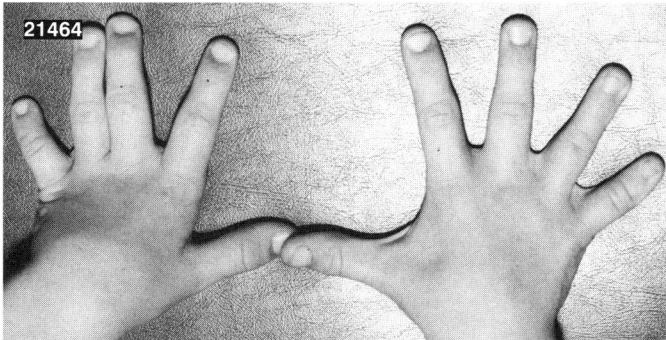

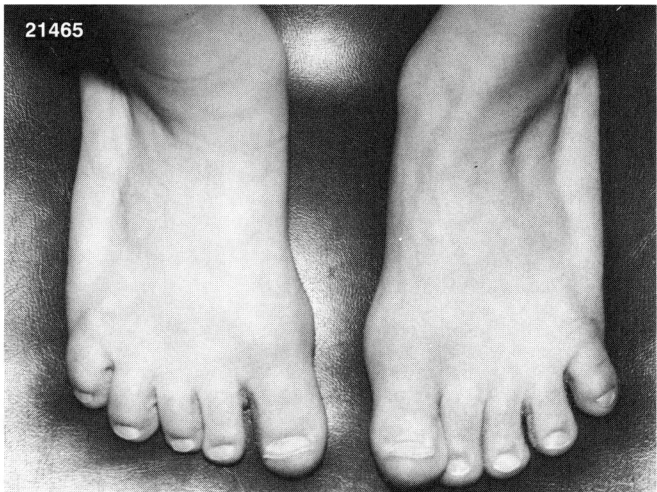

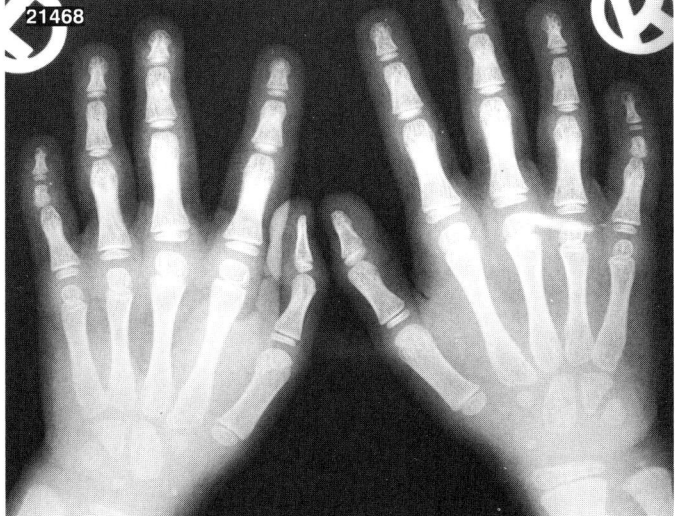

2355C-21464–65: Brachydactyly, syndactyly and broad short nails. 21468: X-ray shows brachydactyly, brachymesophalangy V and retarded bone age.

Complications: Susceptibility to upper respiratory infections or to otitis media in infancy (60%) followed sometimes by hearing impairment. Scoliosis usually develops with age.

Associated Findings: Precocious puberty (23%) in female infants, congenital heart diseases and great vessel anomalies (32%).

Etiology: Most cases have been sporadic. No parental consanguinity has been observed among 62 couples except for four cases. Parental ages are not higher than those of children in general population. There is no common history during pregnancy particular to every case such as radiation exposures, drug intakes, or infections. Karyotypes are normal in most patients, even with high-resolution bandings, except for three patients. One patient had inv(Y)(p11.2q11.23) and the other two had r(X)(p11.2q13) or r(Y)(p11.2q11.2). Niikawa et al (1988) speculated pseudoautosomal dominant inheritance. Halal et al (1989) reported a familial case suggestive of autosomal dominant inheritance.

Pathogenesis: Unknown. The fingertip pads, as observed in three-fourth of patients, have not previously been described in live born individuals and are the remnant of the fingerpads descernible in fetuses at the sixth week of gestation. Normally they begin to regress during the 10th and 12th weeks, to be gradually replaced by the primary dermal ridges that are formed between the 13th and 18th weeks. Therefore, the presence of the pads may reflect a developmental disturbance by the 18th week of gestation.

MIM No.: 14792

POS No.: 3541

Sex Ratio: M1:F1

Occurrence: More than 70 cases have been reported; 62 in Japan, three Canadians from one family, one each from Latin-American, Italian, and Germany, a Libyan Arab, and a United States citizen of English-Irish ancestry.

Risk of Recurrence for Patient's Sib:
See Part I, *Mendelian Inheritance.*

Risk of Recurrence for Patient's Child:
See Part I, *Mendelian Inheritance.*

Age of Detectability: At birth, by physical examination.

Gene Mapping and Linkage: KMS (Kabuki make-up syndrome) is unassigned.

Prevention: None known. Genetic counseling indicated.

Treatment: Orthopedic management may be indicated; physical therapy to prevent scoliosis. Detection and management of possible recurrent otitis.

Prognosis: Unknown.

Detection of Carrier: Unknown.

References:
Kuroki Y, et al.: A new malformation syndrome of long palpebral fissures, large ears, depressed nasal tip, and skeletal anomalies associated with postnatal dwarfism and mental retardation. J Pediatr 1981; 99:570–573.
Niikawa N, et al.: Kabuki make-up syndrome: a syndrome of mental retardation, unusual facies, large and protruding ears, and postnatal growth deficiency. J Pediatr 1981; 99:565–569. * †
Niikawa N, et al.: The dermatoglyphic pattern of the Kabuki make-up syndrome. Clin Genet 1982; 21:315–320.
Kaiser-Kupfer MI, et al.: The Niikawa-Kuroki (Kabuki make-up) syndrome in an American black. Am J Ophthalmol 1986; 102:667–668.
Niikawa N, et al.: Kabuki make-up (Niikawa-Kuroki) syndrome: a study of 62 patients. Am J Med Genet 1988; 31:565–589. *
Halal F, et al.: Autosomal dominant inheritance of the Kabuki make-up (Niikawa-Kuroki) syndrome. Am J Med Genet 1989; 33:376–381.

NI010   **Norio Niikawa**

Kahler disease
See CANCER, MULTIPLE MYELOMA

KALLMANN SYNDROME 2301

Includes:
DeMorsier dysplasia olfactogenitalis
Dysplasia olfactogenitalis of DeMorsier
Hypogonadotropic hypogonadism with anosmia or
hyposmia
Olfactogenital dysplasia

Excludes:
Ataxia-hypogonadism syndrome (0093)
Gonadal dysgenesis (all forms)
Gonadotropin deficiencies (0438)
Hypogonadotropic hypogonadism (2300)
Klinefelter syndrome (0556)

Major Diagnostic Criteria: Luteinizing hormone (LH) and follicle-stimulating hormone (FSH) levels of <5 mIU/ml and anosmia or hyposmia.

Clinical Findings: LH and FSH levels are below the levels of clinical detection with current assay specificity. Biologic effects reflect the amount of total gonadotropin function and usually result in failure of the gonad to function and allow pubertal development. In addition, patients have decreased or absent ability to smell due to absent olfactory bulbs either unilaterally or bilaterally secondary to defective development of the rhinencephalon. Males may be cryptorchid.

In both sexes, somatic anomalies may exist.

Complications: Lack of gonadal stimulation in both sexes results in failure of secondary sexual development and sterility.

Females exhibit estrogen deficiency syndrome, including vaginal atrophy with resultant dyspareunia, osteoporosis, hot flashes after initial estrogen replacement and sudden withdrawal.

Cryptorchidism imposes the risk of decreased spermatogenesis and testicular tumors.

Associated Findings: Borderline normal intelligence; cleft lip and palate; hearing loss and deafness; renal anomalies, particularly unilateral agenesis; cardiac anomalies; diabetes mellitus; choanal atresia; short fourth metacarpal.

Etiology: Genetic heterogeneity. The disorder may be inherited differently in different families; thus, counseling will depend on presence or absence of other affected relatives and their relationship to the proband. Autosomal dominant, X-linked recessive, and autosomal recessive inheritance have all been observed. Relative proportions of the three modes are unknown. There is no evidence that different modes differ clinically.

Pathogenesis: Abnormal development of the rhinencephalon results in interference in the communication of the hypothalamus with the pituitary. Disordered gonadotropin releasing hormone (GNRH) signals to the pituitary result in absence of LH and FSH. In turn, this results in failure of gonadal stimulation and therefore absence of the subsequent development stimulated by gonadal steroids, namely, secondary sex characteristics and reproductive processes.

MIM No.: *14795, *24420, *30870

POS No.: 4216

Sex Ratio: M5:F1

Occurrence: 1:10,000 in males and 1:50,000 in females; prevalence is 1:25 hyposmic or anosmic patients and 1:30 46,XY individuals with hypogonadism.

Risk of Recurrence for Patient's Sib:
See Part I, *Mendelian Inheritance.* Varies with etiology. The disorder may be inherited differently in different families; thus, counseling depends on other affected relatives in the pedigree.

Risk of Recurrence for Patient's Child:
See Part I, *Mendelian Inheritance.* The disorder may be inherited differently in different families; thus counseling depends on other affected relatives in the pedigree. If no other relative is affected, risk could be as high as 50%.

Age of Detectability: During puberty, unless anosmia is diagnosed in childhood.

Gene Mapping and Linkage: KAL (Kallmann syndrome) has been mapped to Xp22.32.
Linkage to HLA has been excluded.

Prevention: None known. Genetic counseling indicated.

Treatment: Hormonal replacement to stimulate development and to maintain integrity of secondary sex characteristics and sexual function.

Gonadal steroid replacement is necessary for the initiation and maintenance of secondary sex characteristics and sexual function.

Fertility may be achieved in both sexes by administration of pulsatile GNRH. Most patients are unresponsive to single-dose GNRH administration unless first primed by multiple doses. Repeated hCG injections in males and hMG in females may also be used to stimulate gametogenesis. Clomiphene citrate is ineffective in treatment of these patients.

Prognosis: Life span is normal. Reproduction depends on the success of therapy to stimulate spermatogenesis or oogenesis.

Detection of Carrier: Unknown.

References:
Santen RJ, Paulsen CA: Hypogonadotropic eunuchoidism: clinical study of the mode of inheritance. J Clin Endocrinol 1973; 36:47–54.
Santen RJ, Paulsen CA: Hypogonadotropic eunuchoidism: gonadal responsiveness to exogenous gonadotropins. J Clin Endocrinol Metab 1973; 36:55–63.
Wegenke JD, et al.: Familial Kallmann syndrome with unilateral renal aplasia. Clin Genet 1975; 7:368–381.
Lieblich JM, et al.: Syndrome of anosmia with hypogonadotropic hypogonadism (Kallmann syndrome): clinical and laboratory studies in 23 cases. Am J Med 1982; 73:506–519.
White BJ, et al.: The syndrome of anosmia with hypogonadotropic hypogonadism: a genetic study of 18 new families and a review. Am J Med Genet 1983; 15:417–435.
Pawlowitzki IH, et al.: Estimating frequency of Kallmann syndrome among anosmic patients. Am J Med Genet 1987; 26:473–479.

CA041 **Sandra Ann Carson**

Kanamycin, fetal effects
See FETAL AMINOGLYCOSIDE OTOTOXICITY
Kandori fleck retina
See RETINA, FLECKED KANDORI TYPE
Kanner disease
See AUTISM, INFANTILE
Kantrex^, fetal effects
See FETAL AMINOGLYCOSIDE OTOTOXICITY
Kaposi dermatosis
See XERODERMA PIGMENTOSUM
Kappa light chain of immunoglobulin
See SERUM ALLOTYPES, HUMAN
Kartagener syndrome
See DEXTROCARDIA-BRONCHIECTASIS-SINUSITIS SYNDROME
Kasabach-Merritt syndrome
See HEMANGIOMA-THROMBOCYTOPENIA SYNDROME
Kasabach-Merritt syndrome (some cases)
See HEMANGIOMAS OF THE HEAD AND NECK
Kaufman syndrome
See OCULO-CEREBRO-FACIAL SYNDROME, KAUFMAN TYPE
Kaufman-McKusick syndrome
See VAGINAL SEPTUM, TRANSVERSE

KBG SYNDROME 0554

Includes: Short stature-facial/skeletal anomalies-retardation-macrodontia

Excludes: Malformation-mental retardation syndromes (other)

Major Diagnostic Criteria: Rounded face, bow-shaped narrow lips, macrodontia, and broad eyebrows in a short, mentally retarded person combined, with X-ray abnormalities of ribs, vertebrae, hips, and hands.

Clinical Findings: Shows great variability in expression. Findings in the majority of patients include shortness of stature (below 3rd percentile), moderate mental retardation, biparietal prominence, brachycephaly, round face, telecanthus (75–90%), broad

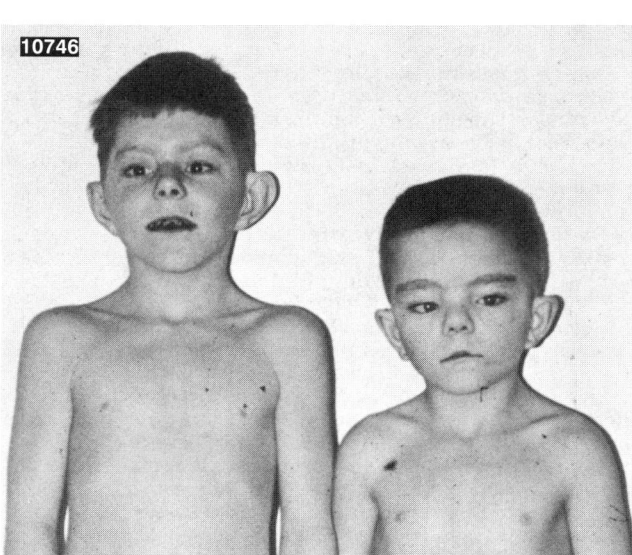

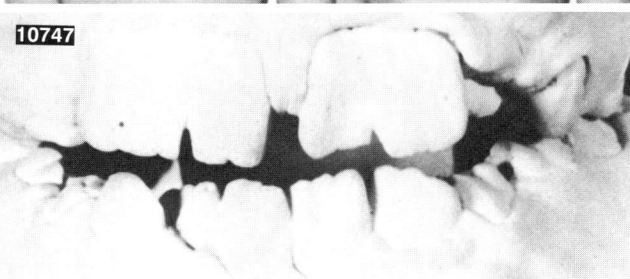

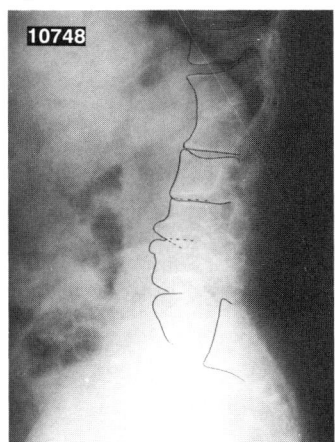
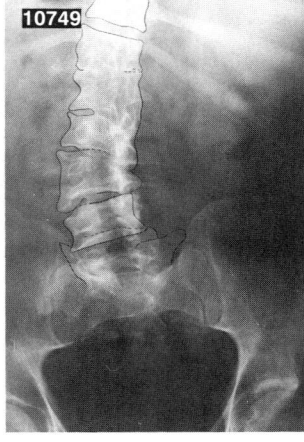

0554-10746: Characteristic round facies with bow-shaped lips and thick eyebrows with pectus excavatum. **10747:** Model of teeth shows macrodontia. **10748-49:** Block vertebrae from T12-L2, deformed and partially collapsed L3-5 vertebral bodies and short femoral necks.

eyebrows, short alveolar ridges, macrodontia, cervical ribs, abnormal vertebrae, short femoral necks, short tubular bones in hands, delayed bone age, syndactyly of toes 2–3, palmar distal axial triradius and simian crease. The EEG was abnormal in two cases investigated. Other significant low-frequency findings include pectus excavatum, hip dysplasia, hexadactyly, and hearing deficit.

Complications: Deformities and pain secondary to skeletal manifestations. Crowding and noneruption of teeth.

Associated Findings: None known.

Etiology: Autosomal dominant inheritance. There have been no instances to date of sibs born to unaffected parents. Sporadic cases may represent new mutations.

Pathogenesis: Undetermined. Many of the manifestations seem related to skeletal defects.

MIM No.: *14805

POS No.: 3270

Sex Ratio: Presumably M1:F1, although actual reports show a greater percentage of males.

Occurrence: At least five kindreds, with nine cases, have been reported.

Risk of Recurrence for Patient's Sib:
See Part I, *Mendelian Inheritance.*

Risk of Recurrence for Patient's Child:
See Part I, *Mendelian Inheritance.*

Age of Detectability: At birth.

Gene Mapping and Linkage: Unknown.

Prevention: None known. Genetic counseling indicated.

Treatment: Supportive and symptomatic; including especially orthopedic surgery for spine or hip problems, dental care, hearing aid, and speech therapy.

Prognosis: Apparently good for life span; dependent on degree of mental retardation and skeletal manifestations.

Detection of Carrier: Unknown.

Special Considerations: The designation KBG syndrome followed from John Opitz's practice of naming conditions after the initials of the affected families' surnames.

References:

Herrmann J, et al.: The KBG syndrome: a syndrome of short stature, characteristic facies, mental retardation, macrodontia and skeletal abnormalities. BD:OAS;XI(5). New York: National Foundation-March of Dimes, 1975:7–18.

Parloir C, et al.: Short stature, craniofacial dysmorphism and dento-skeletal abnormalities in a large kindred: a variant of KBG syndrome or a new mental retardation syndrome. Clin Genet 1977; 12:263–266.

Novembri A, et al.: K.B.G. syndrome: review of the literature and presentation of a case. Arch Put Chir Org Mo 1983; 33:423–430.

Fryns JP, Hospeslagh M: Mental retardation, short stature, minor skeletal anomalies, craniofacial dysmorphism and macrodontia in two sisters and their mother. Clin Genet 1984; 26:69–72.

Tollard I, et al.: Dento-maxillo-facial anomalies in the KBG syndrome. Minerva Stomatol 1984; 33:437–446.

GR021   **Arthur W. Grix**
HE023   **Jürgen Herrmann**

KEARNS-SAYRE DISEASE	2070

Includes:
    Kearns-Sayre syndrome, typical (KSS)
    Kearns-Shy syndrome
    Kiloh-Nevin dystrophy of the external ocular muscles
    Mitochondrial cytopathy
    Mitochondrial encephalomyopathy
    Oculocraniosomatic neuromuscular disease
    Ophthalmoplegia-pigmentary degeneration of retina-cardiomyopathy
    Ophthalmoplegia plus syndrome
    Partial Kearns-Sayre syndrome (PKSS)
    Stephens syndrome (ophthalmoplegia-ataxia-peripheral neuropathy)

Excludes:
    Ataxia
    Diplegia, congenital facial (0376)
    Encephalopathy, necrotizing (0344)

Machado-Joseph disease (2996)
Muscular dystrophy, oculopharyngeal (0692)
**Myopathy-metabolic, mitochondrial cytochrome C oxidase
    deficiency** (2707)
Myopathy, myotubular (0695)
Ocular myasthenia gravis
Ophthalmoplegia, progressive external (0752)
Optic atrophy, Leber type (0579)
Poliodystrophia cerebri progressiva

Major Diagnostic Criteria: Ophthalmoparesis, pigmentary retinal dystrophy, and cardiac conduction disorders are three major necessary clinical symptoms. Since age of onset varies from infancy to advanced adult years, other findings have been variably added through the years: cerebellar ataxia, proximal-axial muscle weakness, hearing loss, and/or vestibular dysfunction. Body undergrowth and polyglandular abnormalities include hypoparathyroid and hypothyroid states. The original laboratory finding of an increased CSF protein often includes abnormal plasma or CSF resting state lactate/pyruvate levels in 50%. Folic acid deficiency in CSF causes a high plasma:CSF ratio. Serum creatine kinase (CK) is normal in 75%, as are standard hematologic and urine examinations. Histologic, structural, or functional defects in mitochondria from muscle or fibroblasts may be identified without specific correlation to clinical findings, as well as many secondary biochemical effects in plasma and CSF, including amino acids and, in urine, organic acids. Plasma and tissue total and free carnitine may be altered. Phosphorus (^{31}P) magnetic resonance spectroscopy (MRS) in the noncarnitine forms of mitochondrial myopathy may show a reduced muscle energy state. Cerebral, cerebellar, and brainstem hypodense lesions occasionally suggesting vascular infarcts are seen by CT scanning, along with calcifications or hypodense lesions of the basal ganglia (50%). Reduced vision (40%) or optic atrophy may be observed as the condition progresses. Seizures are uncommon.

Electrophysiologic responses of retinal function (ERGs), visual-evoked potentials (VERs) with P100 latencies, somatosensory-evoked responses (SSERs), and muscle electromyograms (EMGs), as well as conduction velocities of peripheral motor and sensory nerves, may be altered. Specific saccadic velocity patterns in chronic progressive extraocular muscle paralysis (CPEO) by direct current electrooculogram (dc-EOG) may differentiate disorders of neurophthalmic motility. There is clinical evidence that peripheral neuropathy causes hyporeflexia and sensory loss in a few patients.

Clinical Findings: Often ptosis and extraocular motor abnormalities are the presenting symptom under age 20 years, and not infrequently under age five years, especially CPEO. Onset of an asymmetric ocular paresis preceded by ptosis then leads to total ophthalmoplegia without a pupillary defect in 90% of patients. A pigmentary retinopathy of fine, diffuse, granular character, centrally located, in some patients followed by CPEO, occurs over decades. Diminished visual acuity or night blindness occurs in 40% with rare corneal dystrophic opacities. Saccadic and smooth pursuit extraocular eye movements are restricted and slowed, causing a pendular opticokinetic nystagmus. Palatal and tongue movements may be limited, causing dysarthric speech and mild dysphagia accentuated by cerebellar involvement. Tongue bulk may be reduced, but fasciculations are not observed. Bilateral peripheral facial paralysis and sensorineural deafness may be evident initially in 54% of patients. Vestibular dysfunction occurs in one-third of patients. Temporal and masseter muscle bulk and strength are normal. Neck muscle strength reduction occurs especially in the flexor group, including the sternocleidomastoids, and may be detected early. The distribution of muscle involvement may be similar to **Muscular dystrophy, facio-scapulo-humeral**; **Muscular dystrophy, oculopharyngeal**; and **Diplegia, congenital facial**.

Facial sensation and corneal reflexes are intact. Occasionally abnormal facial (snout) and head-neck reflexes (head retraction) occur. Although myopathic extraocular muscle changes are observed, the structural changes in the central nervous system suggest that the pathogenesis of CPEO is of neurogenic origin. Proximal muscle paresis and hypotonia are seldom prominent initially. Weakness is proximal and especially axial. Upper extremities are involved first, then the shoulder-neck region, and later the proximal lower extremities, causing great difficulty in walking. Muscle bulk is symmetrically reduced, proximally early in life, suggesting a dysmorphic appearance as in a congenital myopathy (myotubular or centronuclear forms). The clinical findings are of a myopathic process without distal atrophy, fasciculations, or symptomatic or percussion myotonia, although myotonia and muscle hypertrophy have been observed. Motor function examination reveals cerebellar ataxia (40–70%), with truncal titubation, action tremors, occasionally "wing-beating," extremity dysmetria, dysdiadochokinesia, and extrapyramidal movements (chorea or dystonia) occurring singly or in combination.

Speech and gait slowly deteriorate with weakness as does coordination, limiting ambulation. A static or subtly progressive encephalopathy in children presents as mental retardation. Cognitive, intellectual, and behavioral deficiencies may be identified by history and neurologic and psychologic examination (40%). Intellectual function is normal (80%) in many. Sensory examination is most often normal. Reflexes are quite variable, with hypoactive responses and significant muscle weakness. Hyperactive reflexes, including bilateral Babinski signs, occur in the progressive disorder. Other systemic symptoms and signs are common, especially in partial Kearns-Sayre syndrome (PKSS). Cardiac conduction defects, including complete atrioventricular (AV) heart block appearing early, may remain asymptomatic for decades. Most patients are affected with serious cardiac involvement, including sudden death (in about two-thirds). The cardiomyopathy may be related to carnitine deficiency. Cardiac-related syncope is found in about one-half. Disordered endocrine system function may be polyglandular, including hypoparathyroidism, hypothyroidism, diabetes, pubertal delay, and hypercholesterolemia. Generalized seizures occur with hypocalcemia, but are not otherwise common (10%). A short stature observed in over two-thirds of patients occurs with delayed puberty in one-third.

In 1968 Drachman (see Berenberg et al, 1977) assembled these heterogeneous features of conditions surrounding progressive external ophthalmoplegia (PEO) into the *Ophthalmoplegia-Plus syndrome*. In 1975 Rowland suggested an eponym to recognize Kearns and Sayre (1958) and Daroff for their original clinical and pathologic findings of ophthalmoparesis and spongy degeneration in the brain. Descriptions of infantile, juvenile, and adult forms may relate to partial expression of typical KSS (TKSS). However, mild and moderate forms are not always progressive in family studies. The appellation *oculocraniosomatic syndrome* held only a brief popularity. In 1977 Berenberg et al attempted to resolve the complex issues of nosology in a careful analysis of 35 patients with "typical" Kearns-Sayre syndrome (TKSS), suggesting this eponym. Rowland later reaffirmed an "invariant triad": PEO, pigmentary retinopathy, and one additional finding of either heart block, a cerebellar syndrome, or a CSF protein over 100 mg/dl. Some authors add age of onset as a fourth criterion. While neuromuscular abnormalities occurred in other family members, there were no recorded instances of more than one "typical" KSS in any family.

Another review (see Petty et al, 1986) added 13 more patients with less restrictive major symptoms and accepted a positive family history that indicated a dominant mode of inheritance. The recognition of mitochondrial structural and functional defects associated with clinical and metabolic abnormalities with some response to treatment, including documented familial recurrence, may justify a "disease" concept.

Complications: The heterogeneous features of KSS, without a specific cause, accounts for the difficulty in separating primary from secondary complications. Several effects appear to be the result of the underlying disease process: Heart block with Stokes-Adams attacks occurs in 50% of patients. Conduction heart block accompanies cardiac muscle and conduction system mitochondrial abnormalities. One-half require cardiac pacemakers. Heart failure and cardiac arrest occur in one-third. One-third of affected patients die of cardiac complications. Proximal muscle weakness interferes with motor function, limiting ambulation as well as pulmonary function. Abrupt neurologic deterioration of sudden onset, especially in children, with coma and death may occur with or without cardiac findings. The therapeutic use of steroids potentiates this risk with a fatal ketotic or nonketotic metabolic acidosis and hyperglycemia. There appears to be an underlying unexplained CNS lactate-pyruvate metabolic defect in nonsteroid-treated patients as well. A separate or partial expression of an underlying mitochondrial defect associated with encephalopathy, lactic acidosis, and stroke-like episodes is known as the "MELAS" syndrome. Another syndrome with myoclonic seizures, optic atrophy, and sensory neural hearing loss, known as "Fukuhara disease" (MERRF), has similarities to KSS. There is also a characteristic pathologic cerebral, cerebellar, and brainstem spongiform encephalopathy in this group.

Associated Findings: The inclusion of many findings, possibly epiphenomena, in a less restrictive definition or "partial" expression of KSS may have utility, since the characteristic progressive systemic and neurologic deterioration alters clinical presentation at all ages. Many infrequent clinical and laboratory findings are of unknown significance. Some authors consider KSS to be merely a cluster of a more generic mitochondrial group of disorders and suggest that a rational classification on clinical grounds is not possible. Peripheral neuropathies are absent in typical KSS. Degenerative peripheral nerve demyelination (*Stephens syndrome*), and inclusions similar to Hirano bodies have been documented in less complete forms of KSS. Optic atrophy and optic neuritis have been reported. CPEO and parkinsonism, dementias, **Ataxia, Friedreich type, Machado-Joseph disease**, and Charcot-Marie-Tooth disease have been noted. Rarely hypoplastic anemias and renal dysfunction occur in children. Arachnodactyly, sternal deformities, high-arched palates, and myopia are rare dysmorphic features. Low CSF folate levels compared with plasma levels, resulting in a high plasma:CSF ratio, may be useful in diagnosis and as a guide to treatment. Folic acid deficiency rather than malabsorption may contribute to muscle carnitine reduction. Malabsorption in megaloblastic anemias is known to be associated with symptoms of mental retardation and calcification of the basal ganglia. Folic acid deficiencies may secondarily alter CSF neurotransmitters. Regional bilateral subcortical hypodense lesions in the thalamus, similar to those described in **Encephalopathy, necrotizing**, are associated with hypersomnia and altered nocturnal sleep patterns.

Histopathologic examination shows some muscle-fiber atrophy, and, on histochemical staining, a vacuolar myopathy with lipid or glycogen accumulation initially suggested a slow virus infection. Gomori trichrome stain shows abnormal structure or number of subsarcolemmal mitochondrial aggregations and paracrystalline inclusions identified as "ragged red fibers" (RRF) in type I fibers. This mitochondrial proliferation and the abnormalities in earlier reports suggested a "pleoconial" or "megaconial" myopathy. However, over 10% of myopathies demonstrate RRFs, while 5–25% of KSS muscle biopsy materials contain these abnormal aggregates. Intramitochondrial paracrystalline inclusions by electron microscopy are of unknown biochemical nature, and the pathophysiologic significance is undetermined. Similar structural abnormalities are found in cardiac muscle cells and in some cells of the conduction system. The role of mitochondria in brain is unknown. Skin and conjunctival biopsy may assist identification during life.

Low state III (to NAD- and FAD-linked substrates) respiration rates on polarographic studies and histochemically uncoupled respiration (Mg^{2+}-activated ATPase) suggest mitochondrial dysfunction with reduced glycolytic energy production. Reduced cytochrome oxidase (c, aa_3/b/cc1) and a decreased ratio of cytochrome oxidase/succinate-cytochrome c, normal monoamine oxidase, depend on the presence or absence of RRFs.

NADH-Coenzyme Q reductase may be low in muscle and fibroblasts. Mitochondrial metabolic malfunctions are variable and may affect complexes I, II, III, IV, or V (ATPase). Several malfunctions include muscle carnitine deficiency with normal plasma levels and reduced palmitoyl-CoA synthetase. Patients may also have normal cellular responses. Lactate and pyruvate elevations in plasma and CSF, with or without glucose loading, suggest a disorder of pyruvate utilization in the citric-acid cycle. Typically CSF protein is elevated over 100 mg/dl, while lower amounts may

relate to partial disorders. Abnormalities in albumin, IgG, oligoclonal bands, and tau fractions with normal myelin basic protein are rarely reported. Muscular and humoral immunologic abnormalities and circulating immune complexes also are rarely observed.

Etiology: The decision to confine to TKSS three (occasionally four) clinical manifestations and to designate as partial forms or as separate syndromes the less consistent features is based on the state of knowledge regarding underlying etiology. Viral infections, immunologic disorders, and, more recently, metabolic defects of mitochondrial function have all been considered. Genetic issues are unclear. Some studies of TKSS found no families with more than one person with characteristic KSS, suggesting the pseudogenetic mechanisms of acquired disease and leading to the statement that there is no evidence of genetic abnormality or metabolic defect in this syndrome. Autosomal dominant inheritance has been observed in an only minimally less complete form of KSS, with 15 members of one family reported to be affected in two generations. Careful examinations of all family members have not always been achieved. The age differences of family members adds to the variable degree and number of clinical manifestations. Autosomal recessive inheritance, X-linked recessive inheritance, and an X-linked dominant inheritance have also been suggested.

The mitochondrial myopathies may be viewed as secondary to as yet unknown primary defects in different syndromes or as heterogeneous polygenetic syndromes. There is evidence for a disturbance of mitochondrial DNA (mtDNA) caused by defects of a mitochondrial genome and transmitted by maternal inheritance, with mitotic segregation accounting for mutual phenotypes.

Pathogenesis: The pathogeneses of TKSS and PKSS are unknown. Disorders of folic acid metabolism, confirmed in separate studies, and treatment responses to coenzymes, including coenzyme Q (CoQ), involved in the mitochondrial electron transport chain, along with the supplemental use of folic acid and carnitine, suggest basic metabolic mechanisms. Recent reports identify mitochondrial abnormalities associated with disordered metabolism of folic acid, mitochondrial enzymes, substrate, and transport defects. Functional and structural abnormalities in skeletal and cardiac muscle, liver, pancreas, and brain have been documented with a CNS spongy degeneration, especially in the brainstem. Abrupt neurologic deterioration may be an independent and sudden cause of death unrelated to cardiac failure.

MIM No.: 16510

POS No.: 3747

Sex Ratio: M1:F1

Occurrence: About 80 cases have been reported. No ethnic or demographic characteristics. Rare among the neuromusclar disorders. Needs consideration among conditions associated with congenital lactic acidoses, CPEO, and disorders of folic acid metabolism, although molecular mechanisms are not established. CT hypodense lesions and basal ganglion calcification especially with a pigmentary retinopathy are also suggestive.

Risk of Recurrence for Patient's Sib: No genetic risk known in TKSS, but probably as high as 1:2 (50%) if parent affected, as in some partial mitochondrial syndromes. There may be some unestablished risk if any family members in recent generations are affected.

Risk of Recurrence for Patient's Child: Depending on interpretation of complete and incomplete syndromes, may be as high as 1:2 for some, and probably no risk for others.

Age of Detectability: Infancy through adult years.

Gene Mapping and Linkage: Deletions of mtDNA have recently been identified (Zeviani et al, 1988).

Prevention: None known. Genetic counseling indicated.

Treatment: Folic acid (oral folinic acid) when the plasma or CSF folate ratio is low as determined by measurement of plasma or CSF folate ratios. Reduced muscle tissue carnitine to be supplemented by oral L-carnitine. The lactic-pyruvic acid abnormalities, resting or after oral glucose, may respond to the oral administration of CoQ. CSF protein may decrease as clinical improvement occurs. Cardiac pacemakers for conduction defects are essential. Tarsofrontalis surgical suspensions improve obstructed vision, but must be performed with extreme caution to avoid lagophthalmos and corneal exposure. Independent therapy for hypoparathyroidism, hypothyroidism, and diabetes may be required. Steroid use is to be carefully considered in view of the reports of steroid-associated acute neurologic deterioration with coma and death.

Prognosis: A progressive deterioration of all neuromuscular functions is expected without effective treatment. Limited physical function may require orthopedic equipment. Cardiac death may be avoidable by early studies of cardiac competence and use of a pacemaker. Acute neurologic deterioration occurs at any time, unprovoked and not related to cardiac status. Survival into adult years is likely with long-term supportive therapy.

Detection of Carrier: Carriers cannot be distinguished at this time. Careful examination of all family members, however, is warranted to delineate epidemiology.

Special Considerations: As in many neurologic conditions, there is an overlap among these disorders. Careful clinical, medical, and neurologic family examinations and comprehensive laboratory studies are appropriate. Confusion to date is largely related to the reports of individual families or patients in past decades studied by the then available procedures. DNA analysis may help separate the disorders. Magnetic resonance imaging (MRI) in early consideration of this diagnosis is potentially the most sensitive for spongy generalized or regional brain changes. Metabolic studies during and after acute illness should include electrolytes, plasma and urine organic acids, muscle and tissue biopsies for structural and functional mitochondrial abnormalities, CSF proteins, lactate-pyruvate, plasma and CSF folates, and carnitine. Clinical monitoring of supplemental therapies, including CoQ therapy, are needed in long-term care.

References:

Kearns TP, Sayre GP: Retinitis pigmentosa, external ophthalmoplegia, and complete heart block. Arch Ophthal 1958; 60:280–289.

Berenberg RA, et al.: Lumping or splitting? Ophthalmoplegia-Plus or Kearns-Sayre syndrome? Ann Neurol 1977; 1:37–54. *

Schnitzler ER, et al.: Familial Kearns-Sayre syndrome. Neurology 1979; 29:1172–1174.

Coulter DL, Allen RJ: Abrupt neurological deterioration in children with Kearns-Sayre syndrome. Arch Neurol 1981; 38:247–250.

Allen RJ, et al.: Kearns-Sayre syndrome with reduced plasma and cerebrospinal fluid folate. Ann Neurol 1983; 13:679–682.

Rowland LP: Molecular genetics, pseudogenetics, and clinical neurology. Neurology 1983; 33:1179–1195.

Arnold DL, et al.: Investigation of human mitochondrial myopathies by phosphorus magnetic resonance spectroscopy. Ann Neurol 1985; 18:189–196.

DiMauro S, et al.: Mitochondrial myopathies. Ann Neurol 1985; 17:521–528.

Ogasahara S, et al.: Improvement of abnormal pyruvate metabolism and cardiac conduction defects with coenzyme Q_{10} in Kearns-Sayre syndrome. Neurology 1985; 35:372–377.

Petty RKH, et al.: The clinical features of mitochondrial myopathy. Brain 1986; 109:915–938. *

Holt IJ, et al.: Deletions of mitochondrial DNA in patients with mitochondrial myopathies. Nature 1988; 331:717–719.

Rowland LP, et al.: Kearns-Sayre syndrome in twins: lethal dominant mutation or acquired disease? Neurology 1988; 38:1399–1402.

Moraes CT, et al.: Mitochondrial DNA deletions in progressive external ophalmoplegia and Kearns-Sayre syndrome. New Engl J Med 1989; 320:1293–1299. *

AL028   **Richard J. Allen**

KERATOSIS PALMARIS ET PLANTARIS OF UNNA-THOST   3264

Includes:

  Epidermolytic hyperkeratosis
  Greither keratoderma
  Keratoderma, palmoplantar, Norrbotten recessive type
  Keratosis of Greither
  Palmo-plantar keratoderma, hereditary epidermolytic
  Palmo-plantar keratodermia, diffuse hereditary
  Thost-Unna disease
  Tylosis

Excludes:

  Acrokeratoelastoidosis (3068)
  Howell Evans syndrome (3290)
  Hyperkeratosis palmoplantaris-periodontoclasia (0494)
  Mal de Meleda (3289)

Major Diagnostic Criteria: Diffuse palmoplantar keratoderma without involvement of the dorsal surfaces of the hands and feet or distal sites.

Clinical Findings: Onset is usually evident after birth, and consists of slight thickening of the palms and soles. It is usually well-developed by the sixth to twelfth month and persists throughout life. The keratoderma is limited to either the palms, soles, or both; stopping abruptly at the lateral margins and often with an erythematous rim.

The skin lesions consists of a dense, homogenous hyperkeratosis with a whitish or yellow hue in a bilateral and symmetrical distribution.

Hyperhidrosis is present in most of the cases causing maceration and fissuring of the affected areas. The nails may be thickened, opaque, or curved. The hair and teeth are normal.

The histologic picture is not specific, consisting of hyperkeratosis, hypergranulosis, acanthosis, and a mild inflammatory infiltrate in the upper dermis.

Recently, many cases have been reported with the peculiar histologic feature of *epidermolytic hyperkeratosis*. At this time there is a debate whether this form, which is clinically indistinguishable from the Unna-Thost disease, is a separate entity.

Complications: Development of painful fissures as well as secondary dermatophyte infections have been frequently reported.

Associated Findings: Deafness has been reported in some kindred.

Etiology: Usually autosomal dominant inheritance, although a severe recessive form has been suggested.

Pathogenesis: Unknown.

MIM No.: *14840, 24485.

Sex Ratio: M1:F1

Occurrence: The incidence varies depending on geographic location, being 1:40,000 in Northern Ireland; 1:12,000 in Yugoslavia; and 1:200 in Northern Sweden.

Risk of Recurrence for Patient's Sib:
See Part I, *Mendelian Inheritance*.

Risk of Recurrence for Patient's Child:
See Part I, *Mendelian Inheritance*.

Age of Detectability: Usually shortly after birth.

Gene Mapping and Linkage: Unknown.

Prevention: None known. Genetic counseling indicated.

Treatment: Keratolytic agents can be useful to soften the hyperkeratotic skin. Recent studies have shown some effectiveness with oral synthetic retinoids.

Prognosis: Life span is not affected.

Detection of Carrier: Unknown.

Special Considerations: Some authors consider the recessive *Greither keratoderma* to be a distinct entity, which has the same clinical and histological features as Unna-Thost disease, but also involves the knees and elbows. Others, however, feel that this merely describes a severe variant of the Unna-Thost type of keratoderma.

References:
Unna PG: Uber das keratoma palmare et plantare ereditarium. Wochenschr Dermatol 1883; 10:231–274.
Kansky A, Arzensek J: Is palmoplantar keratoderma of Greither's type a separate nosologic entity? Dermatologica 1979; 158:244–248.
Bergfeld WF, et al.: The treatment of keratosis palmaris et plantaris with isotretinoin: a multicenter study. J Am Acad Dermatol 1982; 6:727–731.
Hatamochi A, et al.: Diffuse palmoplantar keratoderma with deafness. Arch Dermatol 1982; 118:605–607.
Camisa C, William H: Epidermolytic variant of hereditary palmoplantar keratoderma. Br J Dermatol 1985; 112:221–225.
Gamborg Neilsen P: Hereditary palmoplantar keratoderma in the northern most county of Sweden. Acta Derm Venereol (Stockh) 1985; 65:224–229.

MI038   **Giuseppe Micali**

Keratosis palmoplantaris transgrediens
See MAL DE MELEDA
Keratosis palmoplantaris-corneal dystrophy
See TYROSINEMIA II, OREGON TYPE
Keratosis rubra figurata
See SKIN, ERYTHROKERATODERMIA, VARIABLE

Keratosis, focal palmoplantar and gingival
See SKIN, HYPERKERATOSIS, FOCAL PALMOPLANTAR AND GINGIVAL
Keto acid decarboxylase deficiency
See MAPLE SYRUP URINE DISEASE
Ketotic hyperglycinemia I
See ACIDEMIA, PROPIONIC

KEUTEL SYNDROME   0263

Includes:
  Brachytelephalangy-peripheral pulmonary stenoses-deafness
  Calcification of cartilages-brachytelephalangy-pulmonary stenosis
  Deafness-peripheral pulmonary stenoses-brachytelephalangy
  Pulmonary stenoses (peripheral)-brachytelephalangy-deafness

Excludes:
  Chondrodysplasia punctata, X-linked dominant type (2730)
  Heart, cor triatriatum (0204)
  Fetal rubella syndrome (0384)
  Pulmonary stenoses, familial multiple

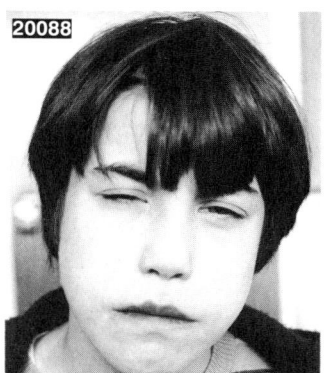
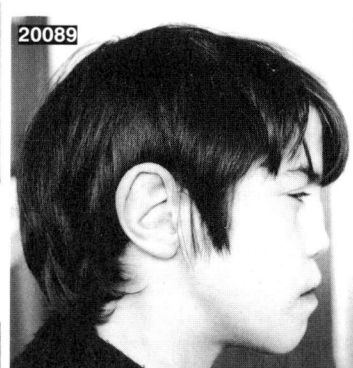
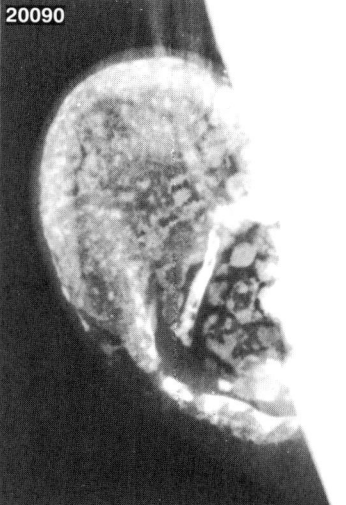

0263-20088: Characteristic dysmorphic facies with midface hypoplasia. **20089:** Note small depressed nose and midface hypoplasia on lateral view of face. **20090:** Cartilage calcifications in the ear.

Major Diagnostic Criteria: Brachytelephalangy, multiple peripheral pulmonary stenoses, mixed or conductive hearing loss, calcification of cartilage and typical craniofacial dysmorphism with small, depressed nose and midfacial hypoplasia.

Clinical Findings: Cormode et al. (1986) have summarized the clinical findings in the six reported patients. Two of these were sibs.

Facies: In one of the sibs, the face was described as coarse. In four other patients, the face was characteristic with midface hypoplasia, depressed nasal bridge, and small alae nasi.

Hands and feet: Brachytelephalangy was present in six of six patients. This includes short, malformed terminal phalanges, partial fusion of epiphyseal-metaphyseal joints, short nails, and interphalangeal webbing.

Cartilage: Widespread, diffuse calcifications throughout the nose, auricles, larynx, epiglottis, trachea, bronchial rings, and ribs were noted as early as age three years. Stippling of the epiphyses was seen as early as age 1.5 years. The ears especially were tough and showed perichondral and endochondral ossifications.

Cardiovascular system: Peripheral pulmonary artery stenoses, most frequently at the bifurcation of the pulmonary arteries, were present in three of six patients. One of these also had a ventricular septal defect (VSD).

Hearing loss: Mixed or conductive hearing loss was present in five of six patients, ranging from 30 to 70 db. Ossicular malformation was reported in one patient.

Growth: Delayed in the patient with VSD; normal in the other four patients for whom information was reported.

Intellectual ability: Mental retardation noted in two patients (one with VSD). Normal ability reported for three other patients.

Respiratory system: Chronic upper respiratory infections or wheezing noted in five of six patients.

Complications: Language delay secondary to hearing loss. Failure to thrive.

Associated Findings: Nasal speech possibly due to short palate, but without clefting.

Etiology: Probably autosomal recessive inheritance. Consanguinity noted in three of the five families reported.

Pathogenesis: Unknown.

MIM No.: *24515

POS No.: 3675

Sex Ratio: M1:F1

Occurrence: Six cases from five families have been reported.

Risk of Recurrence for Patient's Sib:
See Part I, *Mendelian Inheritance.*

Risk of Recurrence for Patient's Child:
See Part I, *Mendelian Inheritance.*

Age of Detectability: By X-ray in the first years of life.

Gene Mapping and Linkage: Unknown.

Prevention: None known. Genetic counseling indicated.

Treatment: Control of peripheral stenoses. Surgery as appropriate for cardiovascular defects. Amplification and speech and language therapy as needed for hearing loss. Educational intervention if intellectual impairment is present.

Prognosis: Apparently normal life span unless significant heart defect is present.

Detection of Carrier: No evidence of hearing loss or calcifications in obligate carriers.

References:
Keutel J, et al.: A new autosomal recessive syndrome: peripheral pulmonary stenoses, brachytelephalangism, neural hearing loss and abnormal cartilage calcifications-ossification. In: BD:OAS; VIII(5). New York: March of Dimes Birth Defects Foundation, 1972:60–68.
Say B, et al.: Unusual calcium deposition in cartilage associated with short stature and peculiar facial features: a case report. Pediatr Radiol 1973; 1:127–129.
Walbaum R, et al.: Le syndrome de Keutel. Ann Pediatr 1975; 51:461.

Temtamy S, McKusick V: The genetics of hand malformation. New York: Alan R. Liss, 1978:264.
Fryns JP, et al.: Calcification of cartilages, brachytelephalangy and peripheral pulmonary stenosis: confirmation of the Keutel syndrome. Eur J Pediatr 1984; 142:201–203.
Cormode EJ, et al.: Keutel syndrome: clinical report and literature review. Am J Med Genet, 1986; 24:289–294. * †

FR030   **Jean-Pierre Fryns**
SM008   **Shelley D. Smith**

Kidney disease, autosomal recessive polycystic
See HEPATIC FIBROSIS, CONGENITAL
Kidney, adult polycystic disease of
See KIDNEY, POLYCYSTIC DISEASE, DOMINANT
Kidney, clear cell sarcoma
See CANCER, WILMS TUMOR
Kidney, congenital solitary
See RENAL AGENESIS, UNILATERAL

KIDNEY, GLOMERULOCYSTIC   3146

Includes:
> Glomerular cysts
> Glomerulocystic kidney
> Glomerulocystic renal dysplasia
> Hypoplastic glomerulocystic kidney, familial

Excludes:
> **Kidney, polycystic disease, dominant** (0859)
> **Kidney, polycystic disease, recessive** (2003)
> **Meckel syndrome** (0634)
> Tuberous sclerosis-cystic kidneys

Major Diagnostic Criteria: Glomerular cysts are usually discovered by examination of biopsy or postmortem specimens of kidney tissue obtained from patients with unexplained chronic renal failure or dysmorphic syndromes. The presence of glomerular cysts does not define or characterize any single disease entity, but may be found in several disparate conditions. The glomeruli may be small and primitive, and several small glomerular tufts may be seen within a large, dilated Bowman capsule. Proximal tubules may be dilated. Both kidneys are involved, and they may be large, normal, or small. The interstitium may be distorted and sclerosed.

Glomerulocystic kidney is characterized by the occurrence of chronic renal failure, small kidneys, absent renal papillae, and glomerular cysts. There are no major extrarenal malformations, and there is no associated hepatic fibrosis.

Clinical Findings: Familial hypoplastic glomerulocystic kidney disease presents with chronic renal failure during the first months of life. The renal function tends to be stable over several decades. Patients may fail to thrive. Two patients have had marked prognathism.

Complications: Chronic renal failure, hypertension, and failure to thrive.

Associated Findings: Glomerular cysts have also been seen in kidneys of patients with obstructive uropathy, **Chromosome 13, trisomy 13**, **Kidney, polycystic disease, dominant**, **Renal dysplasia-retinal aplasia, Loken-Senior type**, and in association with malformations of various organs.

Etiology: Presumably autosomal dominant inheritance. Glomerular cysts may also occur sporadically or in association with other defined syndromes that have dominant or recessive modes of inheritance.

Pathogenesis: Unknown.

MIM No.: 13792

Sex Ratio: M4:F8 (observed).

Occurrence: Twelve patients from four families have been documented in the literature.

Risk of Recurrence for Patient's Sib:
See Part I, *Mendelian Inheritance.*

Risk of Recurrence for Patient's Child:
See Part I, *Mendelian Inheritance*.

Age of Detectability: Patients can be detected when they present with chronic renal failure. Glomerulocystic kidneys have been detected *in utero* by ultrasonography at eight months gestation.

Gene Mapping and Linkage: Unknown.

Prevention: None known. Genetic counseling indicated.

Treatment: Chronic hemodialysis or continuous peritoneal dialysis. Renal transplantation.

Prognosis: All documented patients have survived but have mild-to-moderate, fairly stable or slowly progressive chronic renal failure.

Detection of Carrier: Unknown.

References:
Roos A: Polycystic kidney: report of a case studied by reconstruction. Am J Dis Child 1941; 61:116–127.
Rizzoni G, et al.: Familial hypoplastic glomerulocystic kidney: a new entity? Clin Nephrol 1982; 18:263–268.
Melnick SC, et al.: Cortical microcystic disease of the kidney with dominant inheritance: a previously undescribed syndrome. J Clin Pathol 1984; 37:494–499.
Fitch SJ, Stapleton FB: Ultrasonographic features of glomerulocystic disease in infancy: similarity to infantile polycystic kidney disease. Pediatr Radiol 1986; 16:400–402.
Barratt TM, et al.: Autosomal dominant hypoplastic glomerulocystic kidney disease. Am J Hum Genet 1987; 41:A45 only.

KA042   **Bernard S. Kaplan**

KIDNEY, HORSESHOE   2004

Includes:
Horseshoe kidneys
Kidneys connected by a fibrous or parenchymatous isthmus

Excludes:
Kidney, fusion anomalies of, other
Kidney, true ectopic

Major Diagnostic Criteria: Physical examination may detect an abdominal mass. Urine examination may be normal or show pyuria, hematuria, proteinuria or positive bacterial cultures if infection or stones are present; excretory urography shows relatively low-lying kidneys, downward convergence of the renal axis, medially located and malrotated pelvis and high insertion of ureters from the anterior or lateral aspects of the kidney. Other confirmatory studies include retrograde pyelography, ultrasonography, or computed tomography.

Clinical Findings: Horseshoe kidney is the most common fusion anomaly of the kidneys. The kidneys are connected across the midline by a fibrous or parenchymatous isthmus which, in 40% of the patients, lies at the level of the fourth lumbar vertebra. In 95% of the cases the kidneys are joined at the lower pole. It is seen twice as often in males as in females. Approximately one-third of all patients are asymptomatic. Clinical symptoms are usually related to secondary complications such as infections, hydronephrosis, or calculus formation. The most common symptoms are abdominal or flank pain (approximately 33%), symptoms of urinary tract infection such as dysuria, hematuria, pyuria, and frequency (between 22–33%), renal calculi (approximately 20%), and palpable abdominal mass (approximately 5–10%). Ureteropelvic junction obstruction causing significant hydronephrosis is not uncommon; it is believed to be secondary to high insertion of the ureter in the renal pelvis, the abnormal course of the ureter and anomalous blood supply. The horseshoe kidney, even when asymptomatic, is frequently associated with other congenital anomalies. Boatman, et al reported that nearly one-third of 96 patients he studied had at least one other abnormality. The organ systems most commonly involved include: skeletal, cardiovascular, genitourinary, gastrointestinal, and central nervous systems. Horseshoe kidneys are frequently found in chromosomal abnor-

mality syndromes, e.g. **Turner syndrome** or **Chromosome 18, trisomy 18**. The clinical manifestations may be dominated by the associated anomalies of other organ systems. The diagnosis of horseshoe kidney is confirmed by excretory urography.

Complications: Most commonly related to malrotated renal pelvis causing urinary stasis, leading to infection and renal calculus. Ureteropelvic obstruction may cause hydronephrosis.

Associated Findings: The incidence of associated congenital anomalies in horseshoe kidney is high: approximately one-third of affected individuals have at least one other anomaly, which most frequently involves the cardiovascular system, the skeletal system, the central nervous system, or the genitourinary system. Genitourinary anomalies include ureteral duplication (10%); vesicoureteral reflux; in the male, hypospadias (4%); undescended testicles (4%); in the female, abnormalities of the vagina or uterus (7%). Central nervous system abnormalities include **Hydrocephaly**, **Meningomyelocele** or both as well as cerebral cortical atrophy and mental retardation. The cardiovascular anomalies, multiple and severe in nature, are varied and often lead to early death. The gastrointestinal findings include anorectal malformations, fistulas, a malrotated bowel, and **Meckel diverticulum**. Musculoskeletal anomalies include spina bifida, hip dislocation, webbed neck, **Polydactyly**, cleft lip, cleft palate, and clubfoot. Inguinal, umbilical and diaphragmatic hernias are also reported, as well as two patients with congenital deformity of the iris. Horseshoe kidney is seen in 60% of patients with **Turner syndrome** and 21% of patients with **Chromosome 18, trisomy 18**.

Renal cancer, **Cancer, renal cell carcinoma**, and **Cancer, Wilms tumor** are reported with higher incidence in association with horseshoe kidney. **Kidney, polycystic disease** has also been reported with horseshoe kidney.

Etiology: An embryologic abnormality which occurs between the fourth and sixth week of gestation. The exact cause is undetermined. Horseshoe kidney has been reported in identical twins, and among several siblings within the same family. Possibly the result of a genetic expression with a low penetrance.

Pathogenesis: Partial or complete fusion of the kidney results from failure of the metanephric cell mass to separate at the 5–8 mm. stage of embryogenesis; this occurs between 4–6 weeks of gestation, prior to renal rotation. Although the cause is unknown, it is theorized that deviation of the point of origin of the umbilical artery or other local mechanical factors may cause primary fusion by interfering with the normal upward growth of ureteral buds.

CDC No.: 753.320

Sex Ratio: M2:F1

Occurrence: 1:400–600 in the general population. Autopsy finding in 1:300 to 1:1000 autopsies. No particular ethnic distribution.

Risk of Recurrence for Patient's Sib: Presumably not significantly increased.

Risk of Recurrence for Patient's Child: Presumably not significantly increased.

Age of Detectability: Present at birth.

Gene Mapping and Linkage: Unknown.

Prevention: None known. Genetic counseling indicated.

Treatment: Asymptomatic horseshoe kidney requires no treatment. Urinary tract infection is treated with appropriate antibiotics. Complications such as ureteropelvic obstruction, hydronephrosis, and renal calculi may require surgical intervention.

Prognosis: Good for asymptomatic patients. Progression to renal failure is rare, and related to secondary complications. An increased incidence of renal cancer has been observed. If the horseshoe kidney is associated with other congenital anomalies, the severity of the involvement of other systems may determine the clinical course, and often lead to significant morbidity or early death.

Detection of Carrier: Unknown.

Special Considerations: The frequent association of horseshoe kidney with multiple congenital anomalies and certain chromosome abnormalities should prompt the physician to search for evidence of such association; and vice versa, a patient with birth defects should be investigated for the presence of horseshoe kidney.

Support Groups: New York; National Kidney Foundation

References:
Boatman DL, et al.: Congenital anomalies associated with horseshoe kidney. J Urol 1972; 107:205–207.
Perlmutter AD, et al.: Horseshoe kidney. In: Walsh PC, et al, eds: Campbell's urology, 5th ed, vol 2. Philadelphia: Saunders, 1986: 1686–1692.
Pitts WR, Muecke EC: Horseshoe kidneys: a 40 years experience. J Urol 1975; 113:743–746.
Kissane JM: Congenital malformations. In: Heptinstall RH, ed: Pathology of the kidney, 3rd ed., vol 1. Boston: Little, Brown, 1983:94–95.

SA008
BI012

Inge Sagel
Nesrin Bingol

KIDNEY, MEDULLARY SPONGE KIDNEY   3019

Includes:
  Cystic dilation of renal collecting tubules
  Cystic disease of renal pyramids
  Medullary sponge kidney
  Precalyceal canalicular ectasia
  Sponge kidney
  Tubular ectasia

Excludes:
  Kidney, nephronophthisis-medullary cystic desease (3018)
  Kidney, polycystic disease, dominant (0859)
  Kidney, polycystic disease, recessive (2003)

Major Diagnostic Criteria: The patient is usually asymptomatic but may present with nephrolithiasis (80%), nephrocalcinosis, urinary tract infections, and hematuria. The combination of multiple pyramidal or calyceal calculi with cystic and ectatic medullary pyramidal changes on X-ray examination is diagnostic.

Clinical Findings: The patient is generally asymptomatic. Calculus formation and infection are usually responsible for the majority of symptoms: ureteral colic or loin pain (50–60%), nephrocalcinosis (40–60%), urinary tract infection and pyelonephritis (20–33%), and gross hematuria (10–30%). Few patients may be diagnosed incidentally on intravenous pyelogram (IVP) done to investigate a microscopic hematuria or pyuria, mild proteinuria, or enuresis. Hypertension is unusual. Progression to end-stage renal disease and death are rare, although a decrease in glomerular filtration rate (GFR) may be observed. Defective urinary solute-concentrating ability is present in the majority of patients; urinary dilution is unimpaired. Diagnosis is usually done by IVP. Renal ultrasound may show well-defined, highly echogenic pyramids due to multiple small cysts or pyramidal nephrocalcinosis.

Complications: Renal calculi (usually calcium phosphate, calcium oxalate, and ammonium magnesium phosphate); urinary tract infections; pyelonephritis; renal acidification and concentration defects; hematuria; absorptive (59%) and renal (18%) hypercalciuria; enhanced fractional excretion of sodium; interstitial nephritis; secondary renal failure; proteinuria; hyperuricemia.

Associated Findings: **Ehlers-Danlos syndrome**, **Hemihypertrophy**, congenital pyloric stenosis, adult polycystic kidney disease, pyeloureterocystitis cystica, renal ectopia and malrotation, **Kidney, horseshoe**, ureteral duplication, bifid ureter, calyceal diverticulae, megaureter, **Artery, renal fibromuscular dysplasia**, **Hyperparathyroidism**, parathyroid adenoma, distal renal tubular acidosis, **Meckel syndrome**, **Marfan syndrome**, hypokalemic paralysis, and **Gout**.

Etiology: Unknown. The disorder is considered to be a congenital abnormality. Most cases are sporadic, although the disease has been described in sibs and family members of successive generations.

Pathogenesis: Although the disease is considered to be a congenital abnormality, a variety of physical, chemical, and genetic factors may contribute to dysembryoplastic development. The most often-cited pathogenetic mechanism is dysplastic, cystic dilation of the first few generations of the metanephric duct arborizations within nephrogenic tissue early in embryonic development. This may represent a renal expression of more generalized abnormality of connective tissue.

CDC No.: 753.150

Sex Ratio: M1:F1

Occurrence: Incidence is estimated to be 1:1,000 to 1:5,000 cases in the population. The disease is reported to occur in 3.5–17% of stone formers. There is no racial preponderance.

Risk of Recurrence for Patient's Sib: Unknown.

Risk of Recurrence for Patient's Child: Unknown.

Age of Detectability: The disease usually presents in the fourth to fifth decade, although it has been observed at all ages.

Gene Mapping and Linkage: Unknown.

Prevention: None known. Genetic counseling indicated.

Treatment: Asymptomatic patients require no specific treatment except for yearly urinalysis. Treatment of symptomatic patients consists of high fluid intake and, when indicated, antibiotics. Renal calculi are managed conservatively. Urolithotomy and partial or total nephrectomy may be needed occasionally. Hypercalciuria may be treated with thiazides.

Prognosis: The course of uncomplicated medullary sponge kidney disease is benign and does not affect longevity. About 10% of symptomatic patients may have a poor long-term prognosis, urolithiasis, septicemia and renal failure.

Detection of Carrier: Unknown.

Special Considerations: *Medullary sponge kidney* should not be confused with **Kidney, nephronophthisis-medullary cystic desease** which is a distinctly different condition. The alternate terms of *precalyceal canalicular ectasia, cystic dilation of renal collecting tubules,* or *tubular ectasia* are more appropriate, but are not as widely accepted.

Support Groups: New York; National Kidney Foundation

References:
Morris RC, et al.: Medullary sponge kidney. Am J Med 1965; 38:883–892.
Kuiper JJ: Medullary sponge kidney. In: Gardner KD, ed: Cystic diseases of the kidney. New York: John Wiley & Sons, 1976:151–171. *
Backman U, et al.: Clinical and laboratory findings in patients with medullary sponge kidney. In: Smith LH, et al., eds: Urolithiasis: clinical and basic research. New York: Plenum, 1980:113–120.
O'Neill M, et al.: Metabolic evaluation of nephrolithiasis in patients with medullary sponge kidney. J Am Med Asso 1981; 245:1233–1236.
Yendt ER: Medullary sponge kidney and nephrolithiasis. New Engl J Med 1982; 306:1106–1107.

BA065

Amin Y. Barakat

KIDNEY, NEPHRONOPHTHISIS-MEDULLARY CYSTIC DISEASE   3018

Includes:
  Cystic disease of the renal medulla
  Cysts of the renal medulla, congenital
  Fanconi nephronophthisis
  Kidney, uremic sponge
  Medullary cystic disease-nephronophthisis
  Medullary cystic kidney disease
  Microcystic disease of the renal medulla
  Nephritis, salt-losing
  Nephronophthisis, familial juvenile
  Nephronophthisis-medullary cystic disease
  Polycystic kidney disease, medullary type
  Renal medulla, familial disease
  Tubulointerstitial nephropathy, chronic idiopathic

Excludes:
   Kidney, medullary sponge kidney (3019)
   Kidney, polycystic disease, dominant (0859)
   Kidney, polycystic disease, recessive (2003)
   Renal dysplasia-retinal aplasia, Loken-Senior type (2687)

Major Diagnostic Criteria: Anemia, renal salt wasting, hyposthenuria, polyuria, scanty urinary abnormalities, and progressive renal failure. Histologic features consist of renal medullary or corticomedullary cysts (73%), relatively preserved glomeruli, interstitial fibrosis, and atrophied tubules.

Clinical Findings: The disease presents early in the second decade in the juvenile and sporadic types and late in the third decade in the adult type with polyuria, enuresis, and polydipsia (80%); normochromic, normocytic anemia (76%); azotemia (75%); renal sodium wasting (68%); weakness and pallor (60%); short stature in children (40%); hypertension (30%); abnormal bone metabolism and osteodystrophy (28%); asymptomatic relatives of patients (15%); and signs of azotemia (10%). Urinalysis may be normal in 32%; scanty urine findings (mild proteinuria, few blood cells, and an occasional cast) may be seen in 61% of patients.

Complications: Chronic renal failure.

Associated Findings: Eye changes consisting of **Retinitis pigmentosa**, tapetoretinal degeneration, and cataracts; **Bardet-Biedl syndrome**; red hair; **Kidney, horseshoe**; hepatic fibrosis; skeletal abnormalities; cerebellar ataxia, **Asphyxiating thoracic dysplasia**; **Ehlers-Danlos syndrome**.

Etiology: The evidence for two modes of inheritance suggests more than one etiology. Juvenile nephronophthisis by autosomal recessive inheritance; adult medullary cystic disease by autosomal dominant inheritance. Sporadic cases have been described.

Pathogenesis: Unknown. A nephrotoxic substance, probably the product of an inborn enzymatic defect and leading to early tubular dysfunction, has been suggested. An embryonal developmental anomaly in which the primary generation of uriniferous tubules do not undergo complete degeneration but persist as degenerating cysts; hypokalemia, and infection have been incriminated also in the pathogenesis of this disease. A primary defect in the renal tubular basement membrane of these patients has been described by Cohen and Hoyer (1986).

MIM No.: *17400, *25610,

CDC No.: 753.150, 753.140

Sex Ratio: M1:F1

Occurrence: Juvenile nephronophthisis occurs in about 1:50,000 births. Most reports describe affected Caucasians or do not mention race.

Risk of Recurrence for Patient's Sib:
See Part I, *Mendelian Inheritance.*

Risk of Recurrence for Patient's Child:
See Part I, *Mendelian Inheritance.*

Age of Detectability: In the early second decade in the juvenile and sporadic types and in late third decade in the adult type.

Gene Mapping and Linkage: Unknown.

Prevention: None known. Genetic counseling indicated.

Treatment: Chronic renal failure is treated symptomatically, eventually by renal transplantation. Changes of medullary cystic disease have not been observed in the transplanted kidney.

Prognosis: In untreated patients, death due to renal failure occurs in the second decade in the juvenile and sporadic types and in the fourth decade in the adult type.

Detection of Carrier: Asymptomatic family members of patients with nephronophthisis and tapetoretinal degeneration (see **Renal dysplasia-retinal aplasia, Loken-Senior type**) have been detected by electro-oculographic and retinographic studies.

Special Considerations: *Nephronophthisis* and *medullary cystic disease* are similar, clinically and histologically. However, the first is characterized by early onset, relatively longer course, and autosomal recessive inheritance; while in the second there is late onset, rapid progression, and autosomal dominant inheritance.

Most authors agree that these are very closely related entities and refer to them as the *nephronophthisis-medullary cystic disease complex.*

Support Groups: New York; National Kidney Foundation

References:
Gardner KD: Juvenile nephronophthisis and renal medullary cystic disease. In: Gardner KD, ed: Cystic disease of the kidney. New York: John Wiley & Sons, 1976:173–185. *
Chamberlin BC, et al.: Juvenile nephronophthisis and medullary cystic disease. Mayo Clin Proc 1977; 52:485–491.
Steele BT, et al.: Nephronophthisis. Am J Med 1980; 68:531–538.
Zerres K, et al.: Cystic kidneys: genetics, pathologic anatomy, clinical picture, and prenatal diagnosis. Hum Genet 1984; 68:104–135. *
Barakat AY, et al.: Nephronophthisis-medullary cystic disease. In: The kidney in genetic disease. Edinburgh: Churchill Livingstone, 1986: 30–32.
Cohen AH, Hoyer JR: Nephronophthisis: a primary tubular basement membrane defect. Lab Invest 1986; 55:564–572.

BA065   **Amin Y. Barakat**

KIDNEY, POLYCYSTIC DISEASE, DOMINANT   0859

Includes:
   Adult polycystic kidney disease (APKD)
   Kidney, adult polycystic disease of
   Polycystic renal disease, adult type (Potter type III)
   Potter type III polycystic kidney disease
   Renal disease, polycystic adult type

Excludes:
   Kidney, medullary sponge kidney (3019)
   Kidney, nephronophthisis-medullary cystic desease (3018)
   Kidney, polycystic disease, recessive (2003)
   Kidney, renal dysplasia, Potter type II (3028)
   Medullary cystic disease
   Multilocular renal cysts
   Nephrosis, congenital (0709)
   Renal cortical cysts (Simple)

Major Diagnostic Criteria: Familial occurrence of bilateral flank masses with or without hypertension, proteinuria and/or hematuria. X-ray features are characteristic, and show large kidneys with lobulated margins and multiple cysts.

Clinical Findings: Dominant polycystic kidney disease occurs in both sexes and is characterized by progressive cystic enlargement of the kidneys, with eventual renal insufficiency. The vast majority of cases that become clinically apparent do so during the fourth decade. One-third of the individuals who have autosomal dominant polycystic kidney disease are asymptomatic. Fewer than 10% of cases present during the first decade of life. The entity occasionally presents in the newborn. Death from renal insufficiency usually occurs in the sixth decade of life in patients who have clinical manifestations, unless dialysis is instituted.

The presenting feature is often the feeling of abdominal fullness, discomfort, or pain. Bilateral abdominal masses may be detected on examination. Hypertension, proteinuria, hematuria, and headache are also important symptoms and signs. Pyuria and bacteriuria may be present. Loss of renal concentrating ability may be an early sign. Blood chemistries may be normal or may indicate renal impairment. Anemia is common, and polycythemia is observed occasionally. Some patients have ureteral colic resulting from passage of a blood clot from a ruptured cyst. Subarachnoid hemorrhage from a ruptured aneurysm can occur.

Diagnosis of polycystic disease may be confirmed by ultrasonography or intravenous pyelogram (IVP) which shows enlarged kidneys with lobulated margins. The cysts cause expansion of the renal cortex and displacement of the calyces. Occasionally, kidney size may be asymmetric or normal. In these instances nephrotomography may sometimes help define cysts as small as 1 cm in diameter. Ultrasound or computerized tomography (CT) scan may be able to define cysts that cannot be seen by nephrotomograms. Isotopic studies may be helpful to assess kidney size and contour. Ultrasound is a useful noninvasive technique to define cystic structures within the kidneys and to assess and follow kidney size.

Complications: Patients with polycystic kidney disease are prone to pyelonephritis (50- 75%) and arteriolar nephrosclerosis. Rupture of cysts and hemorrhage into cysts may occur. Renal colic due to renal calculi or blood clots are not infrequent. Renal calculi occur in 10–20% of patients. Compression of the ureter by the large kidney may lead to hydronephrosis.

Attacks of gout often precede symptoms of significant uremia. Approximately 8% of patients show a number of bone problems such as demineralization, trabeculation, and spontaneous fractures secondary to hyperparathyroidism.

Subarachnoid hemorrhage secondary to rupture of cerebral aneurysm occurs in 3–10% of patients.

The prevalence of neoplasms (carcinoma, sarcoma) in polycystic kidneys is a topic of controversy.

Associated Findings: Approximately one-third of patients with adult polycystic renal disease have one or more cysts of the liver. Cysts are found in the pancreas (10%), spleen, and lungs (5%); cysts of the ovary, endometrium, seminal vesicles, epididymis, bladder, and thyroid have been reported. Twenty-two percent of patients with polycystic kidney disease were found to have cerebral aneurysms on autopsy. Cardiovascular abnormalities such as dilatation of aortic root and annulus with aortic regurgitation and **Mitral valve prolapse** are found in 18% of patients. Echocardiogram may be a useful screening procedure.

Etiology: Autosomal dominant inheritance. In 25% of cases there is no family history of polycystic kidney disease; these are presumably new mutations.

Pathogenesis: Theories favor a developmental malformational abnormality; however, intrarenal obstruction may play a role. More recently, it has been suggested that a toxic or other intermediate factor may lead to cyst formation in a susceptible host. None of these theories is generally accepted. Cystic disease of kidneys may be induced in animals by intrauterine obstruction of ureters and by several chemicals including diphenylamine, diphenylthiazoles, lithium chloride, and corticosteroids.

In polycystic kidney disease, the kidney tissue is displaced by many cysts of varying size, which are scattered throughout the parenchyma; the cysts are dilated nephrons and collecting ducts. Cyst fluid composition indicates that the cyst walls are metabolically active; depending on whether they arise from proximal or distal nephron structures, the fluid composition resembles plasma or urine. The cystic structures slowly become more distended, gradually leading to gross enlargment of the kidneys and to progressive renal failure.

MIM No.: *17390

CDC No.: 753.120

Sex Ratio: M1:F1

Occurrence: Estimates for hospital populations generally range from between 1:3,000 to 1:5,000 patients. No ethnic group variation has been reported. Polycystic kidney disease is responsible for end-stage renal disease in the United States in 5%, and in Europe in 8%, of patients receiving renal dialysis.

Risk of Recurrence for Patient's Sib:
See Part I, *Mendelian Inheritance.*

Risk of Recurrence for Patient's Child:
See Part I, *Mendelian Inheritance.*

Age of Detectability: Usually after the fourth decade of life clinically, as early as 30 weeks gestation in utero by ultrasound. Prenatal diagnosis is possible by restriction fragment length polymorphism and linkage analysis of fetal DNA obtained by chorionic villus sampling.

Gene Mapping and Linkage: PKD1 (polycystic kidney disease 1 (autosomal dominant)) has been mapped to 16p13.

Prevention: None known. Genetic counseling indicated.

Treatment: Conservative management of renal insufficiency (protein-restricted diet, correction of electrolyte and acid-base imbalance, control of hypertension) and of cardiovascular complications and infection. Dialysis treatment and renal transplantation are needed for patients in end-stage renal failure.

Prognosis: The cystic conversion of renal parenchyma progresses, and uremia gradually develops. There are wide variations in the course of the disease. Some remain asymptomatic, while others have a slow progression of the disease. Once the renal function is impaired, most patients develop end-stage renal disease requiring dialysis within 3 years. Myocardial infarcts, congestive heart failure, and cerebral hemorrhage contribute significantly to mortality.

Detection of Carrier: In affected families urinalysis and ultrasound and/or IVP with nephrotomogram should be obtained on each family member to identify a carrier.

Support Groups:
MO; Kansas City; Polycystic Kidney Research (PKR) Foundation
NY; New York; National Kidney Foundation

References:
Kissane JM: Congenital malformations. In: Heptinstall RH, ed: Pathology of the kidney. Boston: Little Brown, 1974:3:89–93.
Danovitch GM: Clinical features and pathophysiology of polycystic kidney disease in man. In: Gardner KD Jr, ed: Cystic diseases of the kidney. New York: Wiley, 1976:125–150.
Baer JC, et al.: Age at clinical onset and at ultrasonographic detection of adult polycystic disease: data for genetic counseling. Am J Med Genet 1984; 18:45–53.
Reeder ST, et al.: A highly polymorphic DNA marker linked to adult polycystic kidney disease on chromosome 16. Nature 1985; 317:542–544.
Reeder ST, et al.: Prenatal diagnosis of autosomal dominant polycystic kidney disease with a DNA probe. Lancet 1986; II:6–7.
Sedman A, et al.: Autosomal dominant polycystic kidney disease in childhood: a longitudinal study. Kidney Int 1987; 31:1000–1005.

SA008   **Inge Sagel**
BI012   **Nesrin Bingol**
WA034   **Edward Wasserman**
KA042   **Bernard S. Kaplan**

KIDNEY, POLYCYSTIC DISEASE, RECESSIVE   2003

Includes:
Cystic kidney, type I
Hepatic fibrosis, congenital
Infantile polycystic disease (IPCD)
Potter type I infantile polycystic kidney disease
Polycystic disease of infancy and childhood
Polycystic disease of the newborn
Renal-hepatic-pancreatic dysplasia (one form)

Excludes:
Kidney, polycystic disease, dominant (0859)
Kidney, renal dysplasia, Potter type II (3028)
Liver, congenital cystic dilatation of intrahepatic ducts (3155)
Renal cortical cysts
Renal cysts in hereditary syndromes
Renal medullary cysts

Major Diagnostic Criteria: Palpable enlarged kidneys in the infant are a prominent physical finding. Oligohydramnios sequence and "Potter face" ('squashed' nose, micrognathia, and large floppy low-set ears; resembling a face pressed against a window pane) may be present in the newborn. A family history of cystic kidney disease, or early death from kidney disease, or a history of oligohydramnios in the newborn suggest the diagnosis. Oliguria, anuria, proteinuria, pyuria and low specific gravity are found. Other laboratory data may indicate renal insufficiency. Excretory urography usually confirms the diagnosis, producing an irregularly mottled nephrogram and linear opacifications. It shows poor functioning in the newborn by the retention of the contrast medium within dilated collecting ducts. In older children uroradiographic findings are more variable. One may see variable renal enlargement and cyst formation. A characteristic finding is medullary tubular ductal ectasia. Ultrasonography and other radiographic techniques may be helpful in establishing the diagnosis. In an occasional patient, confirmation rests on kidney and especially liver biopsy.

Clinical Findings: Affects both the kidney and the liver. The clinical findings are age related and variable. Blyth and Ockenden characterized four subgroups according to age of onset and predominance of renal versus hepatic involvement.

Perinatal: Presentation at birth and with 90% of renal tubules dilated.

Neonatal: Presentation within the first month of life and with 60% of renal tubules dilated.

Infantile: Presentation between 3–6 months of age and with 25% of tubules dilated.

Juvenile: Presentation after the first year of life and less than 10% of tubules dilated.

The perinatal and neonatal forms of the disease are characterized by massive diffuse renal enlargement and oliguria. Many infants have the facial features of Potter syndrome and a history of oligohydramnios and dystocia. The abdomen is distended and the kidneys are palpable. Respiratory distress, apparently secondary to pulmonary hypoplasia, is common. Liver enlargement is variable. Hematuria is common. Death within the first few days of life is usually due to pulmonary rather than renal insufficiency.

The clinical picture in older children is more variable, with less severe initial renal enlargement, sometimes with progressive reduction in renal size with stabilization around 4–5 years. The kidneys are usually palpable. Renal insufficiency begins in early childhood, but its progression is very variable. Hypertension is almost always present, often leading to heart failure. Other nonspecific symptoms include nausea, abdominal pain, vomiting and growth retardation.

Hepatic involvement is always present, and is usually more pronounced in the older child, but rarely leads to functional impairment. The finding of marked hepatic fibrosis and portal hypertension with only mild renal involvement is referred to as congenital hepatic fibrosis. Hepatosplenomegaly and ascites may be present in these patients.

Complications: Hypertension is found in almost all patients and heart failure is common. Advancing renal insufficiency may lead to anemia and secondary hyperparathyroidism; this may result in skeletal involvement and growth failure. In patients with significant hepatic involvement, hepatocellular dysfunction and portal hypertension may be found. Hemorrhage from esophageal varices is not uncommon in these patients.

Associated Findings: Cystic lesions of the pancreas are occasionally found, but are asymptomatic. Hypoplasia rather than cystic changes are found in the lungs of newborns.

Etiology: Autosomal recessive inheritance.

Pathogenesis: The exact cause of cyst formation is not clear. Faulty embryologic development has been cited, but not proven. The association of characteristic cystic changes in the kidney and intrahepatic biliary system is suggestive of a generalized metabolic abnormality which affects both organs. A primary defect in the supporting structures of tubules and bile ducts, or a primary defect in the renal and biliary epithelium has also been suggested. None of these theories is proven or generally accepted. The kidneys are enlarged; more so in neonates than older children. The essential morphologic abnormality appears to be enlargement of the collecting tubules. Microdissections have shown a normal number of nephrons and other nephron structures, suggesting that the abnormality is acquired later in gestation. Although older children have less cystic dilatation than neonates, the fact that they have more peritubular fibrosis may be related to progressive tubular damage. It has been suggested that progressive tubular damage rather than cyst formation is responsible for progressive renal failure. The enlarged and fibrotic portal areas in the liver contain an increased number of bile ducts and periductal collagen; this abnormality leads to vascular obstruction and portal hypertension.

MIM No.: *26320

POS No.: 3368

CDC No.: 753.110

Sex Ratio: M1:F1

Occurrence: Estimated to be between 1:20,000 and 1:60,000.

Risk of Recurrence for Patient's Sib:
See Part I, *Mendelian Inheritance.*

Risk of Recurrence for Patient's Child:
See Part I, *Mendelian Inheritance.*

Age of Detectability: At birth for neonatal and perinatal form. Variable in older children. Prenatal detection is possible.

Gene Mapping and Linkage: Unknown.

Prevention: None known. Genetic counseling indicated.

Treatment: Medical therapy is supportive. Hypertension and heart failure may require antihypertensive drugs and digitalis. In end stage renal failure, hemodialysis and renal transplantation are indicated. Portal hypertansion, the principal hepatic complication, is currently treated by surgical portocaval shunt.

Prognosis: In the perinatal and neonatal form, death in the first few days or weeks of life often occurs, and is frequently related to pulmonary complications as well as renal failure. In older children, the course is variable as far as the development of renal insufficiency is concerned, although close to one-half now survive to at least 15 years of age. For those who survive their first year, the number alive at age 15 increases to 79%. Complications such as hypertension and heart failure contribute to mortality. In older children renal involvement is frequently mild and hepatic fibrosis dominates. Liver dysfunction is unusual; if portal hypertension exists, hemorrhage from esophageal varices may be a fatal complication.

Detection of Carrier: Unknown.

Special Considerations: There is marked clinical variability in this condition. While the disease is known to be transmitted as an autosomal recessive inheritance and the basic pathology in regard to cystic dilatation of renal collecting tubules and involvement of the intrahepatic biliary system is observed in all patients, the age of onset, the extent of renal and hepatic involvement and the rate of progression vary greatly.

The condition occurs in animals other than man; in goldfish (Grassius Auratus), mice (FWw strain), rats (Gunn strain) and rabbits.

Chronic administration of lithium chloride produced cystic kidneys in dogs.

Support Groups:
New York; National Kidney Foundation
MO; Kansas City; Polycystic Kidney Research (PKR) Foundation

References:
Blythe H, Ockenden BG: Polycystic disease of kidneys and liver presenting in childhood. J Med Genet 1971; 8:257.
Morin PR, et al.: Prenatal detection of the autosomal recessive type of polycystic kidney disease by trehalase assay in amniotic fluid. Prenatal diagn 1981; 1:75–79.
Zerres K, et al.: Cystic kidneys: genetics, pathologic anatomy, clinical picture and prenatal diagnosis. Hum Genet 1984; 68:104–135.
Bernstein J, et al.: Renal-hepatic-pancreatic dysplasia: a syndrome reconsidered. Am J Med Genet 1987; 26:391–403.
Kaariainen H: Polycystic kidney disease in children: a genetic and epidemiological study of 82 Finnish patients. J Med Genet 1987; 24:474–481.
Wirth B, et al.: Autosomal recessive and dominant forms of polycystic kidney disease are not allelic. Hum Genet 1987; 77:221–222.
Kaplan BS, et al.: Variable expression of autosomal recessive polycystic kidney disease and congenital hepatic fibrosis within a family. Am J Med Genet 1988; 29:639–647.
Kaplan BS, et al.: Autosomal recessive polycystic kidney disease. Pediatr Nephrol 1989; 3:43–49.

SA008   **Inge Sagel**
BI012   **Nesrin Bingol**
KA042   **Bernard S. Kaplan**

KIDNEY, POLYCYSTIC DISEASE-CATARACT-BLINDNESS 3288

Includes:
    Blindness-polycystic kidney disease-cataract
    Cataract-polycystic kidney disease-blindness
    Cystic kidney disease-cataract-blindness

Excludes:
    Cataract-renal tubular necrosis-encephalopathy, Crome type (2162)
    Oculo-cerebro-renal syndrome (0736)
    Renal dysplasia-retinal aplasia, Loken-Senior type (2687)

Major Diagnostic Criteria: Congenital blindness, cystic kidney disease and cataracts.

Clinical Findings: Patients usually present with congenital blindness and renal disease mainly proteinuria. Hypertension, renal failure and findings suggestive of renal tubular disease may be present. Central cataracts, myopia and retinal dystrophy may also be present. Kidney abnormalities described include polycystic kidney disease, medullary cystic disease, pyramidal cysts, and microcystic renal dysplasia.

Complications: Chronic renal failure.

Associated Findings: Microcornia; retinal dysplasia, hypoplasia or aplasia; absence of ciliary body and nystagmus.

Etiology: Possibly autosomal recessive inheritance.

Pathogenesis: Possibly an antenatal dysgenetic process.

MIM No.: 26310

Sex Ratio: M1:F4 (observed).

Occurrence: Five cases have been documented in the literature.

Risk of Recurrence for Patient's Sib:
    See Part I, *Mendelian Inheritance.*

Risk of Recurrence for Patient's Child:
    See Part I, *Mendelian Inheritance.*

Age of Detectability: At any age. Congenital blindness may suggest the diagnosis.

Gene Mapping and Linkage: Unknown.

Prevention: None known. Genetic counseling indicated.

Treatment: Diagnosis and treatment of recurrent urinary tract infections and renal calculi help to prevent deterioration in renal function. The cataracts and chronic renal failure are treated as indicated.

Prognosis: Varies with the severity of the renal disease. Renal failure can occur in childhood.

Detection of Carrier: Unknown.

Special Considerations: Since polycystic kidney disease, medullary cystic disease, **Kidney, medullary sponge kidney**, and microcystic renal dysplasia have been described in patients with this syndrome, the term *cystic kidney disease* is more appropriate than "polycystic kidney" in the title.

References:
Fairley KF, et al.: Familial visual defects associated with polycystic kidney and medullary sponge kidney. Brit Med J 1963; 1:1060–1063.
Pierson M, et al.: Une curieuse association malformative congenitale et familiale atteignant l'oeil et le rein. J Genet Hum 1963; 12:184–213.

BA065
                 Amin Y. Barakat

Kidney, renal cell carcinoma
See CANCER, RENAL CELL CARCINOMA

KIDNEY, RENAL DYSPLASIA, POTTER TYPE II 3028

Includes:
    Cystic dysplasia
    Cystic hydrocalicosis, congenital
    Multicystic kidney, congenital unilateral
    Multicystic renal dysplasia
    Potter type II renal dysplasia

Excludes:
    Kidney, polycystic disease, dominant (0859)
    Kidney, polycystic disease, recessive (2003)
    Renal dysplasia with primitive renal tubules

Major Diagnostic Criteria: The diagnosis of multicystic renal dysplasia should be suspected by the presence of multiple, irregular anechoic renal cysts in renal ultrasonographic examinations. Radionuclide renal scans demonstrate absence of blood flow and excretory function in affected kidneys. Histologic features include primitive epithelial ductal structures surrounded by fibrous tissue with islands of metaplastic, cartilage-scattered immature tubules, or glomeruli occasionally identified in otherwise disorganized mesenchyme.

Clinical Findings: Most patients are identified when an asymptomatic flank mass is palpated in the newborn nursery. Multicystic renal dysplasia is the most common unilateral flank mass in newborns and involves the left kidney more commonly than the right. Occasionally, multicystic renal dysplasia is bilateral and results in anuria and early death. The urinalysis is generally normal in neonates with unilateral multicystic renal dysplasia.

Complications: Rarely, hypertension may accompany unilateral multicystic renal dysplasia (Chen et al., 1985). Bilateral multicystic renal dysplasia results in pulmonary hypoplasia and shares the facial and cranial features of Potter syndrome.

Associated Findings: Obstruction of the contralateral kidney occurs in 30% of patients with unilateral multicystic renal dysplasia. Multicystic renal dysplasia is also frequently associated with ectopic kidney or **Kidney, horseshoe**. The ureter of a multicystic dysplastic kidney is usually not patent. Cystic dysplasia may be associated with cerebral malformation, including **Hydrocephaly**, **Polydactyly**, and hepatic dysgenesis (Simopoulos syndrome), Dandy-Walker malformation, **Meckel syndrome**, and Miranda syndrome. Biliary dysgenesis and multicystic renal dysplasia (usually bilateral) occurs in Meckle syndrome and in Jeune **Asphyxiating thoracic dysplasia**. Other syndromes that include bilateral multicystic renal dysplasia are **Asplenia syndrome**, **De Lange syndrome**, and **Short rib-polydactyly syndrome**.

Etiology: In most instances, multicystic renal dysplasia (particularly when unilateral) is sporadic. Rarely, bilateral multicystic renal dysplasia has been reported to occur in sibs, suggesting an autosomal recessive inheritance. Bernstein (1983) reports that renal ultrasonic examination of 51 family members of children with multicystic renal dysplasia revealed only one instance of cystic renal dysplasia; the one familial recurrence was a stillborn male infant with posterior urethral valves.

Pathogenesis: Osathanondh and Potter (1965) attributed multicystic renal dysplasia to inhibition of ampullary branching with failure to induce normal nephrogenesis in metanephric tissue. Bernstein (1971) proposed that most multicystic renal dysplasia is the result of injury following nephron induction and that the most plausible injury is ureteral obstruction.

POS No.: 3368

Sex Ratio: Presumably M1:F1, although some investigators report a male preponderance.

Occurrence: Unknown. There is no known racial difference, and incidence figures are not available.

Risk of Recurrence for Patient's Sib: Two percent (observed), although autosomal recessive inheritance (25%) has been suggested for some families with multiple affected sibs (Cole et al, 1976).

Risk of Recurrence for Patient's Child: Unknown. No instances of affected offspring have yet been reported.

Age of Detectability: During the third trimester.

Gene Mapping and Linkage: Unknown.

Prevention: None known. Genetic counseling indicated.

Treatment: Surgical removal of a unilateral multicystic renal dysplastic kidney may be required for abdominal discomfort, hypertension, or, rarely, infection.

Prognosis: Usually good.

Detection of Carrier: Unknown.

Support Groups: New York; National Kidney Foundation

References:
Osathanondh V, Potter EL: Pathogenesis of polycystic kidneys. Arch Pathol 1965; 77:459–512.
Bernstein J: The morphogenesis of renal parenchymal maldevelopment (renal dysplasia). Pediatr Clin North Am 1971; 18:395–407.
Cole BR, et al.: Bilateral renal dysplasia in three siblings: report of a survivor. Clin Nephrol 1976; 5:83–87.
Kissane JM: The morphology of renal cystic disease. In: Gardener KG, ed: Cystic diseases of the kidney. New York: John Wiley & Sons, 1976:31–63.
Bernstein J: Renal dysplasia: morphologic and family studies. In: Brodehl J, Ehrich JHH, eds: Pediatric nephrology. Berlin: Springer-Verlag, 1983:353–355.
Chen Y-H et al.: Neonatal hypertension from a unilateral multicystic dysplastic kidney. J Urol 1985; 133:664–665.

ST055   **F. Bruder Stapleton**

Kidney, uremic sponge
See KIDNEY, NEPHRONOPHTHISIS-MEDULLARY CYSTIC DESEASE
Kidney-liver disease, adult type polycystic
See LIVER, POLYCYSTIC AND MULTICYSTIC DISEASE, ADULT TYPE
Kidneys connected by a fibrous or parenchymatous isthmus
See KIDNEY, HORSESHOE
Kidneys, absence of
See RENAL AGENESIS, BILATERAL
Kidneys, congenital bilateral absence of
See RENAL AGENESIS, BILATERAL
Kidneys, cystic-retinal aplasia-Joubert syndrome
See JOUBERT SYNDROME
Killian syndrome
See PALLISTER-KILLIAN MOSAIC SYNDROME
Kiloh-Nevin dystrophy of the external ocular muscles
See KEARNS-SAYRE DISEASE
Kindler-Weary syndrome
See POIKILODERMA, HEREDITARY ACROKERATOTIC, KINDLER-WEARY TYPE

KING SYNDROME   2492

Includes:
King-Denborough syndrome
Malignant hyperthermia-Noonan-like phenotype
Noonan-like phenotype-malignant hyperthermia

Excludes:
Kniest dysplasia (0557)
Muscular dystrophy, facio-scapulo-humeral (2049)
Myopathy, central core disease type (0134)
Myopathy, malignant hyperthermia (2710)
Noonan syndrome (0720)
Pterygium syndrome, multiple (2186)

Major Diagnostic Criteria: A Noonan-like phenotype and malignant hyperthermia. Absence of webbed neck, congenital heart defects and mental retardation, as well as presence of muscle weakness, differentiate King from **Noonan syndrome**. Its sporadic occurrence is another differentiating feature.

Clinical Findings: The most common major features are the Noonan-like facies, short stature, and episodes of malignant hyperthermia. Based on 11 reported patients, the approximate frequency of the clinical features is as follows: hyperthermia (11/11), short stature (9/11), transient delay of motor development (8/11), normal intelligence (11/11), muscle weakness (7/11), downward slant of palpebral fissures (7/11), ptosis (6/11), midface hypoplasia (9/11), micrognathia (11/11), low-set ears (7/11), **Pectus carinatum** (10/11), kyphoscoliosis and/or lordosis (11/11), and cryptorchidism (8/9).

The dysmorphic signs are usually apparent in early infancy. The short stature becomes evident in early childhood. The malignant hyperthermia is a pharmacogenetic feature which manifests when exposed to depolarizing skeletal muscle relaxants and/or volatile hydrocarbon anesthetics. End tidal carbon dioxide rises very early in the development of the hyperthermia and capnography during anesthesia appears useful for the early detection of this sign.

Complications: The life-threatening feature is the malignant hyperthermia. The muscle weakness is mild and appears to be non-progressive.

Associated Findings: Contractures have been reported in three of the 11 patients.

Etiology: While all cases have been sporadic, in four there was a family history of elevated serum creatine kinase (CK) levels in several relatives without the characteristic dysmorphic phenotypic features of the syndrome. Etiologic heterogeneity of the syndrome has been suggested by a family sibs with King-like phenotype, including hyperthermia. The parents in this family did not have any of the phenotypic features, and had normal CK levels.

Pathogenesis: The pathogenesis of the malignant hyperthermia appears similar to that of other malignant hyperthermias. Several studies of hyperthermias have implied disrupted intracellular calcium movement and enhanced calcium release, as well as tubular, mitochondrial, and sarcolemmal dysfunctions. Elevated levels and enhanced activity of phospholipase A in the muscles appear to represent another component of the pathogenetic mechanism. In another patient, CT scan of the extremities showed myopathic changes within certain muscle groups. The changes consisted of areas of degeneration and fatty infiltration. Thus CT scan of the extremities may be of diagnostic help.

MIM No.: *14560

POS No.: 4183

Sex Ratio: M5:F1

Occurrence: Fewer than a dozen cases have been documented.

Risk of Recurrence for Patient's Sib: If the syndrome is indeed sporadic, the risk should not be increased. In the families with elevated CK levels, the risk for malignant hyperthermia may be as high as 50%.

Risk of Recurrence for Patient's Child: Unknown.

Age of Detectability: Variable, but can be detected in infancy or whenever the malignant hyperthermia is encountered.

Gene Mapping and Linkage: Unknown.

Prevention: Capnography during anesthesia and prompt administration of dantrolene have already reduced the mortality of malignant hyperthermia from 70% to 10%. Muscle biopsy for a caffeine contracture test prior to anesthesia may detect a predisposition to hyperthermia. Elevated CK levels in relatives are found in only about 30% of those tested, making this a less reliable test. Exposure of platelet-rich plasma from patients with malignant hyperthermia to halothane produces a significant decrease in the platelet ATP pool compared to controls. Control patients who had hyperthermia, hyperkalemia, acidosis, or myopathy not related to malignant hyperthermia had nucleotide profiles that were indistinguishable from those of normal persons. Thus the platelet test appears to be specific for malignant hyperthermia. It can be done within 45 minutes and appears promising for the prevention of hyperthermia.

Treatment: Prompt administration of dantrolene for treatment of malignant hyperthermia is crucial. Physical therapy for the muscle weakness appears beneficial.

Prognosis: Shortened life span if fatal malignant hyperthermia occurs. If prevention or successful treatment of this feature occurs, there are no other clinical features in the syndrome expected to shorten the life span.

Detection of Carrier: Determination of CK levels in the families with sporadic King syndrome may detect relatives at risk for malignant hyperthermia.

References:
King JO, Denborough MA: Anesthetic-induced malignant hyperpyrexia in children. J Pediatr 1973; 83:37–40.
McPherson EW, Taylor CA: The King syndrome: malignant hyperthermia, myopathy, and multiple anomalies. Am J Med Genet 1981; 8:159–165.
Koussseff BG, Nichols P: A new autosomal recessive syndrome with Noonan-like phenotype, myopathy with congenital contractures and malignant hyperthermia. BD:OAS XXI(2). New York: March of Dimes Birth Defects Foundation, 1985:111–117.
Qazi QH, et al.: King syndrome with focal myopathic involvement demonstrated by C-T scan. Pediatr Res 1985; 19:329A.

K0018 **Boris G. Koussseff**

King-Denborough syndrome
See KING SYNDROME
Kinky hair disease
See MENKES SYNDROME
Kirghizian dermato-osteolysis
See DERMATO-OSTEOLYSIS, KIRGHIZIAN TYPE
Kitamura acropigmentatio reticularis
See SKIN CREASES, RETICULATE PIGMENTED FLEXURES, DOWLING-DEGOS TYPE
Kjer optic atrophy
See OPTIC ATROPHY, KJER TYPE
Klebcil∧, fetal effects
See FETAL AMINOGLYCOSIDE OTOTOXICITY
Kleeblattschadel craniosynostosis
See CRANIOSYNOSTOSIS, KLEEBLATTSCHADEL TYPE
Klein-Waardenburg syndrome
See WAARDENBURG SYNDROMES

KLINEFELTER SYNDROME 0556

Includes:
　　Chromosome XXY
　　Hypergonadotropic hypogonadism
　　Primary hypogonadism
　　Seminiferous tubule dysgenesis
　　True Klinefelter syndrome

Excludes:
　　Gonadotropin deficiencies (0438)
　　Hypogonadism (other forms)
　　Sertoli cell-only syndrome (3163)

Major Diagnostic Criteria: X-chromatin-positive male with phenotypic male genitalia; small, firm testes; and karyotype usually 47,XXY, elevated serum; and urinary gonadotropins.

Clinical Findings: Most affected individuals appear normal as neonates and in early infancy, except when the testes are found to be significantly smaller than normal. As first described by Klinefelter, Reifenstein and Albright in 1942, the characteristic clinical features that become evident at adolescence are small atrophic testes, small penis, gynecomastia, incomplete virilization, variable eunuchoidism, and tendency to dull mentality. Tall stature occurs with the syndrome (an average 10 cm taller than XY males), and altered body proportions, i.e. low upper to lower segment ratio and span less than or equal to height.

The testes remain less than 2.5 cm in length even into adulthood and often less than 1.5 cm. Cryptorchidism, gynecomastia, and incomplete virilization occur in more than one-half of the cases. Plasma and urinary gonadotropins are increased. Plasma testosterone is often less than the normal range for men. Later disturbances of sexual function occur, i.e. complete infertility, impotence, and lack of libido.

The number of spermatogonia is decreased as early as infancy compared to normal 46,XY males of the same age. At and after puberty, progressive sclerosis and hyalinization of seminiferous

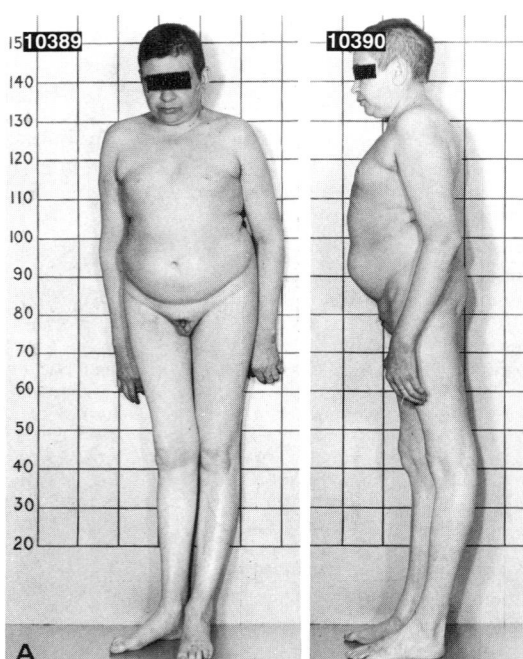

0556-10389–90: Tall stature with relatively long limbs and truncal obesity.

tubules leads to loss of germinal tissue with consequent secondary clumping ("nodular hyperplasia") of Leydig cells, which are ultimately also lost in a process of progressive fibrosis and atrophy.

Behavioral problems and personality disturbances are common in the syndrome but may not be evident until school age. The true frequency of such manifestations is unknown since patients with behavioral problems appear in treatment more frequently than those without.

Complications: Psychologic and psychiatric complications of a person with less than average intelligence, hypogonadism, and impotence. Vertebral collapse sometimes occurs secondary to osteoporosis. Increased predisposition to breast cancer has been reported in Klinefelter syndrome. Also, varicose veins appear to be more common in this syndrome.

Associated Findings: Multiple minor anomalies are common in the Klinefelter syndrome: brachycephalic skull configuration, at times with low nuchal hairline, minor defects of differentiation of auricles, clinodactyly of fifth fingers at times with only one flexion crease on that finger, simian creases and other variations of palmar crease patterns, decreased total ridge count of fingertip dermatoglyphic patterns, and increased incidence of hypothenar patterns with distal axial palmar triradius. Radioulnar synostosis occurs with increased incidence in this syndrome. In individuals with more complex sex chromosome aneuploidy (48,XXXY; 49XXXXY; 49,XXXYY, etc.) multiple somatic anomalies and mental retardation are common. Scoliosis during adolescence has been noted. Incidence of diabetes mellitus and thyroid dysfunction is increased in this syndrome.

Etiology: More complex meiotic nondisjunction in either parent results in 47,XXY, while mitotic nondisjunction after fertilization results in mosaicism, of which 46,XY/47,XXY is the most common.

Pathogenesis: Pathogenesis of seminiferous tubule dysgenesis is unknown. Eunuchoidism and other manifestations of hypogonadism presumably are due to progressive testicular sclerosis with loss of germinal and endocrine tissue.

About 2/3 of 47,XXY cases are of the X^MX^MY type, 1/3 are

XᴹXᴾY, (M = maternal, P = paternal source). In the former group, increased maternal age supports the hypothesis of maternal meiotic nondisjunction; maternal age is not increased in the mosaic or XᴹXᴾY cases.

MIM No.: 23832, 25730

POS No.: 3107

CDC No.: 758.7

Sex Ratio: M1:F0

Occurrence: Buccal smear survey: incidence of males with X-chromatin: 1:590 live-born males (1:1250 to 1:110 live-born infants). Neonatal chromosome surveys: approximately 1:500 live-born males.

Prevalence estimated at 1:1000, primarily in the general Caucasian populations. In institutions for the mentally retarded; around 1:100 male patients.

Among populations of infertile men: 1:77 to 1:24 of all infertile men; 1:9 to 1:5 for men with high grades of infertility (i.e. azoospermia or sperm count less than 1 x 10⁶/ml).

Among men in psychiatric institutions: 1:169.

Risk of Recurrence for Patient's Sib: Presumably not significantly increased.

Risk of Recurrence for Patient's Child: Only four fertile 46,XY/47,XXY mosaics are known; one child was a 47,XXY male; all other offspring were presumably normal. All 47,XXY patients are infertile.

Age of Detectability: Prenatally in the second trimester by amniocentesis and cytogenetic analysis of amniotic cells.

Gene Mapping and Linkage: HHG (hypergonadotropic hypogonadism) is ULG5.

Prevention: None known. Genetic counseling indicated.

Treatment: Treatment of hypogonadism. Supportive psychotherapy for emotional complications. Testosterone replacement therapy, beginning at age 11 to 12 years, is indicated to bring about adolescent development and prevent some of the features of adult Klinefelter syndrome. Depo-testosterone 50–100 mg every 3 weeks until adult dosage of 150–200 mg is achieved at age approximately 17 years.

Prognosis: Life span is presumably normal.

Detection of Carrier: Unknown.

Special Considerations: The patients with more complex sex chromosome aneuploidy (48,XXXY; 49,XXXX; 48,XXYY; 49,XXXYY, etc.) are usually ascertained on the basis of mental retardation, generally with multiple anomalies. 47,XYY individuals do not have Klinefelter syndrome.

References:
Klinefelter HF, et al.: Syndrome characterized by gynecomastia, aspermatogenesis without aleydigism and increased secretion of follicle-stimulating hormone (gynecomastia). J Clin Endocrinol Metab 1942; 2:615.
Becker KL, et al.: Klinefelter's syndrome. Arch Intern Med 1966; 118:314.
Caldwell PD, Smith DW: The XXY syndrome in childhood detection and treatment. J Pediatr 1972; 80:250.
Laron Z: Klinefelter's syndrome: early diagnosis and treatment. Hosp Pract 1972; 7:135.
Williams RH, ed: Textbook of endocrinology. 6th ed. Philadelphia: W.B. Saunders, 1981.

BU007
HU010
SA024

Bruce A. Buehler
Carol A. Huseman
Warren Sanger

KLIPPEL-FEIL ANOMALY 2032

Includes:
  Brevicollis, congenital
  Cervical vertebral fusion, congenital
  Klippel-Feil syndrome

Excludes:
  Cervico-oculo-acoustic syndrome (0142)
  Eye, Duane retraction syndrome (3180)
  Spondylocostal dysplasia (0896)
  Spondylothoracic dysplasia (0900)

Major Diagnostic Criteria: Congenital fusion of cervical vertebrae is the only constant sign, with typical patients presenting the clinical triad of short neck, limitation of head and neck movement, and low posterior hairline.

Clinical Findings: According to Feil's classification, there are three morphological types of vertebral fusion: *type I* is an extensive cervical and upper thoracic vertebral fusion; *type II* is a localized fusion of one or two pairs of cervical vertebrae, often accompanied by hemivertebrae and occipitoatlantal fusion; and *type III* is a combination of cervical and lower thoracic or lumbar fusion. Since

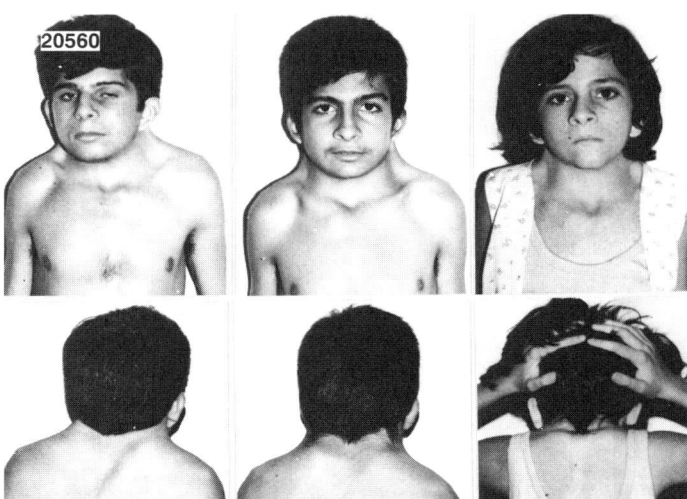

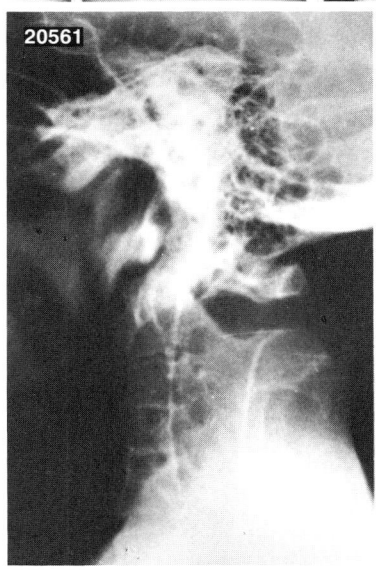

2032-20560: Note short neck and low posterior hairlines. 20561: Fusion of vertebrae C2-5.

this classification does not encompass all the reported cases of Klippel-Feil anomaly, a type IV fusion was recently proposed for patients with cervical, upper thoracic, lower thoracic and/or lumbar vertebral fusions. The classical cases of Klippel-Feil anomaly have a short webbed neck, limitation of head and neck, motion, and low posterior hairline. Usually, the neck motion is better preserved in the flexion and extension than in the lateral and rotational planes. Patients with the type II pattern of fusion, which is considered the most frequent and the less severe form, may have a normal or almost normal appearance.

A wide variety of anomalies has been associated with Klippel-Feil anomaly. Scoliosis or kyphoscoliosis is found in about 60% of the patients, and spina bifida occulta in 45%. Urinary anomalies also appear to be very frequent. The combined data of three large series showed that 55% of the patients (57/103) had urinary anomalies, one-half (29 cases) being **Renal agenesis, unilateral**. Other abnormalities include absence of both kidneys, renal dysgenesis or hypoplasia, ectopic kidney, horseshoe kidney, malrotation of kidney, absence of ureter, double collecting system, and hydronephrosis. Genital abnormalities are less frequent, but not uncommon; they are observed mostly in female patients and include absent vagina, absent or rudimentary uterus, absent or hypoplastic fallopian tube, and bicornuate uterus; **Hypospadias** and cryptorchidism are found in some male patients. Sprengel deformity, deafness (conductive, sensorineural, or mixed), and rib anomalies (mainly rib fusion) are found in 30% of the cases. Variable ocular defects (**Eye, microphthalmia/coloboma**, **Eyelid, ptosis, congenital**, **Eye, hypertelorism**, nystagmus, rectus palsy, and others), craniofacial asymmetry, fixed torticollis, and synkinesia (mirror movement) are observed in 20%; **Cleft palate** in 15%; and heart defects (mainly interventricular septal defects) in about 8%.

Complications: The most important complications are neurologic symptoms of cervical spinal cord injury (such as pain, easy fatigability, spasticity, hyperreflexia, paresthesia, hypesthesia, hemiparesis, and quadriplegia) as a consequence of occipitocervical instability. In many patients, these symptoms occur either spontaneously or after minor trauma. Sudden death after minor trauma has been reported. The complications are not directly derived from the fused cervical vertebrae, but result from adjacent unfused segments with the free joints becoming hypermobile and being subjected to an excessive stress, which can lead to a cervical instability and/or degenerative changes. A C2-C3 fusion with occipitalization of the atlas, for example, may lead to an atlantoaxial instability. The onset of these problems usually occurs between the second and third decades of life.

Associated Findings: **Meningocele, Encephalocele**, enlargement or narrowing of the cervical canal, **Brain, Arnold-Chiari malformation** basilar impression, **Syringomyelia, Cleft lip, Hydrocephaly, Microcephaly**, external ear anomalies, **Pectus carinatum, Pectus excavatum**, ectopic lungs, **Situs inversus viscerum**, enteric cysts and duplications, congenital megacolon, anal atresia, and upper extremity abnormalities. Short stature and mental retardation also were reported.

Etiology: Klippel-Feil anomaly appears to be etiologically heterogeneous. Most cases are sporadic. Environmental or multifactorial causes may be involved in many cases. In some families, an affected mother and daughter, father and daughter, and father and son have been described. In other families, including a large one with 12 cases, affected sibs of both sexes with normal consanguineous parents were reported. Based on these data, at least two single-gene forms of Klippel-Feil anomaly must be recognized: one autosomal dominant and the other autosomal recessive.

Pathogenesis: Congenital fusion of cervical vertebrae results from abnormal segmentation of the cervical somites between the fourth and eighth weeks of fetal life. A theory of vascular etiology has also been proposed (see **Poland syndrome**).

MIM No.: *11810, 14886, 14887, *14890, 21430

POS No.: 3274

CDC No.: 756.110

Sex Ratio: M1:F1.5 (approximately).

Occurrence: The reported incidence of about 1:40,000 live births which appears in the literature is probably an underestimate, since many mildly affected cases would not be diagnosed because of lack of significant symptoms.

Risk of Recurrence for Patient's Sib:
See Part I, *Mendelian Inheritance.*

Risk of Recurrence for Patient's Child:
See Part I, *Mendelian Inheritance.*

Age of Detectability: At birth.

Gene Mapping and Linkage: Unknown.

Prevention: None known. Genetic counseling indicated.

Treatment: Limited mostly to the complications and associated anomalies. In the presence of cervical spinal cord compression (usually due to cervical instability), decompression or stabilization surgical procedures are required. Patients with Klippel-Feil anomaly, especially those with extensive cervical synostosis, should be guided to avoid activities potentially harmful to the cervical spine. Corrective surgery of associated anomalies may be indicated; for example surgical correction of Sprengel deformity, in properly selected patients, may provide cosmetic and functional improvement.

Prognosis: Normal life span in the absence of serious complications and associated anomalies, especially renal abnormalities and scoliosis.

Detection of Carrier: Unknown.

Special Considerations: Klippel-Feil anomaly, with its wide constellation of associated anomalies, may represent a group of several related but distinct conditions, such as the **Cervico-oculo-acoustic syndrome** (which is virtually limited to females). Some female patients reported as having Klippel-Feil anomaly with associated deafness were possibly cases of **Cervico-oculo-acoustic syndrome**, and the mentioned excess of females with Klippel-Feil anomaly may not be realistic. The association of **Mullerian aplasia** with fused cervical vertebrae and other defects probably constitutes another distinct entity.

References:

Klippel M, Feil A: Un cas d'absence des vertébres cervicales avec cage thoracique remontant jusqu'á la base du crâne (cage thoracique cervicale). Nou Iconogr Saloet 1912; 25:223–250.
Gunderson CH, et al.: The Klippel-Feil syndrome: genetic and clinical reevaluation of cervical fusion. Medicine 1967; 46:491–512.
Hensinger RN, et al.: Klippel-Feil syndrome: a constellation of associated anomalies. J Bone Joint Surg 1974; 56A:1246–1253. *
Helmi C, Pruzansky S: Craniofacial and extracranial malformations in the Klippel-Feil syndrome. Cleft Palate J 1980; 17:65–88. †
da-Silva EO: Autosomal recessive Klippel-Feil syndrome. J Med Genet 1982; 19:130–134. *
Nagib MG, et al.: Identification and management of high-risk patients with Klippel-Feil syndrome. J Neurosurg 1984; 61:523–530.
Shaver KA, et al.: Deafness, facial asymmetry and Klippel-Feil syndrome in five generations. (Abstract) Am J Hum Genet 1986; 39:A81 only.

DA025   **Elias O. da-Silva**

Klippel-Feil anomaly-deafness-abducens palsy
See CERVICO-OCULO-ACOUSTIC SYNDROME
Klippel-Feil syndrome
See KLIPPEL-FEIL ANOMALY
Klippel-Trenaunay-Weber syndrome (KTW)
See ANGIO-OSTEOHYPERTROPHY SYNDROME

KNEE, GENU RECURVATUM 2938

Includes: Hyperextension of the knee

Excludes: Knee, dislocation

Major Diagnostic Criteria: Anterior overextension of the knee, generally present immediately after birth. Genu recurvatum may occur unilaterally, but is usually found bilaterally.

Clinical Findings: Hyperextension of the knee can be present as an isolated anomaly. In such circumstances the infants were generally constrained *in utero*, especially in full knee extension breech position, or confined to a bicorneate uterus. Other constraint-induced deformities of the legs and facies are often associated. Hyperextension of the knee may also occur because of primary malformations of ligament, bone and joint, or neuromuscular system. The overall physical examination and the gestational history will almost always suggest the deformational or malformational origin in this disorder.

Complications: When genu recurvatum is left untreated in the newborn period it may progress to dislocation of the knee, with secondary changes then occurring in the bones, ligaments, and muscles. Distortion of the distal femoral epiphysis and shortening or fibrosis of the quadriceps both occur frequently.

Associated Findings: Genu recurvatum of deformational origin is often associated with dislocated hip, plantar position of the forefoot, and flattening of the face. Infants with congenitally small patellas or the **Nail-patella syndrome** often have genu recurvatum or knee dislocations. Joint hyperextension and dislocations including the knee are seen in conditions of ligamentous laxity, such as the **Ehlers-Danlos syndrome**. **Meningomyelocele, Arthrogryposes,** and other intrinsic neuromuscular conditions can produce unusual muscle pull about the knee and hyperextension or dislocation.

Etiology: Heterogeneous, with both deformational and primary and secondary malformational causes.

Pathogenesis: The shape and growth of the knee, like any joint, is determined by a balanced interplay between intrinsic properties of bone and soft tissues and by extrinsic biomechanical forces. Intrinsic factors include the biochemical structure of the bones, their growth potential, and physical properties, while extrinsic factors include muscle pull and dynamic stress applied by the fetal confines.

CDC No.: 754.430

Sex Ratio: M1:F1

Occurrence: Estimated at 2:10,000 births.

Risk of Recurrence for Patient's Sib: Recurrence is unlikely when deformation occurred without evidence of a primary central nervous system process in the infant except when there is a maternal uterine process (like fibroids or a bicornate structure), which predisposes subsequent infants to constraint. When genu recurvatum is due to a primary or secondary malformation, specific risk recurrence for that causal disorder will apply.

Risk of Recurrence for Patient's Child: Recurrence is unlikely when deformation occurred without evidence of a primary central nervous system process in the infant except when there is a maternal uterine process (like fibroids or a bicornate structure), which predisposes subsequent infants to constraint. When genu recurvatum is due to a primary or secondary malformation, specific risk recurrence for that causal disorder will apply.

Age of Detectability: Immediately after birth.

Gene Mapping and Linkage: Unknown.

Prevention: None known. Genetic counseling indicated.

Treatment: Genu recurvatum can be managed conservatively in the neonatal period with manipulation and mild pressure immobilization toward the normal joint position.

Prognosis: The prognosis for correction of genu recurvatum is fully dependent on the cause. Deformations of the knee should respond well to repositioning. Malformational hyperextension may respond to repositioning, but often requires surgery. In some cases of severe bony anomaly or neuromuscular imbalance, surgery may not be fully corrective or capable of preventing recurrence.

Detection of Carrier: Unknown.

References:

Niebauer JT, King DE: Congenital dislocation of the knee. J Bone Joint Surg 1960; 42A:207–225.

Laurence M: Genu recurvatum congenitum. J Bone Joint Surg 1967; 49B:121–134.

Smith DW: Recognizable patterns of human deformation. Philadelphia: W.B. Saunders, 1981. †

CL006   **Sterling K. Clarren**

Kniest disease
See KNIEST DYSPLASIA

KNIEST DYSPLASIA 0557

Includes:

Dwarfism, metatropic, type II
Kniest disease
Metatropic dysplasia, type II
Pseudometatropic dwarfism
Swiss-cheese cartilage syndrome

Excludes:

Dwarfism, dyssegmental, Rolland-Desbuquois type (2690)
Dwarfism, dyssegmental, Silverman-Handmaker type (2935)
Metatropic dysplasia (0656)
Mucopolysaccharidosis IV (0678)
Spondyloepiphyseal dysplasia congenita (0897)
Spondyloepiphyseal dysplasia, late (0898)

Major Diagnostic Criteria: Disproportionate dwarfism with typical X-ray changes in the skeleton, frequently myopia and typical flat facies. Characteristic chondroosseous histopathology may be used to verify the diagnosis.

Clinical Findings: Disproportionate dwarfism and kyphoscoliosis associated with flat facies and prominent eyes, cleft palate, hearing loss, myopia, and limited joint motion. The skeletal abnormalities are recognizable at birth with shortening and deformity of the limbs and stiff joints. Marked lumbar lordosis and kyphoscoliosis develop in childhood resulting in disproportionate shortening of the trunk. Walking is delayed and difficult. The long bones are short and bowed and the joints appear enlarged. There is limitation of joint motion with pain, stiffness and flexion contractures of the major joints. The flexion contractures in the hips produce a characteristic stance. The fingers appear long and knobby, and flexion is limited resulting in an inability to form a fist. The face is flat and dish-shaped with prominent wide-set eyes, flat nasal bridge and a broad mouth. There is severe myopia which frequently leads to retinal detachment. Umbilical and inguinal herniae are common. Cleft palate may lead to chronic otitis media and both conductive and neurosensory hearing loss

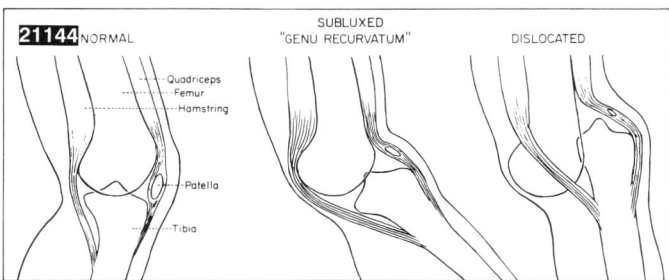

2938-21144: The subluxed knee is an intermediate pattern of anatomic distortion when compared to the normal or dislocated knee.

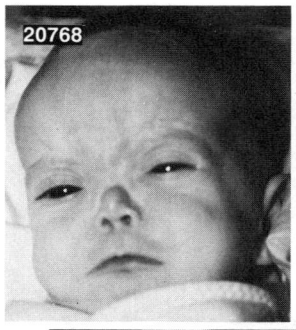
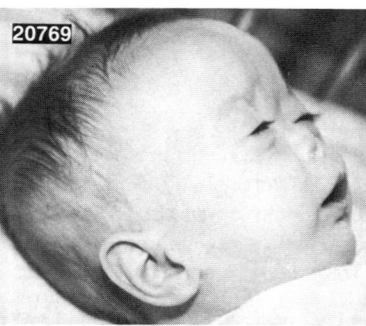
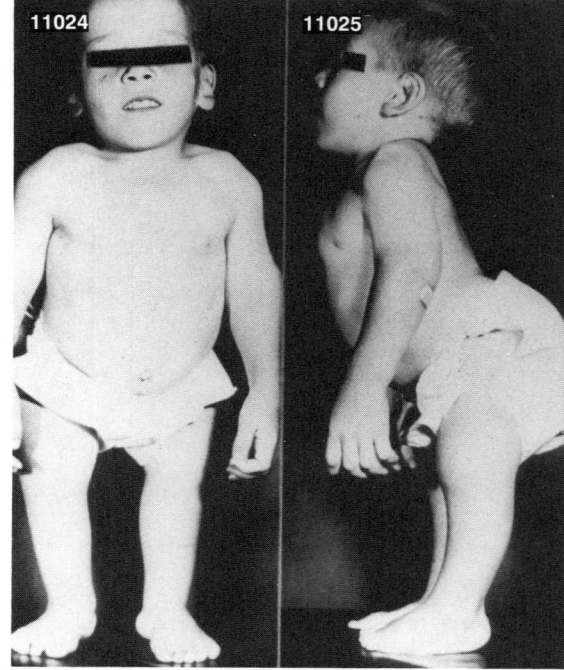
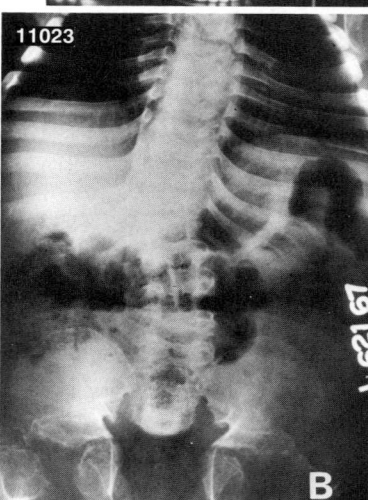
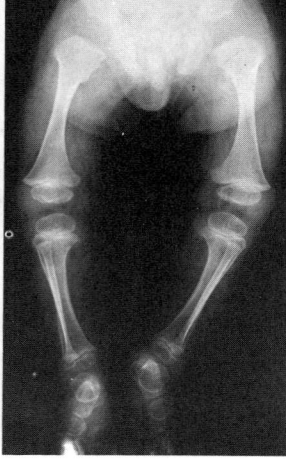

are common. Recurrent respiratory distress with tracheomalacia may occur in infancy. Motor milestones and speech development may be delayed, but intelligence usually is normal.

The characteristic X-ray abnormalities during the newborn period include dumbbell-shaped femora, hypoplastic pelvic bones, vertical clefts of the vertebrae, and platyspondyly. In infancy and childhood one sees a dessert-cup shaped pelvis, increased soft tissue densities around the joints, enlarged epiphyses, cloud-like calcifications near the epiphyseal plates, and flat elongated vertebral bodies with cloud-like calcifications. The bones of the hands are osteoporotic and show delay in formation of epiphyses; soft tissue swelling occurs near the joints. There are fragmented accessory ossification centers and joint spaces are narrowed. The femoral heads show a marked delay in ossification and may not appear until mid-childhood. In adult life, there is rhizomelic short stature but the cloud calcifications disappear after epiphyseal fusion. Hands show a bulbous enlargement of the ends of the short tubular bones, short thumb tufts, and a flat and squared appearance of the metacarpal-phalangeal joints.

Complications: Myopia may lead to retinal detachment. Shortened and deformed bones and limitation of joint motion may lead to severe orthopedic complications. Cleft palate may lead to speech impairment and chronic otitis media.

Associated Findings: Ocular findings include vitreoretinal degeneration, rhegmatogenous retinal detachment, dislocated lenses, and blepharoptosis.

Etiology: Presumably autosomal dominant inheritance.

Pathogenesis: The chondro-osseous histopathology is abnormal and distinctive. Resting cartilage contains large cells, a loosely woven matrix with irregular staining, and many "holes" which have been likened to "swiss-cheese cartilage." The growth plate contains hypercellular cartilage with ballooned chondrocytes and sparse matrix. The condition is characterized by an apparent abnormal processing of the C-propeptide of type II cartilage collagen, resulting in imperfect fibril assembly.

MIM No.: *15655

POS No.: 3272

Sex Ratio: M1:F1

Occurrence: Undetermined. Established literature.

Risk of Recurrence for Patient's Sib:
See Part I, *Mendelian Inheritance.*

Risk of Recurrence for Patient's Child:
See Part I, *Mendelian Inheritance.*

Age of Detectability: Prenatal diagnosis by ultrasound.

Gene Mapping and Linkage: Unknown.

Prevention: None known. Genetic counseling indicated.

Treatment: Orthopedic surgery for joint contractures, kyphoscoliosis, and epiphyseal dysplasia; repair of cleft palate, frequent regular ophthalmologic examinations for detection and prevention of retinal detachment.

Prognosis: Apparently normal for life.

Detection of Carrier: Unknown.

Special Considerations: This condition had been confused with **Metatropic dysplasia** in the past because of the similar dumbbell appearance of the long bones in the newborn. These disorders can be readily distinguished on the basis of skeletal X-rays and clinical features. Recently several distinct Kniest-like skeletal dysplasias have been reported which also appear to be autosomal recessive.

References:
Maroteaux P, Spranger J: La maladie de Kniest. Arch Fr Pediatr 1973; 30:735–750.
Rimoin DL, et al.: Metatropic dwarfism, the Kniest syndrome, and the pseudoachondroplastic dysplasias. Clin Orthop 1976; 114:70–82.
Sconyers SM, et al.: A distinct chondrodysplasia resembling Kniest dysplasia. J Pediatr 1983; 103:898–904.
Friede H, et al.: Craniofacial and mucopolysaccharide abnormalities in Kniest dysplasia. J Craniofac Genet Devel Biol 1985; 5:267–276.

0557-20768–69: Kniest dysplasia; note hypertelorism, flat facies, hemangioma on the glabella and low-set ears. **11024–25:** Note round facies; shortening of trunk and limbs. Pelvis and trunk are bent forward secondary to flexion contractures of the hip. **11023:** Moderately severe thoracolumbar scoliosis, decreased vertical diameter of ilia. **20650:** Lower limbs in a 1-year-old; note the short long bones, wide metaphyses, the large femoral distal epiphyses and the tibial proximal epiphyses contrasting with the femoral head which is not visible.

Maumenee IH, Traboulsi EI: The ocular findings in Kniest dysplasia. Am J Ophthal 1985; 100:155–160.

Poole AR, et al.: Kniest dysplasia is characterized by an apparent abnormal processing of the C-propeptide of type II cartilage collagen, resulting in imperfect fibril assembly. J Clin Invest 1988; 81:579–589.

B0025
LA006

Zvi Borochowitz
Ralph S. Lachman
David L. Rimoin

Kniest, severe neonatal form
See KNIEST-LIKE DYSPLASIA

KNIEST-LIKE DYSPLASIA   2799

Includes:

    Chondrodysplasia, Kniest-like
    Chondrodysplasia, micromelic (misnomer)
    Kniest-like dysplasia with pursed lips and ectopia lentis
    Kniest, severe neonatal form
    Skeletal dysplasia, Kniest-like

Excludes:

    Dwarfism, dyssegmental, Rolland-Desbuquois type (2690)
    Kniest dysplasia (0557)
    Thanatophoric dysplasia (0940)
    Thanatophoric dysplasia, Glasgow type (2821)

Major Diagnostic Criteria: Differentiation of this condition from other forms of neonatally lethal short-limbed dwarfisms is based on X-ray and histologic findings.

Clinical Findings: Both known cases were born prematurely, following a pregnancy complicated by hydramnios. Birth weights were normal, but birth lengths were at the 25th or less percentile, and head circumferences at or greater than the 90th percentile. The face was described as flat with wide-set-appearing eyes. **Cleft palate** was present in one, and an "unusual" pharynx in another. The ears were malformed and low set. Both infants also had severe rhizomelia, short neck, narrow thorax, talipes equinovarus, and edema. One had cardiac arrhythmia; the other had **Atrial septal defects** and **Ductus arteriosus, patent**.

X-ray findings included dumbbell-shaped long bones with flared, irregular metaphyses and markedly shortened diaphyses; platyspondyly with wide vertebral clefts; wide, shortened ribs; and hypoplastic ilia. Histologically, the cartilage was similar to the "Swiss-cheese" appearance described in **Kniest dysplasia**; however, there was also a "frayed" appearance to the matrix between chondrocytes. Ultrastructurally, the chondrocyte endoplasmic reticulum was not dilated as it is in Kniest dysplasia.

Complications: Pulmonary hypoplasia may be the result of small thoracic size. Hydrops may occur as a result of in utero cardiac arrhythmia.

Associated Findings: Pursed lips and ectopia lentis were reported in two siblings by Burton et al (1986). Upper limbs were normal, and histologic examination of bone did not show a Swiss cheese appearance.

Etiology: Possibly autosomal recessive inheritance.

Pathogenesis: Although this condition is a chondrodysplasia, the basic genetic defect is unknown. While the term "micromelic chondrodysplasia" has been applied to this group of disorders, the designation is generally considered inappropriate.

MIM No.: 24519

POS No.: 4510

Sex Ratio: Presumably M1:F1.

Occurrence: Reported in two sibs from California.

Risk of Recurrence for Patient's Sib:
    See Part I, *Mendelian Inheritance.*

Risk of Recurrence for Patient's Child:
    See Part I, *Mendelian Inheritance.*

Age of Detectability: At birth. Prenatal diagnosis by ultrasound may also be possible.

Gene Mapping and Linkage: Unknown.

Prevention: None known. Genetic counseling indicated.

Treatment: Unknown.

Prognosis: Both children died within one week of birth.

Detection of Carrier: Unknown.

References:

Stevenson RE: Micromelic chondrodysplasia: further evidence for autosomal recessive inheritance. Proc Greenwood Genet Center 1982; 1:52–57.

Sconyers SM, et al.: A distinct chondrodysplasia resembling Kniest dysplasia: clinical, roentgenographic, histologic, and ultrastructural findings. J Pediatr 1983; 103:898–904.

Burton BK, et al.: A new skeletal dysplasia: clinical, radiologic and pathologic findings. J Pediatr 1986; 109:642–648.

T0007

Helga V. Toriello

Kniest-like dysplasia with pursed lips and ectopia lentis
See KNIEST-LIKE DYSPLASIA

KNUCKLE PADS-LEUKONYCHIA-DEAFNESS   0558

Includes:

    Bart-Pumphrey syndrome
    Deafness, knuckle pads and leukonychia
    Knuckle pads-leukonychia-deafness, keratosis palmoplantaris
    Leukonychia, knuckle pads and deafness

Excludes:

    Deafness-keratopachydermia-digital constrictions (0259)
    Deafness without appropriate cutaneous findings
    Keratopachydermia-digital constriction-deafness
    Knuckle pads without deafness
    Nails, leukonychia (0589)

Major Diagnostic Criteria: Deafness, leukonychia (nails need not be dead white), and knuckle pads (thickened areas of skin over the knuckles).

Clinical Findings: Sensorineural deafness occurs in all cases but may require audiometric studies to confirm. Conductive hearing loss may be present in some cases. Increased whiteness of finger and toenails is seen in all cases studied. Knuckle pads are usually found and keratoderma palmare et plantare frequently occurs.

All patients have sensorineural loss, with the defect in the cochlea. Some patients have a superimposed conductive loss which may or may not be associated with structural abnormalities of the middle ear. Whether hearing loss may be progressive in some patients is not known. Keratoderma palmare et plantare is more commonly found in adults with the syndrome than in affected children.

Complications: Unknown.

Associated Findings: None known.

Etiology: Autosomal dominant inheritance with complete penetrance but variable expressivity.

Pathogenesis: Unknown.

MIM No.: *14920

POS No.: 4267

Sex Ratio: M1:F1

Occurrence: Two pedigrees have been reported. In addition, an isolated case with all the features of the syndrome has been reported; other members of the family had various abnormalities, but none was deaf.

Risk of Recurrence for Patient's Sib:
    See Part I, *Mendelian Inheritance.*

Risk of Recurrence for Patient's Child:
See Part I, *Mendelian Inheritance.* Reproductive fitness probably unimpaired.

Age of Detectability: Hearing loss and knuckle pads can be first observed in infancy or early childhood. Leukonychia probably begins in early childhood.

Gene Mapping and Linkage: Unknown.

Prevention: None known. Genetic counseling indicated.

Treatment: That appropriate for the degree of hearing loss, including hearing aid and speech therapy.

Prognosis: Normal life span and intelligence.

Detection of Carrier: Unknown.

References:
Schwann J: Keratosis palmaris et plantaris cum surditate congenita et leuconychia totali unguium. Dermatologica 1963; 126:335–353.
Bart RS, Pumphrey RE: Knuckle pads, leukonychia and deafness: a dominantly inherited syndrome. New Engl J Med 1967; 276:202–207.
Konigsmark BW: Hereditary childhood hearing loss and integumentary system disease. J Pediatr 1972; 80:909–919.
Crosby EF, Vidurrizaga RH: Knuckle pads, leukonychia, deafness, and keratosis palmoplantaris: report of a family. Johns Hopkins Med J 1976; 139:90–92.
Paller A, Herbert AA: Knuckle pads in children. Am J Dis Child 1986; 140:915–917.

MI038   **Giuseppe Micali**

KUSKOKWIN SYNDROME   0560

Includes: Arthrogryposis-like disorder
Excludes: Arthrogryposes (0088)
Major Diagnostic Criteria: Multiple joint contractures, often severely affecting the knees and ankles, with either atrophy or compensatory hypertrophy of associated muscle groups. Intelligence is normal. There is evidence for an autosomal recessive mode of inheritance.
Clinical Findings: Multiple joint contractures develop early with severe involvement of the knees and ankles and accompanying atrophy or compensatory hypertrophy of associated muscle groups. Gait is a duck-like waddle, or is accomplished by walking on the knees. Flexion contractures also are seen at the elbows but are less severe. Pigmented nevi and decreased corneal reflexes have been noted in several patients. Intelligence is normal. Laboratory studies, including serum muscle enzymes, calcium, and phosphorus measurements, and tests for urinary amino acids and mucopolysaccharides, are normal. Electromyography with nerve conduction velocities and muscle biopsies do not show any abnormalities; histochemical studies of frozen sections are also unremarkable. X-rays demonstrate hypoplasia of the first or second lumbar vertebral body, progressive elongation of the pedicles of the 5th lumbar vertebra, producing spondylolisthesis, cathedral chest, osteolytic areas in the outer clavicle and proximal humerus (particularly in children), and hypoplasia of the patella associated with knee contractures.
Complications: The patella, normally placed at birth, migrates proximally through attenuation elongation of the patella tendon, which becomes a yellowish, amorphous mass, blending into the retinaculum of the knee. The quadriceps femoris consistently migrates to the proximal one-third of the thigh. Equinus and planovalgus foot deformities commonly occur.
Associated Findings: None known.
Etiology: Probably autosomal recessive inheritance.
Pathogenesis: Kuskokwim syndrome is differentiated from **Arthrogryposes** by its mode of inheritance, lack of laboratory evidence of abnormalities of muscles or nerves around affected joints, and characteristic X-ray changes. Abnormal muscle attachment, predominantly involving the tendons of the extensor muscles which are under constant strain, is believed to be a primary defect.
MIM No.: *20820
POS No.: 4283
Sex Ratio: M1:F1
Occurrence: Less than 20 cases have been reported, all in Eskimos in the Kuskokwim River delta of southwestern Alaska. Cases are thinly distributed in this limited geographic area of isolated villages.
Risk of Recurrence for Patient's Sib:
See Part I, *Mendelian Inheritance.*
Risk of Recurrence for Patient's Child:
See Part I, *Mendelian Inheritance.*
Age of Detectability: At birth.
Gene Mapping and Linkage: Unknown.
Prevention: None known. Genetic counseling indicated.
Treatment: Advanced deformities are often treated with osteotomies and muscle transfer. Early treatment with selected casting and bracing with passive manipulation will circumvent some of the severe contractures seen in adults.
Prognosis: Normal for life span and intelligence; functional ambulation is variable.
Detection of Carrier: Unknown.
References:
Petajan JH, et al.: Arthrogryposis syndrome (Kuskokwim syndrome) in the Eskimo. J.A.M.A. 1969; 209:1481–1486.
Wright DG, Aase J: The Kuskokwim syndrome: an inherited form of

arthrogryposis in the Alaskan Eskimo. BD:OAS;V(3). New York: The National Foundation March of Dimes, 1969:91–95.

G0043

Donald P. Goldsmith

KYPHOMELIC DYSPLASIA 2754

Includes:
    Bowing, congenital, with short bones
    Familial congenital bowing with short bones
    Short-limbed campomelic syndrome, normocephalic type
    Skeletal dysplasia, kyphomelic dysplasia

Excludes:
    Campomelic dysplasia (0122)
    Cortical hyperostosis, infantile (0221)
    Femoral hypoplasia-unusual facies syndrome (2027)

Major Diagnostic Criteria: Dwarfism; predominant shortening and bowing of the femora, with metaphyseal abnormalities; skin dimples; and micrognathia.

Clinical Findings: Dwarfism with severely angulated, shortened femora are cardinal features. Other tubular bones are less affected. The trunk is shortened. Skin dimples are present and are located over the greater trochanters (100%). Restricted abductions and extension of the hip joints results in a waddling gait. The chest is narrow (100%) and may be deformed or flattened (60%), giving rise to respiratory distress in the neonate. Midfacial hypoplasia, a small anteverted nose, and micrognathia are clinical features that manifest early and revert to normality in mid-childhood.

On X-ray, all the long bones are bowed and broadened, especially the femora. Irregularity of the lower femoral metaphyses is usually present. The ribs are shortened with flared ends (100%), and absence of one pair of ribs sometimes occurs (40%). Platyspondyly (87%), underossification of the proximal tibial epiphyses (43%), hypoplastic fibulae and acetabulae, and sacral anomalies are less common findings.

Complications: Unknown.

Associated Findings: Small midfacial and eyelid hemangiomas are infrequently reported.

Etiology: Probable autosomal recessive inheritance as evidenced by the report of two sibs in two separate kindreds. Four of the eight known cases have been sporadic.

Pathogenesis: Unknown.

MIM No.: 21135

POS No.: 3930

Sex Ratio: M5:F1 (sex undetermined in two individuals).

Occurrence: Eight cases have been reported.

Risk of Recurrence for Patient's Sib:
See Part I, *Mendelian Inheritance.*

Risk of Recurrence for Patient's Child:
See Part I, *Mendelian Inheritance.*

Age of Detectability: At birth, or prenatally by ultrasound.

Gene Mapping and Linkage: Unknown.

Prevention: None known. Genetic counseling indicated.

Treatment: Orthopedic procedures to straighten limb bowing and aid hip joint mobility may be indicated.

Prognosis: Normal intelligence and life span.

Detection of Carrier: Unknown.

Special Considerations: Nosologic confusion between kyphomelic dysplasia and **Femoral hypoplasia-unusual facies syndrome** (FH-UFS) exists. FH-UFS can be diagnosed clinically in that the proximal portions of the femora are very hypoplastic. FH-UFS is sporadic, patients have persistent facial dysmorphology throughout life, and a history of maternal diabetes can often be obtained.

References:
Khajavi A, et al.: Heterogeneity in the campomelic syndromes: long- and short-bone varieties. Pediatr Radiol 1976; 120:641–647.

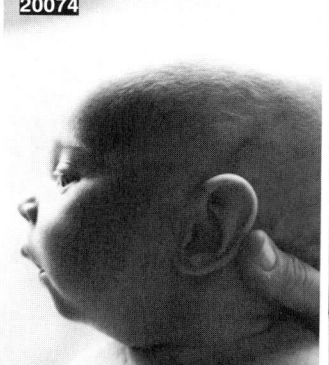 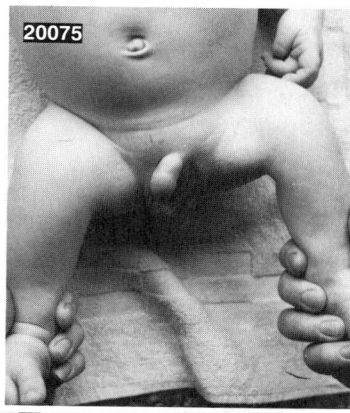

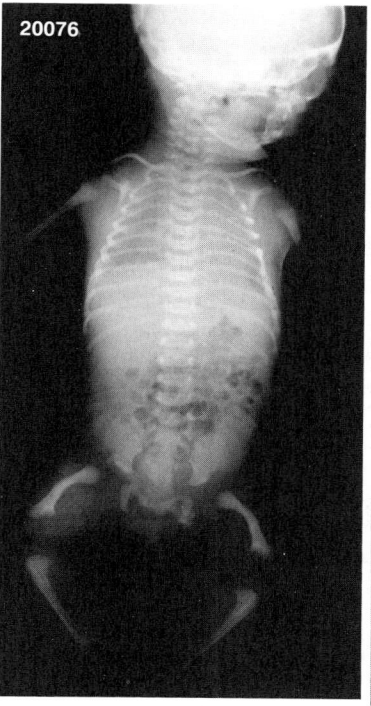 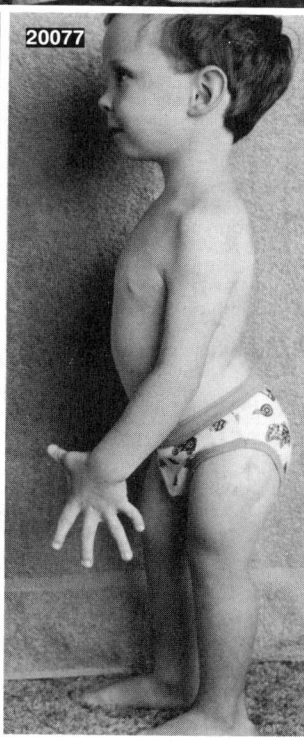

2754-20074: Note small upturned nose and micrognathia. **20075:** Short and bowed lower limbs. **20076:** Bowed femora, hypoplastic acetabulae, under-ossified pubic symphysis and abnormally segmented sacrum. **20077:** Note clinodactyly, lumbar lordosis and surgical scar over the trochanteric region in this 4-year-old boy.

Hall BD, Spranger JW: Familial congenital bowing with short bones. Pediatr Radiol 1979; 132:611–614.
Maclean RN, et al.: Skeletal dysplasia with short, angulated femora (kyphomelic dysplasia). Am J Med Genet 1983; 14:373–380. *
Viljoen D, Beighton P: Kyphomelic dysplasia-further delineation of the phenotype. Dysmorphol Clin Genet 1988; 1:136–141. †

VI005

Denis L. Viljöen

Kyrle disease
See SKIN, KYRLE DISEASE

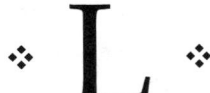

L-5-hydroxytryptophan induced scleroderma
  See SCLERODERMA, FAMILIAL PROGRESSIVE
L-transposition with situs solitus
  See VENTRICLES, INVERTED WITH TRANSPOSITION OF GREAT
    ARTERIES
L-xylulose reductase deficiency
  See PENTOSURIA
L-xylulosuria
  See PENTOSURIA
Laband syndrome
  See GINGIVAL FIBROMATOSIS-DIGITAL ANOMALIES
Labile factor deficiency
  See FACTOR V DEFICIENCY
Labyrinthine otosclerosis
  See OTOSCLEROSIS
Labyrinthine otosclerosis-fixed stapes footplate
  See OTOSCLEROSIS

LACRIMAL CANALICULUS ATRESIA   0563

Includes:
  Lacrimal canaliculus with or without punctum absence
  Lacrimal canaliculus with or without punctum atresia

Excludes: Obstructed nasolacrimal duct at the valve of Hasner

Major Diagnostic Criteria: In cases of aplasia of the canaliculus there is coexistent aplasia of the punctum. In cases of aplasia of the punctum the canaliculus may be variably present.

Clinical Findings: Symptoms relate to epiphora (tearing) if the lower punctum or canaliculus is incompletely represented. Absence of the entire lacrimal drainage system may occur secondary to midline facial anomalies, such as cyclopia or arrhinencephaly, or to eyelid malformations, such as cryptophthalmos or colobomas.

Complications: Chronic epiphora.

Associated Findings: May be seen in **Ectrodactyly-ectodermal dysplasia-clefting syndrome** and **Branchial arch-premature aging syndrome.**

Etiology: Usually sporadic. Hereditary cases may be autosomal dominant with variable penetrance and expression.

Pathogenesis: Deficiency in outbudding of the superior end of the ectodermal core.

MIM No.: *14970

CDC No.: 743.640

Sex Ratio: M1:F1 in hereditary cases.

Occurrence: Undetermined.

Risk of Recurrence for Patient's Sib:
  See Part I, *Mendelian Inheritance*. Not all cases are hereditary.

Risk of Recurrence for Patient's Child:
  See Part I, *Mendelian Inheritance*. Not all cases are hereditary.

Age of Detectability: At birth.

Gene Mapping and Linkage: Unknown.

Prevention: None known. Genetic counseling indicated.

Treatment: Surgery. In cases with minimal disruption of the canaliculus or punctum, Quickert silicone intubation may prove sufficient. In cases with significant disruption conjunctivorhinostomy may prove necessary.

Prognosis: Good, following surgical correction.

Detection of Carrier: By examination.

References:
Lumbroso BD: On a case of congenital atresia of the lacrimal ducts with familial characteristics. Acta Genet Med Gemellol 1960; 9:290–295.
Waardenburg P, et al.: Genetics and ophthalmology, Vol 1. Oxford: Blackwell Scientific, 1961:293.
Werb A: The management of canalicular occlusion. Trans Ophthalmol Soc NZ 1976; 28:41.
Kohn R: Textbook of ophthalmic plastic and reconstructive surgery. Philadelphia: Lea & Febiger, 1988:261–262.

K0025   **Roger Kohn**

Lacrimal canaliculus with or without punctum absence
  See LACRIMAL CANALICULUS ATRESIA
Lacrimal canaliculus with or without punctum atresia
  See LACRIMAL CANALICULUS ATRESIA
Lacrimal gland, aberrant
  See LACRIMAL GLAND, ECTOPIC
Lacrimal gland, congenital dislocation of
  See LACRIMAL GLAND, ECTOPIC

LACRIMAL GLAND, ECTOPIC   0564

Includes:
  Lacrimal gland, aberrant
  Lacrimal gland, congenital dislocation of

Excludes: Prolapse of normal lacrimal gland

Major Diagnostic Criteria: Presence of lacrimal gland tissue anywhere distant from its normal location in the lacrimal fossa.

Clinical Findings: Congenital lobulated fleshy tumor usually found beneath the conjunctiva near the limbus, at the lateral canthal region, or within the orbit distant from the lacrimal fossa. Intraocular involvement is rare. Lacrimal gland tissue, situated normally or ectopically, is subject to inflammatory or neoplastic changes; therefore, biopsy of symptomatic expanding lesion is indicated. Ectopic lacrimal gland tissue should be considered when evaluating intraocular or intraorbital mass.

Complications: Epibulbar lesions may distort the cornea or cause strabismus by impinging upon extraocular muscle. Intraorbital tumors may become symptomatic as a result of inflammation or neoplastic transformation. Computed tomographic scanning is useful to detect intraorbital involvement.

Associated Findings: Blepharochalasis, coloboma of the lids. Intraorbital vascular malformations.

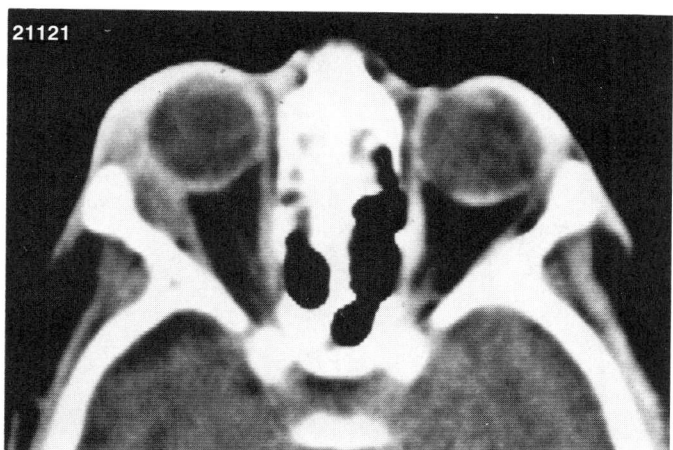

0564A-21121: Orbital CT scan (image viewed from below) shows ectopic lacrimal gland along the superotemporal aspect of the right orbit.

Etiology: Unknown.

Pathogenesis: Unknown.

CDC No.: 743.660

Sex Ratio: M1:F1

Occurrence: Undetermined but presumed rare.

Risk of Recurrence for Patient's Sib: Unknown.

Risk of Recurrence for Patient's Child: Unknown.

Age of Detectability: At birth.

Gene Mapping and Linkage: Unknown.

Prevention: None known. Genetic counseling indicated.

Treatment: Surgical removal for cosmesis and histologic confirmation of the diagnosis. When lesion distorts cornea, induces orbital inflammation, undergoes growth, or compromises intraocular structures, removal is indicated.

Prognosis: Good; no visual impairment occurs.

Detection of Carrier: Unknown.

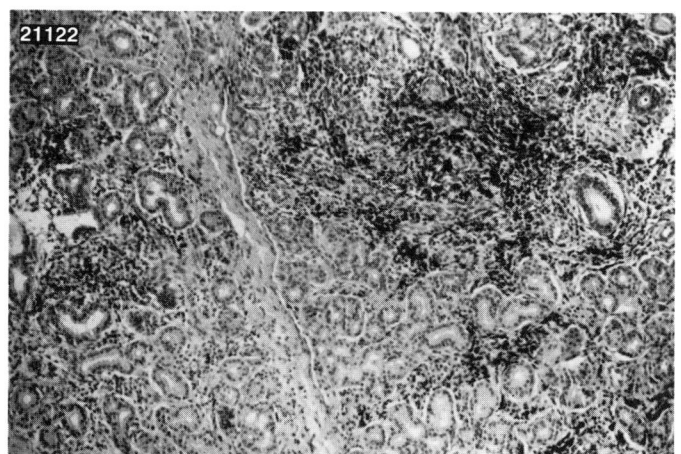

0564B-21122: Histopathologic specimen of orbital mass shows ectopic lacrimal gland infiltrated with inflammatory cells.

References:

Christiansen L, Anderson ED: Aberrant intraocular adenomata and epitheliazation of the anterior chamber. Arch Ophthalmol 1952; 48:19–29.

Green WR, Zimmerman LE: Ectopic lacrimal gland tissue: report of 8 cases with orbital involvement. Arch Ophthalmol 1967; 78:318–327.

Appel N, Som PM: Ectopic lacrimal gland tissue. J Comput Assist Tomogr 1982; 6:1010–1012.

Margo CE, et al.: Ectopic lacrimal gland tissue of the orbit and sclerosing dacryoadenitis. Ophthalmic Surg 1985; 16:178–181.

WE035   **Avery H. Weiss**

Lacrimal passage ectasia
  See LACRIMAL SAC FISTULA
Lacrimal puncta, absence of
  See ALACRIMA-APTYALISM

LACRIMAL SAC FISTULA   **0565**

Includes: Lacrimal passage ectasia

Excludes:
  Lacrimal canaliculus atresia (0563)
  Supernumerary puncta and canaliculi

Major Diagnostic Criteria: Abnormal opening (fistulous tract) from the lacrimal sac to the skin.

Clinical Findings: Lacrimal fistula present as a small opening at the inner canthus through which tears (sometimes purulent) drain. This is caused by an underlying obstruction at the nasolacrimal duct.

Complications: Dacryocystitis from the obstruction at the nasolacrimal duct.

Associated Findings: None known.

Etiology: Unknown.

Pathogenesis: Obstruction at the nasolacrimal duct.

CDC No.: 743.660

Sex Ratio: Presumably M1:F1

Occurrence: Undetermined. Somes estimates as high as 1:4,000 live births.

Risk of Recurrence for Patient's Sib: Low. Familial cases seldom reported.

Risk of Recurrence for Patient's Child: Low. Familial cases seldom reported.

Age of Detectability: At birth or during the neonatal period.

Gene Mapping and Linkage: Unknown.

Prevention: Resolution of the underlying obstruction at the nasolacrimal duct.

Treatment: Resolution of the underlying obstruction along with excision of the fistulous tract. Treatment of inflammation, if present.

Prognosis: Life span not reduced. Repeated inflammation may occur.

Detection of Carrier: Unknown.

References:

Masi A: Congenital fistula of the lacrimal sac. Arch Ophthalmol 1969; 81:701.

Kohn R: Textbook of ophthalmic plastic and reconstructive surgery. Philadelphia: Lea & Febiger, 1988:274.

K0025   **Roger Kohn**

Lacrimal system, impatency of the
  See NASOLACRIMAL DUCT OBSTRUCTION

LACRIMO-AURICULO-DENTO-DIGITAL SYNDROME   2180

Includes:
    LADD syndrome
    Levy-Hollister Syndrome
    Limb malformations-dento-digital syndrome

Excludes: Ectrodactyly-ectodermal dysplasia-clefting syndrome (0337)

Major Diagnostic Criteria: Upper limb malformations (most commonly radial defects) are a constant feature. Variable features include lacrimal malformations, small cupped ears, hearing loss, dental anomalies, absent salivary glands, aberrant dermal ridge patterns, and genitourinary anomalies.

Clinical Findings: Based on 12 individuals, upper limb malformations were present in 100%. The typical upper limb anomaly was a radial ray defect, with absent or hypoplastic radius and digitalization or hypoplasia of the thumb and second finger. Other upper limb anomalies included shortening of the radius and ulna, **Radial-ulnar synostosis**, triphalangeal thumb, preaxial polydactyly, duplication of the distal phalanx of the thumb, and **Syndactyly** of the second and third fingers, and clinodactyly of the fifth finger.

Although small, simple, cupped pinnae have been noted in 80% of affected patients, only 60% have a hearing loss. The hearing loss was of a mixed conductive and sensorineural nature. Audiometric studies in one family suggested otosclerosis or abnormalities of the ossicular chain. The pinnae were described as having a short helix and an underdeveloped antihelix.

Lacrimal malformations were present in 75% of affected individuals, and included nasolacrimal duct obstruction, hypoplasia or aplasia of the lacrimal puncta, and nasolacrimal duct fistulae.

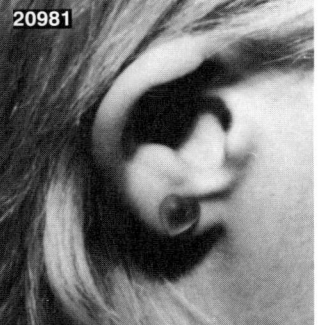

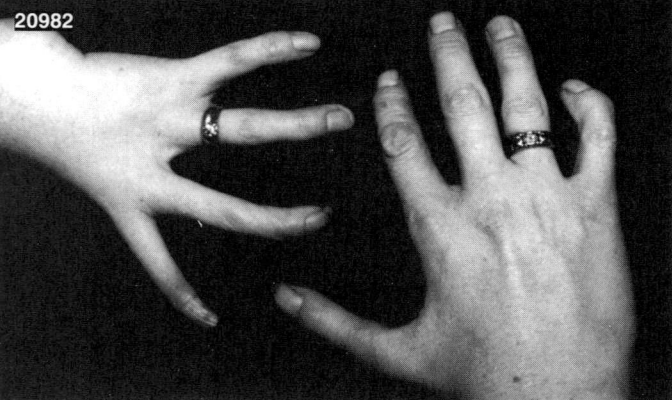

2180-20980: Lacrimo-auriculo-digital-dental syndrome; note the nasolacrimal duct fistula. **20981:** Small, cupped pinna. **20982:** Typical upper limb malformations; note the left radial aplasia and the hypoplastic thenar eminence, digitalized thumb, and fifth finger clinodactyly on the right.

Dental anomalies have been documented in 80% of patients and included hypodontia, enamel dysplasia with variations of premolar cusp patterns, peg-shaped maxillary lateral incisors, excessive wear patterns, tooth darkening, and enamel thinning, suggestive of a mild amelogenesis imperfecta-like defect.

Two (20%) of the patients described had unusual dermal ridge patterns with a predominance of low arch patterns. Two individuals previously described have had genitourinary malformations. One had **Renal agenesis, unilateral**, and the other had **Hypospadias** and nephrosclerosis.

Complications: Lacrimal malformations cause epiphora, chronic dacryocystitis, conjunctivitis, and keratoconjunctivitis. Renal anomalies may lead to hypertension and/or chronic renal disease.

Associated Findings: None known.

Etiology: Autosomal dominant inheritance.

Pathogenesis: Unknown.

MIM No.: *14973

POS No.: 3546

Sex Ratio: M1:F1

Occurrence: About a dozen cases have been described, most from Mexican-American and Caucasian-American populations.

Risk of Recurrence for Patient's Sib:
See Part I, *Mendelian Inheritance.*

Risk of Recurrence for Patient's Child:
See Part I, *Mendelian Inheritance.*

Age of Detectability: In infancy.

Gene Mapping and Linkage: Unknown.

Prevention: None known. Genetic counseling indicated.

Treatment: Ophthalmic surgery may be indicated to correct the lacrimal apparatus malformation and prevent further ophthalmologic complications. Regular dental care is indicated. Hearing aids may be successful in ameliorating the associated mixed hearing loss. Surgical correction of renal anomalies may also be indicated.

Prognosis: Normal for life span and intelligence.

Detection of Carrier: Unknown.

Special Considerations: All of the features of this syndrome have been reported as isolated genetically determined traits inherited in an autosomal dominant fashion. The radial ray defects characteristic of this disorder serve to distinguish it from **Ectrodactyly-ectodermal dysplasia-clefting syndrome**, in which digital anomalies consisting of a split hand and/or foot are found in conjunction with lacrimal, auricular, and dental anomalies.

References:
Levy WJ: Mesoectodermal dysplasia: a new combination of anomalies. Am J Ophthalmol 1967; 63:978–982.
Hollister D, et al.: The lacrimo-auriculo-dento-digital syndrome. J Pediatr 1973; 83:438–444. * †
Shiang EL, Holmes LB: The lacrimo-auriculo-dento-digital syndrome. Pediatrics 1977; 59:927–930. * †
Thompson E, et al.: Phenotypic variation in LADD syndrome. J Med Genet 1985; 22:382–385.
Wiedemann H-R, Drescher J: LADD syndrome: report of new cases and review of the clinical spectrum. Eur J Pediatr 1986; 144:579–582.
Kreutz JM, Hoyme HE: The Levy-Hollister syndrome. Pediatrics 1988; 82:96–99.

H0040   **H. Eugene Hoyme**

Lactase deficiency, adult
See LACTASE DEFICIENCY, PRIMARY

LACTASE DEFICIENCY, CONGENITAL 0566

Includes:
Alactasia, congenital
Alactasia, early onset
Disaccharide intolerance II
Lactase insufficiency, hereditary

Excludes:
Glucose-galactose malabsorption (0419)
Lactase deficiency, acquired
Lactase deficiency, primary (0567)
Lactase deficiency, secondary
Lactose intolerance (0569)
Monosaccharide intolerance
Sucrase-isomaltase deficiency (0920)

Major Diagnostic Criteria: Fermentative diarrhea from birth with lactose ingestion, and not with other carbohydrates. Deliberate feeding of measured dose of lactose yields flat serum glucose curve, abdominal discomfort, and explosive stool of pH below 5.0 containing reducing sugars. These findings do not occur on feeding glucose, galactose, or sucrose. If one is certain that the condition is hereditary, these criteria may suffice if the patient's condition precludes peroral biopsy. In all other instances, it is essential to demonstrate normal intestinal histology with decreased or absent lactase activity.

Clinical Findings: Symptoms of fermentative diarrhea (100%), and failure to thrive (100%), begin with initial ingestion of lactose (in human or cow's milk) at birth. Infants almost always have abdominal distention, suffer crampy abdominal pain, and vomit sporadically. They usually appear to be very hungry, despite diarrhea, unless the debilitating effects of secondary dehydration, acidosis, and inanition supervene. Diarrhea clears as soon as lactose is removed from the diet.

The stool is fluid and quite frothy from contained gas as it is passed, usually explosively. The pH of fresh stool is always below 5.0 if lactose has been ingested; such stool usually contains reducing sugars that can be identified as one or more of the following: lactose, glucose, and galactose. Lactosuria occurs in about one-third of the patients. Ingestion of a standard dose of lactose (1.5–2.0 g/kg or 45–60 g/m^2) after an overnight fast is always associated with a flat 3-hour "tolerance curve" for serum glucose; the test dose almost universally produces clinical discomfort and explosive diarrhea during the 3-hour observation period. Accordingly, the oral loading test should be performed in a diarrhea-free period.

Hydrogen breath analysis, following the oral lactose dose, is a simple alternative. Samples of expired air are obtained before and at 30-minute intervals after administration of the lactose test dose. A rise of hydrogen excretion exceeding 20 parts per million above baseline is considered abnormal and indicates probable lactose malabsorption. Since the hydrogen is elaborated from colonic bacterial activity, false negative tests occur in patients taking oral antibiotics or in infants whose diarrhea stools are so acid that they inhibit hydrogen production by the flora. In many normal newborns, sufficient lactose reaches the colon in undigested form so as to give false positive tests by this method.

Peroral biopsy specimen of the upper small intestinal mucosa is histologically normal, but contains decreased β glycosidase (lactase) activity when compared with the activity of the maltose, sucrose, or isomaltose-digesting enzymes, or when assayed in relation to unit weight of tissue, or to protein content of the tissue.

Complications: Dehydration, electrolyte, and acid-base disturbance in almost all cases.

Associated Findings: Failure to thrive, or death, in all cases if correct diagnosis is not made or if treatment instituted early enough.

Etiology: Probably autosomal recessive inheritance.

Pathogenesis: Ingested lactose is not hydrolyzed to the component monosaccharides in the upper small intestine as in normal individuals, and therefore passes undigested to the colon. Here the disaccharide is hydrolyzed and fermented, and the resultant mixture contains two and three carbon volatile acids, glucose and galactose, and often some undigested lactose. The increase in osmolarity of the colonic contents induces net flux of water into the lumen. A combination of the irritant effect of excessive fermentation, increased colonic gas, and distension of the bowel walls by the increase in fluid results in explosive passage of the loose stool.

MIM No.: *22300

Sex Ratio: Presumably M1:F1

Occurrence: A relatively common disorder in Finland, with 16 of the approximately 35 patient reported representing 17 years of Finnish experience. Rarer outside of Finland.

Risk of Recurrence for Patient's Sib:
See Part I, *Mendelian Inheritance.*

Risk of Recurrence for Patient's Child:
See Part I, *Mendelian Inheritance.*

Age of Detectability: At birth, by lactose loading test and assay of enzymes in intestinal mucosal biopsy specimen.

Gene Mapping and Linkage: LCT (lactase) has been provisionally mapped to 2.

Prevention: None known. Genetic counseling indicated.

Treatment: Avoidance of lactose in the diet. This includes all forms of mammalian milk and milk products. Fluid and electrolyte support may be necessitated during the diarrhea, which results from upsets with lactose ingestion.

Prognosis: Current indications are for normal life span if patient is diagnosed and treated early. If not recognized in infancy, patients may die of severe inanition and electrolyte disturbances.

Detection of Carrier: Unknown.

Special Considerations: The condition must be distinguished from two closely allied conditions. Durant (1958) described, and others also reported, infants with diarrhea on ingestion of lactose. These patients additionally displayed excessive vomiting, lactosemia, lactosuria, other urinary sugars, aminoaciduria, or renal acidosis. Lactase activity was not studied in these patients and the outcomes varied from clearance of the intolerance to lactose to death in infancy (See **Lactose intolerance**). Infants may also develop transitory lactose intolerance in the course of acute diarrhea of presumed infectious origin. These infants also display lactosemia and lactosuria. Although confirmatory biopsy is not available in all cases, it is assumed that the defect in lactose absorption is secondary to temporary mucosal damage and secondary loss of enzyme activity, which returns to normal after a number of weeks or months on a lactose-free diet.

It is generally difficult to differentiate congenital lactase deficiency from secondary defects in the young infant. However, lactosemia, lactosuria, presence of other urinary sugars, histologically abnormal intestinal mucosal specimens, and development of tolerance to lactose after a period of its withdrawal from the diet all point away from the diagnosis of congenital lactase deficiency.

References:
Prader A, Auricchio S: Defects of intestinal disaccharide absorption. Annu Rev Med 1965; 16:345.
Davidson M: Disaccharide intolerance. Pediatr Clin North Am 1967; 14:93.
Hozel A: Sugar malabsorption and sugar intolerance in childhood. Proc R Soc Med 1968; 61:1095
Levin B. et al.: Congenital lactose malabsorption. Arch Dis Child 1970; 45:173.
Gray GM: Intestinal disaccharidase deficiencies and glucose-galactose malabsorption. In; Stanbury JB, et al, eds: The metabolic basis of inherited disease, 5th ed. New York: McGraw-Hill, 1983:1729.
Savilahti E, et al.: Congenital lactase deficiency. Arch Dis Child 1983; 58:246–252.
Semeneza G, Auricchio S: Small intestinal disaccharides. In: Scriver CR, et al, eds: The metabolic basis of inherited disease, 6th ed. New York: McGraw-Hill, 1989:2975–2992.

DA017 **Murray Davidson**

LACTASE DEFICIENCY, PRIMARY 0567

Includes:
Alactasia, late-onset
Disaccharide intolerance III
Hypoactasia, primary
Lactase deficiency, adult
Lactase insufficiency, noncongenital isolated
Lactose intolerance, adult
Racial lactase deficiency

Excludes:
Lactase deficiency, acquired
Lactase deficiency, congenital (0566)
Lactase deficiency, secondary
Lactose intolerance (0569)
Monosaccharide intolerance
Sucrase-isomaltase deficiency (0920)

Major Diagnostic Criteria: Patients must have a history of normal tolerance to mammalian milk in infancy with development of clinical intolerance to lactose-containing foods in later childhood or adult life. The discomfort, bloating, and fermentative diarrhea which occurs with lactose ingestion should be absent with other carbohydrates. Ingestion of a standard dose of lactose (1.5–2.0 g/kg or 45–60 g/m^2) is always associated with a flat 3-hour "tolerance curve" for serum glucose; in some reports the clinical discomfort and explosive diarrhea, usually associated with the test among children with congenital lactase deficiency, was not observed at these doses among adults with primary lactase deficiency. However, feeding of 100 gm/m^2 produces symptoms more uniformly. The loose stools are pH below 5.0, and contain any or all of lactose, glucose and galactose. These findings do not occur on feeding glucose, galactose or sucrose.

Peroral biopsy is necessary to distinguish patients from those with secondary forms of insufficiency. Peroral biopsy specimen of the upper small intestinal mucosa is histologically normal, but it contains decreased β-glycosidase (lactase) activity when compared with the activity of the maltose, sucrose, or isomaltose digesting enzymes, or when assayed in relation to unit weight of tissue or to protein content of the tissue.

Clinical Findings: Ingestion of milk or other lactose-containing foods usually causes abdominal bloating, cramping, and sometimes diarrhea. The difficulty is absent in infants and appears in childhood or in adult life. Individuals with primary lactase deficiency are frequently asymptomatic, if it is their normal pattern not to ingest significant quantities of milk and milk products.

The syndrome has been reported from a number of laboratories to occur in Caucasian adults, as an explanation for "milk allergy." In the United States the adult deficiency is reported with increased frequency among Blacks and Orientals.

Complications: While dehydration, and electrolyte and acid base disturbances, as well as failure to thrive are theoretically possible in individuals with primary lactase deficiency (similar to those of individuals with congenital lactase deficiency), these are not reported. A combination of larger body size, less dependence on milk as an important dietary constituent, and less total diminution of lactase activity than in patients affected with congenital lactase deficiency may account for the differences in incidence of these complications.

Associated Findings: None known.

Etiology: Autosomal dominant inheritance. It is not clear if these are distinct infantile and adult lactases, or if lactose tolerance and intolerance represent differences in the regulation of a single locus.

Pathogenesis: Reduction in production of this enzyme with aging ultimately reduces lactase activity below a threshold level. From this time on, ingested lactose is not hydrolyzed to the component monosaccharides in the upper small intestine, as in normal individuals, and passes undigested to the colon. In this organ, the disaccharide is hydrolyzed and fermented and the resultant mixture contains two and three carbon volatile acids, glucose and galactose, and often some undigested lactose. The increase in osmolality of the colonic contents induces net flux of water to the lumen. A combination of the irritant effect of the excessive fermentation, increased colonic, gas and distention of the bowel wall by the increase in fluid, results in explosive passage of the loose stool.

MIM No.: *22310

Sex Ratio: Presumably M1:F1

Occurrence: Adult lactase deficiency affects 5–20% of whites and 70–75% of Blacks in North America. Other affected populations include American Indians (83–95%), Chinese (87%), and Thai (97%).

Risk of Recurrence for Patient's Sib:
See Part I, *Mendelian Inheritance.*

Risk of Recurrence for Patient's Child:
See Part I, *Mendelian Inheritance.*

Age of Detectability: Whereas lactose intolerance is usually first symptomatic in the teens in North American whites, it may become evident in younger children in other populations, and may appear in the first four years and even in the first six months in Africans. Not all lactase deficient individuals are lactose intolerant, and some classified as heterozygotes may be symptomatic. The condition appears to develop at approximately three years of age in populations in which more than one-half of the adults are affected.

Gene Mapping and Linkage: Unknown.

Prevention: None known. Genetic counseling indicated.

Treatment: Avoidance of lactose in the diet. This includes all forms of mammalian milk and milk products, unless they are pretreated *in vitro* with a commercially available lactase enzyme preparation. Small amounts of milk solids in foods may be tolerated by some patients. Patients and their physicians should be aware of the common use of lactose as the major component of most medicinal pills. Fluid and electrolyte support may be necessitated during the diarrheal activity that results from upsets with lactose ingestion.

Prognosis: Excellent for life and freedom from morbidity if lactose is avoided in the diet.

Detection of Carrier: Unknown.

Special Considerations: Secondary lactase deficiency may be differentiated from the primary defect by four distinguishing criteria: 1) Mucosal biopsy specimens from patients with primary lactase deficiency are normal on histologic examination but are distorted in accordance with the appropriate underlying condition among patients with secondary lactase deficiency. 2) In primary lactase deficiency, reduction of lactase activity in mucosal specimens is isolated, while in secondary deficiencies there is loss of activity of all disaccharidases. With ingestion of lactose, both groups would demonstrate flat serum glucose curves and GI intolerance. 3) However, lactosemia, lactosuria and presence of other urinary sugars are reported only with secondary deficiencies. 4) Development of tolerance to lactose after a period of its withdrawal from the diet, or after treatment for an underlying malabsorptive condition, precludes the diagnosis of primary lactase deficiency.

References:
Bayless TM, Rosensweig NS: A racial difference in incidence of lactase deficiency: a survey of milk intolerance and lactase deficiency in healthy adult males. J.A.M.A. 1966; 197:968–972.
Dahlqvist A, Lindquist B: Lactose intolerance and protein malnutrition. Acta Paediatr Scand 1971; 60:488.
Kretchmer N: Lactose and lactase: a historical perspective. Gastroenterology 1971; 61:805–813.
Ransome-Kuti O, et al.: A genetic study of lactose digestion in Nigerian families. Gastroenterology 1975; 68:431.
Welsh JD, et al.: Intestinal disaccharidase activities in relation to age, race, and mucosal damage. Gastroenterology 1978; 75:847.
Simoons FJ: Age of onset of lactose malabsorption. Pediatrics 1980; 66:646.
Ho MW, et al.: Lactase polymorphism in adult British natives. Am J Hum Genet 1982; 34:650–657.

Potter J, et al.: Human lactase and the molecular basis of lactase persistence. Biochem Genet 1985; 23:423–439.

DA017 **Murray Davidson**

Lactase insufficiency, hereditary
See LACTASE DEFICIENCY, CONGENITAL
Lactase insufficiency, noncongenital isolated
See LACTASE DEFICIENCY, PRIMARY
Lactate dehydrogenase - A
See LACTATE DEHYDROGENASE ISOZYMES
Lactate dehydrogenase - B
See LACTATE DEHYDROGENASE ISOZYMES
Lactate dehydrogenase - C
See LACTATE DEHYDROGENASE ISOZYMES
Lactate dehydrogenase - K
See LACTATE DEHYDROGENASE ISOZYMES

LACTATE DEHYDROGENASE ISOZYMES 0568

Includes:
Lactate dehydrogenase - A
Lactate dehydrogenase - B
Lactate dehydrogenase - C
Lactate dehydrogenase - K
Nicotinamide adenine dinucleotide and oxidoreductase

Excludes: N/A

Major Diagnostic Criteria: Electrophoretic techniques are available for determining the isozyme composition of tissues and body fluids. In normal serum, lactate dehydrogenase (LDH) isozymes are present in the following proportions: LDH-2 > LDH-1 > LDH-3 > LDH-4 > LDH-5. A variety of diseases exhibit unique changes in serum isozyme patterns. LDH-1 is markedly increased in myocardial infarction, and LDH-5 in infectious hepatitis.

Clinical Findings: Abnormal elevation or depression of lactate dehydrogenase isozymes are associated with certain disease states but are not proven causes. Lactate dehydrogenase (LDH) is an enzyme of the Embden-Myerhoff pathway, which catalyzes the interconversion of pyruvate and lactate. Nicotinamide adenine dinucleotide (NAD) is a specific cofactor, NAD being formed during the reduction of pyruvate and reduced nicotinamide adenine dinucleotide (NADH) during the oxidation of lactate.

LDH exists in multiple molecular forms (isozymes) in the somatic and gametic tissues of many mammalian and avian species. Five molecular forms of LDH are present in human somatic tissues: LDH-1, LDH-2, LDH-3, LDH-4, and LDH-5. The type and amount of the molecular forms vary for each tissue. In adult human heart and kidney, the major forms are LDH-1, LDH-2 and LDH-3, whereas in adult human muscle and liver the dominant form is LDH-5. Multiple forms of LDH may exist in single cells. Thus hemolysates of thoroughly washed erythrocytes exhibit three isozymes, LDH-1, LDH-2, and LDH-3. A 6th isozymic form of LDH (LDH-X) appears in testis at the time of puberty. LDH-X is the predominant form of LDH in sperm.

The relative distribution of isozymes in each human tissue changes during development. In heart, for example, the pattern exhibited by adults is not attained until 3 years of age. In testis, the adult complement of isozymes appears at the time of puberty. Thus each tissue exhibits a unique profile of isozyme development.

A variety of diseases exhibit unique changes in serum isozyme patterns. LDH-1 is markedly increased in myocardial infarction, and LDH-5 in infectious hepatitis. Analysis of tissue isozyme patterns may also have diagnostic application. In chickens and humans a form of muscular dystrophy is associated with a failure of development of the adult isozyme pattern. Whether this abnormality is a primary or secondary event is unknown. These findings suggest that isozymic analyses may be helpful in determining at what period of development a metabolic abnormality occurs.

Complications: Unknown.

Associated Findings: A disturbed LDH pattern may indicate one of a variety of diseases e.g. myocardial infarction, infectious hepatitis, hemolytic disorders, meningitis and **Muscular dystrophy**.

Etiology: Autosomal dominant inheritance of isozymes. Discovery of polypeptide A and B variants in human and animal tissues, together with appropriate genetic studies, showed that the synthesis of A and B polypeptides is controlled by two separate nonallelic genes. Observations on pigeon testes have shown that the synthesis of the LDH-X subunit (C) is controlled by a 3rd genetic locus in the pigeon. The total complement of LDH isozymes can be explained on the basis of the activity of genes at three loci, A, B, and C, each being responsible for the synthesis of a corresponding polypeptide. The C locus, in contrast to the other loci, is not activated until pubescence in the male and remains inactive in the female.

Pathogenesis: Unknown.

MIM No.: *15000, *15010, *15015, 15016

Sex Ratio: For LDH-1, -2, -3, -4 and -5: M1:F1; for LDH-X: M1:F0

Occurrence: Each isozyme normally present at proper age and in appropriate tissue.

Risk of Recurrence for Patient's Sib:
See Part I, *Mendelian Inheritance.*

Risk of Recurrence for Patient's Child:
See Part I, *Mendelian Inheritance.*

Age of Detectability: Adult isozyme pattern in heart at age three, and LDH-X in testis at puberty.

Gene Mapping and Linkage: LDHA (lactate dehydrogenase A) has been mapped to 11p15.1-p14.
LDHB (lactate dehydrogenase B) has been mapped to 12p12.2-p12.1.
LDHC (lactate dehydrogenase C) has been provisionally mapped to 11.

Prevention: Not applicable.

Treatment: Not applicable.

Prognosis: Normal life span.

Detection of Carrier: Electrophoresis can determine LDH isozyme pattern.

Special Considerations: Molecular forms of lactate dehydrogenase (LDH) in heart and kidney are to a large extent different from those in muscle and liver. Each tissue exhibits characteristic changes of the isozyme patterns during development, and in at least one tissue, the testis, an entirely new isozyme appears at the time of puberty. Isozymic analysis of tissues and body fluids may aid in diagnosing certain diseases - myocardial infarction, infectious hepatitis, hemolytic disorders, meningitis, etc. Also further studies on the molecular heterogeneity of LDH, as well as other enzymes, will increase our understanding of the biochemical processes that accompany growth and development.

References:
Wroblewski F, Gregory KK: Lactic dehydrogenase isozymes and their distribution in normal tissues and plasma and in disease states. Ann NY Acad Sci 1961; 94:912–921.
Zinkham WH: Lactate dehydrogenase isozymes of testis and sperm: biological and biochemical properties and genetic control. Ann NY Acad Sci 1968; 151:598–609.
Mayeda K, et al.: Localization of the human lactate dehydrogenase B gene on the short arm of chromosome 12. Am J Hum Genet 1974; 26:59–64.
Francke U, Busby N: Assignments of the human genes for lactate dehydrogenase-A and thymidine kinase to specific chromosomal regions. Cytogenet Cell Genet 1975; 14:313–319.
Markert CH, et al.: Evolution of a gene. Science 1975; 189:102–114.
Anderson GR, Kovacik WP Jr: LDH (k), an unusual oxygen-sensitive lactate dehydrogenase expressed in human cancer. Proc Natl Acad Sci 1981; 78:3209–3213.
Benz C, et al.: Lactic dehydrogenase isozymes, 31P magnestic resonance spectroscopy, and in vitro antimitochondrial tumor toxicity with gossypol and rhodamine 123. J Clin Invest 1987; 79:517–523.

ZI000 **William H. Zinkham**

Lactate dehydrogenase, M isozyme
  See GLYCOGENOSES
Lactate transporter
  See GLYCOGENOSES
Lactate transporter defect, myopathy due to
  See ERYTHROCYTE, LACTATE TRANSPORTER DEFECT
Lactate transporter deficiency
  See ERYTHROCYTE, LACTATE TRANSPORTER DEFECT
Lactate transporter myopathy, metabolic
  See ERYTHROCYTE, LACTATE TRANSPORTER DEFECT
Lactic acidemia without hypoxemia
  *See PYRUVATE CARBOXYLASE DEFICIENCY WITH LACTIC
  ACIDEMIA*
Lactic acidosis
  *See MYOPATHY, MITOCHONDRIAL-ENCEPHALOPATHY-LACTIC
  ACIDOSIS-STROKE*
Lactic and pyruvic acidemia with carbohydrate sensitivity
  See PYRUVATE DEHYDROGENASE DEFICIENCY
Lactic and pyruvic acidemia with episodic ataxia and weakness
  See PYRUVATE DEHYDROGENASE DEFICIENCY

LACTOSE INTOLERANCE   0569

Includes:
> Gastrogen lactose intolerance
> Lactose intolerance with lactosuria, congenital
> Lactosuria, idiopathic

Excludes:
> Disaccharidase deficiency syndromes due to celiac disease
> **Lactase deficiency, congenital** (0566)
> Monosaccharide malabsorption
> Protein malnutrition (kwashiorkor)
> **Sucrase-isomaltase deficiency** (0920)

Major Diagnostic Criteria: Vomiting, failure to thrive, lactosuria, sucrosuria, and aminoaciduria. Lactose tolerance test results in a normal increase in blood glucose, but severe lactosuria appears. A normal glucose response to sucrose loading with sucrosuria is also seen.

In contrast, nolactosuria and sucrosuria occur when the lactose or the sucrose are given intraduodenally. Intestinal lactase and sucrase are normal.

Small intestinal biopsy shows a villous mucosa with slightly reduced height or a normal mucosa. Light and electron-microscopy of gastric mucosa from the fundus and corpus region are apparently normal. The morphology of the antral mucosa has not been studied. Lactose and sucrose are not normally found in the blood, and their presence may have toxic effects.

Clinical Findings: The disorder manifests soon after birth. Affected infants are characteristically critically ill, with vomiting and failure to thrive; diarrhea is uncommon. Dehydration develops quickly. Disacchariduria, aminoaciduria, and tubular acidosis indicate renal damage. Lactosuria is the most striking feature and can be profuse as long as milk intake persists. Pronounced sucrosuria may be also present on a diet rich in sucrose. The lactose and sucrose concentrations in urine are occasionally up to 100 times greater than normally found at this age.

The infant's general condition deteriorates rapidly and may be fatal unless lactose intake is curtailed. On a lactose-free diet, lactose intolerance disappears at 6 to 18 months after onset. Reintroduction of lactose in the diet before this period can be fatal.

Complications: Malnutrition; liver damage with bleeding tendency and renal damage are probably secondary phenomena caused by the disaccharides. Lactose malabsorption due to lactase deficiency can develop later in childhood.

Associated Findings: Pyloric stenosis and cataracts have been present in some infants.

Etiology: The cause of severe lactose intolerance is unknown. Familial incidence and consanguinity among the parents of the patients suggest a hereditary factor.

Pathogenesis: A gastrogenic origin of the disorder, with abnormal absorption of disaccharide likely; lactose passes through an abnormally permeable gastric mucosa and leading to lactosuria and sucrosuria. The gastric defect appears to be temporary.

MIM No.: 15022

Sex Ratio: M1:F1

Occurrence: More than 20 cases documented in the literature.

Risk of Recurrence for Patient's Sib: Unknown.

Risk of Recurrence for Patient's Child: Unknown.

Age of Detectability: First month of life.

Gene Mapping and Linkage: Unknown.

Prevention: None known. Genetic counseling indicated.

Treatment: In the acute phase, use of a formula free from disaccharides, or intraduodenal feeding with a disaccharide containing formula. Supportive measures such as intravenous fluid and electrolyte replacement are needed in infants with severe dehydration.

Prognosis: Timely removal of lactose from the feeding formula will assure recovery. Diet is well tolerated.

Detection of Carrier: Unknown.

References:
Durand P: Lattosuria idiopatica in una paziente con diarrea cronica ed acidosi. Minerva Pediatrica 1958; 10:706–711.
Durand P, et al.: Disorders due to intestinal defective carbohydrate digestion and absorption. New York: Grune and Stratton, 1964.
Russo G, et al.: Congenital lactose intolerance of gastrogen origin associated with cataracts. Acta Paediatr Scand 1974; 63:457–460.
Berg NO, et al.: A boy with severe infantile gastrogen lactose intolerance and acquired lactase deficiency. Acta Paediatr Scand 1979; 68:751–758.
Hirashima Y, et al.: Lactose intolerance associated with cataracts. Eur J Pediat 1979; 130:41–45.
Hoskova A, et al.: Severe lactose intolerance with lactosuria and vomiting. Arch Dis Child 1980; 55:304–316.

DU010   **Paolo Durand**

Lactose intolerance with lactosuria, congenital
  See LACTOSE INTOLERANCE
Lactose intolerance, adult
  See LACTASE DEFICIENCY, PRIMARY
Lactosuria, idiopathic
  See LACTOSE INTOLERANCE
LADD syndrome
  See LACRIMO-AURICULO-DENTO-DIGITAL SYNDROME
Lafora body disease
  See SEIZURES, PROGRESSIVE MYOCLONIC, LAFORA TYPE
Lafora disease
  See SEIZURES, PROGRESSIVE MYOCLONIC, LAFORA TYPE
Lakuregebee
  See ANEMIA, SICKLE CELL
LAMB syndrome
  See NEVI-ATRIAL MYXOMA-MYXOID NEUROFIBROMAS-EPHELIDES
Lambdoid suture closure, premature
  See CRANIOSYNOSTOSIS
Lambert type ichthyosis
  See NEVUS, EPIDERMAL NEVUS SYNDROME
Lamellar cataract
  See CATARACT, AUTOSOMAL DOMINANT CONGENITAL
Lamellar exfoliation of the newborn
  See ICHTHYOSIS
  also ICHTHYOSIS, LAMELLAR RECESSIVE
  also ICHTHYOSIS, CONGENITAL ERYTHRODERMIC
Lamellar ichthyosis, autosomal dominant form
  See ICHTHYOSIS, LAMELLAR DOMINANT
Lamellar ichthyosis, classical
  See ICHTHYOSIS, LAMELLAR RECESSIVE
Lamellar ichthyosis, nonbullous congenital
  See ICHTHYOSIS, LAMELLAR DOMINANT
Landouzy-Dejerine muscular dystrophy
  See MUSCULAR DYSTROPHY, FACIO-SCAPULO-HUMERAL
Lane disease
  See SKIN, PALMO-PLANTAR ERYTHEMA
Lange-Nielsen syndrome
  See CARDIO-AUDITORY SYNDROME
Langer type mesomelic dwarfism
  See MESOMELIC DYSPLASIA, LANGER TYPE

Langer-Giedion syndrome
See TRICHO-RHINO-PHALANGEAL SYNDROME, TYPE II
Langer-Saldino achondrogenesis
See ACHONDROGENESIS, LANGER-SALDINO TYPE
Language-induced epilepsy
See EPILEPSY, REFLEX
Laron pituitary dwarfism
See DWARFISM, LARON

LARSEN SYNDROME   0570

Includes:

Desbuquois syndrome
Joint dislocations-unusual facies-skeletal abnormalities
Skeletal anomalies-joint dislocations-unusual facies

Excludes:
Arthrogryposes (0088)
Larsen syndrome, lethal type (2800)

Major Diagnostic Criteria: Flat facies with depressed nasal bridge, wide-spaced eyes, and prominent forehead; dislocations of multiple major joints and cylindrical, nontapering fingers with multiple carpal ossification centers.

Clinical Findings: Congenital joint dislocations, usually bilateral, involving the elbows, hips, and knees (typically anterior dislocation of the tibia or the femur); subluxation of the shoulders; cylindrical fingers; broad, spatulate thumbs; short metacarpals; a juxtacalcaneal accessory ossification center, short nails; equinovarus or valgus feet; unusual facies characterized by a prominent or bossed forehead, flat and depressed nasal bridge and wide-set eyes. Most affected individuals are mentally normal.

Complications: In early infancy decreased rigidity of the cartilage of the rib cage, epiglottis, arytenoid, and possibly trachea may cause respiratory difficulties.

Associated Findings: Congenital heart disease, cleft palate without cleft lip, **Hydrocephaly**, and abnormal spinal segmentation.

Etiology: Genetic heterogeneity is present, with both autosomal dominant and autosomal recessive inheritance reported. Differentiation between the two forms may be difficult, but the recessive form is generally more severe.

Pathogenesis: Undetermined. May be related to mesenchymal connective tissue.

MIM No.: *15025, *24560, 22188

POS No.: 3275

CDC No.: 755.810

Sex Ratio: M1:F1

Occurrence: Undetermined but presumed rare. Established literature.

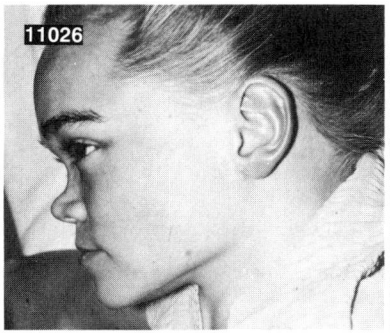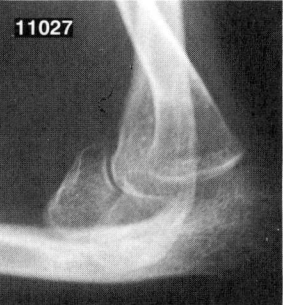

0570-11026: Profile shows depressed nasal bridge. 11027: Lateral view of right elbow shows joint dislocation, underdeveloped bones and accessory ulnar ossicle.

Risk of Recurrence for Patient's Sib:
See Part I, *Mendelian Inheritance.*

Risk of Recurrence for Patient's Child:
See Part I, *Mendelian Inheritance.*

Age of Detectability: Usually at birth by physical examination, but mild cases may not be noticed until adulthood.

Gene Mapping and Linkage: Unknown.

Prevention: None known. Genetic counseling indicated.

Treatment: Early, intensive and continued orthopedic care.

Prognosis: Physically handicapped to a variable degree, depending on nature and extent of patient's condition and results of orthopedic surgery.

Detection of Carrier: Unknown.

Special Considerations: Cases of Larsen syndrome have been reported under other names, primarily centering on the striking knee deformities: genu recurvatum; congenital hyperextension and subluxation of the knee. *Desbuquois syndrome* is a possible variant in which supernumerary carpal ossification centers cause deviation of the fingers. This is discernible only during the first year or so of life, along with coronal clefts of the vertebrae (Beighton et al, 1988),

References:

Larsen LJ, et al.: Multiple congenital dislocations associated with characteristic facial abnormality. J Pediatr 1950; 37:574–581.
Latta RJ, et al.: Larsen's syndrome: a skeletal dysplasia with multiple joint dislocations and unusual facies. J Pediatr 1971; 78:291–298.
Steel HH, Kohl H: Multiple congenital dislocations associated with other skeletal anomalies (Larsen's syndrome) in three siblings. J Bone Joint Surg 1972; 54A:75–82.
Gorlin RJ, et al.: Syndromes of the head and neck. New York: McGraw-Hill, 1976.
de Nazar MM: Larsen's syndrome: Clinical and genetic aspects. J Genet Hum 1980; 28:83–88.
Houston CS, et al.: Separating Larsen's syndrome from the 'arthrogryposis basket'. J Canad Assoc Radiol 1981; 32:206–214.
Tsang MCK, et al.: Oral and craniofacial morphology of a patient with Larsen syndrome. J Craniofac Genet Dev Biol 1986; 6:357–362.
Beighton P, et al.: International nosology of heritable disorders of connective tissue, Berlin, 1986. Am J Med Genet 1988; 29:581–594.

MY001   **Terry L. Myers**

LARSEN SYNDROME, LETHAL TYPE   2800

Includes:

Joint dislocations, multiple, lethal, Larsen-like
Lethal, Larsen-like, multiple joint dislocations

Excludes: **Larsen syndrome** (0570)

Major Diagnostic Criteria: Multiple congenital dislocations of joints, severe short stature, cleft soft palate, skeletal abnormalities, abnormal dermal collagen bundles, pulmonary insufficiency due to laryngotracheomalacia and lung hypoplasia, and early death. X-rays confirm clinical impressions of joint dislocations and skeletal abnormalities. Histochemical and electron microscopy show abnormalities of cartilage matrix, collagen bundles of joint capsules, and hyaline cartilage of the trachea.

Clinical Findings: At birth, body length is short. A poor cry, severe hypotonia, and respiratory metabolic acidosis are present shortly after birth. Pulmonary insufficiency rapidly ensues due to laryngotracheomalacia and lung hypoplasia, leading to early death.

Congenital dislocations may involve shoulders, hips, knees, ankles, elbows, and wrists. X-rays confirm the multiple dislocations and may, in addition, reveal hypoplasia of the fibulae and of the distal ends of the humeri, cervical kyphosis, coronal clefts of the lower lumbar vertebrae, small proximal tarsal bones, and talipes equinovarus. Rhizomelic shortening of the upper limbs may be present.

Craniofacial features include a prominent forehead, large posterior fontanelle, flat nasal bridge, **Eye, hypertelorism**, cleft of soft

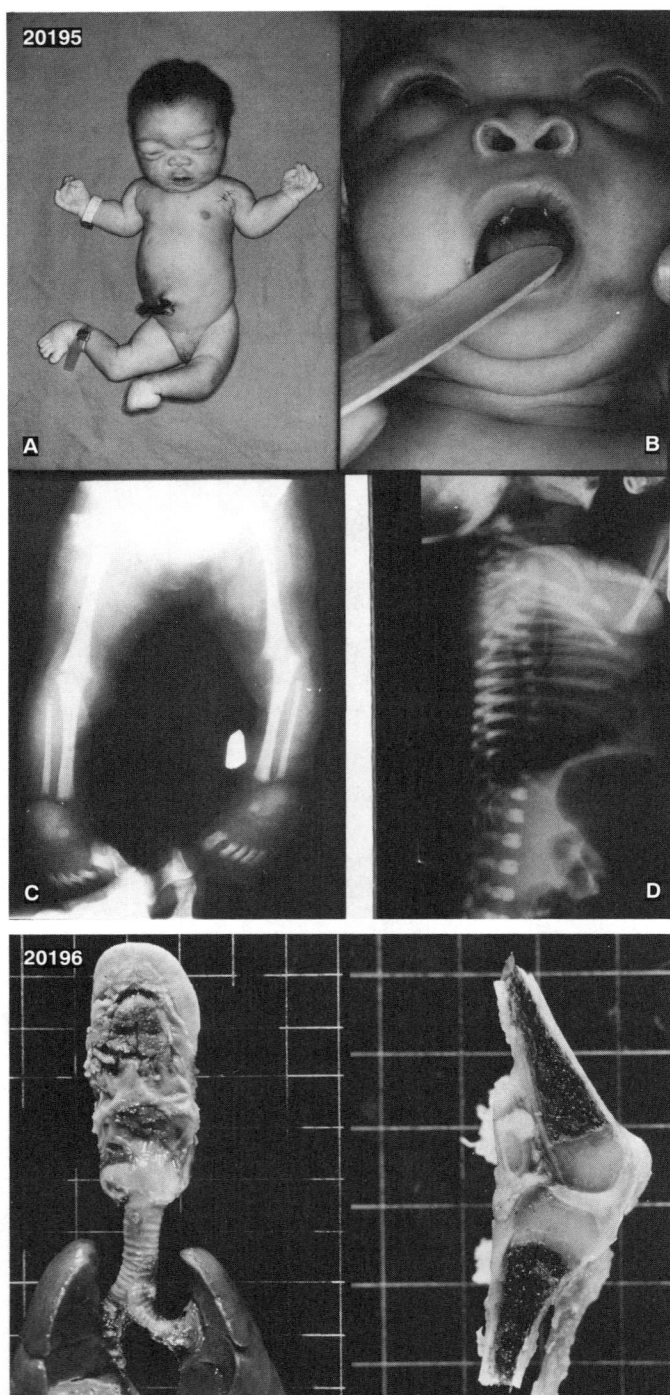

2800-20195: A) Gross view of a patient with Larsen syndrome, lethal type II. B) Close-up view of facial appearance and cleft palate. C) PA view of lower extremities, showing small proximal tarsal bones and hypoplasia of the fibulae. D) Lateral X-ray of lumbar spine showing coronal clefts of the lower lumbar vertebrae. **20196:** A) Gross view of the respiratory tract showing collapsed and soft trachea and hypoplastic lungs. B) Lateral view of the cross section of the knee showing thin fibrous ligament supporting the posterior aspect of the knee joint.

palate, small mouth, and low-set ears. In addition, short neck may be present due to an excess of subcutaneous tissue.

Dense, mature collagen bundles may be strikingly deficient, especially in the flexor aspects of the tendon sheath at the knees and shoulders. Dermal connective tissue, the matrix of tracheal and articular hyaline cartilages, and joint capsules may have abnormal histochemical properties; the dermal collagen bundles may appear broad and smudgy. Electron microscopic study may reveal loss of uniformity in the size of collagen fibers due to the presence of many small fibers in the hyaline cartilage of the trachea.

Complications: Pulmonary insufficiency due to laryngotracheomalacia and pulmonary hypoplasia is the main cause of death. Spinal instability due to vertebral anomalies may also be a cause of death.

Associated Findings: Signs and symptoms secondary to collagen dysmaturity.

Etiology: Probably autosomal recessive inheritance. Two reported cases have been sporadic with no family history.

Pathogenesis: Abnormal histochemical properties and morphologic findings of connective tissue fibers strongly suggest a disorder of connective tissue, possibly dysmaturity of collagen fibers with a predilection to joint capsules, tracheal cartilage, and possibly nasal cartilage. A striking deficiency of dense mature collagen bundles, especially in the flexor aspects of the tendon sheath at the knees and shoulders may be responsible for anterior dislocation of the tibia at the knee and lateral dislocation of the shoulder.

The significance of the decreased lysyl hydroxylase activity of cultured fibroblasts is unknown. However, the values are not in the range of lysyl hydroxylase deficiency that is seen in the type VI (ocular) **Ehlers-Danlos syndrome**.

MIM No.: 24565

POS No.: 3372

CDC No.: 755.810

Sex Ratio: Presumably M1:F1 (M0:F3 observed).

Occurrence: Three isolated females have been documented.

Risk of Recurrence for Patient's Sib:
See Part I, *Mendelian Inheritance.*

Risk of Recurrence for Patient's Child:
See Part I, *Mendelian Inheritance.*

Age of Detectability: At birth.

Gene Mapping and Linkage: Unknown.

Prevention: None known. Genetic counseling indicated.

Treatment: Symptomatic treatment for respiratory failure.

Prognosis: Death due to pulmonary insufficiency.

Detection of Carrier: Unknown.

References:
Chen H, et al.: A lethal, Larsen-like multiple joint dislocation syndrome. Am J Med Genet 1982; 13:149–161. †
Clayton-Smith J, Donnai D: A further patient with the lethal type of Larsen syndrome. J Med Genet 1988; 25:499–500.

CHO15   **Harold Chen**

Laryngeal abductor paralysis
See VOCAL CORD PARALYSIS

LARYNGEAL ABDUCTOR PARALYSIS-MENTAL RETARDATION 3045

Includes:
Plott syndrome
Vocal cord dysfunction, familial

Excludes: X-linked mental retardation (other)

Major Diagnostic Criteria: Inspiratory stridor due to laryngeal abductor paralysis is necessary to make the diagnosis.

Clinical Findings: All affected individuals have had inspiratory stridor from birth, with cyanosis occasionally occurring in the neonatal period. Subsequent growth and development are slow, with mental retardation being a constant finding. The facial expression is described as "blank," but with normal facial movement. Speech and swallowing difficulties also occur, suggesting involvment of ninth, tenth, and twelfth cranial nerves. The less severely affected individuals are described as clumsy, whereas the more severely affected individuals have hypotonia, severe cyanosis, and death.

Complications: Unknown.

Associated Findings: One boy also had optic atrophy and nystagmus.

Etiology: Presumably X-linked recessive inheritance.

Pathogenesis: Unknown. The cause of the laryngeal abductor defect is thought to be an abnormality of nucleus ambiguus function. However, the gene also apparently affects the brain in that retardation is also one of the findings.

MIM No.: 30885

POS No.: 4008

Sex Ratio: M7:F0 (observed).

Occurrence: Two families, both from North America, have been reported in detail.

Risk of Recurrence for Patient's Sib:
See Part I, *Mendelian Inheritance.*

Risk of Recurrence for Patient's Child:
See Part I, *Mendelian Inheritance.*

Age of Detectability: At birth, by inspiratory stridor.

Gene Mapping and Linkage: Unknown.

Prevention: None known. Genetic counseling indicated.

Treatment: Tracheostomy may be indicated.

Prognosis: Death occurred in the neonatal period in two individuals; mental retardation was present in all survivors, with measured IQs of 56–73.

Detection of Carrier: Unknown.

References:
Plott D: Congenital laryngeal-abductor paralysis due to nucleus ambiguus dysgenesis in three brothers. New Engl J Med 1964; 271:593–597.
Watters GV, Fitch N: Familial laryngeal abductor paralysis and psychomotor retardation. Clin Genet 1973; 4:429–433.

T0007 **Helga V. Toriello**

Laryngeal aerocele
See LARYNGOCELE
Laryngeal and skeletal anomalies-motor and sensory neuropathy
See NEUROPATHY, CONGENITAL MOTOR & SENSORY-SKELETAL-LARYNGEAL DEFECTS
Laryngeal atresia, congenital
See LARYNX, ATRESIA
Laryngeal chondromalacia, congenital
See LARYNGOMALACIA
Laryngeal hernia
See LARYNGOCELE
Laryngeal mucocele
See LARYNGOCELE
Laryngeal papillomatosis, juvenile
See PAPILLOMA VIRUS, CONGENITAL INFECTION

LARYNGEAL PARALYSIS 3080

Includes:
Abductor vocal cord paralysis
Adductor vocal cord paralysis
Gerhardt syndrome
Plott syndrome
Vocal cord dysfunction

Excludes: Laryngeal abductor paralysis-mental retardation (3045)

Major Diagnostic Criteria: Laryngoscopy reveals bilateral adductor or abductor vocal cord paralysis, either partial or complete.

Clinical Findings: Hoarseness, usually since birth; however, it may develop later in life. The severity of hoarseness may be progressive throughout life. Laryngoscopy reveals bilateral adductor or abductor vocal cord paralysis, either partial or complete. Aspiration is not significant due to intact afferent laryngeal innervation.

Complications: Unknown.

Associated Findings: None known.

Etiology: Usually autosomal dominant inheritance, although X-linked recessive forms have been reported.

Pathogenesis: Unknown. No postmortem examinations have been performed on affected individuals. The cause of paralysis is probably neuronal, but may be due to a muscular abnormality of the adductor muscle itself (Mace et al., 1978).

MIM No.: *15026, *15027, 30885

Sex Ratio: Presumably M1:F1, but a male preponderance has been observed.

Occurrence: Some seven kinships have been reported.

Risk of Recurrence for Patient's Sib:
See Part I, *Mendelian Inheritance.*

Risk of Recurrence for Patient's Child:
See Part I, *Mendelian Inheritance.*

Age of Detectability: At birth, or when speech problems become apparent.

Gene Mapping and Linkage: Unknown.

Prevention: None known. Genetic counseling indicated.

Treatment: If aspiration becomes a problem, vocal cord medialization may be indicated.

Prognosis: Normal life span.

Detection of Carrier: Unknown.

Special Considerations: *Gerhardt syndrome* refers to an autosomal dominant form of laryngeal abductor paralysis, while *Plott syndrome* is an X-linked form of laryngeal abductor paralysis.

References:
Mace M, et al.: Autosomal dominantly inherited adductor laryngeal paralysis-a new syndrome with a suggestion of linkage to HLA. Clin Genet 1978; 14:265–270.
Morelli G, et al.: Familial laryngeal abductor paralysis with presumed autosomal dominant inheritance. Ann Otol Rhinol Laryngol 1982; 91:323–324.
Cunningham MJ, et al.: Familial vocal cord dysfunction. Pediatrics 1985; 76:750–753.

WI061 **Brian Wiatrak**
MY003 **Charles M. Myer III**

Laryngeal pouch
See LARYNGOCELE
Laryngeal pyocele
See LARYNGOCELE
Laryngeal retention cyst
See EPIGLOTTIS, VALLECULAR CYST
Laryngeal stridor, congenital
See LARYNGOMALACIA
Laryngeal ventricle prolapse
See LARYNX, VENTRICLE PROLAPSE

LARYNGO-TRACHEO-ESOPHAGEAL CLEFT 0577

Includes:
Cleft larynx
Esophagotrachea, persistent
Larynx and trachea, congenital posterior cleft of
Tracheo-laryngo-esophageal cleft

Excludes: Tracheoesophageal fistula (0960)

Major Diagnostic Criteria: Direct endoscopic visualization of a congenital posterior cleft of the larynx and trachea with persistent esophagotrachea.

Clinical Findings: Symptoms depend on the size of the defect in the posterior laryngeal and tracheal wall. The most common finding is respiratory embarrassment with feeding; this includes cyanosis, choking, and aspiration. Additionally, abnormal voice, increased oral secretions, and stridor, predominantly expiratory due to aspirated oral secretions, are noted.

Complications: Repeated episodes of aspiration pneumonia and respiratory distress. Poor feeding results in nutritional deficiency and growth failure.

Associated Findings: Increased incidence of esophageal abnormalities, including atresia and various tracheoesophageal fistulas. Higher incidence of other tracheobronchial abnormalities.

Etiology: Unknown.

Pathogenesis: An arrest in the rostral advancement of the tracheoesophageal septum, which then prevents the dorsal fusion of the cricoid cartilages.

POS No.: 4341

CDC No.: 748.385, 748.390

Sex Ratio: M1:F1

Occurrence: Approximately 150 cases have been reported. However, four clefts were found in a series of 2,000 consecutive autopsies at a pediatric hospital.

Risk of Recurrence for Patient's Sib: Two instances of affected sibs have been reported.

Risk of Recurrence for Patient's Child: Unknown.

Age of Detectability: At birth.

Gene Mapping and Linkage: Unknown.

Prevention: None known. Genetic counseling indicated.

Treatment: Gastrostomy, tracheostomy, and surgical closure of defect have been successful when the lesion is limited to the cervical region.

Prognosis: Normal life span, intelligence, and function if surgical repair is successful.

Detection of Carrier: Unknown.

References:
Blumberg JB, et al.: Laryngotracheoesophageal cleft, the embryologic implications: review of the literature. Surgery 1965; 57:559–566.
Delahunty JE, Cherry J: Congenital laryngeal cleft. Ann Otol Rhinol Laryngol 1969; 78:96.
Imbrie JD, Doyle PJ: Laryngotracheoesophageal cleft: report of a case and review of the literature. Laryngoscope 1969; 79:1252–1274.
Cohen SR: Cleft larynx: a report of seven cases. Ann Otol 1975; 84:747–756.
Cotton RT, Schreiber JT: Management of laryngotracheoesophageal cleft. Ann Otol Rhinol Laryngol 1981; 90:401–405.

JA013   **R. Kirk Jackson**

LARYNGOCELE 0575

Includes:
Diverticulum of larynx
Laryngeal aerocele
Laryngeal hernia
Laryngeal mucocele
Laryngeal pouch
Laryngeal pyocele
Laryngoceles: internal, external or combined
Ventricular cyst of larynx

Excludes:
Larynx, cysts (0572)
Larynx, ventricle prolapse (0573)

Major Diagnostic Criteria: A ventricular cystic mass or neck mass over the thyrohyoid membrane is the major clinical finding. Direct visualization by endoscopy establishes the diagnosis and rules out the possibility of a coexistent disease.

Clinical Findings: A cyst-like mass is present in the neck and laryngeal ventricle. The external component may enlarge with straining but decrease with rest; it may collapse with gentle pressure. This lesion arises as a saccular dilatation of the saccus or

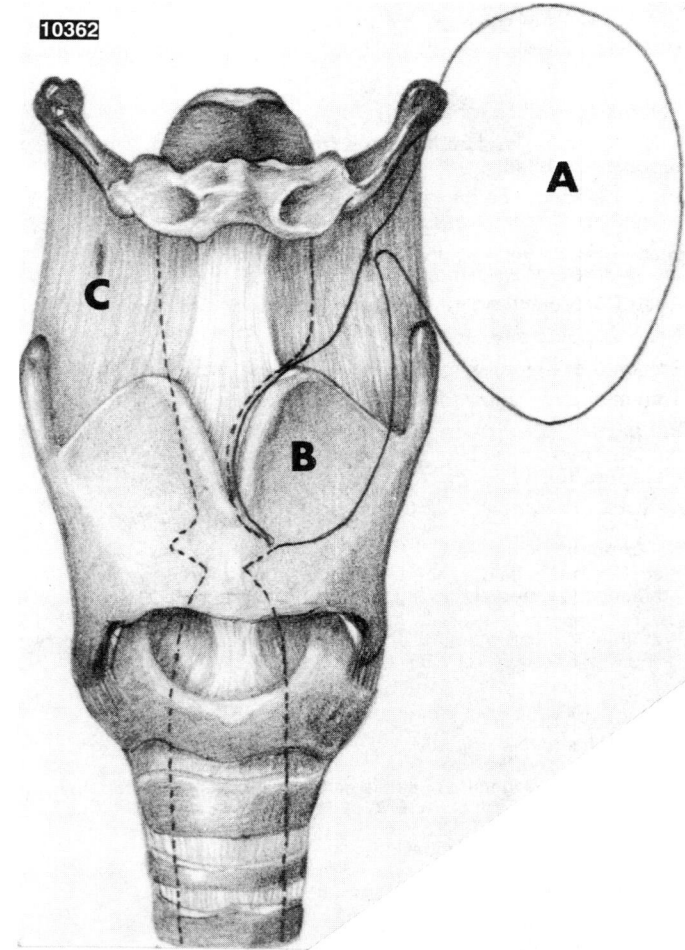

0575-10362: Laryngocele within larynx. External component (A) is connected with internal component (B) through thyrohyoid membrane at perforation of neurovascular bundle (C).

appendix of the laryngeal ventricle or the sinus of Morgagni. Herniation of mucosa occurs upward from the ventricle and lateral to the false vocal cord. This cystic mass remains within the interior of the larynx or passes through the thyrohyoid membrane at the perforation site of the neurovascular bundle (superior laryngeal nerve and vessels). Laryngoceles are subsequently classified by location as internal, external, or combined. Their classification by content is aerocele, pyocele, or mucocele.

The laryngeal appendix is larger in Caucasians than in other racial groups. In other primates it may extend into the neck, across the chest, and into the axilla. In the orangutan, a structure similar to a laryngocele is thought to be an air reservoir for use during climbing and phonation.

The clinical symptoms vary with the extent and location of the lesion. In one series, the initial symptoms were strider (90%), dyspnea (55%), feeding problems (50%), and coughing (20%). Seven of 20 children were premature, and five required ventilation for RDS. Emergency tracheotomy was needed in 20% of these cases.

The patient's voice may be normal, hoarse, or aphonic. A cystic swelling of the neck between the hyoid bone and the thyroid cartilage often occurs. Compression of the mass may produce gurgling and hissing in the throat (Bryce sign). The mass may also increase with straining and decrease with rest. Dysphagia and aspiration often develop with large lesions. Airway obstruction and asphyxiation are potential dangers. Small laryngoceles may be entirely asymptomatic.

The relationship between laryngoceles and laryngeal carcinoma has been studied by Micheau, et al (1978). Laryngoceles are found in approximately 2% of normal larynges; however, they may be found in 18% of laryngeal carcinoma specimens. It has been suggested that laryngeal carcinoma may play a role in the genesis of a laryngocele. Carcinoma may develop in laryngoceles in as many as 50% of patients. Pre-existing laryngoceles might provide a preferential site for tumor development.

Complications: Infection, hoarseness, aspiration, obstruction, and carcinoma of larynx may occur.

Associated Findings: None known.

Etiology: Undetermined. Subglottic cysts have resulted from the trauma of intubation.

Pathogenesis: Increased intraluminal laryngeal pressure in persons with congenitally large ventricular appendices are the major considerations in this disease. The laryngeal appendix becomes dilated with an increase in intraluminal pressure from straining, coughing, singing, glass blowing, and the playing of wind instruments. This dilated saccus (saccular cyst) then expands up into the false cord, or the aryepiglottic fold, or both; it passes into the neck through the perforation of the neurovascular bundle in the thyrohyoid ligament. These cysts are lined with ciliated respiratory epithelium that contain mucous-secreting glands. Varying degrees of inflammatory reactions occur in the wall of the cyst.

CDC No.: 748.300

Sex Ratio: M1:F1

Occurrence: Anout 200 cases have been documented.

Risk of Recurrence for Patient's Sib: Unknown.

Risk of Recurrence for Patient's Child: Unknown.

Age of Detectability: Mitchell (1987) reported the clinical findings of 20 patients with laryngeal cysts that were treated at the Hospital for Sick Children in London between 1969 and 1984. Forty percent of the cysts were apparent the first day of life, and 95% were discovered before six months of age.

Gene Mapping and Linkage: Unknown.

Prevention: None known. Genetic counseling indicated.

Treatment: In patients with a symptomatic laryngocele, a one-stage surgical excision of the lesion through an external incision may be necessary as well as a treatment of infections with antibiotics. Although incision and drainage should be avoided, they may be necessary with an acute infection. Tracheotomy may be necessary when airway obstruction or aspiration are problems.

Airway obstruction in children is a dangerous and life threat-ening situation. Booth and Birck (1981) report two infants, one with a saccular cyst and the other with a laryngocele, who presented with respiratory difficulty. Symptoms of both of these conditions are non-specific and can be confused with the symptoms of laryngomalacia. Early recognition and treatment is important because of the small airway. Surgical approach to laryngocele and large saccular cysts is usually by the external approach and tracheotomy. In infants, however, an endoscopic method of dealing with these conditions is preferred. Marsupialization of the dome and stripping of the cyst wall with laryngeal forceps is usually sufficient. The carbon dioxide laser may be useful in selected cases. Post-operatively, the endotracheal tube should be left in place approximately 72 hours to act as a stent.

Prognosis: With adequate treatment, the outlook for normal life span, intelligence, and functioning is good.

Detection of Carrier: Unknown.

References:

English GM, DeBlanc GB: Laryngocele: a case presenting with acute airway obstruction. Laryngoscope 1968; 78:386–398.

Harrison DFN: Saccular mucocele and laryngeal cancer. Arch Otolaryngol 1977; 103:232–234.

Holinger LD, et al.: Laryngocele and saccular cysts. Ann Otol Rhinol Laryngol. 1978; 87:675–685. *

Micheau C, et al.: Relationship between laryngoceles and laryngeal carcinomas. Laryngoscope 1978; 88:680–688.

Donegan JO, et al.: Internal laryngocele and saccular cysts in children. a comparative account of symptoms, diagnosis, and management. Ann Otol Rhinol Laryngol 1980; 89:409.

Booth JB, Birck HG: Operative treatment and postoperative management of saccular cyst and laryngocele. Arch Otolaryngol 1981; 107:500–502.

Baker HL, et al.: Manifestations and management of laryngoceles. Head Neck Surg 1982; 4:450–456. *

Mitchell DB: Cysts of the infant larynx. J Laryngol Otol 1987; 101:833–837.

EN002   **Gerald M. English**

Laryngoceles: internal, external or combined
See LARYNGOCELE

LARYNGOMALACIA   0576

Includes:

> Croup, congenital
> Laryngeal chondromalacia, congenital
> Laryngeal stridor, congenital
> Larynx, congenital flaccid
> Stridor, congenital

Excludes:

> Croup (other)
> Laryngismus stridulous
> Larynx, atresia (0571)

Major Diagnostic Criteria: Persistent stuttering, inspiratory respirations with episodes of cyanosis, especially during feeding; neck, chest, and esophageal X-rays negative for possible thyroglossal duct cyst, tracheal compression, mediastinal mass, and vascular ring. Direct laryngoscopy shows fluttering arytenoids; curled or tubular epiglottis, and it demonstrates absence of other laryngeal or tracheal obstruction.

Clinical Findings: Stridorous, noisy, inspiratory crowing respirations, which may be associated with intermittent episodes of hypoxia and cyanosis, accompanied by indrawing at the suprasternal notch and epigastrium. Usually begins shortly after birth and increases in severity, lasting 6–18 months, then gradually subsides. Direct or flexible laryngoscopy shows flaccidity of all supraglottic structures; the epiglottis is often curled or tubular and soft, as are the arytenoids and aryepiglottic folds, which all flutter during inspiration. Cord motility is normal. Symptoms are often exacerbated during feeding, supine positioning, or agitation.

Exaggerated or persistent infantile features of the larynx, tubular longitudinal folding of the epiglottis, and inward rolling of the

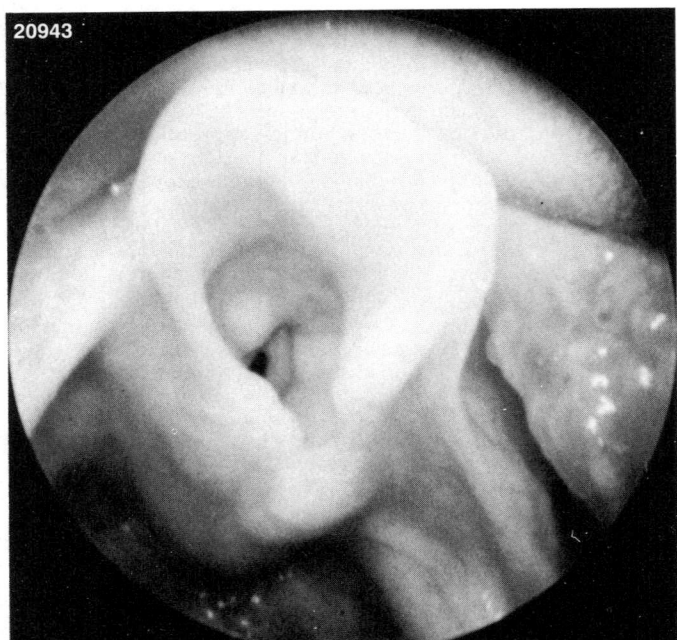

0576-20943: Laryngomalacia.

arytenoids and aryepiglottic folds have been recorded as postmortem findings. Histologically, edema and a slight increase in the lymphatic and polymorphonuclear cellular elements of the submucosa were found. Kelemen (1953) describes cartilages found to be about one-half the thickness of control specimens, and Shulman (1976) describes cartilages with unusual matrix staining.

Complications: Failure to gain weight, in severe cases. Pectus excavatum associated with the constant epigastric indrawing. Hypoxia and cyanosis may be found in addition to obstructive sleep apnea.

Associated Findings: Micrognathia, macroglossia.

Etiology: In one kindred, the mother of three affected sibs had respiratory problems in infancy, suggesting the possibility of autosomal dominant inheritance.

Pathogenesis: Unknown.

MIM No.: 15028

CDC No.: 748.300

Sex Ratio: M2:F1

Occurrence: Most common of congenital laryngeal anomalies, constituting 650 of a series of 866 laryngeal anomalies.

Risk of Recurrence for Patient's Sib: Unknown.

Risk of Recurrence for Patient's Child: Unknown.

Age of Detectability: At one to six months by direct or flexible laryngoscopy.

Gene Mapping and Linkage: Unknown.

Prevention: None known. Genetic counseling indicated.

Treatment: Interrupt feeding frequently to assist breathing; place infant in position of least obstruction. Surgical trimming of epiglottis and aryepiglottic folds may be effective in selective circumstances. Tracheotomy only in severe involvement.

Prognosis: Normal for life span, intelligence, and function.

Detection of Carrier: Unknown.

Special Considerations: Stridor is the auditory evidence of upper airway obstruction; therefore, laryngomalacia must be differentiated from all other causes of stridor in infants. Direct laryngos-

copy usually shows a curled and flaccid epiglottis, with soft, edematous-appearing arytenoids that are drawn into the glottis with a fluttering appearance with each inspiration. The symptom is exaggerated when the infant is on its back and decreases in severity when the infant lies on its abdomen. The noise is increased with total relaxation, as during sleep, or with vigorous crying. Bronchoscopy often shows an associated, similar tracheo- and bronchomalacia.

References:

Schwartz L: Congenital laryngeal stridor (inspiratory laryngeal collapse): new theory as to its underlying cause and desirability of a change in terminology. Arch Otolaryngol 1944; 39:403.

Finlay HVL: Familial congenital stridor. Arch Dis Child 1949; 24:219.

Kelemen G: Congenital laryngeal stridor. Arch Otolaryngol 1953; 58:245.

Holinger PH, Brown WT: Congenital webs, cysts, laryngoceles and other anomalies of the larynx. Ann Otol Rhinol Laryngol 1967; 76:744.

Shulman JB, et al.: Familial laryngomalacia: a case report. Laryngoscope 1976; 86:84–91.

Belmont JR, Groundfast K: Congenital laryngeal stridor (laryngomalacia): etiologic factors and associated disorders. Ann Otol Rhinol Laryngol 1984; 93:430–437.

MY003   **Charles M. Myer III**

Larynx and trachea, congenital posterior cleft of
See LARYNGO-TRACHEO-ESOPHAGEAL CLEFT
Larynx cancer
See CANCER, LUNG, FAMILIAL

LARYNX, ATRESIA   0571

Includes:
 Atresia of larynx, types I, II and III
 Glottic atresia
 Laryngeal atresia, congenital
 Stenosis at the conus elasticus

Excludes:
 Laryngocele (0575)
 Laryngomalacia (0576)
 Larynx, cysts (0572)
 Larynx, web (0574)

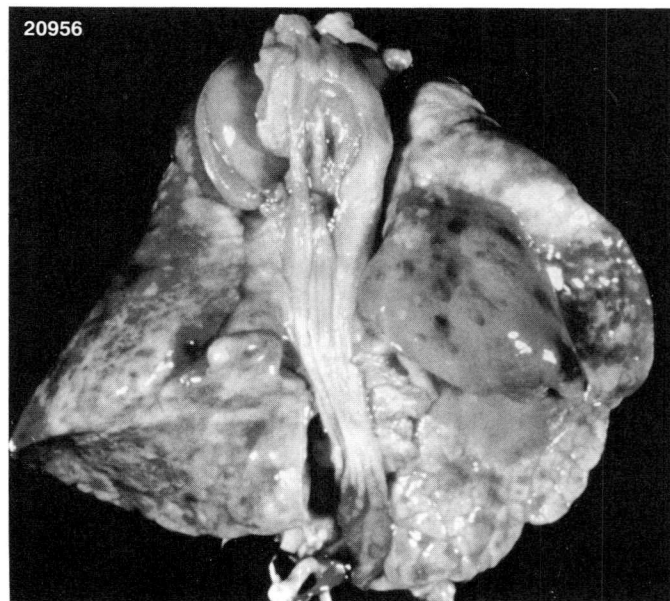

0571-20956: Laryngeal atresia.

Subglottic stenosis (0919)
Tracheoesophageal fistula (0960)

Major Diagnostic Criteria: Asphyxia neonatorum or stridor at birth, with complete or partial laryngeal obstruction.

Clinical Findings: Incompatible with life unless it is recognized immediately at birth and steps are taken at once to establish an airway. When the obstruction is incomplete, the signs and symptoms are related to the functioning diameter of the stenosed lumen. Marked respiratory effort without air exchange or stridor at birth, with or without cyanosis, depending on the severity of the stenosis, is the first sign of laryngeal obstruction.

Direct laryngoscopy will reveal a complete or partial membranous occlusion of the larynx. Smith and Bain (1965) distinguish three types of atresia:
Type I: supraglottic and infraglottic parts are atretic
Type II: atresia is infraglottic
Type III: atresia is glottic

Complications: The risk of neonatal death is extremely high with complete laryngeal atresia. In mild cases (i.e. stenosis or partial atresia) recurrent episodes of "croup" and repeated superimposed respiratory infections simulating laryngotracheobronchitis are common. Complications associated with tracheotomy in the newborn must also be considered. Chances of complications would be high in most instances because of the emergent nature of the situation should accidental decannulation occur.

Associated Findings: About one-half the cases reported in the literature had other potentially fatal malformations. Malformations include the CNS (hydrocephaly, malformations of the aqueduct); alimentary system (esophageal atresia, bronchoesophageal fistula, tracheoesophageal fistula and atresia); urogenital system (hypoplasia of kidney, hydroureter, urethral atresia, vesicovaginal fistula, bicornuate uterus), and skeletal system (varus deformity of feet, partial absence of cervical vertebrae, absence of radius, syndactyly).

Etiology: Presumably autosomal dominant inheritance.

Pathogenesis: The various types of atresia are the result of arrest of development. A chromosomal basis has also been suggested (Lewandowski and Yunis, 1977).

MIM No.: 15030

CDC No.: 748.300

Sex Ratio: Presumably M1:F1

Occurrence: Undetermined but presumed rare.

Risk of Recurrence for Patient's Sib:
See Part I, *Mendelian Inheritance.*

Risk of Recurrence for Patient's Child:
See Part I, *Mendelian Inheritance.*

Age of Detectability: At birth.

Gene Mapping and Linkage: Unknown.

Prevention: None known. Genetic counseling indicated.

Treatment: Establishment of immediate diagnosis and provision of immediate airway (i.e. tracheostomy). Treatment of secondary infections and stridor.

Prognosis: The vast majority of newborns with complete laryngeal atresia die because the condition is not recognized and not treated immediately or because of other life threatening anomalies. If the child survives the neonatal period, with proper surgical and medical treatment he or she will have a normal life span, unless the condition is complicated by serious associated malformations.

Detection of Carrier: Unknown.

Special Considerations: There is little doubt that atresia of the larynx is closely related to laryngeal webs, not only in its presenting signs and pathologic findings, but also in its mode of genesis. Most authors feel that the condition has not been recognized in many infants and, as webs are not uncommon, it is safe to assume that atresia too is no rarity. Baker and Savetsky (1966) believe that heredity is a factor in "congenital partial atresia of the larynx" (study includes laryngeal webs and other types of laryngeal

stenosis), as was demonstrated in a mother and her two children, all of whom had this entity.

References:
Smith II, Bain AD: Congenital atresia of the larynx. Ann Otol Rhinol Laryngol 1965; 74:338–349.
Baker DC Jr, Savetsky L: Congenital partial atresia of the larynx. Laryngoscope 1966; 78:616–620.
Holinger PH, Brown W: Congenital webs, cysts, laryngoceles and other anomalies of the larynx. Ann Otol Rhinol. Laryngol 1967; 76:744.
Jackson C: Anomalies of the larynx. In: Maloney WH, ed: Otolaryngology. vol. 4. Hagerstown: Harper & Row, 1969.
Holinger PH, et al.: Pediatric laryngology. Otolaryngol Clin North Am 1970; 3:625.
Lewandowski RC Jr, Yunis JJ. Phenotypic mapping in man. In: Yunis JJ, ed: New chromosomal syndromes. New York: Academic Press, 1977:369–394.

MY003   **Charles M. Myer III**

Larynx, congenital flaccid
See LARYNGOMALACIA

LARYNX, CYSTS   0572

Includes:
Cysts, glottic
Cysts, saccular
Excludes:
Cysts, mucosal retention
Laryngocele (0575)
Thyroglossal duct remnant (0945)

Major Diagnostic Criteria: A cyst located in the larynx usually causing respiratory symptoms, which may result in feeding difficulties and an abnormal cry. A lateral X-ray of the neck may help with the diagnosis, but it is only made with certainty by direct laryngoscopy.

Clinical Findings: Saccular cysts of the larynx are non-air-containing, fluid-filled structures that do not communicate with the laryngeal lumen. They result from cystic distention of the laryngeal ventricle and lie beneath normal mucosa. They are usually sessile, but may be pedunculated. Most cysts are confined to the immediate area of the ventricular appendix. There are two types of cysts: 1) Anterior, which are located near the saccular orifice of the ventricle. They may bulge from deep within the ventricle and overhang the glottis. Some may be large enough to fill the entire ventricle. 2) Lateral cysts are typically located on the lateral wall of the supraglottic larynx or epiglottis. They may extend from the aryepiglottic fold and arytenoid downward to and including the ventricle, laterally into the pyriform sinus, or even through the thyrohyoid membrane into the neck.

Symptoms vary depending on the location, size, and age at presentation. In infants, respiratory distress, usually with inspiratory stridor, is the most common symptom because of the small size of the larynx. Cyanosis and use of the accessory muscles of respiration may be present. A change in the degree of obstruction can also occur with a change in head position. Dysphagia and an abnormal cry, which may be muffled, shrill, hoarse, feeble, or inaudible, are also common. Tracheostomy or endotrachial intubation is required for the severely compromised airway.

In an older child, hoarseness or a weak voice may be the presenting symptom.

Complications: Asphyxia at birth, respiratory distress, dysphagia, and an abnormal voice.

Associated Findings: Funnel chest may develop due to prolonged epigastric indrawing.

Etiology: Unknown.

Pathogenesis: Unknown. Several theories have been postulated; 1) a pinching off of some of the cells that normally form the appendix of the laryngeal ventricle, 2) failure of an epithelial cord of cells to hollow out between the fetal ventricle and laryngeal lumen, and 3) branchial derivation. Some investigators believe it need not be considered an actual malformation of the larynx, but simply a secondary disturbance in development.

CDC No.: 748.380

Sex Ratio: M1:F4

Occurrence: Undetermined but presumed rare.

Risk of Recurrence for Patient's Sib: Unknown.

Risk of Recurrence for Patient's Child: Unknown.

Age of Detectability: At birth for severe cases causing symptoms; otherwise, at any age if symptoms occur and laryngeal examination is warranted.

Gene Mapping and Linkage: Unknown.

Prevention: None known. Genetic counseling indicated.

Treatment: Aspiration under direct laryngoscopy. The cysts tend to recur and eventually may need to be unroofed and the frayed edges removed. Sometimes marsupialization is the initial procedure. Temporary tracheostomy may be required. Large cysts are treated by submucous resection through an external approach.

Prognosis: A cyst causing complete obstruction at birth will result in death unless an airway is secured. Once cysts are diagnosed and treated, life spain is normal.

Detection of Carrier: Unknown.

Special Considerations: Ductal cysts form at any site in the larynx where there are mucous glands. This excludes only the gland-free area on the free edge of the true cords. Obstruction of the ducts, with retention of mucus and dilation of the glands, is thought to be the origin of these cysts.

Intralaryngeal true branchiogenic cysts and a thyroid cartilage foraminal cyst have been described in the literature.

Congenital cysts and laryngoceles have a similar development, but laryngoceles differ from congenital cysts in that they communicate with the lumen of the larynx and become clinically perceptible only when swollen by air forced into them or when filled with a collection of fluid.

References:
DeSanto LW, et al.: Cysts of the larynx: classification. Laryngoscope 1970; 80:145–176. *
Hollinger LD, et al.: Laryngocoele and saccular cysts. Ann Otol 1978; 87:675–685. †
Donegan JO, et al.: Internal laryngocele and saccular cysts in children. A comparative account of symptoms, diagnosis, and management. Ann Otol Rhinol Laryngol 1980; 89:409. *
Abramson AL, Zeilinski B: Congenital laryngeal saccular cyst of the newborn. Laryngoscope 1984; 94:1580–1582.

K0023
B0049

**Frederick K. Kozak
Valerie L. Boswell**

LARYNX, VENTRICLE PROLAPSE 0573

Includes:
Eversion of sacculus
Eversion of ventricle
Laryngeal ventricle prolapse
Prolapse of laryngeal ventricle

Excludes:
Chronic laryngitis
Hyperplasia of larynx
Laryngeal polyp
Laryngocele (0575)
Reinke edema

Major Diagnostic Criteria: Intermittent hoarseness and a dry, irritating cough are produced by the prolapse of the ventricle. Direct laryngoscopic examination, manipulation of the mass to determine its site of origin, and biopsy to establish its histopathologic characteristics are necessary to establish the diagnosis.

Clinical Findings: An irritating, nonproductive cough and intermittent hoarseness are the usual symptoms when a mass of prolapsed tissue extends onto the true vocal cords. The degree of hoarseness varies depending on the size of the mass. Pain is rare, and airway obstruction becomes a problem only after the mass reaches a size that occludes the glottic airway.

Idiopathic or true eversion of the ventricular mucosa is rare because this tissue is normally firmly attached to underlying structures. An associated disease that contributes to the development of saccular eversion should always be suspected. Eversion of the sacculus has been detected in persons from the 2nd to the 6th decades of life and is more common in men than in women. In one third of reported cases the lesion was bilateral, with the remainder of the cases divided nearly equally between the right and left sides of the larynx.

Examination reveals a smooth, pear-shaped, pale red mass, protruding from the ventricle onto the true vocal cord. This mass moves freely when palpated during direct laryngoscopy and can usually be pushed back into the ventricle. It should not be difficult to determine that the mass originates from the ventricle and not from the vocal cords. Aspiration during direct laryngoscopy may be required to distinguish this lesion from a cyst. Biopsies should be obtained to rule out possibility of a neoplasm.

Complications: Neoplasms, recurrent airway obstruction, hoarseness, cough.

Associated Findings: None known.

Etiology: Undetermined. Infections of the larynx, cysts of the false vocal cord, aryepiglottic fold and ventricle, neoplasms of the larynx, chronic cough from pulmonary disease, and external laryngeal trauma have all been implicated. No known familial incidence exists. Seid, et al (1979), report that children may develop protrusion or prolapse of the laryngeal ventricle subsequent to endotracheal tube intubation. In these cases, the prolapsed ventricle caused airway obstruction necessitating tracheostomy. The prolapsed ventricle subsequently resolved and decannulation was possible.

Pathogenesis: Eversion of the sacculus, or appendix of the ventricle, or a portion of the ventricular mucosa produces a mass that lies upon the true vocal cord. The prolapsed sacculus is lined with ciliated pseudostratified columnar epithelium resting on an intact basement membrane. Scott (1976) reports an anatomic study of 111 larynges from both sexes. He determined the dimensions of the laryngeal saccule and sinus, relative to the height and width of the larynx in the two sexes, and found pouches that were asymptomatic in two patients. The male saccule tended to be relatively shallower than the female.

CDC No.: 748.300

Sex Ratio: M5:F1

Occurrence: Undetermined.

Risk of Recurrence for Patient's Sib: Unknown.

Risk of Recurrence for Patient's Child: Unknown.

Age of Detectability: Usually during early adulthood by indirect mirror examination of the larynx. Flexible laryngoscopy may allow earlier diagnosis in children.

Gene Mapping and Linkage: Unknown.

Prevention: None known. Genetic counseling indicated.

Treatment: Surgical excision during direct laryngoscopy is recommended as well as appropriate treatment of associated diseases. Tracheostomy may be required when airway obstruction occurs or if there is excessive surgical trauma. An open surgical approach may be necessary in some cases.

Prognosis: The prognosis is good when the mass is completely excised; however, any underlying disease may require more extensive therapy. In these patients the prognosis will depend on the success or failure of treatment for these disorders.

Detection of Carrier: Unknown.

References:
Freedman AO: Diseases of the ventricle of Morgagni; with special references to pyocele of congenital air sac of ventricle. Arch Otolaryngol 1938; 28:329–343.

Scott GBD: A morphometric study of the laryngeal saccule and sinus. Clin Otolaryngol 1976; 1:115–122.

Seid AB, et al.: Protrusion of the laryngeal ventricle in a pediatric patient following nasotracheal tube intubation. Otolaryngol Head Neck Surg 1979; 87:199–202.

Barnes DR, et al.: Prolapse of the laryngeal ventricle. Otolaryngol Head Neck Surg 1980; 88:165–171. *

Canalis RF: Laryngeal ventricle. Ann Otol Rhinol Laryngol 1980; 89:184–187. *

Weissler MC, et al.: Laryngopyocele as a cause of airway obstruction. Laryngoscope 1985; 95:1345–1351.

EN002   **Gerald M. English**

LARYNX, WEB   0574

Includes:
>   Glottic web
>   Subglottic web
>   Supraglottic web

Excludes:
>   Acquired webs of larynx
>   **Larynx, atresia** (0571)
>   **Subglottic stenosis** (0919)

Major Diagnostic Criteria: Diagnosis is based on the presence of a membranous web partially occluding the lumen in the supraglottic, glottic, or subglottic larynx. The diagnosis must be confirmed by direct laryngoscopy; indirect laryngoscopy may be used in those patients old enough to cooperate.

Clinical Findings: A laryngeal web or other laryngeal anomaly must be considered in a newborn with evidence of upper airway obstruction or dysphonia. Seventy-five percent of congenital laryngeal webs are present at birth. In the young child, this defect may go undetected until the cause of recurrent croup, tracheobronchitis, or pneumonia is sought. In adults or older children, hoarseness or dyspnea on exertion may be due to a laryngeal web.

The webs are usually grayish-white and glistening in appearance, but may be grayish-yellow or pink. Some of the reported webs have consisted of only a thin translucent membrane, but they are usually thin posteriorly and up to 1.5 cm thick anteriorly. Glottic webs are classified according to degree of occlusion of the lumen: type 1, 35% covering the anterior glottis, with the true vocal cords easily seen; type 2, 35–50% occlusion of the lumen, with the true vocal cords usually visible; type 3, 50–75% occlusion, with the vocal cords possibly visualized; type 4, 75–90% occlusion, with the vocal cords not seen. Type 3 is the most common type of glottic web. Subglottic webs may occur with or without cricoid involvement. Congenital interarytenoid fixation is included in the supraglottic web group.

Ninety-eight percent of all webs of the larynx are anterior, and 2% are posterior. The location and frequency of laryngeal webs are approximately: supraglottic 12.5%; glottic 75%; and subglottic, 12.5%.

Histologically, the superior surface of the web is lined by squamous epithelium, with the inferior surface covered by respiratory epithelium. The majority have a considerable mesodermal element of dense connective tissue, mucous glands, striated muscle, fat, and cartilage.

The severity of the symptoms is dependent upon the extent of the web. In infants, the most common signs, in the order of frequency, are aphonia, inspiratory and expiratory stridor, difficulty in feeding, and attacks of dyspnea. The most common symptoms in older children and adults are hoarseness; dyspnea on exertion or with respiratory tract infections; a weak, high-pitched voice, or easy tiring of the voice.

Complications: Minor manipulation of the airway or infections may lead to severe airway obstruction in patients with previously undetected webs.

Associated Findings: As many as 10–15% of individuals with laryngeal webs have other congenital anomalies, with one-third of these having associated abnormalities of the respiratory tract. The following anomalies have been reported: tetralogy of Fallot, ventricular septal defect, choanal atresia, bronchopulmonary dysplasia, cleft palate, bifid uvula and submucous cleft of the soft palate, tracheoesophageal fistula, adherent lingual frenulum, ptosis of eyelids, preauricular sinus, subglottic hemangioma, subglottic stenosis, nevus flammeus, mental retardation, seizure disorders, syndactyly, and urogenital anomalies.

Etiology: Unknown.

Pathogenesis: Differentiation of the larynx occurs between the 4th and 10th weeks of gestation. In the development of the larynx there is epithelial fusion between the two sides, which is thought to dissolve at about the 10th week of gestation. A laryngeal web is the result of incomplete recannulization of the primitive larynx between the 7th and 8th weeks of gestation.

CDC No.: 748.2

Sex Ratio: M1:F1

Occurrence: Five percent of congenital anomalies of the larynx are webs. The overall occurrence of laryngeal webs is unknown.

Risk of Recurrence for Patient's Sib: Undetermined. Familial reports exist.

Risk of Recurrence for Patient's Child: Unknown.

Age of Detectability: At birth by direct laryngoscopy or later when symptoms present.

Gene Mapping and Linkage: Unknown.

Prevention: None known. Genetic counseling indicated.

Treatment: Treatment of a web is dependent upon its thickness, extent, and location. For severe airway compromise, establishment of an adequate airway by intubation or tracheostomy is required. Simple webs may respond to division with microsurgical scissors and repeated dilation with the bougienge. CO_2 laser techniques have recently been used, but long-term results are not available. Tracheostomy may or may not be required for extensive webs. The larger and thicker webs are amenable to external laryngofissure, in which the thyroid cartilage is divided in the midline, the larynx entered, and the web resected. Intralaryngeal stents or keels have been used to prevent restenosis in glottic webs.

Speech improvement is achieved, but restoration of normal speech is often not possible.

Prognosis: Normal life span if airway obstruction is adequately treated.

Detection of Carrier: Unknown.

References:
McHugh HE, Loch WE: Congenital webs of the larynx. Laryngoscope 1942; 52:43–65.

Cotton RT, Richardson MA: Congenital laryngeal anomalies. Otolaryngol Clin North Am 1981; 14:203–218.

Benjamin B: Congenital laryngeal webs. Ann Otol Rhinol Laryngol 1983; 92:317–326. †

Cohen S: Congenital glottic webs in children. A retrospective review of 51 patients. Ann Otol Rhinol Laryngol (Suppl) 1985; 121:2–16. * †

Hardingham M, Walsh-Waring GP: The treatment of a congenital laryngeal web. J Laryngol Otol 1985; 89:273–279.

B0049   **Valerie L. Boswell**
K0023   **Frederick K. Kozak**

LAURENCE-MOON SYNDROME   0578

Includes: Laurence-Moon-Bardet-Biedl syndrome (some cases)

Excludes:
   Acrocephalopolysyndactyly (0013)
   Alstrom syndrome (0041)
   Bardet-Biedl syndrome (2363)
   Biemond II syndrome (2169)
   Cohen syndrome (2023)
   Prader-Willi syndrome (0823)
   Vasquez syndrome

Major Diagnostic Criteria: Hypogenitalism, mental retardation, retinitis pigmentosa, spastic paraplegia.

Clinical Findings: Hypogenitalism is present at birth but may not be noticed until later when normal genital growth is not observed. Postpubertal studies show hypogonadotrophic hypogonadism. Slow development, night blindness, mental retardation, and ataxic gait are noticed in turn during childhood. Ophthalmic examination then may show only retinal mottling due to thinning of the retina, leading to increased visibility of choroid. Retinal pigment accumulations are noticed peripherally in late childhood and gradually encroach on the central retina, accompanied by progressive optic atrophy. The ataxia slowly progresses to spastic paraplegia by early adulthood.

Complications: The retinitis pigmentosa leads to blindness. The mental defect is quite limiting, and the spastic paraplegia culminates in a bedridden state.

Associated Findings: None known.

Etiology: Presumably autosomal recessive inheritance.

Pathogenesis: Failure of normal embryologic development. The progressive nature suggests a metabolic error that interferes with development and continues after birth in some differentiated cells.

MIM No.:   24580

POS No.:   3113

CDC No.:   759.820

Sex Ratio: M1:F1

Occurrence: Presumably rare. Reportedly of increased frequency in the Arab population of Kuwait. The syndrome described by Laurence and Moon (1866) is a specific entity, while the syndrome described by Bardet and Biedl (see **Bardet-Biedl syndrome** is a different disorder. Shortly after the report of these two syndromes, the medical literature became confused, grouping many different disorders under the terms *Laurence-Moon-Biedl* syndrome or *Laurence-Moon-Bardet-Biedl* syndrome. Very few case descriptions truly fit into either the Bardet-Biedl syndrome or the Laurence-Moon syndrome. Most descriptions appear to represent either isolated cases or quite distinct syndromes rather than variants of either of the two classic syndromes. The **Bardet-Biedl syndrome** and the Laurence-Moon syndrome both breed true, as do several of the other disorders that have been grouped with them.

Risk of Recurrence for Patient's Sib:
   See Part I, *Mendelian Inheritance.*

Risk of Recurrence for Patient's Child:
   See Part I, *Mendelian Inheritance.* Most affected individuals are infertile.

Age of Detectability: Evident at birth, although definitive diagnosis is difficult until late childhood.

Gene Mapping and Linkage: Unknown.

Prevention: None known. Genetic counseling indicated.

Treatment: Unknown.

Prognosis: A deteriorating, handicapping condition due to mental retardation, progressive vision loss, and progressive spastic paraplegia.

Detection of Carrier: If genealogic studies identify the underlying cause as parental consanguinity stemming from membership in a small genetic isolate, normal relatives have as high as 50% chance of heterozygosity.

Support Groups: MD; Lexington Park; Laurence-Moon-Biedl Syndrome (LMBS) Support Network

References:

Laurence JZ, Moon RC: Four cases of retinitis pigmentosa occurring in the same family and accompanied by general imperfection of development. Ophthalmol Rev 1866; 2:32–41.
Roth AA: Familial eunuchoidism: the Laurence-Moon-Biedl syndrome. J Urol (Baltimore) 1947; 57:427–445.
Bowen P, et al.: The Laurence-Moon syndrome. Association with hypogonadotrophic hypogonadism and sex-chromosome aneuploidy. Arch Intern Med 1965; 116:598–604.
Schachat AP, Maumenee IH: The Bardet-Biedl syndrome and related disorders. Arch Ophthal 1982; 100:285–288.
Farag TI, Teebi AS: Bardet-Biedl and Lawrence-Moon syndromes in a mixed Arab population. Clin Genet 1988; 33:78–82.

TH017
UR001

T.F. Thurmon
S.A. Ursin

Laurence-Moon-Bardet-Biedl syndrome (some cases)
   See LAURENCE-MOON SYNDROME
Laurence-Moon-Bardet-Biedl syndrome (some)
   See BARDET-BIEDL SYNDROME
Lawrence syndrome
   See LIPODYSTROPHY SYNDROME, BERARDINELLI TYPE
LCAT deficiency
   *See LECITHIN-CHOLESTEROL ACYL TRANSFERASE DEFICIENCY
   also ANEMIA, HEMOLYTIC, RED CELL MEMBRANE DEFECTS*
LDL-receptor disorder
   See HYPERCHOLESTEREMIA
Lead poisoning, susceptibility to
   See DELTA-AMINOLEVULINIC ACID DEHYDRASE DEFICIENCY
Lead, effects of postnatal exposure
   See FETAL EFFECTS FROM MATERNAL LEAD EXPOSURE
Lead, fetal effects from maternal exposure
   See FETAL EFFECTS FROM MATERNAL LEAD EXPOSURE
Leaky red cell syndrome
   See ANEMIA, HEMOLYTIC, RED CELL MEMBRANE DEFECTS
Leber hamartoma
   See LIVER, HAMARTOMA
Leber miliary aneurysms
   See RETINA, COATS DISEASE
Leber optic atrophy
   See OPTIC ATROPHY, LEBER TYPE
Lecithin-cholesterol acyl transferase (LCAT) deficiency
   See ANEMIA, HEMOLYTIC, RED CELL MEMBRANE DEFECTS

LECITHIN-CHOLESTEROL ACYL TRANSFERASE
DEFICIENCY   0580

Includes:
   Alpha LCAT deficiency
   Alpha and beta LCAT deficiency
   Corneal opacities-dyslipoproteinemia
   Fish eye disease (obsolete; pejorative)
   LCAT deficiency
   Lecithin: cholesterol acyltransferase (LCAT) deficiency
   Norum disease
   Plasma cholesteryl ester deficiency, familial

Excludes:
   Apolipoprotein A-I and C-III deficiency states (3165)
   Analphalipoproteinemia (0048)
   Cholesteryl ester storage disease (0151)
   Hypoalphalipoproteinemia (3096)
   Wolman disease (1003)

Major Diagnostic Criteria: In familial lecithin:cholsterol acyltransferase (LCAT) deficiency, there is corneal opacities, proteinuria, and slight anemia, and a marked reduction in plasma cholesteryl esters and the activity of LCAT (both beta and alpha LCAT). In "fish eye disease", a variant of LCAT deficiency, marked corneal opacification, and deficiencies of HDL cholesterol and alpha LCAT activity are present.

Clinical Findings: In familial LCAT deficiency, marked changes in plasma lipids are invariable. All patients have low absolute and relative levels of cholesteryl esters, and increased levels of unesterified cholesterol. Plasma lecithin is increased and lysolecithin usually decreased. Most patients have increased levels of plasma triglycerides. Patients have low levels of high-density lipoproteins (HDL), and high levels of very-low-density lipoproteins (VLDL). Electron microscopy of lipoproteins reveals several abnormalities, the most frequent being disk-shaped HDL and the presence of chylomicron remnants in the VLDL fraction. Proteinuria, with late renal failure, is common. Several patients have died in renal failure. All patients have corneal opacities, and most have a slight normochromic anemia. There are no neurologic symptoms.

In "fish eye disease", there is a marked decrease in plasma HDL constituents, especially cholesterol esters, and also marked corneal opacification.

Complications: Disturbances in lipoprotein metabolism may give accelerated atherosclerosis. Cholesterol deposits in the kidney give rise to renal failure, which is the most severe complication. Corneal opacification affecting vision is a complication of both familial LCAT deficiency and "fish eye disease".

Associated Findings: None known.

Etiology: Autosomal recessive inheritance. Related disorders may exist because of a lack of LCAT or the presence of inhibitors of LCAT. Some patients have a very low level of normal LCAT, and others have a low level of abnormal LCAT.

Pathogenesis: LCAT has a role in normal cholesterol metabolism and turnover. One may therefore suggest that lack of the enzyme leads to decreased flux and transport of cholesterol from peripheral tissues to the liver. This may explain the increased unesterified cholesterol in the red blood cells and the accelerated atherosclerosis. A lack of LCAT may also cause cholesterol deposits in the glomerular tuft in the kidney, starting the events leading to renal failure. In familial LCAT deficiency there is decreased alpha and beta LCAT activity, while in "fish eye disease", only alpha LCAT activity is decreased.

MIM No.: *24590

Sex Ratio: M1:F1

Occurrence: Familial LCAT disease was first described in Norway, where most of the early patients were detected. Today patients are described in all parts of the world, including Japan and Germany, and more than 50 cases have been published. Alpha LCAT deficiency ("fish eye disease") has been described in several Swedish kindreds.

Risk of Recurrence for Patient's Sib:
See Part I, *Mendelian Inheritance.*

Risk of Recurrence for Patient's Child:
See Part I, *Mendelian Inheritance.*

Age of Detectability: The corneal opacities are usually detectable early in life. Proteinuria occurs usually from puberty. The enzyme defect is detectable from birth.

Gene Mapping and Linkage: LCAT (lecithin-cholesterol acyltransferase) has been mapped to 16q22.1.

Prevention: None known. Genetic counseling indicated.

Treatment: Dietetic to reduce plasma cholesterol. Secondary treatment of the renal failure may include kidney transplantation. No therapeutic effect has been obtained by infusions of purified enzyme or by transfusions of fresh plasma. Corneal transplantation can be used to treat the corneal opacification, but opacification can recur in the new cornea.

Prognosis: In familial LCAT deficiency, more than 50% of patients develop renal failure, which may lead to death. Some patients live into old age. In alpha LCAT deficiency, the prognosis is good except for the development of severe corneal opacification affecting vision.

Detection of Carrier: Heterozygotes have about 50% of the normal amount of LCAT. However, since the methods for detecting LCAT (both enzyme activity and enzyme protein) are somewhat difficult and uncertain, testing is normally confined to at-risk families.

References:
Norum KR, Gjone E: Familial lecithin:cholesterol acyltransferase deficiency: biochemical study of a new inborn error of metabolism. Scand J Clin Lab Invest 1967; 20:231–243.

Glomset JA: The plasma lecithin:cholesterol acyltransferase reaction. J Lipid Res 1968; 9:155–166.

Carlson LA, Philipson B: Fish eye disease: a new familial condition with massive corneal opacification and dyslipoproteinemia. Lancet 1979; II:921–923.

Norum KR: Familial lecithin:cholesterol acyltransferase deficiency. In: Miller NE, Miller GJ, eds: Clinical and metabolic aspects of high-density lipoproteins. New York: Elsevier Science Publisher, 1984: 297–324.

Carlson LA, Holmquist L: Evidence for deficiency of high density lipoprotein lecithin:cholesterol acyltransferase activity (alpha-LCAT) in fish eye disease. Acta Med Scand 1985; 218:189–196.

Norum KR, et al.: Familial lecithin:cholesterol acyltransferase deficiency, including fish eye disease. In: Scriver CR, et al, eds: The metabolic basis of inherited disease, 6th ed. New York: McGraw-Hill, 1989:1181–1194.

N0006   **Kaare R. Norum**

LENS AND PUPIL, ECTOPIC 0583

Includes: Pupil and lens, ectopic

Excludes: Lens, ectopic (0584)

Major Diagnostic Criteria: Dislocation of the pupil and lens.

Clinical Findings: Incomplete dislocation (subluxation) of both lenses with ectopic pupils is present at birth. Usually the lenses and pupils are displaced in opposite directions with the lenses most frequently displaced inferiorly. The direction may vary, however, and rare patients exhibit considerable asymmetry in the 2 eyes. The pupil is often oval or slit-shaped. Vision is often reduced and monocular diplopia may be present. Aphakic vision is sometimes seen. Transillumination of the iris is sometimes but not always present.

Complications: Aphakia, **Glaucoma, congenital**, retinal detachment.

Associated Findings: None known.

Etiology: Autosomal recessive inheritance.

Pathogenesis: Unknown.

MIM No.: *22520

CDC No.: 743.440

Sex Ratio: M1:F1

Occurrence: Undetermined but presumed rare.

Risk of Recurrence for Patient's Sib:
See Part I, *Mendelian Inheritance*.

Risk of Recurrence for Patient's Child:
See Part I, *Mendelian Inheritance*.

Age of Detectability: At birth.

Gene Mapping and Linkage: Unknown.

Prevention: None known. Genetic counseling indicated.

Treatment: Optical iridectomy or lens extraction may (rarely) be needed.

Prognosis: Normal life span, ocular prognosis dependent upon degree of defect.

Detection of Carrier: Unknown.

References:
Franceschetti A: Ectopia lentis et pupillae congenita als rezessives Erbleiden und ihre Manifestierung durch Konsanguinität. Klin Monatsbl Augenheilkd 1927; 78:351–362.
Lueffers JA, et al.: Iris transillumination and variable expression in ectopic lens and pupil. Am J Ophthalmol 1977; 83:647–656.
Cross HE: Ectopic lens and pupil. Am J Ophthalmol 1979; 88:381–384. *

CR012 **Harold E. Cross**

Lens opacities
See CATARACTS
Lens, aniridia
See ANIRIDIA

LENS, APHAKIA 0084

Includes: Aphakia

Excludes: Surgical aphakia

Major Diagnostic Criteria: Complete absence of the lens or presence of remnants.

Clinical Findings: Aphakia, or absence of the lens, may be divided into primary and secondary types. Primary aphakia is very rare and more serious than the secondary form because it is usually accompanied by gross malformations of the eye such as aplasia of the anterior segment, severe microphthalmia, or anophthalmia.

Secondary aphakia implies degeneration or rupture and absorption of the lens. This may occur without other eye disorders. Lens capsule remnants, often vascularized with fibrous tissue formation, are visualized along with ill-formed zonules within the pupil, which generally dilates poorly.

Complications: Visual impairment.

Associated Findings: Anterior segment anomalies, microphthalmia, anophthalmia, cataract in the opposite eye, facial malformations, retinal colobomas, nystagmus, congenital retinal folds, harelip, cleft palate, strabismus, and mental retardation; also seen in **Oculo-mandibulo-facial syndrome** and chromosomal aberrations.

Etiology: Undetermined. Possible intrauterine inflammation, teratogenic agents, or chromosomal abnormality. Occurs also in rats and pigs.

Pathogenesis: In primary aphakia an arrest or failure of development of the lens plate has been postulated. Secondary aphakia results from reabsorption of the lens. This may follow spontaneous rupture of an abnormally thin lens capsule or abnormality in either the surface ectoderm or lens fibers.

CDC No.: 743.300

Sex Ratio: Presumably M1:F1

Occurrence: Secondary more common than primary, but exact occurrence undetermined.

Risk of Recurrence for Patient's Sib: Unknown.

Risk of Recurrence for Patient's Child: Unknown.

Age of Detectability: Primary: at birth. Secondary: at birth or postnatally.

Gene Mapping and Linkage: Unknown.

Prevention: None known. Genetic counseling indicated.

Treatment: Correct refractive error whenever possible. Enucleation may be necessary if eye is grossly abnormal and cosmetically disfiguring. An oculoprothesis is inserted after enucleation.

Prognosis: Vision adequate-to-good in the presence of an otherwise normal eye. Vision guarded-to-poor dependent upon associated eye anomalies.

Detection of Carrier: Unknown.

References:
Mann I: Developmental abnormalities of the eye. Philadelphia: J.B. Lippincott, 1957:301–303.
Manschot WA: Primary congenital aphakia. Arch Ophthalmol 1963; 69:571.

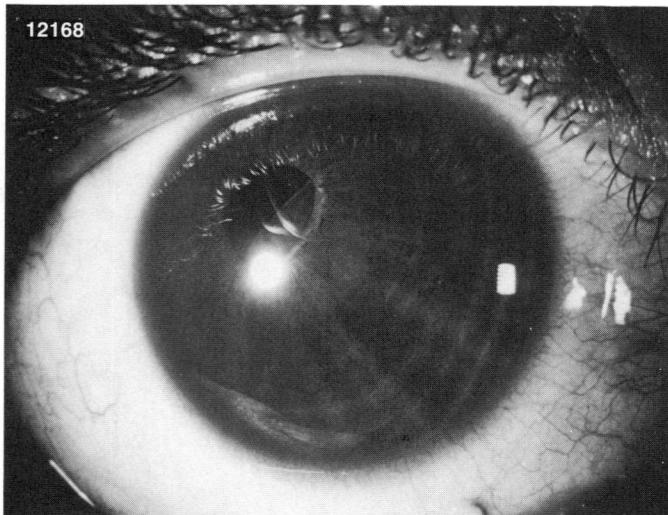

0583-12168: Ectopic lens and pupil.

Pratt JC, Richards RD: Bilateral secondary congenital aphakia. Arch Ophthalmol 1968; 80:420.

RA004   Elsa K. Rahn

LENS, ECTOPIC   0584

Includes:
Ectopia lentis, congenital
Ocular lens, dislocation of
Subluxation of lens

Excludes:
Aciduria, sulfite oxidase deficiency (0921)
Homocystinuria (0474)
Lens and pupil, ectopic (0583)
Marfan syndrome (0630)
Spherophakia-brachymorphia syndrome (0893)

Major Diagnostic Criteria: Dislocation of lens; if minimal, may require dilated slit-lamp biomicroscopy for diagnosis.

Clinical Findings: Isolated incomplete dislocation (subluxation) of the lens may be present at birth or occur later. The patient may have no symptoms or may complain of poor vision and monocular diplopia. Physical signs include iridodonesis, irregularly deep anterior chambers and uncorrected poor visual acuity in some cases. Bilateral dislocation is the rule. The lens is usually displaced upward and temporally.

Complications: **Glaucoma, congenital, cataract**, detached retina.

Associated Findings: **Cataract, Myopia, congenital**, astigmatism, **Aniridia**, persistent pupillary membrane, colobomas. Joint stiffness and dolichostenomelia have also been reported in one Black and one white family.

Etiology: Autosomal dominant inheritance. Most likely, heterogeneity exists with at least two recognizable disorders: simple ectopia lentis as a congenital, usually benign abnormality, and spontaneous late subluxation which is usually detected after the 3rd decade of life and often complicated by glaucoma.

Pathogenesis: Structural defect of lens zonules which may relate to persistence of the vascular tunic of the lens. Histologic studies show an absence of zonular fibers at the capsular attachments.

MIM No.: *12960

CDC No.: 743.330

Sex Ratio: M1:F1

Occurrence: Undetermined. Established literature.

Risk of Recurrence for Patient's Sib:
See Part I, *Mendelian Inheritance.*

Risk of Recurrence for Patient's Child:
See Part I, *Mendelian Inheritance.*

Age of Detectability: Usually at birth.

Gene Mapping and Linkage: Unknown.

Prevention: None known. Genetic counseling indicated.

Treatment: Optical iridectomy; cataract extraction when indicated.

Prognosis: Normal life span, ocular prognosis guarded.

Detection of Carrier: Unknown.

References:
Jaureguy BM, Hall JG: Isolated congenital ectopia lentis with autosomal dominant inheritance. Clin Genet 1979; 15:97–109. *
Nelson LB, Maumenee IH: Ectopic lentis: survey. Ophthalmology 1982; 27:143–160.
Stevenson RE, et al.: Dislocated lens, dolichostenomelia, and joint stiffness. Proc Greenwood Genet Center 1982; 1:16–22.

CR012   **Harold E. Cross**

LENS, MICROSPHEROPHAKIA   0663

Includes:
Microphakia and spherophakia, congenital
Microspherophakia

Excludes:
Acquired microphakia and spherophakia
Spherophakia-brachymorphia syndrome (0893)

Major Diagnostic Criteria: Small spherical lens within a dilated pupil.

Clinical Findings: Microphakia and spherophakia are usually concurrent. The lens has a smaller than normal diameter and is spherical in shape. The anterior-posterior measurement is increased and may cause the lens to protrude forward into the anterior chamber. This forward protrusion and close apposition of the lens to the iris may, in later life, result in glaucoma. Glaucoma in infancy is generally concomitant with abnormalities within the anterior chamber. The periphery of the lens is readily outlined with the pupil dilated. The zonules can also be visualized as radial strands between the pupillary and lens margins. Subluxation or luxation of the lens may occur from rupture of poorly developed, elongated and weakened zonules. Microspherophakia usually occurs bilaterally as an isolated phenomenon.

Complications: Myopia, cataract, glaucoma, subluxation or luxation of the lens.

Associated Findings: None known.

Etiology: Affected siblings and parental consanguinity suggest autosomal recessive inheritance of isolated defect. May be sporadic. When associated with other syndromes, it follows the inheritance mode of that symptom complex.

Pathogenesis: Arrest in development of the lens between the fifth or sixth fetal month. It has been postulated that an inadequate blood supply from the vascular tunic of the lens, or improper support secondary to faulty zonular development are possible mechanisms of pathogenesis.

MIM No.: 25175

CDC No.: 743.310

Sex Ratio: M1:F1

Occurrence: Undetermined, but literature over the past 70 years suggest that the condition is rare.

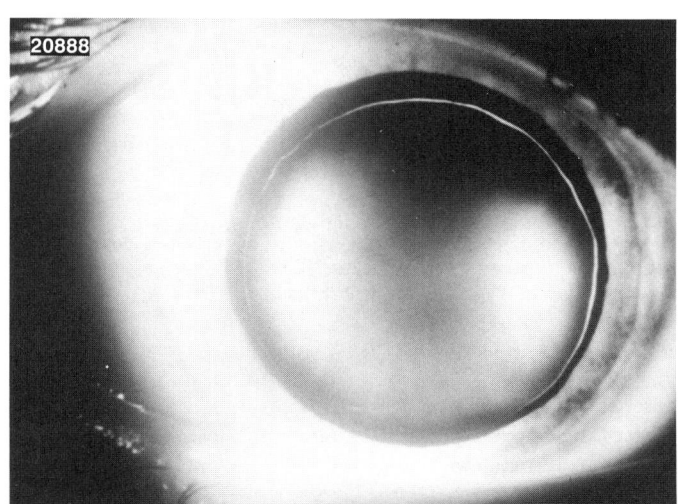

0663-20888: Spherophakia; note the edge of the lens is seen within the pupil.

Risk of Recurrence for Patient's Sib:
See Part I, *Mendelian Inheritance.*

Risk of Recurrence for Patient's Child:
See Part I, *Mendelian Inheritance.*

Age of Detectability: At birth.

Gene Mapping and Linkage: Unknown.

Prevention: None known. Genetic counseling indicated.

Treatment: Correction of existing refractive errors, usually myopia, due to the increased anterior-posterior diameter. Surgery is indicated if glaucoma occurs as a complication.

Prognosis: Generally good.

Detection of Carrier: Unknown.

References:

Waardenburg PJ, et al.: Genetics and ophthalmology. vol. 1. Springfield: Charles C Thomas, 1961.
Duke-Elder S: System of ophthalmology. vol. 3, part 2. Congenital deformities. London: Henry Kimpton, 1963:694.

RA004   **Elsa K. Rahn**

LENTICONUS   0585

Includes: N/A

Excludes:
Cornea, megalocornea (0637)
Eye, keratoconus (0552)

Major Diagnostic Criteria: Protrusion of the anterior or posterior surface of the lens in either a conical (conus) or a spherical (globus) shape. Slit-lamp exam can confirm protruded lens surface.

Clinical Findings: The anterior variety usually presents as bilateral localized thickenings of the anterior lens cortex. The central lens may be clear. Although probably present at birth, the youngest described patient was 4 years old. The deformity may be progressive leading to further diminution of vision.

An oil globule appearance is characteristic of the posterior variety. Central high myopia is also found. On slit-lamp examination there is a ring reflex. This condition is usually unilateral. Visual acuity may be poor due to opacification of the posterior lens capsule. A remnant of the hyaloid artery is often seen attached.

Complications: Anterior polar cataracts may develop in anterior lenticonus, and posterior cateracts in posterior lenticonus.

Associated Findings: Posterior polar lens opacities are common (80%) concomitant features of posterior lentiglobus. Other associations include uveal colobomas, microphthalmos, lens colobomas, oxycephaly, deafness, hypertelorism and **Nephritis-deafness (sensorineural), hereditary type.** Associated defects are rare in anterior lenticonus, although it has been reported with **Fetal rubella syndrome** and a variety of forms of congenital cataract.

Etiology: Most cases are isolated, although rare families have been reported. Bilateral involvement is more common in familial cases. Both autosomal dominant and autosomal recessive inheritance have been reported.

Pathogenesis: Delayed separation of the lens vesicle from the surface epithelium in anterior lenticonus, and posterior hyaloid artery persistence with a weak posterior capsule or overgrowth of lens fibers in posterior lentiglobus have been suggested to be the mechanisms responsible for the defects.

CDC No.: 743.380

Sex Ratio: Lenticonus M1F<1; Lentiglobus M2:F3

Occurrence: Estimated at 1:100,000 births. Anterior lenticonus is rarer than posterior lentiglobus.

Risk of Recurrence for Patient's Sib: Unknown.

Risk of Recurrence for Patient's Child: Unknown.

Age of Detectability: At birth.

Gene Mapping and Linkage: Unknown.

Prevention: None known. Genetic counseling indicated.

Treatment: Lens extraction where indicated.

Prognosis: Life span normal; visual prognosis variable.

Detection of Carrier: Unknown.

References:

Howitt D, Hornblass A: Posterior lenticonus. Am J Ophthalmol 1968; 66:1133–1136.
Pollard ZF: Familial bilateral posterior lenticonus. Arch Ophthalmol 1983; 101:1238–1240.
Felt D, et al.: Infantile leucocoria caused by posterior lenticonus. Ann Ophthalmol 1984; 16:679–684.

CR012   **Harold E. Cross**

Lenticular cataract
See CATARACT, AUTOSOMAL DOMINANT CONGENITAL

LENTIGINES SYNDROME, MULTIPLE   0586

Includes:
Cardiocutaneous syndrome
Cardiomyopathic lentiginosis
Generalized lentigo
Lentiginosis profusa syndrome
Leopard syndrome
Multiple lentigines syndrome
Progressive cardiomyopathic lentiginosis

Excludes:
Mitral regurgitation-deafness-skeletal defects (0667)
Nevi-atrial myxoma-myxoid neurofibromas-ephelides (2572)
Noonan syndrome (0720)
Pulmonic stenosis-cafe-au-lait spots, Watson type (2776)
Unilateral lentigo

Major Diagnostic Criteria: The diagnosis should be considered in a patient with some combination of multiple lentigines, EKG conduction defect, **Eye, hypertelorism**, **Pulmonary valve, stenosis**, growth retardation, sensorineural hearing loss, and genital defects.

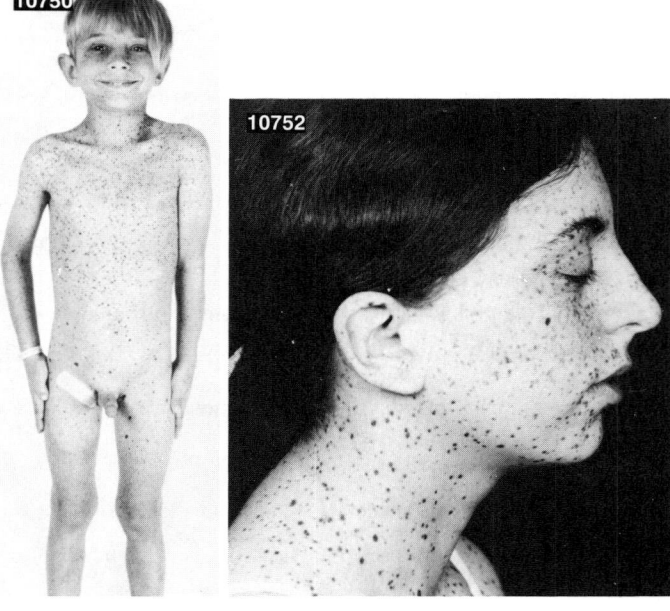

0586-10750–52: Multiple lentigines are present in a universal distribution.

Clinical Findings: The syndrome consists of multiple lentigines that are 2–8 mm in diameter and scattered over the face, scalp, neck, trunk, genitalia, upper limbs, palms and soles. They are sparser below the knees (ca. 80%) and the mucous membranes are spared; café "noir" spots occur in 20%. The lentigines may present at birth or during childhood and increase in number and darken with age. Biopsy of the lentigines reveals intracellular giant pigment granules similar to those found in neurofibromatosis. EKG abnormalities indicate axis deviations, unilateral or bilateral hypertrophy, and conduction abnormalities (prolonged P-R interval, hemiblock, bundle branch block, complete heart block) of varying severity in 60%. Other findings include ocular hypertelorism (ca. 25%); pulmonary stenosis, either valvular or infundibular (ca. 50%); aortic or mitral stenosis, obstructive cardiomyopathy (20%); abnormalities of the genitalia, such as cryptorchidism (ca. 15%); retardation of growth (ca. 35%) and sensorineural hearing loss (ca. 20%). Mild mental retardation has been noted in about 30% of cases, while oculomotor deficits occur in about 50%.

Complications: Sterility, if cryptorchidism is bilateral; speech difficulties.

Associated Findings: Other less common findings include triangular face with biparietal bossing, eyelid ptosis, delayed primary dentition, delayed puberty and various skeletal abnormalities such as kyphoscoliosis, **Pectus carinatum** or **Pectus excavatum**, winging of scapulae, and multiple granular cell myoblastomas.

Etiology: Autosomal dominant inheritance with variable expressivity.

Pathogenesis: Undetermined. Possibly a neurocristopathy.

MIM No.: *15110

POS No.: 3277

Sex Ratio: M1:F1

Occurrence: About 75 cases reported in the literature.

Risk of Recurrence for Patient's Sib:
See Part I, *Mendelian Inheritance.*

Risk of Recurrence for Patient's Child:
See Part I, *Mendelian Inheritance.* Affected males may have a somewhat reduced reproductive fitness due to cryptorchidism.

Age of Detectability: Four to 5 years of age, since lentigines usually become abundant by this time; possibly earlier if there is an involved sib.

Gene Mapping and Linkage: Unknown.

Prevention: None known. Genetic counseling indicated.

Treatment: Surgical correction of cryptorchidism and possibly of cardiac lesion.

Prognosis: Good, the pulmonary stenosis is rarely seriously disabling. Intellectual deficit occurs infrequently, and speech difficulties may be caused by deafness.

Detection of Carrier: Detailed examination will usually allow detection of affected individuals who do not have lentigines.

References:
Gorlin RJ, et al.: Multiple lentigines syndrome: complex comprising multiple lentigenes, electrocardiographic conduction abnormalities, ocular hypertelorism, pulmonary stenosis, abnormalities of genitalia, retardation of growth, sensorineural deafness and autosomal dominant hereditary pattern. Am J Dis Child 1969; 117:652–662.
Gorlin RJ, et al.: The LEOPARD (multiple lentigines) syndrome revisited. BD:OAS;VII(4). Baltimore: The Williams & Wilkins Co. for The National Foundation - March of Dimes, 1971:110–115.
Polani PE, Moynahan EJ: Progressive cardiopathic lentigines. Q J Med 1972; 41:205–225.
Seuanez H, et al.: Cardio-cutaneous syndrome (the "LEOPARD" syndrome): review of the literature and a new family. Clin Genet 1976; 9:266–276.
Voron DA, et al.: Multiple lentigines syndrome: case report and review of the literature. Am J Med 1976; 60:447–456.
Weiss LW, Zelickson AS: Giant melanosomes in multiple lentigines syndrome. Arch Dermatol 1977; 113:491–494.
St. John Sutton MG, et al.: Hypertrophic obstructive cardiomyopathy and lentiginosis: a little known neural ectodermal syndrome. Am J Cardiol 1981; 47:214–217.

G0038   **Robert J. Gorlin**

Lentigines-peptic ulcer/hiatal hernia-hypertelorism-myopia
See GASTROCUTANEOUS SYNDROME
Lentiginosis profusa syndrome
See LENTIGINES SYNDROME, MULTIPLE
Lenz dysmorphogenetic syndrome
See LENZ MICROPHTHALMIA SYNDROME
Lenz dysplasia
See LENZ MICROPHTHALMIA SYNDROME

LENZ MICROPHTHALMIA SYNDROME   **3171**

Includes:
    Anophthalmos with associated anomalies
    Lenz dysplasia
    Lenz dysmorphogenetic syndrome
    Microphthalmia with associated anomalies

Excludes:
    Charge association (2124)
    Anophthalmia-limb defects, Waardenburg type (2784)

Major Diagnostic Criteria: Microphthalmos is present in all cases. Other abnormalities include developmental retardation in 92% of cases, external ear abnormalities in 83% of cases, **Microcephaly** in 83% of cases, blepharoptosis (see **Eyelid, ptosis, congenital**) in 75% of cases, skeletal abnormalities in 67% of cases, dental abnormalities of number and position in 67% of cases, digital anomalies in 58% of cases, urogenital anomalies in 50% of cases and **Cleft lip**/**Cleft palate** abnormalities in one-third of patients.

Clinical Findings: The various congenital malformations associated with this syndrome are discovered at birth. The microphthalmos is usually bilateral and asymmetrical, colobomatous or non-colobomatous, and may even be extreme with clinical anophthalmia. The earlobes are usually large and protruding with thin hypoplastic antihelices, but may be small and hypoplastic. Teeth may be crowded or widely spaced. Skeletal abnormalities are most prominent in the thoracic cage, which is barrel-shaped

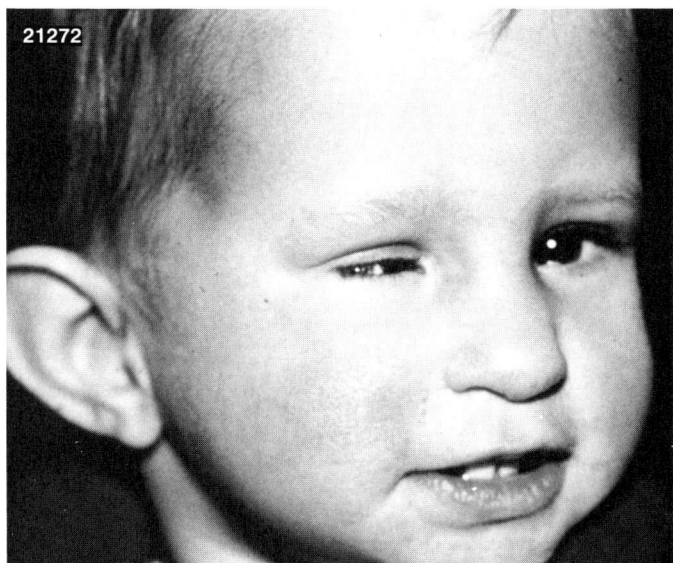

3171-21272: Three-year-old boy with the Lenz microphthalmia syndrome; note the bilateral microphthalmia more severe on the right, and the thin, anteverted protruding earlobes.

with kyphoscoliosis and occasional gibbus formation. Thinning of the lateral third of the clavicles is a particular finding in some patients. **Microcephaly** is present in a majority of patients, and developmental retardation ranging from mild to profound seems to be a universal finding. Digital anomalies, though found in only 58% of cases, are helpful in differentiating this syndrome from other malformation syndromes featuring microphthalmia; clino-dactyly, **Camptodactyly**, and **Syndactyly** are most commonly observed, however thumb duplication has been noted in some patients. Clinically evident heart disease is not a feature of this syndrome, but autopsy on Lenz's original patient revealed a bicuspid arotic valve. Urogenital anomalies include cryptorchidism, renal hypoplasia and renal aplasia.

Complications: Retinal detachment has been observed in one patient.

Associated Findings: Cardiac anomalies, imperforate anus, hearing loss, spastic diplegia, sacral pits, webbed neck, and abnormal dermatoglyphs.

Etiology: X-linked recessive inheritance.

Pathogenesis: Unknown.

MIM No.: *30980

POS No.: 3277

Sex Ratio: M1:F0

Occurrence: Twelve documented cases have been reported.

Risk of Recurrence for Patient's Sib:
See Part I, *Mendelian Inheritance.*

Risk of Recurrence for Patient's Child:
See Part I, *Mendelian Inheritance.*

Age of Detectability: At birth. Fetal ultrasonography may detect major malformations in a fetus who has an affected sibling.

Gene Mapping and Linkage: MAA (microphthalmia or anophthalmia and associated anomalies) has been mapped to X.

Prevention: None known. Genetic counseling indicated.

Treatment: Surgical correction of malformations as indicated.

Prognosis: Good for life; poor for vision. Mental retardation is a universal finding, though mild in some cases.

Detection of Carrier: Carrier females may have digital anomalies, microcephaly and short stature.

References:
Lenz W: Recessivgeschlechtsgebundene mikrophtalmie mit multiplen Missbildunger. Z Kinderheilkd 1955; 77:384–390.
Hoefnagel D, et al: Heredofamilial bilateral anophthalmia. Arch Ophthalmol 1963; 69:760–764.
Goldberg MF, McKusick VA: X-linked colobomatous microphthalmos and other congenital anomalies: a disorder resembling Lenz's dysmorphogenetic syndrome. Am J Ophthalmol 1971; 71:1128–1133.
Traboulsi EI, et al: The Lenz microphthalmia syndrome. Am J Ophthalmol 1988; 105:40–45. * †

TR009   **Elias I. Traboulsi**

Lenz-Majewski hyperostotic dwarfism
See CRANIODIAPHYSEAL DYSPLASIA, LENZ-MAJEWSKI TYPE
Leopard syndrome
See LENTIGINES SYNDROME, MULTIPLE

LEPRECHAUNISM	0587

Includes:
    Donohue syndrome
    Insulin receptor, defect in
    Insulin resistance, familial severe

Excludes:
    Skin, acanthosis nigricans (0005)
    Chromosome 8, trisomy 8 (0157)
    Cockayne syndrome (0189)
    Diabetes mellitus, maturity onset of the young (MODY) (2326)
    Diabetes mellitus, non-insulin dependent type (2327)

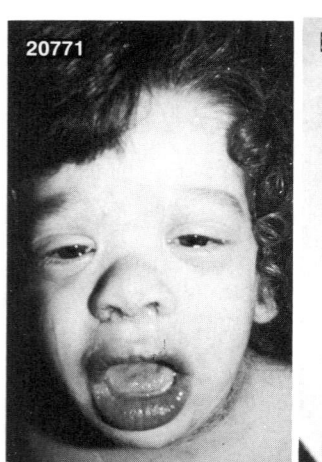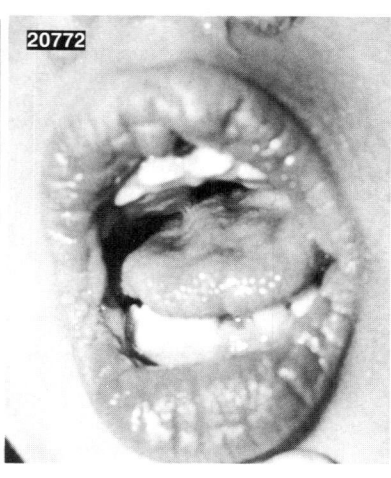

0587A-20771: Leprechaunism; note coarse facies with thick lips, coarse hair, hirsutism. **20772:** Furrowed tongue and lips.

    Lipodystrophy-coarse facies-acanthosis nigricans, Miescher type (2423)
    Lipodystrophy, familial limb and trunk (2614)
    Myotonic dystrophy (0702)
    Skin, acanthosis nigricans (0005)

Major Diagnostic Criteria: A diagnosis of leprechaunism is made on the basis of clinical and laboratory findings. A presumptive clinical diagnosis of leprechaunism may be made if a newborn presents as small for gestational age with failure to thrive; elfin facies; thick lips; pachyderma; hirsutism; and relatively prominent breasts, hands, feet; **Skin, acanthosis nigricans**; and external genitalia. The clinical diagnosis is supported by the laboratory dem-

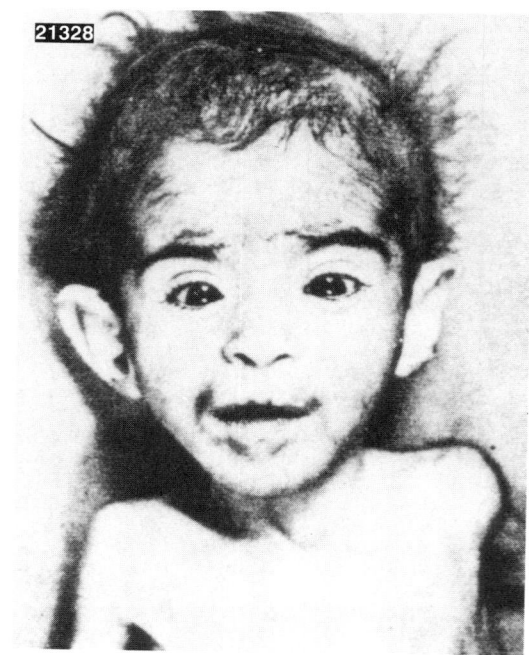

0587B-21328: Small face with prominent eyes, wide nostrils, large mouth, large ears, and hirsutism.

onstration of insulin resistance with hyperinsulinemia, fasting hypoglycemia, and postprandial hyperglycemia. Absence of antibodies to insulin and the insulin receptor is included. Pathohistology includes increased hepatic glycogen, hyperplasia of the endocrine pancreas, and ovarian cystic changes.

Laboratory diagnosis requires finding markedly decreased binding of insulin to the patient's cultured cells.

Clinical Findings: Leprechaunism is characterized by continued small stature; elfin facies, with a flat nasal bridge and flaring nostrils; thick lips; hirsutism; pachyderma, acanthosis nigricans; and breast enlargement. Because of small size, there is relative prominence of the clitoris and labia minora or penis, as well as ears, hands, and feet. There is a deficiency of subcutaneous tissue leading to the presence of excessive folding of the skin (pachyderma). Motor and mental retardation and severe failure to thrive are common sequelae.

Other less frequently noted features include **Microcephaly**, hypertelorism, high or narrowly arched palate, cardiac murmur, umbilical and inguinal herniae or diastasis recti, cryptorchidism, poor muscle tone, unusually large hands and feet, and delayed skeletal maturation.

Complications: Susceptibility to infection, hypoglycemia, early death.

Associated Findings: Intrauterine growth restriction.

Etiology: Autosomal recessive inheritance. Decreased-to-absent high-affinity insulin binding can be used as a genetic discriminant in cultured dermal fibroblasts. Several different mutant alleles involving the alpha subunit (insulin binding domain) of the insulin receptor gene have been identified.

Pathogenesis: A primary mutation in the insulin receptor gene results in decreased utilization of secreted insulin and end-organ resistance to insulin binding and signaling. The growth-promoting, embryologic effects of insulin are blunted, producing intrauterine growth restriction. Many different mutations with variably altered end-organ resistance are described. One mutation has absent insulin binding to the fibroblast insulin receptor with increased, noninsulin-responsive glucose transport. This may account for recurrent hypoglycemia in the presence of normal glycogen stores.

MIM No.: *24620

POS No.: 3278

CDC No.: 759.870

Sex Ratio: M1:F1

Occurrence: About 50 cases reported in the literature.

Risk of Recurrence for Patient's Sib:
See Part I, *Mendelian Inheritance.*

Risk of Recurrence for Patient's Child:
See Part I, *Mendelian Inheritance.* Most affected individuals do not survive to reproduce.

Age of Detectability: During early infancy. Prenatal monitoring using restriction fragment length polymorphism analysis of the insulin receptor gene is available.

Gene Mapping and Linkage: Mutations in the insulin receptor gene (19p13.2→13.3).

Prevention: None known. Genetic counseling indicated.

Treatment: Various complications, particularly infections and hypoglycemia, should be treated as indicated. Utilization of gastrostomy feedings has been of benefit in some cases.

Prognosis: Most classic patients have died in early childhood. A few, who are compound heterozygotes for two different alleles, survive childhood.

Detection of Carrier: By decreased insulin binding or DNA analysis if the exact mutation is known. Some severe mutations may be expressed in the heterozygote as **Diabetes mellitus, non-insulin dependent type.** Type A insulin resistance with acanthosis nigricans has been associated with mutations in the insulin receptor gene. Insulin binding may be normal in these patients.

References:
D'Ercole AJ, et al.: Leprechaunism: studies of the relationship among hyperinsulinism, insulin resistance, and growth retardation. J Clin Endocrinol Metab 1979; 48:495.
Elsas LJ, et al.: Leprechaunism: an inherited defect in insulin-receptor interaction. In: Wapnir RA, ed: Congenital metabolic diseases: diagnosis and treatment. New York: Marcel Dekker, 1985:301–334.
Elsas LJ, et al.: Leprechaunism: an inherited defect in a high-affinity insulin receptor. Am J Hum Genet 1985; 37:73–88.
Yang-Feng TL, et al.: Gene for human insulin receptor: localization to site on chromosome 19 involved in pre-β cell leukemia. Science 1985; 228:728–730.
Cantani A, et al.: A rare polydysmorphic syndrome: leprechaunism - review of 49 cases reported in the literature. Ann Genet 1987; 30:221–227.
Elsas LJ, Longo N: Impaired insulin binding and excess glucose transport in fibroblasts from a patient with leprechaunism. Enzyme 1987; 38:184–193.
Endo F, et al.: Structural analysis of normal and mutant insulin receptors in fibroblasts cultured from families with leprechaunism. Am J Hum Genet 1987; 4:102–106.
Elsas LJ, et al.: Comparison of the insulin receptor gene and insulin binding in families with severe insulin resistance. Trans Asso Am Phys 1988; CI:137–148.
Kadowaki T, et al.: Two mutant alleles of the insulin receptor gene in a patient with extreme insulin resistance. Science 1988; 240:787–790.
Kahn CR, Goldstein BJ: Molecular defects in insulin action. Science 1989; 245:13–14.
Taira M, et al: Human diabetes associated with deletion of the tyrosine kinase domain of the insulin receptor. Science 1989; 245:63–65.

EL009   **Louis J. Elsas, II**

LERI PLEONOSTEOSIS SYNDROME   **2102**

Includes: Pleonosteosis

Excludes:
   Dyschondrosteosis (0308)
   Mucopolysaccharidosis

Major Diagnostic Criteria: Limitation of joint movement and flexion contractures of interphalangeal joints.

Clinical Findings: Broad, deformed, thumbs and great toes; short stature; and flattened facies. Enlargement of the posterior neural arches of the cervical vertebrae has been reported as a significant diagnostic X-ray finding.

Complications: Cervical cord compression due to stenosis of the cervical canal has been reported. Carpal tunnel compression of the median nerve and Morton metatarsalgia have also been reported.

Associated Findings: Blepharophimosis and microcornea have been reported.

Etiology: Autosomal dominant inheritance with variable expression.

Pathogenesis: Unknown.

MIM No.: *15120

POS No.: 3615

Sex Ratio: M1:F1

Occurrence: Over 20 cases have been reported.

Risk of Recurrence for Patient's Sib:
See Part I, *Mendelian Inheritance.*

Risk of Recurrence for Patient's Child:
See Part I, *Mendelian Inheritance.*

Age of Detectability: In early childhood.

Gene Mapping and Linkage: Unknown.

Prevention: None known. Genetic counseling indicated.

Treatment: Conservative, symptomatic treatment in most cases.

Prognosis: Normal intelligence and life span.

Detection of Carrier: Possibly on the basis of X-ray changes.

References:

Leri A: Une maladie congenitale et hereditaire de l'ossification: la pleonosteose familiale. Bull Soc Med Paris 1921; 45:1228.

Watson-Jones R: Leri's pleonosteosis, carpal tunnel compression of the median nerves and Morton's metatarsalgia. J Bone Joint Surg 1949; 31B:560–571.

Rukavina JG, et al.: Leri's pleonosteosis: a study of a family with a review of the literature. J Bone Joint Surg 1959; 41A:397–408.

Hilton RC, Wentzel J: Leri's pleonosteosis. Q J Med 1980; 49:419–429.

Friedman M, et al.: Leri's pleonosteosis. Brit J Radiol 1981; 54:517–518.

Metcalfe RA, Butler P: Spinal cord compression in Leri's pleonosteosis. Brit J Radiol 1985; 58:1117–1119.

GRO11   **Frank Greenberg**

Leri-Weill disease
See DYSCHONDROSTEOSIS
Leroy disease
See MUCOLIPIDOSIS II

LESCH-NYHAN SYNDROME   0588

Includes:

> Hyperuricemia, X-linked primary
> Hypoxanthine guanine phosphoribosyl transferase (HGPRT) deficiency
> Uric acid metabolism-central nervous system disorder

Excludes:

> **Adenine phospho-ribosyl-transferase (APRT) deficiency** (3104)
> **Gout** (0441)
> HGPRT, partial variants of

Major Diagnostic Criteria: Patients with complete absence of hypoxanthine guanine phosphoribosyl transferase (HGPRT) activity with resulting hyperuricemia (see **Gout**) and evidence of cerebral dysfunction; choreoathetosis, **Cerebral palsy**, mental retardation, and self-mutilation.

Clinical Findings: Patients appear normal at birth but develop progressive choreoathetosis and spastic cerebral palsy. Mental

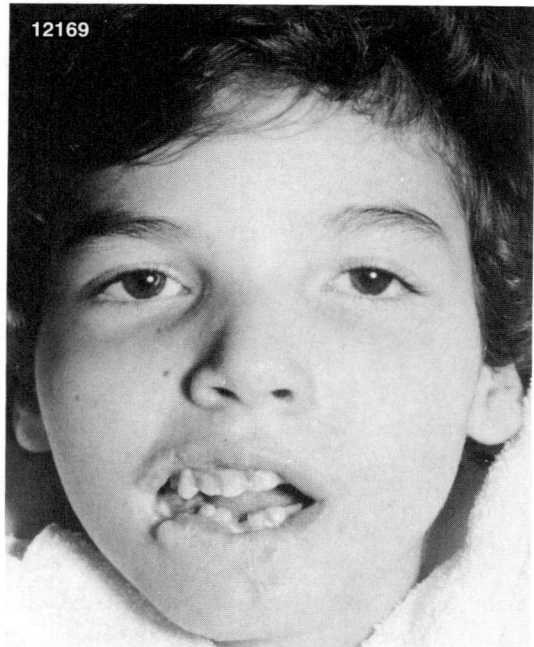

0588-12169: Lesch-Nyhan syndrome. Note self-mutilation of lips.

retardation and motor defects are such that these patients do not walk and few can sit without assistance. They are characterized by bizarre aggressive behavior; its most prominent manifestation is self-mutilation, usually by biting. In addition to the features relevant to the nervous system, these patients have all the clinical findings of gout, including hyperuricemia, hematuria, crystalluria, urinary tract stones, nephropathy, tophi, and acute arthritis. Mild anemia may be encountered and megaloblasts are occasionally seen in the marrow.

Complications: Nephropathy; renal failure; athetoid dysphagia is extreme and vomiting is prominent; thus these patients are hard to feed. They may die of inanition or aspiration and pneumonia, as well as of renal failure.

Associated Findings: None known.

Etiology: X-linked recessive inheritance.

Pathogenesis: Absence of hypoxanthine guanine phosphoribosyl transferase (HGPRT) activity. The manner in which this leads to the cerebral manifestations of the disease is unknown.

MIM No.: *30800

POS No.: 3279

Sex Ratio: M1:F0

Occurrence: About 1:100,000 births.

Risk of Recurrence for Patient's Sib:
See Part I, *Mendelian Inheritance.*

Risk of Recurrence for Patient's Child:
See Part I, *Mendelian Inheritance.*

Age of Detectability: At birth; it is now possible to detect prior to birth by assay of the enzyme in cultured cells obtained by amniocentesis. Gibbs et al (1984) have reported the use of chorionic villus biopsy and employed enzyme assay to diagnose Lesch-Nyhan syndrome in the first trimester.

Gene Mapping and Linkage: HPRT (hypoxanthine phosphoribosyltransferase) has been mapped to Xq26.

Prevention: None known. Genetic counseling indicated.

Treatment: As for gout, Allopurinol is excellent therapy for the management of hyperuricemia. It will prevent all of those manifestations of this disease that are direct consequences of elevated concentrations of uric acid. It does not prevent or alleviate the cerebral manifestations. Appropriate restraint binding of hands or elbows to prevent mutilation of hands is necessary.

Prognosis: In the absence of allopurinol most patients have died under five years of age. A few long survivors have lived to 20 years.

Detection of Carrier: Culture of fibroblasts from the skin and cloning have yielded two populations of cells from the maternal heterozygote. One population has normal enzyme activity and the other is completely deficient like the patient's. This identifies the carrier and is consistent with the Lyon hypothesis. Hair follicles are also largely clonal and they are the most practical method for the detection of the heterozygote by analysis of the enzyme activity in hair roots. The blood cannot be used for this purpose as the blood of the maternal carrier of this disease is always normal.

References:

Lesch M, Nyhan WL: A familial disorder of uric acid metabolism and central nervous system function. Am J Med 1964; 36:561–570. *

Bland J, ed: Proceedings of the seminars on the Lesch-Nyhan syndrome. Fed Proc 1968; 27:1019–1112.

Christie R, et al.: Lesch-Nyhan disease: clinical experience with nineteen patients. Develop Med Child Neurol 1982; 24:293–306.

Gibbs DA et al.: First trimester diagnosis of Lesch-Nyhan syndrome. Lancet 1984; 2:1180–1183.

Gibbs RA, Caskey CT: Identification and localization of mutations of the Lesch-Nyhan locus by ribonuclease A cleavage. Science 1987; 236:303–305.

Nyhan WL: Diagnostic recognition of genetic disease. Philadelphia: Lea & Febiger, 1987:1–8. *

NY000   **William L. Nyhan**

Lethal congenital contracture syndrome
See CONTRACTURES, CONGENITAL LETHAL FINNISH TYPE
Lethal multiple pterygium syndrome
See PTERYGIUM SYNDROME, MULTIPLE LETHAL
Lethal osteopetrosis
See OSTEOPETROSIS, MALIGNANT RECESSIVE
Lethal, Larsen-like, multiple joint dislocations
See LARSEN SYNDROME, LETHAL TYPE

LETTERER-SIWE DISEASE   2181

Includes:
Histiocytosis, acute disseminated
Reticuloendotheliosis, nonlipoid
Reticulosis, familial histiocytic

Excludes:
Eosinophilic granuloma of bone
Hand-Schuler-Christian disease
Immunodeficiency, reticuloendotheliosis with eosinophilia
(2688)

Major Diagnostic Criteria: 1) Onset in first year of life; 2) skin lesions, although variable in nature, often of the scalp; 3) organomegaly of liver and spleen; 4) adenopathy; and 5) pulmonary infiltration. The microscopic picture of the lesions shows a nodular or spreading infiltration containing numerous large histiocytes.

Clinical Findings: 1) Onset of signs in first year of life; 2) diffuse, papulous eruption of a vesicular nature; 3) scaly and petechial dermatitis, particularly on the forehead and trunk; 4) moist, denuded involvement in intertriginous areas; 5) seborrheic eruption of scalp and in ear canals; 6) stomatitis; 7) pulmonic infiltrations; 8) general adenopathy; 9) hepatomegaly; 10) splenomegaly; 11) fever; and 12) lytic osseous lesions, often of the cranium. Laboratory studies show only the nonspecific effects to be expected from the organ or tissue involvement. Anemia is common, and leukocytosis may occur.

Complications: General exhaustion, toxemia, bone marrow depletion, septicemia, and **Diabetes insipidus**.

Associated Findings: None known.

Etiology: Autosomal recessive inheritance with reduced (7/8ths) penetrance.

Pathogenesis: Progressive granulomatous process.

MIM No.: *24640

Sex Ratio: M1:F1

Occurrence: Extensive literature. No geographic predilection. One study found over 50 deaths per year in the United States from this condition.

Risk of Recurrence for Patient's Sib:
See Part I, *Mendelian Inheritance.*

Risk of Recurrence for Patient's Child:
See Part I, *Mendelian Inheritance.*

Age of Detectability: Within the first year of life.

Gene Mapping and Linkage: Unknown.

Prevention: None known. Genetic counseling indicated.

Treatment: None specific except for pitressin in the event of diabetes insipidus. Radiotherapy may affect individual bone lesions, skin eruptions, and large lymph nodes.

Prognosis: Fatal outcome when general process becomes advanced. Spontaneous recovery has been reported.

Detection of Carrier: Unknown.

Special Considerations: This or a similar disorder was reported by Kloepfer et al (1972) in an inbred triracial group in Louisiana known as the "Redbones".

References:
Schoeck VW, et al.: Familial occurrence of Letterer-Siwe disease. Pediatrics 1963; 32:1055–1063.
Juberg RC, et al.: Genetic determination of acute disseminated histiocytosis X (Letterer-Siwe syndrome). Pediatrics 1970; 45:753–765. * †

Kloepfer HW, et al.: Fulminating disseminated histiocytosis simulating Letterer-Siwe disease. BD:OAS VIII(3). New York: March of Dimes Birth Defects Foundation, 1972:112–114.
Frisell E, et al.: Familial occurrence of histiocytosis. Clin Genet 1977; 11:163–170.

JU000   **Richard C. Juberg**

Leucine metabolism, defect in
See ACIDEMIA, 3-HYDROXY-3-METHYLGLUTARIC
Leucine-sensitive hypoglycemia of infancy, familial
See HYPOGLYCEMIA, FAMILIAL NEONATAL

LEUKEMIA, ACUTE LYMPHOCYTIC, FAMILIAL   3073

Includes:
Acute lymphocytic leukemia (ALL)
J. Chain
Lymphocytic leukemia, cell type-childhood acute

Excludes: Cytogenetic and other syndromes that predispose to leukemia

Major Diagnostic Criteria: Two or more first-degree relatives with childhood (onset under age 15 years) acute lymphocytic leukemia.

Clinical Findings: Although the annual age-adjusted incidence of childhood leukemia is low (40 cases of leukemia per one million children under age 15 years), this malignancy accounts for 30% of childhood cancer. In Western countries, incidence rates of acute lymphocytic leukemia (ALL) are three times higher than those for acute nonlymphocytic leukemia (ANLL) among children, although ANLL comprises a substantially higher proportion of childhood leukemia in Japanese and other Asian children of all ages. Despite the relatively rare occurrence, familial childhood leukemia, particularly ALL, has been recognized for several decades. Familial aggregation of a number of types has been described, including a 20–25% concordance for ALL among identical twins following occurrence in one member of the pair; significantly increased risk of ALL among sibs of an affected child; and association with a number of congenital conditions characterized by chromosomal abnormalities and other hereditary disorders.

The clinical symptoms and course are usually indistinguishable from nonfamilial ALL of childhood, with the exception of the often striking similarity of age of onset (within a few months and usually in infancy) and age at death for concordant ALL in identical twins. Although four immunologic subtypes have become widely recognized since the advent of immunologic and enzymatic phenotyping in the 1970s, use of standardized immunophenotyping techniques has only recently become widespread. Separate examination of postulated risk factors by leukemia histologic cell type (ALL vs. ANLL) has only recently begun to occur in reports of epidemiologic studies, and the new immunologic subgroups have not been used in such studies.

Complications: Similar to sporadic childhood ALL, familial childhood ALL usually causes death by infection or hemorrhage. In the last couple of decades, survivorship has greatly improved due to increasingly effective combination chemotherapy and treatment prophylaxis with chemotherapy and radiation specifically directed at the central nervous system.

Associated Findings: None known.

Etiology: A number of postulated genetic, immunologic, and environmental factors have been identified. Clinical reports have implicated familial and nonfamilial congenital chromosomal abnormalities (including the Philadelphia or Ph[1] chromosome, inv(11)(p15q13), ring chromosomes, and others). Unlike the associations of **Retinoblastoma** and some cases of **Cancer, Wilms tumor** with specific constitutional chromosome abnormalities, no one specific chromosome deletion or other abnormality has been exclusively linked with childhood ALL, although **Chromosome 21, trisomy 21** has been associated with an increased risk of childhood ALL. Two large U.S. death certificate studies of 4,670 and 10,390 leukemia cases demonstrated a concordance of 20 to 25% for ALL among identical (probably monozygotic) twins. A similar study in England and Wales failed to identify any concordant pairs among 5,763 with childhood cancer (numbers of leukemia deaths not separately reported).

An excess risk of childhood leukemia has been observed among children with several hereditary conditions characterized by a tendency to chromosomal abnormalities or breaks, including **Chromosome 21, trisomy 21** (risk of leukemia of both major histologic types estimated as 1:74), **Bloom syndrome** (risk estimated as 1:8 before age 26 years), **Ataxia-telangiectasia** (1:8 before age 25 years), and **Pancytopenia syndrome, Fanconi type** (1:12 before age 21 years). Due to the rare nature of virtually all of the above conditions and the lack of population-based studies, the cumulative risk of subsequent childhood leukemia among subjects with each of these rare conditions represents an estimate, based on literature review.

As further evidence of a possible genetic basis of childhood ALL, aggregation of childhood leukemia in sibships can be demonstrated when the sample size is large enough (>1,000 sibs). A fourfold excess risk has been estimated from at least one large population-based study. Acute leukemia may also aggregate among sibs in families with other heritable leukemia-prone disorders, such as Bloom, Fanconi, and so forth. Thus, if leukemia occurs among two or more sibs, cytogenetic and immunologic tests should be undertaken within the family. The affected cases should also be studied in detail to determine if the morphology or natural history of childhood ALL in these families differs from usual. HLA studies suggest that the genetic background of patients with ALL may have restricted heterogeneity; there appears to be an increased occurrence of haplotype sharing in parents of patients with ALL. HLA genotypes of patients with ALL and those with acute myelocytic leukemia have been found more frequently than the expected 25% among their sibs. Although the HLA antigen types A2 and B12 have been associated in some reports with childhood ALL, these findings are not consistent, nor are associations with specific haplotypes.

There have been reports of familial childhood ALL occurring in families with many consanguineous marriages. One group of investigators has suggested that closer degrees of consanguinity are associated with leukemia onset at younger ages. Childhood leukemia has been occasionally linked with occurrence of congenital anomalies in case mothers. Although some investigators attribute multiple occurrences of ALL in a sibship to a rare recessive gene with high penetrance, such occurrences are extremely rare, and other investigators have discounted the likelihood of a homozygous recessive mechanism.

A number of studies examining immunologic characteristics of first-degree relatives of patients with ALL have shown a variety of differences between family members of cases and controls. Mothers of children with leukemia have been reported to have a significantly lower number of monocytes, higher levels of gamma globulin, IgA, IgG, and IgM; both fathers and mothers have been found to have higher numbers of basophils. Some investigators have noted a history of an increased occurrence of autoimmune disorders, including **Arthritis, rheumatoid**, **Thyrotoxicosis**, Hashimoto thyroiditis, rheumatic fever, and other conditions among parents of patients compared with parents of controls, although these findings have not been consistent. Several studies have indicated that parents of patients have suffered an excess of serious or life-threatening infections compared with parents of controls. Atopy has also inconsistently been reported more commonly among parents of patients. The inconsistency of these findings may reflect small numbers, selected case groups, and differences between studies in types of controls. Nevertheless, there is some support for the observation that there may be an underlying immune system dysfunction among a proportion of mothers, and possibly fathers, of childhood ALL patients. Further studies of immunologic function ought to be undertaken among parents of patients compared with those of parents of controls within the context of large-scale, population-based, case-control studies of childhood ALL.

It is interesting to note that **Chromosome 21, trisomy 21**, associated with an excess risk of ALL, is also characterized by a number of immunologic abnormalities, including increased levels of IgG, elevated numbers of basophils, and decreased IgM, as well as a decreased response for delayed hypersensitivity to bacterial and viral antigens and a decreased response to phytohemagglutinin. Several maternal reproductive and pregnancy-related disorders have been linked to ALL, including higher birth weight, birth order (first), and maternal age (older), although these findings have not been consistent across studies. Postnatal exposure to high levels of ionizing radiation and prenatal exposure to diagnostic ionizing radiation are the most consistently demonstrated associations. A number of parental occupational exposures have also been implicated, although findings have been inconsistent and specific exposures not isolated. Childhood environmental exposures and medically related conditions have also been implicated, including pesticides, certain viral disorders (particularly varicella during fetal development; see **Fetal effects from varicellazoster**), and use of chloramphenicol.

Among the several non-random chromosomal translocations associated with childhood ALL are t(q;22) (q34;q11) found in six percent of cases (primarily pre-B and B-cell precursors, ALL and T-ALL); t(4;11) (q21;q23) linked with five percent of childhood cases, particularly non-T, non-B ALL; t(1;19) (q23;p13.3) associated with pre-B ALL; t(11;14) (p13;q13) found in T-ALL , and three translocations unique to B-ALL including t(8;14) (q24;q32), t(2;8) (p11–13;q24), and t(8;22) (q24;q11).

Pathogenesis: The cause(s) of familial childhood ALL are unknown, although interactions of underlying genetic or immunogenetic disorders with a number of environmental variables is probable. Some familial cases appear to be associated with various chromosomal abnormalities, others with heritable disorders characterized by increased chromosomal abnormalities or breakage. The relationship of familial ALL to the apparently increased haplotype sharing among parents or to underlying immunologic dysfunction among mothers, and perhaps fathers, requires further study. The basis of the high concordance rate for leukemia in identical twins under age six years seems to be intrauterine transfusion (via placental anastomosis; see **Fetal monozygous multiple pregnancy dysplacentation effects**) of leukemia cells from one fetus to the co-twin.

MIM No.: *14779

Sex Ratio: M1.3:F1.0. There appears to be no difference in the sex ratio of familial ALL cases compared with the sex ratio of sporadic cases.

Occurrence: Although concordance among identical twins is 20–25% overall, and certain rare disorders are associated with an exceptionally high subsequent risk of childhood leukemia, a relatively small fraction of childhood ALL cases are familial. Data are not available to quantify prevalence or incidence of familial ALL.

Risk of Recurrence for Patient's Sib:
See Part I, *Mendelian Inheritance*. Surveys have suggested a fourfold excess risk.

Risk of Recurrence for Patient's Child:
See Part I, *Mendelian Inheritance*.

Age of Detectability: Virtually all cases among identical twins are diagnosed before ten years of age.

Gene Mapping and Linkage: IGJ (immunoglobulin J polypeptide) has been provisionally mapped to 4q21.

Prevention: Data from the United Kingdom and from the Connecticut Tumor Registry suggest an increase in childhood ALL over the last four decades. The underlying reasons for this rise in incidence are not known. Epidemiologic studies have failed to identify consistently major environmental risk factors other than postnatal exposure to high levels of ionizing radiation and prenatal exposure to diagnostic ionizing radiation. Children with **Chromosome 21, trisomy 21** or a number of other rare heritable disorders and sibs of affected persons are at increased risk, and genetic counseling may be of benefit to parents of such children.

Treatment: As with non-familial ALL.

Prognosis: As with non-familial ALL.

Detection of Carrier: Unknown.

Support Groups: New York; Leukemia Society of America

References:
Vidabaek A: Heredity in human leukemia and its relation to cancer: a genetic and clinical study of 209 probands. London: HK Lewis and Co., 1947.

Miller RW: Down's syndrome (monogolism), other congenital malformations and cancers among sibs of leukemic children. New Engl J Med 1963; 268:393–401.

MacMahon B, Levy MA: Prenatal origin of childhood leukemia: evidence from twins. New Engl J Med 1964; 270:1082–1085.

Miller RW: Relation between cancer and congenital defects: an epidemiologic evaluation. JNCI 1968; 40:1079–1085. *

Zuelzer WW, Cox DE: Genetic aspects of leukemia. Semin Hematol 1969; 6:228–249.

Miller RW: Deaths from childhood leukemia and solid tumors among twins and other sibs in the United States, 1960–1967. JNCI 1971; 46:203–209. *

Gunz GW, et al.: Familial leukemia: a study of 909 families. Scand J Haematol 1975; 15:117–131. *

Koshland ME: The coming of age of the immunoglobulin J chain. Ann Rev Immun 1985; 3:425–453.

Pendergrass TW: Epidemiology of acute lymphoblastic leukemia. Semin Oncol 1985; 12:80–91.

Max EE, et al.: Human J chain gene: chromosomal localization and associated restriction fragment length polymorphisms. Proc Nat Acad Sci 1986; 83:5592–5596.

Neglia JP, Robison LL: Epidemiology of childhood acute leukemias. Pediatr Clin N Am 1988; 35:675–692.

LI029   **Martha S. Linet**

Leukemia, chronic granulocytic
See LEUKEMIA, CHRONIC MYELOID (CML)
Leukemia, chronic lymphatic
See LEUKEMIA/LYMPHOMA, B-CELL
Leukemia, chronic lymphatic type II
See LEUKEMIA/LYMPHOMA, B-CELL
Leukemia, chronic lymphatic, type 2
See LYMPHOMA, NON-HODGKIN

LEUKEMIA, CHRONIC MYELOID (CML)   3092

Includes:
> Breakpoint cluster region-1
> Granulocytic leukemia, chronic
> Leukemia, chronic granulocytic

Excludes:
> Erythroleukemia
> **Gaucher disease** (0406)
> Leukemoid reaction
> Myelofibrosis
> Polycythemia vera
> Thrombocytopenia, primary

Major Diagnostic Criteria: Bone marrow is hyperplastic. There is an increased number of immature granulocytes. The ratio of granulocytes/erythrocytes is 10–50:1 rather than 2–5:1, as seen in the normal bone marrow. In nearly all cases, the Philadelphia (Ph) chromosome has been found cytogenetically in the granulocytes. In a blood film from CML cases, there is granulocytic leukocytosis. The white count is elevated (avg. 200,000/dl with a range of 15,000/dl to 600,000/dl). The platelet count is above 450,000/dl in about 50% of the cases.

Clinical Findings: The basic abnormality is granulocytic leukocytosis. The blood film gives a picture of granulocytes in all stages of differentiation but which appear to be morphologically normal. The composition of the granulocytes found in the blood are 50% neutrophils, 22% myelocytes, less than 10% are promyelocytes and blast cells, and the eosinophils and basophils are less than 5%. The mature neutorphils appear to function normally. There is an associated anemia that is normocytic and normochromic, having an average hemoglobin level of 9–12 g/dl. The platelets are functionally and morphologically abnormal. The metabolic rate is increased in CML cases, leading to weight loss, fever and increased sweating. Occasionally the bone marrow and spleen presents with lipid-containing histocytes resembling those observed in **Gaucher disease**.

The level of glucocerebrosidase is elevated in CML cases rather than deficient, as is observed in **Gaucher disease**. The level of uric acid is elevated in untreated CML cases. Neutrophil alkaline phosphatase is markedly decreased in CML cases. There is a considerable elevation of serum vitamin B_{12} and serum lactic dehydrogenase in CML cases. During the chronic phase, hepatosplenomegaly is often observed, but lymphadenopathy is rare. The presence of lymphadenopathy should alert one to the involvement of the disease to the terminal stage or an extramedullary myeloblastoma.

Complications: The terminal phase of CML could present either as a "myeloproliferative acceleration" or as a "blastic transformation." This phase can occur at any point during the chronic phase of the disease. The "myeloproliferative acceleration" leads to a progressive leukocytosis. The disease becomes refractory to previously effective treatment. In approximately 33% of the cases, myelofibrosis occurs. There is an increased basophilia at the terminal phase. During the terminal phase, there is weakness due to progressive anemia, weight loss and an increase in pain due to splenomegaly. In the "blastic transformation" approximately 30–40% of the cells in the bone marrow are blasts which may be lymphoid or myeloid in origin, but the presence of anemia and thrombocytopenia are also necessary for this diagnosis. The lymphatic cells are differentiated by their cytoplasmic TdT (terminal deoxynucleotidyl transferase) expression. These patients respond to chemotherapy effective for lymphoid leukemias.

Approximately 50% of the CML cases at this phase will have cytogenetic abnormalities, especially aneuploidy, usually being trisomic for chromosomes 1, 8, 17, isochromosome of the long arm of chromosome 17, or an additional Ph chromosome.

Associated Findings: None known.

Etiology: An increased incidence of CML has been observed after exposure to significant amounts of ionizing radiation.

Pathogenesis: Considered to be a neoplastic disease of the pluripotent stem cell in the bone marrow.

MIM No.: *15141

Sex Ratio: M1:F<1

Occurrence: CML is rarely found in children; only about 1–3% of childhood leukemias are CML. The median age is 40–45 years for CML. About 20% of all the leukemias in the Western countries are CML.

Risk of Recurrence for Patient's Sib: Unknown.

Risk of Recurrence for Patient's Child: Unknown.

Age of Detectability: At any age.

Gene Mapping and Linkage: BCR (breakpoint cluster region) has been mapped to 22q11.

Nearly all CML cases have the Ph chromosome present in their hemopoietic cells. By using glucose-6-phosphate dehydrogenase isozyme analyses, the clonal nature of the cells containing the Ph chromosome has been demonstrated. The neoplastic cells most probably derived from a Ph chromosome containing pluripotential stem cell. The consistent chromosomal translocation associated with CML is t(9:22)(q34;q11), which results in the Ph chromosome. The c-abl oncogene which is located at 9q34 is translocated to chromosome 22q11 when the t(9;22) occurs. The breakpoint on chromosome 22 is clustered around a 5.8 kb region identified as the "breakpoint cluster region" (bcr). This bcr-abl fusion gene is expressed at the transcriptional level, giving rise to a fusion mRNA of 8 kb in size, and also at the translational level, giving rise to a fusion bcr-abl protein of 210 kd. The role of this fusion protein is unknown. Occasionally a Ph negative CML case appears, but at the molecular level there is a rearrangement at 22q11 at the location of bcr; thus these cases contain a masked Ph chromosome.

Prevention: None known. Genetic counseling indicated.

Treatment: The chronic phase of the disease can be controlled by oral chemotherapeutic drugs such as hydroxyurea or busulfan. This treatment is stopped once the white cell count drops to 10,000/dl. New therapeutic trials with high dose chemotherapy and autologous bone marrow or allogenic bone marrow transplantation for curative approaches are being analyzed.

Prognosis: The median survival time after the diagnosis ranges from 36 months to four years for the chronic phase. In the terminal phase, the median survival time is about 2–3 months. A white cell count of less than 100,000/mm3, the presence of less than 1% myeloblasts and erythroid precursors in the peripheral blood and the absence of hepatosplenomegaly are good prognostic indicators, with median survival time of approximately 60 months.

Detection of Carrier: Unknown.

Support Groups: New York; Leukemia Society of America

References:
Williams WJ, et al: Hematology, ed. 3. New York: McGraw-Hill, 1983. *
Yunis JJ: The chromosomal basis of human neoplasia. Science 1983; 221:227–236.
Reich PR: Hematology, ed. 2. Boston: Little, Brown & Co, 1984. †
DeVita VT Jr, et al: Cancer: principles and practice of oncology, ed. 2. Philadelphia: J.B. Lippincott Co, 1985. †
Haluska FG, et al: Oncogene activation by chromosome translocation in human malignancy. Ann Rev Genet 1987; 21:321–345. *

L0016
CR024

Elaine Louie
Carlo M. Croce

LEUKEMIA/LYMPHOMA, B-CELL 3097

Includes:
B-cell chronic lymphocytic leukemia
B-cell prolymphocytic leukemia
Follicular lymphoma
Leukemia, chronic lymphatic
Leukemia, chronic lymphatic type II
Lymphoma, B-cell
Non-Hodgkin lymphoma of B-cell type
Oncogene B-cell leukemia
Small cell lymphocytic lymphoma

Excludes:
Leukemia/lymphoma, T-cell (3095)
Lymphoma, non-Hodgkin (3107)

Major Diagnostic Criteria: In B-cell chronic lymphocytic leukemia (CLL), there is peripheral lymphocytosis, lymphoadenopathy and, splenomegaly. Minimal requirements leading to this diagnosis are the presence of 40% or greater lymphocytosis in the bone marrow and an absolute lymphocytosis of greater than 15,000/dl. The B-cells in CLL have a restricted Ig class, IgG subclass and light chain type. Distinction between lymphocytic leukemia and lymphocytic lymphoma is based mainly on the distribution of the abnormal B-cells.

Clinical Findings: In chronic lymphocytic leukemia there is an accumulation and proliferation of abnormal, relatively immature B-cells in the bone marrow, lymph nodes and spleen. There is a generalized lymphadenopathy, and 75% of the cases have splenomegaly. Normocytic and normochromic anemia and/or enlarged lymph nodes are also present. The peripheral lymphocytes are uniformly small cells with condensed nuclei. Surface immunoglobulin of a specific light chain and heavy chain isotype identifies the clonal nature of the neoplastic B-cells. B-cells are functionally abnormal, leading to an immunodeficiency state. Prolymphocytic leukemia of B-cells is considered to be a rare variant of B-cell chronic lymphocytic leukemia, with an increased expression of membrane immunoglobulin. There is massive splenomegaly, while lymphoadenopathy is minimal. The total peripheral lymphocyte count is greater than 100 x 10⁹/L. In small cell lymphocytic leukemia, there is a diffuse growth pattern in the lymph nodes. The majority of the cells are similar to those seen in chronic lymphocytic leukemia. These lymphomas are considered

to be the solid tumor counterpart of chronic lymphocytic leukemia.

Complications: There is an increased risk of all types of infections due to the impaired immune state of the patient. The final stage can lead to a refractory anemia, splenomegaly, leukemic cells replacing the bone marrow and hypogammaglobulinemia which leads to fatal septicemia. Rarely is a blastic stage seen in chronic lymphocytic leukemias.

Associated Findings: There is an increased risk in developing other cancers such as skin cancer, melenoma, sarcoma and lung cancer.

Etiology: There is a tendency of closely-related persons to have CLL, but no well-defined mode of inheritance has been found.

Pathogenesis: A clonal proliferation of neoplastic B-cells at a relatively immature stage in differentiation.

MIM No.: *15140, *15143

Sex Ratio: M3:F1

Occurrence: This is the commonest leukemia in Western countries. The median age is 60 years, and it occurs in adults older than 30 years. Chronic lymphocytic leukemia is rare in Japan.

Risk of Recurrence for Patient's Sib: There appears to be a slight increase in risk for patient's sib.

Risk of Recurrence for Patient's Child: There appears to be a slight increase in risk for patient's child.

Age of Detectability: At any age.

Gene Mapping and Linkage: BCL1 (B cell CLL/lymphoma 1) has been mapped to 11q13.3.
BCL2 (B cell CLL/lymphoma 2) has been mapped to 18q21.3.
In 10% of B-cell chronic lymphocytic leukemias, the leukemic cells carry t(11;14)(q13;q32). This translocation is present in certain small cell lymphomas as well. The translocation involves the immunoglobulin heavy chain locus and a putative oncogene on chromosome 11 called bcl-1 (B-cell leukemia/lymphoma 1). The breakpoints on the chromosome is clustered around the 5' ends of the joining regions (J region) of the immunoglobulin heavy chain locus. The clustering of the breakpoint on chromosome 14 occurs near sequences involved in the normal V-D-J rearrangement seen during normal B-cell differentiation. This association has suggested that the translocation observed in the leukemia may represent an aberrant V-D-J joining event.

Prevention: None known. Genetic counseling indicated.

Treatment: Intensive therapy is rarely used because of the advanced age of the patients and the indolent nature of the disease. The symptomatic enlarged lymph node is treated effectively with involved field radiation therapy. For systemic treatment, steroids and alkylating agents such as chlorambucil have been employed.

Prognosis: The median survival time is greater than 70 months if anemia or thrombocytopenia is absent. Patients who present with thrombocytopenia in addition to anemia, splenomegaly, and lymphadenopathy have a median survival time of less than 2 years.

Detection of Carrier: Unknown.

Support Groups: New York; Leukemia Society of America

References:
Williams WJ, et al: Hematology, ed 3. New York: McGraw-Hill 1983. *
Yunis JJ: The chromosomal basis of human neoplasia. Science 1983; 221:227–236.
Reich PR: Hematology, ed 2. Boston: Little, Brown & Co, 1984. †
DeVita VT Jr., et al: Cancer: principles and practice of oncology, ed 2. Philadelphia: J.B. Lippincott Co, 1985. †
Milo JV, et al: Relationship between chronic lymphocytic leukemia and prolymphocytic leukemia. J Haematol 1986; 3:377–387.
Chenevix-Trench G: The molecular genetics of human non-Hodgkin's lymphoma. Cancer Genet Cytogenet 1987; 27:191–213.
Haluska FG, et al: Oncogene activation by chromosome translocation in human malignancy. Ann Rev Genet 1987; 21:321–345. *

L0016
CR024

Elaine Louie
Carlo M. Croce

LEUKEMIA/LYMPHOMA, T-CELL   3095

Includes:
- Cutaneous T-cell lymphomas
- Diffuse T-cell lymphoma
- Mycosis fungoides
- Non-Hodgkin lymphoma of T-cell type
- Sezary syndrome
- T-cell antigen receptor, alpha subunit (TCRA)
- T-cell chronic lymphocytic leukemia
- T-cell leukemia/lymphoma, adult
- T-cell prolymphocytic leukemia

Excludes:
- **Leukemia/lymphoma, B cell (3097)**
- **Lymphoma, non-Hodgkin (3107)**

Major Diagnostic Criteria: In adult T-cell chronic lymphocytic leukemia, there is erythroderma, hepatosplenomegaly and neurological involvement. The neoplastic cells are negative for surface immunoglobulin but instead have the mature T-cell phenotype. Characteristically the cells are large and have convoluted nuclei. The deep paracortex of the lymph nodes and the skin is infiltrated by these T-cells. In *cutaneous T-cell lymphomas* (*Mycosis fungoides* and *Sezary syndrome*), the skin (both epidermis and upper dermis) is infiltrated by T lymphocytes. During the later stages of this disease there is also systemic organ involvement. The neoplastic cells are pleiomorphic, their nuclei are highly convoluted, and they have the phenotype of T-cells.

Clinical Findings: The patient presents with hepatosplenomegaly, neutropenia and skin infiltration, but not with lymphadenopathy. Leukemic cells are positive for T-cell surface antigens, negative for surface immunoglobulin, and they form rosettes with sheep red blood cells. The karyotype in the leukemic cells is usually aneuploid. Adult T-cell leukemia/lymphoma have been associated with HTLV-1 (human T-cell leukemia/lymphoma virus-1). The leukemic cells have surface antigens of mature immunocompetent T-cells. There is infiltration of the skin by these T-cells, hypercalcemia, lymphadenopathy and hepatosplenomegaly. The cells are large and pleiomorphic. The T-cells are usually OKT-4 positive with a high density of T-cell receptors, but they function abnormally.

Complications: In T-cell leukemias, involvement of the central nervous system is characteristic.

Associated Findings: None known.

Etiology: Adult T-cell leukemia/lymphoma is associated with HTLV-1 but no etiological factors have been identified.

Pathogenesis: An uncontrolled expansion of monoclonal T-cells.

MIM No.: *18688

Sex Ratio: M1:F<1

Occurrence: Adult T-cell leukemia/lymphoma is endemic to certain regions of Japan and the Caribbean. Both of these diseases are rare in developed countries. *Cutaneous T-cell lymphoma* is not very common, having a rate of 2–3 cases per million in the United States. Usually it occurs in patients 30 years or older; it rarely occurs in patients less than 30 years.

Risk of Recurrence for Patient's Sib: Unknown.

Risk of Recurrence for Patient's Child: Unknown.

Age of Detectability: At any age.

Gene Mapping and Linkage: TCRA (T cell receptor, alpha (V,D,J,C)) has been mapped to 14q11.2.

TAL1 (T cell acute lymphoblastic leukemia 1) has been mapped to 11p15.

Some T-cell leukemias and lymphomas exhibit specific nonrandom chromosomal traslocations which frequently involve 14q11, where the alpha and delta chains of the T-cell receptor are located. The most frequent chromosomal abnormalities are inversions -- inv(14) -- and translocations -- t(14;14)(q11;q32), t(8;14)(q24;q11), t(10;14)(q24;q11), or t(11;14)(p13;q11). The T-cell receptor genes are organized in a similar manner to the immunoglobulin genes, and during normal cellular differentiation the gene undergoes rearrangement at the DNA level in a manner similar to the immunoglobulin loci. Putative oncogenes have been hypothesized to exist at or near the site of the breakpoint on chromosomes 14q32, 11p13 and 10q24, called *tcl*-1, *tcl*-2 and *tcl*-3, respectively (T-cell leukemia/lymphoma-1, -2 and -3). In the case of the t(8;14)(q24;q11), the T-cell alpha locus on chromosome 14 translocates into the 3' end of the proto-oncogene c-*myc* locus on chromosome 8. Thus, the T-cell receptor alpha locus is split between the Vα and Jα regions, and the c-*myc* locus remains intact.

The question of whether c-*myc* is deregulated in cells containing the t(8;14) has been approached using somatic cell hybrids. These experiments demonstrate that only the translocated intact c-*myc* locus is expressed, which suggests that the T-cell receptor alpha locus can activate the transcription of a juxtaposed oncogene *in cis*. The inv(14) and other translocations specific for T-cell leukemias and lymphomas may have the T-cell receptor loci activate *in cis* a newly-juxtaposed gene in the vicinity of the chromosomal breakpoint. It should be noted that the T-cell receptor beta chain locus and T-cell receptor gamma chain locus which maps to chromosome 7q35 and 7p13, respectively, are also sites of chromosomal translocations in T-cell leukemias and lymphomas but at a lesser frequency than 14q11.

Prevention: None known. Genetic counseling indicated.

Treatment: The T-cell leukemias and lymphomas do not respond well to therapy. Therapy is usually palliative using radiotherapy or combination chemotherapy. In cutaneous T-cell lymphoma, application of nitrogen mustard, combined ultraviolet A light and psoralen therapy, whole body irradiation with an electron beam, or systemic chemotherapy are often used to control the skin lesions that arise from this disease.

Prognosis: Survival time is less than one year.

Detection of Carrier: Unknown.

Support Groups: New York; Leukemia Society of America

References:
Williams WJ, et al: Hematology, ed. 3. New York: McGraw-Hill, 1983. *
Yunis JJ: The chromosomal basis of human neoplasia. Science 1983; 221:227–236.
Reich PR: Hematology, ed. 2. Boston: Little, Brown & Co, 1984. †
DeVita VT Jr, et al: Cancer: principles and practive of oncology, ed. 2. Philadelphia: J.B. Lippincott Co, 1985. †
Chenevix-Trench G: The molecular genetics of human non-Hodgkin's lymphoma. Cancer Genet Cytogenet 1987; 27:191–213.
Haluska FG, et al: Oncogene activation by chromosome translocation in human malignancy. Ann Rev Genet 1987; 21:321–345. *

L0016   **Elaine Louie**
CR024   **Carlo M. Croce**

Leukocyte adherence deficiency
See GRANULOCYTE GLYCOPROTEIN CD11/CD18 DEFICIENCY
Leukocyte interferon deficiency
See INTERFERON DEFICIENCY

LEUKOCYTE, MAY-HEGGLIN ANOMALY 2681

Includes:
May-Hegglin anomaly
Megathrombocytopenia
Nephritis-megathrombocytopenia-deafness
Platelet, May-Hegglin anomaly
Thrombocytopenia-Dohle bodies in neutrophils

Excludes:
Alder anomaly
Chediak-Higashi syndrome (0143)
Dohle bodies, transient, from infections or chemotherapy
Nephritis-deafness (sensorineural), hereditary type (0708)
Toxic granulation of neutrophils

Major Diagnostic Criteria: The presence of bizarre giant platelets in the circulation and basophilic inclusions (Döhle bodies) within a large portion of the granulocytes (neutrophils, eosinophils, and basophils) and in occasional monocytes. These inclusions are large (2–5 μm) RNA-containing granules located in the cytoplasm (usually one per cell) which stain sky blue with Wright stain. Under the electron microscope the Döhle bodies are spindle-shaped and consist of linear arrays of 7–10 nm filaments. Approximately 50% of the reported patients have had platelet counts of <75,000/mm³, sometimes associated with a mild bleeding tendency. The survival time and function of the platelets are normal. Döhle bodies caused by infection can appear transiently in neutrophils but are not associated with giant platelets.

Clinical Findings: Mild hemorrhagic manifestations have been the only specific clinical problem encountered. In a review of all 89 documented cases in the literature by Godwin and Ginsburg (1974), 43% had features of abnormal bleeding, including recurrent epistaxis, easy bruisability, gingival bleeding, menorrhagia, and excessive bleeding following dental extraction, tonsillectomy, or trauma. This bleeding tendency was associated with a platelet count of <75,000/mm³ in 86% of the symptomatic patients. The remaining patients cited in this review were entirely asymptomatic. No increased incidence of bacterial or fungal infections due to the granulocyte inclusions has been reported.

There is some variability in the expression of the morphologic and thrombocytopenic manifestations of the disorder. Even within a given family, not all members will necessarily have thrombocytopenia and some will have transitory decreases in the platelet count. Similarly, the percentage of granulocytes containing Döhle bodies can vary within a family and can be as low as <10%.

Complications: Severe bleeding can potentially occur in those patients with the lowest platelet counts.

Associated Findings: Hereditary nephritis and deafness associated with the May-Hegglin anomaly.

Etiology: Autosomal dominant inheritance.

Pathogenesis: The defect responsible for the formation of the Döhle bodies is unknown, although the finding that cytotoxic drugs can also cause this abnormality suggests that a metabolic disorder could be responsible. The giant platelets are thought to arise from abnormal maturation and fragmentation of normal-appearing megakaryocytes in the bone marrow. The reason for this abnormality or how it relates to the granulocyte inclusions is unknown.

MIM No.: *15510

Sex Ratio: M1:F1

Occurrence: In their 1974 report, Godwin and Ginsburg were able to find 83 patients reported in the literature of whom 22 belonged to a single kinship.

Risk of Recurrence for Patient's Sib:
See Part I, *Mendelian Inheritance.*

Risk of Recurrence for Patient's Child:
See Part I, *Mendelian Inheritance.*

Age of Detectability: During infancy. In one report, a child was diagnosed at age five months.

Gene Mapping and Linkage: Unknown.

Prevention: None known. Genetic counseling indicated.

Treatment: Patients with severe thrombocytopenia may require platelet transfusions for surgical procedures or severe trauma.

Prognosis: Normal life span.

Detection of Carrier: Due to the dominant mode of inheritance, carriers exhibit the May-Hegglin anomaly.

Special Considerations: This condition is distinct from Alport syndrome associated with macrothrombocytopenia (Peterson et al, 1985), and Döhle bodies and leukemia (Goudsmit et al, 1971).

References:
Oski FA, et al.: Leukocytic inclusions-Döhle bodies-associated with platelet abnormality (the May-Hegglin anomaly): report of a family and review of the literature. Blood 1962; 20:657–667. *
Jordan SW, Larsen WE: Ultrastructural studies of the May-Hegglin anomaly. Blood 1965; 25:921–932. †
Goudsmit R, et al.: Dohle bodies and acute myeloblastic leukemia in one family: a new familial disorder. Brit J Haemat 1971; 20:557–562.
Cawley JC, Hayhoe FGJ: The inclusions of the May-Hegglin anomaly and Döhle bodies of infection: an ultrastructural comparison. Br J Haematol 1972; 22:491–496. †
Godwin HA, Ginsburg AD: May-Hegglin anomaly: a defect in megakaryocyte fragmentation? Br J Haematol 1974; 26:117–128. *
Brivet F, et al.: Hereditary nephritis associated with May-Hegglin anomaly. Nephron 1981; 29:59–62. †
Peterson L, et al.: Fechtner syndrome: a variant of Alport's syndrome with leukocyte inclusions and macrothrombocytopenia. Blood 1985; 65:397–406. †

CU012

John T. Curnutte

Leukocytes, granulation anomaly of
See CHEDIAK-HIGASHI SYNDROME
Leukoderma acquisitum centrifugum of Sutton
See SKIN, VITILIGO
Leukoderma, primary
See SKIN, VITILIGO

LEUKODYSTROPHY, ADULT-ONSET PROGRESSIVE DOMINANT TYPE 2975

Includes: Adult-onset leukodystrophy, hereditary

Excludes:
Adrenoleukodystrophy, X-linked (2533)
Brain, spongy degeneration (0115)
Cerebro-hepato-renal syndrome (0139)
Leukodystrophy, globoid cell type (0415)
Metachromatic leukodystrophies (0651)
Multiple sclerosis, familial (2598)
Multiple systems atrophies: Shy-Drager syndrome
Olivopontocerebellar atrophy
Pelizaeus-Merzbacher syndrome (0803)

Major Diagnostic Criteria: Steadily progressive symptoms of cerebellar, pyramidal, and autonomic nervous system dysfunction with onset in the early thirties to late forties. Leg pain, weakness, postural hypotension, neurogenic bladder, rectal incontinence, progressive loss of balance, spasticity, and slurred speech are accompanied by little or no mental deterioration. Death occurs within 15–25 years. X-ray findings show symmetric decrease in white matter density.

Clinical Findings: Of the two kindreds reported, one is of Irish and the other of Scots-Irish origin. The clinical picture is that of an adult-onset (ranging from early fourth to late fifth decade), slowly progressive multisystem nondementing neurologic disorder that, in some aspects, resembles multiple sclerosis. The most common initial symptoms include lower extremity pain, weakness, gait disturbance, vertigo, loss of fine motor control, orthostatic hypotension, and lower back pain. As the disease progresses, affected individuals often have slurred speech, diaphoresis, intermittent rigidity, spasticity, paraplegia, bladder and bowel incontinence, and impotence. Personality and orientation remain intact, but patients are usually bedridden prior to death. The immediate cause of death is most frequently bronchopneumonia or "stroke."

Cranial CT scans and magnetic resonance imaging have shown symmetric atrophy of white matter in affected individuals and in at least one presymptomatic affected woman whose mother was affected.

Pathologic studies of the brains of some of the affected individuals revealed white matter degeneration of the cerebral hemispheres and cerebellum. There was little involvement of the internal capsule, brainstem, and cervical cord and no involvement of the subcortical tracts. Microscopic examination showed spongiform leukoencephalopathy with no gliosis, inflammation, or storage.

Laboratory findings include theta activity showing on EEG in three affected family members, abnormalities of central conduction on somatosensory evoked potentials, which evolved over a period of two years in the presymptomatic daughter of the affected mother mentioned above, abnormal brainstem evoked auditory response, and abnormal visual evoked response. Laboratory testing for known metabolic diseases has been repeatedly uninformative.

Complications: Postural hypotension is usually associated with severe vertigo. Progression of symptoms leads to increasing disability through incontinence, spasticity, and inability to walk. Patients are usually bedridden prior to death and require 24-hour nursing care.

Associated Findings: None known. The clinical picture is relatively consistent, and affected individuals in both kindreds have had remarkably similar clinical courses. A personality change was described in one of the patients, but it is more probable that it was caused by frustration and emotional reaction to the disease.

Etiology: Autosomal dominant inheritance. In each kindred there are at least four consecutive generations of affected individuals. While the families described have been referred to as having **Pelizaeus-Merzbacher syndrome**, their condition does not cause dementia.

Pathogenesis: A demyelinating process is suspected, and symmetric white matter degeneration has been documented through imaging as well as at autopsy.

MIM No.: *16950

Sex Ratio: M1:F1

Occurrence: Two kinships have been documented. Extensive efforts have not resulted in the discovery of a common ancestor of the two families, although the possibility has not been completely ruled out. The families are of Irish and Scots-Irish origin. Two other families, one American and the other German, were reported previously with a disorder that had a similar clinical course to that described here; however, the patients also deteriorated intellectually, so it is unclear whether all four kindreds have the same disorder.

Risk of Recurrence for Patient's Sib:
See Part I, *Mendelian Inheritance.*

Risk of Recurrence for Patient's Child:
See Part I, *Mendelian Inheritance.*

Age of Detectability: Ranges from the early thirties to late forties, although presymptomatic identification of affected individuals may be possible through imaging or electrophysiologic techniques. No prenatal detection known. It is possible that presymptomatic individuals could be identified (if they desire) with imaging or electrophysiologic techniques.

Gene Mapping and Linkage: Unknown.

Prevention: None known. Genetic counseling indicated.

Treatment: Symptomatic only. Emotional support for patients and families similar to that available to families with **Huntington disease**.

Prognosis: The clinical course is slowly progressive; death occurs usually within 10–25 years of onset of symptoms and follows a period of severe disability.

Detection of Carrier: Unknown.

Support Groups: IL; Sycamore; United Leukodystrophy Foundation

References:
Eldridge R, et al.: Hereditary adult-onset leukodystrophy simulating chronic progressive multiple sclerosis. New Engl J Med 1984; 331:948–953.
Laxova R, et al.: A new autosomal dominant adult onset progressive leukodystrophy. Am J Hum Genet 1985; 37:A65.

LA033 **Renata Laxova**

Leukodystrophy, Alexander disease
See ALEXANDER DISEASE

LEUKODYSTROPHY, GLOBOID CELL TYPE 0415

Includes:
 Galactosylceramidase deficiency
 Galactosylceramide beta-galactosidase deficiency
 Globoid cell leukodystrophy
 Krabbe disease
 Psychosine lipidosis

Excludes:
 Adrenoleukodystrophy, X-linked (2533)
 Alexander disease (2712)
 Brain, spongy degeneration (0115)
 Encephalopathy, necrotizing (0344)
 Metachromatic leukodystrophies (0651)
 Paraplegia, familial spastic (0295)
 Phytanic acid oxidase deficiency, infantile type (2278)
 Sudanophilic leukodystrophy

Major Diagnostic Criteria: Definitive antemortem diagnosis can be established only by profound deficiency of galactosylceramidase activity in serum, leukocytes, fibroblasts, cultured amniotic fluid cells, chorionic villi, and solid tissues. Diagnosis should be suspected in infants with early hyperirritability, rapidly progressive neurologic signs, particularly of the white matter, and elevated spinal fluid protein. Postmortem examination of the central nervous system can also provide the definite diagnosis. The white matter is almost completely devoid of myelin, which is replaced by severe astrocytic gliosis and the unique, multinucleated, PAS-positive globoid cells.

Clinical Findings: The onset of clinical symptoms in typical cases is between ages 3 and 6 months. Rarely, the clinical onset can be immediately after birth. The initial symptoms are usually vague and nonspecific, such as episodic fever of unknown origin, hyperirritability, and hypersensitivity to external stimuli. Vomiting and feeding difficulty with or without seizures may occur as initial clinical symptoms. Rapidly progressive severe mental and motor deterioration follows. Neurologic signs are largely referrable to the central white matter and to the peripheral nerves. There is marked hypertonicity with extended and crossed legs, flexed arms, and opisthotonus. Tendon reflexes are hyperactive. Cherry red spots have been reported. Optic atrophy and sluggish pupillary reflexes are common. Toward the terminal stage, the patients are often blind, deaf, decerebrate, and have no contact with the surroundings. The early hyperactive reflexes are replaced by diminished or absent reflexes. Because of their severity, clinical signs of the white matter lesions often overshadow signs of the pathologically less-involved gray matter. Signs of peripheral nervous system involvement, such as reduced nerve conduction velocity, are almost always present except in the very early stages of the disease.

Radiologic findings can trace the evolution of the disease. At first, discrete and symmetric dense areas on CT are found in deep gray matter of the cerebral hemispheres, thalamus, posterior limb of the internal capsule, quadrigeminal plate and cerebellum, and also in the periventricular and capsular white matter. MRI shows decreased T1 values with normal or slilghtly decreased T2 values in white matter of the centrum semiovale. Later, both CT and MRI show diffuse reduction in gray matter and, more profoundly, in the white matter mass.The spinal fluid protein is highly elevated from the early stages. Systemic organs are usually not affected. Typically patients die before two years of age.

However, the exceedingly rare, late-onset form of the disease shows more variable clinical features and is probably heterogeneous genetically. The clinical onset can be in late infancy, childhood, or even later. Visual impairment due to cortical blindness and optic atrophy, spasticity with pyramidal signs, and difficulty walking are common manifestations. Clinical signs of peripheral nervous system involvement are not obvious. The spinal fluid protein is normal or only slightly elevated. Clinical diagnosis of the late-onset form is difficult to impossible without galactosylceramidase assays.

Complications: Blindness, deafness, spasticity (early), difficulty feeding, contracture of the limbs, decerebration.

Associated Findings: Macrocephaly, **Hydrocephaly**, infantile spasms.

Etiology: Autosomal recessive inheritance of deficient activity of galactosylceramidase.

Pathogenesis: The affected enzyme, galactosylceramidase, normally hydrolyzes galactosylceramide, which is quantitatively almost exclusively localized in the myelin sheath. This explains the highly restricted pathology to the myelin-containing tissues. The plausible hypothesis concerning the biochemical pathogenesis of the disease postulates that a toxic side-product of the involved metabolic pathway causes destruction of the myelin-forming cells, the oligodendrocytes in the CNS, and the Schwann cells in the PNS (the psychosine hypothesis). Galactosylsphingosine (psychosine) can be formed as a by-product of galactosylceramide synthesis. It is also a substrate for galactosylceramidase. Patients with this disease therefore cannot catabolize galactosylsphingosine. Psychosine is highly cytotoxic and destroys the cells in which it accumulates due to the genetic defect. Because galactosylceramide is almost exclusively localized in myelin, the above events take place only in the myelin-generating cells, resulting in the destruction of the oligodendrocytes and Schwann cells.

MIM No.: *24520

Sex Ratio: M1:F1

Occurrence: The disease is pan-ethnic, and the geographic distribution is widespread. The incidence appears to be higher in the Scandinavian countries. An incidence of 2–4:100,000 births has been reported for Sweden, and the calculated figure for Japan was 2–3 per 1 million births. Incidence in most other countries is probably closer to that in Japan. An exceedingly high frequency of 6:1,000 births was recently reported for a large inbred Druze isolate in Israel.

Risk of Recurrence for Patient's Sib:
See Part I, *Mendelian Inheritance.*

Risk of Recurrence for Patient's Child:
See Part I, *Mendelian Inheritance.* Few affected individuals survive to reproduce.

Age of Detectability: Definitive diagnosis is possible at 7–8 weeks of gestation by the galactosylceramidase assay on biopsied chorionic villi and several weeks later by the same assay on cultured amniotic fluid cells. The enzyme assay can also establish the diagnosis at any age after birth.

Gene Mapping and Linkage: GALC (galactosylceramidase) has been provisionally mapped to 17.

Prevention: None known. Genetic counseling indicated.

Treatment: No effective treatment is known.

Prognosis: A vast majority of patients die within 2–3 years of birth. Patients with the late-onset form are exceedingly rare, and only a few have been reported to survive into their teens.

Detection of Carrier: Carrier detection is possible by galactosylceramidase assays on leukocytes, serum, or cultured fibroblasts. No large-scale statistical data are available concerning the accuracy of carrier detection. A zone of uncertainty of ±10% would seem to be a reasonable estimate of the reliability.

Special Considerations: A genetic deficiency of galactosylceramidase is known to occur in other mammalian species, including the dog, mouse, and sheep. They all exhibit clinical and pathologic features similar to those of the human disease. The dog model was used extensively for research of this disease, but it is no longer available on a regular basis. The more recently discovered mouse model (the twitcher mutant) has been increasingly popular as a research tool. Transplantation of normal bone marrow to affected mice has been shown to prolong the life span of the hosts from the usual 30–40 days to over 100 days, although it did not prevent or arrest the disease process.

Support Groups: IL; Sycamore; United Leukodystrophy Foundation (ULF)

References:
Krabbe K: A new familial infantile form of diffuse brain-sclerosis. Brain 1916; 39:74–114.
Suzuki K, Suzuki Y: Globoid cell leucodystrophy (Krabbe's disease): deficiency of galactocerebroside β-galactosidase. Proc Natl Acad Sci USA 1970; 66:302–309.
Loonen MCB, et al.: Late-onset globoid cell leucodystrophy. Neuropediatrics 1985; 16:137–142.
Harzer K, et al.: Prenatal enzymatic diagnosis and exclusion of Krabbe's disease (globoid-call leukodystrophy) using chorionic villi in five risk pregnancies. Hum Genet 1987; 77:342–344.
Suzuki K, Suzuki Y: Galactosylceramide lipidosis: globoid cell leukodystrophy (Krabbe's disease). In: Scrivner CR, et al., eds: The metabolic basis of inherited disease, ed 6. New York: McGraw-Hill, 1989:1699–1720.

SU021   **Kunihiko Suzuki**

Leukodystrophy, sudanophilic
See PELIZAEUS-MERZBACHER SYNDROME
Leukokeratosis, hereditary mucosal
See MUCOSA, WHITE FOLDED DYSPLASIA
Leukomelanoderma-hypodontia-hypotrichosis-retardation
See BERLIN SYNDROME
Leukomelanoderma-infantilism-retardation-hypodontia-hypotrichosis
See BERLIN SYNDROME
Leukonychia totalis
See ULCER-LEUKONYCHIA-GALLSTONES
also NAILS, LEUKONYCHIA
Leukonychia, knuckle pads and deafness
See KNUCKLE PADS-LEUKONYCHIA-DEAFNESS
Leukonychia-short stature-hypolipidemia
See HOOFT DISEASE
Leukonychia-ulcer-gallstones
See ULCER-LEUKONYCHIA-GALLSTONES
Leung syndrome
See MICROCEPHALY-LYMPHEDEMA
Levin syndrome
See CRANIO-ECTODERMAL DYSPLASIA
Levine-Critchley syndrome
See ACANTHOCYTOSIS-NEUROLOGIC DEFECTS
Levy-Hollister Syndrome
See LACRIMO-AURICULO-DENTO-DIGITAL SYNDROME
Leyden-Moebius muscular dystrophy
See MUSCULAR DYSTROPHY, LIMB-GIRDLE
Leydig cell agenesis
See LEYDIG CELL HYPOPLASIA
Leydig cell differentiation, abnormality of
See LEYDIG CELL HYPOPLASIA
Leydig cell hypofunction
See LEYDIG CELL HYPOPLASIA
Leydig cell hypogenesis
See LEYDIG CELL HYPOPLASIA

LEYDIG CELL HYPOPLASIA   2298

Includes:

 Gonadotropin unresponsiveness
 Leydig cell agenesis
 Leydig cell differentiation, abnormality of
 Leydig cell hypofunction
 Leydig cell hypogenesis

Excludes:
 Agonadia (0029)
 Androgen insensitivity syndrome, incomplete (0050)
 Anorchia (0068)
 Gonadal dysgenesis, XY type (0437)
 Gonadotropin deficiencies (0438)
 Hermaphroditism, true (0971)
 Hypogonadotropic hypogonadism (2300)
 Kallmann syndrome (2301)
 Steroid 5 alpha-reductase deficiency (3062)
 Steroid 3 beta-hydroxysteroid dehydrogenase deficiency (0909)
 Steroid 17 alpha-hydroxylase deficiency (0903)
 Steroid 17-ketosteroid reductase deficiency (2299)
 Steroid 17,20-desmolase deficiency (0904)
 Steroid 20–22 desmolase deficiency (0907)

Major Diagnostic Criteria: Absence or severe reduction in Leydig cells in 46,XY individuals.

Clinical Findings: In Leydig cell hypoplasia the primary defect involves absence or hypoplasia of Leydig cells.

Affected individuals show female or ambiguous external genitalia despite their normal male chromosomal complement. Sometimes the clitoris may be normal for females, with the urethra located in the normal position for the female. In most affected individuals, however, labial fusion exists and a urogenital sinus is present. Sometimes the single perineal orifice leads anteriorly to the bladder and posteriorly to a (vaginal) pouching. In other cases separate perineal orifices lead to both the urethra and a blindly ending vagina. Testes are similar in size to that of normal testes and typically are palpable at the inguinal canal. Spermatogenesis to the stage of spermatocytes is demonstrable. The interstitial area contains few if any completely mature Leydig cells. Epididymides and vasa deferentia are usually present. As would be predicted for 46,XY individuals, no female internal organs are present. Specifically, the uterus and fallopian tubes are absent.

Testosterone is low despite elevated FSH and LH levels. Administration of human chorionic gonadotropin (hCG) does not increase testosterone production. Secondary sexual development thus does not occur. Somatic anomalies do not coexist.

Complications: Lack of testosterone results in genital differentiation inappropriate for the genetic sex. Lack of hormonal secretion at puberty further results in inadequate secondary sexual development. Eventually, osteoporosis and other signs of estrogen deficiencies occur.

Associated Findings: None known.

Etiology: Possibly autosomal recessive inheritance, based on 1) one family with affected multiple sibs and 2) observations of parental consanguinity. Other etiologies are not excluded.

Pathogenesis: Absence or early destruction of Leydig cells results in lack of testosterone synthesis by fetal testes. Androgen-dependent steps in differentiation are thus inhibited, either partially or completely. Embryonic differentiation not dependent on testosterone or its derivatives remains undisturbed. The actual mechanism responsible for hypoplasia of Leydig cells remains uncertain. It could be secondary to abnormalities in trophic hormones or it could involve Leydig cell differentiation per se.

MIM No.: 23344

Sex Ratio: M1:F0

Occurrence: Fewer than a dozen cases have been reported.

Risk of Recurrence for Patient's Sib:

 See Part I, *Mendelian Inheritance.* In as much as this condition is male-limited, risk is 1:8 for any sib, or 1:4 for male sibs. However, X-linked recessive inheritance is not excluded.

Risk of Recurrence for Patient's Child: Affected individuals are sterile.

Age of Detectability: Usually at birth. Cases with female external genitalia may not be detected until puberty.

Gene Mapping and Linkage: Unknown.

Prevention: None known. Genetic counseling indicated.

Treatment: Reconstructive surgery is applicable to assure female sex of rearing and sexual adaptation. Administration of sex steroids to prevent osteoporosis and to enhance secondary sexual development and function.

Prognosis: Intelligence and life span are probably normal, assuming proper hormonal treatment. Fertility is not possible, but secondary sexual development can be achieved with hormones. Reconstructive surgery can enhance sexual adaptation.

Detection of Carrier: Unknown.

References:
Berthezene F, et al.: Leydig-cell agenesis: a cause of male pseudohermaphroditism. New Engl J Med 1976; 295:969–972.
Perez-Palacios G, et al.: Inherited male pseudohermaphroditism due to gonadotropin unresponsiveness. Acta Endocrinol 1981; 98:148–155.
Lee PA, et al.: Leydig cell hypofunction resulting in male pseudohermaphroditism. Fertil Steril 1982; 37:675–679.
Rogers RM, et al.: Leydig cell hypogenesis: a rare cause of male pseudohermaphroditism and a pathological model for the understanding of normal sexual differentiation. J Urol 1982; 128:1325–1329.
El-Awady MK, et al.: Familial Leydig cell hypoplasia as a cause of male pseudohermaphroditism. Hum Hered 1987; 37:36–40.
Saldenha PH, et al.: A clinico-genetic investigation of Leydig cell hypoplasia. Am J Med Genet 1987; 26:337–344.

SI018   **Joe Leigh Simpson**

LFA-1 (CD11a/CD18) deficiency
 See GRANULOCYTE GLYCOPROTEIN CD11/CD18 DEFICIENCY
LH deficiency, isolated
 See HYPOGONADOTROPIC HYPOGONADISM
Li-Fraumeni syndrome (some cases)
 See CANCER, BREAST, FAMILIAL
Librium^, fetal effects
 See FETAL BENZODIAZEPINE EFFECTS
Lichen acuminatus
 See SKIN, PITYRIASIS RUBRA PILARIS
Lichen ruber acuminatus
 See SKIN, PITYRIASIS RUBRA PILARIS

LIDDLE SYNDROME   0590

Includes:

 Nephropathy, potassium-losing with low aldosterone
 Potassium-losing nephropathy with low aldosterone
 Pseudoaldosteronism

Excludes: Hypokalemic alkalosis-renal potassium loss-hyperaldosteronism

Major Diagnostic Criteria: Polydipsia, polyuria and hypertension secondary to a potassium-losing nephropathy with subnormal-to-low aldosterone secretion.

Clinical Findings: Hypokalemic alkalosis, hypertension, and renal potassium wasting of as much as 80 mEq of K+ daily. Growth is unaffected. Polydipsia, polyuria, and an inability to concentrate urine are also present. In contrast to expectations, aldosterone secretion is low and does not increase with sodium deprivation even when potassium stores are repleted. Neither spironolactone, that which blocks the renal tubular effects of aldosterone, nor a drug (SU9055) that blocks aldosterone biosynthesis, modifies the renal loss of electrolytes. Renin levels are normal or high, which differs from the situation in primary hyperaldosteronism where renin levels are low. There is a satisfactory renal response to ammonium chloride, acetezolamide, and exogenous aldosterone. Renal function appears normal apart from the potassium loss.

Triamterene, which blocks renal tubular exchange of potassium for sodium, is effective; it corrects the high blood pressure, hypokalemic alkalosis, and the increasing sodium excretion.

Complications: Related to the degree of hypokalemia.

Associated Findings: None known.

Etiology: Probably autosomal dominant inheritance.

Pathogenesis: Presumably related to membrane transport of sodium at the renal tubular level, perhaps reflecting a generalized membrane defect affecting other tissues and sites.

MIM No.: 17720

Sex Ratio: M1:F1

Occurrence: Undetermined but presumed rare.

Risk of Recurrence for Patient's Sib:
See Part I, *Mendelian Inheritance.*

Risk of Recurrence for Patient's Child:
See Part I, *Mendelian Inheritance.*

Age of Detectability: From birth.

Gene Mapping and Linkage: Unknown.

Prevention: None known. Genetic counseling indicated.

Treatment: Triamterene is effective in correcting blood pressure, potassium loss and alkalosis. This therapy should be maintained since the clinical findings return on discontinuation of treatment.

Prognosis: The prognosis appears normal for life span if treated.

Detection of Carrier: Unknown.

References:

Liddle CW, et al.: A familial renal disorder simulating primary aldosteronism but with negligible aldosterone secretion. In: Baulieu EE, Robel P, eds: Aldosterone, a symposium. Oxford: Blackwell Scientific, 1964:353–368.
Aarskog D, et al.: Hypertension and hypokalemic alkalosis associated with underproduction of aldosterone. Pediatrics 1967; 39:884–890.
Gardner JD, et al.: Abnormal membrane sodium transport in Liddle's syndrome. J Clin Invest 1971; 50:2253–2258.
Hyman PE, et al.: Liddle syndrome. J Pediatr 1979; 95:77–78.
Levine LB, et al.: Hypertension in childhood. In: Lavin N, ed: Manual of endocrinology and metabolism. Boston: Little Brown, 1986:169.

SP004   **Mark A. Sperling**

Ligamentous laxity-cutis laxa-delayed development
See CUTIS LAXA-DELAYED DEVELOPMENT-LIGAMENTOUS LAXITY
Light, sensitivity to
See PORPHYRIA, PROTOPORPHYRIA
Ligneous conjunctivitis
See EYE, LIGNEOUS CONJUNCTIVITIS

LIMB AND SCALP DEFECTS, ADAMS-OLIVER TYPE   0459

Includes:
Absence defects of limbs, scalp, and skull
Adams-Oliver syndrome
Amniotic bands complex
Aplasia cutis congenita-terminal, transverse defects of limbs
Hemimelia-scalp skull defects
Scalp defect-ectrodactyly
Scalp, skull, and limbs; absence defect of Adams-Oliver

Excludes:
Ectrodactyly (0336)
Ectrodactyly-ectodermal dysplasia-clefting syndrome (0337)
Skin, localized absence of (0608)
Tibial hypoplasia/aplasia-ectrodactyly (2388)

Major Diagnostic Criteria: Terminal transverse defects (TTD) of hands, and sometimes feet, with skull and scalp defects.

Clinical Findings: Central skull and scalp defects present at birth, such as denuded ulcerated area or areas on the vertex of the scalp associated with underlying bony defects of the skull. The scalp defect ranges from 2.5mm by 5mm to 7cm by 9cm. The skull and scalp defects usually heal spontaneously and completely in the first few months of life. In a few cases, plastic surgery was required. The limb deformity affects one or more limbs and varies from aphalangia, adactylia or acheiria, and apodia, to transverse hemimelia. Usually the feet are more severely affected. The terminal phalanges are sometimes short. Association of the congenital scalp defect and post-axial **Polydactyly** A has been described in two cases. Cutis marmorata and markedly dilated and tortuous scalp veins are also found.

Complications: Dilated and tortuous scalp veins, which can be injured in cases of head trauma. Scalp defects may lead to infection.

Associated Findings: Congenital heart defects, club feet, cryptorchidism, cleft lip.

Etiology: Probably autosomal dominant inheritance with complete penetrance and variable expression. Some observations suggest reduced penetrance. Reports suggestive of autosomal recessive inheritance were made. Almost one-half of the reported cases have been sporadic.

Pathogenesis: Aplasia cutis congenita (ACC) is also observed in cases of congenital ring constrictions, in epidermolysis bullosa, in focal dermal hypoplasia, in **Chromosome 13, trisomy 13**, and in cases of deletion of chromosome four. These findings illustrate the etiologic heterogeneity of skull and scalp defects of which ACC associated with TTD represents a distinct genetic entity. TTD is not simply inherited except in the rare acheiropody trait. The finding of ACC in patients with TTD, not associated with congenital ring constrictions, is a useful clue to inheritance. The cutis marmorata could be part of the syndrome and could be interpreted as a pleiotropic effect of the mutant gene.

Some observers have suggested that the TTD results from *constricting* or *amniotic bands*. While this general concept has been in and out of favor (Gellis, 1977), it has been used to explain a wide range of fetal "amputation" malformations (Pauli et al, 1985).

MIM No.: *10030, 21710

POS No.: 3250

CDC No.: 756.080

Sex Ratio: M1:F1

Occurrence: Thirty-eight cases have been reported in the literature of which 19 were familial and 19 sporadic.

Risk of Recurrence for Patient's Sib:
See Part I, *Mendelian Inheritance.*

Risk of Recurrence for Patient's Child:
See Part I, *Mendelian Inheritance.*

Age of Detectability: At birth.

Gene Mapping and Linkage: Unknown.

Prevention: None known. Genetic counseling indicated.

Treatment: Plastic surgery to scalp, if required, and appropriate surgery and/or prosthesis for limbs. Helmet for head when engaged in physical activities if marked dilation of scalp veins is present.

Prognosis: Normal life span and intelligence. Variable for function.

Detection of Carrier: Unknown.

References:

Adams FH, Oliver CP: Hereditary deformities in man due to arrested development. J Hered 1945; 36:3–7.
Scribanu N, Temtamy SA: Syndrome of aplasia cutis congenita with terminal transverse defects of limbs. J Pediatr 1975; 87:79–82. †
Gellis SS: Constrictive bands in the human. BD:OAS;XIII(1). New York: March of Dimes Birth Defects Foundation, 1977:259–268.
McMurray BR, et al.: Hereditary aplasia cutis congenita and associated defects: three instances in one family and a survey of reported cases. Clin Pediatr 1977; 16:610–614.
Bonafede RP, Beighton P: Autosomal dominant inheritance of scalp defects with ectrodactyly. Am J Med Genet 1979; 3:35–41.
Shapiro SD, Escobedo MK: Terminal transverse defects with aplasia

cutis congenita (Adams-Oliver syndrome). BD:OAS;XXI(2). New York: March of Dimes Birth Defects Foundation, 1985:135–142.

Pauli RM, et al.: Familial recurrence of terminal transverse defects of the arm. Clin Genet 1985; 27:555–563.

Sybert VP: Aplasia cutis congenita: a report of 12 new families and review of the literature. Pediatr Dermatol 1985; 3:1–14. * †

Fryns JP: Congenital scalp defects with distal limb reduction anomalies. J Med Genet 1987; 24:493–496.

Kuster W, et al.: Congenital scalp defects with distal limb anomalies (Adams-Oliver syndrome): report of ten cases and review of the literature. Am J Med Genet 1988; 31:99–115.

SC052
GU008

Nina Scribanu
Alan E. Guttmacher

Limb anomalies (upper)-Waardenburg syndrome
See WAARDENBURG SYNDROMES

LIMB DEFECT WITH ABSENT ULNA/FIBULA   2822

Includes:
    Fibular and ulnar absence with severe limb deficiency
    Limb deficiency-thoracic dystrophy-unusual facies
    Ulnar and fibular absence with severe limb deficiency

Excludes:
    Fibula, congenital absence of (2229)
    Mesomelic dysplasia, Reinhardt-Pfeiffer type (0648)
    Roberts syndrome (0875)

Major Diagnostic Criteria: Absent ulnae and fibulae, hypoplastic femora, absence of some ulnar and foot rays. Minor facial abnormalities with thoracic and pelvic dystrophy.

Clinical Findings: Defects are evident at birth with severe deficiency of the four limbs, less severe in the upper limbs. Elbow joints have not functioned, with contracture deformities at the site with absent ulna and some ulnar rays in both hands. Absence defects are variable. Nails are absent or vestigial. The lower limbs are useless, and the appendages very short, consisting of one deformed long bone (tibia) and rudimentary or absent femora with some tarsal bones and foot rays. The anomalies in both lower limbs are also variable. The patients' facies are unusual and looked different from their parents and normal sibs. Facies are elongated with a broad nasal bridge and bulbous nose, epicanthic folds, and broad necks. Development and intelligence is normal.

Complications: Thoracic dystrophy with barrel-shaped chest and prominent sternum, thoracic kyphosis, lumbar lordosis, and marked pelvic deformities. Patients tend to be shy.

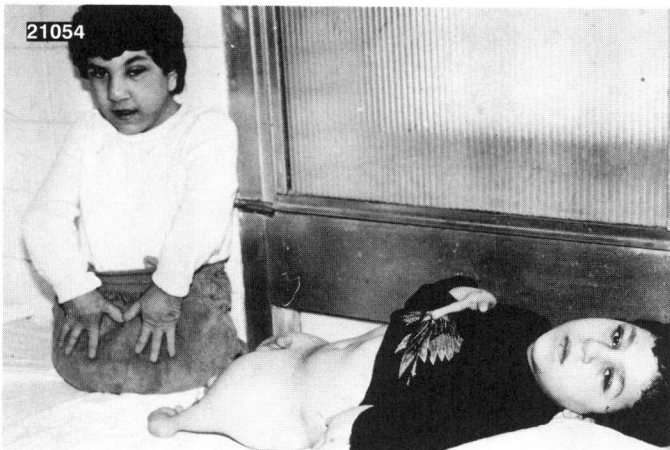

2822A-21054: Severe lower limb deficiencies with milder upper limb defects and mildly dysmorphic facies.

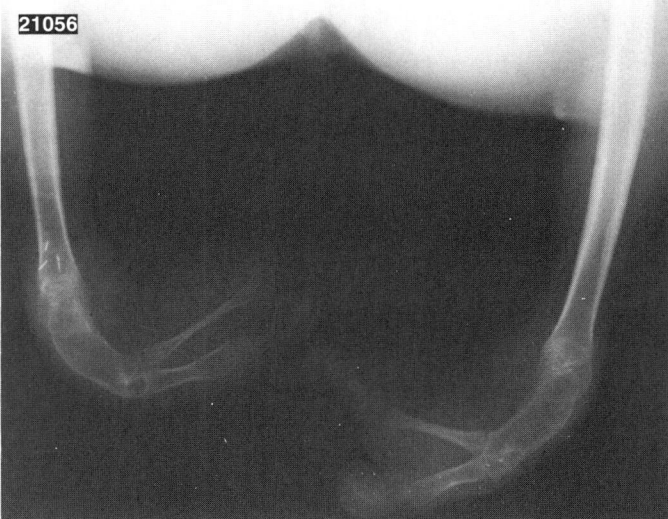

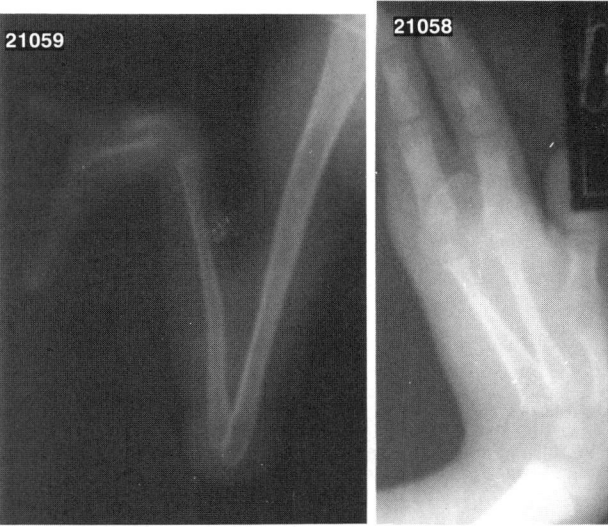

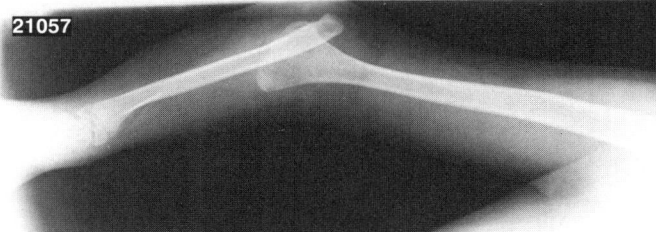

2822B-21056-59: Note the degree and severity of the absence defects in these limbs.

Associated Findings: None known.

Etiology: Probable autosomal recessive inheritance, based on parental consanguinity and affected sibs of both sexes. Expression is variable.

Pathogenesis: Unknown.

MIM No.: 27682

POS No.: 3294

Sex Ratio: Presumably M1:F1.

Occurrence: A brother and sister of consanguineous Palestinian Arab parents have been documented, and at least two other Jewish patients have been reported. A similar phenotype restricted to the lower limbs has been reported in a man from the endogamous Malay community of Cape Town (a relative of a patient with rhizomelic dysplasia reported in Viljoen et al, 1987). This is *not* a private syndrome and may be diagnosed in isolates with a high rate of intermarriage.

Risk of Recurrence for Patient's Sib:
See Part I, *Mendelian Inheritance*.

Risk of Recurrence for Patient's Child:
See Part I, *Mendelian Inheritance*.

Age of Detectability: Clinically evident at birth. Prenatal diagnosis is feasible by ultrasonography which can be performed in the second trimester.

Gene Mapping and Linkage: Unknown.

Prevention: None known. Genetic counseling indicated.

Treatment: Rehabilitation and physical therapy, artificial limbs.

Prognosis: Probably normal for life span. Physical handicaps lead to a change in life-style. Intelligence is normal.

Detection of Carrier: Unknown.

References:
Pfeiffer RA: Bectrag Zur erblichen Verkuerzung von Ulna und Fibula. In: Wiedemann HR, ed: Dysostosen. Stuttgart: Gustav Fischer Verlag, 1966.

Langer LO Jr: Mesomelic dwarfism of the hypoplastic ulna, fibula, mandible type. Radiology 1967; 89:654–660.

Al-Awadi SA, et al.: Profound limb deficiency, thoracic dystrophy, unusual facies, and normal intelligence: a new syndrome. J Med Genet 1985; 22:36–38.

Viljoen D, et al.: Familial rhizomelic dysplasia: phenotypic variation or heterogeneity? Am J Med Genet 1987; 62:941–947.

AL030
TE012

S. A. Al-Awadi
Ahmad S. Teebi

Limb deficiency-splenogonadal fusion
See SPLENOGONADAL FUSION-LIMB DEFECT
Limb deficiency-thoracic dystrophy-unusual facies
See LIMB DEFECT WITH ABSENT ULNA/FIBULA
Limb malformations-dento-digital syndrome
See LACRIMO-AURICULO-DENTO-DIGITAL SYNDROME

LIMB REDUCTION DEFECTS   3285

Includes:
Amelia
Amputation, congenital
Central ray defects
Dysmelia
Hemimelia
Hypoplasia, limb
Intercalary defects
Limb, absence of
Micromelia
Phocomelia
Reduction defects of limb
Terminal longitudinal defects
Terminal transverse defects

Excludes:
Amniotic bands syndrome (ADAM complex) (0874)
Hand, radial club hand (2409)
Hand, ulnar and fibular ray deficiency, Weyers type (2292)
Hand, ulnar drift (2410)
Poland syndrome (0813)
Skeletal dysplasia
Thrombocytopenia-absent radius (0941)
Limb defects, syndromes with (other)

Major Diagnostic Criteria: Complete or partial absence of a limb bone or bones.

Clinical Findings: Limb reduction defects are heterogeneous defects that range from mild absence of a limb bone to total absence of the limb (amelia). Several classifications systems exist but none has gained universal acceptance. In general, defects can be divided into *amelia*, i.e. total absence of a limb, or *meromelia*, i.e. partial absence of a limb. Partial absence is further classified as being either terminal or intercalary. A *terminal defect* is characterized by partial or total absence of limb bones distal from the defect named, i.e. no normal parts exist distal to the defect. An *intercalary defect* consists of partial or total absence of the proximal or distal segments of a limb with significant or relatively normal distal parts. The distal parts need not be completely normal.

Defects are further subclassified as *transverse*, i.e. the defect extends across the total width of the limb, or *longitudinal*, i.e. the defect occurs lengthwise along the limb. If known, the precise missing bone is included in the classification.

Hypoplasia is a term used to describe a generalized reduction in limb size when the defect can not easily be identified more specifically. *Central ray defects* are used to describe defects of the 2, 3 and 4th phalanges. *Phocomelia* is used to describe limbs with relatively normal distal parts and absent or nearly absent proximal and medial parts.

Terminal transverse defects are more common than transverse longitudinal defects. Seventy-five percent of limb defects involve the upper limb, 25% the lower limb. There is no evidence of a predilection for a particular side.

Complications: Vary with the site and extent of the defect.

Associated Findings: About half of affected individuals have other defects, usually in the muscular skeletal system, e.g. **Foot, congenital clubfoot**, dislocated hip, and congenital contracture. Other systems that may have associated congential defects include the cardiovascular system, the gastrointestinal system, and the genitourinary system.

Etiology: Unknown. Probably heterogeneous. A vascular accident is also a possible etiology.

Pathogenesis: Unknown.

Sex Ratio: M>1:F1.

Occurrence: 5.97:10,000 live births (1:1,1692 live births) in British Columbia.

Risk of Recurrence for Patient's Sib: Unknown. In the British Columbia study, 6.5% had another family member with a limb defect.

Risk of Recurrence for Patient's Child: Unknown.

Age of Detectability: By ultrasound examination at 16 weeks gestation. Most are apparent at birth or within the first year of life.

Gene Mapping and Linkage: Unknown.

Prevention: None known. Genetic counseling indicated.

Treatment: Orthopedic, rehabilitative, and reconstructive therapy is indicated depending on the nature and extent of the defect.

Prognosis: Death occurs in 12.9–20% within the first year of life, but of these, 85% had additional defects. Overall prognosis depends on the size and location of the defect.

Detection of Carrier: Unknown.

References:
Frantz CH, O'Rahilly R: Congenital skeletal limb deficiency. J Bone Joint Surg 1961; 430A:1202–1224.

Henkel L, et al.: Dysmelia: a classification and a pattern of malformation in a group of congenital defects of the limbs. J Bone Joint Surg 1969; 51B:399–414.

Smith ESO, et al.: An epidemiological study of congenital reduction deformities of the limbs. Br J Prev Soc Med 1977; 31:39–41.

Kallen B, et al.: Infants with congenital limb reduction registered in the Swedish register of congenital malformations. Teratology 1984; 29:73–85.

Froster-Iskenius, UG, Baird P: Limb reductions defects in over one million consecutive livebirths. Teratology 1989; 39:127–135.

BU032   **Mary Louise Buyse**

LIMB REDUCTION-ICHTHYOSIS   2019

Includes:

    CHILD syndrome
    Ectromelia, unilateral-psoriasis-CNS anomalies
    Hemidysplasia-ichthyosis, congenital
    Ichthyosiform erythryoderma, unilateral-ipsilateral
      malformations
    Ichthyosis-limb reduction
    Limbs, absence deformity of-ichthyosiform erythryoderma

Excludes:

    Chondrodysplasia punctata
    Incontinentia pigmenti (0526)
    Nevus, epidermal nevus syndrome (0593)

Major Diagnostic Criteria: Unilateral skin erythema and scaling, with ipsilateral limb defects.

Clinical Findings: All affected individuals have unilateral ichthyosiform erythroderma affecting the trunk and limbs, but generally sparing the face. The nails are often hyperkeratotic, and alopecia occasionally occurs on the same side. Ipsilateral limb anomalies, ranging from hypoplastic phalanges and metacarpals to absent limbs, are also a constant finding. Skeletal hypoplasia of the trunk and head also occur, but less consistently. Ipsilateral visceral anomalies are also common, and include unilateral brain hypoplasia, cardiac defects, unilateral renal agenesis, and unilateral lung hypoplasia. Punctate calcification of the cartilage on X-rays disappears by two years of age. Histologic examination has shown acanthotic epidermis with thickened, parakeratotic stratum corneum, and a broadened or absent granular layer. In 20 affected individuals, the right side was affected in 14, and the left in six. A few individuals also had skin lesions, skeletal anomalies, and/or visceral defects on the contralateral side.

Complications: Scoliosis may occur as a result of either limb asymmetry or vertebral defects. Mild mental retardation, presumably secondary to unilateral brain hypoplasia, has also been reported.

Associated Findings: **Cleft lip**, bilateral mild hearing loss, **Hernia, umbilical**, **Hydrocephaly**, and **Meningomyelocele** have each been reported as occasional findings.

Etiology: Possibly X-linked dominant inheritance.

Pathogenesis: The basic gene defect is unknown. Lyonization is unable to account for the unilateral distribution of anomalies without invoking an auxiliary hypothesis.

MIM No.: 30805

POS No.: 3457

CDC No.: 755.2

Sex Ratio: M1:F28

Occurrence: At least 29 cases from different parts of the world have been described.

Risk of Recurrence for Patient's Sib:
    See Part I, *Mendelian Inheritance.*

Risk of Recurrence for Patient's Child:
    See Part I, *Mendelian Inheritance.*

Age of Detectability: At birth, by the presence of limb defects. Severe limb defects may also be detectable in utero by ultrasound. Skin defects are usually present at or soon after birth, but may not appear until later.

Gene Mapping and Linkage: Unknown.

Prevention: None known. Genetic counseling indicated.

Treatment: Topical skin ointment occasionally improves the skin condition; orthopedic treatment may also be indicated.

Prognosis: If visceral anomalies are not present, then life span is not affected. Intellectual development is usually normal, although mild mental retardation has also been reported. The skin condition can improve, or alternatively can improve and worsen.

Detection of Carrier: Unknown.

References:
Cullen SI, et al.: Congenital unilateral ichthyosiform erythroderma. Arch Dermatol 1969; 99:724–729. †
Tang TT, McCreadie SR: Congenital hemidysplasia with ichthyosis. BD:OAS X(5). New York: March of Dimes Birth Defects Foundation, 1974::257–260.
Happle R, et al.: The CHILD syndrome. Europ J Pediatr 1980; 134:27–33. *
Wettke-Schafer R, Kantner G: X-linked dominant inherited diseases with lethality in hemizygous males. Hum Genet 1983; 64:1–23.
Hebert AA, et al.: The CHILD syndrome: histologic and ultrastructural studies. Arch Derm 1987; 123:503–509.

T0007   **Helga V. Toriello**

LIMB REDUCTION-MENTAL RETARDATION   3128

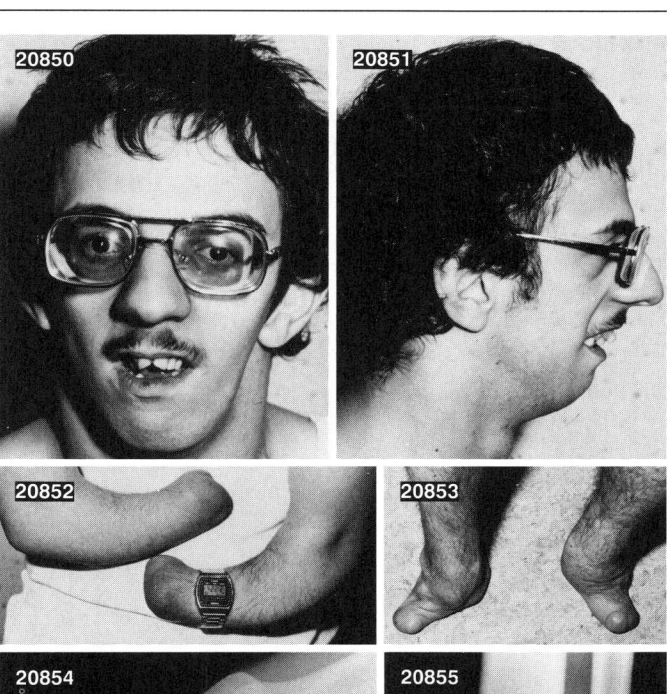

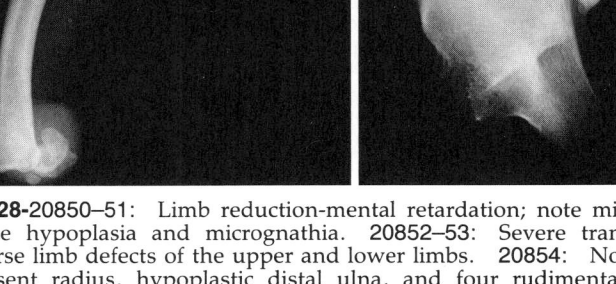

3128-20850–51: Limb reduction-mental retardation; note midface hypoplasia and micrognathia. 20852–53: Severe transverse limb defects of the upper and lower limbs. 20854: Note absent radius, hypoplastic distal ulna, and four rudimentary carpal bones. 20855: Synostosis of the rudimentary calcaneus and talus.

Includes: Mental retardation-limb deficiency

Excludes: **Hypoglossia-hypodactylia** (0451)

Major Diagnostic Criteria: The combination of transverse limb reduction defect, oral anomalies, and mental retardation.

Clinical Findings: In the reported sibs (one male, one female), both had limb anomalies of all extremities, with the limb defects resembling transverse terminal defects, but actually being a paraxial radial/preaxial limb defect. In addition, both had maxillary hypoplasia, micrognathia, small mouth with highly arched palate, normal tongue, and mild-to-moderate mental retardation. One sib also had myopia and oligomeganephronia; the other also had short stature.

Complications: Unknown.

Associated Findings: None known.

Etiology: Possibly autosomal recessive inheritance.

Pathogenesis: Unknown.

Sex Ratio: M1:F1

Occurrence: Documented in one pair of Greek sibs.

Risk of Recurrence for Patient's Sib:
See Part I, *Mendelian Inheritance.*

Risk of Recurrence for Patient's Child:
See Part I, *Mendelian Inheritance.*

Age of Detectability: At birth, although prenatal diagnosis using ultrasound may be possible.

Gene Mapping and Linkage: Unknown.

Prevention: None known. Genetic counseling indicated.

Treatment: Orthopedic intervention for the limb defects.

Prognosis: Mental retardation is variable, being mild in one sib and moderate in the other. Life span is presumably normal.

Detection of Carrier: Unknown.

References:
Buttiens M, Fryns JP: Apparently new autosomal recessive syndrome of mental retardation, distal limb deficiencies, oral involvement, and possible renal defect. Am J Med Genet 1987; 27:651–660.

T0007

Helga V. Toriello

Limb, absence of
See LIMB REDUCTION DEFECTS

LIMB, REDUCTION DEFORMITIES OF UPPER LIMBS   2885

Includes: Bone aplasias-hypoplasias of the upper extremities

Excludes: **Acheiropody** (2486)

Major Diagnostic Criteria: Multiple, extensive, and variable reduction deformities of the upper limbs.

Clinical Findings: Unilateral amelia; unilateral amelia with bidactyly; modification of the configuration of the articular elements of the shoulder and elbow, bowed humerus, aplasia of radius (with associated defects such as a short, thick, and bent ulna), absence of some carpal bones, absence of the first radial ray and manus vara; hypoplasia of the humerus, whose remaining part (with irregular contours) is disarticulated from the glenoid fossa, aplasia of the radius, bowed ulna, absence of some carpal bones, absence of first and second radial rays, and manus vara; hypoplasia of both clavicles and scapulas, absence of the glenoid fossae, unilateral amelia, presence of a rounded prominence constituted of soft tissues; unilateral amelia with the presence of only one finger with two phalanges, and some bones without precise X-ray characteristics.

Complications: The highly mutilating nature of this anomaly may affect social life and marriage.

Associated Findings: None known.

Etiology: Reduction deformities of the limbs are generally sporadic and due to unknown etiology. However, a minority of them

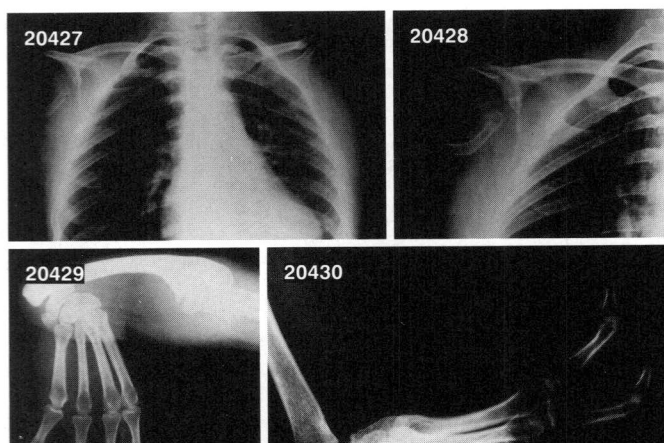

2885-20427: X-ray of an affected woman; note total absence of the left arm and a few remaining bones of the right arm (see fig. 20428). **20428:** Detail of the remaining left arm of an affected woman. **20429:** Right forearm and hand of an affected man; note absence of radius; short, thick and bent ulna; absence of five carpal bones and of the first radial ray; and manus vara. **20430:** Left forearm and hand of the man shown in fig. 20429; note the absence of first and second radial rays, and manus vara among other defects.

are due to either autosomal dominant or autosomal recessive inheritance.

Pathogenesis: Unknown.

Sex Ratio: Presumably M1:F1.

Occurrence: One Brazilian kindred with two men and two women belonging to three sibships has been reported in the literature.

Risk of Recurrence for Patient's Sib:
See Part I, *Mendelian Inheritance.* Recurrence risk ranges from a low of zero to 25–50% for reduction deformities in general.

Risk of Recurrence for Patient's Child:
See Part I, *Mendelian Inheritance.*

Age of Detectability: At birth, or prenatally by ultrasound.

Gene Mapping and Linkage: Unknown.

Prevention: None known. Genetic counseling indicated.

Treatment: Orthopedic care as indicated.

Prognosis: Normal for life span and reproduction. Three of the four affected individuals married and had children.

Detection of Carrier: A heterozygote was born with aplasia of the right thumb and the corresponding metacarpal.

References:
Birch-Jensen A: Congenital deformities of the upper extremities. Copenhagen: Ejnar Munksgaard, 1949.
Freire-Maia N, et al.: Hereditary bone aplasias and hypoplasias of the extremities. Acta Genet Stat Med 1959; 9:33–40.
Freire-Maia N, Freire-Maia A: Multiple congenital abnormalities. Lancet 1964; I:113–114.
Freire-Maia N, Freire-Maia A: Recurrence risks of bone aplasias and hypoplasias of the extremities. Acta Genet Stat Med 1967; 17:418–421.
Freire-Maia N, Azevedo JBC: Skeletal limb deficiencies. Lancet 1968; II:1296 only.
Freire-Maia N: Congenital skeletal limb deficiencies: a general view. BD:OAS V(3). New York: March of Dimes Birth Defects Foundation, 1969:7–13.

Freire-Maia N: A heterozygote expression of a "recessive" gene? Hum Hered 1975; 25:302–304.

FR033   **Newton Freire-Maia**

LIMB, UPPER HYPOPLASIA-MULLERIAN DUCT DEFECTS   2932

Includes:
> Hypomelia with Mullerian duct anomalies
> Limb-uterus syndrome
> Mullerian duct defects-upper limb hypoplasia
> Uterus-limb syndrome

Excludes:
> **Acro-renal-mandibular syndrome** (2778)
> **Aredyld syndrome** (2785)
> Camptobrachydactyly
> Cryptophthalmos
> **Ectrodactyly-ectodermal dysplasia-clefting syndrome** (0337)
> **Hand-foot-genital syndrome** (2570)
> **Meckel syndrome** (0634)
> **Renal-genital-middle ear anomalies** (0860)
> **Vaginal septum, transverse** (0985)

Major Diagnostic Criteria: Upper limb hypoplasia with Müllerian duct anomalies.

Clinical Findings: The association of upper limb anomalies with genital defects was described in five members of a French Canadian family. Two of the three affected women had upper limb anomalies and Müllerian duct defects, and one had only a Müllerian duct anomaly. The two affected males had both upper limb or acral malformation, and one had a genital anomaly (micropenis). Limb anomalies varied in expression from postaxial **Polydactyly,** to ectrodactyly (ulnar ray defect), to severe upper limb hypoplasia with split hand. Genital anomalies varied from a complete duplication of the uterus and vagina in two individuals, to only a vaginal septum in one female.

All affected individuals examined had a distal loop in the hallucal area, two had a hypothenar pattern, and one had distal axial triradii.

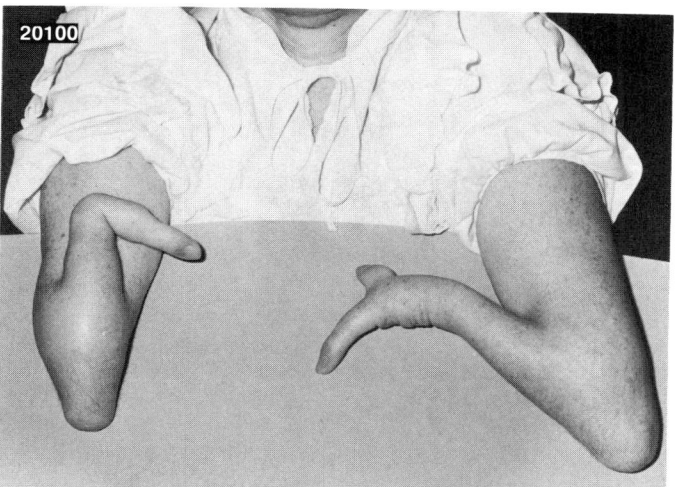

2932-20100: The hypoplastic forearms are tightly flexed over the arms. On the right, she has one digit with fixed radial deviation and on the left she has a split hand with a thumb and one other digit.

Complications: The two individuals with split hand had hypoplastic forearms. The latter were tightly flexed over the arms, allowing very little passive and active extension.

Associated Findings: Bilateral mild tubular ectasia in one individual. Hypothyroidic goiter in one affected female and euthyroidic goiter in another.

Etiology: Probably autosomal dominant inheritance with variable expressivity.

Pathogenesis: Unknown.

MIM No.: 14616

POS No.: 3896

CDC No.: 755.2

Sex Ratio: Presumably M1:F1 (M2:F3 observed).

Occurrence: Reported in five members of three generations of a French Canadian family.

Risk of Recurrence for Patient's Sib:
> See Part I, *Mendelian Inheritance.*

Risk of Recurrence for Patient's Child:
> See Part I, *Mendelian Inheritance.*

Age of Detectability: At birth. Prenatal diagnosis of limb anomalies is possible by ultrasonography.

Gene Mapping and Linkage: Unknown.

Prevention: None known. Genetic counseling indicated.

Treatment: Prosthetic replacement of severely malformed limbs.

Prognosis: Normal life span.

Detection of Carrier: Gynecologic examination of female relatives for evidence of the trait (vaginal or uterine septum), since Müllerian duct anomaly can be present without limb defects.

References:
Halal F: A new syndrome of severe upper limb hypoplasia and Müllerian duct anomalies. Am J Med Genet 1986; 24:119–126.

HA074   **Fahed Halal**

Limb-blood syndrome
> *See WT SYNDROME*

Limb-face syndrome (one form)
> *See CHARLIE M SYNDROME*

Limb-girdle muscular dystrophy
> *See MUSCULAR DYSTROPHY, LIMB-GIRDLE*

LIMB-OTO-CARDIAC SYNDROME   0592

Includes:
> Cardiac-limb-oto syndrome
> Facioauriculoradial dysplasia
> Oto-limb-cardiac syndrome
> Phocomelia-ectrodactyly-oto-sinus arrhythmia syndrome

Excludes:
> **Fetal thalidomide syndrome** (0386)
> **Heart-hand syndrome** (0455)
> **Acrofacial dysostosis, Nager type** (2167)

Major Diagnostic Criteria: Hypoplasia of upper limbs, malformed external ear, conduction deafness, vertebral anomalies.

Clinical Findings: Dysmorphic facial features include mid-face hypoplasia, a long philtrum, and flattened nasal bridge. Hypoplasia of the upper limbs, sinus arrhythmia, malformed external ears, profound conduction deafness, and vertebral anomalies have been reported in two families. The malformation of the upper limbs is characterized by the absence of the radius, hypoplasia of the humerus, and metacarpophalangeal hypoplasia. Lumbar vertebral abnormalities and fibular hypoplasia have been variably present. Short stature was present in two instances. Malformation of the middle ear was characterized by the absence of the incus and stapes and an aplasia of the oval window.

Complications: Unknown.

Associated Findings: None known.

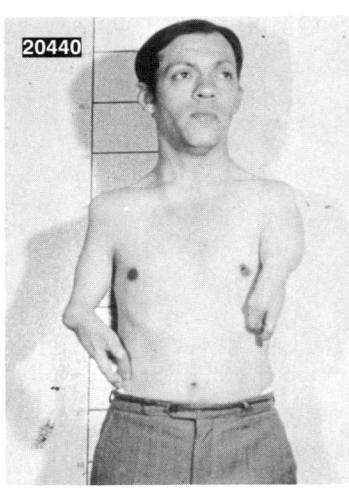
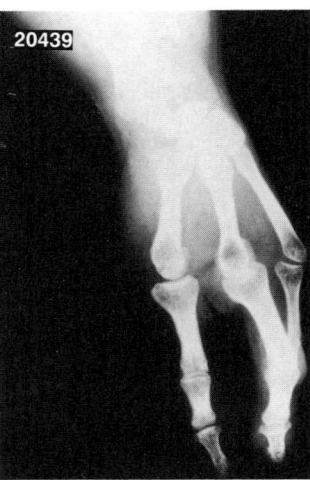

0592-20440: Hypoplasia of the upper limbs. 20439: Absent carpals, metacarpals, and digits.

Etiology: Presumably autosomal dominant inheritance.

Pathogenesis: Unknown.

MIM No.: 17148

POS No.: 3280

Sex Ratio: M2:F3

Occurrence: Two reported families with two affected males, a father and son, and three females (two sisters and one daughter).

Risk of Recurrence for Patient's Sib:
See Part I, *Mendelian Inheritance.*

Risk of Recurrence for Patient's Child:
See Part I, *Mendelian Inheritance.*

Age of Detectability: Limb anomalies may be detectable by ultrasound or fetoscope prenatally; otherwise at birth.

Gene Mapping and Linkage: Unknown.

Prevention: None known. Genetic counseling indicated.

Treatment: Surgery. Because of the absence of the oval window, reconstructive middle ear surgery was impossible in these cases. Arrhythmias reported in some cases may be normal sinus arrhythmias.

Prognosis: Probably normal life span; intelligence is normal.

Detection of Carrier: Unknown.

References:
Stoll C, et al.: L'association phocomélie-ectrodactylie, malformations des oreilles avec surdité, arythmie sinusale: constitue-t-elle un nouveau syndrome héréditaire? Arch Fr Pediatr 1974; 31:669–680.
Harding AE, et al.: Autosomal asymmetric radial dysplasia, dysmorphic facies, and conductive hearing loss (facioauriculoradial dysplasia). J Med Genet 1982; 19:110–115.

MU020

Jeff Murray
Cor W.R.J. Cremers

LIMBS, SUPERNUMERARY   2494

Includes:
    Limbs, duplicated
    Limbs, ectopic
    Twins, parasitic conjoined without spinal columns

Excludes:
    Spinal tail
    Twins, conjoined (0202)

Major Diagnostic Criteria: An extra limb, including all tissue layers, long bones with an intercalated joint, and a terminal digital structure, in the absence of duplication of the spinal column.

Clinical Findings: The most common situation, conjoined twins with duplications of the spinal cord, is excluded as representing a complete central duplication. Otherwise, extra limbs are unusual, but can be seen in several situations: 1) So-called "parasitic conjoined twins" which typically involve bilateral (although not always symmetrical) limbs on both sides of the midline, but lack any indications of a head or spinal column. 2) Duplicated limbs, which are unilateral and in situ. They may be relatively complete, polydactylous, or abortive with only a few digits. There is no duplication of spinal elements. 3) True ectopic limbs, which are single midline posterior structures. Again, they may be relatively complete or terminally abortive or polydactylous.

Complications: Those due to mechanical problems from the physical presence of the extra limb(s).

Associated Findings: Other midline problems are common. Heart and spinal anomalies, and teratomatous structures ranging

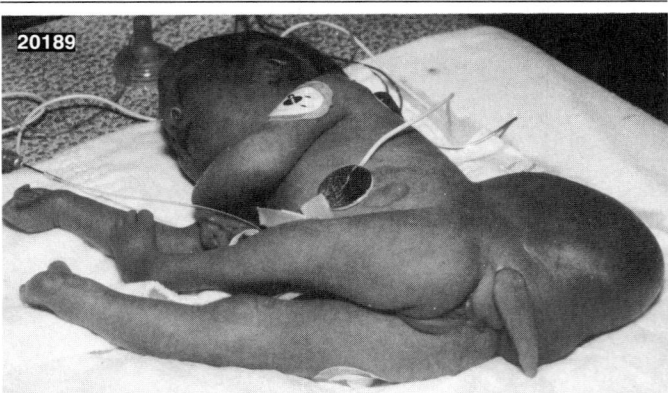
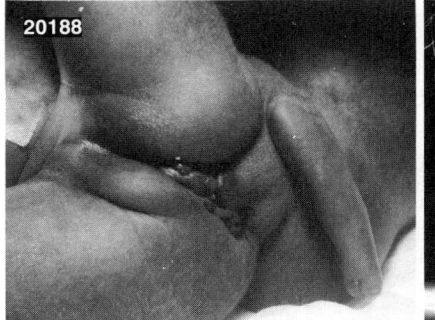
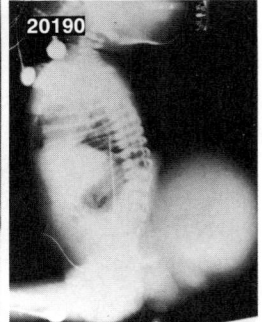

2494-20189: The additional limb is attached to the myelomeningocele sac. 20188: Additional limb and duplication of the external genitalia. 20190: X-ray view of the third limb and the myelomeningocele sac.

from dermoid cysts to malignant teratomas can be seen, mostly with types 2 and 3.

Etiology: Unknown. Maternal trauma has been suggested, but is unproved. Factors predisposing to duplications or midline disruptions may be involved.

Pathogenesis: For parasitic conjoined twins, duplication of the Wolffian ridges has been suggested. However, the origins of the bilaterality of these structures is difficult to understand under this hypothesis. A spectrum including "typical" conjoined twins is possible, but it is likely that these are pathogenetically different. Duplications in situ often are found with vertebral defects and may represent the induction of a second limb bud near the site of the first. True ectopic limbs are difficult to explain with any variant of normal embryology. Their invariable midline location suggests a pathogenetic relationship that somehow involves this area. A case of formed digits with nails, phalanges, and metacarpals within a sacrococcygeal teratoma is instructive; nerves to the digits came from the sacral nerves of the host. Teratomas are certainly capable of full differentiation given the proper circumstances. Rarely, this may occur in situ, perhaps with an atypical inductive stimulus supplied by a disrupted spinal cord.

Sex Ratio: Undetermined but presumably M1:F1.

Occurrence: Undetermined but presumed rare.

Risk of Recurrence for Patient's Sib: Unknown, but there are no reported familial cases.

Risk of Recurrence for Patient's Child: Unknown.

Age of Detectability: Presumably prenatally by ultrasound, although interpretation would probably be very difficult.

Gene Mapping and Linkage: Unknown.

Prevention: None known. Genetic counseling indicated.

Treatment: Surgical removal and repair of the primary anomaly and of any associated problems. Awareness of possible malignant teratoma.

Prognosis: Depends on associated anomalies. Reports of unoperated cases indicate that long-term survival and good overall function are possible, although obviously psychosocial difficulties can be great.

Detection of Carrier: Unknown.

Special Considerations: These are rare and poorly characterized anomalies about which little is certain. The relationship to other teratologia, such as conjoined twins and midline "tails", is unknown. Any cases should be well studied anatomically and reported if possible.

A possible mouse model for these anomalies is the semidominant mutant, Disorganization. This gene causes a wide range of anomalies, including limb duplications and hamartomas. The latter often resembled limbs and digits. Extra limbs can be seen, usually close to normal limbs, but limb-like projections can be found elsewhere, particularly on the ventral abdomen.

References:
Nicholson GW: A sacro-coccygeal teratoma with three metacarpal bones and digits. Guy's Hosp Rep 1937; 87:46.
Hummel KP: Developmental anomalies in mice resulting from action of the gene, disorganization, a semi-dominant lethal. Pediatrics 1959; 23:212.
Stephens TD, et al.: Parasitic conjoined twins, two cases, and their relation to limb morphogenesis. Teratology 1982; 26:115.
Saul RA, Stevenson RE: Limb amputation/autotransplantation: follow-up. Proc Greenwood Genet Cen 1985; 4:78.

LU001   **Mark Lubinsky**

Limit dextrinosis
See GLYCOGENOSIS, TYPE III
Lindau disease
See VON HIPPEL-LINDAU SYNDROME
Linear nevus sebaceous syndrome
See NEVUS, EPIDERMAL NEVUS SYNDROME
Linear porokeratosis
See SKIN, POROKERATOSIS

Linear sebaceous nevus syndrome
See NEVUS, EPIDERMAL NEVUS SYNDROME
Linear sebaceous nevus-mental retardation-seizures
See PROTEUS SYNDROME
Lingua fissurata types I, II, and III
See TONGUE, FISSURED
Lingua plicata
See TONGUE, GEOGRAPHIC
Lingual thyroid
See THYROGLOSSAL DUCT REMNANT
Lip pits or mounds and cleft lip or palate
See CLEFT LIP/PALATE-LIP PITS OR MOUNDS

LIP, CHEILITIS GLANDULARIS   0144

Includes:

Baelz syndrome
Cheilitis glandularis apostematosa
Lip, enlargement of lower

Excludes:

Blepharochalasis-double lip-nontoxic goiter (0111)
Cheilitis exfolitiva
Cheilitis granulomatosa, Melkersson-Rosenthal type (2083)

Major Diagnostic Criteria: Enlargement of lower lip, increased secretion of mucus, vesicle-like lesions, or palpable enlargement of mucous glands.

Clinical Findings: There is enlargement of the lower lip and increased secretion of mucus on the lower lip, resulting in a wet, sticky lip; collection of mucus in dilated mucous ducts beneath the mucosa gives vesicle-like cystic lesions; there is protrusion and eversion of the lower lip; and nodular enlargement of mucous glands of the lip can be detected by palpation. All of these features are present in the well-developed stage, but earlier changes consist of enlargement of the lower lip and excess mucous secretion with or without vesicle-like lesions.

Complications: Mucous cyst (mucocele) formation is due to traumatic rupture of mucous ducts, and this complication is common. In Caucasians, 18–35% of patients reported with cheilitis glandularis have developed squamous cell carcinoma. This complication is due presumably to protrusion of the lip, making it susceptible to solar radiation and other irritations such as smoking. Secondary bacterial infection may occur with fistula formation.

Associated Findings: None known.

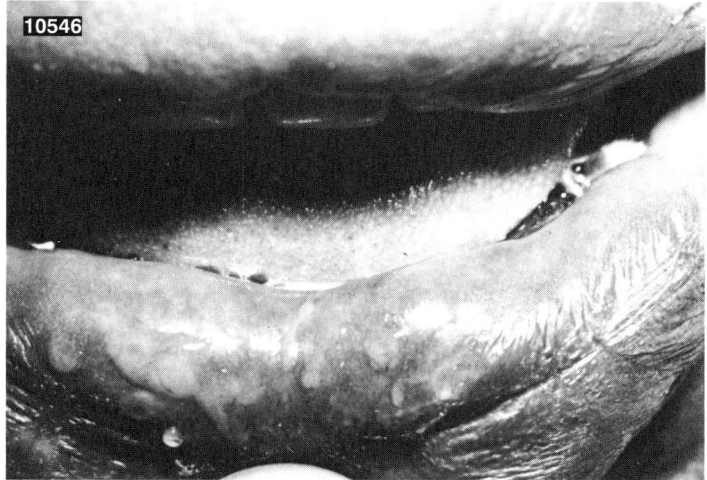

0144-10546: Cheilitis glandularis.

Etiology: Possibly autosomal dominant inheritance. The majority of patients with cheilitis glandularis recognized in the past have not been reported as having a hereditary form of the disease.

Pathogenesis: The gross structural defect in the fully developed condition includes enlargement of lower lip two to four times normal size, enlargement of mucous glands up to 12 mm in size, dilation of the mucous ducts in the mucosa or submucosa, a marked hypertrophy of the mucous glands, chronic inflammation involving the stroma of the mucous glands consisting mainly of plasma cells and fibrosis, and edema of the stroma. It is probable that the glandular hypertrophy with increased mucous secretion occurs as the initial change, with secondary changes of partial obstruction resulting in dilatation of ducts and inflammation.

MIM No.: 11833

CDC No.: 750.270

Sex Ratio: Presumably M1:F1 (males predominate in reported cases).

Occurrence: Over one hundred cases reported.

Risk of Recurrence for Patient's Sib:
See Part I, *Mendelian Inheritance.*

Risk of Recurrence for Patient's Child:
See Part I, *Mendelian Inheritance.*

Age of Detectability: Usually between 5 and 10 years by enlargement of lower lip, increased mucous secretion of lip, and vesicle-like lesions.

Gene Mapping and Linkage: Unknown.

Prevention: None known. Genetic counseling indicated.

Treatment: Partial excision of the lower lip with removal of enlarged mucous glands. This will prevent complications and give a cosmetically and functionally satisfactory result.

Prognosis: If treated, there is minimal morbidity and normal life span. If untreated, complications may cause moderate morbidity, and if squamous cell carcinoma develops and is not treated, death may occur.

Detection of Carrier: Unknown.

References:
Doku HC, et al.: Cheilitis glandularis. Oral Surg 1965; 20:563–571.
Weir TW, Johnson WC: Cheilitis glandularis. Arch Dermatol 1971; 103:433–437.
Rada DC, et al.: Cheilitis glandularis: a disorder of ductal ectasia. J Dermatol Surg Oncol 1985; 11:4:372–375.

J0009   **Waine C. Johnson**

Lip, cleft
See CLEFT LIP

LIP, DOUBLE   0594

Includes:
Duplicate labiale
Lip, double upper or lower
Midline maxillary double lip

Excludes:
Blepharochalasis-double lip-nontoxic goiter (0111)
Lip, cheilitis glandularis (0144)
Lip, pits or mounds (0596)
Macrocheilia

Major Diagnostic Criteria: The appearance of two vermilion borders of the upper or lower lip when smiling in a patient without blepharochalasis and nontoxic thyroid enlargement.

Clinical Findings: The vermilion border of the lip is divided into two parts by a transverse furrow (horizontal sulcus) so that the inner portion of the lip, the pars villosa, sags below the outer portion, the pars glabra. When the lip is drawn tightly across the teeth in smiling, it gives the impression of two vermilion margins of the lip and two masses of hyperplastic tissue on either side of the midline. In most cases only the upper lip is involved, but

deformity is bilateral and involves the upper lip alone; rarely both upper and lower lips show the deformity. Unilateral and midline deformities have been described.

Complications: May be of cosmetic concern to the patient.

Associated Findings: May occur as one sign of **Blepharochalasis-double lip-nontoxic goiter**.

Etiology: Most cases are sporadic, has been observed in sibs, and autosomal dominant inheritance has been suggested.

Pathogenesis: The defect has ben ascribable to displacement of the orbicularis oris fibers because of hypertrophy of the mucous gland ducts and submucous tissues, resulting in the herniation of submucosa. Endocrine and allergic factors have been postulated.

CDC No.: 750.270

Sex Ratio: M1:F1

Occurrence: Chileans, 1:480; Caucasians in Utah in the United States, 1:200. Overall incidence data is, however, undetermined, and is not assumed to be as high as that shown for Chile and Utah.

Risk of Recurrence for Patient's Sib: Unknown.

Risk of Recurrence for Patient's Child: Unknown.

Age of Detectability: Usually during infancy.

Gene Mapping and Linkage: Unknown.

Prevention: None known. Genetic counseling indicated.

Treatment: Surgery.

Prognosis: Of cosmetic concern only; general health is not impaired.

Detection of Carrier: Unknown.

References:
Guerrero-Santos J, Altamirano JT: The use of W-plasty for correction of double lip deformity. Plast Reconstr Surg 1967; 39:478–481.
Witkop CJ Jr: The face and oral structures. In: Rubin A, ed: Handbook of congenital malformations. Philadelphia: W.B. Saunders, 1967: 103–139.
Rintala AE: Congenital double lip and Ascher syndrome: II. Relationship to the lower lip sinus syndrome. Br J Plast Surg 1981; 34:31–34.
Lamster IB: Mucosal reduction for correction of a maxillary double lip. Oral Surg 1983; 55:457–458.

BL002   **Will Blackburn**

Lip, double upper or lower
See LIP, DOUBLE
Lip, double-blepharochalasis-goiter
See BLEPHAROCHALASIS-DOUBLE LIP-NONTOXIC GOITER
Lip, enlargement of lower
See LIP, CHEILITIS GLANDULARIS
Lip, indentations of upper
See CLEFT LIP

LIP, MEDIAN CLEFT OF UPPER   0595

Includes:
Median cleft of upper lip
True median cleft

Excludes:
Agnathia-holoprosencephaly (2780)
Cebocephaly
Chondroectodermal dysplasia (0156)
Face, median cleft face syndrome (0635)
Oro-facio-digital syndrome (all)

Major Diagnostic Criteria: Midline cleft of the upper lip.

Clinical Findings: Midline cleft of the upper lip.

Complications: Unknown.

Associated Findings: Midline cleft of the upper lip may be present alone, or in association with **Face, median cleft face syndrome**.

Etiology: Unknown.

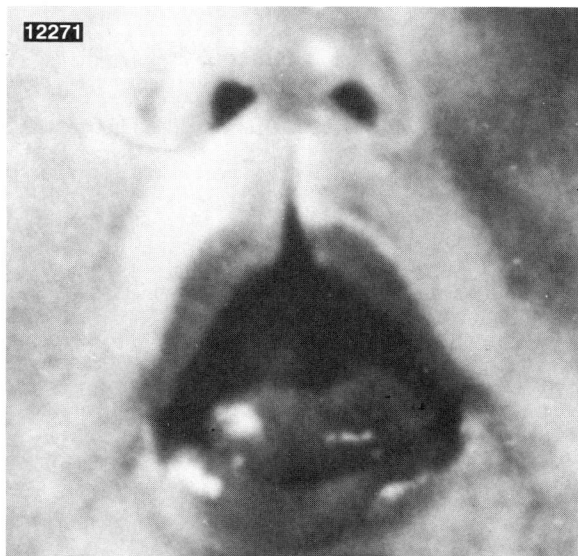

0595-12271: Median cleft of upper lip.

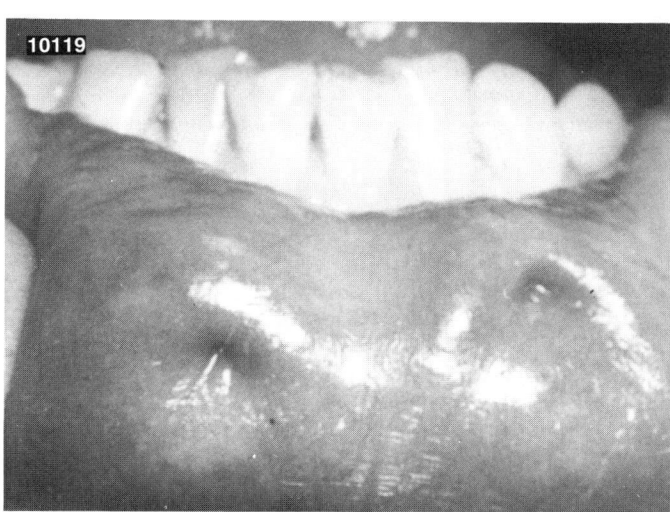

0596-10119: Lower lip pits.

Pathogenesis: Midline mesenchymal filling defect with persistent infranasal furrow.

Sex Ratio: Presumably M1:F1

Occurrence: Undetermined but presumed rare.

Risk of Recurrence for Patient's Sib: Unknown.

Risk of Recurrence for Patient's Child: Unknown.

Age of Detectability: At birth.

Gene Mapping and Linkage: Unknown.

Prevention: None known. Genetic counseling indicated.

Treatment: Surgical closure of the cleft.

Prognosis: Full recovery following surgery.

Detection of Carrier: Unknown.

References:
Millard DR, Williams S: Median lip clefts of the upper lip. Plast & Reconstr Surg 1968; 42:4–14. *
Lehman JA, Cuddapah S: The true hare lip: a case report. Cleft Palate J 1974; 11:497–498. †
Nakamuna J, et al.: True median cleft of the upper lip associated with three pedunculated club-shaped skin masses. Plast Reconst Surg 1985; 75:727–731.

J0027

Ronald J. Jorgenson
Hermine M. Pashayan

LIP, PITS OR MOUNDS   0596

Includes:
   Commissural lip pits (isolated trait)
   Paramedian pits of lower lip (isolated trait)
   Pits of upper lip

Excludes:
   Cleft lip/palate-filiform fusion of eyelids (0176)
   Cleft lip/palate-lip pits or mounds (0177)
   Oro-facio-digital syndrome (0770)
   Pterygium syndrome, popliteal (0818)

Major Diagnostic Criteria: Presence of pits on the vermilion border of lips.

Clinical Findings: *Commissural lip pits* are small openings or fistulas on the lip vermilion at the angles of the lips. They are either bilateral or unilateral. The pits do not cause any discomfort or cosmetic problems.
   Paramedian pits of the lower lip are usually bilateral, or occasionally unilateral, fistulas located lateral to the midline on the vermilion border of the lower lip. The openings may be minute but occur in the center of a mound of lip tissue; they may be openings of fistulas 10 to 15 mm deep, which excrete mucous. Rarely, a single centrally located pit may be present.
   Pits of the upper lip are exceedingly rare and are usually unilateral openings on the vermilion border.
   While kindreds are known in which individuals have had only paramedian lip pits, in general, these are not extensive kindreds. Kindreds more fully documented have individuals with clefts of lip and palate. For this reason, individuals or families with paramedian pits should be viewed as also having a high risk for clefts of lip or palate.

Complications: Rarely, infection may occur.

Associated Findings: Commissural lip pits are associated with aural sinuses (auricular pits) in 4% of cases. Paramedian lip pits are associated with cleft lip/palate syndromes, cleft lip or palate and filiform fusion of eyelids, and with popliteal pterygium syndrome. Pits of upper lip are associated with cysts in line of fusion of premaxilla and maxillary processes.

Etiology: *Commissural lip pits:* No genetic study has been published but there are reports of familial occurrence suggesting autosomal dominant transmission (father and son, mother and two sons, father and two daughters, mother, son and daughter, and transmission through three generations).
   Paramedian pits of the lower lip: Reported in kindreds showing autosomal dominant transmission, and with no known relative with cleft lip/palate. However, data are still insufficient to say with certainty whether this occurs as an isolated trait or whether it is always part of the cleft lip or palate and lip pits syndromes. Shprintzen et al (1980) observed penetrance to be 100%.
   Pits of the upper lip: Probably of nongenetic origin.

Pathogenesis: *Commissural lip pits* originate from epithelial rests in the line of the embryonal furrow between maxillary and mandibular processes.
   Paramedian pits of the lower lip originate as vestigial remnants of the "lateral sulci" appearing in the embryonic mandible at the 7.5–12.5 mm long stage.
   Pits of the upper lip are due to failure of complete fusion of premaxilla and maxillary processes.

MIM No.: 12050, 15163

CDC No.: 750.260

Sex Ratio: *Commissural lip pits:* M1:F1 in Caucasians, American blacks, and North American Indians (Chippewa).
Paramedian pits of the lower lip: M1:F1 in Caucasians.
Pits of the upper lip: Undetermined.

Occurrence: *Commissural lip pits:* Caucasians: 1:500 to 1:83; American blacks: 1:48; North American Indians (Chippewa): 1:110.
Paramedian pits of the lower lip: Undetermined.

Risk of Recurrence for Patient's Sib: Unknown.

Risk of Recurrence for Patient's Child: Unknown.

Age of Detectability: At birth.

Gene Mapping and Linkage: Unknown.

Prevention: None known. Genetic counseling indicated.

Treatment: *Commissural lip pits:* No treatment necessary. *Paramedian pits of the lower lip:* Plastic surgery. *Pits of the upper lip:* Surgical excision.

Prognosis: Normal for life span and intelligence when an isolated trait.

Detection of Carrier: Unknown.

References:

Everett FG, Wescott WB: Commissural lip pits. Oral Surg 1961; 14:202–209.
Witkop CJ: Genetic diseases in the oral cavity. In: Tiecke RW, ed: Oral pathology. New York: McGraw-Hill, 1965:786–843.
Baker BR: Pits of the lip commissures in caucasoid males. Oral Surg 1966; 21:56–60.
Cervenka J, et al.: The syndrome of pits of the lower lip and cleft lip and/or palate: genetic considerations. Am J Hum Genet 1967; 19:416–432.
Fenner von W, v der Leyen, U-E: Über die kongenitale Oberlippenfistel. Dtsch Zahnaerztl Z 1969; 24:963–968.
Shprintzen RJ, et al.: The penetrance and variable expression of the Van der Woude syndrome. Implications for genetic counseling. Cleft Palate J 1980; 17:52–57.

CE003 **Jaroslav Červenka**

LIPA deficiency
See CHOLESTERYL ESTER STORAGE DISEASE
Lipa deficiency
See WOLMAN DISEASE
Lipase D deficiency
See HYPERCHYLOMICRONEMIA

LIPASE, CONGENITAL ABSENCE OF PANCREATIC 0597

Includes:
Pancreatic lipase deficiency, congenital
Pancreatic lipase deficiency, congenital isolated

Excludes:
Co-lipase deficiency
Lipase/co-lipase deficiency, isolated congenital
Pancreatic exocrine insufficiency, generalized

Major Diagnostic Criteria: Steatorrhea is the only significant clinical finding. Basal and secretin-stimulated pancreatic juices are deficient in lipase activity. Peptidase, amylase and co-lipase activities are normal. Absent lipase has recently been demonstrated by an immunologic technique which improves specificity.

Clinical Findings: Steatorrhea is the only significant clinical finding. All patients have had the onset of oily, slightly foul stools in early infancy. The oil separates from the bulk movement and will solidify at room temperature. Soiling of clothing with oil is common.

Normal growth and development is the rule. Abdominal distention is unusual. Basal and secretin-stimulated pancreatic juices obtained by peroral duodenal intubation are found to contain normal activities of peptidase and amylase but to be deficient in lipase. Lipase assays are reliable only if performed by experienced investigators. Reproducibility is marginal, and incubation conditions are critical. Newer immunologic assay provides improved specificity.

Co-lipase is necessary for optimal function of lipase in the conditions present in the intestinal lumen. In vivo, co-lipase deficiency could masquerade as lipase deficiency. Recently a patient with deficiencies of both lipase and co-lipase has been described.

Complications: Steatorrhea.

Associated Findings: None known.

Etiology: Autosomal recessive inheritance.

Pathogenesis: Pancreatic lipase is essential for optimal fat absorption. Hydrolysis of triglycerides to α-fatty acids and β-monoglycerides occurs at the surface of emulsified fat globules by the action of pancreatic lipase in the presence of bile salts and co-lipase. In the absence of lipase, limited hydrolysis occurs as a result of the action of gastric lipolytic activity and pancreatic esterase. The coefficient of fat absorption in the lipase deficient patient is 50–80%.

MIM No.: *24660

Sex Ratio: M3:F1 (observed in four cases in which sex was reported)

Occurrence: Fewer than 20 cases have been documented.

Risk of Recurrence for Patient's Sib:
See Part I, *Mendelian Inheritance.*

Risk of Recurrence for Patient's Child:
See Part I, *Mendelian Inheritance.*

Age of Detectability: In infancy.

Gene Mapping and Linkage: Unknown.

Prevention: None known. Genetic counseling indicated.

Treatment: Treatment with orally administered pancreatic enzyme replacement improves fat absorption but does not usually normalize function. Dietary fat restriction is necessary to abolish steatorrhea. Medium-chain triglycerides may be used as a fat substitute when needed for nutrition in the infant.

Prognosis: Excellent.

Detection of Carrier: Unknown.

References:

Sheldon W: Congenital pancreatic lipase deficiency. Arch Dis Child 1964; 39:268–271.
Figarella C, et al.: Congenital pancreatic lipase deficiency. J Pediatr 1980; 96:412–416.
Ghishan FK, et al.; Isolated congenital lipase-colipase deficiency. Gastroenterology 1984; 86:1580–1582.

WH007 **Peter F. Whitington**

Lipid histiocytosis of spleen
See THROMBOCYTOPENIC PURPURA AND LIPID HISTIOCYTOSIS

LIPID TRANSPORT DEFECT OF INTESTINE 3226

Includes:
Anderson disease
Apoprotein in intestinal cells-hypobetalipoproteinemia
Chylomicron retention disease
Hypobetalipoproteinemia-apoprotein in intestinal cells
Intestine, lipid transport defect

Excludes:
Abetalipoproteinemia (0002)
Hypobetalipoproteinemia (2386)
Normotriglyceridemic abetalipoproteinemia

Major Diagnostic Criteria: Failure of enterocytes to secrete chylomicrons in response to the absorption of dietary lipid. In contrast to abetalipoproteinemia in which enterocyte apo B is reduced or absent in the face of cellular steatosis, fasting enterocytes in this disorder reveal increased apo B immunostaining in association with accumulation of intracellular lipid droplets. Apo B-48 and associated chylomicrons of intestinal origin are not detectable in plasma after fat-feeding. Plasma triglyceride levels are within the normal range, but the total plasma cholesterol concentration is reduced. Plasma lipoprotein isolation reveals increased VLDL cholesterol and decreased LDL and HDL cholesterol. The plasma apo B level is mildly reduced and is present exclusively as the larger liver-derived apo B-100 form.

Clinical Findings: Diarrhea and failure to thrive associated with fat malabsorption with onset usually in the first year of life are the prominent clinical features of this disorder. Neurologic and ophthalmologic findings typical of **Abetalipoproteinemia** are usually absent or very mild in this disease. Atypical retinitis pigmentosa has not been described, although mild subclinical retinal electrophysiologic abnormalities may occur. As in abetalipoproteinemia, these findings, when present, may be secondary to vitamin E deficiency. Acanthocytosis of circulating red blood cells, a diagnostic feature of abetalipoproteinemia, is absent. If treated with dietary long chain fat restriction supplemented with essential and medium chain fatty acids and fat-soluble vitamins, growth has been reported to normalize, and neurologic symptoms, if present, may improve or resolve.

Complications: If untreated, diarrhea and steatorrhea with associated growth failure will persist. Mild neurologic and ophthalmologic dysfunction, if present, may persist in the untreated patient.

Associated Findings: None known.

Etiology: Autosomal recessive inheritance. Since intestinal synthesis of apo B and uptake and esterification of long chain fatty acids appear to be unimpaired in in vitro studies, a defect in the final assembly and secretion of chylomicrons has been proposed. Whether the enterocyte secretory block is at the pre- or post-Golgi level is controversial at present. A defect in glycosylation of apo B has been observed in jejunal explants.

Pathogenesis: Unknown.

MIM No.: 24670

Sex Ratio: M11:F5

Occurrence: Sixteen well-described cases have been reported in the literature.

Risk of Recurrence for Patient's Sib:
See Part I, *Mendelian Inheritance.*

Risk of Recurrence for Patient's Child:
See Part I, *Mendelian Inheritance.*

Age of Detectability: Many patients reported with symptoms in the first month of life.

Gene Mapping and Linkage: Unknown.

Prevention: None known. Genetic counseling indicated.

Treatment: Restriction of long chain dietary fat and supplementation of essential and medium chain fats and fat soluble vitamins, particularly vitamin E.

Prognosis: Long-term follow-up into adulthood has not been reported. However, since response to treatment is usually favorable, long term prognosis is probably good.

Detection of Carrier: Unknown.

References:
Anderson CM, et al.: Unusual causes of steatorrhea in infancy and childhood. Med J Aust 1961; 2:617–622.
Bouma M-E, et al.: Hypobetalipoproteinemia with accumulation of an apoprotein B-like protein in intestinal cells: immunoenzymatic and biochemical characterization of seven cases of Anderson's disease. J Clin Invest 1986; 78:398–410.
Levy E, et al.: Intestinal apo B synthesis, lipids, and lipoproteins in chylomicron retention disease. J Lipid Res 1987; 28:1263–1274.
Roy CC, et al.: Malabsorption, hypocholesterolemia, and fat-filled enterocytes with increased intestinal apo B. Gastroenterology 1987; 92:390–399.
Bouma M-E, Infante R: Chylomicron retention disease. Gastroenterology 1988; 94:554–556.

BL025   **Dennis D. Black**

Lipid, deficiency of
See *HYPERCHYLOMICRONEMIA*
Lipid-storage myopathy secondary to SCAD
See *ACYL-CoA DEHYDROGENASE DEFICIENCY, SHORT CHAIN TYPE*
Lipidosis, late infantile systemic
See *G(M1)-GANGLIOSIDOSIS, TYPE 2*
Lipidosis, sulfatide
See *METACHROMATIC LEUKODYSTROPHIES*
Lipidosis-thrombocytopenia-angiomata of the spleen
See *THROMBOCYTOPENIC PURPURA AND LIPID HISTIOCYTOSIS*
Lipoatrophic diabetes with dominant transmission, familial
See *LIPODYSTROPHY, FAMILIAL LIMB AND TRUNK*
Lipoatrophic diabetes, congenital
See *LIPODYSTROPHY SYNDROME, BERARDINELLI TYPE*
Lipodermoid
See *EYE, DERMOLIPOMA*

LIPODYSTROPHY SYNDROME, BERARDINELLI TYPE   2038

Includes:
   Berardinelli-Seip syndrome
   Gigantism, acromegaloid-lipodystrophy
   Lawrence syndrome
   Lipoatrophic diabetes, congenital
   Seip syndrome
   Total lipodystrophy-acromegaloid gigantism

Excludes:
   De Lange syndrome (0242)
   Diabetes, insulin-resistant with acanthosis nigricans
   Leprechaunism (0587)
   Lipodystrophy, familial limb and trunk (2614)
   Partial lipodystrophy syndromes

Major Diagnostic Criteria: The diagnosis is made clinically, based upon growth characteristics, physical features, and laboratory data. The index findings are absence of clinically apparent adipose tissue and hepatomegaly. Patients are tall and thin as infants and children, with advanced dental and skeletal maturation. However, their ultimate height potential is limited. Insulin-resistant, non-ketotic diabetes mellitus with hyperlipidemia develops with age and supports the diagnosis.

Clinical Findings: Affected patients have abundant, often curly scalp hair and a gaunt, triangular face. Skin pigmentation is increased, generalized hypertrichosis may be found, and acanthosis nigricans may be present in the axillae, groin, or other intertriginous regions. Significant hepatomegaly is usually present, and splenomegaly and genitomegaly are frequent findings. Muscles and veins are prominent, and abdominal distension with umbilical herniation is common. Stature is increased in childhood but may be decreased in adults; the extremities may appear enlarged. Weight is normal but is usually low in relation to height. Skeletal maturation is advanced for chronologic age and for height age in childhood. X-ray features can include sclerotic and angiomatous lesions of the long bones and hands, and cardiomegaly. Laboratory findings include hyperglycemia, hypercholesterolemia, hypertriglyceridemia, hyperinsulinemia, and hyperglucagonemia. Liver function tests are often abnormal. Other endocrine investigations have not shown consistent abnormalities.

Complications: Patients develop the typical microvascular manifestations of chronic diabetes mellitus, as well as premature atherosclerosis. Fatty infiltration of the liver may evolve into overt cirrhosis, with portal hypertension and gastrointestinal hemorrhage.

Associated Findings: Protracted vomiting with failure to thrive in infancy has been reported. Renal involvement manifests with proteinuria or frank nephrotic syndrome. The central nervous system can be affected, and findings can include dilated ventricles and mental retardation. Polycystic ovaries and oligomenorrhea have been described. Corneal opacities may be found.

Etiology: Although total lipodystrophy is a heterogeneous condition, there is a high incidence of parental consanguinity in the

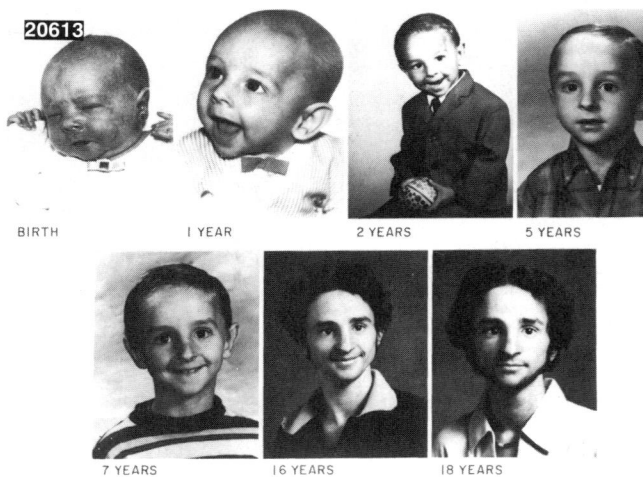

BIRTH   I YEAR   2 YEARS   5 YEARS

7 YEARS   16 YEARS   18 YEARS

2038-20613: Lipodystrophy, Berardinelli type; note the development of a gaunt, triangular facial appearance in these serial photographs of an affected subject.

families of patients with the congenital form, strongly suggesting autosomal recessive inheritance. At present, this causation should be ascribed only to patients with features of the classical phenotype present at birth.

Pathogenesis: Patients are hypermetabolic with increased fat catabolism, markedly decreased fat storage, and fatty infiltration of the liver. Hypothalamic dysfunction has been postulated, but structural lesions are not usually demonstrable. Hyperglycemia and hyperinsulinemia are present without insulin antibodies; in some patients, decreased binding by insulin receptors has been noted. The receptor defect appears to be heterogeneous even within the group of patients with the congenital form. The number of fat cells in adipose tissue is probably normal, but intracellular fat deposits are markedly reduced. Muscular prominence is partly due to reduced subcutaneous fat, but there may be an element of primary muscular hypertrophy or hyperplasia with excess glycogen deposition as well. The pathogenesis and natural history of liver and cardiac involvement are not well understood.

MIM No.: *26970

POS No.: 3439

Sex Ratio: M1:F1 in the congenital form; M1:F2–3 in the acquired form.

Occurrence: Undetermined but presumed rare. Established literature. No particular ethnic group, with the possible exception of the Portuguese, appears to be at additional risk.

Risk of Recurrence for Patient's Sib:
See Part I, *Mendelian Inheritance.*

Risk of Recurrence for Patient's Child:
See Part I, *Mendelian Inheritance.*

Age of Detectability: At birth for the congenital form.

Gene Mapping and Linkage: Unknown.

Prevention: None known. Genetic counseling indicated.

Treatment: Without a clear understanding of the pathogenesis of the syndrome(s) of total lipodystrophy, treatment has been symptomatic, empirical, and largely unsatisfactory. The treatment of the diabetic syndrome and its related lipemia is made difficult by profound resistance to exogenous insulin observed in many patients. Fortunately, ketoacidosis is infrequent. Salutory effects of a neuroleptic diphenylbutylpiperidine, (pimozide), have been reported in a few patients but have not been sustained at puberty. Improvement in some of the characteristic endocrine and metabolic abnormalities has been noted with short-term caloric restric-

tion but this approach is obviously impractical in gaunt, undernourished patients. Recently, improvement has been reported in one patient during eucaloric feeding with medium-chain triglycerides substituted for dietary long-chain fatty acids. The efficacy of medium chain triglyceride feeding has not been examined in other patients.

Prognosis: Patients have a shortened life expectancy as a result of inanition, premature atherosclerosis, gastrointestinal hemorrhage secondary to cirrhosis, and the development of microvascular complications of diabetes mellitus.

Detection of Carrier: Unknown.

Special Considerations: The lipodystrophies as a group are quite heterogeneous with respect to age of onset, degree of involvement, and associated findings. The above discussion is limited to one subset of these conditions, namely that which is total, involving all body regions. Although clinical features were present at birth in the patients described by Berardinelli (1954) and Seip (1959), many of the somatic clues to the diagnosis and abnormal laboratory findings evolve with age, and a period of observation may be necessary to reach a secure diagnosis. Lawrence (1946) originally described a form of total lipodystrophy that differs in its later onset (often following a systemic illness or infection) and absence of reported parental consanguinity. This suggests different causation for these closely related conditions, but, because of significant clinical similarities they must currently be classified together.

Support Groups: New York; American Diabetes Association

References:
Lawrence RD: Lipodystrophy and hepatomegaly with diabetes, lipaemia, and other metabolic disturbances. Lancet 1946; I:724–731, 733–775.
Berardinelli W: An undiagnosed endocrinometabolic syndrome: report of two cases. J Clin Endocr 1954; 14:193–204. * †
Seip M: Lipodystrophy and gigantism with associated endocrine manifestation. Acta Paediat 1959; 48:555–574.
Senior B, Gellis SS: The syndromes of total lipodystrophy and of partial lipodystrophy. Pediatrics 1964; 33:593–612. *
Rossini AA, Cahill GF Jr: Lipatrophic diabetes. In: DeGroot LJ, ed: Endocrinology. New York: Grune & Stratton, 1979:1093–1098.
Wachslicht-Rodbard H, et al.: Heterogeneity of the insulin-receptor interaction in lipoatrophic diabetes. J Clin Endocrinol Metab 1981; 52:416–425.
Wilson DE, et al.: Eucaloric substitution of medium chain triglycerides for dietary long-chain fatty acids in acquired total lipodystrophy: effects on hyperlipoproteinemia and endogenous insulin resistance. J Clin Endocrinol Metab 1983; 57:517–523.

J0012   **John P. Johnson**
WI060   **Dana E. Wilson**

LIPODYSTROPHY, FAMILIAL LIMB AND TRUNK   2614

Includes:
> Dunnigan syndrome
> Koebberling-Dunnigan syndrome
> Limbs and trunk, familial lipodystrophy of
> Lipodystrophy, reverse partial
> Lipoatrophic diabetes with dominant transmission, familial
> Partial lipodystrophy-lipoatrophic diabetes-hyperlipidemia

Excludes:
> Barraquer-Simons disease
> Diabetes, acquired lipoatrophic
> Fetthals
> Launois-Bensaude adenolipomatosis
> Lipoatrophic diabetes, congenital
> Lipoatrophy secondary to insulin hypersensitivity, acquired
> Lipodystrophy, cephalo-thoracic
> Lipodystrophy, partial with familial C3 deficiency
> **Lipodystrophy-rieger anomaly-short stature-diabetes** (2834)
> **Lipodystrophy syndrome, Berardinelli type** (2038)
> **Nevi-atrial myxoma-myxoid neurofibromas-ephelides** (2572)

Major Diagnostic Criteria: Partial lipodystrophy involving the limbs (which may extend to the trunk), diabetes mellitus, and hyperlipidemia.

Clinical Findings: Females have been described with diabetes commencing in the first or second decade, symmetric atrophy of fat in the arms and legs, preservation of subcutaneous fat over the neck, face and shoulders. Muscle bulk and power may resemble masculine body habitus and true muscular hypertrophy has been reported. Lean, muscular limbs with apparent fat accumulation around the neck, shoulders, and face may simulate the appearance of **Nevi-atrial myxoma-myxoid neurofibromas-ephelides. Hyperlipoproteinemia** Type IIb, III or IV, as well as hyperuricemia, have been reported. Associated skin lesions include tuberoeruptive xanthomata over the elbows and knees, acanthosis nigricans in the axillae, and thin skin with increased visibility of subcutaneous veins. Hepatosplenomegaly does not occur to the extent seen in acquired total lipodystrophy.

Complications: Diabetic microangiopathic retinopathy and peripheral vascular disease.

Associated Findings: None known.

Etiology: Autosomal dominant inheritance with sex limitation. One male patient was reported by Burn and Baraitser (1986). The predominance of female patients has been attributed to the more extensive distribution of fat in females, but X-linked dominant inheritance with lethality in hemizygous males has also been suggested.

Pathogenesis: Unknown.

MIM No.: *15166

POS No.: 3439

Sex Ratio: M<1:F1.

Occurrence: Several sibships and at least one isolated case has been reported.

Risk of Recurrence for Patient's Sib:
See Part I, *Mendelian Inheritance.*

Risk of Recurrence for Patient's Child:
See Part I, *Mendelian Inheritance.*

Age of Detectability: Late childhood or early adult life. Lipodystrophy usually appears at puberty.

Gene Mapping and Linkage: Unknown.

Prevention: None known. Genetic counseling indicated.

Treatment: Insulin as indicated for diabetes. Insulin resistance requiring high dosage, as seen in total acquired lipodystrophy, is rare.

Prognosis: Lipodystrophy is not reversible in affected areas. Otherwise, prognosis is that of the associated diabetes, and is generally good.

Detection of Carrier: Unknown.

Support Groups: New York; American Diabetes Association. NJ; Elizabeth; National Lipid Diseases Foundation

References:
Dunnigan MG, et al.: Familial lipoatrophic diabetes with dominant transmission: a new syndrome. Quart J Med 1974; 43:33–48.
Kobberling J, et al.: Lipodystrophy of the extremities: a dominantly inherited syndrome associated with lipoatrophic diabetes. Humangenetik 1975; 29:111–120.
Wettke-Schafer R, Kantner G: X-linked dominant inherited diseases with lethality in hemizygous males. Hum Genet 1983; 64:1–23.
Burn J, Baraitser M: Partial lipoatrophy with insulin resistant diabetes and hyperlipiaemia (Dunnigan's syndrome). J Med Genet 1986; 23:128–130.
Kobberling J, Dunnigan MG: Familial partial lipodystrophy: two types of an X linked dominant syndrome, lethal in the homizygous state. J Med Genet 1986; 23:120–127.

LE050   **Raymond M. Lewkonia**

Lipodystrophy, reverse partial
See LIPODYSTROPHY, FAMILIAL LIMB AND TRUNK

LIPODYSTROPHY-COARSE FACIES-ACANTHOSIS NIGRICANS, MIESCHER TYPE   2423

Includes:
Bloch-Miescher syndrome
Mendenhall syndrome
Miescher syndrome
Rabson-Mendenhall syndrome

Excludes:
Insulin resistance-acanthosis nigricans, types A and B (Kahn)
Leprechaunism (0587)
Lipodystrophy syndrome, Berardinelli type (2038)
Lipodystrophy (others)

Major Diagnostic Criteria: Lipodystrophy, coarse facies, dental anomalies, acanthosis nigricans, and lanugo-type hypertrichosis. An additional and important feature is insulin-resistant diabetes.

Clinical Findings: The earliest manifestation, typically present at birth or shortly thereafter, is an augmented pigmentation, which later in childhood develops into acanthosis nigricans with typical localization (neck; nape; and axillary, inguinal, and genital regions). In the severe form, acanthosis nigricans is complicated by multiple skin tags. Premature dentition also occurs in the first months of life. Longitudinal growth and bone maturation can be temporarily accelerated; however, some of the patients showed a slight growth retardation. Mental retardation is *not* present. In addition, the patients are dysmorphic, and in the severe form of the disorder lipatrophy develops. These described characteristics cause children and youth to appear older than the corresponding chronologic age.

Further characteristics are coarse facies with prominent upper and lower jaw, full lips, and relatively large ears. Irregular and supernumerary, often carious, teeth are striking and can be abnormally large (macrodontia). The tongue is furrowed. A lanugo-type hypertrichosis is seen early in life, and scalp hair is often abundant. On the other hand, females in early adulthood may have alopecia. Hands and feet may be short and plump, with thickened nails. A prominent abdomen and enlarged phallus (especially in females) can occur.

During childhood or later in youth, a mild diabetes with only slight tendency toward ketosis may develop. The basal plasma insulin concentration can increase 100-fold. Examination of the insulin receptors shows a pathologic diminished binding capacity. Although the total number of the receptors is normal, there appears to be a complete absence of receptors with high affinity. Additional characteristics in females are menstrual disorders (oligomenorrhea or amenorrhea) and reduced fertility.

There is strikingly variable expression of clinical manifestations, not only interfamilial but also among patients of the same sibship.

Complications: Patients are prone to benign tumors in the thyroid gland and to polycystic ovaries. Even in childhood, recurrent gastric and duodenal ulcers can appear. The diabetes leads to diminished resistance against possibly fatal infections. Late complications of the diabetes, such as retinopathy or neuropathy, have been documented.

Associated Findings: A pathogenetically obscure hyperplasia of the pineal body was demonstrated in some patients at autopsy.

Etiology: Autosomal recessive inheritance with variable expression.

Pathogenesis: There is no current theory to explain all the manifestations of this homozygous autosomal recessive gene, but hyperinsulinism per se (in different types of insulin-resistant diabetes) apparently leads to characteristics such as lipodystrophy, acanthosis nigricans, hypertrichosis, polycystic ovaries, and reduced fertility.

MIM No.: *26219, *24309

POS No.: 3741

Sex Ratio: M1:F1

Occurrence: Possibly a dozen or more cases, under various designations, have been reported in the literature.

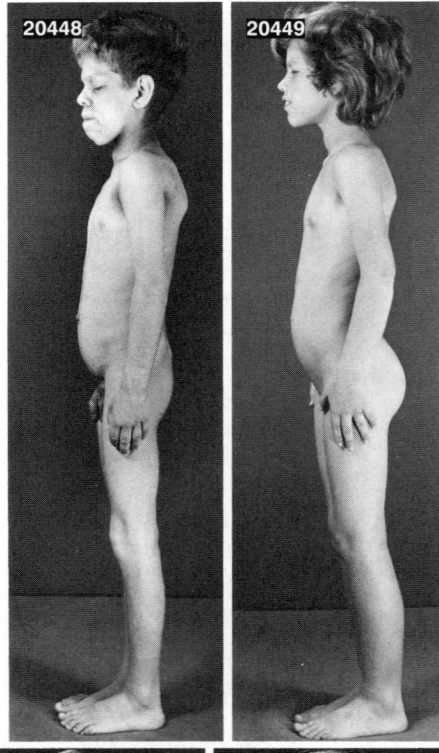

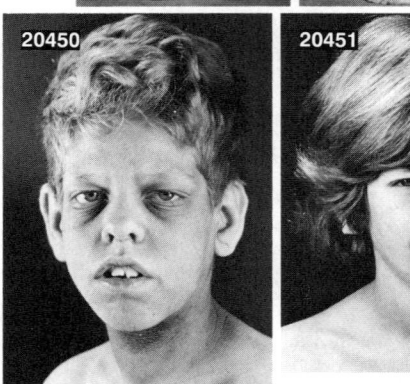
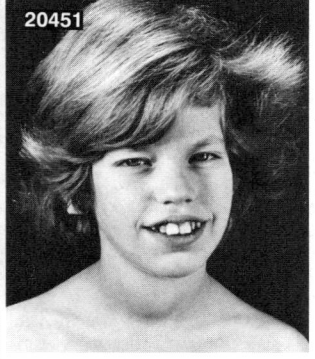

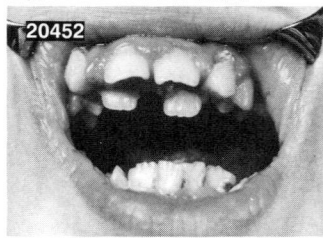
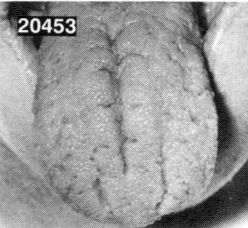

2423-20448–20453: Characteristics in a pair of sibs with variably expressed lipodystrophy, Miescher type. The boy is 13.5 years old, the girl 11.5 years old. **20448–49:** Note lipodystrophy and hypertrichosis, more pronounced in the brother. **20450–51:** Coarse facial features; note also acanthosis nigricans, macrodontia, and abundant scalp hair. **20452:** Note large, supernumerary (double row), and carious teeth in the male patient. **20453:** Furrowed tongue in the male patient.

Risk of Recurrence for Patient's Sib:
See Part I, *Mendelian Inheritance.*

Risk of Recurrence for Patient's Child:
See Part I, *Mendelian Inheritance.*

Age of Detectability: During the first year of life.

Gene Mapping and Linkage: Unknown.

Prevention: None known. Genetic counseling indicated.

Treatment: Treatment of the diabetes is only possible with high doses of insulin and therefore is hardly practicable. A therapy with biguanides can be successful, because it leads to an increased number of insulin receptors. Further treatment is symptomatic and is confined to surgical procedures in cases of recurrent gastric or duodenal ulcers and to orthodontic measures. In the case of hirsutism, cosmetic measures are indicated.

Prognosis: Life span may be diminished by later complications of diabetes, but precise data are not available. On the other hand, there are several reports on partial remission of the disorder; diabetes and acanthosis nigricans tend to improve in adulthood. Affected women showed reduced fertility, but pregnancies are possible.

Detection of Carrier: Clinical examination to detect those who are only mildly affected.

Special Considerations: The extraordinary complexity of this syndrome may be the cause for the correspondingly large number of different designations in the literature. This has led to considerable difficulties in nosologic classification. The early reports on the same pair of sibs by Bloch in 1920 and by Miescher in 1921, both in German, remained largely unknown in the English literature. It was not until about 30 years later that Mendenhall (1950) and Rabson and Mendenhall (1956) described three typically affected sibs in the American literature. Since then there have been a number of publications in the American but also in the European literature, most of which have been cited by Wiedemann et al (1985).

Since about the mid-1970s, insulin-resistant diabetes has gained special attention. For example, Kahn et al (1976) described types A and B of insulin-resistant diabetes with acanthosis nigricans. Whereas type A shares several of the characteristics with the above mentioned syndrome but is probably a different disorder, type B is an immunologic disorder with circulating antibodies to the insulin receptors. The type A literature, however, came to include reports by Rüdiger et al (1981) and further by Rüdiger et al (1983) concerning the same sibship. They described three adult sibs with mild diabetes, acanthosis nigricans, dental anomalies, dystrophy, mild acral hypertrophy, and excessively elevated fasting plasma insulin levels. Insulin binding was defective as a result of a complete lack of receptors with high affinity. Two of these patients (then children) had been described by Wiedemann et al. (1968) in the German pediatric literature. Comparable receptor studies such as those by Rüdiger et al. have been done by several authors, e.g. Taylor et al (1981). An exact interpretation of these results seems still to be controversial (Taylor, 1982).

Lastly, there are some striking parallels between this syndrome and **Leprechaunism** in respect to nosology. However, these are distinct entities.

References:
Rabson SM, Mendenhall EN: Familial hypertrophy of pineal body, hyperplasia of adrenal cortex and diabetes mellitus. Am J Clin Pathol 1956; 26:283–290.
Kahn CR, et al.: The syndromes of insulin resistance and acanthosis nigricans: insulin-receptor disorders in man. New Engl J Med 1976; 294:739–745.
Rüdiger HW, et al.: Insulin resistant diabetes mellitus due to a genetic defect of the insulin receptor. Jerusalem: Sixth Int Cong Hum Genet, 1981:255.
Taylor SI, et al.: Decreased insulin binding in cultured lymphocytes from two patients with extreme insulin resistance. J Clin Endocrinol Metab 1982; 54:919–930.
Rüdiger HW, et al.: Familial insulin-resistant diabetes secondary to an affinity defect of the insulin receptor. Hum Genet 1983; 64:407–411. *

Wiedemann HR, et al.: An atlas of characteristic syndromes: a visual aid to diagnosis, ed 2. London: Wolfe Medical Publications, 1985. * †

ME008
WI003
Peter Meinecke
Hans-Rudolf Wiedemann

LIPODYSTROPHY-RIEGER ANOMALY-SHORT STATURE-DIABETES 2834

Includes:

Aarskog lipodystrophy syndrome
Diabetes-Rieger anomaly-lipodystrophy-short stature
Rieger anomaly-lipodystrophy-short stature-diabetes
Short stature-Rieger anomaly-lipodystrophy-diabetes

Excludes:

Aarskog syndrome (0001)
Lipodystrophy, familial limb and trunk (2614)
Lipodystrophy syndrome, Berardinelli type (2038)
Lipodystrophy, partial sporadic
Short syndrome (2098)

Major Diagnostic Criteria: Facial lipodystrophy, Rieger anomaly, and short stature.

Clinical Findings: Lipodystrophy is present from infancy, affecting the face and limited areas of the buttocks and without progression. In the one known family, the condition was present in a grandfather, two of his daughters, and the propositus, son of one of the daughters. All affected persons had short stature and Rieger anomaly. Additional features were retarded bone age, delayed puberty, midface hypoplasia, large anteverted ears, hypospadias, and hypotrichosis. The propositus developed diabetes mellitus at age 14 years, his mother at age 39 years, and the maternal aunt had glucose intolerance at age 55 years.

Complications: Unknown.

Associated Findings: None known.

Etiology: Probably autosomal dominant inheritance.

Pathogenesis: Unknown.

MIM No.: 15168

POS No.: 3496

Sex Ratio: M1:F1

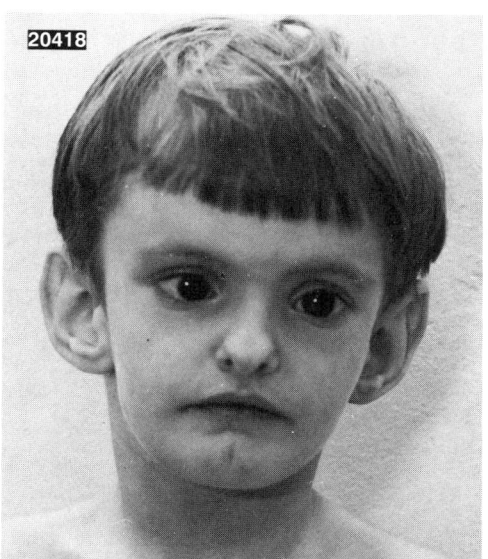

2834-20418: Note paucity of facial fat, deep-set eyes, pinched nose, wide mouth and large ears.

Occurrence: One family from the Lofoten Islands of Norway has been reported in which four persons in three generations were affected.

Risk of Recurrence for Patient's Sib:
See Part I, *Mendelian Inheritance.*

Risk of Recurrence for Patient's Child:
See Part I, *Mendelian Inheritance.*

Age of Detectability: During infancy or early childhood.

Gene Mapping and Linkage: Unknown.

Prevention: None known. Genetic counseling indicated.

Treatment: Treatment of the possible manifestation of diabetes mellitus.

Prognosis: Bone age is delayed, and growth might continue into the late teenage years. Puberty is delayed but otherwise normal. The ultimate prognosis depends on the development of diabetic complications.

Detection of Carrier: Unknown.

References:
Gorlin RJ: A selected miscellany. In: BD:OAS XI(2). New York: March of Dimes Birth Defects Foundation, 1975:46–48.
Sensenbrenner JA, et al.: A low birth weight syndrome? Rieger syndrome. In: BD:OAS XI(2). New York: March of Dimes Birth Defects Foundation, 1975:423–426.
Aarskog D, et al.: Autosomal dominant partial lipodystrophy associated with Rieger anomaly, short stature, and insulinopenic diabetes. Am J Med Genet 1983; 15:29–38.
Köbberling J, Dunnigan MG: Familial partial lipodystrophy: two types of an X-linked dominant syndrome, lethal in the hemizygous state. J Med Genet 1986; 23:120–127.

AA002
Dagfinn Aarskog

Lipoglycoproteinosis
See SKIN, LIPOID PROTEINOSIS

LIPOGRANULOMATOSIS 0598

Includes:

Ceramidase deficiency
Ceramide deficiency
Disseminated lipogranulomatosis
Farber disease

Excludes:

Arthritis, rheumatoid (2517)
Histiocytosis
Lipoid dermatoarthritis
Sarcoid arthritis

Major Diagnostic Criteria: The hallmark of this syndrome is the clinical triad of discrete lumpy masses over the wrists and ankles, combined with joint deformities and hoarseness. Diagnosis is confirmed by demonstrating deficient activity of acid ceramidase. Biopsy lesion material shows foam cells that contain characteristic inclusions and infiltration by histiocytes, lymphocytes, and fibroblasts.

Clinical Findings: Typical cases develop normally for the first weeks or months, until parents note that movement of fingers, wrists, or ankles may be painful, that these joints are tender, and that there are subcutaneous nodules near these joints or over pressure points. A second and nearly constant feature is that the child's cry is hoarse. The nodules enlarge, and the joint deformities progress. There is difficulty in feeding and swallowing, progressive inanition, intermittent fever, and respiratory disturbances due to pulmonary infiltrates that may cause death during the first year. The liver is enlarged in about one-fourth of the cases. Central nervous system function is relatively intact, but may be difficult to assess due to the severe systemic illness. One-third of the patients have peripheral nerve involvement, evidenced by diminished or absent deep tendon reflexes and signs of denervation in neurometric studies. The retina may show

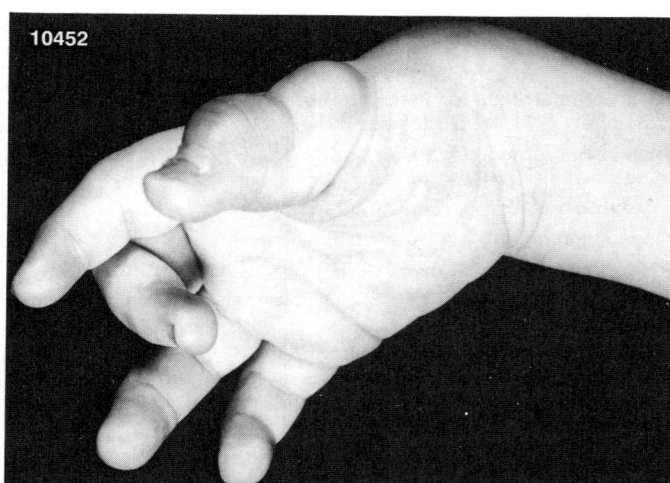

0598-10452: Lipogranulomatosis of hand.

diffuse grayish opacification about the foveola, with a cherry-red spot.

Several variant forms are now recognized. These include a mild variant in which four patients are in stable condition in their second or third decade. They show moderate arthropathy, subcutaneous nodules, hoarseness, and moderate psychomotor retardation. They appear free of pulmonary or hepatic disease. Intermediate degrees of involvement are shown by children 4–10 years old who have severe arthropathy and prominent nodules, as well as seizures and signs of CNS involvement but no lung involvement. Two other variants have been described recently. In three children the presenting signs were hepatosplenomegaly and osteolytic lesions during the first few weeks of life, leading to the diagnosis of malignant histiocytosis. Subcutaneous nodules were absent in one patient and not prominent in the other two. In the other variant form the presenting signs were progressive psychomotor retardation and retinal cherry-red spots. Subcutaneous nodules and hoarseness were present but mild.

Laboratory diagnosis depends on demonstration of deficient acid ceramidase activity in leukocytes or cultured skin fibroblasts and on evidence of ceramide storage by biochemical or microscopic techniques. Abnormally high ceramide levels may be present in urine, but some cases have failed to show this. Biochemical assays of nodule biopsy material show high levels of ceramide (up to 30% of total lipids). Under the electron microscope these nodules show characteristic inclusions, which have been referred to as *Farber bodies*.

Momoi et al (1982) have proposed that N-(1-^{14}C) lauroylsphingosine may be a better substrate for the diagnosis of Farber disease than N-(1-^{14}C) oleoylsphingosine. A different and valuable approach to the enzymatic diagnosis of Farber disease has been provided by Kudoh and Wenger (1982). These investigators incubated cultured skin fibroblasts with [^{14}C] stearic acid-labeled cerebroside sulfate and measured its rate of degradation. Cells from Farber disease patients had a deficient capacity (15% of control) to degrade the ceramide that is formed from cerebroside-sulfate.

Complications: The laryngeal involvement may lead to difficulties with breathing and swallowing. Pulmonary infiltrates due to alveolar lipid infiltrates cause respiratory insufficiency and are difficult to distinguish from pneumonia. The nodules and joint involvement cause discomfort and limit mobility and well-being. The osteolytic lesions may cause hypercalcemia. Neurologic involvement may cause seizures, ataxia, weakness, and dementia.

Associated Findings: None known.

Etiology: Autosomal recessive inheritance.

Pathogenesis: The defective function of acid ceramidase leads to tissue accumulation of ceramide within lysosomes. This causes cell damage and an inflammatory response manifest by nodule formation and arthropathy. Ceramides have important roles (water barrier) in skin and form the "core" of gangliosides and sphingoglycolipids. Impaired capacity to degrade this "core" leads to its accumulation in the nervous system.

MIM No.: *22800

POS No.: 3436

Sex Ratio: M1:F1

Occurrence: Thirty-eight cases have been reported or identified. High incidence of consanguinity in parents. No predilection in any particular group.

Risk of Recurrence for Patient's Sib:
See Part I, *Mendelian Inheritance.*

Risk of Recurrence for Patient's Child:
See Part I, *Mendelian Inheritance.* No affected individuals are known to have reproduced.

Age of Detectability: In typical cases, signs and symptoms permit strong clinical suspicion during the first few months of life, and this can be confirmed by laboratory studies. Prenatal diagnosis has been made by demonstrating deficient activity of acid ceramidase in cultured amniocytes.

Gene Mapping and Linkage: Unknown.

Prevention: None known. Genetic counseling indicated.

Treatment: Tracheostomy may be required for airway obstruction. In mildly involved older patients unsightly nodules may be removed by plastic surgery. Other therapies are symptomatic. The more mildly involved Farber disease patients may be candidates for bone marrow transplantation. Enzymatically competent circulating bone marrow-derived cells may be able to clear the unmetabolized ceramide that appears to be the cause of the disabling nodules and infiltrates. The relatively mild or absent CNS involvement would also favor such an approach. Up to now this procedure has not been used in any Farber disease patients. In the severely ill young children with pulmonary involvement the procedure would be extremely hazardous.

Prognosis: The patients with typical Farber disease usually die before age two years due to pulmonary involvement, sometimes with general inanition. A second group of somewhat more mildly involved patients live to ages 5–10 years. These patients appear not to have lung involvement and succumb to the combination of joint involvement and progressive neurologic disease.

The most mildly involved patients appear in relatively stable condition in their teens or early adulthood. This group has been defined only recently, and information about the long-term outlook is lacking.

Detection of Carrier: Carriers have approximately 50% of normal acid ceramidase activity in leukocytes or cultured skin fibroblasts. The enzyme assay requires a synthetic substrate that is not commercially available and must be performed under carefully controlled conditions in a laboratory that has experience with the procedure.

Support Groups: NJ; Elizabeth; National Lipid Diseases Foundation

References:
Farber S, et al : Lipogranulomatosis: a new lipo-glyco-protein storage disease. J Mt Sinai Hosp 1957; 24:816.
Crocker AC, et al.: The "lipogranulomatosis" syndrome; review with report of patient showing milder involvement. In: Aronson SM, Volk BW, eds: Inborn disorders of sphingolipid metabolism. Oxford: Pergamon, 1967:485.
Dulaney JT, Moser HW: Farber's disease (lipogranulomatosis). In Glew RH, Peters SP, eds: Practical enzymology of the sphingolipidoses. New York: Alan R. Liss, Inc., 1977:283–296.
Fenson AH, et al.: Prenatal diagnosis of Farber's disease. Lancet 1979; II:990–992.
Kudoh T, Wenger DA: Diagnosis of metachromatic leukodystrophy, Krabbe disease, and Farber disease after uptake of fatty acid-labeled cerebroside sulfate into cultured skin fibroblasts. J Clin Invest 1982; 70:89–97.

Momoi T, et al.: Substrate-specificities of acid and alkaline cerami-
dases in fibroblasts from patients with Farber disease and controls.
Biochem J 1982; 205:419–425.
Antonarakis S, et al.: Phenotypic variability in siblings with Farber
disease. J Pediatr 1984; 104:406–409.
Moser HW, et al.: Ceramidase deficiency: Farber lipogranulomatosis.
In: Scriver CR, et al., eds: The metabolic basis of inherited disease,
ed 6. New York: McGraw-Hill, 1989:1645–1654.

M0038   **Hugo Moser**

Lipoid adrenal hyperplasia with male pseudohermaphroditism
See STEROID 20-22 DESMOLASE DEFICIENCY

LIPOMAS, FAMILIAL SYMMETRIC   0600

Includes:
Lipomas, multiple circumscribed
Lipomatosis, multiple familial

Excludes:
Adiposis dolorosa
Launois-Bensaude syndrome
Lipomatosis, multiple symmetric
Lipomatosis, benign diffuse symmetric
Neck/face, lipomatosis (0601)

Major Diagnostic Criteria: Presence of multiple encapsulated
subcutaneous lipomas spread over the extremities and torso in
association with a positive family history.

Clinical Findings: Multiple lipomas may be present anywhere on
the torso or extremities in a symmetric pattern. Generally, they
have developed by the third or fourth decade. They gradually
increase in size and number and may be associated with pain
during the growth phase. The number of lipomas may range from
a few up to several hundred. They are generally less than 5 cm in
size. Rarely, spontaneous regression occurs.

Complications: Pain or neurologic symptoms related to nerve
compression; cosmetic deformity.

Associated Findings: Multiple telangiectases or angiomas, multiple endocrine abnormalities, diaphyseal aclasis, hyperkeratosis
of the palms and soles, hypercholesterolemia.

Etiology: Autosomal dominant inheritance.

Pathogenesis: Unknown.

MIM No.: *15190

CDC No.: 214.800

Sex Ratio: M2:F1 (the higher proportion of males is unexplained).

Occurrence: Several large kindreds have been reported.

Risk of Recurrence for Patient's Sib:
See Part I, *Mendelian Inheritance.*

Risk of Recurrence for Patient's Child:
See Part I, *Mendelian Inheritance.*

Age of Detectability: The lipomas usually begin in early adulthood but have been described as early as age nine years.

Gene Mapping and Linkage: Unknown.

Prevention: None known. Genetic counseling indicated.

Treatment: Excision if lipomas are causing pain or nerve compression and for cosmetic indications.

Prognosis: Normal for life span and intelligence.

Detection of Carrier: Examination for evidence of lipomas in
family members.

Special Considerations: Some lipomas may follow the course of
peripheral nerves but do not appear to arise from the neural
sheath. Inheritance may be difficult to assess. The disorder may
have variable severity within a given family, the lipomas may not
present until after age 35 years. Unrelated, solitary lipomas are not
an uncommon finding in the general population. Multiple lipomas
may occur in the GI tract, but do not appear to have a familial
tendency and are most likely unrelated to this disorder. Benign

diffuse symmetric lipomatosis may be differentiated from this
disorder by the presence of unencapsulated subcutaneous symmetric fat deposits on the trunk and neck, in a typical horse collar
distribution, as well as deep accumulations of adipose tissue. It
has been reported that chromosomal abnormalities, often involving chromosome 12, in the region (q13-q14), are found in some
lipomas. However, no such association has yet been made with
the lipomas of this disorder.

References:
Kurzweg FT, Spencer R: Familial multiple lipomatosis. Am J Surg
1951; 82:762–765.
Osment LS: Cutaneous lipomas and lipomatosis. Surg Gynecol Obstet
1968; 127:129–132.
Rabbiosi G, et al.: Familial multiple lipomatosis. Acta Dermatol
Venereol 1977; 57:265–267.
Mandahl N, et al.: Lipomas have characteristic structural chromo-
somal rearrangements of 12q13-q14. Int J Cancer 1987; 39:685–688.

FI032   **Janice Finkelstein**
JA014   **Ethylin Wang Jabs**

Lipomas, multiple circumscribed
See LIPOMAS, FAMILIAL SYMMETRIC
Lipomatosis of face and neck
See NECK/FACE, LIPOMATOSIS
Lipomatosis of pancreas, congenital
See SHWACHMAN SYNDROME
Lipomatosis, benign symmetric
See NECK/FACE, LIPOMATOSIS
Lipomatosis, multiple familial
See LIPOMAS, FAMILIAL SYMMETRIC
Lipomatosis-angiomatosis-macrencephalia
See OVERGROWTH, BANNAYAN TYPE
Lipomembranous osteodystrophy
*See OSTEODYSPLASIA, LIPOMEMBRANOUS POLYCYSTIC-
DEMENTIA*

LIPOMENINGOCELE   0602

Includes:
Cauda equina lipoma
Intraspinal lipomas
Lumbosacral lipoma
Spinal dysraphism syndrome

Excludes:
Dermal sinus tract
Meningomyelocele (0693)

Major Diagnostic Criteria: A visible mass present over the vertebral column, accompanied by spina bifida occulta and widening of
interpedicular distances, is the usual presentation. Myelogram
will show widened subarachnoid space, with filling defect of
lipoma, at termination of spinal cord.

Clinical Findings: A skin-covered mass in the lumbosacral region
is noted at birth. This mass may have an associated angioma or
tuft of hair. Neurologic function is normal for legs and sphincters,
or there may be minor deficits. X-rays indicate the presence of a
spina bifida. As the child grows, scoliosis and neurologic loss may
occur, as they do in diastematomyelia. Asymmetry of the lower
extremities may be present. In some cases lipomeningocele has
been associated with cloacal exstrophy.

Complications: Progressive neurologic and sphincter loss; progressive orthopedic deformity.

Associated Findings: Minor dysraphic changes in spinal cord,
i.e. enlarged central canal.

Etiology: Unknown.

Pathogenesis: Displaced or heterotopic adipose tissue.

Sex Ratio: M1:F>1

Occurrence: Unknown.

Risk of Recurrence for Patient's Sib: Varies with ethnic group
and geographic location. In the range of 2–6%.

Risk of Recurrence for Patient's Child: Varies with ethnic group and geographic location. In the range of 2–6%.

Age of Detectability: At birth.

Gene Mapping and Linkage: Unknown.

Prevention: None known. Genetic counseling indicated.

Treatment: An exploration and excision of lipomatous tissue, particularly the tissue connecting the skin mass to the cord, so that the spinal cord may ascend with growth. Neurologic loss can be stabilized by surgery and may possibly be prevented by early surgery.

Prognosis: Good.

Detection of Carrier: Unknown.

References:
Dubowitz V, et al.: Lipoma of the cauda equina. Arch Dis Child 1965; 40:207.
James CCM, Lassman L: Spina bifida occulta. New York: Grune & Stratton, 1981.

SH007   **Kenneth Shapiro**

Lipomucopolysaccharidosis
See MUCOLIPIDOSIS I
Lipoprotein deficiency, familial high-density
See ANALPHALIPOPROTEINEMIA
Lipoprotein lipase deficiency, familial
See HYPERCHYLOMICRONEMIA
Lipoproteinemia-hyperchylomicronemia, hyperprebeta
See HYPERLIPOPROTEINEMIA V
Lipoproteinemia-hyperprebeta
See HYPERTRIGLYCERIDEMIA
Lipoproteinosis
See SKIN, LIPOID PROTEINOSIS
Liposarcoma
See CANCER, SOFT TISSUE SARCOMA
Lips, thick-oral mucosa
See ACROMEGALOID FACIAL APPEARANCE SYNDROME
Lisinopril, possible fetal effects
See FETAL ANGIOTENSIN CONVERTING ENZYME (ACE) INHIBITION RENAL FAILURE
Lissencephaly sequence
See LISSENCEPHALY SYNDROME

LISSENCEPHALY SYNDROME   0603

Includes:
    Chromosome 17, deletion 17p13
    Chromosome 17, monosomy 17p13
    Lissencephaly sequence
    Miller-Dieker syndrome
    Norman-Roberts syndrome

Excludes:
    Brain, schizencephaly (3001)
    Fetal retinoid syndrome (2261)
    Neu-laxova syndrome (2092)
    Walker-Warburg syndrome (2869)

Major Diagnostic Criteria: Lissencephaly (smooth brain) with absence of the gyri (agyria) or pachygyria. The appearance of the brain on CT scan is that of a figure eight with failure of opercularization. There is a wide cortical mantle and posterior enlargement of the ventricles (colpocephaly). This is combined with characteristic facial features and monosomy for the distal portion of the short arm of chromosome 17 in most of the cases studied.

Clinical Findings: *Prenatal:* polyhydramnios, decreased fetal movement.
Perinatal: low Apgar score, prolonged jaundice, low birth weight.
Brain: lissencephaly, heterotopias, colpocephaly, ventricular enlargement, hypoplasia of the corpus callosum, midline calcifications.
Neurologic function: profound mental retardation, early hypotonia, subsequent hypertonia, poor feeding, seizures, decreased spontaneous activity.

Head: congenital microcephaly, bitemporal hollowing, high forehead, prominent occiput.
Face: broad nasal bridge with epicanthal folds, upturned nares, malformed and/or malpositioned ears, abnormal irides, tortuous fundal vessels, micrognathia, long thin upper lip, late eruption of primary teeth, prominent palatine ridges. There is sometimes an unusual vertical wrinkling of the forehead.
Other: abnormal palmar creases, clinodactyly, camptodactyly, polydactyly, cryptorchidism, inguinal hernia, sacral dimple, rudimentary tail, congenital heart defects, other visceral defects.

Complications: Failure to thrive, apneic and cyanotic spells, and infantile spasms with hypsarrhythmia. Seizures may be refractory to anticonvulsant drugs, ACTH, or steroids.

Associated Findings: Duodenal atresia, urinary tract abnormalities.

Etiology: Most patients who have been adequately studied have monosomy of the distal short arm of chromosome 17. These chromosome deletions arise as de novo terminal deletions, inherited or de novo unbalanced translocations involving 17p, or unbalanced inversions of chromosome 17. However, there are some patients who have normal prophase chromosome studies. Whether these cases represent submicroscopic deletions of 17p or a phenocopy is currently unknown.

The Miller-Dieker lissencephaly/monosomy 17p13 syndrome is one of several conditions with type I lissencephaly. Type I lissencephaly is defined as agyria with or without pachygyria in conjunction with a wide cortical mantle and minimal or no hydrocephalus. A form of type I lissencephaly with sloping forehead and other facial features was described in a consanguineous family and is distinct from the Miller-Dieker type. This condition has been designated the Norman-Roberts syndrome and is felt to be autosomal recessive. Some cases of type I lissencephaly are not associated with monosomy 17p13 or with the features of Miller-Dieker syndrome or the Norman-Roberts syndrome. These cases have been described as having isolated lissencephaly sequence, which is of unknown etiology.

Patients with lissencephaly can be categorized into one of the

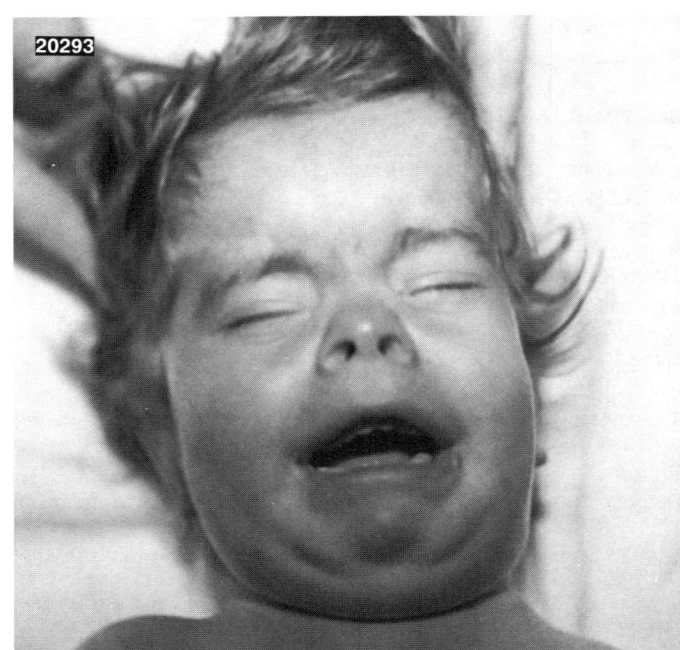

0603A-20293: Lissencephaly syndrome; note wrinkling of the forehead, broad nasal bridge, anteverted nares, long, thin upper lip, and low-set ears.

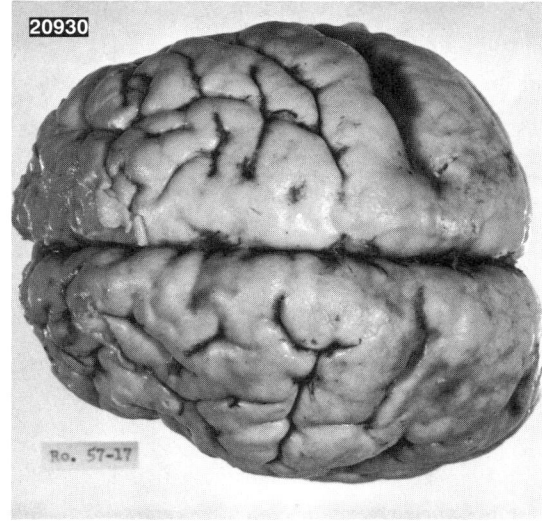

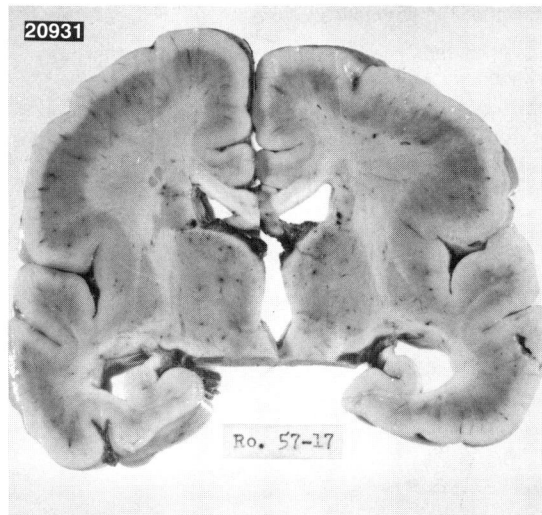

0603B-20930: Cerebral hemispheres, top view; there is a simple, convolutional pattern formed by broad gyri. **20931:** Coronal section through both hemispheres shows reduction in the number of sulci and convolutions.

above conditions based on clinical, X-ray, and cytogenetic findings. Unless a chromosomal etiology can be found, couples should probably be given a recurrence risk as high as 25% for an autosomal recessive condition.

Pathogenesis: Lissencephaly appears to be due to defect in neuronal migration with four rather than six layers in the cortex.

MIM No.: *24720

POS No.: 3134

CDC No.: 742.240

Sex Ratio: M8:F18

Occurrence: About a dozen kinships, as well as sporadic cases, have been reported.

Risk of Recurrence for Patient's Sib:
See Part I, *Mendelian Inheritance.* Probably low if de novo deletion or translocation. As high as 25% if caused by inherited translocation from one parent or if chromosome studies are normal.

Risk of Recurrence for Patient's Child:
See Part I, *Mendelian Inheritance.* Affected individuals are not expected to survive to reproduce.

Age of Detectability: Monosomy 17p13 can be detected prenatally by amniocentesis or chorionic villus sampling. Otherwise, it is usually detected postnatally based on clinical features and CT scan appearance.

Gene Mapping and Linkage: MDCR (Miller-Dieker syndrome chromosome region) has been mapped to 17p13.3.

Prevention: None known. Genetic counseling indicated.

Treatment: Supportive.

Prognosis: Patients are usually severely mentally retarded and have a reduced life span. Most affected children die by five years of age.

Detection of Carrier: Chromosome analysis.

References:
Jones KL, et al.: The Miller-Dieker syndrome. Pediatrics 1980; 66:277–281. * †
Dobyns WB, et al.: Miller-Dieker syndrome: lissencephaly and monosomy 17p. J Pediatr 1983; 102:552–558. * †
Dobyns WB, et al.: Syndromes with lissencephaly. I: Miller-Dieker and Norman-Roberts syndromes and isolated lissencephaly. Am J Med Genet 1984; 18:509–526. * †
Stratton RF, et al.: New chromosomal syndromes: Miller-Dieker syndrome and monosomy 17p13. Hum Genet 1984; 67:193–200. * †
Greenberg F, et al.: Familial Miller-Dieker syndrome associated with pericentric inversion of chromosome 17. Am J Med Genet 1986; 23:853–859.

GR011   **Frank Greenberg**

Lissencephaly syndrome II
  See WALKER-WARBURG SYNDROME
Lithium induced goiter
  See GOITER, GOITROGEN INDUCED
Lithium, fetal effects
  See FETAL LITHIUM EFFECTS
  also TRICUSPID VALVE, EBSTEIN ANOMALY
Lithobid^ induced goiter
  See GOITER, GOITROGEN INDUCED
Lithobid^, fetal effects
  See TRICUSPID VALVE, EBSTEIN ANOMALY
  also FETAL LITHIUM EFFECTS
Lithone^ induced goiter
  See GOITER, GOITROGEN INDUCED
Lithone^, fetal effects
  See FETAL LITHIUM EFFECTS
  also TRICUSPID VALVE, EBSTEIN ANOMALY
Livedo reticularis
  See CUTIS MARMORATA
Liver cholesteryl ester storage
  See CHOLESTERYL ESTER STORAGE DISEASE
Liver cyst, solitary but multilocular
  See LIVER, CYST, SOLITARY
Liver disease-erythrohepatic protoporphyria
  See PORPHYRIA, PROTOPORPHYRIA
Liver disease-neuronal degeneration of childhood
  See ALPERS DISEASE
Liver fibrosis and cirrhosis, adult
  See ALPHA(1)-ANTITRYPSIN DEFICIENCY
Liver glycerol kinase deficiency-hypertriglyceridemia
  See GLYCEROL KINASE DEFICIENCY
Liver glycerol kinase deficiency-pseudohypertriglyceridemia
  See GLYCEROL KINASE DEFICIENCY
Liver phosphorylase deficiency
  See GLYCOGENOSIS, TYPE VI
Liver phosphorylase kinase deficiency
  See GLYCOGENOSIS, TYPE IXa

LIVER, ACCESSORY LOBE 0467

Includes:
    Accessory hepatic lobes
    Hepatic lobes, accessory
    Hepatic lobes anomalous

Excludes: Liver anomalies (other)

Major Diagnostic Criteria: Evidence of additional hepatic lobe.

Clinical Findings: The lobes of the liver may vary in size and shape with either one being absent, or there may be more than two. The Reidel lobe is a tongue-like downward projection of liver tissue from the right lobe. This may resemble a large or mobile right kidney and rarely causes concern as a possible hepatic neoplasm.

Accessory lobes are not uncommonly seen in cases of anterior abdominal wall defects (i.e. omphalocele), where liver tissue may project through the defect.

Complications: Unknown.

Associated Findings: Omphalocele.

Etiology: Unknown.

Pathogenesis: Unknown.

CDC No.: 751.620

Sex Ratio: Presumably M1:F1.

Occurrence: Unknown.

Risk of Recurrence for Patient's Sib: Unknown.

Risk of Recurrence for Patient's Child: Unknown.

Age of Detectability: Unknown.

Gene Mapping and Linkage: Unknown.

Prevention: None known. Genetic counseling indicated.

Treatment: Unknown.

Prognosis: Unknown.

Detection of Carrier: Unknown.

References:
Abernathy J: Account of two instances of uncommon formation of the viscera of the human body. Philos Trans Royal Soc London [Biol] 1793; 83:59–66.

GR022   **Jay L. Grosfeld**
CL007   **H. William Clatworthy, Jr.**

LIVER, AGENESIS 0463

Includes: Hepatic agenesis

Excludes: Biliary atresia (0110)

Major Diagnostic Criteria: Complete absence of liver.

Clinical Findings: Agenesis of the liver is incompatible with life. This finding has been reported in stillborn fetuses, usually in association with other severe anomalies.

Complications: Unknown.

Associated Findings: None known.

Etiology: Failure of development of hepatic bud from foregut; causes unknown.

Pathogenesis: Unknown.

CDC No.: 751.600

Sex Ratio: Presumably M1:F1.

Occurrence: Unknown.

Risk of Recurrence for Patient's Sib: Unknown.

Risk of Recurrence for Patient's Child: Unknown.

Age of Detectability: In stillborn.

Gene Mapping and Linkage: Unknown.

Prevention: Unknown.

Treatment: Unknown.

Prognosis: Incompatible with life.

Detection of Carrier: Unknown.

Support Groups:
    NJ; Cedar Grove; American Liver Foundation
    NJ; Maplewood; The Children's Liver Foundation, Inc.

References:
Weichert RF, 3rd, et al.: Atrophy of the right lobe of the liver: case report and review of the syndromes associated with atrophy or agenesis of the liver. Am Surg 1970; 36:667–673.

GR022   **Jay L. Grosfeld**
CL007   **H. William Clatworthy, Jr.**

LIVER, ARTERIAL ANOMALIES 0464

Includes: Hepatic arterial anomalies

Excludes:
    Liver, hemangiomatosis (0466)
    Liver, venous anomalies (0468)

Major Diagnostic Criteria: Direct visualization either by angiography or at operation.

Clinical Findings: The common hepatic artery arises from the celiac axis and bifurcates into a right and left hepatic artery in the great majority of cases. The right hepatic artery divides into anterior and posterior segmental branches and the left hepatic artery into the medial and lateral branches to supply their appropriate lobes and segments.

In 17% of people, the right hepatic artery arises in an aberrant fashion from the superior mesenteric artery. In 14–23% of cases, the left hepatic artery originates directly from the left gastric artery. The recognition of these aberrant vessels is of great importance during the performance of hepatobiliary or gastric operations.

Complications: Unknown.

Associated Findings: None known.

Etiology: Unknown.

Pathogenesis: Unknown.

CDC No.: 751.620

Sex Ratio: Presumably M1:F1

Occurrence: Unknown.

Risk of Recurrence for Patient's Sib: Unknown.

Risk of Recurrence for Patient's Child: Unknown.

Age of Detectability: Unknown.

Gene Mapping and Linkage: Unknown.

Prevention: Unknown.

Treatment: Unknown.

Prognosis: Unknown.

Detection of Carrier: Unknown.

References:
Michels N: The hepatic, cystic and retroduodenal arteries and their relation to the biliary ducts. Ann Surg 1951; 133:503.
Michels N: Blood supply and the anatomy of the upper abdominal organs. Philadelphia: J.B. Lippincott, 1955.

GR022   **Jay L. Grosfeld**
CL007   **H. William Clatworthy, Jr.**

LIVER, CONGENITAL CYSTIC DILATATION OF INTRAHEPATIC DUCTS 3155

Includes:
Caroli disease
Nonobstructive dilation of the intrahepatic biliary tree

Excludes:
Bile duct choledochal cyst (0149)
Cystic fibrosis (0237)
Hepatic cyst, isolated primary
Kidney, polycystic disease, recessive (2003)

Major Diagnostic Criteria: Demonstration of fusiform, saccular, or cystic dilation of intrahepatic bile ducts in the absence of obstruction and portal fibrosis.

Clinical Findings: Patients present at any age with fever and right upper quadrant pain. These symptoms usually result from cholangitis, which frequently complicates this condition. The symptom may also result from acute obstruction from stones, which may form in ducts. Hepatomegaly and jaundice are infrequent. Transaminases are usually normal, whereas alkaline phosphates and gamma-glutamyltranspeptidase levels are elevated.

Ultrasound and computed tomography of the liver will reveal multiple enlarged ducts or cystic structures. Cholangiogram, either percutaneous transhepatic or endoscopic retrograde, will demonstrate the typical ductular dilation. Filling defects represent intraductal stones.

Complications: Cholangitis results from stagnation of bile. Infection can cause acute febrile episodes and worsening of liver function. Hepatic abcess can result. Liver failure is infrequent, and can be treated with orthotopic hepatic transplantation. Cholangiocarcinoma occurs at increased frequency.

Associated Findings: Occasional patients will have renal lesions as in congenital hepatic fibrosis (see **Kidney, polycystic disease, recessive**). **Bile duct choledochal cyst** has also been reported.

Etiology: Sporadic; no known familial incidence.

Pathogenesis: During early organogenesis, when ductular elements are proliferating, an uncontrolled overproliferation of cellular elements may occur. During subsequent canalization, redundant ductular epithelium results in dilated or cystic ducts.

MIM No.: *26320

Sex Ratio: M1:F1

Occurrence: Fewer than 50 cases have been documented.

Risk of Recurrence for Patient's Sib: Presumably not increased.

Risk of Recurrence for Patient's Child: Presumably not increased.

Age of Detectability: Clinically, from infancy to old age.

Gene Mapping and Linkage: Unknown.

Prevention: None known. Genetic counseling indicated.

Treatment: Acute episodes of cholangitis are treated with intravenous antibiotics. Acute obstructions are managed by surgical drainage. If one lobe is particularly involved, partial hepatectomy may be performed. Orthotopic liver transplantation is curative.

Prognosis: Variable. Recurrent cholangitis can result in rapid progression to liver failure.

Detection of Carrier: Unknown.

References:
Caroli J, et al.: La dilatation polykystique congenitale desvoies biliares intra-hepatiques: essai de classification. Sem Hop Paris 1958; 34:128–135.
Murray-Lyon IM, et al.: Non-obstructive dilatation of the intrahepatic biliary tree with cholangitis. Q J Med 1972; 41:477–489.
Hermansen MC, et al.: Caroli disease: the diagnosis approach. J Pediatr 1979; 94:879–882.
Thung SN, Gerber MA: Caroli's disease: a rarely recognized entity. Arch Pathol Lab Med 1979; 103:650–652.
Fagundes-Nato U, et al.: Caroli's disease in childhood: report of two new cases. J Pediatr Gastro Nutr 1983; 2:708–711.

WH007   **Peter F. Whitington**

LIVER, CYST, SOLITARY 0465

Includes:
Cysts, solitary liver
Hepatic cyst, nonparasitic
Hepatic cyst, solitary
Hepatic cyst, unilocular
Liver cyst, solitary but multilocular

Excludes:
Bile duct choledochal cyst (0149)
Liver, hamartoma (0604)
Liver, hepatic fibrosis, congenital (0605)
Parasitic cysts

Major Diagnostic Criteria: A mass in right upper quadrant makes solitary hepatic cyst a possible diagnosis.

Clinical Findings: Solitary hepatic cysts are unilocular (90%) or multilocular (10%), and are usually located in the anteroinferior margin of the right lobe. While most of these cysts are slow growing and asymptomatic, pain and the presence of a mass are common findings. Pain may be due to distention of the liver capsule, resulting from torsion of a pedunculated cyst, or hemorrhage into the cyst. A solitary hepatic cyst is occasionally seen associated with abdominal wall defect (omphalocele). Ultrasonography, radioisotopic scintiscans, and CAT scan may be useful diagnostic adjuncts.

Complications: Torsion of a pedunculated tumor, hemorrhage, infection, and rarely, portal hypertension.

Associated Findings: Strangulation due to torsion of a pedunculated lesion, rupture and hemorrhage into the abdominal cavity, and rarely, development of portal hypertension with bleeding varices.

Etiology: Undetermined. It is thought that these cysts arise from aberrant bile ducts obstructed as a result of congenital malformation.

Pathogenesis: The solitary hepatic cyst is non-calcified and lined with an inner layer of cuboidal epithelial cells or a dense fibrous layer. The outer layer often contains portions of bile duct remnants. The cyst has low internal tension and fluid that contains albumin, cholesterol, mucin, and epithelial elements. Infection, hemorrhage into, and torsion of the cysts may occur.

CDC No.: 751.610

Sex Ratio: M1:F4

Occurrence: 1:1000 autopsies.

Risk of Recurrence for Patient's Sib: Not demonstrably increased.

Risk of Recurrence for Patient's Child: Not demonstrably increased.

Age of Detectability: The majority of these cysts are asymptomatic and usually do not become apparent until the fourth or fifth decade or are incidental findings at necropsy studies. Solitary hepatic cysts (nonparasitic) are rarely observed in childhood. Although often asymptomatic throughout life, the cyst is potentially dangerous.

Gene Mapping and Linkage: Unknown.

Prevention: None known. Genetic counseling indicated.

Treatment: Simple excision of the cyst is the treatment of choice when possible, with internal drainage as an alternative. Under certain conditions, hepatic lobectomy may be required. Marsupialization is an alternative for non-resectable lesions as the cyst secretions can be absorbed by the peritoneum. However, if a biliary radical enters the cyst, marsupialization should be avoided because it may result in persistent bile drainage and the risk of biliary peritonitis.

Prognosis: Good. Many remain asymptomatic throughout life and are noted only as an autopsy finding. Others are usually amenable to operative extirpation. Overall mortality rate due to the cyst is 2.4–5.0%, related perhaps to portal hypertension and its complications.

Detection of Carrier: Unknown.

References:

Henson SW Jr, et al.: Benign tumors of the liver. III. Solitary cysts. Surg Gynecol Obstet 1956; 103:607.

Clark DD, et al.: Solitary hepatic cysts. Surgery 1967; 61:687.

Longmire WP Jr. Hepatic surgery: trauma, tumors and cysts. Ann Surg 1965; 161:1.

GR022   **Jay L. Grosfeld**
CL007   **H. William Clatworthy, Jr.**

Liver, diffuse capillary or cavernous hemangioma of
See LIVER, HEMANGIOMATOSIS

LIVER, HAMARTOMA   0604

Includes:

Cystic hamartoma of liver
Hamartoma of liver
Hepatic hamartoma
Leber hamartoma
Mesenchymal hamartoma of liver

Excludes:

Hepatic adenoma
Hepatic nodular hyperplasia
Liver, cyst, solitary (0465)
Liver, hemangiomatosis (0466)

Major Diagnostic Criteria: Large, asymptomatic, right-upper quadrant mass in an infant. Actual histologic evaluation is necessary for a final diagnosis.

Clinical Findings: Mesenchymal hamartoma of the liver is a rare benign tumor of infancy that is usually asymptomatic, except for the presence of a mass. Most are located in the right lobe of the liver; in one-third of the cases the mass is on a pedicle. These tumors may be exceptionally large and may occupy much of the peritoneal cavity.† They are more common in patients with hemihypertrophy.

Complications: Respiratory embarrassment from diaphragmatic elevation due to large mass; rarely, torsion of tumor on pedicle.

Associated Findings: None known.

Etiology: Unknown.

Pathogenesis: The tumor is composed of collagenous tissue thought to arise from primitive mesenchyme and small cystic areas having distorted hepatic tissue components. Grossly, the lesion appears as a reddish-brown, firm, elastic tumor that is solitary and spherical. It is quite large, weighing between 1,500–3,000 gm. There are two types: one in which loose collagenous fibrous stroma predominate, and one in which multiple small cysts predominate. The cyst walls may be of bile duct or lymphangiomatous origin. Smaller cysts have a single layer of lining cells, while larger cysts are usually devoid of lining cells.

CDC No.: 751.620

Sex Ratio: Presumably M1:F1.

Occurrence: Undetermined but presumed rare.

Risk of Recurrence for Patient's Sib: Unknown.

Risk of Recurrence for Patient's Child: Unknown.

Age of Detectability: Usually detected within the first two years of life.

Gene Mapping and Linkage: Unknown.

Prevention: None known. Genetic counseling indicated.

Treatment: The therapy of choice for mesenchymal hamartoma of the liver is surgical resection. This is simple if a pedicle is

present (1/3 of cases), since it is not necessary to resect beyond the tumor into normal liver when the diagnosis can be established at the time of operation. When such a distinction cannot be made, hepatic lobectomy is indicated.

Prognosis: Excellent when resection is possible.

Detection of Carrier: Unknown.

Special Considerations: Mesenchymal hamartoma of the liver is an interesting congenital lesion that only recently has been appreciated as an entity. This lesion should be differentiated from hemangiomatosis (which is a more diffuse lesion with skin components and heart failure) and from solitary cysts and polycystic disease of the liver. It is important to separate this entity from true hepatic adenomas and focal nodular hyperplasia. True hepatic adenomas are very rare; they and consist of normal-appearing or atypical liver cells arranged in cords and, occasionally, forming bile ducts. Portal triads and central veins are absent. Hepatic adenomas are usually solitary and occur in otherwise normal livers. Focal nodular hyperplasia is a "tumor-like" condition that is seen with regeneration following liver injury. The cause of this disorder is unknown; however, some type of injury to the liver and interference with and diminution of the blood supply has been suggested. Many of these tumors and conditions have a strikingly similar gross appearance, so differentiation by appearance alone is unreliable, and careful microscopic analysis is important.

References:

Edmondson HA: Differential diagnosis of tumors and tumor-like lesions of the liver in infancy and childhood. Am J Dis Child 1956; 91:168–186.

Ishida M, et al.: Mesenchymal hamartoma of the liver. Ann Surg 1966; 164:175–182.

GR022   **Jay L. Grosfeld**
CL007   **H. William Clatworthy, Jr.**

LIVER, HEMANGIOMATOSIS   0466

Includes:

Liver, diffuse capillary or cavernous hemangioma of
Hepatic hemangiomatosis
Hepatic infantile hemangioendothelioma

Excludes:

Liver, hamartoma (0604)
Solitary hepatic hemangioma

Major Diagnostic Criteria: Consider hepatic hemangiomatosis in any infant in the first six months of life with hepatomegaly, congestive heart failure, and cutaneous hemangiomas. Confirm with hepatic scintiscan and celiac angiogram.

Clinical Findings: Hepatic hemangiomatosis of infancy is usually seen with the triad of progressive hepatomegaly (100%), congestive heart failure (93%), and multiple cutaneous hemangiomas (86%). These lesions attain their maximum growth rate in the first six months of life. Due to their immense size, they may trap platelets causing thrombocytopenia, produce arteriovenous shunting leading to cardiac failure, or may cause symptoms by compressing adjacent viscera. Hepatic hemangiomatosis is a diffuse process usually involving the entire organ. A wide pulse pressure, bounding peripheral pulses, and a systolic bruit and thrill over the liver can usually be observed. Jaundice is rare and ascites has not been observed. Dilutional anemia may be noted as a result of compensatory expansion of plasma volume. Flat-plate and erect abdominal X-rays may show an enlarged liver shadow. Hepatic scintiscan will show a large filling defect. Celiac angiogram shows a characteristic arteriovenous blush within the liver with a large celiac axis and hepatic artery. A decrease in the circumference of the abdominal aorta beyond the celiac axis consistent with the diversion of blood flow through the liver is also seen. Computerized axial tomography may be a useful diagnostic aid.

Complications: Thrombocytopenia due to platelet trapping, congestive heart failure due to arteriovenous shunting, hemorrhage due to rupture of hemangioma.

Associated Findings: Multiple cutaneous hemangiomas.

Etiology: These tumors represent a congenital vascular malformation composed of endothelial-lined channels of capillary size and are very cellular. Capillary hemangiomas usually involve the skin, but may be of multicentric origin, which helps explain occurrence in the liver.

Pathogenesis: The pathophysiology of hepatic hemangiomatosis includes a wide-open conduit between the hepatic artery and veins. The arteriovenous (A-V) fistula increases the venous return to the heart, and raises the cardiac output with subsequent increase in right atrial pressure as congestive failure occurs. The severity of the symptoms corresponds to the natural history of the tumor and its growth pattern.

CDC No.: 751.620

Sex Ratio: M1:F2

Occurrence: Unknown.

Risk of Recurrence for Patient's Sib: Unknown.

Risk of Recurrence for Patient's Child: Unknown.

Age of Detectability: Usually within the first six months of life.

Gene Mapping and Linkage: Unknown.

Prevention: None known. Genetic counseling indicated.

Treatment: Corticosteroid therapy, radiation, and hepatic-artery ligation have all been employed with some degree of success. Transangiographic catheter embolization with gel-foam has been occasionally successful. Steroids are also useful if thrombocytopenia is present. Congestive heart failure develops within six weeks of birth in 50% of cases. The failure of digitalis and diuretics in the past makes other avenues of therapy a most important consideration. Since the liver is diffusely involved by hemangioendothelioma, hepatic lobectomy is also an ineffective form of treatment.

Steroids have caused noticeable regression of hemangioma within two weeks of therapy. Although the mechanism of steroid therapy is unknown, it is suggested that the rapidly proliferating endothelium in the hemangioma is sensitive to circulating steroids. The frequency of response to steroids has not been documented.

Although radiotherapy is a somewhat controversial method of therapy, occasional reports of its effectiveness have been recorded. Catheter embolization may be useful.

Hepatic-artery ligation has been successfully employed when accomplished proximal to the collateral branches so that obliteration of all arterial inflow is prevented.

All of these adjuncts to therapy hopefully are employed to "buy time" until spontaneous involution and shrinkage of the tumor occurs.

Digitalis derivatives and diuretics alone do not improve most infants in failure because of the large A-V shunts.

Prognosis: Mortality is greater than 90% if diuretics or digitalis alone are employed. In all fatal cases, death occurs within six months of birth during the rapid growth of the lesion and prior to spontaneous involution.

Detection of Carrier: Unknown.

References:
DeLorimier AA, et al.: Hepatic-artery ligation for hepatic hemangiomatosis. New Engl J Med 1967; 277:333.
Fost NC, Esterly, NB: Successful treatment of juvenile hemangiomas with prednisone. J Pediatr 1968; 72:351.
Goldberg SJ, Fonkalsrud EW: Successful treatment of hepatic hemangioma with corticosteroids. J.A.M.A. 1969; 208:2473.
Larcher V, et al.: Hepatic artery ligation in hepatic hemangioma. Arch Dis Child 1981; 56:7.

GR022
CL007

Jay L. Grosfeld
H. William Clatworthy, Jr.

LIVER, POLYCYSTIC AND MULTICYSTIC DISEASE, ADULT TYPE　　3201

Includes:
　Hepatic (liver) cysts
　Kidney-liver disease, adult type polycystic
　Multiple autosomal dominant liver-kidney cystic disease

Excludes:
　Hepatic cysts, secondary and infectious
　Kidney, polycystic adult type (0859)
　Kidney, polycystic disease infantile potter type I (2003)
　Kidney, renal dysplasia, Potter type II (3028)
　Liver, congenital cystic dilatation of intrahepatic ducts (3155)
　Liver, cyst, solitary (0465)
　Liver, hepatic fibrosis, congenital (0605)

Major Diagnostic Criteria: Demonstration by ultrasound or computerized tomography of multiple cysts in the liver and/or kidney in an individual with positive family history.

Clinical Findings: The peak age of detection is about 50 years. There is usually no liver dysfunction, and the lesions are often found at autopsy. About one-half of patients have symptoms, which include dull pain, a sense of fullness and a mass in the right upper abdominal quadrant. Fifty to 70 percent of patients will have coexistant polycystic kidneys, and about one-sixth of all patients will be seen first for renal symptoms, particularly hypertension.

Any of the newer imaging techniques, which include ultrasound, computerized X-ray tomography and nuclear magnetic resonance imaging, can be used to demonstrate multiple cysts in the liver and kidneys. The number of cysts vary from fewer than ten to many hundreds. Cysts vary in size from <1 to >12 cm. diameter.

The cysts are filled with thin, straw-colored fluid, *not* bile. Bile-filled cysts are biliary in origin and communicate with functional bile ducts, which is an important differentiation from polycystic disease. Pathologic examination reveals a thin cuboidal lining of uncertain origin. About a third of cases will have associated von Meyenberg complexes, which are thought to originate from biliary epithelium.

Complications: Significant complications are rare. Portal hypertension with esophageal varices have been reported. Post-traumatic rupture with bleeding and infection also occur.

Associated Findings: Fifty to seventy percent have polycystic kidneys; 4:70 in one series had intracranial arterial aneurysms; occasional cysts in other glandular organs and lungs; rarely intestinal duplication.

Etiology: Autosomal dominant inheritance.

Pathogenesis: The cell or tissue origin of the cysts is uncertain. The presence of many organic anions and proteins in the fluid suggests that transport of solutes into the cyst space drives the accumulation of fluid. Bile salts do not enter the space, which suggests that these cysts do not communicate with or share the functions of the excretory system of the liver.

MIM No.: 17405

CDC No.: 751.610

Sex Ratio: M1:F1

Occurrence: Undetermined. 1:687 autopsies in Michigan, and 29 cases in the surgical pathology files of the Mayo Clinic from 1907–1954, suggest the probable frequency.

Risk of Recurrence for Patient's Sib:
　See Part I, *Mendelian Inheritance.*

Risk of Recurrence for Patient's Child:
　See Part I, *Mendelian Inheritance.*

Age of Detectability: As early as first decade, usually during the fifth and sixth decades.

Gene Mapping and Linkage: Unknown.

Prevention: None known. Genetic counseling indicated.

Treatment: Excisional therapy is impractical and often impossible because of the diffuse hepatic involvement. Aspiration and incision have the disadvantage of high recurrence. More permanent relief can be obtained by internal drainage if the cysts can be fenestrated to communicate with the liver surface. Instances of polycystic disease that are asymptomatic need no treatment. Portal hypertension, when present, can be treated with conventional medical and surgical techniques. Rarely orthotopic liver transplantation will be required for management.

Prognosis: Usually excellent, with polycystic disease of the liver having no impact on longevity. Associated findings, particularly renal disease, may produce significant morbidity.

Detection of Carrier: Possibly by ultrasound of the liver and kidneys.

Support Groups:
MO; Kansas City; Polycystic Kidney Research (PKR) Foundation
NY; New York; National Kidney Foundation

References:
Melnick PJ: Polycystic liver. Arch Pathol 1955; 59:162–172.
Henson SW, et al.: Benign tumors of the liver: polycystic disease of surgical significance. Surg Gynecol Obstet 1957; 104:63–67.
Fisher J, et al.: Polycystic liver disease: studies on the mechanisms of cyst fluid formation. Gastroenterology 1974; 66:423–428.
Luoma PV, et al.: Low high-density lipoprotein and reduced antipyrine metabolism in members of a family with polycystic liver disease. Scand J Gastroent 1980; 15:869–873.
Berrebi G, et al.: Autosomal dominant polycystic liver disease: a second family. Clin Genet 1982; 21:342–347.
Karhunen PJ, Tenhu M: Adult polycystic liver and kidney diseases are separate entities. Clin Genet 1986; 30:29–37.

WH007   **Peter F. Whitington**

Liver, steatosis of
See VISCERA, FATTY METAMORPHOSIS

LIVER, TRANSPOSITION   0606

Includes:
Hepatic situs inversus
Transposition of liver

Excludes: N/A

Major Diagnostic Criteria: The liver is found in the left side of the abdomen.

Clinical Findings: Mirror-image transposition places the liver on the left side, rather than its usual right-upper-quadrant position. Abdominal situs inversus may be complete or partial and is usually associated with dextrocardia. This anomaly should be suspected if the abdominal X-ray shows the gastric air bubble on the right.

Complications: Unknown.

Associated Findings: Findings are related to associated congenital malformations: congenital heart disease (tetralogy of Fallot, transposition of great vessels, pulmonic stenosis) and intra-abdominal anomalies (duodenal atresia or stenosis, incomplete bowel fixation prone to midgut volvulus), preduodenal portal vein, biliary atresia, asplenia, polysplenia syndrome, and Kartagener triad of bronchitis, sinusitis, and situs inversus.

Etiology: Unknown.

Pathogenesis: Related to presence of associated malformations.

CDC No.: 751.620

Sex Ratio: M1.5:F1

Occurrence: Undetermined. 1:11,000 in an X-ray survey.

Risk of Recurrence for Patient's Sib: Undetermined, but is more common in sibs of patients with situs inversus.

Risk of Recurrence for Patient's Child: Unknown.

Age of Detectability: Some 46% are detected in the first month of life.

Gene Mapping and Linkage: Unknown.

Prevention: None known. Genetic counseling indicated.

Treatment: Operations are often required for associated correctable intraabdominal anomalies such as duodenal atresia, biliary atresia, etc. Because of situs inversus, the abdominal incision should be placed in the proper location. The frequent association of cardiovascular and GI anomalies must be emphasized in these infants. Individuals in whom dextrocardia is observed should be carefully evaluated for a heart lesion, and, in addition, they should have X-ray studies of the abdomen for possible abdominal manifestations of situs inversus. Similarly, in the newborn with intestinal obstruction, the presence of dextrocardia on chest X-ray should alert the surgeon to place the incision on the appropriate side of the abdomen. In regard to the liver itself, biliary atresia has been reported in approximately 8% of the cases of situs inversus. The prognosis of the biliary atresia is not altered by the left-sided hepatic position.

Prognosis: This depends on the presence and severity of associated anomalies of the cardiovascular and GI systems, in which case mortality may be greater than 50%.

Detection of Carrier: Unknown.

References:
Merklin RJ, et al.: Situs inversus and cardiac defects: a study of 111 cases of reversed asymmetry. J Thorac Cardiovasc Surg 1963; 45:334–342.
Fonkalsrud EW, et al.: Abdominal manifestations of situs inversus in infants and children. Arch Surg 1966; 92:791–795.

GR022   **Jay L. Grosfeld**
CL007   **H. William Clatworthy, Jr.**

LIVER, VENOUS ANOMALIES   0468

Includes:
Anterior duodenal portal vein
Cavernous transformation of portal vein
Hepatic venous anomalies
Portal-vein atresia
Preduodenal portal vein
Total anomalous hepatic venous return

Excludes:
Liver, arterial anomalies (0464)
Liver, hemangiomatosis (0466)

Major Diagnostic Criteria: Specific criteria vary by type of anomaly.

Clinical Findings: *Preduodenal portal vein* is a rare congenital anomaly that occurs when the embryonic caudal branch persists between 2 primitive vitelline veins while the middle and cephalic branches atrophy, placing the portal vein anterior to the pancreas and duodenum. Preduodenal portal vein is of surgical significance since it may readily cause difficulties in operations involving the duodenum and biliary tract. Its presence should be observed and care taken not to divide it inadvertently.

Portal-vein atresia: excessive obliteration of the fetal umbilical vein and ductus venosus may lead to involvement of the portal vein resulting in atresia or stenosis. The atresia may involve the whole extent of the vein or may be localized to the portion just proximal to its division into its 2 main branches in the porta hepatis.

Cavernous transformation of portal vein: controversy exists whether this anomaly represented by spongy trabeculated venous lakes involving the portal vein is an angiomatous tumor or a result of portal vein thrombosis with recanalization and compensatory enlargement of collateral capillaries and veins. This is frequently associated with portal hypertension, splenomegaly, and bleeding esophageal varices.

Other hepatic vein anomalies: rarely, the portal vein may enter directly into the vena cava by-passing the liver or may enter directly into the right atrium. Duplication of the portal vein has been seen, but is quite rare.

In certain cases of total anomalous hepatic venous return, the pulmonary veins may drain directly into the portal vein or the ductus venosus. The pulmonary plexus drains into a common channel closely associated with the esophagus, and pierces the diaphragm entering the portal venous system. Eighty-three percent of these cases occur in male infants.

Complications: Unknown.

Associated Findings: Biliary atresia, situs inversus, complete bowel rotation, dextrocardia, and most frequently, **Duodenum, atresia or stenosis** are associated with preduodenal portal vein. Portal hypertension, splenomegaly, and rarely, variceal hemorrhage may be associated with portal-vein atresia or cavernous transformation of portal vein.

Etiology: Unknown.

Pathogenesis: Unknown.

CDC No.: 747.480

Sex Ratio: Presumably M1:F1.

Occurrence: Unknown.

Risk of Recurrence for Patient's Sib: Unknown.

Risk of Recurrence for Patient's Child: Unknown.

Age of Detectability: Unknown.

Gene Mapping and Linkage: Unknown.

Prevention: None known. Genetic counseling indicated.

Treatment: Unknown.

Prognosis: Unknown.

Detection of Carrier: Unknown.

References:
Boles ET Jr, et al.: Preduodenal portal vein. Pediatrics 1961; 28:805.
Marks C: Developmental basis of the portal venous system. Am J Surg 1969; 117:671.
Rudolph AM: Hepatic and ductus venosus blood flows during fetal life. Hepatology 1983; 2:254–258.
Whitington PF: Portal hypertension in children. Pediatr Ann 1985; 14:494–499.
Abramson SJ, et al.: Biliary atresia and noncardiac polysplenic syndromes and surgical considerations. Radiology 1987; 163:377.
McCarten K, Tule R: Preduodenal portal vein: venography, ultrasonography, and review of the literature. Ann Radiol 1978; 21:155.

GR022   **Jay L. Grosfeld**
CL007   **H. William Clatworthy, Jr.**

LUNG, ABERRANT LOBE   0611

Includes:
  Accessory lung arising from bronchial tree, esophagus, and stomach
  Accessory lung with foregut communication
  Bronchus, aberrant
  Esophageal lobe of the lung
  Lobe of lung, aberrant
  Tracheal lobe of the lung

Excludes:
  Accessory lobe(s) caused by accessory fissures
  Azygous lobe of the lung
  Lung, lobe sequestration (0612)
  Subcardiac lobe of the lung

Major Diagnostic Criteria: Demonstration of aberrant bronchus originating from trachea or esophagus.

Clinical Findings: *Aberrant lobe* generally refers to either a tracheal or esophageal lobe. Tracheal lobe is associated with an aberrant or extra bronchus arising from the lateral wall of the trachea. Patients usually present by age five years. About 50% present with recurrent pneumonia. Stridor is another frequent clinical sign. At least two cases have occurred in children with **Chromosome 21, trisomy 21**. There is an increased incidence of associated malformations (vide infra).

Esophageal lobe refers to the abnormal origin of a mainstem bronchus from the esophagus. Therefore, there is no ventilation of the involved lung. Blood supply is from the pulmonary artery.

Complications: Infection and hemorrhage.

Associated Findings: In one series 14/18 cases of tracheal lobe had associated malformations. Five patients had hypoplastic, fused, or extra fibs. Two patients had **Chromosome 21, trisomy 21**, one with associated duodenal web. **Klippel-Feil anomaly**, tracheoesophageal fistula, **Larynx, web**, omphalocele, and **Ventricular septal defect** were also reported in individual patients.

Etiology: Unknown.

Pathogenesis: The theory suggests a failure of regression of extra tracheal buds during embryogenesis of the foregut. Another theory is local disruption of normal embryogenesis, with the high incidence of associated malformation cited as supporting evidence.

CDC No.: 748.690

Sex Ratio: M1:F1

Occurrence: Undetermined. Established literature.

Risk of Recurrence for Patient's Sib: Unknown.

Risk of Recurrence for Patient's Child: Unknown.

Age of Detectability: At birth. Depending on symptoms, child may present during infancy, childhood, or, less commonly, adulthood.

Gene Mapping and Linkage: Unknown.

Prevention: None known. Genetic counseling indicated.

Treatment: Surgery is indicated in symptomatic cases. Lobectomy, or segmental resection in some cases, removes the aberrant lobe.

Prognosis: Normal. In one series surgery (lobectomy in all but one case) was performed in 10/18 patients.

Detection of Carrier: Unknown.

Special Considerations: The differentiation of esophageal lobe from **Lung, lobe sequestration** is important. The latter does not frequently involve the entire lung, and the trachea branches normally. The arterial supply in sequestration is anomalous, arising from the descending or, rarely, abdominal aorta.

Support Groups: New York; American Lung Association

References:
Young LW: Anomalous apical bronchus of the right upper lobe. Am J Dis Child 1980; 134:615–616.
Lacina S, et al.: Esophageal lung with cardiac abnormalities. Chest 1981; 79:468–470.
McLaughlin FJ, et al.: Tracheal bronchus: association with respiratory morbidity in childhood. J Pediatr 1985; 106:751–755.

BI009   **Robert M. Bilenker**

LUNG, BRONCHOGENIC CYST   2702

Includes: Bronchogenic cyst

Excludes:
  Lung, aberrant lobe (0611)
  Lung, congenital lobar adenomatosis (2501)
  Lung, extralobar sequestration
  Lung, intralobar sequestration
  Lung, lobe sequestration (0612)

Major Diagnostic Criteria: Extrapulmonary unilobular cystic lesion adherent to left main stem bronchus or carina.

Clinical Findings: Infants with obstructing bronchogenic cysts present with symptoms of moderate or severe respiratory distress and clinical signs such as wheezing, stridor, and cyanosis. Chest X-ray may show emphysema or severe obstructive atelectasis with a mediastinal shift. Bronchoscopy is thought to be too dangerous and is usually not recommended. Barium swallow will suggest the preoperative diagnosis. In the rare instance of a juxtadiaphragmatic lesion, evaluation of the lower thorax and upper abdomen with computed tomography (CT) to diagnose a "dumbell" bronchogenic cyst is of value. CT is a standard part of evaluation of lung cysts.

Complications: Infection in the cyst or adjacent atelectatic lung segments. Rhabdomyosarcoma arising in the wall of a bronchogenic cyst has been reported twice.

Associated Findings: None known.

Etiology: Undetermined. In view of associated malignancy, Krous and Sexaur (1981) recommend screening family members.

Pathogenesis: Abnormal diverticulum of a lung bud in the fifth week of gestation. The cyst is lined by ciliated columnar epithelium and has a fibrous tissue wall with nests of cartilage and sometimes bronchial glands. The cyst does not have its own blood supply. Distal structures, such as alveoli, do not form.

CDC No.: 748.480

Sex Ratio: M1:F1

Occurrence: Undetermined but presumed rare.

Risk of Recurrence for Patient's Sib: Unknown.

Risk of Recurrence for Patient's Child: Unknown.

Age of Detectability: Most cases are detected from the neonatal period to childhood. Age at presentation depends on location, size, and symptoms.

Gene Mapping and Linkage: Unknown.

Prevention: None known. Genetic counseling indicated.

Treatment: Surgical removal is the only effective treatment and is almost always indicated.

Prognosis: Excellent for complete recovery.

Detection of Carrier: Unknown.

Support Groups: New York; American Lung Association

References:
Crawford TJ, Cahill JL: The surgical treatment of pulmonary cystic disorders in infancy and childhood. J Pediatr Surg 1971; 6:251–255.
Krous HF, Sexauer CL: Embryonal rhabdomyosarcoma arising within a congenital bronchogenic cyst in a child. J Pediatr Surg 1981; 16:506–508.
Amendola MA, et al.: Transdiaphragmatic bronchopulmonary foregut anomaly: "dumbell" bronchogenic cyst. Am J Radiol 1982; 138:1165–1167.
Mendelson DS, et al.: Bronchogenic cysts with high CT numbers. Am J Radiol 1983; 149:463–465.

BI009   **Robert M. Bilenker**

LUNG, CONGENITAL LOBAR ADENOMATOSIS   2501

Includes:
  Cystic adenomatoid dysplasia of the lung
  Cystic adenomatoid malformation of the lung
  Lobar adenomatosis, lung, congenital

Excludes:
  Bronchiectasis
  Bronchopulmonary dysplasia
  Bullous emphysema
  Diaphragmatic hernia (0289)
  Lung, bronchogenic cyst (2702)
  Lung, emphysema congenital lobar (2703)
  Lung, lobe sequestration (0612)
  Lymphangiectasia, congenital pulmonary
  Mesothelial cysts
  Pneumatocele
  Pneumothorax

Major Diagnostic Criteria: In the neonatal period, a classical X-ray pattern of a cystic mass with a mediastinal shift is the key to the diagnosis.

Clinical Findings: In the neonatal period, respiratory distress, characterized by tachypnea and cyanosis. Chest X-rays show an expansible multicystic lesion with shift of the mediastinum toward the contralateral side. Because the condition has been reported in preterm hydropic stillborns (Aslam et al, 1970), sonar examination should be added to the prenatal diagnostic tools and carried out in all pregnancies complicated by hydramnios (Oster and Fortune, 1978).

Complications: Respiratory failure following progressive respiratory distress in the neonatal period, or persistent and recurrent

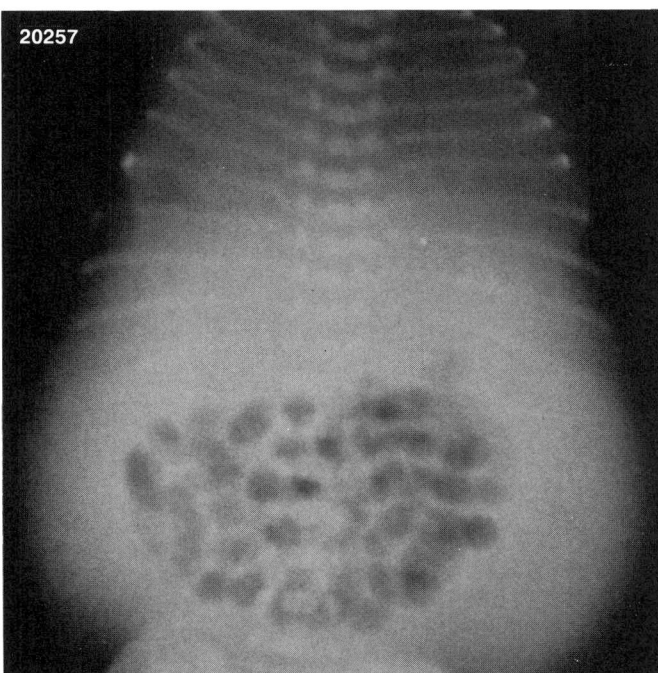

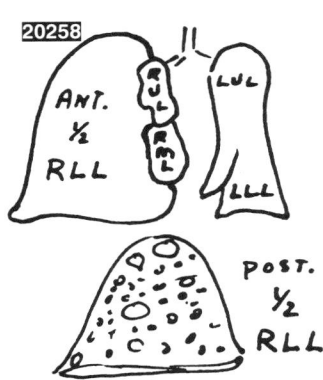
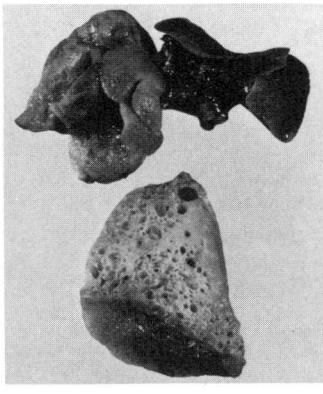

2501-20257: X-ray of the chest and abdomen showing right lower lobe cystic mass and ascites. **20258:** Pathological specimens of the lungs and an artist's drawing of the cystic adenomatoid malformation of the right lower lobe of the lung.

pneumonic processes in the affected segment of the lung in the older child.

Associated Findings: Compression of the heart and vena cava by the mass may result in fetal hydrops (Elhassani and Webb, 1984). **Pectus excavatum** occurred in four of 32 patients reported by Wolf et al (1980). Other overall associated anomalies were present in 26% of the infants described by Stoker et al (1970). Such anomalies include **Renal agenesis, bilateral** or dysgenesis and **Diaphragmatic hernia.**

Etiology: Unknown.

Pathogenesis: Cystic, solid, or mixed masses typically involving one pulmonary lobe. According to the histologic appearance of the lesion, three classes are recognized: *type I* is characterized by multiple large cysts; *type II*, by smaller and more numerous cysts; and *type III*, by a bulky, firm mass with evenly spaced small cysts (Stoker et al, 1978).

CDC No.: 748.580

Sex Ratio: M1:F1

Occurrence: About 150 cases have been reported in the literature.

Risk of Recurrence for Patient's Sib: Presumably not increased.

Risk of Recurrence for Patient's Child: Presumably not increased.

Age of Detectability: Although the majority of patients develop respiratory distress in the first week of life, the condition may be overlooked in asymptomatic children.

Gene Mapping and Linkage: Unknown.

Prevention: None known. Genetic counseling indicated.

Treatment: Surgical resection of the involved area of the lung.

Prognosis: Unknown.

Detection of Carrier: Unknown.

Support Groups: New York; American Lung Association

References:
Aslam PA, et al.: Congenital cystic adenomatoid malformation of the lung. J Am Med Asso 1970; 212:622–624.
Stoker JT, et al.: Congenital cystic adenomatoid malformation of the lung: classification and morphological spectrum. Hum Pathol 1977; 8:156–171.
Ostor AG, Fortune DW: Congenital cystic adenomatoid malformation of the lung. Am J Clin Pathol 1978; 70:595–604.
Stoker JT, et al.: Cystic and congenital lung disease in the newborn. Perspect Pediatr Pathol 1978; 4:93–154.
Wolf SA, et al.: Cystic adenomatoid dysplasia of the lung. J Pediatr Surg 1980; 15:925–930.
Avitabile IM, et al.: Congenital cystic adenomatoid malformations of the lung in adults. Am J Surg Pathol 1984; 8:193–202.
Elhassani SB, Webb CM: Right lower lobe congenital adenomatosis of the lung with anasarca. J Calif Perinat Assoc 1984; 4:59–60.

EL013   **Sami B. Elhassani**

LUNG, EMPHYSEMA CONGENITAL LOBAR   2703

Includes:
  Emphysema, congenital lobar
  Emphysema, localized congenital
  Lobar emphysema, infantile
  Lobar tension emphysema in infancy

Excludes:
  Atelectasis with compensatory emphysema
  Lung cyst, congenital
  Mucous plug, isolated

Major Diagnostic Criteria: Hyperinflated, emphysematous lung lobe with persistence of lung markings (vessels) seen on chest X-ray.

Clinical Findings: Affected infants present with respiratory distress of variable severity precipitated by crying, feeding, or respiratory infection. Left upper lobe is most often involved, followed by right middle lobe. The thoracic wall over the involved lobe(s) may be prominent, with hyperresonance on percussion and decreased breath sounds. Apical beat may be shifted away from the involved side. Chest X-ray shows the hyperinflated lobe with mediastinum displaced away from the affected side. Differential diagnosis often includes pneumothorax, pneumatocele, and congenital lung cyst. These disorders, however, all have absent lung markings in involved areas on X-ray.

Complications: Infection. Pneumothorax is rare.

Associated Findings: Cardiac defects present in a higher percentage (14% in one series) of cases in this disease than in other congenital cystic disorders of the lungs. Most often found are **Ventricular septal defect** and **Ductus arteriosus, patent. Pectus excavatum** deformities have been related to presence of congenital localized emphysema (CLE). Approximately 70% have some degree of segmental **Bronchomalacia.**

Etiology: Unknown. Sporadic in the vast majority of cases. Possible autosomal recessive inheritance has been reported twice, and dominant transmission once.

Pathogenesis: CLE is the result of several possible pathogenetic mechanisms. Lesion is most often attributed to deficient bronchial cartilage in the affected main stem bronchus. This causes endobronchial proliferation of mucous membrane, with subsequent obstruction, or extrinsic compression of a bronchus by an anomalous vessel. In 50% of cases no cause is demonstrated. In these cases an alveolar wall defect in quality, quantity, or distribution of collagen or elastin has been theorized.

MIM No.: 13071

CDC No.: 748.580

Sex Ratio: M1:F1

Occurrence: Undetermined but presumed rare.

Risk of Recurrence for Patient's Sib:
See Part I, *Mendelian Inheritance.*

Risk of Recurrence for Patient's Child:
See Part I, *Mendelian Inheritance.*

Age of Detectability: During the newborn period.

Gene Mapping and Linkage: Unknown.

Prevention: None known. Genetic counseling indicated.

Treatment: Lobectomy is generally advocated with excellent results. Segmental resection may be curative in some cases.

Prognosis: Excellent in almost all cases.

Detection of Carrier: Unknown.

Support Groups: New York; American Lung Association

References:
DeMuth GR, Sloan H: Congenital lobar emphysema: long term effects and sequelae in treatment cases. Surgery 1961; 59:601–607.
Hendren WH, McKee DM: Lobar emphysema of infancy. J Pediatr Surg 1966; 1:24–39.
Eigen H, et al.: Congenital lobar emphysema: long term evaluation of surgically conservatively treated children. Am Rev Respir Dis 1976; 113:823–831.
Wall MA, et al.: Congenital lobar emphysema in a mother and daughter. Pediatrics 1982; 70:131–133.

BI009   **Robert M. Bilenker**

Lung, hypoplastic-systemic arterial supply-venous drainage
See SCIMITAR SYNDROME

LUNG, LOBE SEQUESTRATION   0612

Includes:
Aortic pulmonary lobe
Pulmonary sequestration, extralobar
Pulmonary sequestration, intralobar

Excludes: N/A

Major Diagnostic Criteria: Extralobar sequestration is a nonfunctional pulmonary tissue mass with its own pleural covering and systemic blood supply, often associated with bronchial or gastrointestinal malformations, presenting in the thoracic or, rarely, the retroperitoneal cavity.

Intralobar sequestration is found as a mass within an existing lobe of the lung, consisting of nonfunctional pulmonary tissue not connected to the tracheobronchial tree and commonly receiving its own systemic blood supply.

Clinical Findings: Findings vary depending on the type of sequestration. Extralobar lesions present earlier, with approximately one-half found at less than age one year. Earlier age at discovery is often associated with other malformations. Approximately one-half of intralobar sequestrations are initially diagnosed in adults. Patients present with infection from contiguous or hematogenous spread. A mass is seen on X-ray with further information available from computed tomographic (CT) scanning. Aor-

tography may be used to demonstrate the aberrant systemic blood supply in either form of the disorder.

Establishing the diagnosis has been enhanced with CT scanning supplemented by selective angiography to demonstrate aberrant vascular supply and drainage.

Complications: Infection is frequent in intralobar but is unusual in extralobar (own pleural sac); hemorrhage is rare in both types.

Associated Findings: Diaphragmatic hernia may be associated on the ipsilateral, usually left, side with extralobar lesions. Foregut duplication, fistulous connection, aberrant pancreatic tissue, bronchial isomerism, and congestive heart failure have been reported with intralobar sequestration.

Etiology: Unknown.

Pathogenesis: There are two general theories of aberrant development. First, accessory budding from lung buds or from distal esophagus (in cases of bronchoesophageal fistula). Timing of the budding determines the type of sequestration. Early accessory budding causes intralobar sequestration and late accessory budding extralobar sequestration. The second theory is persistence of a pulmonary branch of the dorsal aorta predominating when the pulmary artery fails to vascularize the periphery of the lower lobe.

CDC No.: 748.520

Sex Ratio: Intralobar, M1:F1; extralobar, M4:F1

Occurrence: Less than 10% of congenital pulmonary malformations. General incidence not known.

Risk of Recurrence for Patient's Sib: Unknown.

Risk of Recurrence for Patient's Child: Unknown.

Age of Detectability: From birth onward for both types. One-half of extralobar lesions found before age one year. One-half of intralobar lesions are found in adults.

Gene Mapping and Linkage: Unknown.

Prevention: None known. Genetic counseling indicated.

Treatment: Lobectomy for intralobar lesions. Segmental resection for extralobar lesions, with medical and surgical treatment for associated findings as indicated.

Prognosis: Normal.

Detection of Carrier: Unknown.

Support Groups: New York; American Lung Association

References:
Smith RA: A theory of the origin of intralobar sequestration of lung. 1956; Thorax 11:10–24.
de Parades CG, et al.: Pulmonary sequestration in infants and children: a 20 year experience and review of the literature. J Pediatr Surg 1970; 5:136–147.
Lilly JR, et al.: Segmental lung resection in the first year of life. Ann Thorac Surg 1976; 22:16–22.

BI009   **Robert M. Bilenker**

Lung, unilobular-polydactyly-sex reversal-renal hypoplasia
See SMITH-LEMLI-OPITZ SYNDROME, TYPE II
Lupus erythematosis, neonatal, arrhythmia from
See ARRHYTHMIA, FROM MATERNAL AUTOIMMUNE DISEASE, CONGENITAL

LUPUS ERYTHEMATOSUS, SYSTEMIC   2515

Includes: Systemic lupus erythematosis (SLE)

Excludes:
Complement component 1, deficiency of (3210)
Discoid lupus erythematosus
Drug-induced lupus
Mixed connective tissue disease
Subacute cutaneous lupus erythematosus

Major Diagnostic Criteria: Revised criteria for the classification of systemic lupus erythematosus (SLE) have been established by the American Rheumatism Association (Tan et al, 1982). A person is said to have SLE if any four or more of the following 11 criteria are present serially or simultaneously during any time period: malar rash, discoid rash, photosensitivity, oral ulcers, arthritis, serositis, renal disorder, neurologic disorder, hematologic disorder, immunologic disorder, and the presence of antinuclear antibody.

Clinical Findings: Systemic lupus erythematosus (SLE) is a systemic connective tissue disease with marked and varied immunologic abnormalities. Systemic symptoms include fever, weight loss, and fatigue. The majority (85%) of affected individuals have cutaneous lesions, the most common being an erythematous butterfly rash of the face and a maculopapular rash that develops on exposed surfaces after exposure to sunlight. Alopecia is common (67%). Joint involvement with arthritis, arthralgia, and myalgia is the most common manifestation of SLE. Nonerosive arthritis associated with pain on motion, swelling, or effusion is common (75%). The arthritis is symmetric and commonly involves the proximal interphalangeal, metacarpophalangeal, knee, and wrist joints, with less involvement of the ankle, elbow, hip, and distal interphalangeal joints. Clinically evident renal disease is present in approximately 50% of individuals with SLE, while the majority (>90%) have immunopathologic changes on renal biopsy. Focal (mild) proliferative, diffuse (severe) proliferative, or membranous and mesangial (minimal) lupus nephritis can occur. Serosal involvement leads to clinically evident cardiac and pulmonary changes, the most common of which are pericarditis (25%), pleurisy (46%), and pleural effusion (40%). Nervous system involvement may be central or peripheral, as with a peripheral neuropathy. Central nervous involvement may lead to psychiatric abnormalities, seizures, long tract signs, and cranial nerve abnormalities.

Nearly all affected individuals have hematologic changes, including anemia of chronic disease, leukopenia with an absolute lymphopenia, and a mild thrombocytopenia. Hemolytic anemia with reticulocytosis and severe thrombocytopenia are infrequent. The eye, liver, and gastrointestinal tract can be involved.

SLE is an autoimmune disease in which antibodies are directed against a variety of nuclear, cytoplasmic, and cell membrane self-antigens. No antibody is specific for SLE. The fluorescent antinuclear antibody test has been the established screening test for SLE, since most affected individuals will have one or more of these antibodies, but the lack of specificity has reduced its usefulness. Antibodies directed against specific antibodies, including native DNA (positive in 80%) and the Sm nuclear antigen (positive in less than 50%), are more confirmatory. Reduced hemolytic complement (CH_{50}) levels and hypergammaglobulinemia are found with active disease.

Complications: These depend on the organ system involved. For example, severe renal involvement may lead to acute or chronic renal failure. Treatment with steroids and cytotoxic agents can lead to other complications such as opportunistic infections. Pregnancy in a woman with SLE leads to special problems, both for the mother and the child. Pregnancy may exacerbate the activity of the disease, and the fetus can develop neonatal lupus erythematosus, presenting as skin lesions and/or congenital heart block. Transplacental transfer of maternal autoantibodies directed

Table 2515-1 Revised Criteria for Lupus Erythematosus, Systemic (SLE)

Criterion	Definition
Malar rash	Fixed erythema, flat or raised, over the malar eminences, tending to spare nasolabial folds.
Discoid rash	Erythematous raised patches with adherent keratotic scaling and follicular plugging; atrophic scarring may occur in older lesions.
Photosensitivity	Skin rash as a result of unusual reaction to sunlight, by patient history or physician observation.
Oral ulcers	Oral or nasopharyngeal ulceration, usually painless, observed by physician.
Arthritis	Nonerosive arthritis involving two or more peripheral joints, characterized by tenderness, swelling, or effusion.
Serositis	1. Pleuritis—Convincing history of pleuritic pain or rub heard by a physician or evidence of pleural effusion. *or* 2. Pericarditis—Documented by ECG or rub or evidence of pericardial effusion.
Renal disorder	1. Persistent proteinuria greater than 0.5 g per day of greater than 3+ if quantitation not performed. *or* 2. Cellular casts—May be red cell, hemoglobin, granular, tubular, or mixed.
Neurologic disorder	1. Seizures—In the absence of offending drugs or known metabolic derangements (e.g., uremia, ketoacidosis, or electrolyte imbalance). *or* 2. Psychosis—In the absence of offending drugs or known metabolic derangements (e.g., uremia, ketoacidosis, or electrolyte imbalance).
Hematologic Disorder	1. Hemolytic anemia—With reticulocytosis. *or* 2. Leukopenia—Less than 4,000/mm³ total on two or more occasions. *or* 3. Lymphopenia—Less than 1,500/mm³ on two or more occasions. *or* 4. Thrombocytopenia—Less than 100,000/mm³ in the absence of offending drugs.
Immunologic disorder	1. Positive LE cell preparation. *or* 2. Anti-DNA—Antibody to native DNA in abnormal titer. *or* 3. Anti-Sm—Presence of antibody to Sm nuclear antigen. *or* 4. False-positive serologic test for syphilis known to be positive for at least 6 months and confirmed by *Treponema pallidum* immobilization or fluorescent treponemal antibody absorption test.
Antinuclear antibody	An abnormal titer of antinuclear antibody by immunofluorescence or an equivalent assay at any point in time and in the absence of drugs known to be associated with "drug-induced lupus" syndrome

SOURCE: Tan EM, Cohen AS, Fries JF, et al; The 1982 revised classification of SLE. *Arthritis Rheum* 25:1271, 1982. Reprinted from ARTHRITIS AND RHEUMATISM Journal, copyright 1982. Used by permission of the American College of Rheumatology.

against the SS-A (Ro) antigen is thought to be the responsible mechanism for neonatal lupus.

Associated Findings: Spontaneous abortion, premature birth, and newborns who are small for gestational age are more common with maternal SLE.

Etiology: Undetermined. Probably multifactorial with genetic, environmental and endocrine factors playing some part. The genetic susceptibility is related to histocompatibility antigens, complement, and immunoglobulin allotypes by unknown mechanisms.

Approximately 1–2% of the first-degree relatives of an affected individual have SLE, and the frequency of those with antinuclear antibodies and hypergammaglobulinemia is greater. Impressive pedigrees with many affected members have been published. Concordance for SLE in monozygotic twins is approximately 50–70%. Rare inherited deficiencies of C2, C1q, C1r, C1s, C4, C5, C8, and C1 esterase inhibitor are associated with the development of SLE, the most common being a deficiency of C2. The frequencies of HLA-B8, HLA-DR3, and HLA-DR2 are increased in affected individuals when compared with a control population. The C4A null allele is in linkage disequilibrium with HLA-B8 and HLA-DR3 and is found in excess in SLE. Family studies to determine haplotype sharing and linkage between HLA and a possible SLE susceptibility gene (or genes) are inconclusive. An association between SLE and the immunoglobulin (Gm) allotypes has been established, and studies have suggested an interaction between Gm and HLA that is important in the genetic predisposition to lupus nephritis.

Pathogenesis: SLE is probably not a single disease but a syndrome. Genetic, hormonal, and environmental factors (e.g. sunlight, drugs, infections) all seem to play a role. The occurrence of a variety of autoantibodies, the presence of circulating immune complexes, demonstration of immune complexes in affected organs, and consumption of complement suggest that the clinical manifestations of the disease is mediated by immune complexes. However, it is not clear whether the primary defect is with the uncontrolled function of B-cells or with defects in T-cell regulation of B-cells.

MIM No.: 15270

Sex Ratio: M1:F3 in children, increasing to M1:F8–9 in young adults (aged 20–30 years) and falling to M1:F3 after ages 40–50 years. The altered sex ratio and the fact that SLE has been described in **Klinefelter syndrome** suggest that hormone balance may be important in the development of SLE.

Occurrence: Worldwide. Annual incidence is 6–7:100,000 for low-risk populations and up to 35:100,000 for high-risk populations. SLE is three times more common in American Blacks and Orientals than in American Caucasians. Certain Amerindian tribes (Sioux, Crow, Arapahoe) have a high incidence.

Risk of Recurrence for Patient's Sib:
See Part I, *Mendelian Inheritance.*

Risk of Recurrence for Patient's Child:
See Part I, *Mendelian Inheritance.*

Age of Detectability: Usually clinically evident by ages 20–30 years of age. Neonatal lupus can be a complication of maternal SLE.

Gene Mapping and Linkage: Unknown.

Prevention: None known. Genetic counseling indicated. Detection of a slow acetylator phenotype may be helpful in predicting an increased susceptibility to drug-induced SLE.

Treatment: Variable, depending on the systems involved and the severity of the condition. Nonsteroidal anti-inflammatory drugs, hydroxychloroquin, steroids, and cytotoxic agents have been used.

Prognosis: Dependent on the organ systems involved. Genetic factors do not clearly predict severity of disease or prognosis.

Detection of Carrier: Unknown. Autoantibodies are common in healthy relatives of an affected individual and do not identify those individuals who will develop clinical disease.

Special Considerations: It is unlikely that SLE is a single disease; rather, it is a genetically heterogeneous group of disorders with a common phenotype. The component responsible for the genetic susceptibility will differ from family to family, as will the responsible environmental component(s).

Many of the immunologic, genetic, and hormonal factors in this disease have been studied extensively in the murine counterpart of human SLE (NZB/NZW F_1 mice).

Support Groups:
New York; Systemic Lupus Erythematosus Foundation
CA; Torrance; American Lupus Society
CA; Van Nuys; National Lupus Erythematosus Foundation
DC; Washington; The Lupus Foundation of America

References:
Block SR, et al.: Studies of twins with systemic lupus erythematosus: a review of the literature and presentation of 12 additional sets. Am J Med 1975; 59:533–552.
Russell AS: Genetic factors in systemic lupus erythematosus. Semin Arthritis Rheu 1981; 10:255–263.
Tan EM, et al.: The 1982 revised criteria for the classification of systemic lupus erythematosus. Arthritis Rheum 1982; 25:1271–1277.
Rothfield N: Clinical features of systemic lupus erythematosus. In: Kelley WN, et al, eds: Textbook of rheumatology, ed 2. Philadelphia: W.B. Saunders, 1985:1070–1097.
Agnello V: Lupus diseases associated with hereditary and acquired deficiencies of complement. Springer Semin Immunopathol 1986; 9:161–178.
Howard PF, et al.: Relationship between C4 null genes, HLA-D region antigens, and genetic susceptibility to systemic lupus erythematosus in Caucasian and black Americans. Am J Med 1986; 81:187–193.
Mintz G, et al.: Prospective study of pregnancy in systemic lupus erythematosus. Results of a multidisciplinary approach. J Rheumatol 1986; 13:732–739.
Stenszky V, et al.: Interplay of immunoglobulin G heavy chain markers (Gm) and HLA in predisposing to systemic lupus nephritis. J Immunogenet 1986; 13:11–17.
McCune AB, et al.: Maternal and fetal outcome in neonatal lupus erythematosus. Ann Intern Med 1987; 106:518–523.
Greer JM, Panush RS: Incomplete lupus erythematosus. Arch Intern Med 1989; 149:2473–2476.

KI007   **Richard A. King**

LYMPHEDEMA I   0614

Includes:

Edema (vs. Lymphedema)
Lymphedema, congenital hereditary
Lymphedema, early-onset
Microcephaly-lymphedema-normal intelligence
Milroy disease
Nonne-Milroy type hereditary lymphedema

Excludes:

Acquired lymphedema (post radiation, surgical, infectious)
Lymphedema II (0615)
Lymphedema-hypoparathyroidism (2801)

Major Diagnostic Criteria: Usually present at birth; a firm or brawny edema usually of the lower extremity, distal to Poupart's ligament. May be generalized to the leg or limited to portions of a foot or toes.

Lymphedema and "edema" are not the same and should not be confused (Watts, 1985).

Clinical Findings: Congenital hereditary lymphedema is one of two principal types of chronic hereditary lymphedema (see **Lymphedema II**) This form is equivalent to that originally described by Milroy, earlier and independently by Nonne. Milroy's valuable 35 year follow up (1928) of his original family discussed and distinguished the possibly variant form now known as Meige disease, or late-onset chronic hereditary lymphedema. Schroeder and Helweg-Larsen (qua Schroeder infra) (1950) considered these as variants of one process. The paper marking the modern era of study is that of (Esterly, 1965), which contains a still useful review of earlier reports. Esterly distinguished the two types. There are differences in manifestation, other than the age of effective clinical onset, which suggest some value in continuing to consider chronic hereditary lymphedema as having two subtypes, pending further studies. Nevertheless, the overlap is such that classification of the various lymphedema can not be done simply or with certainty.

In most forms of lymphedema, the edema pits with ease (Esterly, 1965) and shows diurnal fluctuation, with lessening at night (Schroeder and Helweg-Larsen, 1950). The swelling is neither painful or tender (Milroy, 1928). Temperature differences of skin surface may be found. A high tissue fluid flow rate has been demonstrated, possibly explaining Esterly's observation of tachycardia in an adult with congenital hereditary lymphedema. While usually found in the legs, clinically and pathologically significant cases occur with isolated arm involvement (Merrick, et al. 1971).

Under the designation of "primary lymphedema" (Dale, 1985) reported four anatomic subtypes according to lymphographic findings:

Distal hypoplasia: a reduced number and/or size of lymph channels.

Proximal hypoplasia: vessels and nodes too small or too few in groins and pelvis. This is associated with dilated and tortuous, numerous distal vessels.

Distal and proximal hypoplasia: a combination of the above.

Hyperplasia: large, numerous, dilated, and tortuous vessels in leg, groin or pelvis with or without megalymphatics. The latter are usually unilateral whereas hyperplasia is often bilateral.

Generally, systemic pathophysiologic manifestations are absent or not well documented. Hypotonia is often seen in the congenital form.

In making a diagnosis in an infant, other forms of extremity enlargement, such as in hemihypertrophy, would need to be distinguished. In adults with apparent congenital lymphedema, local causes of lymphatic obstruction would need to be ruled out, such as postinfectious states, radiation fibrosis, metastatic or primary tumor in regional lymph nodes, or after surgical interruption as in mastectomy.

Complications: Poor healing of the tissues following minor trauma would seem to be a possibility but the literature is silent on this. Milroy cited Hope and French as describing acute "attacks" characterized by shivering, emesis, onset of pain over the lymphedema, tachycardia, fever, tachypnea, and an acute redness, added swelling, and increased tenderness too painful to attempt pitting. Milroy pointed out that none of his cases ever showed this peculiar finding. Subsequent literature has failed to comment on the matter. The attacks were self limited and never fatal, points which, given the era of the report by Hope and French (1907), would seem to rule out superimposed infection.

A significant longer term complication is the occurrence of malignant disease within the involved extremity. This has been mainly lymphangiosarcoma (Dubin, et al 1974) but squamous (epidermoid) carcinoma has also been described (Epstein and Mendelsohn, 1984). In three cited cases the interval between diagnosis of the lymphedema and the appearance of tumor was 52 years for lymphangiosarcoma in an arm showing congenital lymphedema, 53 years for squamous carcinoma of the foot of the leg with congenital lymphedema, and 28 years for another case of lymphangiosarcoma following on lymphedema first diagnosed at age 6 months. Both sarcomas were fatal, with survival post diagnosis of 30 and 9 months respectively. A larger series indicated a 50% mortality rate within 24 months after diagnosis of lymphangiosarcoma (Woodward, et al 1972). A man with squamous carcinoma had nonhealing ulcers 15 and 10 years earlier treated by excision and skin grafting, to no avail.

Associated Findings: Most lesions are isolated findings. Recently, however associated syndromes with other heritable conditions have been described. The most consistent has been the combination of microcephaly and lymphedema with normal intelligence (Robinow et al, 1970; Crowe & Dickerman, 1986; Leung, 1985, 1987; Meinecke, 1987) (see also **Microcephaly-lymphedema**). Intestinal lymphangiectasis (Vardy, et al 1975) and extradural cysts (Chynn, 1981) have been described in association with lymphedema I. When distichiasis occurs with primary lymphedema the latter is of the bilateral hyperplastic type (Dale, 1987) (see also **Distichiasis-lymphedema syndrome**).

Etiology: Autosomal dominant inheritance with variable expressivity approaching 50%. Father to son inheritance has been reported.

Pathogenesis: There is usually a slow, asymptomatic progression in the severity of the edema with age. Attempts to visualize lymphatics in involved areas have been unsuccessful. For this reason, the edema appears to be due to a defect in the development of lymphatic drainage rather than increased filtration, which may be secondary to edema of any type.

MIM No.:   *15310

CDC No.:   757.000

Sex Ratio: M1:F3 (Dale, 1985) to M1:F1 (Esterly, 1965; sequential generations) or M1:F2 (Esterly; skipped generations). There is nonuniform passage by sex.

Occurrence: Estimated 1:6,000. Association with microcephaly is expected in 1–2:50,000.

Risk of Recurrence for Patient's Sib:

See Part I, *Mendelian Inheritance*. About 10% risk by the time the sibling is five years older than when the proband was first diagnosed. The risk to siblings of a male proband is about 50% greater than for a female proband.

Risk of Recurrence for Patient's Child:

See Part I, *Mendelian Inheritance*. About 10% risk by the time the sibling is five years older than when the proband was first diagnosed. The risk to siblings of a male proband is about 50% greater than for a female proband.

Age of Detectability: At birth. Lymphedema II is usually diagnosed around puberty, while lymphedema diagnosed after age 30 is most likely acquired.

Gene Mapping and Linkage: Unknown.

Prevention: None known. Genetic counseling indicated.

Treatment: Resection of subcutaneous tissues with subsequent skin autografts have been performed with variable results. Diuretics and bed rest are partially and temporarily effective. Chronic lymphedema is primarily a cosmetic handicap. The potential complications of a proposed therapy should be evaluated accordingly. Reports of lymphangiosarcoma indicate that attempts to reduce the lesions by radiotherapy are contraindicated because of enhanced risk of carcinogenesis.

Prognosis: Normal life span and intelligence. Some degree of disability may result from edema of lower limbs. Many members of the Omaha family studied by Milroy were prominent in public and professional life. Malignant transformation, especially into vascular sarcoma, is a grave complication with a very poor prognosis thereafter.

Detection of Carrier: By clinical examination. Strong familial penetrance warrants close observation of apparently unaffected relatives (Esterly, 1965; Leung, 1985; Opitz, 1986).

Support Groups: MA; Cambridge; National Lymphatic and Venous Diseases

References:

Hope WB, French H: Persistant hereditary oedema of the legs with acute exacerbations: Milroy's disease. Quart J Med 1907–08; 1:312–330.

Milroy WF: Chronic hereditary edema: Milroy's disease. J Am Med Assoc 1928; 91:1172–1175.

Schroeder E, Helweg-Larson HF: Congenital hereditary lymphedema (Nonne-Milroy-Meige's disease). Acta Med Scand 1950; 137:198.

Esterly JR: Congenital hereditary lymphoedema. J Med Genet 1965; 2:93–98.

Merrick TA, et al.: Lymphangiosarcoma of a congenitally lymphedematous arm. Arch Pathol 1971; 91:365–371.

Woodward AH, et al.: Lymphangiosarcoma arising in chronic lymphedematous extremities. Cancer 1972; 30:562–572.

Dubin HV, et al.: Lymphangiosarcoma and congenital lymphedema of the extremity. Arch Dermatol 1974; 110:608–614.

Vardy AH, et al.: Lymphangiosarcoma arising in chronic lymphedematous extremities. Cancer 1972; 30:562–572.

Chynn K: Congenital spinal extradural cyst in two siblings. Clin Genet 1981; 20:25–27.

Epstein JI, Mendelsohn G: Squamous carcinoma of the foot arising in association with long-standing verrucous hyperplasia in a patient with congenital lymphedema. Cancer 1984; 54:943–947.

Leung AK: Dominantly inherited syndrome of microcephaly and congenital lymphedema. Clin Genet 1985; 27:611–612.

Watts GT: Lymphedema (non-pitting) and simple (pitting) edema are different. Lancet 1985; II:1414–1415.

Crowe CA, Dickerman LH: A genetic association between microcephaly and lymphedema. Am J Med Genet 1986; 24:131–135.

Opitz JM: On congenital edema. (Editorial) Am J Med Genet 1986; 24:127–129.

Dale RF: Primary lymphedema when found with distichiasis is of the type defined as bilateral by lymphograph. J Med Genet 1987; 24:170–171.

Leung AKC: Dominantly inhherited syndrome of microcephaly and congenital lymphedema with normal intelligence. (Letter) Am J Med Genet 1987; 26:231 only.

Meinecke P: A genetic association between microcephaly and lymphedema. (Letter) Am J Med Genet 1987; 26:233 only.

SH054
ES003

Douglas R. Shanklin
John R. Esterly

LYMPHEDEMA II   0615

Includes:

> Lymphedema forme tarde
> Lymphedema, idiopathic
> Lymphedema, late-onset
> Lymphedema praecox
> Lymphedema, primary non-inflammatory
> Lymphedema with multiple congenital malformations
> Lymphedema with onset after childhood, familial
> Meige type lymphedema
> Yellow nail syndrome with familial late-onset lymphedema

Excludes:

> Distichiasis-lymphedema syndrome (2039)
> Lymphangiosarcoma in chronic lymphedema of the lower limb
> Lymphedema of the Turner or Bonnevie-Ullrich syndrome

Lymphedema I (0614)
Lymphedema-hypoparathyroidism (2801)
Secondary lymphedema from multiple causes
Tumorigenic lymphedema

Major Diagnostic Criteria: The diagnosis is clinical, with onset of limb edema occuring between the second and fifth decade. A positive family history is helpful and all forms of secondary lymphedema should be ruled out. If the edema presents after the age of 40 years, an underlying malignant lesion should be suspected.

Lymphangiographic studies can be helpful in considering the differential diagnosis and, in cases of idiopathic lymphedema, these may show aplasia, hypoplasia, or dilated lymph trunks.

Clinical Findings: Late-onset lymphedema II may make its appearance as early as the teens, but the most common time of onset is between ages 20 and 40 years. Upper and lower limbs may be involved, but in the vast majority of cases it is the lower limbs that are affected. In one series of 131 cases only five patients had upper limb involvement. Bilateral lower limb lymphedema occurred in approximately half of those cases with lower limb involvement. The degree of involvement can be quite variable and may be so minimal as to go undetected, or, in contrast, it may be so extensive that ambulation is a problem. Since there is no specific laboratory test to diagnose this form of lymphedema, it becomes imperative that all causes of secondary lymphedema be excluded. Namely, such processes as infection, postphlebitic lymphedema, postlymphangitic lymphedema, and neoplasia should be excluded. In general, other genetic abnormalities have not been associated with the hereditary form of late-onset lymphedema II. However, in 1966 Wells described a family with affected members showing dystrophic yellow nails and lymphedema involving both lower limbs and, occasionally, the hands and face. Whether these two findings are related or represent a coincidental occurrence is not known.

Recently, a three-year-old male child was reported with congenital lymphedema of the hands and feet and having other skeletal and facial deformities: macrocephaly, frontal bossing, depressed nasal bridge, anteverted nares and a high-arched palate.

Complications: The most common complication is single or recurrent episodes of lymphangitis or cellulitis, and these may lead to ulceration. Trichophytosis has been found in approximately 10% of the cases. Lymphangiosarcoma may develop, but this occurs in less than 1% of the cases.

Associated Findings: Cleft palate. Possibly yellow, dystrophic nails.

Etiology: Most forms are sporadic, or by autosomal dominant inheritance.

Pathogenesis: Undetermined. Anatomically, there seems to be a hypoplasia of the lymphatic system in all genetic forms of lymphedema.

MIM No.: *15320, 15330

CDC No.: 757.000

Sex Ratio: Typically M1:F1. However, it is M1:F10 in lymphedema praecox and lymphedema forme tarde.

Occurrence: About a half-dozen kindreds reported with inherited forms. Primary types are more common than the genetic.

Risk of Recurrence for Patient's Sib:
See Part I, *Mendelian Inheritance*.

Risk of Recurrence for Patient's Child:
See Part I, *Mendelian Inheritance*.

Age of Detectability: Late-onset lymphedema II, around puberty. Yellow nail syndrome with lymphedema, middle age. Primary form, detectable between the ages of 10 and 40 years, most common between 20 and 30 years.

Gene Mapping and Linkage: Unknown.

Prevention: None known. Genetic counseling indicated.

Treatment: Either type of edema may partially respond to a pararubber bandage or an elastic stocking. Some patients have been reported to have had a reduction of the edema with the use of a diuretic. When the lymphedema is severe and uncontrollable, surgery may be indicated.

Prognosis: The lymphedema per se does not alter the normal life span or intelligence. However, complications such as lymphangitis or the development of lymphangiosarcoma may result in an early death. If the edema is extreme with an unsightly appearance, problems in ambulation, coupled with various emotional difficulties, are usually present.

Detection of Carrier: Unknown.

Support Groups: MA; Cambridge; National Lymphatic and Venous Diseases

References:

Goodman RM: Familial lymphedema of the Meige's type. Am J Med 1962; 32:651–656.

Schirger A, et al.: Idiopathic lymphedema: review of 131 cases. JAMA 1962; 182:14–22.

Samman PD, White WF: The "yellow nail" syndrome. Brit J Derm 1964; 76:153–157.

Wells GC: Yellow nail syndrome: with familial primary hypoplasia of lymphatics, manifest late in life. Proc R Soc Med 1966; 59:447 only.

Wheeler ES, et al.: Familial lymphedema praecox: Meige's disease. Plast Reconst Surg 1981; 67:362–364.

Figueroa AA, et al.: Meige disease (familial lymphedema praecox) and cleft palate: report of a family and review of the literature. Cleft Palate J 1983; 20:151–157.

Herbert FA, Bowen PA: Hereditary late-onset lymphedema with pleural effusion and laryngeal edema. Arch Int Med 1983; 143:913–915.

G0026   **Richard M. Goodman**

Lymphedema praecox
  See LYMPHEDEMA II
Lymphedema with multiple congenital malformations
  See LYMPHEDEMA II
Lymphedema with onset after childhood, familial
  See LYMPHEDEMA II
Lymphedema, congenital hereditary
  See LYMPHEDEMA I
Lymphedema, early-onset
  See LYMPHEDEMA I
Lymphedema, idiopathic
  See LYMPHEDEMA II
Lymphedema, late-onset
  See LYMPHEDEMA II
Lymphedema, primary non-inflammatory
  See LYMPHEDEMA II
Lymphedema-distichiasis
  See DISTICHIASIS-LYMPHEDEMA SYNDROME

LYMPHEDEMA-HYPOPARATHYROIDISM   2801

Includes:

Hypoparathyroidism-lymphedema-nephropathy
Nephropathy-hypoparathyroidism-lymphedema

Excludes:

Noonan syndrome (0720)
Parathyroid hormone resistance (0830)

Major Diagnostic Criteria: The combination of congenital lymphedema, hypoparathyroidism, nephropathy, mitral valve prolapse, and brachytelephalangy.

Clinical Findings: Each of the documented cases had a history of developing lymphedema soon after birth. They also had short stature; dry, thickened skin; and an unusual facial appearance consisting of medial eyebrow flare, broad nasal bridge, telecanthus, and hypertrichosis of the face and forehead; **Mitral valve prolapse; Brachydactyly;** and increased carrying angle. One boy also had cataracts at age 19 years and ptosis. Laboratory studies indicated both nephropathy and hypoparathyroidism in that hemoglobin, calcium, phosphate, magnesium, serum creatinine, parathyroid hormone, and blood urea nitrogen levels were all abnormal. Intravenous pyelogram demonstrated small, inade-

quately functioning kidneys in each sib. Chest X-rays indicated that pulmonary lymphangiectasia was also likely to be present.

Complications: Hypertension and cellulitis each occurred as a complication.

Associated Findings: None known.

Etiology: Possibly autosomal recessive or X-linked inheritance.

Pathogenesis: Unknown.

MIM No.: 24741

POS No.: 3599

Sex Ratio: M2:F0 (observed).

Occurrence: Reported in two adult male sibs in the United States.

Risk of Recurrence for Patient's Sib:
  See Part I, *Mendelian Inheritance.*

Risk of Recurrence for Patient's Child:
  See Part I, *Mendelian Inheritance.*

Age of Detectability: Soon after birth by the development of lymphedema.

Gene Mapping and Linkage: Unknown.

Prevention: None known. Genetic counseling indicated.

Treatment: Renal transplantation may be indicated. Vitamin D and calcium carbonate for hypoparathyroidism, penicillin V or other antibiotics for cellulitis, and propranolol and methyldopa for hypertension are all possible treatments for the symptoms.

Prognosis: Intellectual development appears to be normal; life span may be shortened because of renal failure.

Detection of Carrier: Unknown.

Support Groups: MA; Cambridge; National Lymphatic and Venous Diseases

References:

Dahlberg PJ, et al.: Autosomal or X-linked recessive syndrome of congenital lymphedema, hypoparathyroidism, nephropathy, prolapsing mitral valve, and brachytelephalangy. Am J Med Genet 1983; 16:99–104.

T0007   **Helga V. Toriello**

Lymphedema-microcephaly
  See MICROCEPHALY-LYMPHEDEMA
Lymphoblast interferon deficiency
  See INTERFERON DEFICIENCY
Lymphocytes, natural killer, defect in
  See CHEDIAK-HIGASHI SYNDROME
Lymphocytic leukemia, cell type-childhood acute
  See LEUKEMIA, ACUTE LYMPHOCYTIC, FAMILIAL
Lymphocytophisis
  See IMMUNODEFICIENCY, X-LINKED SEVERE COMBINED

LYMPHOHISTIOCYTOSIS, FAMILIAL ERYTHROPHAGOCYTIC   2946

Includes:

Erythrophagocytic lymphohistiocytosis, familial
Familial hemophagocytic lymphohistiocytosis
Immunodeficiency, erythrophagocytic lymphohistiocytosis
Reticulosis, familial histocytic

Excludes:

Histiocytosis X
Immunodeficiency, reticuloendotheliosis with eosinophilia (2688)
Langerhans cell histiocytosis
Malignant histiocytosis
Viral-associated hemophagocytic syndrome

Major Diagnostic Criteria: In the absence of an infectious etiology, the diagnosis is supported by lymphohistiocytic infiltration of lymph nodes and other tissues. The diagnosis is strongly supported by a positive family history of the disease. Care must be taken to exclude other similar diseases by histopathologic evaluation of biopsy specimens.

Clinical Findings: Familial erythrophagocytic lymphohistiocytosis (FEL) is a systemic disease that commonly presents with irritability, recurrent fevers, hepatosplenomegaly, and failure to thrive.

Laboratory findings may include abnormal liver function tests, hypofibrinogenemia, anemia, and intermittent leukopenia and thrombocytopenia. Hyperlipidemia (of types I, IV, and V) is a characteristic finding. Familial erythophagocytic lymphohistiocytosis is characterized by an immunologic deficiency syndrome that includes defects in both humoral and cellular immunity and a plasma inhibitor of immune function. Defects in humoral immunity include low natural antibody titers, low titers to antigens to which patients had previously been immunized, and poor responses to polysaccharide antigens. Cellular defects include defective T-cell cytotoxic function, monocyte antibody-dependent cellular cytotoxicity, and antigen-specific lymphocyte proliferative responses. Associated with the hyperlipidemia in FEL is plasma-mediated suppression of normal cellular immune responses in vitro.

Clinical onset may occur any time within the first several years of life, and the course thereafter is usually relentlessly progressive, culminating rapidly in death usually caused by infection.

Complications: Seizures and cortical blindness may result secondary to central nervous system involvement. The infections that frequently are the ultimate cause of death may be secondary to the immunodeficiency.

Associated Findings: None known.

Etiology: Autosomal recessive inheritance.

Pathogenesis: One hypothesis suggests that the expression of a primary genetic defect is triggered by an environmental stimulus (e.g., an infection or an unknown antigen) that results in the lymphohistiocytosis seen on histopathologic examination of affected tissues. The abnormal immune response contributes to the ultimate death by infection.

MIM No.: *26770

Sex Ratio: M1:F1

Occurrence: Approximately 150 cases have been reported since the initial description by Farquhar & Claireaux in 1952.

Risk of Recurrence for Patient's Sib:
See Part I, *Mendelian Inheritance.*

Risk of Recurrence for Patient's Child:
See Part I, *Mendelian Inheritance.* Affected individuals are not expected to survive to reproduce.

Age of Detectability: Only upon the onset of clinical symptoms, which may occur from the neonatal period on. The latest documented onset is age five years.

Gene Mapping and Linkage: Unknown.

Prevention: None known. Genetic counseling indicated.

Treatment: Treatment remains experimental and has included cytotoxic chemotherapy, repeated plasmaphereses remove immunosuppresive activity and thereby ameliorate the defective immune responses, and bone marrow transplantation.

Prognosis: Ultimately fatal, usually within months of the onset of clinical symptoms, which is between birth and age five years.

Detection of Carrier: Unknown.

Special Considerations: It is extremely important to differentiate familial erythrophagocytic lymphohistiocytosis from several other clinically similar syndromes, which have markedly different prognoses and treatment approaches. These are Langerhans cell histiocytosis (characterized by Birbeck granules seen in the lesional cells by electron microscopy), malignant histiocytosis, which has clearly malignant morphologic characteristics, and the viral-associated hemophagocytic syndrome, which can be expected to resolve in most cases if immunosuppressive therapy is avoided.

References:
Farquhar JW, Claireaux AE: Familial haemophagocytic reticulosis. Arch Dis Child 1952; 27:519–525.

Ladisch S, et al.: Immunodeficiency in familial erythrophagocytic lymphohistiocytosis. Lancet 1978; I:581–583.
Ladisch S, et al.: Immunologic and clinical effects of repeated blood exchange in familial erythrophagocytic lympho-histiocytosis. Blood 1982; 60:814–821.
Janka GE: Familial hemophagocytic lymphohitiocytosis. Eur J Pediatr 1983; 140:221–230.

LA039

Stephan K. Ladisch

Lymphoma, B-cell
See LEUKEMIA/LYMPHOMA, B-CELL

LYMPHOMA, BURKITT TYPE 3089

Includes:
    African Burkitt lymphoma
    Burkitt-like lymphoma
    Diffuse undifferentiated lymphoma
    Endemic Burkitt lymphoma
    Non-African Burkitt lymphoma
    Non-Hodgkin lymphoma of the B-cell type
    Protooncogene homologous to myelocytomatosis virus
    Small non-cleaved cell lymphoma
    Sporadic Burkitt lymphoma
    Transformation gene:ONC:MYC

Excludes:
    Fetal toxoplasmosis syndrome (0387)
    Lymph node hyperplasia
    Lymphoma, non-Hodgkin (3107)
    Lymphoma, pleiomorphic variant

Major Diagnostic Criteria: *African Burkitt lymphoma* may present with either the involvement of the mandible, maxilla, or with bulky masses within the abdomen. The non-African *Burkitt lymphoma* presents in the ileocecal area of the gastrointestinal tract or in the cervical nodes. Frequently, there is involvement of the lymphatic system, while this is rare in African Burkitt lymphoma. The neoplastic B-cells in the lymph nodes have uniform sized nuclei with prominent nucleoli, and the cytoplasm is more baosophilic. Frequent mitotic figures are present, and when there are macrophages present, it gives the lymph node biopsy a "starry sky" appearance. The use of imprint preparations helps in distinguishing this type of lymphoma from lymphoblastic types. Immunological studies have demonstrated the presence of membrane and cytoplasmic monoclonal immunoglobulin in the abnormal B-cells.

Clinical Findings: An association has been found between *African Burkitt lymphoma* and Epstein-Barr virus (EVB), but this association is rare in non-African Burkitt lymphoma. *Burkitt lymphoma* is a very aggressive neoplasma. Frequently, the bone marrow and central nervous system also becomes involved. An increase in serum lactic dehydrogenase, uric acid, and antibodies to EBV early antigen are observed. These increases correlate with the stage and are indicators of the prognosis of the disease.

Complications: Obstruction in the respiratory, urinary and gastrointestinal tracts due to enlarged lymph nodes is a frequent complication. Hyperuricemia and lactic acidosis are common.

Associated Findings: None known.

Etiology: An association with EBV, but no other etiological factors have been identified.

Pathogenesis: A solid neoplasm of the B-cell of the immune system.

MIM No.: *19008

Sex Ratio: M1:F<1 in both the African and non-African Burkitt lymphomas.

Occurrence: *African Burkitt lymphoma* is a childhood disease found endemically in tropical Africa and New Guinea. In the non-African Burkitt lymphoma, there is a wider age range (up to 35 years). A higher mean age exists in non-African Burkitt versus African Burkitt lymphoma (11 versus 7 years).

Risk of Recurrence for Patient's Sib: Presumably not increased.

Risk of Recurrence for Patient's Child: Presumably not increased.

Age of Detectability: At any age.

Gene Mapping and Linkage: MYC (avian myelocytomatosis viral (v-myc) oncogene homolog) has been mapped to 8q24.

Approximately 75% of Burkitt lymphomas, independent of whether they are African or non-African types, carry the typical t(8;14) chromosomal translocation. The variant t(8;22) and t(2;8) translocations are present in 16% and 9% of Burkitt lymphomas, respectively. Recently, it has been shown that the immunoglobulin loci are involved in these translocations. It involves either chromosomes 14q32, 22q11 or 2p12 where immunoglobulin heavy chain locus (IgH), immunoglobulin light chain lambda or kappa loci are mapped, respectively, and the protooncogene c-myc is located on chromosome 8q24. In the t(8;14) (q24;q32), the breakpoints on both chromosomes 8 and 14 are very heterogeneous. Breakpoints in the IqH locus have been found within the D_H segments, upstream of the $S\mu$ region and also within the $S\mu$ region, $S\gamma$ region and $S\alpha$ region. In the variant translocations, the breakpoints may occur within the Vk or Jk segments on chromosome 2 or 5' of $C\delta$ on chromosome 22. Breakpoints on chromosome 8 may occur far 5' of c-myc, immediately upstream of the first exon of c-myc or within the first intron when the translocation occurs with chromosome 14. When the translocation occurs with either chromosome 2 or 22, the breakpoint on chromosome 8 occurs at variable distances 3' of the c-myc coding regions. The cellular event which appears to be of primary importance to Burkitt lymphoma is the loss of ability to regulate c-myc expression. Various hypotheses have been suggested: trans-acting control of c-myc expression is interrupted; the feedback control by the c-myc gene itself is interrupted; an increased stability in mRNA transcripts from translocated genes; an escape from translational suppression due to translocation; importance of nucleotide changes in the non-coding or coding region of c-myc; and finally, cis-acting enhancer or enhancer-like elements of the Ig loci which are brought in by the translocation act upon c-myc. Most of these hypotheses have evidence supporting them based on experiments performed on cell lines derived from Burkitt lymphoma, but rarely has fresh biopsy material been used. It should be noted that the molecular complexity underlying the Burkitt lymphoma translocation may be indicative that more than one hypothesis is necessary to explain the phenomenon of constitutive expression of c-myc in Burkitt lymphoma at levels similar to those seen in proliferating but normal cells.

Prevention: None known.

Treatment: This condition is highly sensitive to chemotherapeutic drugs such as cyclophosphamide. Intermittent high dose cyclophosphamide in combination with high dose glucocorticoids, vincristine, methotrexate and central nervous system prophylaxis with chemotherapy or ratiotherapy has been found to be effective.

Prognosis: Over 50% of the cases survive up to two years.

Detection of Carrier: Unknown.

Support Groups: Atlanta; American Cancer Society

References:
Williams WJ, et al: Hematology, ed. 3. New York: McGraw-Hill, 1983. *
Yunis JJ: The chromosomal basis of human neoplasia. Science 1983; 221:227–236.
Reich PR: Hematology, ed. 2. Boston: Little, Brown & Co, 1984. †
DeVitta VT Jr, et al: Cancer: principles and practice of oncology, ed. 2. Philadelphia: JB Lippincott Co, 1985. †
Chenevix-Trench G: The molecular genetics of human non-Hodgkin's lymphoma. Cancer Genet Cytogenet 1987; 27:191–213.
Haluska FG, et al: Oncogene activation by chromosome translocation in human malignancy. Ann Rev Genet 1987; 21:321–345. *

L0016
CR024

Elaine Louie
Carlo M. Croce

LYMPHOMA, NON-HODGKIN   3107

Includes:
    Follicular lymphoma
    Follicular small cleaved lymphoma
    Follicular mixed small cleaved and large cell lymphoma
    Follicular large cell lymphoma
    Leukemia, chronic lymphatic, type 2
    Oncogene B-cell leukemia-2

Excludes: Lymphoma (other)

Major Diagnostic Criteria: Follicular small cleaved lymphoma presents with a follicular growth pattern on the lymph nodes. The cells are small, have an irregular, angular-shaped nuclei with a small nucleoli. The frequency of mitotic figures is low. Follicular mixed small cleaved and large cell lymphoma is similar to follicular small cleaved lymphoma. But an even mixture of two cell types, centrocytes and centroblasts, small germinal center cells and large germinal center cells, respectively, are present. Follicular large cell lymphoma has a majority of large germinal center cells (centroblasts), and the follicular pattern of growth becomes diffuse in the lymph node.

Clinical Findings: These lymphomas originate from a corresponding B-cell type found in the normal germinal center follicles of lymph nodes. The abnormal cells have monoclonal surface IgM and complement receptors, as is also present in their normal counterparts. These abnormal B-cells can circulate throughout the blood, lymphatic tissue and bone marrow, leading to peripheral areas of adenopathy. Abdominal involvement is observed in greater than 60% of the cases. The abdominal nodes most often involved are the mesenteric, portal, para-aortic and celiac ones. The affected lymph node will lose its normal architecture and show a diffuse pattern. Greater than 60% of the cases will also have bone marrow involvement, and approximately 90% will have the retroperitoneal nodes involved upon lymphangiography. Follicular lymphomas are composed of three types: the small cleaved cell type which represents 20% of all non-Hodgkin lymphomas; the mixed small and large cell types which represent another 20% of all non-Hodgkin lymphomas; and the large cell type which represents only 3–10% of all non-Hodgkin lymphomas.

Complications: About two-thirds of the patients with follicular lymphoma will proceed to diffuse large cell lymphoma.

Associated Findings: None known.

Etiology: Unknown.

Pathogenesis: A solid neoplasm involving the B-cells characteristically found in the germinal center follicles of lymph nodes.

MIM No.: *15143

Sex Ratio: M1:F1

Occurrence: Unknown. Primarily found in the middle-aged and elderly population.

Risk of Recurrence for Patient's Sib: Unknown.

Risk of Recurrence for Patient's Child: Unknown.

Age of Detectability: At any age, but usually at or after middle age.

Gene Mapping and Linkage: BCL2 (B cell CLL/lymphoma 2) has been mapped to 18q21.3.

A consistent chromosomal translocation, the t(14;18)(q34;q21), is associated with follicular lymphoma in approximately 80–90% of the cases. The molecular cloning and analysis of a number of these translocations have revealed that the breakpoint on chromosome 14 is clustered tightly 5'of the J_H segments of the immunoglobulin heavy chain locus located on chrosegments of the immunoglobulin heavy chain locus located on chrosegments of the immunoglobulin heavy chain locus located on chromosome 14q32. On chromosome 18, in 60–70% of the translocations the breakpoint interupts a 100 base pair region immediately 3' of the gene that is involved, and less frequently the breakpoint occurs further 3' downstream from the gene or 5' of the first exon of the gene. The gene, a putative oncogene, on chromosome 18 has been disegnated as *bcl*-2 (B-cell leukemia/lymphoma-2). The *bcl*-2 gene is composed of 2 exons and is expressed in several B-cell lines, but the highest levels occur in cells carrying the t(18;14). Three different size mRNA transcripts have been found (.5, 5.5 and 3.5 kb). These mRNAs are generated by either differential splicing or polyadenylation. The 8.5 and 5.5 kb mRNA give rise to a protein of 239 amino acids long, and the 3.5 kb mRNA gives rise to a protein 205 amino acids long, called bcl-2 α and bcl-2 β, respectively. The function of these two proteins is unknown. As yet, the function of the bcl-2 gene in normal B-cells or in follicular lymphoma is unknown.

Prevention: None known.

Treatment: Careful staging of the disease is necessary before any therapy is given. Radiation therapy is used to manage localized disease. The more aggressive lymphoma, follicular lymphoma of the large cell type, requires the use of chemotherapeutic drugs such as a combination of cyclophosphamide, vincristine, methotrexate and Prednisone. Current treatment protocols that include high dose chemotherapy with autologous bone marrow transplantation are in progress.

Prognosis: Follicular lymphoma is usually an indolent disease. A good prognosis exists for the patient if there is a greater amount of nodularity in comparison to the amount of diffuse pattern in the lymph nodes.

Detection of Carrier: Unknown.

Support Groups: Atlanta; American Cancer Society

References:
Williams WJ, et al: Hematology, ed 3. New York: McGraw-Hill, 1983. *
Yunis JJ: The chromosomal basis of human neoplasia. Science 1983; 221:227–236.
Reich PR: Hematology, ed 2. Boston: Little, Brown & Co, 1984. †
DeVita VT Jr., et al: Cancer: principles and practice of Oncology, ed 2. Philadelphia: J.B. Lippincott Co, 1985. †
Chenevix-Trench G: The molecular genetics of human non-Hodgkin's lymphoma. Cancer Genet Cytogenet 1987; 27:191–213.
Haluska FG, et al: Oncogene activation by chromosome translocation in human malignancy. Annual Review of Genetics 1987; 21:321–345. *

L0016
CR024

Elaine Louie
Carlo M. Croce

❖ M ❖

Machado disease
See MACHADO-JOSEPH DISEASE

MACHADO-JOSEPH DISEASE 2996

Includes:
Azorean neurologic disease (pejorative)
Joseph disease
Machado disease
Motor system degeneration, autosomal dominant
Neurological disease, Machado-Joseph type
Nigrospinodentatal degeneration with nuclear ophthalmoplegia
Spinopontine atrophy
Striatonigral degeneration, autosomal dominant

Excludes:
Dentatorubropallidoluysian degeneration, hereditary (3283)
Olivopontocerebellar atrophy
Striatonigral degeneration, nongenetic

Major Diagnostic Criteria: Cerebellar ataxia, pyramidal signs, and progressive external ophthalmoplegia (PEO). Dystonia, contraction fasciculations of the face and tongue, and bulging eyes are very specific signs.

Clinical Findings: Onset is always with an unsteady gait. Cerebellar signs, PEO, and fasciculation-like movements (after contraction of the periorbital and perioral muscles and tongue) are virtually always present. Other findings may vary.
Type 1 - 14.7% of cases: Patients with an earlier onset who tend to develop a marked dystonic-rigid extrapyramidal syndrome.
Type 2 - 45.0% of cases: In these intermediate cases, cerebellar and pyramidal signs dominate.
Type 3 - 40.3% of cases: Tend to show striking peripheral amyotrophies and (on occasion) mild sensory loss and to have a later onset.
Different types may be seen in sibs. Mental deterioration is typically absent. CNS involvement is highly variable; structures most often involved include the substantia nigra, dentate, pontine, and motor cranial nerve nuclei, anterior horn cells, Clarke columns, and spinal root ganglia. Bulbar olives are always spared.

Complications: Pulmonary infections (the major cause of death).

Associated Findings: Diabetes and hyperuricemia have been described.

Etiology: Autosomal dominant inheritance.

Pathogenesis: Unknown.

MIM No.: *10915

Sex Ratio: M1.16:F1. The slight preponderance of males may reflect preferential ascertainment.

Occurrence: Found mostly in the Azores Islands (1:3,900) and in people of Azorean extraction in the United States (1:6,000) and Canada; also found in non-Azorean Portuguese, United States Blacks, Japanese, Indians, Italians, French, Brazilians, Spanish,

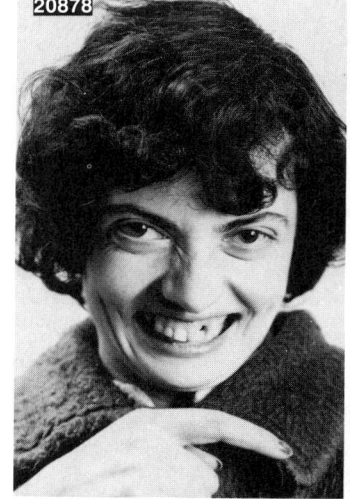
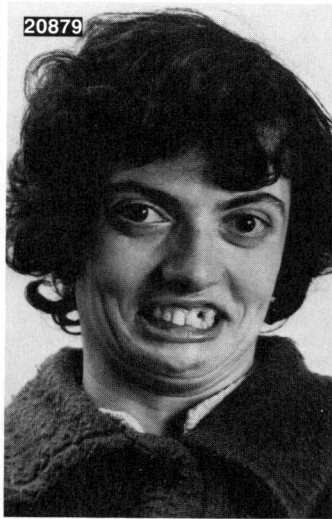
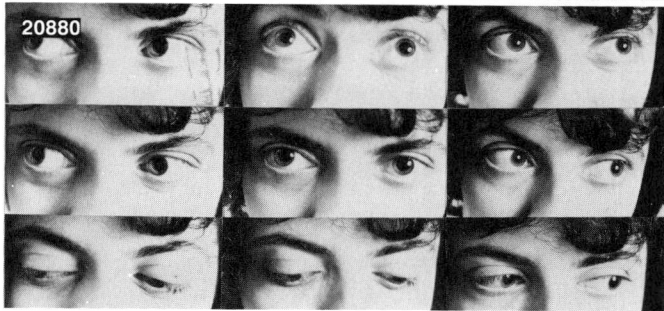

2996-20878–79: Machado-Joseph disease; note dystonic posturing in a woman with subphenotype 1. 20880: Progressive external ophthalmoplegia. This is a constant finding that first affects the gaze upwards, then horizontally, and later downwards. Typical bulging, injected eyes are also evident.

Russian, and Chinese. Close to one thousand cases have been documented.

Risk of Recurrence for Patient's Sib:
See Part I, *Mendelian Inheritance.* Penetrance is virtually complete by the eighth decade. Age-dependent correction based on 377 patients: about 40% risk at age 31, 20% at age 48, and 10% at age 55 years.

Risk of Recurrence for Patient's Child:
See Part I, *Mendelian Inheritance.*

Age of Detectability: Range, 1–73 years; mean, 37.44 years; SD, 14.10 years.

Gene Mapping and Linkage: MJD (Machado-Joseph disease) is unassigned.

Unconclusive (loose linkage with PGM1 on chromosome 1 has been reported, but not confirmed).

Prevention: None known. Genetic counseling indicated.

Treatment: None known to affect progression or prognosis.

Prognosis: Variable (most serious in type 1, better in type 3), though poor in general. The typical patient will be confined to a wheel-chair within a few years, and later bedridden; death occurs 15–20 years (on average) after onset.

Detection of Carrier: Unknown.

Special Considerations: Two cases of presumed homozygotes, with extreme phenotype and early age of onset (six and eight years) have been reported. Rare asymptomatic heterozygotes (as old as age 90) have been documented.

Support Groups: CA; Livermore (Box 2550); International Joseph Diseases Foundation, Inc.

References:
Nakano KK, et al.: Machado disease: an hereditary ataxia in Portuguese emigrants to Massachusetts. Neurology 1972; 22:49–55.
Woods BT, Schaumburg HH: Nigro-spino-dentatal degeneration with nuclear ophthalmoplegia. In: Vinken PJ, Bruyn G, eds: Handbook of clinical neurology, vol 22. Amsterdam: North Holland, 1975:157–176.
Rosenberg RN, et al.: Autosomal dominant striatonigral degeneration: a clinical, pathologic, and biochemical study of a new genetic disorder. Neurology 1976; 26:703–714.
Coutinho P, Andrade C: Autosomal dominant system degeneration in Portuguese families of the Azores Islands: a new genetic disorder involving cerebellar, pyramidal, extrapyramidal and spinal cord motor functions. Neurology 1978; 28:703–709.
Rosenberg RN, et al.: Joseph's disease: an autosomal dominant neurological disease in the Portuguese of the United States and the Azores Islands. In: Kark RAP, et al., eds: Advances in neurology 21 (The inherited ataxias). New York: Raven, 1978:33–57.
Lima L, Coutinho P: Clinical criteria for diagnosis of Machado-Joseph disease: report of a non-Azorean Portuguese family. Neurology 1980; 30:319–322.
Coutinho P, et al.: The pathology of Machado-Joseph disease: report of a possible homozygous case. Acta Neuropathol (Berlin) 1982; 58:48–54.
Barbeau A, et al.: The natural history of Machado-Joseph disease: an analysis of 138 personally examined cases. Can J Neurol Sci 1984; 11:510–525.
Fowler HL: Machado-Joseph-Azorean disease: a ten-year study. Arch Neurol 1984; 41:921–925.
Sequeiros J, Murphy EA: Age of onset and genetic counseling in Machado-Joseph disease. Am J Hum Genet 1984; 36:126S.
Myers SM, et al.: Machado-Joseph disease: linkage analysis between the loci for the disease and 18 protein markers. Cytogenet Cell Genet 1986; 43:226–228.
Sequeiros J, Suite NDA: Spinopontine atrophy disputed as a separate entity: the first description of Machado-Joseph disease. Neurology 1986; 36:1408.

SE020
C0069

Jorge Sequeiros
Paula Coutinho

Macrocephaly
See MEGALENCEPHALY
Macrocephaly, benign familial
See MEGALENCEPHALY
Macrocephaly-diffuse hamartomas
See OVERGROWTH, BANNAYAN TYPE
Macrocephaly-hemangioma
See OVERGROWTH, MACROCEPHALY-HEMANGIOMA, RILEY-SMITH TYPE
Macrocephaly-multiple lipomas-hemangiomata
See OVERGROWTH, BANNAYAN TYPE

Macrocephaly-pseudopapilledema-multiple hemangiomata
See OVERGROWTH, MACROCEPHALY-HEMANGIOMA, RILEY-SMITH TYPE
Macroencephaly
See MEGALENCEPHALY
Macrogenitosomia praecox
See STEROID 21-HYDROXYLASE DEFICIENCY

MACROGLOSSIA   0618

Includes:
> Muscular macroglossia
> Tongue gigantism
> Tongue, isolated congenital enlarged
> Tongue, large and protruding

Excludes:
> **Amyloidosis**
> **Beckwith-Wiedemann syndrome** (0104)
> **Chromosome 21, trisomy 21** (0171)
> **Glycogenosis, type IIa** (0011)
> Hypothyroidism, congenital
> **Mucolipidosis**
> **Mucopolysaccharidosis**
> **Neurofibromatosis** (0712)

Major Diagnostic Criteria: An excessively large and protruding tongue.

Clinical Findings: At birth, large and protruding tongue causing stridor, transient cyanosis, and feeding difficulties. From early infancy, there may be mouth breathing with later articulation difficulties, tongue interposition between the teeth during daytime, snoring, indentations along the tongue border, retruded maxillary incisors, and a class III molar relationship (Angle classification).

Complications: Macroglossia secondary to hemangioma, lymphangioma, or neurofibroma can involve the tongue and the floor of the mouth and can extend to contiguous structures in the neck and oral area. If the macroglossia persists until the age of five years, such problems as malocclusion, open bite, drooling, and difficulty with speech are encountered. Occasionally superficial ulcerations may appear and become infected, specifically in hemangiomatous and lymphangiomatous macroglossia. Psychosocial impact due to large and protruding tongue.

Associated Findings: None known.

Etiology: Two kinships with 18 cases have been reported with autosomal dominant inheritance. All other cases appear sporadic or in association with syndromes.

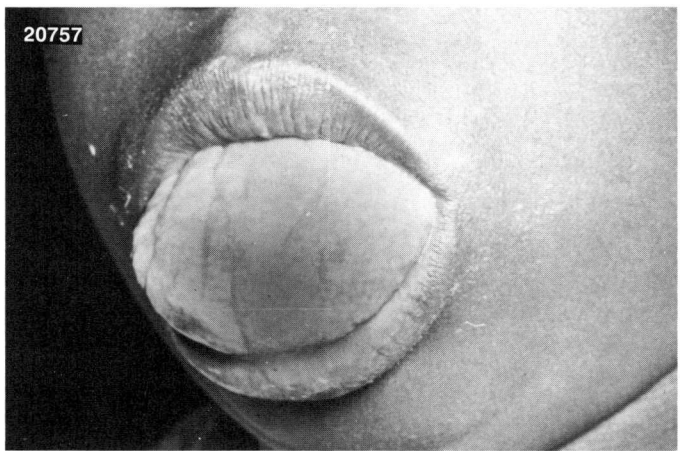

0618A-20757: Tongue, macroglossia.

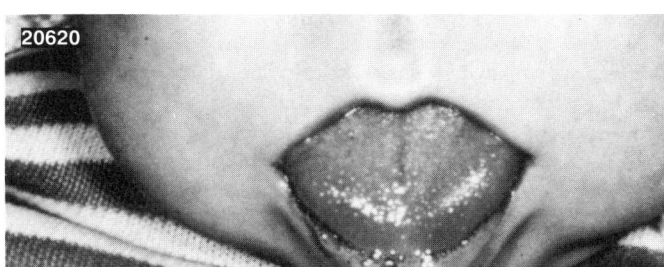

0618B-20620: Tongue, macroglossia.

Pathogenesis: Depends upon the type of macroglossia. Hemangiomatous and lymphangiomatous macroglossia result from hamartomatous overgrowth of vascular and lymphatic tissue, respectively. Hypertrophy of muscle fibers is noted in muscular macroglossia.

MIM No.: *15363

CDC No.: 750.120

Sex Ratio: Presumably M1:F1.

Occurrence: Two kindreds with inherited form have been reported.

Risk of Recurrence for Patient's Sib:
See Part I, *Mendelian Inheritance.*

Risk of Recurrence for Patient's Child:
See Part I, *Mendelian Inheritance.*

Age of Detectability: At birth.

Gene Mapping and Linkage: Unknown.

Prevention: None known. Genetic counseling indicated.

Treatment: Early surgical treatment should be avoided, as sometimes with facial growth, the tongue fits inside the mouth. If by the age of four or five years the macroglossia causes malocclusion, open bite, drooling, and interferes with social acceptance, surgical reduction can be carried out. This usually means marginal wedge excision sometimes accompanied by an anterior wedge excision.

Prognosis: Life expectance is unimpaired in uncomplicated cases.

Detection of Carrier: Unknown.

Special Considerations: Macroglossia as a mendelian trait should be distinguished from syndromes with associated anomalies, mainly those with autosomal dominant inheritance. The genetic basis for other forms of uncomplicated macroglossia, such as those due to hamartomatous overgrowth of vascular and lymphatic tissue, remains undetermined.

References:
Warkany J: Congenital malformations. Notes and comments. Chicago: Year Book Medical Publishers, 1971:662–663.
Massengill R, Pickrell K: Surgical correction of macroglossia. Pediatrics 1978; 61:485–488.
Kharbanda OP, et al.: Isolated true macroglossia. J Ind Med Assoc 1984; 82:29–30.
Rizer FM, et al.: Macroglossia: etiologic considerations and management techniques. Int J Ped Otorhinolaryngol 1985; 8:225–236. *
Reynoso MC, et al.: Autosomal dominant macroglossia in two unrelated families. Hum Genet 1986; 74:200–202.

RE027   **Martha Celina Reynoso**
CA011   **José María Cantú**
J0027   **Ronald J. Jorgenson**

Macroglossia-omphalocele-visceromegaly syndrome
See BECKWITH-WIEDEMANN SYNDROME
Macrosomia associated with polydactyly and craniosynostosis
See ACROCEPHALOPOLYDACTYLOUS DYSPLASIA
Macrostomia
See FACIAL CLEFT, LATERAL

Macrostomia-ablepharon
See ABLEPHARON-MACROSTOMIA
Macrothrombopathia-deafness-nephritis
See DEAFNESS-NEPHRITIS-MACROTHROMBOPATHIA
Macrotia
See EAR, MACROTIA

MACULAR COLOBOMA-BRACHYDACTYLY   0621

Includes:
Apical dystrophy
Brachydactyly and macular coloboma
Sorsby syndrome

Excludes:
Brachydactyly (0114)
Fetal toxoplasmosis syndrome (0387)

Major Diagnostic Criteria: Congenital macular coloboma and demonstration of digital malformation.

Clinical Findings: Characterized by 1) bilateral pigmented macular colobomata of 5 to 6 DD by 3 to 4 DD, with the larger diameter horizontally placed, and 2) an apical dystrophy of hands and feet. The latter consists of rudimentary nails on the index finger of each hand and hallux of each foot, plus an abnormal appearance of the terminal part of the thumb and big toe, which varies from extreme broadness to complete bifurcation. X-rays reveal diminution or actual suppression of the second phalanx of the little finger, a variable bifurcation of the terminal phalanx of thumb and hallux, with a considerable atrophy of all terminal phalanges of both hands and feet. Absence of the small toe is a variable feature.

Complications: Horizontal pendular nystagmus and decreased visual acuity (maximally 10/200 corrected).

Associated Findings: None known.

Etiology: Possibly autosomal dominant inheritance.

Pathogenesis: Unknown.

MIM No.: 12040

Sex Ratio: M1:F1

Occurrence: One family has been described.

Risk of Recurrence for Patient's Sib:
See Part I, *Mendelian Inheritance.*

Risk of Recurrence for Patient's Child:
See Part I, *Mendelian Inheritance.*

Age of Detectability: Neonatal period.

Gene Mapping and Linkage: Unknown.

Prevention: None known. Genetic counseling indicated.

Treatment: Unknown.

Prognosis: Normal for life span and intelligence. Visual acuity is in the legally blind range.

Detection of Carrier: Unknown.

References:
Sorsby A: Congenital coloboma of the macula, together with an account of the familial occurrence of bilateral macular coloboma in association with apical dystrophy of hands and feet. Br J Ophthalmol 1935; 19:65–90.
Smith RD, et al.: Congenital macular colobomas and short-limb skeletal dysplasia. Am J Med Genet 1980; 5:365–371.

MA054   **Irene H. Maumenee**

Macular corneal dystrophy
See CORNEAL DYSTROPHY, MACULAR TYPE
Macular degeneration and fundus flavimaculatus
See RETINA, FUNDUS FLAVIMACULATUS
Macular degeneration, polymorphic vitelliruptive
See RETINA, MACULAR DEGENERATION, VITELLIRUPTIVE
Macular dystrophy, atypical vitelliform
See RETINA, MACULAR DEGENERATION, VITELLIRUPTIVE
Macular pseudocysts
See RETINA, MACULAR DEGENERATION, VITELLIRUPTIVE

Madarosis
See EYELID, MADAROSIS
Madelung deformity
See DYSCHONDROSTEOSIS
Madelung disease
See NECK/FACE, LIPOMATOSIS
Maffucci syndrome
See ENCHONDROMATOSIS AND HEMANGIOMAS
Magnesium, defect in renal tubular transport of
See HYPOMAGNESEMIA, PRIMARY
Magnocellular nevus
See OPTIC DISK, MELANOCYTOMA
Majewski short rib-polydactyly syndrome
See SHORT RIB-POLYDACTYLY SYNDROME, TYPE II
Major affective disorders
See MOOD AND THOUGHT DISORDERS

MAL DE MELEDA   3289

Includes:
> Keratodermia palmoplantaris transgrediens
> Keratosis palmoplantaris transgrediens
> Meleda disease
> Mljet disease
> Siemens disease

Excludes:
> **Howel Evans syndrome** (3290)
> **Keratosis palmaris et plantaris of Unna-Thost** (3264)
> **Skin** (other)

Major Diagnostic Criteria: Diffuse, progressive palmoplantar keratoderma with involvement of the dorsal surfaces (transgrediens).

Clinical Findings: Onset is usually evident after birth and consists of palmoplantar erythema followed by hyperkeratosis and thickening. The disease is usually well developed by the second-to-third year of life. With time, the thickening of the skin extends to the dorsal surfaces of the hand and feet, including fingers and toes. In some patients, especially in those reported in geographic areas other than the Island of Meleda, the erythema may persist.

Gradually, the hyperkeratosis becomes progressive involving the wrists, forearms, and knees. The trunk and the axillary region are rarely involved. Some patients may show a non-keratotic perioral erythema.

The skin lesions consist of yellow brown hyperkeratotic plaques, in a symmetrical and bilateral distribution. Sometimes the hyperkeratotic lesions may be isolated, resembling lichenoid plaques.

Marked hyperkeratosis with malodor is present in almost all cases. The nails are always affected, presenting longitudinal striae, koilonychia, pachyonychia, and onychogryphosis. Brachyphalangia of the fingers has been reported. Hair and teeth are unaffected. Histology shows marked hyperkeratosis, acanthosis, hypergranulosis and moderate perivascular chronic inflammatory infiltration.

Complications: Development of painful fissures as well as constriction bands of the distal phalanx has been described.

Associated Findings: Macroglossia, lingua plicata, partial **Syndactyly**, and in males hair growth over the thenar area and the sole, have been reported.

Etiology: Autosomal recessive inheritance.

Pathogenesis: Unknown.

MIM No.: *24830

Sex Ratio: M1:F1

Occurrence: Mal de Meleda received its name from the Dalmatian island of Mljet (Yugoslavia) where it was originally observed. In the past, most of the cases described were originally from that region. In the past two decades, many cases have been reported in different countries.

Risk of Recurrence for Patient's Sib:
> See Part I, *Mendelian Inheritance*.

Risk of Recurrence for Patient's Child:
> See Part I, *Mendelian Inheritance*.

Age of Detectability: Usually shortly after birth.

Gene Mapping and Linkage: Unknown.

Prevention: None known. Genetic counseling indicated.

Treatment: Keratolytic agents may be helpful to soften the hyperkeratosis. The oral synthetic retinoids have been used successfully for the relief of significant discomfort.

Prognosis: The disease persists throughout life. Life span is not affected.

Detection of Carrier: Unknown.

References:
Kogoj FR; Die Krankheit von Mljet (Mal de Meleda). Acta Derm Venereol (Stock) 1934; I5:264–299.
Schnyder UW, et al.: La Maladie de Meleda autochtone. Ann Derm Syph Paris 1969; 96:517–530.*†
Reed ML, et al.: Mal de Meleda treated with 13-cis-retinoid acid. Arch Derm 1979; 115:605–608.
Jee SH, et al.: Report of a family with Mal de Meleda in Taiwan. Dermatologica 1985; 171:30–37.
Salomon T: Hairgrowth over thenar and the sole in Mal de Meleda (Mljet disease). Acta Derm Venereol 1985; 65:352–353.†

MI038   **Giuseppe Micali**

Malabsorption of vitamin B(12) (two types)
See VITAMIN B(12) MALABSORPTION
Malabsorption, methionine
See METHIONINE MALABSORPTION
Malabsorption-ectodermal dysplasia-nasal alar hypoplasia
See JOHANSON-BLIZZARD SYNDROME
Maladie de Gelineau
See NARCOLEPSY
Malaria, susceptibility to vivax malaria
See MALARIA, VIVAX, SUSCEPTIBILITY TO

MALARIA, VIVAX, SUSCEPTIBILITY TO   3065

Includes:
> Duffy blood group positive
> Benign tertian malaria
> Plasmodium vivax malaria
> Haemamoeba vivax malaria
> Malaria, susceptibility to vivax malaria

Excludes: Malaria, susceptibility to other types

Major Diagnostic Criteria: All individuals with erythrocytic Duffy antigens Fy^a and or Fy^b are susceptible to vivax malaria. The presence of vivax malaria is unequivocally diagnosed by the identification of characteristic species-specific morphologic features of schizonts and gametocytes in erythrocytes from thin and thick peripheral blood smears stained with Romanowsky type stains. Paroxysms of fever and chills occurring every 48 hours are indicative of *P. vivax* malaria.

Clinical Findings: Duffy factor has no known ill effects on erythrocytic morphology or physiology. When vivax malaria does occur, classical paroxysms of fever, chills and sweating occur at intervals of 48 hours. These are the most prominent features. However, myalgia, anorexia and nausea are commonly associated. Developing immunity alters the classical findings to produce irregular fever and chills. Anemia, leukopenia and thrombocytopenia commonly occur. Thick or thin peripheral blood smears will show schizonts in synchronous development depending on when the blood sample is taken. Urine may contain protein indicative of immune complex deposition in glomerulus. The presence of hemoglobinuria is indicative of excessive hemolysis with elevated direct and indirect serum bilirubin.

Complications: Duffy factor alone has no untoward effects. In vivax malaria, anemia is commonly seen. Death is seldom seen in vivax malaria.

Associated Findings: None known.

Etiology: Autosomal condominant inheritance: Duffy alleles, Fª, Fyᵇ.

Pathogenesis: Duffy factor (Fyª or Fyᵇ) on red blood cell membranes acts as ligand for receptor on *P. vivax* merozoites (trophozoites) to allow entry into erythrocytes and parasitization. Development of schizonts in erythrocytes leads to destruction of these cells. The Duffy Fy⁴ antigen does not seem to act as a ligand as all Fy(a-b-) erythrocytes are positive for Fy⁴ antigen but refractory to *P. vivax* infection.

MIM No.: *11070

Sex Ratio: M1:F1

Occurrence: Fyª and Fyᵇ alleles are found throughout the world. In whites, the gene frequencies are: Fyª 0.425; Fyᵇ 0.557; and Fy 0.002. The less defined Fyˣ has a frequency of 0.016. Fyª is very frequent in Southeast Asia, Korea, Japan, Melanesia and Micronesia. However, the gene frequencies in Blacks are: Fyª 0.0646; Fyᵇ 0.1130; and Fy 0.8224.

Risk of Recurrence for Patient's Sib:
See Part I, *Mendelian Inheritance.*

Risk of Recurrence for Patient's Child:
See Part I, *Mendelian Inheritance.*

Age of Detectability: Fyª and Fyᵇ antigens are found in red blood cells in fetuses from six weeks onwards and well-developed at birth. The course of Fy⁴ antigen development is undetermined.

Gene Mapping and Linkage: FY (Duffy blood group) has been mapped to 1q21-q25.

Duffy factor was first blood group system to be localized on an autosome. Duffy group is linked to uncoiler-1 (1qh); an inherited visible deformity of the lone arm of autosome no. 1, close the centromere. Close linkage of Duffy system with "congenital zonular, pulverulent cataract" was determined by higher mathematics and computer analysis. Linkage of Fy with amylase, pancreatic (AmP) and amylase, salivary (AmS) was identified in 1972.

Prevention: None known. Genetic counseling indicated. Prevention of vivax malaria by chemoprophylaxis is possible with chloroquine in endemic areas. Additional prevention by personal strategies to reduce exposure to potentially infective anopheline mosquito bites.

Treatment: None needed for Duffy factor. Treatment of vivax malaria with chloroquine and primaquine.

Prognosis: Life span not affected.

Detection of Carrier: Duffy factor, Fyª and or Fyᵇ detected by erythrocyte agglutination assays using anti-Fyª and anti-Fyᵇ antibodies.

References:
Sanger R, et al: The Duffy blood groups in New York Negroes: the phenotype Fy (a-b-). Brit J Haematol 1958; 1:370–374. *

Renwick JH, Lawler SD: Probable linkage between a congenital cataract locus and the Duffy blood group locus. Ann Hum Genet 1963; 27:67–84.

Donahue RP, et al: Probably assignment of the Duffy blood group locus to chromosome 1 in man. Proc Natl Acad Sci USA 1968; 61:949–955. *

Kamaryt J, et al: Possible linkage between uncoiler chromosome Un 1 and amylase polymorphism Amy 2 loci. Humangenetik 1971; 11: 218–220.

Benzad O, et al: A new anti-erythrocyte antibody in the Duffy system: anti-Fy⁴. Vox Sang 1973; 24:337–342.

Merritt AD, et al: Human amylase loci: genetic linkage with the Duffy blood group locus and assignment to linkage group 1. Am J Hum Genet 1973; 25:523–538.

Race RR, Sanger R: Blood Groups in Man, ed. 6. Oxford, Blackwell, 1975.

Miller LH, et al: The resistance factor to Plasmodium vivax in blacks: the Duffy-blood-group genotype, FyFy. New Engl J Med 1976; 295:302–304. *

Mourant AE, et al: The distribution of the human blood groups and other polymorphisms, ed. 2. London: Oxford University Press, 1976.

HI014   **Gene I. Higashi**

Malattia levantinese
See OCULAR DRUSEN
Malaysian-Melanesian elliptocytosis
See ELLIPTOCYTOSIS
Male hypogonadism-mental retardation-skeletal anomalies
See SHOVAL-SOFFER SYNDROME
Male pattern baldness
See HAIR, BALDNESS, COMMON
Male pseudo-precocious puberty
See STEROID 21-HYDROXYLASE DEFICIENCY
Male pseudohermaphroditism due to 17-KSR deficiency
See STEROID 17-KETOSTEROID REDUCTASE DEFICIENCY
Male pseudohermaphroditism due to 5 alpha reductase deficiency
See STEROID 5 ALPHA-REDUCTASE DEFICIENCY
Male Turner syndrome
See NOONAN SYNDROME
Malignant acanthosis nigricans (AN)
See SKIN, ACANTHOSIS NIGRICANS
Malignant congenital osteopetrosis
See OSTEOPETROSIS, MALIGNANT RECESSIVE
Malignant fibrous histiocytoma
See CANCER, SOFT TISSUE SARCOMA
Malignant hyperpyrexia
See MYOPATHY, MALIGNANT HYPERTHERMIA
Malignant hyperthermia
See MYOPATHY, MALIGNANT HYPERTHERMIA
Malignant hyperthermia-Noonan-like phenotype
See KING SYNDROME
Malignant melanoma
See CANCER, MALIGNANT MELANOMA, FAMILIAL
Malignant melanoma, site-specific aggregation of
See CANCER, MALIGNANT MELANOMA, FAMILIAL
Malignant rhabdoid tumor of the kidney (MRTK)
See CANCER, WILMS TUMOR
Maloschisis
See FACIAL CLEFT, OBLIQUE
Malpuech facial clefting syndrome
See FACIAL CLEFTING SYNDROME, GYPSY TYPE
Malrotation
See INTESTINAL ROTATION, INCOMPLETE
Malrotation of midgut
See INTESTINAL ROTATION, INCOMPLETE
Mammary gland tissue without nipple or areola
See BREAST, POLYTHELIA
Mammary glands, complete supernumerary
See BREAST, POLYTHELIA
Mammary-ulnar syndrome
See ULNAR-MAMMARY SYNDROME

MANDIBLE, TORUS MANDIBULARIS   0958

Includes:
Mandibular enlargement
Torus mandibular

Excludes: N/A

Major Diagnostic Criteria: A bony swelling that interrupts the smooth curvature of the lingual surface of the mandible.

Clinical Findings: An enlargement of bone on the lingual surface of the mandible above the mylohyoid line and usually opposite the cuspid and premolar teeth. They may have single or multiple lobes.

Complications: Only if swelling grows so large as to interfere with mastication or the wearing of a denture.

Associated Findings: None known.

Etiology: Autosomal dominant inheritance with variable expression and incomplete penetrance according to sex. It has been suggested that this condition is due to the same gene responsible for **Palate, torus palatinus.**

Pathogenesis: Unknown.

MIM No.: *18970

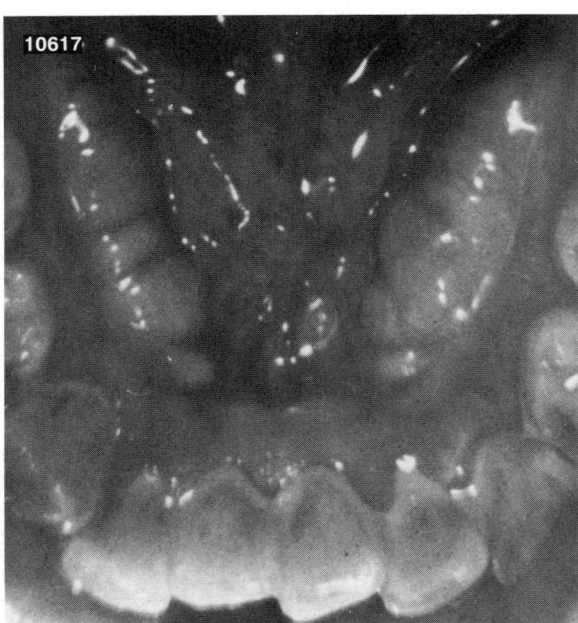

0958-10617: Torus mandibularis.

CDC No.: 750.280

Sex Ratio: M0.7:F1

Occurrence: United States whites: 1:13 over 15 years of age; United States Blacks: 1:9; Chileans: 1:2,000; Peruvians: 1:290; American Indians: 1:7; Eskimos: 1:2.5; Aleuts: 1:1.7.

Risk of Recurrence for Patient's Sib:
See Part I, *Mendelian Inheritance*. If parent is affected, about 1:3 for sons and 1:2 for daughters. Negligible for all sibs if patient is the result of a fresh mutation.

Risk of Recurrence for Patient's Child:
See Part I, *Mendelian Inheritance*. About 1:3 for sons (assuming 70% penetrance in males), and about 1:2 for daughters. These figures exclude children under 15 years of age.

Age of Detectability: Usually by 15 years of age.

Gene Mapping and Linkage: Unknown.

Prevention: None known. Genetic counseling indicated.

Treatment: Surgical removal, if interfering with oral functions.

Prognosis: Excellent. Does not recur after removal.

Detection of Carrier: By clinical examination of first degree relatives.

References:
Suzuki M, Sakai T: A familial study of torus palatinus and torus mandibularis. Am J Phys Anthropol 1960; 18:263–272.
Austin JE, et al.: Palatal and mandibular tori in the Negro. NY Dent J 1965; 31:187.
Johnson CC, et al.: Torus mandibularis: a genetic study. Am J Hum Genet 1965; 17:433–439.
Axelsson G, Hedegard B: Torus mandibularis among Icelanders. Am J Phys Anthropol 1981; 54:383–389.

J0011   **Clinton C. Johnson**

Mandibular cleft, median
See CLEFTS, LOWER MEDIAN LIP, MANDIBLE AND TONGUE
Mandibular enlargement
See MANDIBLE, TORUS MANDIBULARIS

MANDIBULAR PROGNATHISM   0626

Includes:
Hapsburg jaw
Progenie
Prognathism, mandibular
Skeletal malocclusion, class III

Excludes:
Dental malocclusion, class III
Maxillary retrognathism

Major Diagnostic Criteria: Overgrowth of the mandible.

Clinical Findings: With overgrowth of the mandible, the lower teeth are carried forward and interdigitate more anteriorly than normal with the upper teeth. This is a Class III relationship and is usually judged on the basis of molar interdigitation. The chin protrudes and the lower lip assumes a pouting configuration in mandibular prognathism. The angle between the ascending portion of the condyle and the body of the mandible is more obtuse than usual.

Complications: Dental malocclusion.

Associated Findings: None known.

Etiology: Multifactorial, autosomal dominant inheritance.

Pathogenesis: Besides an inherent discrepancy of mandibular growth, a number of factors contribute to mandibular prognathism. Enlarged tonsils and nasal obstruction may interfere with normal breathing and lead to abnormal posture of the mandible and subsequently to prognathism. Trauma, irregular eruption or loss of teeth, and endocrine disturbances may also lead to mandibular prognathism.

MIM No.: *17670

Sex Ratio: M1.5:F1

Occurrence: 1:25 to 1:50.

Risk of Recurrence for Patient's Sib: 10% for sisters, 20% for brothers.

Risk of Recurrence for Patient's Child: 20 to 25%.

Age of Detectability: Mandibular prognathism is rarely evident at birth, but becomes obvious with eruption of the teeth. Some cases are progressive.

Gene Mapping and Linkage: Unknown.

Prevention: None known. Genetic counseling indicated.

Treatment: Orthodontics may suffice for mild cases, but orthognathic surgery is needed in some.

Prognosis: Normal life span.

Detection of Carrier: Unknown.

Special Considerations: Mandibular prognathism was transmitted through several generations of the European Hapsburg royal family. It has also been observed in at least one Black family. The condition is a feature of the XXY, XXXY, and XXXXY syndromes, progressing as the number of X chromosomes increases. Nevertheless, the trait is not X-linked.

References:
Stiles KA, Luke JE: The inheritance of malocclusion due to mandibular prognathism. J Hered 1953; 44:241–245.
Horowitz SL, et al.: Craniofacial relationships in mandibular prognathism. Arch Oral Biol 1969; 14:121–131.
Litton SF, et al.: A genetic study of class III malocclusion. Am J Orthod 1970; 58:565–577. *

J0027   **Ronald J. Jorgenson**

Mandibular-acro-renal syndrome
See ACRO-RENAL-MANDIBULAR SYNDROME
Mandibulo-facial-oculo syndrome
See OCULO-MANDIBULO-FACIAL SYNDROME
Mandibulo-melic dwarfism with corneal clouding
See OPHTHALMO-MANDIBULO-MELIC DWARFISM

MANDIBULOACRAL DYSPLASIA 2082

Includes:
> Acromandibular dysplasia
> Craniomandibular dermatodysostosis

Excludes:
> **Cleidocranial dysplasia** (0185)
> **Hajdu-Cheney syndrome** (2022)
> **Pyknodysostosis** (0846)

Major Diagnostic Criteria: The combination of micrognathia, atrophic skin, joint limitation, and hypoplastic terminal phalanges.

Clinical Findings: Birth weight and length are normal. Facial changes often do not appear until after infancy. Clinical findings in 11 reported cases include micrognathia (11/11); short, broad terminal phalanges (11/11); atrophic skin (10/11); protruding eyes (7/11); decreased amount of subcutaneous fat on extremities (6/11); increased facial fat (6/11); brown skin mottling (6/11); beaked nose (6/11); dysplastic, brittle nails (5/11); short stature (5/11); hardening of subcutaneous tissue (5/11); and scanty hair (4/11).

X-ray findings have included hypoplastic distal phalanges, thought to be acroosteolysis (11/11); widening of cranial sutures (10/11); absent or hypoplastic clavicles (10/11); wormian bone in sutures (9/11); coxa valga (7/11); hypoplastic ramus of the mandible (5/11); and narrow chest (5/11).

Complications: Complications have included joint limitation secondary to skin defect; and dental crowding and respiratory obstruction secondary to the micrognathia.

Associated Findings: Findings present in only one or two affected individuals have included increased subcutaneous fat on the trunk (2/11); cortical sclerosis of the long bones on X-ray (2/11); delayed onset of puberty (2/11); highly arched palate (1/11); relative macrocephaly (1/11); scoliosis (1/11); and deformed medial condyles on X-ray (1/11).

Etiology: Autosomal recessive inheritance.

Pathogenesis: The tissues involved are mainly of mesodermal origin, although the basic defect is unknown.

MIM No.: *24837

POS No.: 3161

Sex Ratio: Presumably M1:F1 (M8:F3 observed).

Occurrence: At least nine reported families; five of which are Italian (possibly due to a founder effect).

Risk of Recurrence for Patient's Sib:
> See Part I, *Mendelian Inheritance.*

Risk of Recurrence for Patient's Child:
> See Part I, *Mendelian Inheritance.*

Age of Detectability: The somatic changes usually occur by the age of 6–7 years, although one child was diagnosed at 18 months of age.

Gene Mapping and Linkage: Unknown.

Prevention: None known. Genetic counseling indicated.

Treatment: Orthopedic management may be indicated.

Prognosis: Life span and intellect are apparently not impaired. The oldest reported patient was 37 years of age, and was healthy at the time of the report. It is unknown whether males are fertile; one affected female has reproduced, and, of ten pregnancies, five resulted in spontaneous abortions.

Detection of Carrier: Unknown.

References:
Young LW, et al: New syndrome manifested by mandibular hypoplasia, acro-osteolysis, stiff joints, and cutaneous atrophy (mandibulacral dysplasia) in two unrelated boys. BD:OAS VII(7). New York: March of Dimes Birth Defects Foundation, 1971:291–297.
Danks DM, et al: Craniomandibular dermatodysostosis. BD:OAS X(12). New York: March of Dimes Birth Defects Foundation, 1974: 99–105.
Welsh O: Study of a family with a new progeroid syndrome. BD:OAS XI(5). New York: March of Dimes Birth Defects Foundation, 1975: 25–38.
Palotta R, Morgese G: Mandibuloacral dysplasia: a rare progeroid syndrome. Clin Genet 1984; 26:133–138. *
Tenconi R et al. Another Italian family with mandibuloacral dysplasia: why does it seem more frequent in Italy? Am J Med Genet 1986; 24:357–364. * †

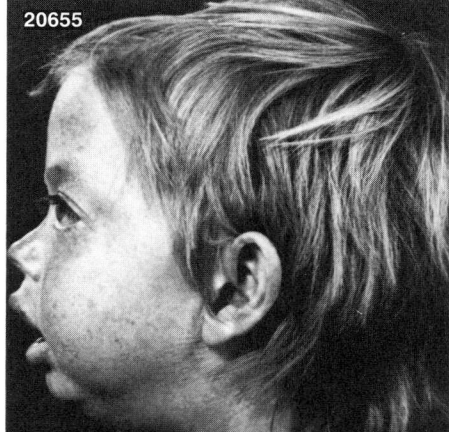 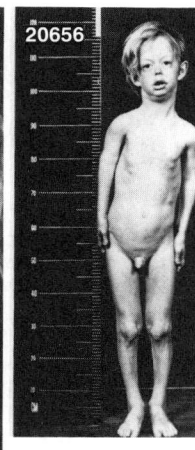

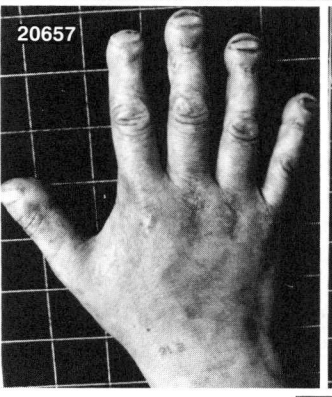 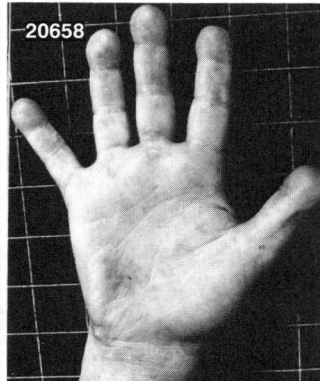

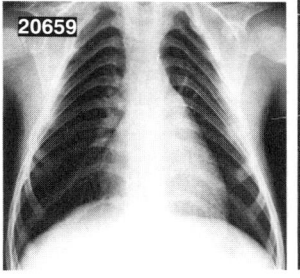 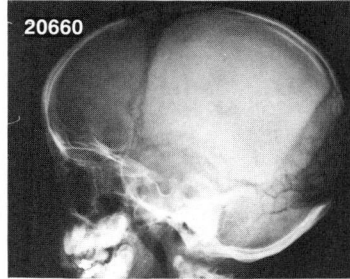

2082-20655–56: Mandibuloacral dysplasia in subject aged 8 years; note micrognathia, prominent eyes and increased buccal fat with short stature, proximal arm shortening, chest wall deformity, scarring and atrophy of the skin, abnormal pigmentation. **20657–58:** Note short distal phalanges and scarring with abnormal pigmentation. The larger scars on the hands are at sites of spontaneous subcutaneous calcification followed by extrusion of the calcified lump. **20659:** Chest X-ray shows rib-cage abnormality and absent clavicles. **20660:** Skull X-ray shows greatly delayed closure of the sutures and multiple wormian bones.

Helga V. Toriello

MANDIBULOFACIAL DYSOSTOSIS   0627

Includes:
> Dysostosis mandibulofacial
> Franceschetti-Klein syndrome
> Treacher Collins syndrome
> Treacher Collins-Franceschetti syndrome

Excludes:
> Achard syndrome
> **Acrofacial dysostosis, Nager type (2167)**
> **Cervico-oculo-acoustic syndrome (0142)**
> **Mandibulofacial dysostosis, Treacher Collins type, recessive**
> (2802)
> **Oculo-auriculo-vertebral anomaly (0735)**

Major Diagnostic Criteria: Findings include microtia, hearing loss, midface hypoplasia, downward slant of palpebral fissures, colobomata of lower lids, and micrognathia.

Clinical Findings: Downward slant of palpebral fissures (89%); malar hypoplasia (81%); micrognathia (78%); lower lid coloboma (69%); partial or total absence of lower eyelashes medial to the coloboma (53%); microtia (77%); external ear canal defect (36%); conductive hearing loss (40%); cleft palate (35%); projection of scalp hair onto lateral cheek (26%).

An affected person may be misdiagnosed as being mentally retarded because of an associated severe hearing loss. Respiratory and/or feeding problems may be present in the neonatal period because of severe micrognathia. In such cases obstructive sleep apnea may be a persistent problem in the older infant and young child.

Complications: Unknown.

Associated Findings: Microphthalmia (very rare), macrostomia, choanal atresia, blind fistulas, and skin tags between the auricle and the angle of mouth.

Etiology: Autosomal dominant inheritance with high penetrance and variable expressivity. About half of the cases represent fresh mutations, some of which have been found to be associated with advanced paternal age. An excess of affected offspring from affected females and of normal offspring from affected males has been reported. For a recessive form of this condition, see **Mandibulofacial dysostosis, Treacher Collins type, recessive**.

Pathogenesis: Balestrazzi et al (1983) reported a girl with a de novo balanced translocation and decreased level of hexosaminidase. The malformations produced in mice by isotretinoin have been suggested as a model by Sulik et al (1987). Lungarotti et al (1987) speculated on a maternal hyposensitivity to vitamin A.

MIM No.: *15450

POS No.: 3283

CDC No.: 756.045

Sex Ratio: M1:F1

Occurrence: Undetermined. Several large multi-generation kindreds have been documentaed.

Risk of Recurrence for Patient's Sib:
See Part I, *Mendelian Inheritance.*

Risk of Recurrence for Patient's Child:
See Part I, *Mendelian Inheritance.*

Age of Detectability: At birth, by physical examination. Prenatal diagnosis has been accomplished by ultrasound.

Gene Mapping and Linkage: Unknown.

Prevention: None known. Genetic counseling indicated.

Treatment: Orthodontic and surgical correction of the facial deformities. Hearing aids at an early age if hearing loss is present.

Prognosis: Good when hearing loss is diagnosed and treated early. In rare cases where severe micrognathia leads to respiratory problems or sleep apnea, serious consideration to tracheotomy should be given.

Detection of Carrier: Unknown.

Special Considerations: One name for this condition is drawn from the author of the original paper; Dr. E. Treacher Collins who first described cases in the Transactions of the Ophthalmology Society of the United Kingdom in 1933. The frequent practice of hyphenating the name is, therefore, incorrect.

Support Group: NH; Concord; (P.O. Box 5) Treacher Collins Foundation

References:
Franceschetti A, Klein D: Mandibulo-facial dysostosis: new hereditary syndrome. Acta Ophthalmol 1949; 27:141–224.
Roven S, et al.: Mandibulofacial dysostosis: a family study of five generation. J Pediat 1964; 65:215–221.
Frazen L, et al.: Mandibulo-facial dysostosis (Treacher-Collins syndrome). Am J Dis Child 1967; 113:405–410.
Herring SW, et al.: Anatomical abnormalities in mandibulofacial dysostosis. Am J Med Genet 1979; 3:225–259.
Balestrazzi P, et al.: Franceschetti syndrome in a child with a de novo balanced translocation (5;13)(q11;p11) and significant decrease of hexosaminidase B. Hum Genet 1983; 64:305–308.
Crane JP, Beaver HA: Midtrimester sonographic diagnosis of mandibulofacial dysostosis. Am J Med Genet 1986; 25:251–255.
Lungarotti MS, et al.: Multiple congenital anomalies associated with apparently normal maternal intake of vitamin A. Am J Med Genet 1987; 27:245–248.
Sulik KK, et al.: Mandibulofacial dysostosis (Treacher Collins syndrome): a new proposal for its pathogenesis. Am J Med Genet 1987; 27:359–372.
Kay ED, Kay CN: Dysmorphogenesis of the mandible, zygoma, and middle ear ossicles in hemifacial microsomia and mandibulofacial dysostosis. Am J Med Genet 1989; 32:27–31.

J0027   **Ronald J. Jorgenson**
                                             Hermine M. Pashayan

0627-12204–05: Microtia, downward slanting palpebral fissures, and maxillary hypoplasia.

Mandibulofacial dysostosis, recessive type
See MANDIBULOFACIAL DYSOSTOSIS, TREACHER COLLINS TYPE, RECESSIVE

MANDIBULOFACIAL DYSOSTOSIS, TREACHER COLLINS TYPE, RECESSIVE   2802

Includes:
Mandibulofacial dysostosis, recessive type
Treacher Collins mandibulofacial dysostosis, recessive type

Excludes: Mandibulofacial dysostosis (0627)

Major Diagnostic Criteria: The combination of down-slanting palpebral fissures, lower lid coloboma, absent eyelashes, malar hypoplasia, malformed ears, deafness, and absence of a positive family history.

Clinical Findings: The clinical findings are the same as in **Mandibulofacial dysostosis**, autosomal dominant type, and consist of down-slanting palpebral fissures, lower lid colobomas, absent eyelashes, malar and mandibular hypoplasia, malformed ears, auditory canal narrowing or stenosis, conductive deafness, cleft hard palate, cleft soft palate and projection of scalp hair onto the lateral cheek.

Complications: Delayed speech development secondary to conductive hearing loss.

Associated Findings: None known.

Etiology: Presumably autosomal recessive inheritance.

Pathogenesis: The basic defect is thought to be an abnormality of the first and second branchial arch placodes.

It has been suggested by Reynolds et al (1986) that mandibulofacial dysostosis is a developmental field defect and can therefore have several causes. If this is so, then it would not be unusual to find both an autosomal recessive and autosomal dominant form of the same condition. However, germinal mosaicism could also explain the occurrence of affected sibs to normal parents.

MIM No.: 24839

POS No.: 3283

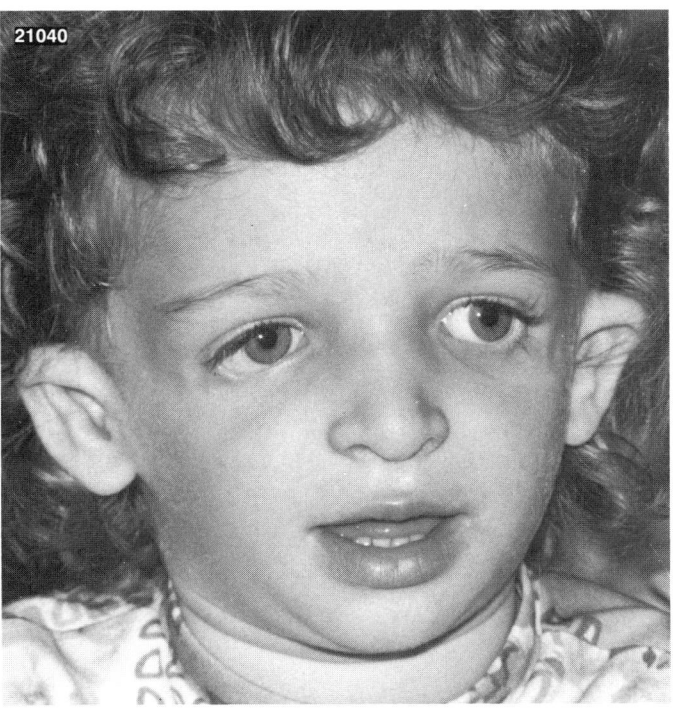

2802-21040: Proband has downward slanting palpebral fissures, lower lid coloboma, malar hypoplasia, and abnormal pinnae.

CDC No.: 756.045

Sex Ratio: M1:F1

Occurrence: Reported in sibs in a Hutterite population. There are eight other reports of affected sibs born to apparently unaffected parents from different parts of the world.

Risk of Recurrence for Patient's Sib:
See Part I, *Mendelian Inheritance.*

Risk of Recurrence for Patient's Child:
See Part I, *Mendelian Inheritance.*

Age of Detectability: At birth by physical examination.

Gene Mapping and Linkage: Unknown.

Prevention: None known. Genetic counseling indicated.

Treatment: Hearing loss can be treated with hearing aids.

Prognosis: Intellectual development, growth, and life span are normal.

Detection of Carrier: Unknown.

Special Considerations: Gonadal mosaicism for autosomal dominant mandibulofacial dysostosis (Treacher Collins) could also account for the findings described above.

References:
Lowry RB, et al.: Mandibulofacial dysostosis in Hutterite sibs: a possible recessive trait. Am J Med Genet 1985; 22:501–512.
Reynolds JF, et al.: A new autosomal dominant acrofacial dysostosis syndrome. Am J Med Genet 1986; Suppl 2:143–150.

T0007   **Helga V. Toriello**

Mandibulofacial dysostosis, Treacher Collins type-limb anomalies
See ACROFACIAL DYSOSTOSIS, NAGER TYPE
Manic-depressive (bipolar) disorders
See MOOD AND THOUGHT DISORDERS
Mannen-Balcom syndrome
See SARCOIDOSIS

MANNOSIDOSIS   2079

Includes:
Alpha-mannosidosis
Lysosomal alpha-mannosidase A and B deficiencies
Lysosomal alpha-D-mannosidase deficiency
Mannosidosis, type I
Mannosidosis, type II

Excludes: N/A

Major Diagnostic Criteria: Psychomotor retardation, coarse facies resembling that of the Hurler syndrome, dysostosis multiplex, hepatosplenomegaly, hearing loss, and recurrent infections. Confirmation of the diagnosis is made by demonstration of deficiency of alpha-mannosidase A and B activities in plasma, leukocytes, or cultured skin fibroblasts assayed at the appropriate acidic pH.

Clinical Findings: The more severe infantile phenotype is referred to as type I, characterized by severe disease with hepatosplenomegaly, severe recurrent infections, and early death, usually between three and 10 years of age. Type II patients have a milder, or juvenile-adult, phenotype, which is characterized by hearing loss, mental retardation, milder dysostosis multiplex, and survival into adulthood.

Clinical findings that can be seen in either phenotype include psychomotor retardation, a coarse facies, hernias, lenticular or corneal opacities, and hepatosplenomegaly. Hearing loss is particularly prominent in type II patients. The skeletal dysplasia includes thickening of the calvaria, abnormalities of the vertebral bodies, gibbus deformity, and bony abnormalities of the metacarpals. The vertebral bodies are prominently involved and can be ovoid, flat, hypoplastic, or recessed with anteroinferior beaking. The skeletal abnormalities are more severe in type I patients.

Laboratory findings include vacuolated lymphocytes in the peripheral blood, storage cells ("foamy macrophages") in the bone marrow, and the accumulation of mannose-rich oligosaccharides in the urine and in neural and visceral tissues. Decreased serum IgG and a shortened PR interval on EKG have been reported.

Complications: The recurrent infections seen in affected patients are felt to be due to abnormalities of neutrophil function. Studies in one type I patient revealed depressed chemotactic responsiveness, delayed phagocytosis of bacteria, and decreased response of lymphocytes to phytohemagglutinin. Hearing loss may lead to speech and language delay.

Associated Findings: Megalencephaly, muscular hypotonia, and tall stature.

Etiology: Autosomal recessive inheritance of a deficiency of acidic alpha-mannosidase A and B.

Pathogenesis: Deficiency of lysosomal acidic alpha-mannosidase A and B activities results in the lysosomal accumulation of mannose-rich oligosaccharides in neural and visceral tissues. This lysosomal storage results in the clinical abnormalities seen.

MIM No.: *24850

Sex Ratio: M1:F1

Occurrence: Over 75 cases have been reported in the literature.

Risk of Recurrence for Patient's Sib:
See Part I, *Mendelian Inheritance.*

Risk of Recurrence for Patient's Child:
See Part I, *Mendelian Inheritance.*

Age of Detectability: Can be detected clinically in the first year of life, or prenatally. Confirmation of diagnosis can be made by enzyme assay in plasma, leukocytes, or cultured fibroblasts.

Gene Mapping and Linkage: MANB (mannosidase, alpha B, lysosomal) has been mapped to 19cen-q13.1.

Prevention: None known. Genetic counseling indicated.

Treatment: No means presently available for correction of the enzymatic defect or for stimulation of residual enzyme activity.

Prognosis: Patients with type I disease usually die in childhood, often between three and 10 years of age. Patients with type II disease survive into adulthood.

Detection of Carrier: The enzymatic identification of heterozygotes has been difficult. The ratio of alpha-mannosidase to total beta-hexosaminidase activities at pH 4.4 has been used in heterozygote detection, but does not always discriminate heterozygotes. Multiple determinations of acidic alpha-mannosidase activity in several different sources may be required.

References:
Öckerman PA: A generalized storage disorder resembling Hurler's syndrome. Lancet 1967; II:239–241.
Masson PK, et al.: Mannosidosis: detection of the disease and of heterozygotes using serum and leukocytes. Biochem Biophys Res Commun 1974; 56:296–303.
Desnick RJ, et al.: Mannosidosis: clinical, morphologic, immunologic, and biochemical studies. Pediatr Res 1976; 10:985–996.
Poenaru L, et al.: Antenatal diagnosis in three pregnancies at risk for mannosidosis. Clin Genet 1979; 16:428–432.
Spranger J, et al.: The radiographic features of mannosidosis. Radiology 1976; 119:401–407.
Montgomery TR, et al.: Mannosidosis in an adult. Johns Hopkins Med J 1982; 151:113–117.
Press OW, et al.: Pancytopenia in mannosidosis. Arch Int Med 1983; 143:1266–1268.
Warner TG, et al.: Alpha-mannosidosis: analysis of urinary oligosaccharides with high performance liquid chromatography and diagnosis of a case with unusually mild presentation. Clin Genet 1984; 25:248–255.

IR000   **Mira Irons**

Mannosidosis, type I
See MANNOSIDOSIS
Mannosidosis, type II
See MANNOSIDOSIS
Map-dot-fingerprint corneal dystrophy
See CORNEAL DYSTROPHY, RECURRENT EROSIVE

MAPLE SYRUP URINE DISEASE   0628

Includes:
Branched-chain alpha-keto acid dehydrogenase deficiency
Branched-chain ketoaciduria
Branched-chain ketonuria
Intermittent branched-chain ketonuria
Keto acid decarboxylase deficiency
Thiamine-responsive MSUD

Excludes: Hypervalinemia (0509)

Major Diagnostic Criteria: Elevation of the branched-chain amino acids (BCAA), leucine, isoleucine, and valine, and/or the respective keto acids (BCKA) in blood and in urine is almost diagnostic. The presence of alloisoleucine, not normally detectable in blood, is an important diagnostic aid. The diagnosis is confirmed by demonstrating a reduction in BCKA decarboxylase activity in leukocytes or cultured skin fibroblasts. Screening programs of newborn infants to detect serum elevations of BCAA exist in many states and in Europe.

In the mildest variants, the plasma BCAA may be normal during asymptomatic periods. The enzymatic deficiency is always demonstrable.

Clinical Findings: The "classical" or most severe type of MSUD causes symptoms with onset during the first week of life. These are poor feeding, vomiting, shrill cry, lethargy, convulsions, coma, and possibly death. The only specific sign is that of a maple syrup-like odor in urine and other secretions. The untreated child that survives is neurologically damaged.

Many variants have been described and classified according to symptomatology (classic, intermediate, intermittent). A more useful approach to clinical classification derives from the tolerance to dietary BCAA. In the classic form, the ability to degrade the BCAA is extremely limited, so dietary intake may not far exceed the maintenance and growth requirements without symptoms. As a result, a purified amino acids diet is required. With greater dietary tolerance, symptoms may be delayed and more subtle. Limitation of protein intake without amino acid supplements may be adequate. In the mildest variants, patients may tolerate a normal diet without elevations in the BCAA or BCKA. They are at risk of "decompensating" either unpredictably or with acute infections or surgery, at which time plasma BCAA and BCKA increase, neurological symptoms appear, and death may occur.

A thiamine-responsive type of MSUD has been reported. Thiamine is a cofactor in the first step of the oxidative-decarboxylase series of reactions.

Complications: Unknown.

Associated Findings: Acidosis, hypoglycemia.

Etiology: Autosomal recessive inheritance involving a mutation of the decarboxylase of the three BCKA.

Pathogenesis: The first two steps in the degradation of the BCAA, leucine, isoleucine, and valine are transamination to the respective keto acids followed by oxidative-decarboxylation to isovaleric acid, 2-methylbutyric acid and isobutyric acid. Two inborn errors of metabolism, hypervalinemia and hyperleucine-isoleucinemia, suggest that there are two specific transaminases. The evidence is that one decarboxylase is effective against the three BCKA. The many clinical variants, which reproduce within families, indicate a variety of enzymatic mutations.

The acute and chronic consequences of MSUD can be avoided by controlling the intake of BCAA, making it clear that the cause of the symptoms is the elevation of the BCAA and their metabolites. Clinical and experimental studies suggest that ketoisocaproic acid (keto-leucine) is the most "toxic" of the metabolites. The compound causing the maple syrup odor has not been identified but appears to be related to isoleucine.

MIM No.: *24860

POS No.: 3784

CDC No.: 270.300

Sex Ratio: M1:F1

Occurrence: Reported variously as 1:125,000 to 1:300,000 live births. Described in many ethnic groups and in many geographic locations.

Risk of Recurrence for Patient's Sib:
See Part I, *Mendelian Inheritance.*

Risk of Recurrence for Patient's Child:
See Part I, *Mendelian Inheritance.*

Age of Detectability: The enzyme defect is demonstrable at any age, including antepartum. Increased concentrations of BCAA and BCKA become evident in severe cases within the first few days of life.

Gene Mapping and Linkage: Unknown.

Prevention: None known. Genetic counseling indicated.

Treatment: Dietary therapy with control of BCAA intake to meet nutritional requirements and not exceed tolerance. In the severe form of the disease, diagnosis must be made very early in life, and dietary treatment must be started promptly if neurological sequelae are to be avoided. Early diagnosis has been facilitated by screening programs. In the acutely decompensated case, intravenous fluids, reduction of protein intake, and peritoneal dialysis may be life-saving. Dietary care must be maintained for life. Thiamine has been reported to lower BCAA levels in some of the mildly affected cases but has not succeeded in replacing dietary control.

Prognosis: Very poor if untreated. Death occurs almost invariably before the end of the second year. With careful dietary control, normal growth and development are possible.

Detection of Carrier: Unknown. There is a great deal of genetic heterogeneity.

Special Considerations: Dihydrolipoyl dehydrogenase deficiency (E3) may also be associated with elevated levels of BCAA and BCKA. This is accompanied by a massive lactic aciduria and some elevation of ketoglutarate excretion.

Support Groups: IN; Goshen; Maple Syrup Urine Disease Support Group (Joyce Brubacher 24806 SR 119, Zip 46526)

References:

Dancis J, et al.: Enzyme activity in classical and variant forms of maple syrup urine disease. J Pediatr 1972; 81:312–320.
Wendel IJ, Cloussen U: Antenatal diagnosis of maple-syrup-urine disease. Lancet 1979; 1:161–162.
Chuang DT, et al.: Activities of branched-chain 2-oxo acid dehydrogenase and its components in skin fibroblasts from normal and classical maple syrup urine disease subjects. Biochem J 1981; 200:59–67.
Chuang DT, et al.: Biochemical basis of thiamin-responsive maple syrup urine disease. Trans Asso Am Phys 1982; 95:196–204.
Duran M, Wadman SK: Thiamine-responsive inborn errors of metabolism. J Inherit Metab Dis 1985; 8(suppl. 1):70–75.
Snyderman SE: Maple syrup urine disease. In: Wapnir RA, ed: Congenital metabolic diseases. New York: Marcel Dekker, 1985:153–168.
Snyderman SE: Newborn screening for maple syrup urine disease. J Pediatr 1985; 107:259–261.

SN005
DA003

Selma Snyderman
Joseph Dancis

Marble bone disease
See OSTEOPETROSIS, BENIGN DOMINANT
also OSTEOPETROSIS, MALIGNANT RECESSIVE
Marble brain disease
See OSTEOPETROSIS, MALIGNANT RECESSIVE
also RENAL TUBULAR ACIDOSIS-OSTEOPETROSIS SYNDROME
Marble skin
See CUTIS MARMORATA
Marbling effect of newborn skin
See CUTIS MARMORATA
Marburg (AI) apolipoprolipoprotein variants
See HYPOALPHALIPOPROTEINEMIA
Marcus Gunn phenomenon
See JAW-WINKING SYNDROME

MARDEN-WALKER SYNDROME 0629

Includes: Connective tissue disorder, Marden-Walker type

Excludes: Chondrodystrophic myotonia, Schwartz-Jampel type (0155)

Major Diagnostic Criteria: Distinctive facies consisting of blepharophimosis, flat nasal bridge, micrognathia, fixed facial expression, cleft or high-arched palate, low-set ears, joint contractures, reduced muscle mass, psychomotor and growth retardation.

Clinical Findings: Micrognathia, ptosis, hypertelorism, and muscle hypotonia are common. Microcephaly is often present, but the head circumference was increased in a few newborn and in one 5 year old. There may be heart, genitourinary, or bony abnormalities. Deep tendon reflexes may be decreased or absent.

Electromyography is usually abnormal. There may be myopathic changes in the form of many small-amplitude, short-duration motor unit potentials. Muscle biopsy specimens usually show that some fibers (types I and II) are reduced in size. Electron microscopy of muscle material from one patient showed replacement of myofibrils by glycogen particles and massive subsarcolemmal accumulation of glycogen. There was also subsarcolemmal accumulation of vesicular profiles and invasion by macrophages.

Pneumocephalogram in one case showed enlarged cisterna magna, medullary cistern, fourth ventricle, and suprapineal recess. Ventriculography in another infant showed moderate dilation of the lateral ventricles and basal cisterns and widening of the cerebral sulci.

Complications: Kyphosis, scoliosis, pectus excavatum or carinatum, and osteoporosis may be due to joint and muscle abnormalities.

Associated Findings: Preauricular tag, small mouth, short neck, low hairline, abnormal eyelashes, microphthalmos, Zollinger-Ellison syndrome, pyloric stenosis, duodenal bands, and pancreatic insufficiency have been reported.

Etiology: Autosomal recessive inheritance.

Pathogenesis: The abnormal muscles may be secondary to CNS abnormalities.

MIM No.: *24870

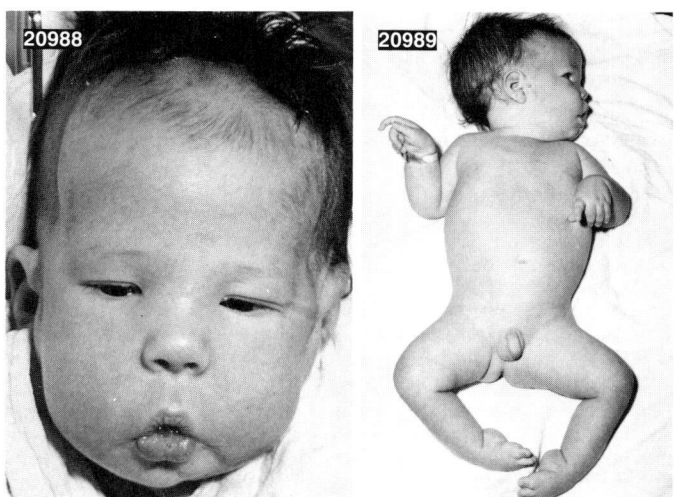

0629-20988: Marden-Walker syndrome; facies at birth includes blepharophimosis, small, pursed mouth with everted lower lip and sagging cheeks. **20989:** Congenital contractures and preauricular tags.

POS No.: 3284

Sex Ratio: M11:F3 (observed).

Occurrence: About twenty cases reported in the literature.

Risk of Recurrence for Patient's Sib:
See Part I, *Mendelian Inheritance.*

Risk of Recurrence for Patient's Child:
See Part I, *Mendelian Inheritance.*

Age of Detectability: Newborn period.

Gene Mapping and Linkage: Unknown.

Prevention: None known. Genetic counseling indicated.

Treatment: Supportive.

Prognosis: Severe psychomotor and growth retardation, with one exception reported as having normal intelligence.

Detection of Carrier: Unknown.

Special Considerations: Two reports of microphthalmos suggest that it is important to study the eyes, because microphthalmos may be the cause of blepharophimosis and also may indicate early disturbance in brain development.

References:

Younessian S, Amman F: Deux cas de malformations cranio-faciales: microphthalmie ("nanisme oculo-palpebral") avec dysostose craniofaciale et status dysraphique; 2. Dysmorphie mandibulo-oculofaciale (syndrome d'Hallermann-Streiff). Ophthalmologica 1964; 147:108–117.

Marden PM, Walker WA: A new generalized connective tissue syndrome. Am J Dis Child 1966; 112:225–228. *

Fitch N, et al.: Congenital blepharophimosis, joint contractures, and muscular hypotonia. Neurology 1971; 21:1214–1220.

King CR, Magenis E: The Marden-Walker syndrome. J Med Genet 1978; 15:366–369.

Abe K, et al.: Zollinger-Ellison syndrome with Marden-Walker syndrome. Am J Dis Child 1979; 133:735–738.

Ferguson SD, et al.: Congenital myopathy with oculo-facial and skeletal abnormalities. Dev Med Child Neurol 1981; 23:237–242.

Howard FM, Rowlandson P: Two brothers with the Marden-Walker syndrome: case report and review. J Med Genet 1981; 18:50–53.

Jaatoul NY, et al.: The Marden-Walker syndrome. Am J Med Genet 1982; 11:259–271. †

Gossage D, et al.: A 26-month-old child with Marden-Walker syndrome and pyloric stenosis. Am J Med Genet 1987; 26:915–919.

FI020
MA030

Naomi Fitch
Philip Marden

MARFAN SYNDROME 0630

Includes:

Marfanoid hypermobility syndrome
Contractural arachnodactyly (some cases)

Excludes: Homocystinuria (0474)

Major Diagnostic Criteria: Arachnodactyly, dolichostenomelia, scoliosis, anterior chest deformity, ectopia lentis, dilatation of the ascending aorta. When a first-degree relative has documented Marfan syndrome, characteristic features must be present in two organ systems; when the family history is negative, three systems must be affected. More diagnostic weight is given to features uncommon in the general population (ectopia lentis, aortic dilation, aortic dissection, and dural ectasia) than to common abnormalities (e.g., tall stature, myopia, and mitral valve prolapse). No laboratory test is available for definitive diagnosis.

Clinical Findings: Skeletal features include tall stature, arachnodactyly, dolichostenomelia, highly arched palate, vertebral column deformity (scoliosis, thoracic lordosis), and deformity of the anterior chest. Joints may be hypermobile or congenitally contracted. The ocular features are ectopia lentis in 50–60%, myopia, flattening of the cornea and retinal detachment, the latter most likely when the lens has been removed. Spontaneous pneumothorax occurs in about 5%. The cardiovascular features are progressive dilation of the ascending aorta and mitral valve prolapse.

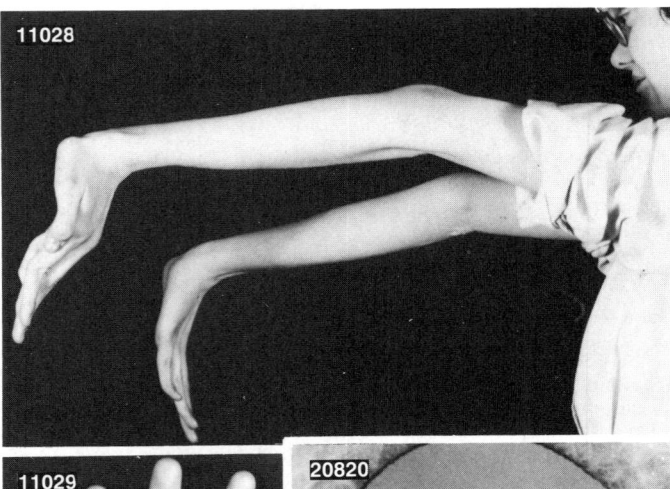

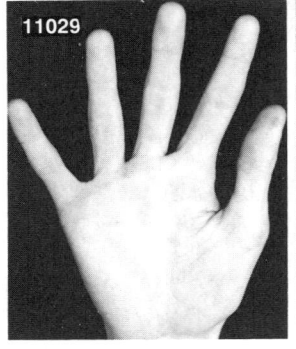

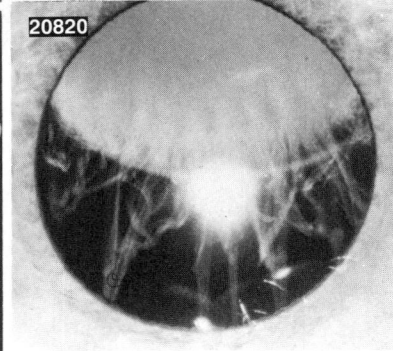

0630-11028: Joint hyperextensibility and long arms. 11029: Arachnodactyly. 20820: Upward dislocation of the lens.

Other features include ectasia of the dura, especially in the lumbosacral region, striae atrophicae, inguinal hernias, reduced subcutaneous tissue and muscle hypoplasia, and neuropsychologic problems, especially attention deficit disorder and verbal performance discrepancy on cognitive function tests.

Complications: Joint instability, severe thoracic deformity and restrictive lung disease, loss of vision, aortic regurgitation, mitral regurgitation, aortic dissection, sudden death, bacterial endocarditis, learning disability. Without treatment, life span reduced by 30–50% on average.

Associated Findings: None known.

Etiology: Autosomal dominant inheritance with complete penetrance but highly variable expression; undoubtedly genetically heterogeneous.

Pathogenesis: A recently discovered glycoprotein, fibrillin, which is a major component of microfibrils, may be the common pathogenetic link among the pleiotropic manifestations.

MIM No.: *15470, 15474, 15475

POS No.: 3285

CDC No.: 759.860

Sex Ratio: M1:F1

Occurrence: Prevalence at least 1:10,000 in most populations.

Risk of Recurrence for Patient's Sib:
See Part I, *Mendelian Inheritance.*

Risk of Recurrence for Patient's Child:
See Part I, *Mendelian Inheritance.*

Age of Detectability: Usually apparent clinically in infancy if suspected, but often not detected until second or third decade.

Gene Mapping and Linkage: MFS (Marfan syndrome) is unassigned.

Studies using blood group markers, serum protein polymorphisms, and candidate gene probes for procollagens (alpha1(I), alpha2(I), alpha1(II), and alpha1(III)) and elastin have excluded close linkage.

Prevention: None known. Genetic counseling indicated.

Treatment: Chronic treatment with a beta-adrenergic blocking drug (atenolol or propranolol) retards the rate of aortic dilation and the occurrence of dissection; treatment should be started before the aorta is widely dilated. Replacement of the aortic root with a valved conduit should be strongly considered whenever the ascending aortic diameter reaches 60 mm regardless of symptoms. Early detection and bracing of scoliosis may prevent severe deformity. In females, early induction of puberty with hormones can avert excessive height and possibly retard scoliosis. Correction of anterior chest deformity should be delayed until near skeletal maturity unless cardiopulmonary compromise is present. Early ophthalmologic evaluation is essential to correct visual acuity and to prevent amblyopia. Removal of the lens should be avoided. Spontaneous pneumothorax tends to recur unless the apical bleb is resected. Antibiotic prophylaxis for endocarditis should be recommended. Physical activity should be restricted: no body contact sports, exertion at maximal capacity, isometric exercise, or heavy weight lifting.

Prognosis: Markedly variable; infants have died from severe aortic or mitral regurgitation, whereas some patients have survived into the eighth decade. The average age of death in a retrospective series of patients who died before 1970 was the fourth decade for males and the fifth decade for females; when a cause of death could be ascribed, aortic complications accounted for over 90%.

Detection of Carrier: N/A

Support Groups: NY; Port Washington; National Marfan Foundation

References:
Pyeritz RE, McKusick VA: The Marfan syndrome: diagnosis and management. New Engl J Med 1979; 300:772–777.
Pyeritz RE, Wappel MA: Mitral valve dysfunction in the Marfan syndrome. Am J Med 1983; 74:797–807.
Sisk HE, et al.: The Marfan syndrome in early childhood: analysis of 15 patients diagnosed at less than 4 years of age. Am J Cardiol 1983; 52:353–358.
Gott VL, et al.: Surgical treatment of aneurysm of the ascending aorta in the Marfan syndrome: result of composite repair in 50 patients. New Engl J Med 1986; 314:1070–1074.
Beighton P, et al.: International nosology of heritable disorders of connective tissue, Berlin, 1986. Am J Med Genet 1988; 29:581–594.
Hofman KJ, et al.: Marfan syndrome: neuropsychologic aspects. Am J Med Genet 1988; 31:331–338.
Pyeritz RE, et al.: Dural ectasia is a common feature of the Marfan syndrome. Am J Hum Genet 1988; 43:726–732.
Hollister DW, et al.: Marfan syndrome: abnormalities of the microfibrillar fiber array detected by immunohistopatholgic studies. (Abstract) Am J Med Genet 1989; 32:244 only.
Pyeritz RE: Effectiveness of beta-adrenergic blockade in the Marfan syndrome: experience over 10 years. (Abstract) Am J Med Genet 1989; 32:245 only.
Pyeritz RE, ed: Conference report: first international symposium on the Marfan syndrome. Am J Med Genet 1989; 32:233–238.

PY000   **Reed E. Pyeritz**

Marfanoid habitus and X-linked mental retardation
See X-LINKED MENTAL RETARDATION, MARFANOID HABITUS TYPE
Marfanoid hypermobility syndrome
See MARFAN SYNDROME
Marfanoid mental retardation syndrome
See FACIO-NEURO-SKELETAL SYNDROME
Marie Unna type hypotrichosis
See HAIR, HYPOTRICHOSIS
Marie-Sainton disease
See CLEIDOCRANIAL DYSPLASIA

Marie-Strumpell spondylitis
See ANKYLOSING SPONDYLITIS
Marinesco-Garland syndrome
See MARINESCO-SJOGREN SYNDROME

MARINESCO-SJOGREN SYNDROME   2031

Includes:
Ataxia, hereditary cerebellar-childhood cataracts
Cerebello-lental degeneration with mental retardation
Oligophrenic cerebello-lental degeneration
Marinesco-Garland syndrome
Marinesco-Sjogren-Garland syndrome
Marinesco-Sjogren syndrome-hypergonadotropic hypogonadism
Marinesco-Sjogren syndrome-myopathy
Marinesco-Sjogren syndrome-neuropathy
Moravcsik-Marinesco-Sjogren syndrome
Myopathy-Marinesco-Sjogren syndrome

Excludes:
Ataxia, Friedreich type (2714)
Oculo-cerebro-renal syndrome (0736)
Sjogren syndrome (2101)

Major Diagnostic Criteria: Cerebellar ataxia, hypotonia, mental subnormality, cataracts in infancy or childhood, myopathy, hypergonadotropic hypogonadism, and skeletal defects.

Clinical Findings: The most common reported features are cataracts in infancy or childhood, cerebellar ataxia, and mental retardation. Dysarthria, nystagmus, and squint are also common. The most prominent clinical features are cerebellar ataxia (100%), cataracts (100%), nystagmus (90%), dysarthria (90%), mental retardation (85%), squint (65%), myopathy (50%), hypotonia (50%), spasticity (35%), microcephaly (30%), contractures (30%), short stature (30%), skeletal defects (30%), and hypergonadotropic hypogonadism (20%).

The clinical course is characteristic. At birth, the cardinal feature is hypotonia. Affected infants have normal lenses and subsequently develop cataracts (mainly nuclear). In infancy, cerebellar ataxia, delayed psychomotor development, and bilateral cataracts become apparent. Biochemical and histologic evidence of myopathy are present in infancy. Muscle weakness is progressive, and although most patients are ambulatory during childhood, by adulthood most need wheelchairs. The signs of cerebellar ataxia are clearcut. Some patients also have a Babinski sign, which may later dissipate. Puberty is delayed, and hypergonadotropic hypogonadism is common. In the teens, skeletal deformations become evident. A bulging sternum with or without scoliosis is most common. Scoliosis can be severe and has been successfully treated surgically. Asymmetric and variable shortening of metacarpals and metatarsals are common. Most patients stabilize in their late twenties, some with signs of end-stage muscle disease. Limb motion is barely possible against gravity, and serum creatinine kinase returns to normal. Most adults are able to walk with crutches, although there are patients who may be less severely affected. IQ is generally between 60 and 70.

Additional clinical features include short stature; pes planovalgus valgoplanus; long, slender limbs; and increased carrying angle in adults. These features may reflect the combination of muscle weakness and sexual infantilism. Skeletal defects seen include scoliosis; bulging sternum; variable-symmetric shortening of the metacarpals (44%), metatarsals (67%), and phalanges; gracile long bones (71%); cubitus valgus (67%); and coxa valga (50%). The percentages shown have been reported to shift significantly between patient populations.

Computerized tomography (CT) and magnetic resonance imaging (MRI) may show cerebellar hypoplasia, particularly of the vermis. Supratentorial abnormalities have occasionally been found and may be incidental; cerebral atrophy and agenesis of the corpus callosum have been observed. Muscle biopsy, even of young children, reveals marked variation of myofiber size, internalization of nuclei, focal myofibril degeneration and regeneration. Electron micrographs demonstrate subsarcolemmal accumulation of membranous inclusions and abnormally enlarged and distorted mitochondria separating the myofibrils. Peripheral nerve biopsies have generally been uninformative, but some investigators have found nerve conduction studies to be suggestive of a neuropathic component.

Complications: Weakness is severe, and most patients need wheelchairs. Visual acuity problems are common.

Associated Findings: Hypotrichosis and cryptorchidism have been occasionally noted, and some have reported signs of peripheral neuropathy. Seizures are reported in occasional patients and unaffected relatives.

Etiology: Autosomal recessive inheritance.

Pathogenesis: Electron microscopic studies have shown enlarged lysosomes with inclusion bodies in fibroblasts. This may represent a type of lysosomal storage disease.

MIM No.: *24880

POS No.: 3438

Sex Ratio: M1:F1

Occurrence: Over 100 cases have been documented. There appears to be an increased frequency in Scandinavia, Italy, and in a tri-racial isolated population in Mobile and Washington counties in southern Alabama in the United States.

Risk of Recurrence for Patient's Sib:
See Part I, *Mendelian Inheritance.*

Risk of Recurrence for Patient's Child:
See Part I, *Mendelian Inheritance.* Many patients suffer from hypogonadism and do not reproduce.

Age of Detectability: At birth or in infancy. Prenatal examination of the posterior fossa may reveal cerebellar hypoplasia.

Gene Mapping and Linkage: MSS (Marinesco-Sjogren syndrome) is ULG5.

Prevention: None known. Genetic counseling indicated.

Treatment: Treatment for individual clinical problems as they occur, including resection of cataracts, correction of scoliosis and other orthopedic problems, special education, and orthopedic appliances as needed.

Prognosis: Life span is normal or may be slightly shortened. Complications from progressive scoliosis, myopathy, immobilization, weakness, and visual loss may be significant.

Detection of Carrier: Unknown.

Special Considerations: Only a few of the reported patients have had detailed electrophysiologic, electron microscopic, nerve, muscle, and skin biopsy studies. These studies have suggested lysosomal storage in fibroblasts (Walker et al, 1985) and segmental demyelination in peripheral nerves (Hakamada et al, 1981). Thus further studies are warranted, particularly in homozygotes and obligate carriers.

In 1904, Moravcsik described this syndrome a quarter century prior to Marinesco in 1931. Occasional investigators have elicited signs suggestive of peripheral neuropathy, but peripheral nerve biopsies have been generally normal. The presence of Babinski signs, with subsequent reversal, were noted, and may relate to the occasional presence of calcifications in the upper cervical cord and brain stem. Such signs may be sequelae of inflammatory events in these sites. Streak ovaries and testicular tubular atrophy have been documented in a few patients.

Six of 17 patients from one kindred underwent muscle biopsies. Active myopathy was evident at the ages of 1.5, two, 21, 24, and 29 years, while one patient had end stage myopathy at the age of 26 years. Elevated serum CK and myopathic EMGs appear to be the rule. These changes may be present at birth. Signs of abnormal mitochondrial morphology were noted, and may provide a clue to pathogenesis. Clinical variability was extensive, and one 45 year old patient remained ambulatory.

References:
Todorov A: Le syndrome de Marinesco-Sjögren: premiere etude anatomo-clinique thesis. Geneva: Editions Medicine et Hygiene, 1964.

Ron MA, Pearce J: Marinesco-Sjögren-Garland syndrome with unusual features. J Neurol Sci 1971; 13:175–179.

Skre H, Berg K: Linkage studies on the Marinesco-Sjögren syndrome and hypergonadotropic hypogonadism. Clin Genet 1977; 11:57–66.

Hakamada S, et al.: Peripheral neuropathy in Marinesco-Sjögren syndrome. Brain Dev 1981; 3:403–406.

Walker PD, et al.: Marinesco-Sjögren syndrome: evidence for a lysosomal storage disorder. Neurology 1985; 35:415–419.

Superneau DW, et al.: Myopathy in Marinesco-Sjogren syndrome. Eur Neurol 1987; 26:8–16.

K0018   **Boris G. Kousseff**
WE029   **W. Wertelecki**

Marinesco-Sjogren syndrome-hypergonadotropic hypogonadism
See *MARINESCO-SJOGREN SYNDROME*
Marinesco-Sjogren syndrome-myopathy
See *MARINESCO-SJOGREN SYNDROME*
Marinesco-Sjogren syndrome-neuropathy
See *MARINESCO-SJOGREN SYNDROME*
Marinesco-Sjogren-Garland syndrome
See *MARINESCO-SJOGREN SYNDROME*
Maroteaux rhizomelic dysplasia
See *OMODYSPLASIA*
Maroteaux-Lamy syndrome
See *MUCOPOLYSACCHARIDOSIS VI*
Maroteaux-Martinelli-Campailla acromesomelic dysplasia
See *ACROMESOMELIC DYSPLASIA, MAROTEAUX-MARTINELLI-CAMPAILLA TYPE*
Marshall syndrome
See *DEAFNESS-MYOPIA-CATARACT-SADDLE NOSE, MARSHALL TYPE*
Marshall syndrome, accelerated skeletal maturation type
See *MARSHALL-SMITH SYNDROME*

MARSHALL-SMITH SYNDROME   2193

Includes:
Accelerated skeletal maturation syndrome
Marshall syndrome, accelerated skeletal maturation type
Shurtleff syndrome
Skeletal maturation (fast)-dysmorphic facies-failure to thrive

Excludes:
Cebebral gigantism (0137)
Deafness-myopia-cataract-saddle nose, Marshall type (0261)
Weaver syndrome (2036)

Major Diagnostic Criteria: The syndrome should be suspected in infants or children with early overgrowth but subsequent growth failure, dysmorphic facial features, chronic pulmonary disease, and advanced skeletal maturation ("bone age").

Clinical Findings: The most frequent dysmorphic facial findings in 14 reported patients include prominent eyes (13), low nasal bridge (13), upturned nose (11), micrognathia (11), prominent forehead (10), metopic suture ridging (7), and blue sclerae (7). Hypertrichosis (8) and **Hernia, umbilical** (7) are also consistent features.

Respiratory complications are a major component of this syndrome. Anatomical abnormalities of the respiratory tract include choanal atresia or stenosis. **Laryngomalacia**, and unusual laryngeal positioning causing intubation to be difficult. Functional consequences include stridor, lingual airway obstruction, and chronic neck hyperextension as a compensatory posture to maintain airway patency. Recurrent aspiration, atelectasis, hemorrhagic pneumonia, and pulmonary hypertension are serious pulmonary sequelae.

X-ray features are helpful and essential for diagnosis of the syndrome. These include increased skull radiodensity; craniofacial disproportion with predominance of the cranial vault; slender tubular bones; wide, bullet-shaped proximal and middle phalanges of the hand; and a striking advancement of bone age beyond 2 SDs above the mean for the patient's age. At birth, the bone age often exceeds that normal for a two year old.

Complications: Most of the reported patients have developed respiratory distress in the first few months of life and have required extensive hospitalization. Attempts to maintain an open airway, including tracheostomy, suturing of the tongue to the lip, and fixing the mandible to the hyoid bone, have generally been unsuccessful. Failure to thrive is an accompanying problem at least partly due to the respiratory symptomatology. Birth weight is average, length average is at the 90th percentile, and head circumference is at the 75th percentile. Thereafter, weight gain is significantly below normal with length often maintained in the normal range.

Development is significantly retarded. Central nervous system complications, such as intracranial hemorrhage and hydrocephalus, contribute to this problem. Eleven of the 14 cases have died in the first two years of life due to pulmonary and central nervous system debilitation. Reported weights at death have been far below the third percentile for age, lengths have been in the third to tenth percentile, and head circumference has been at the third percentile.

Associated Findings: Occasional findings include sagittal or metopic synostosis; **Hydrocephaly**; low-set, large, and/or dysplastic ears; hypo- or hypertelorism with up- or downslanting palpebral fissures; megacornea; small nose; long philtrum; high palate; long thin hands and feet; **Camptodactyly**; low-set thumbs; clinodactyly; prominent heels; deep foot creases; narrow thorax; scoliosis; cryptorchidism; hydronephrosis; **Omphalocele**; and congenital heart disease.

Etiology: Unknown. Karyotypes and standard metabolic studies are normal. There are 16 unaffected siblings to the 14 reported cases. One mother was treated with thyroxine and another, addicted to heroin, was withdrawn on methadone during pregnancy. There have been no other significant maternal complications of pregnancy, and mean parental age is within the normal range (mother 25.4, father 30.1). Autopsy findings have been unrevealing.

Pathogenesis: The pulmonary problems appear to derive primarily from respiratory obstruction with both congenital and functional components as described above. Aspiration, with resulting chemical and superimposed bacterial pneumonia, is a common problem. This may be further complicated by congenital heart defects (**Atrial septal defects**, **Ductus arteriosus, patent**), and a frequent end result is right heart failure with pulmonary hypertension.

One patient demonstrated a deficiency in absolute number of T cells as well as in the suppressor T-cell fraction. The significance of this finding is unknown. Reported immunoglobulin levels have been normal, and thymic hypoplasia in one patient was felt to be a secondary finding. The contribution of subtle immunodeficiency to the pulmonary pathology is therefore undetermined.

POS No.: 3316

Sex Ratio: M1:F1

Occurrence: Some 14 cases have been documented.

Risk of Recurrence for Patient's Sib: Unknown.

Risk of Recurrence for Patient's Child: Unknown.

Age of Detectability: At birth.

Gene Mapping and Linkage: Unknown.

Prevention: None known. Genetic counseling indicated.

Treatment: Supportive care for respiratory distress and pulmonary infection is required. In one case, tracheostomy was beneficial, though this procedure and other methods of maintaining the airway were not successful in other patients.

Prognosis: Eleven of the 14 patients have died at reported ages of seven days to 20 months. The living patients were aged nine months, 30 months, and three years when described. All of the patients have exhibited significant development retardation, though the patient treated successfully with tracheostomy was subsequently showing improvement at age 30 months.

Detection of Carrier: Unknown.

Special Considerations: Careful attention to airway anatomy and function both pre- and postmortem may contribute to the understanding of this disorder. Likewise, investigation of immune function would be helpful to determine the incidence and significance of immunodeficiency.

References:
Marshall R, et al.: Syndrome of accelerated skeletal maturation and relative failure to thrive: a newly recognized clinical growth disorder. J Pediatr 1971; 78:95–101.
Fitch N: The syndromes of Marshall and Weaver. J Med Genet 1980; 17:174–178. *
LaPenna R, Folger GM Jr: Extreme upper airway obstruction with the Marshall syndrome. Clin Pediatr 1982; 21:507–510.
Johnson JP, et al.: Marshall-Smith syndrome: two case reports and a review of pulmonary manifestations. Pediatrics 1983; 71:219–223. * †

J0012 **John P. Johnson**

Martin-Bell X-linked mental retardation
See X-LINKED MENTAL RETARDATION, FRAGILE X SYNDROME

MARTSOLF SYNDROME 2556

Includes:
    Cataract-mental retardation-hypogonadism-microcephaly
    Hypogonadism-cataract-mental retardation-microcephaly

Excludes:
    Borjeson-Forssman-Lehmann syndrome (2272)
    Cohen syndrome (2023)
    Retinopathy-microcephaly-mental retardation (2846)

Major Diagnostic Criteria: Cataracts, mental retardation, hypergonadotropic hypogonadism, and microcephaly.

Clinical Findings: In 50% or more of the cases, the following physical and laboratory findings were evident: cataracts developing between ages two months and 14 years, severe mental retardation, hypergonadotropic hypogonadism, short stature, **Microcephaly**, brachycephaly, premature aged appearance, maxillary retrusion, malaligned teeth, broad and flat sternum, broad fingertips, lax finger joints, short palms, abnormal finger and palm ratios, lumbar lordosis, and talipes valgus.

In less than one-half of the cases, the following clinical and laboratory findings were evident: short philtrum, furrowed tongue, pouting lower lip, sparse facial hair, low posterior hairline, prominent nipples, ulnar deviation of fingers 2 and 3, excess palmar creases, abnormal toenails, hypotelorism, short ulna, prognathism, delayed bone age, and cardiopathy.

Extensive biochemical, metabolic, X-ray, and enzymatic laboratory tests did not show any specific findings except for elevated FSH and LH levels, and relatively low testosterone, delayed bone age, and pneumoencephalographic evidence of cerebral atrophy. Chromosome studies were normal. Cases described by Mikati et al (1985) are distinctly different due to the absence of cataracts and the presence of genua valga and cubiti valgi.

Complications: Visual problems secondary to the presence of cataracts, as well as lenticular opacification from residual pupillary membranes that were present from previous cataract aspirations. Secondary orthopedic problems may develop from the marked lordosis. Dental hygiene and orthodontic problems are expected because of the malaligned and crowded teeth in conjunction with the prognathism.

Associated Findings: None known.

Etiology: Although the majority of reported patients to date have been males, autosomal recessive inheritance is suggested by consanguinity in the initial cases, possible consanguinity in subsequent cases, and the occurrence in females.

Pathogenesis: Unknown.

MIM No.: 21272

POS No.: 3497

Sex Ratio: Presumably, M1:F1; (M7:F2 observed).

Occurrence: Nine cases have been observed; two Polish Jews, two Sephardic Jews, one in nonspecified non-Jewish population, two Dutch-Belgian, and two Pakistanian.

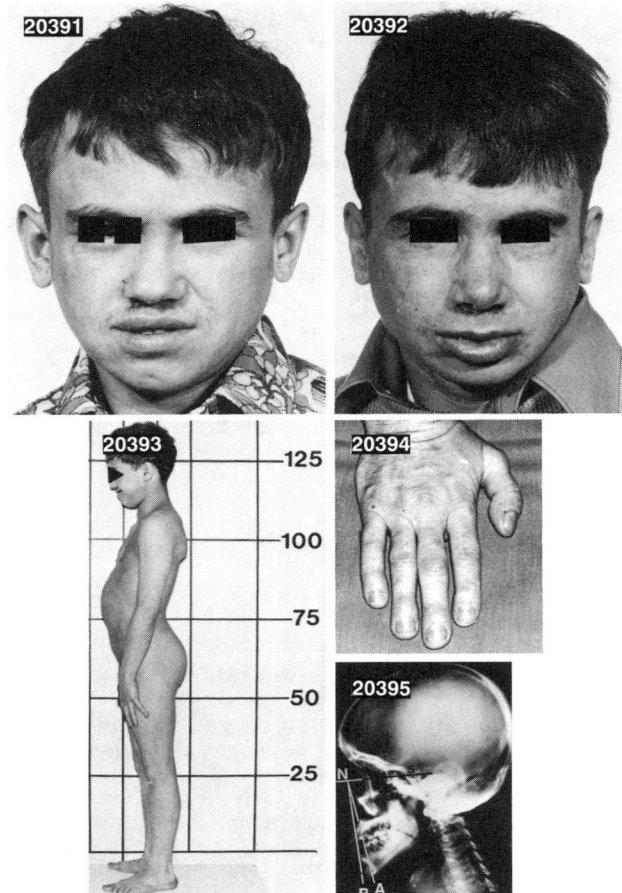

2556-20391-92: Two brothers with Martsolf syndrome; note prominent antitragus, mild maxillary hypoplasia, short philtrum, pouting lower lip, and sparse facial hair. The brother on the left has an opacity in the right eye. 20393: Lateral view shows maxillary hypoplasia, prominent nipples and increased lumbar lordosis. 20394: Note the bulbous fingertips and mild distal clinodactyly of several fingers. 20395: Skull X-ray marked for cephalometric analysis; note maxillary hypoplasia and relative prognathism.

Risk of Recurrence for Patient's Sib:
See Part I, *Mendelian Inheritance.*

Risk of Recurrence for Patient's Child:
See Part I, *Mendelian Inheritance.* There is no reported case of affected individuals reproducing. With the small testicles and the hypogonadism, decreased fertility is expected.

Age of Detectability: The disorder is usually clinically evident by ages 10–20 years, but developmental retardation and the cataracts may be present earlier during childhood.

Gene Mapping and Linkage: Unknown.

Prevention: None known. Genetic counseling indicated.

Treatment: Special education programs, cataract removal, dental care, and general supportive measures as indicated.

Prognosis: Severe mental retardation, but life span is normal.

Detection of Carrier: Unknown.

Special Considerations: The cases reported by Mikati et al (1985) are similar but do not have cataracts and do have genua valga and cubiti valgi, and are therefore considered a different condition.

References:
Cuendet JF, et al.: Association de cataracte congenitale et d'oligophrenie. Bull Mem Soc Fr Ophtalmol 1976; 87:164–168.
Martsolf JT, et al.: Severe mental retardation, cataracts, short stature, and primary hypogonadism in two brothers. Am J Med Genet 1978; 1:291–299.
Mikati MA, et al.: Microcephaly, hypergonadotropic hypogonadism, short stature, and minor anomalies: a new syndrome. Am J Med Genet 1985; 22:599–608.
Sanchez JM, et al.: Two brothers with Martsolf's syndrome. J Med Genet 1985; 22:308–310.
Hennekam RCM, et al.: Martsolf syndrome in a brother and sister: clinical features and pattern of inheritance. Europ J Pediatr 1988; 147:539–543.
Strisciuglo P, et al.: Martsolf's syndrome in a non-Jewish boy. J Med Genet 1988; 25:267–269.
Harbord MG, et al.: Microcephaly, mental retardation, cataracts, and hypogonadism in sibs: Martsolf's syndrome. J Med Genet 1989; 26:397–406.

MA043 **John T. Martsolf**

Mason type diabetes
See DIABETES MELLITUS, MATURITY ONSET OF THE YOUNG (MODY)
Mast cell disease
See URTICARIA PIGMENTOSA (UP)
Mastocytosis
See URTICARIA PIGMENTOSA (UP)
Maternal hyperphenylalaninemia
See FETAL EFFECTS FROM MATERNAL PKU
Maternal hyperthermia, fetal effects from
See FETAL EFFECTS FROM MATERNAL HYPERTHERMIA
Maternal phenylketonuria
See FETAL EFFECTS FROM MATERNAL PKU
Maturity-onset diabetes of the young (MODY)
See DIABETES MELLITUS, MATURITY ONSET OF THE YOUNG (MODY)
Maturity-onset type hyperglycemia of the young (MOHY)
See DIABETES MELLITUS, MATURITY ONSET OF THE YOUNG (MODY)
Maumenee congenital corneal edema
See CORNEAL DYSTROPHY, ENDOTHELIAL, CONGENITAL HEREDITARY
Maumenee corneal dystrophy
See CORNEAL DYSTROPHY, ENDOTHELIAL, CONGENITAL HEREDITARY

MAXILLA, MEDIAN ALVEOLAR CLEFT   0631

Includes: Cleft, maxillary median alveolar

Excludes:
    Lip, median cleft of upper (0595)
    Maxillary bone, failure of formation of premaxillary portion

Major Diagnostic Criteria: X-ray evidence of a cleft in the pre-maxilla that measures at least 2 mm. The maxillary incisors must be or must have been present.

Clinical Findings: X-ray evidence of a cleft in the midline of the premaxillary portion of the maxilla. There may be a diastema between the central incisors. A divergence of the roots of the central incisors may be present.

Complications: Orthodontic movement of the maxillary central incisors could cause the loss of teeth because of lack of bone support.

Associated Findings: None known.

Etiology: Postulated by Stout and Collett (1969) to be entrapment of epithelial nests which prevents fusion of the center of calcification of the premaxilla.

Pathogenesis: Failure of fusion of the primary ossification center of the premaxilla during early embryonic development.

Sex Ratio: Undetermined. M0:F5 observed.

Occurrence: Undetermined but presumed rare.

Risk of Recurrence for Patient's Sib: Unknown.

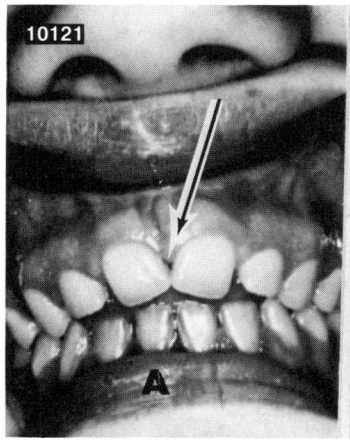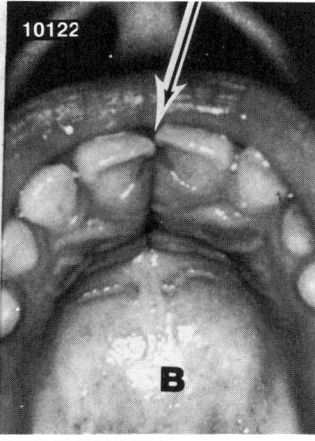

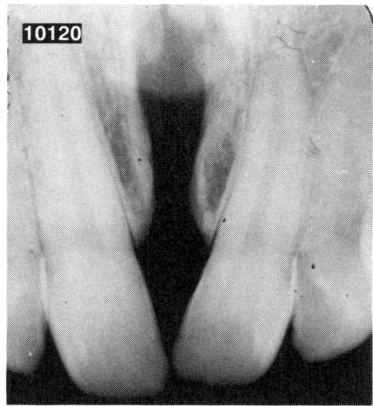

0631-10121: Maxillary median alveolar cleft. **10122:** Intraoral view of cleft. **10120:** Periapical X-ray of maxillary median alveolar cleft.

Risk of Recurrence for Patient's Child: Unknown.

Age of Detectability: Earliest reported case detected at seven years on routine X-ray examination. This condition can now be diagnosed only when all four maxillary incisors are present, indicating that there has been at least primary formation of the premaxillary portion of the maxilla.

Gene Mapping and Linkage: Unknown.

Prevention: None known.

Treatment: None indicated. Orthodontic movement is not recommended.

Prognosis: Normal life span and function.

Detection of Carrier: Unknown.

References:
Gier RE, Fast TB: Median maxillary anterior alveolar cleft: case reports and discussion. Oral Surg 1967; 24:496–502.
Miller AS, et al.: Median maxillary anterior cleft: report of three cases. J Am Dent Assoc 1969; 79:896–897.
Stout FW, Collett WK: Etiology and incidence of median maxillary anterior alveolar cleft. Oral Surg 1969; 28:66–72.

GI004   **Ronald E. Gier**

Maxillary hypoplasia-metaphyseal dysplasia-brachydactyly
See METAPHYSEAL DYSPLASIA-MAXILLARY HYPOPLASIA-BRACHYDACTYLY
Maxillary incisor, single central
See TEETH, FUSED

Maxillary lateral incisor, hypodontia of
See TEETH, PEGGED OR ABSENT MAXILLARY LATERAL INCISOR
Maxillary lateral incisor, pegged or missing
See TEETH, PEGGED OR ABSENT MAXILLARY LATERAL INCISOR

MAXILLOFACIAL DYSOSTOSIS   2512

Includes: Hypoplasia of the maxilla, primary familial

Excludes:
   Acrodysostosis (0016)
   Acrofacial dysostosis (0017)
   Mandibulofacial dysostosis (0627)

Major Diagnostic Criteria: All reported patients have presented with maxillary hypoplasia, delayed development of speech and language skills with dysarthria in the absence of hearing loss, and normal or near-normal intelligence.

Clinical Findings: The most consistent malformations seen in maxillofacial dysostosis include anteroposterior shortening of the maxilla, occasionally resulting in a relative mandibular prognathism; downslanting palpebral fissures; minor malformations of the auricles; and severely delayed onset of speech, with poor vocabulary development and poorly connected discourse, as well as nonfluent and inarticulate speech, including prolonged hesitations, vowel and consonant substitutions, omissions, and distortions.

Other clinical findings include flat occiput, maxillary hypoplasia, flat nasal bridge, narrow beaked nose, ptosis of eyelids, nystagmus, strabismus, **Pectus excavatum**, and hypoplastic nipples.

Cephalometric analysis confirms a small anterior cranial fossae and a decreased anteroposterior size of the maxilla.

Complications: Unknown.

Associated Findings: Most of these patients have had normal or near-normal intelligence; however, because of their speech difficulties, teachers and school officials have thought them to be mentally retarded.

Etiology: Autosomal dominant inheritance.

Pathogenesis: A genetic disorder that induces branchial arch developmental delay. This delay also affects the neuronal pathways connecting Brocca and Wernicke areas in the brain, producing a clinical condition similar to conduction aphasia.

MIM No.: *15500

POS No.: 3921

Sex Ratio: M1:F1

Occurrence: About a dozen cases have been reported.

Risk of Recurrence for Patient's Sib:
   See Part I, *Mendelian Inheritance.*

Risk of Recurrence for Patient's Child:
   See Part I, *Mendelian Inheritance.*

Age of Detectability: At birth, with affected individuals showing maxillary hypoplasia and eye and ear anomalies.

Gene Mapping and Linkage: Unknown.

Prevention: None known. Genetic counseling indicated.

Treatment: If the facial malformations are severe, plastic reconstructive surgery and orthodontic treatment may be helpful. It is important not to interfere with growth centers, because this syndrome's facial features improve with age, giving a close to normal profile in adulthood. The patients seen by Melnick and Eastman (1977) and by Escobar et al (1977) all responded positively to speech therapy.

Prognosis: Speech developmental delay, which may hamper intellectual achievement and school progress. Life span does not seem to be impaired.

Detection of Carrier: Clinical examination.

References:
Villaret M, Desoille H: L'hypoplasie primitive familiale du maxillaire superieur. Ann Med 1932; 32:378–381.

Peters A, Hovels O: Die Dysostosis maxillo-facialis, eine erbliche, typische Fehlbildung des 1. Visceralbogens Z Menschl Vererb. Konstitutionsl 1960; 35:434–444.
Escobar V, et al.: Maxillofacial dysostosis. J Med Genet 1977; 14:355–358.
Melnick M, Eastman JR: Autosomal dominant maxillofacial dysostosis. BD:OAS XII(3B). New York: March of Dimes Birth Defects Foundation, 1977:39–44.

ES000   **Victor Escobar**

Maxillonasal dysostosis
See MAXILLONASAL DYSPLASIA, BINDER TYPE

MAXILLONASAL DYSPLASIA, BINDER TYPE   2235

Includes:
> Binder syndrome
> Maxillonasal dysostosis
> Nasomaxillary hypoplasia
> Nasomaxillovertebral syndrome

Excludes:
> **Aarskog syndrome** (0001)
> **Chondrodysplasia**
> **Deafness-myopia-cataract-saddle nose, Marshall type** (0261)
> **Fetal warfarin syndrome** (0389)
> **Robinow syndrome** (0876)
> Syphilis, congenital

Major Diagnostic Criteria: Collapsed nasal pyramid lacking cartilaginous support; short nose with a flat bridge; acute nasolabial angle; short and hypoplastic columella; hypoplastic alar cartilages; and atrophic nasal mucosa with normal sense of smell. X-ray findings including hypoplasia of the frontal process of the maxilla with absence of the anterior nasal spine, thinness of the alveolar bone labial to the maxillary incisors, and obtuse nasofrontal angle and obtuse gonial angle.

Clinical Findings: The face is characterized by nasomaxillary hypoplasia with a flat nose, absence of the nasal septum, short columella, and hypoplastic perialar areas. The external nares may have a "cat's ear" shape or "half moon" appearance. The sense of smell and intelligence are normal. Dental findings usually include an Angle Class III malocclusion with proclination of the maxillary incisors.

X-ray findings include Class III facial skeletal pattern with a retrognathic maxilla, absence of the anterior nasal spine, thinness of the alveolar bone labial to the maxillary incisors, obtuse nasofrontal angle, acute nasolabial angle, and obtuse gonial angle. Less frequent findings include abnormalities of the cervical spine (53%).

Complications: Frequent upper respiratory infections; psychosocial consequences of unusual facial appearance.

Associated Findings: Neonatal respiratory distress; labiomaxillary cleft.

Etiology: Both sporadic and inherited (dominant and recessive) cases have been described. Maxillonasal dysplasia also occurs as a finding in several syndromes.

Pathogenesis: A defect in cartilage development during weeks five to six has been proposed as the mechanism for the simultaneous occurrence of anomalies in the cervical spine and maxillonasal complex.

MIM No.: 15505

POS No.: 3330

Sex Ratio: Presumably M1:F1.

Occurrence: Over 100 cases have been reported in the literature.

Risk of Recurrence for Patient's Sib: If the patient represents a new occurrence in the family, the risk to the sib is near zero. However, given inheritance patterns in some families, a careful family history is needed before assigning risk figures.

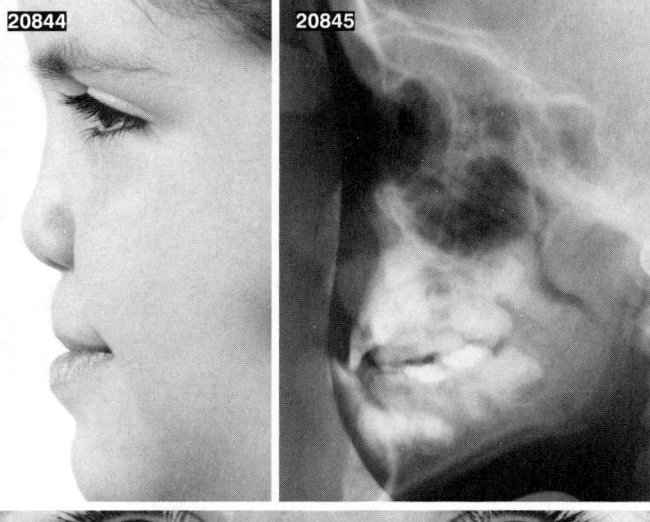
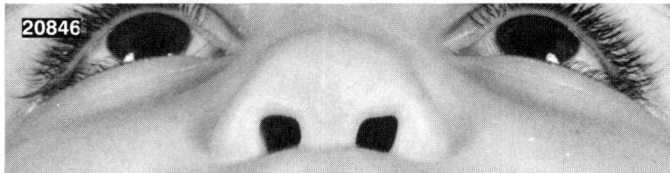
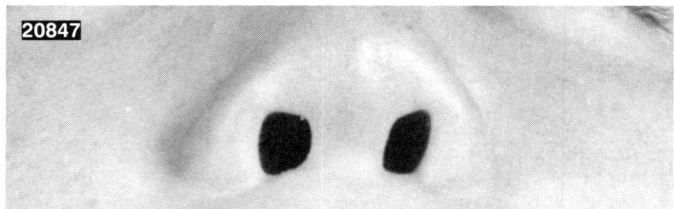
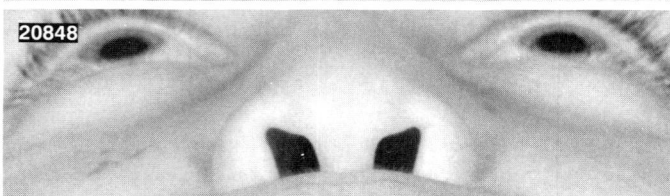
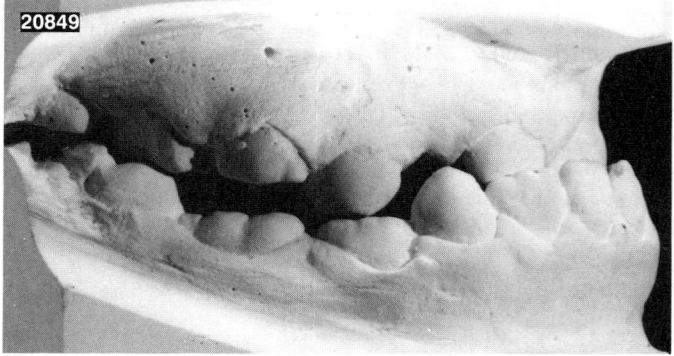

2235-20844: Maxillonasal dysplasia, Binder type; note characteristic facial profile. **20845:** X-ray shows the bony dysplasia in the maxilla and the nasal bones. **20846–48:** Note different nasal shapes seen in maxillonasal dysplasia. **20849:** Dental cast shows the relative positions of the maxilla and the mandible.

Risk of Recurrence for Patient's Child: Recent reports suggest autosomal dominant inheritance with variable expression in some families. If so, the risk to the child may be as high as 1:2.

Age of Detectability: At birth.

Gene Mapping and Linkage: Unknown.

Prevention: None known. Genetic counseling indicated.

Treatment: Nasal bone grafts, surgical and/or orthopedic maxillary advancement, orthodontic and/or prosthodontic treatment.

Prognosis: Good.

Detection of Carrier: Unknown.

Special Considerations: Maxillonasal dysplasia is a finding, not a diagnosis, and therefore is likely to be heterogeneous.

References:
Binder KH: Dysostosis maxillo-nasalis, ein arinencephaler Missbildungskomplex. Deutsch Zahnaerztl A 1962; 17:438–444.
Munro IR, et al.: Maxillonasal dysplasia (Binder's syndrome). Plast Reconstr Surg 1979; 63:657–663.
Delair J, et al.: Clinical and radiologic aspects of maxillonasal dysostosis (Binder syndrome). Head Neck Surg 1980; 3:105–122. *
Resche F, et al.: Craniospinal and cervicospinal malformations associated with maxillonasal dysostosis (Binder syndrome). Head Neck Surg 1980; 3:123–131.
Gross-Kieselstein E, et al.: Familial variant of maxillonasal dysplasia? J Craniofacial Genetics and Developmental Biology 1986; 6:331–334.
Horswell BB, et al.: Maxillonasal dysplasia (Binder's syndrome): a critical review and case study. J Oral Maxillofac Surg 1987; 45:114–122. *

EV002   **Carla A Evans**
H0058   **Lili K. Horton**

Maxillopalpebral synkinesis
See JAW-WINKING SYNDROME
May-Hegglin anomaly
See LEUKOCYTE, MAY-HEGGLIN ANOMALY
Mayer-Rokitansky-Kuster (MRK) anomaly
See MULLERIAN APLASIA
McArdle disease
See GLYCOGENOSIS, TYPE V
McCune-Albright syndrome
See FIBROUS DYSPLASIA, POLYOSTOTIC

MCDONOUGH SYNDROME   0632

Includes: Noonan-like McDonough syndrome

Excludes:
Noonan syndrome (0720)
Turner syndrome (0977)

Major Diagnostic Criteria: The combination of mental retardation, short stature, kyphoscoliosis, pectus carinatum/excavatum, cardiac defect, diastasis recti, cryptorchidism, and a possibly altered facial appearance.

Clinical Findings: Only two families have been reported; features present in affected individuals of both families include short stature (third to 25th percentile), mental retardation, synophrys, strabismus, malocclusion, anteverted auricles, kyphoscoliosis, **Pectus carinatum** or **Pectus excavatum**, cardiac defect (including **Atrial septal defects** or **Ventricular septal defect** with pulmonic stenosis and aortic stenosis), diastasis recti, and cryptorchidism. Further delineation of the phenotype is difficult, however, since in each family, unaffected family members shared some of the variant features with affected individuals. In the first reported family (Neuhauser and Opitz, 1975), additional features included upslanting palpebral fissures, grooved tongue, micrognathia, single transverse palmar crease, hypoplastic toenails, and clinodactyly. In the second reported family (Garcia-Sagredo et al, 1984), features included sparse or bristly hair, apparent **Eye, hypertelorism**, ptosis, large nose, short philtrum, and prognathism. In one family, one affected individual had an XXY karyotype apparently inherited from his XY/XXY father; in the second family a

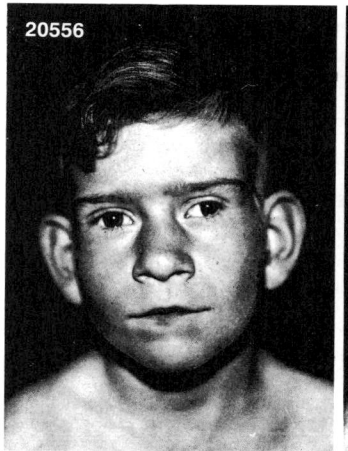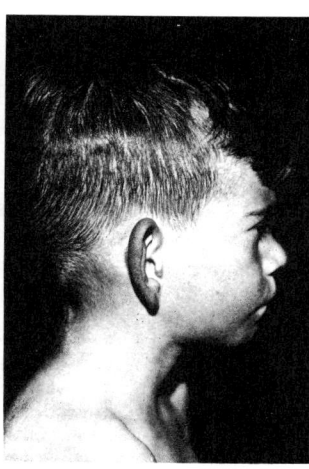

0632-20556: McDonough syndrome; note anteverted auricles, upward slanting palpebral fissures and synophrys in this boy who also had a 47, XYY chromosome constitution.

balanced X;20 translocation was found in one affected child and his mother.

Complications: Heart failure, scoliosis.

Associated Findings: None known.

Etiology: Possibly autosomal recessive inheritance.

Pathogenesis: Unknown.

MIM No.: 24895

POS No.: 3286

Sex Ratio: Presumably M1:F1

Occurrence: Two families have been reported; one from the United States and one from Spain.

Risk of Recurrence for Patient's Sib:
See Part I, *Mendelian Inheritance.*

Risk of Recurrence for Patient's Child:
See Part I, *Mendelian Inheritance.*

Age of Detectability: Soon after birth by the presence of the cardiac defect.

Gene Mapping and Linkage: Unknown.

Prevention: None known. Genetic counseling indicated.

Treatment: Treatment of the kyphoscoliosis may be indicated, as well as surgical correction of the cardiac defect and cryptorchidism.

Prognosis: All affected individuals have been mentally retarded, with IQs between 47 and 71. Prognosis is undetermined, although life span should be normal.

Detection of Carrier: Unknown.

References:
Neuhauser G, Opitz JM: Studies of malformation syndromes in man. XXXX: multiple congenital anomalies/mental retardation syndrome or variant familial developmental pattern; differential diagnosis and description of the McDonough syndrome (with XXY son from XY/XXY father). Z Kinderheilkd 1975; 120:231–242.
Garcia-Sagredo JM, et al.: Mentally retarded siblings with congenital heart defect, peculiar facies and cryptorchidism in the male: possible McDonough syndrome with coincidental (X;20) translocation. Clin Genet 1984; 26:117–124.

T0007   **Helga V. Toriello**
NE012   **Gerhard Neuhäuser**

McKusick-Kaufman syndrome
See VAGINAL SEPTUM, TRANSVERSE

McLeod phenotype
See ANEMIA, HEMOLYTIC, RED CELL MEMBRANE DEFECTS

MECKEL DIVERTICULUM   0633

Includes:
    Omphalomesenteric duct
    Vitelline duct, remnant

Excludes: Intestinal duplication (0532)

Major Diagnostic Criteria: Positive diagnosis can only be made by the gross anatomic findings made at operation or autopsy. The diverticulum can vary in size, both in diameter and length, and arises from the antimesenteric border of the ileum, usually within 100 cm of the ileocecal valve (90%). Ectopic gastric or pancreatic tissue is present in approximately two-thirds of the diverticula; the lesion presents most frequently in the pediatric age group with massive gastrointestinal hemorrhage, and in the older patients with inflammation or intestinal obstruction.

Clinical Findings: Asymptomatic, except if a complication occurs. Fifteen percent to 20% become symptomatic, and the rest are asymptomatic. The presenting symptoms are related to the complication and include, in the pediatric age group, hemorrhage, intestinal obstruction, inflammation (simulating appendicitis), peritonitis, and umbilical drainage. Rarely, carcinoma can arise in a Meckel diverticulum. Hemorrhage results from a peptic ulcer in the diverticulum or in the adjacent ileum and is associated with gastric mucosa in the diverticulum. Intestinal obstruction can result from congenital bands, either mesodiverticular or omphalomesenteric, previous inflammatory adhesion, intussusception (ileo-ileo with the diverticulum as the lead point), and from the incarceration of the diverticulum in a hernia: the so-called Littre hernia. Inflammation is related to obstruction of the mouth of the diverticulum, as in appendicitis, or in association with a foreign body such as a fish-bone stuck in the diverticulum. Perforation results from diverticulitis or from perforation of an ulcer. Umbilical drainage results from an omphalomesenteric duct sinus or fistula. The sinus may present only as an umbilical polyp of intestinal mucosa. Very rarely, the diverticulum can be demonstrated by ordinary X-ray examinations, such as a small bowel series or a barium enema with reflux into the ileum. A 99 m$_{Tc}$-pertechnetate scan of the abdomen may demonstrate a Meckel diverticulum by showing gastric mucosa, present in 50% of symptomatic diverticula. Asymptomatic diverticula are usually found incidentally at celiotomy for some other reason. Symptomatic patients usually present with one of the four following condition: an omphalomesenteric duct remnant recognized as such on examination of the umbilicus; an acute surgical abdomen of uncertain origin, but signifying inflammation with peritonitis or obstruction of the small bowel; gross rectal bleeding, or intermittent abdominal pain. Sixty percent of symptomatic diverticula present in childhood, and 50% manifest in the first three years of life. Of the symptomatic patients, 75% are male.

Complications: Hemorrhage (40%), obstruction (25%), inflammation (23%), perforation (5%), or umbilical discharge (5%). The above percentages are for the pediatric age group; older patients present more commonly with obstruction and inflammation.

Associated Findings: There is an increased incidence of a Meckel diverticulum in children born with a major malformation of the umbilicus, alimentary tract, and nervous and cardiovascular systems (in descending order of frequency). For omphalocele and gastroschisis the association is 25%; for esophageal atresia it is 12%.

Etiology: Unknown.

Pathogenesis: Meckel diverticulum, or its variants, develops as a gross structural defect of the yolk sac, vitelline duct and/or omphalomesenteric duct, which are a normal structures of the 5–9 mm embryo. At this stage (the end of the fifth week), the yolk stalk or vitelline duct constricts and separates from the intestine and disappears. A persistence of the yolk stalk appears in several forms. The stalk may remain patent and continuous, forming an umbilical-intestinal fistula. It may be patent at the outer end, producing a sinus. A cyst will form if the central portion is patent. Most commonly, a blind pouch occurs on the ileum, free in the abdomen except for its attachment to the ileum or sometimes connected to the umbilicus by a fibrous band. The diverticulum is a true diverticulum showing all layers of the intestinal wall. Some diverticula contain gastric mucosa or pancreatic tissue. One of the vitelline arteries persists as a branch of the terminal superior mesenteric artery to form the arterial blood supply to the diverticulum. The other vitelline artery can form a mesodiverticular band.

CDC No.: 751.010

Sex Ratio: M1:F1

Occurrence: 1:60 live births.

Risk of Recurrence for Patient's Sib: Unknown.

Risk of Recurrence for Patient's Child: Unknown.

Age of Detectability: By complications that occur more commonly before the age of three years (50%), but can occur at any age.

Gene Mapping and Linkage: Unknown.

Prevention: None known. Genetic counseling indicated.

Treatment: Excision of the diverticulum by means of a wedge diverticulectomy is the usual surgical treatment. In certain complications of a Meckel diverticulum, such as obstruction or bleeding from an ileal ulcer, it may be necessary to do an ileal resection and ileo-ileal anastomosis. An incidental resection of a Meckel diverticulum at the time of laparotomy may be done to prevent the subsequent complications of the diverticulum if good surgical judgment calls for its removal. Elective resection may be considered advisable if there are atypical features, such as abnormal bands or attachments, or heterotopic tissue, noted on inspection and palpation of the diverticulum. The evidence of heterotopic tissue is indirect and consists of mucosal or submucosal nodules, evidence of inflammation, and serosal scarring and adhesions. Other risk factors for future symptoms are age of the patient and length of the diverticulum. The younger the patient, the more likely he or she is to be symptomatic. And the longer diverticula are more symptomatic than the shorter ones; 2 cm is the critical differential point. The diameter and the position of the diverticulum are not factors significant for future symptoms. It is estimated that 5% of incidentally found Meckel diverticula lead to symptoms during a lifetime.

Prognosis: Excellent with recovery from surgical treatment. Most deaths occur from a delayed recognition of a perforation and obstruction in infants.

Detection of Carrier: Unknown.

Special Considerations: In the newborn there occurs a distinct form of the anomaly, known as giant Meckel diverticulum. This type of diverticulum can measure 4–8 cm in diameter, and presents as a palpable or viable abdominal mass and as intestinal obstruction. Surgical resection is urgently required to relieve the obstruction.

References:

Kiesewetter WB: Meckel's diverticulum in children. Arch Surg 1957; 75:914–919.

Craft AW, et al.: Giant Meckel's diverticulum causing intestinal obstruction of newborn. J Pediatr Surg 1976; 11:1037–1038.

Simms MH, Corkery JJ: Meckel diverticulum: association with congenital malformation and the significance of atypical morphology. Br J Surg 1980; 67:216–219.

Williams RS: Management of Meckel's diverticulum. Br J Surg 1981; 68:477–480.

Cooney DR, et al.: The abdominal technetium scan (a decade of experience). J Pediatr Surg 1982; 17:611–619.

Mackey WC, Dineen P: A fifty year experience with Meckel's diverticulum. Surg Gynec Obstet 1983; 153:56–64.

Paul W. Johnston

MECKEL SYNDROME 0634

Includes:
    Dysencephalia splanchnocystica
    Gruber syndrome
    Meckel-Gruber syndrome

Excludes:
    Chromosome 13, trisomy 13 (0168)
    Oculo-encephalo-hepato-renal syndrome (3242)
    Smith-Lemli-Opitz syndrome (0891)

Major Diagnostic Criteria: Cystic dysplasia of the kidneys with fibrotic changes of the liver, occipital encephalocele, or some other CNS malformation plus other frequently seen anomalies such as polydactyly, cleft lip and/or palate, microcephaly, small or ambiguous genitalia.

Clinical Findings: Microcephaly is commonly associated with occipital encephalocele. On occasion there may be hydrocephaly or anencephaly. The facies is described as Potter-like, especially in cases with severe oligohydramnios. Facial characteristics include a

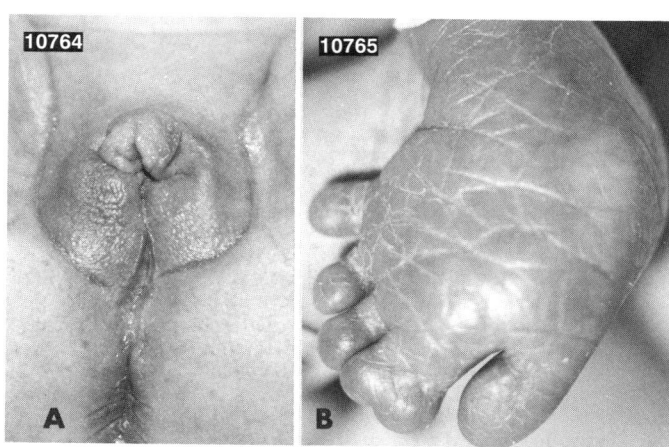

0634B-10764: Hypoplastic phallus with dorsal prepuce, urethral opening at base of phallus, and fusion of labioscrotal swellings. 10765: Short 1st toe, postaxial hexadactyly, complete cutaneous syndactyly of 2nd and 3rd toes, and severe valgus deformity.

shape that is broad and round, low sloping forehead, broad cheeks, small chin, hypertelorism, upslanted palpebral fissures, broad flattened nose, wide mouth, full lips, and low-set ears. The neck is often short. Other associated craniofacial malformations include microphthalmia, colobomata, cataracts, cleft lip and more commonly cleft palate, natal teeth, small lobulated or cleft tongue with or without papillomatous processes, and buccal frenula.

Renal dysplasia is almost always bilateral. Both kidneys are usually grossly enlarged, but on occasion slightly enlarged, normal, or smaller than normal. Kidneys usually have macroscopic cysts. On histologic examination they invariably show cystic

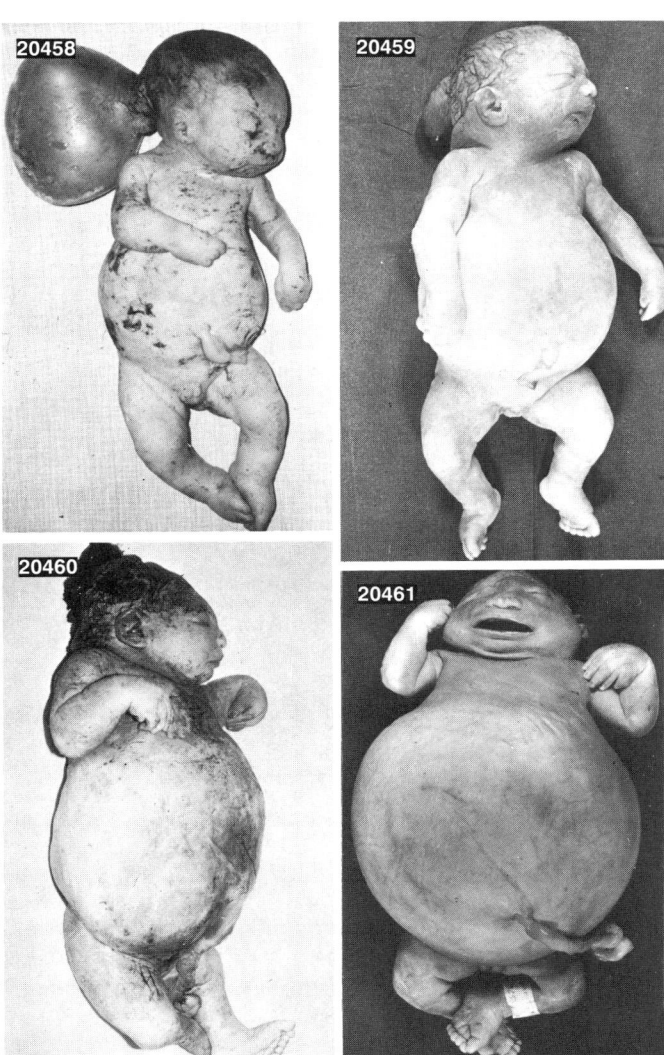

0634A-20458–61: Meckel syndrome; note occipital encephalocele, polydactyly, and abdominal enlargement from megacystic kidneys.

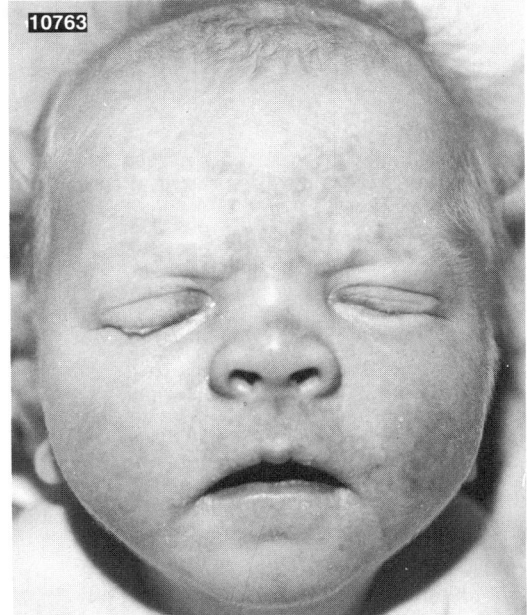

0634C-10763: Facial features include overlapping eyelids, capillary hemangiomas on forehead, bridge and top of the nose; downturned corners of the mouth.

dysplastic changes with very little normal parenchyma. Anomalies of the urinary tract are common, including hypoplastic ureters, hypoplastic bladder, bladder not connected to the urethra, or an absent urethra.

CNS malformations are varied, with occipital encephalocele being the most common. Occipital holes are found in the skull, which may be connected by an occipitoschisis with the foramen magnum. The encephalocele is usually accompanied by microcephaly, and on occasion, hydrocephaly. There are various grades of aplasia/hypoplasia of the cerebrum, cerebellum, and olfactory lobes and microencephaly.

Limb malformations are also common. Polydactyly is present in the vast majority of cases, such that previous reports required minimal criteria to include two out of three features; occipital encephalocele, cystic kidneys, and polydactyly. One or two extra digits are present postaxially, almost always bilaterally on both hands and feet. There may be partial or total syndactyly involving fingers and toes. Ulnar deviation of the hands and clubfeet are also common. Short limbs have been described. Genital anomalies are also a common feature. Ambiguous genitalia often turn out to be cases of male pseudohermaphroditism with testes or 46,XY karyotype. Both testes and ovaries have been, rarely, found.

Other internal organ defects include cardiac, gastrointestinal, and pulmonary abnormalities. The liver is usually too large for gestational age, up to twice the normal size. Microscopic cysts are often present. Bile ducts may be dilated, and the gall bladder may be absent. Microscopically, the liver shows fibrosis of the portal areas with ductal proliferation and dilation of the liver. Heart anomalies consist of atrial septal defect, **Ventricular septal defect**, and other complex malformations. There may be an accessory spleen, absent spleen, splenomegaly, and absent or hypoplastic adrenals. Hypoplasia of the lungs is common, assumed to be secondary to the enlarged abdomen and oligohydramnnios.

All cases are stillborn or die within a few hours after birth, due to renal insufficiency, with or without pulmonary or cardiac complications. A long term survival of one week is reported with death due to renal failure.

Complications: Breech presentation is frequent. Caesarean section is common because of hydrocephaly, abnormal fetal position or fetal distress. Oligohydramnios is also common.

Associated Findings: None known.

Etiology: Autosomal recessive inheritance.

Pathogenesis: Unknown.

MIM No.: *24900

POS No.: 3287

CDC No.: 759.890

Sex Ratio: M1:F1

Occurrence: Found world-wide, but particularly prevalent in Finland (1:9,000 births), among the Tatars of the Soviet Union, and among Gujarati Indians.

Risk of Recurrence for Patient's Sib:
See Part I, *Mendelian Inheritance.*

Risk of Recurrence for Patient's Child:
See Part I, *Mendelian Inheritance.* Affected individuals are not expected to survive to reproduce.

Age of Detectability: Prenatal diagnosis using ultrasonography and alpha fetoprotein determination is well documented. The condition is often suspected because of a previous affected sibling. Sonography often detects the occipital encephalocele or cystic dysplastic kidneys. Maternal serum and amniotic fluid alpha fetoprotein is often elevated from the associated encephalocele or anencephaly. These findings are present in midtrimester. The syndrome is also diagnosable at birth.

Gene Mapping and Linkage: Unknown.

Prevention: None known. Genetic counseling indicated.

Treatment: Unknown.

Prognosis: Invariably fatal within the first hours or days of life.

Detection of Carrier: Unknown.

Special Considerations: This condition is named after Johann Friedrich Meckel who first described it in 1822. G.B. Gruber, who termed the condition dysencephalia splanchnocystica, published his findings in 1934. In 1984, the American Journal of Medical Genetics devoted much of its volume 18 to the proceedings of a Meckel symposium organized by John M. Opitz on the bicentennial of Meckel's death.

References:
Opitz JM, Howe JJ: The Meckel syndrome (dysencephalia splanchnocystica, the Gruber syndrome). BD:OAS V(2). New York: The National Foundation-March of Dimes, 1969:167–179.
Meckel S, Passarge E: Encephalocele, polycystic kidneys and polydactyly as an autosomal recessive trait simulating certain other disorders: the Meckel syndrome. Ann Genet 1971; 14:97–103.
Hsia YE, et al.: Genetics of the Meckel syndrome (dysencephalia splanchnocystica). Pediatrics 1971; 48:237–247.
Johnson VP, et al.: Prenatal diagnosis of Meckel syndrome: case reports and literature review. Am J Med Genet 1984; 18:699–711.
Salonen R: The Meckel syndrome: clinicopathologic findings in 67 patients. Am J Med Genet 1984; 18:671–689.
Rapola J, Salonen R: Visceral anomalies in the Meckel syndrome. Teratology 1985; 31:193–201.

J0010
Virginia P. Johnson

Meckel-Gruber syndrome
See MECKEL SYNDROME
Meconium ileus, isolated
See INTESTINAL ILEUS, ISOLATED MECONIUM ILEUS
MED-IDDM syndrome
See EPIPHYSEAL DYSPLASIA, MULTIPLE-DIABETES MELLITUS
Medial coronary sclerosis of infancy
See ARTERY, CORONARY CALCINOSIS
Medial fibroplasia
See ARTERY, RENAL FIBROMUSCULAR DYSPLASIA
Median cleft face syndrome
See FACE, MEDIAN CLEFT FACE SYNDROME
Median cleft of upper lip
See LIP, MEDIAN CLEFT OF UPPER
Median clefts of lower lip, mandible and tongue
See CLEFTS, LOWER MEDIAN LIP, MANDIBLE AND TONGUE
Median incisal diastema
See TEETH, DIASTEMA, MEDIAN INCISAL
Median rhomboid glossitis
See GLOSSITIS, MEDIAN RHOMBOID
Mediterranean anemia
See THALASSEMIA
Mediterranean fever, familial (FMF)
See FEVER, FAMILIAL MEDITERRANEAN (FMF)
Medium-chain acyl-CoA dehydrogenase deficiency (MCAD)
See ACYL-CoA DEHYDROGENASE DEFICIENCY, MEDIUM CHAIN TYPE
Medullary cystic disease-nephronophthisis
See KIDNEY, NEPHRONOPHTHISIS-MEDULLARY CYSTIC DESEASE
Medullary cystic kidney disease
See KIDNEY, NEPHRONOPHTHISIS-MEDULLARY CYSTIC DESEASE
Medullary sponge kidney
See KIDNEY, MEDULLARY SPONGE KIDNEY
Medullary thyroid carcinoma and pheochromocytoma syndrome
See ENDOCRINE NEOPLASIA, MULTIPLE TYPE II
Medullary thyroid carcinoma syndrome (most cases)
See ENDOCRINE NEOPLASIA, MULTIPLE TYPE II
Medulloblastoma
See CNS NEOPLASMS
Meesmann corneal dystrophy
See CORNEAL DYSTROPHY, JUVENILE EPITHELIAL, MEESMANN TYPE
Mefenamic acid, fetal effects
See FETAL EFFECTS OF NONSTEROIDAL ANTI-INFLAMMATORY DRUGS (NSAIDS)
Megacolon, aganglionic
See COLON, AGANGLIONOSIS
Megacolon, idiopathic
See INTESTINAL PSEUDO-OBSTRUCTION SYNDROMES
Megacystis, idiopathic
See INTESTINAL PSEUDO-OBSTRUCTION SYNDROMES

MEGACYSTIS-MEGADUODENUM SYNDROME 2316

Includes:
Intestinal pseudo-obstruction, idiopathic
Megaduodenum-megacysts syndrome
Visceral myopathy, familial
Visceral myopathy, hereditary hollow

Excludes:
Colon, aganglionosis (0192)
Colon, atresia or stenosis (0193)
Colon, duplication (0194)
Duodenum, atresia or stenosis (0300)
Intestinal atresia or stenosis (0531)
Intestinal hypoperistalsis, megacystis-microcolon type (2317)
Pyloric stenosis (0848)
Stomach, pyloric atresia (0910)

Major Diagnostic Criteria: Familial megaduodenum and/or megacystis without evidence of organic obstruction in the gastrointestinal or urinary tracts. Intestinal activity is intermittently abnormal with reverse peristalsis. The severity of the symptoms is variable.

Clinical Findings: May present as intermittent abdominal pain with constipation or diarrhea. Vomiting is a common sign. The abdomen is distended. The esophagus may show aperistalsis or other disturbance of motility. The esophagus, stomach, colon, or small bowel may be dilated. Symptoms are progressive and may remit and relapse. Hydronephrosis secondary to a neurogenic bladder with reflux has been reported. Examination of the bladder has revealed a thickening of the wall with fibrosis. Some patients have a normal number and appearance of ganglion cells, while others have shown hyperplasia or a decrease in the number of ganglion cells.

Complications: Malnutrition and weight loss may lead to death.

Associated Findings: The smooth muscle of the iris (pupillary sphincter) may be involved, as evidenced by mydriasis.

Etiology: Autosomal dominant inheritance. There are also pedigrees with similar clinical findings consistent with X-linked and autosomal recessive inheritance, even though most show dominant inheritance. Sporadic cases have also been reported.

Pathogenesis: Histologic studies of families with apparent autosomal dominant inheritance found normal number and appearance of ganglion cells and smooth muscle fibers. Reports of patients with decreased number of ganglion cells and nerve fibers by silver stain indicated a neuronal disorder. Another group of patients had fiber loss, degeneration, and fibrosis of the longitudinal intestinal muscle layer. The circular muscle layer may be similarly affected. Silver staining produced no evidence of ganglion cell or nerve fiber involvement; thus, a primary myopathy was considered. It may be due to alteration in contractile protein synthesis. Neuronal and smooth muscle abnormalities have been reported in one patient. Manometric studies showed a decrease in the total contractual activity of the bowel, including rhythmic short and propulsive (type III) waves.

MIM No.: *15531

POS No.: 4259

Sex Ratio: Unknown. A predominance of affected females was reported in one family without clear male-to-male transmission, suggesting heterogeneity with X-linked inheritance as a possibility.

Occurrence: Over 100 cases have been reported, including patients of German, Italian, and American-Black extraction.

Risk of Recurrence for Patient's Sib:
See Part I, *Mendelian Inheritance.*

Risk of Recurrence for Patient's Child:
See Part I, *Mendelian Inheritance.*

Age of Detectability: The gastrointestinal symptoms of the condition usually become manifest by late childhood or early adolescence, even though occurrence in middle age has been reported. The signs and symptoms may be progressive. The urinary tract is surprisingly asymptomatic, despite the underlying anomalies; it may become symptomatic, however, at varying ages.

Gene Mapping and Linkage: Unknown.

Prevention: None known. Genetic counseling indicated.

Treatment: Chronic abdominal pain and nausea may be assuaged by bed rest, intravenous fluids, and analgesics. Nasogastric suction and hyperalimentation may be used to treat the episodes of hypoperistalsis. Surgery may be of help in a few patients. Ileo-colic anastomosis has been of temporary benefit. Laparotomy may determine whether or not an anatomic obstruction exists in the proband; resection is not necessary. Further laparotomies may not be necessary in other affected family members. If bacterial overgrowth contributes to the abdominal distention, antibiotics may be helpful. Persistence of the hypoperistalsis requires hyperalimentation.

Prognosis: Growth and development do not appear to be significantly affected. Life span does not appear to be shortened, except in acute severe cases.

Detection of Carrier: Asymptomatic family members should be examined, especially for silent megaduodenum or renal abnormalities.

Special Considerations: Intestinal pseudo-obstruction can occur either as a primary or as a secondary condition. It may be due to **Scleroderma**, **Amyloidosis**, **Myotonic dystrophy**, or Chagas disease. Tricyclic antidepressants and phenothiazine may cause intestinal pseudo-obstruction. Patients without underlying disease are considered to have the heterogeneous "chronic idiopathic intestinal pseudo-obstruction" (CIIP), due to sporadic or familial *visceral neuropathy or myopathy*. The lack of an underlying condition, and the evidence of autosomal dominant mode of inheritance, are indicative of megacystis microcolon syndrome, which appears to be the most common cause of primary chronic intestinal pseudo-obstruction.

References:
Law DH, Ten Eyck EA: Familial megaduodenum and megacystis. Am J Med 1962; 33:911–922.
Faulk DL, et al.: A familial visceral myopathy. Ann Intern Med 1978; 89:600–606.
Roy AD, et al.: Idiopathic intestinal pseudo-obstruction: a familial visceral neuropathy. Clin Gen 1980; 18:291–297.
Schuffler MD, et al.: Chronic intestinal pseudo-obstruction: a report of 27 cases and review of the literature. Medicine 1981; 60:173–196. *
Mitros FA, et al.: Pathologic features of familial visceral myopathy. Hum Pathol 1982; 13:825–833.
Smout AJPM, et al.: Chronic idiopathic intestinal pseudo-obstruction: coexistence of smooth muscle and neuronal abnormalities. Dig Dis Sci 1985; 30:282–287.

HA069 **James K. Hartsfield, Jr.**

MEGALENCEPHALY 2319

Includes:
  Macrocephaly
  Macrocephaly, benign familial
  Macroencephaly
  Megalobarencephaly
  Megalocephaly

Excludes:
  Brain edema
  Cebebral gigantism (0137)
  CNS Neoplasms(0188)
  Hydrocephaly (0481)
  Megalencephaly due to metabolic causes
  Specific syndromes with anatomic megalencephaly

Major Diagnostic Criteria: The patient must have an occipitofrontal circumference (OFC) greater than 2 SD above the mean, and normal-sized or slightly enlarged but not enlarging ventricles, with no evidence of a metabolic cause for megalencephaly.

Clinical Findings: The question of megalencephaly arises when the patient's OFC exceeds 2 SD above the mean. It may be present at birth or discovered first as the head increases too rapidly after birth. If the patient has no neurologic deficits, the diagnosis is benign (and often familial) anatomic megalencephaly, or the patient may have any neurologic manifestation of a congenitally abnormal brain, such as retardation, seizures, or any variety of motor signs from hypotonia to spasticity. Although some megalencephalic infants have a normal birth weight, many have a birthweight in the 4,000–5,000g range. Some infants, as they grow, will become huge in stature, but many also have a dwarfed stature.

In spite of the increasing head size, the infant usually does not show symptoms and signs of increased intracranial pressure in the form of vomiting, or bulging fontanelle, but some may have a slight separation of skull sutures. The development of megalencephalic infants with neurologic deficits will fall behind the normal time table, but will not show a developmental peak followed by retrogression, which would characterize metabolic megalencephaly, increasing **Hydrocephaly**, or other lesions that progressively impair neurologic function.

Complications: Learning disabilities, mental retardation, seizures.

Associated Findings: A variety of mostly minor skeletal or visceral dysplasias may occur with megalencephaly. These include abnormal head shape, single palmar creases, ambiguous genitalia, heterotropia, and either gigantism or dwarfism.

Etiology: Usually autosomal dominant inheritance, in contrast to the metabolic megalencephalies, which tend to have an autosomal recessive pattern. No consistent chromosomal error is reported. In many instances, no genetic pattern is apparent. No exogenous teratogens are known to cause megalencephaly in man.

Pathogenesis: The enlarged brain has cells that are too large or too numerous. Whether this overgrowth in size or number affects neuronal and glial elements equally is unknown. While many large brains have a normal surface, some of the larger brains have distinct disorders of the gyral pattern. Some will show neuronal heterotopias and other evidence of a disturbance in the migration of neuroblasts from the periventricular proliferative zone to the cerebral surface. These patients will have severe impairment of mental and motor functions. No consistent biochemical error is known.

MIM No.: 24800

CDC No.: 742.400

Sex Ratio: M4:F1

Occurrence: Undetermined but presumed uncommon.

Risk of Recurrence for Patient's Sib:
  See Part I, *Mendelian Inheritance.*

Risk of Recurrence for Patient's Child:
  See Part I, *Mendelian Inheritance.*

Age of Detectability: Neonatal period or early infancy.

Gene Mapping and Linkage: Unknown.

Prevention: None known. Genetic counseling indicated.

Treatment: Unknown.

Prognosis: Depends on the functional capacity of the patient's brain.

Detection of Carrier: Measurement of OFC.

Special Considerations: The term, *megalocephaly* refers to any head with an excessive occipitofrontal circumference, without regard to the case or brain size. While some use the term *megalocephaly* or *macrocephaly* to describe megalencephaly, we urge all to use the most specific term possible. Also, it is wise not to interchange the terms, as a large head may contain a large brain as in megalencephaly; a dilated cerebrum as in **Hydrocephaly**; a small cerebrum (*micrencephaly*); or no cerebrum as in severe **Hydranencephaly**. *Macrocephaly* and its antonym, *microcephaly* refer only to the size of the cranium itself, while megalencephaly and its antonym, *micrencephaly* refer to an abnormal brain size. All of these quantitative terms denote size without regard to cause.

Major problems in differential diagnosis include how to classify the patient with a small body and an OFC that may remain within the upper border of normal, but is disproportionately large, or those huge-framed individuals who occupy the upper reaches of the normal distribution curve whose large head and brain merely reflect extremes of normal variation (these individuals have benign (asymptomatic) familial megalencephaly. When the diagnosis of megalencephaly is considered, the OFC of all available family members should be measured and any neurologic deficits that may exist should be determined. Whenever the suspicion arises of a neurologic deficit in a patient with megalencephaly, a CT or MRI scan should be ordered. If the patient has neurologic retrogression, a scan and a full workup for lysosomal enzyme defects and a metabolic type of megalencephaly may be necessary. Patients with benign familial anatomic megalencephaly have normal karyotypes.

References:
Portnoy HD, Croissant PD: Megalencephaly in infants and children: the possible role of increased dural sinus pressure. Arch Neurol 1978; 35:306–316.
Lorber J, Priestley BL: Children with large heads: a practical approach to diagnosis in 557 children, with special reference to 109 children with megalencephaly. Dev Med Child Neurol 1981; 23:494–504.
Lewis BA, et al.: Language and motor findings in benign megalencephaly. Ann Neurol 1983; 14:364 only.
Gooskens RH, et al.: Cerebrospinal fluid dynamics and cerebrospinal fluid infusion in children: clinical application of lumbar cerebrospinal fluid infusion in children with macrocephaly and normal growth rate of the head circumference. Neuropediatrics 1985; 16:121–125.
Alvarez LA, et al.: Idiopathic external hydrocephalus: natural history and relationship to benign familial macrocephaly. Pediatrics 1986; 77:901–907.
DeMyer W: Megalencephaly: types, clinical syndromes, and management. Pediatr Neurol 1986; 2:321–328.

DE007   **William DeMyer**

Megalencephaly-cranial sclerosis-osteopathia striata
  See OSTEOPATHIA STRIATA-CRANIAL SCLEROSIS-MEGALENCEPHALY
Megalencephaly-intestinal polyposis-pigmentary changes of genitali
  See OVERGROWTH, RUVALCABA-MYHRE-SMITH TYPE
Megalobarencephaly
  See MEGALENCEPHALY
Megalocephaly
  See MEGALENCEPHALY
Megalocornea
  See CORNEA, MEGALOCORNEA

MEGALOCORNEA-MENTAL RETARDATION SYNDROME　　0638

Includes:
　　Cerebral palsy, hypotonic-seizures-megalocornia
　　MMR syndrome
　　Seizures-hypotonic cerebral palsy-megalocornea-mental
　　　retardation

Excludes:　Marfan syndrome (0630)

Major Diagnostic Criteria: Megalocornea, short stature, and mental retardation.

Clinical Findings: Short stature and mental retardation of moderate-to-severe range. Hypotonic cerebral palsy consisting of delayed motor development, muscular hypotonia, and ataxia was present in most affected persons. Choreoathetotic movements were seen occasionally. Epileptic seizures occurred in most patients and EEG anomalies with generalized or focal discharges were noted. Megalocornea was present in all children, with a corneal diameter greater than 12–15 mm and accompanied by deep anterior chamber (anterior megalophthalmus), iris hypoplasia, and iridodonesis. Most patients were microcephalic from birth. Minor anomalies of the face included prominent forehead, telecanthus, epicanthus, and micrognathia.

Complications: Glaucoma, cataracts.

Associated Findings: None known.

0638-20558: Megalocornea-mental retardation syndrome; note megalocornea, prominent forehead, telecanthus, epicanthal folds and micrognathia in these affected siblings.

Etiology: Autosomal recessive inheritance.

Pathogenesis: Unknown.

MIM No.: *24931

POS No.: 3734

Sex Ratio: M1:F1

Occurrence: The syndrome has been observed in two boys and one girl of non-consanguineous parents, and in at least eight sporadic cases.

Risk of Recurrence for Patient's Sib:
　　See Part I, *Mendelian Inheritance.*

Risk of Recurrence for Patient's Child:
　　See Part I, *Mendelian Inheritance.*

Age of Detectability: Infancy or early childhood.

Gene Mapping and Linkage: Unknown.

Prevention: None known. Genetic counseling indicated.

Treatment: Early treatment of increased intraocular pressure and cataracts; physiotherapy and anticonvulsant medication.

Prognosis: Many patients are severely retarded.

Detection of Carrier: Unknown.

References:
Frank Y, et al.: Megalocornea associated with multiple skeletal anomalies-new genetic syndrome. J Genet Hum 1973; 21:67–72.

Neuhäuser G, et al.: Syndrome of mental retardation, seizures, hypotonic cerebral palsy and megalocorneae, recessively inherited. Z Kinderheilk 1975; 120:1–18.

Schmidt R, Rapin I: The syndrome of mental retardation and megalocornea. Am J Hum Genet 1981; 33:90A.

Del Giudice E, et al.; Megalocornea and mental retardation syndrome: two new cases. Am J Med Genet 1987; 26:417–420.

Gronbech-Jensen M: Megalocornea and mental retardation syndrome: a new case. Am J Med Genet 1989; 32:468–469.

NE012　　　　　　　　　　　　　　　　**Gerhard Neuhäuser**

Megathrombocytopenia
　　See LEUKOCYTE, MAY-HEGGLIN ANOMALY
Meige type lymphedema
　　See LYMPHEDEMA II
Meischer cheilitis (oligosymptomatic forms)
　　See CHEILITIS GRANULOMATOSA, MELKERSSON-ROSENTHAL
　　　TYPE
Melanesian ovalocytosis
　　See ELLIPTOCYTOSIS
Melanin formation, reduction or absence
　　See ALBINISM
Melanoblastosis cutis linearis
　　See INCONTINENTIA PIGMENTI
Melanocytic nevus, congenital
　　See NEVUS, CONGENITAL NEVOMELANOCYTIC
Melanocytic nevus, giant congenital
　　See NEVUS, CONGENITAL NEVOMELANOCYTIC
Melanocytic nevus, small congenital
　　See NEVUS, CONGENITAL NEVOMELANOCYTIC
Melanocytoma, optic disk
　　See OPTIC DISK, MELANOCYTOMA
Melanoderma, familial generalized
　　See SKIN, CUTANEOUS MELANOSIS, DIFFUSE
Melanodermic leukodystrophy
　　See ADRENOLEUKODYSTROPHY, X-LINKED
Melanoleucoderma
　　See BERLIN SYNDROME
Melanoma, benign of optic nerve head
　　See OPTIC DISK, MELANOCYTOMA
Melanophoric nevus
　　See ECTODERMAL DYSPLASIA, NAEGELI TYPE
Melanosis oculi, congenital
　　See EYE, MELANOSIS OCULI, CONGENITAL
Melanosis retinae
　　See RETINA, GROUPED HYPERTROPHY OF RETINAL PIGMENT
　　　EPITHELIUM
Melanosis retinae, congenital grouped
　　See RETINA, GROUPED HYPERTROPHY OF RETINAL PIGMENT
　　　EPITHELIUM

Melanosis, neurocutaneous
 See *NEUROCUTANEOUS MELANOSIS*
Melanosis, universal
 See *SKIN, HYPERPIGMENTATION, FAMILIAL*
Melanotic ameloblastoma
 See *JAW, NEUROECTODERMAL PIGMENTED TUMOR*
Melanotic neuroectodermal tumor of infancy
 See *JAW, NEUROECTODERMAL PIGMENTED TUMOR*
Melanotic odontoma
 See *JAW, NEUROECTODERMAL PIGMENTED TUMOR*
Melanotic progonoma
 See *JAW, NEUROECTODERMAL PIGMENTED TUMOR*
MELAS
 See *MYOPATHY, MITOCHONDRIAL-ENCEPHALOPATHY-LACTIC
 ACIDOSIS-STROKE*
Meleda disease
 See *MAL DE MELEDA*
Melkersson-Rosenthal syndrome
 See *CHEILITIS GRANULOMATOSA, MELKERSSON-ROSENTHAL
 TYPE*
Melnick-Fraser syndrome
 See *BRANCHIO-OTO-RENAL DYSPLASIA*
Melnick-Needles osteodysplasty
 See *OSTEODYSPLASTY*

MELORHEOSTOSIS   0641

Includes:
 Flowing hyperostosis
 Melorheostosis Leri
 Osteosis eburnisans monomelica

Excludes:
 Diaphyseal dysplasia (0290)
 Endosteal hyperostosis (0497)

Major Diagnostic Criteria: This rare unilateral hyperostosis causes pain and joint stiffness and is diagnosed from the typical X-ray changes resembling melting wax dripping down from the side of a candle.

Clinical Findings: This disorder is a rare form of hyperostosis, which has a linear distribution along the major axis of the long

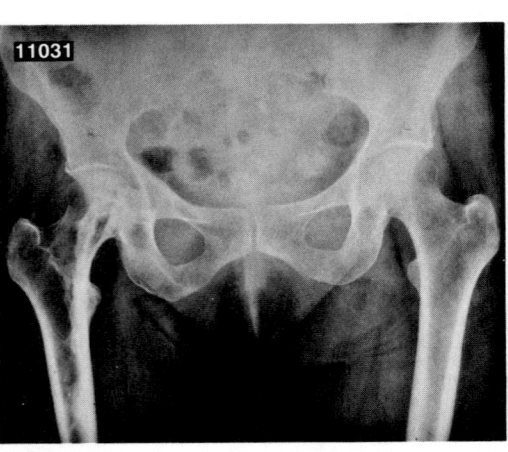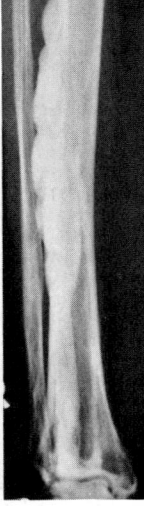

0641-11031: Longitudinal bands of increased density beginning in the femoral head. **11032:** Striking streaks of increased density in the right tibia.

bones. On X-ray, the hyperostosis resembles melting wax dripping down the side of a candle, hence the term, melorheostosis, from the Greek words *melos* (member) and *rhein* (flow). The disease is almost always unilateral in its distribution, and usually affects a single limb. It is usually first detected in childhood or young adulthood, but it has been diagnosed at birth because of deformities of the fingers. Patients usually present because of progressive pain, stiffness, and limitation of motion, or deformity such as contractures of the fingers. The pain ranges from a dull to sharp ache; it is not constant, and is often aggravated by activity. The overlying skin is often normal in appearance, but may be tense, shiny, or erythematous. Linear scleroderma has been described. The subcutaneous tissues are often indurated and edematous, and the overlying muscles may be atrophic and weak. The adjacent joints may be intermittently warm and swollen with eventual limitation of joint motion due to soft tissue fibrosis. The affected limb may be shorter or, less commonly, longer. It usually appears larger in circumference, and may be angulated or curved.

X-rays reveal the typical molten wax appearance, with streaked sclerotic thickening of the side of the long bone. This irregular linear opacity runs along the major axis of the long bone, and may extend from one bone to an adjacent bone. The limb girdle is usually involved as well. The sclerosis may extend into the epiphyseal regions as streaks, but the articular areas are usually unaffected. The hyperostosis may not be prominent in infancy or childhood, but becomes more apparent with age.

Biopsies of affected sclerotic bones have revealed irregularly arranged Haversian systems, with dense thickened trabeculae and occasional islands of cartilage. Cellular fibrotic tissue is seen in the marrow spaces. Fibrosis of the subcutaneous tissues and skeletal muscle atrophy have been described. Degenerative, inflammatory, and obliterative changes have been noted in the surrounding blood vessels.

Complications: This disorder can lead to painful limitation of motion and weakness of the affected limb, as well as fibrous contractures of the adjacent joints.

Associated Findings: Some reports have described associated disorders such as scleroderma, **Neurofibromatosis**, lymphedema, hemangioma, vascular nevus, and A-V aneurysms, and localized osteopecilia.

Etiology: Possibly autosomal dominant inheritance.

Pathogenesis: Approximation of the anatomical distribution to the sclerotomes suggests a major, if not primary, role for the sensory nerve.

MIM No.: 15595

Sex Ratio: M1:F1

Occurrence: Unknown.

Risk of Recurrence for Patient's Sib: Undetermined. All cases to date have been sporadic.

Risk of Recurrence for Patient's Child: Unknown.

Age of Detectability: From birth by medical imaging. Usually not diagnosed until late childhood or early adulthood, when a limb is X-rayed because of pain symptoms or joint immobility.

Gene Mapping and Linkage: Unknown.

Prevention: None known. Genetic counseling indicated.

Treatment: Orthopedic procedures to prevent or correct limb deformities.

Prognosis: Apparently normal for life span. The pain and disability are usually progressive.

Detection of Carrier: Unknown.

References:
Morris JM, et al.: Melorheostosis. J Bone Joint Surg [Am] 1963; 45A:1191–1206.
Patrick JH: Melorheostosis associated with arteriovenous aneurysm of the left arm and trunk. J Bone Joint Surg [Br] 1969; 51B:126–129.

Murry RO, McCredi E: Melorheosteosis and the sclerotomes: a radiological correlation. Skeletal Radiol 1979; 4:57–71.

B0025
Zvi Borochowitz
David L. Rimoin

Melorheostosis Leri
See *MELORHEOSTOSIS*
Meltzer-Franklin syndrome
See *CRYOGLOBULINEMIA*
Membranous cataract
See *CATARACT, AUTOSOMAL DOMINANT CONGENITAL*
Membranous choanal atresia, anterior
See *NOSE, ANTERIOR ATRESIA*
Membranous choanal atresia, posterior
See *NOSE, POSTERIOR ATRESIA*
Membranous conjunctivitis
See *EYE, LIGNEOUS CONJUNCTIVITIS*
Membranous lipodystrophy
See *OSTEODYSPLASIA, LIPOMEMBRANOUS POLYCYSTIC-DEMENTIA*
Membranous septal defect
See *VENTRICULAR SEPTAL DEFECT*
Membranous subaortic stenosis
See *HEART, SUBAORTIC STENOSIS, FIBROUS*
MEN II syndrome
See *ENDOCRINE NEOPLASIA, MULTIPLE TYPE II*
MEN IIa syndrome
See *ENDOCRINE NEOPLASIA, MULTIPLE TYPE II*
MEN IIb syndrome
See *ENDOCRINE NEOPLASIA, MULTIPLE TYPE III*
Mendenhall syndrome
See *LIPODYSTROPHY-COARSE FACIES-ACANTHOSIS NIGRICANS, MIESCHER TYPE*
Mendes da Costa syndrome
See *SKIN, ERYTHROKERATODERMIA, VARIABLE*
Meningeal capillary angiomatosis
See *STURGE-WEBER SYNDROME*
Meningitis-polyarthritis-lymphadenitis-pulmonary hemosiderosis
See *INFLAMMATORY DISEASE, NEONATAL BATES-LORBER TYPE*

MENINGOCELE 0642

Includes:
Cranial meningoceles
Neural-tube defect
Spina bifida cystica without neurologic deficit

Excludes:
Encephalocele (0343)
Lipomeningocele (0602)
Meningomyelocele (0693)
Myelorachischisis
Schisis association (2249)
Spina bifida occulta

Major Diagnostic Criteria: Translucent skin mass over the vertebral column or cranium, with spina bifida and widening of interpedicular distance seen on X-ray.

Clinical Findings: Most commonly seen in the lumbar area, a skin-covered mass of soft tissue occurs either over the midline of the back or slightly off to one side of the midline. Herniation of the meninges can occur over the midline of the cervical spine and cranium. In the latter location they are called cranial meningoceles. The overlying skin may have an angiomatous or hairy patch. There is no paralysis or sensory loss. The head circumference is normal; hydrocephaly rarely is associated. On X-ray, spina bifida underlies the mass.

Complications: Breakdown of the skin covering. Rarely, nerve roots are trapped in the sac, causing leg weakness.

Associated Findings: May be a component of many other syndromes.

Etiology: Polygenic.

Pathogenesis: Failure of complete midline fusion of the vertebral arches, with cystic distention of the meninges, but without neural tissue in the sac. Gardner's (1968) theory is based upon the existence of hydrocephalus and hydromyelia as a normal condition in early embryonic life: a result of fluid first secreted by the neural epithelium and then by the choroid plexus. By preventing the normal circulation of cerebrospinal fluid, the delay or failure of permeation of the roof of the fourth ventricle will produce all grades of anomalies seen in the dysraphic states. A meningocele results when the internal hydromyelia becomes external; the expanding subarachnoid space then bulges beneath cutaneous ectoderm impeding, at the same time, proper mesodermal closure.

POS No.: 3720

Sex Ratio: M1:F1

Occurrence: Estimated 1:20,000 live births.

Risk of Recurrence for Patient's Sib: Depends on ethnic group and geographic location. Can vary between 2–6%, as in other neural tube defects.

Risk of Recurrence for Patient's Child: Depends on ethnic group and geographic location. Can vary between 2–6%, as in other neural tube defects.

Age of Detectability: Prenatally in second trimester by amniography, fetoscopy and, ultrasonography, which shows a U-shaped deformity of the fetal spine, with a sonolucent area.

Gene Mapping and Linkage: Unknown.

Prevention: Mulinare et al (1988) have presented data showing that preconceptional use of multivitamins can reduced the risk of neural tube defects.

Treatment: Repair of cystic mass during first year of life.

Prognosis: Good.

Detection of Carrier: Unknown.

Support Groups:
MD; Rockville; Spina Bifida Association of America (SBAA)
CANADA: Manitoba; Winnipeg; Spina Bifida Association of Canada
SWEDEN: Stockholm; International Federation for Hydrocephalus and Spina Bifida

References:
Gardner WJ: Myelocele: rupture of the neural tube? Clin Neurosurg 1968; 15:57.
Shulman K, Shapiro K: Defects of closure of the neural plate. In: Rudolph A, ed: Pediatrics. 16th ed. New York: Appleton-Century-Crofts, 1977:1757.
Mulinare J, et al.: Periconceptional use of multivitamins and the occurrence of neural tube defects. JAMA 1988; 260:3141–3145.
Mills JL, et al.: The absence of a relationship between the periconceptional use of vitamins and neural-tube defects. New Engl J Med 1989; 321:430–435.

SH007
Kenneth Shapiro

Meningocele, anterior sacral
See *TERATOMA, PRESACRAL-SACRAL DYSGENESIS*

MENINGOCELE-CONOTRUNCAL HEART DEFECT, KOUSSEFF TYPE 2266

Includes:
Sacral meningocele-conotruncal heart defects-head/neck anomalies
Kousseff syndrome

Excludes:
Heart, transposition of great vessels (0962)
Heart, truncus arteriosus (0972)
Hydrocephaly (0481)
Meningocele (0642)
Meningomyelocele (0693)
Schisis association (2249)

Major Diagnostic Criteria: Characteristic head and neck anomalies, conotruncal heart defects, and sacral meningoceles.

Clinical Findings: Findings in four known cases included depressed nasal tip (1), retrognathia (4) short neck/excess neck skin (3), minimally low-set ears (4); conotruncal cardiac defects (3); sacral **Meningocele** / **Meningomyelocele** (4); unilateral renal agenesis (1).

Birth weight, length, and occipito-frontal circumference are all normal.

Complications: **Hydrocephaly** occurrred in three cases, seizures in one case.

Associated Findings: None known.

Etiology: The occurrence of this syndrome is sibs of each sex is strongly suggestive of autosomal recessive inheritance.

Pathogenesis: Unknown.

MIM No.: 24521

POS No.: 3172

Sex Ratio: M3:F1 (observed).

Occurrence: Undetermined. May account for as much as 1% of spina bifida cases. Four cases have been reported.

Risk of Recurrence for Patient's Sib:
See Part I, *Mendelian Inheritance.*

Risk of Recurrence for Patient's Child:
See Part I, *Mendelian Inheritance.*

Age of Detectability: At birth by physical examination. In the one case in which prenatal diagnosis was attempted, serum alpha feto-protein levels were normal; amniotic alpha feto-protein levels were slightly elevated. An increased number of rapidly adhering cells were also observed from the amniotic sample. Ultrasound at 15, 17, and 22 weeks did not detect any defects (although this infant was subsequently found to be affected).

Gene Mapping and Linkage: Unknown.

Prevention: None known. Genetic counseling indicated.

Treatment: When indicated, surgical repair of the cardiac and sacral defects; shunting for the **Hydrocephaly**.

Prognosis: Unknown.

Detection of Carrier: Unknown.

Support Groups:
MD; Rockville; Spina Bifida Association of America (SBAA)
CANADA: Manitoba; Winnipeg; Spina Bifida Association of Canada
SWEDEN: Stockholm; International Federation for Hydrocephalus and Spina Bifida

References:
Kousseff BG: Sacral meningocele with conotruncal heart defects: a possible autosomal recessive trait. Pediatrics 1984; 74:395–398. *
Toriello HV, et al.: Autosomal recessive syndrome of sacral and contruncal developmental field defects (Kousseff syndrome). Am J Med Genet. 1985; 22:357–360. †

T0007   **Helga V. Toriello**

MENINGOMYELOCELE   0693

Includes:
Myelomeningocele
Myeloschisis
Neural-tube defect
Spina bifida cystica with paralysis
Valproic acid, fetal effects

Excludes:
Hydrocephaly (0481)
Lipomeningocele (0602)
Meningocele (0642)

Major Diagnostic Criteria: Midline spinal defect with neurologic deficit.

Clinical Findings: A visible sac or epithelial defect over the spine, caudal to the level of the lesion in which nerve tissue can be seen,

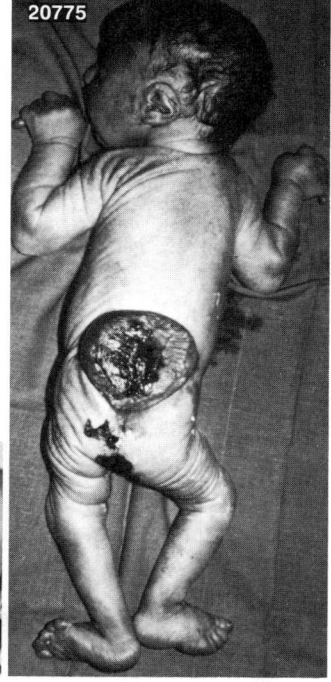

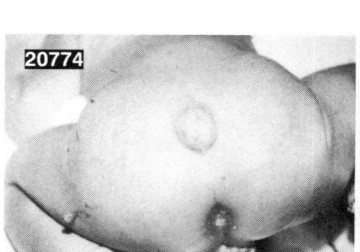

0693-20774: Meningomyelocele, small lumbar-sacral meningomyelocele. **20775:** Lumbar meningomyelocele.

---

and associated with neurologic deficit. The surface lesion varies from one that is almost completely skin covered to a fully exposed lower spinal cord and cauda equina. In myeloschisis, the paravertebral muscle mass is also exposed. Neurologic loss is generally of the lower motor neuron type, with absent reflexes and segmental sensory loss. However, spotty sensory deficit may be seen. Bowel and bladder sphincter loss is usual. Myelomeningocele occurs most frequently in the lumbosacral area followed by the cervical area. An enlarged head indicating hydrocephaly associated with the Arnold-Chiari malformation is often found.

Complications: *Nervous system*: Hydrocephalus is present in about 90% of patients secondary to the **Brain, Arnold-Chiari malformation**. Lower cranial nerve abnormalities and long tract signs also may complicate the Arnold-Chiari malformation. Mental retardation is noted in about 10% of children.

Urologic: Neurogenic bladder may be complicated by recurrent urinary tract infection or hydronephrosis. Urinary incontinence is usually found.

Orthopedic: Foot, knee, and/or hip deformities may be found, depending upon the level of the spinal cord defect. Scoliosis develops frequently.

Associated Findings: Structural GU anomalies and, less frequently, cardiac, craniofacial, and limb anomalies.

Etiology: Multifactorial. Nutritional factors may play a role. Some children with **Chromosome 18, trisomy 18** have neural tube defects. Recent data suggest maternal exposure to valproic acid may cause this defect (see **Fetal valproate syndrome**).

Pathogenesis: Failure of neural tube closure at four weeks gestation or later. Cleft formation and cord splitting due to central cord distention with overgrowth of neural elements.

POS No.: 3720

CDC No.: 741

Sex Ratio: M1:F>1. Slightly more common in females.

Occurrence: 1:500 to 1:2,000 live births. Spina bifida occured in 4.3:10,000 live births in the United States in 1987. There is wide geographic and ethnic variation, and "epidemics" have been well documented. The condition is associated with low socioeconomic status; the rate in Appalachia is more than twice the United States national average, and the rate in rural China is about nine times that in the United States.

Risk of Recurrence for Patient's Sib: 2–5% depending on family history, ethnic group, and geographic location.

Risk of Recurrence for Patient's Child: 2–5% depending on family history, ethnic group, and geographic location.

Age of Detectability: Prenatally in second trimester by amniography, fetoscopy, and ultrasonography; which show a U-shaped deformity of fetal spine with a sonolucent area. In the amniotic fluid, there are elevated levels of alpha-fetoprotein (AFP), and acetylcholinesterase, as well as other substances. AFP is elevated in maternal serum.

Gene Mapping and Linkage: Unknown.

Prevention: Recent research suggests a possible relationship between maternal nutrition or vitamin deficiency and neural tube defects (Mulinare et al, 1988).

Treatment: Repair of open defects to prevent meningitis and loss of neural function. Treatment of hydrocephaly. Treatment of urologic, orthopedic, and CNS complications.

Prognosis: Good in patients with minimal neurologic defects without hydrocephaly. Prognosis in others varies with extent of lesion and presence of complications. The number of children surviving with spina bifida is increasing. Of about 13,600 American children born with the condition between 1980 and 1987, an estimated 9,800 were alive in 1987.

Detection of Carrier: Unknown.

Support Groups:
MD; Rockville; Spina Bifida Association of America (SBAA)
CANADA: Manitoba; Winnipeg; Spina Bifida Association of Canada
SWEDEN: Stockholm; International Federation for Hydrocephalus and Spina Bifida

References:
Holmes LB, et al.: Etiologic heterogenicity of neural tube defects. New Engl J Med 1976; 294:365.
Black PM: Selective treatment of infants with myelomeningocele. Neurosurgery 1979; 5:334.
Colgan MT: The child with spina bifida. Am J Dis Child 1981; 135:854.
Toriello HV, Higgins JV: Occurrence of neural tube defects among first-, second-, and third-degree relatives of probands: results of a United States study. Am J Med Genet 1983; 15:601.
Mulinare J, et al.: Periconceptional use of multivitamins and the occurrence of neural tube defects. JAMA 1988; 260:3141–3145.
Mills JL, et al.: The absence of a relationship between the preconceptional use of vitamins and neural-tube defects. New Engl J Med 1989; 321; 430–435.
Milunsky A, et al.: Multi-vitamin/folic acid supplementation in early pregnancy reduces the prevalence of neural tube defects. J Am Med Asso 1989; 262:2847–2852.

SH007
BA039

Kenneth Shapiro
Louis E. Bartoshesky

MENKES SYNDROME 0643

Includes:
Copper transport disease
Kinky hair disease
Sex-linked neurodegenerative disease associated with monilethrix
Steely hair disease
Trichopoliodystrophy
X-linked copper malabsorption

Excludes:
Aciduria, argininosuccinic (0087)

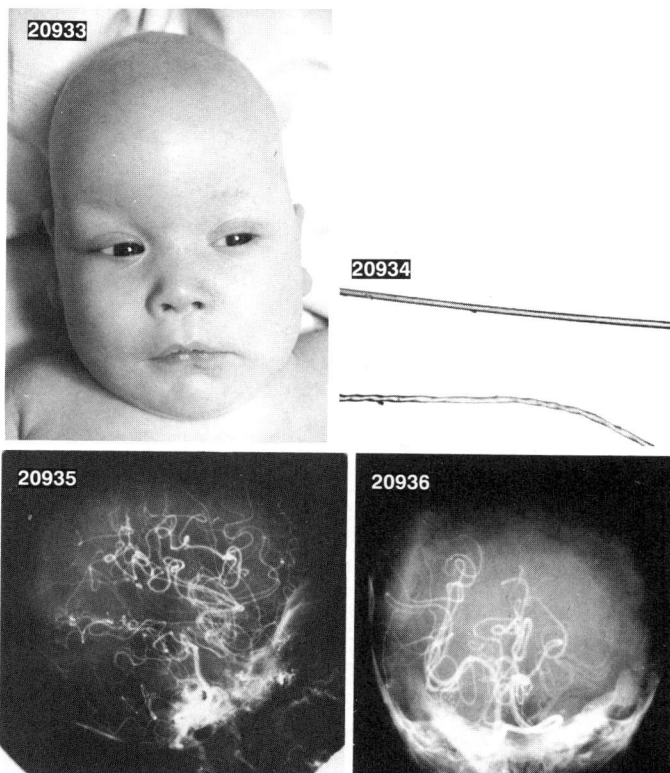

0643A-20933: Menkes syndrome; note the cherubic appearance of the face and the sparse, brittle scalp hair and lashes. 20934: Spiral, twisted microscopic appearance of the scalp hair (lower) from the child shown in 20933 compared with a straight, normal hair (upper). 20935: Lateral view of cerebral arteriogram showing tortuous, winding vessels. 20936: Vertebral cerebral arteriogram shows tortuous vessels.

Biotinidase deficiency (2591)
Nutritional copper deficiency

Major Diagnostic Criteria: Male sex, abnormal hair, seizures, developmental retardation, low serum copper and ceruloplasmin, abnormalities as they appear on X-rays and EEG.

The relatively unique clinical feature of Menkes syndrome is the coarse, colorless, sparse, friable secondary scalp hair, with variable microscopic abnormalities, of which pili torti (twisting of the shaft) is most common, but also including monilethrix (variations in diameter) or trichorrhexis nodosa (fragmentation).

Seizures are the most common initial symptom and have a peak incidence at age 3 months. After age five months the EEG pattern often resembles hypsarrhythmia. The typical facial appearance has been described as cherubic with pudgy cheeks, irregular eyebrows, micrognathia, and expressionless facies. The course is progressively fatal and is characterized by developmental failure or regression. Bone changes may lead to the misdiagnosis of child abuse.

Average birth weight is 2,660 grams. Neuropathological findings consist of widespread cortical neuronal loss, demyelination and gliosis of the white matter, and profound reduction of all elements of the cerebellum.

Clinical Findings: Percentages calculated from review by French (1977), N=37.
Clinical findings: Progressively fatal course (100%); male sex [X-linked inheritance] (100%); seizures (95%); abnormal secondary hair (94%); developmental regression or failure after earlier devel-

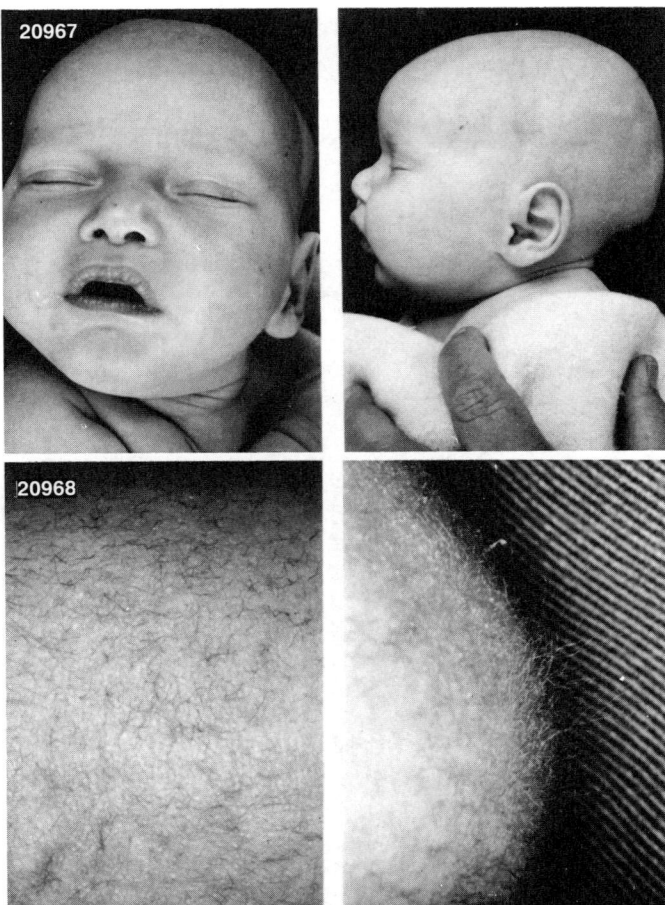

0643B-20967: Menkes syndrome; note sparse, fine, brittle hair and decreased eyebrows and eyelashes. **20968:** Close-up of sparse, brittle, wiry hair which is depigmented and lacks lustre. The short stubbles of broken hair are characteristic.

opmental progress (81%); abnormal muscle tone [hyperreflexia and spasticity most common - 38%] (68%); prematurity [gestational age 34–37 weeks] (55%); terminal or intermittent respiratory infections (49%); micrognathia (46%); thermal instability [intermittent or persistent] (43%); oral abnormalities [high-arched palate, failure or delay of tooth eruption] (32%); microcephaly [less than second percentile] (32%); abnormal neonatal adaptation [depressed Apgar, meconium staining, lethargy, respiratory problems, feeding problems, thermal instability] (30%); weight less than third percentile (30%); variable congenital malformations [pectus excavatum, talipes, hernias, undescended testes, etc.] (30%); intracranial subdural fluid collections and/or membranes (22%); neonatal icterus (19%); gastrointestinal symptoms [emesis, gastroenteritis, feeding difficulty] (19%); abnormal skull or facial shape [asymmetry, bossing, etc.] (16%); neuro-ophthalmic deficits [disc pallor; dysplastic optic disks; horizontal nystagmus; episodic, rapid, vertical eye movements; nystagmoid eye movements] (16%); survival past age two years (12%); neonatal-onset developmental failure (11%); and growth failure (common but percentage undetermined).

Other findings: Low serum copper (100%); low serum ceruloplasmin (97%); abnormal EEG at some time during life (97%); tortuous, abnormal cerebral arteries [based on 6 of 7 cases with cerebral angiograms] (86%); metaphyseal spurring or fractures [with or without periosteal thickening or new bone formation (19/24)] (80%); long bone metaphyseal cupping or anterior rib end flaring [based on 20 of 27 patients X-rayed] (80%). Additional findings for which percentages are unknown include abnormal visual evoked responses; abnormal electroretinogram; tortuous systemic arteries; anemia, usually hypochromic; wormian bones; bladder diverticuli; hydroureters, and ureteric reflux.

Complications: Developmental failure or regression, death.

Associated Findings: Seborrheic dermatitis (16%), simian creases (15%), pyogenic leptomeningitis (8%), macrocephaly, neonatal occurrence of "kinky hair" (one reported case) or "steely, depigmented hair" (2 cases), early infancy vascular collapse (one reported case).

Etiology: X-linked inheritance of copper malabsorption.

Pathogenesis: Evidence suggests that the basic defect in Menkes syndrome is a selective defect in tissue uptake or retention of copper, or abnormal copper transport. This concept is supported by an incomplete gastrointestinal absorption defect (10–25% of normal) when patients are given oral ^{67}Cu, while duodenal biopsies have shown increased copper concentration. Intravenous copper therapy can normalize serum copper levels but not brain copper levels. In spite of hypocupremia in untreated patients, erythrocyte copper concentration is normal. This is in contrast to normal children with nutritional copper deficiency in whom erythrocyte copper is depleted. The findings of characteristic hair abnormalities, elevated blood copper and ceruloplasmin, decreased hepatic copper levels, and increased urinary copper excretion in two newborns with Menkes syndrome who subsequently had a decrease in blood copper levels is further evidence for the presence of adequate transplacental copper transport combined with in utero selective deficits of copper transport, or tissue uptake or retention. These selective defects may account for the failure of simple parenteral copper therapy.

Most of the clinical and laboratory deficits are postulated to be caused by dysfunction of the numerous copper-dependent enzyme systems. These enzyme systems are involved in connective tissue synthesis and cross linkage (lysyoxidase), melanin synthesis (tyrosinase), catabolism of superoxide (superoxide dismutase), neurotransmitter synthesis (dopamine-β-hydroxylase), nicotinic acid synthesis (hepatic tryptophan pyrollase), and mitochondrial function (cytochrome c oxidase). Hypoceruloplasminemia may lead to deficient ferroxidase activity and may disrupt ascorbic acid oxidation.

MIM No.: *30940

POS No.: 3290

CDC No.: 759.870

Sex Ratio: M1:F0

Occurrence: Incidence in Australia 29:1,000,000. Less than 40 cases documented in the literature.

Risk of Recurrence for Patient's Sib:
See Part I, *Mendelian Inheritance*.

Risk of Recurrence for Patient's Child:
See Part I, *Mendelian Inheritance*. Affected individuals are not expected to survive to reproduce.

Age of Detectability: Prenatally by amniotic fibroblast copper incorporation studies, or at birth by finding elevated serum copper and ceruloplasmin, decreased hepatic copper levels, increased urinary copper excretion.

Gene Mapping and Linkage: MNK (Menkes syndrome) has been mapped to Xcen-q13.

Prevention: None known. Genetic counseling indicated.

Treatment: Administration of parenteral copper or oral copper chelated to trisodium nitrilotriacetate or histidine has resulted in increased ceruloplasmin levels and normal blood and liver copper levels, but the copper level in the brain has remained low. There is currently no effective treatment; however, copper therapy may improve seizure control (Grover et al, 1982). To be successful, initiation of therapy in utero may be required. Treatment of complications includes anticonvulsants for seizures, drainage for subdural fluid collections, antibiotics for meningitis, and iron for iron-deficiency anemia.

Prognosis: Death usually occurs within two years and is commonly associated with pneumonia.

Detection of Carrier: Mothers or sisters of some boys with Menkes syndrome have had microscopic hair abnormalities. Scanning electron microscopy of the hair may aid carrier identification. If hair abnormalities are not present, there is no reliable method of carrier detection. The sister of a Black American boy had mottled skin. Fibroblast copper concentration has been elevated in all tested children with Menkes syndrome. Fibroblast copper concentration was elevated in one of two possible maternal heterozygotes; however, in another study, two presumed heterozygote mothers had copper concentration values indistinguishable from controls.

Special Considerations: The concept of allelic variation with differing manifestations or genetic heterogeneity is supported by cases of Menkes disease with a milder course (Procopis et al, 1981).

A disorder of copper metabolism with X-linked inheritance was studied by Haas et al (1981) in two brothers. The boys were thought to have a disorder distinct from Menkes syndrome because of several features unlike the typical Menkes profile; i.e., prolonged survival, hypotonia, choreoathetosis, and the absence of hair, skin, facial, or bony changes. However, the possibility that these cases represent an allelic variant of Menkes is strengthened by several factors: hair changes become less prominent with age in untreated Menkes syndrome; hair abnormalities (pili torti) present by scanning electron microscope may not be discernible by light microscope (Taylor and Green, 1981); cases occur with hypotonia (Grover et al, 1979); and finally, the presence of choreoathetosis in the patients of Haas et al may be due to their long survival (choreoathetosis in their patients was not commented on until the ages of two and nine years). DNA linkage studies may clarify these issues.

Support Groups: VA; Dumfries; Wilson's Disease Association

References:

Danks DM, et al.: Menkes' kinky hair syndrome; an inherited defect in copper absorption with widespread effects. Pediatrics 1972; 50:188–201.

Horn N: Copper incorporation studies on cultured cells for prenatal diagnosis of Menkes' disease. Lancet 1976; I:1156–1158.

French JH: X-chromosome-linked copper malabsorption. In: Vinken PJ, Bruyn GW, eds: Handbook of clinical neurology. vol. 29. Amsterdam: North Holland Publishing, 1977:279–309.

Grover WD, et al.: Clinical and biochemical aspects of tricho-poliodystrophy. Ann Neurol 1979; 5:65–71.

Haas RH, et al.: An X-linked disease of the nervous system with disordered copper metabolism and features differing from Menkes disease. Neurology 1981; 31:852–859.

Procopis P, et al.: A mild form of Menkes steely hair syndrome. J Pediatr 1981; 98:97–99.

Taylor CJ, Green SH: Menkes's syndrome (trichopoliodystrophy): use of a scanning electron microscope in diagnosis and carrier identification. Develop Med Child Neurol 1981; 23:361–368.

Grover WD, et al.: A defect in catecholamine metabolism in kinky-hair disease. Ann Neurol 1982; 12:263–266.

Kuivaniemi H, et al.: Type IX Ehlers-Danlos syndrome and Menkes syndrome: the decrease in lysyl oxidase activity is associated with a corresponding deficiency in the enzyme protein. Am J Hum Genet 1985; 37:798–808.

Leone A, et al.: Menkes' disease: abnormal metallothionein gene regulation in response to copper. Cell 1985; 40:301–309.

Moore CM, Howell RR: Ectodermal manifestations in Menkes disease. Clin Genet 1985; 28:532–540.

Tonnesen T, et al.: Measurement of copper in chorionic villi for first trimester diagnosis of Menkes disease (letter) Lancet 1985; I:1038–1039.

Beighton P, et al.: International nosology of heritable disorders of connective tissue, Berlin, 1986. Am J Med Genet 1988; 29:581–594.

Danks DM: The mild form of Menkes disease: progress report on the original case. Am J Med Genet 1988; 30:859–864.

KA008
DS000

Raymond S. Kandt
Bernard D'Souza

MENTAL RETARDATION, HEMOGLOBIN H RELATED   3103

Includes:

Chromosome 16, interstitial deletions at alpha-globin loci
Hemoglobin H disease-mental retardation-multiple anomalies

Excludes:

Alpha-thalassemia, silent carrier and trait forms of Hemoglobin H disease without mental retardation

Major Diagnostic Criteria: Developmental delay and hemoglobin H disease with or without congenital anomalies.

Clinical Findings: The mental retardation is moderate to severe, with reported IQ scores ranging from 76 to <50. Congenital anomalies and features reported in over one-half of cases include hypotonia, **Microcephaly**, telecanthus, onset of seizures in childhood, foot deformity, and cryptorchidism. One child also had **Hypospadias** and **Ductus arteriosus, patent**. In the one reported female patient, no associated congenital anomalies were noted.

In all reported cases studied by DNA analysis, one parent had a normal alpha-globin genotype ($\alpha\alpha/\alpha\alpha$) while the other was heterozygous for alpha-thalassemia 2 ($\llcorner\alpha/\alpha\alpha$). This is different from the usual form of hemoglobin H disease in which offspring result from matings between alpha-thal 2 and alpha-thal 1 heterozygotes ($[\llcorner\alpha/\alpha\alpha]$ X $[\llcorner\!\!\llcorner/\alpha\alpha]$). All karyotypes performed were normal.

Complications: Unknown.

Associated Findings: None known.

Etiology: Hemoglobin H-related mental retardation appears to be a sporadic event arising from matings between an alpha-thalassemic and a non-alpha-thalassemic parent. Thus, it may result from *de novo* interstitial deletions of portions of chromosome 16 contiguous to and including the alpha-globin loci.

Pathogenesis: The effect of this hypothesized acquired abnormality of chromosome 16 is unclear. It has been proposed that this disorder may result from intrauterine anoxia secondary to deficient alpha-globin synthesis in the fetus, but this seems unlikely since the association is not reported in the Oriental and Mediterranean populations where familial hemoglobin H disease is relatively more common.

MIM No.: 14175

Sex Ratio: M4:F1 (observed).

Occurrence: Hemoglobin H-related mental retardation has been reported in four unrelated male children and one female child of Northern European origin. Hemoglobin H disease is a form of alpha-thalassemia that usually occurs in persons of Oriental or Mediterranean origin and only rarely in Northern Europeans. As a rule, affected individuals are the offspring of matings between alpha-thal 2 and alpha-thal 1 heterozygotes ($[\llcorner\alpha/\alpha\alpha]$ X $[\llcorner\!\!\llcorner/\alpha\alpha]$). Patients with hemoglobin H and mental retardation are unusual, not only for their Northern European background but also because each had one parent without alpha-thalassemia. Restriction endonuclease mapping demonstrated one child to be ($\llcorner\!\!\llcorner/\alpha$) from a de novo cis deletion on the paternally derived chromosome 16 paired with the single alpha-globin gene inherited from the mother. While this child had the genotype typically seen in Oriental and Mediterranean populations affected with hemoglobin H disease, two other patients evaluated by restriction endonuclease mapping showed no deletion in either the affected children or the parents, indicating they had nondeletion forms of the disease ($\alpha\alpha^T/\alpha^T\alpha^T$). In these three patients a spontaneous mutation or unequal crossing-over event affecting alpha-globin gene expression is implied since at least one parent does not have alpha-thalassemia. The effects of these mutations on contiguous gene(s) may cause the associated mental retardation and congenital anomalies.

Risk of Recurrence for Patient's Sib: Unknown. *De novo* deletions implied.

Risk of Recurrence for Patient's Child: Unknown. *De novo* deletions implied.

Age of Detectability: During infancy.

Gene Mapping and Linkage: Presumably the affected gene(s) are contiguous with the alpha-globin loci on chromosome 16.

Prevention: None known. Genetic counseling indicated.

Treatment: Management of clinical symptoms as indicated.

Prognosis: All affected individuals have had moderate-to-severe mental retardation. Life span is undetermined.

Detection of Carrier: Unknown.

References:
Ronisch P, Kleihauer E: Alpha-thalassamie mit HbH und Hb Bart's in einer deutschen familie. Klin Wochenschr 1967; 45:1193–1200.

Borochovitz D, et al.: Hemoglobin-H disease in association with multiple congenital abnormalities. Clin Pediatr 1970; 9:432–435.

Phillips JA III, et al.: Unequal crossing-over: a common basis of single alpha-globin genes in Asians and American blacks with hemoglobin-H disease. Blood 1980; 55:1066–1069.

Weatherall DJ, et al.: Hemoglobin H disease and mental retardation: a new syndrome or a remarkable coincidence? New Engl J Med 1981; 305:607–612. †

Schmickel RD: Contiguous gene syndromes: a component of recognizable syndromes. J Pediat 1986; 109:231–241.

ST056
PH003

Stephen M. Strakowski
John A. Phillips, III

Mental retardation, Smith-Fineman-Myers type
See SMITH-FINEMAN-MYERS SYNDROME
Mental retardation, X-linked-marXq28
See X-LINKED MENTAL RETARDATION, FRAGILE X SYNDROME
Mental retardation-alopecia
See ALOPECIA-MENTAL RETARDATION
Mental retardation-alopecia-skeletal anomalies-short stature
See ALOPECIA-SKELETAL ANOMALIES-SHORT STATURE-MENTAL RETARDATION
Mental retardation-aplasia-shuffling gait-adducted thumbs (MASA)
See X-LINKED MENTAL RETARDATION-CLASPED THUMB
Mental retardation-ears (malformed)-deafness
See DEAFNESS-MALFORMED EARS-MENTAL RETARDATION
Mental retardation-growth/hearing/genetal defects, X-linked
See X-LINKED MENTAL RETARDATION-GROWTH-HEARING AND GENITAL DEFECTS

MENTAL RETARDATION-HEART DEFECTS-BLEPHAROPHIMOSIS 3132

Includes:
Blepharophimosis-blepharoptosis-heart defects-mental retardation
Heart defects-blepharophimosis-mental retardation
Ohdo-Madokoro-Hayakawa syndrome

Excludes:
Blepharoptosis-blepharophimosis-epicanthus inversus-telecanthus (2103)
Marden-Walker syndrome (0629)
Mutchinick syndrome (3274)

Major Diagnostic Criteria: The combination of blepharophimosis, ptosis, hypoplastic teeth, cardiac defect, and mental retardation.

Clinical Findings: In the three reported girls, blepharophimosis and ptosis were present at birth. One girl had an **Atrial septal** defect, and another had a **Ventricular septal defect** (in neither case was the diagnosis made at birth). Other anomalies also became apparent with age, including small, conical teeth; amblyopia; and mental retardation.

Complications: Unknown.

Associated Findings: Microphthalmia (1/3); narrow ear canals (1/3); and mild short stature (2/3).

Etiology: Possibly autosomal recessive or autosomal dominant inheritance with reduced penetrance, or a small chromosome rearrangement.

Pathogenesis: Unknown.

MIM No.: 24962

POS No.: 3875

Sex Ratio: M0:F3 (observed).

Occurrence: One family from Japan with two female sibs and an affected cousin has been documented.

Risk of Recurrence for Patient's Sib: Unknown. May be as high as 50%.

Risk of Recurrence for Patient's Child: Unknown. May be as high as 50%.

Age of Detectability: At birth, by the presence of blepharophimosis and ptosis.

Gene Mapping and Linkage: Unknown.

Prevention: None known. Genetic counseling indicated.

Treatment: Cosmetic surgery for the blepharophimosis and ptosis; corrective lens for amblyopia.

Prognosis: Mental retardation is severe, with IQs of 37–42 in the three reported girls. Life span is undetermined, although unlikely to be impaired to a significant degree.

Detection of Carrier: Unknown.

References:
Ohdo S, et al.: Mental retardation associated with congenital heart disease, blepharoptosis, and hypoplastic teeth. J Med Genet 1986; 23:242–244.

T0007

Helga V. Toriello

Mental retardation-limb deficiency
See LIMB REDUCTION-MENTAL RETARDATION
Mental retardation-osteodystrophy, Ruvalcaba type
See OSTEODYSTROPHY-MENTAL RETARDATION, RUVALCABA TYPE
Mental retardation-retinopathy-microcephaly
See RETINOPATHY-MICROCEPHALY-MENTAL RETARDATION
Mental retardation-seizures-adenoma sebaceum
See TUBEROUS SCLEROSIS
Mental retardation-sexual maturity (delayed)-short stature
See SHORT STATURE-MENTAL RETARDATION-DELAYED SEXUAL MATURITY
Mental retardation-spondyloepiphyseal dysplasia
See SPONDYLOEPIPHYSEAL DYSPLASIA-MENTAL RETARDATION
Mental retardation-unusual facies-intrauterine growth retardation
See DWARFISM-DYSMORPHIC FACIES-RETARDATION, PITT TYPE
Mental retardation-xeroderma pigmentosum
See XERODERMA PIGMENTOSUM-MENTAL RETARDATION
Mephenytoin, fetal effects of
See FETAL HYDANTOIN SYNDROME
Meretoja-type amyloidosis
See AMYLOIDOSIS, FINNISH TYPE
MERRF
See MYOCLONIC EPILEPSY-RAGGED RED FIBERS
Merten-Singleton syndrome
See SINGLETON-MERTEN SYNDROME
Mesangial sclerosis, diffuse renal-ocular abnormalities
See RENAL MESANGIAL SCLEROSIS-EYE DEFECTS
Mesantoin^, fetal effects of
See FETAL HYDANTOIN SYNDROME
Mesenchymal dysplasie of Puretic
See FIBROMATOSIS, JUVENILE HYALINE
Mesenchymal hamartoma of liver
See LIVER, HAMARTOMA

MESENTERIC CYSTS 0645

Includes:
    Cystic hygroma of mesentery
    Lymphangioma of mesentery
    Lymphatic cyst of mesentery

Excludes: Intestinal duplication (0532)

Major Diagnostic Criteria: A cystic mass in the mesentery, which does not share a wall with the intestine, has no muscular lining of its wall, and has an alkaline content.

Clinical Findings: Presenting complaints may include an abdominal mass, pain, partial or complete intestinal obstruction, or fever of unknown etiology. They may appear alone or in combination.

Complications: Infection, rupture, intestinal obstruction.

Associated Findings: None known.

Etiology: Unknown.

Pathogenesis: Anomaly of the lymphatic tissue in the mesentery, with obstructed lymphatics and cyst formation.

Sex Ratio: M1:F1

Occurrence: 8:820,000 admissions at Mayo Clinic; 3:12,425 admissions at Children's Hospital, Los Angeles.

Risk of Recurrence for Patient's Sib: Unknown.

Risk of Recurrence for Patient's Child: Unknown.

Age of Detectability: Any age; 25% occur in first decade.

Gene Mapping and Linkage: Unknown.

Prevention: None known.

Treatment: Resection of the cyst from the mesentery, with or without adjacent bowel, depending on the blood supply to the cyst. Marsupialization of cyst generally results in recurrence or ascites.

Prognosis: Excellent for complete recovery with resection.

Detection of Carrier: Unknown.

References:
Colodny AH: Mesenteric and omental cysts. In: Welch KJ, et al, eds: Pediatric surgery, 4th ed, vol 2. Chicago: Year Book Medical Publishers, 1986:921–925.

SE006   **John H. Seashore**

MESOMELIC DYSPLASIA, LANGER TYPE 0646

Includes:
    Homozygous dyschondrosteosis
    Langer type mesomelic dwarfism
    Mesomelic dwarfism, hypoplastic ulna, fibula, and
        mandible type
Excludes:
    Acrodysostosis (0016)
    Acromesomelic dysplasias
    Chondroectodermal dysplasia (0156)
    Dyschondrosteosis (0308)
    Mesomelic dysplasia (other)
    Robinow syndrome (0876)

Major Diagnostic Criteria: Severe dwarfism, with shortening maximal in the radius and tibia, both of which are curved, and aplasia or severe hypoplasia of the ulna and fibula.

Clinical Findings: Disproportionate dwarfism with shortening of the forearms and lower legs is characteristic. Adult height seldom exceeds 130 cm. Movement at the elbows is restricted in extension, as is pronation and supination of the forearms. Increase in lumbar lordosis is present, and the mandible is variably hypoplastic. The hands and feet are displaced laterally, and mild brachydactyly may be a feature. By X-ray, severe hypoplasia or aplasia of the ulna and fibula is present with bowing. The radius is short, thick, and laterally curved, while the tibia is usually straight but foreshortened. Apart from the lumbar lordosis, the remainder of the skeleton is normal.

Complications: Unknown.

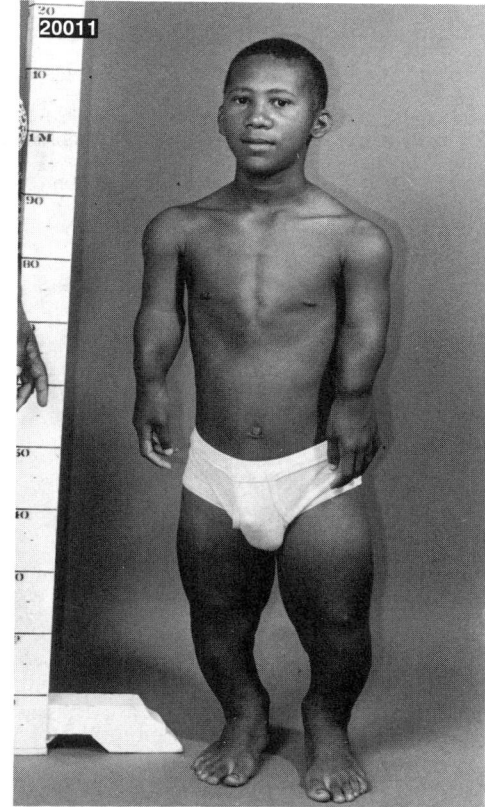

0646-20011: Note 16-year-old male with disproportionate short stature and short limbs with marked shortening of the middle segment of the limbs.

Associated Findings: None known.

Etiology: Presumably autosomal recessive inheritance. The homozygous state is expressed as mesomelic dysplasia, and the heterozygote state manifests as **Dyschondrosteosis**.

Pathogenesis: Unknown.

MIM No.: 24970

POS No.: 3292

Sex Ratio: M1:F1

Occurrence: About ten kindreds have been documented.

Risk of Recurrence for Patient's Sib:
See Part I, *Mendelian Inheritance.* Fifty percent for **Dyschondrosteosis**.

Risk of Recurrence for Patient's Child:
See Part I, *Mendelian Inheritance.* One-hundred percent for dyschondrosteosis.

Age of Detectability: At birth. Ultrasonographic prenatal detection may be possible.

Gene Mapping and Linkage: Unknown.

Prevention: None known. Genetic counseling indicated.

Treatment: Orthopedic procedures and physiotherapy can relieve the ulnar deviation of the hands.

Prognosis: Normal intelligence and life span.

Detection of Carrier: Clinical and X-ray examination of the forearms will enable detection of **Dyschondrosteosis** and is recommended for the spouse of a patient with this condition.

Special Considerations: Evidence for **Dyschondrosteosis** representing the heterozygous state of this condition has been forthcoming from several sources (see Fryns and van der Bergh, 1979; Goldblatt et al, 1987). It is possible that the mandibular manifestation is a syndromic component of Langer mesomelic dysplasia.

References:
Langer LO: Mesomelic dwarfism of the hypoplastic ulna, fibula, mandible type. Radiology 1967; 89:654–660.
Kaitila II, et al.: Mesomelic skeletal dysplasias. Clin Orthop 1976; 114:94–103. *
Fryns JP, van der Berghe H: Langer type of mesomelic dwarfism as the possible homozygous expression of dyschondrosteosis. Hum Genet 1979; 46:21–27.
Goldblatt J, et al.: Heterozygous manifestations of Langer mesomelic dysplasia. Clin Genet 1987; 31:19–24. †
Evans MI, et al.: Prenatal diagnosis and fetal pathology of Langer mesomelic dwarfism. Am J Med Genet 1988; 31:915–920.

VI005   **Denis L. Viljöen**

MESOMELIC DYSPLASIA, NIEVERGELT TYPE   0647

Includes: Nievergelt syndrome

Excludes:
 Acrodysostosis (0016)
 Acromesomelic dysplasia
 Chondroectodermal dysplasia (0156)
 Dyschondrosteosis (0308)
 Mesomelic dysplasia
 Robinow syndrome (0876)

Major Diagnostic Criteria: Mesomelic shortening of the limbs, with a rhomboid appearance of the tibia and fibula on X-ray.
 Restricted mobility of the elbows due to radioulnar luxation or subluxation of the redial head.

Clinical Findings: Moderate to severe disproportionate dwarfism occurs in which there exists specific deformities of the radius, ulna, tibia and fibula. Physical examination reveals bony protuberances with cutaneous dimples present at both medial and lateral aspects of the lower legs. Moderate valgus deformity is present at the knees. Atypical club feet with prominent equinovarus deformity may be present. Extension at the elbows and supination of the forearms are moderately limited, and the hands

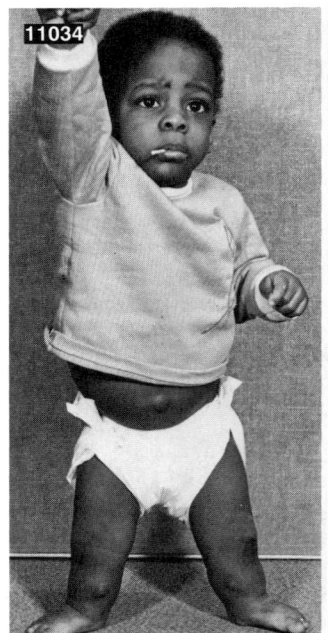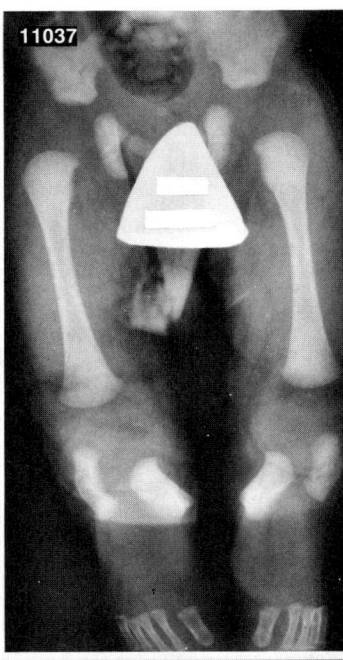
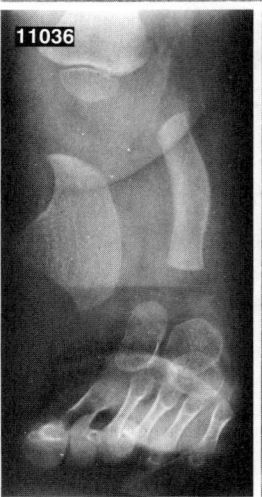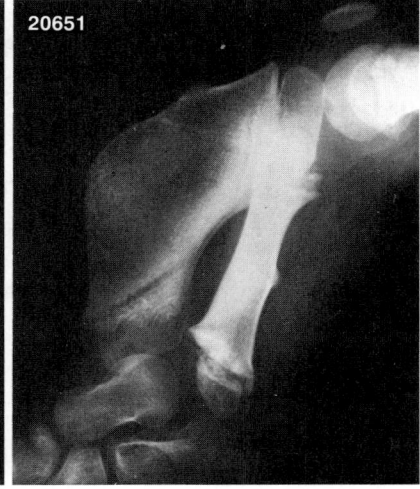

0647-11034: Note bilateral medial protuberances of the underlying tibial apices at age 2 years. **11037:** X-ray of pelvis and lower limbs in neonatal period; note normal variant "strip defect" in pubic rami and lack of ossification of talis and calcanei. **11036:** Tibial profile at 2 years; note the triangular configuration and vertically oriented "post-growth arrest" type lines suggesting sidewards growth. **20651:** Short tibia and fibula and triangular configuration of the tibia in a 7-year-old.

---

deviate medially at the wrists. Adult height is reported to be 135–147 cm and intelligence is normal.
 X-ray findings are very specific. The middle segment bones, especially the tibia and fibula, are rhomboid in appearance. The proximal head of the radius and often the ulna are dislocated and may be synostotic. Metatarsal synostosis is common. The growth plates of the tibia and fibula are severely slanted. There is considerable clinical variability.

Complications: Walking is delayed.

Associated Findings: None known.

Etiology: Autosomal dominant inheritance with variable expressivity. Sporadic cases have been reported.

Pathogenesis: The severely disturbed development of the tubular bones, with anomalous slanting of the growth plates in the middle segment of the limbs, results in marked growth retardation and deformity of the bones.

MIM No.: *16340

POS No.: 3293

Sex Ratio: M1:F1

Occurrence: Several kindreds, as well as sporadic cases, have been reported.

Risk of Recurrence for Patient's Sib:
See Part I, *Mendelian Inheritance.*

Risk of Recurrence for Patient's Child:
See Part I, *Mendelian Inheritance.*

Age of Detectability: At birth.

Gene Mapping and Linkage: Unknown.

Prevention: None known. Genetic counseling indicated.

Treatment: Orthopedic surgery and physiotherapy for correction of the atypical clubfeet and possibly of the malaligned growth plates of the tibia and fibula.

Prognosis: Normal life span with orthopedic problems.

Detection of Carrier: Unknown.

References:

Nievergelt K: Positiver Vaterschaftsnachweis auf Grund erblicher Missbildungen der Extremitäten. Arch Julius Klaus-Stiftung Vererbungsforsch 1944; 19:157 only.

Solonen KA, Sulamaa M: Nievergelt syndrome and its treatment: a case report. Ann Chir Gynaecol Fenn 1958; 47:142–147.

Spranger, et al.: Bone Dysplasias. W. B. Saunders, 1974:222–223.

Young LW, Wood BP: Nievergelt syndrome (mesomelic dwarfism-type Nievergelt). BD:OAS X(5). Miami: Symposia Specialists for The National Foundation-March of Dimes, 1974:81–86.

Hess OM, et al.: Familiaerer mesomeler Kleinwuchs (Nievergelt-syndrom). Schweiz Med Wschr 1978; 108:1202–1206.

KA004
GR044

Ilkka I. Kaitila
Gisele A. Greenhaw

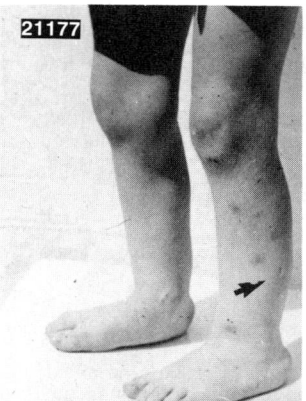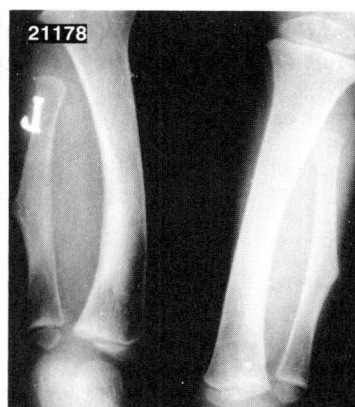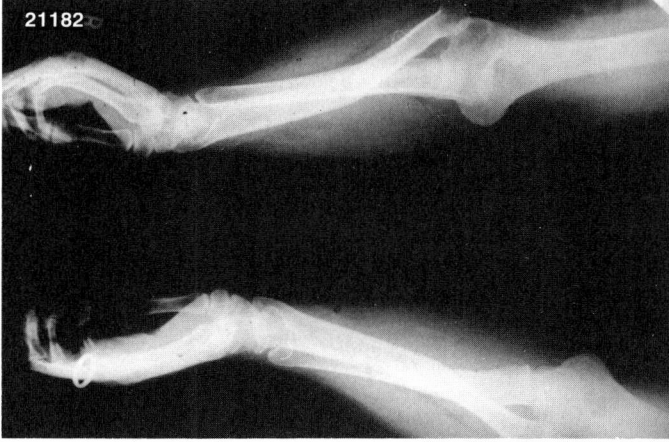

0648-21177: Typical dimple above the curvature of the fibula (see arrow). **21178:** Short, triangular fibula. **21182:** Bowed radius, dysplastic distal ulna and subluxed elbow.

MESOMELIC DYSPLASIA, REINHARDT-PFEIFFER TYPE   0648

Includes:
Reinhardt-Pfeiffer mesomelic dysostosis
Ulna and fibula, hypoplasia of

Excludes:
Dyschondrosteosis (0308)
Mesomelic dysplasia (other)
Skeletal dysplasia, boomerang dysplasia (2522)

Major Diagnostic Criteria: Hypoplasia of ulna and fibula in the absence of constant skeletal dysplasia elsewhere.

Clinical Findings: In the presence of a mildly retarded body stature, there are normal upper arms and legs while lower arms and legs are shortened symmetrically. Pro- and supination of the arms are diminished. The ulna is short and broad. The radius is bowed anteriorly and radially; the radial head is dislocated in the same directions. Usually, a radioulnar joint is not formed; the bones do not touch. There is a fork-like abnormality of the wrist. Slight deformations of elbows and dislocations of carpal bones appear to be secondary. In 12 of 14 patients the abnormalities of the lower arm are as severe as those of the lower leg; in the remaining two, the lower arm is more severely affected. The fibula is hypoplastic, the fibular head does not reach the tibial head, but is displaced dorsally. In the middle part of the tibial diaphysis there is a triangular exostosis, pointing laterally. The distal part of the fibular bone is also hypoplastic; the fibulotalar joint may be missing. The middle-third part of the fibula is broad and anteriorly angulated, leading to a skin identation with a central dark brown pigmentation. Deformations of knee joint and tarsus are secondary. There may be severe valgus feet with more or less marked talus and calcaneus changes on X-ray.

Complications: The radial bowing may become more severe during growth; a slight valgus deformity of the tibia may also develop.

Associated Findings: One quarter of the patients had -5D myopia and strabismus.

Etiology: Probably autosomal dominant inheritance with full penetrance and very variable expression.

Pathogenesis: Unknown.

MIM No.: 19140

POS No.: 3294

Sex Ratio: M1:F2.7.

Occurrence: Fifteen cases known; fourteen in Western Germany, one in France.

Risk of Recurrence for Patient's Sib:
See Part I, *Mendelian Inheritance.*

Risk of Recurrence for Patient's Child:
See Part I, *Mendelian Inheritance.*

Age of Detectability: May be present at birth. Detection by prenatal ultrasound may be possible.

Gene Mapping and Linkage: Unknown.

Prevention: None known. Genetic counseling indicated.

Treatment: Orthopedic treatment for triangular angulation of the lower leg.

Prognosis: Normal life span. Occasionally patients do have difficulties in ambulation.

Detection of Carrier: Careful clinical and X-ray examination of all relatives will help indicate those who are minimally affected.

Special Considerations: It has been suggested that this disorder is allelic to **Dyschondrosteosis**. The absence of major radial and tibial dysplasias makes it possible to differentiate this condition from **Mesomelic dysplasia, Nievergelt type**.

References:

Pfeiffer RA: Beitrag zur erblichen Verkuerzung von Ulna und Fibula. In: Wiedemann H-R, ed: Dysostosen. Stuttgart: Gustav Fischer Verlag, 1966.

Reinhardt K, Pfeiffer RA: Ulno-fibulare Dysplasie. Eine autosomal-dominant vererbte Mikromesomelie aehnlich dem Nievergeltsyn-drom. Fortschr Rontgenstr 1967; 107:379–391. * †

Maroteaux P, Spranger J: Essai de classification des chondrodysplasies a predominance mesomelique. Arch Fr Pediatr 1977; 34:945–958.

Lewin SO, Opitz JM: Fibular a/hypoplasia: review and documentation of the fibular developmental field. Am J Med Genet 1986; (Suppl 2):215–238. *

BE006   **Frits A. Beemer**

Mesomelic dysplasia, type Robinow
See ROBINOW SYNDROME

MESOMELIC DYSPLASIA, WERNER TYPE   0649

Includes:

    Eaton-McKusick syndrome
    Femoral duplication
    Mesomelic dwarfism of hypoplastic tibia and radius
    Tibia, absece of, with polydactyly
    Tibia, bilateral aplasia of with polydactyly and absent
        thumbs
    Tibia, hypoplasia of, with polydactyly

Excludes:

    Acrodysostosis (0016)
    Acromesomelic dysplasia
    Chondroectodermal dysplasia (0156)
    Dyschondrosteosis (0308)
    Mesomelic dysplasia
    Robinow syndrome (0876)
    Tibial hypoplasia/aplasia-ectrodactyly (2388)
    Tibia, unilateral aplasia of with polydactyly and absent
        thumbs

Major Diagnostic Criteria: Absent or hypoplastic tibia bilaterally with **Polydactyly** and absent thumbs.

Clinical Findings: Dwarfism that is due to marked shortening of the lower legs. In most cases, there is aplasia or severe hypoplasia of the tibia. There may be preaxial polydactyly of hands and feet and all digits may be triphalangial. The forearms are usually normal, but the carpal bones may be fused; range of movement is limited at the wrists. There may be pedunculated postminimi.

On X-ray, the tibia is rudimentary or totally absent and has no growth plates. The proximal head of the fibula is posteriorly and laterally dislocated and lies lateral to the middle shaft of the femur. The distal end of the fibula extends down to the lateral side of the foot. The patellae are hypoplastic. The bones in the ankle are deformed, and the number of metatarsals and phalanges is increased. In the hand, even the extra fingers appear normal, with three phalanges and normal metacarpal bones. There are no thumbs.

Complications: Those associated with orthopedic problems. Walking is delayed.

Associated Findings: Generally, no other associated defects have been described. However, there is one report of an infant born with absent tibias, preaxial polydactyly of the feet and

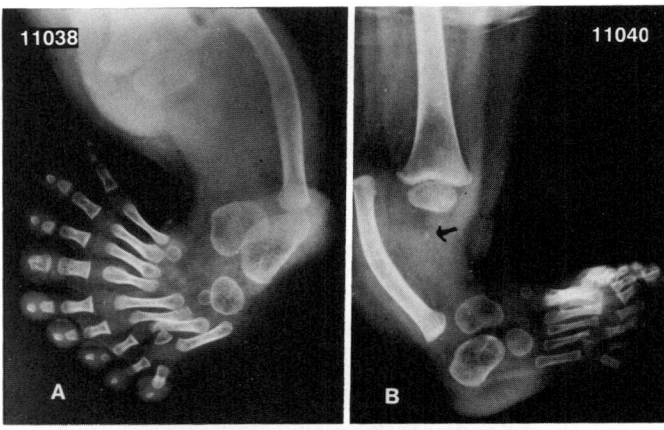

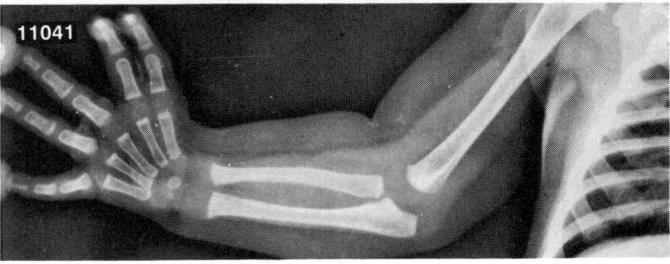

0649-11038: Preaxial polydactyly with 4th toe from medial aspect appearing as the hallux; postaxial polydactyly with a trapezoidal 8th metatarsal. **11040:** Absent tibia with rudimentary calcified proximal remnant; bowed and dislocated fibula. **11041:** Digitalized thumb with syndactyly of the 1st and 2nd digits.

---

normal thumbs who had multiple other congenital malformations, including **Cleft lip**, **Ventricular septal defect**, micrognathia, and wormian bones. Another report describes a child with **Polydactyly**, tibial dysplasia, **Ventricular septal defect**, and **Colon, aganglionosis**.

Etiology: Autosomal dominant inheritance with marked variability in phenotypic expression.

Pathogenesis: The short stature presumably results from the absence of growth plates of the tibia. The cause of the digital anomalies is unknown.

MIM No.: *15623, *18877, 18874

POS No.: 3295

Sex Ratio: M1:F1

Occurrence: Undetermined but presumed rare. The variability of this condition makes definitive diagnosis difficult.

At least six kindreds have been described with variable presentation in family members. For example, the father of two identically affected daughters with severly hypoplastic tibias and with polydactyly and absent thumbs had identical manifestations in his hands whereas his tibiae were completely normal. In another kindred, a father and two sons had varying degrees of tibial and radial hypoplasia without polydactyly.

Risk of Recurrence for Patient's Sib:
    See Part I, *Mendelian Inheritance.*

Risk of Recurrence for Patient's Child:
    See Part I, *Mendelian Inheritance.*

Age of Detectability: At birth. Prenatal diagnosis by ultrasound may be possible.

Gene Mapping and Linkage: Unknown.

Prevention: None known. Genetic counseling indicated.

Treatment: Orthopedic surgery to remove the supernumerary digits may be recommended to improve upper extremity function.

In cases of complete tibial agenesis, disarticulation at the knee with prosthetic replacement has been advocated to give the best functional result. In cases of partial tibia absence, transfer of the fibula into the tibial remnant can be considered.

Prognosis: Normal life span.

Detection of Carrier: Clinical and X-ray examination.

References:
Werner P: Ueber einen seltenen Fall von Zwergwuchs. Arch Gynakol 1915; 104:278–300.
Eaton GO, McKusick VA: A seemingly unique polydactyly-syndactyly syndrome in four persons in three generations. BD:OAS V(3). New York: March of Dimes Birth Defects Foundation, 1969:221–225.
Pashayan H, et al.: Bilateral aplasia of the tibia, polydactyly and absent thumbs in father and daughter. J Bone Joint Surg [Br] 1971; 53:495–499.
Ho CH, et al.: Congenital malformations: Cleft palate, congenital heart disease, absent tibia and polydactyly. Am J Dis Child 1975; 129:714–716.
LeRoy JG, et al.: Dominant mesomelic dwarfism of the hypoplastic tibia, radius type. Clin Genet 1975; 7:280–286.
Tetamy S, McKusick VA: The genetics of hand malformations. New York: Alan R. Liss, 1978.
Hall CM: Werner's mesomelic dysplasia with ventricular septal defect and Hirschsprung's disease. Ped Radiol 1981; 10:247–249.
Lamb PW, et al.: Five-fingered hand associated with partial or complete tibial absence and pre-axial polydactyly. J Bone Joint Surg 1983; 65:60–63.
Canun S, et al.: Absent tibia, triphalangeal thumbs and polydactyly: description of a family and prenatal diagnosis. Clin Genet 1984; 25:182–186.
Cordeiro I, Maroteaux HS: Congenital absence of the tibae and thumbs with polydactyly. Ann de Genet 1986; 29:275–277.
Al-Awadi SA, et al.: Hypoplastic tibiae with postaxial polysyndactyly: a new dominant syndrome. J Med Genet 1987; 23:367–372.
Bodurtha J, et al.: Femoral duplication: a case report. Am J Med Genet 1989; 33:165–169.
Kohn G, et al.: Aplasia of the tibia with bifurcation of the femur and ectrodactyly. Am J Med Genet 1989; 33:172–175.
Pavone L, et al.: Two rare developmental defects of the lower limbs with confirmation of the Lewin and Opitz hypothesis on the fibular and tibial developmental fields. Am J Med Genet 1989; 33:161–164.

KA004
GR044
Ilkka I. Kaitila
Gisele A. Greenhaw

Mesotaurodontism
See TEETH, TAURODONTISM
Mesothelial cysts-squamous metaplasia
See SPLEEN, CYSTS
Metabolic craniopathy
See HYPEROSTOSIS FRONTALIS INTERNA
Metacarpal 4-5 fusion
See SYNDACTYLY

METACHONDROMATOSIS   0650

Includes: N/A

Excludes:
    Enchondromatosis (0345)
    Exostoses, multiple cartilaginous (0685)

Major Diagnostic Criteria: Both exostoses and enchondromata in the same patient. This disorder must be distinguished from both **exostoses, multiple cartilaginous** and **enchondromatosis**. The presence of both lesions in the same patient, and the fact that the exostoses point toward the epiphyses, frequently occurring in the hands, are differentiating features of this disorder.

Clinical Findings: Exostotic lesions occur in the hands and long bones of a person who is unusually short. In contrast to multiple exostoses, the osteochondromata point toward the joint. Furthermore, they frequently regress and may disappear. Both exostoses and enchondromata are seen on X-rays. The exostoses frequently involve the hands, as well as the long bones, and the enchondro-

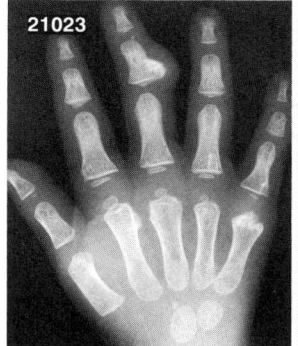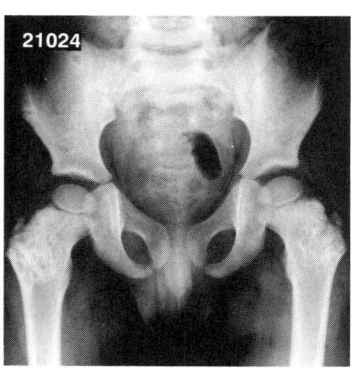

0650-21023–24: Metachondromatosis; note exostoses and enchondromata.

---

mata are in various growth plates. The spine may have irregular vertebral end plates.

Complications: Short stature secondary to enchondromata in the growth plates of the long bones. Deformity and limitation of function of fingers due to exostoses.

Associated Findings: None known.

Etiology: Presumably autosomal dominant inheritance.

Pathogenesis: Iliac crest biopsy has demonstrated typical lobulated enchondromata. The exostoses are histopathologically indistinguishable from both solitary and multiple exostoses.

MIM No.: 15625

POS No.: 4015

Sex Ratio: Presumably M1:F1.

Occurrence: About 20 cases documented.

Risk of Recurrence for Patient's Sib:
    See Part I, *Mendelian Inheritance.*

Risk of Recurrence for Patient's Child:
    See Part I, *Mendelian Inheritance.*

Age of Detectability: Infancy to early childhood.

Gene Mapping and Linkage: Unknown.

Prevention: None known. Genetic counseling indicated.

Treatment: Orthopedic surgery to remove exostoses if they produce pain, deformity, or limitation of function.

Prognosis: Undetermined. No malignancies have been reported.

Detection of Carrier: Unknown.

References:
Maroteaux P: La metachondromatose. Z Kinderheilk 1971; 109:246–261.
Lachman RS, et al.: Metachondromatosis. BD:OAS X(9). Miami: Symposia Specialists for The National Foundation-March of Dimes, 1974:171–178.
Kennedy LA: Metachondromatosis. Radiology 1983; 148:117–118.
Bassett GS, Cowell HR: Metachondromatosis: report of four cases. J Bone Joint Surg 1985; 67A:811–814.

B0025
LA006
Zvi Borochowitz
Ralph S. Lachman

Metachromatic form of diffuse cerebral sclerosis
See METACHROMATIC LEUKODYSTROPHIES

METACHROMATIC LEUKODYSTROPHIES 0651

Includes:
Arsacerebroside sulfatase deficiency
Arylsulfatase A deficiency
Cerebral sclerosis, degenerative diffuse, Scholz type
Cerebroside sulfatidosis
Lipidosis, sulfatide
Metachromatic form of diffuse cerebral sclerosis
Multiple sulfatase deficiency
Pseudo-arylsulfatase A deficiency
Sulfatide lipidosis
Sulfatidosis, juvenile, Austin type (some forms)

Excludes:
Leukodystrophy, globoid cell type (0415)
Leukodystrophy, sudanophilic type
Pelizaeus-Merzbacher syndrome (0803)
Other leukodystrophies of nervous system

Major Diagnostic Criteria: The three known clinical forms are named for their usual age of presentation. In the late infantile form, affected children usually present in the second year of life with delayed development and progressive weakness. The juvenile form usually presents later with ataxia and progressive gait involvement. In the adult form, dementia is progressive, and there is evidence of basal ganglial or long tract involvement. All may be suspected on the basis of the clinical picture plus increased CSF protein, prolonged nerve conduction times, or the demonstration of metachromatic material in a peripheral nerve biopsy. In all forms of the disease, the diagnosis is established by demonstration of the enzymatic defect in white cells or skin fibroblasts. MRI and CT scans may direct attention to distinct degenerative changes in white matter. These are more diffuse in younger patients, and multifocal in older patients.

Clinical Findings: The three clinical forms of metachromatic leukodystrophy (MLD) are late infantile, juvenile, and adult:
Late infantile metachromatic leukodystrophy: the child is usually normal until approximately 12–16 months of life. Early symptoms and signs include delayed motor development, particularly in terms of the lower limbs, followed by a progressive loss of the ability to walk. With a genu recurvatum, the child then regresses to hanging onto objects to stand. Following these symptoms, there is involvement of the upper limbs. Some patients may show nystagmus. By the age of 2 or 2 1/2 years, the patient is unable to pull himself to a sitting position, has dysarthria, is hypotonic, and may have difficulty with swallowing. Since both the central and peripheral nervous systems are involved, the child may have spasticity and hyperreflexia or hypotonicity and hyporeflexia. At times, there are combinations of both the decreased reflexes in the lower limbs and increased reflexes in the upper limbs. Eventually the child loses speech, and it is difficult to tell if the child is in contact with his surroundings. However, prior to the loss of speech, intellect seems to be relatively preserved, and seizures are an uncommon phenomenon. There may be involvement of the retina with optic atrophy or retinal changes.
Juvenile metachromatic leukodystrophy: is more likely to present as ataxia. There is then progressive involvement of gait and a slower progression than seen in the late infantile form.
Adult metachromatic leukodystrophy: presents as a dementia or an involvement of basal ganglia and long-tract findings. The progression is one of increasing dementia, often with behavioral disturbance.
Arylsulfatase A screening tests are useful, but the finding of "low" arylsulfatase A activity per se does not suffice to make a diagnosis of MLD. The demonstration of a cerebroside sulfatase deficiency and of increased sulfatide excretion in urine are much more specific tests.

Complications: Progressive loss of motor function, aspiration pneumonia, urinary tract infections, and a bedridden patient.

Associated Findings: None known.

Etiology: Autosomal recessive inheritance and possibly X-linked inheritance.

Pathogenesis: The basic defect is a failure to split sulfatide (the sulfate ester of galactocerebroside). The enzymatic defect is the lack of activity of the lysosomal enzyme, cerebroside sulfatase. Rarely, an activator protein is defective.
Sulfatide catabolism is abnormally slow. The defective cerebroside sulfatase activity causes a widespread increase in sulfatides, notably in the brain, peripheral nerves, and gallbladder. Associated with the sulfatide accumulation is the progressive breakdown of membranes of the myelin sheath, which contains abnormal amounts of sulfatide.

MIM No.: 25000, *25010, 25020, 30270, *27220

POS No.: 3775

Sex Ratio: M1:F1

Occurrence: 1:40,000–50,000 births in northern Sweden.

Risk of Recurrence for Patient's Sib:
See Part I, *Mendelian Inheritance.*

Risk of Recurrence for Patient's Child:
See Part I, *Mendelian Inheritance.* Late infantile and juvenile forms are lethal prior to reproductive age.

Age of Detectability: In utero by demonstration of the enzymatic defect in amniotic cells, as well as at birth from leukocytes or from skin fibroblasts.

Gene Mapping and Linkage: ARSA (arylsulfatase A) has been mapped to 22q13.31-qter.

Prevention: None known. Genetic counseling indicated.

Treatment: Supportive as indicated.

Prognosis: Late infantile form: death 2–4 years after diagnosis. Juvenile form: death 4–6 years after diagnosis. Adult form unknown.

Detection of Carrier: The heterozygote can be detected by enzymatic assay of leukocytes or skin fibroblasts using the arylsulfatase assay. Carriers have 40–60% of the activity of control patients.

Special Considerations: In a special form of this disease, multiple sulfatase deficiency (MLD), a variant of *sulfatidosis, juvenile, Austin type*; a condition which combines the enzyme deficiency and phenotypic features of several other conditions (Kihara, 1982), not only do sulfatides accumulate, but also sulfated steroids, sulfated mucopolysaccharides, and gangliosides in cerebral cortex. The accumulated sulfated mucopolysaccharide resembles heparan sulfate. These patients have skeletal abnormalities, ichthyosis and deafness. They also show a distinctive granulation abnormality in their leukocytes and have a deficiency not only of sulfatase A, but also of sulfatase B and sulfatase C.
A "pseudodeficiency" allele at the arylsulfatase A locus has been delineated by Schaap et al (1981). Otherwise healthy relatives of MLD patients may show ARSA levels in the range with MLD patients, but cultured fibroblasts from such relatives catabolize cerebroside sulfate; fibroblasts from MLD patients do not.

References:
Schaap T, et al.; The genetics of the aryl sulfatase A locus. Am J Hum Genet 1981; 33:531–539.
Kihara H: Genetic heterogeneity in metachromatic leukodystrophy. Am J Hum Genet 1982; 34:171–181.
Skomer C, et al.: Metachromatic leukodystrophy (MLD). XV: adult MLD with focal lesions by computed tomograph. Arch Neurol 1983; 40:354–355.
McKhann G: Metachromatic leukodystrophy: clinical and enzymic parameters. Neuropediatrics 1984; 15(suppl):4–10.
Farrell K, et al.: Pseudoarylsulfatase-A deficiency in the neurologically impaired patient. Can J Neurol Sci 1985; 12:274–277.
Waltz G, et al.: Adult metachromatic leukodystrophy: value of computed tomographic scanning and magnetic resonance imaging of the brain. Arch Neurol 1987; 44:225–227.
Austin J: Metachromatic leukodystrophy. In: Rowland L, ed: Merritt's textbook of neurology, 8th ed. Philadelphia: Lea and Febiger, 1988. *
Kolodny E: Metachromatic leukodystrophy and multiple sulfatase

deficiency. In: Scriver CR, et al, eds: The metabolic basis of inherited disease, 6th ed. New York: McGraw-Hill, 1989:1721–1750.

AU002
K0010

James H. Austin
Edwin H. Kolodny

METAPHYSEAL CHONDRODYSPLASIA WITH THYMOLYMPHOPENIA 0655

Includes:

Achondroplasia, so-called, and Swiss-type agammaglobulinemia
Adenosine deaminase deficiency
Agammaglobulinemia, variant form of Swiss type
Dwarfism-immunodeficiency, Swiss type
Immunodeficiency, Swiss type-dwarfism
Lymphopenic agammaglobulinemia-short limbed dwarfism
Metaphyseal dysostosis with Swiss type agammaglobulinemia

Excludes:

Hypoparathyroidism
Metaphyseal chondrodysplasia (other)
Metaphyseal osteochondrodystrophies
Rickets
Swiss type agammaglobulinemia without bone disease
Other immunologic conditions

Major Diagnostic Criteria: Recurrent, severe infections in a child with ectodermal dysplasia, absence of thymic-dependent and thymic-independent lymphoid tissue, and metaphyseal chondrodysplasia.

Clinical Findings: At birth, short-limbed short stature, and ectodermal dysplasia; cutis laxa, scalp alopecia; ichthyosiform dermatosis. Within weeks, failure to thrive and recurrent bacterial, fungal and viral infections. Severe combined immune deficiency (lymphopenia, total or selective immunoglobulin deficiency). On X-ray, metaphyseal chondrodysplasia, pelvic dysplasia (flat acetabulae); flaring of the anterior ends of the ribs, osteoporosis; absent tonsils, adenoids, and thymus. Accumulation of toxic metabolites can disturb neurologic functions.

Complications: Recurrent severe infections.

Associated Findings: Lymphopenia with none of the B-cells and T-cell surface markers. After maternal antibodies are cleared, hypogammaglobulinemia, and negative skin test reactions to infectious and chemical agents. Very low or immeasurable levels of adenosine deaminase.

Etiology: Presumably autosomal recessive inheritance; one-third of severe combined immunodeficiency cases are inherited as a recessive trait caused by adenosine deaminase deficiency.

Pathogenesis: A deficiency of adenosine deaminase leads to accumulation of adenosine in the cells and disruption of cellular proliferation of lymphoid and cartilage tissues.

MIM No.: 20090

POS No.: 3299

CDC No.: 756.450

Sex Ratio: M1:F1

Occurrence: About 50 families have been identified.

Risk of Recurrence for Patient's Sib:
See Part I, *Mendelian Inheritance.*

Risk of Recurrence for Patient's Child:
See Part I, *Mendelian Inheritance.* No probands have survived to reproduce.

Age of Detectability: Deficient adenosine deaminase activity in cultured amniotic fluid cells or chorionic villus biopsy; in neonatal period with appropriate methods.

Gene Mapping and Linkage: Unknown.

Prevention: None known. Genetic counseling indicated.

Treatment: Bone marrow transplantation can result in complete immune reconstitution. Enzyme replacement therapy may improve function.

Prognosis: Death in infancy, unless protective measures are taken.

Detection of Carrier: Carriers have about one-half the normal levels of erythrocyte adenosine deaminase.

References:
Alexander WJ, Dunbar JS: Unusual bone changes in thymic alymphoplasia. Ann Radiol [Paris] 1968; 11:389–394.
Gatti RA, et al.: Hereditary lymphopenic agammaglobulinemia associated with a distinctive form of short-limbed dwarfism and ectodermal dysplasia. J Pediatr 1969; 75:675–684.
Sutcliffe J, Stanley P: Metaphyseal chondrodysplasias. Progr Pediatr Radiol 1973; 4:250–269.
Meuwissen HJ, et al.: Combined immunodeficiency disease associated with adenosine deaminase deficiency. J Pediatr 1975; 86:169–181. * †
Spranger JW: Metaphyseal chondrodysplasia. Postgrad Med J 1977; 53:480–486.
Young LW, et al.: Severe combined immunodeficiency associated with adenosine deaminase deficiency. Am J Dis Child 1978; 132:621–622.
Kredich NM, Hershfield MS: Immunodeficiency disease caused by adenosine deaminase deficiency and purine nucleoside phosphorylase deficiency. In: Scriver CR, et al, eds: The metabolic basis of inherited disease, 6th ed. New York: McGraw-Hill, 1989:1045–1076.

K0021

K.S. Kozlowski

METAPHYSEAL CHONDRODYSPLASIA, TYPE JANSEN 0652

Includes:

Jansen metaphyseal dysostosis
Murk Jansen metaphyseal chondrodysplasia

Excludes:

Enchondromatosis (0345)
Enchondromatosis and hemangiomas (0346)
Hypophosphatasia (0516)

Major Diagnostic Criteria: Dwarfism and peculiar facies, with severe metaphyseal chondrodysplasia.

Clinical Findings: Progressive, short-limb dwarfism with contractural deformities of the joints and expansion of the ends of the long bones. Adult height about 120 cm. Facies are dysmorphic. Often elevated serum calcium levels. Diagnostic X-ray findings: severe, generalized metaphyseal changes. The metaphyses are expanded and irregularly mottled (an expression of severely disorganized enchondral ossification). The short tubular bones show marked cupping. Additional characteristic findings include shortening of the diaphyses and progressive sclerosis; particularly of the base of the skull. Minor spinal and epiphyseal changes may also be noted.

Complications: Severe, early progressive osteoarthritic changes, kyphoscoliosis.

Associated Findings: None known.

Etiology: Autosomal dominant inheritance.

Pathogenesis: Disorganized metaphyseal ossification with presence of irregular masses of abnormal cartilage in the metaphyseal regions.

MIM No.: *15640

POS No.: 3296

CDC No.: 756.450

Sex Ratio: M1:F1

Occurrence: About 20 verified cases have been reported.

Risk of Recurrence for Patient's Sib:
See Part I, *Mendelian Inheritance.*

Risk of Recurrence for Patient's Child:
See Part I, *Mendelian Inheritance.*

Age of Detectability: In infancy, by X-ray.

Gene Mapping and Linkage: Unknown.

Prevention: None known. Genetic counseling indicated.

Treatment: Physiotherapy; orthopedic treatment. It is important to distinguish this disorder from metabolic disorders, especially rickets, as in presence of hypercalcemia, vitamin D therapy may be harmful.

Prognosis: Normal life span.

Detection of Carrier: Unknown.

References:

Jansen M: Über atypische chondrodystrophie (achondroplasie) und über eine noch nicht beschriebene angeborene wachstumsstörung des knochensystems: metaphysäre dysostose. Z Orthop Chir 1934; 61:253–286.

Ozonoff MB: Metaphyseal dysostosis of Jansen. Radiology 1969; 93:1047–1050.

De Haas WHD, et al.: Metaphyseal dysostosis. A late follow-up of the first reported case. J Bone Joint Surg 1969; 51B:290–299.

Sutcliffe J, Stanley P: Metaphyseal chondrodysplasias. Prog Pediatr Radiol 1973; 4:250–269.

Holthusen W, et al.: The skull in metaphyseal chondrodysplasia, type Jansen. Pediatr Radiol 1975; 3:137–144. †

Silverthorn KG, et al.: Murk Jansen's metaphyseal chondrodysplasia with long term follow-up. Pediatr Radiol 1987; 17:119–123. *

K0021   **K.S. Kozlowski**

METAPHYSEAL CHONDRODYSPLASIA, TYPE MCKUSICK   0653

Includes:

Agammaglobulinemia-lymphopenia-dwarfism
Cartilage-hair hypoplasia
Dwarfism-lymphopenia-agammaglobulinemia
Immunodeficiency, cartilage-hair hypoplasia
Lymphopenia-agammaglobulinemia-dwarfism

Excludes:

Dyschondrosteosis (0308)
Hypochondroplasia (0510)
Hypophosphatasia (0516)
Hypophosphatemic rickets and other types of "renal rickets"
Immunodeficiency, adenosine deaminase deficiency (2196)
Shwachman syndrome (0885)

Major Diagnostic Criteria: Short-limb dwarfism with fine sparse hair. Metaphyseal chondrodysplasia with predominant peripheral involvement. Cellular immunodeficiency may be noted, particularly a marked impairment of T-cell function due to an intrinsic defect in cell proliferation.

Clinical Findings: Progressive short-limb dwarfism with predominant peripheral involvement. Fine, sparse, usually light-colored hair, eyebrows, and lashes, otherwise normal head and skull. Adult height about 120 cm. Characteristic X-ray findings include metaphyseal chondrodysplasia with predominant hand, foot, and knee involvement; cupping of the anterior ends of the ribs and little change in the proximal femoral and humeral metaphyses. There is considerable variability of expressivity, not only in X-ray findings but in possible associated cellular immunodeficiency.

Complications: Early osteoarthritic changes. Equinovarus deformity of the feet subsequent to overgrowth of the fibula.

Associated Findings: Malabsorption, Hirschsprung disease and impaired cellular immunity with chronic neutro- and lymphopenia sometimes reported. Varicella, anemia, and various malignancies have been reported, as have dental anomalies.

Etiology: Autosomal recessive inheritance.

Pathogenesis: Relation between ectodermal and bone defects, immunodeficiency, and associated diseases is unclear.

MIM No.: *25025

POS No.: 3061

CDC No.: 756.450

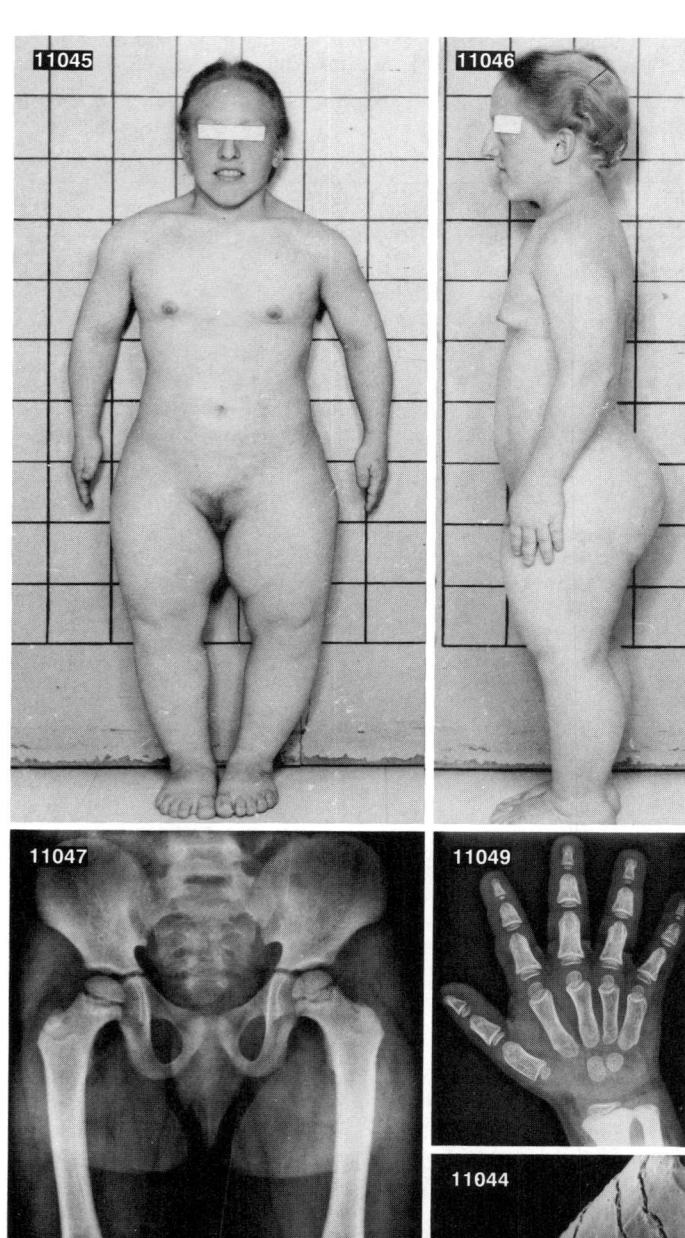

0653-11045–46: Mild bowing of the femurs and tibiae, excessively long fibulae, and sparse, short blond hair which has never been cut. **11047:** Long bones are short with flared ends; metaphyseal zones of provisional calcification are scalloped and irregular but of normal density. **11049:** Carpal ossification is delayed; phalanges are relatively wide with mild metaphyseal cupping. **11044:** Scanning electron micrograph of hair.

Sex Ratio: M1:F1

Occurrence: With exception of some inbred groups, presumed rare. 170:100,000 among Amish population in the United States. Increased gene frequency in some areas in Finland.

Risk of Recurrence for Patient's Sib:
See Part I, *Mendelian Inheritance.*

Risk of Recurrence for Patient's Child:
See Part I, *Mendelian Inheritance.*

Age of Detectability: Sometimes in infancy, usually early pre-school age.

Gene Mapping and Linkage: Unknown.

Prevention: None known. Genetic counseling indicated.

Treatment: Physiotherapy; orthopedic treatment. Affected individuals should avoid smallpox vaccinations and be guarded against all viral infections. Leukocyte interferon has been proposed as a treatment for patients who also have varicella. Serial transfusions and steroids have been used in cases with associated congenital anemia.

Prognosis: Usually a normal life span if treated. One patient with severe combined immunodeficiency died despite thymus transplantation.

Detection of Carrier: Unknown.

References:
McKusick VA, et al.: Dwarfism in the Amish. II. Cartilage-hair hypoplasia. Bull Johns Hopkins Hosp 1965; 116:285–326. * †
Lux SE, et al.: Chronic neutropenia and abnormal cellular immunity in cartilage-hair hypoplasia. New Engl J Med 1970; 282:231–236.
Ray HC, Dorst JP: Cartilage-hair hypoplasia. Prog Pediatr Radiol 1973; 4:270–298.
Kartila I, Perheentupa J: Cartilage-hair hypoplasia (CHH). In: Eriksson AW, et al., eds: Population structure and genetic disorders. New York: Academic Press, 1980:588–591.
Harris RE, et al.: Cartilage-hair hypoplasia, defective T-cell function, and Diamond-Blackfan anemia in an Amish child. Am J Med Genet 1981; 8:291–297.
Polmar SH, Pierce GF: Cartilage-hair hypoplasia: immunological aspects and their clinical implications. Clin Immunol Immunopathol 1986; 40:87–93.

K0021
WI024

K.S. Kozlowski
Golder N. Wilson

METAPHYSEAL CHONDRODYSPLASIA, TYPE SCHMID　0654

Includes: Schmid metaphyseal dysostosis

Excludes:
　Dyschondrosteosis (0308)
　Hypochondroplasia (0510)
　Hypophosphatasia (0516)
　Hypophosphatemic rickets and other types of "renal" rickets

Major Diagnostic Criteria: Moderate shortening of stature, normal head circumference, and bowed legs. Bony changes of moderately severe metaphyseal chondrodysplasia are found in X-rays, which show expanded cupped metaphyses and disorganized metaphyseal ossification.

Clinical Findings: Moderate, progressive shortening of stature with bowed legs and waddling gait. Adult height is about 140 cm. Characteristic X-ray findings show expanded, cupped metaphyses with disorganized metaphyseal ossification. There is often coxa vara and genu varum deformity of the hips, and cupping of the anterior ends of the ribs. The density and texture of the bones is normal (an important differential diagnostic sign with all forms of rickets). The spinal, epiphyseal, and diaphyseal changes are minimal. The skull is normal.

Complications: Coxa and genua vara; early progressive osteoarthritis.

Associated Findings: None known.

Etiology: Autosomal dominant inheritance.

Pathogenesis: Disorganized metaphyseal ossification, biochemical defect not defined.

MIM No.: *15650

POS No.: 3298

CDC No.: 756.450

Sex Ratio: M1:F1

Occurrence: Several large kindreds have been documented.

Risk of Recurrence for Patient's Sib:
See Part I, *Mendelian Inheritance.*

Risk of Recurrence for Patient's Child:
See Part I, *Mendelian Inheritance.*

Age of Detectability: Early preschool age.

Gene Mapping and Linkage: Unknown.

Prevention: None known. Genetic counseling indicated.

Treatment: Physiotherapy; orthopedic treatment. It is important to distinguish this disorder from metabolic diseases, especially rickets, as vitamin D therapy is unnecessary and may be harmful.

Prognosis: Normal life span.

Detection of Carrier: Unknown.

References:
Schmid F: Beitrag zur Dysostosis enchondralis metaphysarea. Monatsschr Kinderheilkd 1949; 97:393–397.
Rosenbloom AL, Smith DW: The natural history of metaphyseal dysostosis. J Pediatr 1965; 66:857–868.
Sutcliffe J, Stanley P: Metaphyseal chondrodysplasias. Prog Pediatr Radiol 1973; 4:250–269.
Beluffi G, et al.: Metaphyseal dysplasia type Schmid: Early X-ray detection and evolution with time. Ann Radiol 1983; 26:237–243. * †

K0021

K.S. Kozlowski

Metaphyseal dysostosis with Swiss type agammaglobulinemia
See METAPHYSEAL CHONDRODYSPLASIA WITH THYMOLYMPHOPENIA

METAPHYSEAL DYSOSTOSIS-DEAFNESS　0250

Includes:
　Deafness-metaphyseal dysostosis
　Metaphyseal dysostosis-mental retardation-conductive deafness
　Skeletal dysplasia-deafness

Excludes:
　Metaphyseal chondrodysplasia (other)
　Other disorders associated with metaphyseal dysostosis

Major Diagnostic Criteria: Metaphyseal dysostosis, conductive hearing loss, and mental retardation.

Clinical Findings: A kindred has been reported in which all three sibs were found to have short-limbed dwarfism, metaphyseal dysostosis, conductive hearing loss, and mild mental retardation. The parents were fourth cousins. The skeletal disorder can be classified as "metaphyseal dysostosis," since the major lesions consist of widening and fragmentation of the metaphyses of the long bones with relative sparing of the skull, spine, and epiphyses. Coxa vara, genua vara, scoliosis, or lumbar lordosis were noted. The feet and hands were short and broad, and the fingers were loose-jointed. Two sibs were hyperopic and had alternating esotropia. Anterior polar cataract was present in one sib. Polytomography revealed bilateral low placement of the ossicles in all three sibs. There was a striking upward angulation of the internal auditory canals. Audiologic examination in the three boys demonstrated a moderate bilateral conductive hearing deficit.

Complications: Unknown.

Associated Findings: None known.

Etiology: Autosomal recessive inheritance.

Pathogenesis: Unknown.

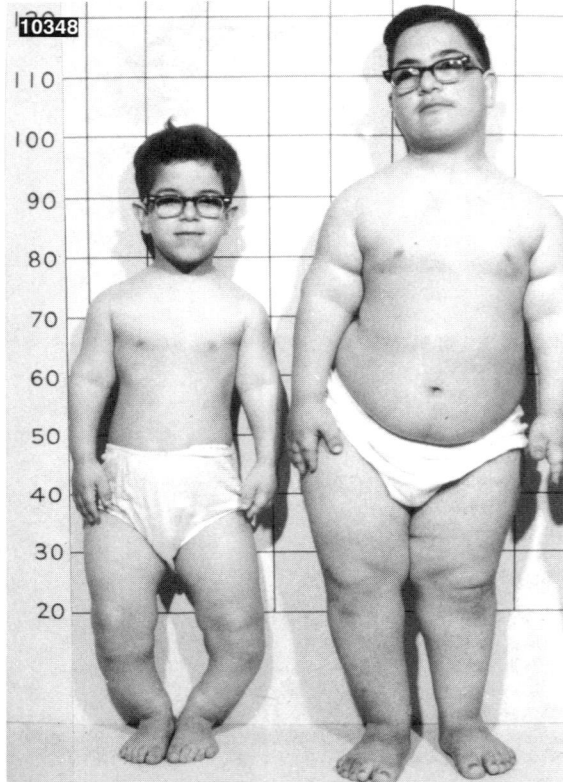

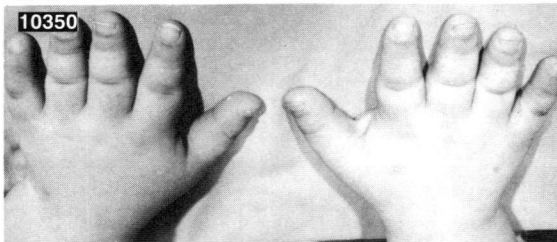

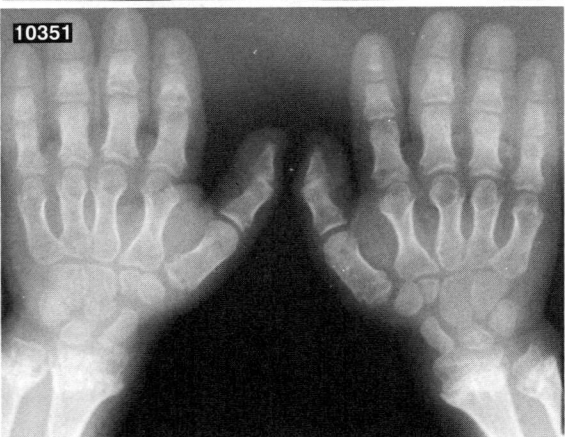

0250-10348: Short stature, coxa vara, genua vara and scoliosis in two brothers. **10350:** Short, stubby hands with squared-off nails. **10351:** Short tubular bones with widened metaphyses.

MIM No.: 25042

POS No.: 3194

Sex Ratio: M3:F0 (observed)

Occurrence: One reported family with three affected sibs.

Risk of Recurrence for Patient's Sib:
See Part I, *Mendelian Inheritance.*

Risk of Recurrence for Patient's Child:
See Part I, *Mendelian Inheritance.*

Age of Detectability: Early childhood.

Gene Mapping and Linkage: Unknown.

Prevention: None known. Genetic counseling indicated.

Treatment: Orthopedic therapy and a hearing aid may be useful.

Prognosis: Probably normal life span.

Detection of Carrier: Unknown.

References:
Rimoin DL, McAlister WH: Metaphyseal dysostosis, conductive hearing loss, and mental retardation: a recessively inherited syndrome. In: BD:OAS; VII(4). Baltimore: Williams & Wilkins, for The National Foundation-March of Dimes, 1971:116–122.

MU020
Jeff Murray
Cor W.R.J. Cremers

Metaphyseal dysostosis-mental retardation-conductive deafness
See METAPHYSEAL DYSOSTOSIS-DEAFNESS
Metaphyseal dysplasia
See PYLE DISEASE

METAPHYSEAL DYSPLASIA-MAXILLARY HYPOPLASIA-BRACHYDACTYLY   2768

Includes:
Brachydactyly-maxillary hypoplasia-metaphyseal dysplasia
Maxillary hypoplasia-metaphyseal dysplasia-brachydactyly

Excludes:
Cranio-diaphyseal dysplasia (0224)
Craniometaphyseal dysplasia (0228)
Diaphyseal dysplasia (0290)
Dysosteosclerosis (0310)
Frontometaphyseal dysplasia (0394)
Oculo-dento-osseous dysplasia (0737)
Pyle disease (0847)

Major Diagnostic Criteria: Metaphyseal dysplasia with maxillary hypoplasia and **Brachydactyly.**

Clinical Findings: Metaphyseal flaring, a constant finding in affected individuals, is symmetric and mild. It is most obvious in the proximal humeri, distal femora, and proximal tibiae. Aside from a few wormian bones and mild hyperostosis of the inner frontoparietal area of the skull in some affected persons, the cranium was normal. Changes in the spine varied from severe osteoporosis with several spontaneous fractures and platyspondyly to no abnormalities. The majority of affected individuals (4/6) were short.

Facial changes of small head circumference (proportionate to short stature), beaked nose or high nasal bridge, short philtrum, thin lips, maxillary hypoplasia with relative prognathism, and yellow dystrophic deciduous and permanent teeth with dental extraction in adolescence were present in most affected individuals. A part of the maxillary hypoplasia may be secondary to early loss of teeth. There was a suggestion of mild hypoplasia of the malar bones in at least one affected individual.

Acral anomalies were present in (4/5) affected individuals with available hand X-rays (the index patient did not have hand anomalies). These consisted of severe bilateral shortness of metacarpal 5 with or without shortness of the middle phalanx of fingers 2 and 5. The Poznanski hand pattern profile failed to show any other significant changes in the hand bones of affected persons.

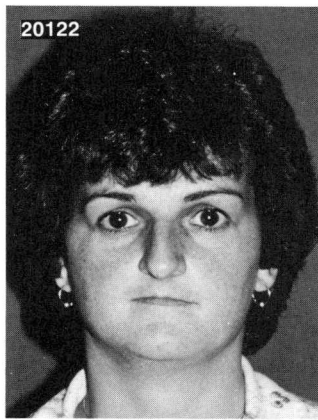
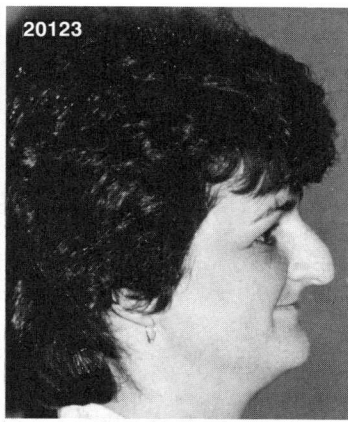
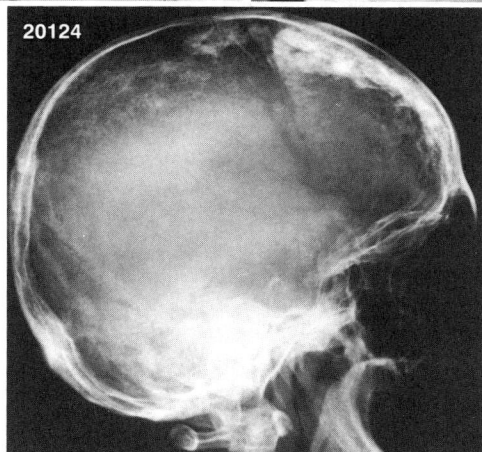
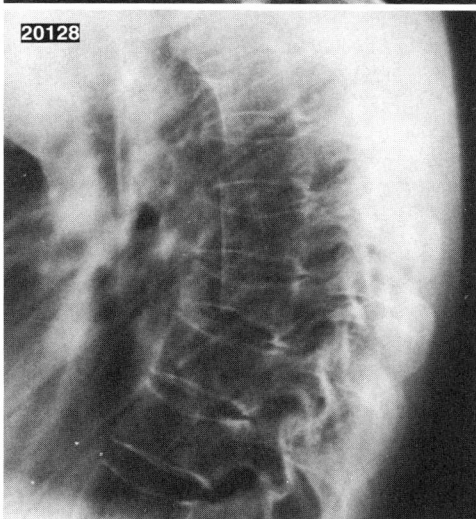

2768-20122–20123: Note beaked nose, short philtrum, thin lips, and maxillary hypoplasia with relative prognathism. 20124: Mild hyperostosis of inner frontal and parietal areas of the skull. 20128: Platyspondyly, multiple spontaneous small vertebral fractures, and osteoporosis of the spine.

Complications: Spontaneous fractures of the vertebrae, severe back pain, the need for dental extraction at adolescence.

Associated Findings: Mild **Camptodactyly** of DIP joints of fifth fingers in one affected female.

Etiology: Possibly autosomal dominant inheritance with variable expression.

Pathogenesis: Unknown. Serum levels of calcium; phosphorus; alkaline phosphatase; vitamin D; 25(OH) vitamin D; 24,25(OH)$_2$ vitamin D; 1,25(OH)$_2$ vitamin D; and parathormone were normal in two affected individuals.

MIM No.: 15651

POS No.: 3947

CDC No.: 756.450

Sex Ratio: Presumably M1:F1.

Occurrence: Reported in four generations of a French Canadian family.

Risk of Recurrence for Patient's Sib:
See Part I, *Mendelian Inheritance.*

Risk of Recurrence for Patient's Child:
See Part I, *Mendelian Inheritance.*

Age of Detectability: The youngest patient was diagnosed five years of age. X-ray manifestations could probably be present at an earlier age.

Gene Mapping and Linkage: Unknown.

Prevention: None known. Genetic counseling indicated.

Treatment: Physiotherapy. Orthopedic intervention if necessary. Avoid competitive sports to decrease the risk of fractures.

Prognosis: Normal life span.

Detection of Carrier: By skeletal survey.

References:
Halal F, et al.: Metaphyseal dysplasia with maxillary hypoplasia and brachydactyly. Am J Med Genet 1982; 13:71–79.

HA074   **Fahed Halal**

Metaphyseal dysplasia-pancreatic hypoplasia-marrow dysfunction
See SHWACHMAN SYNDROME
Metatarsus adductus
See FOOT, CONGENITAL CLUBFOOT
Metatarsus varus
See FOOT, CONGENITAL CLUBFOOT
Metatarsus varus, type I
See FOOT, METATARSUS VARUS
Metatropic dwarfism
See METATROPIC DYSPLASIA

METATROPIC DYSPLASIA   0656

Includes:
Chondrodystrophy, hyperplastic form
Dwarfism, metatropic
Metatropic dwarfism

Excludes:
Achondroplasia (0010)
Asphyxiating thoracic dysplasia (0091)
Kniest dysplasia (0557)
Mucopolysaccharidosis IV (0678)

Major Diagnostic Criteria: Skeletal dysplasia with tongue-like flattening of the vertebral bodies, short ribs, progressing kyphoscoliosis, crescent-like iliac wings, osseous hyperplasia of the trochanteric region and the metaphyses of the tubular bones, irregular metaphyses and epiphyses, normal cranial vault and viscerocranium, and dysplastic skull base.

Clinical Findings: In infancy, long narrow thorax and relatively short limbs; rapidly progressing kyphoscoliosis. In later infancy and childhood, reversion of body proportions, with development of short-spine dwarfism. On X-ray, severe spondyloepimetaphyseal dysplasia of the skeleton.

Complications: Severe progressive kyphoscoliosis, and early arthroses.

Associated Findings: None known.

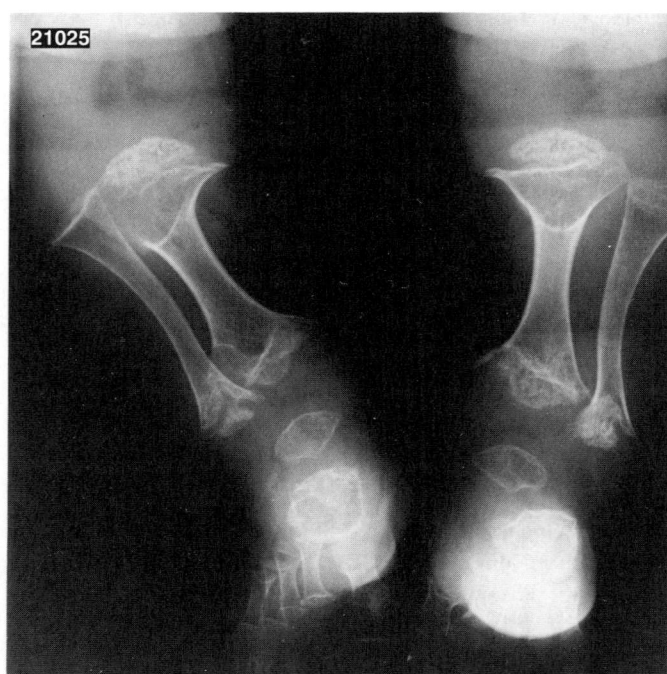

0656-21025: Metatropic dysplasia; note short long bones and osseous hyperplasia.

Etiology: Both autosomal dominant and autosomal recessive inheritance has been reported.

Pathogenesis: Presumed shortening of the tubular bones with irregular metaphyseal and epiphyseal ossification. Irregular arrangement of bone trabeculae, which contain islands of cartilage. Endochondral ossification processes are grossly reduced in quantity. Boden et al (1987), after study of bone samples, concluded that there had been an uncoupling of endochondral and perichondral growth, which explained the dumbbell-shaped changes in the metaphysis.

MIM No.: *25060

POS No.: 3300

CDC No.: 756.446

Sex Ratio: M1:F1

Occurrence: Undetermined but presumed rare.

Risk of Recurrence for Patient's Sib:
See Part I, *Mendelian Inheritance.*

Risk of Recurrence for Patient's Child:
See Part I, *Mendelian Inheritance.*

Age of Detectability: At birth, by X-ray, especially lateral view of the spine.

Gene Mapping and Linkage: Unknown.

Prevention: None known. Genetic counseling indicated.

Treatment: Intensive orthopedic care to prevent kyphoscoliosis and secondary positional defects.

Prognosis: Guarded, because of incapacitating physical deformities. Death frequently occurs in early infancy. Surviving patients may reach at least their third decade of life. Ultimate body height between 110 and 120 cm.

Detection of Carrier: Unknown.

Special Considerations: Cases of "hyperplastic chondrodystrophy" of the older literature probably had metatropic dwarfism. There exist one or more closely related, though ill-defined, conditions (pseudometatropic dwarfism) necessitating the obser-

vance of rigid diagnostic criteria. No criteria are available to distinguish the autosomal recessive from the autosomal dominant form.

References:

Maroteaux P, et al.: Der metatropische Zwergwuchs. Arch Kinderheilkd 1966; 173:211–226.

Spranger J, et al.: Bone dysplasias. Philadelphia: W.B. Saunders, Co., 1974.

Beck MM: Heterogeneity of metatropic dysplasia. Eur J Pediatr 1983; 140:231–237.

Boden SD, et al.: Metatropic dwarfism: uncoupling of endochondral and perichondral growth. J Bone Joint Surg 1987; 69A:174–184.

SP007 **Jürgen W. Spranger**

Metatropic dysplasia, type II
See KNIEST DYSPLASIA
Methemoglobin reductase deficiency
See METHEMOGLOBINEMIA, NADH-DEPENDENT DIAPHORASE DEFICIENCY

METHEMOGLOBINEMIA, NADH-DEPENDENT DIAPHORASE DEFICIENCY 2682

Includes:
Diaphorase deficiency
Methemoglobin reductase deficiency
NADH cytochrome b5 reductase deficiency

Excludes:
Cytochrome b5, deficiency of
Glucose-6-phosphate dehydrogenase deficiency (0420)
Hb M and other hemoglobin variants that produce cyanosis
NADPH-dependent methemoglobin reductase deficiency
Toxic methemoglobinemia

Major Diagnostic Criteria: Increased levels of methemoglobin (ferrihemoglobin) in the erythrocytes (typically between 10 and 40%) with NADH-dependent diaphorase activity of less than 20% of normal.

Clinical Findings: Affected individuals characteristically exhibit cyanosis, which is apparent at birth or shortly afterward, with an absence of demonstrable cardiac or pulmonary disease. The abnormality is ordinarily not accompanied by accelerated hemolysis or other hematologic changes; however, mild erythrocytosis has been observed in some affected individuals. The disorder has a characteristically benign course (but see below). Affected women have not experienced adverse obstetric events. Three clinical phenotypes of NADPH-dependent diaphorase deficiency have been described:

Type I: The abnormality is apparently confined to the erythrocytes and has benign methemoglobinemia as its only clinical abnormality. Most known individuals with NADPH-dependent diaphorase deficiency fall within this group.

Type II: Represents a more generalized abnormality in which the enzyme deficiency involves the leukocytes, platelets, fibroblasts, and other tissues. In addition to methemoglobinemia, affected individuals exhibit severe progressive encephalopathy with neurologic abnormalities, **Microcephaly**, and retardation. Approximately 10% of individuals with NADPH-dependent diaphorase deficiency are estimated to have this severe syndrome.

Type III: Associated with a deficiency of NADH-dependent diaphorase demonstrable in platelets and leukocytes as well as erythrocytes, but apparently not in other tissues. Affected individuals in the two reported families with this type did not exhibit any neurologic abnormalities.

Complications: Individuals with this enzyme deficiency are presumed to be at increased risk of developing toxic methemoglobinemia following exposure to drugs and chemicals that are known to produce methemoglobinemia in normal persons; care to prevent exposure to these agents is therefore advised. Levels of methemoglobin greater than 25% may produce mild fatigue and dyspnea. Cosmetic consequences of the accompanying cyanosis may also sometimes result in psychologic difficulties.

Associated Findings: None known.

Etiology: Autosomal recessive inheritance.

Pathogenesis: The NADH-dependent diaphorase is the physiologically active methemoglobin reductase in the erythrocytes, and in normal individuals it functions to maintain methemoglobin levels of less than 1%. The enzyme catalyzes the reduction of methemoglobin (ferrihemoglobin), which is incapable of binding oxygen, to the deoxyferrohemoglobin form. NADH and cytochrome b_5 are necessary cofactors, with the diaphorase functioning to catalyze the transfer of electrons from NADH to the cytochrome b_5. Cytochrome b_5 appears to reduce methemoglobin by a nonenzymatic mechanism. A deficiency of cytochrome b_5 has also been shown to produce congenital methemoglobinemia.

MIM No.: *25080

Sex Ratio: M1:F1

Occurrence: Numerous electrophoretic variants, deficiency forms, and stability variants have been described. The occurrence of affected homozygous or compound-heterozygous individuals with cyanosis is undetermined but nevertheless presumed rare.

Risk of Recurrence for Patient's Sib:
See Part I, *Mendelian Inheritance.*

Risk of Recurrence for Patient's Child:
See Part I, *Mendelian Inheritance.*

Age of Detectability: Junien et al. (1981) have reported successful prenatal diagnosis of the severe type II syndrome by measurement of cytochrome b_5 reductase activity in amniocytes.

Gene Mapping and Linkage: DIA1 (diaphorase (NADH) (cytochrome b-5 reductase)) has been mapped to 22q13.31-qter.

Prevention: None known. Genetic counseling indicated.

Treatment: Cosmetic improvement of the accompanying cyanosis may be achieved by treatment with methylene blue (100–300 mg/day), ascorbic acid (0.5 g/day), or riboflavin (20 mg/day). No effective treatment is known for the encephalopathic manifestations of the type II syndrome.

Prognosis: *Types I and III:* normal growth, development, and life span. *Type II:* severe and progressive neurologic dysfunction, poor growth, and mental retardation, often with a fatal outcome during infancy or childhood.

Detection of Carrier: Carriers of deficiency variants with altered electrophoretic mobility are readily identified by electrophoretic diaphorase analysis of red cell lysates. Enzyme activity in heterozygous carriers is approximately one-half of normal.

References:
Jaffe ER, et al.: Hereditary methemoglobinemia with and without mental retardation: a study of three families. Am J Med 1966; 41:42–55.
Hsieh H-S, Jaffe ER: Electrophoretic and functional variants of NADH-methemoglobin reductase in hereditary methemoglobinemia. J Clin Invest 1971; 50:196–202.
Jaffe ER, Hsieh H-S: DPNH-methemoglobin reductase deficiency and hereditary methemoglobinemia. Semin Hematol 1971; 8:417–437.
McAlpine PJ, et al.: Is the DIA-1 locus linked to the P blood group locus? Cytogenet Cell Genet 1978; 22:629–632.
Junien C, et al.: Prenatal diagnosis of congenital enzymopenic methaemoglobinaemia with mental retardation due to generalized cytochrome b_5 reductase deficiency: first report of two cases. Prenatal Diagn 1981; 1:17–24.
Hegesh E, et al.: Congenital methemoglobinemia with a deficiency of cytochrome b_5. New Engl J Med 1986; 314:757–761.

H0024   **George R. Honig**

Methimazole, fetal effects, scalp and urachal
See FETAL EFFECTS FROM METHIMAZOLE AND CARBIMAZOLE
Methionine 111 amyloidosis
See AMYLOIDOSIS, DANISH CARDIAC TYPE
Methionine 30 amyloidosis
See AMYLOIDOSIS, TRANSTHYRETIN METHIONINE-30 TYPE

METHIONINE MALABSORPTION   0657

Includes:
    Malabsorption, methionine
    Oast-house urine disease
    Smith-Strang disease

Excludes: Hartnup disorder (0453)

Major Diagnostic Criteria: This rare condition is associated with convulsions, mental retardation, and a sweet odor of body fluids in a child with fair hair and blue eyes. Diagnosis is suspected by detection of increased α-hydroxybutyric acid in urine and feces in amounts related to methionine intake.

Clinical Findings: Mental retardation with normal physical development. Clinical findings included white hair, blue eyes, convulsions, intermittent diarrhea, and an intermittent sweet odor to the urine and the patient. The level of dietary intake of protein determined the presence or absence of intestinal symptoms, seizures, and odor; a high protein intake provoked symptoms.

Alpha-hydroxybutyric acid is found in urine and feces in amounts related to the methionine intake. This compound is believed to account for the peculiar odor. Its formation occurs in the intestine from bacterial degradation of methionine. Methionine excretion is increased in feces but not in the urine under usual endogenous conditions. Oral loading with methionine increases fecal excretion of many amino acids; loading with branched-chain compounds does not affect methionine excretion.

Complications: Diarrhea, seizures, and mental retardation seem related to metabolic disorder; whether they are incidental findings cannot be ruled out, but this seems unlikely.

Associated Findings: None known.

Etiology: Autosomal recessive inheritance.

Pathogenesis: Proposed deficiency of specific intestinal membrane transport system for L-methionine.

MIM No.: *25090

Sex Ratio: Presumably M1:F1.

Occurrence: Two or three families reported in the literature, including English and Belgian cases.

Risk of Recurrence for Patient's Sib:
See Part I, *Mendelian Inheritance.*

Risk of Recurrence for Patient's Child:
See Part I, *Mendelian Inheritance.*

Age of Detectability: Presumably at birth.

Gene Mapping and Linkage: Unknown.

Prevention: None known. Genetic counseling indicated.

Treatment: Low methionine intake, e.g., low animal protein or soy protein diet, improves symptoms and EEG.

Prognosis: Unknown.

Detection of Carrier: Evidence for partial intestinal transport defect.

Special Considerations: The Belgian male proband was the youngest of 12 children. Both parents showed partial trait. Smith and Strang's (1958) female infant with "oasthouse" odor had similar appearance and clinical symptoms. Her urine contained α-hydroxybutyric acid, but phenylpyruvic acid was also present, plus many hydroxy-, keto-, and amino acids. She is the only case of "oasthouse urine syndrome" reported to date, but probably similar to a case reported by Hooft et al. (1968).

References:
Jepson JB, et al.: An inborn error of metabolism with urinary excretion of hydroxyacids, ketoacids, and aminoacids (Letter). Lancet 1958; II:1334–1335.
Smith AJ, Strang LB: An inborn error of metabolism with the urinary excretion of alpha-hydroxy-butyric acid and phenylpyruvic acid. Arch Dis Child 1958; 33:109–113.

Hooft C, et al.: Further investigations in the methionine malabsorption syndrome. Helv Paediatr Acta 1968; 23:334–349.

SC050   **Charles R. Scriver**

Methotrexate, fetal effects of
See FETAL AMINOPTERIN SYNDROME

METHYLCOBALAMIN DEFICIENCY   2605

Includes:

Anemia, megaloblastic-homocystinuria
B(12) responsive homocystinuria without methylmalonic
    aciduria
Cobalamin E disease (cb1E)
Cobalamin G disease (cb1G)
Homocystinuria-megaloblastic anemia due to cobalamin
    defect

Excludes:

B(12) responsive homocystinuria with methylmalonic
    aciduria
Cobalamin C disease (cb1C)
Cobalamin D disease (cb1D)
Homocystinuria (0474)
Methylene-tetrahydrofolate reductase deficiency

Major Diagnostic Criteria: Homocystinuria with normal organic acid quantitation, megaloblastic anemia with normal serum B_{12}, folate, and orotic acid levels. Biochemical assay documenting failure of production of methylcobalamin.

Clinical Findings: Feeding difficulties, developmental delay, seizures, megaloblastic anemia, cortical atrophy, and **Microcephaly**.

Complications: Mental retardation, seizure disorders, failure to thrive, infections, cerebral atrophy, and death.

Associated Findings: None known.

Etiology: Autosomal recessive inheritance.

Pathogenesis: Inborn error of metabolism.

MIM No.: *23627

Sex Ratio: Cobalamin E: M5:F0 observed; Cobalamin G: M3:F4 observed.

Occurrence: Twelve cases have been documented in the literature.

Risk of Recurrence for Patient's Sib:
See Part I, *Mendelian Inheritance.*

Risk of Recurrence for Patient's Child:
See Part I, *Mendelian Inheritance.*

Age of Detectability: At birth, or by prenatal diagnosis by measurement of B_{12} distribution and methyl-tetrahydrofolate incorporation in amniocytes.

Gene Mapping and Linkage: Unknown.

Prevention: None known. Genetic counseling indicated.

Treatment: Pharmacologic doses of hydroxycobalamin. Two patients have been maintained with cyanocobalamin, but in others, response to cyanocobalamin has been poor. Methylcobalamin, betaine, and folinic acid have been used. Prenatal treatment of an affected fetus has been reported.

Prognosis: Appears to be good if treatment is begun early. The anemia has been easier to correct than the neurologic manifestations.

Detection of Carrier: Unknown.

Special Considerations: Heterogeneity exists among patients with methylcobalamin deficiency. At present, two complementation groups have been demonstrated. This implies that there are multiple mutations capable of producing methylcobalamin deficiency, which may not be allelic. Methionine synthase has been localized to chromosome 1 using human-hamster hybrids; the relationship to the cb1E and cb1G loci is not clear.

References:

Rosenblatt DS, et al.: Altered vitamin B12 metabolism in fibroblasts from a patient with megaloblastic anemia and homocystinuria due to a new defect in methionine biosynthesis. J Clin Invest 1984; 74:2149–2156.
Schuh S, et al.: Homocystinuria and megaloblastic anemia responsive to vitamin B-12 therapy. New Engl J Med 1984; 310:686–690. *
Rosenblatt DS, et al.: Prenatal vitamin B-12 therapy of a fetus with methylcobalamin deficiency (cobalamin E disease). Lancet 1985; I:1127–1129.
Rosenblatt DS, et al.: Vitamin B-12 responsive homocystinuria and megaloblastic anemia: heterogeneity in methylcobalamin deficiency. Am J Med Genet 1987; 26:377–383.
Tuchman M, et al.: Vitamin B-12 responsive megaloblastic anemia, homocystinuria, and transient methylmalonic aciduria in cb1E disease. J Pediatr 1988; 113:1052–1056.
Watkins D, Rosenblatt DS: Genetic heterogeneity among patients with methylcobalamin deficiency. J Clin Invest 1988; 81:1690–1694. * (cb1G)

FL001   **David B. Flannery**
WA053   **David Watkins**
R0052   **David S. Rosenblatt**

Methylenetetrahydrofolate reductase (MTHFR) deficiency
See HOMOCYSTINURIA, N(5,10) METHYLENE
    TETRAHYDROFOLATE DEFICIENCY TYPE
Methylmalonic acidemia
See ACIDEMIA, METHYLMALONIC
Methylmalonic aciduria
See ACIDEMIA, METHYLMALONIC
Methylmalonic aciduria due to B release defect
See VITAMIN B(12) LYSOSOMAL TRANSPORT DEFECT
Methylmercury, organic, fetal effects of
See FETAL METHYLMERCURY EFFECTS
Mevalonate kinase deficiency
See ACIDEMIA, MEVALONIC
Mevalonic aciduria
See ACIDEMIA, MEVALONIC
Mexican cardiomelic dysplasia
See HEART-HAND SYNDROME IV
Michail-Matsoukas-Theodorou-Rubinstein-Taybi syndrome
See RUBINSTEIN-TAYBI BROAD THUMB-HALLUX SYNDROME
Michel malformation of inner ear
See EAR, LABYRINTH APLASIA

MICHELIN TIRE BABY SYNDROME   2642

Includes:

Skin creases, multiple benign circumferential of the limbs
Skin, generalized folded with an underlying lipomatous
    nevus

Excludes:

Amniotic bands syndrome (0874)
Cutis verticus gyrata (2295)
Deafness-keratopachydermia-digital constrictions (0259)
Disruption complex
Skin, generalized folded in short-limb dwarfism

Major Diagnostic Criteria: Generalized symmetric folding of skin around arms, legs, and trunk without symptoms of strangulation.

Clinical Findings: Multiple benign ring-shaped skin creases on all extremities, fingers, toes, and the trunk without amputations or limb deformities.

Complications: Unknown.

Associated Findings: Findings in only one affected individual each: such minor anomalies as epicanthic folds, upward-slanting palpebral fissures, hypertelorism, median **Cleft palate**, neuroblastoma; micrognathia, malformed ears, ureteroceles; febrile convulsions, slight mental retardation; left hemihypertrophy; and idiopathic scarring of the skin. Underlying lipomatous nevus and a median cleft were observed in two patients.

Etiology: Autosomal dominant inheritance. Heterogeneity may exist.

Pathogenesis: Unknown.

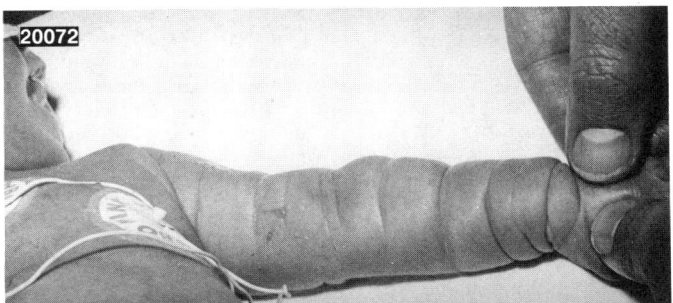

2642-20072: Note the multiple, irregular ring-shaped skin creases on the arm of this 6-day-old infant.

MIM No.: *15661

POS No.: 4404

Sex Ratio: M8:F7 (observed).

Occurrence: Several sibships have been reported. Wiedemann (1987) pointed out that the condition appears in a bronze representation on the door of the cathedral of Hildesheim in northwestern Germany.

Risk of Recurrence for Patient's Sib:
See Part I, *Mendelian Inheritance.*

Risk of Recurrence for Patient's Child:
See Part I, *Mendelian Inheritance.*

Age of Detectability: At birth by physical examination.

Gene Mapping and Linkage: Unknown.

Prevention: None known. Genetic counseling indicated.

Treatment: Unknown.

Prognosis: In all familial cases, the circular skin alterations almost disappeared in later life.

Detection of Carrier: Unknown.

References:
Ross CM: Generalized folded skin with an underlying lipomatous nevus. Arch Dermatol 1969; 100:320–323.
Gardner EW, et al.: Folded skin associated with underlying nevus lipomatous. Arch Dermatol 1979; 115:978–979.
Wallach D, et al.: Naevus musculaire généralisé avec aspect clinique de "Bébé Michelin." Arch Dermatol Venereol 1980; 107:923–927.
Burgdorf WH, et al.: Folded skin with scarring: Michelin tire baby syndrome? J Am Acad Dermatol 1982; 7:90–93.
Kunze J, et al.: A new genetic disorder: autosomal-dominant multiple benign ring-shaped skin creases. Eur J Pediatr 1982; 138:301–303.
Niikawa N, et al.: The "Michelin tire baby" syndrome: an autosomal dominant trait. (Letter) Am J Med Genet 1985; 22:637–638.
Kunze J: The "Michelin tire baby syndrome": an autosomal-dominant trait. Am J Med Genet 1986; 25:169 only.
Niikawa N, et al.: Letter to the editor: response to Dr. Kunze. Am J Med Genet 1986; 25:171 only.
Wiedemann H-R: Multiple benign circumferential skin creases on limbs: a congenital anomaly existing from the begining of mankind. (Letter) Am J Med Genet 1987; 28:225–226.

KU008   **Jürgen Kunze**

Microcephalic primordial dwarfism
See SECKEL SYNDROME
Microcephalic primordial dwarfism, type II
See DWARFISM, OSTEODYSPLASTIC PRIMORDIAL, MAJEWSKI-RANKE TYPE

MICROCEPHALY   0659

Includes: Microencephaly

Excludes:
Congenital diplegia with small head
Cranial sutures, premature closure of
Fetal cytomegalovirus syndrome (0381)
Fetal rubella syndrome (0384)
Fetal toxoplasmosis syndrome (0387)
Microcephaly, autosomal recessive with normal intelligence (2838)
Microcephaly, isolated autosomal dominant type (2334)
Microcephaly (other)
Relative microcephaly associated with cerebral lesions of infancy

Major Diagnostic Criteria: Head circumference is very small; in infancy, normal open sutures are seen on X-ray. Mental retardation is usually present.

Clinical Findings: A heterogeneous state in which head circumference is smaller than 2 SD below the mean for age. A narrow, sloping forehead, often with a flat occiput. Varying degrees of mental retardation occur, although severe amentia is the most common. In infancy, X-rays show that the cranial sutures are open. Skull thickness may be normal or increased. EEG is frequently normal. Seizures are present in a small percentage of affected individuals. Care must be taken to distinguish microcephaly secondary to degenerative brain disorders from microcephaly as a primary inherited disorder.

Complications: Mental retardation.

Associated Findings: Cataracts, short stature.

Etiology: Usually autosomal recessive inheritance. This condition may follow a degenerative brain disorder, birth trauma, intrauterine infection, or exposure to X-rays in utero. Rarely, autosomal dominant inheritance is reported (see **Microcephaly, isolated autosomal dominant type**).

Pathogenesis: Microcephaly is the result of failure of normal growth of the brain. The brain may show various abnormalities of sulcation and gyration, or an essentially normal pattern.

MIM No.: *25120

POS No.: 3301

CDC No.: 742.100

Sex Ratio: Presumably M1:F1

Occurrence: 1:250,000 based on Netherlands studies.

Risk of Recurrence for Patient's Sib:
See Part I, *Mendelian Inheritance.*

Risk of Recurrence for Patient's Child:
See Part I, *Mendelian Inheritance.*

Age of Detectability: In infancy. Ultrasound shows abnormal fetal head growth rate, fetal chest and abdominal diameters greater than biparietal diameter, biparietal diameter and head area greater than 3 SD below mean, no midline fetal brain echo, oligohydramnios.

Gene Mapping and Linkage: Unknown.

Prevention: None known. Genetic counseling indicated.

Treatment: Unknown.

Prognosis: Varies with degree of mental retardation.

Detection of Carrier: Unknown.

The author wishes to thank Kenneth Shulman for his contribution to a previous version of this article.

References:
Cowie V: The genetics and sub-classification of microcephaly. J Ment Defic Res 1960; 4:42–47.
Qazi QH, Reed TE: A possible major contribution to mental retardation in the general population by the gene for microcephaly. Clin Genet 1975; 7:85.

Haslam RHA, Smith DW: Autosomal dominant microcephaly. J Pediatr 1979; 95:701–705.
Ramirez ML, et al.: Silent microcephaly. Clin Genet 1983; 23:281–286.
Tolmie JL, et al.: Microcephaly: genetic counseling and antenatal diagnosis after the birth of an affected child. Am J Med Genet 1987; 27:583–594.

SH007   **Kenneth Shapiro**

MICROCEPHALY WITH CHORIORETINOPATHY   **2333**

Includes:
Chorioretinopathy-congenital microcephaly
Pseudotoxoplasmosis syndrome

Excludes:
Craniosynostosis (0230)
Fetal cytomegalovirus syndrome (0381)
Fetal rubella syndrome (0384)
Fetal toxoplasmosis syndrome (0387)
Microcephaly (0659)
Microcephaly, in other syndromes
Relative microcephaly associated with cerebral lesions of infancy

Major Diagnostic Criteria: Congenital microcephaly and chorioretinal degeneration.

Clinical Findings: Congenital microcephaly; chorioretinal dysplasia with retinal pigmentation and a progressive visual deficiency evident during childhood; choroidal and optic atrophy; embryonic remnants, pale optic disks, and cataracts sometimes with microphthalmia; nystagmus; delayed psychomotor development; and variable degrees of mental deficiency. Normal intelligence is also found in affected individuals.

X-ray studies show that all the cranial diameters are diminished. There may be craniofacial disproportion without calcifications or closed sutures. The EEG suggests encephalodysplasia. Serologic studies for toxoplasmosis, rubella, cytomegalovirus, and herpes infection are negative.

This is a distinct microcephaly consistently accompanied by chorioretinal dysplasia. There is widely variable expressivity in patients with the autosomal dominant form ranging from normocephaly to microcephaly, from normal eyes to chorioretinal dysplasia, and from normal intelligence to mental retardation.

Complications: Decreased visual acuity. Mental retardation probably due to microcephaly.

Associated Findings: In the autosomal recessive form, early nanosomy, **Cutis marmorata**, nystagmus, and severe neurologic problems can also be found. Embryonic remnants, mainly persistence of primary vitreous, may be present in both autosomal dominant and recessive forms.

Etiology: Autosomal dominant or autosomal recessive inheritance.

Pathogenesis: Unknown.

MIM No.: 15659, *25127

POS No.: 3240

Sex Ratio: M1:F1

Occurrence: Reported in eight kinships and a Mennonite sect.

Risk of Recurrence for Patient's Sib:
See Part I, *Mendelian Inheritance.*

Risk of Recurrence for Patient's Child:
See Part I, *Mendelian Inheritance.*

Age of Detectability: At birth.

Gene Mapping and Linkage: Unknown.

Prevention: None known. Genetic counseling indicated. Given the similarity between chorioretinopathy and toxoplasmosis, at-risk individuals should be managed with care (Daffos et al, 1988).

Treatment: Surgery, as needed, for ophthalmologic abnormalities.

Prognosis: Normal life span.

Detection of Carrier: Unknown.

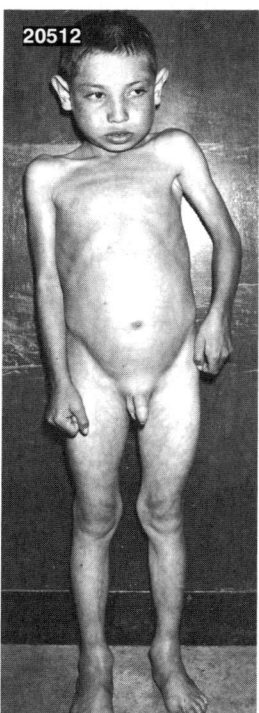

2333-20512: Note microcephaly, short stature, cutis marmorata in this boy with chorioretinal degeneration.

References:
McKusick VA, et al.: Chorioretinopathy with hereditary microcephaly. Arch Ophthalmol 1966; 75:597–600. †
Schmidt B, et al.: Ein mikrozephalie-syndrom mit atypischer tapetoretinaler Degeneration bei 3 Geschwister. Klin Mbnatsbl Augenheilkd 1968; 150:188–196.
Cantú JM, et al.: Autosomal recessive microcephaly associated with chorioretinopathy. Hum Genet 1977; 36:243–247. *
Alzial C, et al.: Microcephalie ''vraie'' avec dysplasie chorioétinienne a hérédite dominante. Ann Genet (Paris) 1980; 23:91–94. * †
Tenconi R, et al.: Chorio-retinal dysplasia, microcephaly and mental retardation: an autosomal dominant syndrome. Clin Genet 1981; 20:347–351.
Parke JT, et al.: A syndrome of microcephaly and retinal pigmentary abnormalities without mental retardation in a family with coincidental autosomal dominant hyperreflexia. Am J Med Genet 1984; 17:585–594.
Daffos F, et al.: Prenatal management of 746 pregnancies at risk for congenital toxoplasmosis. New Engl J Med 1988; 318:271–275.

CR023   **Diana García-Cruz**
CA011   **José María Cantú**

Microcephaly without mental retardation
See MICROCEPHALY, ISOLATED AUTOSOMAL DOMINANT TYPE

MICROCEPHALY, AUTOSOMAL RECESSIVE WITH NORMAL INTELLIGENCE   2838

Includes: Microcephaly, nonsyndromal with normal intelligence

Excludes:
> **Chromosome instability, Nijmegen type** (2551)
> **Dwarfism, microcephalic primordial with cataracts** (2584)
> **Microcephaly** (0659)
> Microcephaly, familial with normal intelligence
> **Microcephaly, isolated autosomal dominant type** (2334)
> **Seckel syndrome** (0881)

Major Diagnostic Criteria: **Microcephaly** significantly below the third percentile for age, peculiar facies, normal stature or stature at the lower limit of normal, and normal psychomotor development and intelligence.

Clinical Findings: At birth, head circumference is small (between 30 and 32 cm) but with normal length and body weight. Affected persons show a low receding forehead with normal scalp hair, unlike patients with autosomal recessive "true" microcephaly, whose foreheads incline acutely and scalp may be excessively furrowed. Facial features also include prominent eyes with an upward slant, epicanthic folds, long and straight nose, high nasal bridge, widely spaced teeth with or without malocclusion, and receding chin. Affected individuals often reach normal developmental milestones with no clinical evidence of immunodeficiency. There is no neurologic deficit. Data indicate that none had mental retardation, often with fairly good scholastic performance but were not "clever" compared to their normal sibs. Only one had borderline intelligence.

Interfamilial variability is minimal. Careful examination of parents is essential to rule out the possibility of **Microcephaly, isolated autosomal dominant type**. The condition must be distinguished from that with immunodeficiency and risk for lymphoreticular malignancies (see **Chromosome instability, Nijmegen type**). In both of these conditions, the facies are similar.

Complications: Affected individuals are usually "shy" and lack self-confidence. A sporadic case 1 1/2 years of age was hyperactive.

Associated Findings: None known.

Etiology: Probably autosomal recessive inheritance. All known sibships with affected individuals have consanguineous parents.

Pathogenesis: Unknown.

MIM No.: *25126

Sex Ratio: Presumably M1:F1; M2:F1 observed.

Occurrence: Ten cases have been reported; a kindred with eight affected individuals, and two sporadic cases.

Risk of Recurrence for Patient's Sib:
> See Part I, *Mendelian Inheritance*. Observed frequency is 30 percent.

Risk of Recurrence for Patient's Child:
> See Part I, *Mendelian Inheritance*.

Age of Detectability: Usually clinically evident at birth. Confirmation by age 1–2 years when adequate intelligence testing can be performed. IQ is around 100.

Gene Mapping and Linkage: Unknown.

Prevention: None known. Genetic counseling indicated.

Treatment: Assurance of patients and parents of this condition's benign nature. Special attention to those with borderline intelligence.

Prognosis: Out of ten patients reported, two died in early life during the early 1970s in areas with limited medical care, one with postmeasles bronchopneumonia and the other with leukemia. Two patients lived for 60 and 65 years and had normal reproductive lives. No physical handicaps. In general, life span and function are probably normal.

Detection of Carrier: Unknown.

Special Considerations: Though allelism is not exluded between this entity and **Chromosome instability, Nijmegen type**, genetic heterogeneity remains a possibility in the patients with microcephaly and normal intelligence in general, which includes in addition to these two autosomal recessive types, **Microcephaly, isolated autosomal dominant type** and **Seckel syndrome**.

References:
Teebi AS, et al.: Autosomal recessive nonsyndromal microcephaly with normal intelligence. Am J Med Genet 1987; 26:355–359.

TE012   **Ahmad S. Teebi**

MICROCEPHALY, ISOLATED AUTOSOMAL DOMINANT TYPE   2334

Includes:
> Microcephaly without mental retardation
> Silent microcephaly

Excludes:
> Microcephaly with mental retardation
> Microcephaly, all other forms
> "True" microcephaly

Major Diagnostic Criteria: A cephalic circumference below the third percentile or 2 SD below the mean for the corresponding age and sex, with normal skull by X-ray studies, and average intelligence.

Clinical Findings: Microcephaly as the sole trait can be recognized by the occipitofrontoal circumference (OFC) below the third percentile. The facies are not dysmorphic and are proportional to the small head. Normal stature, behavior, and scholastic performance are the rule. Neurologic and psychometric evaluations, and X-rays of the skull, are also normal.

Complications: Unknown.

Associated Findings: Short stature was reported in a Black family (Burton, 1981).

Etiology: Autosomal dominant inheritance.

Pathogenesis: Unknown.

MIM No.: *15658

POS No.: 3600

Sex Ratio: M1:F2 (observed).

Occurrence: Over a dozen kinships have been documented, including several Italian families and at least one Black family.

Risk of Recurrence for Patient's Sib:
> See Part I, *Mendelian Inheritance*.

Risk of Recurrence for Patient's Child:
> See Part I, *Mendelian Inheritance*.

Age of Detectability: Usually at birth.

Gene Mapping and Linkage: Unknown.

Prevention: None known. Genetic counseling indicated.

Treatment: Unknown.

Prognosis: Good for life span and intelligence.

Detection of Carrier: Unknown.

References:
Burton BK: Dominant inheritance of microcephaly with short stature. Clin Genet 1981; 20:25–27.
Ramírez ML, et al.: Silent microcephaly: a distinct autosomal dominant trait. Clin Genet 1983; 23:281–286.
Rossi LN, et al.: Autosomal dominant microcephaly without mental retardation. Am J Dis Child 1987; 141:655–659.

RA021   **Maria Lourdes Ramírez**
CA011   **José María Cantú**

Microcephaly, nonsyndromal with normal intelligence
> *See MICROCEPHALY, AUTOSOMAL RECESSIVE WITH NORMAL INTELLIGENCE*

Microcephaly, X-linked
> *See X-LINKED MENTAL RETARDATION-GROWTH-HEARING AND GENITAL DEFECTS*

Microcephaly-albinism-digital defects
See ALBINISM-MICROCEPHALY-DIGITAL DEFECTS
Microcephaly-branchial arch, X-linked
See BRANCHIAL ARCH SYNDROME, X-LINKED
Microcephaly-chemotactic defect-transient hypogammaglobulinemia
See MICROCEPHALY-RETARDATION-SKELETAL AND IMMUNE DEFECTS
Microcephaly-growth/mental retardation-unusual facies-cleft palate
See WEAVER-WILLIAMS SYNDROME

MICROCEPHALY-HIATUS HERNIA-NEPHROSIS, GALLOWAY TYPE 2755

Includes:
> Galloway syndrome
> Hiatus hernia-microcephaly-nephrosis, Galloway type
> Nephrosis-microcephaly-hiatus hernia, Galloway type

Excludes:
> **Hernia, hiatal** (0471)
> **Microcephaly** (0659)
> **Nephrosis, congenital** (0709)
> **Nephrosis, familial type** (0710)

Major Diagnostic Criteria: **Microcephaly** is evident at birth. **Hernia, hiatal** may be suspected because of recurrent vomiting, and confirmed by X-ray studies. Nephrotic syndrome appears within a few days to two years after birth.

Clinical Findings: Pregnancies were uneventful, and birth weights ranged between 2,240 and 3,100 g. Striking **Microcephaly** was observed at birth associated with a peculiarly shaped head with narrow and receding forehead, flat occiput, and flat vertex. Head size grew very little with age. Skull X-rays showed asymmetry and secondary craniosynostosis but no calcifications. Neurologic observations included poor head control; marked generalized hypotonia; lack of interest in surroundings; nonexistence of purposeful movements of eyes, hands, and feet; absence of any motor development even at age three years; and profound psychomotor retardation. Neck retraction episodes and seizures were common.

Recurrent and sometimes projectile vomiting episodes began very early, leading to suspicion of hiatus hernia, which was confirmed by contrast X-ray studies in three of five patients.

Proteinuria associated with microscopic hematuria was noted as early as the first week of life in two patients, but was delayed until age two years in one. These findings, along with periorbital and dependent edema, hypoalbuminemia, and anemia were consistent with the diagnosis of the nephrotic syndrome. There was no associated aminoaciduria.

Autopsy information is available on three of five patients reported to date. Brain weights were considerably smaller than that expected for age. In one patient microscopic studies showed lack of cortical stratification, hypomyelination of the brainstem and the spinal cord, complete absence of the internal granular layer of the cerebellum and dentate gyrus within the hippocampal formation, and hypoplasia of the olivary nuclei. Kidneys were large; histologic observations included hypercellularity, microcystic dysplasia, and focal glomerulosclerosis. In one patient the biopsy findings were interpreted as being similar to those observed in the "Finnish-type" nephrotic syndrome. Hiatus hernia was not seen at autopsy in two patients, although it had been demonstrated premortem by X-ray.

Complications: Severe psychomotor retardation, hypotonia, failure to thrive, massive edema, hypoalbuminemia, and early death due to renal failure.

Associated Findings: Large floppy ears (low and posteriorly set), micrognathia, high-arched palate, **Eye, hypertelorism**, calcifications in intervertebral disk, failure of cleavage of anterior chamber of the eye, and optic atrophy.

Etiology: Autosomal recessive inheritance.

Pathogenesis: Unknown.

MIM No.: *25130

POS No.: 3985

Sex Ratio: M1:F1

Occurrence: Five patients have been reported in three families; two Caucasian and one Black American.

Risk of Recurrence for Patient's Sib:
See Part I, *Mendelian Inheritance.*

Risk of Recurrence for Patient's Child:
See Part I, *Mendelian Inheritance.* Affected individuals are not expected to survive to reproduce.

Age of Detectability: Of the three obligatory features of the syndrome, small head with peculiar shape is readily evident at birth. Hiatus hernia may be suspected in the first weeks because of recurrent vomiting. Onset of nephrosis may be delayed for several months.

Gene Mapping and Linkage: Unknown.

Prevention: None known. Genetic counseling indicated.

Treatment: Supportive for seizures and nephrotic syndrome. The hiatus hernia could be treated surgically.

Prognosis: All reported patients have died between ages two weeks and three years. Severe psychomotor retardation is the rule.

Detection of Carrier: Unknown.

References:
Galloway WH, Mowat AP: Congenital microcephaly with hiatus hernia and nephrotic syndrome in two sibs. J Med Genet 1968; 5:319–321. *
Shapiro LR, et al.: Congenital microcephaly, hiatus hernia and nephrotic syndrome: an autosomal recessive syndrome. BD:OAS XII(5). New York: March of Dimes Birth Defects Foundation, 1976; 275–278. †
Qazi QH, et al.: Galloway syndrome in a black infant. Pediatr Res 1985; 19:252A.
Roos RAC, et al.: Congenital microcephaly, infantile spasms, psychomotor retardation, and nephrotic syndrome in two sibs. Europ J Pediat 1987; 146:532–536.
Kozlowski PB, et al.: Brain morphology in the Galloway syndrome. Clin Neuropathol 1989; 8:85–91.

QA000   **Qutub H. Qazi**

Microcephaly-immunodeficiency-lymphoreticular malignancy
See CHROMOSOME INSTABILITY, NIJMEGEN TYPE

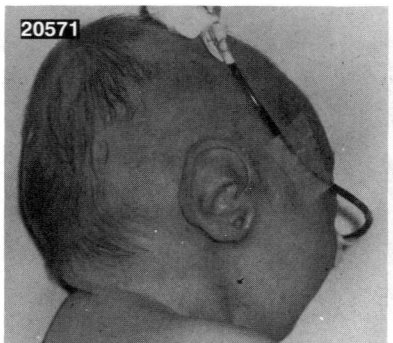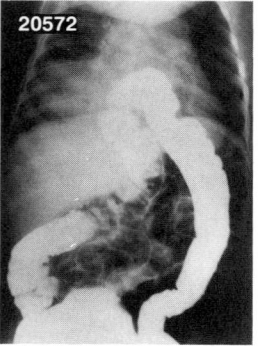

2755-20571: Large floppy ears and microcephaly. 20572: Hiatal hernia of the colon.

MICROCEPHALY-LYMPHEDEMA 2639

Includes:
Leung syndrome
Lymphedema-microcephaly

Excludes:
Distichiasis-lymphedema syndrome (2039)
Fabry disease (0373)
Lymphedema I (0614)
Microcephaly (0659)

Major Diagnostic Criteria: The combination of congenital **Microcephaly** and **Lymphedema** of the lower limbs in the absence of other findings.

Clinical Findings: Affected individuals have congenital **Microcephaly** (OC ≥2 SD below the mean) and congenital lymphedema of the lower limbs. The lymphedema apparently disappears with age, although the propositus in one reported family still had pitting edema of the feet at age one year, and an affected individual in another family had intermittent swelling of feet and legs his entire life. Minor facial anomalies, including epicanthal folds, flat nasal bridge, micrognathia, and prominent ear helix can also be present. These minor anomalies have been termed the "congenital lymphedema face" by Opitz (1986).

Complications: Unknown.

Associated Findings: None known.

Etiology: Probably autosomal dominant inheritance.

Pathogenesis: Unknown.

MIM No.: *15295

POS No.: 3754

Sex Ratio: M1:F1

Occurrence: Four generations of one Canadian family of Chinese ethnic origin, and at least two members of a second family, have been reported.

Risk of Recurrence for Patient's Sib:
See Part I, *Mendelian Inheritance.*

Risk of Recurrence for Patient's Child:
See Part I, *Mendelian Inheritance.*

Age of Detectability: At birth, although prenatal diagnosis by ultrasound may be possible.

Gene Mapping and Linkage: Unknown.

Prevention: None known. Genetic counseling indicated.

Treatment: Unknown.

Prognosis: Life span and intellect are not affected.

Detection of Carrier: Unknown.

References:
Leung AKC: Dominantly inherited syndrome of microcephaly and congenital lymphedema. Clin Genet 1985; 27:611–612.
Crowe CA, Dickerman LH: A genetic association between microcephaly and lymphedema. Am J Med Genet 1986; 24:131–135.
Opitz JM: On congenital lymphedema. (Editorial) Am J Med Genet 1986; 24:127–129.
Leung AKC: Dominantly inherited syndrome of microcephaly and congenital lymphedema with normal intelligence. (Letter) Am J Med Genet 1987; 26:231 only.

T0007   **Helga V. Toriello**

Microcephaly-lymphedema-normal intelligence
See LYMPHEDEMA I
Microcephaly-mental retardation-retinopathy
See RETINOPATHY-MICROCEPHALY-MENTAL RETARDATION
Microcephaly-microphthalmia-falciform retinal folds
See RETINAL FOLD
Microcephaly-multiple congenital anomalies
See CEREBRO-OCULO-FACIO-SKELETAL SYNDROME
Microcephaly-nephrosis-hiatal hernia
See NEPHROSIS-HYDROCEPHALUS-THIN SKIN-BLUE SCLERA-GROWTH DEFECT

MICROCEPHALY-RETARDATION-SKELETAL AND IMMUNE DEFECTS 3131

Includes:
Immunodeficiency-microencephaly-retardation-skeletal defects
Microcephaly-chemotactic defect-transient hypogammaglobulinemia
Say-Barber-Miller syndrome

Excludes:
Dwarfism, osteodysplastic primordial, Majewski-Ranke type (2582)
Dwarfism, osteodysplastic primordial, Majewski-Winter type (2581)

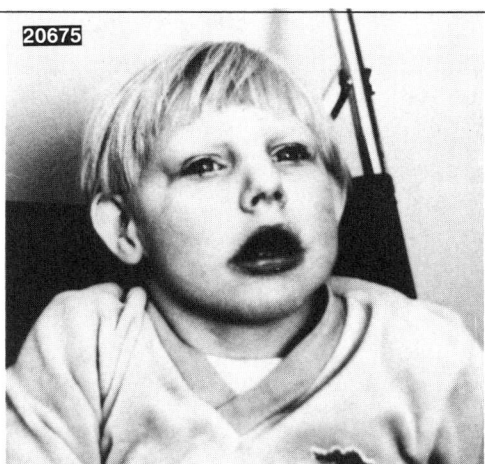

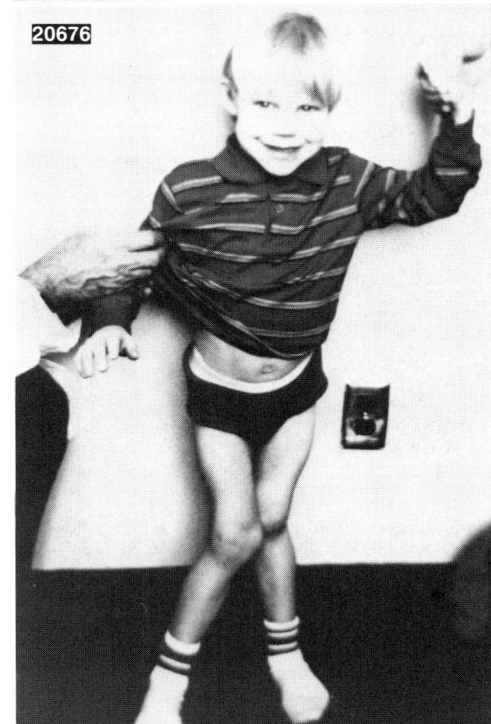

3131-20675: Microcephaly-retardation-skeletal and immune defects; note affected proband at 6 years of age. Craniofacial features include sloping forehead, prominent beaked nose, prominent ears, and micrognathia. 20676: Affected sib at age 4 years; note similar craniofacial features, dislocated hip, and decreased subcutaneous fat. Both boys had retinitis pigmentosa.

Immunodeficiency, thymic agenesis (0943)
Oculo-mandibulo-facial syndrome (0738)
Seckel syndrome (0881)

Major Diagnostic Criteria: The combination of hypogammaglobulinemia, **Microcephaly**, growth delay, skeletal anomalies, and hypogenitalism.

Clinical Findings: The reported affected sibs both had normal birth weights, with postnatal growth deficiency. Craniofacial features included **Microcephaly**, sloping forehead, prominent beaked nose with a high nasal bridge, highly arched palate, micrognathia, and large protruding ears. Other anomalies included small genitalia, scoliosis, hypoplastic patellae, decreased subcutaneous fat. Frequent respiratory infections and eczema affected both boys. Immune deficiency was characterized by transient hypogammaglobulinemia, with defective chemotaxis. Mental retardation was severe in the older boy and mild in the younger boy.

Complications: Frequent respiratory infections, herpes, eczema, and otitis media secondary to the immune defect.

Associated Findings: In one of the children, craniosynostosis of the left coronal suture, posterior aspect of the sagittal sutures, hypodontia, anal stenosis, and hip dislocation.

Etiology: Presumbably either autosomal or X-linked recessive inheritance.

Pathogenesis: Unknown.

MIM No.: 25124

POS No.: 3899

Sex Ratio: M2:F0 observed.

Occurrence: One family with two affected male sibs has been reported.

Risk of Recurrence for Patient's Sib:
See Part I, *Mendelian Inheritance.*

Risk of Recurrence for Patient's Child:
See Part I, *Mendelian Inheritance.*

Age of Detectability: At birth, by physical examination.

Gene Mapping and Linkage: Unknown.

Prevention: None known. Genetic counseling indicated.

Treatment: Symptomatic.

Prognosis: Mental retardation is progressive in that development becomes more delayed over time. Life span is undetermined; the oldest boy was aged 6.5 years at the time of the last report.

Detection of Carrier: Unknown.

References:
Say B, et al.: Microcephaly, short stature, and developmental delay associated with a chemotactic defect and transient hypogammaglobulinemia in two brothers. J Med Gent 1986; 23:355–359.

T0007 **Helga V. Toriello**

Microcephaly-syndactyly-mental retardation, Filippi type
See SYNDACTYLY-MICROCEPHALY-MENTAL RETARDATION, FILIPPI TYPE
Microcephaly-vitreoretinal dysplasia
See NORRIE DISEASE
Microcornea-cataract
See CATARACT-MICROCORNEA SYNDROME
Microcystic disease of the renal medulla
See KIDNEY, NEPHRONOPHTHISIS-MEDULLARY CYSTIC DESEASE
Microcystic dystrophy
See CORNEAL DYSTROPHY, RECURRENT EROSIVE
Microcystic renal disease
See NEPHROSIS, CONGENITAL
Microcythemia
See THALASSEMIA
Microdontia
See TEETH, MICRODONTIA

Microdontia, generalized
See TEETH, AMELOGENESIS IMPERFECTA
Microencephaly
See MICROCEPHALY
Microepiphyseal dysplasia
See EPIPHYSEAL DYSPLASIA, MULTIPLE RIBBING TYPE
Microgastria
See STOMACH, HYPOPLASIA
Micrognathia-cleidocranial dysplasia
See YUNIS-VARON SYNDROME
Micrognathia-glossoptosis-cleft palate
See CLEFT PALATE-MICROGNATHIA-GLOSSOPTOSIS
Micrognathia-limb deficiency-splenogonadal fusion
See SPLENOGONADAL FUSION-LIMB DEFECT
Microgyria
See BRAIN, MICROPOLYGYRIA
Micromelia
See LIMB REDUCTION DEFECTS
Micromelia (lethal)-spondylocostal dysostosis-skeletal anomalies
See SPONDYLOCOSTAL DYSOSTOSIS-VISCERAL DEFECTS-DANDY WALKER CYST
Micromesomelia, Campailla-Martinelli
See ACROMESOMELIC DYSPLASIA, CAMPAILLA-MARTINELLI TYPE
Micropenis, isolated
See ANDROGEN INSENSITIVITY (RESISTANCE), MINIMAL
Microphakia and spherophakia, congenital
See LENS, MICROSPHEROPHAKIA
Microphthalmia with associated anomalies
See LENZ MICROPHTHALMIA SYNDROME
Microphthalmia, colobomatous isolated
See EYE, MICROPHTHALMIA/COLOBOMA
Microphthalmia-cataract
See CATARACT, POLAR AND CAPSULAR
Microphthalmia-gingival fibromatosis-depigmentation
See GINGIVAL FIBROMATOSIS-DEPIGMENTATION-MICROPHTHALMIA
Microplasmin
See PLASMINOGEN DEFECTS
Micropolygyria
See BRAIN, MICROPOLYGYRIA
Micropolygyria-muscular dystrophy
See MUSCULAR DYSTROPHY, CONGENITAL WITH MENTAL RETARDATION
Microspherophakia
See LENS, MICROSPHEROPHAKIA
Microstomia-agnathia-synotia
See AGNATHIA-MICROSTOMIA-SYNOTIA
Microtia from exposure to retinoids
See FETAL RETINOID SYNDROME
Microtia-atresia
See EAR, MICROTIA-ATRESIA
Microtia-facial clefting-hypertelorism
See HYPERTELORISM-MICROTIA-FACIAL CLEFT-CONDUCTIVE DEAFNESS
Microtia-meatal atresia-conductive deafness
See EAR, MICROTIA-ATRESIA
Microvillus atrophy, congenital
See MICROVILLUS INCLUSION DISEASE

MICROVILLUS INCLUSION DISEASE 3222

Includes:
Brush border, congenital disorganization of
Diarrhea with hypoplastic microvillus atrophy
Davidson disease
Enteropathy, familial
Microvillus atrophy, congenital

Excludes:
Autoimmune enteropathies and hypersensitivity
Diarrhea, congenital chloride (0148)
Enteropathy, infectious or post-infectious

Major Diagnostic Criteria: Typically, severe secretory diarrhea in these infants begins shortly after birth, no later than one week of age.
The initial small bowel biopsy shows hypoplastic microvillus atrophy with abnormal surface enterocytes lacking brush border definition and showing vacuolation of apical cytoplasm. Transmission electron microscopy (essential for confirmation of diagno-

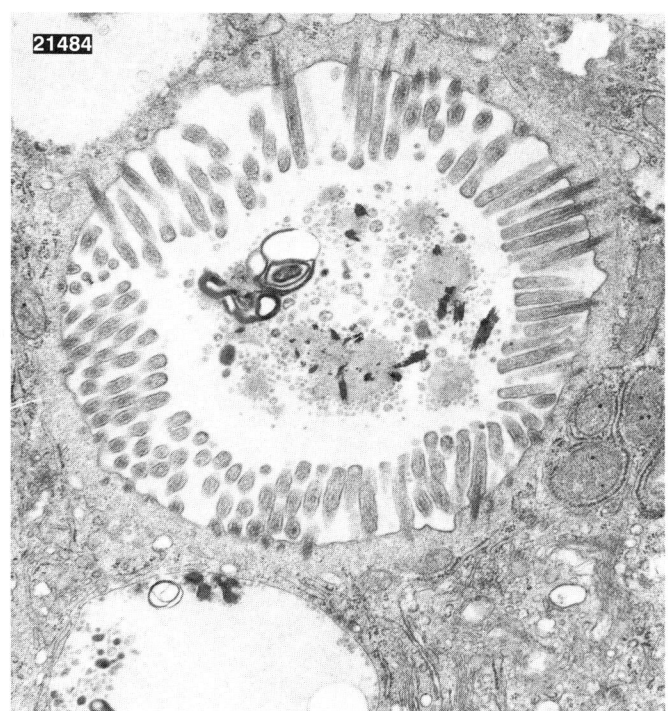

3222-21484: Electron microscopic appearance of small bowel enterocyte in microvillus inclusion disease. Microvillus inclusion with inwardly facing brush border microvilli. Core filaments and the terminal web appear to be well developed. The lumen of the inclusion has an aggregate of small vesicles, patches of moderately electron-dense floccular material, and myelin-like figures.

sis) shows a combination of the following three diagnostic features, confined mainly to the surface enterocytes: 1) absent or sparse and disorganized microvilli on apical membrane; 2) intracytoplasmic, cyst-like inclusions ("microvillus inclusions") enclosed by well-formed brush border microvilli (microvillus inclusions are seen only in some cells); and 3) numerous pleomorphic vesicular inclusion bodies, lined by a single limiting membrane, which may sometimes show an occasional microvillus, and containing floccular to homogeneous material of moderate to high electron density. The inclusions do not appear to be phagosomes, as originally proposed, because they are bound by only one membrane (that of the brush border) and because acid phosphatase, a lysosomal marker, has not been localized in larger vesicular bodies or microvillus inclusions.

Rectal (colonic) biopsies appear normal by light microscopy, but on electron microscopy the apical cytoplasm of proximal colonocytes contains microvillus inclusions similar to those in the small intestine as well as numerous clear vesicular bodies.

Clinical Findings: Severe watery diarrhea with stool volumes usually more than 80 ml/kg/d beginning during the first week of life results from impaired absorption across the enterocyte brush border. Stools are similar in electrolyte composition to normal small intestinal juice (Na > 75 mM, K < 30 mM). Affected infants tolerate less than 10 cal/kg/day of enteral feeding.

The small intestine of all patients shows diffuse villus atrophy, crypt hypoplasia, and normal or decreased numbers of inflammatory cells in the lamina propria. An abnormal distribution of periodic acid-schiff positive material in in apical cytoplasm of proximal enterocytes is in contrast to normal PAS staining which is confined to the brush border membrane (glycocalyx). Several lines of evidence suggest that this material represents intracytoplasmic sequestration of glycocalyx material.

Electron microscopy confirms the lack of well formed brush border microvilli and provides further evidence that microvillus

inclusions are unlikely to form by surface invaginations of apical membrane. The most severe ultrastructural changes are confined to proximal (most mature) enterocytes; mid and upper crypt cells may show early changes, whereas immature crypt cells, goblet, Paneth and enteroendocrine cells show no abnormalities. A similar pattern of cellular involvement is observed in colonic (rectal) mucosa.

Complications: Severe dehydration and acidosis result from fluid and electrolyte loss. Malnutrition is usually responsive only to total parenteral nutrition, which can be complicated by catheter-related septicemia and hepatobiliary disease. Growth delay is also a problem.

Associated Findings: None known. Maternal polyhydramnios is not usually observed.

Etiology: Four families have now been described in which more than one sibling was affected. Sex of the affected siblings has been different. Because the disease is lethal, the pattern conforms best to autosomal recessive inheritance.

Pathogenesis: The possible pathogenic mechanisms proposed include: 1) a defect in crypt cell maturation; 2) a disorder of cytoskeletal proteins, namely myosin; and 3) an inborn error of intracellular vesicular transport leading to abnormal assembly of the microvillus membrane on the inner surface of intracytoplasmic vesicles rather than at the apical cell surface. Similar aberrant assembly of the brush border has been induced in experimental models in rodents by administration of colchicine or in human fetal intestinal organ cultures by adding cytochalasin.

Sex Ratio: Presumably M1:F1.

Occurrence: A total of 15 infants with this condition have been described. During a six year period at a large children's hospital, of the eight infants diagnosed with severe congenital watery diarrhea, six had microvillus inclusion disease. Patients with this condition have now been described in Canada, Great Britain, France, and the United States. Some patients reported were originally from the Middle East (Lebanon, Eqypt).

Risk of Recurrence for Patient's Sib:
See Part I, *Mendelian Inheritance.*

Risk of Recurrence for Patient's Child:
See Part I, *Mendelian Inheritance.*

Age of Detectability: Days 1–3 of life, on rectal biopsy examined by electron microscopy.

Gene Mapping and Linkage: Unknown.

Prevention: None known. Genetic counseling indicated.

Treatment: Typically, massive amounts of intravenous electrolytes are required for replacement (e.g., Na, 25 mEq/kg/day). Total parenteral nutrition is required. Attempts to stimulate small bowel growth with human colostrum, glucocorticoids, pentagastrin, and epidermal growth factor have not been successful. In one patient, a reduction in stool output from 250 to 180 ml/kg/day occurred in response to twice-daily injections of the long-acting somatostatin analogue octreotide. Subtotal enterectomy to alleviate and stabilize the massive fluid losses has not been tried. Multiorgan transplant including liver and bowel in one patient was not successful (R. Jaffe, personal communication).

Prognosis: All patients described to date except one have died before their second birthday.

Detection of Carrier: Unknown.

Special Considerations: Heterogeneity may exist. A single patient, presenting after two months of life with microvillus inclusions in small intestinal and rectal biopsies, experienced a milder clinical course (Carruthers et al, 1986).

References:
Davidson GP, et al.: Familial enteropathy: a syndrome of protracted diarrhea from birth, failure to thrive, and hypoplastic villus atrophy. Gastroenterology 1978; 75:783–790. *
Phillips AD, et al.: Congenital microvillous atrophy: specific diagnostic features. Arch Dis Child 1985; 60:135–140. †
Carruthers L, et al.: Disorders of the cytoskeleton of the enterocyte. Clinics in Gastroenterology 1986; 15:105–120. * †

Drumm B, et al.: Urogastrone/epidermal growth factor in treatment of congenital microvillous atrophy. Lancet 1988; I:111–112.

Lake BD, et al.: Microvillus inclusion disease: specific diagnostoc features shown by alkaline phosphatase histochemistry. J Clin Pathol 1988; 41:880–882.

Cutz E, et al.: Microvillus inclusion disease: an inherited defect of brush-border assembly and differentiation. New Engl J Med 1989; 320:646–651. * †

RH005
CU015

J. Marc Rhoads
Ernest Cutz

Middle ear aneurysm of internal carotid artery
See EAR, ANEURYSM OF INTERNAL CAROTID ARTERY
Middle ear malformations with hearing loss
See EAR, OSSICLE AND MIDDLE EAR MALFORMATIONS
Midface retraction-X-ray and renal anomalies-hypertrichosis
See SCHINZEL-GIEDION SYNDROME
Midfrequency nerve loss, hereditary
See DEAFNESS (SENSORINEURAL), MIDFREQUENCY
Midfrequency sensorineural deafness
See DEAFNESS (SENSORINEURAL), MIDFREQUENCY
Midline defects
See SCHISIS ASSOCIATION
Midline diastema
See TEETH, DIASTEMA, MEDIAN INCISAL
Midline maxillary double lip
See LIP, DOUBLE
Midsystolic click-late systolic murmur syndrome
See MITRAL VALVE PROLAPSE
Miescher elastoma
See SKIN, ELASTOSIS PERFORANS SERPIGINOSA
Miescher syndrome
See LIPODYSTROPHY-COARSE FACIES-ACANTHOSIS NIGRICANS, MIESCHER TYPE

MIETENS-WEBER SYNDROME   2013

Includes: Mental retardation syndrome, Mietens-Weber type

Excludes:
> Arachnodactyly, contractural Beals type (0085)
> Arthrogryposes (0088)

Major Diagnostic Criteria: The combination of mental retardation, eye findings (e.g., corneal opacity, nystagmus), and upper limb anomalies (flexion contractures of the elbow, short radius, and ulna).

Clinical Findings: The clinical findings in the six reported cases were corneal opacity (6); nystagmus, horizontal and rotational (6); strabismus (6); small, pointed nose (6); short radius and ulna with elongated humerus (6); flexion contractures of the elbows (6); pes valgus planus (5); short stature (5); mental retardation (IQ 70–80) (6); and clinodactyly (4).

Anomalies noted on X-ray include dislocated radial head (5), absence of epiphysis of the radial head (3), and hypoplastic upper third of the radius (1).

The growth failure seems to be progressive, in that the youngest child had a normal length at five months of age. The corneal opacities and elbow contractures are likely congenital.

Complications: Blindness secondary to corneal opacity.

Associated Findings: Low birth weight, microphthalmia, hip dislocation, and small testes were each noted in one or two of the affected children.

Etiology: Affected siblings of normal, consanguineous parents suggest autosomal recessive inheritance.

Pathogenesis: Unknown.

MIM No.: 24960

POS No.: 3317

Sex Ratio: M1:F3 (observed in the four reported cases).

Occurrence: One family with four affected children, and two sporadic cases, have been reported.

Risk of Recurrence for Patient's Sib:
See Part I, *Mendelian Inheritance.*

Risk of Recurrence for Patient's Child:
See Part I, *Mendelian Inheritance.*

Age of Detectability: At birth, by physical examination.

Gene Mapping and Linkage: Unknown.

Prevention: None known. Genetic counseling indicated.

Treatment: Unknown.

Prognosis: All affected individuals have been retarded (IQ 70–80); Life span seems unaffected.

Detection of Carrier: Unknown.

References:
Mietens C, Weber H: A syndrome characterized by corneal opacity, nystagmus, flexion contractures of the elbows, growth failure, and mental retardation. J Pediatr 1966; 69:624–629.

Carnevale A, Ruiz Garcia FJ: Sindrome de Mietens-Weber: descripcion de un nuevo caso. Rev Invest Clin (Medico) 1976; 28:347–351.

Nagano A, et al.: Mietens' syndrome. Arch Orthop Unfall-Chir 1977; 89:81–86.

T0007

Helga V. Toriello

Migeon syndrome
See ADRENOCORTICAL UNRESPONSIVENESS TO ACTH, HEREDITARY

MIGRAINE   3223

Includes:
> Basilar migraine
> Benign exertional headache
> Benign sexual headache
> Classic migraine
> Coital headache
> Common migraine
> Childhood migraine
> Exertional headache, benign
> Headache, benign exertional
> Headache, benign sexual
> Headache, migraine
> Migraine, familial hemiplegic
> Migraine, complicated
> Ophthalmoplegic migraine
> Sexual headache, benign
> Transformational migraine
> Transient migraine accompaniments

Excludes:
> Headache, cluster
> Headache secondary to structural, metabolic, or infectious disease
> Headache, tension

Major Diagnostic Criteria: Since 1962, the report of the Ad Hoc Committee on the Classification of Headache has served as the basis for the diagnostic criteria for migraine. Presently, the classification and diagnostic criteria for headache (and migraine) are undergoing transition, with a new but preliminary international classification currently being circulated. The following represent consensus opinion with respect to diagnostic criteria.

Migraine without aura (formerly "common migraine") is an idiopathic, chronic, recurring head pain disorder, with each attack lasting 4–72 hours (untreated or unsuccessfully treated) or longer, and separated by pain-free intervals. Features typical of migraine include unilateral or bilateral discomfort with a pulsating quality and moderate to severe intensity; nausea and/or vomiting; photophobia and/or phonophobia; aggravation by physical activity; and absence of an organic cause for headache.

Migraine with aura (formerly "classic migraine") is an idiopathic, chronic, recurring headache disorder which is manifested by headache episodes preceded by neurological symptoms unequivocally localizable to the cerebral cortex or brainstem. The neurological symptoms develop over 15–20 minutes, usually lasting less than 60 minutes. Headache, nausea, photophobia, and other symptoms generally follow the neurological (aura) symptoms directly or after an interval of less than one hour. Neurological and physical examinations do not suggest the presence of organic disease.

Familial hemiplegic migraine is a variant of migraine (with aura), the primary neurological symptom being hemiparesis in which at least one first degree relative has identical attacks.

Basilar migraine is a migraine (with aura) variant originating in the brainstem or from both occipital lobes, and may include symptoms of dysarthria, vertigo, tinnitis, ataxia, decreased consciousness, and bilateral neurological symptoms.

Ophthalmoplegic migraine is a migraine (with aura) variant with paresis of one or more ocular cranial nerves.

Transformational migraine is a pattern of migraine which reflects the evolutive or transformational transition seen in some patients with migraine, in which intermittent migraine (without aura) episodes evolve to a daily or almost daily pattern. Mild to moderate pain occurs on a daily basis and paroxysmal (episodic) more intense attacks (fulfilling migraine without aura criteria) develop less often. It is believed that over one-half of those who have this transformational syndrome have accompanying depression and sleep disturbances.

Transient migraine accompaniments are neurological symptoms (usually visual) in the absence of headache, occurring periodically and which first develop after age 50.

Benign sexual headache consists of three patterns of headache which may occur in association with sexual exertion or masturbation. The most common pattern occurs in about 70% of reported cases, beginning shortly before or after orgasm. This consists of a high-intensity pain, usually frontal or occipital in location, and may have an explosive or throbbing quality, lasting for a few minutes to several hours.

A second pattern, occurring in about 25% of cases, begins early in the course of intercourse, is occipital or diffuse in location, and has a dull, aching quality which intensifies at the time of orgasm. The form occurring least often is an occipital headache present when the patient is standing, and is often associated with nausea and vomiting. A low CSF pressure has been considered a probable cause, perhaps occurring as a consequence of a dural tear from exertion during sexual activity. No consistent biological factor has been identified as a cause for these headache phenomena, but a relationship to migraine or mechanical alteration of the CSF dynamics has been postulated. Aneurysm, intracranial mass lesion, or structural abnormality must be ruled out. Treatment consists of a variety of drugs, many of which are useful in migraine, including beta adrenergic blockade and indomethacin treatment.

Clinical Findings: Migraine may begin at any time in life, with over 21% of patients reporting the first headache prior to age 10 and over 50% of patients before age 20. Later life onset (after age 40) is noted in up to 8% of patients. Although it is assumed that migraine attacks will cease over the course of years, little data can confirm this belief. Periodic and recurring episodes may span the entire lifetime of some patients, cease permanently after childhood or at some other milestone (hormonal, etc.), or return after a period of remission, decades after the last attack.

Though not all attacks of migraine are associated with headache, most migraine episodes, by diagnostic criteria, reflect episodic attacks of head pain accompanied by one or more symptoms, including, but not limited to, neurological events; nausea and vomiting (87% and 56% respectively); sensitivity to light and/or sound (82%); visual disturbances (36%); paresthesias (33%); lightheadedness (72%); and dizziness (33%). Autonomic disturbances, i.e., vasomotor changes and edema, and mental and mood disturbances are common.

In women, migraine attacks are often influenced by various hormonal milestones, including menarche, menstruation, pregnancy, and menopause. The use of oral contraceptives, exogenous estrogen, or other hormonal manipulations usually adversely affect the course.

The location of pain is variable, as is the intensity. Some attacks are characterized by occipital (neck pain) discomfort, but most

have a hemicranial or transcranial expression. Facial pain can occur during migraine.

Throughout the years of vulnerability, the pattern and frequency of attacks may be influenced by hypothalamic (chronobiological) factors which alone or in conjunction with external provoking factors (activating, precipitating factors) incite the onset of the attack. Among the well known migraine activating events are dietary factors, head trauma, stress and anxiety, hormonal fluctuation, sleep cycles, weather changes, physical exertion, and others.

The natural history of migraine is variable. Current attention focuses upon the transformational, evolutive phenomenon in which periodic migraine events evolve to a daily or almost daily pain pattern. Cervical/occipital, and/or frontal pain occurs on a daily basis, and episodic, intense, "typical" migraine attacks develop periodically.

Currently available diagnostic tests are normal in migraine, and the diagnosis rests upon the absence of other identifiable causes for head pain.

Childhood migraine, the most common of the recurring headaches in childhood, affects males more than females and is usually characterized by briefer attacks (than in adults), with prominent GI symptoms, sleep disturbance, and a generally favorable prognosis, particularly for males. Migraine "equivalents" (symptoms of migraine in the absence of headache in children) include episodic vertigo, dizziness, abdominal pain and cyclical vomiting, and episodic mood disturbance. Typical adult-type migraine attacks are also common in children.

Complications: Complications of migraine are of two forms: iatrogenic (treatment-related) and natural (physiological) attributed to the disease process itself.

Iatrogenic complications reflect the consequences of excessive treatment with a variety of pharmacological agents. These include GI, liver, and renal disturbances secondary to excessive use of mixed analgesic preparations; addictive disease resulting from dependency upon narcotic analgesics or addicting tranquilizers; and vascular complications arising from excessing use of ergotamine tartrate and other vasoconstrictive preparations.

The natural risks of migraine include the persistence of hemiplegic, aphasic, hemianopic, and retinal sequelae of individual migraine (with aura) attacks. When persistent, it is called *complicated migraine*. Though rare, numerous examples are documented in the literature. It is currently believed that complicated migraine may result from nonischemic impairment of brain rather than from occlusive, ischemic disease. Recently, several cases of brain hemorrhage during migraine have been reported, though a certain linkage between acute migraine and hemorrhage into the brain is yet to be confirmed.

Many migraine sufferers experience accompanying depression and sleep disturbance, which may reflect the primary factors related to the pathogenesis of the illness.

Associated Findings: Few associated findings have been confirmed, although a higher than expected incidence of depression and sleep disturbance has been tentatively noted in transformational migraine. Moreover, 60% of migraineurs report motion sickness (sometimes severe) during early childhood, and over 60% of adult migraine patients report unrelated episodes of motion sickness from time to time, compared to 11% of controls. Migraine occurs with a higher-than-chance frequency in children with primary familial dyslipoproteinemia. **Raynaud disease** and labile hypertension are also noted in many migraine sufferers and may be related to autonomic disturbances.

Etiology: Autosomal dominant inheritance with incomplete penetrance. In familial hemiplegic migraine; autosomal dominant inheritance. A family history of migraine is obtained in 60–91% of patients with migraine.

Pathogenesis: Attitudes regarding the pathogenesis of migraine are currently in transition and dispute. Traditional considerations had focused upon overactive vasomotor systems, resulting in excessive cranial and extracranial vascular responses. The most favored current concept suggests that migraine is caused by a central (brain) disturbance involving neurotransmission (serotonergic and monoaminergic) within the upper brainstem and diencephalic pathways.

MIM No.: 15730

Sex Ratio: In childhood, boys and girls seem equally affected (perhaps slightly more males than females). In adults, the male-to-female ratio is M1:F7.5.

Occurrence: Because precise diagnostic criteria for migraine and its classification are not universally agreed upon, determinations of actual incidence and prevalence are varied and remain uncertain. The most reliable current data on recent prevalence in the Western world is 30% of women between the ages of 21 and 34 (declining to 10% in those 75 years or older) and 17% of men (declining to 5% in those 75 years or older). Approximately 40% of individuals in the United States and Europe have reported severe headaches at some point in their lives. No apparent relationship exists between migraine and intelligence, social class, race, or educational background. It may be higher in the United States and Europe than in China and rural Ecuador.

Risk of Recurrence for Patient's Sib:
See Part I, *Mendelian Inheritance.*

Risk of Recurrence for Patient's Child:
See Part I, *Mendelian Inheritance.*

Age of Detectability: Migraine has been reported in two and three year-olds. Between 20% and 35% of children with headache are under five years of age when symptoms begin. Over 90% of all patients with migraine have experienced their first attack before the age of 40.

Gene Mapping and Linkage: Unknown.

Prevention: None known. Genetic counseling indicated.

Treatment: The treatment of migraine consists of non-medical and medical interventions. *Non-medical therapies* include avoidance of provoking factors, biofeedback and stress management techniques, improving general health and leisure aspects of life, and regulating day-to-day routines such as time of retiring and arising each day and taking meals. *Pharmacological techniques* address both acute attacks and prevention of recurring attacks. Acute attacks are treated with a variety of agents, including analgesics, specific migraine preparations (such as ergotamine tartrate, dihydroergotamine, etc.), nonsteroidal anti-inflammatory drugs (NSAID), hypnotics, and tranquilizers.

Preventive therapy for recurring attacks employs a long list of pharmacological agents, including β-adrenergic blocking agents, calcium channel antagonists, methysergide, antidepressants, nonsteroidal anti-inflammatory agents (NSAID), and many others.

It is believed that most effective agents act through a mechanism involving central serotonergic or mono-aminergic pathways.

Prognosis: Variable. In its natural untreated state, migraine will vary in intensity and frequency throughout the life span, with periods of remission and exacerbation. Cyclical patterns are noted. With treatment, the natural history is not altered, but control of recurring episodes of pain can be achieved in over 75% of those treated.

Detection of Carrier: The diagnosis is established through delineation of the history and the exclusion of organic disease.

Special Considerations: The concepts and perspectives on migraine are changing rapidly. Many respected authorities now believe that most chronic recurring headaches, with the possible exception of cluster headache and its variants, are actual variations of migraine. Central (brain) disturbances are now believed to be the primary pathogenetic process, and reactions of blood vessels and muscles are secondary events or epiphenomena. The periodicity of migraine may be determined by hypothalamic, chronobiological influences. The vulnerability to migraine is though to result primarily from a genetically-determined disturbance, either activated or in some cases acquired from "perturbation" of critical brain regions.

Among the external factors which may "perturb" or influence migraine are: mild to moderate head trauma, prolonged emotional duress, metabolic or infectious illness, or neuronal stimulation

from pathological processes along the course of the fifth cranial nerve. The most effective treatments appear to influence central mechanisms rather than extracranial targets as has traditionally been assumed. Comprehensive outpatient and special hospital treatment units (the first of its kind in Ann Arbor, Michigan, in 1978) have been developed to address the most resistent cases.

References:
Allan W: Inheritance of migraine. Arch Intern Med 1928; 42:590–599.
Goodell H, et al.: The familial occurrence of migraine headache: a study of heredity. Arch Neurol Psychiat 1954; 72:325–334.
Refsum S: Genetic aspects of migraine. In: Vinken PJ, Bruyn GW, eds: Handbook of Clinical Neurology, Vol. 5. Amsterdam: North Holland Publishing, 1968:258–270.
Paulson GW, Klawans HL: Benign orgasmic cephalgia. Headache 1974; 13:181–187.
Lance, JW: Mechanism and management of headache, 4th ed. Boston: Butterworth, 1982. *
Saper JR: Headache disorders: current concepts and treatment strategies. Boston: Wright-PSG Medical Publishers, 1983. *
Johns DR: Benign sexual headache within a family. Arch Neurol 1986; 43:1158–1160.
Saper JR: Changing perspectives in headache treatment. Clin J Pain 1986; 2:19–28.
Waters WE: Headache (series in clinical epidemiology). London: Croom Helm, 1986.
Saper JR: Drug treatment of headache: changing concepts and treatment strategies. Semin Neurol 1987; 7:178–191.
Raskin NH: Headache. New York: Churchill-Livingstone, 1988. *

SA047   **Joel R. Saper**

Migraine, complicated
See MIGRAINE
Migraine, familial hemiplegic
See MIGRAINE
Mikulicz disease
See PAROTITIS, PUNCTATE
Mikulicz syndrome
See SJOGREN SYNDROME
Milano (Al) apolipoproprolipoprotein variants
See HYPOALPHALIPOPROTEINEMIA
Miller syndrome
See ACROFACIAL DYSOSTOSIS, POSTAXIAL TYPE
Miller-Dieker syndrome
See LISSENCEPHALY SYNDROME
Milroy disease
See LYMPHEDEMA I
Minamata disease
See FETAL METHYLMERCURY EFFECTS
Mineralocorticoid-receptor deficiency
See ALDOSTERONE RESISTANCE
Minimal pigment albinism
See ALBINISM, OCULOCUTANEOUS, MINIMAL PIGMENT TYPE
Minkowski-Chauffard syndrome
See SPHEROCYTOSIS
Minkowski-Chauffard syndrome (obsolete)
See ANEMIA, HEMOLYTIC, RED CELL MEMBRANE DEFECTS
Minoxidil, fetal effects
See FETAL EFFECTS FROM MATERNAL VASODILATOR
Miosis and partial ptosis
See HORNER SYNDROME
Mirhosseini-Holmes-Walton syndrome
See RETINOPATHY-MICROCEPHALY-MENTAL RETARDATION
Mitochondrial acetoacetyl-CoA thiolase deficiency
See ACIDEMIA, 3-KETOTHIOLASE DEFICIENCY
Mitochondrial ALDH deficiency
See ALCOHOL INTOLERANCE
Mitochondrial cytopathy
See KEARNS-SAYRE DISEASE
also OPHTHALMOPLEGIA, PROGRESSIVE EXTERNAL
Mitochondrial encephalomyopathy
See KEARNS-SAYRE DISEASE
Mitochondrial myopathy
See MYOPATHY, MITOCHONDRIAL-ENCEPHALOPATHY-LACTIC ACIDOSIS-STROKE
also MYOPATHY, METABOLIC
Mitochondrial myopathy due to cytochrome C oxidase deficiency
See MYOPATHY-METABOLIC, MITOCHONDRIAL CYTOCHROME C OXIDASE DEFICIENCY

Mitral insufficiency due to isolated clefts of the valve leaflets
See MITRAL VALVE INSUFFICIENCY
Mitral regurgitation, congenital
See MITRAL VALVE INSUFFICIENCY

MITRAL REGURGITATION-DEAFNESS-SKELETAL DEFECTS — 0667

Includes:
Deafness-mitral regurgitation-skeletal malformations
Skeletal malformations-heart disease-conductive hearing loss

Excludes:
Arthro-ophthalmopathy, hereditary, progressive, Stickler type (0090)
Lentigines syndrome, multiple (0586)
Mitral valve prolapse (0668)
Pulmonic stenosis-deafness

Major Diagnostic Criteria: Conductive hearing loss, mitral regurgitation, and osseous abnormalities.

Clinical Findings: Three relatives have been described with conductive hearing loss, mitral regurgitation, and osseous abnormalities. All three were of short stature and normal intelligence, had similar facies, and prominent freckling over the face and shoulders. External auditory canals were narrow and oblique; middle ear exploration in two cases revealed a fixed footplate. Audiograms prior to surgery demonstrated a conductive hearing loss with normal cochlear function. X-rays showed varying degrees of fusion of the cervical vertebrae, carpal and tarsal bones; the phalanges appeared shortened. All had mild degrees of mitral regurgitation of unclear cause; whether mitral stenosis was also present was not addressed. The EKG showed an incomplete right-bundle branch block and cardiac catheterization showed normal hemodynamics. Karyotypes were normal.

Complications: Language delay may result from the hearing loss. The long-term course of the mitral valve abnormality is undetermined.

Associated Findings: One child had a left exotropia. A high-arched palate and crowded dentition were present. The thyroid was palpable in each case, but thyroid function studies were normal.

Etiology: Presumably autosomal dominant inheritance with variable expression.

Pathogenesis: Unknown.

MIM No.: 15780

POS No.: 3303

Sex Ratio: Undetermined. All three reported cases were female.

Occurrence: Undetermined; three cases reported.

Risk of Recurrence for Patient's Sib:
See Part I, *Mendelian Inheritance.*

Risk of Recurrence for Patient's Child:
See Part I, *Mendelian Inheritance.*

Age of Detectability: Theoretically diagnosable at birth by physical examination and audiogram. The murmur and conductive hearing loss may easily be missed on initial examination and newborn audiometric screening.

Gene Mapping and Linkage: Unknown.

Prevention: None known. Genetic counseling indicated.

Treatment: Middle ear surgery may improve hearing, although amplification may be necessary prior to surgery. Cardiac surgery could correct severe valvular problems.

Prognosis: Good.

Detection of Carrier: Unknown.

References:
Forney WR, et al.: Congenital heart disease, deafness and skeletal malformations: a new syndrome? J Pediatr 1966; 68:14–26.

PY000 **Reed E Pyeritz**

MITRAL VALVE ATRESIA — 0665

Includes: Atresia, mitral valve

Excludes:
Mitral atresia associated with other major cardiac anomalies

Major Diagnostic Criteria: Clinical presentation varies depending on the anatomical features but may include cyanosis, systolic murmur or congestive heart failure. Echocardiography is suggestive with selective left atrial angiocardiography being diagnostic. Ventriculography will delineate the associated anatomic abnormalities.

Clinical Findings: Mitral atresia is represented by a complete fusion of the mitral valve leaflets with no entry into the left ventricle. The left ventricle is almost always hypoplastic with a small cavity. The left atrium is similarly reduced in size. The communication between the atria is usually a patent foramen ovale rather than a defect of the secundum or primum variety. The atrial septum is rarely (<10%) intact and, under these circumstances, entry into the right side of the heart is via a levocardinal vein. The hemodynamic alterations are dependent on the presence or absence of pulmonary stenosis and the size of the atrial communication. Oxygenated blood in this malformation returns from the lungs into the left atrium and then passes into the right atrium via the foramen ovale or atrial defect to mix with the caval return. Following right ventricular filling, both great arteries receive blood: the pulmonary artery from the right ventricle, and the aorta through a VSD and the LV, or through a patent ductus arteriosus. The size of the aorta and pulmonary artery reflects the proportion of right ventricular output directed into each major vessel as determined by pulmonary and systemic vascular resistances.

The age of presentation and clinical picture depend largely on the size of the atrial patency and the status of pulmonary blood flow. In those patients with diminished pulmonary blood flow, ie associated pulmonary stenosis, cyanosis is the main finding. Auscultation in this group reveals a harsh systolic ejection murmur along the left sternal border secondary to pulmonary outflow tract obstruction. There is a single second heart sound. Signs of congestive heart failure are not present. In the group with augmented pulmonary blood flow or pulmonary venous obstruction, congestive heart failure is the dominant feature. Tachypnea and hepatomegaly are then the chief presenting findings along with nonspecific murmurs. On occasion, a continuous murmur has been described along the left upper sternal margin secondary to flow from the high pressure left atrium to the lower pressure right atrium.

No specific X-ray picture has been described, and the findings vary according to the hemodynamic alterations present. In patients with increased pulmonary blood flow, cardiac enlargement with prominent pulmonary vascular markings is seen. If the size of the atrial communication is small, a predominantly pulmonary venous obstructive pattern will be noted. When pulmonary stenosis is present, the heart is usually of normal size and the vascularity of the lungs diminished. In cases with associated transposition of the great arteries, a narrow cardiac base has been observed.

The EKG commonly shows right axis deviation, right atrial enlargement and severe right ventricular hypertrophy. The latter is associated with a QR pattern in the right precordial leads.

The echocardiogram shows absence of the mitral leaflet motion pattern, a variable-sized left atrium and a dilated right ventricle, exaggerated tricuspid motion, a slit-like or absent left ventricular cavity and, generally, a hypoplastic aortic root in the anterior-posterior and superior-inferior echocardiographic axes. The echocardiogram, when all of the above are noted, is definitive in this diagnosis. (See also **Aortic valve atresia**).

Cardiac catheterization with selective left atrial angiocardiography is crucial for the confirmation of the diagnosis. A left-to-right shunt is usually present at the atrial level. The right ventricular and pulmonary artery pressures are elevated to systemic levels in the absence of pulmonary stenosis. The left atrial pressure is variably increased, depending on the size of the left atrial communication and the magnitude of the pulmonary blood flow. Large prominent a waves are generally found. When a large opening exists, the pressures in both atria tend to be equal. Injection of contrast material into the left atrium will show a direct passage of the contrast media into the right atrium, right ventricle, and then simultaneous opacification of both great arteries. Right ventricular injection may also be helpful in the delineation of the origin of the great arteries and the presence or absence of pulmonary stenosis.

Complications: Death is usually secondary to congestive heart failure or hypoxemia.

Associated Findings: **Aorta, coarctation** or **Aortic arch interruption**, **Heart, transposition of great vessels**, and **Ventricular septal defect** or single ventricle; a high incidence (40%) of noncardiac malformations has been reported. They are of wide variety, including horseshoe kidney, ectopic pancreas, and **Cleft lip**.

Etiology: Unknown.

Pathogenesis: Congenital mitral atresia is due to fusion of left AV primordia at an early age. It has also been suggested by some authors that premature closure of the foramen ovale in utero is the primary event and the consequent hemodynamic changes result in the left ventricular underdevelopment.

CDC No.: 746.505

Sex Ratio: M1:F>1

Occurrence: 5:1,000 cases of autopsied congenital heart disease.

Risk of Recurrence for Patient's Sib: 1:50 (2%) for each sibling to be affected.

Risk of Recurrence for Patient's Child: Affected individuals are not expected to survive to reproduce.

Age of Detectability: From birth, by cardiac catheterization and selective angiocardiography.

Gene Mapping and Linkage: Unknown.

Prevention: None known. Genetic counseling indicated.

Treatment: If the patient is in congestive heart failure, digitalis, diuretics, etc should be promptly instituted. Pulmonary artery banding is frequently required. In children with decreased pulmonary blood flow, an appropriate aorticopulmonary shunt is necessary. Attempt should be made during cardiac catheterization to enlarge the atrial septum using the balloon atrial septostomy technique as this is often a site of obstruction.

Prognosis: The overall prognosis is poor. In selective cases, palliation with pulmonary artery banding and atrial septostomies as well as systemic pulmonary artery shunts can lead to long-term survival.

Detection of Carrier: Unknown.

References:
Meyer RA, Kaplan S: Echocardiography in the diagnosis of hypoplasia of the left or right ventricles in the neonate. Circulation 1972; 46:55–65.
Baylen BG, Criley JM: Diseases of the mitral valve. In: Adams FH, Emmanouilides GC, eds: Heart disease in infants, children, and adolescents. Baltimore: Williams & Wilkins, 1983:516–526.

N0003   **James J. Nora**

MITRAL VALVE INSUFFICIENCY   0666

Includes:
> Chordae tendineae, anomalous shortened
> Heart, arcade formation of the leaflets and chordae
> Heart, shortened or defective valve tissue
> Mitral insufficiency due to isolated clefts of the valve leaflets
> Mitral regurgitation, congenital
> Mitral valve, double orifice

Excludes:
> Endocardial cushion defects, partial or complete
> Mitral insufficiency, acquired
> Mitral insufficiency associated with metabolic defects
> Mitral insufficiency secondary to anomalous left coronary artery
> **Mitral valve prolapse** (0668)
> Rheumatic mitral insufficiency

Major Diagnostic Criteria: Auscultation of a harsh holosystolic murmur at the cardiac apex with radiation to the axilla and back indicates the presence of mitral insufficiency. Echocardiography using two-dimensional and pulsed Doppler is the diagnostic modality of choice to confirm the diagnosis. Cardiac catheterization is frequently needed to assess the severity of insufficiency.

Clinical Findings: The presentation of mitral insufficiency is extremely variable due to the multiple etiologies of this disorder. It is also complicated by the high frequency of other associated cardiac defects. An isolated lesion of the mitral valve may consist of single or multiple clefts in the anterior or posterior leaflet. Shortening of the chordae tendineae with abnormalities of the papillary muscles also results in varying degrees of mitral insufficiency. Occasionally these form an "arcade" type appearance to the anterior leaflet. As isolated defects these lesions are extremely rare. More commonly these defects occur in association with other cardiac defects. In these circumstances, the finding of mitral insufficiency may be obscured by the coexisting lesions.

Secondary mitral insufficiency may also result in the presence of normal valve anatomy. Idiopathic hypertrophic obstructive cardiomyopathy has resulted in mitral insufficiency in severe cases. Anomalous origin of the left coronary artery from the pulmonary artery frequently results in left ventricular and papillary muscle dysfunction with resultant mitral insufficiency. Various metabolic disorders result in degeneration of the mitral valve and subsequent insufficiency. Most common of these are **Marfan syndrome** and **Mucopolysaccharidosis** types I and II. Myxomatous degeneration of valve tissue, and rarely cardiac tumor, are also causes of mitral insufficiency.

The age of presentation may range from early infancy to late adulthood. The clinical findings and age of presentation will vary with the severity of the insufficiency and presence of associated defects. The patient may present with an asymptomatic murmur in cases of mild insufficiency. In severe cases, a history of easy fatigue, poor growth, or respiratory abnormalities may be elicited. In isolated mitral insufficiency, apical activity is increased. A palpable apical thrill may also be present. A high frequency harsh holosystolic murmur is audible with radiation to the axilla and back. The split of the second heart sound will be narrowed with an increased pulmonic component in the presence of significant pulmonary hypertension. With severe insufficiency, a low pitched diastolic rumble (Carey-Coombs murmur) may be heard. The electrocardiogram in the presence of significant mitral insufficiency shows left ventricular hypertrophy and left atrial enlargement. Chest X-ray shows left ventricular and left atrial enlargement. In the presence of severe insufficiency, pulmonary vascular markings are also increased. Echocardiography is a useful diagnostic modality to diagnose mitral insufficiency. Clefts and abnormalities of the chordae are visualized well with two-dimensional echocardiography. Parasternal short axis views will show clefts in both anterior and posterior mitral valve leaflets. This view also allows visualization of the papillary muscle size and location. Parasternal long axis and especially the apical four-chamber views allow evaluation of the chordal structure and attachments. These views may show valve tissue prolapse into the left atrium. Doppler echocardiography is very sensitive in identifying the presence of insufficiency. Mapping of the regurgitant jet with Doppler in the apical four-chamber and parasternal long view has been used to estimate the degree of severity from mitral insufficiency. This is limited by the angle of the Doppler beam and remains only a qualitative estimate of the severity of the insufficiency. Color Doppler may be found to be more useful for this purpose but remains unvalidated at this time. Cardiac catheterization is therefore indicated when the degree of mitral insufficiency is uncertain. Direct measurement of the left atrial pressure and left ventricular angiography are used to establish the severity of the mitral insufficiency. High pulmonary artery capillary wedge pressures with large V waves are usually present in cases of mitral insufficiency. Because prominent V waves can occur in the absence of significant mitral insufficiency, direct measurement of the left atrial pressure pattern is preferable. Pulmonary arterial pressure may also be elevated in the face of severe insufficiency with left ventricular failure. Left ventricular angiography will show systolic regurgitation of contrast into the left atrium and depending upon the severity, into the pulmonary veins as well. The degree of left atrial and ventricular dilation and the rapidity of clearing of the dye from the left atrium is used to evaluate the severity of the insufficiency.

Complications: Severe, chronic mitral insufficiency will result in left ventricular volume overload and left ventricular failure. Pulmonary venous congestion results in pulmonary hypertension and right heart failure. Infective endocarditis may occur. This risk is greatest in very abnormal valves with some degree of concomitant mitral stenosis.

Associated Findings: Mitral insufficiency presents only rarely as an isolated defect. It is seen with other cardiac defects especially secundum atrial septal defect, **Ductus arteriosus, patent, Aortic valve stenosis**, and **Aorta, coarctation**. Mitral regurgitation has been reported in association with **Turner syndrome**. Secondary mitral regurgitation occurs with idiopathic hypertrophic cardiomyopathy and anomalous origin of the left coronary artery from the pulmonary artery. Mitral insufficiency is also seen in connective tissue disorders such as **Marfan syndrome** and various **Mucopolysaccharidosis**.

Etiology: Probably multifactorial inheritance.

Pathogenesis: An isolated cleft probably represents a form of **Heart, endocardial cushion defects**, despite the absence of other components normally seen in endocardial cushion type defects.

MIM No.: 12100

CDC No.: 746.600

Sex Ratio: Presumably M1:F1

Occurrence: Less than 1:1,000

Risk of Recurrence for Patient's Sib: Unknown.

Risk of Recurrence for Patient's Child: Unknown. Presumably in the range of two to five percent.

Age of Detectability: From birth with two-dimensional and pulsed Doppler echocardiography.

Gene Mapping and Linkage: Unknown.

Prevention: None known. Genetic counseling indicated.

Treatment: In infants and children, treatment should be conservative with attempts to avoid surgical intervention if possible. Valvuloplasty is surgical procedure of choice in children. Valve replacement may be necessary in severe cases, especially in adults and adolescents.

Prognosis: Variable depending upon etiology and associated lesions. Excellent surgical results in older children can be obtained with valvuloplasty or replacement. Management of infants and young children remains difficult with a high mortality.

Detection of Carrier: Unknown.

References:

Titus JL: Congenital malformations of the mitral and aortic valves and related structures. Dis Chest 1969; 55:358–367.

Friedensohn A, et al.: An unusual form of mitral insufficiency accompanying atrial septal defect. Clin Cardiol 1979; 2:158–161.

Baylen BG, Criley MJ: Diseases of the mitral valve. In: Adams FM, Emmanoulides GC, eds: Moss's heart disease in infants, children and adolescents. 3rd ed. Baltimore: Williams & Wilkins, 1983:516–526. *

Segni ED, et al.: Isolated cleft mitral valve: a variety of congenital mitral regurgitation identified by 2-dimensional echocardiography. Am J Cardiol 1983; 51:927–931.

Barth CW, et al.: Mitral valve cleft without cardiac septal defect causing severe mitral regurgitation but allowing long survival. Am J Cardiol 1985; 55:1229–1231.

PA045

BR014

Stephen M. Paridon

J. Timothy Bricker

MITRAL VALVE PROLAPSE 0668

Includes:

Balloon or billowing mitral valve

Barlow syndrome

Click-murmur syndrome

Floppy mitral valve

Midsystolic click-late systolic murmur syndrome

Mitral valve regurgitation, familial

Excludes:

Heart, endocardial cushion defects (0347)

Rheumatic and other acquired types of mitral valve insufficiency

Major Diagnostic Criteria: An apical midsystolic click, particularly if it is followed by a late systolic murmur of mitral insufficiency, suggests the diagnosis. Echocardiography can be diagnostic in the mitral valve prolapse syndrome by demonstrating the displacement of the mitral leaflets above the mitral anulus. Selective left ventricular angiocardiography may be used to confirm the diagnosis and to establish the degree of valvar insufficiency.

Clinical Findings: An aneurysmal protrusion of the posterior or anterior mitral valve leaflet, or both, into the left atrium, usually late in ventricular contraction. Patients with isolated mitral valve prolapse are asymptomatic, or complain of mild exercise intolerance or vague chest pain. Upon physical examination there is an apical midsystolic click or a late systolic murmur of mitral valve insufficiency. Both auscultatory findings are highly influenced by postural changes and often can only be detected in the left reclining or upright position. Chest X-rays usually are normal, but thoracic skeletal anomalies are common: "straight back," scoliosis or pectus excavatum. The EKG may show an indeterminate or left QRS axis and, particularly, biphasic or negative T waves in leads aVF or III.

Mitral valve prolapse sometimes is associated with atrial septal defects of the ostium secundum or sinus venosus type. These patients have all the clinical and radiologic findings of an atrial septal defect. In addition, an apical click or a late systolic murmur of mitral insufficiency may be present. When an ASD coexists, the EKG shows right ventricular hypertrophy and sometimes an indeterminate QRS axis or mild left axis deviation. Abnormal T waves in leads aVF or III may be found.

The M-mode echocardiogram can support the clinical diagnosis of a prolapsing mitral valve by demonstrating an abrupt posterior dip in late systole. Pansystolic "hammock" type displacement of the mitral leaflets is sometimes seen but can be a technical artifact. Two-D echocardiography using multiple views can also demonstrate the abnormal prolapse motion of either leaflet in systole. Strict diagnostic criteria should be used to avoid overdiagnosis.

Selective left ventriculography will confirm the prolapsing of the valve leaflets into the left atrium during ventricular contraction. In some instances there is a mild-to-moderate degree of mitral valve insufficiency. Frequently, the left ventricle will show an asymmetric contraction with a convex bulging in the mid-aspect of the anterolateral wall, or a localized protrusion of the posteroinferior wall into the left ventricular cavity ("ballerina" slipper configuration).

Complications: Little is known about the natural history of a congenital prolapsing mitral valve identified in childhood. Adults, however, have been found to have significant complications as a result of similarly malformed atrioventricular valves. Dysfunction of the mitral apparatus may produce insufficiency that, once established, may become progressively worse. Infective endocarditis has been reported even when the valve is competent. In rare instances, sudden death is presumably caused by significant cardiac arrhythmias, mostly of ventricular origin.

Associated Findings: Findings include other congenital heart defects, particularly **Atrial septal defects** of the ostium secundum or sinus venosus type, as well as thoracic skeletal anomalies ("straight back" syndrome, scoliosis and **Pectus excavatum**. Similarly, malformed mitral valves have been reported in both **Marfan syndrome** and **Ehlers-Danlos syndrome**.

Etiology: The majority of cases are sporadic. Several families have been described with autosomal dominant inheritance, with increased expression among females.

Pathogenesis: Myxomatous-type degeneration of the valve leaflets, or stretching of the mitral annulus resulting in disjunction between the atrium and ventricle.

MIM No.: *15770

Sex Ratio: M1:F2

Occurrence: Undetermined, but mitral valve prolapse may be the most commonly diagnosed cardiac valvar abnormality.

Risk of Recurrence for Patient's Sib:
See Part I, *Mendelian Inheritance.*

Risk of Recurrence for Patient's Child:
See Part I, *Mendelian Inheritance.* Depends on etiology; low recurrence risk in most cases.

Age of Detectability: From infancy, with echocardiography or selective angiocardiography.

Gene Mapping and Linkage: Unknown.

Prevention: None known. Genetic counseling indicated.

Treatment: The susceptibility of these patients to bacterial endocarditis warrants prophylactic antibiotics for dental or surgical procedures. Antiarrhythmic therapy for symptomatic patients with signs of ventricular irritability may be required. Mitral valve annuloplasty or replacement may be necessary in case of severe insufficiency.

Prognosis: Good, particularly during childhood and adolescence.

Detection of Carrier: Unknown.

References:
Barlow JB, et al.: Late systolic murmurs and non-ejection ("mid-late") systolic clicks: an analysis of 90 patients. Brit Heart J 1968; 30:203–218. *
Rizzon P, et al.: Familial syndrome of midsystolic click and late systolic murmur. Br Heart J 1973; 35:245–259.
Victorica BE, et al.: Ostium secundum atrial septal defect associated with balloon mitral valve in children. Am J Cardiol 1974; 33:668–673.
Salomon J, et al.: Thoracic skeletal abnormalities in idiopathic mitral valve prolapse. Am J Cardiol 1975; 36:32–36.
Sahn DJ, et al.: Echocardiographic spectrum of mitral valve motion in children with and without mitral valve prolapse. Am J Cardiol 1977; 39:422–431.
Jeresaty RM: Mitral valve prolapse. New York: Raven Press, 1979. *
Venkatesh A, et al.: Mitral valve prolapse in anxiety neurosis (panic disorder). Am Heart J 1980; 100:302–305.
Malcolm AD: Mitral valve prolapse associated with other disorders: casual coincidence, common link, or fundamental genetic disturbance. Brit Heart J 1985; 53:353–362.
Hutchins GM, et al.: The association of floppy mitral valve with disjunction of the mitral annulus fibrosus. New Eng J Med 1986; 314:535–541.

VI001   **Benjamin E. Victorica**

Mitral valve regurgitation, familial
See MITRAL VALVE PROLAPSE

MITRAL VALVE STENOSIS 0669

Includes:
  Parachute mitral valve
  Supramitral ring

Excludes:
  Lutembacher syndrome
  Rheumatic and other forms of acquired mitral stenosis
  Scimitar syndrome (0879)
  Ventricle, endocardial fibroelastosis of left ventricle (0348)
  Ventricle, endocardial fibroelastosis of right ventricle (0349)

Major Diagnostic Criteria: The presence on auscultation of loud first and second heart sounds accompanied by a low pitched apical diastolic murmur in an infant or child exhibiting signs or symptoms of congestive heart failure should raise the possibility of congenital mitral stenosis. Echocardiography and cardiac catheterization establish the diagnosis.

Clinical Findings: The anatomic findings in congenital mitral stenosis are variable and may include one or more of the following: thickened, rolled valve leaflets; shortened, thickened chordae tendineae; fused chordae; partial obliteration of interchordal spaces by fibrous tissue; abnormal or underdeveloped papillary muscles. Occasionally a double orifice of the mitral valve may be associated with stenosis. In the parachute mitral valve, the chordae (usually shortened and thickened) insert into one papillary muscle. Accummulation of connective tissue in a circumferential ring arising from the atrial insertions of the mitral valve leaflets may encroach on the mitral orifice producing obstruction. The left atrium in all forms of significant obstruction is enlarged, often with evidence of wall thickening and fibroelastosis. Dilatation and hypertrophy of the right ventricle and atrium are present in varying degrees depending on the severity of obstruction to left ventricular inflow.

Obstruction to flow across the mitral valve results in elevation of left atrial pulmonary venous, capillary and arterial pressures with pulmonary hypertension. The right ventricle hypertrophies and, with long standing mitral stenosis, may fail. In severe mitral stenosis, cardiac output may be diminished.

The age at which symptoms develop varies with the degree of stenosis and with the presence and type of associated cardiac defects. Infants often present with recurrent pulmonary infections, poor growth and tachypnea. Other symptoms include diaphoresis and dyspnea with feeds, chronic cough and irritability. Cyanosis is usually a late finding. Older children present with exertional dyspnea, fatigue and orthopnea. Syncope, hemoptysis and aphonia occur rarely. Symptoms tend to occur earlier in patients with associated cardiac anomalies.

On physical examination, pulses are normal except with severe stenosis. A right ventricular impulse is often palpable at the left sternal border. The first heart sound is loud. The second sound is narrowly split with a loud pulmonary component. In most patients, a low pitched, long diastolic murmur is audible at the apex, often with a presystolic component. Fifteen percent of patients have no murmur. An opening snap may be heard, but is not common. When right heart failure is present, jugular venous pulsations and hepatomegaly may be evident. Other physical findings may be present with associated cardiac anomalies.

Mild to marked cardiomegaly is evident on chest X-ray. There is often left atrial enlargement, pulmonary venous congestion (ranging from redistribution of flow to Kerley B lines), a prominent pulmonary trunk, and right-sided cardiac enlargement.

The electrocardiogram usually demonstrates a frontal plane QRS axis between $+90°$ and $+150°$. Right ventricular hypertrophy, left atrial enlargement and sometimes right atrial enlargement are evident. The presence of left ventricular hypertrophy suggests an additional cardiac defect.

M-mode echocardiography may show qualitative abnormalities of mitral stenosis. Anterior (instead of posterior) diastolic motion of the posterior mitral leaflet, decreased E-F slope, absent A wave, and left atrial enlargement are the typical findings, but M-mode is unreliable in assessing either the severity or the site of stenosis. Two-dimensional echocardiography may be helpful in determining the site and type as well as the severity of obstruction. Evaluation of the supravalvar region may reveal a supramitral ring, while views of the valve and subvalve regions may reveal abnormal papillary muscle anatomy and parachute mitral valve. The severity of stenosis can be evaluated by estimating the valve orifice area and by measuring the maximal transmitral inflow velocity by Doppler interrogation. In addition, two-dimensional echocardiography may reveal associated cardiac defects.

At cardiac catheterization, pulmonary artery and capillary wedge pressures are elevated. The left atrial mean as well as Á wave pressures are also elevated with a diastolic pressure gradient between the left atrium and left ventricle. Cineangiography demonstrates left atrial enlargement and may show delayed emptying of the left atrium with dilated pulmonary veins. Thickened leaflets with decreased mobility may be seen with valve stenosis, or an hourglass left ventricular filling defect may be seen with parachute mitral valve.

Complications: Pulmonary hypertension with pulmonary vascular disease may develop, leading to right heart failure. Death occurs due to severe congestive heart failure or recurrent pulmonary infections.

Associated Findings: Congenital mitral stenosis occurs uncommonly as an isolated defect. It often occurs in association with obstructive lesions of the aorta and aortic valve. Shone syndrome or complex includes four potentially obstructive left-sided anomalies that have a tendency to coexist: parachute mitral valve, supravalvular ring of the left atrium, subaortic stenosis and **Aorta, coarctation**. Other anomalies associated with congenital mitral stenosis include patent ductus arteriosus, **Ventricular septal defect, Heart, tetralogy of Fallot, Heart, transposition of great vessels**, and double outlet right ventricle.

Etiology: Unknown.

Pathogenesis: The pathogenesis varies with the type of stenosis present. Abnormal development of any of the major components of the valve (leaflets, chordae tendineae, papillary muscles, annulus) may produce obstruction to left ventricular inflow).

MIM No.: 12100

CDC No.: 746.500

Sex Ratio: M1.5–2.2:F1

Occurrence: 6–12:1,000 cases of autopsied congenital heart disease; 2–4:1,000 cases in clinical series.

Risk of Recurrence for Patient's Sib: Unknown.

Risk of Recurrence for Patient's Child: Unknown.

Age of Detectability: From birth, with echocardiography and cardiac catheterization.

Gene Mapping and Linkage: Unknown.

Prevention: None known. Genetic counseling indicated.

Treatment: Medical treatment with diuretics and digoxin may be effective in patients with mild to moderate stenosis. Intractable congestive heart failure, pulmonary edema or systemic pulmonary hypertension are indications for surgery, mitral valvotomy or mitral valve replacement (or resection of supravalvar tissue in supramitral ring).

Prognosis: The prognosis depends on the severity of the obstruction and the nature of associated cardiac defects. The median age at death varies with the type of obstruction: parachute mitral valve: 9 11/12 years; supramitral ring: 5 6/12 years; typical congenital mitral valve stenosis: 6 months. Fifty-three percent of all patients live to age 10, 42% of those managed medically and 56% of the surgical patients.

Detection of Carrier: Unknown.

References:
Shone JD, et al.: The developmental complex of "parachute mitral valve", supravalvular ring of left atrium, subaortic stenosis, and coarctation of aorta. Am J Cardiol 1963; 11:714–725.
Van der Horst RL, Hastreiter AR: Congenital mitral stenosis. Am J Cardiol 1967; 20:773–783.
Collins-Nakai RL, et al.: Congenital mitral stenosis. a review of 20 years' experience. Circulation 1977;56:1039–1047.
Baylen BG, Criley JM: Diseases of the mitral valve. In: Adams FH, Emmanoulides OC, eds: Heart disease in infants, children and adolescents. Baltimore: Williams & Wilkins, 1983:516–526. *
Grenadier E, et al.: Two-dimensioanl echo Doppler study of congenital disorders of the mitral valve. Am Heart J 1984; 107:319–325.
Vitarelli A, et al.: Echocardiographic assessment of congenital mitral stenosis. Am Heart J 1984; 108:523–531.
Kveselis DA, et al.: Balloon angioplasty for congenital and rheumatic mitral stenosis. Am J Cardiol 1986; 57:348–350.

BR014
TA007

J. Timothy Bricker
Lloyd Tani

MOLYBDENUM CO-FACTOR DEFICIENCY 2412

Includes:
> Sulfite oxidase/xanthine dehydrogenase/aldehyde oxidase deficiency
> Xanthine dehydrogenase/sulfite oxidase/aldehyde oxidase deficiency
> Aldehyde oxidase/sulfite oxidase/xanthine dehydrogenase deficiency

Excludes: Aciduria, sulfite oxidase deficiency (0921)

Major Diagnostic Criteria: Facial dysmorphia, encephalopathy with **Microcephaly**, hypertonia with hypertonic seizures, bilateral ocular lens dislocation. Low serum uric acid. Low urinary uric acid with increased urinary S-sulfo-cysteine. Urinary sulfite thiosulfate taurine, xanthine, and hypoxanthine are also elevated. Sulfate excretion is diminished.

Clinical Findings: This condition generally presents in the first or second week of life but one case has been reported as late as five years of age. The findings are similar to those of **Aciduria, sulfite oxidase deficiency**, probably because this is the most important enzyme defect in that condition. The patients present with dysmorphic features, psychomotor retardation, extensive neurologic dysfunction, and seizures. Dislocation of the ocular lens may not be present in the first few weeks of life, but generally appears by the third month.

Complications: Progressive cerebral dysfunction and death.

Associated Findings: None known.

Etiology: Autosomal recessive inheritance.

Pathogenesis: There is a deficiency of a molybdenum containing cofactor. An unusual pterin is also found in this cofactor. The absence of this cofactor leads to a deficiency of the enzymes sulfite oxidase (sulfite-oxygen oxido reductase E.C. 1.8.2.1) and xanthine oxidase (E.C. 1.2.3.2).

MIM No.: *25215

Sex Ratio: M1:F1

Occurrence: About 15 cases cases have been reported in the literature.

Risk of Recurrence for Patient's Sib:
See Part I, *Mendelian Inheritance.*

Risk of Recurrence for Patient's Child:
See Part I, *Mendelian Inheritance.* Affected individuals are not expected to survive to reproduce.

Age of Detectability: As early as the first day of life, or by amniocentesis. The amniocentesis fluid is analysed for S-sulfocysteine and amniotic cells analysed for sulfite oxidase.

Gene Mapping and Linkage: Unknown.

Prevention: None known. Genetic counseling indicated.

Treatment: Unknown.

Prognosis: Most patients die within one year of diagnosis, although one was reported alive at five years of age.

Detection of Carrier: Unknown.

References:
Duran M, et al.: Combined deficiency of xanthine oxidase and sulfite oxidase: a defect of molybdenum metabolism or transport. J Inherit Metab Dis 1978; 1:175.

Johnson JL, et al.: Characterization of the molybdenum cofactor of sulfite oxidase, xanthine oxidase and nitrate reductase. J Biol Chem 1980; 255:1783.

Wadman SK, et al.: Absence of hepatic molybdenum cofactor: an inborn error of metabolism leading to a combined deficiency of sulfite oxidase and xanthine dehydrogenase. J Inherit Metab Dis 1983; 6(Suppl 1):78.

Desjacques P, et al.: Combined deficiency of xanthine and sulfite oxidase: diagnosis of a new case followed by an antenatal diagnosis. J Inherit Metab Dis 1985; 8(Suppl 2):117.

Roth A, et al.: Anatomo-pathological findings in a case of combined deficiency of sulfite oxidase and xanthine oxidase with a defect of molybdenum cofactor. Virchows Arch [Pathol Anat] 1985; 405:379.

Roesel RA, et al.: Combined xanthine and sulphite oxidase defect due to a deficiency of molybdenum cofactor. J Inherit Metab Dis 1986; 9:343–347.

Johnson JL, Wadman SK: Molybdenum cofactor deficiency. In: Scriver CR, et al, eds: The metabolic basis of inherited disease, 6th ed. New York: McGraw-Hill, 1989:1463–1477.

CR006   **John C. Crawhill**

MOOD AND THOUGHT DISORDERS   1532

Includes:
  Affective personality disorders
  Bipolar affective disorder
  Depressive disorders
  Manic-depressive (bipolar) disorders
  Major affective disorders
  Panic disorder
  Schizophrenic disorders

Excludes:
  Attention-deficit hyperactivity disorder (ADHD) (3240)
  Autism, infantile (2128)
  Neurologically determined behavioral disorders (other)
  Tourette syndrome (2305)

Major Diagnostic Criteria: Major affective disorders are characterized by a significant disturbance in mood: depressed or excited/elated (manic). Schizophrenic disorders are characterized by some combination of impaired thought processes, disturbed thought content, disturbed perceptual processes (e.g. hallucinations), and flattened or inappropriate emotional tone.

Clinical Findings: Major affective disorders display a high degree of phenotypic variability, even within a given family. In addition to the spectrum of classic bipolar and unipolar manic-depressive disorders, certain types of personality disorders, anxiety disorders, and eating disorders also aggregate in affective disorder families and respond to affective disorder medications. Onset of symptomatology can occur at any age and symptoms can change or progress from mild to severe over time. A cyclical pattern of episodes is frequent and may follow the seasons.

Manic symptomatology may include: elated, excited or irritable mood; increased activity and decreased sleep; expanded "flight of ideas" and rapid, pressured talking; and over-inflated grandiosity with impulsive acting-out (e.g. buying sprees). Manic episodes may be of psychotic proportions (e.g. grandiose delusions).

A severe depression may include depressed mood and a loss of interest or pleasure in life's activities; depressive ideation with excessive self-reproach or guilt; thoughts of death or suicide; fatigue; diminished concentration; and vegetative signs and symptoms such as disturbed sleep, appetite, psychosomatic, or psychomotor activity. Again, episodes can be psychotic.

Schizoaffective disorders display, in addition to the affective components discussed above, a disorder of thought. The schizoaffective diagnosis is genetically heterogeneous, present in schizophrenic families as well as affective disorder families.

Schizophrenic symptomatology is classified as positive or negative. Negative symptoms can include a poverty of thought and speech, flattened affect, and psychomotor retardation or catatonia. Hallucinations, delusions, bizarre or inappropriate affect, and excited behavior are examples of positive symptoms. Onset may be sudden or insidious. Onset occurs at any age and peaks in early adulthood.

Complications: Self-destructive behaviors. Impaired adaptation to life.

Associated Findings: None known.

Etiology: Major affective disorders and schizophrenia probably consist of a collection of disorders with heterogeneous etiologies. Genetics as well as environmental factors and development play etiological roles.

Pathogenesis: Dysregulations of numerous neuroendocrine, circadian, neurotransmitter and neuropeptidergic systems have been demonstrated in some patients with major affective disorders. Catecholaminergic hypotheses have been intensely pursued, in part, because of the known interactions of antidepressant medications with catecholaminergic systems.

Dysfunctional dopaminergic systems are implicated in the pathogenesis of schizophrenia. Most antipsychotic medications are potent dopamine antagonists.

MIM No.: *12548, *30920, 18150, 16787

Sex Ratio: M1:F1 for bipolar disorders and schizophrenia. M1:F2 for major depression.

Occurrence: Bipolar disorder prevalence ranges from 0.5 to 1.2% of the general population. Lifetime prevalence rates for major depression in males range from 3% to 10%; females 6% to 20%. The lifetime prevalence of schizophrenia is approximately 1%.

Risk of Recurrence for Patient's Sib:
See Part I, *Mendelian Inheritance*. Major affective disorders and schizophrenia often display reduced penetrance.

Risk of Recurrence for Patient's Child:
See Part I, *Mendelian Inheritance*. Major affective disorders and schizophrenia often display reduced penetrance.

Age of Detectability: May be diagnosed at any age. Most frequently detected after puberty for bipolar disorders and after late adolescence for schizophrenia. Behavioral manifestations of affective disorder are being increasingly recognized in childhood.

Gene Mapping and Linkage: MAFD1 (major affective disorder 1) has been mapped to 11p15.5 [in one Old Order Amish family only.] Subsequent studies on this same family have demonstrated insignificant mild positive linkage to the 11p15.5 probes (Barinaga, 1989)].
MAFD2 (major affective disorder 2) has been mapped to Xq27-q28 [in some families].
SCZD2 (schizophrenia disorder 2) is unassigned.
BDM (behavior disorder modifier) has been provisionally mapped to X.
While there have been recent attempts to gene map mood and personality variables, most have provided interesting but inconclusive findings.

Prevention: None known. Genetic counseling indicated.

Treatment: A variety of psychopharmacological interventions are successful in the treatment of major affective illness (e.g. antidepressants, lithium carbonate) and schizophrenia (e.g. dopamine blocking neuroleptics). Electroconvulsive treatment is beneficial in certain cases of major depression. Psychotherapy is beneficial in many cases.

Prognosis: Extremely variable.

Detection of Carrier: Clinical assessment.

Support Groups:
VA; Alexandria; National Mental Health Association
DC; Washington; National Alliance for the Mentally Ill

References:
DeLong GR: Lithium carbonate treatment of select behavior disorders in children suggesting manic-depressive illness. J Pediat 1978; 93:689–694.
Weissman MM, et al.: Family-genetic studies of psychiatric disorders. Arch Gen Psychiatry 1986; 43:1104–1116.
Baron M, et al.: Genetic linkage between X-chromosome markers and bipolar affective illness. Nature 1987; 326:289–292.
Egeland JA, et al.: Bipolar affective disorders linked to DNA markers on chromosome 11. Nature 1987; 325:783–787.
Hodgkinson S, et al.: Molecular genetic evidence for heterogeneity in manic depression. Nature 1987; 325:805–806.
Diagnostic and Statistical Manual of Mental Disorders - Revised (DSM-III-R) APA Press, 1988.
Kennedy JL, et al.: Evidence against linkage of schizophrenia to markers on chromosome 5 in a northern Swedish pedigree. Nature 1988; 336:167–170.
Sherrington R, et al.: Localization of a susceptibility locus for schizophrenia on chromosome 5. Nature 1988; 336:164–167.
Barinaga M: Manic depression gene put in limbo. Science 1989; 246:886–887.
Weissman MM, et al.: Suicidal ideation and suicide attempts in panic disorder and attacks. New Engl J Med 1989; 321:1209–1214.

LE057   **James E. Lee**

Moore-Federman syndrome
See DWARFISM-STIFF JOINTS
Moravcsik-Marinesco-Sjogren syndrome
See MARINESCO-SJOGREN SYNDROME

MUCOLIPIDOSIS I   0671

Includes:
Cherry-red spot-myoclonus syndrome
Glycoprotein neuraminidase, deficiency of
Lipomucopolysaccharidosis
Myoclonus syndrome-cherry red spot
Neuraminidase deficiency
Sialidase deficiency
Sialidosis

Excludes:
Dentatorubropallidoluysian degeneration, hereditary (3283)
Mucolipidosis II (0672)
Mucolipidosis III (0673)
Mucopolysaccharidosis

Major Diagnostic Criteria: The primary means of diagnosis is the demonstration of an isolated deficiency of the lysosomal enzyme neuraminidase (sialidase), which can be accomplished in peripheral leukocytes or cultured fibroblasts. Other lysosomal enzymes need to be shown to be at normal levels to exclude the diagnosis of mucolipidosis (ML) II or III. In all three forms of ML, there is an increased urinary excretion of bound sialic acid that can be used as a simple screening test. If excessive urinary bound-sialic acid is found, measurement of serum hexosaminidase will give normal results in ML I and markedly elevated levels in ML II and III.

Clinical Findings: Lysosomal storage diseases are noted for a series of phenotypes associated with deficiency of the same enzyme; this is carried to the extreme in ML I in which, in general, the disease in each family appears to result in a distinct phenotype. Lowden and O'Brien (1979) have suggested two major categories, defined as dysmorphic and nondysmorphic sialidosis; *Hurler-like* and *non-Hurler-like* are more descriptive designations.
The Hurler-like forms of ML I occur as infantile (death between ages one and six years) and childhood (a slower progressing

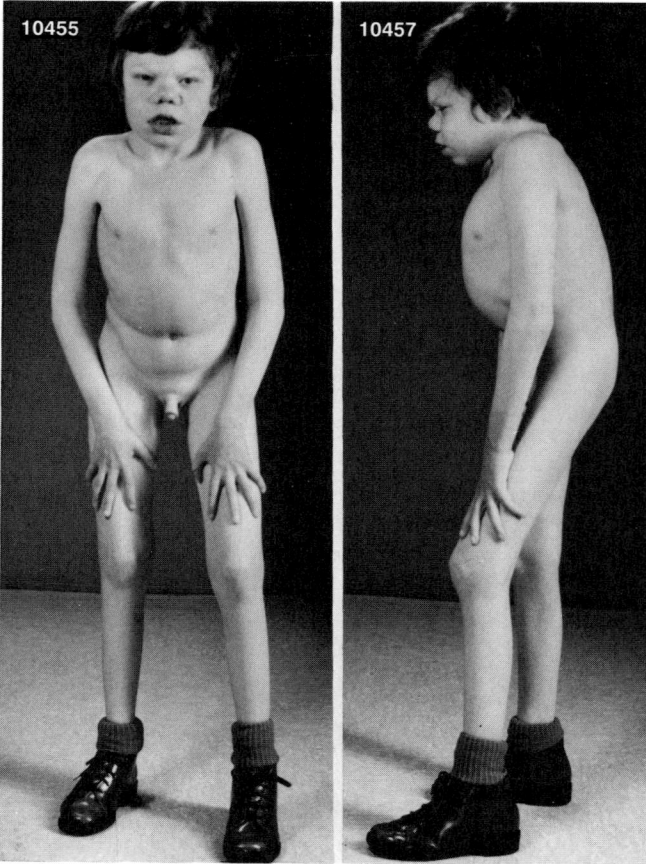

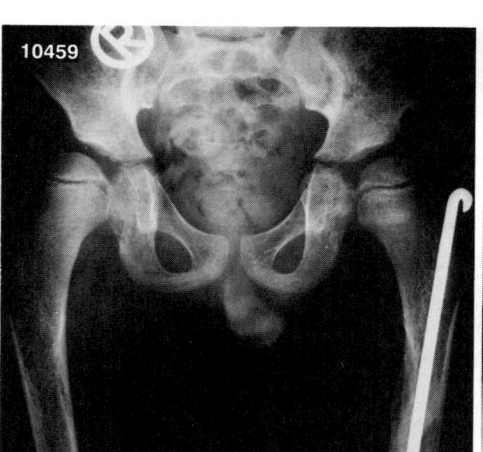

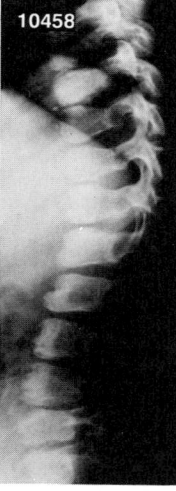

0671-10455–57: Stature is short due to shortened and deformed trunk. **10459:** Mild hypoplasia of basilar portion of ilia. Subluxed femoral heads, small epiphyses, and necks in valgus position. Note the pathologic fracture in the left femoral shaft. **10458:** Vertebral bodies are rounded and dorsally wedged. There are hook-shaped deformities of L1-L4.

disorder with survival into young adulthood) types. As implied by the term *Hurler-like*, the disorder involves multiple organ systems with skeletal, ocular, CNS, and visceral manifestations. The infantile form may be as clinically striking as ML II (I-cell disease) with coarse facies, severe skeletal contractures, marked hepatosplenomegaly, and an early onset of mental decline. Early deaths have occurred secondary to renal, hepatic, and cardiac complications. The childhood form was the first form described clinically and was designated *ML I* by Spranger et al. (1977).

The non-Hurler-like form of ML I is better known as the *cherry-red spot myoclonus syndrome* with an onset in the late teen or early adult years. It follows a slowly progressive course thereafter. A cherry-red spot of the macula may be seen with several forms of childhood lysosomal storage diseases, but it is virtually unique in adulthood to ML I.

Complications: The multisystem involvement of ML I leads to a preponderance of clinical manifestations varying with individual patients from renal, hepatic, or cardiac failure in infantile forms to skeletal and mental decline dominating childhood forms. The adult forms are compatible with reasonably good health, while slow mental regression occurs over a number of years.

Associated Findings: While one organ system pathology may dominate the course of individual patients, this occurs against the background of a progressive, multisystem disease.

Etiology: Autosomal recessive inheritance for mutations at the structural gene locus for neuraminidase. The different phenotypes occur as the result of combinations of different mutant neuraminidase alleles.

Pathogenesis: The accumulation of sialic acid-rich oligosaccharides in many tissues leads to local cell death and dysfunction. The phenotypic difference among individual patients apparently reflects differences in residual enzyme activity and accumulation of different compounds, depending on the age of the patient and the kinetics of the mutant enzyme toward its natural substrates.

MIM No.: *25240, *25655

POS No.: 3305

Sex Ratio: M1:F1

Occurrence: Collectively, the mutations resulting in the varying forms of ML I lead to an incidence of roughly 1:250,000

Risk of Recurrence for Patient's Sib:
See Part I, *Mendelian Inheritance.*

Risk of Recurrence for Patient's Child:
See Part I, *Mendelian Inheritance.* No recorded instances of reproduction by an affected individual, but dependent on frequency of carrier state, which is presumably low.

Age of Detectability: The infantile form may be clinically apparent in the newborn, whereas the other forms vary with the cherry red spot-myoclonus syndrome not apparent clinically until early adulthood. The biochemical abnormality can be detected at any age, including assays of cultured amniotic fluid cells and chorionic villi.

Gene Mapping and Linkage: NEU (neuraminidase) has been inconsistently mapped to 10pter-q23 or 6.

Prevention: None known. Genetic counseling indicated.

Treatment: As with all lysosomal diseases, no specific therapy exists, and symptomatic care of the patient and support of the family are important.

Prognosis: Varies with individual cases, and the course must be established by follow-up of individual patients.

Detection of Carrier: By enzyme assay in peripheral leukocytes, but overlap between carriers and noncarriers is observed.

Support Groups: NJ; Elizabeth; National Lipid Diseases Foundation

References:
Spranger JW, et al.: Lipomucopolysaccharidose. Z Kinderheilkd 1968; 103:285–306.
Spranger JW, Wiedemann HR: The genetic mucolipidoses: diagnosis and differential diagnosis. Humangenetik 1970; 9:113–139.

Kelly TE, Graetz GS: Isolated acid neuraminidase deficiency: a distinct lysosomal storage disease. Am J Med Genet 1977; 1:31–46. †

Spranger JW, et al.: Mucolipidosis I-a sialidosis. Am J Med Genet 1977; 1:21–29.

O'Brien JS: Neuraminidase deficiency in the cherry red spot-myoclonus syndrome. Biochem Biophys Res Commun 1977; 79:1136–1140.

Lowden JA, O'Brien JS: Sialidosis: a review of human neuraminidase deficiency. Am J Hum Genet 1979; 31:1–18.

Kelly TE, et al.: Mucolipidosis I (acid neuraminidase deficiency): three cases and delineation of the variability of the phenotype. Am J Dis Child 1981; 135:703–708.

Young ID, et al.: Neuraminidase deficiency: case report and review of the phenotype. J Med Genet 1987; 24:283–290.

KE012   **Thaddeus E. Kelly**

MUCOLIPIDOSIS II   0672

Includes:
> I-cell disease
> Leroy disease
> N-acetylglucosamine-1-phosphotransferase deficiency

Excludes:
> **Fucosidosis** (0398)
> **G(M1)-gangliosidosis, type 1** (0431)
> **G(M1)-gangliosidosis, type 2** (0432)
> **Mannosidosis** (2079)
> **Mucolipidosis III** (0673)
> **Mucolipidosis** (other)
> **Mucopolysaccharidosis**

Major Diagnostic Criteria: The clinical presentation includes a pseudo-Hurler phenotype with an absence of urinary excretion of mucopolysaccharides. Clinical findings include coarse facies, severe skeletal changes including kyphoscoliosis, lumbar gibbus, anterior vertebral breaking and wedging, wide ribs, and joint contractures. Cardiomegaly and congestive heart failure are common and may be present at birth. Serum levels of a variety of lysosomal acid hydrolases are elevated; these include beta-N-acetylhexosaminidase and arylsulfatase A, iduronate sulfatase, glycosidases, and the like. There is a corresponding deficiency of these enzymes in cultured fibroblasts. Some cells do not show this deficiency (leukocytes) or show it minimally (nerve cells and hepatocytes). Prominent phase-dense inclusion bodies are present in cultured fibroblasts. In trophoblasts, the enzyme most conspicuously deficient is beta-galactosidase.

Clinical Findings: Pseudo-Hurler phenotype with growth and psychomotor retardation. Cardiomegaly, congestive heart failure, and respiratory infections are potentially lethal complications. Hepatomegaly is also exaggerated by heart failure. Corneal clouding may be present, but this is not generally a prominent feature that can aid early diagnosis. The skin is tight and puffy; this can be very dramatic around the eyes. Gum hyperplasia may also be striking. Clinical onset is quite early, and most patients have obvious problems by six months of age.

Complications: Congestive heart failure, orthopedic deformities, and psychomotor retardation.

Associated Findings: Frequent respiratory infections.

Etiology: Autosomal recessive inheritance.

Pathogenesis: There is an absence or deficiency of N-acetyl-glucosamine phosphotransferase. In the absence of this enzyme, the acid hydrolases that are intended for the lysosomes lack the recognition marker, mannose-6-phosphate. The enzymes are secreted instead of being trapped within the lysosome. Ordinarily, these acid hydrolases are further "processed" in the lysosomes. Because they are not trapped in this organelle, the resultant secreted acid hydrolases differ from the "normal, trapped" lysosomal enzymes.

MIM No.: *25250

POS No.: 3306

Sex Ratio: M1:F1

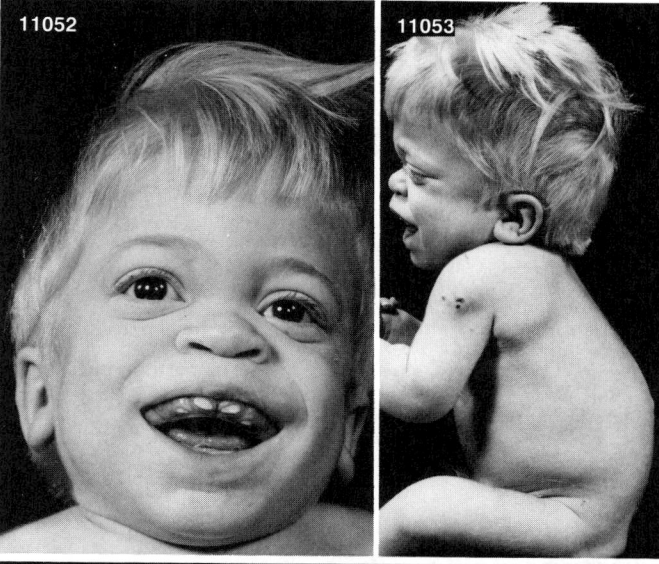

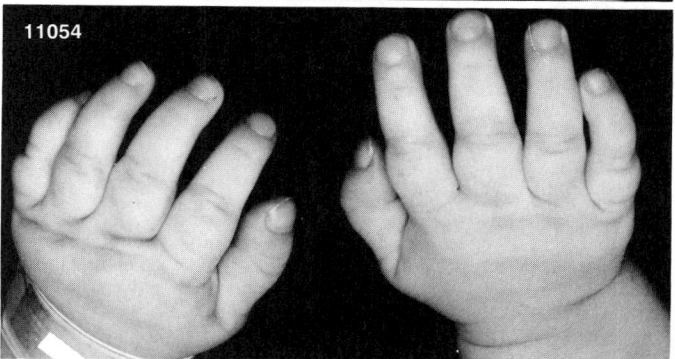

0672-11052–53: Coarse facies with proptotic eyes; open, wide mouth; hyperplastic gingiva; abundant hair; scaphocephaly and gibbus. 11054: Short digits and the beginning of a claw-hand deformity.

Occurrence: More than 30 reported cases; many from Japan.

Risk of Recurrence for Patient's Sib:
See Part I, *Mendelian Inheritance.*

Risk of Recurrence for Patient's Child:
See Part I, *Mendelian Inheritance.* Affected individuals are not expected to survive to reproduce.

Age of Detectability: Clinically, in early infancy. Prenatal diagnosis can be made from amniocytes obtained by conventional amniocentesis and from trophoblasts at 10 weeks menstrual (8 weeks embryonic) age.

Gene Mapping and Linkage: GNPTA (UDP-N-acetylgluco.-lysosomal-enzyme N-acetylglucosaminephosphotrans.) has been provisionally mapped to 4q21-q23.

Prevention: None known. Genetic counseling indicated.

Treatment: Supportive therapy.

Prognosis: Usually death by five years of age.

Detection of Carrier: No reproducible abnormalities have been identified in heterozygotes.

Support Groups: NJ; Elizabeth; National Lipid Diseases Foundation

References:
Sly WS and Fischer HD: The phosphomannosyl recognition system for intracellular and intercellular transport of lysosomal enzymes. J Cell Biochem 1982; 18:67–85.
Whelan DT, et al.: Mucolipidosis II: the clinical, radiological and biochemical features in three cases. Clin Genet 1983; 24:90–96.
Okada S, et al.: I-cell disease: clinical studies of 21 Japanese cases. Clin Genet 1985; 28:207–215.
Kornfeld S: Trafficking of lysosomal enzymes in normal and disease states. J Clin Invest 1986; 77:1–6.
Herzog V, et al.: Thyroglobulin, the major and obligatory exportable protein of thyroid follicle cells, carries the lysosomal recognition marker mannose-6-phosphate. EMBO J 1987; 6:555–560.
Ben-Yoseph Y, et al.: First trimester prenatal evaluation for I-cell desease by N-acetyl-glucosamine 1-phosphototransferase assay. Clin Genet 1988; 33:38–43.
Nolan CM, Sly WS: I-cell disease and pseudo-Hurler polydystrophy. In: Scriver CR, et al, eds: The metabolic basis of inherited disease, 6th ed. New York: McGraw-Hill, 1989:1589–1602.

AM001
                                                        R. Stephan S. Amato

MUCOLIPIDOSIS III   0673

Includes:
> Pseudo-Hurler polydystrophia
> Pseudopolysystrophy

Excludes:
> **Mucolipidosis II** (0672)
> **Mucopolysaccharidosis**

Major Diagnostic Criteria: Early onset of painless joint stiffness and decreased mobility, short stature, some coarseness of the facial features suggesting a mild mucopolysaccharidosis, mild mental retardation, no excess urinary acid mucopolysaccharides, and X-ray evidence of dysostosis multiplex. Ten to twenty-fold elevations (compared to intracellular fibroblast levels) of beta-

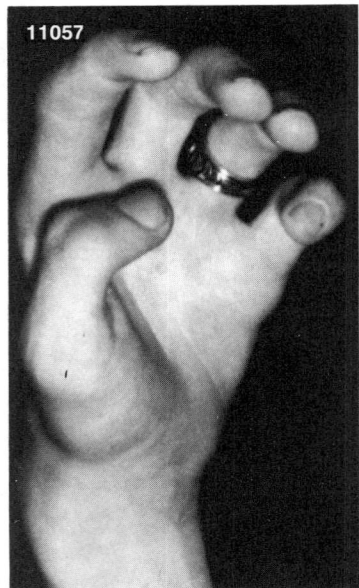

0673B-11057:   Joint contractures.

hexosaminidase, iduronate sulfatase, and aryl-sulfatase A are found in plasma (as they are in I-cell disease).

Clinical Findings: Early childhood onset of joint stiffness; limitation of mobility is slowly progressive but seems to become stationary after puberty. Other characteristics are corneal opacities detected by slit-lamp examination; short stature with short trunk

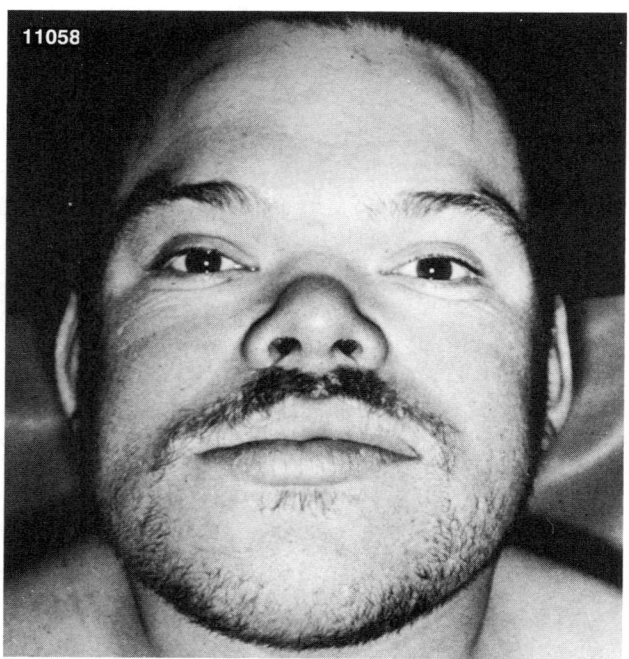

0673A-11058:   Note coarse facial features.

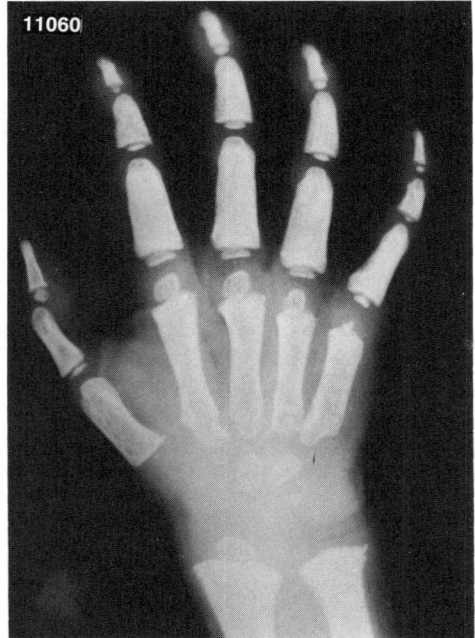

0673C-11060:   X-ray at age 7 years shows rather mild Hurler-like changes of the hand skeleton: reduction of carpal space, misshaped metacarpals, expanded diaphyses of proximal and middle phalanges, and hypoplastic distal phalanges.

and relatively long extremities; and mild mental retardation in some patients. Liver and spleen are usually not enlarged. The urinary excretion of acid mucopolysaccharides is normal; that of sialyloligosaccharides is excessive. Skin fibroblast cultures are metachromatic; the I-cell phenomenon is found too. Peripheral leukocytes are normal in light microscopic appearance, although they have a deficiency of the enzyme. Vacuolated plasma cells are found in the bone marrow. X-ray of the skeleton shows abnormalities that resemble milder forms of the mucopolysaccharidoses, except for severe pelvic dysplasia; vertebral anomalies are common. There is generalized osteoporosis.

Complications: Easy fatigability. Congestive heart failure may occur. Carpal tunnel compression is occasional.

Associated Findings: Aortic valvular disease, carpal tunnel compression.

Etiology: Autosomal recessive inheritance. Deficiency of UDP-N-acetylglucosamine-1-phosphotransferase.

Pathogenesis: The primary deficiency of mucolipidosis (ML) III is in UDP-N-acetylglucosamine-1-phosphatotransferase. In normal fibroblasts, acid hydrolases are glycosylated and phosphorylated. UDP-N-acetylglucosamine phosphatase brings the phosphate to the oligosaccharide chain of the lysosomal enzymes. Subsequently, the glucosamine is removed and leaves the phosphate attached to the mannose. This acts like a recognition marker that finds the receptor in the endoplasmic reticulum or Golgi apparatus and drives the enzyme to the lysosome. There the enzymes acquire their mature form by limited proteolysis. Normally, very little of the enzymes is secreted outside of the cell, and they can be recovered by endocytosis. In ML III, the partial lack of phosphorylation deprives acid hydrolases of the recognition marker, and they are secreted after additional carbohydrate modifications (sialization). They cannot be taken up by endocytosis and thus remain in the extracellular spaces or in the serum, increasing their concentration to the levels previously noted.

MIM No.: *25260

POS No.: 3307

Sex Ratio: M1:F1

Occurrence: A few dozen cases have been documented, including four original French cases (Maroteaux and Lamy, 1966), and two Cape Coloured cases.

Risk of Recurrence for Patient's Sib:
See Part I, *Mendelian Inheritance.*

Risk of Recurrence for Patient's Child:
See Part I, *Mendelian Inheritance.*

Age of Detectability: Joint stiffness has been noted as early as 13 months, but usually manifests itself after the second year of life. Prenatal diagnosis is possible by measuring the levels of lysosomal enzymes, especially hexosaminidases, in the amniotic fluid and in the amniocytes and by the analysis of the specific enzyme UDP-N-acetylglucosamine-1-phosphotransferase.

Gene Mapping and Linkage: GNPTA (UDP-N-acetylglucosamine-lysosomal-enzyme N-acetylglucosaminephosphotransferase) has been provisionally mapped to 4q21-q23.

Prevention: None known. Genetic counseling indicated.

Treatment: Symptomatic.

Prognosis: Joint stiffness typically is evident by age 2–4 years. This can cause a significant handicap for the adult. Progressive destruction of the hip joints results in the most disabling problems for these individuals by late teens. Mental retardation, if present, is mild and not progressive. Survival to age 50 years is known, but there is little information available on the course of the disease in adulthood.

Detection of Carrier: Heterozygote detection has been reported using [32P]UDP-G1cNAc and 3H or 14C labeled UDP-G1cNAc as the donor substrate for the UDP-N-acetylglucosamine-1-phosphotransferase. These reports show some overlap between the activity ranges of presumed heterozygotes and normals.

Special Considerations: The finding of three different complementation groups in fibroblasts suggests the heterogeneous nature of ML III and could be due to either allelic variation in the expression of defects in a single gene, or mutations in distinct genes. Varki et al (1981) found that fibroblasts from two sibs with ML III had normal enzyme activity when measured with the assay using alpha methyl-mannose as acceptor, but a low activity when assayed with endogenous acceptor. The diagnosis of the condition is made by recognition of the clinical and developmental signs previously noted, by the highly elevated levels of lysosomal enzymes in serum, and by the demonstration of the deficiency of the enzyme UDP-N-acetylglucosamine-1-phosphotransferase.

Support Groups: NJ; Elizabeth; National Lipid Diseases Foundation

References:
Maroteaux P, Lamy M: La pseudo-polydystrophie de Hurler. Presse Med 1966; 74:2889–2892.
Reitman ML, et al.: Fibroblast from patients with I-cell disease and pseudo-Hurler polydystrophy are deficient in uridine 5'-diphosphate-N-acetylglucosamine: glycoprotein N-acetylglucosaminylphosphotransferase activity. J Clin Invest 1981; 67:1574–1578.
Varki AP, et al.: Identification of a variant of mucolipidosis III: a catalytically active N-acetylglucosaminyl-phosphotransferase that fails to phosphorylate lysosomal enzymes. Proc Natl Acad Sci USA 1981; 78:7773–7777.
Neufeld EF, McKusick VA: Mucolipidosis III. In: Stanbury JB, et al., eds: The metabolic basis of inherited disease. 5th ed. New York: McGraw-Hill, 1983.
Little LE, et al.: Heterogeneity of N-acetylglucosmine 1-phosphotransferse within mucoloipidosis III. J Biol Chem 1986; 261:733–735.
Traboulsi EI, Maumenee IH: Ophthalmologic findings in mucolipidosis III (pseudo-Hurler polydystrophy). Am J Ophthal 1986; 102:592–597.
Mueller OT, et al.: Chromosomal assignment of N- acetylglucosaminylphospho-transferase, the lysosomal hydrolase trageting enzyme deficient in mucolipodosis II and III. (Abstract) Cytogenet Cell Genet HGM9, 1987.
Nolan CM, Sly WS: I-cell disease and pseudo-Hurler polydystrophy. In: Scriver CR, et al, eds: The metabolic basis of inherited disease, 6th ed. New York: McGraw-Hill, 1989:1589–1602.

TR008   **Carlos J. Trujillo-Botero**

MUCOLIPIDOSIS IV   2251

Includes:
Ganglioside neuraminidase deficiency
Ganglioside sialidase deficiency
Neuraminidase deficiency

Excludes:
Mucolipidosis (other)
Mucopolysaccharidosis
Niemann-Pick disease (0717)

Major Diagnostic Criteria: Corneal clouding; slowly progressive neurologic degeneration with mental retardation; normal urinary mucopolysaccharides; cytoplasmic inclusions seen with electron microscopy (EM) in conjunctival biopsies, skin fibroblasts, and cultured amniotic fluid cells. Skeletal changes and hepatosplenomegaly are usually absent.

Clinical Findings: Corneal opacities, slowly progressive pyramidal tract signs with hypotonia and extrapyramidal involvement. Corneal opacities were reported in 100% of cases, but may vary with age in the same patient. Visual acuity was diminished, sometimes profoundly, and an abnormal electroretinogram (ERG) was found in one-half. Strabismus was noted in 7%. Facial coarsening was subtle, but milder cases have been reported.

Bone marrow and leukocytes were normal. Electron microscopy (EM) of skin biopsies and/or conjunctiva were abnormal in all cases and showed both single membrane-bound granular inclusions and lamellar concentric bodies. These were also noted in cultured fibroblasts, amniocytes, and in liver, muscle, and brain. All phospholipids were increased in liver, skin fibroblasts, and urine, and only phosphatidylcholine in brain. Lysobisphosphatidic acid (LBPA) was markedly increased in these tissues, but was the only lipid stored in muscle. A mild increase in gangliosides has been reported in urine, brain white matter, and cultured fibroblasts.

Complications: Photophobia associated with corneal clouding and diminished visual acuity.

Associated Findings: None known.

Etiology: Autosomal recessive inheritance.

Pathogenesis: A partial ganglioside sialidase deficiency has been found in cultured fibroblasts. Whether this is the primary enzyme defect is doubtful. Increased phospholipids have now been reported in urine (2/6) and fibroblasts (5/6) from six unrelated patients. The nature of a putative defect in lysosomal membrane turnover remains undetermined.

MIM No.: *25265

POS No.: 3548

Sex Ratio: M11:F6 (observed).

Occurrence: Prevalence <1:100,000. About 20 cases, including three pairs of siblings, have been reported: eight in Ashkenazi Jews and nine in non-Jewish families.

Risk of Recurrence for Patient's Sib:
See Part I, *Mendelian Inheritance.*

Risk of Recurrence for Patient's Child:
See Part I, *Mendelian Inheritance.*

Age of Detectability: From one to two months of age; or prenatally from study of cultured fibroblasts.

Gene Mapping and Linkage: Unknown.

Prevention: None known. Genetic counseling indicated.

Treatment: A corneal graft was attempted without success in one case.

Prognosis: Age of oldest known patient is in the mid-twenties.

Detection of Carrier: Unknown.

Support Groups:
NY; Moncey; The Children's Association for Research on Mucolipidosis IV
NJ; Elizabeth; National Lipid Diseases Foundation

References:
Tellez-Nagel I, et al.: Mucolipidosis IV: clinical, ultrastructural, histochemical and chemical studies of a case, including a brain biopsy. Arch Neurol 1976; 33:828–835.
Philippart M, et al.: Mucolipidosis IV: a phospholipidosis. Trans Am Soc Neurochem 1980; 11:72.
Caimi L, et al.: Mucolipidosis IV: a sialolipidosis due to ganglioside sialidase deficiency. J Inherit Metab Dis 1982; 5:218–224.
Crandall BF, et al.: Mucolipidosis IV. Am J Med Genet 1982; 12:301–308. *
Lake BD, et al.: A mild variant of mucolipidosis type 4 (ML4). BD:OAS (XVIII(6). New York: March of Dimes Birth Defects Foundation, 1982:391–404.
Riedel KG, et al.: Ocular abnormalities in mucolipidosis IV. Am J Ophthal 1985; 99:125–136.
Amir N, et al.: Mucolipidosis type IV: clinical spectrum and natural history. Pediatrics 1987; 79:953–959.
Ornoy A, et al.: Early prenatal diagnosis of mucolipidosis IV. (Letter) Am J Med Genet 1987; 27:983–985.
Bargal R, et al.: Phospholipids accumulation in mucolipidosis IV cultured fibroblasts. J Inherit Metab Dis 1988; 11:144–150.
O'Brien JS: Beta-galactosidase deficiency. In: Scriver CR, et al, eds: The metabolic basis of inherited disease, 6th ed. New York: McGraw-Hill, 1989:1797–1806.

CR018
PH000

Barbara Crandall
Michel Philippart

Mucopolysaccharidosis (MPS) III, types A, B, C and D
See MUCOPOLYSACCHARIDOSIS III
Mucopolysaccharidosis (MPS) IV, types A and B
See MUCOPOLYSACCHARIDOSIS IV
Mucopolysaccharidosis F
See FUCOSIDOSIS

MUCOPOLYSACCHARIDOSIS I-H   0674

Includes:
Alpha-L-iduronidase deficiency
Gargoylism (obsolete/pejorative)
Hurler syndrome
Hurler-Pfaundler syndrome
Hurler-Scheie syndrome
Mucopolysaccharidosis I-H/I-S compound

Excludes:
G(M1)-gangliosidosis, type 1 (0431)
Mucolipidosis II (0672)
Mucolipidosis III (0673)
Mucopolysaccharidosis (other)

Major Diagnostic Criteria: Coarse facies, corneal clouding, joint contractures and hepatosplenomegaly. Excess mucopolysacchariduria occurs, but for confirmation, laboratory studies must demonstrate either 1) deficient α-L-iduronidase in leukocytes or fibroblasts, or 2) abnormal sulfate incorporation and degradation by cultured fibroblasts which can be "corrected" by addition of "Hurler factor." Metachromatic staining of fibroblasts and leukocyte inclusions are non-specific findings.

Clinical Findings: Normal appearance at birth but may have excessive birth weight. In early months of life, onset of progressive coarsening of facial features, depressed nasal bridge, corneal clouding, hepatosplenomegaly, joint stiffness, and thoracolumbar kyphosis. Other constant features seen by age two years include inguinal or umbilical herniae; abundance of fine body hair, particularly over extensor areas and back; enlarged and scaphoid head; large tongue and lips; small, widely spaced teeth; mucoid rhinorrhea; noisy respiration; and limitation of joint mobility, especially at phalanges, elbows, shoulders, and hips. Later signs include cardiac murmurs, deafness, blindness, and short stature. Growth is normal or excessive during first year, with decline thereafter. Short stature is apparent by three years. Motor and mental development reach a peak before two years and deteriorate thereafter.

X-ray findings include scaphocephaly; "shoe-shaped" and enlarged sella; diaphyseal widening of tubular bones, most pro-

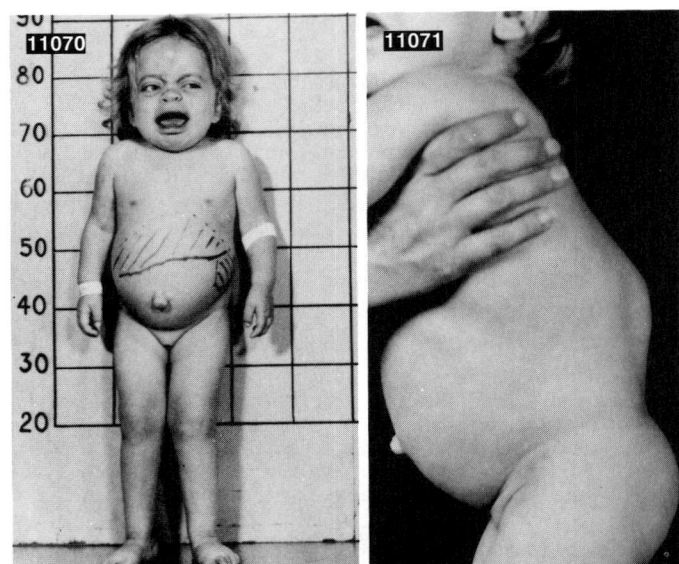

0674-11070: Coarse facial features and hepatosplenomegaly are evident in this young child. **11071:** Umbilical hernia, protruding abdomen and gibbus.

nounced in upper limbs; expansion of shaft of the ribs; and anterior beaking of the vertebrae.

Laboratory findings include mucopolysacchariduria, with excessive excretion of dermatan sulfate and heparan sulfate. Deficiency of the lysosomal enzyme, α-L-iduronidase is demonstrable in fibroblasts or leukocytes. Fibroblasts have abnormal sulfate kinetics in culture, incorporating excessive sulfate from the media and failing to normally degrade sulfated mucopolysaccharide when grown in sulfate-deficient media. Leukocytes and fibroblasts show metachromatic staining granules.

Complications: Loss of vision because of corneal clouding and retinal degeneration; mental deterioration because of deposits in CNS and hydrocephaly; cardiac decompensation from mucopolysaccharide deposits in intima of coronary vessels and valves; deafness; skeletal incapacitation because of joint limitation; and death, usually from cardiorespiratory decompensation.

Associated Findings: None known.

Etiology: Autosomal recessive inheritance.

Pathogenesis: The Hurler features develop because of progressive deposition of acid mucopolysaccharide (AMPS) in various tissues. Deficient function of α-L-iduronidase, an enzyme responsible for degradation of AMPS underlies this condition.

MIM No.: *25280

POS No.: 3308

CDC No.: 277.510

Sex Ratio: M1:F1

Occurrence: Incidence probably about 1:100,000 live births; described in Caucasians, Orientals, and Blacks. Prevalence less because of early death.

Risk of Recurrence for Patient's Sib:
See Part I, *Mendelian Inheritance.*

Risk of Recurrence for Patient's Child:
See Part I, *Mendelian Inheritance.* Affected individuals are not expected to survive to reproduce.

Age of Detectability: At 10 weeks gestation, by iduronidase assay of chorionic villi. Clinically detectable in the first year of life.

Gene Mapping and Linkage: IDUA (iduronidase, alpha-L-) has been provisionally mapped to 22pter-q11.

Prevention: None known. Genetic counseling indicated.

Treatment: Curative therapy is not available. Surgical correction of joint contractures, corneal transplantation, and cardiac valvular replacement do not give lasting benefits. Umbilical and inguinal hernias often require surgical correction but may recur. None of these surgical measures impede mucopolysaccharide deposition or progressive deterioration. Physical therapy and special education, with attention to deafness, visual difficulties, and physical handicaps, are necessary. Enzyme replacement therapies have shown no clinical benefits to date. Bone marrow transplanation is now being evaluated.

Prognosis: Physical and mental deterioration leads to death before age 10 years in most patients. Death results from pneumonia or cardiac decompensation.

Detection of Carrier: The heterozygote can be identified by assay of α-L-iduronidase in leukocytes, and in cultured fibroblasts.

Special Considerations: In the truest sense, the mucopolysaccharidoses are storage diseases. The signs are progressive, developing parallel to the accumulation of tissue mucopolysaccharide. In addition to the seven generally acknowledged types of mucopolysaccharidoses (MPS), occasional patients are seen in whom the combination of clinical, X-ray, and laboratory findings prevent easy classification.

MPS I (I-H) and MPS V (I-S) have deficiency of the same enzyme, α-L-iduronidase; hence the suggestion that they are allelic conditions. In keeping with this hypothesis, a group of patients has been identified with iduronidase deficiency who have intermediate clinical features. These patients, thought to have one Hurler mutant gene and 1 Scheie mutant gene, have the onset of signs between ages one and two years, normal or near normal

intelligence, and intermediate progression of signs. The oldest patient is in her 20s. This condition has been termed *Hurler-Scheie compound* or *Mucopolysaccharidoses I-H/I-S compound.*

Other patients with intermediate phenotypes may represent the homozygous state for a third mutation of the iduronidase gene.

Support Groups:
NY; Hicksville; National Mucopolysaccharidoses (MPS) Society
CANADA: Manitoba; Flin Flon Society for Mucopolysaccharide Diseases

References:
Maroteaux P, Lamy M: Hurler's disease, Morquio's disease and related mucopolysaccharidoses. J Pediatr 1965; 67:312–322.
Leroy JG, Crocker AC: Clinical definition of the Hurler-Hunter phenotypes. Am J Dis Child 1966; 112:518–530.
McKusick VA: Heritable disorders of connective tissue, 4th ed. St. Louis: C.V. Mosby Co., 1972.
Pennock CA, Barnes IC: Review article: the mucopolysaccharides. J Med Genet 1976; 13:169–181.
Stevenson RE, et al.: The iduronidase deficient mucopolysaccharidoses: clinical and roentgenographic features. Pediatrics 1976; 57: 111–122. * †
Roubicek M, et al.: The clinical spectrum of alpha-L-iduronidase deficiency. Am J Med Genet 1985; 20:471–481.
Whitley CB, et al.: A nonpathologic allele (I-W) for low alpha-L-iduronidase enzyme activity via-a-vis prenatal diagnosis of Herler syndrome. Am J Med Genet 1987; 28:233–243.
Schuchman EH, Desnick RJ: Mucopolysaccharidosis type I subtypes: presence of immunologically cross-reactive material and in vitro enhancement of the residual alpha-L-iduronidase activities. J Clin Invest 1988; 81:98–105.
Neufeld EF, Muenzer J: The mucopolysaccharidoses. In: Scriver CR, et al., eds: The metabolic basis of inherited disease, ed 6. New York: McGraw-Hill, 1989:1565–1588.

ST021   **Roger E. Stevenson**

Mucopolysaccharidosis I-H/I-S compound
See MUCOPOLYSACCHARIDOSIS I-H

MUCOPOLYSACCHARIDOSIS I-S   0675

Includes:
Mucopolysaccharidosis V
Scheie syndrome

Excludes:
G(M1)-gangliosidosis, type 1 (0431)
G(M1)-gangliosidosis, type 2 (0432)
Mucolipidosis III (0673)
Mucopolysaccharidosis (other)

Major Diagnostic Criteria: Corneal clouding, mild or absent intellectual impairment, variable but generally mild somatic features plus mucopolysacchariduria plus 1) specific abnormal sulfate kinetics in fibroblast culture, or 2) deficiency of α-L-iduronidase activity in fibroblasts or leukocytes. The distinction from the severe mucopolysaccharidosis (MPS) I-H, and the moderately severe MPS I-H/I- S compound is clinical; all three types having the same laboratory findings.

Clinical Findings: Corneal clouding and herniae may be present at birth or soon thereafter; otherwise, signs of mucopolysaccharide disease are absent during infancy. By early school age, joint stiffness with limitation of phalanges, elbows, and shoulders. Genu valgum is the rule. Cardiac murmurs, often aortic in origin, appear; corneal clouding, retinal degeneration, and skeletal involvement increase; auditory and visual acuity decrease, and carpal tunnel signs and psychotic episodes may develop; hepatosplenomegaly, mental retardation, and stunting of growth are not features. Hurler-like features, if present at all, are mild.

X-ray findings include mild changes of dysostosis multiplex. Laboratory findings include excessive heparan sulfate and dermatan sulfate excretion in the urine; fibroblasts and leukocyte inclusions may stain metachromatically; leukocytes and fibroblasts have deficient α-L-iduronidase activity.

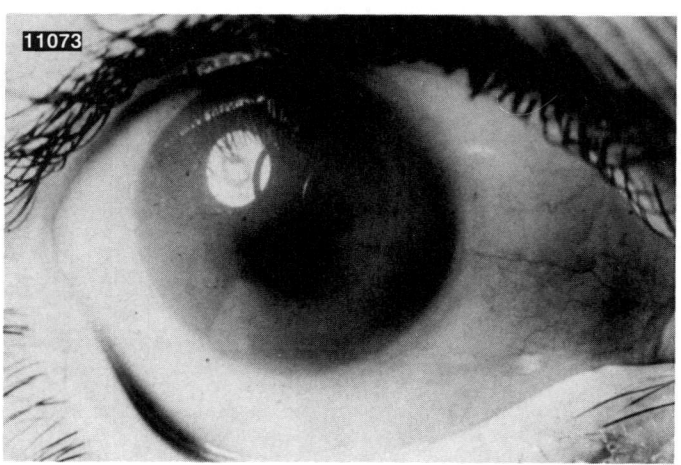

0675-11073: Diffuse corneal clouding involving the entire stroma.

Complications: Aortic regurgitation, carpal tunnel syndrome, blindness from corneal clouding and retinal degeneration, hearing loss, and psychotic episodes.

Associated Findings: Unknown.

Etiology: Autosomal recessive inheritance.

Pathogenesis: Deficiency of α-L-iduronidase, one of the lysosomal enzymes responsible for mucopolysaccharide degradation, leading to deposition of acid mucopolysaccharide in soft tissues and interruption of normal bone development.

MIM No.: *25280

POS No.: 3312

Sex Ratio: M1:F1

Occurrence: Undetermined, but presumed rare.

Risk of Recurrence for Patient's Sib:
See Part I, *Mendelian Inheritance.*

Risk of Recurrence for Patient's Child:
See Part I, *Mendelian Inheritance.*

Age of Detectability: At 10 weeks gestation, by assay of α-L-iduronidase using chorionic villi.

Gene Mapping and Linkage: IDUA (iduronidase, alpha-L-) has been provisionally mapped to 22pter-q11.

Prevention: None known. Genetic counseling indicated.

Treatment: Curative treatment is not available. Surgical correction of hernias, joint contractures, and carpal tunnel compression is beneficial. Corneal transplantation has provided at least temporary benefit. Physical therapy for joint contractures, hearing aids, and medical or surgical management of aortic valve disease may be necessary.

Prognosis: The few patients reported have survived into adulthood.

Detection of Carrier: Carriers have intermediate levels of α-L-iduronidase in leukocytes and cultured fibroblasts.

Special Considerations: Scheie syndrome is considered allelic to Hurler syndrome because both lack α-L-iduronidase.

Support Groups:
NY; Hicksville; National Mucopolysaccharidoses (MPS) Society
CANADA: Manitoba; Flin Flon Society for Mucopolysaccharide Diseases

References:
Scheie HG, et al.: A newly recognized forme fruste of Hurler's disease (gargoylism). Am J Ophthalmol. 1962; 53:753–769.

Wiesmann UN, Neufeld EF: Scheie and Hurler syndromes: apparent identity of the biochemical defect. Science 1970; 169:72–74.

McKusick VA, et al.: Allelism, nonallelism and genetic compounds among the mucopolysaccharidoses. Lancet 1972; I:993–996.

Stevenson RE, et al.: The iduronidase-deficient mucopolysaccharidoses: clinical and roentgenographic features. Pediatrics 1976; 57: 111–122. * †

McKusick VA, et al.: The mucopolysaccharide storage diseases. In: Stanbury JB, et al, eds: Metabolic basis of inherited disease, 4th ed. New York: McGraw-Hill, 1978:1282–1307. * †

Neufeld EF, Muenzer J: The mucopolysaccharidoses. In: Scriver CR, et al, eds: The metabolic basis of inherited disease, 6th ed. New York: McGraw-Hill, 1989:1565–1588.

ST021   **Roger E. Stevenson**

MUCOPOLYSACCHARIDOSIS II   0676

Includes:
Hunter syndrome
Mucopolysaccharidosis II, types A and B
Sulfatidosis, juvenile, Austin type (Some forms)
Sulfo-iduronate sulfatase deficiency

Excludes:
G(M1)-gangliosidosis, type 1 (0431)
G(M1)-gangliosidosis, type 2 (0432)
Mannosidosis (2079)
Mucolipidosis
Mucopolysaccharidosis (other)

Major Diagnostic Criteria: Affected males have normal or impaired intellect, clear corneas, hernias, hepatosplenomegaly, skin nodules, progressive stiffening of joints, thickening of skin, coarsening of facies, and mucopolysacchariduria. Diagnosis can be confirmed by cultured fibroblasts, corrected by Hunter factor, or demonstration of sulfoiduronate sulfatase deficiency in fibroblasts, serum, or leukocytes.

Clinical Findings: Appearance is normal at birth with normal or excessive growth during first 1–2 years. During infancy few clinical signs occur except for respiratory symptoms (noisy breathing from upper airway obstruction, recurrent rhinorrhea), large scaphoid head, and herniae (inguinal and umbilical). Coarsening of facial features, with thickening of the nostrils, lips, and tongue; joint stiffness, growth failure, excessive growth of fine body hair, and hepatosplenomegaly become obvious at about age two years and progress in severity. Thick skin, short neck, widely spaced teeth, hearing loss of some degree, and papilledema are commonly present; nodular skin lesions on the arms or posterior chest wall, retinal pigmentation, mild pectus excavatum, pes cavus, mucoid diarrhea and seizures are less common. The spine is straight; corneas are clear grossly; and intellect may be normal, but with a tendency to disruptive, destructive behavior. Mentation, valvular and coronary heart disease, hearing, and joint mobility slowly deteriorate.

Two more or less distinctive types of mucopolysaccharidosis (MPS) II are recognized clinically: in the "mild form" (MPS II-B) mentation may be normal, and deterioration of mental function only slowly progressive; in the "severe form" (MPS II-A) profound mental retardation becomes obvious by late childhood. Other clinical features may be the same, but with slower progression in the "mild form." With rare exception, the subtypes "breed true" within a family.

X-ray findings include scaphoid skull, enlarged sella with anterior excavation, skeletal findings of dysostosis multiplex, minimal vertebral changes, and precocious osteoarthritis of femoral head.

Laboratory findings include acid mucopolysacchariduria with excessive excretion of dermatan sulfate and heparan sulfate; leukocytes and fibroblasts are deficient in the enzyme sulfoiduronate sulfatase; metachromatic staining of leukocyte granules and fibroblasts; cultured fibroblasts accumulate sulfated mucopolysaccharides at an enhanced rate and can be "corrected" with purified

Hunter factor or with fibroblast secretion from non-Hunter individuals.

Complications: Coronary and valvular cardiac disease from AMPS deposition, myelopathy due to meningeal thickening, hydrocephaly, progressive hearing loss, immobilization by joint contractures, and degenerative hip disease.

Associated Findings: None known.

Etiology: Usually X-linked recessive inheritance. The possibility of a rare autosomal recessive form has not been excluded, but may represent cases of *sulfatidosis, juvenile, Austin type* (Burch et al, 1986).

Pathogenesis: Accumulation of acid mucopolysaccharide in tissues underlies most of the observed clinical features. The block in mucopolysaccharide metabolism has been shown to be a deficiency of the enzyme sulfoiduronate sulfatase.

MIM No.: *30990, *27220

POS No.: 3309

Sex Ratio: M1:F0. Females have rarely been affected, the presumed result of nonrandom lyonisation or selection for cells whose active X chromosome bore the mutant (Hunter) gene.

Occurrence: Estimated 1:100,000 live births in Caucasians, blacks, Orientals, and American Indians. Prevalence lower than birth frequency because of early death, particularly in severe type.

Risk of Recurrence for Patient's Sib:
See Part I, *Mendelian Inheritance.*

Risk of Recurrence for Patient's Child:
See Part I, *Mendelian Inheritance.*

Age of Detectability: At 9–11 weeks gestation, by studies of chorionic villous samples. Karyotypic analysis should accompany such tests to confirm sex of fetus.

Gene Mapping and Linkage: IDS (iduronate 2-sulfatase (Hunter syndrome)) has been mapped to Xq27.3-q28.

Prevention: None known. Genetic counseling indicated.

Treatment: No curative treatment is available. Attempts at enzyme replacement with plasma or leukocyte infusions have not produced definite benefits. Supportive measures include hearing devices, physical therapy, and special education. Surgical correction of hernias, joint contractures, myelopathy, carpal tunnel syndrome, and hydrocephaly may become necessary.

Prognosis: Compatible with survival to adult life. However, the majority of patients with the severe subtype (MPS II-A) die prior to age 20 years of cardiac decompensation, pulmonary infection, or neurologic complications. Several patients with the mild subtype (MPS II-B) have survived beyond age 60 years, and a number have reproduced.

Detection of Carrier: May be identified by enzyme assay or sulfate incorporation studies of fibroblasts. Utilizing cloning techniques, two cell lines, one with the mucopolysaccharide abnormality and the other normal, can be discerned. Carrier identification may also be made by demonstrating a mosaic pattern of enzyme activity in the hair bulbs and, in many cases, by reduced enzyme activity in serum.

Special Considerations: Individuals with MPS I and MPS II excrete the same acid mucopolysaccharides qualitatively and quantitatively; yet they are quite distinct genetically and clinically. MPS II has all the features of MPS I; but to a remarkably milder degree, the corneal changes can be seen only with the slit-lamp; intellect may be normal, at least initially; the skeletal changes are less severe, and outlook for longevity is greater. The mild and severe subtypes of MPS II both lack the same enzyme; hence they are probably allelic conditions.

Sulfatidosis, juvenile, Austin type is an autosomal recessive disorder which combines features of metachromatic leukodystrophy and mucopolysaccharidosis. The condition combines the enzyme deficiency and phenotypic features of a number of other conditions (Burch et al, 1986).

Support Groups:
NY; Hicksville; National Mucopolysaccharidoses (MPS) Society

CANADA: Manitoba; Flin Flon Society for Mucopolysaccharide Diseases

References:
Leroy JG, Crocker AC: Clinical definition of the Hurler-Hunter phenotypes. Am J Dis Child 1966; 112:518–530. * †
Erickson R, et al.: Biochemical differentiation of two forms of mucopolysaccharidosis II (Hunter's disease). Am J Hum Genet 1972; 24:26A.
McKusick VA: Heritable disorders of connective tissue. ed. 4. St. Louis: CV Mosby, 1972. * †
Bach G, et al.: The defect in the Hunter syndrome: deficiency of sulfoiduronate sulfatase. Proc Natl Acad Sci 1973; 70:2134–2138.
Yatziv D, et al.: Mild and severe Hunter syndrome (MPS II) within the same sibships. Clin Genet 1977; 11:319–326.
Hobolth N, Pedersen C: Six cases of a mild form of the Hunter syndrome in five generations: three affected males with progeny. Clin Genet 1978; 13:121 only.
Tonnesen T, et al.: Diagnosis of Hunter's syndrome carriers: radioactive sulphate incorporation into fibroblasts in the presence of fructose 1-phosphate. Hum Genet 1982; 60:167–171.
Zlotogora J, et al.: Hunter syndrome among Ashkenazi Jews in Israel; evidence for prenatal selection favoring the Hunter allele. Hum Genet 1985; 71:329–332.
Burch M, et al.: Multiple sulphatase deficiency presenting at birth. Clin Genet 1986; 30:409–415.

ST021   **Roger E. Stevenson**

Mucopolysaccharidosis II, types A and B
See MUCOPOLYSACCHARIDOSIS II

MUCOPOLYSACCHARIDOSIS III   **0677**

Includes:
Acetyl CoA:alpha-glucosaminide N-acetyltransferase deficiency
Heparan sulfate sulfatase deficiency
Mucopolysaccharidosis (MPS) III, types A, B, C and D
N-acetyl-alpha-D-glucosaminidase deficiency
N-acetylglucosamine-6-sulfate sulfatase deficiency
Polydystrophia oligophrenia
Sanfilippo syndrome

Excludes:
G(M1)-gangliosidosis, type 2 (0432)
Mucolipidosis
Mucopolysaccharidosis (others)

Major Diagnostic Criteria: Severe mental deterioration, mild Hurler-like somatic defects, and the urinary excretion of heparan sulfate alone are findings sufficient for the diagnosis of MPS III. Metachromatic staining is non-specific. Confirmatory enzyme assay or sulfate kinetic studies on cultured fibroblasts are necessary to distinguish the four types currently delineated.

Clinical Findings: Normal appearance at birth, initial developmental milestones normal. Slowing of development, usually obvious within one to two years, may not become apparent until early school age. Mental and motor development reach a peak by early school age, followed by behavioral disturbances and dramatic intellectual decline. Mental and motor skills are lost, and the often agitated, demented patient becomes bedridden. Growth is minimally affected, the head enlarged, hirsutism present. The mild coarsening of facial features, limitation of joint mobility, and hepatosplenomegaly never become prominent features. Deafness, although hard to evaluate, is thought to occur. Corneal clouding and cardiac abnormalities are not to be expected, although both have been seen in individual patients. The A, B, C, and D subtypes are not clinically separable but can be distinguished by enzymatic assays.

All bone changes on X-ray, except for the skull, are similar but milder than in MPS I. The calvarium is remarkably thickened, and sellar enlargement is not pronounced.

Laboratory findings show urinary excretion of heparan sulfate. Sanfilippo A, the more common of the subtypes, lacks heparan

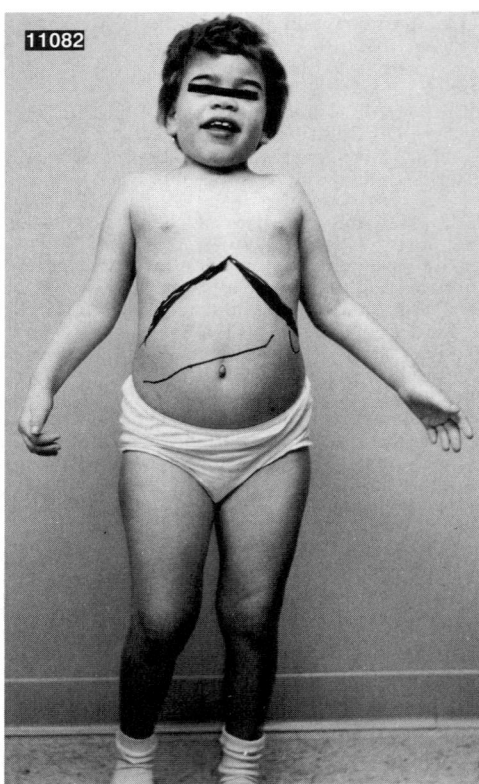

0677-11082: MPS III; note mild coarsening of facial features, hepatosplenomegaly.

sulfate sulfatase; Sanfilippo B lacks N-acetyl-α-glucosaminidase; Sanfilippo C lacks acetyl CoA:α-glucosaminide N-acetyltransferase; Sanfilippo D lacks N-acetyl-α-glucosamine-6-sulfate sulfatase. Fibroblasts and lymphocyte granules stain metachromatically.

Complications: Severe mental deterioration.

Associated Findings: None known.

Etiology: Autosomal recessive inheritance.

Pathogenesis: An enzymatic error in degradation of acid mucopolysaccharide underlies each subtype. Unlike the enzymes in the A, B, and D subtypes, the enzyme in Sanfilippo C is not hydrolytic but transfers an acetyl group from acetyl CoA to the free amino portion of a glucosamine residue.

MIM No.: *25290, *25292, *25293, *25294

POS No.: 3310

Sex Ratio: M1:F1

Occurrence: About 1:25,000. Sanfilippo A is the more common subtype. Prevalence less than incidence because of early death.

Risk of Recurrence for Patient's Sib:
See Part I, *Mendelian Inheritance.*

Risk of Recurrence for Patient's Child:
See Part I, *Mendelian Inheritance.* Affected individuals are not expected to survive to reproduce.

Age of Detectability: At 10 weeks gestation by enzyme assay of chorionic villi.

Gene Mapping and Linkage: GNS (N-acetylglucosamine-6-sulfatase (Sanfilippo disease IIID)) has been provisionally mapped to 12q14.

Prevention: None known. Genetic counseling indicated.

Treatment: No curative treatment is available. Attempts at enzyme replacement therapy have produced no clinical benefits.

Prognosis: Death in bedridden, severely demented state by age 20. Few survivors to age 30.

Detection of Carrier: Intermediate enzyme levels in asymptomatic carriers.

Special Considerations: MPS III carries the grave prognosis of severe CNS involvement but is largely spared the pronounced skeletal, corneal, and visceral involvement of the other mucopolysaccharidoses. The four subtypes presently known, although identical clinically, are separable biochemically.

Support Groups:
NY; Hicksville; National Mucopolysaccharidoses (MPS) Society
CANADA: Manitoba; Flin Flon Society for Mucopolysaccharide Diseases

References:
Sanfilippo SJ, et al.: Mental retardation associated with acid mucopolysacchariduria (heparitin sulfate type). J Pediatr 1963; 63:837–838.
Maroteaux P, Lamy M: Hurler's disease, and related mucopolysaccharidoses. J Pediatr 1965; 67:312–322.
Andria G, et al.: Sanfilippo B syndrome (MPS III B): mild and severe forms within the same sibship. Clin Genet 1979; 15:500–504.
Bartsocas C, et al.: Sanfilippo type C disease: clinical findings in four patients with a new variant of mucopolysaccharidosis III. Eur J Pediatr 1979; 130:251–258.
Kresse H, et al.: Sanfilippo disease type D: deficiency of N-acetylglucosamine-6-sulfate sulfatase required for heparan sulfate degradation. Proc Natl Acad Sci USA 1980; 77:6822–6826.
van de Kamp JJP, et al.: Genetic heterogeneity and clinical variability in the Sanfilippo syndrome (types A, B, and C). Clin Genet 1981; 20:152–160. * †
Beratis NG, et al.: Sanfilippo disease in Greece. Clin Genet 1986; 29:129–132.
Kaplan P, Wolfe LS: Sanfilippo syndrome type D. J Pediatr 1987; 110:267–271.

ST021   **Roger E. Stevenson**

MUCOPOLYSACCHARIDOSIS IV   0678

Includes:
   Brailsford syndrome
   Chondroosteodystrophy
   Galactosamine-6-sulfatase deficiency
   Keratansulfaturia
   Morquio syndrome
   Morquio-Üllrich syndrome
   Mucopolysaccharidosis (MPS) IV, types A and B

Excludes:
   Beta-galactosidase deficiency
   Dwarfism, other forms of short-trunk
   G(M1)-gangliosidosis, type 1 (0431)
   Mucolipidosis
   Mucopolysaccharidosis (other)

Major Diagnostic Criteria: Short-trunk dwarfism with normal intellect, cloudy corneas, and lax joints, plus pathognomonic X-ray findings and keratansulfaturia. Confirmation by enzyme assay (6-sulfate sulfatase).

Clinical Findings: The normal intrauterine growth and development continues during the early postnatal months. By age 18 months, growth retardation and skeletal changes (genu valgum, flaring of lower ribs, kyphoscoliosis) become obvious. Intellectual development proceeds at a normal pace and may remain relatively normal despite progressive somatic changes: marked growth retardation, diffuse steamy corneal clouding, prominent lower face, enamel hypoplasia in deciduous and secondary teeth, short neck, pectus carinatum, exaggerated lumbar lordosis, laxity and subluxation of joints (e.g. wrists), and flat feet. Hearing loss present in many patients, and cardiac signs (aortic insufficiency) are found in a minority.

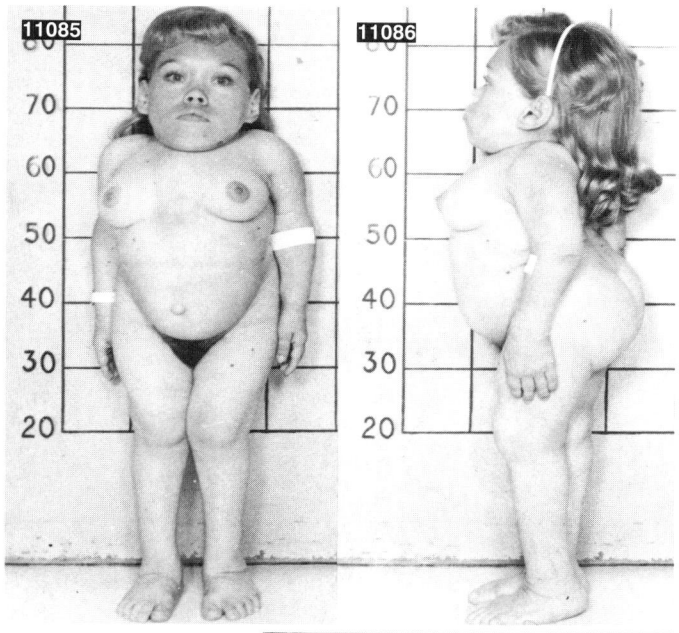

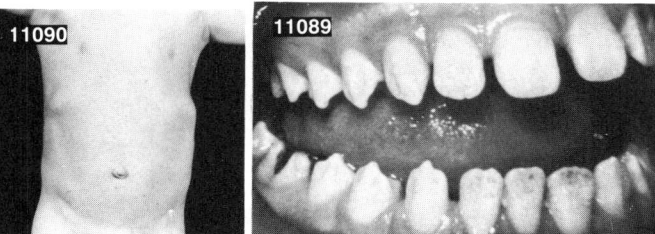

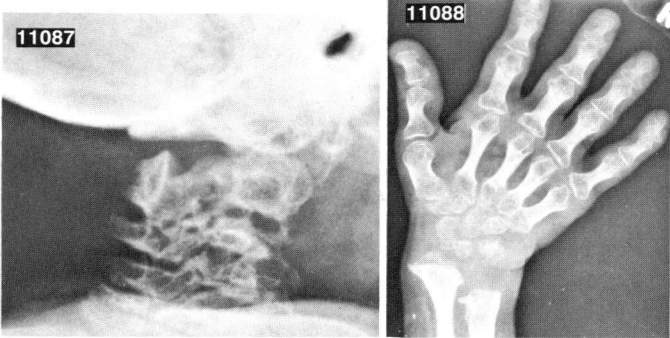

0678-11085–86: Prominent lower face, short neck, short-trunk dwarfism and skeletal deformities. 11090: Young male showing flaring of the lower ribs. 11089: Enamel hypoplasia. 11087: Cervical spine shows rudimentary dens and the atlas closely applied to the occiput. 11088: Small, extremely irregular carpals; short ulna and ulnar deviation; short metacarpals and phalanges with wide ends but well constructed shafts.

X-ray findings predate clinical abnormalities and progressively worsen. Vertebral flattening with central anterior projections occurs in the thoracic area, and hook-shaped projections are found in the lumbar area. The odontoid is hypoplastic. Other findings include increased intervertebral spaces, delayed ossification centers, irregular epiphyses, proximal pointing of metacarpals, wide ribs and generalized osteoporosis. A normal skull is present.

Laboratory findings include keratansulfaturia, with normal or increased total urinary AMPS excretion. Deficiency of N-acetyl-galactosamine-6-sulfate sulfatase is demonstrated in cultured fibroblasts. Granular inclusions are found in a small percentage of granulocytes.

Clinically similar but milder findings have been found in several patients with β-galactosidase deficiency. This condition has been designated as MPS IV-B to distinguish it from sulfate sulfatase deficiency, which is designated MPS IV-A . The enzyme defect(s) are yet to be identified in other patients who have mild features, with or without keratansulfaturia.

Complications: Neurologic signs from spinal cord and nerve root compression, hearing loss, aortic regurgitation, and compensatory hyperpnea. Atlantoaxial subluxation due to aplasia of the odontoid and ligamentous laxity may lead to acute or chronic neurologic signs. Weakness in the legs usually results, and paraplegia is frequent.

Associated Findings: None known.

Etiology: Autosomal recessive inheritance.

Pathogenesis: In MPS IV-A, a deficiency of n-acetyl-galactosamine-6-sulfate sulfatase leads to lysosomal accumulation of keratan sulfate in susceptible tissues. In MPS IV-B, a deficiency of β-galactosidase underlies the abnormal tissue storage of mucopolysaccharide.

MIM No.: *25300, 25301

POS No.: 3311

Sex Ratio: M1:F1

Occurrence: Probably <1:100,000.

Risk of Recurrence for Patient's Sib:
See Part I, *Mendelian Inheritance.*

Risk of Recurrence for Patient's Child:
See Part I, *Mendelian Inheritance.* Few patients have reproduced. Offspring would be obligate carriers.

Age of Detectability: Prenatally by enzyme assay of amniocyte culture or chorionic villi in both types; postnatally prior to one year of age by X-ray changes and keratansulfate excretion.

Gene Mapping and Linkage: The locus for the enzyme N-acetyl-galactosamine-6-sulfate sulfatase is not known; the β-galactosidase locus is on chromosome 3.

Prevention: None known. Genetic counseling indicated.

Treatment: No curative therapy is available. Surgical correction of herniae; upper cervical spinal fusion to avert or remedy spinal cord compression. Corneal transplantation not helpful, cardiac valve replacement not appropriate. Physical therapy and hearing aids may be helpful.

Prognosis: May survive to early adulthood; many die prior to age 20 years from cardiac or neurologic complications. Few survive to an advanced age. Greater longevity is seen in less severely affected individuals.

Detection of Carrier: Unknown.

Special Considerations: Designation of Morquio disease as a mucopolysaccharidosis is based on urinary excretion of keratan-sulfate. Excessive keratansulfaturia may occur in the absence of elevated total urinary mucopolysaccharides. Keratansulfaturia may decrease or disappear entirely in older patients. Study of the kinetics of sulfate metabolism has not been useful in the diagnosis of MPS IV. At least two subtypes exist: the classic form described above, and a type with less severe features without excessive mucopolysacchariduria. Additionally, a group of patients with very mild clinical features and keratansulfaturia and β-galactosidase deficiency have been designated MPS IV-B.

A three-part set of articles by Nelson and colleages, published in volume 33 of Clinical Genetics (1988, pages 111–130), was devoted to the issue of heterogeneity in Morquio disease.

Support Groups:
NY; Hicksville; National Mucopolysaccharidoses (MPS) Society
CANADA: Manitoba; Flin Flon Society for Mucopolysaccharide Diseases

References:
Langer LO Jr, Carey LS: The roentgenographic features of the KS mucopolysaccharidosis of Morquio (Morquio-Brailsford' disease). Am J Roentgenol Radium Ther Nucl Med 1966; 97:1–20.

Arbisser AI, et al.: Morquio-like syndrome with beta-galactosidase deficiency and normal hexosamine sulfatase activity: mucopolysaccharidosis IV B. Am J Med Genet 1977; 1:195–205.

Groebe H, et al.: Morquio syndrome (mucopolysaccharidosis IV-B) associated with beta-galactosidase deficiency: report of two cases. Am J Hum Genet 1980; 32:258–272.

Holzgreve W, et al.: Morquio syndrome: clinical findings in 11 patients with MPS IV A and 2 patients with MPS IV B. Hum Genet 1981; 57:360–365. * †

Yuen M, Fensom AH: Diagnosis of classic Morquio's disease. J Inherit Metab Dis 1985; 8:80–86.

ST021   **Roger E. Stevenson**

Mucopolysaccharidosis V
See MUCOPOLYSACCHARIDOSIS I-S

MUCOPOLYSACCHARIDOSIS VI   0679

Includes:
   Arylsulfatase B deficiency
   Maroteaux-Lamy syndrome

Excludes:
   G(M1)-gangliosidosis, type 1 (0431)
   Mucolipidosis
   Mucopolysaccharidosis (other)

Major Diagnostic Criteria: Severe Hurler-like somatic features, such as growth retardation, cloudy corneas, coarse facies, joint contractures, hepatosplenomegaly, and kyphosis develop progressively in early childhood. Intelligence is normal. Laboratory findings include urinary dermatan sulfate excess, arylsulfatase B deficiency, and abnormal sulfate kinetics in cultured fibroblasts.

Clinical Findings: Normal appearance at birth. Mental development is normal or nearly so. Growth retardation is noted by two to three years. Progressive clouding of corneas, hearing loss, joint stiffness, coarsening of facial features with thick nostrils and lips, are obvious by early school age. Hepatosplenomegaly, lumbar kyphosis, genu valgum, herniae, carpal tunnel, cervical spinal cord compression, and hip dysplasia also occur. Mild, intermediate, and severe forms of this condition exist.

X-rays show calvaria with greatly enlarged sella, fragmented epiphyses, mild flattening of vertebrae with anterior wedging of lumbar vertebrae, and expanded ribs.

Laboratory findings include urinary excretion of dermatan sulfate, and metachromatic staining of fibroblasts and leukocyte inclusions. Fibroblasts and leukocytes have deficient arylsulfatase B (N-acetylgalactosamine-4-sulfatase) activity.

Complications: Visual loss, progressive hearing loss, cardiac and respiratory decompensation, hydrocephaly, cervical spinal cord compression from atlantoaxial subluxation or thickened dura.

Associated Findings: None known.

Etiology: Autosomal recessive inheritance.

Pathogenesis: Deficiency of arylsulfatase B prevents normal lysosomal degradation of mucopolysaccharide, allowing accumulation of AMPS in soft tissues, and disruption of bone development.

MIM No.: *25320

POS No.: 3313

Sex Ratio: M1:F1

Occurrence: Undetermed but presumed rare. Prevalence less than incidence because of early death.

Risk of Recurrence for Patient's Sib:
See Part I, *Mendelian Inheritance.*

Risk of Recurrence for Patient's Child:
See Part I, *Mendelian Inheritance.* Pregnancy has occurred in several females.

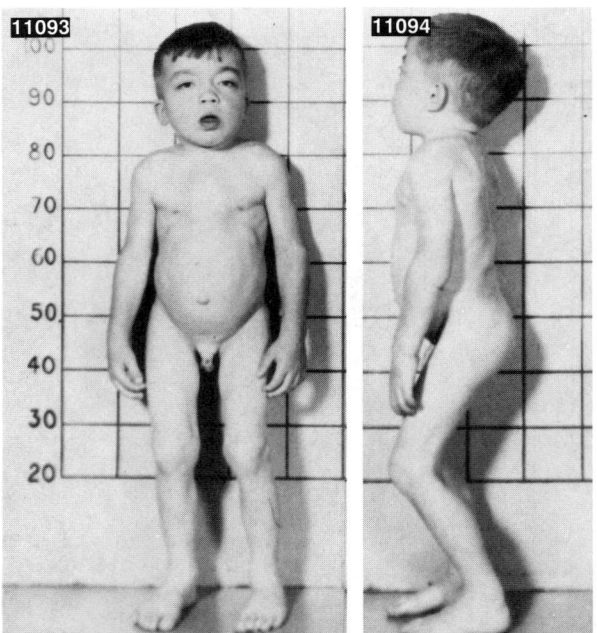

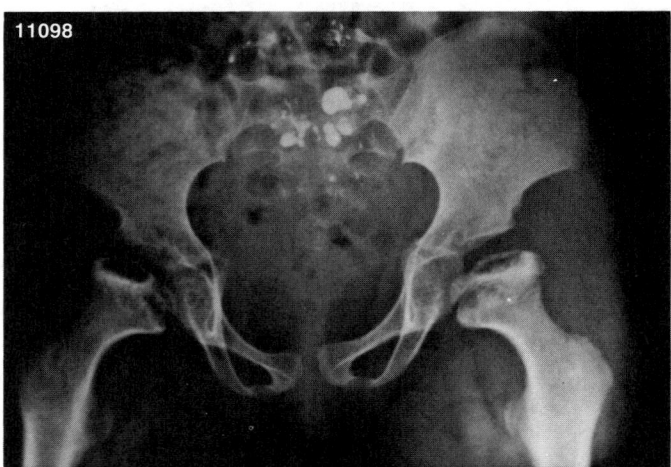

0679-11093–94: Short stature, coarse facies, protruding tongue, short neck, deformed chest and semicrouching stance. **11098:** Flat femoral capital epiphyses with large, cyst-like radiolucencies; surrounding sclerosis; narrow necks; gracile pelvic bones; oblique acetabular roofs.

Age of Detectability: At 10 weeks gestation by study of chorionic villi.

Gene Mapping and Linkage: ARSB (arylsulfatase B) has been mapped to 5p11-q13.

Prevention: None known. Genetic counseling indicated.

Treatment: Curative therapy is not available. Surgical correction of herniae, joint contractures, cardiac valves, carpal tunnel compression, hydrocephaly, and cervical spinal cord compression benefit patients. Physical therapy and hearing devices may be helpful.

Prognosis: Death prior to 20 years, generally of cardiorespiratory complications in the severe subtype. Patients with the mild subtype are productive and intelligent in mid-adult life, but can develop significant myelopathy or cardiovascular problems.

Detection of Carrier: Possible by enzyme (arylsulfatase B) assay of leukocytes or cultured fibroblasts.

Special Considerations: There appears to be a milder form that is less common than the classic form described above. One patient with the mild subtype and normal stature has been reported. Sulfate incorporation, "correction" studies, and enzyme analysis, indicate the two subtypes to be allelic. Intermediate forms may represent compound conditions.

Support Groups:
NY; Hicksville; National Mucopolysaccharidoses (MPS) Society
CANADA: Manitoba; Flin Flon Society for Mucopolysaccharide Diseases

References:
Maroteaux P, Lamy M: Hurler's disease, Morquio's disease, and related mucopolysaccharidoses. J Pediatr 1965; 67:312–323.
McKusick VA: Heritable disorders of connective tissue, 4th ed. St. Louis: C.V. Mosby, 1972. * †
Beratis NG, et al.: Arylsulfatase B deficiency in Maroteaux-Lamy syndrome: cellular studies and carrier identification. Pediatr Res 1975; 9:475–480.
Levy LA, et al.: Ultrastructures of Reilly bodies (metachromatic granules) in the Maroteaux-Lamy syndrome (mucopolysaccharidosis VI): a histochemical study. Am J Clin Pathol 1980; 73:416–422.
Saul RA, et al.: Atypical presentation with normal stature in Maroteaux-Lamy syndrome (MPS VI). Proc Greenwood Genet Ctr 1984; 3:49–52.
Black SH, et al.: Maroteaux-Lamy syndrome in a large consanguineous kindred: biochemical and immunological studies. Am J Med Genet 1986; 25:273–279.

ST021
SA030

Roger E. Stevenson
Robert A. Saul

MUCOPOLYSACCHARIDOSIS VII   0680

Includes:
Beta-glucuronidase deficiency
GUSB deficiency
Sly syndrome

Excludes:
Aspartylglucosaminuria (2042)
Fucosidosis (0398)
Mannosidosis (2079)
Mucolipidosis
Mucopolysaccharidosis (others)

Major Diagnostic Criteria: At least two phenotypes may be present. One has early onset of coarse facies, hepatosplenomegaly, corneal clouding, and other features consistent with the Hurler phenotype. Onset of this first form has been reported in the second decade of life. The other form begins in the second decade with mild skeletal abnormalities, corneal opacities, aortic regurgitation, and normal growth and mentation. Hepatosplenomegaly is not present. Diagnosis is established by demonstrating β-glucuronidase deficiency in tissues, fibroblasts, leukocytes, or serum. Although a mucopolysaccharidosis (MPS) screen is usually positive, no diagnostic pattern of MPS excretion has been identified.

Clinical Findings: The clinical description is based on the first 20 described cases of MPS VII. Although this disease is not yet well defined, two major groups appear to be emerging. Some patients (13 cases) have had clinical signs at birth or within the first years of life. These patients exhibit coarsened facies, hepatosplenomegaly, corneal clouding, frequent respiratory infections, umbilical or additional inguinal herniae, leukocyte inclusions, short stature, and developmental retardation. Three of these patients were affected at birth. Non-immune hydrops fetalis has been reported in two patients. The X-ray features of the early-onset form include moderate-to-severe bony abnormalities with J-shaped sella, vertebral beaking and broadening of the tubular bones (dysostosis multiplex). A second form, presenting in the second decade of life, has been recognized in six cases. In these

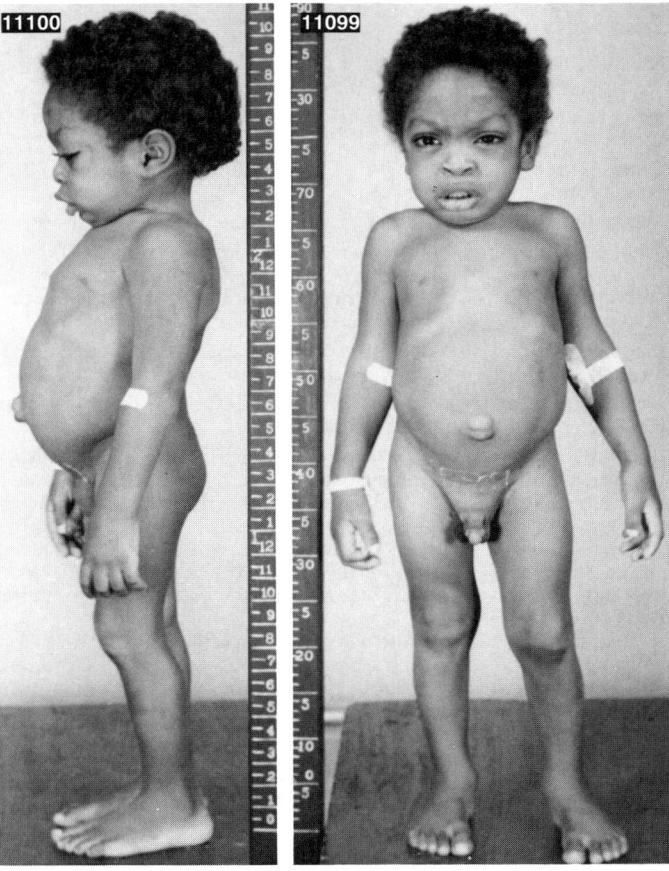

0680A-11099–11100: Short stature, coarse facial features, abdominal protuberance from hepatosplenomegaly, chest configuration including pigeon breast and flared ribs and umbilical hernia are present by age 3 years. By his late teens his main problems were orthopedic including kyphoscoliosis, odontoid hypoplasia and progressive hip deformity. His mental retardation has been moderate but non-progressive.

patients, mild bony changes, little facial coarsening, normal growth and mentation, and no hepatosplenomegaly is seen. Fibromuscular dysplasia with aortic regurgitation was noted in one case.

A final reported case that does not fit well into the above two classifications was noted to have somatic features much like the early-onset form but presented at 13 years of age.

Complications: Moderate mental retardation in early onset cases; orthopedic problems include joint contractures and spinal malformations. Severe aortic infiltration results in fibromuscular dysplasia and aortic regurgitation.

Associated Findings: Frequent respiratory illnesses and dislocated hips.

Etiology: Autosomal recessive inheritance.

Pathogenesis: Absence of lysosomal enzyme β-glucuronidase in all tissues examined and storage of mucopolysaccharides in various organs. The clinical variability is not yet explained.

MIM No.: *25322

POS No.: 3314

Sex Ratio: M8:F12 (observed).

Occurrence: At least 20 cases reported to date.

Risk of Recurrence for Patient's Sib:
See Part I, *Mendelian Inheritance.*

Risk of Recurrence for Patient's Child:
See Part I, *Mendelian Inheritance.*

Age of Detectability: At 10 weeks gestation by study of chorionic villi.

Gene Mapping and Linkage: GUSB (glucuronidase, beta) has been mapped to 7q21.2-q22.

Prevention: None known. Genetic counseling indicated.

Treatment: Prenatal diagnosis; enzyme replacement therapy is being investigated but is not yet feasible. Surgical procedures for correction of herniae, and orthopedic, ophthalmologic, and cardiac problems.

Prognosis: The disease course exhibits marked variability and, as such, accurate prediction of the prognosis is not yet possible.

Detection of Carrier: Possible by fibroblasts or leukocyte assays for β-glucuronidase activity.

Special Considerations: Mucopolysaccharidosis VII differs from the other mucopolysaccharidoses in that it was defined as a biochemical entity as quickly as it was clinically recognized. Subsequent cases, therefore, were identified on biochemical grounds and not on the basis of clinical findings. It has been suggested that the clinical forms represent allelic disorders; however, the genetic and molecular basis for phenotypic heterogeneity is unknown.

Two siblings were found to have marked clinical variability. Cultured fibroblasts from four early-onset cases showed antigenically cross-reactive material to β-glucuronidase. All four showed different titration patterns suggesting even further heterogeneity.

Support Groups:
NY; Hicksville; National Mucopolysaccharidoses (MPS) Society
CANADA: Manitoba; Flin Flon Society for Mucopolysaccharide Diseases

References:
Sly WS, et al.: Beta-glucuronidase deficiency: report of clinical, radiologic and biochemical features of a new mucopolysaccharidosis. J Pediatr 1973; 82:249–257. †
Beaudet AL, et al.: Variation in the phenotypic expression of β-glucuronidase deficiency. J Pediatr 1975; 86:388–394.

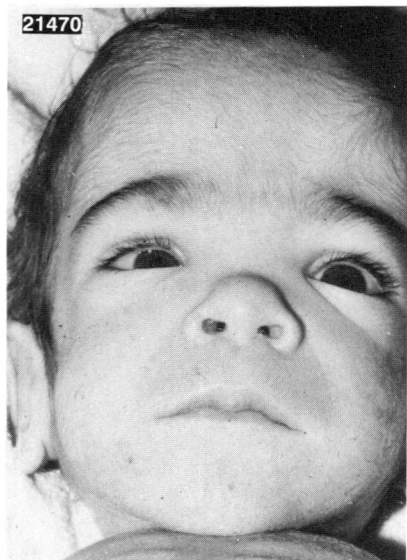

0680B-21470: Coarsening of the facies in this affected 7-month-old.

Francke U: The human gene for beta glucuronidase is on chromosome 7. Am J Hum Genet 1976; 28:357–362.
Bell CE Jr, et al.: Human beta-glucuronidase deficiency mucopolysaccharidosis: identification of cross-reactive antigen in cultured fibroblasts of deficient patients by enzyme immunoassay. J Clin Invest 1977; 59:97–105.
Hoyme HE, et al.: Presentation of mucopolysaccharidosis VII (beta-glucuronidase deficiency) in infancy. J Med Genet 1981; 18:237–239.
Lee JES, et al.: Beta-glucuronidase deficiency: a heterogeneous mucopolysacchiridosis. Am J Dis Child 1985; 139:57–59. *
Neufeld EF, Muenzer J: The mucopolysaccharidoses. In: Scriver CR, et al, eds: The metabolic basis of inherited disease, 6th ed. New York: McGraw-Hill, 1989:1565–1588.

AL006   **Kirk Aleck**

Mucopolysaccharidosis, 'focal'
See GELEOPHYSIC DWARFISM

MUCOSA (ORAL/EYE), INTRAEPITHELIAL DYSKERATOSIS, BENIGN   0538

Includes:
Benign intraepithelial dyskeratosis
Dyskeratosis, intraepithelial
Intraepithelial dyskeratosis

Excludes:
Dermal hypoplasia, focal (0281)
Dyskeratosis congenita (2024)
Focal epithelial hyperplasia of oral mucosa
Leukoplakia
Mucosa, white folded dysplasia
Nails, pachyonychia congenita (0789)
Skin, vitiligo (0993)

Major Diagnostic Criteria: Perilimbal gelatinous plaques on a hyperemic bulbar conjunctiva with white shaggy lesions of oral mucosa occurs. Diagnosis is made on Papanicolaou-stained smear, with compatible history or tissue section.

Clinical Findings: Affected persons have white, soft shaggy lesions of oral mucosa. Gelatinous perilimbal plaques occur in the bulbar conjunctiva with a hyperemic base. Temporary blindness occurs in summer in about one-fourth of cases due to vernal exacerbation and autumnal remissions. Vascularization of cornea with loss of vision results by the fifth to sixth decade. Occasional involvement occurs in the lid conjunctiva with white plaques. X-ray findings are normal. Exfoliative cytologic smears of oral and eye lesions stained with Papanicolaou stain are characterized by two types of cells: elongated waxy orangeophilic cells (resembling the grains of keratosis follicularis) and a cell-within-cell body consisting of a central abnormal cell and a normal appearing epithelial cell that surrounds it. Central cell is dyskeratotic, orangeophilic with abnormal nucleus. The surrounding cell appears normal but with an eccentric nucleus and refractile hyaline membrane separating normal cells from the central cell. Histologic characteristics show a thickened stratum spinosum containing many dyskeratotic waxy appearing cells with elongated nuclei and cell-within-cell dyskeratotic bodies. No basal lacuna or inflammation occurs in the lamina propria, but dilated vessels may occur.

Complications: Temporary blindness in about one-fourth of cases in summer. Vascularization of cornea in late adulthood with loss of vision.

Associated Findings: None known.

Etiology: Autosomal dominant inheritance with moderate variation in expressivity. The severity of manifestation of the eye lesion possibly depends on the response to unknown environmental factors. This may explain the vernal exacerbations and autumnal remissions.

Pathogenesis: Primary protein defect is unknown. However, by analogy with the fact that identical cellular lesions can be produced experimentally in man by use of agents affecting nucleic acid integrity (X-radiation, methotrexate, 5-fluorouracil) the gene

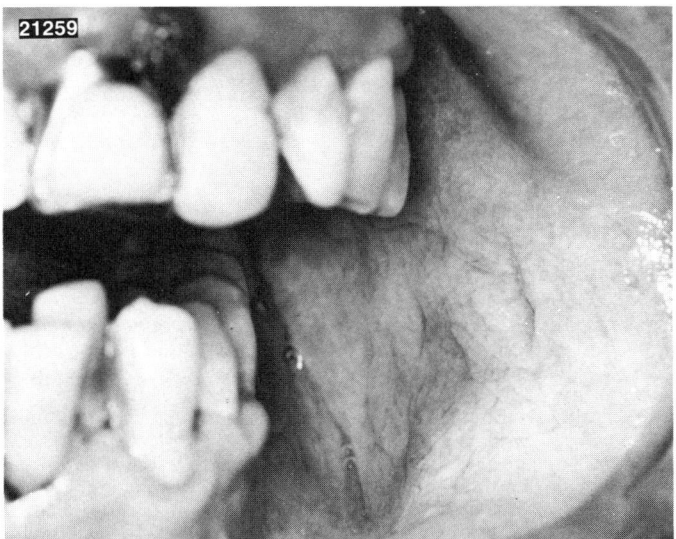

0538-21259: Intraepithelial dyskeratosis affecting the buccal mucosa is a soft non-indurated white lesion which accompanies similar white gelatenous lesions of the sclera with prominent underlying vascular dilation. The presence of the eye lesions differentiates the oral lesions from leukoplakia, white folded dysplasia of the mucosa, leukoedema and lichen planus.

defect appears to result in nucleic acid damage to epithelial cell nuclei. These damaged cells are then surrounded by normal epithelial cells and exfoliated. Electron microscopic features show degenerated cell surrounded by a more normal-appearing epithelial cell. Included cell shows dense bundles of tonofibrils and nuclear fragments.

MIM No.: *12760

Sex Ratio: M1:F1

Occurrence: Only three large kindreds are known. Among "Haliwa" (from Halifax and Warren counties) Indians of North Carolina, however, 1:52.

Risk of Recurrence for Patient's Sib:
See Part I, *Mendelian Inheritance.*

Risk of Recurrence for Patient's Child:
See Part I, *Mendelian Inheritance.*

Age of Detectability: By visual examination most cases detected by one year of age. Confirmed by exfoliative cytology or biopsy.

Gene Mapping and Linkage: Unknown.

Prevention: None known. Genetic counseling indicated.

Treatment: Avoidance of sunlight and dust reduces the severity of eye lesions.

Prognosis: No reduced longevity. Lesion does not appear to predispose to neoplastic change. Blindness from vascularization of cornea in fifth to sixth decade occurs in about 50% of affected persons.

Detection of Carrier: Unknown.

Special Considerations: Must be differentiated from white folded dysplasia of mucosa, especially if such patients also have pterygia, and histologically from keratosis follicularis, which shows basilar clefting absent in benign intraepithelial dyskeratosis. Cortisone eye drops temporarily reduce the hyperemia of conjunctivae but do not alter the basic lesion. Penetrating keratoplasty may benefit corneal opacification.

References:
Von Sallmann L, Paton D: Hereditary benign intraepithelial dyskeratosis. I. Ocular manifestations. Arch Ophthalmol 1960; 63:421–429.
Witkop CJ Jr, et al.: Hereditary benign intraepithelial dyskeratosis. II. Oral manifestations and hereditary transmission. Arch Pathol 1960; 70:696–711. *
Sadeghi EM, Witkop CJ Jr: Ultrastructural study of hereditary benign intraepithelial dyskeratosis. Oral Surg 1977; 44:567–577.
Reed JW, et al.: Corneal manifestations of hereditary benign intraepithelial dyskeratosis. Arch Ophthalmol 1979; 97:297–300. †

WI043   **Carl J. Witkop, Jr.**

MUCOSA, ORAL INCLUSION CYSTS OF THE NEWBORN   3236

Includes:
Bohn nodules
Cysts, inclusion of the oral mucosa of the newborn
Dental lamina cyst
Epstein pearls
Gingival cyst of the newborn
Inclusion cysts of the oral mucosa in the newborn

Excludes:
Alveolar ridges, lymphangioma (0613)
Eruption cysts
Teeth, natal or neonatal (0933)

Major Diagnostic Criteria: White nodules located in the mucosa overlying the alveolar ridges or hard palate.

Clinical Findings: Inclusion cysts generally present as multiple, small, 1–3 mm diameter, white-yellow, raised, firm mucosal nodules on the palate or alveolar ridges. Most are incomspicuous. Occasionally a solitary inclusion cyst is observed. Palatal cysts ("Epstein's pearls" and "Bohn's nodules") are more common than alveolar ridge cysts. Dental lamina cysts are more common in the anterior aspects of the maxilla or mandible.

All three entities represent epithelial inclusion cysts of the oral mucosa. Histologically they are all true cysts lined by a thin layer of stratified squamous epithelium surrounding a keratin-filled lumen.

Inclusion cysts are asymptomatic and, generally, do not cause discomfort. They rupture spontaneously and usually exfoliate within the first weeks to three months of age. Occasionally they present and/or persist later in infancy or childhood.

Complications: These cysts exfoliate spontaneously and do not interfere with tooth eruption.

Associated Findings: Inclusion cysts of the oral mucosa in the newborn have been observed in stillborns (80%), and in infants with congenital anomalies including **Cleft lip** and **Cleft palate** (58%).

Etiology: Gingival cysts of the newborn (dental lamina cyst) arise from postfunctional dental lamina epithelium and are found on the crest, buccal and lingual surfaces of the maxillary and mandibular alveolar ridges.

Epstein pearls are found only in the midline of the hard palate and are thought to represent entrapped epithelial remnants in the line of fusion of the palate during embryological development.

Bohn nodules were originally described on the hard and soft palate arising from epithelial remnants of the developing salivary glands. In the literature, Bohn nodules also refer to epithelial inclusion cysts of the buccal and lingual aspects of the maxillary and mandibular alveolar ridges and probably represent, in this location, dental lamina cysts arising from postfunctional dental lamina or, less likely, ectopic remnants of salivary gland ductal epithelium.

Pathogenesis: During embryogenesis ectoderm forms the oral epithelium that covers the palatal processes and also differentiates into dental lamina and salivary gland primordia. Entrapped epithelium may degenerate or persist between the lines of palatal fusion. Following odontogenesis, remnants of dental lamina may degenerate or persist. Persistent epithelial rests may undergo cystic degeneration resulting in inclusion cysts of the oral mucosa.

Sex Ratio: M1:F1

Occurrence: 76.8% of Caucasian babies. 62.0% of black babies.

Risk of Recurrence for Patient's Sib: Unknown.

Risk of Recurrence for Patient's Child: Unknown.

Age of Detectability: May be present at birth. Often appear and spontaneously exfoliate, usually within the first three months of life.

Gene Mapping and Linkage: Unknown.

Prevention: None known. Genetic counseling indicated.

Treatment: None necessary. The inclusion cysts enlarge and rupture when in contact with the oral mucosal epithelium. Healing occurs rapidly.

Prognosis: Excellent.

Detection of Carrier: Unknown.

References:
Fromm A: Epstein's pearls, Bohn's nodules and inclusion-cysts of the oral cavity. J Dent Child 1967; 34:275–287.
Maher WP, et al.: Etiology and vascularization of dental lamina cysts. Oral Surg 1970; 29:590–597.
Cohen RL: Clinical perspectives on premature tooth eruption and cyst formation in neonates. Pediatric Dermatol 1984; 1:301–306.
Gilhar A, et al.: Gingival cysts of the newborn. Int J Dermatol 1988; 27:261–262.

ZU002 **Susan L. Zunt**

MUCOSA, WHITE FOLDED DYSPLASIA 0681

Includes:
Leukokeratosis, hereditary mucosal
White folded dysplasia of mucosa
White sponge nevus of Cannon

Excludes:
Dermal hypoplasia, focal (0281)
Dyskeratosis congenita (2024)
Focal epithelial hyperplasia of oral mucosa
Mucosa (oral/eye), intraepithelial dyskeratosis, benign (0538)
Leukoedema
Leukoplakia
Oral epithelial nevus of Cooke
Nails, pachyonychia congenita (0789)

Major Diagnostic Criteria: A congenital, soft, white, folded hyperplastic lesion occurs in the mucosa of the oral, and possibly

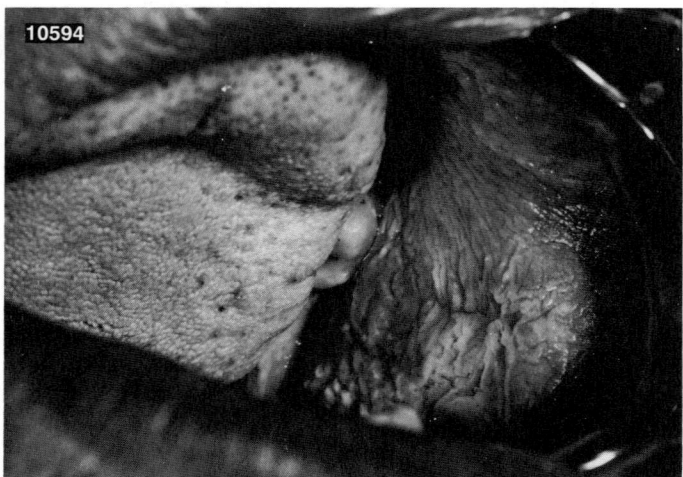

0681-10594: Mucosa, white folded dysplasia.

vagina, rectum and nasal cavities. No eye involvement is present. There may be a history of similar mucosal lesions in other family members.

Clinical Findings: Congenital, asymptomatic, white, folded, soft, hyperplastic mucosal lesions are reported to involve the following mucosal sites in the percentages given: oral mucosa (100%); vaginal mucosa (60%); anal mucosa (40%); penile mucosa (30%); and nasal mucosa (10%). It is not known if all sites listed were examined in all cases.

There are no X-ray changes. Cytologic smears (Papanicolaou stain) show that the majority of mucosal cells contain a perinuclear or cytoplasmic condensation in the cytoplasm (by electron microscopy, tonofibrils) that stain intensely (hematoxylin & eosin, and Papanicolaou). Tissue sections demonstrate hyperplasia of prickle-cell layer, moderate acanthosis, and intracellular edema which give a "chicken wire" appearance to the section. Perinuclear or cytoplasmic condensations are best seen on Papanicolaou or Periodic acid-Schiff stains, and show little or no change in lamina propria or submucosa.

Must be differentiated from leukoedema, which is acquired, usually found in debilitated conditions, and usually not folded; from leukoplakia, which is acquired, not congenital and usually is a firm hard lesion of the mucosa. (Any patient with atypical vaginal "leukoplakia" should be examined for lesions at other mucosal sites, as a possible example of this condition, and radical therapy should be avoided.) Must also be differentiated from focal hyperplasia of oral mucosa, which is the same color as the adjacent normal mucosa and histologically shows only increased thickness of the epithelial cell layer.

This condition must also be differentiated from intraepithelial dyskeratosis, which has perilimbal gelatinous plaques of the bulbar conjunctivae, and from oral epithelial nevus of Cooke which is not familial and histologically has a basket weave pattern of the superficial cornified layer, and a granular layer absent in normal oral mucosa. Diagnosis of this condition can be made on smears which show the perinuclear or cytoplasmic condensations, giving this disease the designation of the "spotted cell disease." Distribution of cytoplasmic condensation is the opposite of that seen in pemphigus, which has a perinuclear halo and peripheral cytoplasmic condensation.

Complications: Iatrogenic effects resulting from surgical or X-ray therapy for supposed precancerous lesion, when treatment was initiated while the lesion was mistaken for leukoplakia, especially in response to vaginal involvement.

Associated Findings: None known.

Etiology: Autosomal dominant inheritance.

Pathogenesis: An intracellular lesion with alterations in the cytoplasmic distribution of tonofibrils in epithelial cells.

MIM No.: *19390

Sex Ratio: M1:F1

Occurrence: Over 100 reported cases.

Risk of Recurrence for Patient's Sib:
See Part I, *Mendelian Inheritance.*

Risk of Recurrence for Patient's Child:
See Part I, *Mendelian Inheritance.*

Age of Detectability: Diagnosed in neonatal period by visual examination confirmed by cytologic or histologic examination. Most cases are not diagnosed until late childhood.

Gene Mapping and Linkage: Unknown.

Prevention: None known. Genetic counseling indicated.

Treatment: Undetermined. Stripping and other surgical procedures, especially for vaginal and penile lesions, should be avoided. There is no indication that this is a precancerous lesion.

Prognosis: Excellent. Does not predispose to malignant disease. There is no demonstrable reduction in reproductive fitness or longevity. The main complications result when lesions are treated by surgery or radiation on the basis of a mistaken diagnosis.

Detection of Carrier: Unknown.

References:
Zegarelli EV, et al.: Familial white folded dysplasia of the mucous membranes. Arch Dermatol 1959; 80:59–65.
Witkop CJ Jr, Gorlin RJ: Four hereditary mucosal syndromes: comparative histology and exfoliative cytology of Darier-White's disease, hereditary benign intraepithelial dyskeratosis, white sponge nevus, and pachyonychia congenita. Arch Dermatol 1961; 84:762–771. *
Browne WG, et al.: White sponge naevus of the mucosa: clinical and linkage data. Ann Hum Genet 1969; 32:271–282.
Whitten JB: The electron microscopic examination of congenital keratoses of the oral mucous membranes. I. White sponge nevus. Oral Surg 1970; 29:69–84.
Jorgenson RJ, Levin S: White sponge nevus. Arch Dermatol 1981; 117:73–76.

WI043   **Carl J. Witkop, Jr.**

Mucosal neuroma syndrome
  See ENDOCRINE NEOPLASIA, MULTIPLE TYPE III
Mucosulfatidosis
  See SULFATASE DEFICIENCY, MULTIPLE
Mucoviscidosis
  See CYSTIC FIBROSIS
Muir-Torre (MT) syndrome
  See CANCER, SEBACEOUS GLAND TUMOR-MULITPLE VISCERAL CARCINOMA
Mulberry molars
  See TEETH, ENAMEL HYPOPLASIA
Mulibrey nanism
  See DWARFISM, MULIBREY TYPE

MÜLLERIAN APLASIA   0682

Includes:
  Mayer-Rokitansky-Kuster (MRK) anomaly
  Mullerian duct failure
  Rokitansky-Kuster-Hauser syndrome
  Rokitansky sequence
  Uterus, congenital absence of
  Vagina, congenital absence of
  Vaginal atresia
  Von Mayer-Rokitansky-Kuster anomaly

Excludes:
  Androgen insensitivity syndrome, complete (0049)
  Mullerian fusion, incomplete (0684)
  Spinal cord, neurenteric cyst (0894)
  Transverse vaginal septum, incomplete

Major Diagnostic Criteria: Congenital absence of the uterus in a 46,XX individual with normal ovarian development and normal female external genitalia. Müllerian remnants or fallopian tubes may persist.

Clinical Findings: Individuals with Müllerian aplasia show normal sexual development, except for absence of Müllerian derivatives; thus, fallopian tubes, uterine corpus, uterine cervix, and the upper portion of the vagina are absent. Often fibromuscular remnants or even rudimentary fallopian tubes persist. The external genitalia are those of a normal female. The hymen is intact, but the vagina ends blindly. At puberty, normal female secondary sexual development occurs, including breast enlargement, pubic and axillary hair, and an appropriate increase in the size of external genitalia. The presenting symptom is most often primary amenorrhea. Pelvic examination at puberty reveals a blindly ending vaginal pouch, usually 4–5 cm long, but occasionally no more than 1–2 cm long. Ovaries are normal; sex steroid levels are normal, and plasma gonadotropin levels respond appropriately to normal feedback control. Urologic anomalies are associated with Müllerian aplasia more frequently than expected; the most frequent are unilateral renal aplasia, pelvic kidney, and renal ectopia. The frequency of certain skeletal abnormalities, particularly vertebral abnormalities, is increased.

Complications: Lack of adequate vaginal length may cause difficulties with coitus; infertility.

Associated Findings: Renal and vertebral anomalies.

Etiology: Cytogenetic studies are normal, and no teratogenic factors have been demonstrated. There are several reports of multiple affected sibs. Recurrence risk is very low, despite Shokeir's (1978) suggestion that this may be a sex-limited autosomal dominant disorder. Multifactorial inheritance is more likely.

Pathogenesis: The Müllerian ducts differentiate into the fallopian tubes, uterus, uterine cervix, and upper portion of the vagina. The lower portion of the vagina is derived from invaginations of the urogenital sinus. Thus, the phenotype observed in these individuals can be explained completely by absence or aplasia of Müllerian ducts. Cramer et al (1987) have suggested that maternal deficiency of galactose-1-phosphate uridyl transferase may be a factor in the pathogenesis.

MIM No.: 15833, 27700

Sex Ratio: M0:F1

Occurrence: About 20% of women with primary amenorrhea have Müllerian aplasia, which is a more common explanation for "absence of uterus" than complete **Androgen insensitivity syndrome, complete**.

Risk of Recurrence for Patient's Sib: Probably 1–2%.

Risk of Recurrence for Patient's Child: All affected individuals are infertile.

Age of Detectability: At puberty, on the basis of primary amenorrhea.

Gene Mapping and Linkage: Unknown.

Prevention: None known. Genetic counseling indicated.

Treatment: Construction of artificial vagina may be necessary, but often dilators and other nonsurgical methods can produce normal vaginal depth. Hormonal therapy is not necessary, nor is laparotomy or laparoscopy necessary to confirm the diagnosis.

Prognosis: Presumably normal life span, unless renal abnormalities are severe.

Detection of Carrier: Unknown.

Special Considerations: In many affected individuals there persist rudimentary Müllerian structures--relatively undifferentiated fibromuscular elements, rudimentary fallopian tubes, or, occasionally, a small uterine-like structure. If such Müllerian remnants persist, many investigators apply the term Rokitansky-Küster-Hauser syndrome. It seems likely that Müllerian aplasia and the Rokitansky-Küster-Hauser syndrome represent the same entity.

A separate group of individuals show absence of the lower portion of the vagina. The caudal portion is replaced by 2–3 cm of fibrous tissue, superior to which lie a well-differentiated upper vagina, uterine cervix, uterine corpus, and fallopian tubes. These individuals have vaginal atresia.

A phenotypic female with normal secondary sexual development, but without a uterus, has either Müllerian aplasia or complete androgen insensitivity (testicular feminization). These two disorders are readily distinguished by cytogenetic studies, with the former being more common.

References:
Jones HW Jr, Mermut S: Familial occurrence of congenital absence of the vagina. Am J Obstet Gynecol 1972; 114:1100–1106.
Simpson JL: Disorders of sexual differentiation: Etiology and clinical delineation. New York: Academic Press, 1976:342–345.
Sarto GE, Simpson JL: Abnormalities of the Müllerian and Wolffian duct systems. BD:OAS XIV(6c) New York: Alan R. Liss, Inc for The National Foundation-March of Dimes, 1978:37–54.
Shokeir MHK: Disorders of sexual differentiation: etiology and clinical delineation. BD:OAS XIV(6c). New York: Alan R. Liss, Inc for The National Foundation-March of Dimes, 1978:147–165.
Carson SA, et al.: Heritable aspects of uterine anomalies: genetic analysis of Müllerian aplasia. Fertil Steril 1983; 40:86–90.
Jones HW Jr, Rock JA: Reparative and constructive surgery of the female generative tract. Baltimore: Williams & Wilkins, 1983; 146–158.
Cramer DW, et al.: Mullerian aplasia associated with maternal deficiency of galactose-1-phosphate uridyl transferase. Fertil Steril 1987; 47:930–934.

Opitz JM: Vaginal atresia in hereditary renal adysplasia. (Editorial) Am J Med Genet 1987; 26:873–876.

Pavanello R deC M, et al.: Relationship between Mayer-Rokitansky-Kuster (MRK) anomaly and hereditary renal adysplasia (HRA). Am J Med Genet 1988; 29:845–849.

SI018   **Joe Leigh Simpson**

MÜLLERIAN DERIVATIVES IN MALES, PERSISTENT   0683

Includes:
Hernia uteri inguinale syndrome
Mullerian inhibitor factor, deficiency of
Oviducts in males, persistence of
Pseudohermaphroditism, male internal
Persistent oviduct syndrome
Tubular male pseudohermaphroditism
Uterine hernia syndrome
Uterine inguinal hernia syndrome

Excludes:
Chromosome mosaicism, 45x/46,XY type (0173)
Hermaphroditism, true (0971)
Male pseudohermaphroditism, all other forms of

Major Diagnostic Criteria: 46,XY individual, with normal male external genitalia and testes, who has a uterus and fallopian tubes.

Clinical Findings: A uterus and fallopian tubes are present in otherwise normal males. Affected individuals have normal male external genitalia, normal Wolffian derivatives (vasa deferentia, epididymides, and seminal vesicles), and usually anatomically normal testes. No somatic anomalies are present. At puberty virilization occurs. Endocrine studies produce results expected of a normal male. The disorder is often detected because the uterus and fallopian tubes prolapse into an inguinal hernia; thus, these patients are often said to have the uterine inguinal hernia syndrome. However, many affected individuals do not have inguinal herniae.

Complications: Herniation of the uterus and fallopian tubes into the inguinal canal; neoplastic transformation of cryptorchid testes.

Associated Findings: Infertility.

Etiology: Probably X-linked recessive inheritance, based upon one report of affected maternal half-sibs. Sex-limited autosomal recessive inheritance is also possible.

Pathogenesis: Undetermined. Müllerian derivatives presumably fail to regress, either because of failure of the fetal testes to elaborate anti-Müllerian hormone (AMH) or because of the inability of the Müllerian ducts to the AMH. If the disorder is X-linked recessive, location of the locus for AMH on an autosome (19p13.3) suggests that pathogenesis involves not synthesis of AMH, but perhaps a receptor.

MIM No.:   *26155

Sex Ratio: M1:F0

Occurrence: Undetermined and presumably rare. Many cases may remain undetected.

Risk of Recurrence for Patient's Sib:
See Part I, *Mendelian Inheritance*.

Risk of Recurrence for Patient's Child:
See Part I, *Mendelian Inheritance*.

Age of Detectability: Usually after puberty or later in life, when herniation occurs.

Gene Mapping and Linkage: AMH (anti-Müllerian hormone) has been provisionally mapped to 19p13.3.

Prevention: None known. Genetic counseling indicated.

Treatment: Inguinal herniorrhaphy. Uterus and fallopian tubes should be removed if discovered. Orchiopexy may be necessary if testes are intra-abdominal.

Prognosis: Presumably normal life span, provided neoplastic transformation does not occur.

Detection of Carrier: Unknown.

References:
Armendares S, et al.: Two male sibs with uterus and fallopian tubes: a rare probably inherited disorder. Clin Genet 1973; 4:291–296.

Brook CGD, et al.: Familial occurrence of persistent Müllerian structures in otherwise normal males. Br Med J 1973; 1:771–773.

Sloan WR, Walsh PC: Familial persistent Müllerian duct syndrome. J Urol 1976; 115:459–461.

Malamayaman D, et al.: Male pseudohermaphroditism with persistent Müllerian and Wolffian structures complicated by intra-abnormal seminoma. Urology 1984; 24:67–69.

Naguib KK, et al.: Familial uterine hernia syndrome: report of an Arab family with four affected males. Am J Med Genet 1989; 33:180–181.

SI018   **Joe Leigh Simpson**

Mullerian duct defects-upper limb hypoplasia
See LIMB, UPPER HYPOPLASIA-MULLERIAN DUCT DEFECTS
Mullerian duct failure
See MULLERIAN APLASIA
Mullerian duct-renal-cervicothoracic and upper limb defects
See MURCS ASSOCIATION

MÜLLERIAN FUSION, INCOMPLETE   0684

Includes:
Arcuate uterus
Bicornuate uterus
"Double uterus" (misnomer)
Rudimentary uterine horn
Uterus arcuatus
Uterus bicornus
Uterus bicornus unicollis
Uterus bilocularis
Uterus bipartitus
Uterus didelphys
Uterus pseudodidelphys
Uterus subseptus
Uterus unicornus

Excludes:
Hymen, imperforate (0483)
Mullerian aplasia (0682)
True duplication of Müllerian ducts
Vaginal septum, transverse (0985)

Major Diagnostic Criteria: Broadening and medial depression of the superior portion of the uterine septum (arcuate uterus) or more severe fusion defects in a 46,XX individual with normal ovarian and external genital development. Diagnosis should be confirmed by X-ray studies, or by hysteroscopic or laparoscopic visualization.

Clinical Findings: Failure of fusion of the paired Müllerian ducts results in two hemiuteri; each hemiuterus has a single fallopian tube. Sometimes one Müllerian duct fails to contribute to the definitive uterus or produces only a rudimentary horn. The extent of Müllerian fusion may vary from slight broadening and medial depression of the superior portion of the uterine septum (arcuate uterus) to completely separated hemiuteri with separate cervices, vaginas, and perineal orifices. The most frequent types of incomplete Müllerian fusion include uterus arcuatus, uterus unicornus (absence of one uterine horn), uterus septus (persistence of the entire uterine septum), uterus bicornis unicollis (two hemiuteri, each leading to the same cervix), and uterus bicornis bicollis (two hemiuteri, each leading to separate cervices). Vaginal septa and paired perineal orifices are relatively uncommon.

The external genitalia usually are normal, but a vaginal septum may be present. Ovarian development and puberty are normal.

Complications: A rudimentary uterine horn may retain blood, produce pain, and possibly rupture. Pregnancy in a rudimentary uterine horn may lead to uterine rupture or missed abortion.

Pregnancies may be complicated by an increase in the incidences of second trimester abortion and premature labor. Malpresentations are not uncommon. Following delivery, the placenta may fail to separate readily from the uterus.

Associated Findings: Urologic anomalies may occur ipsilateral to a rudimentry or absent uterine horn. Incomplete Müllerian fusion may be present in the **Meckel syndrome, Ectrodactyly-ectodermal dysplasia-clefting syndrome**, and the **Hand-foot-genital syndrome**.

Etiology: Reported familial aggregates have included several kindreds with multiple affected sibs, and several kindreds in which both mother and daughter were affected. Only one formal study has been conducted, with low recurrence risks (3%) for female sibs most consistent with polygenic or multifactorial etiology.

Pathogenesis: The Müllerian ducts are originally paired organs that fuse and subsequently canalize to form the upper vagina, uterus, and fallopian tubes. Failure of fusion or canalization results in uterine septa or hemiuteri, each associated with no more than one fallopian tube. More extensive failure of fusion results in persistence of vaginal septa.

MIM No.: 19200, 19205

Sex Ratio: F1:M0

Occurrence: About 1:1,000 females, although very minor uterine anomalies have been claimed in as many as 2–3% of women whose uteri are examined immediately following delivery. A relatively high proportion of the latter have uterus arcuatus or uterus subseptus.

Risk of Recurrence for Patient's Sib: Estimated at 1–5%.

Risk of Recurrence for Patient's Child: Estimated at 1–5%.

Age of Detectability: Variable. Retention of menstrual blood in rudimentary horns may produce symptoms shortly after puberty, but affected individuals are usually detected at a later age because of recurrent second trimester abortions, abnormal uterine contour during labor, or other intrapartum or postpartum abnormalities. Many affected individuals are probably never detected, particularly those with uterus arcuatus or uterus subseptus.

Gene Mapping and Linkage: Unknown.

Prevention: None known. Genetic counseling indicated.

Treatment: Many patients with hemiuteri or septal defects have normal pregnancies and require no treatment. Extirpation of a rudimentary uterine horn may be necessary. Reunification of paired hemiuteri or removal of a septum may permit full-term pregnancy; however, in general, surgery should not be undertaken unless the patient has had a least one second trimester abortion.

Prognosis: Normal life span, provided rupture of a uterine horn does not lead to life-threatening complications.

Detection of Carrier: Unknown.

Special Considerations: Incomplete Müllerian fusion should be distinguished from true Müllerian duplication, an anomaly that probably results from division of one or both Müllerian ducts early in embryogenesis. Such individuals have two separate uteri, each of which may have two fallopian tubes.

Several unusual clinical situations may result from the presence of a rudimentary horn. Menstrual blood may be retained, producing a pelvic mass and pelvic pain. Pregnancy occurring in a rudimentary tube that communicates with the uterus may terminate in uterine rupture or missed abortion; the latter may lead to lithopedion formation. A canal between hemiuteri may exist, even if a septum extends to the cervix or if two cervices are present. A vaginal septum bulging with blood from a rudimentary horn may obscure the cervix, mimicking Müllerian aplasia.

References:
Jones HW Jr, Wheeless CR: Salvage of the reproductive potential of women with anomalous development of the Müllerian ducts: 1868–1968–2068. Am J Obstet Gynecol 1969; 104:348–364.

Simpson JL: Disorders of sexual differentiation: etiology and clinical delineation. New York: Academic Press, 1976:351–354.

Wiersma AF, et al.: Uterine anomalies associated with unilateral renal agenesis. Obstet Gynecol 1976; 47:654–657.

Jones HW Jr, Rock JA: Reparative and constructive surgery of the female generative tract. Baltimore: Williams & Wilkins, 1983:164–185.

Verp MS, et al.: Heritable aspects of Müllerian anomalies. I. Three familial aggregates with Müllerian fusion anomalies. Fertil Steril 1983; 40:80–85.

Elias S, et al.: Genetic studies in incomplete Müllerian fusion. Obstet Gynecol 1984; 63:276–279.

SI018   **Joe Leigh Simpson**

Mullerian inhibitor factor, deficiency of
  See *MULLERIAN DERIVATIVES IN MALES, PERSISTENT*
Multicentric osteolysis
  See *OSTEOLYSIS, ESSENTIAL*
Multicentric osteolysis with recessive transmission
  See *OSTEOLYSIS, RECESSIVE CARPAL-TARSAL*
Multicentric osteosarcoma
  See *OSTEOSARCOMA*
Multicystic kidney, congenital unilateral
  See *KIDNEY, RENAL DYSPLASIA, POTTER TYPE II*
Multicystic renal dysplasia
  See *KIDNEY, RENAL DYSPLASIA, POTTER TYPE II*
Multiple Acyl-CoA Dehydrogenation (MAD) disorders, mild variants
  See *ACIDEMIA, ETHYLMALONIC-ADIPIC*
Multiple acyl-CoA dehydrogenation deficiency (MADD)
  See *ACIDEMIA, GLUTARIC ACIDEMIA II*
Multiple acyl-CoA dehydrogenation deficiency, severe variants
  See *ACIDEMIA, GLUTARIC ACIDEMIA II*
Multiple autosomal dominant liver-kidney cystic disease
  See *LIVER, POLYCYSTIC AND MULTICYSTIC DISEASE, ADULT TYPE*
Multiple carboxylase deficiency, infantile
  See *BIOTINIDASE DEFICIENCY*
Multiple carboxylase deficiency, juvenile-onset
  See *BIOTINIDASE DEFICIENCY*
Multiple carboxylase deficiency, late-onset
  See *BIOTINIDASE DEFICIENCY*
Multiple carboxylase deficiency, neonatal or early onset form
  See *CARBOXYLASE DEFICIENCY, HOLOCARBOXYLASE DEFICIENCY TYPE*
Multiple cartilaginous exostoses
  See *EXOSTOSES, MULTIPLE CARTILAGINOUS*
Multiple cysts anomaly, abnormal karyotype other than 45,X
  See *FETAL MULTIPLE CYSTS ANOMALY*
Multiple enchondromatosis
  See *ENCHONDROMATOSIS*
Multiple epiphyseal dysplasia, flat epiphyses type
  See *EPIPHYSEAL DYSPLASIA, MULTIPLE RIBBING TYPE*
Multiple epiphyseal dysplasia, mild
  See *EPIPHYSEAL DYSPLASIA, MULTIPLE RIBBING TYPE*
Multiple exostoses
  See *EXOSTOSES, MULTIPLE CARTILAGINOUS*
Multiple hamartoma syndrome
  See *GINGIVAL MULTIPLE HAMARTOMA SYNDROME*
Multiple hemangiomata-macrocephaly-pseudopapilledema
  See *OVERGROWTH, MACROCEPHALY-HEMANGIOMA, RILEY-SMITH TYPE*
Multiple lentigines syndrome
  See *LENTIGINES SYNDROME, MULTIPLE*
Multiple lipoprotein-type hyperlipidemia
  See *HYPERLIPOPROTEINEMIA, COMBINED*
Multiple myeloma
  See *CANCER, MULTIPLE MYELOMA*

MULTIPLE SCLEROSIS, FAMILIAL   2598

Includes:
  "Creeping paralysis" (obsolete, pejorative)
  Demyelinating disease
  Disseminated sclerosis

Excludes:
  Adrenoleukodystrophy, X-linked (2533)
  Alexander disease (2712)
  Amyotrophic lateral sclerosis (2067)
  Behcet syndrome
  Brainstem neoplasms-arteriovenous malformations-infections
  Cerebral arteritis
  Degenerative neurological disorders
  Encephalopathy, necrotizing (0344)
  Leukodystrophy

Lupus erythematosus, neuropsychiatric forms
Meningovascular syphilis
Olivopontocerebellar atrophy

Major Diagnostic Criteria: 1) demonstration of lesions reflecting mainly white matter dysfunction disseminated in time and space; 2) objective abnormalities on neurologic examination; 3) either two clear-cut episodes of significant worsening, each lasting over 24 hours and separated by at least one month, or slow progression of the same pattern over a minimum of six months; 4) determination by an appropriately experienced physician that no other disease process better explains the signs and symptoms.

Tests to aid in the diagnosis include evoked potentials, computed tomography (CT scan), magnetic resonance imaging (MRI), and analysis of cerebrospinal fluid (CSF) to identify abnormalities such as oligoclonal banding and an increased gamma globulin fraction in the total protein.

Clinical Findings: Within families, there is great variability in symptoms, age at onset, and disease course, even among close relatives such as siblings, parents, and children. In a series of 742 patients, the most common initial symptoms were motor symptoms (52%), sensory symptoms in limbs or face (32%), optic neuritis (14%), brainstem symptoms such as vertigo and diplopia (9%), gait disturbance (10%), bladder disturbance (2%), l'hermitte sign (1%), acute transverse myelitis (1%), and pain (1%). Ninety percent of patients were monosymptomatic at onset; 10% were polysymptomatic.

Complications: Sensory problems such as numbness or tingling, optic neuritis, diplopia, l'hermitte sign (sudden electric-like shocks extending down the spine upon flexion of the head), motor weakness (acute or chronic), bladder and/or bowel disturbances, acute transverse myelitis, vertigo, cerebellar ataxia of a limb, nonspecific gait disturbance, slurred speech, and pain. Fatigue can make daily living extremely difficult. Cognitive changes may occur late in the disease course.

Associated Findings: Iritis, ocular venous sheathing, and depression are frequently experienced by patients and require appropriate treatment. Recent data indicate that the suicide rate among patients is higher compared with that for the age-matched general population.

Etiology: Not definitively established. Heredity appears to play an important role in disease susceptibility. At a critical age, perhaps puberty, it has been suggested that in a genetically susceptible individual there may be infection by an environmental agent, e.g., a virus, that either becomes latent or initiates a cyclic immune regulatory defect. During an incubation period postulated to last from 5–20 years, repeated challenges to the immune system may result in the development of an autoimmune process. Subsequent to this, an environmental trigger, such as infection or trauma, or an endogenous trigger such as stress or other disease, may result in the first major episode of demyelination and clinically evident disease.

Pathogenesis: It is generally considered that multiple sclerosis exclusively affects the central nervous system (CNS). It was previously believed that indications of peripheral nerve involvement were secondary to the CNS pathology or incidental. However, there is growing evidence that distal demyelination may be present in the peripheral nervous system.

The individual plaques or lesions are characterized by demyelination with relative preservation of the axon. It is unclear whether the destruction of the myelin represents a primary attack against normal myelin or is secondary to previously injured and/or abnormal myelin. The earliest lesions are probably inflammatory. As the plaques age and develop, the amount of inflammation decreases and gliosis begins. With time, there is less axonal preservation, and eventually there is demyelination of entire tracts secondary to axonal loss. Plaques occur most often in the optic nerves, spinal cord, and cerebral hemispheres. In chronic cases, eventually there will be very few areas of central nervous system white matter that are not involved. Demyelination is often symmetric. Many plaques are apparently neurologically asymptomatic.

MIM No.: 12620, *16950

Sex Ratio: Ranges from M1:F1.5 to M1:F2

Occurrence: Varies with ethnic group and geographic location. Most frequent among Caucasians of central and northern European ancestry. Areas of high prevalence (at least 50:100,000 population) include northern and central Europe, northern North America, New Zealand, Japan, and parts of southern Australia. In well-documented series, 20% of patients have at least one other relative affected.

Risk of Recurrence for Patient's Sib: The risks given below are age-corrected, lifetime risks. The risk for brothers of female patients is 2.27±0.71%, and for sisters is 5.65±1.10%. The risk for brothers of male patients is 4.15±1.28%, and for sisters is 3.46±1.14%. These rates are computed on the British Columbia population with a prevalence of 1:1,000 population. The concordance rate for monozygotic twins is 25.9%, compared with a rate of 2.3% for dizygotic twins.

Risk of Recurrence for Patient's Child: The risk for children of female patients is 2.58±1.14%. The risk for children of male patients is 2.47±1.72%. These rates are for the British Columbia population with a prevalence of 1:1,000 population. There appears to be a greatly reduced father-son concordance rate, controlling for the observed sex ratio in the condition. Mother-daughter, mother-son, and father-daughter concordance rates are as expected, controling for the sex ratio.

Age of Detectability: Onset ranges from 10–60 years of age, with the majority having onset between 20–40 years of age.

Gene Mapping and Linkage: Reportedly a multiple sclerosis susceptibility gene exists in the HLA complex in linkage disequilibrium with HLA-D (Francis et al, 1987).

Prevention: None known. Genetic counseling indicated.

Treatment: Adrenocorticotropic hormone (ACTH) or corticosteroids are used when acute relapses produce disabling symptoms. Due to their relative ease of administration, oral steroids such as prednisone may be preferable to intravenous ACTH. Long-term steroid treatment should be avoided for patients following a remitting and relapsing course or for patients with chronic progressive disease. Bed rest is recommended only when fatigue is a significant factor in the relapse. In patients with chronic progressive disease, immunosuppressive agents may be effective. Specific symptoms such as spasticity, bladder and bowel problems, pain, and excessive fatigue may be treated on an individual basis.

Prognosis: The course of the disease is highly variable. At opposite extremes are a benign course, which occurs in 4–20% of cases, and a malignant course with death within five years of onset, which occurs in approximately 3% of cases. About 18% of patients have chronic progressive disease from the onset. The majority of patients initially undergo episodes of relapses and remissions, and the average length of time that patients follow this pattern is 6.8 years, after which the disease commonly becomes chronic progressive. Five and 11 years after onset, 30% and 50% of patients, respectively, are in a chronically progressive phase of their illness.

There are no fully reliable prognostic indicators, although age at onset and severity after five years may give some indication about the future course. Females with early onset of sensory symptoms, optic neuritis, or vertigo may have a relatively good prognosis. Conversely, males with late-onset disease who have significant pyramidal or cerebellar signs and symptoms either at onset or early in the disease seem to have a relatively poor prognosis. Gait disorder at onset also appears to be a poor prognostic sign for both sexes.

In terms of life expectancy, 90% of patients are alive 10 years after disease onset; about 75% at 20 years; and approximately 68% at 25 years. In general, there appears to be a significant increase in mortality 10–15 years after the onset of clinical disease.

Detection of Carrier: Unknown.

Support Groups: New York; National Multiple Sclerosis Society

References:
Antel JP, ed: Symposium on multiple sclerosis. Neurol Clin 1983; 1:571–785.
Paty DW, et al.: The diagnosis of multiple sclerosis. New York: Thieme-Stratton, 1984. *
Matthews WB, et al.: McAlpine's multiple sclerosis. New York: Churchill Livingstone, 1985. *
Ebers GC, et al.: A population-based study of multiple sclerosis in twins. New Engl J Med 1986; 315:1638–1642.
Hashimoto SA, Paty DW: Multiple sclerosis. Disease-a-Month 1986; 32:518–589.
Francis DA, et al.: HLA genetic determinants in familial MS: a study from the Grampian region of Scotland. Tissue Antigens 1987; 29:7–12.
Sadovnick AD, et al.: Multiple sclerosis: updated risks for relatives. Am J Med Genet 1988; 29:533–541.

BA011   **Patricia A. Baird**
SA043   **Adele D. Sadovnick**

Multiple sulfatase deficiency
See METACHROMATIC LEUKODYSTROPHIES
Multisynostotic osteodysgenesis-long bone fractures
See ANTLEY-BIXLER SYNDROME

MURCS ASSOCIATION   2406

Includes: Mullerian duct-renal-cervicothoracic and upper limb defects
Excludes:
    Klippel-Feil anomaly (2032)
    Mullerian aplasia (0682)
    Noonan syndrome (0720)
    Renal agenesis, bilateral (0856)
    Renal agenesis, unilateral (0857)
    Turner syndrome (0977)
    Vater association (0987)

Major Diagnostic Criteria: Cervicothoracic vertebrae, rib, and/or upper limb malformations in association with uterovaginal anomalies and renal agenesis and/or ectopy.

Clinical Findings: The usual clinical presentation occurs in young adult females with primary amenorrhea, vaginal agenesis, and short stature but with normal development of secondary sexual characteristics. Diagnosis of the MURCS association can be established by identification of the Rokitansky sequence (96%) in association with renal agenesis and/or ectopy (88%) and dysmorphic cervicothoracic vertebrae (80%) and/or rib or upper limb abnormalities, and a normal female karyotype (46,XX).

Complications: Urinary tract infection, obstruction, or failure; growth deficiency (adult stature is usually less than 152 cm).

Associated Findings: Moderate occurrence: Sprengel scapular anomaly. Infrequent occurrence: deafness, dysmorphic ears, facial asymmetry, cleft lip and/or palate, micrognathia, hemifacial microsomia, and gastrointestinal anomalies.

Etiology: Has occurred sporadically in otherwise normal families.

Pathogenesis: A hypothesis has been proposed that attributes the major components of the MURCS Association to an alteration of the blastema of the lower cervical and upper thoracic somites, arm buds, and pronephric ducts, all of which have an intimate spatial inter-relationship late in the fourth embryonic week.

POS No.: 3535

Sex Ratio: M0:F1 (Sex-limited).

Occurrence: About 40 cases have been reported.

Risk of Recurrence for Patient's Sib: Presumably not significantly increased.

Risk of Recurrence for Patient's Child: Probands are infertile.

Age of Detectability: Shortly after puberty.

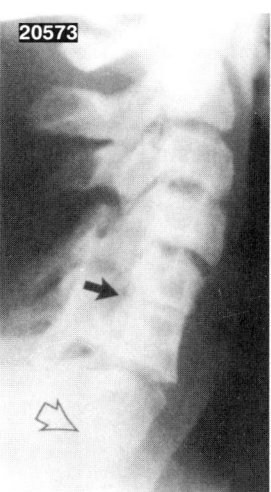 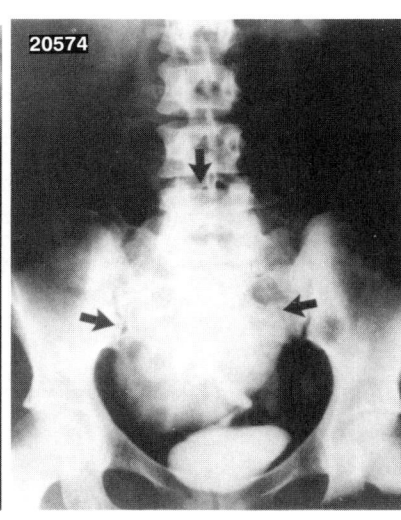

2406-20573: Complete and incomplete asymptomatic fusions of the cervical vertebrae. 20574: Solitary pelvic kidney demonstrated by intravenous pyelography.

Gene Mapping and Linkage: Unknown.

Prevention: None known. Genetic counseling indicated.

Treatment: Corrective surgery for genitourinary and limb complications. Medical management of renal complications.

Prognosis: Normal for life span unless renal complications are severe. Affected individuals are infertile, intelligence is not affected.

Detection of Carrier: Unknown.

Special Considerations: MURCS is an acronym for Müllerian duct (MU); Renal (R); Cervicothoracic vertebrae, rib and upper limb (CS) anomalies.

References:
Duncan PA, et al.: The MURCS Association: müllerian duct aplasia, renal aplasia, and cervicothoracic somite dysplasia. J Pediatr 1979; 95:399–402. *
Duncan PA, Shapiro LR: MURCS and VATER associations: vertebral and genitourinary malformations with distinct embryologic pathogenetic mechanisms. Teratology 1979; 19:24A only.
Winer-Muram HT, et al.: The concurrence of facioauriculovertebral spectrum and the Rokitansky syndrome. Am J Obstet Gynecol 1984; 149:569–570.
Greene RA, et al.: MURCS association with additional congenital anomalies. Hum Pathol 1986; 17:88–91.
Lo Iudice G, et al.: The MURCS association: clinical, radiological, endocrinological and familial data in a 40-year-old patient. Minerva Endocrinol 1986; 11:205–209.
Jones KL: Smith's recognizable patterns of human malformation, 4rd ed. Philadelphia: W.B. Saunders Company, 1988:604–605.

DU003   **Peter A. Duncan**
SH009   **Lawrence R. Shapiro**

Murk Jansen metaphyseal chondrodysplasia
See METAPHYSEAL CHONDRODYSPLASIA, TYPE JANSEN
Murray syndrome
See FIBROMATOSIS, JUVENILE HYALINE
Murray-Puretic syndrome
See FIBROMATOSIS, JUVENILE HYALINE
Murray-Puretic-Drescher syndrome
See FIBROMATOSIS, JUVENILE HYALINE
Muscle adenosine monophosphate (AMP) deaminase deficiency
See MYOPATHY-METABOLIC, MYOADENYLATE DEAMINASE DEFICIENCY

Muscle adenylate deaminase deficiency
  See MYOPATHY-METABOLIC, MYOADENYLATE DEAMINASE
  DEFICIENCY
Muscle atrophy-contractures-oculomotor apraxia
  See CONTRACTURES-MUSCLE ATROPHY-OCULOMOTOR APRAXIA
Muscle atrophy-mental retardation, X-linked-contractures-apraxia
  See X-LINKED MENTAL RETARDATION-MUSCLE ATROPHY-
  CONTRACTURES-APRAXIA
Muscle carnitine deficiency
  See MYOPATHY-METABOLIC, CARNITINE DEFICIENCY, PRIMARY
  AND SECONDARY
Muscle glycogen phosphorylase deficiency
  See GLYCOGENOSIS, TYPE V
Muscle phosphofructokinase deficiency
  See GLYCOGENOSIS, TYPE VII

MUSCLE WASTING OF HANDS-SENSORINEURAL DEAFNESS   0450

Includes:
  Arthrogryposis-like hand anomaly-sensorineural deafness
  Deafness, sensorineural-hand muscle wasting
  Hands, muscle wasting-sensorineural deafness

Excludes:
  Arthrogryposes (isolated or with syndromes)
  Cranio-carpo-tarsal dysplasia, whistling face type (0223)
  Hand anomalies associated with dwarfism
  Synostosis, multiple synostosis syndrome (2312)

Major Diagnostic Criteria: Congenital flexion contractures and atrophy of thenar, hypothenar and, interosseous muscles in a patient with congenital sensorineural hearing loss and normal joints by X-ray are characteristic of the condition.

Clinical Findings: Familial congenital bilateral or unilateral sensorineural hearing losses of varying degrees. A congenital hand abnormality is seen in both normal-hearing and deaf patients. There are congenital flexion contractures of the digits and wasting of the thenar, hypothenar, and interosseous muscles which is nonprogressive. Flexion creases over the interphalangeal joints are absent. Active and passive flexion and extension of the fingers is limited. Some of the fingers may show ulnar deviation. There may be muscle weakness, most marked in the distribution of the ulnar nerve. There is no pain; there are no other neurologic deficits; nerve conduction studies and electromyography are normal. Dermatoglyphics show a striking vertical orientation of the palmar digital lines. X-rays in both adults and children show normal joints. Petrous pyramid polytomography, electronystagmography, and various laboratory tests (CBC, urinalysis, serum electrolytes, BUN, blood glucose, serum glutamic oxalic transaminase, aldolase, CPK, urine and plasma amino acid screening, urine mucopolysaccharide screening, EKG, and karyotype) are normal.

Complications: Failure to acquire speech and language in a patient with profound hearing loss. Articulation errors and poor school progress occur in patients with lesser degrees of hearing loss.

Associated Findings: Limitation of motion of other joints has been seen. These include the wrist, toes, forearm pronation and supination, and elbow extension. Clubfoot, acetabular dysplasia, coxa vera may also be present.

Etiology: Autosomal dominant inheritance with complete penetrance but variable expressivity.

Pathogenesis: Unknown.

MIM No.: 10820

POS No.: 3486

Sex Ratio: M1:F1

Occurrence: Undetermined. One reported kindred had 12 affected persons in five generations.

Risk of Recurrence for Patient's Sib:
  See Part I, *Mendelian Inheritance.*

Risk of Recurrence for Patient's Child:
  See Part I, *Mendelian Inheritance.*

Age of Detectability: The hand abnormality is detectable at birth and if bilateral, the hearing loss may be detected at birth also, unless the loss is mild. A unilateral loss may escape detection for years.

Gene Mapping and Linkage: Unknown.

Prevention: None known. Genetic counseling indicated.

Treatment: Hearing loss, if significant, should be treated by hearing aids and special speech training. Less severe losses may be managed by preferential seating in school, lip-reading training, and the use of hearing conservation (regular otologic and audiologic checkups, avoidance of acoustic trauma, and ototoxic drugs). Mumps immunization might be desirable in susceptible patients with unilateral hearing loss. Physical therapy may be of benefit in patients with more severe contractures. An infant with the characteristic hand abnormality should have audiometric evaluation and periodic follow-up to rule out hearing loss. The hearing loss is the only potential serious disability, as the hand abnormality seems not to hinder patients in their daily activities and occupations.

Prognosis: Normal for life expectancy and intelligence. There is some evidence to suggest that the inner ears in these patients may be more susceptible to injury from febrile illnesses.

Detection of Carrier: Unknown.

References:
Stewart J, Bergstrom L: Familial hand abnormality and sensori-neural deafness: new syndrome. J Pediatr 1971; 78:102–110.
Akbarnia BA, et al.: Familial arthrogrotic-like hand abnormality and sensorineural deafness. Am J Dis Child 1979; 133:403–405.
Martinon F, et al.: Sindrome de Stewart y Bergstrom: anales españoles de pediatria. 1979; 12:549–552.
Drachman DB, Banker BQ: Arthrogryposis multiplex congenita. Arch Neurol 1961; 5:77–93.

BE028   **LaVonne Bergstrom**
                                                    Janet M. Stewart

Muscle wasting-deafness-vitiligo
  See DEAFNESS-VITILIGO-MUSCLE WASTING
Muscle weakness
  See SINGLETON-MERTEN SYNDROME

MUSCLE-EYE-BRAIN SYNDROME   3047

Includes:
  Brain-muscle-eye syndrome
  Eye-muscle-brain syndrome

Excludes: **Facio-neuro-skeletal syndrome** (2339)

Major Diagnostic Criteria: The combination of severe hypotonia, mental retardation, and visual failure is sufficient to suggest the diagnosis.

Clinical Findings: Abnormal findings are confined to muscle, eye, and brain. Muscular anomalies present in all include severe early hypotonia and subsequently retarded motor development and reduced or absent deep tendon reflexes. Diagnostic studies in all patients indicated myopathic EMG, elevated serum CK, and histologic features of muscular dystrophy. Eye anomalies include visual failure in all affected children, with myopia described as severe in 10/14 and mild in 4/14; in addition, glaucoma (8/11), optic disk hypoplasia or pallor (7/10), and retinal hypoplasia (9/10) have also been described. The brain anomalies are mental retardation and slight spasticity (14/14), mild **Hydrocephaly** (7/11), and myoclonic jerks or convulsions (6/11). Abnormal electroencephalograms were found in children thus investigated.

Complications: Unknown.

Associated Findings: None known.

Etiology: Autosomal recessive inheritance.

Pathogenesis: Unknown.

MIM No.: *25328

POS No.: 3589

Sex Ratio: M1:F1

Occurrence: Some 14 affected individuals have been reported, all from Finland.

Risk of Recurrence for Patient's Sib:
See Part I, *Mendelian Inheritance.*

Risk of Recurrence for Patient's Child:
See Part I, *Mendelian Inheritance.*

Age of Detectability: Soon after birth by the presence of severe hypotonia.

Gene Mapping and Linkage: Unknown.

Prevention: None known. Genetic counseling indicated.

Treatment: Treatment of glaucoma as indicated; regular physiotherapy may also be useful.

Prognosis: Mental retardation is a constant finding; prognosis for life span is unknown.

Detection of Carrier: Unknown.

References:
Raitta C, et al.: Ophthalmological findings in a new syndrome with muscle, eye and brain involvement. Acta Ophthalmol (Copenh) 1978; 56:465–472.
Santavuori P, Leisti J: Muscle, eye and brain disease (MEB). In: Eriksson AW, et al., eds: Population structure and genetic disorders. New York: Academic, 1980:647–651.

T0007 **Helga V. Toriello**

Muscular atrophy, adult spinal
See SPINAL MUSCULAR ATROPHY
Muscular atrophy, juvenile spinal
See SPINAL MUSCULAR ATROPHY
Muscular atrophy, progressive
See AMYOTROPHIC LATERAL SCLEROSIS, FAMILIAL ADULT AND JUVENILE TYPES
also AMYOTROPHIC LATERAL SCLEROSIS

MUSCULAR ATROPHY, SPINAL AND BULBAR, X-LINKED KENNEDY TYPE   2493

Includes:
Bulbospinal muscular atrophy, X-linked
Calves, hypertrophy of-spinal muscular atrophy
Kennedy type spinal and bulbar muscular atrophy
Kennedy-Stefanis disease
Spinal muscular atrophy-hypertrophy of the calves
X-linked adult onset spinobulbar muscular atrophy
X-linked adult spinal muscular atrophy

Excludes:
Adrenoleukodystrophy, X-linked (2533)
Spinal muscular atrophy (0895)

Major Diagnostic Criteria: Facial, bulbar, and spinal proximal muscle atrophy with fasiculations; especially around the lips, chin, and tongue. Cramps, tremor, sexual dysfunction, and gynecomastia are common findings. The age of onset ranges from 15–59 years of age. The inheritance pattern is X-linked recessive.

Clinical Findings: Based on over 50 patients: onset age > 15 years (100%); facial weakness (75%); bulbar symptoms (75%); muscle fasiculations (90%); gynecomastia (50%); sexual dysfunction (75%); X-linked family history (95%).

Complications: Slow progression of muscular disease. Although patients have normal sexual function prior to onset of the disease, they develop decreased libido and impotence after onset. In addition, sperm production diminishes with decreasing fertility as the disease progresses.

Associated Findings: None known.

Etiology: X-linked inheritance.

Pathogenesis: There appears to be some overlap with X-linked adrenomyeloneuropathy (see **Adrenoleukodystrophy, X-linked)**, which is associated with abnormalities in long chain fatty acid metabolism and peroxisomal dysfunction.

MIM No.: *31320

Sex Ratio: M1:F0

Occurrence: Over 50 cases have been reported. Represents about 3% of all spinal muscular atrophy patients in one center.

Risk of Recurrence for Patient's Sib:
See Part I, *Mendelian Inheritance.*

Risk of Recurrence for Patient's Child:
See Part I, *Mendelian Inheritance.*

Age of Detectability: Usually in adulthood.

Gene Mapping and Linkage: SBMA (spinal and bulbar muscular atrophy (Kennedy disease)) has been mapped to Xq13-q22.

Prevention: None known. Genetic counseling indicated.

Treatment: Supportive.

Prognosis: Life span and intelligence are not affected.

Detection of Carrier: Unknown.

References:
Kennedy WR, et al.: Progressive proximal spinal and bulbar muscular atrophy of late onset, a sex-linked recessive trait. Neurology (Minneap) 1968; 18:671–680.
Papapetropoulos T, Panayotopoulos CP: X-linked spinal and bulbar muscular atrophy of late onset (Kennedy-Stefanis disease?). Eur Neurol 1981; 20:485–488.
Hausmanova-Petrusewicz I, et al.: X-linked adult form of spinal muscular atrophy. J Neurol 1983; 229:175–188.
Fischbeck KH, et al.: X-linked neuropathy: gene localization with DNA probes. Annals Neurol 1986; 20:527–532.
Mukai E, Yasuma T: A pedigree with protanopia and bulbospinal muscular atrophy. Neurology 1987; 37:1019–1021.

GR011 **Frank Greenberg**

Muscular atrophy, spinal, intermediate type
See SPINAL MUSCULAR ATROPHY
Muscular atrophy-mental retardation, X-linked
See X-LINKED MENTAL RETARDATION-MUSCULAR WEAKNESS-AWKWARD GAIT
Muscular central core disease
See MYOPATHY, CENTRAL CORE DISEASE TYPE
Muscular dystrophy
See MYOPATHIES
Muscular dystrophy (Duchenne type)-glycerol kinase deficiency
See GLYCEROL KINASE DEFICIENCY
Muscular dystrophy I
See MUSCULAR DYSTROPHY, LIMB-GIRDLE
Muscular dystrophy without central nervous system damage
See MUSCULAR DYSTROPHY, CONGENITAL WITH ARTHROGRYPOSIS

MUSCULAR DYSTROPHY, ADULT PSEUDOHYPERTROPHIC   0687

Includes:
Becker muscular dystrophy
Muscular dystrophy, benign X-linked recessive
Muscular dystrophy, pseudohypertrophic adult type

Excludes:
Muscular dystrophy, autosomal recessive pseudohypertrophic (0688)
Muscular dystrophy, childhood pseudohypertrophic (0689)
Muscular dystrophy, limb-girdle (0691)

Major Diagnostic Criteria: Pelvic muscle weakness accompanied by pseudohypertrophy of the calf muscles. Onset is in late childhood, followed by a slow progressive course, allowing the patients to reach adult age. Highly elevated serum creatine kinase. Positive family history.

Clinical Findings: This disease was identified by the German geneticist Becker. Weakness is first apparent in the proximal muscles of the lower extremities and usually manifests itself by difficulty in running, rising from the floor, or climbing stairs. The age of onset in about 75% of the patients is between four and 19 years of age, with a mean age of 12 years. The patients are almost always able to walk until at least the age of 16 and this has been used as the differentiating point between the diagnosis of adult and childhood pseudohypertrophic muscular dystrophy. Of 144 patients with adult type, only 28.5% were confined to a wheelchair, 60.4% were alive and mobile at the time of the investigations, and 11.1% died while still ambulatory.

Neurologic evaluation shows waddling gait, with increased lordosis, and positive Gowers and Trendelenburg signs. There is mild to moderate atrophy and weakness of the gluteals, iliopsoas, tibialis anterior, supraspinati, infraspinati, serratus anterior, and sternocleidomastoids. Other muscles such as pectoralis, biceps, and brachioradialis show only very mild atrophy and weakness. Marked pseudohypertrophy of the calves is present in all patients. The Achilles tendons are contracted bilaterally and cannot be dorsiflexed beyond neutral position. Deep tendon reflexes are usually present or decreased.

Serum creatine kinase is highly elevated, with values of 10,000 to 20,000 IU (normal 50–200 IU). The creatine kinase isozymes show a 90–97% predominance of MM and MB isozymes. The electromyogram usually demonstrates a pattern of short duration, small amplitude, polyphasic potentials with some fibrillation potentials. Nerve conduction velocities are normal. Muscle biopsy reveals marked random variation in fiber size (many atrophic and some hypertrophic fibers), internal displacement of nuclei, split fibers, necrosis, phagocytosis, regeneration and endomysial fibrosis. According to some observers, about half the biopsies demonstrate neurogenic atrophy or denervation atrophy in addition to myopathic changes. However, some of the "neurogenic changes," such as fiber type grouping, could be caused by muscle

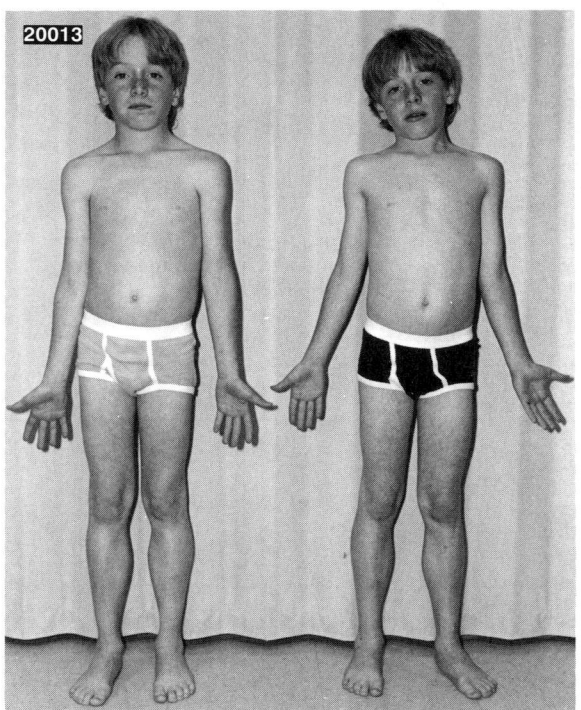

0687-20013: The twin patients (propositi) at 12 years of age show identical phenotype. Significant calves pseudohypertrophy is present in both.

fiber splitting. The EKG may be abnormal (right ventricular or combined ventricular hypertrophy) in 46% of patients.

Complications: Congestive heart failure secondary to cardiomyopathy may be present. Wheelchair confinement occurs in about one-third of the patients, when in an advanced stage of the disease.

Associated Findings: Unknown.

Etiology: X-linked recessive inheritance. Becker muscular dystrophy (BMD) described here, and Duchenne muscular dystrophy (DMD) (See **Muscular dystrophy, childhood pseudohypertrophic**) are allelic disorders. Affected males may represent new mutations (one-third of BMD cases). The DMD/BMD gene has been cloned and its protein product, called *dystrophin*, has been identified. Mutations involving the dystrophin gene are 60–70% intragenic deletions. Several studies have tried to explain the phenotypical characteristics of DMD (severe muscular dystrophy with less than 2% of normal dystrophin) and BMD (mild muscular dystrophy with qualitative abnormality of dystrophin; larger or smaller protein) by the location and/or size of the deletion and the mutation's effect on translational reading frame. Medori et al (1989) have suggested that deletions at the 5' end of the gene are associated with BMD while those in the central portion are associated with DMD. By contrast, Baumbach et al (1989) conclude that the size and location of the deletion does not account for differences between DMD and BMD.

Monaco et al (1988) and Hoffman (1988) suggest that the effect of the mutation on translational reading frame may account for the differences between DMD and BMD. BMD deletions remove nucleotides in exact multiples of three so that the reading frame (three nucleotides for each amino acid) is preserved. DMD deletions were found to remove an odd number of nucleotides, which shift the reading frame and make the remaining message beyond the site of the mutation meaningless. However, a later study by Malhotra et al (1988) showed exceptions to this rule, with deletions in some BMD patients producing shifts in the reading frame similar to those found in DMD patients. A significant number of DMD/BMD families (30–40%) have no detectable deletions, and must be studied by RFLP linkage.

Pathogenesis: Dystrophin is associated with sarcolemma of skeletal muscle. The abnormality of dystrophin may account for the increased permeability of sarcolemma resulting in high levels of serum creatine kinase in BMD patients.

MIM No.: *31020

Sex Ratio: M1:F0

Occurrence: In a 12-year prospective study in the Campania region of southern Italy, the incidence of Becker adult pseudohypertrophic muscular dystrophy was found 3.2:100,000, which is one-seventh the incidence of **Muscular dystrophy, childhood pseudohypertrophic** in the same region.

Risk of Recurrence for Patient's Sib:
See Part I, *Mendelian Inheritance.*

Risk of Recurrence for Patient's Child:
See Part I, *Mendelian Inheritance.*

Age of Detectability: Prenatal diagnosis relies on dystrophin cDNA probes for deletion identification in the male fetus, and on genetic linkage between the Becker gene and DNA intragenic markers. The condition can be diagnosed clinically at between four and 19 years of age.

Gene Mapping and Linkage: DMD (muscular dystrophy, Duchenne and Becker types) has been mapped to Xp21.3-p21.1.

Prevention: None known. Genetic counseling indicated.

Treatment: Physical therapy to prevent contractures (stretching exercises). Appropriate orthoses (braces) may be helpful. Treatment of congestive heart failure secondary to cardiomyopathy usually induces only a short improvement.

Prognosis: Decreased life expectancy to 30–55 years. For function, progressive decrease in muscular strength and difficulty in ambulation. Almost one-third of patients need a wheelchair in the last ten years of life.

Detection of Carrier: Based on both serum creatine kinase (elevated in 50% of carriers), dystrophin cDNA probes for deletion identification (Darras et al, 1988), and linkage between Becker locus and cloned DNA markers mapped in the area of Xp21.

Support Groups:
New York; Muscular Dystrophy Association (MDA)
ENGLAND: London; Muscular Dystrophy Group of Great Britain

References:
Becker PE: Two new families of benign sex linked recessive muscular dystrophy. Rev Can Biol 1962; 21:551–556.
Bradley WG, et al.: Becker type muscular dystrophy. Muscle Nerve 1978; 1:111–132. *
Nigro G, et al.: Prospective study of X-linked progressive muscular dystrophy in Campania. Muscle Nerve 1983; 6:253–262.
Kunkel LM, et al.: Analysis of deletions in DNA from patients with Becker and Duchenne muscular dystrophy. Nature 1986; 323:73–77.
Darras BT, et al.: Direct method for prenatal diagnosis and carrier detection in Duchenne/Becker muscular dystrophy using the entire dystrophin cDNA. Am J Med Genet 1988; 29:713–726.
Hoffman EP: Characterization of dystrophin in muscle biopsy specimen from patients with Duchenne's or Becker's muscular dystrophy. New Engl J Med 1988; 318:1363–1368.
Ionasescu V, et al.: Becker muscular dystrophy: recombinant DNA studies in identical twins. Muscle Nerve 1988; 11:287–290.
Malhotra SB, et al.: Frame shift deletions in patients with Duchenne and Becker muscular dystrophy. Science 1988; 242:755–759.
Monaco AP, et al.: An explanation of the phenotypic differences between patients bearing partial deletions of the DMD locus. Genomics 1988; 2:90–95.
Baumbach LL, et al.: Molecular and clinical correlation of deletions leading to Duchenne and Becker muscular dystrophies. Neurology 1989; 39:465–474.
Medori R, et al.: Genetic abnormalities in Duchenne and Becker dystrophies: clinical correlations. Neurology 1989; 39:461–465.

I0000   **Victor V. Ionasescu**

MUSCULAR DYSTROPHY, AUTOSOMAL RECESSIVE PSEUDOHYPERTROPHIC   0688

Includes:
Duchenne-like autosomal recessive muscular dystrophy
Pseudohypertrophic muscular dystrophy

Excludes:
Muscular dystrophy, adult pseudohypertrophic (0687)
Muscular dystrophy, childhood pseudohypertrophic (0689)

Major Diagnostic Criteria: Occurrs in both male and female children, with progressive proximal weakness and atrophy of the legs, hypertrophy of the calf muscles, high serum creatine kinase, and dystrophic alterations confirmed on muscle biopsy.

Clinical Findings: Onset before five years of age, with pelvic muscle weakness, pseudohypertrophy of the calves, and contractures of Achilles tendons in both boys and girls, or only in girls. Progression of the disease is variable, usually slower with ability to walk until adult age. However, a severe form has been reported in Tunisia, where wheelchair confinement with flexion contractures occur between ages 10 and 20 years. Cardiac involvement with congestive heart failure is common in advanced cases. Intellectual functions are normal.

The serum creatine kinase activity is markedly high in the first stages of the disease. There is a necrotic regenerative pattern shown on muscle biopsy. Electromyography shows short duration, small amplitude, multiphasic potentials. Chromosomal studies show normal findings.

Complications: Hip-girdle weakness may contribute to accidents.

Associated Findings: None known.

Etiology: Autosomal recessive inheritance, often associated with consanguinity in the parents. The 28 kindreds from Tunisia included 45 pairs of parents with dystrophic children. Seventy-six percent of the parental pairs were closely consanguineous, compared with consanguinity rates of 16–23% in the general population.

Pathogenesis: Undetermined. The progressive deterioration of the proximal muscles of the extremities resembles limb-girdle muscular dystrophy. Laboratory studies (serum creatine kinase, electromyography, and muscle biopsy) are not helpful in the differential diagnosis.

MIM No.: *25370

Sex Ratio: M1:F1

Occurrence: Most frequent in Tunisia and Sudan. Ninty-three cases have been reported in Tunisia, and 15 in the Sudan.

Risk of Recurrence for Patient's Sib:
See Part I, *Mendelian Inheritance.*

Risk of Recurrence for Patient's Child:
See Part I, *Mendelian Inheritance.*

Age of Detectability: Varies from three to 15 years.

Gene Mapping and Linkage: Unknown.

Prevention: None known. Genetic counseling indicated.

Treatment: Physical therapy for prevention of contractures, and orthopedic surgery for correction of scoliosis.

Prognosis: Guarded because of cardiac involvement and possible severe motor handicap.

Detection of Carrier: Unknown.

Support Groups:
New York; Muscular Dystrophy Association (MDA)
ENGLAND: London; Muscular Dystrophy Group of Great Britain

References:
Ionasescu V, Zellweger H: Duchenne muscular dystrophy in young girls? Acta Neurol Scand 1974; 50:619–630.
Ben Hamida M, et al.: Severe childhood muscular dystrophy affecting both sexes and frequent in Tunisia. Muscle Nerve 1983; 6:469–480.
Salih M, et al.: Severe autosomal recessive muscular dystrophy in an extended Sudanese kindred. Dev Med Child Neurol 1983; 25:43–52.
Somer H, et al.: Duchenne-like muscular dystrophy in two sisters with normal karyotypes: evidence for autosomal recessive inheritance. Clin Genet 1985; 28:151–156.

I0000   **Victor V. Ionasescu**

Muscular dystrophy, benign X-linked recessive
See MUSCULAR DYSTROPHY, ADULT PSEUDOHYPERTROPHIC

MUSCULAR DYSTROPHY, CHILDHOOD PSEUDOHYPERTROPHIC   0689

Includes:
Childhood pseudohypertrophic muscular dystrophy
Duchenne muscular dystrophy
Muscular dystrophy, classic X-linked recessive
Muscular dystrophy, pseudohypertrophic progressive, Duchenne type
Progressive muscular dystrophy of childhood

Excludes:
Glycerol kinase deficiency (2310)
Muscular dystrophy, adult pseudohypertrophic (0687)
Muscular dystrophy, autosomal recessive pseudohypertrophic (0688)
Muscular dystrophy (other)

Major Diagnostic Criteria: Pelvic weakness and atrophy accompanied by pseudohypertrophy of the calves and tight heelcords in a male child, manifested between 3–5 years of age; highly elevated serum creatine kinase.

Clinical Findings: While most newborn boys who inherit Duchenne muscular dystrophy (DMD) do not show clinical evidence of the disease during infancy, a more or less pronounced hypotonia is noticeable in others. Some children remain symptom free for a number of years, whereas others acquire the milestones of motor development at a slow pace; they walk late and fall frequently. At about the age of 3–5 years, weakness of the pelvic muscles is obvious in all cases. Squatting and climbing stairs are difficult; running and jumping are impossible. The patient shows a waddling gait, with increased lordosis on his toes. Neurologic evaluation at this stage reveals positive Gowers and Trendelenburg signs related to weakness of gluteus maximus and gluteus medius, respectively. Neck flexors (sternocleidomastoids) and back muscles (rhomboids, lower trapezius, latissimus dorsi) are also weak. Enlargement of the calves (pseudohypertrophy, i.e. related to fibrous tissue and fat infiltration) and Achilles tendon contractures are other early findings. Weakness of the shoulder girdle and arms follows, but distal muscles are preserved for a longer period of time. Deep tendon reflexes become depressed or absent.

Between nine and 14 years of age, DMD patients cease to ambulate. Various contractures of iliopsoas, hamstrings, forearm flexors, and finger flexors, and severe pes equinovarus develop in many patients. Severe paralytic thoracolumbar scoliosis becomes prominent. The arms, thighs, and pectoral muscles become atrophic. Intercostals become weak, and the lungs are hypoventilated and easily infected, causing pneumonia and bronchopneumonia. Death occurs between ages 20 and 25 years in 90% of the patients.

The disease process of DMD is not limited to skeletal musculature; the heart muscle is affected as well (cardiomyopathy), and death due to congestive heart failure is common. About one third of the DMD patients are mentally subnormal. Verbal IQ seems to be particularly affected, and many patients have reading problems. The overall IQ is between 70 and 85. The mental retardation is static and does not progress with the muscle involvement. Some DMD patients are of normal or even superior intelligence. Behavioral abnormalities, such as stubbornness, negativism, and selective mutism, are also reported.

Laboratory tests that are of value include the serum creatine kinase (CK), the electrocardiogram (EKG), electromyogram (EMG), and muscle biopsy. Elevated levels of CK are always seen in the early stages of the illness; reaching 10,000–40,000 IU (normal 50–200 IU). There is no well documented case of a patient with a normal CK during the first year of life who later develops DMD; thus, a normal CK is strong presumptive evidence against the possibility of the disease. As the illness progresses, the levels of CK fall, although they never attain normal values. The CK remains in the hundreds even in the patient who is severely disabled and in a wheelchair. Abnormalities in the EKG are common in DMD in the neighborhood of 70–90%. There are tall, right precordial R waves and deep limb lead and precordial Q waves. Arrhythmias and persistent tachycardias have been noted in patients with DMD. Many different explanations have been postulated for all of these EKG changes, but none has been entirely satisfactory. Correlation of EKG, echocardiogram and autopsy studies of the heart demonstrated replacement fibrosis of the wall of the left ventricle.

Electromyography shows small polyphasic potentials and increased recruitment of motor units. In the advanced stages, there may be additional changes such as fibrillations.

The muscle biopsy is characteristic, even early in the disease. There is increased fibrosis. Most of the fibers are circular rather than the usual polygonal shape. There is evidence of necrosis and phagocytosis and, in particular, small groups of basophilic fibers. Often large circular fibers demonstrating very dark staining, the so-called "opaque" hypercontracted fibers are present. Many type 2C or undifferentiated fibers are noted, often leading to poor separation into type 1 and type 2 fibers with the routine ATPase stains. Dystrophin evaluation (by immunoblotting or by immunofluorescence) demonstrates absence of the protein in the muscle biopsy.

Complications: Congestive heart failure secondary to cardiomyopathy; thoracolumbar scoliosis secondary to weakness of back muscles; and respiratory failure secondary to pulmonary hypoventilation and intercostal muscle weakness.

Associated Findings: Mild mental retardation with learning disability, particularly dyslexia.

Etiology: Usually X-linked recessive inheritance. The entire 14kb cDNA of the DMD gene has been cloned (Koenig et al, 1987) and its protein product, called *dystrophin*, has been identified (Hoffman et al, 1987). Mutations involving the dystrophin gene can cause either severe DMD or the milder allelic form such as Becker Muscular Dystrophy (BMD) (see **Muscular dystrophy, adult pseudohypertrophic**). Affected males may represent new mutations (one-third of the DMD cases). The majority of mutations (60–70%) are intragenic deletions clustered in a region near the center of the gene, or less frequently near the 5' end. There have been several reports (about 10% of cases) of germ line mosaicism in mothers of sons with DMD deletions. Therefore, it is possible that the mother could have two populations of ova; only one population carrying the deletion. No detectable deletions have been found in 30–40% of DMD families, and these must studied by RFLP linkage analysis using intragenic DNA markers. Other genetic defects in DMD include duplications which are seen in six percent (Den Dunnen et al, 1989), and insertions.

An estimated 6.8% of DMD cases are thought to be autosomal recessive (Zatz et al, 1989). The possibility of an autosomal DMD mutation should be suspected when the cytogenetic and molecular genetic (deletions, RFLP linkage analysis) screenings are negative, and when dystrophin evaluation of the muscle biopsy demonstrates normal size and abundance by immunoblotting (Francke et al, 1989).

Pathogenesis: Dystrophin protein is localized in the sarcolemma of human muscle (Zubrzycka-Gaarn et al, 1988), and the absence of dystrophin in the sarcolemma could explain the leakage of soluble sarcoplasmic enzymes, such as creatine kinase, in the serum of DMD affected individuals. The transcript of the DMD gene and the amino terminal of the encoded protein differ in brain and muscle. This difference may account for the mental retardation which is present only in 30% of DMD patients (Nudel et al, 1989).

MIM No.: *31020

Sex Ratio: M1:F>0. There are unusual situations in which DMD is expressed in females: manifesting heterozygotes, females with X chromosomal abnormalities, and in autosomal recessive DMD. Cytogenetic evaluations should be made of all female DMD patients.

Occurrence: Incidence varies between 1:1,700 and 1:7,700 live born boys. The average incidence for the United States, Japan, and Australia is 1:3,300 live born boys. In a 12-year prospective study in the Campania region of Southern Italy, the incidence of DMD was 21.7:100,000 live births. DMD monozygotic twins with deletion of the dystrophin gene have been reported (Ionasescu et al, 1989).

Risk of Recurrence for Patient's Sib:
See Part I, *Mendelian Inheritance.*

Risk of Recurrence for Patient's Child:
See Part I, *Mendelian Inheritance.* DMD patients are usually infertile. There is only one case report in the literature of a DMD patient who fathered a normal son.

Age of Detectability: Prenatal diagnosis is preceded by fetal sex determination. Prenatal diagnosis uses dystrophin cDNA probes for deletion identification and genetic linkage between intragenic DNA markers and the DMD gene. The condition can be recognized clinically between two and six years of age.

Gene Mapping and Linkage: DMD (muscular dystrophy, Duchenne and Becker types) has been mapped to Xp21.3-p21.1.

Prevention: None known. Genetic counseling indicated.

Treatment: Physical therapy to prevent contractures (stretching exercises). Night splints may be helpful for a limited period of time. Surgical treatment of scoliosis will help prevent severe restrictive lung syndrome. Management of end-stage respiratory failure is based on overnight mouth intermittent positive pressure. Life expectancy is improved following treatment, and in one patient death occurred at 30 instead of 20 years. Treatment of congestive heart failure using digitalis and diuretics produces only mediocre results.

Prognosis: Invariably fatal, usually by age 20. For function, progressive decline in muscular capability with wheelchair confinement by age 10–12.

Detection of Carrier: Based on both serum CK (elevated in 60% of carriers), dystrophin cDNA probes for screening of deletions, and linkage between DMD locus and cloned genomic DNA sequences mapped on the short arm of the X chromosome.

Support Groups:
New York; Muscular Dystrophy Association (MDA)
ENGLAND: London; Muscular Dystrophy Group of Great Britain

References:
Monaco AP, et al.: Detection of deletions spanning the Duchenne muscular dystrophy locus using a tightly linked DNA segment. Nature 1985; 316:842–845.
Heitmancik JF, et al.: Carrier diagnosis of Duchenne muscular dystrophy using restriction fragment length polymorphisms. Neurology 1986; 86:1553–1562.
Kunkel LM, et al.: Analysis of deletions in DNA from patients with Becker and Duchenne muscular dystrophy. Nature 1986; 322:73–77. *
Hoffman EP, et al.: Dystrophin: the protein product of the Duchenne muscular dystrophy locus. Cell 1987; 51:919–928.
Koenig M, et al.: Complete cloning of the Duchenne muscular dystrophy (DMD) cDNA and preliminary genomic organization of the DMD gene in normal and affected individuals. Cell 1987; 50:509–517.
Darras BT, et al.: Direct method for prenatal diagnosis and carrier detection in Duchenne/Becker muscular dystrophy using the entire dystrophin cDNA. Am J Med Genet 1988; 29:713–726.
Zubrzycka-Gaarn EK, et al.: The Duchenne muscular dystrophy gene product is localized in sarcolemma of human muscle. Nature 1988; 333:466–469.
LeRoy BS, et al.: Identification of carriers of Duchenne muscular dystrophy: value of molecular analysis. Am J Med Genet 1988; 31:709–721.
Den Dunnen JT, et al.: Topography of the Duchenne Muscular Dystrophy (DMD) gene: FIGE and cDNA analysis of 194 cases reveals 115 deletions and 13 duplications. Am J Hum Genet 1989; 45:835–847.
Francke U, et al.: Brother/sister pairs affected with early onset, progressive muscular dystrophy: molecular studies reveal etiologic heterogeneity. Am J Hum Genet 1989; 45:63–72.
Ionasescu V, et al.: Duchenne muscular dystrophy in monozygotic twins: deletion of 5' fragments of the gene. Am J Med Genet 1989; 33:113–116.
Nudel V, et al.: Duchenne muscular dystrophy gene product is not identical in muscle and brain. Nature 1989; 337:76–78.
Zatz M, et al.: Estimate of the proportion of Duchenne muscular dystrophy with autosomal recessive inheritance. Am J Med Genet 1989; 32:407–410.

I0000   **Victor V. Ionasescu**

Muscular dystrophy, classic X-linked recessive
See MUSCULAR DYSTROPHY, CHILDHOOD PSEUDOHYPERTROPHIC

MUSCULAR DYSTROPHY, CONGENITAL WITH ARTHROGRYPOSIS   2706

Includes:
Arthrogryposis multiplex congenita-muscle involvement
Atonic sclerotic muscular dystrophy, Ullrich type
Muscular dystrophy without central nervous system damage
Myosclerosis, Lowenthal type

Excludes: Myopathies, congenital, with characteristic pathology

Major Diagnostic Criteria: Affected infants are usually hypotonic and weak at birth. Many display multiple joint contractures. Mental development is usually normal. The disease is nonprogressive.

Clinical Findings: The infants show generalized muscular weakness, more severe proximally than distally. Facial, neck, and chest muscles are variably involved, and extraocular muscles are spared. The tendon reflexes are usually depressed or absent. Contractures of the joints, particularly of the elbows, hips, knees, and ankles, occur at birth. During the course of the illness, there is very little loss of functions already gained. The patients have normal intelligence and do well in school. These children may adapt without difficulty to braces or devices such as "stand in" tables, which will allow them to stand. Some patients develop kyphoscoliosis as they grow older.

The laboratory findings are the same as in other muscular dystrophies. Serum creatine kinase is usually mildly increased. The EMG is abnormal, revealing brief, small-amplitude, low-duration, polyphasic potentials. Fibrillation potentials are usually not detected. Muscle biopsy shows increased fibrosis with random variability in the size of the muscle fibers. There is often type 1 fiber predominance, as there is in many other congenital muscle diseases. Necrosis of single muscle fibers is usually not detected. Ultrastructural changes serve only to amplify the above muscle alterations.

Complications: Paralytic kyphoscoliosis can become a troublesome problem. Respiratory infections are common.

Associated Findings: Dysmorphic features such as high-arched palate, deformed chest, and posterior displacement of the calcaneum have been noted.

Etiology: Autosomal recessive inheritance has been reported in several kindreds. In a series of 24 children with congenital muscular dystrophy, there were three sets of affected sibs, including two sisters, a brother and sister, and one set of female twins. Sporadic cases have also been reported.

Pathogenesis: The abundance of collagen and its structural appearance suggested that an abnormality of collagen synthesis is basic to this disease.

MIM No.: *25390, 25560

Sex Ratio: M1:F1

Occurrence: About a half-dozen kindreds have been reported.

Risk of Recurrence for Patient's Sib:
See Part I, *Mendelian Inheritance.*

Risk of Recurrence for Patient's Child:
See Part I, *Mendelian Inheritance.*

Age of Detectability: During the first three years of life. Prenatal ultrasound diagnosis may show absence or decreased movement of the extremities (Baty et al, 1988; Gorczyca et al, 1989).

Gene Mapping and Linkage: Unknown.

Prevention: None known. Genetic counseling indicated.

Treatment: Symptomatic and supportive, based on physiotherapy and orthopedic surgery for correction of contractures.

Prognosis: Kyphoscoliosis and recurrent upper respiratory infections may generate high mortality.

Detection of Carrier: Unknown.

Support Groups: New York; Muscular Dystrophy Association (MDA)

References:
Banker BQ, et al.: Arthrogryposis multiplex due to congenital muscular dystrophy. Brain 1957; 80:319–334.
Fidzianska A, et al.: Congenital muscular dystrophy: a collagen formative disease? J Neurol Sci 1982; 55:79–86.
McMenamin JB, et al.: Congenital muscular dystrophy: a clinicopathologic report of 24 cases. J Pediatr 1982; 100:692–697.
Banker BQ: Congenital muscular dystrophy. In: Engel AG, Banker BQ, eds: Myology, vol 2. New York: McGraw-Hill, 1986:1367–1382. †
Socol ML, et al.: Prenatal diagnosis of congenital muscular dystrophy producing arthrogryposis. (Letter) New Engl J Med 1986; 313: 1230 only.
Baty BJ, et al.: Prenatal diagnosis of distal arthrogryposis. Am J Med Genet 1988; 29:501–510.

Gorczyca DP, et al.: Arthrogryposis multiplex congenita: prenatal ultrasonographic diagnosis. J Clin Ultrasound 1989; 17:40–44.

I0000   **Victor V. Ionasescu**

Muscular dystrophy, congenital with central nervous involvement
See MUSCULAR DYSTROPHY, CONGENITAL WITH MENTAL RETARDATION

MUSCULAR DYSTROPHY, CONGENITAL WITH MENTAL RETARDATION   2705

Includes:

Cerebromuscular dystrophy, Fukuyama type
Fukuyama disease
Muscular dystrophy, congenital with central nervous involvement
Micropolygyria-muscular dystrophy

Excludes: Myopathies (other)

Major Diagnostic Criteria: Onset before nine months of age, with generalized muscle weakness, hypotonia, and mental retardation. Many patients have seizures. More than 95% are Japanese. Electroencephalogram (EEG) and CT scan of the head show abnormalities. Muscle biopsy and electromyography (EMG) reveal myopathic alterations.

Clinical Findings: Mothers are often aware that fetal movements of affected infants are diminished. The children are born floppy, suck and swallow poorly, and have a weak cry. A funnel chest is noted in about 30% of patients. Weakness is generalized, but proximal muscles are affected more than distal muscles. Facial and neck weakness is also present. Mild contractures at knees and elbows are often reported early or develop by age three. Hip dislocations are not uncommon. Tendon reflexes are decreased or absent. Affected children are severely mentally retarded, the development of speech is affected, and many children have seizures; either grand mal or petit mal. Few of the children learn to walk and most lead a passive existence and die by ten years of age.

Laboratory studies demonstrate elevation of the serum creatine kinase (CK), lactic dehydrogenase, and glutamic oxaloacetic transaminase. After the age of six, these values begin to decline. The EEG shows a diffuse and marked decrease in the frequency of brain waves and abnormal focal paroxysmal discharges of spikes mostly in the frontoparietal zones. CT scan of the head reveals poor cortical gyral development as well as prominent sylvian fissures. The lateral ventricles are dilated and there is an increased lucency of the cerebral white matter particularly in the periventricular areas. The findings are consistent with such developmental defects as pachygyria and polymicrogyria. The EMG demonstrates a myopathic pattern consisting of low-amplitude, short-duration motor units and no spontaneous discharges. Muscle biopsy shows marked variation in the size of the fibers, and all are embedded in fibrous tissue, (endomysial and perimysial fibrosis). There is no remarkable change in the fiber types, although occasional type 1 predominance and numerous type 2 C fibers are noted. The cortex is thick and the sulci are shallow or absent (lissencephaly). In many cases, there is micropolygyria and agyria with distortion of the architecture of both the cerebral and cerebellar cortices. The changes are in general dysplastic.

Complications: Status epilepticus occurs occasionally and may result in death.

Associated Findings: Myocardial fibrosis was reported in one case.

Etiology: Autosomal recessive inheritance, with high rates of consanguinity in the parents of the patients, was reported by a genetic study in Japan on 153 families with 186 cases. Consanguineous marriage of the parents was found in 41 families (26.80%). Inbreeding coefficients in the patients was 10 times higher than in the general population. No single parent of the patients was affected. Recurrence among sibs was frequent: nine out of 41 sibs in offspring of related parents and 18 out of 110 sibs in offspring of unrelated parents were affected. The segregation ratio was 23.91–27.08% in offspring of related parents and 10.00–22.94% in offspring of unrelated parents. These values are not significantly different from the 25% expected for autosomal recessive mode of inheritance. Two twin pairs were part of the analyzed sample of patients, of which one male twin pair was identical. Sporadic cases were not significantly more numerous than expected. All these data indicate that the disorder is caused by homozygosity of an autosomal recessive gene.

Pathogenesis: Undetermined. The major changes in the central nervous system represent an arrest in the migration and differentiation of neurons early in the course of fetal development. This defect is expressed as **Microcephaly**, polymicrogyria, pachygria, lissencephaly and heterotopias. The occurrence of lissencephaly and polymicrogyria in siblings suggests that the underlying defect in the migration and differentiation of neurons is transmitted genetically. The disorder of muscle is characterized by an active degeneration of the muscle fibers. The fact that both systems are involved would indicate that the genetic factor responsible for the brain developmental defect is also responsible for the active progressive degeneration of muscle. A pleiotropic gene accounting for the lesions of muscle and central nervous system was postulated.

Follow-up studies of CT scan of the head revealed that the cerebral white matter low density areas were most apparent around the age of one year, and decreased or disappeared at 2–3 years of age. From these observations, delayed myelination was suspected for the pathogenesis of the low density areas (Yoshioka & Saiwai, 1988).

MIM No.: *25380

Sex Ratio: M1.1:F1

Occurrence: This condition been almost completely confined to Japan, where it reaches relative high frequency. Recently, several Caucasian patients were also reported. Frequency of the gene in Japan was estimated to be 5.2 to 9.7×10^{-3} and frequency of the patients $6.9-11.9 \times 10^{-5}$. In Japan the ratio of **Muscular dystrophy, childhood pseudohypertrophic** to Fukuyama congenital muscular dystrophy is 2.1:1. Mutation rate was estimated to be $6.9 - 11.0 \times 10^{-5}$.

Risk of Recurrence for Patient's Sib:
See Part I, *Mendelian Inheritance.*

Risk of Recurrence for Patient's Child:
See Part I, *Mendelian Inheritance.*

Age of Detectability: During infancy.

Gene Mapping and Linkage: Unknown.

Prevention: None known. Genetic counseling indicated.

Treatment: Anticonvulsants are necessary to control the seizures. Physiotherapy is helpful in preventing contractures. In infants with aqueductal obstruction, shunt procedures may be necessary to prevent the progressive enlargement of the ventricular system.

Prognosis: Guarded; short life expectancy.

Detection of Carrier: Unknown.

References:

Dambaka M, et al.: Cerebro-oculo-muscular syndrome: variant of Fijuyama congenital cerebro-muscular dystrophy. Clin Neuropath 1982; 1:93–98.

Nonaka I, et al.: Muscle histochemistry in congenital muscular dystrophy with central nervous system involvement. Muscle Nerve 1982; 5:102–106.

Fukuyama Y, Ohsawa M: A genetic study of the Fukuyama type of congenital muscular dystrophy. Brain Dev 1984; 6:373–390.

Takada K, et al.: Cortical dysplasia in congenital muscular dystrophy with central nervous system involvement (Fukuyama type). J Neuropath Exp Neurol 1984; 43:395–407.

Miura K, Shirasawa H: Congenital muscular dystrophy of the Fukuyama type (FCMD) with severe myocardial fibrosis. Acta Path Jpn 1987; 37:1823–1835.

Yoshioka M, Saiwai S: Congenital muscular dystrophy (Fukuyama type): changes in the white matter low density on CT. Brain Dev 1988; 10:41–44.

I0000   **Victor V. Ionasescu**

MUSCULAR DYSTROPHY, DISTAL   0690

Includes:
  Distal muscular dystrophy
  Gowers form of dystrophy
  Muscular dystrophy, late distal hereditary
  Myopathy, late distal hereditary
  Swedish type distal myopathy
  Welander type of muscular dystrophy

Excludes:
  Charcot-Marie-Tooth disease
  Neuropathy, hereditary motor and sensory
  Distal spinal muscular atrophy
  Myopathy, malignant hyperthermia (2710)
  Myopathy, myotubular (0695)
  Myopathy, nemaline (0696)
  Myotonic dystrophy (0702)

Major Diagnostic Criteria: Weakness of distal limb muscles. Electromyogram and muscle biopsy consistent with myopathy. Positive family history.

Clinical Findings: *Autosomal dominant form (Welander)*: Onset is in late adult life (usually after age 40). The initial symptoms are clumsiness and weakness of hand movements, such as fastening buttons, handling needles, or typing. Slow progression, with weakness spreading proximally to the forearm, whereas the leg muscles are spared or involved later. Weakness of foot extensors, steppage gait, and twisting of ankles, were present initially in only nine of 249 patients. The deep tendon reflexes are relatively preserved in the early stage of the disease, but become decreased or absent after many years. Sensation is not impaired, in contrast to **Neuropathy, hereditary motor and sensory**. The disorder does not shorten life expectancy.
Autosomal recessive form: Onset is in early adult life. The involvement of distal leg muscles is first noticed with weakness and atrophy of peroneal muscles and subsequent rapid progression to thigh and hand muscles. Neurologic evaluation may include absent Achilles and patellar reflexes in a few patients, but the majority have intact deep tendon reflexes. Cardiomyopathy may occur.
  Laboratory studies in distal muscular dystrophy show moderate to striking elevation of serum creatine kinase. Electromyographic studies are compatible with myopathy; e.g. brief duration, small amplitude, and abundant motor unit potentials. No myotonic discharges are recorded. Motor and sensory nerve conductions are normal in both arms and legs. Muscle biopsy is characterized by marked variation in fiber size with frequent splitting, occasional degenerating fibers with secondary vacuolar degenerations, necrotic fibers with associated phagocytosis, numerous internal nuclei, and occasional basophilic fibers. These histologic features are characteristic for muscular dystrophy.

Complications: Unknown.

Associated Findings: None known.

Etiology: The autosomal dominant form of inheritance is variable in expression. The autosomal recessive form may appear to be sporadic when only one person is affected in a small family.

Pathogenesis: Unknown.

MIM No.: *16050

Sex Ratio: M1:F1

Occurrence: The autosomal dominant (Welander) form is frequent in Sweden, where 249 affected persons distributed in 72 kindreds were originally reported. The trait had 80% penetrance in males and 69% penetrance in females. The autosomal recessive form has been reported in the United States, Italy, and Japan. The exact incidence is not known.

Risk of Recurrence for Patient's Sib:
See Part I, *Mendelian Inheritance.*

Risk of Recurrence for Patient's Child:
See Part I, *Mendelian Inheritance.*

Age of Detectability: Between 30–40 years of age.

Gene Mapping and Linkage: Unknown.

Prevention: None known. Genetic counseling indicated.

Treatment: There is no specific treatment. Patients with distal leg weakness can be helped with bilateral ankle-foot orthoses. Molded polypropylene orthoses are usually the most successful.

Prognosis: Good for life, but guarded for ambulation in autosomal recessive form.

Detection of Carrier: Examination of relatives for evidence of the trait.

Support Groups:
  New York; Muscular Dystrophy Association (MDA)
  ENGLAND: London; Muscular Dystrophy Group of Great Britain

References:
Eastrom L: Histochemical and histopathological changes in skeletal muscle in late-onset hereditary distal myopathy. J Neurol Sci 1975; 26:147–157. *
Markesbery WR, et al.: Distal myopathy: electron microscopic and histochemical studies. Neurology 1977; 27:727–735. *
Matsubara S, Tanabe H: Hereditary distal myopathy with filamentous inclusions. Acta Neurol Scand 1982; 65:363–365.
Scoppetta C, et al.: Distal muscular dystrophy with autosomal recessive inheritance. Muscle Nerve 1984; 7:478–481.

I0000   **Victor V. Ionasescu**

MUSCULAR DYSTROPHY, FACIO-SCAPULO-HUMERAL   2049

Includes:
  Facio-scapulo-humeral dystrophy
  Facio-scapulo-humeral dystrophy, infantile
  Landouzy-Dejerine muscular dystrophy

Excludes:
  Myopathies with facial muscle weakness, other congenital
  Myopathy, central core disease type (0134)
  Myopathy, myotubular (0695)
  Myopathy, nemaline (0696)
  Myotonic dystrophy (0702)
  Spinal muscular atrophy (0895)

Major Diagnostic Criteria: Facial and scapular muscle weakness is apparent clinically. The diagnosis is confirmed by EMG evidence of a myopathy and histologic evidence of dystrophy (phagocytosis, necrosis, internal nuclei in about 20% of fibers). Serum creatinine phosphokinase may be elevated.

Clinical Findings: Clinical signs may manifest anytime in the first two decades of life. Facial weakness is the earliest sign and produces difficulty in activities such as blowing or puckering the lips. As the facial muscle weakness progresses, by adolescence there may be a characteristic mask-like facial expression with horizontal movement of lips during an effort to smile and an inability to close the eyes during sleep.
  An early clinical sign of shoulder girdle involvement is the inability to lift the arms and hands above the head. The neck and the scapular muscles become weak and wasted with relative sparing of deltoid muscles. Further involvement of the shoulder girdle is characterized by progressive loss of function. Some affected individuals are unable to raise their arms to eye level because of their inability to fixate the scapula. Wrist-drop may occur. The dystrophy may also involve the hip girdle muscles. The more severely affected individuals are unable to walk because of hip-girdle muscle weakness. Muscle involvement may be asymmetric.
  Clinical variability is common; the muscle weakness may be moderately or very slowly progressive, or it may even be static

with involvement of a few muscles. Penetrance is generally complete, although there may be wide intrafamilial variability in clinical expression of the trait. For example, in a single kindred there may be an individual with profound weakness requiring a wheelchair, while facial weakness may be the only manifestation in another relative. Careful examination of all family members is essential. *A severe, early onset form* of facioscapulohumeral dystrophy has been described. Clinical expression is evident in infancy, and it progresses rapidly, leading to profound muscle weakness requiring the use of a wheelchair by age ten. This severe infantile type disease has been described in families where one parent might have only minimal facial weakness (Bailey, 1986).

Complications: Lordosis, foot drop and gait abnormalities are sometimes seen. Muscle weakness can make some activities of daily living difficult. For example, combing the hair may be difficult or impossible. Hip girdle weakness may contribute to accidents. Heart muscle involvement and congestive heart failure are rare.

Associated Findings: Sensorineural hearing loss is found in 5–15%. Fitzsimmons et al (1987) noted retinal capillary abnormalities, and suggested that capillary anomalies may play a role in the pathogenesis of the disease.

Etiology: Autosomal dominant inheritance with variability in expression. Heterogeneity may exist. An autosomal recessive variant of facioscapulohumeral dystrophy has been postulated, but this condition could be a variant of **Muscular dystrophy, limb-girdle** involving the facial muscles.

Pathogenesis: Current theory postulates a defect in the muscle membrane, possibly related to capillary anomalies.

MIM No.: *15890

POS No.: 3229

Sex Ratio: M1:F1

Occurrence: In general, this muscular dystrophy is less common than the Duchenne type. However, the incidence varies with ethnic group and geographic location. There are high incidences in southern Germany and in Utah, presumably from a few large affected kindreds. Mutations are thought to be rare. The mutation rate was estimated to be between 4.7×10^{-6} and 5×10^{-7}. The prevalence was estimated by Morton (1959) to be 2:1,000,000, but this may be an underestimate.

Risk of Recurrence for Patient's Sib:
See Part I, *Mendelian Inheritance.*

Risk of Recurrence for Patient's Child:
See Part I, *Mendelian Inheritance.*

Age of Detectability: Usually clinically evident by 10–20 years of age; however, it may be present as early as the first year of life.

Gene Mapping and Linkage: FMD (facioscapulohumeral muscular dystrophy) has been tentatively mapped to unassigned.

Prevention: None known. Genetic counseling indicated.

Treatment: Physical therapy to prevent contractures. Appropriate orthoses may be helpful depending upon disability. Surgical fixation of scapula allows use of the proximal muscles of upper extremities.

Prognosis: Normal life expectancy in 98%. Physical handicaps leading to a change in lifestyle occurs in about 5–10%. Intelligence is normal.

Detection of Carrier: Careful clinical muscle examination and history for all relatives will help indicate those who are minimally affected.

Support Groups:
New York; Muscular Dystrophy Association (MDA)
ENGLAND: London; Muscular Dystrophy Group of Great Britain

References:
Morton NE, Chung CS: Formal genetics of muscular dystrophy. Am J Med Genet 1959; 11:360–379.
Carroll JH, Brooke MH: Infantile facioscapulohumeral dystrophy. In: Serratrice G, Roux H, eds: Peroneal atrophies and related disorders. New York: Masson USA, 1979.
Ionasescu V, Zellweger H: Genetics in neurology. New York: Raven Press, 1983:412–413.
Bailey RO, et al.: Infantile facioscapulohumeral muscular dystrophy: new observations. Acta Neurol Scand 1986; 74:51–58.
Bodensteiner JB, Schochet SS: Facioscapulohumeral muscular dystrophy: the choice of a biopsy site. Muscle Nerve 1986; 9:544–547.
Brooke MH: A clinician's view of neuromuscular diseases, 2nd ed. Baltimore: Williams & Wilkins, 1986:158–170.
Fitzsimmons RB, et al.: Retinal vascular abnormalities in facioscapulohumeral muscular dystrophy: a general association with genetic and therapeutic implications. Brain 1987; 110:631–648.

RU013   **Barry S. Russman**

Muscular dystrophy, late distal hereditary
See MUSCULAR DYSTROPHY, DISTAL

MUSCULAR DYSTROPHY, LIMB-GIRDLE   0691

Includes:
> Erb muscular dystrophy
> Leyden-Moebius muscular dystrophy
> Limb-girdle muscular dystrophy
> Muscular dystrophy I
> Pelvofemoral muscular dystrophy

Excludes:
> **Glycogenosis, type IIb** (2873)
> **Muscular dystrophy, adult pseudohypertrophic** (0687)
> **Muscular dystrophy, childhood pseudohypertrophic** (0689)
> **Muscular dystrophy, facio-scapulo-humeral** (2049)
> **Myopathy** (others)
> **Spinal muscular atrophy** (0895)

Major Diagnostic Criteria: Onset in second decade. Findings include weakness of proximal muscles in hip and shoulder area; "myopathic" electromyogram; muscle biopsy consistent with a "dystrophy" pattern (phagocytosis, split fibers, internal nuclei), and elevation of serum creatine kinase.

Clinical Findings: Patient first complains of difficulty climbing stairs; will use railing during this activity. In some cases, primary complaint will be difficulty holding hands above head. Onset of symptoms typically begins in the second decade of life, but the patient may not seek medical help until the third decade. Physical findings include weakness of proximal leg muscles and shoulder muscles; the biceps and brachioradialis muscles are weaker than the triceps muscle. Pseudohypertrophy of calf muscles is seen in 20% of patients. Serum creatine kinase is mildly elevated, but may be normal. Twenty percent of the patients will develop severe, intractable low back pain.

Complications: Low back pain, rarely contractures.

Associated Findings: Heart failure, which may occur late in the course of the disease (10%).

Etiology: Usually autosomal recessive inheritance; there have been few reports of an autosomal dominant transmission with complete penetrance and partial expression.

Pathogenesis: Presumably a defect of muscle membrane.

MIM No.: *25360

Sex Ratio: M1:F1

Occurrence: There is a high occurrence of this condition in the Amish community of Indiana. Studies (Jackson, 1961) traced this to descendents from Swiss Canton (Berne).

With new techniques of muscle biopsy analysis, specifically histochemical staining, it is anticipated that this category of muscular dystrophy will become less frequent. For the present, an individual who has proximal weakness of extremities and no facial weakness, with a complete muscle biopsy analysis showing necrosis, internal nuclei, and split fibers may, be placed in this category. With a totally negative family history, including physical examination and CPK testing, it may be difficult to exclude

Muscular dystrophy, adult pseudohypertrophic (Becker) in male patients except on the basis of X chromosome genetic linkage.

Risk of Recurrence for Patient's Sib:
See Part I, *Mendelian Inheritance.*

Risk of Recurrence for Patient's Child:
See Part I, *Mendelian Inheritance.*

Age of Detectability: Clinically, at 10–25 years of age.

Gene Mapping and Linkage: LGMD2 (limb girdle muscular dystrophy 2 (autosomal recessive)) is unassigned.

Prevention: None known. Genetic counseling indicated.

Treatment: Physical therapy to minimize contractures and use of orthoses as indicated.

Prognosis: Normal life span. May need wheelchair eventually. Occasionally, onset may be later than usual, with rapid progression leading to wheelchair over a three year period of time.

Detection of Carrier: Unknown.

Support Groups:
New York; Muscular Dystrophy Association (MDA)
ENGLAND: London; Muscular Dystrophy Group of Great Britain

References:
Jackson CE, Carey JH: Progressive muscular dystrophy: autosomal recessive type. Pediatrics 1961; 28:77–84.
DeCoster W, et al.: A late autosomal dominant form of limb-girdle muscular dystrophy. Neurology 1974; 12:159–172.
Cöers C, Telerman-Toppet N: Differential diagnosis of limb-girdle muscular dystrophy and spinal muscular atrophy. Neurology 1979; 29:957–972.
Fowler WM, Nayak NN: Slowly progressive proximal weakness: limb-girdle syndromes. Arch Phys Med Rehabil 1983; 64:527–538.
Yates JRW, Emery AEH: A population study of adult onset limb-girdle muscular dystrophy. J Med Genet 1985; 22:250–257.
Chutkow JG, et al.: Adult-onset autosomal dominant limb-girdle muscular dystrophy. Ann Neurol 1986; 20:240–248.
Norman A, et al.: Distinction of Becker from limb-girdle muscular dystrophy by means of dystrophin cDNA probes. Lancet 1989; I:466–468.

RU013 **Barry S. Russman**

MUSCULAR DYSTROPHY, OCULO-GASTROINTESTINAL 2016

Includes:
Intestinal pseudo obstruction-external ophthalmoplegia
Muscular dystrophy, oculogastrointestinal
Oculogastrointestinal muscular dystrophy
Ophthalmoplegia-intestinal pseudo-obstruction
Visceral myopathy-external ophthalmoplegia

Excludes:
Kearns-Sayre disease (2070)
Ophthalmoplegia, progressive external (0752)
Muscular dystrophy, oculopharyngeal (0692)

Major Diagnostic Criteria: Ptosis, external ophthalmoplegia, and progressive intestinal pseudo-obstruction leading to malnutrition. Autosomal recessive inheritance.

Clinical Findings: The clinical syndrome becomes apparent between childhood and age 50 years, and is manifested by ptosis and external ophthalmoplegia followed by gastrointestinal symptoms. The latter include postprandial abdominal distension and pain, chronic diarrhea, malnutrition with severe weight loss and rarely, nausea and vomiting. Physical evaluation shows peristaltic waves visible over the abdominal wall, hyperactive bowel sounds, mild-to-moderate proximal limb muscle weakness and atrophy, ptosis and external ophthalmoplegia. Peripheral facial weakness, peripheral neuropathy with distal weakness, hypesthesia and decreased deep tendon reflexes may also occur. Heterogeneity of the disease is suggested by the presence of two clinical forms. The childhood onset of the disease has a rapid progression with death before age 30 years.

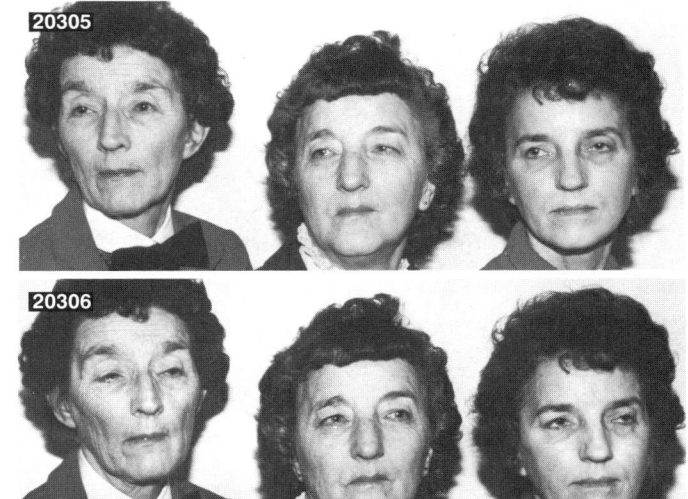

2016A-20305: Note marked limitation of eye movements and ptosis in extreme right gaze. 20306: Limitation in extreme left gaze.

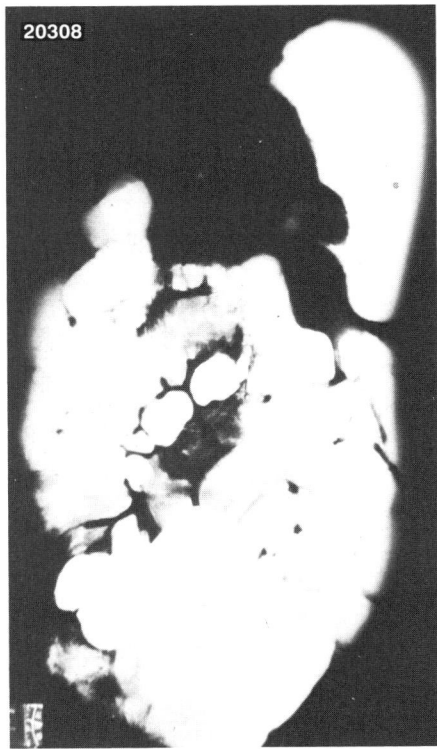

2016B-20308: Upper gastrointestinal X-ray shows presence of barium in the stomach after 8 h, jejunal dilatation and jejunal diverticula.

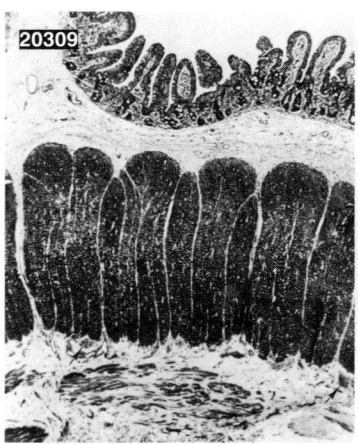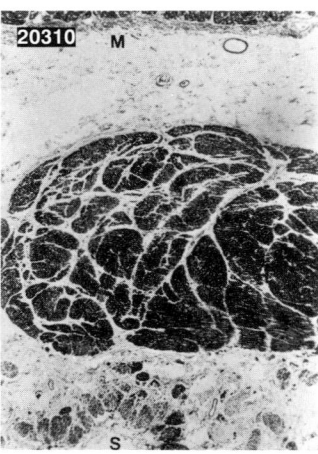

2016C-20309: Full thickness section of the stomach shows muscle atrophy and fibrosis affecting the more external muscle bundles located near the serosa (S); the mucosa, including muscularis mucosa (M) appears to be intact. Trichrome stain, original magnification × 20. **20310:** Section of jejunum reveals severe atrophy of the longitudinal muscle layer while circular muscle layer is intact. The atrophic muscle fibers are replaced by connective tissue. Trichrome stain, original magnification × 25.

The late adult-onset type (around age 50 years) has a mild course. Upper gastrointestinal X-rays shows delayed gastric emptying, jejunal dilation, and diverticulosis. Autopsy pathologic studies in two cases showed primary myopathic lesions of the smooth muscle of the stomach and intestine with severe atrophy and fibrosis, while the neurogenic structures (myenteric plexus and vagus nerves) were intact. Jejunal mucosal biopsy showed preserved villus architecture, without inflammatory changes. Absorption tests for fat, protein, carbohydrate, folic acid and vitamin B_{12} are normal. Mild-to-moderate myopathic changes are seen in the biopsy of proximal limb muscles and include variability of fiber size, atrophic fibers of both types I and II and several "moth-eaten" fibers. A neurogenic component of the disease was documented only in one case and consisted of demyelinating and axonal peripheral neuropathy as well as spongiform degeneration of the posterior columns.

Complications: Intestinal pseudo-obstruction was present in 56% of cases as the result of severe smooth muscle myopathic involvement of both stomach and jejunum.

Associated Findings: Prolapse of the mitral valve in one case.

Etiology: Autosomal recessive inheritance has been suggested. The disease was originally described in three sibships of an inbred kindred of German extraction. Three of four affected persons were products of consanguineous marriages and the proportion of diseased sibs approached 25%, consistent with autosomal recessive inheritance. The father of the proposita had ptosis and died of spontaneous rupture of the esophagus. This may be an example of pseudodominance. The second reported family had three diseased sisters with unaffected, nonconsanguineous parents and four unaffected sibs.

Pathogenesis: Biochemical studies of contractile proteins (myosin, actin and tropomyosin) in the fresh and cultured smooth muscle cells of one patient obtained at the time of gastrectomy showed a 50–75% decrease in the synthesis of different contractile proteins. Turnover of contractile proteins and synthesis and turnover of collagen showed normal values. The reduction in synthesis of contractile proteins may account for the weak peristalsis, and be a factor in the pathogenesis of the intestinal pseudo-obstruction.

MIM No.: 27732

POS No.: 3996

Sex Ratio: M1:F6

Occurrence: Undetermined. Seven cases in two families have been reported.

Risk of Recurrence for Patient's Sib:
See Part I, *Mendelian Inheritance.*

Risk of Recurrence for Patient's Child:
See Part I, *Mendelian Inheritance.*

Age of Detectability: Varies from childhood to late adulthood.

Gene Mapping and Linkage: Unknown.

Prevention: None known. Genetic counseling indicated.

Treatment: No specific treatment is available. Surgical treatment (partial gastrectomy and gastrojejunostomy) was tried unsuccessfully in one case.

Prognosis: Good for life span only in the late adult-onset type. Guarded prognosis in the early-onset type, where life expectancy may be significantly reduced.

Detection of Carrier: Unknown.

Support Groups: New York; Muscular Dystrophy Association (MDA)

References:
Ionasescu VV: Oculogastrointestinal muscular dystrophy. Am J Med Genet 1983; 15:103–112. *
Ionasescu VV, et al.: Inherited ophthalmoplegia with intestinal pseudo-obstruction. J Neurol Sci 1983; 59:215–228. †
Ionasescu VV, et al.: Late onset oculogastrointestinal muscular dystrophy. Am J Med Genet 1984; 18:781–788.

I0000   **Victor V. Ionasescu**

Muscular dystrophy, oculogastrointestinal
See MUSCULAR DYSTROPHY, OCULO-GASTROINTESTINAL

MUSCULAR DYSTROPHY, OCULOPHARYNGEAL   0692

Includes:
Oculopharyngeal muscular dystrophy
Oculopharyngeal myopathy
Pharyngeal muscular dystrophy

Excludes:
Bulbar weakness and ptosis, other causes of
Muscular dystrophy (other)
Myasthenia gravis
Myotonic dystrophy (0702)

Major Diagnostic Criteria: Adult onset of ptosis and pharyngeal muscle weakness, along with a positive family history of this condition, or a muscle biopsy disclosing myopathic or dystrophic features, with rimmed vacuoles and intra-nuclear filamentous inclusion.

Clinical Findings: Late-onset bilateral ptosis of the eyelids and progressive dysphagia. The onset of weakness of those involved muscle groups may occur anywhere from the fourth to eighth decades. There may be progressive ptosis, necessitating correction of the ptotic defect. Dysphagia often proves to be progressive with increasing difficulty in handling solid foods and eventually in handling fluids. After being present for 1–2 decades in the above mentioned muscle groups, mild evidence of proximal muscle weakness develops in the shoulder and pelvic girdles.

There are no definitive laboratory tests aside from muscle biopsies that are helpful in this condition. Serum enzymes, such as creatine kinase (CK), are invariably normal or only mildly elevated. Electromyography of the involved muscles may disclose a "myopathic pattern", but this type of study is rarely done.

Complications: Aspiration pneumonitis or other problems associated with serious swallowing difficulty may supervene at any time, especially late in the course of the disease.

Associated Findings: **Ophthalmoplegia, Retinitis pigmentosa,** and distal wasting.

Etiology: Autosomal dominant inheritance.

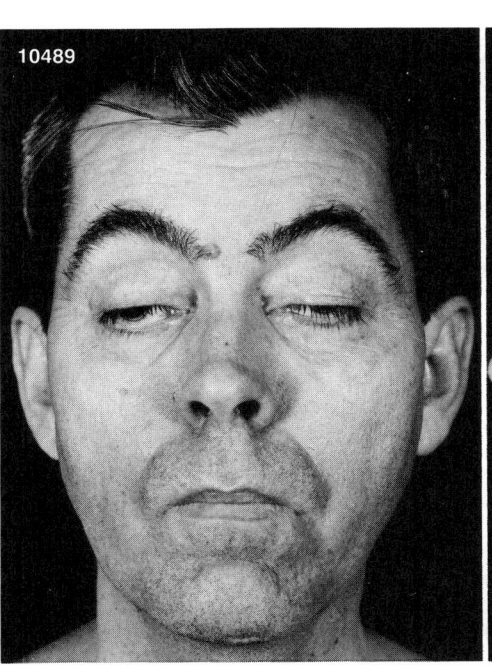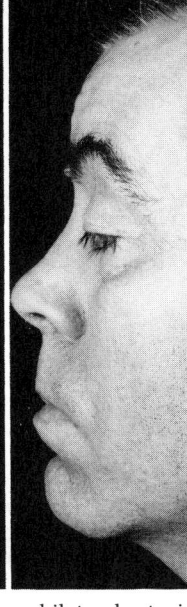

0692-10489–90: Muscular weakness produces bilateral ptosis and an expressionless face.

Pathogenesis: Progressive deterioration of the muscle fibers.

MIM No.: *16430

POS No.: 4328

Sex Ratio: M1:F1

Occurrence: Undetermined. Many affected individuals are of French Canadian descent, and can be traced to one common ancestor who landed in Quebec in 1634. Also reported in Melanesian and Swiss families.

Risk of Recurrence for Patient's Sib:
See Part I, *Mendelian Inheritance.*

Risk of Recurrence for Patient's Child:
See Part I, *Mendelian Inheritance.*

Age of Detectability: Clinically, by the third to fifth decade of life.

Gene Mapping and Linkage: Unknown.

Prevention: None known. Genetic counseling indicated.

Treatment: Supportive measures, such as eyelid crutches to overcome ptotic defect. Operative partial correction of ptosis. Careful nursing and other management to avoid spillover aspiration pneumonitis from dysphagia.

Prognosis: Generally good for life span unless the patient develops aspiration pneumonia associated with the dysphagia problem.

Detection of Carrier: Unknown.

Support Groups:
New York; Muscular Dystrophy Association (MDA)
ENGLAND: London; Muscular Dystrophy Group of Great Britain

References:
Victor M, et al.: Oculopharyngeal muscular dystrophy: a familial disease of late life characterized by dysphagia and progressive ptosis of the eyelids. New Engl J Med 1962; 267:1267–1272. *
Murphy SF, Drachman DB: The oculopharyngeal syndrome. JAMA 1968; 203:1003–1008.
Morgan-Hughes JA, Mair WGP: Atypical muscle mitochondria in oculo-skeletal myopathy. Brain 1973; 96:215–224.

Schmitt HP, Krause KH: An autopsy study of a familial oculopharyngeal muscular dystrophy (OPMD) with distal spread and neurogenic involvement. Muscle Nerve 1981; 4:296–305.
Fukuhara N, et al.: Oculopharyngeal muscular dystrophy and distal myopathy. Acta Neurol Scand 1982; 65:458–467.
Scrimgeour EM, Mastaglia FL: Oculopharyngeal and distal myopathy. Am J Med Genet 1984; 17:763–771.

I0000

Victor V. Ionasescu
Walter G. Bradley

Muscular dystrophy, pseudohypertrophic adult type
See MUSCULAR DYSTROPHY, ADULT PSEUDOHYPERTROPHIC
Muscular dystrophy, pseudohypertrophic progressive, Duchenne type
See MUSCULAR DYSTROPHY, CHILDHOOD PSEUDOHYPERTROPHIC
Muscular dystrophy, tardive with contractures
See EMERY-DREIFUSS SYNDROME
Muscular dystrophy-cataract-hypogonadism
See MYOPATHY-CATARACT-GONADAL DYSGENESIS
Muscular dystrophy-cerebrooocular dysplasia
See WALKER-WARBURG SYNDROME
Muscular dystropy-muscular shortening
See HAUPTMANN-THANHAUSER SYNDROME
Muscular macroglossia
See MACROGLOSSIA
Muscular septum, defects in various portions of
See VENTRICULAR SEPTAL DEFECT
Muscular shortening and dystrophy
See HAUPTMANN-THANHAUSER SYNDROME
Muscular subaortic stenosis
See HEART, SUBAORTIC STENOSIS, MUSCULAR
Muscular torticollis
See TORTICOLLIS
Musculo-skeletal-oto-oculo syndrome
See OTO-OCULO-MUSCULO-SKELETAL SYNDROME
Musicogenic epilepsy
See EPILEPSY, REFLEX

MUTCHINICK SYNDROME 3274

Includes: Mental retardation, Buenes Aires type

Excludes:
Dwarfism, osteodysplastic primordial, Majewski-Winter type (2581)
Seckel syndrome (0881)

Major Diagnostic Criteria: The combination of short stature, **Microcephaly**, facial anomalies, mental retardation, and mild cardiac and renal anomalies.

Clinical Findings: Both of the female sibs in which this condition has been reported had marked short stature, microcephaly, **Eye, hypertelorism**, downslanting palpebral fissures, long and curly eyelashes, broad nose with prominent nasal bridge, wide downturned mouth, highly arched palate, malocclusion, prognathism, large ears, clinodactyly, hyperconvex thumb nails, spasticity, and mental retardation. Both girls had dilation of one or both renal calyces; rotated right kidney was present in one, and dilated right ureter was present in the other as well. Both girls also had **Atrial septal defects**, although one also had right bundle branch block and valvular pulmonic stenosis. Light blonde hair, blue irides, and photophobia were also present in both, which is unusual given the ethnic origin of these children.

Complications: Unknown.

Associated Findings: None known.

Etiology: The presence of consanguinity in the parents suggests that autosomal recessive inheritance is most likely.

Pathogenesis: The basic defect is unknown, although a melanin defect as a part of the pleiotropic effect of the gene was suggested by the authors.

MIM No.: 24963

Sex Ratio: M1:F1

Occurrence: One family from Argentina has been described.

Risk of Recurrence for Patient's Sib:
See Part I, *Mendelian Inheritance.*

Risk of Recurrence for Patient's Child:
See Part I, *Mendelian Inheritance.*

Age of Detectability: At birth, by physical examination.

Gene Mapping and Linkage: Unknown.

Prevention: None known. Genetic counseling indicated.

Treatment: Supportive.

Prognosis: Mental retardation is present, and the IQ in one child was 42. Life span is unknown since both girls were under the age of eight years at the time of the report.

Detection of Carrier: Unknown.

References:
Mutchinick O: A syndrome of mental and physical retardation, speech disorders, and peculiar facies in two sisters. J Med Genet 1972; 9:60–63.

T0007   **Helga V. Toriello**

Mutilating keratoderma
See DEAFNESS-KERATOPACHYDERMIA-DIGITAL CONSTRICTIONS
Myasthenia gravis, familial infantile
See MYASTHENIC SYNDROME, FAMILIAL INFANTILE TYPE
Myasthenia, familial infantile
See MYASTHENIC SYNDROME, FAMILIAL INFANTILE TYPE

MYASTHENIC SYNDROME, CONGENITAL SLOW CHANNEL TYPE   2912

Includes: Slow-channel syndrome
Excludes:
Autoimmune myasthenia gravis
Diplegia, congenital facial (0376)
Kearns-Sayre disease (2070)
Lambert-Eaton myasthenic syndrome
Muscular dystrophy, facio-scapulo-humeral (2049)
Muscular dystrophy, limb-girdle (0691)
Myasthenic syndrome, familial infantile type (2913)
Myasthenic syndromes, acquired
Myasthenic syndromes, other
Myotonic dystrophy (0702)
Syringomyelia (0924)

Major Diagnostic Criteria: Abnormal fatigability on exertion; variable weakness of cranial, limb, and trunk muscles; EMG evidence of a repetitive compound muscle action potential evoked by a single nerve stimulus in all rested muscles; abnormally prolonged duration of end-plate potentials and miniature end-plate potentials in all muscles; reduced amplitude of miniature end-plate potentials and a decremental EMG response at 2-Hz stimulation in some muscles.

Acetylcholinesterase activity is intact at all motor end-plates. In clinically affected muscles, the findings include 1) focal degeneration of the junctional folds with concomitant loss of the acetylcholine receptor at the end-plates; 2) degenerative changes in the muscle fibers, most severe near the end-plates; and 3) variable muscle fiber atrophy.

Clinical Findings: Weakness and abnormal fatigability occur in all cases. However, the age of onset, the initial and eventual pattern of muscle involvement, the rate of progression, and the degree of weakness and fatigability may vary from case to case. The disease may present in infancy, childhood, or adulthood. In some patients the disease progresses gradually. In others, it progresses intermittently, remaining stationary for years or decades between periods of worsening. The typical clinical findings consist of selectively severe involvement of cervical, scapular, and finger extensor muscles; mild-to-moderate ptosis and limitation of ocular movements with only occasional diplopia; and variable involvement of masticatory, facial, and other upper extremity, respiratory, and trunk muscles. In some patients the lower limbs are spared or are less severely affected than the upper ones. The

clinically affected muscles are weak and atrophic and fatigue abnormally. The weakness and fatigability can fluctuate, but not as rapidly as in acquired autoimmune myasthenia gravis. The deep tendon reflexes are usually normal, but can be reduced in severely affected limbs. The edrophonium test is negative or gives ambiguous results.

Anticholinesterase drugs are either ineffective or provide only slight subjective improvement. The serum creatine kinase level is normal. Tests for circulating antibodies against the acetylcholine receptor are negative.

Differential diagnoses include **Diplegia, congenital facial,** peripheral neuropathy, radial nerve palsy, motor neuron disease, **Syringomyelia, Kearns-Sayre disease, Muscular dystrophy, limb-girdle, Muscular dystrophy, facio-scapulo-humeral,** and **Myotonic dystrophy.** After careful assessment of the clinical and EMG features, each of the above entities can be excluded. Light microscopic muscle biopsy findings may suggest a primary myopathy or neuropathy. However, the concentration of vacuoles and tubular aggregates near the end-plates should suggest the possibility of neuromuscular transmission defect. Electron microscopic studies reveal structural alterations in postsynaptic regions of end-plates in clinically affected muscles.

Complications: Feeding difficulty from masticatory or pharyngeal muscle weakness; difficulty in holding the head erect; degenerative changes of the cervical spine from abnormal posture; scoliosis and lordosis. Limb muscle weakness makes activities of daily living difficult.

Associated Findings: None known.

Etiology: Autosomal dominant inheritance with variable expression. Sporadic cases, possibly from new mutations, can also occur.

Pathogenesis: Current theory postulates abnormally slow closure (and hence prolonged opening) of the acetylcholine receptor ion channel at the motor end-plate. This results in an abnormal influx of cations, including calcium, into the junctional folds and into the nearby muscle fiber regions. Degeneration of the junctional folds results in acetylcholine receptor loss and a defect in neuromuscular transmission. Degeneration of the muscle fibers results in a permanent myopathy.

MIM No.:   25420

Sex Ratio: M1:F1

Occurrence: Eight cases have been reported in the literature. Encountered much less frequently than acquired autoimmune myasthenic disorders, such as myasthenia gravis or the Lambert-Eaton myasthenic syndrome.

Risk of Recurrence for Patient's Sib:
See Part I, *Mendelian Inheritance.*

Risk of Recurrence for Patient's Child:
See Part I, *Mendelian Inheritance.*

Age of Detectability: EMG abnormalities are probably present from birth in all cases. Weakness and abnormal fatigability begin in infancy, childhood, or adulthood.

Gene Mapping and Linkage: Unknown.

Prevention: None known. Genetic counseling indicated.

Treatment: Appropriate orthoses may be helpful depending on disability. Anticholinesterase medications are ineffective.

Prognosis: Life span is probably not affected. Physical handicaps leading to changes in life style occurred in all affected patients observed to date.

Detection of Carrier: Careful EMG studies to detect a repetitive evoked compound muscle action potential evoked by a single nerve stimulus in well rested muscles will identify affected patients even before the onset of abnormal weakness or fatigability.

Support Groups:
New York; Myasthenia Gravis Foundation (MGF)
New York; Muscular Dystrophy Association (MDA)

References:
Engel AG, et al.: A newly recognized congenital myasthenic syndrome attributed to a prolonged open time of the acetylcholine-induced ion channel. Ann Neurol 1982; 11:553–569.
Engel AG: Myasthenic syndromes. In: Engel AG, Banker BQ, eds: Myology. New York: McGraw-Hill, 1986:1955–1990.
Oosterhuis HJGH, et al.: The slow channel syndrome: two new cases. Brain 1987; 110:1161–1179.

EN005   **Andrew G. Engel**

MYASTHENIC SYNDROME, FAMILIAL INFANTILE TYPE   2913

Includes:
Acetylcholine receptor, defect in
Myasthenia gravis, familial infantile
Myasthenia, familial infantile

Excludes:
Lambert-Eaton myasthenic syndrome
Myasthenia gravis, autoimmune
Myasthenic syndrome, congenital slow channel type (2912)
Myasthenic syndromes, acquired
Myasthenic syndromes, other

Major Diagnostic Criteria: Intermittent myasthenic symptoms from birth associated with crises provoked by stress or fever. A decremental EMG response at 2-Hz stimulation is present only in clinically weak muscles. Weakness can be induced in some, but not all, muscles by exercise or by repetitive indirect stimulation at 10 Hz for a few minutes. The EMG decrement, when present, can be corrected by edrophonium. Tests for antibodies to the acetylcholine receptor are negative. *In vitro* microelectrode studies of neuromuscular transmission demonstrate a normal amplitude of the miniature end-plate potential (MEPP) in rested muscles, but the MEPPs become abnormally small after a 5-minute stimulation at 10 Hz. Ultrastructural studies of the end-plates reveal no abnormalities of the postsynaptic region, and normal amounts of the acetylcholine receptor are present on the junctional folds.

Clinical Findings: The typical history is one of fluctuating ptosis from birth; feeding difficulty during infancy; secondary respiratory infections; easy fatigability on exertion; and episodic crises of increased weakness, hypoventilation, or apnea precipitated by crying, vomiting, or fever. The apnea can cause sudden death during infancy or can lead to anoxic brain injury. Between crises the patients appear unaffected or show minimal weakness of cranial or limb muscles. Weakness can be induced by exercise even between crises. The crises decrease in frequency and the symptoms may improve with age.

Complications: Sudden death or anoxic brain injury from intermittent episodes of apnea are the most serious complications. Secondary respiratory infections can result from respiratory muscle weakness, and the infection and fever can further worsen the defect of neuromuscular transmission. Abnormal fatigability on exertion can make activities of daily living difficult.

Associated Findings: None known.

Etiology: Autosomal recessive inheritance.

Pathogenesis: Current theory postulates a defect in the resynthesis of acetylcholine in the motor nerve terminal or a defect in the packaging of acetylcholine into the synaptic vesicles.

MIM No.: *25421

Sex Ratio: M1:F1

Occurrence: Fewer than 50 cases have been described to date. The disease is encountered much less frequently than acquired autoimmune myasthenic disorders, such as autoimmune myasthenia gravis or the Lambert-Eaton myasthenic syndrome.

Risk of Recurrence for Patient's Sib:
See Part I, *Mendelian Inheritance.*

Risk of Recurrence for Patient's Child:
See Part I, *Mendelian Inheritance.*

Age of Detectability: EMG abnormalities in clinically affected muscles are present from the neonatal period. The symptoms typically present during the neonatal period and occur intermittently thereafter.

Gene Mapping and Linkage: Unknown.

Prevention: None known. Genetic counseling indicated.

Treatment: The muscle weakness, when present, responds well to small or modest doses of anticholinesterase drugs. Some patients are asymptomatic or have only minimal weakness except during crises and require anticholinesterase drugs on an emergency basis only. Parents of affected children must be indoctrinated to anticipate sudden worsening of the weakness and possible apnea with febrile illnesses, excitement, or overexertion. The parents also must be familiar with the use of a hand-assisted ventilatory device and should be able to administer appropriate doses of prostigmine intramuscularly during crises. Patients with a febrile illness and a previous history of crisis should be hospitalized for close observation and ventilatory support as needed.

Prognosis: Guarded because of the possibility of sudden death or anoxic brain damage from episodes of apnea.

Detection of Carrier: Unknown.

Special Considerations: The clinical features of this syndrome have been described in the literature under the rubric of "familial infantile myasthenia." It was recognized as a distinct entity, however, when the autoimmune origin of acquired myasthenia gravis was established and when electrophysiologic and morphologic studies revealed the unique features of this congenital myasthenic syndrome. The differential diagnosis includes autoimmune myasthenia gravis and other congenital myasthenic syndromes. The distinction from autoimmune myasthenia gravis may be difficult if the family history is negative. Although the acetylcholine receptor antibody test is consistently negative in the congenital syndrome, it also can be negative in autoimmune myasthenia gravis, and both disorders respond to anticholinesterase drugs. Careful EMG studies may distinguish between the two entities, but in some patients in vitro studies of neuromuscular transmission and ultrastructural and cytochemical studies of the end-plate are required to clarify the diagnosis.

Support Groups: New York; Myasthenia Gravis Foundation (MGF)

References:
Hart Z, et al.: A congenital, familial, myasthenic syndrome caused by a presynaptic defect of transmitter resynthesis or mobilization. Neurology 1979; 29:556–557.
Robertson WC, et al.: Familial infantile myasthenia. Arch Neurol 1980; 37:117–119.
Engel AG: Myasthenic syndromes. In: Engel AG, Banker BQ, eds: Myology. New York: McGraw-Hill, 1986:1955–1990.
Mora M, et al.: Synaptic vesicle abnormality in familial infantile myasthenia. Neurology 1987; 37:206–214.

EN005   **Andrew G. Engel**

Myoadenylate deaminase deficiency, myopathy due to
See MYOPATHY-METABOLIC, MYOADENYLATE DEAMINASE DEFICIENCY
Myocardial hypertrophy-endocardial fibroelastosis
See VENTRICLE, ENDOCARDIAL FIBROELASTOSIS OF LEFT VENTRICLE
Myoclonic epilepsy, benign
See SEIZURES, MYOCLONIC, JUVENILE JANZ TYPE

MYOCLONIC EPILEPSY-RAGGED RED FIBERS 3225

Includes:
Epilepsy, myoclonic-ragged red fibers
MERRF
Ragged red fibers-myoclonic epilepsy

Excludes:
Dentatorubropallidoluysian degeneration, hereditary (3283)
Kearns-Sayre disease (2070)
Myopathy, mitochondrial-encephalopathy-lactic acidosis-stroke (3224)
Myopathy (other mitochondrial)

Major Diagnostic Criteria: Myoclonus, generalized, or myoclonic seizures; ataxia; and myopathy.

Clinical Findings: Onset of the disease is before age 20 with myoclonus, which is usually the presenting symptom. Cerebellar ataxia, muscle weakness and generalized or myoclonic seizures are the subsequent symptoms. The disease is frequently familial. These patients were originally described as having a combination of "dyssynergia cerebellaris myoclonica" (Ramsay-Hunt syndrome) and mitochondrial myopathy. The individual clinical features of the disease worsen over time for all patients. However, mildly affected patients have not become moderately affected and moderately affected patients have not become severely affected.

Serum lactate and pyruvate may be elevated. Muscle biopsy reveals an excessive number of structurally abnormal mitochondria on electron microscopy, and numerous ragged red fibers on light microscopy. Conventional EEG findings are highly variable, with generalized epileptiform discharges and a background of slow waves. Very high-amplitude visual and somatosensory evoked responses are also reported. Post mortem examination reveals spongy degeneration of the brain.

Complications: Spasticity, hypoventilation.

Associated Findings: Sensorineural hearing loss, vestibular dysfunction.

Etiology: MERRF syndrome is a maternally inherited mitochondrial disease, like **Myopathy, mitochondrial-encephalopathy-lactic acidosis-stroke** and **Myopathy-metabolic, mitochondrial cytochrome C oxidase deficiency**.

Pathogenesis: A mitochondrial enzymatic defect is postulated.

Sex Ratio: M1:F1

Occurrence: Undetermined but presumed rare.

Risk of Recurrence for Patient's Sib: One hundred percent, if the mother is affected.

Risk of Recurrence for Patient's Child: If the mother is affected, 100%. The children of an affected male are not at risk.

Age of Detectability: Usually between 10 and 20 years of age.

Gene Mapping and Linkage: Unknown.

Prevention: None known. Genetic counseling indicated.

Treatment: Symptomatic treatment of seizures and deafness.

Prognosis: Guarded.

Detection of Carrier: Unknown.

References:
Fukuhara N: Myoclonus epilepsy and mitochondrial myopathy. In: Scarlato G, Cerri C, eds: Mitochondrial pathology in muscle diseases. Padova: Piccini Medical Books, 1983:88–110.
Di Mauro S, et al.: Mitochondrial myopathies. Ann Neurol 1985; 17:521–528.

Rosing HS, et al.: Maternally inherited mitochondrial myopathy and myoclonic epilepsy. Ann Neurol 1985; 17:228–237.
Wallace DC, et al.: Familial mitochondrial encephalopathy myoclonic epilepsy and ragged red fibers. Cell 1988; 55:601–610.

10000   **Victor V. Ionasescu**

Myoclonus epilepsy with Lafora bodies progressive
See SEIZURES, PROGRESSIVE MYOCLONIC, LAFORA TYPE
Myoclonus epilepsy, Unverricht-Lundborg type
See SEIZURES, PROGRESSIVE MYOCLONIC, UNVERRICHT-LUNDBORG TYPE
Myoclonus syndrome-cherry red spot
See MUCOLIPIDOSIS I
Myogenic stiff ptosis
See EYELID, PTOSIS, CONGENITAL
Myoglobinuria, idiopathic recurrent
See MYOPATHY-METABOLIC, CARNITINE PALMITYL TRANSFERASE DEFICIENCY
Myopathic ophthalmoplegia externa
See OPHTHALMOPLEGIA, PROGRESSIVE EXTERNAL

MYOPATHIES 1500

Includes:
"Floppy infant"
Muscular dystrophy

The term *myopathy* designates a primary abnormality of muscle in contrast to denervation atrophy in which muscle fiber, lacking innervation, is secondarily affected. Any attempt to understand the many diverse types of myopathies requires that they be classified into several well-defined clinical and pathologic groups.

The *muscular dystrophies* denote a group of inherited progressive degenerations of muscle without known cause. The particular type of dystrophy is determined by the distribution of the weakness and atrophy, age of onset, associated features, and mode of genetic transmission. As a group, the dystrophies demonstrate a constellation of pathologic alterations characteristic of a primary disease of muscle: striking variation in fiber diameter, prominence of centrally placed nuclei, increase in endomysial connective tissue, and degeneration and loss of muscle fibers. More specifically, in the **Muscular dystrophy, childhood pseudohypertrophic / Muscular dystrophy, adult pseudohypertrophic** type of dystrophy, a muscle membrane defect can be detected (Mokri & Engel, 1975).

In *myotonic* dystrophy, centrally placed nuclei, ringbinden, sacroplasmic masses, and often an increased number of intrafusal muscle fibers are characteristic. In **Muscular dystrophy, oculopharyngeal**, rimmed vacuoles can be detected by histochemical and electron microscope techniques. Intranuclear inclusions consisting of tubular filaments that form tangles or palisades can also be observed in muscle fibers (Tomé & Fardeau, 1980).

In contrast to the muscular dystrophies, the *congenital myopathies* are relatively nonprogressive disorders, and possess a number of common characteristics. In most, a clear pattern of inheritance has been defined. Muscular weakness and thinness, the chief clinical manifestations, usually but not always have their onset early in life. Often the clinical presentation is in infancy, with generalized hypotonia and associated weakness (the "floppy infant"). The weakness is symmetric and usually affects the limb-girdle musculature and proximal limb muscles, although in some infants the weakness may be generalized. Certain congenital myopathies are characterized by particular somatic abnormalities, e.g., **Myopathy, myotubular** with ptosis, and **Myopathy, nemaline** with dysmorphic features such as scoliosis, elongated facies, and high-arched palate.

In all congenital myopathies, the deep tendon reflexes are usually decreased or absent. The concentration of serum creatine kinase is usually not elevated, or if it is, the increase is mild in degree. The electromyogram shows short-duration, small-amplitude, polyphasic motor unit potentials. Motor nerve conduction velocities are normal. All of the diseases within this group have distinguishing, but not necessarily specific, morphologic features. Since diagnosis of these disorders cannot be made with confidence on clinical grounds alone, an accurate method of diagnosis is the muscle biopsy and, more specifically, the application of histochemical and electron microscope techniques.

The study of conventional paraffin-embedded material may disclose no alterations or only nonspecific changes. The use of histochemical and ultrastructural methods provides information about the general histologic pattern of the muscle as well as the individual fiber types as defined by their histochemical reactions, distribution, and selective involvement.

The *mitochondrial myopathies* often present as congenital myopathies, but in addition have an often detectable metabolic abnormality. Abnormalities of mitochondrial metabolism are uncommon but are important features of myopathy and of certain diseases that involve systems other than muscle. The mitochondrial myopathies exhibit prominent and selective alterations in the mitochondrial number, activity, and fine structure. The ragged red fibers and intramitochondrial crystalloid inclusions as detected by electron microscopy characterize most of the mitochondrial myopathies.

The *metabolic myopathies* constitute a vast category of muscle diseases characterized by deviations in anabolic and catabolic biochemical reactions. These encompass such groups of disease as the periodic paralyses (see **Paralysis**), disorders of carbohydrate metabolism (see **Glycogenosis**), **Myopathy, malignant hyperthermia**, toxic myopathies, nutritional deficiencies, and diseases associated with myoglobinuria.

The *endocrine myopathies* form a discrete category of muscle disease, the result of the dysfunction of an endocrine gland.

In the *lipid storage myopathies*, abnormal amounts of lipid accumulate in muscle and constitute the predominant pathologic alteration. Triglycerides are abundant in the lipid deposits. The carnitine deficiency syndromes, in which there is insufficient intracellular free carnitine for either transport of long-chain fatty acids into mitochondria, or for modulation of the intramitochondrial coenzyme A/acyl-coenzyme A ratio, are usually included in the lipid myopathy group (Engel, 1986).

References:
Mokri B, Engel AG: Duchenne dystrophy: electron microscopic findings pointing to a basic or early abnormality in the plasma membrane of the muscle fiber. Neurology 1975; 25:1111–1120.
Tomé FMS, Fardeau M: Nuclear inclusions in oculopharyngeal dystrophy. Acta Neuropathol 1980; 49:85–87.
Ionasescu V, Zellweger H: Genetics in neurology. New York: Raven Press, 1983.
Engel AG: Carnitine deficiency syndromes and lipid storage myopathies. In: Engel AG, Banker BQ, eds: Myology. New York: McGraw-Hill, 1986:1663–1696.
Harper PS: The muscular dystrophies. In: Scriver CR, et al, eds: The metabolic basis of inherited disease, 6th ed. New York: McGraw-Hill, 1989:2868–2903. *

BA060   **Betty Q. Banker**

Myopathy (metabolic), lactate transporter defect
 See ERYTHROCYTE, LACTATE TRANSPORTER DEFECT
Myopathy (vacuolar) with glycogen
 See GLYCOGENOSIS, TYPE IIc

MYOPATHY OR CARDIOMYOPATHY DUE TO DESMIN DEFECT   3072

Includes:
 Cardiomyopathy due to desmin defect
 Desmin defect
 Intermediate filament, muscle type
 Myopathy with Mallory body-like inclusions
 Myopathy with sarcoplamic bodies and intermediate
  filaments

Excludes: Myopathy (other)

Major Diagnostic Criteria: Nonspecific clinical symptoms of myopathy with variable localization of weakness and atrophy. Diagnosis is confirmed by morphologic and immunohistologic study of muscle biopsies, which show storage of intermediate filaments containing desmin (DES).

Clinical Findings: This disease is very heterogeneous, with three clinical forms: 1) *Distal myopathy with late onset* starts around age 40 years with weakness of the thenar muscles and the hand flexors. It has a more severe course than **Muscular dystrophy, distal**. 2) *Congenital proximal myopathy* is characterized by weakness of facial, shoulder, and pelvic muscles and kyphoscoliosis. Two of four patients developed pulmonary hypertension and cardiac insufficiency from which they died within one year at ages 11 and 13 years. 3) *Cardiomyopathy* is manifested by complete atrioventricular block requiring implantation of a pacemaker. Concentric and obstructive ventricular hypertrophy are also present.

Laboratory findings include normal or myopathic electromyogram, moderately elevated serum creatine kinase, and abnormal electrocardiogram. Muscle biopsy shows myopathic appearance with considerable variation in fiber diameter, multiple central nuclei, fiber splitting, fibrosis, and stored intermediate filaments. In addition, inclusions composed of granular material and intermediate filaments, rich in DES, can be demonstrated by immunofluorescence studies in all three clinical forms.

Complications: Congestive heart failure.

Associated Findings: None known.

Etiology: Autosomal dominant inheritance in the distal myopathy type. The other two clinical types could follow autosomal recessive inheritance.

Pathogenesis: DES is the muscle-specific subunit of the intermediate filaments. The onset of DES expression during muscle development and the redistribution of DES from free cytoplasmic filaments to the Z disk during the formation of myofibrils suggest a role for this gene in muscle differentiation. Accumulation of DES and lack of contractile activity have been reported in muscular dysgenesis by Tassin et al (1988). An increase of phosphorylated DES (three-fold) and DES isovariants (6 vs 3) have been documented by muscle protein electrophoresis and DES-specific antibodies in four cases with autosomal dominant desmin distal myopathy (Rappaport et al, 1988). Their studies suggest that post-translational events affect, in this condition, both the polymerization and the amount of DES intermediate filaments.

MIM No.: *12566

CDC No.: 756.880

Sex Ratio: M1:F1

Occurrence: Undetermined. One kindred (Goebel et al, 1980) has been extensively studied.

Risk of Recurrence for Patient's Sib:
 See Part I, *Mendelian Inheritance*.

Risk of Recurrence for Patient's Child:
 See Part I, *Mendelian Inheritance*.

Age of Detectability: From birth to age 40 years.

Gene Mapping and Linkage: DES (desmin) has been provisionally mapped to 2.

Prevention: None known. Genetic counseling indicated.

Treatment: Pacemaker implantation is recommended in complete atrioventricular block. Congestive heart failure should be treated by standard procedures.

Prognosis: Variable, depending upon specific symptoms; in particular cardiac involvement can lead to sudden death by acute congestive heart failure (Goebel et al, 1980).

Detection of Carrier: Unknown.

References:
Edstrom L, et al.: A new type of hereditary distal myopathy with characteristic sarcoplasmic bodies and intermediate (skeletin) filaments. J Neurol Sci 1980; 47:171–190.
Goebel HH, et al.: A form of congenital muscular dystrophy. Brain Dev 1980; 2:387–400.
Porte A, et al.: Unusual familial cardiomyopathy with storage of intermediate filaments in the cardiac muscular cells. Virchows Arch [Pathol Anat] 1980; 386:43–58.

Stoeckel ME, et al.: An unusual familial cardiomyopathy characterized by aberrant accumulations of desmin-type intermediate filaments. Virchows Arch [Pathol Anat] 1981; 393:53–60.

Fidzianska A, et al.: Mallory body-like inclusions in a hereditary congenital neuromuscular disease. Muscle Nerve 1983; 6:195–200.

Quax W, et al.: The human desmin and vimentin genes are located on different chromosomes. Gene 1985; 38:189–196.

Rappaport L, et al.: Storage of phosphorylated desmin in a familial myopathy. FEBS Lett 1988; 231:421–425.

Tassin AM, et al.: Unusual organization of desmin intermediate filaments in muscular dysgenesis and tetrodotoxin-treated myotubes. Dev Biol 1988; 129:37–47.

I0000   **Victor V. Ionasescu**

Myopathy with Mallory body-like inclusions
See MYOPATHY OR CARDIOMYOPATHY DUE TO DESMIN DEFECT
Myopathy with sarcoplamic bodies and intermediate filaments
See MYOPATHY OR CARDIOMYOPATHY DUE TO DESMIN DEFECT
Myopathy with storage of glycoproteins and glycosaminoglycans
See MYOPATHY-METABOLIC, GLYCOPROTEIN-GLYCOSAMINOGLYCANS STORAGE TYPE

MYOPATHY, CENTRAL CORE DISEASE TYPE   0134

Includes:
　　Central core disease of muscle (CCD)
　　Muscular central core disease
　　Shy-Magee disease

Excludes:
　　Muscular dystrophy, childhood pseudohypertrophic (0689)
　　Myopathy, myotubular (0695)
　　Myopathy, nemaline (0696)

Major Diagnostic Criteria: Nonprogressive or slowly progressive weakness and hypotonia since birth. Family history is positive. Muscle biopsy has well-demarcated cores within most of the muscle fibers.

Clinical Findings: The onset is noted at or shortly after birth. The patient is floppy, weak, and attains motor milestones slowly. Running and jumping are often impossible. The weakness is diffuse but more prominent in the pelvic muscles. Mild weakness of the face and neck muscles may also be seen. The deep tendon reflexes are normal. Skeletal deformities are not uncommon; hip dislocations and kyphoscoliosis are more frequent. In adult life the patients are often slender and short statured but without any focal muscle atrophy. Serum creatine kinase is not elevated.

Electromyography shows nonspecific findings. The muscle biopsy is strikingly abnormal. The center of most of the fibers contains an area that is unreactive with oxidative enzyme histochemistry. With succinic dehydrogenase and nicotinamide adenine dinucleotide dehydrogenase (NADH), the absence of oxidative enzyme activity in the core contrasts sharply with the normal activity in the surrounding muscle fiber. The lack of activity in the core reflects the absence of mitochondria as proven by electron microscopy. On the "unstructured" cores, the absence of phosphorylase activity correlates with the decrease in glycogen. With the ATPase reaction, the reactivity of the central cores is either decreased or on occasion increased. The term "structured cores" indicates the maintenance of a very precise pattern of cross striation with clear retention of A-, I- and Z-banding. In the "unstructured" cores, the A, I and Z bands can still be traced across the cores, but they are markedly disrupted. The number of cores in the biopsies varies widely, from changes affecting 100% of the fibers to those affecting fewer than 20%. Deeply situated fibers contain more cores than superficial ones. Central cores and type 1 fiber predominance are conjoined in the disease.

Complications: Malignant hyperthermia should always be considered in a patient about to undergo surgery. In vitro muscle contraction studies with caffeine and halothane identify those susceptible to malignant hyperthermia.

Associated Findings: Hip dislocation, kyphoscoliosis and other skeletal malformations.

Etiology: Autosomal dominant inheritance in most cases. Five different sibships in three generations of the original family were affected. There have been reports of sporadic cases as well.

Pathogenesis: There are multiple metabolic deficiencies including oxidative enzymes and phosphorylase within the central cores because of the absence of mitochondria. It is possible that the central core morphologic change may be nonspecific and may occur with other types of myopathy in addition to the specific entity to which the name central core disease can be applied. It has been suggested that core formation may be the result of protein synthesis disturbance in the fetal stage of myogenesis. The similar appearance of central cores and target fibers has given rise to the hypothesis that an abnormality of innervation early in the development of muscle is responsible for central core disease. The relation of central cores to type 1 fiber predominance is still unexplained.

MIM No.: *11700

CDC No.: 756.880

Sex Ratio: M1:F1

Occurrence: Undetermined. Established literature.

Risk of Recurrence for Patient's Sib:
　　See Part I, *Mendelian Inheritance.*

Risk of Recurrence for Patient's Child:
　　See Part I, *Mendelian Inheritance.*

Age of Detectability: Usually within the first year of life.

Gene Mapping and Linkage: Unknown.

Prevention: None known. Genetic counseling indicated.

Treatment: Most patients are so mildly handicapped that no treatment is necessary.

Prognosis: Life expectancy is normal. The disease is non-progressive and is not severely limiting.

Detection of Carrier: Careful clinical muscle evaluation is useful for carrier detection. However, there are documented central core cases by muscle biopsy where the neurologic examinations was normal.

References:
Shy GM, Magee KR: A new congenital non-progressive myopathy. Brain 1956; 79:610–621. *

Ionasescu VV: Miopatie congenite. Prospettive in Pediatria 1975; 5:305–315.

Radu H, et al.: Focal abnormalities in mitochondrial distribution in muscle. Acta Neuropathal (Berl) 1977; 39:25–31.

Frank JP, et al.: Central core disease and malignant hyperthermia syndrome. Ann Neurol 1980; 7:11–17.

Gamstorp I: Non-dystrophic myogenic myopathies with onset in infancy or childhood: a review of some characteristic syndromes. Acta Paediatr Scand 1982; 71:881–886. *

Fidzianska A, et al.: Is central core disease with structural core a fetal defect? J Neurol 1984; 231:212–219.

I0000   **Victor V. Ionasescu**

MYOPATHY, DISPROPORTIONATE FIBER TYPE I   2056

Includes: Fiber-type disproportion myopathy

Excludes:
　　Facio-neuro-skeletal syndrome (2339)
　　Hypotonia, benign congenital
　　Muscular dystrophy (congenital forms)

Major Diagnostic Criteria: The diagnosis can only be made by muscle biopsy using histochemical staining (ATPase reaction) and histographic analysis. Type I fibers are smallest. The largest fibers are Type II. The difference between the mean fiber diameters of the largest and smallest fiber type is always greater than 12% of the value of the mean diameter of the largest fiber type. The variability coefficient (Standard deviation x 1,000 divided by mean fiber diameter) is less than 250 for the largest fibers. Type I fiber predominance is frequently found.

Clinical Findings: Hypotonia and weakness from birth, delayed acquisition of motor milestones (without mental retardation). Hypoflexia or areflexia, highly arched palate, dislocated hips, normal CK, normal or equivocal EMG, normal MNCV.

Complications: Death secondary to respiratory failure/paralysis, kyphoscoliosis.

Associated Findings: Ophthalmoplegia (see **Eye, fibrosis of the extraocular muscles, generalized**).

Etiology: Autosomal recessive inheritance, although sporadic cases have been reported and heterogeneity is likely.

Pathogenesis: Unknown. May be neurogenic.

MIM No.: *25531

CDC No.: 756.880

Sex Ratio: Presumably M1:F1.

Occurrence: Undetermined but presumably rare.

Risk of Recurrence for Patient's Sib: Unknown.

Risk of Recurrence for Patient's Child: Unknown.

Age of Detectability: In infancy, from muscle using the criteria of Dubowitz (1985).

Gene Mapping and Linkage: Unknown.

Prevention: None known. Genetic counseling indicated.

Treatment: Symptomatic, for muscle weakness.

Prognosis: Unknown.

Detection of Carrier: Unknown.

References:
Cavanagh NPC, et al.: Congenital fibre type disproportion myopathy: a histological diagnosis with an uncertain clinical outlook. Arch Dis Child 1979; 54:735–743.
Clancy RR, et al.: Clinical variability in congenital fiber type disproportion. J Neurol Sci 1980; 46:257–266.
Dubowitz V: Muscle biopsy: a practical approach. Philadelphia: W.B. Saunders, 1985:460–462.
Brooke MH: A clinician's view of neuromuscular disease, 2nd ed. Baltimore: Williams and Wilkins, 1986:355–359.
Jaffe M, et al.: Familial congenital fiber type disproportion (CFTD) with an autosomal recessive inheritance. Clin Genet 1988; 33:33–37.

HA015   **Jerome S. Haller**

MYOPATHY, FAMILIAL LYSIS OF TYPE I FIBERS   2059

Includes: Lysis of type I fibers, familial

Excludes: **Myopathy** (others)

Major Diagnostic Criteria: A nonprogressive proximal weakness is present from early infancy. The affected children are slow to pass their motor milestones. Serum creatine kinase may be elevated (2/3). A muscle biopsy, which is essential to establish the diagnosis, and must include histochemical and electron microscopic studies. Nerve conduction studies are normal (1/1). Electromyography may reveal a myopathic pattern (1/2) or may be normal.

Clinical Findings: Affected children are inactive, weak, and hypotonic from birth; they pass their motor milestones very slowly. The weakness is generalized and symmetric and is most marked in the proximal limb muscles. A lumbar lordosis may develop early in life (2/3). The affected muscles are thinned.

Complications: Lumbar lordosis may be observed when the child begins to ambulate.

Associated Findings: The sternocleidomastoid and trapezius muscles may be absent (1/3).

Etiology: Probably autosomal recessive inheritance.

Pathogenesis: The pathologic features of the muscle biopsy specimen are similar in each case (3/3). The diameter of the muscle fibers is either normal or small, and the muscle fibers tend to cluster into these two groups. The cytoplasm of the smaller fibers is divided into a central area containing myofibrils with striations and a peripheral zone that lacks organized contractile substance and appears homogenized. The larger fibers are identified histochemically as type II and the smaller ones as type I. In the involved type I fibers the peripheral zones contain no oxidative enzyme activity, but the myosin ATPase activity is intense. The electron microscopic study of these affected type I fibers demonstrates an absence of myofibrils at the periphery. In such zones, the sarcoplasm consists of a fine granular matrix containing nuclei, scattered mitochondria, and dense granules resembling glycogen. There is an abrupt transition to the more central areas of the muscle fiber where the myofibrils are normal. The structure of the type 2 fibers is normal. It has been postulated that the myofibrils in the peripheral zones of the type I fibers have been lysed.

MIM No.: 25516

CDC No.: 756.880

Sex Ratio: Presumably M1:F1 (M1:F2 observed).

Occurrence: Two reports, covering three cases, have appeared in the literature. In one family, two of six sibs were clinically affected.

Risk of Recurrence for Patient's Sib:
See Part I, *Mendelian Inheritance*. In a family of six sibs, two children (a boy and a girl) were affected. The parents are said to be normal, although there are no descriptions of their examination. The parents have not been subjected to muscle biopsy or to serum creatine kinase testing.

Risk of Recurrence for Patient's Child:
See Part I, *Mendelian Inheritance*.

Age of Detectability: The proximal weakness is discovered when the child begins to ambulate.

Gene Mapping and Linkage: Unknown.

Prevention: None known. Genetic counseling indicated.

Treatment: Prevention of the accentuation of the lordosis.

Prognosis: This disorder appears to be a nonprogressive congenital myopathy.

Detection of Carrier: Unknown.

References:
Cancilla PA, et al.: Familial myopathy with probable lysis of myofibrils in type 1 fibers. Neurology 1971; 21:579–585.
Sahgal V, Sahgal S: A new congenital myopathy: a morphological, cytochemical and histochemical study. Acta Neuropathol 1977; 37:225–230.
Banker BQ: The congenital myopathies In: Engel AG, Banker BQ, eds: Myology. New York: McGraw-Hill, 1986:1570.

BA060   **Betty Q. Banker**

Myopathy, late distal hereditary
  See MUSCULAR DYSTROPHY, DISTAL
Myopathy, lipid storage (one form)
  See OVERGROWTH, RUVALCABA-MYHRE-SMITH TYPE

MYOPATHY, MALIGNANT HYPERTHERMIA   2710

Includes:
  Anesthesia, malignant hyperthermia susceptibility
  Duchenne muscular dystrophy (atypical cases)
  Hyperthermia of anesthesia
  Malignant hyperpyrexia
  Malignant hyperthermia
  Sudden infant death syndrome (SIDS), one theory of

Excludes:
  Hyperthermia associated with hypercalcemia
  Hyperthermia associated with hyperthyroidism
  Hyperthermia associated with polymyositis

Major Diagnostic Criteria: The diagnosis is suspected whenever tachycardia, muscle rigidity, hyperthermia, and metabolic acidosis develop during or after general anesthesia induced by volatile hydrocarbon anesthetics (halothane) and depolarizing muscle relaxants (succinylcholine). Pre-existing neuromuscular disorder and, in particular, a hereditary myopathy are important diagnostic indicators.

Clinical Findings: The characteristic features appear during or shortly after general anesthesia. Masseter spasm may be the only sign; tachycardia (tachyarrythmia), however, is the most common presenting sign and is the forerunner of the forthcoming disaster of hyperthermia, muscle rigidity, and respiratory and metabolic (lactic) acidosis with profound derangement of calcium, potassium, phosphate, and glucose metabolism within the muscle fiber. Rhabdomyolysis with markedly elevated serum creatine kinase (CK) and myoglobin levels and the infrequent disseminated intravascular coagulation are late features. These two features usually indicate a delay in diagnosis and management of the malignant hyperthermia and the preceding myopathy. A history of previous uneventful anesthesia is present in 30% of the patients.

Complications: Cardiac arrest and disseminated intravascular coagulopathy cause the 10% mortality of malignant hyperthermia (down from 70% in the 1970s; early diagnosis and dantrolene therapy are responsible for the reduced mortality).

Associated Findings: Those of the pre-existing myopathy or syndrome. Malignant hyperthermia also occurs more frequently with surgery for ptosis, strabismus, dislocations, and herniorrhaphies. Pre-existing conditions include central core disease of muscle, **Muscular dystrophy, childhood pseudohypertrophic, Kniest dysplasia, King syndrome, Myotonia congenita,** Evans myopathy, and Barnes muscular dystrophy.

Etiology: Usually autosomal dominant inheritance, although cases reflect the heterogeneity of malignant hyperthermia. Families with "isolated" malignant hyperthermia also have demonstrated autosomal dominant inheritance by showing elevated serum CK in several unaffected relatives. **King syndrome** is a sporadic condition, and the sibs with **Noonan syndrome**-like phenotype and contractures imply autosomal recessive inheritance. **Muscular dystrophy, childhood pseudohypertrophic** is an X-linked recessive trait.

Pathogenesis: Malignant hyperthermia is among the best examples of pharmacogenetic disorders. The administration of the anesthetic is necessary for the hypermetabolic state to occur. The skeletal muscle fiber appears to be the site of the primary defect. In addition to the aberrant intracellular calcium metabolism that leads to muscle contractures with catabolic generation of heat, tubular, mitochondrial, and sarcolemmal dysfunctions have also been suggested in some studies; and enhanced activity of phospholipase A has been encountered. The abnormal calcium uptake into the mitochondria leads to uncoupled phosphorylation with a low ATP/ADP ratio. The latter spurs heat production, increases the permeability of the muscle membrane, and diminishes the activity of the calcium pump of the sarcoplasmic reticulum. Extremely stable low-energy myosin-actin complexes (rigor complexes) cause the muscle rigidity.

MIM No.: *14560

POS No.: 4183

CDC No.: 756.880

Sex Ratio: Presumably M1:F1 for the families with "isolated" malignant hyperthermia.

Occurrence: In the United States, accepted incidence figures for malignant hyperthermia are 1:14,000 pediatric anesthesias and 1:40,000 adult anesthesias. These figures may represent underestimates; based on paradoxical increases in masseter tone following succinylcholine administration, the incidence in pediatric anesthesias may be as high as 1:100

Risk of Recurrence for Patient's Sib:
See Part I, *Mendelian Inheritance*. Depends on the etiology of the pre-existing condition; thus, it varies from 0–50%.

Risk of Recurrence for Patient's Child:
See Part I, *Mendelian Inheritance*. Depends on the etiology of the pre-existing condition.

Age of Detectability: Whenever the malignant hyperthermia is encountered. The susceptibility of a particular individual in a family could be determined in advance by *in vitro* testing of the contractibility of skeletal muscle fibers exposed to halothane or caffeine. The testing requires a muscle biopsy and a specialized laboratory, and it is not yet a part of standard medical care.

Gene Mapping and Linkage: Unknown.

Prevention: Determination of malignant hyperthermia susceptibility prior to surgery appears to be the best prevention. CK determinations are the simplest and least reliable testing for malignant hyperthermia susceptibility. *In vitro* muscle fiber response to halothane provides the highest yield (88%). The suggested platelet ATP pool assay appears to be promising, but it requires further testing. Capnography during anesthesia appears to be reliable for the early diagnosis and treatment of malignant hyperthermia. It is based on the early rise of end tidal carbon dioxide in the development of the hyperthermia. According to some reports, oral prophylaxis with dantrolene is an effective preventive measure.

Treatment: Intravenous dantrolene 2.5 mg/kg (mean dose) is life-saving. Intensive symptomatic treatment is also necessary.

Prognosis: The prognosis of malignant hyperthermia has been improved considerably by dantrolene treatment. The mortality rate has been reduced from 70 to 10%. Thus, the long-term prognosis equals that of the underlying pre-existing myopathy or syndrome.

Detection of Carrier: As for the pre-existing conditions. A CT scan of the extremities of patients with **King syndrome** may detect areas of degeneration and fatty infiltration within the muscles.

Special Considerations: The hyperthermia in **Muscular dystrophy, childhood pseudohypertrophic** appears to be somewhat different from the malignant hyperthermia of the other myopathies and syndromes. Bradycardia, instead of tachycardia, is the usual presenting sign, and temperature elevations are rare and small. Rigidity is hardly encountered. Whenever administered, dantrolene did not alter the course of the metabolic catastrophe in these patients. Thus, the anesthetic reactions in this condition may not be a true malignant hyperthermia.

The association of malignant hyperthermia and sudden infant death syndrome (SIDS) is unclear. It is probably not coincidental that five of 15 parents of SIDS victims had muscle membrane dysfunction, despite normal CK levels and muscle electron microscopy. In addition, pathologic findings in the bowel of victims of SIDS have shown similarity to those of heat stroke.

Support Groups: CT; Darien; Malignant Hyperthemia Association of the United States (MHAUS)

References:
Guedel AE: Inhalation anesthesia, ed 2. New York: McMillan, 1951: 110.
Karpati G, Watters GV: Adverse anesthetic reactions in Duchenne dystrophy. In: Angelini C, et al., eds: Muscular dystrophy research: advances and new trends. International Congress Series No. 527. Amsterdam: Excerpta Medica, 1980:206–217.
Denborough MA, et al.: Malignant hyperpyrexia and sudden infant death. Lancet 1982; II:1068–1069.
Ording H, et al.: Investigation of malignant hyperthermia in Denmark and Sweden. Br J Anaesth 1984; 56:1183–1190.
Willner J: Malignant hyperthermia. Pediatr Ann 1984; 13:128–132.
Kousseff BG, Nichols P: A new autosomal recessive syndrome with Noonan-like phenotype, myopathy with congenital contractures and malignant hyperthermia. BD:OAS XXI(2). New York: March of Dimes Birth Defects Foundation, 1985:111–117.
Steenson AJ, Torkelson RD: King's syndrome with malignant hyperthermia: potential outpatient risks. Am J Dis Child 1987; 141:271–273.

K0018   **Boris G. Kousseff**

Myopathy, mitochondrial-cataract
See MYOPATHY-CATARACT-GONADAL DYSGENESIS

MYOPATHY, MITOCHONDRIAL-ENCEPHALOPATHY-LACTIC ACIDOSIS-STROKE
3224

Includes:
Encephalopathy-lactic acidosis-mitochondrial myopathy
Lactic acidosis-mitochondrial myopathy-encephalopathy
MELAS
Strokelike episodes

Excludes:
Brain, spongy degeneration (0115)
Kearns-Sayre disease (2070)
Myoclonic epilepsy-ragged red fibers (3225)
Myopathy (other mitochondrial)

Major Diagnostic Criteria: Patients are usually normal at birth and during the first years of life, then they show stunted growth, episodic vomiting with symptoms of MELAS (seizures, hemiparesis, etc) beginning between ages three and 11 years. Significant cerebellar dysfunction and interictal myoclonus are absent, allowing clinical differential diagnosis from **Myoclonic epilepsy-ragged red fibers.** Heart block, ophthalmoplegia, and retinal pigmentary changes are not found, in contrast to **Kearns-Sayre disease.**

Clinical Findings: Lactate is elevated in the blood and/or cerebrospinal fluid, with values above 4 μm/l. Activities of pyruvate carboxylase and pyruvate dehydrogenase enzyme were reported normal in cultured skin fibroblasts, except in one case (Monnens et al, 1975). Two cases of MELAS syndrome showed NADH-coenzyme Q reductase deficiency (Kobayashi et al, 1987). In all cases, muscle biopsy studies demonstrated ragged red fibers indicative of mitochondrial dysfunction. Computerized axial tomography of the brain revealed low density areas of the cortex and basal ganglia. Post mortem examination showed spongy degeneration of the brain.

Complications: Dementia was reported in many patients.

Associated Findings: Neurosensory hearing loss.

Etiology: The hereditary transmission of MELAS syndrome, as in other primary mitochondrial diseases, is non-Mendelian and based on maternal inheritance. At least two pairs of affected siblings have been reported.

Pathogenesis: It is postulated that MELAS syndrome is related to disturbed energy supply of the brain and muscle caused by a mitochondrial enzyme defect and lactate toxicity. High levels of lactate destroy neurons and cause vessel proliferation or intimal abnormalities of tissues.

CDC No.: 756.880

Sex Ratio: M1:F1

Occurrence: Undetermined but presumed rare.

Risk of Recurrence for Patient's Sib: One hundred percent, if the mother is affected.

Risk of Recurrence for Patient's Child: If the mother is affected, 100%. An affected mother would pass the disease to all her children, but only her daughters would transmit the trait to subsequent generations. The children of an affected male are not at risk.

Age of Detectability: Usually between three and 11 years of age.

Gene Mapping and Linkage: Unknown.

Prevention: None known. Genetic counseling indicated.

Treatment: Symptomatic treatment of seizures, hemiparesis, and deafness.

Prognosis: Guarded.

Detection of Carrier: Unknown.

References:
Monnens L, et al.: A metabolic myopathy associated with chronic lactic acidemia, growth failure and nerve deafness. J Pediatric 1975; 86:983–986.
Pavlakis SG, et al.: Mitochondrial myopathy, encephalopathy, lactic acidosis and strokelike episodes: a distinctive clinical syndrome. Ann Neurol 1984; 16:481–488.
Cohen SR: Why does the brain make lactate? J Theor Biol 1985; 112:429–432.
Di Mauro S, et al.: Mitochondrial myopathies. Ann Neurol 1985; 17:521–528.
Kobayashi M, et al.: Two cases of NADH-coenzyme Q reductase deficiency: relationships to MELAS syndrome. J Pediatr 1987; 110: 223–227.

I0000   **Victor V. Ionassescu**

MYOPATHY, MYOGLOBINURIA-ABNORMAL GLYCOLOSIS, HEREDITARY TYPE
2058

Includes:
Lactic acidosis-myopathy
Myopathy-lactic acidosis

Excludes:
Glycogen storage disease
Lactic acidosis, chronic
Paralysis, hypokalemic periodic (0795)
Paroxysmal myoglobinuria

Major Diagnostic Criteria: Elevated serum lactate and pyruvate with exercise. Muscle biopsy during acute phase shows necrotic fibers and degeneration. In the chronic phase degeneration appears to be complete. No evidence of fatty replacement, increased connective tissue, or glycogen accumulation within muscle fibers.

Clinical Findings: Fatigue, dyspnea, and tachycardia with slight to moderate exercise pain, tenderness, weakness of exercised muscles, hypertrophied calves, nausea, vomiting with complaints beginning in childhood, dark urine present during acute episodes of extreme weakness and severe muscle pain (myoglobinuria).

Complications: Periods of muscle weakness requiring prolonged bed rest for recovery.

Associated Findings: Sideroblastic anemia.

Etiology: Autosomal recessive inheritance.

Pathogenesis: Unknown.

MIM No.: *25515

CDC No.: 756.880

Sex Ratio: Presumably M1:F1.

Occurrence: Fourteen patients from five Swedish families (two with consanguinity) have been described. Two brothers with the same or similar condition have since been reported.

Risk of Recurrence for Patient's Sib:
See Part I, *Mendelian Inheritance.*

Risk of Recurrence for Patient's Child:
See Part I, *Mendelian Inheritance.*

Age of Detectability: Several patients have been identified in their teens.

Gene Mapping and Linkage: Unknown.

Prevention: None known. Genetic counseling indicated.

Treatment: Symptomatic.

Prognosis: Unknown.

Detection of Carrier: Calf hypertrophy has been found in healthy relatives and sibs in 1:5 affected families.

References:
Larsson LE, et al.: Hereditary metabolic myopathy with myoglobinuria due to abnormal glycolysis. J Neurol Neurosurg Psychiat 1964; 27:361–380.
Linderholm H, et al.: Hereditary abnormal muscle metabolism with hyperkinetic circulation during exercise. Acta Med Scand 1969; 185:153–166.
Rawles JM, Weller RO: Familial association of metabolic myopathy, lactic acidosis and sideroblastic anemia. Am J Med 1974; 56:891–897.

HA015   **Jerome S. Haller**

MYOPATHY, MYOTUBULAR 0695

Includes:
Centronuclear myopathy
Myotubular myopathy
Myotubular myopathy, X-linked

Excludes: Myopathy (others)

Major Diagnostic Criteria: Early childhood onset with weakness of extraocular, facial, neck, and limb musculature, and a slow progressive course. Genetic heterogeneity is present; characteristic histopathology consists of predominance of atrophic type I fibers, most of them containing centrally placed nuclei.

Clinical Findings: There are three types of the disease:

Congenital type with an autosomal recessive inheritance is characterized by respiratory distress in the newborn period. Dysmorphic features such as elongated, thin facies and high-arched palate are often present. Ptosis, strabismus, facial weakness, weak crying and sucking, weakness, and atrophy of sternocleidomastoids and of the extremities are the main symptoms. The muscular weakness is diffuse but more severe in a proximal distribution. Speech is often nasal in quality. Talipes equinovarus deformity becomes apparent after the child begins to walk. The deep tendon reflexes are depressed or absent; sensation is entirely normal. In the first 12 years of life, there is usually a slow progression of the weakness and often scoliosis, accentuated lordosis, and winging of the scapulae appear. By adolescence or early adult life, many patients are confined to a wheelchair. Approximately 18% develop seizures which are well controlled by antiepileptic medication.

Congenital X-linked recessive type has similar symptoms to the autosomal recessive phenotype, but is more severe, with high mortality in infancy. Respiratory distress due to weakness of respiratory muscles is usually the main symptom. The affected infants are weak and hypotonic with poor cry, sucking, and coughing; weak neck muscles, and an inability to swallow. Bilateral ptosis, facial diplegia, and limitation of eye movements have been observed in some infants. Deep tendon reflexes are absent but the infant's response to painful stimuli is normal. Maternal polyhydramnios is often noted, and a history of abortions and neonatal death of males is frequent. Cardiomyopathy has also been reported.

Autosomal dominant type has its onset between the first and third decades. The muscular weakness shows limb-girdle distribution with slow progressivity. In addition, the weakness may involve facial musculature, but not ocular or pharyngeal muscles. All patients have increasing difficulty in walking, and are eventually confined to a wheelchair. In some families the disease is manifested only in a mother and daughter.

The diagnosis of centronuclear myopathy types can be made only based on the histologic features of the muscle biopsy. Alterations are present in all muscles. The central position of muscle nuclei, which constitutes the common major feature, can be evaluated by hematoxylin and eosin or Gomori trichrome stain in at least 50% of the muscle fibers. The nuclei are usually surrounded by a clear halo. There are usually two populations of muscle fibers: atrophic type 1 fibers and normal type 2 fibers. Usually the type 1 fibers predominate. The perinuclear halo may lack enzymatic activity and myofibrils. Clusters of mitochondria, lipopigments, glycogen, autophagic vacuoles, rough endoplasmic reticulum, and Golgi complexes are frequently observed in the perinuclear central zone. Post mortem examination of the central and peripheral nervous system in the autosomal recessive and X-linked recessive types showed no abnormalities. Serum creatine kinase level revealed either normal or slightly elevated levels. Electromyographic studies were considered "myopathic" in three reports with brief, small amplitude, polyphasic motor potentials.

Complications: Aspiration pneumonitis, secondary to respiratory distress; congestive heart failure, secondary to cardiomyopathy.

Associated Findings: Epilepsy.

Etiology: Three forms; with autosomal recessive, X-linked recessive, or autosomal dominant inheritance.

Pathogenesis: The primary defect appears to be in the muscle fiber but its nature is unknown.

MIM No.: *16015, 25520, *31040

CDC No.: 756.880

Sex Ratio: M1:F1.5 in autosomal recessive form; M2:F1 in autosomal dominant form, and M1:F0 in X-linked recessive form.

Occurrence: The autosomal recessive form has been described in many parts of the world. In contrast to the other congenital myopathies, there appears to be a higher incidence of involvement of Blacks (seven families reported). The original family of X-linked recessive form described the disorder in five affected males belonging to four sibships connected through females who in two instances showed partial manifestations consistent with carrier state on muscle biopsy. The original pedigree of the autosomal dominant form had sixteen affected members in five generations of a large family. The exact incidence of the disease is not known in any of its three forms.

Risk of Recurrence for Patient's Sib:
See Part I, *Mendelian Inheritance.*

Risk of Recurrence for Patient's Child:
See Part I, *Mendelian Inheritance.*

Age of Detectability: Age one year or less for the autosomal recessive and X-linked recessive form; 10–30 years for the autosomal dominant form.

Gene Mapping and Linkage: MTM1 (myotubular myopathy 1) has been provisionally mapped to Xq27-q28.

Prevention: None known. Genetic counseling indicated.

Treatment: Focused on the respiratory distress syndrome in the autosomal recessive and X-linked recessive forms, with poor results. Antiepileptic medication is used successfully when seizures appear. Supportive treatment with stretching exercises and wheelchair confinement is recommended in the autosomal dominant form.

Prognosis: Very poor in the X-linked recessive form. Most of the patients die in infancy due to the severe weakness of the intercostals and of the diaphragm. the prognosis is fair in the other two forms.

Detection of Carrier: Possible only in the X-linked recessive form by muscle biopsy.

References:

Spiro AJ, et al.: Myotubular myopathy. Arch Neurol 1966; 14:1–14.*
Schochet SS, et al.: Centronuclear myopathy: disease entity or a syndrome? J Neurol Sci 1972; 16:215–228. *
Bruyland M, et al.: Neonatal myotubular myopathy with a probable X-linked inheritance: observations on a new family with a review of the literature. J Neurol 1984; 231:220–222.
Goebel HH, et al.: Centronuclear myopathy with special consideration of the adult form. Eur Neurol 1984; 23:425–434.
Torres CF, et al.: Severe neonatal centronuclear myopathy with autosomal dominant inheritance. Arch Neurol 1985; 42:1011–1014.
Keppen LD, et al.: X-linked myotubular myopathy: intrafamilial variability and normal muscle biopsy in a heterozygous female. Clin Genet 1987; 32:95–99.

I0000   **Victor V. Ionasescu**

MYOPATHY, NEMALINE 0696

Includes:
Nemaline myopathy
Rod body myopathy

Excludes: Myopathy (others)

Major Diagnostic Criteria: Weakness, hypotonia, and dysmorphic features; usually congenital onset and nonprogressive or slowly progressive course. Muscle biopsy with appropriate stains shows nemaline rods.

Clinical Findings: There are three clinical types:
Congenital nonprogressive or slowly progressive myopathy is the

most common type. Clinical signs and symptoms become apparent in infancy and include mild weakness and hypotonia. The weakness is greater in proximal than in distal muscles. Some children have only delayed motor milestones. In others there is involvement of muscles innervated by cranial nerves, particularly the facial and masticatory muscles. The eye muscles are usually spared. The deep tendon reflexes are decreased or absent. The extremities appear slender due to muscle underdevelopment. Dysmorphic features are often present and include elongated face, small jaw, and narrow and highly arched palate. Skeletal malformations, i.e. kyphosis, lordosis, pes cavus, and talipes equinovarus, are sometimes present.

Congenital rapidly fatal myopathy. Infants with this form display severe intercostal and diaphragmatic weakness superimposed on generalized weakness and muscular hypotonia with little spontaneous motor activity. Deep tendon reflexes and Moro response are absent. The infants are often cyanotic and require respiratory assistance. Accumulation of pharyngeal secretions, and feeding difficulties with aspiration, result in frequent bouts of pneumonia and death usually in the first year of life.

Adult onset myopathy is characterized by scapuloperoneal weakness with significant foot-drop. Dysmorphic features are usually absent. Cardiomyopathy has been reported as a prominent feature and may be the cause of sudden death. Otherwise, this form has a slow progression.

Laboratory studies are noncontributory except for muscle biopsy. Only rarely is the serum creatine kinase elevated. Electromyography shows brief duration, small amplitude, and abundant polyphasic motor unit potentials. The muscle biopsy (Bouin or Zenker fixation and phosphotungstic acid hematoxylin staining) shows nemaline rods which measure 1 to 7 μm in length and 0.3 to 3 μm in width. Their distribution is random with a tendency to cluster in subsarcolemmal and paranuclear locations. Most patients also have type 1 fiber predominance (up to 90% of fibers), while type 2 fibers are sparse or absent. There is often type 1 fiber atrophy, particularly in the congenital types. The electron microscopic features consist of the accumulation of nemaline bodies and enlargement and streaming of the Z disks. The rods are contiguous with thin filaments and display periodic lines parallel and perpendicular to their long axis.

Complications: Congestive heart failure secondary to cardiomyopathy, and recurrent pneumonia secondary to weakness of respiratory muscles.

Associated Findings: Mandibular hypoplasia, high-arched palate, kyphoscoliosis, pes cavus, talipes equinovarus.

Etiology: Autosomal dominant inheritance with incomplete penetrance in most cases. The disorder has been well documented in successive generations. The lack of transmission from father to son has been emphasized, and the possibility of an X-linked dominant form has been raised. Autosomal recessive inheritance has been claimed in two families based on the finding that both parents of each index patient had rods, and an increased number of fibers with central nuclei; a presumed heterozygote manifestation.

Pathogenesis: Nemaline rods are thought to originate from the Z disks. Experiments in which electron microscopic studies were combined with biochemical and immunological techniques suggested that a major component of the nemaline rods was alpha-actinin. Desmin, another structural protein of muscle, accumulates at the periphery of the Z disk as well as of nemaline rods. The total amount of muscle alpha-actinin in two patients with congenital nemaline myopathy was increased two-to-three fold. Abnormalities in the light-chain composition of fast myosin, such as absence of LC3F and markedly decreased levels of LC2F and LC1F, were also reported in the muscle of some patients with this illness. There was also evidence of dipeptidyl-peptidase I deficiency, a protease that may participate in post-translational modification of proteins that are to be assembled into Z lines or, alternatively, in the disassembly and degradation of Z-line material.

MIM No.: *16180, *25603

CDC No.: 756.880

Sex Ratio: M1:F>1. The vast majority of patients are female.

Occurrence: Occurs worldwide. The exact incidence and prevalence are not known.

Risk of Recurrence for Patient's Sib:
See Part I, *Mendelian Inheritance.*

Risk of Recurrence for Patient's Child:
See Part I, *Mendelian Inheritance.*

Age of Detectability: Clinically, at early childhood or young adult age.

Gene Mapping and Linkage: Unknown.

Prevention: None known. Genetic counseling indicated.

Treatment: Respiratory assistance in congenital types. Treatment of congestive heart failure in severe cardiomyopathy. Physical therapy using ankle-foot orthosis for the foot-drop.

Prognosis: Guarded for both life span and muscle functions in congenital types. Physical handicaps in adult onset form leading to a change in life style occurs in about 5–10%.

Detection of Carrier: Based on muscle biopsy of the close relatives who are at risk for carrying the gene. The presence of nemaline rods has been described in carriers.

References:
Shy GM, et al.: Nemaline myopathy: a new congenital myopathy. Brain 1963; 86:793–810. *
Afifi AK, et al.: Congenital nonprogressive myopathy: central core

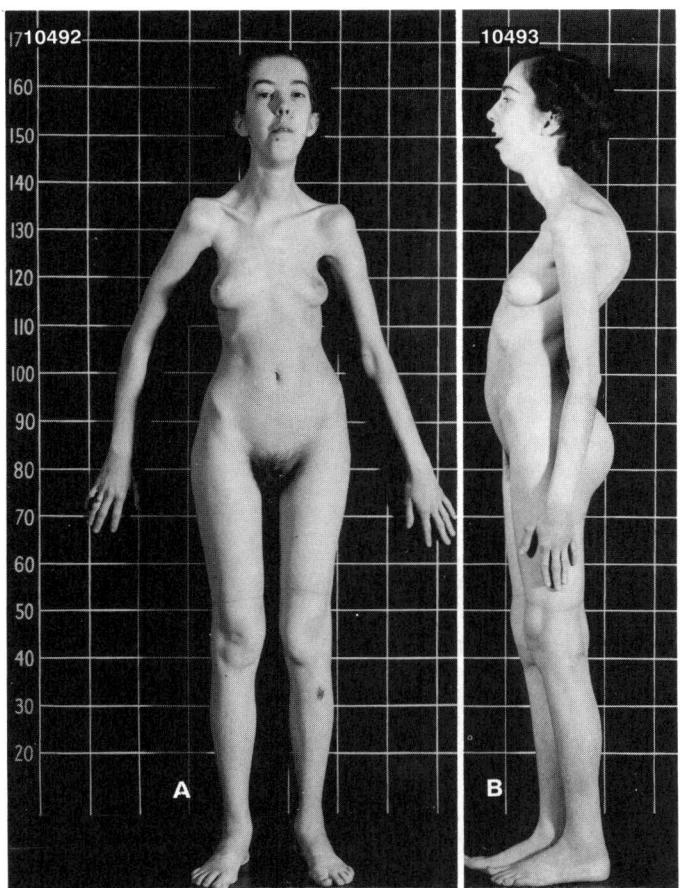

0696-10492: Expressionless facies, muscle loss and extremely narrow thorax. 10493: Marked kyphosis and lordosis.

disease and nemaline myopathy in one family. Neurology 1965; 15:371–381.

Kondo K, Yuasa T: Genetics of congenital nemaline myopathy. Muscle Nerve 1980; 3:308–315. *

Jennekens FGI, et al.: Congenital nemaline myopathy I: defective organization of alpha-actinin is restricted to muscle. Muscle Nerve 1983; 6:61–68.

Meier C, et al.: Nemaline myopathy appearing in adults as cardiomyopathy. Arch Neurol 1984; 41:443–445.

Stauber WT, et al.: Nemaline myopathy: evidence of dipeptidyl peptidase I deficiency. Arch Neurol 1986; 43:39–41.

Schmalbruch H, et al.: Early fetal nemaline myopathy: case report and a review. Dev Med Child Neurol 1987; 29:800–804.

I0000   **Victor V. Ionasescu**

Myopathy, recessive phosphorylase kinase deficiency
See GLYCOGENOSIS, TYPE IXb

MYOPATHY, REDUCING BODY   2062

Includes: Reducing body myopathy

Excludes: Myopathy (other congenital)

Major Diagnostic Criteria: Affected infants have hypotonia and delayed motor milestones but normal intelligence. Progressive weakness involves both proximal and distal muscles. Muscle biopsy reveals characteristic alterations (reducing bodies).

Clinical Findings: Affected infants are weak and hypotonic very early in life. Facial weakness, ptosis, and multijoint contractures may be present. Weakness of the intercostals is severe and results in frequent pneumonias. In some children, death has resulted from pulmonary disease and cardiac failure, but in others the course has been more benign. Five cases have been described thus far. Muscle biopsy material shows distinctive inclusions (intracytoplasmic bodies). These are nonreactive for oxidative enzymes and ATPase, but are able to reduce nitroblue tetrazolium directly when mediated by menandione, hence the suggested name of *reducing body myopathy*. The inclusions are also rich in sulfhydryl groups and contain RNA and glycogen. The electron microscopy is characteristic, the inclusions being round or oval shaped and often in close proximity to a nucleus but separate from it under the sarcolemma. They are composed of closely packed, variably shaped, and moderately basophilic particles measuring 12–16 nm in diameter. The majority of muscle fibers are otherwise normal in structure apart from occasional nonspecific necrotic changes.

The serum CK level was normal in four children and elevated in only one. EMG studies revealed short polyphasic potentials, motor and sensory nerve conduction velocities were normal.

Complications: Pneumonias and congestive heart failure.

Associated Findings: None known.

Etiology: The disorder has been sporadic except for one family in which two sibs were affected. This suggests autosomal recessive inheritance.

Pathogenesis: A partial biochemical characterization of the reducing bodies was done in one patient. Two abnormal proteins of molecular weights of 62,000 and 53,000 were identified. It has been suggested that the reducing bodies have either ribosomal or myofibrillary origin.

CDC No.: 756.880

Sex Ratio: M1:F1

Occurrence: Undetermined but presumed rare.

Risk of Recurrence for Patient's Sib:
See Part I, *Mendelian Inheritance*. Most cases are sporadic.

Risk of Recurrence for Patient's Child:
See Part I, *Mendelian Inheritance*. No affected individuals have reached reproductive age.

Age of Detectability: Within the first four years of age.

Gene Mapping and Linkage: Unknown.

Prevention: None known. Genetic counseling indicated.

Treatment: The complications (pneumonias and congestive heart failure) should be treated.

Prognosis: Guarded.

Detection of Carrier: Unknown.

References:
Brooke MH, Neville HE: Reducing body myopathy. Neurology 1972; 22:829–840.

Dubowitz V, Brooke MH: Muscle biopsy: a modern approach. London: W.B. Saunders, 1973:351 only.

Tome FHS, Fardeau M: Congenital myopathy with "reducing bodies" in muscle fibers. Acta Neuropathol 1975; 31:207–217.

Carpenter S, et al.: New observations in reducing body myopathy. Neurology 1985; 35:207–217.

I0000   **Victor V. Ionasescu**

MYOPATHY, SARCOTUBULAR   2063

Includes: Sarcotubular myopathy

Excludes:
  Muscular dystrophy
  Myopathy (other congenital)

Major Diagnostic Criteria: A nonprogressive proximal weakness is apparent early in life. The electromyogram may be normal (1/2) or may show a myopathic pattern (1/2). Motor and sensory nerve velocities are normal (2/2). Serum creatine kinase may be normal or elevated (1/2). Muscle biopsy is essential to establish the diagnosis. The myopathy is characterized by a structural alteration of the sarcotubular system. This vacuolar change selectively affects the type II muscle fibers.

Clinical Findings: The muscular weakness dates from infancy. Intrauterine movements may be reduced. When the child begins to walk, a proximal weakness is recognized by a waddling gait and difficulty in climbing stairs and rising from a chair. It becomes obvious by the end of the first decade that the child has a symmetric proximal weakness of both upper and lower extremities, with involvement of the flexors of the neck and facial muscles. The muscles of the chest may also be weak and the cough may be feeble. The bulk of the affected muscles is reduced, and the tendon reflexes are hypoactive (1/2). The weakness does not appear to progress.

Complications: Unknown.

Associated Findings: None known.

Etiology: Probably autosomal recessive inheritance, although a sex-linked recessive trait cannot be excluded.

Pathogenesis: When electron cytochemical markers for the transverse tubules and the sarcoplasmic reticulum were applied to biopsied muscle material, the transverse tubules were visualized as displaying a close topographic relationship to the small vacuoles in that they abutted at their periphery or projected into the interior. In addition, the limiting membranes of the vacuoles reacted for sarcoplasmic reticulum-associated ATPase. For these reasons, the disorder is regarded as a segmental vacuolation resulting from the alteration of the sarcotubular system, particularly of the type II muscle fibers.

MIM No.: 26895

CDC No.: 756.880

Sex Ratio: Unknown. Two males have been reported.

Occurrence: Two brothers from an inbred Hutterite colony have been reported.

Risk of Recurrence for Patient's Sib:
See Part I, *Mendelian Inheritance*. Two brothers are affected in a sibship of nine boys and one girl. The parents are Hutterites and are third cousins. Members of two previous generations were not known to have muscle disease.

Risk of Recurrence for Patient's Child:
See Part I, *Mendelian Inheritance*.

Age of Detectability: The proximal weakness can be detected when the child begins to stand and to walk.

Gene Mapping and Linkage: Unknown.

Prevention: None known. Genetic counseling indicated.

Treatment: Avoid excessive exercise and fatigue.

Prognosis: This disorder appears to run a nonprogressive course and to represent a congenital myopathy.

Detection of Carrier: Unknown.

References:
Jerusalem F, et al.: Sarcotubular myopathy: a newly recognized, benign, congenital, familial muscle disease. Neurology 1973; 23:897–906.
Engel AG: Myopathy, sarcotubular In: Myrianthopoulas NC, ed: Handbook of clinical neurology. Neurogenetic directory, Vol 43, Pt 2. Amsterdam: Elsevier/North-Holland, 1982:120–121, 129–130.
Carpenter S, Karpati G: Pathology of skeletal muscle. New York: Churchill Livingstone, 1984:336–342.

BA060 **Betty Q. Banker**

Myopathy, visceral
See INTESTINAL PSEUDO-OBSTRUCTION SYNDROMES

MYOPATHY-CATARACT-GONADAL DYSGENESIS 2052

Includes:
> Cataracts-gonadal dysgenesis-myopathy, familial congenital type
> Gonadal dysgenesis-cataracts-myopathy, familial congenital type
> Muscular dystrophy-cataract-hypogonadism
> Myopathy-cataract-hypogonadism
> Myopathy, mitochondrial-cataract

Excludes:
> **Kearns-Sayre disease** (2070)
> **Myotonic dystrophy** (0702)
> **Myopathy** (others)

Major Diagnostic Criteria: Myopathy, gonadal dysgenesis, and cataracts begin in infancy or early childhood. Electromyogram (EMG), muscle biopsy, gonadotropin, and hormone findings are confirmatory.

Clinical Findings: *Myopathy*: nonprogressive hypotonia, weakness, myopathic facies, and hyporeflexia are present from infancy. Ataxia, myotonia, fasciculations, and spasticity are not found. EMG findings show the pattern of myopathy. Muscle biopsy shows variations in fiber diameter, increased amounts of endomysial connective tissue and no inflammatory cells.
Cataracts appear in early childhood. Ptosis, esotropia, and myopia also occur.
Gonadal dysgenesis: Male and female siblings have been reported by Bassoe (1956), each with hypergonadotropic hypogonadism. The female was 139 cm tall. She had primary amenorrhea, minimal breast development, and scant pubic hair. Her uterus was small and her ovaries fibrous. Gonadotropins were elevated, estrogen decreased. Microscopic examination of the ovaries showed no primary follicles and increased fibrous tissue. The male was 158 cm tall with scant pubic hair, small, soft testes, and a small prostate. Testicular biopsy showed increased hyaline and fibrous tissue, a thick fibrous capsule, clusters of Leydig cells and few Sertoli cells.
IQ appears to be normal.

Complications: Joint contractures, gross motor developmental delay, blindness, short stature, predisposition to respiratory illness.

Associated Findings: Cubitus valgus, short fourth metatarsal, mild osteoporosis.

Etiology: Both autosomal recessive and autosomal dominant inheritance has been suggested.

Pathogenesis: Involvement of skeletal muscle, gonads, lens, and skeletal system suggests a generalized early gestational effect. The biochemical defect is undetermined.

MIM No.: 16055, 25400, 25517

POS No.: 3926

CDC No.: 756.880

Sex Ratio: Presumably M1:F1.

Occurrence: Undetermined but presumed rare. One large kindred has been documented in Norway.

Risk of Recurrence for Patient's Sib:
See Part I, *Mendelian Inheritance.*

Risk of Recurrence for Patient's Child:
See Part I, *Mendelian Inheritance.* Affected individuals appear to be sterile.

Age of Detectability: In infancy.

Gene Mapping and Linkage: Unknown.

Prevention: None known. Genetic counseling indicated.

Treatment: Physical therapy, treatment of respiratory complications, cataract surgery. Replacement of gonadal hormones at age of puberty may be useful in producing secondary sexual characteristics.

Prognosis: Good for survival. Myopathy is apparently not progressive.

Detection of Carrier: Unknown.

Special Considerations: Hereditary myopathy, oligophrenia, cataract, skeletal abnormalities, and hypergonadotropic hypogonadism described in a Swedish family (Lundberg, 1974) differs in that this condition is marked by moderate to severe mental retardation, pyramidal tract involvement, and substantial skeletal deformation and malformation. A myotubular myopathy with cataract (Hawkes and Absolon, 1975) and a familial mitochondrial myopathy with cataract (Pepin et al, 1980) have also been described, and each of these could be distinct entities.

References:
Bassoe HH: Familial congenital muscular dystrophy with gonadal dysgenesis. J Clin Endocrinol 1956; 16:1614–1620.
Lundberg PO: Hereditary myopathy oligophrenia, cataract, skeletal abnormalities, and hypergonadotropic hypogonadism. Eur Neurol 1973; 10:261–280.
Lundberg PO: Hereditary myopathy, oligophrenia, cataract, skeletal abnormalities and hypergonadotropic hypogonadism: a new syndrome. Acta Genet Med Gemellol 1974; 23:245–247.
Hawkes CH, Absolon MJ: Myotubular myopathy associated with cataract and electrical myotonia. J Neurol Neurosurg Psychiatry 1975; 38:761–770.
Pepin B, et al.: Familial mitochondrial myopathy with cataract. J Neurol Sci 1980; 45:191–197.

BA039 **Louis E. Bartoshesky**

Myopathy-cataract-hypogonadism
See MYOPATHY-CATARACT-GONADAL DYSGENESIS
Myopathy-hemolysis
See GLYCOGENOSIS, TYPE VII
Myopathy-lactic acidosis
See MYOPATHY, MYOGLOBINURIA-ABNORMAL GLYCOLOSIS, HEREDITARY TYPE
Myopathy-Marinesco-Sjogren syndrome
See MARINESCO-SJOGREN SYNDROME
Myopathy-metabolic, acid maltase deficiency, infant onset
See GLYCOGENOSIS, TYPE IIa
Myopathy-metabolic, acid maltase deficiency, late onset
See GLYCOGENOSIS, TYPE IIb
Myopathy-metabolic, brancher disease
See GLYCOGENOSIS, TYPE IV

MYOPATHY-METABOLIC, CARNITINE DEFICIENCY, PRIMARY AND SECONDARY   0124

Includes:

Carnitine deficiency, myopathic
Carnitine deficiency, primary
Carnitine deficiency, secondary
Carnitine deficiency, systemic
Muscle carnitine deficiency
Renal reabsorption of carnitine, defect in

Excludes:

Cardiomyopathy (other)
Dicarboxylic aciduria (other)
Lipid myopathy (other)
Mitochondrial myopathies (other)
Myopathy-metabolic, carnitine palmityl transferase deficiency
(0125)
Viscera, fatty metamorphosis (0990)

Major Diagnostic Criteria: Failure to thrive, generalized muscle weakness, hepatomegaly, cardiomyopathy, lowered plasma carnitine levels, lowered muscle carnitine levels, dicarboxylic aciduria, elevated free fatty acids.

Clinical Findings: The clinical picture of L-carnitine deficiency has been evolving since its first description in 1973. Presentation may be primarily myopathic with progressive muscle weakness, myalgias, delayed gross motor development, cardiomyopathy, and biopsy showing lipid myopathy. Systemic signs and symptoms include failure to thrive, recurrent infections, acute Reye-like encephalopathy, and hepatic toxicity with elevated hepatic enzymes, elevated ammonia, hypoglycemia, and lack of ketosis. Dicarboxylic aciduria results from extra mitochondrial oxidation of fats.

Complications: Progressive muscle weakness, cardiomyopathy, hepatic dysfunction, failure to thrive, and hepatic encephalopathy.

Associated Findings: Elevated ammonia, liver enzymes, free fatty acids and dicarboxylic aciduria.

Etiology: Etiology of the deficiency is heterogeneous. The distinction between primary muscle carnitine deficiency with normal plasma, but low muscle carnitine levels and systemic carnitine deficiency where levels are low in both muscle and plasma may be accurate, or may just represent varying severities of the same disorder. Muscle deficiency may be due to an autosomal recessive inherited defect of active transport. The systemic deficiency is usually secondary to another metabolic disorder (liver disease, prolonged parenteral nutrition, poor generalized nutrition or chronic illness). Renal loss secondary to an isolated autosomal recessive renal reabsorption defect of carnitine generalized renal Fanconi syndrome, or increased loss during dialysis can also lead to deficiency. Many inherited organic acidurias result in increase loss of esterified carnitines in the urine.

Pathogenesis: The primary function of L-carnitine is transport of long chain fatty acids across the inner mitochondrial membrane, thus delivering the fatty acids for beta oxidation. There is active transport of L-carnitine into muscle and 98% of the total body L-carnitine is found in muscle. L-carnitine is synthesized from lysine and methionine mainly in the liver and dietary sources include red meats and dairy products. 99% of the L-carnitine loss is via urine and there is active reabsorption of filtered carnitine (>95% filtered). L-carnitine exists in both a free form and an acyl carnitine esterified form. In normal humans, the esters account for 10–20% of the total carnitine measurement in plasma.

Deficiency of L-carnitine results in the failure of delivery of long chain fatty acids for beta oxidation. Since cardiac muscle and skeletal muscle rely heavily on oxidation of fatty acids for energy supply, deficiency of L-carnitine results in muscular weakness, cardiomyopathy and lipid storage.

MIM No.: *21214, *21216
CDC No.: 756.880
Sex Ratio: M>1:F1

Occurrence: Depends on etiology. High with renal Fanconi syndrome, certain organic acidurias, stress states such as illness or starvation, and for infants on total parenteral nutrition. Particular risk is associated with neonates because of poor synthetic capabilities.

Secondary deficiency is more common than once suspected. Certainly highest among pediatric patients presenting with muscle weakness, failure to thrive, hepatic dysfunction, or cardiomyopathy.

Risk of Recurrence for Patient's Sib:
See Part I, *Mendelian Inheritance.*

Risk of Recurrence for Patient's Child:
See Part I, *Mendelian Inheritance.* May be increased in offspring of mothers who are carnitine deficient.

Age of Detectability: Newborn period through maturity.

Gene Mapping and Linkage: Unknown.

Prevention: Supplementation with oral L-carnitine in patients at high risk such as infants on total parenteral nutrition, renal disease states with renal Fanconi syndrome, organic acidurias, or stress states such as pregnancy, chronic illness.

Treatment: Once deficiency occurs, oral L-carnitine therapy at 50–200 mg/kg/day p.o. divided q4-q12h daily. IV L-carnitine also available.

Prognosis: Depends on etiology and treatment. If treated, symptomatic improvement begins shortly after beginning therapy. If primary disease state is under control, complete recovery while being maintained on therapy should be expected. If untreated, progressive muscle weakness, cardiomyopathy and hepatic dysfunction leads to premature death.

Detection of Carrier: Unknown.

References:

Engel AG, Angelini C: Carnitine deficiency of human skeletal muscle with associated lipid storage myopathy: a new syndrome. Science 1973; 179:899.
Cruse RP, et al.: Familial systemic carnitine deficiency. Arch Neurol 1984; 41:301–305.
Engel AG, Rebouche CJ: Carnitine metabolism and inborn errors. J Inherit Metab Dis 1984; 7(Suppl):38–43.
Etzioni A, et al.: Systemic carnitine deficiency exacerbated by a strict vegitarian diet. Arch Dis Child 1984; 59:177–179.
Matsuishi T, et al.: Successful carnitine treatment in two siblings having lipid storage myopathy with hypertrophic cardiomyopathy. Neuropediatrics 1985; 16:6–12.
Treem WR, et al: Primary carnitine deficiency due to a failure of carnitine transport in kidney, muscle, and fibroblasts. New Engl J Med 1988; 319:1331–1336.

WI038   **Susan C. Winter**

MYOPATHY-METABOLIC, CARNITINE PALMITYL TRANSFERASE DEFICIENCY   0125

Includes:

Carnitine palmityl-transferase-A(I) deficiency
Carnitine palmityl-transferase-B(II) deficiency
Hepatic carnitine palmitoyl transferase deficiency (some)
Ibuprofen therapy with carnitine palmityl transferase deficiency
Myoglobinuria, idiopathic recurrent

Excludes:

Myoglobinuria following exertion
Myopathies (other)

Major Diagnostic Criteria: Muscle cramps and myoglobinuria after exercise, fasting, or high fat diets. Hypoglycemia with low plasma ketone bodies. Family history of similar problems. Enzymatic assay of carnitine palmityl transferase A or B deficient in muscle, liver, leukocytes, platelets, lymphoblasts, or fibroblasts.

Clinical Findings: Muscle cramping and myoglobinuria with onset in late childhood or teenage years and being precipitated by strenuous exercise, fasting, or high fat diet. One set of eight-month-old sisters have been described presenting with hypogycemia and lack of ketosis and total absence of this enzyme activity in the liver. Partial deficiency of carnitine palmityl transferase A deficiency has been described with rhabdomyolysis after ibuprofen therapy. This was reported in a 45-year-old woman who developed muscle weakness and tenderness with rhabdomyolsis and respiratory failure after initiation of ibuprofen therapy. Muscle carnitine palmityl transferanse-a deficiency was diagnosed, and persisted after stopping ibuprofen therapy.

Complications: Potential acute renal tubular necrosis secondary to massive myoglobinuria, fibrosis of muscle following repeat attacks, carnitine deficiency.

Associated Findings: On at least two occasions, reduced levels of carnitine acetyl transferase has been found associated with carnitine palmityl transferase deficiency.

Etiology: Probable autosomal recessive inheritance resulting in partial enzyme deficiency or X-linked recessive inheritance.

Pathogenesis: Carnitine palmityl transferase occurs in two isoenzymatic forms. Carnitine palmityl transferase-A is located on the cytosol side of the inner mitochondrial membrane and carnitine palmityl transferase-II is located in the matrix side of the same inner mitochondrial membrane. Deficiency of both enzymes have been described and it is still uncertain as to whether these represent the same or different genetic entities. Evidence points to separate genetic control for these enzymes. There are likely three acyl transferases: a short chain acyl transferase, a C14–16 carnitine palmityl transferase, and a C6–10 octanoyl transferase. **Acyl-CoA dehydrogenase deficiency, short chain type** and **Acyl-CoA dehydrogenase deficiency, medium chain** have been reported.

The carnitine palmityl transferases A and B are involved in transport of C14–16 long chain fatty acyl carnitine esters from the outer surface of the inner mitochondrial membrane to the matrix of the inner mitochondrial membrane. Reduced activity of this enzyme results in reduced palmityl CoA delivered to the inner mitochondrial matrix and this reduced beta oxidation. Therefore, during states which require increased energy production such as fasting or excessive exercise, muscle breakdown and myoglobinuria occurs. In complete absence of the enzyme, hypoglycemia, and lack of ketosis is seen.

MIM No.: *25511, *25512

CDC No.: 756.880

Sex Ratio: M10:F1

Occurrence: Rare, but at least 30 cases reported.

Risk of Recurrence for Patient's Sib:
See Part I, *Mendelian Inheritance.*

Risk of Recurrence for Patient's Child:
See Part I, *Mendelian Inheritance.*

Age of Detectability: Generally early teens to early 20's--as early as infancy. Biochemical measurements could be done shortly after birth and should demonstrate deficiency.

Gene Mapping and Linkage: Unknown.

Prevention: None known. Genetic counseling indicated.

Treatment: High carbohydrate, low fat diet, and avoiding fasting and excessive exercise, and carnitine supplementation.

Prognosis: Unknown.

Detection of Carrier: Enzymatic studies have been done on muscle, liver, fibroblasts, thrombocytes, and leukocytes.

References:

Engel WK, et al.: A skeletal-muscle disorder associated with intermittent symptoms and a possible defect of lipid metabolism. New Engl J Med 1970; 282:697.

DiMauro S, DiMauro PM: Muscle carnitine palmityltransferase deficiency and myoglobinuria. Science 1973; 182:929.

Bougneres PF, et al.: Fasting hypoglycemia resulting from hepatic carnitine palmitoyl transferase deficiency. J Pedaitr 1981; 98:742–746.

Bremer J: Carnitine--metabolism function. Physiol Rev 1983; 63(4).

Coates PM, et al.: Detection of medium-chain acyl CoA dehydrogenase deficiency in leukocytes. Pediatr Res 1983; 17:288A.

Trevisan CP, et al.: Myoglobinuria and carnitine palmityl transferase deficiency: studies with malonyl CoA suggests absence of only CPT. Neurology 1984; 34:3538–3546.

Turnbull DM, et al.: Short-chain acyl-CoA dehydrogenase deficiency associated with a lipid-storage myopathy and secondary carnitine deficiency. New Engl J Med 1985; 311:1232–1236.

Ross NS, Hoppel CL: Partial muscle carnitine palmityltransferase-A deficiency. J Am Med Assoc 1987; 257:62–65.

WI038   **Susan C. Winter**

MYOPATHY-METABOLIC, GLYCOPROTEIN-GLYCOSAMINOGLYCANS STORAGE TYPE   2868

Includes:

Glycoprotein-glycosaminoglycan storage myopathy
Myopathy with storage of glycoproteins and
glycosaminoglycans
Polysaccharide storage cardioskeletal myopathy

Excludes: Glycogen storage myopathies (other)

Major Diagnostic Criteria: Cardioskeletal myopathy with variable onset of weakness and progression. Storage of glycoproteins and glycosaminoglycans can be demonstrated in muscle biopsy and cultured fibroblasts by histochemical and biochemical procedures. Positive family history.

Clinical Findings: Of the five known patients, the first was a women who had slow progressive weakness of the legs manifested at age 21 years and who died at age 31 years with severe involvement of both striated and heart muscle. Eight members of her family, both males and females in two generations, died at an early age from conditions vaguely referred to as pneumonia and heart disease. The most striking histologic abnormality was the infiltration of cardiac and skeletal muscle with a basophilic substance that appeared to be a neutral mucopolysaccharide. The second patient was a 19-year-old man who developed an acute nonobstructive cardiomyopathy with fatal heart failure in one month. His two brothers and sister had died of unidentified heart disease. Chemical analyses of the striated muscle showed low glycogen content and storage of glycosaminoglycans.

The third patient, a 13-year-old male, developed progressive weakness and atrophy of pelvic muscles with enlargement of the calves and diminished deep tendon reflexes. The heart was not affected. Biochemical studies showed accumulation of glycosaminoglycans in both fibrillar structures and intermyofibrillar spaces. The synthesis of glycosaminoglycans was found to be increased. The last two patients (mother and daughter, ages 28 and five years) manifested moderate weakness and atrophy of facial and shoulder muscles with congenital onset and mild progression. The heart was normal. Serum creatine kinase was elevated only in the child. Muscle biopsy material from both patients revealed vacuolar myopathy with storage of granular material. Muscle glycogen values were low-normal, and glycolytic enzymes were normal. Storage of granular material was also identified in fibroblasts that were weakly periodic acid-Schiff-positive, stained metachromatically with toluidine blue, and orthochromatically with alcian blue. Repeated biochemical studies of cultured fibroblasts identified excessive storage of glycoproteins and glycosaminoglycans. The uptake of ^{3}H-glucosamine in cultured fibroblasts was 1.7–3.4 times greater in the patients than in control individuals, while the rate of turnover of the radioisotope was normal.

Complications: Unknown.

Associated Findings: None known.

Etiology: Presumably autosomal dominant inheritance with variability in expression, although the family of patient No. 2 suggested recessive inheritance.

Pathogenesis: Possibly excessive synthesis of glycoproteins and glycosaminoglycans. The specific defect in the synthesis of mucopolysaccharides is undetermined.

MIM No.: 16057

CDC No.: 756.880

Sex Ratio: M1:F1

Occurrence: Five cases have been documented.

Risk of Recurrence for Patient's Sib:
See Part I, *Mendelian Inheritance.*

Risk of Recurrence for Patient's Child:
See Part I, *Mendelian Inheritance.*

Age of Detectability: Between childhood and adulthood.

Gene Mapping and Linkage: Unknown.

Prevention: None known. Genetic counseling indicated.

Treatment: Unknown.

Prognosis: Good, except in cases with cardiomyopathy, which can limit life span.

Detection of Carrier: Unknown.

References:

Holmes JM, et al.: A myopathy presenting in adult life with features suggestive of glycogen storage disease. J Neurol Neurosurg Psychiatry 1960; 23:302–311.

Karpati G, et al.: Peculiar polysaccharide accumulation in muscle in a case of cardioskeletal myopathy. Neurology 1969; 19:553–564.

Radu H, et al.: A new metabolic disorder: myopathy with glycosamino (sialo) glycans accumulation. Eur Neurol 1974; 12:209–225.

Ionasescu VV, et al.: Inherited metabolic myopathy with storage of glycoproteins and glycosaminoglycans. Am J Med Genet 1984; 18:333–343.

I0000   **Victor V. Ionasescu**

MYOPATHY-METABOLIC, MITOCHONDRIAL CYTOCHROME C OXIDASE DEFICIENCY   **2707**

Includes:

Complex IV deficiency of the mitochondrial respiratory chain
Cytochrome c oxidase deficiency
de Toni-Fanconi-Debre syndrome (some cases)
Leigh syndrome (some cases)
Mitochondrial myopathy due to cytochrome c oxidase deficiency

Excludes:

Encephalopathy, necrotizing (0344)
Myopathy (other mitochondrial)

Major Diagnostic Criteria: The most common clinical presentation is severe generalized myopathy, beginning soon after birth and causing respiratory insufficiency, cardiomyopathy, and death before age one year. Lactic acidosis is severe and represents an important diagnostic feature.

Clinical Findings: Clinical phenotypes fall into two main groups, one in which myopathy is the predominant or exclusive manifestation, and another in which brain dysfunction predominates.

Fatal infantile mitochondrial myopathy includes generalized weakness of striated muscles and heart, renal dysfunction (de Toni-Fanconi-Debre syndrome), and lactic acidosis. Only a few patients were overtly weak at birth. In the others, poor cry, difficult sucking and swallowing, and floppiness became apparent after 3–4 weeks of life. Few patients had bilateral ptosis. The respiratory insufficiency related to intercostals and diaphragm weakness required assisted ventilation and caused death before age 4–8 months. In contrast to this dramatic clinical picture, a few patients showed benign infantile mitochondrial myopathy characterized by spontaneous recovery to normal motor function by age two or three years.

Muscle biopsy studies demonstrate ragged-red fibers and ultrastructural alterations of the mitochondria. There is markedly decreased cytochrome c oxidase activity (COX) in crude muscle extracts and histochemically at the level of the ragged-red fibers (Reichmann et al, 1988). Muscle biopsy and serum lactate returned to normal in benign infantile mitochondrial myopathy.

Of the second group of disorders, dominated by involvement of the central nervous system, **Encephalopathy, necrotizing** (Leigh syndrome) is the most common finding. This devastating encephalopathy is characterized clinically by psychomotor retardation, cranial nerve dysfunction, respiratory abnormalities, and seizures. The characteristic neuropathologic alterations are focal, symmetric, necrotic lesions affecting mostly the brainstem. Microscopically, these "spongiform" lesions show demyelination, vascular proliferation, and astrocytosis. Slowly progressive mitochondrial encephalomyopathy characterized by adult onset, weakness and atrophy of limb muscles, sensorineural hearing loss, and complex partial seizures was recently reported in a 52-year-old man. Biochemical studies showed only partial COX deficiency in crude muscle extracts and in isolated mitochondria (44 and 30% of normal, respectively).

Complications: Congestive heart failure and respiratory failure frequently occur in the fatal infantile form.

Associated Findings: Endocrine involvement (hypothyroidism, hypogonadism) was reported by Doriguzzi et al (1989).

Etiology: The hereditary transmission of COX deficiency, as in other primary mitochondrial diseases, is nonmendelian and based on maternal inheritance. The mitochondrion has its own DNA (mtDNA) and its own transcription and translation apparatuses. The mtDNA encodes only about 12 polypeptides, and nuclear DNA controls the synthesis of 90% of all mitochondrial proteins. These include six subunits of complex I of the respiratory chain, the apoprotein of cytochrome b, the three larger subunits of COX (complex IV), and one subunit of ATPase (complex V). In the formation of the zygote, almost all the mitochondria are contributed by the ovum. Therefore, mtDNA is transmitted by maternal inheritance in a "vertical" nonmendelian fashion. In mammalian tissues, COX is composed of 13 different subunits. The complexity of the enzyme structure most likely accounts for the clinical heterogeneity of COX deficiency.

Pathogenesis: The essential properties of the COX enzyme are electron transport and proton translocation. These functions are related to the three larger subunits (I-III), which are encoded by mtDNA. The function of the nuclearly encoded subunits is uncertain, but it has been suggested that they have a regulatory role and confer tissue specificity to COX. The clinical heterogeneity of COX deficiency is accompanied by biochemical heterogeneity. The enzyme defect may be localized to one tissue only (striated muscle) or expand to several other tissues (heart, liver, kidney, brain, fibroblasts). In Leigh syndrome (see **Encephalopathy, necrotizing**), COX deficiency appears to be generalized.

The clinical and biochemical heterogeneity of COX deficiency suggests that different genetic defects are involved. Further studies are needed to determine these defects at the molecular level.

MIM No.: *22011

CDC No.: 756.880

Sex Ratio: M1:F1

Occurrence: Over a dozen cases have been documented in the literature.

Risk of Recurrence for Patient's Sib: 1:1 (100%).

Risk of Recurrence for Patient's Child: If the mother is affected, 100%. An affected mother would pass the disease to all her children, but only her daughters would transmit the trait to subsequent generations. There is no risk of recurrence for the children of an affected male.

Age of Detectability: Varies between infancy (most cases detected at that age) and adulthood. COX deficiency is present in cultured fibroblasts in Leigh syndrome, which may provide a useful tool for prenatal diagnosis.

Gene Mapping and Linkage: Unknown.

Prevention: None known. Genetic counseling indicated.

Treatment: Symptomatic (congestive heart failure and respiratory insufficiency).

Prognosis: Guarded in the severe forms with the total COX deficiency, but good in benign infantile mitochondrial myopathy.

Detection of Carrier: Unknown.

References:
Morgan-Hughes JA, et al.: Mitochondrial encephalomyopathies: biochemical studies in two cases revealing defects in the respiratory chain. Brain 1982; 105:553–582.
Di Mauro S, et al.: Mitochondrial myopathies. Ann Neurol 1985; 17:521–528.
Di Mauro S, et al.: Metabolic myopathies. Am J Med Genet 1986; 25:635–651.
Glerum M, et al.: Abnormal kinetic behavior of cytochrome oxidase in a case of Leigh disease. Am J Hum Genet 1987; 41:584–593.
Zeviani M, et al.: Benign reversible muscle cytochrome c oxidase deficiency: a second case. Neurology 1987; 37:64–67.
Reichmann C, et al.: Enzyme activity measured in single muscle fibers in partial cytochrome c oxidase deficiency. Neurology 1988; 38:244–249.
Doriguzzi C, et al.: Endocrine involvement in mitochondrial encephalomyopathy with partial cytochrome c oxidase deficiency. J Neurol Neurosurg Psychiatry 1989; 52:122–125.

I0000   **Victor V. Ionasescu**

MYOPATHY-METABOLIC, MYOADENYLATE DEAMINASE DEFICIENCY   2709

Includes:
> Muscle adenosine monophosphate (AMP) deaminase deficiency
> Muscle adenylate deaminase deficiency
> Myoadenylate deaminase deficiency, myopathy due to

Excludes: Myopathy-metabolic (other)

Major Diagnostic Criteria: 1) Failure of blood ammonia to increase, despite an adequate lactate increase, on an ischemic forearm exercise test; 2) absence of histoenzymatic staining for adenylate deaminase on a frozen muscle biopsy despite adequate controls; 3) quantitative biochemical assay demonstrating less than 10% normal mean specific activity levels of adenylate deaminase in a properly prepared muscle homogenate.

Clinical Findings: A small proportion of patients manifest infantile hypotonia, which may be marked during the neonatal period, especially in premature infants. The deep tendon reflexes are normal, and the hypotonia regresses gradually and is rarely a problem after childhood. Most patients develop symptoms of exercise intolerance only in adulthood or middle age, with various combinations of muscle cramping and aching, easy fatigue, and slowly progressive weakness that is never incapacitating. About one-third of cases may have an elevated serum creatine kinase level (perhaps 10 times, but not 100 times, the upper normal limit) and sometimes a nonspecifically abnormal EMG. There are no neurologic signs other than muscle weakness and tenderness. Easy fatigue may suggest myasthenia gravis, but the eye muscles are not involved and the fatigue never progresses to paresis. The tenderness and myalgia may suggest polymyositis, while the lack of impressive objective findings may suggest neurasthenia. The enzyme deficiency, unaccompanied by other neuromuscular abnormalities, is not a severe or dangerous disease, and some patients never manifest symptoms.

Complications: Affected patients may have a somewhat increased risk of exercise-induced rhabdomyolysis and malignant hyperthermia susceptibility, but this is still uncertain.

Associated Findings: About one-half of the cases occur in association with other neuromuscular disease, which may be of any type and is then the determining factor in treatment and prognosis. Of this group, about one-half probably represent coincidental association with primary myoadenylate deaminase deficiency, while the other one-half are myoadenylate deaminase heterozygotes whose enzyme level has been depleted to the deficient category secondarily by the associated disease process ("secondary" cases).

Etiology: Autosomal recessive inheritance.

Pathogenesis: During heavy exercise adenylate deaminase within the muscle cell contributes to 1) ameliorating acidosis, 2) maximizing the ATP/ADP ratio, and 3) maintaining adequate levels of Krebs cycle intermediates and carbohydrate fuels. Its absence results in inefficient muscular contraction and metabolism during prolonged heavy exertion.

MIM No.: *25475

CDC No.: 756.880

Sex Ratio: M1:F1

Occurrence: Prevalence in the general population is unknown. In the muscle biopsy population, the frequency of new cases is about 1.0% primary cases plus 0.5% secondary cases. The frequency of carriers is estimated to be 10–15% of muscle biopsies.

Risk of Recurrence for Patient's Sib:
> See Part I, *Mendelian Inheritance.*

Risk of Recurrence for Patient's Child:
> See Part I, *Mendelian Inheritance.* Less than 1:40, assuming carrier incidence in the general population is less than 10%.

Age of Detectability: At any age by surgical or needle muscle biopsy, if frozen properly.

Gene Mapping and Linkage: Unknown.

Prevention: None known. Genetic counseling indicated.

Treatment: The disease is not serious enough to warrant the danger of side effects from long-term analgesic treatment. No drug has been proved to increase muscular performance, although oral ribose has been claimed to benefit a few affected individuals. Counseling the patient to make the necessary psychologic adjustments is probably the most important therapy, along with reassurance.

Prognosis: Normal muscle function and life span are to be expected. In cases with associated neuromuscular disease, the latter will determine the prognosis.

Detection of Carrier: Quantitative biochemical assay of a muscle homogenate can be used to evaluate carrier status. The problem is rendered difficult by 1) variation of enzyme levels from muscle to muscle and within a given muscle by the fiber type distribution encountered, and 2) requirement for specific solution conditions to maintain maximal activity for this enzyme.

Special Considerations: The enzyme level may drop markedly in severe muscle disease of any kind, causing difficulty in separating primary and secondary deficiency states. There is controversy regarding symptomaticity and therapy of both deficient and carrier states.

References:
Fishbein WN, et al.: Myoadenylate deaminase deficiency: a new disease of muscle. Science 1978; 200:545–548.
Fishbein WN, et al.: Levels of adenylate deaminase, adenylate kinase, and creatine kinase in frozen muscle biopsies relative to type 1/type 2 fiber distribution: evidence for a carrier state of myoadenylate deaminase deficiency. Ann Neurol 1984; 15:271–277.
Sabina RL, et al.: Myoadenylate deaminase deficiency: functional and metabolic abnormalities associated with disruption of the purine nucleotide cycle. J Clin Invest 1984; 73:720–730.
Fishbein WN: Myoadenylate deaminase deficiency: inherited and acquired forms. Biochem Med 1985; 33; 158–169. *
Fishbein WN: Myoadenylate deaminase deficiency. In: Engel AG, Banker BQ, eds: Myology, ed 1. New York: McGraw-Hill, 1986: 1745–1762. *
Zöllner N, et al.: Myoadenylate deaminase deficiency: successful symptomatic therapy by high dose oral administration of ribose. Klin Wochenschr 1986; 64:1281–1290.
Sabina RL, et al.: Myoadenylate deaminase deficiency. In: Scriver CR, et al, eds: The metabolic basis of inherited disease, 6th ed. New York: McGraw-Hill, 1989:1077–1084. *

FI028   **William Fishbein**

Myopia (high-grade)-nightblindness
See NIGHTBLINDNESS, CONGENITAL STATIONARY, AUTOSOMAL RECESSIVE

Myopia severe infantile
See MYOPIA, CONGENITAL

MYOPIA, CONGENITAL   0699

Includes:
  Myopia severe infantile
  Myopia

Excludes:
  Retina, amaurosis congenita, Leber type (0043)
  Retinopathy of prematurity (0872)
  Myopia secondary to forceps corneal injury
  Myopia with myelinated nerve fibers and anisometropic amblyopia
  Myopia (in other syndromes)

Major Diagnostic Criteria: Myopia of -5D or more in a child of 6 years of age or less who has a history of assuming nearsighted mannerisms before age 1 year.

Clinical Findings: Myopia at or shortly after birth which persists. A positive family history often alerts the parents to watch for mannerisms of nearsightedness which may be confirmed by retinoscopy after cyclopegia and ophthalmoscopy. The average age at diagnosis is 3 years. Congenital myopia may remain relatively stationary and shows no gender predilection; however, some patients, especially those with a positive family history of myopia, will increase their refractive errors up to -8D. Other patients will show a mild to moderate decrease in their myopia. The average amount of myopia is approximately -8.00 diopters. Visual acuity may be correctable to 20/30 or better; however, typically the visual acuity ranges between 20/50 and 20/60. Not infrequently, strabismus is present also. Fundus changes occur in 50% of cases and include posterior sclerectasia, juxtapapillary choroidal crescents, tilted optic nerve head, tigroid choroidal mottling, pigment thinning, and vitreous syneresis and condensations. Nystagmus is seen in 3–9% of cases.

Complications: Decreased (uncorrected) visual acuity, retinal detachment.

Associated Findings: **Retinopathy of prematurity, Marfan syndrome, Osteogenesis imperfecta, Chromosome 21, trisomy 21, Eye, keratoconus, Arthro-ophthalmopathy, hereditary, progressive, Stickler type, Spondyloepiphyseal dysplasia congenita, Myopathy, malignant hyperthermia,** and other syndromes.

Etiology: Heterogeneity exists; myopia is probably multifactorial. These disorders are usually autosomal dominant, but autosomal recessive inheritance has been argued in cases of consanguineous matings (Karlsson, 1975); at least one X-linked pedigree has been reported (Bartsocas and Kastrantas, 1981).

Pathogenesis: It has been postulated that increased axial length might be related to delayed scleral condensation during embryonic life with resultant stretching of the posterior pole under normal intraocular tension. Contributing factors include corneal curvature and lens structure and position. More recent theories (Kolata, 1985) have drawn on animal models, and it has even been suggested that nearsightedness may be an adaptation to changing environmental demands.

MIM No.: *16070, 25550, 31046

Sex Ratio: M1:F1

Occurrence: High myopia in newborn populations has a prevalence of about 2%.

Risk of Recurrence for Patient's Sib:
  See Part I, *Mendelian Inheritance.*

Risk of Recurrence for Patient's Child:
  See Part I, *Mendelian Inheritance.*

Age of Detectability: Congenital myopia can be detected as early as infancy, usually before age 3, Prevalence of myopia and other reductions in visual acuity tend to increase with age.

Gene Mapping and Linkage: Unknown.

Prevention: None known. Genetic counseling indicated.

Treatment: Correction of refractive error with appropriate lenses, as early as feasible. Avoidance of physically injurious, athletic, or occupational activities is recommended to prevent retinal detachment.

Prognosis: Favorable, since most cases of myopia are stationary. Visually guarded if myopia is progressive or if retinal detachment develops.

Detection of Carrier: Unknown.

References:
Curtin BJ: The pathogenesis of congenital myopia: a study of 66 cases. Arch Ophthalmol 1963;69:166–173.
Hiatt R, et al: Clinical evaluation of congenital myopia. Arch Ophthalmol 1965;74:31–35.
Karlsson JL: Evidence for recessive inheritance of myopia. Clin Genet 1975;7:197–202.
Bartsocas CS, Kastrantas AD: X-linked form of myopia. Hum Hered 1981;31:199–200.
Curtin BJ: The Myopias. Harper and Row, Publishers, Inc. 1985.*
Kolata G: What causes nearsightedness? Science 1985;229:1249–1250.

RA004   **Elsa K. Rahn**

Myopia, unilateral
See EYE, ANISOMETROPIA

Myopia-cataract-saddle nose-hypertelorism-short stature-deafness
See DEAFNESS-MYOPIA-CATARACT-SADDLE NOSE, MARSHALL TYPE

Myopia-cochlear deafness-intellectual impairment
See DEAFNESS-MYOPIA

Myopia-external ophthalmoplegia
See OPHTHALMOPLEGIA EXTERNA-MYOPIA

Myopia-hearing loss
See DEAFNESS-MYOPIA

Myopia-nightblindness, X-linked
See NIGHTBLINDNESS, CONGENITAL STATIONARY, X-LINKED RECESSIVE

Myosclerosis, Lowenthal type
See MUSCULAR DYSTROPHY, CONGENITAL WITH ARTHROGRYPOSIS

MYOSITIS OSSIFICANS PROGRESSIVA   0700

Includes: Fibrodysplasia ossificans progressiva

Excludes: Localized posttraumatic myositis ossificans

Major Diagnostic Criteria: Progressive, widespread ectopic ossification of many muscles, microdactyly (monophalangeal digit) of the great toe and of the thumb, exostoses, broad neck of the femur, abnormal teeth, absence of the two upper incisors, hypogenitalism, baldness of the scalp, absence of lobules of the ears, deafness.

Clinical Findings: Onset in the first decade of life, with firm, warm, and tender subcutaneous masses around the back of the neck and shoulders. Masses progressively shrink and become bony hard in consistency. Muscles of the back, abdominal wall, chest, and extremities are gradually involved. Usually severe restriction of movement of the shoulders and spine occurs by age 10 years. The hips are involved by age 20 years, and most patients are confined to a wheelchair by age 30 years.

Muscle biopsy material shows hemorrhage, inflammation, and proliferation of collagen in the muscle fascia and dermis. New cartilage and bone formation circumscribe and infiltrate the altered tissues, mimicking a fibroma or fibrosarcoma. Eventually columns and plates of bone replace tendons, fascia, ligaments, and muscle.

Complications: Wheelchair confinement occurs in most patients during the advanced stage of the disease.

Associated Findings: Pathologic fractures, absence of the lobules of the ears, and mild mental retardation.

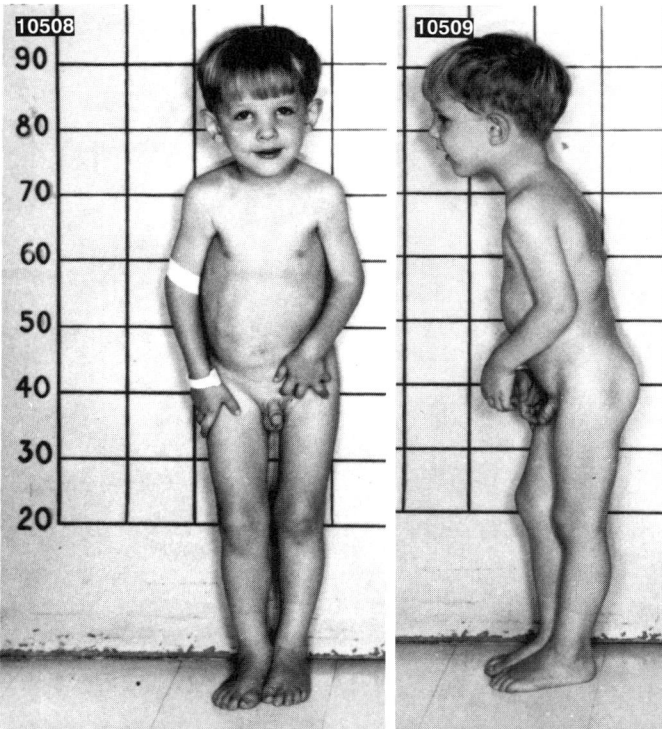

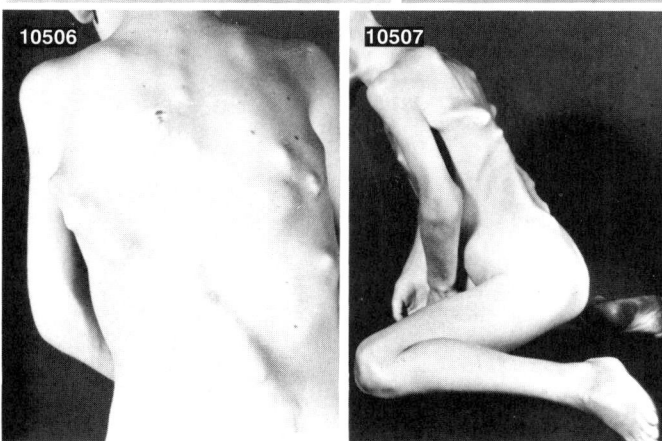

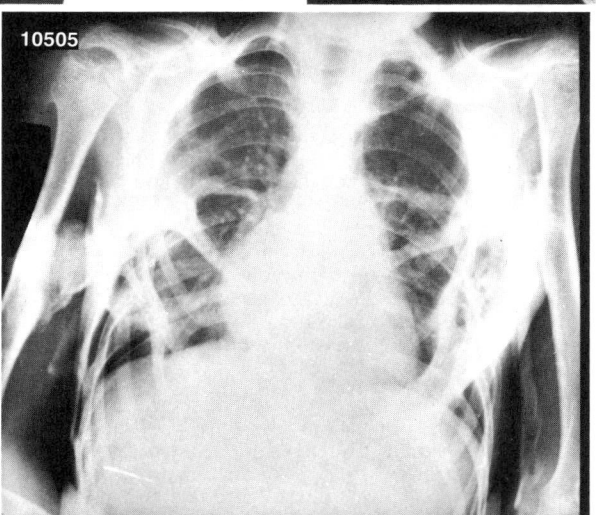

0700-10508–09: Characteristic posture with stiff spine and arms held close to his sides. 10506–07: Bony ridges and nodules are evident along the entire length of the back. 10505: Bony bridges are present between the humerus and the rib cage bilaterally.

Etiology: Autosomal dominant inheritance is postulated based on several instances of parent-to-child transmission, including father-to-son. The disease has complete penetrance but variable expression as shown by some parents who manifest only a skeletal malformation (shortened or monophalangic big toe). Two sets of affected monozygotic twins were reported. Mutation rate is estimated at 1.8 per million gametes per generation. A parental age effect has been noted in sporadic cases.

Pathogenesis: Appears to be excessive proliferation and turn-over of collagen with new bone formation.

MIM No.: *13510

POS No.: 3233

Sex Ratio: M1:F1

Occurrence: Prevalence of 0.61:1,000,000 was found in Great Britain. About 500 cases have been reported in the literature.

Risk of Recurrence for Patient's Sib:
See Part I, *Mendelian Inheritance.*

Risk of Recurrence for Patient's Child:
See Part I, *Mendelian Inheritance.*

Age of Detectability: Usually within the first decade of life.

Gene Mapping and Linkage: Unknown.

Prevention: None known. Genetic counseling indicated.

Treatment: Beneficial effects have been reported in some patients with disodium ethane 1-hydroxy-1, 1-diphosphate (EHDP) in doses of 20 mg/kg of body weight per day. However, progression of the disability in most patients was not influenced by this treatment.

Prognosis: Life span is shortened. The disease is progressive, and severe motor handicap develops after age 30 years. Death occurs around age 40 years.

Detection of Carrier: Unknown.

References:
Bland JH, et al.: Myositis ossificans progressiva. Arch Intern Med 1973; 132:209–212.
Connor JM, Evans DAP: Fibrodysplasia ossificans progressiva: the clinical features and natural history of 34 patients. J Bone Joint Surg 1982; 64B:76–83.
Connor JM, Evans DAP: Genetic aspects of fibrodysplasia ossificans progressiva. J Med Genet 1982; 19:35–39.

I0000   **Victor V. Ionasescu**

Myotonia atrophica
See MYOTONIC DYSTROPHY

MYOTONIA CONGENITA   **0701**

Includes:
　Becker generalized myotonia
　Myotonia, generalized
　Thomsen congenital myotonia

Excludes:
　Chondrodystrophic myotonia
　Myotonic dystrophy (0702)
　Paralysis, hyperkalemic periodic (0794)
　Paramyotonia congenita (0796)

Major Diagnostic Criteria: Dominant congenital myotonia (Thomsen) is characterized by myotonia from infancy and lack of clinical progression. Recessive generalized myotonia (Becker) starts after the age of three years and the clinical course is often progressive.

Clinical Findings: *Dominant congenital myotonia* was described by Thomsen (1876) in his own family. No special muscle groups are involved at first, but later the myotonia produces most symptoms in hands, legs, and eyelids. There is marked variation in severity of myotonia among family members, with males more affected than females. Cold is an aggravating factor, and myotonic symptoms improve after movements of a muscle group. Difficulty with speech, chewing, and swallowing, and transient double vision, are features that result from myotonia of laryngeal, pharyngeal, and ocular muscles. Muscle hypertrophy is frequent, although less marked than in the recessive from. Neurologic evaluation shows normal muscle strength or minimal weakness. Percussion myotonia is obvious, and unlike myotonic dystrophy, it can usually be elicited in many muscle groups as well as in the hands and tongue. A few patients with Thomsen disease, including Thomsen's own son, were considered as malingerers because of their athletic appearance and good muscle strength. One patient was a football player, and his slow, stiff movements related to myotonia were misinterpreted by his coach as "laziness." The patients show no cataracts or any other systemic features of myotonic dystrophy (frontal baldness, diabetes mellitus, testicular atrophy). There is no cardiomyopathy and no smooth muscle involvement.

Recessive generalized myotonia (Becker) is progressive during childhood, beginning in the legs after age three years. Myotonic symptoms may sometimes become severe and mimic rigidity. Muscle hypertrophy can be striking and is more marked than in the dominant form. Neurologic evaluation may detect weakness in addition to myotonia, and this may cause confusion with myotonic dystrophy. Often the nomenclature itself seems confusing. Infants with congenital myotonic dystrophy do not have significant myotonia but have other features such as severe hypotonia and weakness, muscle hypoplasia, and frequent mental retardation. Their mothers are almost always affected.

Electrical myotonia is not influenced by cold, in contrast to *paramyotonia*, in which the prolonged cold state induces electrical silence, with absence of muscle action potentials. Serum creatine kinase is normal or only slightly elevated. Muscle histology is essentially normal, and mild myopathic changes are reported rarely in the recessive type; e.g. increased internal nuclei and lack of 2B muscle fibers with myosin ATPase staining. Similarly, ultrastructural changes are few with no obvious changes in the transverse tubular system, sarcolemma, or sarcoplasmic reticulum.

Complications: Unknown.

Associated Findings: None known.

Etiology: Thomsen congenital myotonia by autosomal dominant inheritance. The disease occurs over multiple generations, usually without skips, although exceptions were reported. Becker generalized myotonia by autosomal recessive inheritance. This condition is characterized by the occurrence of multiple affected sibs with normal but possibly consanguinous parents. Isolated cases have been reported. This recessive form accounts for two-thirds of all sporadic cases.

Pathogenesis: Electrophysiological studies show a decrease in the number of Cl-1 channels, which accounts for most of the symptoms of myotonia congenita. An additional abnormality of Na^+ channel activation has also been also postulated. Fatty acid composition of muscle phospholipids has been reported in recessive generalized myotonia (Becker, 1977). The arachidonic acid (C20:4), oleic acid (C18:1) and linoleic acid (C18:2) levels were significantly decreased; the eicosadienoic (C20:2) and eicosatrienoic acid (C20:3) levels were significantly increased, thus establishing a distinction from the autosomal dominant form (Thomsen).

MIM No.: *16080, *25570

Sex Ratio: M1:F1

Occurrence: The frequency of dominant myotonic congenita (Thomsen) in the Federal Republic of Germany is about 4.4: 1,000,000. The frequency of recessive generalized myotonia (Becker) in the same country is about 2:1,000,000.

Risk of Recurrence for Patient's Sib:
See Part I, *Mendelian Inheritance.*

Risk of Recurrence for Patient's Child:
See Part I, *Mendelian Inheritance.*

Age of Detectability: Early childhood to adult age, based on clinical and electromyographic signs of myotonia.

Gene Mapping and Linkage: Unknown.

Prevention: None known. Genetic counseling indicated.

Treatment: Unlike patients with myotonic dystrophy, the patients with myotonia congenita suffer the effects of myotonia. Some beneficial effects were obtained with 300 mg quinine sulfate (X 3/day) and diphenylhydantoin (Dilantin) (100 mg X 3/day).

Prognosis: Generally excellent for life in Thomsen disease. The patients with recessive generalized myotonia show normal life expectancy, but mild to moderate weakness of proximal limb muscles, in addition to myotonia.

Detection of Carrier: Possibly by electromyography (myotonic discharges) in some asymptomatic cases.

References:
Becker PE: Myotonia congenita and syndromes associated with myotonia. Topics in human genetics. vol. III. Stuttgart: Georg Thieme, 1977. *
Kuhn E, et al.: The autosomal recessive (Becker) form of myotonia congenita. Muscle Nerve 1979; 2:109–117.
Bryant SH: Physical basis of myotonia. In: Schottland DL, ed: Disorders of the motor unit. New York: John Wiley, 1982:381–389.
Subramony SH, et al.: Distinguishing paramyotonia congenita and myotonia congenita by electromyography. Muscle Nerve 1983; 6:374–379.
Sun SF, Streib EW: Autosomal recessive generalized myotonia. Muscle Nerve 1983; 6:143–148.
Ricker K: Myotonia, paramyotonia and periodic paralysis. In: Struppler A, Weindl A, eds: Electromyography and evoked potentials. New York: Springer Verlag, 1985:239–245.

I0000   **Victor V. Ionasescu**

Myotonia congenita intermittens
  See PARAMYOTONIA CONGENITA
Myotonia, generalized
  See MYOTONIA CONGENITA

MYOTONIC DYSTROPHY   0702

Includes:
    Dystrophia myotonica
    Myotonia atrophica
    Steinert disease

Excludes:
    Chondrodystrophic myotonia
    Muscular dystrophy, distal (0690)
    Myopathy (other)
    Myotonia congenita (0701)
    Paralysis, hyperkalemic periodic (0794)
    Paramyotonia congenita (0796)

Major Diagnostic Criteria: *Late onset myotonic dystrophy*: weakness and atrophy of temporalis, facial, neck, oropharyngeal muscles and distal muscles of the extremities. Percussion and voluntary myotonia, cataracts, cardiac involvement, mental retardation, testicular atrophy, and behavior problems. Electromyography shows myotonic discharges and myopathic alterations. Positive family history with autosomal dominant inheritance.

Congenital myotonic dystrophy: myotonic mother, hydramnios in late pregnancy, reduced fetal movements, bilateral facial weakness, hypotonia, neonatal respiratory distress, feeding difficulties, multiple joint contractures with talipes equinus, and mental retardation.

Clinical Findings: *Late onset myotonic dystrophy*: skeletal muscle involvement consists of a combination of muscular weakness, atrophy, and myotonia. The former two symptoms develop in selected muscle groups, such as facial, oropharyngeal muscles, temporalis, masseter, neck flexors and distal muscles of both upper and lower extremities. Finger muscles (flexors, adductors, and abductors), wrist extensors, as well as foot extensors, are often weak; the latter resulting in foot drop, steppage gait, and Achilles tendon contractures. Deep tendon reflexes are present initially, then diminished and even abolished as the disease

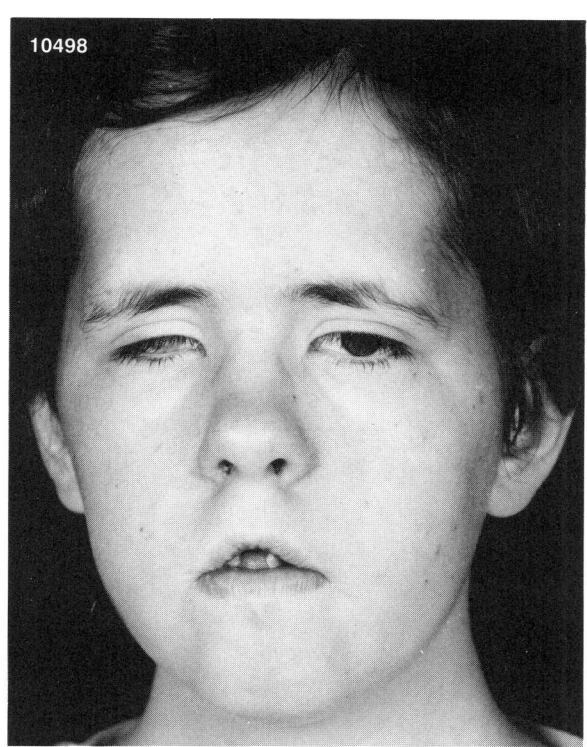

0702-10498: Note expressionless face, ptosis, and corneal opacification OD.

progresses. Deterioration of the condition is insidious, and major incapacitation requiring wheelchair is rarely seen.

Facial diplegia causes a flat and sagging face and, in association with the hollow temples (atrophy of temporalis), a sad and lugubrious expression of the patients. The mouth is frequently kept open, shaped like an inverted V (also called *shark mouth*). Atrophy of the sternocleidomastoid muscles is pronounced; on palpation they often feel like thin, fibrous strands. The neck is thin, the head is bent forward, and kyphosis of the cervical spine may develop. Involvement of the oropharyngeal muscles is recognized by dysphagia and nasal regurgitation. Defective speech (dysarthria) may be a leading symptom and is due to palatal and pharyngeal weakness. Swallowing is altered as well; food particles accumulate and stagnate in the hypopharynx, creating a persistent hazard of food aspiration. Some patients complain of persistent cough and recurrent bronchitis.

Myotonia is usually not as marked as in Thomsen disease (see **Myotonia congenita**). It is limited to some muscles, e.g. hand (thenar muscles) and tongue. Myotonia rarely causes a grave handicap, and most patients interpret it as "stiffness" aggravated by cold. Myotonia is thus a sign that has to be actively sought, and failure to do so is the most common reason for the misdiagnosis of myotonic dystrophy. If a firm grip is followed by the instruction to let go rapidly, this will usually detect active (voluntary) myotonia, while firm percussion of the thenar eminence will show the characteristic delayed relaxation.

Electromyography should always be done. It is valuable when the myotonia is equivocal or absent clinically and the diagnosis is in doubt. The test shows excessive insertional activity and myotonic potentials (discharges). These repetitive potentials wax and wane both in frequency and amplitude and eventually decline, giving a highly distinctive pattern, even more so on auditory recordings ("dive-bomber sound"). Myopathic changes may also be present in the form of short duration, low amplitude, abundant polyphasic potentials.

Muscle biopsy shows central nuclei, often occurring in long chains. Ringed fibers (Ringbinden) are common, being present in at least 70% of biopsies. Ultrastructural studies show sarcoplasmic masses, scattered bundles of myofilaments, free ribosomes and tubular aggregates. Fiber splitting, necrosis, and phagocytosis are less common than in other dystrophies. Histograms demonstrate type 1 fiber atrophy, variation in fiber size, and an enlargement of type 2 muscle fibers. Muscle spindles show an increased number of intrafusal fibers. Serum creatine kinase level is normal or slightly elevated.

Cardiac involvement is common, and present in up to 90% of the patients. Conduction defects (first degree heart block), atrial flutter, other arrhythmias, and mitral valve prolapse are the most frequent cardiac signs. One of our patients with atrial flutter developed cerebral embolism. Cardiomyopathy causing sudden death or congestive heart failure is rare, but can occur at anytime. Postmortem studies of the heart showed atrophy of myocardial fibers, nuclear changes, and replacement of degenerated myofibers by fat and fibrous tissues.

Smooth muscles of various organs, notably upper and lower gastrointestinal tract, gallbladder, and urinary excretory pathways, are affected in some patients with myotonic dystrophy. Achalasia, gastroparesis, constipation, dilatation of the colon with megacolon, gallstones, dysuria, and urinary retention are the clinical syndromes related to smooth muscle pathology.

Lenticular opacities, either iridescent dust or cataracts, are identified by slit-lamp examination in almost every case. The cataracts originate more often in the posterior pole, yet can arise from the anterior pole of the lens as well. It has been proven that apparently unrelated families could be linked by relatives displaying cataracts alone. Other ocular symptoms are ocular hypotonia, ptosis, extraocular weakness, and retinal degenerations (peripheral or macular), with alterations shown on electroretinogram.

Respiratory pathology consists in diaphragmatic and, to a lesser extent, intercostal involvement underlying the chronic alveolar hypoventilation and respiratory distress. Additional respiratory problems include aspiration pneumonia and bronchiectases, while postanesthetic respiratory failure is a serious hazard.

Endocrine disorders include hypogonadism with testicular atrophy due to primary tubular degeneration. Male infertility is a frequent complaint. Overt diabetes is not common even though hyperinsulinism is seen in most patients. Sometimes abnormalities of growth hormone and other pituitary functions may develop. Skin involvement is limited to premature frontal baldness, more pronounced in males than in females. Skeletal abnormalities include cranial hyperostoses, large sinuses, small sella turcica, clubfoot (congenital cases), scoliosis (uncommon), and thin ribs (congenital cases). Severe mental retardation is present in the affected infants. Adults usually show mild mental deterioration. Other signs consistent with central nervous involvement include hypersomnia, which can occur in the absence of detectable respiratory involvement. Some affected individuals were noted to display lack of social responsibility, and they may drop out of work long before physical incapacitation; their social and economic status declines significantly. However, structural changes in the brain are not prominent, even in congenital cases, although CAT scans have shown generalized atrophy and ventricular dilation in some cases.

Congenital myotonic dystrophy: Facial weakness, usually bilateral, is present in over 85% of the cases, and is accompanied by masseter weakness. In older children the immobile facies and open mouth are equally characteristic. Involvement of respiratory muscles is probably the major cause of mortality in affected infants. Hypoplasia of the diaphragm and intercostals was documented histologically, and is responsible for the elevation of the diaphragm and thin ribs. The pulmonary immaturity resulting from reduced intrauterine respiratory action aggravates the respiratory distress caused by primary weakness. Talipes equinus occurs in 50% of the cases and illustrates the selective failure of foot extensors and evertors in utero. A small proportion of patients show other joint contractures, mimicking generalized arthrogryposis. Hypotonia is present in most affected infants, but may disappear within weeks. Myotonia is usually absent, becoming obvious clinically between ages 3–10 years. Motor delay is present in all cases and often improves strikingly during childhood. They may walk unsupported. Mental retardation appears to be present from birth, is static, and usually moderate in degree; IQ levels less than 40 were not reported.

Other symptoms of congenital myotonic dystrophy are swallowing and speech difficulties related to palatal, pharyngeal, and esophageal involvement, as well as strabismus and colonic dilatation. The in utero muscle involvement is manifested by poor fetal movements and hydramnios, the latter being caused by impaired fetal swallowing.

Complications: Malignant hyperthermia was reported in several patients after general anesthesia; halothane, succinylcholine, and thiopental represent particular risks. It has been suggested that local anesthesia be used whenever feasible, and to withhold general anesthesia whenever possible.

Associated Findings: Hernia, undescended testes, congenital hip dislocation, congenital heart defect, and **Hydrocephaly** have been reported in congenital myotonic dystrophy.

Etiology: Autosomal dominant inheritance. The mutant gene is pleiotropic, its expressivity varies, and its penetrance is not always complete. However, in all cases in which both parents were examined, definite signs of the disease are present in one parent. For this reason the mutation rate has been estimated near zero. The recommendation is to base genetic counseling on a case being transmitted as an autosomal dominant trait, even when it is not possible to verify.

The most remarkable phenomenon in the genetics of myotonic dystrophy is the occurrence of congenital myotonic dystrophy exclusively in the offspring of affected mothers.

Anticipation, i.e., earlier onset in more recent generations, has been described in myotonic dystrophy. Anticipation may be an artifact of ascertainment.

Pathogenesis: Myotonia can be defined electrophysiologically as an abnormal tendency of the muscle membrane to discharge trains of repetitive action potentials in response to a voluntary contraction or to direct electrical or mechanical stimulation. This altered excitability persists following alpha-tubocurarine or nerve block. Three different theories on the pathogenesis of late onset myotonic dystrophy have been proposed:

Circulating myotonic factors based on the demonstration that cholesterol-lowering agents such as diazocholesterol were associated with muscle cramping and electrical evidence of myotonia. These chemical compounds appear to change the permeability of the membrane and to cause a decrease in chloride conductivity. The intracellular Na+ concentration in muscle is also abnormally increased, and this leads to an abnormal Na+ channel function;

Missing neural trophic factors theory claims that the muscle membrane in myotonic dystrophy exhibits some of the changes of denervation. However, the involvement of peripheral nerves is rarely significant, according to recent studies. In addition, the widespread tissue alterations in myotonic dystrophy represents evidence against neural trophic factors. It is hard to accept that cardiac, smooth muscle, bone, endocrine glands, lens, and gammaglobulin abnormalities are secondary effects to impaired neural function.

Primary membrane defect theory relies on experimental and clinical data suggesting that human myotonic disorders represent genetically induced primary alterations in the structure and function of cellular membranes. Studies using endogenous protein kinase have shown a significant decrease in phosphorylation of the protein from the red cells and muscle membrane in myotonic dystrophy. It seems unlikely that an alteration in protein kinase represents the primary defect. It is assumed that the altered phosphorylation is related to an unidentified abnormality of a lipid-lipid or lipid-protein complex present in the structure of membranes. Thus, the primary defect of myotonic dystrophy is still unknown. The cloning of the abnormal gene located on chromosome 19 in the near future will allow in vitro translation of the gene product and clarify the pathogenesis of late onset myotonic dystrophy.

The causative factors underlying congenital myotonic dystrophy remain entirely unknown. In all cases of congenital myotonic dystrophy the mother is the affected parent (adult form). Thus, a maternal factor of some type is necessary for the pathogenesis of the disease. An environmental rather than genetic factor was claimed, but this is not likely. No cases of transient congenital myotonic dystrophy were reported as in congenital myasthenia gravis, and affected infants developed progressive myotonia and muscle weakness, indicating that the myotonic dystrophy gene is necessary; finally, at least 50% of children in sibships appear to be entirely normal.

MIM No.: *16090

POS No.: 3193

Sex Ratio: M1:F1

Occurrence: The incidence of the disease varies from 1.2:1,000,000 in England, to 2.4:1,000,000 in Northern Ireland, and 5:1,000,000 in Switzerland. The latter incidence is probably accurate for most European and American populations. Myotonic dystrophy has proved to be the most common adult muscular dystrophy in most of the populations studied, and no racial group is exempt.

Risk of Recurrence for Patient's Sib:
See Part I, *Mendelian Inheritance.*

Risk of Recurrence for Patient's Child:
See Part I, *Mendelian Inheritance.* A number of studies have shown reduced fertility in both sexes to around 75% of normal, although the data are contradictory.

Age of Detectability: Prenatal diagnosis using linkage with ApoC2 and LDR 152 (D19519) in combination with ultrasonography for hydramnios detection characteristic of congenital form. Clinically, from birth to one year of age for congenital form, 10–20 years of age for the adult form.

Gene Mapping and Linkage: DM (dystrophia myotonia) has been mapped to 19q13.2-q13.3.

Prevention: None known. Genetic counseling indicated.

Treatment: Myotonia is usually mild and does not require antimyotonic drugs. Physical therapy and orthopedic measures are helpful in correcting the equinus and other muscle contractures. Surgical resection of advanced cataracts and an external cardiac pacemaker for patients with atrioventricular blocks are also recommended. Myotonic patients should avoid general anesthesia with halothane and succinylcholine because of the risk of developing malignant hyperthermia.

Prognosis: Good for life span, and activity for many years after clinical onset. Sudden death may occur due to cardiac arrythmias.

Detection of Carrier: Based on clinical evaluation, electromyography, ophthalmologic evaluation (slit-lamp, intraocular pressure, electroretinography), and genetic linkage with ApoC2 and LDR 152 (D19519).

References:

Zellweger H, Ionasescu V: Myotonic dystrophy and its differential diagnosis. Acta Neurol Scand 1973; 49(suppl 55):1–28.

Harper P: Myotonic dystrophy. Philadelphia: W.B. Saunders, 1979. *

Nowak TV, et al.: Gastrointestinal manifestations of muscular dystrophies. Gastroenterology 1982; 82:800–810.

Roses AD: Myotonic muscular dystrophy from clinical description to molecular genetics. Arch Intern Med 1985; 45:1487–1492.

Jamal GA, et al.: Myotonic dystrophy: a reassessment by conventional and more recently introduced neurophysiological techniques. Brain 1986; 109:1279–1296.

Spaans, F, et al.: Myotonic dystrophy associated with hereditary motor and sensory neuropathy. Brain 1986; 109:1149–1168.

Bartlett RJ, et al.: A new probe for the diagnosis of myotonic muscular dystrophy. Science 1987; 235:1648–1650.

I0000   **Victor V. Ionasescu**

Myotonic myopathy-dwarfism-chondrodystrophy-eye/face anomalies
See CHONDRODYSTROPHIC MYOTONIA, SCHWARTZ-JAMPEL TYPE

Myotubular myopathy
See MYOPATHY, MYOTUBULAR

Myotubular myopathy, X-linked
See MYOPATHY, MYOTUBULAR
Myriachit
See JUMPING FRENCHMAN OF MAINE
Mysoline, fetal effects of
See FETAL PRIMIDONE EMBRYOPATHY
Myxedematous endemic cretinism
See CRETINISM, ENDEMIC, AND RELATED DISORDERS

MYXOMA, INTRACARDIAC   2160

Includes:
  Atrial, myxoma
  Biatrial myxoma with atrial septal defect
  Left atrial myxoma
  Left ventricular myxoma
  Right atrial myxoma
  Right ventricular myxoma

Excludes:
  Fibroma
  Nevi-atrial myxoma-myxoid neurofibromas-ephelides (2572)
  Rhabdomyoma
  Sarcoma
  Tumors, other intracardiac

Major Diagnostic Criteria: Echocardiographic, angiocardiographic, or necropsy evidence of myxoma.

Clinical Findings: Congestive heart failure; systolic and or diastolic murmurs; arrhythmias; tachycardia; in presence of infection, febrile episodes and bacteremia; EKG evidence of chamber enlargement and various types of heart block; X-ray evidence of cardiomegaly; echocardiographic evidence of mass lesion; angiocardiographic evidence of intracardiac mass. Undiagnosed patients may have infective endocarditis, embolic phenomena (particularly stroke), and symptoms compatible with rheumatic fever.

Complications: Infective endocarditis, cerebral vascular accidents, and other manifestations of embolism. Prolapse and incompetence of the mitral and pulmonary valves.

Associated Findings: Atrial septal defects, Mitral valve prolapse.

Etiology: Possibly autosomal recessive inheritance. Most cases appear to be sporadic, but familial cases have been reported. These include four siblings whose parents were unaffected, and a mother and all three of her sons. Both autosomal recessive and dominant modes of inheritance have been considered. Multifactorial inheritance cannot be ruled out on the basis of the limited number of familial cases studied so far. An environmental relationship to rheumatic fever, as seen in two families, requires further evaluation.

Pathogenesis: Apparently neoplastic.

MIM No.: *25596

Sex Ratio: M1:F1

Occurrence: Undetermined; about 1:12,000 autopsied cases.

Risk of Recurrence for Patient's Sib:
  See Part I, *Mendelian Inheritance.* Most cases are sporadic.

Risk of Recurrence for Patient's Child:
  See Part I, *Mendelian Inheritance.*

Age of Detectability: Patients become symptomatic in late childhood or in adult life. The lesions could probably be detected earlier by echocardiographic examination of first-degree relatives.

Gene Mapping and Linkage: Unknown.

Prevention: None known. Genetic counseling indicated.

Treatment: Surgical excision. Antibacterial therapy for infective endocarditis.

Prognosis: Guarded. The earlier the intervention, the better the outlook, although recurrences are not uncommon.

Detection of Carrier: Echocardiography for preclinical cases and asymptomatic relatives.

Support Groups: Dallas; American Heart Association

References:
Lortscher RH, et al.: Left atrial myxoma presenting as rheumatic fever. Chest 1974; 66:302–303.
Farah MG: Familial atrial myxoma. Ann Intern Med 1975; 83:358–360. *
Grauer K, Grauer MC: Familial atrial myxoma with bilateral recurrence. Heart Lung 1983; 12:600–602.
Dewald GW, et al.: Chromosomally abnormal clones and nonrandom telomeric translocations in cardiac myxomas. Mayo Clin Proc 1987; 62:558–567.

N0003   **James J. Nora**

Myxoma-adrenocortical dysplasia syndrome
See NEVI-ATRIAL MYXOMA-MYXOID NEUROFIBROMAS-EPHELIDES
Myxomas-spotty pigmentation-endocrine overactivity
See NEVI-ATRIAL MYXOMA-MYXOID NEUROFIBROMAS-EPHELIDES

❖ N ❖

N(5,10) methylenetetrahydrofolate reductase deficiency
See HOMOCYSTINURIA, N(5,10) METHYLENE
TETRAHYDROFOLATE DEFICIENCY TYPE
N-acetyl-alpha-D-glucosaminidase deficiency
See MUCOPOLYSACCHARIDOSIS III
N-acetylglucosamine-1-phosphotransferase deficiency
See MUCOLIPIDOSIS II
N-acetylglucosamine-6-sulfate sulfatase deficiency
See MUCOPOLYSACCHARIDOSIS III

N-ACETYLGLUTAMATE SYNTHETASE DEFICIENCY 3170

Includes:
Hyperammonemia III
AGA deficiency
NAGS deficiency

Excludes:
Carbamoyl phosphate synthetase deficiency (3022)
Hyperornithinemia-hyperammonemia-homocitrullinuria (3169)
Ornithine transcarbamylase deficiency (3023)
Transient hyperammonemia of the newborn

Major Diagnostic Criteria: Elevated levels of ammonium in plasma, decreased plasma citrulline and urinary orotate, normal organic acids, deficient activity of N-acetylglutamate synthetase in liver.

Clinical Findings: Episodes of ataxia, vomiting, lethargy/coma, hyperpnea, hypotonicity associated with hyperammonemia.

Complications: The one surviving patient is mentally retarded.

Associated Findings: None known.

Etiology: Presumably autosomal recessive inheritance.

Pathogenesis: N-acetylglutamate is a known activator of the first enzyme in the urea cycle, carbamylphosphate synthetase (the enzyme deficient in hyperammonemia II). Its formation from glutamate and acetyl CoA is catalyzed in the liver by mitochondrial N-acetylglutamate synthetase. In the absence of N-acetylglutamate, activity of carbamylphosphate synthetase is approximately 5% of normal. Thus, the mechanism of hyperammonemia in this disorder is a secondary deficiency of carbamylphosphate synthetase induced by deficient activity of N-acetylglutamate synthetase.

MIM No.: 23731

Sex Ratio: M1:F1

Occurrence: One affected family has been described in which one infant survived with treatment and two of his sibs died without treatment during the newborn period.

Risk of Recurrence for Patient's Sib:
See Part I, *Mendelian Inheritance.*

Risk of Recurrence for Patient's Child:
See Part I, *Mendelian Inheritance.* The one patient described has not reached reproductive age. The risk is likely to be low.

Age of Detectability: At birth by appropriate assays. However, detection in a previously unaffected family is likely to occur only when the child becomes symptomatic.

Gene Mapping and Linkage: Unknown.

Prevention: None known. Genetic counseling indicated.

Treatment: Nitrogen restriction plus supplements with carbamyl glutamate (a congener of N-acetyl glutamate), arginine, sodium benzoate, and sodium phenylacetate.

Prognosis: Guarded. Affected individuals are at risk for recurrent episodes of hyperammonemia associated with dietary indescretions or intercurrent infections.

Detection of Carrier: Unknown.

References:
Bachmann C, et al: N-acetylglutamate synthetase deficiency: diagnosis, clinical observations and treatment. Adv Exp Med Biol 1981; 153:39–46.

BA066

Mark L. Batshaw

N-acetylneuraminic acid storage disease
See SIALIC ACID STORAGE DISEASE, INFANTILE TYPE
N-acetylneuraminic acid storage disease, infantile (one form)
See SALLA DISEASE
N-acetyltransferase polymorphism
See NEUROPATHY, HERITABLE ISONIAZIDE TYPE (INH)
NADH cytochrome b5 reductase deficiency
See METHEMOGLOBINEMIA, NADH-DEPENDENT DIAPHORASE
DEFICIENCY
Naegeli syndrome
See ECTODERMAL DYSPLASIA, NAEGELI TYPE
Naegeli-Franceschetti-Jadassohn syndrome
See ECTODERMAL DYSPLASIA, NAEGELI TYPE
Nager acrofacial dystosis
See ACROFACIAL DYSOSTOSIS, NAGER TYPE
NAGS deficiency
See N-ACETYLGLUTAMATE SYNTHETASE DEFICIENCY
Nail absent
See NAILS, ANONYCHIA, HEREDITARY
Nail dysgenesis and hypodontia
See HYPODONTIA-NAIL DYSGENESIS
Nail dysplasia-curly hair-ankyloblepharon syndrome
See CHANDS
Nail dystrophy and sensorineural deafness
See DEAFNESS-ONYCHODYSTROPHY
Nail-hair-bone-tooth dysplasia
See TRICHO-DENTO-OSSEOUS SYNDROME

NAIL-PATELLA SYNDROME   0704

Includes:
  Anonychia-onychodystrophy
  Arthroosteoonychodysplasia
  Fong disease
  HOOD (hereditary onycho-osteo-dysplasia)
  Iliac horns
  Onychoosteodysplasia
  Turner-Kieser syndrome

Excludes: Turner syndrome (0977)

Major Diagnostic Criteria: Hypoplastic nails and hypoplastic patella.

Clinical Findings: Dysplasia of the nails, absent or hypoplastic patellae, abnormality of the elbows interfering with supination, pronation or extension, and iliac horns. The nails of both hands and feet may be affected; most frequently those of the index and middle fingers and thumb. Hypoplasia, narrowness, and splitting of the nails are the usual findings. Triangular lunulae, sharp and distally pointed at apex, may be present. The patella may be small, tripartite, polygonal, or absent; lateral dislocation of the patella occurs. Iliac horns are seen, arising from the posterior ilium, and if present are pathognomonic for this entity. There may be webbing of the elbow, preventing full extension. Nephropathy occurs in some 30% of patients and may be either glomerulonephritic or nephrotic in type. Scoliosis occasionally occurs.

Complications: Subluxation of the knee, genu varum, early onset osteoarthritis of the knee. Lateral dislocation of the patella may complicate walking, especially down the stairs. The elbow may subluxate. The nephropathy, although usually benign, may cause death at an early age.

Associated Findings: Deformity of sternum, spina bifida occulta, bilateral first rib hypoplasia, shoulder anomalies, anomalies of pectoralis minor, triceps and biceps, hyperostosis frontalis interna, clinodactyly of fifth finger, partial symphalangism of distal interphalangeal joints, hypothyroidism and goiter, mental retardation, cataracts, microcornea, microphthalmia, calcaneal and valgus foot deformities.

Etiology: Autosomal dominant inheritance with variable expressivity.

Pathogenesis: Electron microscopic studies have shown many collagen fibrils in thickened basement membranes and in mesangial matrix of otherwise normal glomeruli, the presence of which is unrelated to demonstrable symptomatic alterations of renal function.

MIM No.: *16120, 10700

POS No.: 3331

CDC No.: 756.830

Sex Ratio: M1:F1

Occurrence: Undetermined; established literature.

Risk of Recurrence for Patient's Sib:
  See Part I, *Mendelian Inheritance.*

Risk of Recurrence for Patient's Child:
  See Part I, *Mendelian Inheritance.*

Age of Detectability: At birth, on the basis of nail defects.

Gene Mapping and Linkage: NPS1 (nail patella syndrome 1) has been mapped to 9q34.

Prevention: None known. Genetic counseling indicated.

Treatment: Orthopedic treatment for problems arising in the knee or elbow. Patients should be repeatedly assessed for renal abnormalities.

Prognosis: The renal complications have caused death as early as eight years of age. About eight percent of patients died of renal disease.

Detection of Carrier: Unknown.

Special Considerations: *Anonychia-onychodystrophy* (Timerman et al, 1969) shows many of the nail characteristics of this syndrome but without the associated manifestations.

References:
Lucas GL, Opitz JM: The nail-patella syndrome. J Pediatr 1966; 68:273–288. * †
Timerman I, et al.: Dominant anonychia and onychodystrophy. J Med Genet 1969; 6:105–106.
Bennett WM, et al.: The nephropathy of the nail-patella syndrome. Am J Med 1973; 54:304–319 *
Garces MA, et al.: Hereditary onchyo-osteo-dysplasia (HOOD syndrome): report of two cases. Skeletal Radiol 1982; 8:55–58.
Yakish SD, Fu FH: Long term follow-up of the treatment of a family with nail-patella syndrome. J Pediatr Orthop 1983; 3:360–363.
Green ST, Natarajan S: Bilateral first-rib hypoplasia: a new feature of the nail-patella syndrome. Dermatologica 1986; 172:323–325. †

ZA000   **Elaine H. Zackai**

Nails (abnormal)-deafness-retardation-seizures-dermatoglyphics
  See DEAFNESS-ONYCHO-OSTEO-DYSTROPHY-RETARDATION-SEIZURES (DOORS)
Nails (hypoplastic)-neutropenia-onychorrhexis
  See ONYCHO-TRICHODYSPLASIA-NEUTROPENIA
Nails, absence of, congenital
  See NAILS, ANONYCHIA, HEREDITARY

NAILS, ANONYCHIA, HEREDITARY   0066

Includes:
  Anonychia
  Nail absent
  Nails, absence of, congenital
  Onychial dysplasia, hereditary

Excludes:
  Ectrodactyly-anonychia (0065)
  Epidermolysis bullosum, type III (2562)
  Nail-patella syndrome (0704)

Major Diagnostic Criteria: Partial or total absence of nails.

Clinical Findings: Characterized by various abnormalities of finger- or toenails and phalanges including complete absence of nail, rudimentary nail matrix at proximal or lateral edge of nail bed, large pointed lunulae, longitudinal furrowing, and thinning or thickening of nail plate. Usually symmetric. May be present at birth or may develop at a later age. Nail beds are present. X-ray

0704-20776: Nail-patella syndrome; note thin, dysplastic nails and dent on the knee due to the absent patella.

studies occasionally show tapering and spatulation of distal phalanges and shortening of phalanges and metacarpal bones.

Complications: Unknown.

Associated Findings: Dental anomalies, aplasia or hypoplasia of upper lateral incisors, spaced teeth, and lack of some molars have been reported. Lymphedema was present in one case.

Etiology: Both autosomal dominant and autosomal recessive inheritance have been reported.

Pathogenesis: Unknown.

MIM No.: *20680

CDC No.: 757.500

Sex Ratio: Presumably M1:F1

Occurrence: Rare.

Risk of Recurrence for Patient's Sib:
See Part I, *Mendelian Inheritance.*

Risk of Recurrence for Patient's Child:
See Part I, *Mendelian Inheritance.*

Age of Detectability: At birth or later.

Gene Mapping and Linkage: Unknown.

Prevention: None known. Genetic counseling indicated.

Treatment: Unknown.

Prognosis: No impact on life span or intelligence.

Detection of Carrier: Unknown.

References:
Cockayne EA: Abnormalities of the nails. In: Inherited abnormalities of the skin and its appendages. London: Oxford University Press, 1933:265–268.
Littman A, Levin S: Anonychia as a recessive autosomal trait in man. J Invest Dermatol 1964; 42:177–178.
Maisels DO: Anonychia in association with lymphoedema. Br J Plast Surg 1966; 19:37–42.
Hopsu-Hava VK, Jensen CT: Anonychia congenita. Arch Derm 1973; 107:752–753.
Freire-Maia N, Pinheiro M: Recessive anonychia totalis and dominant aplasia (or hypoplasia) of upper lateral incisors in the same kindred. J Med Genet 1979; 16:45–48.

MI038   **Giuseppe Micali**

NAILS, KOILONYCHIA   0559

Includes:
Koilonychia, hereditary
Spoon nails

Excludes: Secondary koilonychia

Major Diagnostic Criteria: Concavity of the fingernails. The toenails are commonly concave in normal children and therefore unimportant unless the fingernails are also involved.

Clinical Findings: Concave nail shape with everted edges and thinning of the nail. The thumb is almost always affected; the toenails are involved in over 50%. Not all the nails are involved in each patient. Occasionally, a wide fissure is seen in the center of the nail in addition to spooning. The trait is rarely associated with monilethrix, palmar hyperkeratosis, steatocystoma multiplex, or **Nail-patella syndrome.**

Complications: Unknown.

Associated Findings: None known.

Etiology: Autosomal dominant inheritance with a high degree of penetrance, and variable expressivity in degree of nail involvement. The great majority of isolated cases of koilonychia are not hereditary, but rather traumatic or secondary to a large number of medical disorders.

Pathogenesis: Unknown.

MIM No.: *14930

CDC No.: 757.520

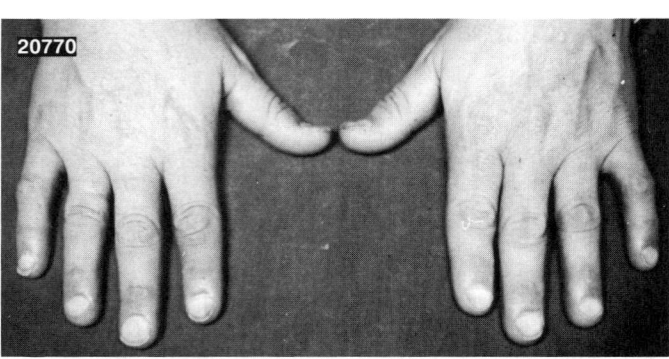

0559-20770: Nails, koilnychia.

Sex Ratio: M1:F1

Occurrence: Six kindreds reported in the literature, including 16 cases over five generations in the family reported by Hellier (1950).

Risk of Recurrence for Patient's Sib:
See Part I, *Mendelian Inheritance.*

Risk of Recurrence for Patient's Child:
See Part I, *Mendelian Inheritance.*

Age of Detectability: At birth or early childhood.

Gene Mapping and Linkage: Unknown.

Prevention: None known. Genetic counseling indicated.

Treatment: Occasionally a deformed toenail that causes discomfort is permanently destroyed surgically.

Prognosis: Normal for life span, intelligence and function.

Detection of Carrier: Unknown.

References:
Hellier FF: Hereditary koilonychia. Br J Dermatol 1950; 62:213–214.
Stone OJ, Maberry JD: Spoon nails and clubbing: review and possible structural mechanisms. Tex State J Med 1965; 61:620–627.
Bergeron JR, Stone OJ: Koilonychia: a report of familial spoon nails. Arch Dermatol 1967; 95:351–353.
Bumpers RD, Bishop ME: Familial koilonychia: a current case history. Arch Derm 1980; 116:845–846.
Stone OJ: Clubbing and koilonychia. Dermatologic Clinics 1985; 3:485–490.

ST030   **Orville J. Stone**

NAILS, LEUKONYCHIA   0589

Includes: Leukonychia totalis

Excludes: Leukonychia, punctate

Major Diagnostic Criteria: White discoloration of the nails.

Clinical Findings: A whitish discoloration of the nails is present, either as a single, broad, or transverse band, one or more narrow bands, a large white area, or a completely white nail. Either the nails of the fingers, toes, or both may be involved. The nails are not brittle or frayed. Nail thickness appears to be average, and no grooves or other irregularities are observed.

Complications: Unknown.

Associated Findings: Reported association with leukotrichia, total alopecia, extensive vitiligo, multiple sebaceous cysts, and renal calculi.

Etiology: Autosomal dominant inheritance.

Pathogenesis: Two major theories propose that the white color is due to opacity of the nail plate. One theory holds that abnormal keratinization of the nail plate is sufficient to cause the opacity, while the other postulates that air must be present within the nail plate.

MIM No.: *15160

CDC No.: 757.530

Sex Ratio: Estimated M1:F1.5

Occurrence: Several kindreds reported in the literature.

Risk of Recurrence for Patient's Sib:
See Part I, *Mendelian Inheritance.*

Risk of Recurrence for Patient's Child:
See Part I, *Mendelian Inheritance.*

Age of Detectability: At birth.

Gene Mapping and Linkage: Unknown.

Prevention: None known. Genetic counseling indicated.

Treatment: Unknown.

Prognosis: Normal life span.

Detection of Carrier: Unknown.

References:
Medansky RS, Fox JM: Hereditary leukonychia totalis. Arch Dermatol 1960; 82:412–414.
Albright SD III, Wheeler CE Jr: Leukonychia: total and partial leukonychia in a single family with a review of the literature. Arch Dermatol 1964; 90:392.
Bushkell LL, Gorlin RJ: Leukonychia totalis, multiple sebaceous cysts, and renal calculi. Arch Derm 1975; 111:899–901.

ME005 **Roland S. Medansky**

NAILS, PACHYONYCHIA CONGENITA   0789

Includes:
Jadassohn-Lewandowsky syndrome
Pachyonychia congenita
Pachyonychia ichthyosiforme
Pachyonychia neonatorum
Polykeratosis congenita

Excludes:
Dyskeratosis congenita (2024)
Onychauxis
Onychogryphosis
Pachyonychia congenita-steatocystoma multiplex (2905)

Major Diagnostic Criteria: Hypertrophy of the nail bed and nail plate, usually involving all 20 digits and associated with other defects. The nails are red to yellow to brown in color and compressed laterally. The diagnosis may be confirmed by a biopsy specimen of the nail unit that reveals epidermal hyperplasia with acanthosis, hyperkeratosis, and focal parakeratosis. There is noted atypical individual cell keratinization of the Malpighian layer cells, which have highly eosinophilic cytoplasm.

Clinical Findings: Nail units are abnormal. These patients have palmar and plantar hyperhidrosis with symmetric focal hyperkeratosis. Follicular hyperkeratosis of the trunk with mildly ichthyosiform skin and hyperpigmentation have occurred. Bullae;

ulcerations; leukokeratosis of the tongue (scalloped) and oral mucous membranes, resembling leukoplakia; and verrucous lesions over the extensor areas as well as buttocks and popliteal fossae have also been reported. Cataracts and corneal dyskeratosis involve the eyes. Steatocystoma multiplex, oral herpes simplex, elevated serum copper and iron, and increased urinary excretion of hexoseamine and hydroxyproline are other associations.

Complications: Unknown.

Associated Findings: Natal and carious teeth with early loss (before age 30 years), other dental anomalies, dry dystrophic alopecia, short stature, mental retardation, epidermolysis bullosa, osteomas, respiratory involvement, and intestinal diverticuli have been reported.

Etiology: Usually autosomal dominant inheritance with incomplete penetrance. An autosomal recessive variant has been reported.

Pathogenesis: Unknown.

MIM No.: *16720, 26013

POS No.: 4181

CDC No.: 757.516

Sex Ratio: Presumably M1:F1.

Occurrence: Several large kindreds have been documented. More frequent among Jewish and Slavic males.

Risk of Recurrence for Patient's Sib:
See Part I, *Mendelian Inheritance.*

Risk of Recurrence for Patient's Child:
See Part I, *Mendelian Inheritance.*

Age of Detectability: Clinically, at about 3–5 months of age, except for natal teeth.

Gene Mapping and Linkage: Unknown.

Prevention: None known. Genetic counseling indicated.

Treatment: Surgical resection of the nail unit with possible matricectomy. Specific and symptomatic therapy for associated defects. Intralesional corticosteroids to the nail unit has been suggested to be a beneficial though inconsistent form of therapy.

Prognosis: Normal life span unless some of the more serious associated defects are present. Patients usually adapt well to the disorder.

Detection of Carrier: Examination of relatives for evidence of the trait.

References:
Chong-Hai T, Rajagopalan K: Pachyonychia congenita with recessive inheritance. Arch Dermatol 1977; 113:685–687.
Zaias N: The nail in health and disease. New York: SP Medical and Scientific Books, 1980.
Franzot J, et al.: Pachyonychia congenita. Dermatologica 1981; 160: 462–472.
Stieglitz JB, Centerwall WR: Pachyonychia congenita: a seventeen-member, four generation pedigree with unusual respiratory and dental involvement. Am J Med Genet 1983; 14:21–28.
Baran R, Dawber RPR: Diseases of the nails and their management. Oxford: Blackwell Scientific, 1984.
Sivasundram A, et al.: Pachyonychia congenita. Int J Dermatol 1985; 24:179–180.

SC060 **Richard K. Scher**

Nails, pachyonychia congenita, Jackson-Lawler type
See PACHYONYCHIA CONGENITA-STEATOCYSTOMA MULTIPLEX
Naito-Oyanagi disease
See DENTATORUBROPALLIDOLUYSIAN DEGENERATION, HEREDITARY
Nakajo nodular erythema with digital changes
See DIGITAL DEFECTS-NODULAR ERYTHEMA-EMACIATION, NAKAJO TYPE
Nakajo syndrome
See DIGITAL DEFECTS-NODULAR ERYTHEMA-EMACIATION, NAKAJO TYPE
Namaqualand hip dysplasia
See HIP, DYSPLASIA, NAMAQUALAND TYPE

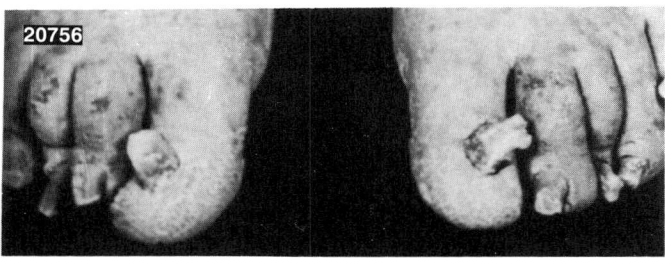

0789-20756: Nails, pachyonychia congenita; note "horn nails."

NAME syndrome
  See NEVI-ATRIAL MYXOMA-MYXOID NEUROFIBROMAS-EPHELIDES
Nance deafness
  See DEAFNESS WITH PERILYMPHATIC GUSHER
Nance-Horan syndrome
  See CATARACTS-OTO-DENTAL DEFECTS
Nance-Insley syndrome
  See OTO-SPONDYLO-MEGAEPIPHYSEAL DYSPLASIA
  also CHONDRODYSTROPHY-SENSORINEURAL DEAFNESS,
    NANCE-INSLEY TYPE
Nance-Sweeney syndrome
  See CHONDRODYSTROPHY-SENSORINEURAL DEAFNESS, NANCE-
    INSLEY TYPE
Nanocephalic dwarf
  See SECKEL SYNDROME
Nape nevus
  See NEVUS FLAMMEUS
Naprosyn^, fetal effects
  See FETAL EFFECTS OF NONSTEROIDAL ANTI-INFLAMMATORY
    DRUGS (NSAIDS)
Naproxen, fetal effects
  See FETAL EFFECTS OF NONSTEROIDAL ANTI-INFLAMMATORY
    DRUGS (NSAIDS)

NARCOLEPSY   3287

Includes:
  Cataplexy
  Maladie de Gelineau
  Narcoleptic syndrome
  Sleep disorder

Excludes:
  Apnea, obstructive sleep
  Encephalitis
  Epilepsy
  Hypersomnia, essential
  Hypoventilation, congenital central alveolar type (2606)
  Klein-Levin hibernation syndrome
  Myoclonus
  Tremor-duodenal ulcer syndrome (0963)

Major Diagnostic Criteria: Chronic daytime somnolence, unavoidable daytime napping, *cataplexy*. Symptoms may also include sleep paralysis and hypnagogic hallucinations. Polygraphic testing with nocturnal recording, followed by daytime multiple sleep latency testing, will find short sleep latencies at each nap; frequent occurence of REM sleep at sleep onset, rather than at a later time during sleep; and nocturnal disrupted sleep.

Clinical Findings: The first symptoms often develop near puberty. The peak age of reported symptoms is between 15–25 years of age, but narcolepsy and other symptoms have been noted at 5–6 years, and a second, smaller peak of onset has been noted between 35–45 years, near menopause in women.

Excessive daytime somnolence and irresistible sleep episodes usually occur as the first symptoms, either independently or associated with one or more other symptoms. They are enhanced by high temperature, indoor activity, and idleness. Symptoms may abate with time but never phase out completely. Attacks of *cataplexy* (an abrupt, reversible decrease or loss of muscle tone, most frequently elicited by strong emotions such as anger or laughter) generally appear in conjunction with abnormal episodes of sleep, but may occur as much as 20 years later. They occasionally, but seldom, occur before the abnormal sleep episodes, in which case they are a major source of difficulty in diagnosis. Episodes can vary in frequency from a few during the subject's entire lifetime to one or several per day.

Hypnagogic hallucinations and sleep paralysis do not affect all subjects and are often transitory. Disturbed nocturnal sleep seldom occurs in the first stages and generally builds up with age.

Complications: Narcolepsy leads to a variety of complications such as driving or machine accidents; difficulties at work resulting in disability, forced retirement or job dismissal; impotence; and depression.

Associated Findings: Sleep apnea is found in ten percent of narcoleptic subjects. Periodic leg movement (PLM) syndrome is also found frequently with the condition. The idea of an association between narcolepsy and **Multiple sclerosis** is conceptually interesting, as both conditions have been hypothesized as possible immune disorders, but the association has not been demonstrated.

Etiology: Multifactorial inheritance strongly influenced by environmental factors. In very limited studies with monozygotic twins, the twins of narcoleptic subjects had an incidence of narcolepsy 6–18 times higher than that of the general population. However, several elderly monozygotic twins have been proven discordant for narcolepsy. The major histocompatibility complex (MHC) antigen HLA-DR2 has been linked to the condition. All known Japanese narcoleptic subjects are HLA-DR2 positive and, secondarily, have the antigen DQw6. Caucasians and Blacks present DR2-negative isolated and familial cases; as many as nine percent of unrelated North American Caucasians with narcolepsy are predicted to be DR2 negative. In more recent studies, a separate gene, *canarc-1*, has been found to be the determinant of the condition in certain dogs. It is postulated that this gene's human analogue is a second genetic factor in the occurence of narcolepsy in humans.

Pathogenesis: Unknown. Special circumstances such as an abrupt change of sleep-wake schedule and/or a severe psychological stress (e.g. death of a relative, divorce) precede the occurence of the first symptom in half of the cases.

MIM No.: *16140

Sex Ratio: M1:F<1

Occurrence: In the San Francisco Bay Area its occurence has been calculated at 0.05%, and in the Los Angeles area at 0.067%. Its prevalence is estimated to be between 0.02 and 0.08% in North American Caucasions.

Risk of Recurrence for Patient's Sib:
  See Part I, *Mendelian Inheritance.* A frequency of narcolepsy among first-degree relatives has been calculated at 0.9%.

Risk of Recurrence for Patient's Child:
  See Part I, *Mendelian Inheritance.* A frequency of narcolepsy among first-degree relatives has been calculated at 0.9%. There was no abnormal dominance of a subgroup (i.e. parents, siblings, or children).

Age of Detectability: Age at onset varies from childhood to the fifth decade, with a peak in the second decade. Signs may be visible as early as 2–3 years of age.

Gene Mapping and Linkage: HLA-DR2 is located on the small arm of the 6th chromosome. The location of canarc-1 is unknown. It is not linked to the major histocompatibility complex.

Prevention: None known. Genetic counseling indicated.

Treatment: Many symptoms will respond to drug therapy. Central nervous system stimulants, especially amphetamines, are effective against excessive daytime somnolence. Tricyclic medications such as protriptyline and clomipramine are often used in the treatment of cataplexy, sleep paralysis, and hypnagogic hallucinations.

Short daytime naps will also help the subject maintain alertness during the day; in fact, it has not been established that stimulant medications are more effective than this simple treatment. Also important for narcoleptic subjects are support groups. Narcolepsy is often poorly understood, and its victims may find rejection from families and other social entities.

Prognosis: Normal life span.

Detection of Carrier: Examination of relatives for evidence of the trait. However, presence of DR2 DQw6 is neither sufficient nor necessary for the development of narcolepsy.

References:
Guilleminault C, et al., eds: Narcolepsy. New York: Spectrum Publications, 1976.
Honda Y, Juji T, eds: HLA in Narcolepsy. Berlin-Heidelberg: Springer-Verlag, 1978

Guilleminault C, et eal.: Familial Patterns of Narcolepsy. Lancet 1989; II:1376–1379.

GU010 **Christian Guilleminault**

Narcoleptic syndrome
See NARCOLEPSY
Nasal agenesis
See NOSE, TURBINATE DEFORMITY
Nasal alar hypoplasia-hypothyroidism-pancreatic achylia-deafness
See JOHANSON-BLIZZARD SYNDROME
Nasal atresia, posterior-lymphedema
See NOSE, CHOANAL ATRESIA-LYMPHEDEMA
Nasal crease
See NOSE, TRANSVERSE GROOVE
Nasal dermoids
See NECK/HEAD, DERMOID CYST OR TERATOMA
Nasal duplication
See NOSE, DUPLICATION
Nasal fundus ectasia
See OPTIC DISK, TILTED
Nasal glioma
See NOSE, GLIOMA
Nasal groove, familial transverse
See NOSE, TRANSVERSE GROOVE
Nasal groove, transverse
See NOSE, TRANSVERSE GROOVE
Nasal hypoplasia-peripheral dysostosis-mental retardation
See ACRODYSOSTOSIS
Nasal septum, absence of
See NOSE/NASAL SEPTUM DEFECTS
Nasal septum, subluxed or dislocated
See NOSE, DISLOCATED NASAL SEPTUM
Nasal stripe, transverse
See NOSE, TRANSVERSE GROOVE
Nasal-fronto-faciodysplasia
See FRONTO-FACIO-NASAL DYSPLASIA
Naso-blepharo-facial syndrome
See BLEPHARO-NASO-FACIAL SYNDROME

NASO-DIGITO-ACOUSTIC SYNDROME, KEIPERT TYPE   2085

Includes:
Deafness-digito-naso syndrome, Keipert type
Digito-naso-acoustic syndrome, Keipert type
Keipert-Fitzgerald-Danks syndrome
Keipert syndrome

Excludes:
Acrocephalosyndactyly type V (2284)
Polysyndactyly-dysmorphic craniofacies, Greig type (2925)
Rubinstein-Taybi broad thumb-hallux syndrome (0119)

Major Diagnostic Criteria: A combination of most of the seven characteristic clinical features should be present for diagnosis.

Clinical Findings: 1. Normal height and weight.
2. Characteristic craniofacial features including a large head circumference (98%), broad face, mildly down-slanted palpebral fissures, broad and high nasal bridge, upturned and prominent nasal alae, large rounded columella, protruding upper lip with a marked cupid's bow configuration, straight lower lip, and open mouth.
3. Intra-oral features of a double upper alveolar margin, narrow and widely spaced teeth, and narrow palate.
4. Unilateral or bilateral severe sensorineural hearing loss.
5. Short and broad distal phalanges of the thumbs, the first, second and third fingers and all of the toes. Clinodactyly and brachydactyly of the fifth fingers. No radial deviations of thumbs were present but a slight tibial deviation of 1st, 2nd, and 3rd toes was present.
6. Neurologic impairment including mental deficiency (present in one out of the two cases).
7. X-ray findings included broad short terminal phalanges, one sib had bifid terminal phalanges in both index index fingers. In the halluces of both patients, the proximal phalanges were short and the terminal phalanges were to the anterior cranial fossa, slender

long bones and coxa valga. Pneumoencephalography had shown mild communicating hydrocephalus in one case.

Complications: Speech delay due to hearing loss, as well as to the global developmental delay.

Associated Findings: None known.

Etiology: Most probably X-linked recessive inheritance, based on affected male siblings and affected maternally related male cousins.

Pathogenesis: Unknown.

MIM No.: 25598

POS No.: 3047

Sex Ratio: M2:F0 (observed).

Occurrence: Two pedigrees have been documented.

Risk of Recurrence for Patient's Sib:
See Part I, *Mendelian Inheritance.*

Risk of Recurrence for Patient's Child:
See Part I, *Mendelian Inheritance.*

Age of Detectability: At birth or in the first year of life.

Gene Mapping and Linkage: Unknown.

Prevention: None known. Genetic counseling indicated.

Treatment: Speech therapy if indicated, hearing aid, as well as referral to special developmental and educational program.

Prognosis: Life span probably not reduced.

Detection of Carrier: Unknown.

References:
Keipert JA, et al.: A new syndrome of broad terminal phalanges and facial abnormalities. Aust Paediatr J 1973; 9:10–13.

G0003 **Mahin Golabi**

Naso-maxillary cleft
See FACIAL CLEFT, OBLIQUE
Naso-ocular cleft
See FACIAL CLEFT, OBLIQUE

NASOLACRIMAL DUCT OBSTRUCTION   0705

Includes:
Dacryostenosis, congenital
Lacrimal system, impatency of the
Nasolacrimal duct, occlusion
Tear duct, blocked

Excludes:
Eyelid abnormalities (other)
Glaucoma, congenital (0414)

Major Diagnostic Criteria: Epiphora with or without a mucoid or purulent discharge is apparent after the first week of life. Regurgitation of mucus or pus through the lacrimal punctum when digital pressure is applied to the lacrimal sac localizes the obstruction to the nasal end of the nasolacrimal duct. Definitive diagnosis is made through attempt at irrigation of the system through one canaliculus and recovery of fluid through the opposite punctum.

Clinical Findings: Presenting signs and symptoms are variable and become evident after the first week of life. Epiphora may be the only symptom, however, it is usually accompanied by a mucoid or purulent discharge. The eyelids are often matted when the infant wakes up. The finding of reflux of muco-purulent material when pressure is applied to the lacrimal sac confirms the diagnosis. The conjunctiva is not injected.
Signs and symptoms may be intermittent or continuous persisting for weeks or months. An upper respiratory tract infection may exacerbate the symptoms. Spontaneous resolution of an obstructed nasolacrimal duct can be expected in up to 90% of cases by twelve months of age.

Complications: Acute and chronic dacryocystitis.

Associated Findings: Other defects of the lacrimal drainage system such as stenosis or occlusion of the puncta and/or canaliculi, and mucocoele of the lacrimal sac. It is a common finding in a number of syndromes and malformations of the head, and is a major manifestation of the **Lacrimo-auriculo-dento-digital syndrome**.

Etiology: Undetermined. Some reports of autosomal dominant inheritance exist when nasolacrimal duct impatency coexists with atresia of the lacrimal puncta or canaliculi.

Pathogenesis: The lacrimal drainage system develops from a core of surface ectodermal cells buried in facial neuroectoderm in a cleft between the maxillary process and lateral nasal process. Outbuddings originate from its upper end to form the canaliculi. A rod of epithelial cells grows upwards to become continuous with the main cord of buried ectodermal cells. At 3 months of gestation, canalization of the passages (puncta, canaliculi, lacrimal sac, and nasolacrimal duct) begins at the upper end and proceeds downwards. At birth, the entire system is patent except the nasal end of the nasolacrimal duct, which may be occluded by a membrane composed of nasal mucosa and the epithelium lining the nasolacrimal duct. The membrane disappears either shortly before or a few weeks after birth. Persistence of the membrane produces the characteristic signs and symptoms of nasolacrimal duct obstruction.

MIM No.: *14970

Sex Ratio: Presumably M1:F1.

Occurrence: Between 2–6% of newborns.

Risk of Recurrence for Patient's Sib: Unknown.

Risk of Recurrence for Patient's Child: Unknown.

Age of Detectability: After the first week of life.

Gene Mapping and Linkage: Unknown.

Prevention: None known. Genetic counseling indicated.

Treatment: Conservative medical management is initially suggested as the method of treatment. The parents are instructed to massage the lacrimal sac and to apply a topical antibiotic ointment if there is purulence.

Lacrimal probing and irrigation are effective means of treating obstructed nasolacrimal ducts. The timing of the initial probing is controversial. Some ophthalmologists advocate probing without sedation or general anesthesia between 3–6 months of age if the signs do not resolve with medical therapy. Others recommend a probing under general anesthesia at 12–13 months as up 90% of cases are expected to improve spontaneously by that age. A second probing should be done in failed cases before considering a silicone intubation of the lacrimal system or a dacryocystorhinostomy.

Prognosis: Excellent.

Detection of Carrier: Unknown.

References:

Veirs ER: Lacrimal disorders diagnosis and treatment. St. Louis, CV Mosby, 1976; 1–53. *

Petersen RA, Robb RM: The natural course of congenital obstruction of the nasolacrimal duct. J Pediat Ophthalmol Strabismus 1978; 15:246–250.

Kushner BJ: Congenital nasolacrimal system obstruction. Arch Ophthalmol 1982; 100:597–600.

Baker JD: Treatment of congenital nasolacrimal duct obstruction. J Pediat Ophthalmol Strabismus 1985; 22:34–5.

Paul TO: Medical management of congenital nasolacrimal duct obstruction. J Pediat Ophthalmol Strabismus 1985; 22:68–70.

Katowitz JA, Welsh MG: Timing of initial probing and irrigation in congenital nasolacrimal duct obstruction. Ophthalmology 1987; 94:698–705. *

P0024   **Robert C. Polomeno**

Nasolacrimal duct, occlusion
See NASOLACRIMAL DUCT OBSTRUCTION
Nasomaxillary hypoplasia
See MAXILLONASAL DYSPLASIA, BINDER TYPE
Nasomaxillovertebral syndrome
See MAXILLONASAL DYSPLASIA, BINDER TYPE

NASOPALPEBRAL LIPOMA-COLOBOMA SYNDROME   3049

Includes:
> Coloboma-nasopalpebral lipoma syndrome
> Palpebral coloboma-lipoma syndrome
> Penchaszadeh-Velasquez-Arwillagi syndrome

Excludes:
> **Face, median cleft face syndrome** (0635)
> **Oculo-auriculo-vertebral anomaly** (0735)

Major Diagnostic Criteria: Nasopalpebral lipomas, upper and lower lid colobomas, telecanthus, maxillary hypoplasia.

Clinical Findings: Anomalies are limited to the face and head. The facial appearance, in six described individuals, consists of broad forehead (6/6); widow's peak (6/6); telecanthus (6/6); laterally displaced outer canthi (5/6); normal interorbital distance (6/6); upper and lower lid colobomas (6/6); sparse, maldirected eyebrows (6/6); misplaced (5/6) or absent (1/6) upper lacrimal punctae; misplaced (1/6) or absent (1/6) lower lacrimal punctae; nasopalpebral lipomas (6/6); abnormal eyelashes (6/6); and midface hypoplasia (6/6).

Complications: Divergent strabismus and exotropia secondary to inner canthal lipomas; conjunctival hyperemia and corneal opacities secondary to chronic corneal exposure.

Associated Findings: Open metopic suture was reported in one affected individual.

Etiology: Autosomal dominant inheritance, based upon the presence of the condition in three generations, with male-to-male transmission.

Pathogenesis: Unknown. A defect in adipose tissue differentiation or neural crest cell migration has been postulated.

MIM No.: *16773

POS No.: 3542

Sex Ratio: M1:F1

Occurrence: Eight members, from three generations, of one family from Venezuela have been documented.

Risk of Recurrence for Patient's Sib:
See Part I, *Mendelian Inheritance.*

Risk of Recurrence for Patient's Child:
See Part I, *Mendelian Inheritance.*

Age of Detectability: At birth by the presence of lipomas and colobomas.

Gene Mapping and Linkage: Unknown.

Prevention: None known. Genetic counseling indicated.

Treatment: Supportive for the ocular defects; cosmetic surgery may also be indicated.

Prognosis: Affected individuals have had normal growth, intellectual development, and life span.

Detection of Carrier: Unknown.

References:

Penchaszadeh VB, The nasopalpebral lipoma-coloboma syndrome: a new autosomal dominant dysplasia-malformation syndrome with congenital nasopalpebral lipomas, eyelid colobomas, telecanthus, and maxillary hypoplasia. Am J Med Genet 1982; 11:397–410.

T0007   **Helga V. Toriello**

Nasopharyngeal atresia
See NOSE, NASOPHARYNGEAL STENOSIS

NASOPHARYNGEAL CYSTS 0706

Includes:
Branchial cleft cysts, Bailey type IV
Cysts of the nasopharynx, congenital
Extra-adenoidal cysts
Intra-adenoidal cysts

Excludes:
Cysts of seromucinous glands with occluded excretory ducts
Interstitial pseudocysts, no epithelium, due to tissue edema
Intra-adenoidal pseudocyst secondary to incomplete adenoidectomy
Pseudocyst secondary to inflammation of fascial envelope
Sealed over crypt secondary to repeated inflammatory episodes

Major Diagnostic Criteria: With the extra-adenoidal cyst, the excised velum of tissue theoretically should show appropriate epithelial coverings on both surfaces, but careful pathologic examinations are rarely carried out in such cases. The true branchial cyst is lateral and often bilateral. Lesions lacking an inner epithelial lining are merely pseudocysts. In as much as the pharyngeal tubercle may hide the essential lesion, direct nasopharyngeal examination is desirable.

Clinical Findings: Symptoms include purulent postnasal discharge not coming through the choanae. Aching pain high in the throat or at the base of the skull, with a feeling of pressure or fullness, periodically relieved by evacuation of secretion.

Intra-adenoidal cysts derive from the medial pharyngeal recess. An elliptical opening on the nether surface of the adenoid, axis anteroposterior, lying in the midline, differing from the usual crypt opening in that it is more regular. Usually there is no special swelling, but pus and debris may be extruded on suction or pressure in the untreated state.

Extra-adenoidal cysts located deep to the pharyngobasilar fascia are derived from bursa pharyngea embryonalis (midline). They will not be diagnosed in children until the adenoid is removed, but, in the adult, they may be seen caudal to the lowermost extent of any adenoid present. Usually no swelling is seen in the nasopharynx, but there is a small hole in the midline, slightly rostral to the pharyngeal tubercle. In the untreated state, this hole may be surrounded by a cuff of granular, inflamed mucosa. It may exude pus intermittently. The hole usually leads to a small cavity, separated from the general nasopharyngeal space by a thin velum of tissue. In rare instances, the space in question can enlarge caudally to the level of the epiglottis. Indentation of the basiocciput has been described but must be quite rare.

Branchial cleft cysts, Bailey type IV are derived from first and dorsal portion of second pharyngeal pouch. They are often paired, and are present on the lateral aspects of the nasopharyngeal wall. The branchial nature is not easy to establish. Cystic nature may be established by injection of radiopaque material, but this may deceive. Lateral location and bilaterality strongly suggest branchial origin. Pathologic findings are more cogent.

It is of the utmost importance to evaluate sinonasal disease as a cause of symptoms. This can only be done with reasonable certainty by careful clinical examination supplemented by X-ray study of the sinuses.

Complications: Chronic or subacute bronchitis; chronic blepharoconjunctivitis; subacute or chronic otitis media, sometimes with conductive hearing loss. Rarely, paranasal sinusitis; fever, and recurring pharyngitis.

Associated Findings: None known.

Etiology: Unknown.

Pathogenesis: The true bursa pharyngea is due to the inductive effect of chorda mesoderm on the pharyngeal epithelium in the fornix region where the bundles of pharyngobasilar fascia do not commingle to form a barrier, as they do more anteriorly, to the extrusion of pharyngeal entoderm.

Intra-adenoidal midline cysts may be due to such an embryonic disturbance of the median pharyngeal recess which, precedes

development of the pharyngeal tonsil itself, but the products of which may be incorporated within the adenoid.

Branchial cleft cysts arise here, as elsewhere, but much more rarely. They are prone to remain intramural (Bailey type IV) and not to migrate into the neck.

Sex Ratio: Presumably M1:F1.

Occurrence: Undetermined but presumed rare.

Risk of Recurrence for Patient's Sib: Unknown.

Risk of Recurrence for Patient's Child: Unknown.

Age of Detectability: Nasopharyngeal cysts are discovered either at the time of adenoid or adenotonsil surgery in childhood; or, less commonly, in adults on careful investigation of postnasal pus which cannot be demonstrated to come from the nose or paranasal sinuses.

Gene Mapping and Linkage: Unknown.

Prevention: None known. Genetic counseling indicated.

Treatment: *Intra-adenoidal cyst* is cured by a thorough adenoidectomy under direct visual control, whether it is of true bursal origin or not.

Extra-adenoidal cyst is usually cured by marsupialization or saucerization.

Branchial cleft cysts are best treated by excision under direct vision.

Aspiration and injection of sclerosing agents or marsupialization temporize only, and recurrence may be expected.

Prognosis: Normal for life span and intelligence; functionally good in all types with proper treatment.

Detection of Carrier: Unknown.

References:
Taylor JNS, Burwell RG: Branchiogenic nasopharyngeal cysts. J Laryngol Otol 1954; 68:677.
Wilson CP: A case of bilateral congenital sinuses of the nasopharynx. Acta Otolaryngol (Stockh) 1957; 48:76.
Wilson CP: Observations on the surgery of the nasopharynx. Ann Otol Rhinol Laryngol 1957; 66:5.
Guggenheim P: Cysts of the nasopharynx. Laryngoscope 1967; 77: 2147–2168.
Toomly JM: Cysts and tumors of the pharynx. In: Paparella MM, Shumrick DA, eds: Otolaryngology, vol 3. Philadelphia: W.B. Saunders, 1980:2323–2324.
Michaels L: Normal anatomy and histology; adenoids; infections; developmental lesions. In: Ear, nose and throat histopathology. New York: Springer-Verlag, 1987:242.

AU005   **Thomas Aufdemorte**

Nasopharyngeal stenosis
See NOSE, NASOPHARYNGEAL STENOSIS
Nasopharyngeal teratomas
See NECK/HEAD, DERMOID CYST OR TERATOMA
Nasu-Hakola disease
See OSTEODYSPLASIA, LIPOMEMBRANOUS POLYCYSTIC-DEMENTIA
Nathalie syndrome
See OTO-OCULO-MUSCULO-SKELETAL SYNDROME
Naumoff type short-rib polydactyly syndrome
See SHORT RIB-POLYDACTYLY SYNDROME, VERMA-NAUMOFF TYPE

NECK, BRANCHIAL CLEFT, CYSTS OR SINUSES 0117

Includes:
Branchial cleft fistula
Cervical cyst or sinus
Pharyngeal cyst or fistula

Excludes:
Branchio-oto-renal dysplasia (2224)
Cavernous hemangioma of neck
Cervical adenopathy
Laryngocele (0575)
Neck/head, dermoid cyst or teratoma (0283)

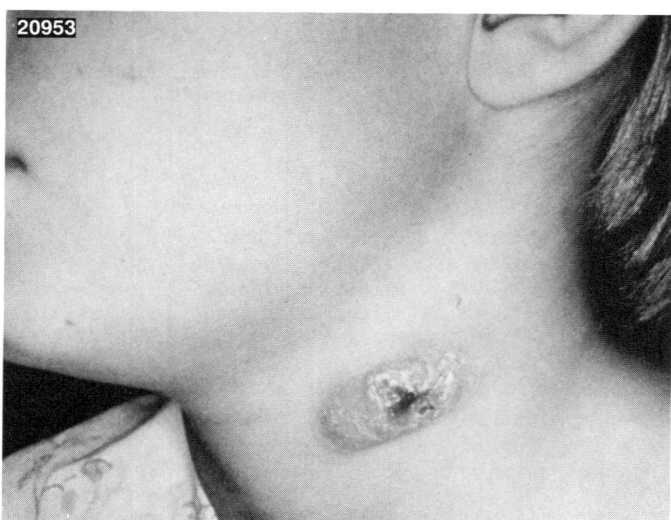

0117A-20953: Branchial cleft sinus (infected).

Pharyngocele
Solitary lymph cysts
Thymic cyst
Thyroglossal duct remnant (0945)
Thyroid cyst

Major Diagnostic Criteria: Histopathologic examination of a cystic mass or sinus medial to the sternocleidomastoid muscle.

Clinical Findings: Either a cyst or a sinus or both can result from abnormal development of the pharyngeal pouches or cervical sinus. These lesions generally appear along the anterior border of the sternocleidomastoid muscle or medial to this muscle. They may also be in the periauricular region.

The branchial cyst is a slowly enlarging, painless mass in the head and neck region that may be present at birth. Pressure and a sense of fullness in the neck with mild dysphagia and hoarseness are frequent symptoms. Children with large cysts may have stridorous breathing and cyanosis. Uncomplicated cysts are characteristically soft, mobile, and transparent when transilluminated. The cyst may vary in size, increasing with infection and decreasing as infection subsides. Neck injuries may cause the cyst to become enlarged, tense, and painful.

Small cysts may be difficult to palpate, particularly those lying medial to the sternocleidomastoid muscle. These may be detected by having the patient push his chin firmly against the examiner's palm. Needle aspiration yields a mucoid material.

A typical sinus has an external opening at the junction of the lower third and upper two-thirds of the sternocleidomastoid muscle. This small pinpoint opening may not be noticed until mucoid material or food particles pass from it. Symptoms of vagal irritation, such as cough, hoarseness, pallor, bradycardia, sweating, and faintness have been elicited by probing the sinus. Persistent cough, drainage into the pharynx, and pain from repeated infections of the external openings are unusual symptoms of a cervical sinus. X-ray examination after injecting the sinus with radiopaque oil reveals a typical smooth-walled tract. A cyst may develop at any point along the sinus tract.

Complications: Upper airway obstruction, dysphagia, aspiration, infection of cyst or sinus, malignant tumor formation.

Associated Findings: None known.

Etiology: Autosomal dominant inheritance. Widstrom et al. (1980) found a 36% positive family history for complete fistulae from the second cleft or pouch and a 10% positive family history with regard to the external sinus. There is no evidence of heredity being associated with lateral neck cysts.

Pathogenesis: Pharyngeal pouches and branchial grooves are present for only a short time during embryonic life. Epithelial rests, incomplete closure of the branchial grooves, rupture of the closing membranes between the pharyngeal pouches and branchial grooves, and persistence of the cervical sinus are thought to be responsible for these abnormalities. The constant relationship between the cyst or sinus and anatomic structures normally formed by the branchial apparatus substantiates this concept.

The question has been raised, do branchial cysts arise from cystic degeneration of cervical lymph nodes? Schewitsch, et al. (1980) presented a series of 82 cysts and sinuses. None of their patients had other developmental abnormalities. All of the cysts contained abundant lymphoid tissue without sinusoids. Lymph nodes were present but separated from the cyst wall by thin, fibrous layers. Histology of the cysts showed columnar ciliated epithelium, consistent with a branchiogenic origin. The authors conclude that it is unlikely that cervical cysts originate from salivary inclusions or lymph nodes. Their data support the classic theory that the majority of lateral cervical cysts originate from embryonic entrapment of epithelial tissue.

MIM No.: *11360

CDC No.: 239.200

Sex Ratio: M3:F1

Occurrence: These are relatively common abnormalities. The occurrence rate is unknown, partly because they may not be apparent until later life.

Risk of Recurrence for Patient's Sib:
See Part I, *Mendelian Inheritance.*

Risk of Recurrence for Patient's Child:
See Part I, *Mendelian Inheritance.*

Age of Detectability: From birth through adulthood, depending on the occurrence of symptoms and clinical findings.

Gene Mapping and Linkage: Unknown.

Prevention: None known. Genetic counseling indicated.

Treatment: Total excision of the cyst and sinus tract will give the patient a complete cure. Stepladder incisions may be indicated to remove the entire sinus tract. When the sinus originates from the tonsillar fossa, a tonsillectomy must be performed to ensure complete excision of the tract. Facial nerve exploration and preservation is necessary for all lesions around the ear.

Prognosis: Normal life span unless rare malignancy occurs.

Detection of Carrier: Unknown.

Special Considerations: The knowledge of embryologic development and related anatomy is essential for understanding branchial cysts and sinuses. There are two types of lateral neck lesions that share the name branchial. One group of cysts are located anterior

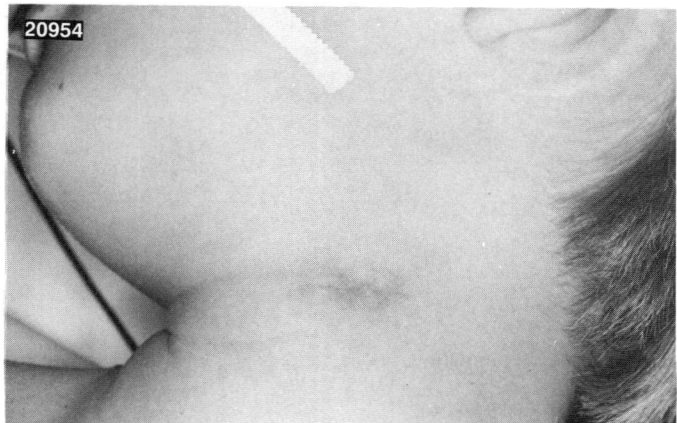

0117B-20954: Branchial cleft sinus.

to the upper part of the sternocleidomastoid muscle. The others are tube-like lesions that open into the skin of the neck. They may be either fistulae with openings at both ends or sinuses with one open end. Howie and Proops (1982) examined 57 lesions that were located in the lateral neck, including cysts, sinuses and fistulae. The lesions fell into two well-defined groups and one miscellaneous group. The first included 46 cysts that presented as a swelling in the neck behind the angle of the mandible and anterior to the junction of the upper third and lower two-thirds of the sternocleidomastoid muscle. In group two, there were four congenital lesions, which were characterized with an opening into the skin of the neck at the anterior border of the sternocleidomastoid. There were seven miscellaneous lesions that had unique features.

A first branchial cleft fistula will be located entirely above the hyoid bone, with its upper end opening into the external auditory canal. The tract is superficial to the mandible and passes through the parotid gland. It may lie deep or superficial to the facial nerve. The lesion may be seen in the periauricular region in the anterior neck.

The second arch sinus begins in the tonsillar fossa. It extends between the internal and external carotid arteries above and superficial to the hypoglossal nerve, glossopharyngeal nerve, and stylopharyngeus muscle. The sinus opens onto the skin along the anterior border of the sternocleidomastoid muscle. The junction of the lower and middle thirds of the muscle is the most common site for this opening. The second arch sinus is the most common of these abnormalities.

A sinus formed from *the third branchial cleft* opens in the same cutaneous region as the second branchial sinus. This tract passes deep to the platysma muscle along the sheath of the common carotid artery, but extends behind the internal carotid artery. The tract is superficial to the vagus nerve and crosses the hypoglossal nerve, but does not ascend above the glossopharyngeal nerve or stylopharyngeus muscle. The internal opening is in the pyriform sinus.

Cysts or sinuses of *the fourth branchial cleft* are theoretically possible, but very few have been reported. The tract would pass below the aorta on the left and the subclavian artery on the right; it ascends into the neck and empties into the upper esophagus after crossing the hypoglossal nerve. Downey and Ward (1969) have described a mediastinal cyst that they believe originated from a fourth branchial cleft. That cyst was lined with squamous and transitional epithelium with islands of lymphoid tissue in its wall. Shugar and Healy (1980) report a patient with the fourth branchial cleft anomaly. This tract extended under the clavicle near the subclavian vessels. Others believe that perithyroidal abscesses occur secondary to infection of a fourth branchial cleft, cyst, or sinus. Contamination is thought to occur from a connection to the apex of the pyriform sinus. This may be demonstrated by a barium esophagram obtained during a quiescent period.

References:
Downey WL, Ward PH: Branchial cleft cysts in the mediastinum. Arch Otolaryngol 1969; 89:762–765. *
Schewitsch I, et al.: Cysts and sinuses of the lateral head and neck. J Otolaryngol 1980; 9:1–6.
Shugar MA, Healy GB: The fourth branchial cleft anomaly. Head Neck Surg 1980; 3:72–75.
Widstrom A, et al.: Aspects on the lateral fistulae and cysts of the neck. J Otolaryngol 1980; 9:291–296.
Chandler JR, Mitchell B: Branchial cleft cysts, sinuses, and fistulas. Otolaryngol Clin North Am 1981; 14:175–186.
Howie AJ, Proops DW: The definition of branchial cysts, sinuses and fistulae. Clin Otolaryngol 1982; 7:51–57.
Albers GD: Congenital sinuses and fistulas of the neck and pharynx. In: English FM, ed: Otolaryngology, ch. 12. Philadelphia: Harper & Row, 1988. *

EN002 **Gerald M. English**

NECK, CYSTIC HYGROMA, FETAL TYPE 2252

Includes:
>Cystic hygroma of the neck (posterior)
Hygroma cervicis
Jugular lymphatic obstruction sequence
Nuchal lymphangioma
Pterygium colli
Turner syndrome phenotype

Excludes:
>**Cystic hygroma** (3284)
Encephalocele (0343)
Hydrops fetalis, non-immune (2198)
Lymphangiomatous malformations localized to other body areas

Major Diagnostic Criteria: A mass on the fetal posterolateral cervical area.

Clinical Findings: A septated, fluid-filled mass or masses occupying the posterolateral cervical area without communication to the brain or to an underlying defect of the fetal skull. Survivors may exhibit redundant nuchal skin or neck webbing.

Failure of the jugular lymphatic sacs to establish venous communication during fetal development leads to massive enlargement of these sacs in the posterolateral cervical areas. The enlarging masses may rotate the axis of the developing auricle posteriorly and elevate the lower pinna. Late communication of the sacs with the internal jugular vein may be manifest by redundancy of posterior nuchal skin or a webbed neck in adult life. Complete obstruction of lymphatic drainage usually results in generalized fetal edema and ascites (hydrops fetalis). The establishment of late or alternative lymphatic drainage may be manifest in survivors by limb edema. Complex cardiac malformations are frequent in affected fetuses, even in cases with euploid chromosome karyotypes (3/10 index cases) or deficient migration of cephalic neural crest cells.

Complications: It has been suggested that intrathoracic distention of lymphatic channels or deficient migration of cephalic neural crest cells in early fetal life might interfere with development of the aortic arch and conotruncal region. **Diaphragmatic hernia** (2/10) has been attributed to the same mechanism.

Associated Findings: None known.

Etiology: The majority of cases are associated with **Turner syndrome** (45,X or 45,X mosaic chromosome constitution). This malformation sequence or its postnatal consequences, nuchal skin

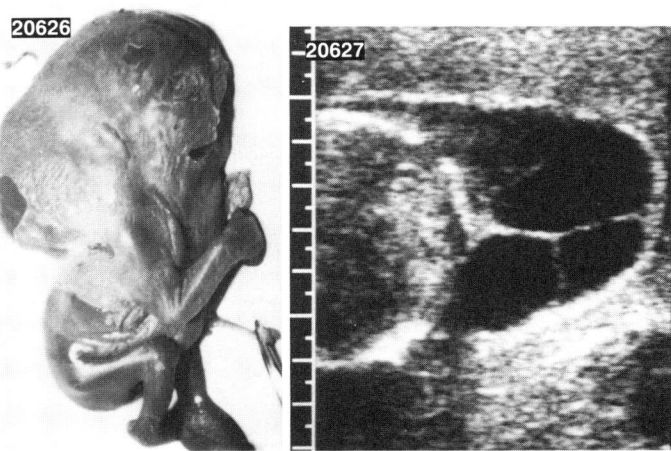

2252A-20626: One of two affected sibs with cystic hygroma. 20627: Ultrasound study of nuchal cystic hygroma with typical septations; fetal head is to the left.

2252B-20949: Cystic hygroma on the right side of this CAT scan.

redundancy and neck webbing, has also been described in association with **Pterygium syndrome, multiple**, **Roberts syndrome** (tetraphocomelia), **Asplenia syndrome**, **Noonan syndrome**, **Fetal alcohol syndrome**, 46,XY gonadal dysgenesis, and chromosomal aneuploidy: +13, +18, +21, +22, 13q-, 18p-, +11p/22q, t6q/12q.

Pathogenesis: Nuchal cystic hygroma is the clinical consequence of delay or absence of the communication that normally develops between the jugular lymph sacs and the internal jugular veins at approximately 40 days gestation. In the course of normal development, the sacs become the terminal portions of the right lymphatic duct and the thoracic duct. The obstructed jugular lymph sacs dilate along the path of least resistance in the posterior and lateral cervical areas, tethered posteromedially by the nuchal ligament and bounded anteriorly by the sternomastoid muscle. The dilated sacs result in the characteristic septated mass or masses, divided posteriorly by the nuchal ligament. Generalized hypoplasia of major lymphatic trunks usually results in fetal edema, ascites, and pleural and pericardial effusions. The absence of fetal hydrops may help to differentiate cystic hygroma associated with a euploid karyotype from that found in cases of Turner syndrome. Localized lymphatic dilatation or tissue edema during early development may lead to the complications noted above.

MIM No.: 25735

CDC No.: 239.200, 744.900

Sex Ratio: M<1:F1. The vast majority are phenotypically female.

Occurrence: 1:875 spontaneous abortions; 1:200 spontaneous abortions with crown-rump length (CRL) > 30 mm.

Risk of Recurrence for Patient's Sib: Depends on associated disorders. If phenotypic male and/or euploid chromosome karyotype noted, autosomal recessive inheritance should be considered (25%).

Risk of Recurrence for Patient's Child: Undetermined. Affected individuals generally do not survive to reproduce.

Age of Detectability: By ultrasound examination at 16 weeks' gestation.

Gene Mapping and Linkage: Unknown.

Prevention: None known. Genetic counseling indicated.

Treatment: Unknown.

Prognosis: Generally lethal in utero when accompanied by hydrops. Prognosis for survivors will depend on etiology of the malformation sequence.

Detection of Carrier: By karyotype in instances of unbalanced translocation.

References:

Graham JM Jr, Smith DW: Dominantly inherited pterygium colli. J Pediatr 1981; 98:664–665.

Cowchock FS, et al.: Not all cystic hygromas occur in the Ullrich-Turner syndrome. Am J Med Genet 1982; 12:327–331. †

Chervenak FA, et al.: Fetal cystic hygroma: cause and natural history. New Engl J Med 1983; 309:822–825. *

Byrne J, et al.: The significance of cystic hygroma in fetuses. Hum Pathol 1984; 15:61–67. †

Miyabara S, et al.: Significance of cardiovascular malformations in cystic hygroma. Am J Med Genet 1989; 34:489–501. †

C0061

Susan Cowchock

Neck, limber-mental retardation
See X-LINKED MENTAL RETARDATION-MUSCULAR WEAKNESS-AWKWARD GAIT

NECK/FACE, LIPOMATOSIS   0601

Includes:
  Adenolipomatosis
  Cervical lipomatosis, familial benign
  Face, diffuse symmetric lipomatosis of
  Lipomatosis, benign symmetric
  Lipomatosis of face and neck
  Madelung disease
  Tongue, Pleomorphic lipoma

Excludes:
  Lipomas, familial symmetric (0600)
  Neurofibromatosis (0712)
  Parotitis, punctate (0799)
  Stiff skin syndrome (2629)

Major Diagnostic Criteria: Symmetric masses in the head and neck region. These masses are clinically and pathologically identical with lipoma.

Clinical Findings: Symmetric fatty growths may involve the neck, parotid area, occipital area, and, in some instances, both the neck and axilla. When the neck, axillary, and orbital regions are affected this condition has been called adenolipomatosis, although lymph nodes are not involved. Telangiectasis and hypertrophy of bone or muscle may accompany the fatty growths. This disorder may be confused with neurofibromatosis. Some cases are associated with an elevated blood cholesterol. Onset is usually in adulthood. In most cases the masses are painless. They remain quiescent for many years but suddenly may enlarge. The major disabilities are cosmetic and respiratory obstruction from lipoma in the neck. Pleomorphic lipoma of the tongue has also been described, and its bulk creates speech impairment. In 145 cases of oral lipoma, 19% were found in the tongue.

Complications: Upper respiratory obstruction.

Associated Findings: Hyperuricemia, diabetes mellitus, elevated plasma triglyceride levels, type 4 lipoprotein pattern, somatic, autonomic and peripheral neuropathy, and renal tubular acidosis. Chemical analysis of the lipoma shows that the neck lipoma contains more lipid than in the buttock and that 39% of the lipid is triglyceride as compared with 3% in other body locations.

Etiology: Undetermined. Affected individuals frequently have a history of alcohol abuse. Possibly autosomal dominant inheritance.

Pathogenesis: This condition is probably only one manifestation of several varieties of hereditary fatty tumors that can involve almost any area of the body. It is not certain now that tumors of the face and neck are a separate entity. This presentation may occur sporadically.

MIM No.: 15180

Sex Ratio: M<1:F1

Occurrence: About 200 cases cases have documented in the literature.

Risk of Recurrence for Patient's Sib:
See Part I, *Mendelian Inheritance.*

Risk of Recurrence for Patient's Child:
See Part I, *Mendelian Inheritance.*

Age of Detectability: Tumors usually become clinically evident after the second decade.

Gene Mapping and Linkage: Unknown.

Prevention: None known. Genetic counseling indicated.

Treatment: Surgical removal is the only effective method to obtain tissue for diagnosis, to improve appearance, and to relieve airway obstruction. The lipoma infiltrates and and readily recurs, so debulking, rather than total excision, should be performed.

Prognosis: Normal for life span.

Detection of Carrier: Unknown.

References:

Pack GT, Ariel IM: Tumors of adipose tissue. In: Tumors of the soft somatic tissues; a clinical treatise. New York: Hoeber-Harper, 1958: 343–365.
McKusick VA: Familial benign cervical lipomatosis. In: Medical genetics, 1961. J Chronic Dis 1962; 15:417–572.
Argenta LC, et al.: Benign symmetrical lipomatosis (Madelung's disease). Head Neck Surg 1981; 3:240–241.
Stevenson RE, et al.: Symmetrical lipomatosis associated with stiff skin and systemic manifestations in four generations. Proc Greenwood Genet Center 1984; 3:56–64.
Enzi G, et al.: Sensory, motor and autonomic neuropathy in patients with multiple symetric lipomatosis. Medicine 1985; 64:388–393.
Gallou L, et al.: Pleomorphic lipoma of the tongue: case report and literature review. J Otolaryngol (Can.) 1986; 15:313–316.

BE028   **LaVonne Bergstrom**

NECK/HEAD, DERMOID CYST OR TERATOMA   0283

Includes:
Bidermoma of head or neck
Cervical teratomas
Dermoid cyst or teratoma of head or neck
Dermoids of the head and neck
Embryoma of head or neck
Epignathus
Hairy cyst on head or neck
Mixed cyst on head or neck
Monodermoma of head or neck
Nasal dermoids
Nasopharyngeal teratomas
Teratoid tumor of head or neck
Teratomas of the orbit
Tridermoma of head or neck

Excludes:
Inclusion cysts of head or neck lined with squamous epithelium
Neck, branchial cleft, cysts or sinuses (0117)
Preauricular tags and cysts
Salivary gland, mixed tumor (0878)
Thyroglossal duct remnant (0945)
Thyroid, dysgenesis (0946)
Other congenital head and neck tumors

Major Diagnostic Criteria: A tumor, cyst, or sinus opening in the head or neck areas. Histopathologic study is necessary to establish the diagnosis.

Clinical Findings: Dermoid cysts or teratomas of the head and neck occur almost exclusively in infants and young children. A review of 103 dermoid cysts of the head and neck revealed the following;

Dermoid Cysts of Head and Neck by Site

Site	No. of Patients	%
Nose	13	12.6
Orbit	51	49.5
Floor of mouth, submental, submaxillary	24	23.3
Occipital, frontal, lip, neck, soft palate	15	14.6

The signs and symptoms depend on the size and location of the tumor.

Nasal dermoids are usually detected shortly after birth. A small midline pit or depression on the bridge of the nose with hair protruding from it may be the only abnormality. This pit represents the opening of a sinus tract that may extend between the nasal bones into the cribriform plate or nasal septum. A CT scan of the skull and facial bones is essential, and injection of the tract with a radiopaque substance before this examination may be helpful in establishing the extent of the sinus tract. Nasal obstruction and rhinorrhea may be present.

Teratomas of the orbit may be associated with a unilateral exophthalmos and some degree of microphthalmos. The patient with a teratoma is usually born with a mass behind the eye, whereas the dermoid cyst may not become apparent until later in life. Orbital teratomas may extend through defects in the orbit or skull into the anterior cranial fossa, middle cranial fossa, temporal fossa, or nasal cavity. Clinical findings will depend upon the size and extensions of the tumor.

Dermoid cysts of the floor of the mouth are congenital inclusion cysts that form along the lines of embryologic fusion. They usually become manifest during the second and third decade of life. These cysts, while characteristically midline, may also be in the lateral neck. Evidence indicates that both midline and lateral dermoid cysts are of common origin and frequently have attachments to the midline of the hyoid bone or mandible. This attachment to the midline may be epithelialized, and failure to follow the tract and excise it completely will result in recurrence.

Cervical teratomas are rare after the age of one year. Equally distributed between the two sexes, most of these tumors are present at birth. A mass in the neck is the usual presentation. Acute respiratory symptoms of stridor, apnea, and cyanosis result from compression or deviation of the trachea. Dysphagia may arise from esophageal compression. Cystic lymphangioma, congenital goiter, branchial cleft cysts, and thyroglossal duct cysts must be considered in the differential diagnosis. These tumors, measuring between 5 and 12 cm, are usually unilateral and quite large. The medial border may extend across the anterior midline in close relation to the thyroid gland and trachea. They may be solid, multiloculated or cystic. The skin overlying the tumor is moveable. The mass may grow to a considerable size, causing cosmetic deformities. X-ray examination of the neck mass may reveal areas of calcification within the tumor. A CT scan should be obtained before excision to assess tumor extent.

Nasopharyngeal teratomas are present at birth and occur in females six times as often as in males. These tumors may be either pedunculated or sessile. Airway obstruction, cough, rhinorrhea, and a nasal or nasopharyngeal tumor are the most common findings. These tumors may be associated with deformities of the skull such as anencephaly, hemicrania, or fissures of the palate.

Complications: Airway obstruction, rhinitis and sinusitis, epistaxis, meningitis, cosmetic deformities, exophthalmos, decreased vision, malignant degeneration.

Associated Findings: The orbital, nasal, and nasopharyngeal teratomas may be associated with cranial defects. Cervical teratomas are not associated with these or other defects.

Etiology: Undetermined. This condition is believed to arise from embryonal disturbances of development. A growth disturbance of the primary axis (the notochord and contiguous structures from Hensen node in the early embryo) has been proposed.

Pathogenesis: There is no sharp delineation between dermoid cysts and simple congenital inclusion cysts. As the cyst enlarges and the patient grows, the lesion may migrate away from its primary location. Dermoid cysts may contain a small percentage of mesodermal elements in addition to predominant dermal elements. Teratomas are much more complex tumors, and their structure varies greatly according to the variety of tissues they contain. Usually they are cystic and the skin-lined cavities contain sebaceous material. The cavities not lined with skin contain mucoid or watery secretions. Skin, hair, bone, cartilage, and teeth may be recognized on gross examination. Microscopically, the tissues within these tumors vary considerably. Skin, hair follicles, sebaceous glands, and sweat glands are common. Respiratory epithelium, intestinal epithelium, nervous tissue, cartilage, bone, and nonstriated muscle are present in varying proportions. Liver, lung, thyroid, and renal tissues are uncommon. Teeth are found in a few tumors. These components are arranged in a chaotic fashion, but they closely resemble their normal counterparts. The benign teratoma and dermoid cyst are usually easy to recognize.

CDC No.: 239.200

Sex Ratio: Nasal dermoid: Slight male preponderance
Orbital dermoid or teratoma: M1:F1
Cervical dermoid or teratoma: M1:F1
Nasopharyngeal teratoma: M1:F6

Occurrence: Unknown.

Risk of Recurrence for Patient's Sib: Unknown.

Risk of Recurrence for Patient's Child: Unknown.

Age of Detectability: Oral: prenatal ultrasonography shows mass attached to fetal head. Hydramnios is also present. Nasal: at birth. Orbital dermoid: childhood. Orbital teratoma: at birth. Cervical: prenatal ultrasonography shows displaced fetal head associated with a large mass. Hydramnios is also present. Nasopharyngeal: at birth.

Gene Mapping and Linkage: Unknown.

Prevention: None known. Genetic counseling indicated.

Treatment: Complete surgical excision is required to prevent recurrences and other complications. Combined ophthalmologic, neurosurgical, and otolaryngologic operations may be needed to successfully treat the orbital tumors. Cervical tumors are usually encapsulated in fibrous tissue, which makes complete surgical excision possible.

Tracheostomy, an extraoral feeding route, antibiotics, and reconstructive procedures for cosmetic deformities may be necessary.

Prognosis: A normal life span can be expected when the tumor is completely excised. Malignant degeneration is rare, except in cases of nasopharyngeal teratoma.

Detection of Carrier: Unknown.

References:
Dekelboum AM: Teratoma of the nasopharynx in the newborn. Otolaryngol Head Neck Surg 1979; 87:628–634.
Leveque H, et al.: Dermoid cysts of the floor of the mouth and lateral neck. Laryngoscope 1979; 89:296–305.
McCaffrey TV, et al.: Dermoid cysts of the nose: review of 21 cases. Otolaryngol Head Neck Surg 1979; 87:52–59.
Hughes GB, et al.: Management of the congenital midline nasal mass: a review. Head Neck Surg 1980; 2:222–233.
Tobey DN, Mangham C: Malignant cervical teratomas. Otolaryngol Head Neck Surg 1980; 88:215–217.
English GM: Embryology and anomalies of the mouth and throat. In: English GM, ed: Otolaryngology. Ch. 5. Philadelphia: Harper & Row, 1983. *

EN002   **Gerald M. English**

Neck/head, hemangiomas
See *HEMANGIOMAS OF THE HEAD AND NECK*
Necrosis of the capital femoral epiphysis-primary coxa plana
See *HIP, OSTEONECROSIS, CAPITAL FEMORAL EPIPHYSIS*
Nemaline myopathy
See *MYOPATHY, NEMALINE*
Neonatal nephrosis
See *NEPHROSIS, CONGENITAL*
Neonatal osseous dysplasia I
See *SKELETAL DYSPLASIA, DE LA CHAPELLE TYPE*
Neonatal seborrheic dermatitis
See *IMMUNODEFICIENCY, PLASMA-ASSOCIATED DEFECT OF PHAGOCYTOSIS*
Neonatal severe primary hyperparathyroidism (NSPH)
See *HYPERPARATHYROIDISM, FAMILIAL*
Neoplasms of CNS
See *CNS NEOPLASMS*
Nephritis, salt-losing
See *KIDNEY, NEPHRONOPHTHISIS-MEDULLARY CYSTIC DESEASE*

NEPHRITIS-DEAFNESS (SENSORINEURAL), HEREDITARY TYPE   0708

Includes:
   Alport syndrome
   Alport syndrome-like hereditary nephritis
   Deafness-nephritis
   Fechtner syndrome
   Hearing loss-nephritis
   Interstitial pyelonephritis, hereditary type
   Nephropathy-deafness, hereditary type

Excludes:
   Deafness-diverticulitis-neuropathy (0265)
   Hematuria, benign familial
   Kidney, nephronophthisis-medullary cystic desease (3018)
   Nephritis (hereditary) without deafness
   Nephropathy-deafness-hyperparathyroidism
   Nephrosis, familial type (0710)

Major Diagnostic Criteria: Hematuria (100%) and proteinuria (70%-80%), at times variable, with sensorineural hearing loss in patient, parent, or sibs, and family history of other members with nephritis, deafness, or both. Renal function may be normal or decreased. Electron microscopy may show patchy glomerular basement membrane thickening and thinning, or thickening and splitting of the basement membrane thought to be pathognomonic for Alport syndrome.

Clinical Findings: When first recognized, it may present with variable hematuria, proteinuria, and occasional pyuria. Initial renal function is usually normal, but progressive deterioration occurs, resulting in renal failure in males by the second or third decade, with a more benign course in females. Abnormal tubular function is rarely seen, and urinary tract infection is unusual. Urinary findings consist of gross or microscopic hematuria; proteinuria; and hyaline, granular, and cellular casts. Renal biopsy in younger children shows thin, irregular basement membrane, which may be due to persistence of fetal or neonatal capillary basement membrane. Diffuse or focal thickening and splitting of the basement membrane predominates in older children and adults.

Bilateral sensorineural hearing loss is present in about half the patients. It may develop within the first few years of life, is more common in males, and is slowly progressive. Audiometric studies show high-tone sensorineural hearing loss with recruitment, high SISI scores, absent tone decay, and type II Bekesy tracings typical of cochlear pathology. Hearing loss and renal involvement may occur separately in affected family members.

Ocular defects occur in about 15% of patients and include anterior or posterior lenticonus, spherophakia, congenital cataracts, and macular or peripheral flecks.

Thrombocytopenia, hypoparathyroidism, polyneuropathy, thyroid antibodies, prolinuria, and ichthyosis have also been described.

The *Fechtner* variant of Alport syndrome is characterized by renal disease, hearing loss, cataracts, and the May Hegglin anomaly (giant platelets, thrombocytopenia, and white blood cell inclusions).

Complications: Those of chronic renal disease.

Associated Findings: Hearing loss in 40–60%; ocular defects in 15%; thrombocytopenia, hypoparathyroidism, polyneuropathy, and ichthyosis in less than 10%.

Etiology: X-linked inheritance with greater severity in males. Some pedigrees have suggested autosomal dominant inheritance. Autosomal recessive transmission has also been reported, though not so well established. The *Fechtner* variant is autosomal dominant with variable expressivity.

Pathogenesis: Unknown. Renal pathology is variable even among members of the same family. Earliest alteration is thickening of glomerular basement membrane. Abnormal antigenicity of the basement membrane has been reported. In some individuals, the histologic pattern is similar to glomerulonephritis; in others, there is periglomerular fibrosis with tubular atrophy and interstitial infiltrates resembling pyelonephritis. Foam cells, although not limited to Alport syndrome, are frequently seen in later stages of disease. The initial renal lesions are mild and tend to progress slowly. Immunofluorescence is negative. Temporal bone histologic findings are inconsistent; atrophy of the organ of Corti and hyalinization and thinning of the tectorial membrane have been described.

MIM No.: *10420, 20378, *30105

CDC No.: 759.870

Sex Ratio: M1:F2 unless autosomal; then M1:F1

Occurrence: Accounts for an estimated one-sixth of familial glomerular disease.

Risk of Recurrence for Patient's Sib:
See Part I, *Mendelian Inheritance.*

Risk of Recurrence for Patient's Child:
See Part I, *Mendelian Inheritance.*

Age of Detectability: As early as the first few weeks of life, by intermittent albuminuria and microscopic hematuria. It might be possible to detect the thrombocytopenia and giant platelets of the *Fechtner* variant through fetal blood sampling.

Gene Mapping and Linkage: ATS (Alport syndrome) has been mapped to Xq21.3-q24.

Prevention: None known. Genetic counseling indicated.

Treatment: Peritoneal or hemodialysis in cases of renal failure. Kidney transplantation has been successful in many patients.

Prognosis: Males have a poor outlook, with death from uremia likely before age 30 and often during adolescence. The condition in females is variable but usually benign, though renal abnormalities persist. While quite uncommon, death from renal failure may occur in females.

Detection of Carrier: Presence of either nephritis or sensorineural deafness with a history of other affected family members.

Special Considerations: An autosomal recessive syndrome of nephropathy, deafness, and hyperparathyroidism has been described in several members of a consangineous Pakistani family (Edwards et al, 1989). The hematuria and proteinuria found in Alport syndrome were, however, lacking.

References:

Myers GJ, Tyler HR: The etiology of deafness in Alport's syndrome. Arch Otolaryngol 1972; 96:333–340.
Gubler M, et al.: Alport's syndrome: report of 58 cases and review of the literature. Am J Med 1981; 70:493–505. * †
Yosikawa N, et al.: Glomerular basal lamina in hereditary nephritis. J Pathol 1981; 135:199–209.
Drayna D, et al.: Genetic mapping of human X chromosome by using RFLPs. Proc Natl Acad Sci USA 1984; 81:2836–2839.
Hasstedt SJ, et al.: Genetic heterogeneity among kindreds with Alport syndrome. Am J Hum Genet 1986; 38:940–953.
Melvin T, et al.: Amyloid P component is not present in the glomerular basement membrane in Alport-type hereditary nephritis. Am J Path 1986; 125:460–464.
Yoshikawa N, et al.: Nonfamilial hematuria associated with glomerular basement membrane alterations charcteristic of hereditary nephritis. J Pediatr 1987; 111:519–524.
Flinter F, et al.: Genetics of classic Alport's syndrome. Lancet 1988; 2:1005–1007. *
Gershoni-Baruch R, et al.: Fechtner syndrome: clinical and genetic aspects. Am J Med Genet 1988; 31:357–367. †
Edwards BD, et al.: A new syndrome of autosomal recessive nephropathy, deafness, and hyperparathyroidism. J Med Genet 1989; 26:289–293.

BA041 **Harold N. Bass**

Nephritis-deafness-macrothrombopathia
See DEAFNESS-NEPHRITIS-MACROTHROMBOPATHIA
Nephritis-megathrombocytopenia-deafness
See LEUKOCYTE, MAY-HEGGLIN ANOMALY
Nephroblastoma
See CANCER, WILMS TUMOR
Nephroblastomatosis
See CANCER, WILMS TUMOR
Nephrogenic diabetes insipidus
See DIABETES INSIPIDUS, VASOPRESSIN RESISTANT TYPES I AND II
Nephronophthisis, familial juvenile
See KIDNEY, NEPHRONOPHTHISIS-MEDULLARY CYSTIC DESEASE
Nephronophthisis-medullary cystic disease
See KIDNEY, NEPHRONOPHTHISIS-MEDULLARY CYSTIC DESEASE
Nephronophtisis-associated ocular anomalies, familial juvenile
See RENAL DYSPLASIA-RETINAL APLASIA, LOKEN-SENIOR TYPE
Nephronophtisis-congenital hepatic
See HEPATIC FIBROSIS, CONGENITAL
Nephropathic cystinosis
See CYSTINOSIS
Nephropathy-deafness, hereditary type
See NEPHRITIS-DEAFNESS (SENSORINEURAL), HEREDITARY TYPE
Nephropathy-diabetes-deafness-photomyoclonus
See DEAFNESS-DIABETES-PHOTOMYOCLONUS-NEPHROPATHY
Nephropathy-hypoparathyroidism-lymphedema
See LYMPHEDEMA-HYPOPARATHYROIDISM
Nephropathy-pseudohermaphroditism-Wilms tumor
See WILMS TUMOR-PSEUDOHERMAPHRODITISM-GLOMERULOPATHY, DENYS-DRASH TYPE

NEPHROSIS, CONGENITAL 0709

Includes:
Finnish nephrosis
Microcystic renal disease
Neonatal nephrosis
Nephrosis, infantile
Pulmonic stenosis-congenital nephrosis

Excludes:
Nephrosis, congenital-diffuse mesangial sclerosis
Nephrosis, familial type (0710)
Nephrotic syndrome, hereditary late
Nephropathies (other)

Major Diagnostic Criteria: Edema, hypoproteinemia, hypoalbuminemia, and proteinuria at birth or shortly thereafter. Onset occurs before the age of four months. Tests are negative for syphilis, malaria, mercury, toxoplasma and cytomegalovirus. Renal biopsy shows cystic dilatation of proximal tubules in cortex.

Clinical Findings: Newborns present with edema, abdominal distention, hypoproteinemia, hypoalbuminemia, and proteinuria. Occasionally the edema is absent at birth, but shortly thereafter it becomes generalized, severe, and persistent. Congenital nephrosis may be suspected when the placenta is large and heavy (25–40% of the weight of the infant) and the infant has a low birth weight. Respiratory distress is often seen in the postnatal period. Laboratory findings consist of proteinuria; hypoproteinemia with serum protein of 2.5–3.7 g/dl; low serum albumin of 0.4–0.9 g/dl. Serum cholesterol may be lower than 200 mg initially, but in most cases, this value varies between 200–400 mg with tendency to rise as high as 800 mg. Many infants die within the first year as a result of infection and, rarely, as the result of renal failure.

Complications: Electrolyte imbalance, infections, renal failure, retardation of growth and development, and coagulation abnormalities.

Associated Findings: Hypothyroidism, pyloric stenosis, and gastroesophageal reflux. One family reported by Fournier et al (1963) had a combination of pulmonary stenosis and congenital nephrosis in the four affected children.

Etiology: Autosomal recessive inheritance. In nearly one-third of the marriages, consanguinity has been noted.

Pathogenesis: Hypothesized inborn error of metabolism that leads to faulty structure of glomerular basal lamina. Decreased heparan sulfate-rich anionic sites have been demonstrated in the lamina rara externa of the glomerular basement membrane. Loss of negatively charged sites may lead to penetration of basement membrane by proteins.

MIM No.: *25630, 26560

Sex Ratio: M1:F1

Occurrence: In Finland, the incidence is 1:10,000 live births. Elsewhere, the incidence is undetermined. Prevalence is undetermined but the greatest number of cases have been reported from Finland and areas outside of Finland where there is a large aggregation of people of Finnish extraction.

Risk of Recurrence for Patient's Sib:
See Part I, *Mendelian Inheritance.*

Risk of Recurrence for Patient's Child:
See Part I, *Mendelian Inheritance.* Affected individuals are not expected to survive to reproduce.

Age of Detectability: At birth or shortly thereafter, by clinical picture. Prenatal detection is available, since mothers at risk of bearing a child with congenital nephrosis have been noted to have markedly elevated alpha-fetoprotein in their own sera and amniotic fluid starting from the 15th week of gestation.

Gene Mapping and Linkage: Unknown.

Prevention: None known. Genetic counseling indicated.

Treatment: Steroid and other immunosuppressive drugs are of no demonstrated value. Successful renal transplantations have been reported. Adequate therapy for infections is necessary.

Prognosis: Very poor without renal transplantation. No recurrences in transplanted kidney. Without transplantation, most succumb within first year of life.

Detection of Carrier: Unknown.

References:
Fournier A, et al.: Syndromes nephrotiques familiaux: syndrome nephrotigue associe a une cardiopathie congenitale chez quatre soeurs. Pediatrie 1963; 18; 677–685.
Hoyer JR, et al.: The nephrotic syndrome of infancy: clinical, morphological and immunological studies of four infants. Pediatrics 1967; 40:233–246.
Hoyer JR, et al.: Successful renal transplantation in 3 children with congenital nephrotic syndrome. Lancet 1973; I:1410–1412.
Aula P, et al.: Prenatal diagnosis of congenital nephrosis in 23 high-risk families. Am J Dis Child 1978; 132:984–987.
Rapola J, Hallman N: A.F.P and congenital nephrosis, Finnish type. Lancet 1979; I:274–275.
Risteli L, et al.: Slow accumulation of basement membrane collagen in kidney cortex in congenital nephrotic syndrome Lancet 1982; I:712–714.
Vernier RL, et al: Heparan sulfate-rich anionic sites in the human glomerular basement membrane: decreased concentration in congenital nephrotic syndrome. New Engl J Med 1983; 309:1001–1009. *
Mahan JD, et al.: Congenital nephrotic syndrome: evolution of medical management and results of renal transplantation. J Pediatr 1984; 105:549–557. *

M0035

Donald I. Moel

NEPHROSIS, FAMILIAL TYPE 0710

Includes:
Nephrotic syndrome occurring postnatally, familial
Nephrotic syndrome-focal glomerular sclerosis

Excludes:
Nephritis-deafness (sensorineural), hereditary type (0708)
Nephritis, other types of hereditary
Nephrosis, congenital (0709)
Nephrosis-nerve deafness-hypoparathyroidism, Barakat type (3026)

Major Diagnostic Criteria: Edema, hypoproteinemia, hypercholesterolemia, and proteinuria. Renal biopsy may reveal findings of minimal change disease, membranoproliferative glomerulonephritis, mesangial sclerosis, and IgM nephropathy. A family history of nephrosis helps to confirm the diagnosis.

Clinical Findings: Onset of familial nephrosis, with the insidious onset of edema, is similar to all types of nephrosis. Anasarca is not present at birth but may appear as early as two months of age. There may be a history of an upper respiratory infection prior to the onset of edema. With increasing edema, there is often history of a decrease in urinary output. Physical examination reveals generalized edema, at times including ascites. Hypertension and hematuria are generally absent at onset. Laboratory studies reveal severe-to-moderate proteinuria, hypoproteinemia, hypercholesterolemia, normal BUN, and no marked reduction in creatinine clearance at onset. Recently, low or absent immunoglobulin levels have been reported in this syndrome. Absence of protective immunoglobulins may contribute to the observed high rate of sepsis in affected infants. Serum complement levels are normal. It is not until the same type of nephrosis develops in a sib that one becomes aware this this is a familial form of nephrosis. Familial nerve deafness is not associated with this form of renal disease and, if present, suggests **Nephritis-deafness (sensorineural), hereditary type** (Alport syndrome).

The course may follow two patterns of response to steroid therapy and outcome. In one group, steroid therapy produces little or no improvement, and death from infection or renal failure ultimately results. Alternatively, the patient responds to steroids, with evidence of complete remission; thereafter the patient may have one or more relapses that respond to steroid therapy, but eventually there is complete recovery. The pattern of response in the second involved member of the family usually follows a course similar to that of the first affected sib.

Complications: Extremely low immunoglobulin levels may predispose the newborn to sepsis. For those who do not respond to steroids, infection or renal failure may be the cause of death. For those who are steroid-responsive, the clinical course may be relatively uncomplicated.

Associated Findings: None known.

Etiology: Undetermined. Autosomal recessive inheritance seems likely.

Pathogenesis: Unknown.

MIM No.: 25635

Sex Ratio: M1:F<1

Occurrence: Undetermined. Established literature.

Risk of Recurrence for Patient's Sib:
See Part I, *Mendelian Inheritance.*

Risk of Recurrence for Patient's Child:
See Part I, *Mendelian Inheritance.*

Age of Detectability: Anytime after the age of two months.

Gene Mapping and Linkage: Unknown.

Prevention: None known. Genetic counseling indicated.

Treatment: Steroid therapy, antibiotics.

Prognosis: The prognosis is favorable for those patients who are steroid-responsive. If there is no response to steroid therapy, the prognosis is unfavorable.

Detection of Carrier: Unknown.

Special Considerations: The pathologic findings vary and do not provide a means to distinguish this form of the nephrotic syndrome from nonfamilial forms. Some may show no abnormalities on routine light microscopy of the kidney; however, on electron microscopy, there is fusion of the foot processes (so-called minimal change). In others, the microscopic features are those of membranous glomerulonephritis, with or without lobular nephritis or focal sclerosing glomerulonephritis. The form with minimal change renal pathology is the steroid-responsive form; with a good outlook for ultimate recovery.

References:

Moncrieff M, et al.: The familial nephrotic syndrome: a clinicopathological study. Clin Nephrol 1973; 1:220–229. *

White R: The familial nephrotic syndrome: a European study. Clin Nephrol 1973; 1:215–219.

Bader P, et al.: Familial nephrotic syndrome. Am J Med 1974; 56:34–43. *

Naruse T, et al.: Familial nephrotic syndrome with focal glomerular sclerosis. Am J Med Sci 1980; 280:109–113.

Chandra M, et al.: Familial nephrotic syndrome and focal segmental glomerulosclerosis. J Pediatr 1981; 98:556–560.

Tejani A, et al.: Familial focal segmental glomerulosclerosis. Int J Ped Nephrol 1983; 4:231–234.

Harris HW, et al.: Altered immunoglobulin status in congenital nephrotic syndrome. Clin Nephrol 1986; 25:308–313.

LI022   **David A. Link**

Nephrosis, infantile
See NEPHROSIS, CONGENITAL
Nephrosis-deafness-digital anomalies
See NEPHROSIS-HYDROCEPHALUS-THIN SKIN-BLUE SCLERA-GROWTH DEFECT

NEPHROSIS-DEAFNESS-URINARY TRACT AND DIGITAL DEFECTS   3122

Includes:

Braun-Bayer syndrome
Deafness-nephrosis-urinary tract and digital defects
Digital defects-nephrosis-deafness urinary tract defects
Urinary tract and digital defects-nephrosis-deafness

Excludes:

Deafness-nephritis-macrothrombopathia (3046)
Nephrosis-nerve deafness-hypoparathyroidism, Barakat type (3026)
Renal tubular acidosis (0862)

Major Diagnostic Criteria: Familial nephrosis, familial deafness, congenital urinary tract abnormalities, digital defects.

Clinical Findings: Nephrotic syndrome, conductive and sometimes perceptive deafness, urinary tract abnormalities (ureterovesical and bladder neck obstruction, duplication of collecting system, hydronephrosis), digital abnormalities (short and bifid distal phalanges of thumbs and big toes), bifurcation of the uvula.

Complications: Hydronephrosis, pyelonephritis.

Associated Findings: Allergic manifestations with bronchial asthma.

Etiology: Presumably either autosomal recessive or X-linked dominant inheritance.

Pathogenesis: Unknown.

MIM No.: 25620

POS No.: 4340

Sex Ratio: M5:F0 (observed).

Occurrence: Five brothers have been reported in the literature.

Risk of Recurrence for Patient's Sib:
See Part I, *Mendelian Inheritance*.

Risk of Recurrence for Patient's Child:
See Part I, *Mendelian Inheritance*.

Age of Detectability: Most patients have been diagnosed before age two years.

Gene Mapping and Linkage: Unknown.

Prevention: None known. Genetic counseling indicated.

Treatment: As per the respective manifestations.

Prognosis: No follow-up of the known affected individuals has been reported.

Detection of Carrier: The deafness and digital anomalies in one brother and the isolated nephrosis in another may represent a variable expression of the same gene.

References:

Braun FC, Jr., Bayer JF: Familial nephrosis associated with deafness and congenital urinary tract anomalies in siblings. J Pediatr 1962; 60:33–41.

BA065   **Amin Y. Barakat**

NEPHROSIS-HYDROCEPHALUS-THIN SKIN-BLUE SCLERA-GROWTH DEFECT   2187

Includes:

Ehlers-Danlos, type IV (possible form)
Growth defect-hydrocephalus-nephrosis-thin skin-blue sclera
Hydrocephalus-nephrosis-thin skin-blue sclera-growth defect
Microcephaly-nephrosis-hiatal hernia
Nephrosis-deafness-digital anomalies
Sclera (blue)-hydrocephalus-nephrosis-thin skin-growth defect
Skin (thin)-hydrocephalus-nephrosis-blue sclera-growth defect

Excludes:

Ehlers-Danlos syndrome (0338)
Microcephaly-hiatus hernia-nephrosis, Galloway type (2755)
Nephrosis-deafness-urinary tract and digital defects (3122)

Major Diagnostic Criteria: Infantile nephrosis; **Hydrocephaly**; thin, transparent skin.

Clinical Findings: Based on two brothers: nephrosis, hydrocephaly, thin skin, blue sclera, growth delay, recurrent infections, and T-cell dysfunction. In addition, both brothers had distinctive facial features, including frontal prominence, narrow midface, thin upper lip, and small ears.

Complications: Both children developed renal failure and died by age three years.

Associated Findings: Recurrent otitis media.

Etiology: Possible autosomal or X-linked recessive inheritance.

Pathogenesis: Possible collagen defect.

POS No.: 3846

Sex Ratio: M2:F0 (observed).

Occurrence: Reported in two brothers of one family.

Risk of Recurrence for Patient's Sib:
See Part I, *Mendelian Inheritance*.

Risk of Recurrence for Patient's Child:
See Part I, *Mendelian Inheritance*. No affected individuals have survived to reproduce.

Age of Detectability: Usually at birth. Prenatal detection theoretically possible in at-risk pregnancies if hydrocephaly or polyhydramnios is detected by ultrasound.

Gene Mapping and Linkage: Unknown.

Prevention: None known. Genetic counseling indicated.

Treatment: Nephrosis has not been responsive to steroids.

Prognosis: Death in both sibs by three years of age. Otherwise, normal development.

Detection of Carrier: Unknown.

Special Considerations: Another two male sibs with nephrosis and neuronal heterotopias (and hydrocephalus in one) were reported by Palm et al. (1986). It is uncertain whether these sibs had the same disorder, since there was no mention of thin skin, blue sclera or similar facial features in the clinical description.

References:
Daentl DL, et al.: Familial nephrosis, hydrocephalus, thin skin, blue sclerae syndrome: clinical, structural, and biochemical studies. BD:OAS XIV(6B). New York: March of Dimes Birth Defects Foundation, 1978:315–339.
Palm L, et al.: Nephrosis and disturbances of neuronal migration in male siblings - a new hereditary disorder? Arch Dis Child 1986; 61:545–548.
Beighton P, et al.: International nosology of heritable disorders of connective tissue, Berlin, 1986. Am J Med Genet 1988; 29:581–594.

GR011   **Frank Greenberg**

Nephrosis-microcephaly-hiatus hernia, Galloway type
See MICROCEPHALY-HIATUS HERNIA-NEPHROSIS, GALLOWAY TYPE

NEPHROSIS-NERVE DEAFNESS-HYPOPARATHYROIDISM, BARAKAT TYPE   3026

Includes:
Barakat syndrome
Deafness (nerve)-nephrosis-hypoparathyroidism
Hypoparathyroidism-nephrosis-nerve deafness

Excludes:
Immunodeficiency, thymic agenesis (0943)
Nephritis-deafness (sensorineural), hereditary type (0708)

Major Diagnostic Criteria: Steroid-resistant nephrotic syndrome, bilateral nerve deafness, hypoparathyroidism.

Clinical Findings: Asymptomatic proteinuria progressing to nephrotic syndrome, severe bilateral nerve deafness, edema, vomiting, lethargy.

Complications: Chronic renal failure, nephrocalcinosis.

Associated Findings: Absent or hypoplastic parathyroid glands.

Etiology: Probably autosomal recessive or X-linked inheritance.

Pathogenesis: Unknown.

MIM No.: 25634

POS No.: 3821

Sex Ratio: M4:F0 observed.

Occurrence: Reported in four brothers, two of whom were twins.

Risk of Recurrence for Patient's Sib:
See Part I, *Mendelian Inheritance.*

Risk of Recurrence for Patient's Child:
See Part I, *Mendelian Inheritance.*

Age of Detectability: During early childhood.

Gene Mapping and Linkage: Unknown.

Prevention: None known. Genetic counseling indicated.

Treatment: Unknown. Kidney transplantation was not attempted.

Prognosis: All four patients died with uremia before eight years of age.

Detection of Carrier: Unknown.

References:
Barakat AY, et al.: Familial nephrosis, nerve deafness, and hypoparathyroidism. J Pediatr 1977; 91:61–64.

BA065   **Amin Y. Barakat**

Nephrotic syndrome occurring postnatally, familial
See NEPHROSIS, FAMILIAL TYPE

Nephrotic syndrome-focal glomerular sclerosis
See NEPHROSIS, FAMILIAL TYPE
Nerve malformations of middle ear
See EAR, OSSICLE AND MIDDLE EAR MALFORMATIONS
Nerve trunk palsies, familial
See NEUROPATHY, HEREDITARY WITH PRESSURE PALSIES
Nervous system endemic cretinism
See CRETINISM, ENDEMIC, AND RELATED DISORDERS
Netherton syndrome
See ICHTHYOSIS, LINEARIS CIRCUMFLEXA
Netilmycin, fetal effects
See FETAL AMINOGLYCOSIDE OTOTOXICITY
Netromycin^, fetal effects
See FETAL AMINOGLYCOSIDE OTOTOXICITY
Nettleship-Falls ocular albinism
See ALBINISM, OCULAR
Neu syndrome
See NEU-LAXOVA SYNDROME

NEU-LAXOVA SYNDROME   2092

Includes: Neu syndrome

Excludes:
Cerebral-arthro digital syndrome
Cerebro-oculo-facio-skeletal syndrome (0140)
Lissencephaly syndrome (0603)
Pena-Shokeir syndrome (2080)
Pterygium syndrome, multiple lethal (2274)

Major Diagnostic Criteria: Should be considered in an infant who is stillborn or dies shortly after birth who has the major features of intrauterine growth retardation, generalized edema, limb contractures, and abnormalities in central nervous system development. Icthyotic-like skin changes are also common.

Clinical Findings: *Pregnancy*: Frequent polyhydramnios (12/14). Third trimester ultrasound abnormalities have included hydramnios, scalp edema, hydrothorax, microcephaly, and growth retardation. *Delivery*: Term (11/14). Short umbilical cord in at least six cases. *Survival*: Stillborn (7/14). 6/14 died within hours. The longest survivor was seven weeks of age.
Physical examination and growth parameters: Affected infants have usually demonstrated extremely low birth weights, lengths, and head circumferences. Reduction in head circumference is, however, the most striking and uniform finding. Head circumferences at term have ranged from 20–26.5 cm. Head circumference may, however, be artifactually increased due to the presence of massive scalp edema. One infant had demonstrated macrocephaly in association with a midline cleft and probable hydranencephaly (Povýšilová, et al (1976).
Craniofacial findings: Sloping forehead and hypertelorism are described in over one-half the cases. Nasal bridge is described as broad and prominent. Eyes have frequently been abnormal. Prominent protuberant eyes with retracted, apparently absent lids and ectropion have been noted in five cases, cataracts in three, and microphthalmia in two. Micrognathia is common, and short neck was specifically noted in eight cases.
Limbs: The limbs frequently have shown contractures of the major joints; a few cases had webbing at the knees and elbows. Fingers are frequently described as overlapping, particularly in those without severe hand edema. Rocker bottom feet are described in several cases. Alteration in palmar creases and camptodactyly and clinodactyly of digits has been noted. Partial syndactyly of fingers and toes have been described in five cases. Hands inflated like yellow rubber gloves have been described in five cases. As seen on pathologic examination, this massive swelling is apparently due to deposition of excessive fat, in addition to the presence of edema fluid.
Skin: Generalized edema of the skin has been a uniform finding in all cases, but the severity has varied dramatically. Myxomatous connective tissue has been noted on sections of subcutaneous tissue in two patients; this is an unusual pathologic finding that may be helpful in the diagnosis of this syndrome. The abnormal deposition of fat described pathologically in a few cases may also be helpful diagnostically. The skin has frequently been described

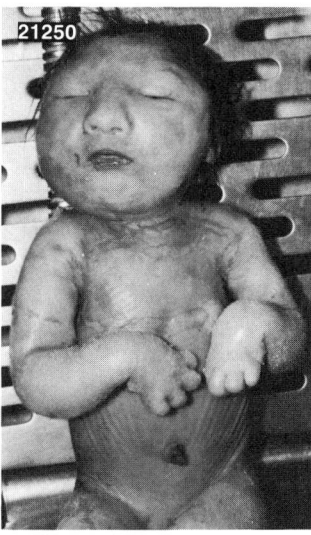
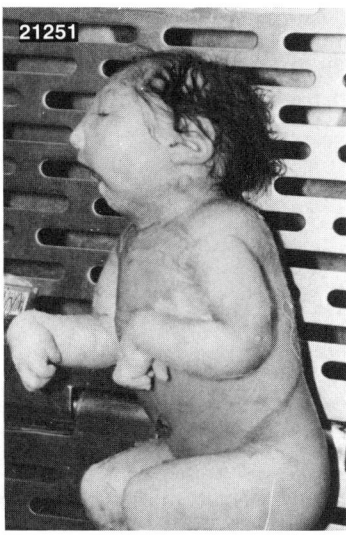
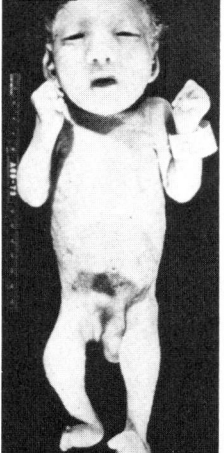
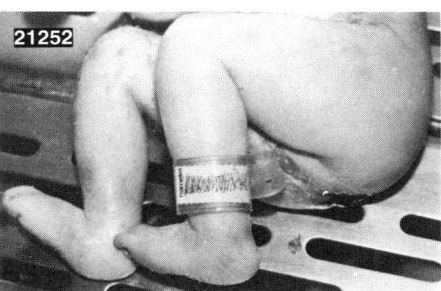

2092-21250–52, 21142: Micrognathia, dysmorphic facies, limb contractures, prominent nasal bridge, sloping forehead, unusual auricles, and edema.

as abnormal, either thin, lemon-colored and scaly; tight, shiny with collodion-like appearance; or ichthyotic. Peeling of the skin and desquamation of the skin in sheets has been a frequent observation. No detailed pathologic examinations of skin have been performed.

X-Ray findings: The skeletal X-rays have generally shown mild undermineralization of the skeleton. Flat acetabular roofs and dysplastic ilia have been noted. Spina bifida occulta at L-5 and S-1 was noted in one case. Intrauterine fractures reported in two cases.

Complications: Lethal.

Associated Findings: Large ventral hernia (1), micropenis (1), and hypoplastic genitalia (2).

Autopsy findings: A neuropathological examinations was performed in nine cases. Hypoplastic cerebellum has been documented in eight, and the absence of the corpus callosum in four. Lissencephaly has been noted in five cases. Several cases have noted dilated lateral ventricles and/or polymicrogyria. Histologic examinations have revealed a thinned cerebral cortex. Other abnormalities at autopsy have included lung hypoplasia, abnor-

mal fetal lobulation of the kidneys, nephroptosis, and gross underdevelopment of skeletal muscle.

Etiology: Autosomal recessive inheritance is presumed on the basis of recurrence in four sibships. Consanguinity has been noted in four reported families.

Pathogenesis: Unknown. No detailed biochemical evaluations of these infants have been performed. It is unlikely that this syndrome is due to a single problem in central nervous system development.

MIM No.: *25652

POS No.: 3326

Sex Ratio: Presumably M1:F1.

Occurrence: About 16 cases have been reported. May be under-diagnosed because of early lethality. Death prior to delivery may also make confirmation of the diagnosis impossible. Three literature reports of Pakistani families (Laxova, 1972, Mueller, 1983) suggests that this gene may be relatively frequent in that population. One family was of Asian-Indian extraction.

Risk of Recurrence for Patient's Sib:
See Part I, *Mendelian Inheritance.*

Risk of Recurrence for Patient's Child:
See Part I, *Mendelian Inheritance.*

Age of Detectability: In utero detection by ultrasound should be possible by the latter half of second trimester, the syndrome is otherwise identified at birth.

Gene Mapping and Linkage: Unknown.

Prevention: None known. Genetic counseling indicated.

Treatment: Unknown.

Prognosis: Lethal.

Detection of Carrier: Unknown.

References:

Neu RL, et al.: A lethal syndrome of microcephaly with multiple congenital anomalies in three siblings. Pediatrics 1971; 47:610–612.

Laxova R, et al.: A further example of a lethal autosomal recessive condition in sibs. J Ment Defic Res 1972: 16:139–143.

Považsilová V, et al.: Letální syndrom mnohočetných malformací u tří sourozenc°u. Ces Pediat 1976; 31:190–194.

Lazjuk GI, et al.: The Neu-Laxova syndrome: a distinct entity. Am J Med Genet 1979; 3:261–267.

Scott C, et al.: Comments on the Neu-Laxova syndrome and the CAD complex. Am J Med Genet 1981; 9:165–175.

Winter RM, et al.: Syndromes of microcephaly, microphthalmia, cataracts and joint contractures. J Med Genet 1981; 18:129–133.

Curry CJR: Further comments on the Neu-Laxova syndrome. Am J Med Genet 1982; 13:441–444.

Fitch N, et al.: The Neu-Laxova syndrome: comments on syndrome identification. Am J Med Genet 1982; 13:445–452.

Karimi-Nejad MH, et al.: Neu-Laxova syndrome: report of a case and comments. Am J Med Genet 1987; 28:17–23.

Muller LM, et al.: A case of the Neu-Laxova syndrome: prenatal ultrasonographic monitoring in the third trimester and the histopathological findings. Am J Med Genet 1987; 26:421–429.

Ostrovskaya TI, Lazjuk GI: Cerebral abnormalities in the Neu-Laxova syndrome. Am J Med Genet 1988; 30:747–756.

CU009   **Cynthia J.R. Curry**

Neural crest, syndrome of
See NEUROPATHY, CONGENITAL SENSORY WITH ANHIDROSIS
Neural deafness, recessive early-onset
See DEAFNESS (SENSORINEURAL), RECESSIVE EARLY-ONSET
Neural tube defects (some)
See SCHISIS ASSOCIATION
Neural tube defects, X-linked
See ANENCEPHALY
Neural-tube defect
See MENINGOMYELOCELE
also MENINGOCELE
Neuralgic amyotrophy, familial
See NEUROPATHY, HEREDITARY RECURRENT BRACHIAL
Neuralgic amyotrophy-brachial predilection, familial
See NEUROPATHY, HEREDITARY RECURRENT BRACHIAL

Neuraminidase deficiency
See MUCOLIPIDOSIS I
also MUCOLIPIDOSIS IV
Neuraminidase deficiency with beta-galactosidase deficiency
See GALACTOSIALIDOSIS
Neuraminidase/beta-galactosidase expression
See GALACTOSIALIDOSIS
Neurenteric cyst
See ESOPHAGUS, DUPLICATION
Neurenteric cyst of spinal cord
See SPINAL CORD, NEURENTERIC CYST
Neuritis with brachial predilection, heredo-familial
See NEUROPATHY, HEREDITARY RECURRENT BRACHIAL
Neuritis, peripheral with isoniazid
See NEUROPATHY, HERITABLE ISONIAZIDE TYPE (INH)

NEURO-FACIO-DIGITO-RENAL SYNDROME 2897

Includes: NFDR syndrome

Excludes: FG syndrome, Opitz-Kaveggia type (0754)

Major Diagnostic Criteria: Limb malformations, renal agenesis, high and prominent forehead, vertical groove on tip of nose, ear abnormalities, **Megalencephaly**, hypotonia, mental retardation, and abnormal EEG.

Clinical Findings: Long thumbs with unilateral triphalangism, broad halluces, flat feet, valgus hips, winging of scapulae, hyperextensible elbows, protruding abdomen, small testes, mandibular prognathism, intrauterine growth retardation, shortness of stature, disproportionately great OFC (see **Megalencephaly**), unilateral renal agenesis, hypotonia, mental retardation, abnormal EEG, high and prominent forehead, vertical groove on tip of nose, frontal upsweep of hairline, bilateral alternating exotropia, epicanthal folds.

Complications: Poor school performance.

Associated Findings: None known.

Etiology: Autosomal recessive or possibly X-linked recessive inheritances.

Pathogenesis: Unknown.

MIM No.: 25669

POS No.: 4336

Sex Ratio: M2:F0 (observed).

Occurrence: Two Brazilian brothers have been reported.

Risk of Recurrence for Patient's Sib:
See Part I, *Mendelian Inheritance.*

Risk of Recurrence for Patient's Child:
See Part I, *Mendelian Inheritance.*

Age of Detectability: At birth, by physical examination.

Gene Mapping and Linkage: Unknown.

Prevention: None known. Genetic counseling indicated.

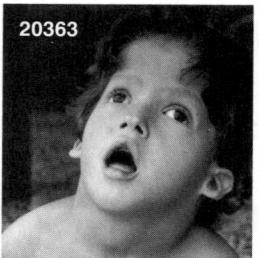 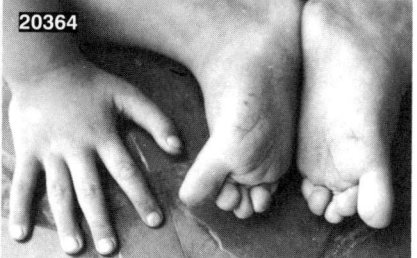

2897-20363: Mouth-breathing facies, small and abnormal auricles, exotropia, vertical groove on tip of the nose and frontal upsweep of the hairline. **20364:** Large halluces and long thumb.

Treatment: Early special education; special medical care mainly in case of problems with the solitary kidney.

Prognosis: Probably normal life span with good medical care.

Detection of Carrier: Unknown.

References:
Freire-Maia N, et al.: The neurofaciodigitorenal (NFDR) syndrome. Am J Med Genet 1982; 11:329–336.

FR033 **Newton Freire-Maia**

Neuro-facio-skeletal syndrome
See FACIO-NEURO-SKELETAL SYNDROME
Neuroacanthocytosis
See ACANTHOCYTOSIS-NEUROLOGIC DEFECTS

NEUROAXONAL DYSTROPHY, INFANTILE 2701

Includes: Seitelberger disease

Excludes:
Alpha-N-acetylgalactosaminidase deficiency (3254)
Brain, spongy degeneration (0115)
Encephalopathy, necrotizing (0344)
Hallervorden-Spatz disease (2526)
Metachromatic leukodystrophies (0651)
Neuroaxonal dystrophy, secondary
Pelizaeus-Merzbacher syndrome (0803)

Major Diagnostic Criteria: The disease can be suspected in an initially normal infant who first exhibits slowing and/or arrest of development, followed by deterioration, with marked hypotonia and visual and auditory impairment, usually unaccompanied by seizures. Confirmation requires demonstration of axonal spheroids either in the brain or via a muscle, skin, or conjunctival biopsy that includes peripheral nerve endings. The electromyo-

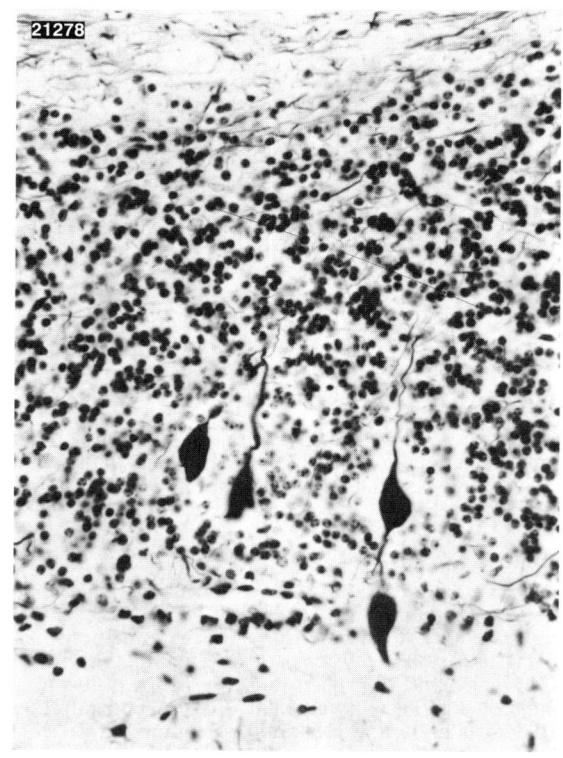

2701-21278: Axonal spheroids in the cerebellum (×400).

gram (EMG) may show denervation changes with normal nerve conduction. Electroretinogram (ERG) findings are normal, but there is a decreased or absent visual envoked response.

Clinical Findings: The most common manifestation is a slowing and/or arrest of development, or a disturbance in gait, between the ages of six months and two years of age, in a previously healthy child. The degree of hypotonia is striking, and may suggest a myopathy, although the children may eventually become spastic. Pyramidal tract signs with upgoing toes and hyperreflexia are characteristic, although reflexes may be decreased due to the marked hypotonia and weakness. Visual impairment is early and significant, and characterized by strabismus, pendular nystagmus, dysconjugate eye movement, and decreased vision with optic atrophy. Hearing and response to tactile stimulation are also impaired.

The clinical course is one of progressive dementia and decerebration, with death before 10 years of age. The central, peripheral, and often autonomic systems are involved. Axonal spheroids are not specific to neuroaxonal dystrophy, and it is the combined clinical and overall pathologic distribution that is diagnostic. The spheroid bodies are widespread in the CNS, especially in the cortex, spinal cord, brainstem, basal ganglia, and peripheral nerve endings in the skin, neuromuscular junctions, and conjunctiva. Atrophy is prominent in the cerebellum, optic pathways, pyramidal tracts, brainstem nuclei, and inferior olivary bodies; there is marked gliosis, especially in the cerebral hemispheres.

Complications: The progressive neurologic deterioration with inanition increases the susceptibility to respiratory disease and aspiration which are commonly the immediate cause of death.

Associated Findings: None known.

Etiology: Autosomal recessive inheritance with very little intrafamilial variation in expression.

Pathogenesis: Undetermined in most cases, but the axonal dystrophy is probably primary. Schindler et al (1989) detected a deficiency of α-N-acetylgalactosamidase in two affected brothers, but the results in eight unrelated patients were normal.

MIM No.: *25660

Sex Ratio: M1:F1

Occurrence: Fewer than 100 cases have been reported. Patients have been reported from most European countries, Israel, the United States, Canada, and Japan.

Risk of Recurrence for Patient's Sib:
See Part I, *Mendelian Inheritance.*

Risk of Recurrence for Patient's Child:
See Part I, *Mendelian Inheritance.* Affected individuals are not expected to survive to reproduce.

Age of Detectability: The typical infantile case shows clinical signs between the ages of six months to two years. A few cases with either earlier or later onset have been reported. The earliest age at which axonal spheroids might be seen on biopsy of peripheral nerve endings is undetermined.

Gene Mapping and Linkage: Unknown.

Prevention: None known. Genetic counseling indicated.

Treatment: Supportive.

Prognosis: Life expectancy is less than ten years, and death usually occurs about five years from onset.

Detection of Carrier: Unknown.

Special Considerations: Several children of both sexes have been reported with prenatal or connatal onset of axonal dystrophy. These children have displayed a rapidly lethal course, with more frequent seizures and less pathologic involvement of the cerebellum. Two male sibs with prenatal onset of neuroaxonal dystrophy manifested a dry peripheral gangrene at two months of age that resulted in autoamputation of the toes and distal fingertips. X-linked recessive inheritance cannot be ruled out for these cases.

References:
Jellinger K: Neuroaxonal dystrophy: its natural history and related disorders. In: Zimmerman HM, ed: Progress in neuropathology, Vol 2. New York: Grune and Stratton, 1973:129–180. *
Aicardi J, Castelein P: Infantile neuroaxonal dystrophy. Brain 1979; 102:727–748. *
Janota I: Neuroaxonal dystrophy in the neonate. Acta Neuropathol 1979; 46:151–154.
Hunter AGW, et al.: Neuroaxonal dystrophy presenting with neonatal dysmorphic features, early onset of peripheral gangrene, and a rapidly lethal course. Am J Med Genet 1987; 28:171–180.
Ramaekers VT, et al.: Diagnostic difficulties in infantile neuroaxonal dystrophy: a clinicopathological study of eight cases. Neuropediatrics 1987; 18:170–175.
Schindler D, et al.: Neuroaxonal dystrophy due to lysosomal α-N-acetylgalactosamidase deficiency. New Engl J Med 1989; 320:1735–1740.

HU008   **Alasdair G.W. Hunter**

Neuroaxonal dystrophy, infantile (one form)
See ALPHA-N-ACETYLGALACTOSAMINIDASE DEFICIENCY
Neuroaxonal dystrophy, late-infantile
See HALLERVORDEN-SPATZ DISEASE
Neuroblastoma and related lesions (all types)
See CANCER, NEUROBLASTOMA
Neuroblastoma, adult
See CANCER, EWING SARCOMA
Neurocutaneous melanosis
See SKIN, NEUROCUTANEOUS MELANOSIS

NEUROCUTANEOUS MELANOSIS   2014

Includes:
  Melanosis, neurocutaneous
  Skin, neurocutaneous melanosis

Excludes:
  Jaw, neuroectodermal pigmented tumor (0711)
  Melanosis coli
  Melanotic neuroectodermal tumor of the brain during infancy
  Skin, cutaneous melanosis, diffuse (2309)
  Skin, hyperpigmentation, familial (2362)

Major Diagnostic Criteria: Congenital giant or multiple melanocytic nevi associated with leptomeningeal melanosis. The skin lesions should be benign, and there should be no presence of malignant melanoma in other organs to assure that the leptomeningeal melanoma is an independent lesion.

Clinical Findings: The skin lesions are characterized by single or multiple giant hairy pigmented nevi, usually assuming a "cape" or "bathing suit" distribution. The multiple large pigmented nevi are usually less common. Both types of lesions represent cosmetic problems. CNS involvement consists of a marked infiltration and pigmentation of melanin-containing cells of the leptomeninges at the base of the brain and over the brainstem. On most of the patients studied the areas frequently affected included the pons, medulla, cerebellum, cerebral peduncles, interpeduncular fossae, and the inferior surfaces of the frontal, temporal, and occipital lobes. A diffuse pigmentation and thickening of the full length of the spinal cord meninges is present in 20% of the cases. A variety of neurologic features may be present depending on the site and the extent of the primary leptomeningeal tumor. These may include epilepsy, psychiatric disturbances, meningeal hemorrhage, cranial nerve palsies, subdural hemorrhage, and intracranial hemorrhage. The first presentation of this disorder, usually occurring during early life, is often the development of hydrocephalus secondary to obstruction of the cerebrospinal fluid (CSF) circulation either at the fourth ventricular outlets or within the basal subarachnoid cisterns. Although the CSF may be normal, the CSF protein content is commonly elevated and glucose concentration decreased. Cytologic examination may show the presence of melanin-containing cells.

Complications: Melanoma and death.

Associated Findings: Progressive **Syringomyelia** has been reported. Seizures, mental retardation, and **Hydrocephaly** have also been reported.

Etiology: Possibly autosomal recessive inheritance.

Pathogenesis: Melanocytes are known to exist normally in the epidermis, hair bulb, uveal tract, retina, and leptomeninges. In these areas they commonly reach sufficient numbers to enable pigmentation to be observed microscopically. Neurocutaneous melanosis is thought to be due to an excessive accumulation of melanin-producing cells in a local or diffuse distribution within both the skin and the leptomeninges. Ultrastructural studies of pigment cells in nevi and meningeal melanosis have shown a marked similarity of cellular structures consistent with a neural crest origin for pigment cells.

Ferris et al (1987) have suggested that this condition could be a consequence of one or more somatic mutations which would result in prenatal lethality if they occurred in the germ line cells.

MIM No.: 24940

POS No.: 3757

Sex Ratio: Presumably M1:F1.

Occurrence: Undetermined but presumably rare.

Risk of Recurrence for Patient's Sib:
See Part I, *Mendelian Inheritance.*

Risk of Recurrence for Patient's Child:
See Part I, *Mendelian Inheritance.*

Age of Detectability: In the first decade of life.

Gene Mapping and Linkage: Unknown.

Prevention: None known. Genetic counseling indicated.

Treatment: Skin lesions can be removed by a plastic surgeon and replaced by a flap or by using skin expanders. Treating hydrocephalus with shunting procedures helps to prevent the dissemination of melanoma; this procedure has only been palliative. There is no effective treatment for primary malignant leptomeningeal melanosis.

Prognosis: Death often usually occurs in early childhood, often as a result of malignant degeneration or occlusion of the ventricular outflow areas.

Detection of Carrier: Unknown.

References:

Reed WB, et al.: Giant pigmented nevi, melanoma, and leptomeningeal melanocytosis: a clinical and histopathological study. Arch Dermatol 1965; 91:100–119.

Lamas E, et al.: Neurocutaneous melanosis: report of a case and review of the literature. Acta Neurochir (Wien) 1977; 36:93–105.

Leaney BJ, et al.: Neurocutaneous melanosis with hydrocephalus and syringomyelia: a case report. J Neurosurg 1985; 62:148–52.

Yu HS, et al.: Neurocutaneous melanosis: electron microscopic comparison of the pigmented melanocytic nevi of skin and meningeal melanosis. J Dermatol (Tokio) 1985; 12:267–276.

Ferris MK, et al.: Neurocutaneous melanosis syndrome. (Abstract) Am J Hum Genet 1987; 41:A57 only.

MI038
M0040

Giuseppe Micali
David M. Mosher

Neuroectodermal melanolysosomal disease
See NEUROECTODERMAL MELANOLYSOSOMAL SYNDROME

NEUROECTODERMAL MELANOLYSOSOMAL SYNDROME 2361

Includes:
Hair (silver)-psychomotor and developmental retardation
Neuroectodermal melanolysosomal disease

Excludes:
Albinism (all types)
Albinism, cutaneous (0031)
Albinism, oculocutaneous, Hermansky-Pudlak type (0033)
Albinoidism (2359)
Chediak-Higashi syndrome (0143)
Gingival fibromatosis-depigmentation-microphthalmia (0413)
Hypopigmentation-immune defect, Griscelli type (2360)

Major Diagnostic Criteria: A striking silver-leaden color of the hair, severe congenital hypotonia, and hypoactive deep tendon reflexes. All known patients have profound psychomotor retardation and hypopigmented skin, with normal growth. The lesions are static and do not suggest a degenerative disorder of the CNS.

Melanin is organized in clumps inside the hair shafts, in both the peripheral and central areas of the hair. Melanosomes are abnormal and have irregular shapes; most of them are incompletely melanized. Some of them have bizarre forms, with fiber in concentric arrangements.

Skin and bone marrow cells show abnormal, round granules that have variable electron density and variable texture of their matrix; they appear to follow a pattern of maturation from a diffuse matrix to a granular one. The "mature granules" are excreted and found in the extracellular space. These granules appear to be derived from lysosomes. Cultured fibroblasts show a prominent Golgi apparatus. These granules show a strongly positive reaction when stained with periodic acid-Schiff, mildly intense with Fontana, and slightly positive with oil red O. They are negative when stained with luxol fast blue, alkaline phosphatase, peroxidase, tyrosinase, and oil red O after extraction with cold acetone, hot acetic acid, or toluidine blue.

Patients do not have visceromegaly, and all signs and symptoms are confined to derivatives of the neuroectoderm.

Clinical Findings: The condition is usually suspected when the infant fails to progress and has a history of congenital hypotonia. The next sign to appear is the lightly colored hair, which progresses to be silver-leaden. The psychomotor retardation is so severe that these infants never speak, sit, or reach any of the developmental milestones completed by normal children aged two years.

There is no special tendency to develop infectious disease, and affected individuals do well regarding common diseases.

When exposed to sunlight, skin shows some degree of tanning. Affected individuals do not show evidence of being blind or deaf. Some patients show severe myopia, signs of myopic degeneration with elongated papillae, normal macula, and normal pigmentation of the fundus.

With age, patients show the consequences of profound hypotonia (probably of prenatal onset), most noticeable in the face, with signs of being hypotonic and "mouth breathers." The chest is flat as a consequence of the almost complete absence of voluntary muscular movements. The joints become stiff and their range of movement limited.

The oldest patient known at last examination was aged 10 years, and she still did not have any type of interaction with those around her.

Complications: The complications seen in these patients can be divided into two major groups: 1) those due to the profound mental retardation, and 2) those due to the severe motor impairment. Patients are completely dependent on others to fulfill their basic needs. The most complex activity shown by one of the patients was to smile.

The consequences of hypotonia and the almost complete absence of voluntary movements are the other source of complications in this condition. The midface is hypoplastic, with crowded teeth and narrow palate; patients are "mouth breathers." The chest is flat, and patients develop respiratory infections that are

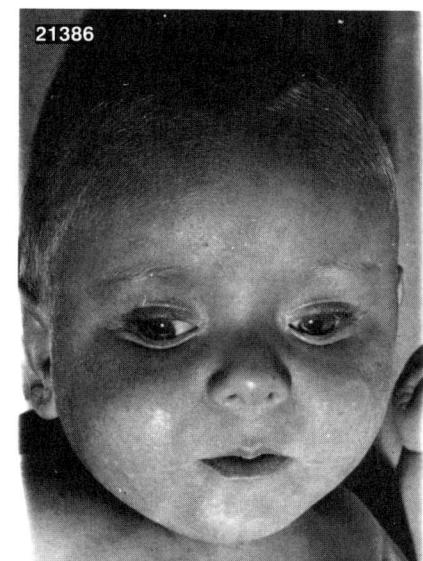

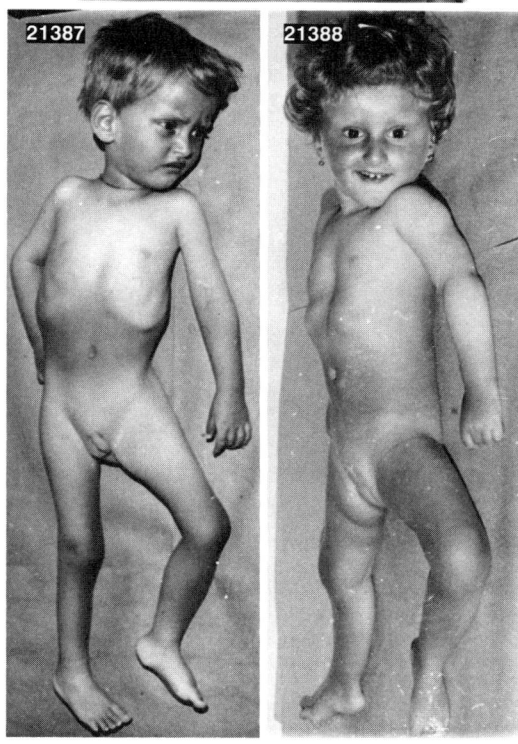

2361A-21386: This young affected infant has a normal appearance and light-colored hair. **21387:** This older affected boy has reduced muscle mass and generalized hypotonia. **21388:** This affected girl shows the hypotonic posture and reduced muscle mass. Her smile is the most advanced developmental milestone that she reached.

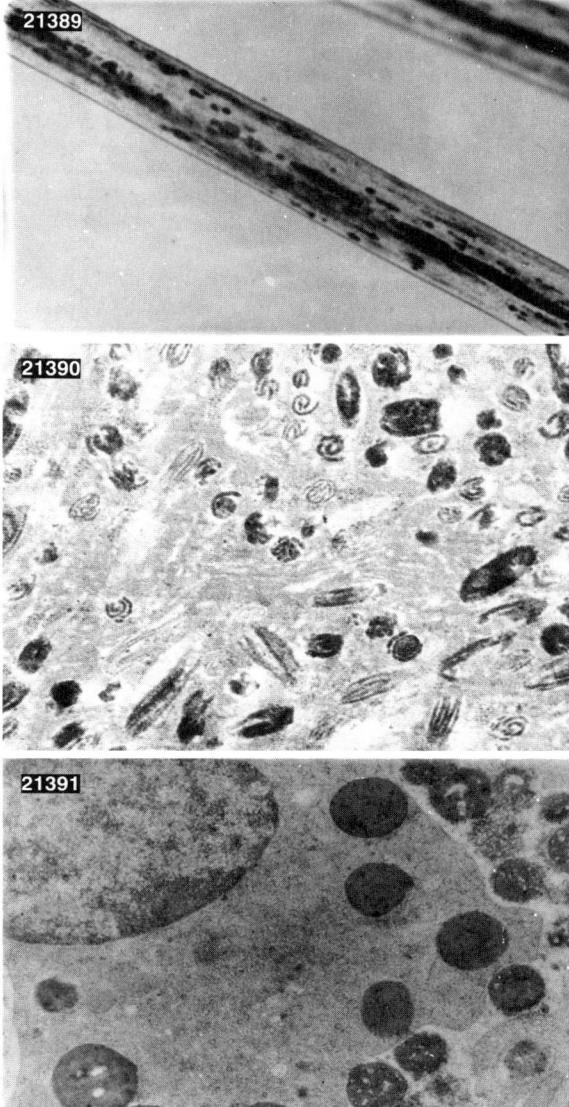

2361B-21389: Microscopic view of a shaft of hair showing the characteristic marked clumping of the melanin in the peripheral and central areas of the hair. This pigment distribution changes the refraction and absorption of light and produces the silver leaden color characteristic of the hair. **21390:** Electron micrograph of a melanocyte from the skin shows the different types of melanosomes. All of the melanosomes are incompletely melanized; the matrix is incompletely formed and disorganized in many of them. **21391:** Electron micrograph of a bone marrow histiocyte contains large round granules with variable electron density and variable texture of the matrix, which varies from very homogenous inside the cells to granulated in the extracellular space. The granules appear to be secreted by the cell; fibroblasts have similar granulations.

more difficult to treat than in normal children. It is necessary to provide physical and occupational therapy. Other complications include plagiocephaly, micrognathia, and respiratory **Pectus excavatum**.

Associated Findings: Absence of upward-slanted palpebral fissures, small hypoplastic nose, upper central incisors, hyperpig-

mented enamel and hypertrophic gingiva, bilateral cryptorchidism, and hypoplastic scrotum.

Etiology: Autosomal recessive inheritance, having pleiotropic effects in different tissues, as demonstrated by segregation analysis in the affected families.

Pathogenesis: The phenotypic characteristics of the condition appear to be the pleiotropic effects of an autosomal recessive gene that preferentially affects the neuroectoderm and some of the tissues derived from it. The hypomelanization of the skin and the lysosomal inclusions in fibroblasts, lymphocytes, and bone marrow cells can be considered autophenes. The severe CNS dysfunction could represent relational pleiotropy. This gene alters the formation of melanosomes and the synthesis of melanin and allows for the fibroblasts and bone marrow cells to produce abnormal lysosomal granules that appear to be related to the formation of the melanosomes.

Possibly the CNS dysfunction is produced by an abnormal neuromelanin as a primary or secondary defect. In the second case it may be related to the dopaminergic system. This possibility is supported by the histochemical similarity of the granules with ceroid and lipofuscin.

MIM No.: *25671

Sex Ratio: M1:F1

Occurrence: Four families have been documented, including an inbred Columbian kindred.

Risk of Recurrence for Patient's Sib:
See Part I, *Mendelian Inheritance.*

Risk of Recurrence for Patient's Child:
See Part I, *Mendelian Inheritance.* Reproduction does not appear to be possible given the profound mental retardation of the patients.

Age of Detectability: At birth or in early childhood.

Gene Mapping and Linkage: Unknown.

Prevention: None known. Genetic counseling indicated.

Treatment: Patients benefit from the types of therapy usually used for profound mental retardation and psychomotor developmental delay.

Prognosis: For those affected, the prognosis is the same as for profoundly mentally retarded individuals. Most do not survive into their teen-age years.

Detection of Carrier: Unknown.

References:
Elejalde BR, et al.: Neuro-ectodermal melanolysosomal disease: an autosomal recessive pigment mutation in man. Am J Hum Genet 1977; 29:39A only.
Elejalde BR, et al.: Mutations affecting pigmentation in man: neuro-ectodermal melanolysosomal disease. Am J Hum Genet 1979; 3:65–80.

EL002
EL014

**B. Rafael Elejalde
Maria Mercedes de Elejalde**

Neuroectodermal pigmented tumor
See JAW, NEUROECTODERMAL PIGMENTED TUMOR

NEUROECTODERMAL SYNDROME, FLYNN-AIRD TYPE   2173

Includes: Flynn-Aird syndrome

Excludes:
   Cockayne syndrome (0189)
   Myotonic dystrophy (0702)
   Phytanic acid storage disease (0810)
   Werner syndrome (0998)

Major Diagnostic Criteria: The combination of deafness, neurologic involvement, and skin and bone defects should suggest the diagnosis.

Clinical Findings: This syndrome has only been described in one family, in which 15 members were affected. Sensorineural deafness was usually the first manifestation of the disorder, which developed in the latter part of the first or the second decade. Other early findings included myopia; ataxia; severe, peripheral neuritic pain; and joint stiffness.

Although severe myopia was the most common ocular finding, cataracts and retinitis pigmentosa also occurred. Epilepsy consisting of episodes of aphasia, blurring of vision, and facial and limb numbness and parasthesia occurred in one third of affected individuals. Although intelligence was unimpaired, change of affect occurred. Another neurologic manifestation was peripheral neuritis, which usually preceded muscular wasting, ataxia, neuritic pain, and joint stiffness. These findings occurred in half of the affected individuals. Skin atrophy and dental caries are other common manifestations. A few individuals developed diabetes (2/15), goiter (4/15), or defective steroid production (2/15).

Most routine laboratory studies have been normal, although in a few cases, elevated cerebrospinal fluid was found following a spinal tap. X-rays have demonstrated increased bone density and cystic areas, particularly of the pelvis. Kyphosis has also been noted in a few individuals. Skin biopsies showed atrophic changes, including generalized hyalinization, sparseness of hair follicles, and marked hyperkeratosis. Autopsies on five individuals were available and demonstrated cardiac and brain involvement in four, adrenal enlargement or cortical atrophy in three, and enlarged thyroid and/or basophilic hyperplasia of the pituitary in two.

Complications: Blindness, osteoporosis, debility, skin ulcers, and kyphoscoliosis have been reported.

Associated Findings: None known.

Etiology: Autosomal dominant inheritance with apparently complete penetrance, but variable expressivity.

Pathogenesis: An enzymatic defect has been suggested, but not identified.

MIM No.: *13630

POS No.: 3437

Sex Ratio: M1:F1

Occurrence: Described in 15 members of one family in North America.

Risk of Recurrence for Patient's Sib:
See Part I, *Mendelian Inheritance.*

Risk of Recurrence for Patient's Child:
See Part I, *Mendelian Inheritance.*

Age of Detectability: By the second decade of life.

Gene Mapping and Linkage: Unknown.

Prevention: None known. Genetic counseling indicated.

Treatment: Supportive.

Prognosis: Life span and intelligence appear unimpaired, although many affected individuals become disabled.

Detection of Carrier: Unknown.

References:
Flynn A, Aird RB: A neuroectodermal syndrome of dominant inheritance. J Neurol Sci 1965; 2:161–182. * †

T0007

Helga V. Toriello

Neuroectodermal syndrome, Johnson type
See ALOPECIA-ANOSMIA-DEAFNESS-HYPOGONADISM, JOHNSON TYPE
Neuroenteric cysts
See INTESTINAL DUPLICATION
Neuroepithelioma
See CANCER, EWING SARCOMA
Neuroepithelioma adenoids
See SCALP, CYLINDROMAS

NEUROFIBROMATOSIS 0712

Includes:
> Intestinal neurofibromatosis
> Mixed central and peripheral neurofibromas
> Neurofibromatosis-pheochromocytoma-duodenal carcinoid syndrome
> NF-1
> von Recklinghausen disease

Excludes:
> **Acoustic neuromata** (0012)
> Phakomatoses (other)
> **Pulmonic stenosis-café-au-lait spots, Watson type** (2776)
> **Tuberous sclerosis** (0975)

Major Diagnostic Criteria: Inclusive criteria include two or more of the following: > 5 café-au-lait spots (standarized criteria vary), with or without intertriginous freckling; multiple discrete neurofibromas or at least one plexiform neurofibroma; iris Lisch nodules; optic pathway glioma; a distinctive bone lesion, such as sphenoid wing dysplasia or tibial pseudarthrosis; a definitely affected first degree relative.

Clinical Findings: Café-au-lait spots and/or axillary freckling may be present at birth. Café-au-lait spots tend to increase in number and size as the child gets older. The diagnosis must be considered if multiple café-au-lait spots are found at any age. The patient's skin color tends to be darker than that of unaffected family members, and freckling becomes more widespread, preferentially involving skin-fold areas. Cutaneous and subcutaneous neurofibromas most usually develop in the second decade, often associated with puberty. They are found on all body segments, but tend

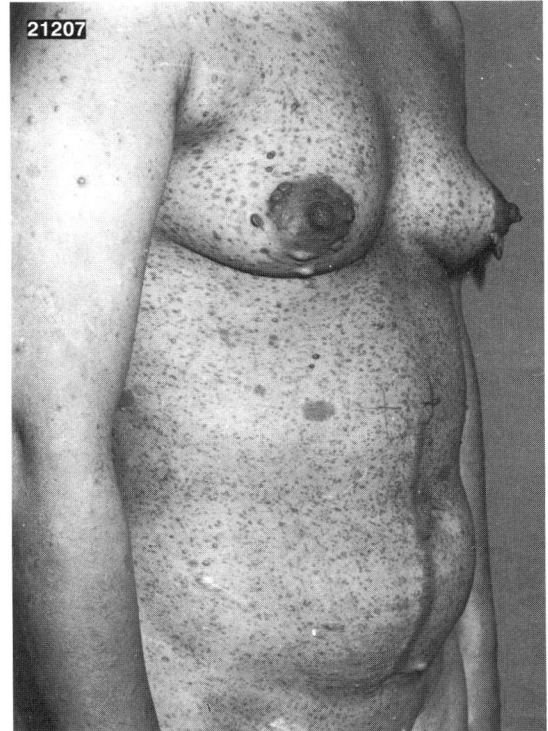

0712B-21207: Multiple neurofibromas and café au lait spots.

to be most numerous on the trunk. Cutaneous neurofibromas may be sessile or pedunculated, and they increase in size with age. Congenital plexiform neurofibromas, with or without overlying hyperpigmentation, may also occur anywhere on the body, and progressive growth is typical, sometimes leading to segmental hypertrophy. Pruritus not infrequently is associated with growing neurofibromas. Paraspinal, mediastinal, and retroperitoneal neurofibromas may cause serious problems. Malignant degeneration to a neurofibrosaracoma probably occurs with a frequency of about 6%, but is very rare before the end of the first decade. Iris Lisch nodules are present in at least 90% of patients over the age of six years, and they increase in number with age; they cause no clinical impairment, but they are very useful for diagnostic purposes. Optic pathway gliomas may occur in upwards of 15% of patients. Astrocytomas may be seen in other intracranial sites as well. Acoustic neuromas do not occur in this disorder. Congenital glaucoma may occur in as many as 1% of patients. A variety of skeletal dysplasias may be seen, including sphenoid wing dysplasia, vertebral dysplasia, and pseudarthrosis, which usually involves the tibia and/or fibula on one side. Scoliosis, with or without cervical-thoracic kyphosis, occurs in at least 5% to 10% of patients. Short stature and macrocephaly are very common. There is a modest excess of seizures of all types, and an even larger number of patients have an asymptomatically abnormal EEG. Hydrocephalus or asymptomatic cerebral ventricular dilation may occur in several percent of patients. Mental retardation may be slightly increased in frequency, but at least 40% of patients have learning disabilities, often associated with speech defects and nonspecific incoordination. Blood vessel involvement, primarily a vascular dysplasia, is seen in all major and medium-sized arteries, particularly those of the brain, the gastrointestinal tract, and the kidneys. The latter may lead to renovascular hypertension. Hypertension may also result from a pheochromocytoma. Biopsies of café-au-lait spots or of tumors merely confirm the nature of the lesion: they do not establish the diagnosis.

Several variations of neurofibromatosis have been described

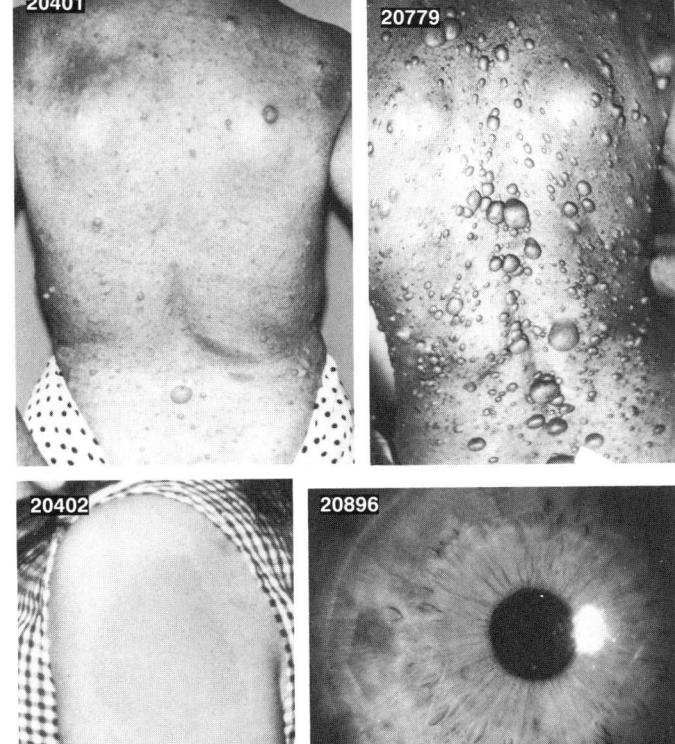

0712A-20401–20779: Cutaneous neurofibromas. 20402: Café au lait spot. 20896: Lisch nodules.

(Riccardi & Eichner, 1986). The classic von Recklinghausen type, described above, has been designated type 1 (*NF-1*). **Acoustic neuromata**, or familial acoustic neuromas, have been designated type 2 (NF-2). A *mixed central and peripheral neurofibromas* has been designated type 3 (NF-3).

In NF-2, bilateral acoustic neuromas, posterior fossa and upper cervical meningiomas, and spinal/paraspinal neurofibromas are characteristic features. Iris Lisch nodules, which occur in close to two-thirds of NF-1 cases, do not occur in NF-2, and optic gliomas have not been reported. CNS tumors appear in the second or third decade and advance rapidly, resulting, unlike NF-1, in a shortened lifespan.

A variant or atypical form has been designated type 4 (NF-4). This is a heterogeneous group, and is distinguished chiefly on the basis of prognosis. Once again, the iris Lisch nodules, characteristic of NF-1, are usually absent.

Familial *intestinal neurofibromatosis* may share the features of NF-1, or may consist simply of multiple intestinal neurofibromatosis without the cutaneous features of NF-1. This rare variation has occurred in sporadic cases or, as with all neurofibromatosis, in an inherited dominant pattern.

A few cases (less than 10) of a *neurofibromatosis-pheochromocytoma-duodenal carcinoid syndrome* have also been reported, as well as a similar number of cases with a neurofibromatosis-Noonan phenotype (See **Noonan syndrome**). Unless otherwise qualified, however, the term neurofibromatosis refers to the classic von Recklinghausen NF-1.

Complications: Blindness may result from optic pathway gliomas. Spinal cord compression may result from paraspinal neurofibromas, vertebral dysplasia and/or severe kyphoscoliosis. Vascular compromise may lead to cerebral or cerebellar infarcts, abdominal angina, or renovascular hypertension. Gastrointestinal neurofibromas may lead to gastrointestinal hemorrhage. A pheochromocytoma may lead to hypertension and death. Death may also result from a neurofibrosarcoma. Pseudarthroses may require amputation proximal to the lesion. Cosmetic disfigurement from facial neurofibromas is common.

Associated Findings: Hyperganglionosis of the large bowel, mimicking **Colon, aganglionosis**. Premature or delayed puberty. **Glaucoma, congenital**. A major psychosocial burden is often seen among patients with NF-1.

Etiology: Autosomal dominant inheritance.

Pathogenesis: Unknown.

MIM No.: *16220, *16222, 16224, 16226, 16227.

POS No.: 3332

CDC No.: 237.700

Sex Ratio: M1:F1

Occurrence: Prevalence about 1:3000. No ethnic differences are noted. There are an estimated 80,000 affected individuals in the United States alone.

Risk of Recurrence for Patient's Sib:
See Part I, *Mendelian Inheritance.*

Risk of Recurrence for Patient's Child:
See Part I, *Mendelian Inheritance.*

Age of Detectability: Often at birth, almost always by the end of the first year, and always by five years of age.

Gene Mapping and Linkage: NF1 (neurofibromatosis 1 (von Recklinghausen disease, Watson disease)) has been mapped to 17q11.2.

Prevention: None known. Genetic counseling indicated.

Treatment: For enlarging or otherwise problematic neurofibromas, surgery is standard treatment; likewise for neurofibrosarcomas, although adjuvant chemotherapy and/or radiation therapy may be used. For optic pathway gliomas, close observation or radiation therapy are standard, though chemotherapy occasionally may have a place. Reparative surgery may be attempted for pseudarthrosis, though amputation is often required. Placement of a Harrington rod or alternative internal fixation procedures are standard for severe or progressive kyphoscoliosis.

Prognosis: Seventy-five percent of patients probably develop at least a moderate level of severity by 30 years of age, but prognosis depends on the presence of the various complications and associated features.

Detection of Carrier: Unknown.

Special Considerations: The Neurofibromatosis Institute, Inc., 715 Bison Drive, Houston, Texas 77079, provides a variety of print and computer-based information services regarding neurofibromatosis (NFormation), including electronic mail, resource identification, over 2,000 NF-related references, annotated bibliographies, an NF-patient database, and an expert system. The Institute, in conjunction with Karger Publishing Co., also produces the journal, *Neurofibromatosis*. NFormation is available on-line at 713/558–9908.

Support Groups:
New York; The National Neurofibromatosis Foundation (NF)
Marland (Washington, D.C. area); Neurofibromatosis, Inc.
AUSTRALIA: NSW; Riverwood; The Neurofibromatosis Association of Australia

References:
Schenkein I, et al.: Increased nerve-growth-stimulating activity in disseminated neurofibromatosis. New Engl J Med 1974; 292:1134–1136.
Bader JL, Miller RW: Neurofibromatosis and childhood leukemia. J Pediatr 1978; 92:925–929.
Kanter WR, et al.: Central neurofibromatosis with bilateral acoustic neuroma: genetic, clinical and biochemical distinctions from peripheral neurofibromatosis. Neurology 1980; 30:851–859.
Riccardi VM, Mulvihill JJ: Neurofibromatosis (von Recklinghausen's disease). In: Advances in neurology, vol. 29. New York: Raven Press, 1981.
Riccardi VM: Von Recklinghausen neurofibromatosis. New Engl J Med 1981; 305:1617–1626.
Riccardi VM, et al.: The pathophysiology of neurofibromatosis. Am J Med Genet 1984; 18:169–176.
Zehavi C, et al.: Iris (Lisch) nodules in neurofibromatosis. Clin Genet 1986; 29:51–55.
Riccardi VM, Eichner JE: Neurofibromatosis: phenotype, natural history and pathogenesis. Baltimore, Johns Hopkins University Press, 1986.
Rubenstein AE, et al.: Neurofibromatosis. Ann New York Acad Sci 1986; 486:1–414.
Fountain JW, et al.: Physical mapping of a translocation breakpoint in neurofibromatosis. Science 1989; 244:1085–1088.

RI000   **Vincent M. Riccardi**

NEURONAL CEROID-LIPOFUSCINOSES (NCL)　　0713

Includes:
Amaurotic familial idiocy
Batten disease
Batten-Mayou disease
Batten-Vogt syndrome
Cerebromacular degeneration, familial
Haltia-Santavuori disease (infantile NCL or INCL)
Jansky-Bielchowsky disease (late infantile NCL or LINCL)
Jansky-Bielchowsky-Hagberg disease (late infantile variant of NCL)
Kufs disease
Spielmeyer-Vogt disease (juvenile NCL or JNCL)
Spielmeyer-Sjogren disease (juvenile NCL)

Excludes:
Alpers disease (3261)
Alzheimer disease, familial (2354)
Cerebro-hepato-renal syndrome (0139)
Dentatorubropallidoluysian degeneration, hereditary (3283)
Hallervorden-Spatz disease (2526)
Huntington disease (0478)
Juvenile metachromatic leukodystrophy
Mucolipidosis I (0671)
Neuroaxonal dystrophy
Neuronal sphingolipidoses
Phytanic acid storage disease (0810)
Seizures, progressive myoclonic, Lafora type (2601)
Seizures, progressive myoclonic, Unverricht-Lundborg type (2602)
Subacute sclerosing panencephalitis

Major Diagnostic Criteria: The neuronal ceroid-lipofuscinoses (NCL) are characterised by progressive motor and cognitive decline, seizures, visual loss due to pigmentary retinal degeneration and the storage of autofluorescent lipopigment in the central nervous system, other organs and skin. The four types are differentiated on the basis of age of onset, temporal relation of visual loss to neurologic deterioration, seizures and electron microscopy of the storage material. A subdivision into infantile (*Haltia-Santavuori*), late-infantile (*Jansky-Bielchowsky*), juvenile (*Spielmeyer-Vogt*), and adult (*Kufs*) is in use. There is overlap between the different types in some patients, especially between late infantile and juvenile symptomatology and pathology.

Clinical Findings: In the *infantile* form, microcephaly, seizures, ataxia, visual impairment with a retinal dystrophy and rapidly progressive developmental delay appear before age 18 months. Seizures common at the beginning disappear by the second year of life. The electroencephalogram (EEG), initially disorganized becomes flat by the end of the second year. The electroretinogram shows progressive decrease in amplitude then abolition. The visual evoked response (VER) is usually flat. CT scan or MRI reveals generalized atrophy and a skull X-ray will show a thickened calvarium. Intralysosomal granular osmiophilic deposits have been found in conjunctival, skin, muscle, or rectal biopsies and brain. They are absent from bone marrow.

In the *late infantile* form, ataxia, seizures (grand mal and myoclonic) and intellectual decline begin between ages 2–4 years and precede retinal degeneration. The EEG shows bursts of diffuse synchronous slow waves. The ERG becomes flat and there is increased amplitude of the VER. CT scan and MRI reveal cerebral and cerebellar atrophy. Intralysosomal curvilinear bodies and occasional fingerprint-like inclusions are seen in conjunctival, skin, muscle, rectal and bone marrow biopsies and brain.

In *juvenile NCL*, pigmentary retinopathy occurs between the ages of 4–10 years. Cognitive decline and seizures (predominantly myoclonic) follow. Some patients show extrapyramidal and cerebellar signs. CT scan or MRI shows thinning of the cortical mantle and MRI shows loss of white matter. Intralysosomal fingerprint-like inclusions associated with curvilinear bodies are seen in conjunctiva, skin, muscle, rectal or bone marrow biopsies and brain and buffy coat preparations.

The clinical findings in *Kufs* disease begin early in the third decade of life and may take the form of cognitive decline and psychotic or motor disturbance. Extrapyramidal signs such as facial dyskinesias and rigidity can be associated. Rarely patients have seizures (myoclonic) and ocular symptoms are notably absent. Brain biopsy is the only definitive way to make the diagnosis and usually granular osmiophilic deposits are seen by electron microscopy.

Elevated urine sediment didohols are a nonspecific finding common to all types.

Complications: Intractable seizures and incapacitating myoclonus are severely debilitating and death occurs from intercurrent illness such as pneumonia.

Associated Findings: **Microcephaly** in the infantile and late infantile variant. Mixed seizure disorder in the late infantile and juvenile types. Behavior problems in the late infantile and juvenile types, and psychiatric disorders in the adult form.

Etiology: Autosomal recessive inheritance. Rare families with autosomal dominantly inherited Kufs disease are described.

Pathogenesis: Pathology suggests a lysosomal storage disease. Brains accumulate large amounts of dolichol oligosaccharides suggesting NCL could be due to faulty glycosylation of proteins. Cathepsin H, a protease, is claimed to be deficient in some late infantile cases.

MIM No.: *25673, 20450, *20420, *20430, *16235

POS No.: 3333

Sex Ratio: M1:F1

Occurrence: Three hundred and sixty children in the United States are registered with the Batten Disease Support and Research Association, most with the juvenile or late infantile form. The incidence of infantile NCL in Finland is 1:13000.

Risk of Recurrence for Patient's Sib:
See Part I, *Mendelian Inheritance.*

Risk of Recurrence for Patient's Child:
See Part I, *Mendelian Inheritance.*

Age of Detectability: Ages at which symptoms first occur are *infantile form*, within the first year of life; *late-infantile*, by three years of age; *juvenile*, between 7–12 years; *adult form*, in the late teens to early 30s. Prenatal diagnosis was accomplished in the sib of a patient with the late-infantile form by electron microscopic examination of amniotic fluid cells.

Gene Mapping and Linkage: BTS (Batten disease) has been provisionally mapped to 16.

Prevention: None known. Genetic counseling indicated.

Treatment: Undetermined for the underlying condition. General supportive care and anticonvulsants are the mainstay of therapy. Neuroleptics for behavior disturbances and anti-Parkinsonian drugs are used when indicated. Antioxidants such as vitamin E and C and selenium have been tried and have not been of great benefit to most patients.

Prognosis: Patients with INCL die in early childhood. Patients with LINCL die in the first decade of life or early teenage years. Patients with JNCL live into their twenties. In Kufs disease the course is slowly progressive and patients may survive into late middle age.

Detection of Carrier: Unknown.

Special Considerations: Metabolic disease with known enzymatic defects must be ruled out in infants and children. It is conjectural whether these diseases are separate entities or due to genetic defects that are different but occurring at the same gene locus (i.e. allelic variants). The late infantile and juvenile forms are more similar than the others, and intermediate forms are recognized (suggesting compound heterozygous status).

Support Groups:
San Francisco; The Children's Brain Diseases Foundation for Research
NY; Brooklyn; Myoclonus Families United
WA; Spanaway; Batten Disease Support and Research Association

References:
Zeman W, et al.: The neuronal ceroid lipofuscinoses. In: Handbook of clinical neurology, leukodystrophies and poliodystrophies, vol. 10 Amsterdam, North Holland, 1970:588–679. * †
Zeman W: Studies in the neuronal ceroid-lipofuscinoses. Presidential address. J Neuropathol Exp Neurol 1974; 33:1–12.
Boustany R-M, et al.: Clinical classification of neuronal ceroid-lipofuscinoses subtypes. Am J Med Genet 1988; 5(suppl):47–58.
Boustany R-M, et al.: The neuronal ceroid-lipofuscinoses: a review. Rev Neurol 1989; 142:105–110.

B0053   **Rose Mary N. Boustany**
H0057   **John H. Holtkamp**
TR009   **Elias I. Traboulsi**

Neuronal degeneration of childhood-liver disease, progressive
See ALPERS DISEASE
Neuronal migration, defective
See HIRSCHPRUNG DISEASE-MICROCEPHALY-COLOBOMA
Neuronopathy, sensorimotor-agenesis of the corpus callosum
See CORPUS CALLOSUM AGENESIS-SENSORIMOTOR NEUROPATHY, FAMILIAL
Neuropathy with liability to pressure palsies, recurrent familial
See NEUROPATHY, HEREDITARY WITH PRESSURE PALSIES

NEUROPATHY, CONGENITAL MOTOR & SENSORY-SKELETAL-LARYNGEAL DEFECTS   3013

Includes:
> Charcot-Marie-Tooth disease with skeletal and laryngeal anomalies
> Laryngeal and skeletal anomalies-motor and sensory neuropathy
> Skeletal and laryngeal anomalies-motor and sensory neuropathy

Excludes:
> **Neuropathy, hereditary motor and sensory, type II** (2105)
> Charcot-Marie-Tooth disease, other

Major Diagnostic Criteria: Neuronal type of motor and sensory neuropathy with prenatal onset. At birth, laryngeal stridor or laryngomalacia, as well as dysmorphic features.

Clinical Findings: A single family with the father and two sons affected has been reported. The two sons presented flexion contractures at birth. All three had delayed motor development, walking after ages 2–4 years, with a widebased and clumsy gait and frequent falls. The course was slowly progressive, and the father's gait improved after surgical lengthening of the Achilles tendons. In adulthood, the picture was that of Charcot-Marie-Tooth disease with atrophy and weakness of peroneal, hand, and feet muscles, pes cavus, absent tendon reflexes, and distal sensory loss. Electromyography revealed a denervation pattern, and motor nerve conduction velocity was normal. Microscopic examination of sural nerves showed loss of predominantly large, myelinated nerve fibers, and demyelinization. One patient had laryngomalacia, and two presented laryngeal stridor in the first months of life.

All three patients showed the following dysmorphic features: high-arched palate, short neck, narrow shoulders, dorsal kyphosis, and protruding chest.

Complications: Unknown.

Associated Findings: None known.

Etiology: Presumably autosomal dominant inheritance.

Pathogenesis: Unknown. A widespread neurologic disorder affecting lower motor neuron axons could explain all findings.

Sex Ratio: Presumably M1:F1; M3:F0 observed.

Occurrence: One family with an affected father and two sons has been reported.

Risk of Recurrence for Patient's Sib:
> See Part I, *Mendelian Inheritance.*

Risk of Recurrence for Patient's Child:
> See Part I, *Mendelian Inheritance.*

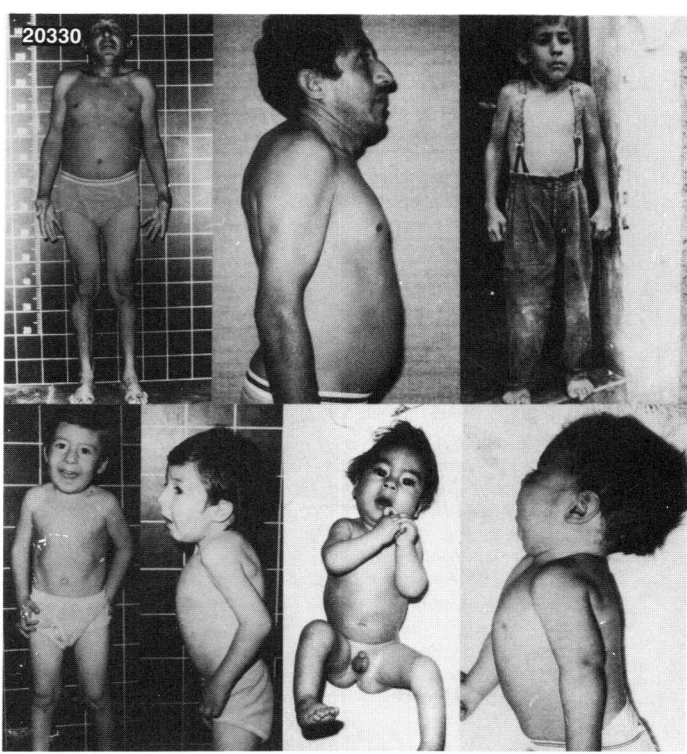

3013-20330: The reported family showing the dysmorphic features. Note the early development of claw hand and late appearance of peroneal atrophy.

Age of Detectability: At birth when flexion contractures are present; otherwise, during the first years of life.

Gene Mapping and Linkage: Unknown.

Prevention: None known. Genetic counseling indicated.

Treatment: Physical therapy reversed most flexion contractures. In one case **Foot, talipes equinovarus (TEV)** required surgery. Surgical lengthening of the Achilles tendon improved the gait in one patient.

Prognosis: Presumably normal life span. The gait disturbance may restrict life-style alternatives.

Detection of Carrier: Unknown.

References:
Ruíz C, et al.: A distinct motor and sensory neuropathy (neuronal type) with dysmorphic features in a father and two sons: a variant of Charcot-Marie-Tooth disease. Clin Genet 1987; 31:109–113.

RU019   **Carlos Ruíz**
CA011   **José María Cantú**

NEUROPATHY, CONGENITAL SENSORY WITH ANHIDROSIS   2390

Includes:
> Analgesia, familial
> Dysautonomia, type II, familial
> Hereditary sensory and autonomic neuropathy IV (HSAN-IV)
> Neural crest, syndrome of
> Pain, insensitivity to, with anhidrosis of Swanson (congenital)

Excludes:
> Biemond congenital and familial analgesia

Dysautonomia I, Riley-Day type (0307)
Lesch-Nyhan syndrome (0588)
Neuropathy, hereditary motor and sensory, type II (2105)
Neuropathy, nonprogressive sensory radicular

Major Diagnostic Criteria: Impaired perception of pain and temperature with normal tactile perception. Autonomic dysfunction manifested by neurogenic anhidrosis, recurrent unexplained fever, vasomotor instability, abnormal intradermal histamine test, self-mutilation, and mental retardation.

Clinical Findings: Clinical findings manifest in the first year of life. Recurrent unexplained fever, blotching, and irritability are some of the earliest manifestations of this disorder. Other features diagnosable early are insensitivity to pain, which is generalized, truncal anhidrosis, and pupillary hypersensitivity to methacholine chloride. Self-mutilation of the tongue, lips, and extremities (fingers) starts as soon as the incisor teeth erupt. Fungiform papillae are present, in contrast to **Dysautonomia I, Riley-Day type** in which fungiform papillae are absent. The skin is parchment-like, especially on the extremities. There is lack of development of erythematous flare on the intradermal histamine test. Deep tendon reflexes are decreased, and the perception of temperature seems to be decreased. The perception of light touch is preserved, as is that of touch. Electroencephalogram and serum catecholamine levels are normal. Hypotonia is a constant feature of the disease. The patient usually functions cognitively in the moderately retarded range and has delayed motor development. Clinical variability is uncommon, and expression is complete.

Complications: Severe lacerations of the tongue and lips, edentulation, scarred excoriations of the fingers, and corneal opacities can be seen due to self-mutilation behavior. Failure to thrive has been reported. Orthopedic complications usually include repeated episodes of osteomyelitis, fractures, and dislocated and neuropathic joints.

Associated Findings: Hyperactive behavior.

Etiology: Autosomal recessive inheritance.

Pathogenesis: Neuropathologic findings show that the brain is normal except for the absence of small neurons in the dorsal ganglia, lack of small fibers in the dorsal roots, absence of the Lissauer tract, and reduction in size of the spinal tract of the trigeminal nerve and its paucity of small fibers. Peripheral (sural) nerve biopsy reveals an almost total absence of nonmyelinated axons and a marked decrease in myelinated axons. Fiber diameters showed an abnormal distribution and an absence of large diameter, and diminution of the number of small myelinated axons.

MIM No.: *25680, 21030

Sex Ratio: M1:F1

Occurrence: About two dozen cases have been reported in the literature.

Risk of Recurrence for Patient's Sib:
See Part I, *Mendelian Inheritance.*

Risk of Recurrence for Patient's Child:
See Part I, *Mendelian Inheritance.*

Age of Detectability: In early infancy.

Gene Mapping and Linkage: Unknown.

Prevention: None known. Genetic counseling indicated.

Treatment: None available for the basic manifestations of the disorder. The infections and orthopedic and ophthalmic complications should be managed appropriately. Plastic surgery on the severely lacerated lower lip of one of the patients with this disorder has been attempted without success due to the continuing self-mutilating behavior.

Prognosis: Guarded, due to the complications, especially the frequent bouts of osteomyelitis. There is not enough information concerning the natural history of this disorder to comment on the life span of the patients.

Detection of Carrier: Unknown.

Special Considerations: *Familial analgesia* has also been described by Biemond (1955) and Freytag and Lindenberg (1967).

Support Groups: New York; The Dysautonomia Foundation, Inc.

References:
Biemond A: Investigations of the brain in a case of congenital and familial analgesia. Proc 11th Intern Cong Neuropath, London, September, 1955.
Swanson AG, et al.: Anatomic changes in congenital insensitivity to pain. Arch Neurol 1965; 12:11–18.
Swanson AG: Congenital insensitivity to pain with anhidrosis: a unique syndrome in two male siblings. Arch Neurol 1963; 8:299–306.
Pinsky L, DiGeorge AM: Congenital familial sensory neuropathy with anhidrosis. J Pediatr 1966; 68:1–13. †
Freytag E, Lindenberg R: Neuropathologic findings in patients of a hospital for the mentally deficient: a survey of 359 cases. Johns Hopkins Med J 1967; 121:379–392.
Scribanu N, Grover-Johnson N: Atypical nerve histology in a case of congenital sensory neuropathy with anydrosis. Neurology 1982; 32:A184.
Dyck PJ, et al.: Not "indifference to pain" but varieties of hereditary sensory and autonomic neuropathy. Brain 1983; 106:373–390.
Axelrod FB, Pearson J: Congenital sensory neuropathies. Am J Dis Child 1984; 138. *
Donaghy M, et al.: Hereditary sensory neuropathy with neurotrophic keratitis. Brain 1987; 110:563–583.

SC052   **Nina Scribanu**

Neuropathy, dominantly inherited hypertrophic
See NEUROPATHY, HEREDITARY MOTOR AND SENSORY, TYPE I

NEUROPATHY, GIANT AXONAL   3140

Includes:
> Giant axonal neuropathy (GAN)
> Neurofilaments (accumulation)-polyneuropathy
> Polyneuropathy-accumulation of neurofilaments

Excludes:
> **Ataxia, Friedreich type** (2714)
> **Dejerine-Sottas disease** (2054)
> **Phytanic acid storage disease** (0810)

Major Diagnostic Criteria: Distal symmetric progressive weakness and sensory loss, cerebellar syndrome, bilateral Babinski sign, kinky hair, normal mental activity, onset at ages 2–3 years. Sural nerve biopsy shows characteristic accumulation of neurofilaments.

Clinical Findings: Onset of polyneuropathy in children at toddler age. Distal weakness and atrophy are accompanied by areflexia and impairment in perceiving touch, position sense, and vibration. Central nervous system involvement, including cerebellar ataxia and corticospinal tract signs with bilateral extensor plantar responses. Tightly curled hair is a common feature.

Light microscopic evaluation of sural nerve biopsy reveals abnormally large masses corresponding to axons that are segmentally enlarged to enormous proportions. Ultrastructurally, axons are distended by masses of tightly woven neurofilaments. Neurofilament masses often begin at a node of Ranvier, and paranodal retraction of myelin can be noticed. Axonal organelles, including mitochondria and vesicles of smooth endoplasmic reticulum, are displaced into a subaxolemmal disposition. The protein composition of neurofilaments that accumulate in this disorder is not appreciably altered.

Complications: Severe distal weakness and cerebellar ataxia lead to wheelchair confinement after several years of progression.

Associated Findings: Distal renal tubular acidosis manifested by metabolic acidosis was reported in one case. Other atypical associations include bilateral vocal cord paralysis due to involvement of laryngeal nerves, skeletal abnormalities (thoracic kyphoscoliosis, **Pectus carinatum**, coxa valga, pes planovalgus), and **Ichthyosis**.

Etiology: Usually autosomal recessive inheritance, although an autosomal dominant form with onset during infancy or childhood, and a congenital form, have also been reported. Parental consanguinity and affected sibs have been reported in several families.

Pathogenesis: One hypothesis assumes a metabolic block of neurofilament transport along axons. A second hypothesis, based on experimental GAN in rats treated with 2,5-hexanedione, claims an acceleration of neurofilament transport (Monaco et al, 1985). Griffin & Watson (1988) also report fast axonal transport through giant axonal swellings in experimental hexacarbon neuropathy.

MIM No.: *25685

Sex Ratio: M1:F1

Occurrence: Approximately 20 cases have been reported worldwide.

Risk of Recurrence for Patient's Sib:
See Part I, *Mendelian Inheritance.*

Risk of Recurrence for Patient's Child:
See Part I, *Mendelian Inheritance.*

Age of Detectability: Age two to seven years. One congenital case has also been reported.

Gene Mapping and Linkage: Unknown.

Prevention: None known. Genetic counseling indicated.

Treatment: Unknown.

Prognosis: Guarded. The disease has a slow progression, over at least ten years in most cases.

Detection of Carrier: Unknown.

References:

Dooley JM, et al.: Clinical progression of giant-axonal neuropathy over a twelve year period. Can J Neurol Sci 1981; 8:321–323.
Duncan ID, et al.: Inherited canine giant axonal neuropathy. Muscle Nerve 1981; 4:223–227.
Ionasescu V, et al.: Giant axonal neuropathy: normal protein composition of neurofilaments. J Neurol Neurosurg Psychiatry 1983; 46:551–554. *
Ionasescu V, Zellweger H: Genetics in neurology. New York: Raven, 1983:386–389. †
Kinney RB, et al.: Congenital giant axonal neuropathy. Arch Pathol Lab Med 1985; 109:636–641. *
Monaco S, et al.: Giant axonal neuropathy: acceleration of neurofilament transport in optic axons. Proc Natl Acad Sci USA 1985; 82:920–924.
Griffin JW, Watson DF: Axonal transport in neurological disease. Ann Neurol 1988; 23:3–13.

10000

Victor V. Ionasescu

NEUROPATHY, HEREDITARY MOTOR AND SENSORY, TYPE I
2104

Includes:
Charcot-Marie-Tooth disease, hypertrophic (some cases)
Charcot-Marie-Tooth disease, slow nerve conduction type
Charcot-Marie-Tooth peroneal muscular atrophy
Foot, claw-absent tendon jerks
Friedreich disease, abortive type
Motor and sensory neuropathy, type I
Motor and sensory neuropathy, X-linked
Neuropathy, dominantly inherited hypertrophic
Peroneal muscular atrophy, axonal type
Peroneal muscular atrophy, hypertrophic
Roussy-Levy syndrome

Excludes:
Abetalipoproteinemia (0002)
Ataxia, Friedreich type (2714)
Charcot-Marie-Tooth disease, sporadic
Dejerine-Sottas disease (2054)
Muscular dystrophy, distal (0690)
Neuropathy, hereditary motor and sensory, type II (2105)

Phytanic acid storage disease (0810)
Spinal muscular atrophy (0895)

Major Diagnostic Criteria: Peroneal muscle weakness and wasting, pes cavus, significantly decreased median nerve conduction velocity and a family history of one or more of these signs.

Clinical Findings: Foot deformities (pes cavus) and scoliosis appear in early childhood. Difficulties in walking and running become prominent in the second decade, while the small muscles of the hand atrophy. As the weakness and atrophy of those small muscles progress, a claw-like hand results. Atrophy of the leg and lower third of the thigh leads to the typical stork leg or inverted champagne bottle appearance.

One fourth of affected persons have palpably enlarged ulnar, radial, peroneal, or posterior auricular nerves. Sensory disturbances are not as severe as the motor deficit. Nerve conduction velocity is strikingly diminished early in life. Sensory nerve action potentials are of long latency if they are elicitable at all.

Complications: The disease is slowly progressive, with moderate ambulation disability and disordered fine motor skills.

Associated Findings: Autonomic changes of decreased sweating in the legs, decreased tear production, and orthostatic hypotension may occur. In some patients an apparent ataxia of lower limbs and tremulousness of the upper extremities is present.

Etiology: Autosomal dominant, autosomal recessive, and X-linked recessive inheritance have all been reported in various kindreds. Sporadic cases have also been reported. There is extreme variability of expression. Dyck (1984) maintains that kinships suggestive of autosomal recessive inheritance probably represent the partial expression of a dominant trait. In support of dominant inheritance, intensive evaluation by a neurologist, including assessment of nerve conduction, has demonstrated abnormalities consistent with type I neuropathy in the parents of some sporadic cases, as well as those thought to be autosomal recessive.

Pathogenesis: The process is essentially one of selective and restricted motor, and to a lesser extent, sensory nerve segmental demyelination. Onion bulb formation and areas of demyelination are prominent in sural nerve biopsies. A biochemical basis for this disorder is unknown.

MIM No.: *11820, *11822, *18080, *21440, *30280

Sex Ratio: M1:F1

Occurrence: Prevalence in western Norway is 36:100,000 for the autosomal dominant form, 1.4:100,000 for the autsomal recessive form, and 3.6:100,000 for the X-linked recessive form. In Newcastle-upon-Tyne, England, 4.7:100,000 for the autosomal dominant form.

Risk of Recurrence for Patient's Sib:
See Part I, *Mendelian Inheritance.*

Risk of Recurrence for Patient's Child:
See Part I, *Mendelian Inheritance.*

Age of Detectability: In a recognized family, it is common to have children diagnosed in the first decade of life. Index cases, however, usually come to medical attention in the second decade.

Gene Mapping and Linkage: CMT1 (Charcot-Marie-Tooth neuropathy 1) has been mapped to 1q.
CMT2 (Charcot-Marie-Tooth neuropathy 2) has been mapped to 17p13.1-q12.
CMTX (Charcot-Marie-Tooth neuropathy, X-linked) has been mapped to Xq11-q13.

Prevention: None known. Genetic counseling indicated.

Treatment: Supportive for the selected weaknesses and sensory deficits.

Prognosis: Variable. Life span is probably not reduced.

Detection of Carrier: The variability of expression in this dominant disorder is extreme. However, mildly affected parents and siblings may show unappreciated skeletal deformities (hammer toes, pes cavus, scoliosis). Median nerve conduction velocities in apparently unaffected parents and other relatives is a reasonably accurate test of the sub-clinical state. In such instances, median nerve conduction velocity will be less than 40 m/sec.

Special Considerations: Although the condition is generally recognized by the second decade of life, a number of children have become clinically affected in infancy. The additional signs of gait ataxia and upper extremity tremor, originally described as a separate entity (the *Roussy-Levy syndrome*, also known as *familial claw-foot with absent tendon jerks* and *abortive type Friedreich disease*), may occur in otherwise typical families.

Support Groups:
Philadelphia; National Foundation for Peroneal Muscular Atrophy
CANADA: Ontario; St. Catharines; Charcot-Marie-Tooth (CMT) International

References:
Buchthal F, Behse F: Peroneal muscular atrophy (PMA) and related disorders. Brain 1977; 100:41–66.
Davis CJF, et al.: The peroneal muscular atrophy syndrome: clinical, genetic and electrophysiologic findings and classification. J Genet Hum 1978; 26:311–349.
Harding AE, Thomas PK: The clinical features of hereditary motor and sensory neuropathy types I and II. Brain 1980; 103:259–280. *
Dyck PJ, et al., eds: Peripheral neuropathy, 2nd ed. Philadelphia: W.B. Saunders, 1984. * †
Hogan-Dann, CM, et al.: Polyneuropathy following vincristine therapy in two patients with Charcot-Marie-Tooth syndrome. J Am Med Asso 1984; 252:2862–2863.
Rozear MP, et al.: Hereditary motor sensory neuropathy, X-linked: a half century follow-up. Neurology 1987; 37:1460–1465. †
Vance JM, et al.: Linkage of Charcot-Marie-Tooth neuropathy type 1a to chromosome 17. Exp Neurol 1989; 104:186–189.

CR011   **Carl J. Crosley**

NEUROPATHY, HEREDITARY MOTOR AND SENSORY, TYPE II   2105

Includes:
Axonal type Charcot-Marie-Tooth disease
Charcot-Marie-Tooth disease, neuronal (some cases)
Motor and sensory neuropathy, hereditary type II
Peroneal muscular atrophy, neuronal

Excludes:
Abetalipoproteinemia (0002)
Ataxia, Friedreich type (2714)
Dejerine-Sottas disease (2054)
Muscular dystrophy, distal (0690)
Neuropathy, hereditary motor and sensory, type I (2104)
Phytanic acid storage disease (0810)
Spinal muscular atrophy (0895)

Major Diagnostic Criteria: Peroneal muscular atrophy, pes cavus, evidence of denervation on electromyography, and mildly decreased median nerve conduction velocity with a family history of one or all of these signs.

Clinical Findings: The onset of weakness is later in this disorder than in **Neuropathy, hereditary motor and sensory, type I** (NHMS I). The peak onset is in the second and third decade with some individuals affected as late as the sixth or seventh decade. Distal weakness of the upper limbs occurs in only 50% of affected persons. Lower limb weakness, on the other hand, tends to be as severe, if not more so, than in NHMS I. Tendon reflexes are only moderately depressed. Muscle atrophy and the characteristic lower extremity deformities (stork leg, pes cavus) remain prominent. Sensory loss (vibration and position sense) is mild. Nerve conduction velocity is abnormal but significantly faster than in NHMS I. The median nerve conduction velocity is greater than 40 m/sec. Nerves are not hypertrophic.

Complications: This disease is very slowly progressive. The onset occasionally may be as late as the sixth or seventh decade. Disability is largely the consequence of leg weakness.

Associated Findings: Tremor of the upper extremities and gait ataxia may be present, but are uncommon findings.

Etiology: Autosomal dominant inheritance.

Pathogenesis: The biopsies of sural nerves reveal loss of large fibers with only occasional segments of demyelination and onion bulb formation. The biochemical basis of this disorder is unknown.

MIM No.: *11821

Sex Ratio: Presumably M1:F1.

Occurrence: Approximately 25% of all peroneal muscular atrophy is thought to be of the type II variety, implying a prevalence of 1–10:100,000.

Risk of Recurrence for Patient's Sib:
See Part I, *Mendelian Inheritance.*

Risk of Recurrence for Patient's Child:
See Part I, *Mendelian Inheritance.*

Age of Detectability: In the first decade of life in 20% of the cases.

Gene Mapping and Linkage: Unknown.

Prevention: None known. Genetic counseling indicated.

Treatment: Largely supportive for complications resulting from progressive leg weakness.

Prognosis: Variable but generally good.

Detection of Carrier: Since nerve conduction velocities may be only mildly depressed, the appreciation of subtle deformities or weakness is essential in recognizing an affected individual.

Support Groups:
Philadelphia; National Foundation for Peroneal Muscular Atrophy
CANADA: Ontario; St. Catharines; Charcot-Marie-Tooth (CMT) International

References:
Buchthal F, Behse F: Peroneal muscular atrophy (PMA) and related disorders. Brain 1977; 100:41–66.
Davis CJF, et al.: The peroneal muscular atrophy syndrome. J Genet Hum 1978; 26:311–349.
Harding AE, Thomas PK: The clinical features of hereditary motor and sensory neuropathy types I and II. Brain 1980; 103:259–280. *
Dyck PJ, et al., eds: Peripheral neuropathy, 2nd ed. Philadelphia: W.B. Saunders, 1984.
Berciano J, et al.: Hereditary motor and sensory neuropathy type II: clinicopathological study of a family. Brain 1986; 109:897–914.

CR011   **Carl J. Crosley**

NEUROPATHY, HEREDITARY RECURRENT BRACHIAL   2071

Includes:
Brachial neuritis, recurrent familial
Brachial neuropathy, familial
Brachial plexopathy, hereditary
Brachial plexus neuropathy, heredo-familial
Neuralgic amyotrophy, familial
Neuralgic amyotrophy-brachial predilection, familial
Neuritis with brachial predilection, heredo-familial

Excludes:
Neuropathy, hereditary with pressure palsies (2108)
Sporadic brachial neuropathies

Major Diagnostic Criteria: Familial recurrent attacks of weakness of the shoulder girdle muscles occur unilaterally or asymmetrically in both arms. Symptoms are frequently preceded by pain and followed by amyotrophy. Early childhood onset and tomaculous (ie, focal thickening of myelin) neuropathy on biopsy are also very characteristic of the condition.

Clinical Findings: Attacks of pain in one arm lasting several days or weeks, followed by the relatively rapid onset of weakness and atrophy of some of the proximal muscles of that arm. The pain often subsides with the onset of the weakness, and in some cases may not occur at all. There may be some sensory loss. The opposite arm may also be asymmetrically involved.

The distribution of the weakness corresponds to that of a nerve, nerve root or plexus, usually proximal. Other peripheral nerve trunks, cranial or autonomic nerves may be involved.

Functional recovery occurs within months, although long-standing residual weakness and atrophy may ensue. The intervals between recurrences may vary from months to years. There is a tendency for attacks to start in early childhood.

Precipitant factors are infections, pregnancy, parturition and, perhaps, strenuous exhertion. Other relapses occur without obvious cause.

Congenital dysmorphology has been described: hypotelorism, small stature, epicanthic folds, facial asymmetry, syndactyly of second-third toes, cleft palate.

Nerve conduction study / electromyogram (NCS/EMG) shows a somewhat patchy sensorimotor polyneuropathy of axonal type, more severe in arm nerves. In some occasions the findings are minor. Sural or radial nerve biopsy shows segmental demyelination-remyelination, with sausage-shaped focal thickenings of myelin (tomaculous neuropathy). These findings are not pathognomonic, and may be absent.

Complications: Permanent arm weakness after one or several attacks may ensue.

Associated Findings: Facial paresis was reported in one case.

Etiology: Autosomal dominant inheritance with variable penetrance.

Pathogenesis: Unknown.

MIM No.: *16210

Sex Ratio: M1:F1

Occurrence: Less than two dozen families have been reported.

Risk of Recurrence for Patient's Sib:
See Part I, *Mendelian Inheritance.*

Risk of Recurrence for Patient's Child:
See Part I, *Mendelian Inheritance.*

Age of Detectability: The first attack usually occurs in early childhood.

Gene Mapping and Linkage: Unknown.

Prevention: None known. Genetic counseling indicated.

Treatment: Prevention of precipitant factors. During the attack: rest, analgesics and physiotherapy. The usefulness of corticosteroids is still controversial. If paralysis develops, physiotherapy.

Prognosis: Unknown.

Detection of Carrier: Unknown.

Special Considerations: The sporadic form of the disease is far more frequent than the familial form. In the sporadic form there is a male predominance, the first attack is not during childhood, there is less tendency to relapses and there are no congenital stigmata. Tomaculae have not been described in the nerve biopsy of sporadic cases. Tomaculous neuropathy and electrically detected generalized neuropathy point to related pathological mechanisms for the familial recurrent brachial neuropathy and **Neuropathy, hereditary with pressure palsies.**

References:
Geiger LR, et al.: Familial neuralgic amytrophy. report of three families with review of the literature. Brain 1974; 97:87–102.
Madrid R, Bradley WG: The pathology of neuropathies with focal thickening of the myelin sheath (tomaculous neuropathy). J Neurol Sci 1975; 25:415–448.
Dunn HG, et al.: Heredofamilial brachial plexus neuropathy (hereditary neuralgic amyotrophy with brachial predilection) in childhood. Dev Med Child Neurol 1978; 20:28–46.
Airaksinen EM, et al.: Hereditary recurrent brachial plexus neuropathy with dysmorphic features. Acta Neurol Scand 1985; 71:309–316.
Phillips, LH, II: Familial long thoracic nerve palsy: a manifestation of brachial plexus neuropathy. Neurology 1986; 36:1251–1253.

M0016

Jesus S. Mora
Walter G. Bradley

NEUROPATHY, HEREDITARY WITH PRESSURE PALSIES 2108

Includes:
> Compression syndrome of peripheral nerves, hereditary
> Mononeuritis, Familial recurrent
> Nerve trunk palsies, familial
> Neuropathy with liability to pressure palsies, recurrent familial
> Polyneuropathy, familial recurrent
> Pressure palsies (hereditary) and neuropathy
> Tomaculous neuropathy

Excludes:
> Neuralgic amyotrophy with brachial plexus predilection
> **Neuropathy, hereditary recurrent brachial** (2071)

Major Diagnostic Criteria: Familial recurrent mononeuropathy or multiple neuropathy, with symptoms triggered by compression or stretching of the nerves, and tomaculous neuropathy in the nerve morphology.

Clinical Findings: Mononeuropathy or multiple neuropathy, with wide variation in symptoms, ranging from paresthesiae, numbness or absent DTR's, to paralysis and objective sensory disturbances. These are triggered by compression or stretching of the nerve trunks, even slightly.

Most frequently affected are peroneal, ulnar, radial and median nerves. Musculocutaneous, axillary, long thoracic, suprascapular, femoral, sciatic, facial or trigeminal nerves are less frequently affected.

Triggering factors include using scissors, knitting, leaning on elbows, squatting, kneeling or crossing legs, wearing tight shoes, etc.

There is recovery within days, weeks or months. Recurrence in the same or in other areas may occur, sometimes leaving permanent damage.

Nerve conduction study/electromyogram (NCS/EMG) shows signs of entrapment neuropathies and peripheral neuropathy. Muscle biopsy shows neurogenic amyotrophy. Teased-nerve studies show sausage-like swellings of the myelin sheaths and extensive demyelination-remyelination, even in non-symptomatic nerves ("tomaculous neuropathy"). These findings are not pathognomonic.

Complications: Permanent nerve trunk damage after one or several recurrences.

Associated Findings: None known.

Etiology: Autosomal dominant inheritance with variable expression.

Pathogenesis: Probable biochemical defect related to the process of myelination. The defect produces lability of the myelin sheath of the peripheral nerves to pressure or stretch. There is aberration of the myelin sheath formation with redundant loops and abnormal irregular thickenings. The remyelination after demyelination is also abnormal.

MIM No.: *16250

Sex Ratio: M1:F1

Occurrence: About 40 families have been described in the literature.

Risk of Recurrence for Patient's Sib:
See Part I, *Mendelian Inheritance.*

Risk of Recurrence for Patient's Child:
See Part I, *Mendelian Inheritance.*

Age of Detectability: Onset varies from four to 67 years of age, but occurs mostly between age 20 and 45.

Gene Mapping and Linkage: Unknown.

Prevention: None known. Genetic counseling indicated.

Treatment: Prevention of the triggering factors; physical therapy if paralysis develops.

Prognosis: Most of the episodes are followed by a good recovery. Some, however, may leave a more permanent deficit.

Detection of Carrier: Unknown.

Special Considerations: The microscopic abnormalities (tomaculae) and the electrophysiologically detected generalized neuropathy are also features of **Neuropathy, hereditary recurrent brachial**. In this condition pain is a frequent feature, and compression is not a specific triggering factor.

References:
De Jong JGY: Over families met hereditaire disposities tot het optreden van neuriteden, gecorreleerd met migraine. Psychiatr Neurol Med Psychol Beih 1947; 50:60–77.

Behse F, et al.: Hereditary neuropathy with liability to pressure palsies: electrophysiological and histopathological aspects. Brain 1972; 95:777–794.

Madrid R, Bradley WG: The pathology of neuropathies with focal thickening of the myelin sheath (tomaculous neuropathy): studies on the formation of the abnormal myelin sheath. J Neurol Sci 1975; 25:415–448.

Debruyne J, et al.: Hereditary pressure-sensitive neuropathy. J Neurol Sci 1980; 47:385–394.

Sellman MS, Mayer RF: Conduction block in hereditary neuropathy with susceptibility to pressure palsies. Muscle Nerve 1987; 10:621–625.

M0016

Jesus S. Mora
Walter G. Bradley

NEUROPATHY, HERITABLE ISONIAZIDE TYPE (INH)   2044

Includes:
Acetylator phenotype, slow
INH (antituberculosis agent) inactivation
Isoniazid inactivation
Isoniazid neuropathy
N-acetyltransferase polymorphism
Neuritis, peripheral with isoniazid
Pyridoxine deficiency induced by isonizid therapy
Tuberculosis, INH inactivation peripheral neuropathy

Excludes:
Acetylator polymorphism (0007)
Ethionamide neuropathy
Hydralazine neuropathy
Neuropathy induced by pyridoxine deficiency
Nutritional neuropathy

Major Diagnostic Criteria: In patients receiving the antituberculosis agent INH, the clinical history and examination are compatible with peripheral neuropathy. Serum pyridoxine levels may be low. These patients demonstrate a genetic phenotype for metabolizing INH slowly.

Clinical Findings: Symptoms include numbness, tingling, or the sensation of "pins and needles" initially in the toes and spreading proximally in a symmetric fashion. There are complaints of muscle aching and soreness, calf tenderness and sometimes burning pain in the skin or muscles. Occasionally, loss of balance, weakness in the legs, and loss of sleep occur.

Examination shows impaired superficial sensation in the legs and weakness of toe movements. Foot plantar and dorsiflexion weakness may be found later or in the more severely affected patients. Dysesthesias in response to contact stimuli are common. Reflexes are decreased at the ankles and occasionally at the knees.

Laboratory findings may show low serum pyridoxine levels. Biochemical evidence of pyridoxine deficiency is indicated by increased urinary excretion of xanthurenic acid or N-methylnicotinamide following tryptophan loading. Slow acetylation of INH and several other drugs can be demonstrated by half-life determinations of plasma INH. A more convenient means of detecting the presence of the slow acetylator phenotype measures the ratio of monoacetyldapsone to dapsone.

Complications: A gradually evolving, predominantly sensory greater than motor neuropathy without rapid deterioration occurs if INH is continued without pyridoxine replacement.

Associated Findings: Seizures, altered behavior (hyperactivity), and dermatologic changes may occur in children with INH-induced pyridoxine deficiency.

Etiology: Autosomal recessive inheritance.

Pathogenesis: Two separate genetic polymorphisms for drug metabolism by acetylation utilizing N-acetyltransferase exist (slow and fast acetylators). The slow acetylation phenotype is autosomal recessive. Acetylation is the first stage of metabolism of INH. INH interferes with pyridoxine metabolism, with increased urinary excretion of pyridoxine. Patients with the slow acetylator phenotype taking INH are more prone to develop pyridoxine deficiency coincident with the peripheral neuropathy. Patients who are fast acetylators may also develop a similar peripheral neuropathy after taking large doses of INH for an extended time period (see **Acetylator polymorphism**).

Light and electron microscopic examinations of sural nerves demonstrate degenerative axonal changes indistinguishable from wallerian degeneration. Both myelinated and unmyelinated fibers are affected. INH is known to enter the endoneurium readily, but the exact mechanism of injury and its relationship to pyridoxine deficiency is unknown.

MIM No.: *24340

Sex Ratio: M1:F1. However, in a study of Swedish men over age 65 years, the ability to acetylate INH decreased as compared with younger men. No similar pattern was found in women.

Occurrence: Undetermined. There is a higher incidence of rapid acetylators among the Japanese than among Europeans. In patients receiving INH 3–5 mg/kg/day, clinical pyridoxine deficiency is reported in 2% of the cases and approximately six months are necessary for clinical manifestations to occur. At 6 mg/kg/day, 10% of patients developed symptoms, often within 3–5 weeks. At 20 mg/kg/day, 40% of patients developed neuropathy.

Risk of Recurrence for Patient's Sib:
See Part I, *Mendelian Inheritance.*

Risk of Recurrence for Patient's Child:
See Part I, *Mendelian Inheritance.*

Age of Detectability: Well-documented in adults, and has been reported in an 11-month-old infant.

Gene Mapping and Linkage: Unknown.

Prevention: The onset of neuropathy varies with dosage and length of therapy. Pyridoxine 150–450 mg daily given in conjunction with INH prevents development of this neuropathy.

Treatment: Early discontinuation of INH when possible will resolve the symptoms, although when treatment was continued for more than a week after the first symptoms appeared, only slight recovery occurred over months.

Pyridoxine supplementation will prevent the development of neuropathy, but has little effect on the speed of recovery.

Prognosis: The neuropathy shows gradual resolution after discontinuation of INH. Except in severely affected patients, recovery is virtually complete but may be delayed for months.

Detection of Carrier: Slow versus rapid inactivators of INH may be determined by half-life determinations of INH. Other methods of detection include dapsone loading with measurement of the ratio of monoacetyldapsone to dapsone. These screening methods demonstrate a bimodal distribution for ability to acetylate both fast and slow. Some investigators suggest that an intermediate heterozygote state also exists.

Special Considerations: Several other drugs are metabolized by the same enzyme system as for acetylation. These include procainamide, hydralazine, sulfamethazine, some sulfonamides, phenelzine, dapsone, and some carcinogenic arylamines. The variability in their metabolism may account for some differences in the incidence of toxic responses to these drugs.

References:
Gammon GD, et al.: Neural toxicity in tuberculous patients treated with isoniazid (isonicotinic acid hydrazide). Arch Neurol Psychiatry 1964; 70:64–69.

Carr K, et al.: Simultaneous analysis of dapsone and monoacetyldapsone employing high performance liquid chromatography: a rapid method for determination of acetylator phenotype. Br J Clin Pharmacol 1978; 6:421–427.

Cavanagh JB: The "dying back" process: a common denominator in many naturally occurring and toxic neuropathies. Arch Pathol Lab Med 1979; 103:659–664.

Clark DWJ: Genetically determined variability in acetylation and oxidation: therapeutic implications. Drugs 1985; 29:342–375.

Paulsen O, Nilsson LG: Distribution of acetylator phenotype in relation to age and sex in Swedish patients. Eur J Clin Pharmacol 1985; 28:311–315.

Pellock JM, et al.: Pyridoxine deficiency in children treated with isoniazid. Chest 1985; 87:658–661.

Nhachi CFB: Polymorphic acetylation of sulphamethazine in a Zimbabwe population. J Med Genet 1988; 25:29–31.

MA075
H0056

Janice M. Massey
Kenneth W. Holmes

Neuropathy, motor sensory, hereditary
See DEJERINE-SOTTAS DISEASE

NEUROPATHY, MYELO-OPTICO, SUBACUTE TYPE   2047

Includes:

Clioquinol induced subacute myelo-optico neuropathy
Myelo-optico neuropathy, subacute
Quinoform induced subacute myelo-optico neuropathy (SMON)
Subacute myelo-optico neuropathy (SMON)

Excludes:

Benign myalgic encephalomyelitis (Iceland disease)
Cervical spondylosis
Encephalomyelitis and viral meningomyelitis
Guillain-Barre syndrome
Multiple sclerosis, familial (2598)
Neuromyelitis optica (Devic disease)
Neurosyphilis
Porphyria
Subacute combined degeneration of the cord
Toxic neuropathies, other

Major Diagnostic Criteria: A characteristic prodromal abdominal disorder, leading to an ascending bilateral sensory disturbance, typically preceded by a history of abdominal complaints treated by clioquinol. Cardinal symptoms include 1) abdominal symptoms as a prodrome, typically preceded by treatment with clioquinol, and 2) neurologic sensory symptoms, often ascending. Other major signs include impaired deep sensation and weakness in the legs, occasional bilateral visual impairment, mental status changes, greenish discoloration of the tongue and feces, sphincter disturbances, protracted course, no significant blood abnormalities (but often increased glucose or amylase), no significant CSF findings except occasional increased protein, and only rare occurrence in children.

Clinical Findings: There is often a recent history of mild GI upset treated with clioquinol. Two to four weeks after clioquinol is given, a separate abdominal prodrome occurs, followed by the onset of neurologic manifestations. Severe abdominal pains, abdominal fullness, and constipation are seen in 70% of the patients and typically last less than two weeks. Fifty percent of the patients have greenish discoloration of the tongue, with elongation of the filiform papillae due to clioquinol-iron complex deposition. Green stool is reported in 8% of patients.

Onset of neurologic dysfunction occurs over several days to about two weeks. Initial symptoms include paresthesias of the feet (72%), numbness and fatigue of the legs (25%), paresthesias of the hands (2%), and blurred vision (1%). There is then an ascending progression of the paresthesias in a bilateral, symmetric fashion. Examination shows normal mental status; decreased visual acuity (27%); motor weakness (50–73%), more prominent in the lower extremities, dermatomal levels below which sensation is lost typically at T10 or lower, with virtually all patients showing sensory loss (light touch, pinprick, and vibration); and variable

deep tendon reflexes. Seventy-five percent of patients have a sensory ataxic gait. Bladder problems occur in 15–20%. Rare cases have unconsciousness, convulsions, or palatal myoclonus. Autonomic disturbances include cold feelings in the feet (68%), edema of the legs and feet (39%), dyshidrosis (36%), and urinary frequency (26%). Following the acute stage, the disease usually takes a chronic course, with symptomatic fluctuation over many months.

Laboratory evaluation shows normal blood chemistries and nonspecific abnormalities (7%). A few patients have shown increased sedimentation rates, C-reactive protein, rheumatoid factor, and SGOT and SGPT levels. Blood sugar and serum amylase are frequently elevated in the initial stages of the disease. Immunoglobulin levels are elevated in 48%, with IgG levels higher than IgA or IgM. The CSF is usually normal, but may show increased protein (10%). Skin biopsy material often shows atrophy of all skin layers. EEG shows bursts of theta activity in 32% of the patients. Slowed motor nerve conduction velocities in the lower extremities are seen in 28–31% of patients. Electromyography of the anterior tibialis occasionally shows fibrillations and positive waves (16–21%) or a decreased interference pattern (37–52%). Sural nerve biopsy shows axonal swelling, demyelination, fibrous proliferation of interstitial tissue, and proliferation of Schwann cells. Axonal degeneration in a "dying back" pattern at 10–14 days after onset is found more prominently than demyelinating changes. Pathologic specimens of the spinal cord show symmetric lesions of the posterior tracts from the sacral to the cervical regions with axonal disruption. The lumbosacral area shows demyelination and gliosis of a secondary degenerative character. There is disintegration of the inner ganglion cells of the retina and bilateral symmetric degeneration throughout almost the entire length of the optic nerve, chiasm, and tract.

Complications: Persistent sensory, abdominal, and visual disturbances are common. Gait problems are also frequent.

Associated Findings: A past history of gastrointestinal diseases (including peptic ulcer disease, hepatitis, and chronic diarrhea), tuberculosis, renal disease, or gynecologic diseases is frequent. Allergic diseases are found in 30–58% of all patients. A history of laparotomy was found in 48% of patients. Appendectomy was eight times as frequent as in the general population.

Etiology: Treatment with quinoform (clioquinol, or 5-chloro-7-iodo-8-hydroxyquinoline) for abdominal discomfort or for *acrodermatitis enteropathica* (a heritable disorder of zinc deficiency, see Gordon et al, 1981) is the most important etiologic factor. The disorder is reproduced by administering quinoform to animals. Although there is a vast amount of epidemiologic data supporting quinoform as the cause of SMON, 4% of patients with clinical SMON have no history of quinoform use. There is no known etiology in these patients, other than for some cases of misdiagnosis. Although the "Inoue-Melnick virus," which has been isolated from the CSF and stool in some patients with SMON and causes a paraplegia in mice, has been raised as a possible cause of SMON, no evidence for any infectious transmission to primates has been found. The pathology in Inoue-Melnick virus mice is not similar to SMON. It is interesting to note that various strains of the Inoue-Melnick virus have been isolated from **Multiple sclerosis** patients in the United States.

Pathogenesis: The toxic effect of clioquinol is not known. Based on the similarity of the disease to subacute combined degeneration of the cord, a possible effect on vitamin B_{12} has been considered. A chelation effect of clioquinol on Co (II) has been proposed to possibly interfere with electron transport in the mitochondria.

It is unclear why the disease was so prevalent in Japan, and not in other countries where clioquinol was also used. The Japanese have had more exposure to metals via environmental pollution than inhabitants of most other countries. Clioquinol can increase the penetration of metallic cations through cellular membranes by forming lipophilic metal chelates, and it has been suggested that the accumulation of these metals in the nervous system may cause the toxicity. There are many similarities between SMON and metal toxicities.

There are also pathologic similarities to phenothiazine toxicity, suggesting abnormal metabolism of nicotinic acid.

The possibility of a metabolic error in amino acid metabolism has been considered based on some similarities of SMON to the megaloneuropathies seen in hepatocerebral diseases associated with increased blood amino acid levels, aminoaciduria, and impaired CSF and urine ceruloplasmin metabolism. No such metabolic error has been discovered in SMON.

MIM No.: *20110

Sex Ratio: M1:F1.8

Occurrence: Undetermined but presumed rare at present. At its peak in 1970 the incidence was 125:100,000 women and 60:100,000 men in Nagoya, Japan, and 35:100,000 women and 18:100,000 men in all of Japan. Nearly 10,000 cases were reported by the early 1970s, but very few since the side-effects of the involved medications have become well known.

Risk of Recurrence for Patient's Sib: Minimal unless also given clioquinol.

Risk of Recurrence for Patient's Child: Minimal unless also given clioquinol.

Age of Detectability: The age of onset usually ranges from nine to 81 years, with the youngest patient having been six months old. Only 0.3% of patients are less than 10 years old.

Gene Mapping and Linkage: N/A

Prevention: The Japanese government officially banned the sale of clioquinol in September 1970.

Treatment: Discontinue clioquinol. General health care, psychologic care to deal with the disability, physical therapy, occupational therapy, and rehabilitation are useful as needed. Treatments proposed for the neurologic and abdominal symptoms have included steroids (methylprednisolone, 30–60 mg/day with taper over months; ACTH), intravenous vitamin B_{12}, pantothenic acid (100–500 mg/day), acupuncture, and hyperbaric oxygen. Warm water lavage often gives symptomatic relief of abdominal complaints. Oral cinnarizine, indomethacin, and imipramine have been reported to decrease dysesthesias.

Prognosis: On follow-up 1.5 to 10 years after onset of symptoms, 6% are cured, one-half to three-fourths are significantly improved, one-third are minimally improved, and 3–6% are dead. The death rates over the 10 years after onset are about twice as high as those for the corresponding age group. Motor recovery is generally very good, but sensory recovery tends to be poor. Chronic abdominal symptoms are present in 50–60%. There is usually no improvement of visual symptoms if optic atrophy is present. Milder visual disturbances improve in 33–49% of patients. A relapse has been reported in 17% of patients, but is related to clioquinol readministration. Fourteen percent need assistance with acts of daily living, and 10% remain unable to walk or unable to walk without an aid. Sixty-five percent returned to work within 12 months.

Detection of Carrier: Unknown.

References:
Kono R: Introductory review of subacute myelo-optico-neuropathy (SMON) and its studies done by the SMON research commission. Jpn J Med Sci Biol 1975; 28:1–21.
Sobue I, et al.: Prognosis of SMON patients. Jpn J Med Sci Biol 1975; 28:203–217.
Shiraki H: Neuropathological aspects of the etiopathogenesis of subacute myelo-optico-neuropathy (SMON). In: Vinken PJ, Bruyn GW, eds: Handbook of clinical neurology, vol. 37. New York: North Holland, 1978:141–197.
Sobue I: Clinical aspects of subacute myelo-optico-neuropathy (SMON). In: Vinken PJ, Bruyn GW, eds: Handbook of clinical neurology, vol. 37. New York: North Holland, 1978:115–139.
Gordon EF, et al.: Zinc metabolism: basic, clinical, and behavioral aspects. J Pediatr 1981; 99:341–349.

H0056
MA075

Kenneth W. Holmes
Janice M. Massey

Neuropathy-deafness-diverticulitis
See DEAFNESS-DIVERTICULITIS-NEUROPATHY
Neuroretinopathy, optic Leber type
See OPTIC ATROPHY, LEBER TYPE
Neurovisceral lipidosis, familial
See G(M1)-GANGLIOSIDOSIS, TYPE 1
Neutral 17-beta-hydroxysteroid oxidoreductase deficiency
See STEROID 17-KETOSTEROID REDUCTASE DEFICIENCY
Neutral lipid storage disease with ichthyosis
See STORAGE DISEASE, NEUTRAL LIPID TYPE

NEUTROPENIA, BENIGN FAMILIAL 2215

Includes:
Idiopathic neutropenia, chronic benign
Neutropenia, ethnic benign

Excludes:
Autoimmune neutropenia
Immunodeficiency, agranulocytosis, infantile Kostmann type (2197)

Major Diagnostic Criteria: Absolute neutropenia with an absolute neutrophil count ranging from 300 to 1,500 cells/ml with no identifiable cause (such as malignancy, drugs, toxins, or connective tissue disease). There may be an accompanying overall leukopenia, but this is not a constant feature. There is no anemia and no thrombocytopenia, and generally there are normal numbers of monocytes, eosinophils, and basophils. Neutrophil morphology is normal.

Clinical Findings: Affected individuals are usually identified serendipitously following routine blood screening. They generally do not display any increased susceptibility to infection, although in some individuals occasional stomatitis and gingivitis are reported. The neutropenia is persistent and not cyclic.

Complications: Unknown.

Associated Findings: None known.

Etiology: Autosomal dominant and autosomal recessive inheritance has been reported. Sporadic cases do occur.

Pathogenesis: Appears to be in the release of neutrophils from the marrow storage pool. Examination of the bone marrow reveals normal cellularity, a normal myeloid to erythroid ratio, and normal maturation of the myeloid cells right up to mature granulocytes. Marrow culture shows normal or, more often, increased numbers of granulocyte colony-forming cells. Therefore this probably is not a stem cell defect. The administration of endotoxin or corticosteroids, both potent stimuli of granulocyte egress from the marrow storage pool, to these individuals results in an increase in their absolute neutrophil count, but the increment is significantly less than that seen in non-neutropenic controls. Studies with ^{32}P-labeled granulocytes do not support either increased margination or increased destruction of the granulocytes as the cause of the neutropenia. The exact nature of this defect in neutrophil release from the bone marrow is not known.

MIM No.: *16270

Sex Ratio: M1:F1

Occurrence: About 20 kinships identified involving well over 100 cases. Most common in Yemenite Jews and American, West Indian, and African Blacks. The true incidence of this condition is unknown because of the mild nature of the defect.

Risk of Recurrence for Patient's Sib:
See Part I, *Mendelian Inheritance*.

Risk of Recurrence for Patient's Child:
See Part I, *Mendelian Inheritance*.

Age of Detectability: In early childhood.

Gene Mapping and Linkage: Unknown.

Prevention: None known. Genetic counseling indicated.

Treatment: None necessary. In particular, corticosteroids, splenectomy, and prophylactic antibiotics are not indicated.

Prognosis: Affected individuals appear to live full, unimpaired lives.

Detection of Carrier: Unknown.

References:
Cutting HO, et al.: Familial benign chronic neutropenia. Ann Intern Med 1964; 61:876–887. *
Mason BA, et al.: Marrow granulocyte reserves in black Americans. Am J Med 1979; 67:201–205.
Schneider M, et al.: Evaluation of bone marrow granulocyte reserves in neutropenic and nonneutropenic Yemenite Jews. Isr J Med Sci 1982; 18:671–674.
Schoenfeld Y, et al.: The mechanism of benign hereditary neutropenia. Arch Intern Med 1982; 142:797–799.
Berrebi A, et al.: Leukopenia in Ethiopian Jews. (Letter) New Engl J Med 1987; 316:549 only.

AX001
B0048

Richard Axtell
Laurence A. Boxer

NEUTROPENIA, CYCLIC   0714

Includes:
  Cyclic neutropenia
  Periodic neutropenia

Excludes:
  Angioedema, hereditary (0054)
  Fever, familial mediterranean (FMF) (2161)
  Thrombocytopenia, Periodic

Major Diagnostic Criteria: Regularly recurrent episodes of profound neutropenia at specific intervals as determined by repeated differential counts.

Clinical Findings: The oscillations of neutrophil counts in cyclic neutropenia have a periodicity of approximately 21 days and are consistent from patient to patient. The peripheral blood neutrophil count is severely depressed and in some cases reaches 0/mm³. Symptoms are minimal when the neutrophil count is greater than 500/mm³. During the neutropenic period, patients may have aphthous stomatitis, fever, malaise, occasional cutaneous and subcutaneous infections and cervical adenopathy. Mild splenomegaly is occasionally observed. The neutrophil counts in the recovery phase attain normal levels in some patients, while in others neutrophil counts remain below normal values.

Complications: Skin infections, chronic gingivitis, abscesses, and oral mucosal ulcers are common. Episodes of recurrent boils, otitis media, cervical adenitis, bronchitis, and pneumonia have been reported.

Associated Findings: Abdominal pain, diarrhea, arthralgia, headache, depression, septicemia, furunculosis, cellulitis, infection of superficial cuts or abrasions with or without lymphangitis. Cyclic neutropenia has also been associated with coincident conditions such as agammaglobulinemia, diabetes insipidus, pancreatic insufficiency, and lymphosarcoma.

Etiology: Possibly autosomal dominant inheritance. May be transferred through bone marrow transplantation (Krance et al, 1982).

Pathogenesis: Peripheral blood neutropenia is always preceded by lower numbers of neutrophil precursors in the bone marrow. Periods of severe neutropenia are also regularly associated with an absolute monocytosis. At the nadir early myeloid precursors in the absence of mature neutrophils may be found in circulation. The disease appears to be due to damage to marrow cells or to a defect in their feedback control mechanisms, the cycle being an expression of deranged control.

MIM No.: 16280

Sex Ratio: M1:F1. A slight preponderance of males has been observed (Wright et al, 1981).

Occurrence: Less than 1:100,000

Risk of Recurrence for Patient's Sib:
See Part I, *Mendelian Inheritance.* About one in three patients have a sib, parent, or child affected with the disease.

Risk of Recurrence for Patient's Child:
See Part I, *Mendelian Inheritance.*

Age of Detectability: From birth through childhood.

Gene Mapping and Linkage: Unknown.

Prevention: None known. Genetic counseling indicated.

Treatment: Timely recognition and prompt treatment of serious infections. Avoidance of activities that cause minor injuries. Careful oral and dental care. Although there is as yet no therapeutic cure for the disease, clinical and hemotologic improvements have been achieved following administration of ACTH, corticosteroids, testosterone, staphylococcal vaccine, and infusion of normal plasma or plasma from a volunteer given typhoid vaccine. Recent studies indicated that lithium carbonate might be an effective and safe therapy. Bone marrow transplantation may provide a definitive cure. Temporary improvement has been associated with neutrophil transfusions.

Prognosis: Although chronic morbidity is characteristic, life-threatening complications are not unusual. Growth, onset of puberty, and intellectual development are normal. Some patients experience a symptom-free state of nearly 2–6 months duration with no spontaneous changes in neutrophil cycling, suggesting a long-term evolution toward milder recurrent illness.

Detection of Carrier: Unknown.

Special Considerations: There is a naturally occurring animal model of cyclic neutropenia in gray collie dogs. In humans, a secondary dip in neutrophil counts about 10–14 days after the period of maximum neutropenia has also been reported. Cycling of other blood elements, such as platelets, eosinophils, monocytes, and reticulocytes, may also be apparent. The presence of reciprocal cycling of T8 lymphocytes has been observed.

References:
Wright DG, et al.: Human cyclic neutropenia: clinical review and long term follow-up of patients. Medicine 1981; 60:1–13.
Krance RA, et al.: Human cyclic neutropenia transferred by allogenic bone marrow grafting. Blood 1982; 60:1263–1266.
Verma DS, et al.: Cyclic neutropenia and T lymphocyte suppression of granulopoiesis: abrogation of the neutropenic cycles by lithium carbonate. Leuk Res 1982; 6:567–576.
Smith JG, et al.: Cyclical neutropenia and T8 lymphocyte mediated stimulation of granulopoiesis. Br J Haematol 1985; 60:481–489.

NA013

Madhavan P. N. Nair

Neutropenia, ethnic benign
  See NEUTROPENIA, BENIGN FAMILIAL
Neutropenia-onychotrichodysplasia
  See ONYCHO-TRICHODYSPLASIA-NEUTROPENIA
Neutrophil differentiation factor
  See IMMUNODEFICIENCY, AGRANULOCYTOSIS, INFANTILE KOSTMANN TYPE
Nevi flammei
  See NEVUS FLAMMEUS

NEVI-ATRIAL MYXOMA-MYXOID NEUROFIBROMAS-EPHELIDES   2572

Includes:
  Adrenocortical nodular dysplasia-Cushing syndrome-cardiac myxomas
  Carney complex
  Carney Syndrome
  Cushing disease-atrial myxoma-pigmentation
  Cushing syndrome, familial
  Endocrine overactivity-spotty pigmentation-myxomas
  LAMB syndrome
  Mucocutaneous lentigines-myxomas-multiple blue nevi
  Myxoma-adrenocortical dysplasia syndrome
  Myxomas-spotty pigmentation-endocrine overactivity
  NAME syndrome
  Pigmented lesions-myxoid neurofibromas-atrial myxoma
  Pigmentation (spotty)-myxomas-endocrine overactivity

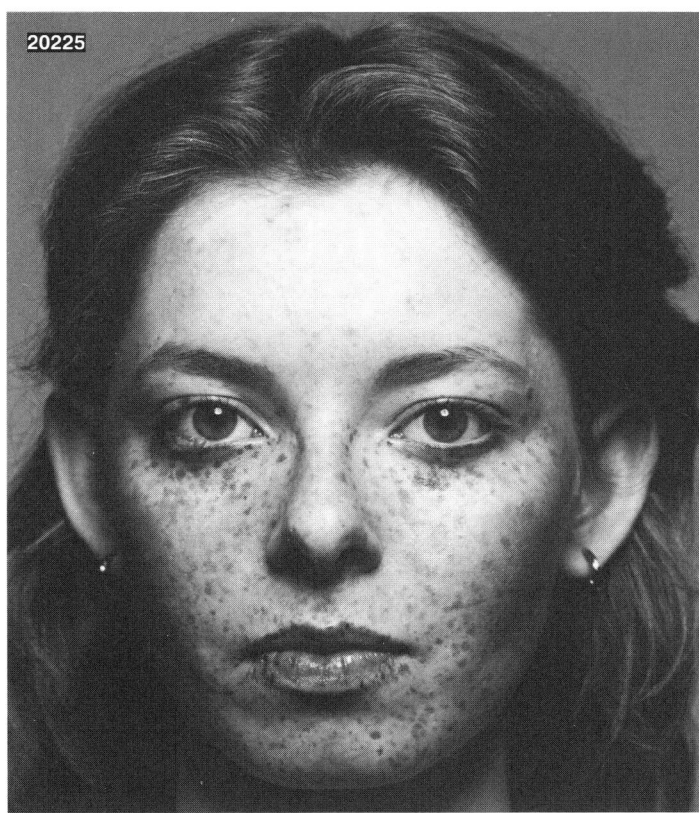

2572-20225: Multiple, non-elevated black-brown spots on face, vermilion border of lips and right upper eyelid. There is a nodule, three times recurrent and histologically a myxoma, on the right-lower eyelid.

Excludes:
Intestinal polyposis, type II (2344)
Lentigines syndrome, multiple (0586)

Major Diagnostic Criteria: Myxoma(s) of the heart, skin, and breast; mucocutaneous lentiginosis and multiple blue nevi; Cushing syndrome, acromegaly or gigantism, and sexual precocity.

Clinical Findings: The cardiac myxoma(s) occur in young patients (mean age, 24 years), tend to be multicentric (45%), and often affect multiple chambers (38%). The cutaneous myxoma(s), often an asymptomatic opalescent papule, typically affects the ears, eyelids, and nipples. Mammary myxoid fibroadenoma(s) tend to be multicentric and bilateral. Lentigines characteristically occur on the face, including the vermilion border of the lips (but infrequently affect the buccal mucosa), the conjunctiva, the trunk and limbs, and the genitalia, especially in the female. The blue nevi have a widespread distribution and are often multiple. Cushing syndrome is due to autonomous adrenocortical overactivity that is caused by a rare bilateral adrenocortical pathology, variously termed *micronodular adrenal disease, primary adrenocortical nodular dysplasia,* and *primary pigmented nodular adrenocortical disease.* The adrenal disorder is unusual in that the total adrenal weight is often normal or less than normal, both adrenal glands being studded with small (<4 mm) black or brown nodules set in an atrophic extranodular cortex. Acromegaly or gigantism is due to a growth hormone-producing pituitary adenoma. Testicular tumors (large-cell calcifying Sertoli cell tumor, Leydig cell tumor, and adrenocortical rest tumor) are bilateral and multicentric and may be associated with sexual precocity (40% of males). Calcifying

melanotic schwannomas, sometimes multicentric, occur in superficial (skin) and deep locations and are usually asymptomatic.

Complications: Acute ischemic phenomena, especially hemiplegia, result from embolization of fragments of cardiac myxoma, a lesion that also may cause acute and chronic heart failure. Morbidity results from multiple operations to excise cardiac myxomas. Partial deafness due to blockage of the external auditory canal by cutaneous myxoma. Osteoporosis due to Cushing syndrome. Growth failure due to Cushing syndrome, testicular tumors, or both.

Associated Findings: None known.

Etiology: Autosomal dominant inheritance with variable expression.

Pathogenesis: Unknown.

MIM No.: *16098

POS No.: 4335

Sex Ratio: M1:F1

Occurrence: Has been reported in North America, Europe, Australia, New Zealand, and Japan. The number of affected Jewish families appears to be disproportionately high.

Risk of Recurrence for Patient's Sib:
See Part I, *Mendelian Inheritance.*

Risk of Recurrence for Patient's Child:
See Part I, *Mendelian Inheritance.*

Age of Detectability: Usually clinically evident by ages 10–20 years. May be present as early as the first year of life.

Gene Mapping and Linkage: Unknown.

Prevention: None known. Genetic counseling indicated.

Treatment: Surgery for excision of myxomas, most importantly cardiac myxoma, keeping in mind that multiple cardiac chambers may be affected. Skin myxomas may need to be excised for diagnostic or cosmetic reasons. Disfiguring lentigines and blue nevi may need to be removed for similar reasons. Bilateral adrenalectomy cures the Cushing syndrome (the Nelson syndrome has not occurred following such surgery). Treatment of the testicular tumors should be conservative; no tumor has yet metastasized. Tumors causing sexual precocity need to be eradicated. The pituitary adenoma is best treated by transphenoidal hypophysectomy. Calcifying melanotic schwannomas are treated by surgical excision.

Prognosis: Long-term outlook is unknown. It may ultimately be found to depend largely on the results of multiple surgical procedures to control multiple episodes of cardiac myxoma. Several patients have had three cardiac operations for removal of recurrent (more likely multicentric) myxomas. About 25% of the patients have died of cardiac myxoma.

Detection of Carrier: Careful clinical examination and history of first-degree relatives together with echocardiogram and study of adrenocortical function.

Special Considerations: The oldest living affected patient (a member of an affected family who has mucocutaneous lentiginosis only) is aged 67 years. The cardiac myxoma has presented as early as age six years and as late as age 58 years (in a patient who was asymptomatic). Abnormalities of steroid metabolism may be present without the clinical features of the Cushing syndrome.

Support Groups: Atlanta; American Cancer Society

References:
Atherton DJ, et al.: A syndrome of various cutaneous pigmented lesions, myxoid neurofibromata and atrial myxoma: the NAME syndrome. Br J Dermatol 1980; 103:421–429.
Rhodes AR, et al.: Mucocutaneous lentigines, cardiomucocutaneous myxomas, and multiple blue nevi: the "LAMB" syndrome. J Am Acad Dermatol 1984; 10:72–82.
Carney JA, et al.: The complex of myxomas, spotty pigmentation, and endocrine overactivity. Medicine 1985; 64:270–283.
Carney JA, et al.: Dominant inheritance of the complex of myxomas, spotty pigmentation, and endocrine overactivity. Mayo Clin Proc 1986; 61:165–172.

Vidaillet HJ, Jr: "Syndrome myxoma": a subset of patients with cardiac myxoma associated with pigmented skin lesions and peripheral and endocrine neoplasms. Brit Heart J 1986; 57:247–255.

Cook CA, et al.: Mucocutaneous pigmented spots and oral myxomas: the oral manifestations of the complex of myxomas, spotty pigmentation, and endocrine overactivity. Oral Surg, Oral Med, Oral Path 1987; 63:175–183.

Danoff A, et al.: Adrenocortical micronodular dysplasia, cardiac myxomas, lentigines, and spindle cell tumors: report of a kindred. Arch Intern Med 1987; 147:443–448.

Kennedy RH, et al.: Ocular pigmented spots and eyelid myxomas. Am J Ophthal 1987; 104:533–538.

Carney JA: Psammomatous melanotic schwannoma. Modern Pathol 1988; 1:15A.

CA042   **J. A. Carney**

NEVO SYNDROME   3273

Includes: Overgrowth-congenital edema-positional defects of the feet

Excludes: Cebebral gigantism (0137)

Major Diagnostic Criteria: The combination of overgrowth with congenital edema and positional defects of the feet.

Clinical Findings: Three affected children (two sibs and their cousin) from an inbred family have been described. Anomalies include excessive birth length (97th centile) (3/3), hypotonia (3/3), congenital edema (2/3), congenital dorsiflexion of the feet (2/3), calcaneovalgus (1/3), dolichocephaly (2/3), highly arched, narrow palate (2/3), large, low-set ears (3/3), kyphosis (3/3), cryptorchidism (2/2 males), clinodactyly (1/3), tapering digits (2/3), single transverse palmar crease (1/3), and advanced bone age (2/3).

Complications: Unknown.

Associated Findings: One child had severe mental retardation, one child developed postnatal **Hydrocephaly.**

Etiology: The presence of the condition in sibs born to consanguineous parents and their double first cousin suggests autosomal recessive inheritance.

Pathogenesis: Unknown.

MIM No.: *11755

Sex Ratio: M1:F1

Occurrence: Documented in one family from Israel.

Risk of Recurrence for Patient's Sib:
See Part I, *Mendelian Inheritance.*

Risk of Recurrence for Patient's Child:
See Part I, *Mendelian Inheritance.*

Age of Detectability: At birth by excessive length and edema.

Gene Mapping and Linkage: Unknown.

Prevention: None known. Genetic counseling indicated.

Treatment: Supportive.

Prognosis: Variable, in that one child died at one month of complications from **Hydrocephaly** (postnatal). Of the two surviving children, one had normal intelligence and one was mentally retarded.

Detection of Carrier: Unknown.

Special Considerations: Although the authors suggested a diagnosis of **Cebebral gigantism** for these children, both the mode of inheritance and the presence of congenital edema, dorsiflexion of the feet, severe kyphosis and normal head circumference are not consistent with such a diagnosis.

References:
Nevo S, et al.: Evidence for autosomal recessive inheritance in cerebral gigantism. J Med Genet 1974; 11:158–165.

T0007   **Helga V. Toriello**

Nevocellular nevus, congenital
See NEVUS, CONGENITAL NEVOMELANOCYTIC

NEVOID BASAL CELL CARCINOMA SYNDROME   0101

Includes:
  Basal cell nevi
  Basal cell nevus syndrome
  Carcinoma, nevoid basal cell syndrome
  Fifth phacomatosis
  Gorlin-Goltz syndrome
  Nevus, basal cell nevus syndrome

Excludes:
  Achrochordons
  Epithelioma adenoides cysticum
  Follicular atrophoderma-hypotrichosis-face and head anhidrosis

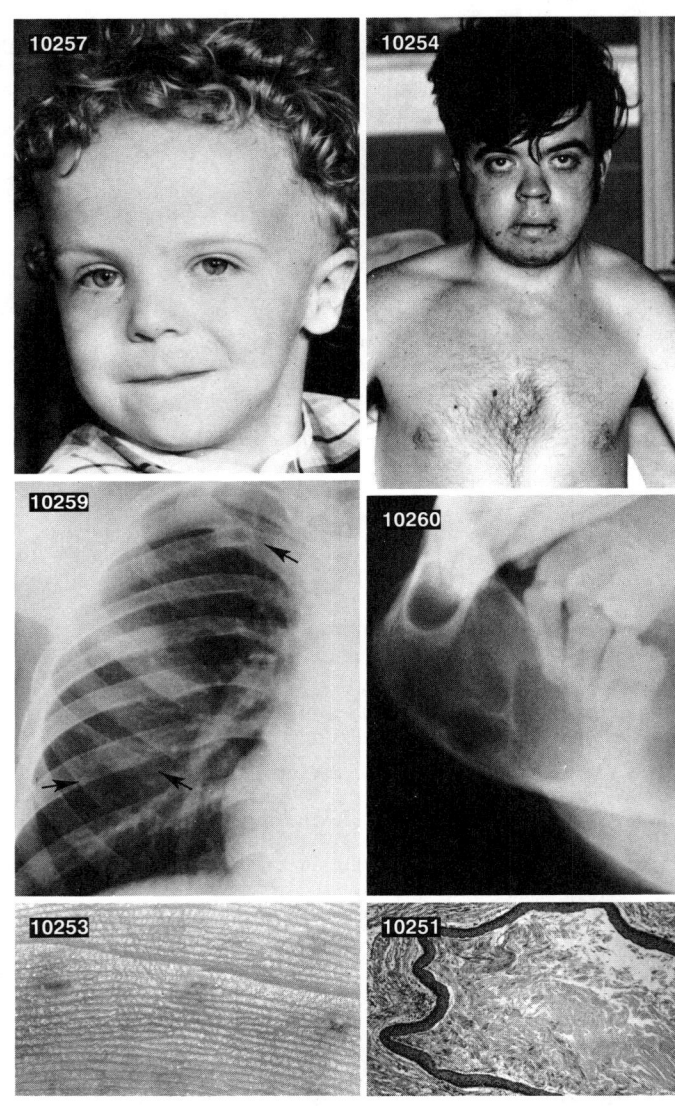

0101-10257: Young affected male with hypertelorism, strabismus, and craniofacial disproportion. **10254:** Older male shows macrocephaly, pectus excavatum, hypertelorism and sunken eyes. **10259:** Chest X-ray shows posterior fusion of ribs 3 and 4 and anterior bifurcation of rib 5. **10260:** Jaw cysts. **10253:** Palmar pits. **10251:** Keratocyst of the jaw; note thin epithelial layer with parakeratinazation.

Linear basal cell nevus
Multiple nevocytic or melanocytic nevi
Neurofibromatosis (0712)
Nevus, epidermal nevus syndrome (0593)
Non-nevus multiple basal cell carcinomas

Major Diagnostic Criteria: Multiple basal cell carcinomas with an early age at onset, epithelium-lined cysts of mandible and maxilla with unique daughter cysts, distinctive pits of the hands and feet, a variety of congenital skeletal anomalies, and ectopic calcification. In the absence of a positive family history, any two major components may be sufficient for diagnosis. With a positive family history, any of the major or a combination of several minor anomalies reflects expression of the syndrome.

Clinical Findings: *Cutaneous:* Multiple basal cell carcinomas (75%); pits of hands and feet (65%); cutaneous keratocysts, numerous milia (20–40%); ectopic calcification of basal cell (?%); carcinomas and subcutaneous tissues (?%).

Osseous: Jaw cysts (mandibular and maxillary) (80%); sellar bridging (75%); vertebral anomalies (spina bifida occulta, scoliosis) (65%); rib anomalies (bifidness, splaying, synostoses) (60%); subcortical cystic changes (long bones and phalanges) (45%); brachymetacarpalism (30%); Sprengel deformity (5%); defective dentition (?%); frontal and biparietal bossing (?%); mandibular prognathism (?%).

Neurologic: Calcification of the falx cerebri (lamellar pattern), tentorium cerebelli, and petroclinoid ligaments (80%); mental aberration, retardation (1–10%); EEG changes (non-specific), various neurological defects (?%); medulloblastoma (50% have onset before age 2 years) (1–5%).

Ophthalmologic: Hypertelorism, dystopia canthorum (25–50%); strabismus (25%); congenital blindness (colobomas, cataracts, glaucoma) (5–10%).

Reproductive: Ovarian fibromas (?%); hypogonadism (?%), ovarian cysts and fibromas; ovarian adenocarcinoma and fibrosarcoma.

Miscellaneous: Lymphatic mesenteric cysts; squamous cell carcinoma of jaw cyst; subconjunctival cysts of eyelids; fibrosarcoma of jaw (radiation-induced following radiation treatment for jaw cysts).

Syndrome may have variable or delayed expressivity. X-rays of skull, mandible, maxilla, ribs, vertebrae, and hands may be helpful in identifying the syndrome, particularly in children, before the basal cell carcinomas become manifest.

Complications: Loss of one or both eyes from basal cell carcinomas of lids and canthi; destruction of skin, scalp, subcutaneous tissue, cartilage, bone, nose, ears, etc. from infiltrating basal cell carcinomas; infection of jaw cysts, with swelling and pain from enlarging jaw cysts, resulting in loss and malposition of teeth; strangulation of mesenteric cyst; death from infiltrating basal cell carcinomas intracranially with or without infection; erosion of sizable blood vessels; or, rarely, metastasis. Death from medulloblastoma, fibrosarcoma, ovarian adenocarcinoma, or squamous cell carcinoma.

Radiation-induced basal cell carcinomas appear as early as 6 months to 3 years after irradiation. Radiation appears to increase the incidence of those tumors that would spontaneously occur in affected individuals. A few female syndrome survivors of medulloblastoma treated with ionizing irradiation have developed multiple ovarian fibrosarcomas and ovarian fibroma.

Associated Findings: None known.

Etiology: Autosomal dominant inheritance with high penetrance of gene (97%) and variable expressivity.

Pathogenesis: Unknown.

MIM No.: *10940

POS No.: 3527

Sex Ratio: M1:F1

Occurrence: Over 300 cases reported in the past decade.

Risk of Recurrence for Patient's Sib:
See Part I, *Mendelian Inheritance.*

Risk of Recurrence for Patient's Child:
See Part I, *Mendelian Inheritance.*

Age of Detectability: At birth, by skeletal anomalies; in childhood, by jaw cysts, defective dentition, skeletal anomalies, or medulloblastoma. In early adult life, by multiple basal cell carcinomas, jaw cysts, pits of hands and feet, skeletal defects of development, and ectopic calcification.

Gene Mapping and Linkage: NBCCS (nevoid basal cell carcinoma syndrome) has been tentatively mapped to 1p.

Prevention: None known. Genetic counseling indicated.

Treatment: Basal cell carcinomas rarely exhibit aggressive biological behavior before puberty. Treatment, therefore, is usually unnecessary until after puberty unless growth of one or several tumors is noted. An exception are children who have received ionizing irradiation for medulloblastoma or other reasons. Radiation-induced tumors appear 6 months to 3 years following treatment. Prevention of problem lesions is desirable by treating nevoid basal cell carcinomas early in their growth phase with surgical excision or open removal using curettage and electrosurgery. Tumors of the eyelids, periorbital and nasomalar areas, and near orifices such as the ear canal should be removed as they appear. Frequent follow-up visits are needed if tumor growth and new tumor development are occurring. Administration of systemic retinoids for retarding tumor growth, preventing new lesions, or treating aggressive lesions, though promising, is still under study and is not practical with available retinoids. Avoid irradiation therapy of tumors as well as modalities not highly curative, e.g., dermabrasion and, 5-fluorouracil.

Other therapy: Cryotherapy of tumors; the Mohs method of excision for problem tumors is very useful. The future value of photoradiation, interferon, and newer retinoids is uncertain.

Prognosis: Generally good for an average life span, but variable depending on location and invasiveness of the basal cell carcinomas and the less common tumors.

Detection of Carrier: Anthropometrics of skull identifies carriers in 85–90% of cases.

References:
Howell JB, Caro MR: The basal cell nevus: its relationship to multiple cutaneous cancers and associated anomalies of development. Arch Dermatol 1959; 79:67–80.
Gorlin RJ, et al.: Multiple basal cell nevi syndrome: an analysis of a syndrome consisting of multiple nevoid basal-cell carcinoma, jaw cysts, skeletal anomalies, medulloblastoma and hyporesponsiveness to parathormone. Cancer 1965; 18:89.
Berlin NI, et al.: Basal cell nevus syndrome. Ann Intern Med 1966; 64:403–421.
Anderson DE, et al.: The nevoid basal cell carcinoma syndrome. Am J Hum Genet 1967; 19:12.
Howell JB, Anderson DE: The nevoid basal cell carcinoma syndrome. In: Andrade R, ed: Cancer of the skin. Philadelphia: W.B. Saunders, 1976:883–898.
Howell JB: The roots of the nevoid basal cell carcinoma syndrome. Clin Exp Dermatol 1980; 5:337–348.
Howell JB, Anderson DE: Commentary: the nevoid basal cell carcinoma syndrome. Arch Dermatol 1982; 118:824–826.
Levine DJ, et al.: Familial subconjunctival epithelial cysts associated with nevoid basal cell carcinoma syndrome. Arch Dermatol 1987; 123:23–24.

H0050   **James B. Howell**
AN017   **David E. Anderson**

Nevoid pigmentation of the retina
See RETINA, GROUPED HYPERTROPHY OF RETINAL PIGMENT EPITHELIUM
Nevomelanocytic nevus, congenital
See NEVUS, CONGENITAL NEVOMELANOCYTIC
Nevus anemicus
See SKIN, VITILIGO

NEVUS FLAMMEUS   0715

Includes:

"Angel's kiss"
"Birthmark" (obsolete)
Capillary hemangioma
Capillary nevus
Erythema nuchae
Nape nevus
Nevi flammei
Nevus flammeus of nape of neck
Nevus planus
Nevus simplex
"Pressure marks" (obsolete)
Port-wine stain
Salmon patch
"Stork bite" mark
Unna nevus

Excludes: Hemangiomas of the head and neck (2514)

Major Diagnostic Criteria: Vascular skin lesions.

Clinical Findings: Nevus flammeus can be divided into two categories: the salmon patch and the port-wine stain. Salmon patches are commonly seen on the nape of the neck, occiput, forehead, glabella, and eyelids. On the forehead and glabella, they usually have a tornado-funnel shape, with the apex pointing downward. Salmon patches of the eyelids, forehead, and glabella generally disappear by the end of the first year of life. A considerable number of those on the occiput and nape of the neck, however, persist.

Port-wine stains consist of pink macules varying in size from one to many centimeters. They can occur anywhere on the body but have a special predilection for the face. The lesion is generally unilateral, and it often approximates a dermatomal pattern. Although both salmon patches and port-wine stains show the same histologic features, ectasia of blood vessels in the superficial dermis without vascular proliferation, port-wine stains do not disappear. With increasing age the vessels become more ectatio and more engorged with erythrocytes. Clinically, a darkening in color and a nodular, "cobblestone" appearence of the skin surface is observed.

Complications: Unknown.

Associated Findings: Glaucoma, phocomelia, **Chromosome 13, trisomy 13, Chromosome 4, monosomy 4p, Beckwith-Wiedemann syndrome,** underlying arteriovenous communication, and possibly congenital heart disease.

Approximately 5% of port-wine stains may be associated with a cavernous hemangioma involving deep dermis, subcutaneous tissue, and even muscle. In some patients, especially those in whom the "cobblestone" pattern is pronounced, there may occur some blood vessel and stromal proliferation.

Etiology: Probably autosomal dominant inheritance, but the high prevalence of salmon patches precludes a definite conclusion regarding these lesions. Nevi flammei of trunk and limbs have also been reported to follow irregularly dominant patterns.

Pathogenesis: Arterial, venous, and capillary circulation of the skin arises from a primitive, pluripotential capillary network. During fetal development certain portions of this network are normally resorbed. Failure or incomplete resorption is thought to result in nevus flammeus.

In their development, appearance, and distribution, nevi flammei may be under neural influences. Phocomelic "thalidomide babies" and infants with various chromosome anomalies have exhibited facial nevi flammei. Rarely, nevi flammei first appear following exposure to intense cold or other physical injury.

It is not known why progressive ectasia of blood vessel walls occurs in port-wine stains. Direct immunofluorescent studies of three major components of blood vessel walls (collagenous basement membrane, fibronectin, and Factor VIII) have shown no differences in the distribution or amount of these materials in either port-wine stains and normal skin. One explanation for these findings is that proteins are antigenically normal but non-

functional. Another possibility may be that the progressive ectasia is not due to an intrinsic abnormality of the vessel itself, but rather to the supporting connective tissue of the dermis.

MIM No.: *16310

CDC No.: 757.380

Sex Ratio: M1:F1 for most types. M>1:F1 in Cobb syndrome.

Occurrence: Salmon patch in over 40% of neonates (i.e. "normal anatomic variants"). Port-wine stains found in 0.3% of 1,058 newborns (80% white). Nape nevi persist in about 30% of adults. Lower figures reported in Blacks, but lesions are less visible.

Risk of Recurrence for Patient's Sib:
See Part I, *Mendelian Inheritance.*

Risk of Recurrence for Patient's Child:
See Part I, *Mendelian Inheritance.*

Age of Detectability: Usually in the neonatal period.

Gene Mapping and Linkage: Unknown.

Prevention: None known. Genetic counseling indicated.

Treatment: Salmon patches are generally not treated.

Treatment of port-wine stains has included cosmetic coverage, excision and graft, laser beam, CO_2 ice, electrodesiccation, tattooing, and various forms of radiotherapy. Both argon and CO_2 laser have been used, but most clinical experience to date has centered on the argon laser. Results have been fair to good, although advances in this technology offer promise (Tan et al, 1989). Excision and grafting, cryotherapy, electrodessication, dermabrasion, and therapeutic tatoo have been used with inconsistent success. Radiotherapy (thorium X, grenz ray, radiophosphorus) has, for the most part, been abandoned. Special opaque cosmetics have been developed for the express purpose of concealing port-wine stains and similar disfiguring lesions, and the use of these cosmetics should be encouraged.

Prognosis: Normal for life span, intelligence, and function when changes are limited to the skin.

Detection of Carrier: Unknown.

Special Considerations: The theory that salmon patches are caused by trauma directly to the lesional area has been dispelled; the expression "pressure marks" and "birthmark" should no longer be used.

Salmon patches are trivial lesions unassociated with other vascular malformations. Port-wine stains, on the other hand, may portend an underlying vascular anomaly, the most serious of which is **Sturge-Weber syndrome.** A number of other eponymic syndromes have been described in which vascular anomalies of the eyes and central nervous system have been inconsistently associated with nevus flammeus. These syndromes are thought by some to be variations of the Sturge-Weber syndrome. Tissue hypertrophy may accompany nevi flammei of the limbs (see **Angio-osteohypertrophy syndrome**), genitalia, lips, and other sites.

References:
Jacobs AH, Walton RG: The incidence of birthmarks in the neonate. Pediatrics 1976; 58:218–222.
Finley JL, et al.: Immunofluorescent staining with antibodies to factor VIII, fibronectin, and collagenous basement membrane protein in normal human skin and port-wine stains. Arch Dermatol 1982; 118:971–975.
Jacobs AH: Vascular nevi. Pediatr Clin North Am 1983; 30:465–482.
Buecker JW, et al.: Histology of port-wine stain treated with carbon dioxide laser. J Am Acad Dermatol 1984; 10:1014–1019.
Finley JL, et al.: Argon laser-port-wine stain interaction. Arch Dermatol 1984; 120:613–619.
Finley JL, et al.: Port-wine stains. Arch Dermatol 1984; 120:1453–1455.
Merlob P, Reisner SH: Familial nevus flammeus of the forehead and unna's nevus. Clin Genetics 1985; 27:165–166.
Tan OT, et al.: Treatment of children with port-wine stains using the flashlamp-pulsed tunable dye laser. New Engl J Med 1989; 320:416–421.

SE014
PE018
                                              Victor J. Selmanowitz
                                              Frederick A. Pereira

Nevus flammeus of nape of neck
See NEVUS FLAMMEUS
Nevus fuscoceruleus ophthalmomaxillaris
See NEVUS OF OTA

NEVUS OF OTA   0716

Includes:
Dermal melanocytosis
Nevus fuscoceruleus ophthalmomaxillaris
Oculocutaneous melanosis
Oculocutaneous pigmentation syndrome
Oculodermal melanocytosis

Excludes:
Conjuctival melanosis
Malignant melanoma
Melanocytoma
Mongolian spot
Nevus, blue rubber bleb nevus syndrome (0113)
Ocular melanosis
Optic disk, melanocytoma (0639)
Precancerous melanosis

Major Diagnostic Criteria: Nevus of Ota is a benign, macular or slightly raised, indistinctly marginated discoloration of the face in the region of innervation of the first and second divisions of the trigeminal nerve. The color of the lesion varies from tan to brown, black, slate-blue, or purple.

Clinical Findings: About one-half of cases of nevus of Ota become apparent in the first year of life. Other cases develop later, and onset or exacerbation during puberty or pregnancy is common. Ninety-five percent of cases are unilateral. Nevus of Ota is associated with ipsilateral ocular hyperpigmentation in one-half to two-thirds of affected patients. Scleral involvement is most common, but hyperpigmentation of the cornea, conjunctiva, uveal tract, optic disk, optic nerve, orbital soft tissue, or periosteum of the bony orbit may occur. Heterochromia of the iris has also been observed. The dermal discoloration may extend beyond the immediate region of the eye to the temple, forehead, cheek, or nose. Pigmentation of the tympanic membrane, palate, and oral or nasal mucosa is commonly associated with nevus of Ota.

Histologically, the nevus of Ota resembles the **Nevus, blue rubber bleb nevus syndrome** and **Skin, cutaneous melanosis: Mongolian spot.** The dermis of affected skin contains heavily pigmented melanocytes with a fusiform, dendritic, or stellate shape.

Complications: A predisposition to development of malignant melanoma (as high as 23% among severe cases) appears to exist with nevus of Ota.

Associated Findings: Persistent mongolian spots on the buttocks or back occasionally are found in adults with nevus of Ota, especially if bilateral. Blue nevi may occur within the nevus of Ota or at neighboring sites. Glaucoma, angiomas, bony anomalies, and neurologic problems have rarely been reported in association with nevus of Ota and may represent coincidental observations.

Etiology: Undetermined. Familial cases are uncommon.

Pathogenesis: Unknown.

CDC No.: 757.380

Sex Ratio: M1:F4, but this may reflect a greater likelihood for females to consult a physician because of a cosmetic lesion on the face.

Occurrence: Undetermed presumably uncommon; more frequent among Orientals (0.2–0.8%) and Blacks than among whites.

Risk of Recurrence for Patient's Sib: Presumably small.

Risk of Recurrence for Patient's Child: Presumably small.

Age of Detectability: The lesion appears in the first year of life in about one-half of cases, and during childhood, adolescence, or early adulthood in the other one-half.

Gene Mapping and Linkage: Unknown.

Prevention: None known. Genetic counseling indicated.

Treatment: Cosmesis.

Prognosis: Nevus of Ota is generally only a cosmetic problem. The lesion is permanent, but may become lighter or darker with aging or hormonal changes.

Detection of Carrier: Unknown.

References:
Kopf AW, Weidman AI: Nevus of Ota. Arch Dermatol 1956; 85:195–208.
Mishima Y, Mevorah B: Nevus Ota and nevus Ito in American Negroes. J Invest Dermatol 1961; 36:133–154.
Hagler WS, Brown CC: Malignant melanoma of the orbit arising in a nevus of Ota. Transact Am Acad Ophthalmol 1966; 70:817–822.
Hidano A, et al.: Natural history of nevus of Ota. Arch Derm 1967; 95:187–195.
Guérin JC, Daudon-Conteaux R: Le naevus de Ota. Arch Ophtalmol (Paris) 1974; 34:359–384.

FR017   **J.M. Friedman**

Nevus planus
See NEVUS FLAMMEUS
Nevus sebaceus of Jadassohn
See NEVUS, EPIDERMAL NEVUS SYNDROME
Nevus simplex
See NEVUS FLAMMEUS
Nevus varicosus osteohypertrophicus
See ANGIO-OSTEOHYPERTROPHY SYNDROME
Nevus, basal cell nevus syndrome
See NEVOID BASAL CELL CARCINOMA SYNDROME

NEVUS, BLUE RUBBER BLEB NEVUS SYNDROME   0113

Includes:
Bean syndrome
Blue rubber bleb nevus of skin and gastrointestinal tract
Hemangiomatosis, generalized cavernous
Hamartoma, venous

Excludes:
Enchondromatosis and hemangiomas (0346)
Fabry disease (0373)
Multiple hemangiomatosis
Solitary cavernous hemangioma
Telangiectasia, osler hemorrhagic (2021)

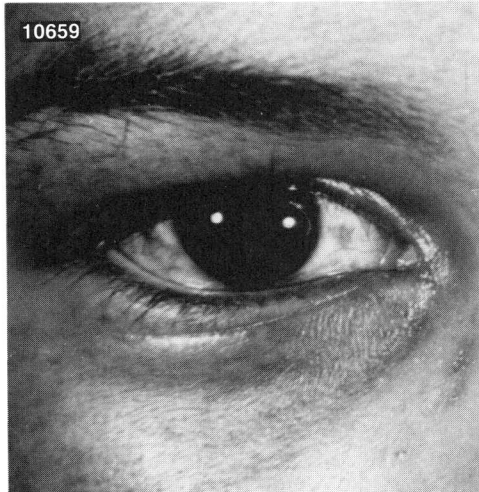

0716-10659: Nevus of Ota.

Major Diagnostic Criteria: Multiple hemangiomas of the skin are present. The hemangiomas range in size from 0.1 to 5.0 cm, are bluish in color, and are characterized by easy compressibility.

Clinical Findings: Multiple cavernous hemangiomas are present in the skin (100%), GI tract (90%), and are less frequently reported to occur in the subcutaneous tissue, mucous membranes, lungs, liver, skeletal muscle, thyroid, brain, spinal cord, meninges, cranial bones, spleen, heart, and kidney. The hemangiomas are 0.2–4 cm in diameter and are bluish to purplish-red to black in color. They are rumpled in appearance when partially emptied by squeezing and slowly refill when pressure is released. Bleeding is common.

Complications: Serious spontaneous GI bleeding and anemia occur frequently. Spontaneous bleeding of the skin lesions is rare, but they may bleed from injury. The skin lesions may produce serious cosmetic problems. Lesions of the soles may interfere with walking. Oozing, irritation, and offensive odor from involvement of the genital area and perianal area may occur.

Associated Findings: Meningioma, medulloblastoma, osteoma, syringomyelia, and cysts of many organs have been reported.

Etiology: Autosomal dominant inheritance. Numerous multi-generation pedigrees have been reported. Sporadic cases may represent new dominant mutations or phenocopies.

Pathogenesis: Microscopically the lesions are thin-walled and filled with blood, with the walls resembling those of veins. Sweat glands are often closely related to vascular lesions.

MIM No.: *11220

POS No.: 4229

CDC No.: 757.380

Sex Ratio: Presumably M1:F1

Occurrence: Rare, but reported in various races.

Risk of Recurrence for Patient's Sib:
See Part I, *Mendelian Inheritance.*

Risk of Recurrence for Patient's Child:
See Part I, *Mendelian Inheritance.*

Age of Detectability: Lesions are usually present at birth.

Gene Mapping and Linkage: Unknown.

Prevention: None known. Genetic counseling indicated.

Treatment: Most troublesome skin lesions may be excised. Anemia due to bleeding from GI lesions should be treated as needed. Carbon dioxide laser treatment has been reported to be effective. Argon laser therapy may also be useful.

Prognosis: Life span may be normal, or patients may die in early adult life from associated conditions or from internal hemorrhage.

Detection of Carrier: Unknown.

The author is indebted to J. Sidney Rice, who authored an earlier version of this article.

References:
Jaffe RH: Multiple hemangiomas of skin and of internal organs. Arch Pathol 1929; 7:44.
Rice JS, Fischer DS: Blue rubber bleb nevus syndrome: generalized cavernous hemangiomatosis or venous hamartoma with medulloblastoma of the cerebellum; case report and review of the literature. Arch Dermatol 1962; 86:503–511.
Morris SJ, et al.: Blue rubber bleb nevus syndrome. JAMA 1978; 239:1887.
McCauley RGK, et al.: Blue rubber bleb nevus syndrome. Radiology 1979; 133:375–377.
Olsen TG, et al.: Laser surgery for blue rubber bleb nevus. Arch Dermatol 1979; 115:81–82.
Munkvad M: Blue rubber bleb nevus syndrome. Dermatologica 1983; 167:307–309.
Satya-Murti S, et al.: Central nervous system involvement in blue-rubber-bleb-nevus syndrome. Arch Neurol 1986; 43:1184–1186.

Virginia P. Sybert

NEVUS, CONGENITAL NEVOMELANOCYTIC 　　　2165

Includes:
　　Giant pigmented hairy nevus (GPHN)
　　Hairy melanocytic nevus, giant congenital
　　Melanocytic nevus, congenital
　　Melanocytic nevus, giant congenital
　　Melanocytic nevus, small congenital
　　Nevocellular nevus, congenital
　　Nevomelanocytic nevus, congenital

Excludes:
　　Nevus, epidermal nevus syndrome (0593)
　　Non-nevomelanocytic congenital nevi

Major Diagnostic Criteria: A congenital nevomelanocytic nevus is a collection of nevus cells in the skin, first apparent at birth.

Clinical Findings: Lesions may be diagnosed on the basis of gross morphology and parental history. Nevomelanocytic nevi are round or oval plaques, pigmented one or more shades or brown, distorting the skin surface by accentuated skin markings or follicles when examined using tangential light, having fine speckling of pigment when examined using bright light and 10X hand lens magnification of the mineral-oil covered lesion surface. Excessive hair may or may not be present. The definition of small is a lesion that can be excised easily and the defect closed primarily without the use of flaps or grafts. Giant is a subset of large, occupying a major portion of a major anatomic site.

Complications: Giant congenital nevomelanocytic nevi have a risk of cutaneous melanoma approaching 10% over a lifetime. Of those giant congenital nevomelanocytic nevi developing cutaneous melanoma, about half the cases are diagnosed in the first three to five years of life. Giant nevi may be the precursor for 0.1% of cutaneous melanomas.

The risk of melanoma associated with small varieties of congenital nevomelanocytic nevi has been estimated to be as high as 5% by age 60 years. Up to 15% of melanomas are alleged to have developed in a small congenital nevus; 2.6% to 8.1% of melanomas may show evidence of a dermal nevus having one or more "congenital" features, in contiguity with the tumor. Although there appears to be a definite risk of melanoma associated with small congenital nevi, the exact magnitude of the risk is regarded as controversial.

Associated Findings: Possibly ear deformities, preauricular appendages, angiomas, and other skin anomalies, according to one study.

Etiology: Possibly autosomal dominant inheritance, in some cases.

Pathogenesis: Presumed dysplasia of neural crest-derived melanoblasts.

MIM No.: 13755, *15560

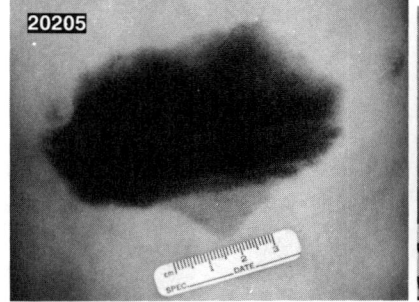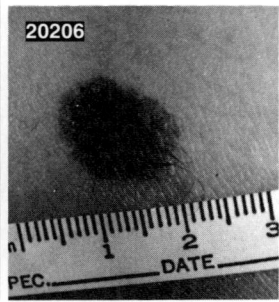

2165-20205: Relatively large congenital nevus on the anterior torso of a 10-month-old male.　**20206:** Small congenital nevus which is uniformly pigmented medium brown with well-demarcated smooth borders and coarse dark hairs on the surface.

CDC No.: 757.380

Sex Ratio: M1:F1

Occurrence: One percent of newborns for small lesions, 1:20,000 newborns for lesions ≥9.9 cm in greatest diameter; 1:500,000 newborns for giant lesions.

Risk of Recurrence for Patient's Sib: Increased, but exact risk not known.

Risk of Recurrence for Patient's Child: Increased, but exact risk not known.

Age of Detectability: At birth.

Gene Mapping and Linkage: CMM (cutaneous malignant melanoma/dysplastic nevus) has been provisionally mapped to 1p36.

Prevention: None known. Genetic counseling indicated.

Treatment: Because of the increased risk of melanoma associated with congenital nevomelanocytic nevi (regardless of size), all such lesions should be evaluated for excision. Melanoma associated with very large lesions may occur even in the first several years of life, so prophylactic excision should be considered early. Melanoma associated with small congenital nevi usually does not occur until after 12 years. Excision of small congenital nevi may be delayed until local anesthesia can be used at the end of the first decade of life, as long as the lesion maintains a benign appearance and lends itself to photographic follow-up. Atypical-appearing nevomelanocytic nevi should be evaluated for immediate excision.

The management of small congenital nevi is considered controversial. Ascertainment of congenital nevomelanocytic nevi in contiguity with cutaneous melanoma has been based on history and histology. Neither of these methods of ascertainment is perfect. The management of congenital nevomelanocytic nevi needs to be individualized. In general, there seems to be little justification for recommending lifetime follow-up for lesions that can be excised easily. The risk of melanoma associated with large lesions is less controversial, but such lesions are more difficult to excise.

Prognosis: Unknown.

Detection of Carrier: Unknown.

References:
Trozak DJ, et al.: Metastatic melanoma in prepubertal children. Pediatrics 1975; 55:191–204.
Walton RG, et al.: Pigmented lesions in newborn infants. Br J Dermatol 1976; 95:389–396.
Lorentzen M, et al.: The incidence of malignant transformation in giant pigmented nevi. Scand J Plast Reconstr Surg 1977; 11:163–167.
Alper J, et al.: Birthmarks with serious medical significance: nevocellular nevi, sebaceous nevi, and multiple cafe au lait spots. J Pediatr 1979; 95:696–700.
Castilla EE, et al.: Epidemiology of pigmented naevi: incidence rates and relative frequency. Br J Dermatol 1981; 104:307–315.
Castilla EE, et al.: Epidemiology of pigmented naevi: risk factors. Br J Dermatol 1981; 104:421–427.
Rhodes AR, et al.: Non-epidermal origin of malignant melanoma associated with giant congenital nevocellular nevi. Plast Reconstr Surg 1981; 67:782–790.
Rhodes AR, et al.: Familial aggregation of small congenital nevomelanocytic nevi. Am J Med Genet 1985; 22:315–326.
Rhodes AR: Neoplasms: benign neoplasms, hyperplasias, and dysplasias of melanocytes. In: Fitzpatrick TB, et al., eds: Dermatology in General Medicine, ed. 3. New York: McGraw Hill, 1987: 902–915.

RH003   **Arthur R. Rhodes**

NEVUS, EPIDERMAL NEVUS SYNDROME   0593

Includes:
     Epidermal nevus syndrome
     Ichthyosis hystrix gravior
     Inflammatory linear verrucous epidermal nevus (ILVEN)
     Jadassohn linear nevus sebaceous syndrome
     Lambert type ichthyosis
     Linear nevus sebaceous syndrome
     Linear sebaceous nevus syndrome
     Nevus sebaceus of Jadassohn
     "Porcupine man"
     Sebaceous nevus syndrome

Excludes:
     Angio-osteohypertrophy syndrome (0055)
     Ichthyosis (all generalized forms)
     Ichthyosis hystrix, Curth-Macklin type (2857)
     Incontinentia pigmenti (0526)
     Limb reduction-ichthyosis (2019)
     Nevus, congenital melanocytic (2165)
     Proteus syndrome (2382)

Major Diagnostic Criteria: At birth or soon after, alopecia with absent or primitive hair follicles and numerous small hypoplastic sebaceous glands with hyperpigmentation and hyperkeratosis. Lesions are usually on the scalp, in the para-midfacial area, from the forehead down into the nasal area. These tend to be linear in distribution, and may also affect the trunk and limbs. At puberty, the lesions become verrucous with hyperplastic sebaceous glands, and tumors may develop. The condition may be associated with

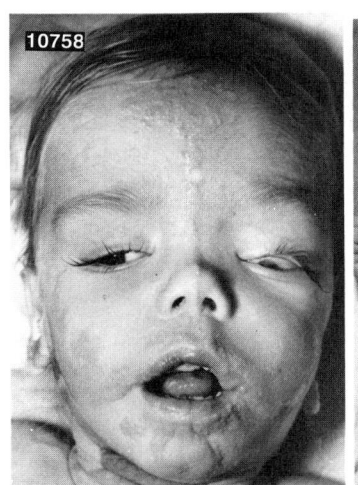
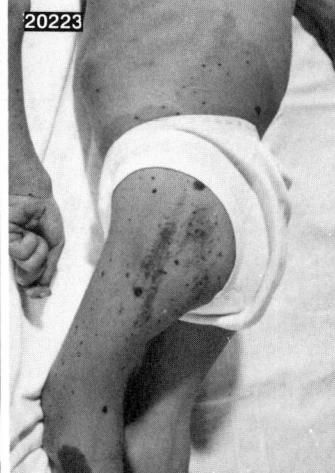
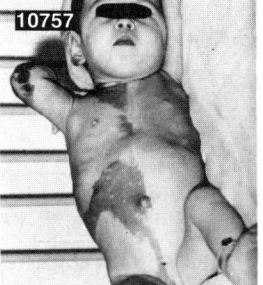
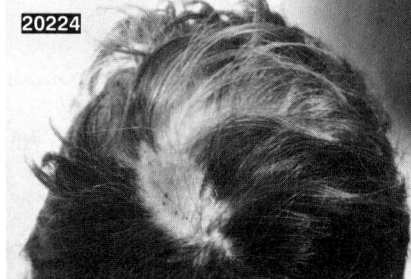

0593-10758: Facial distribution of epidermal nevus. **20223:** Linear distribution on the trunk and leg. **10757:** Note the asymmetry and linear distribution of the skin lesions. **20224:** Orange lesion of the scalp in an area of alopecia.

bony anomalies, ocular anomalies, central nervous system dysfunction, or nevoid anomalies.

Clinical Findings: The first stage consists of alopecia with absent or primitive hair follicles and numerous small hypoplastic sebaceous glands with hyperpigmentation and hyperkeratosis. One or more of the five major types of epidermal nevi may appear (dark, velvety patches; raised warty streaks; scaly streaks on segments of the body; polyp-like masses arranged in a linear manner; or an orange, bald, velvety mass covering part of the scalp, face, eyes, and nose). Lesions often involve the midfacial area, from the forehead down into the nasal area. These tend to be linear in distribution, and may also affect the trunk and limbs. The skin lesions usually progress after birth, altering their size, thickness, and severity with growth and stabilization at age 15–20 years. The lesions tend to become verrucous, and early surgical removal should be considered since there is a risk of tumor; especially basal cell epithelioma.

Other findings can include: epidermal nevus (60%); mental retardation (40%); seizures (33%); skeletal anomalies (70%), including bony hypertrophy; cysts, kyphosis, and scoliosis (28%); ankle, and foot deformities (15%); and ocular abnormalities (33%); including dermolipoid.

Periods of unpredictable rapid growth of the lesions have been reported. Onset of seizures, in cases with central nervous system involvement, has been between two months and two years of age. Intelligence ranges from normal to severe mental retardation.

Inflammatory linear verrucous epidermal nevus (ILVEN) is a related but possibly distinct condition (Hamm and Happle, 1986).

Complications: Oral and ocular involvement with the nevus; severe social and learning problems; with hypertrophic changes, functional problems of walking and using hands may develop. Buying clothes becomes more difficult. Cerebrovascular accidents may be a major problem.

Associated Findings: **Hemihypertrophy**; **Cancer, Wilms tumor**; vitamin D-resistant rickets; vascular defects of skin, bone, brain, and kidney.

Specific ocular findings can include cloudy cornea, coloboma of the eyelid, iris and choroid, esotropia, and lipodermoid of the conjunctiva. Other reported anomalies include asymmetric cortical atrophy, **Hydrocephaly**, **Aorta, coarctation**, **Ventricular septal defect**, hypoplastic teeth, renal hamartomata, and nephroblastoma.

Etiology: Undetermined. Some pedigrees (about two-thirds) suggest autosomal dominant inheritance.

Pathogenesis: Unknown.

MIM No.: 16320, *14660

POS No.: 3215

CDC No.: 757.380

Sex Ratio: M1:F1

Occurrence: Undetermined. About 450 cases have been reported among whites, Blacks, Indians, Orientals, and Hispanics.

Risk of Recurrence for Patient's Sib: Unknown. Available data suggest about a 1% risk.

Risk of Recurrence for Patient's Child: Unknown.

Age of Detectability: For most patients, at birth.

Gene Mapping and Linkage: Unknown.

Prevention: None known. Genetic counseling indicated.

Treatment: Surgical removal of a large lesion is often not possible or does not improve the appearance. Smaller lesions may be surgically removed. Topically, 5–10% lactic acid in 50% aqueous solution of propylene glycol helps somewhat. Propylene glycol absorbed in quantity may be nephrotoxic and caution is advised. Lubricants help somewhat. Topical retinoic acid solution is helpful. Orally administered 13-cis-retinoic acid may help in some patients, but it has many unwanted side effects and its use for this purpose is experimental at this time. Involvement of bones, eyes, and other organs may require attention.

Prognosis: Longevity is occasionally affected because of the relatively high incidence of associated malignancies. (e.g., malignant astrocytoma). In most instances, however, longevity is unaffected. Functional impairment varies with the extent to which the central nervous system, vascular system, kidneys, and skeleton are involved.

Detection of Carrier: Undetermined. Bianchine (1970) reported seizures and/or mental deficiency without skin lesions in first degree relatives of one patient.

Special Considerations: Opinions are divided as to the overlap between this condition and several related disorders. One good example is the famous Lambert pedigree *ichthyosis hystrix gravior*, sometimes called the "porcupine man", discussed in some detail by Anton-Lamprecht (1978).

References:
Solomon LM, et al.: The epidermal nevus syndrome. Arch Dermatol 1968; 97:273–285.
Bianchine JW: The nevus sebaceus of Jadassohn: a neurocutaneous syndrome and a potentially premalignant lesion. Am J Dis Child 1970; 120:223–228.
Lansky LL, et al.: Linear sebaceous nevus syndrome. Am J Dis Child 1972; 123:587–590.
Anton-Lamprecht I: Electron microscope in the early diagnosis of genetic disorders of the skin. Dermatologica 1978; 157:65–85.
Leonidas JC, et al.: Radiographic features of the linear sebaceous syndrome. Am J Roentgenol 1979; 132:277–279.
Monk BE, Vollum DI: Familial naevus sebaceus. J Royal Soc Med 1982; 75:660–661.
Hamm H, Happle R: Inflammatory linear verrucous epidermal nevus (ILVEN) in a mother and her daughter. Am J Med Genet 1986; 24:685–690.
Baker RS, et al.: Neurologic complications of the epidermal nevus syndrome. Arch Neurol 1987; 44:227–232.
Rogers M, et al.: Epidermal nevi and the epidermal nevus syndrome: a review of 131 cases. J Am Acad Derm 1989; 20:476–488.

S0009   **Lawrence M. Solomon**

Nezelof syndrome
    See IMMUNODEFICIENCY, NEZELOF TYPE
NF-1
    See NEUROFIBROMATOSIS
NFDR syndrome
    See NEURO-FACIO-DIGITO-RENAL SYNDROME
Nicotinamide adenine dinucleotide and oxidoreductase
    See LACTATE DEHYDROGENASE ISOZYMES

NIEMANN-PICK DISEASE   0717

Includes:
> Niemann-Pick disease with cholesterol esterification block
> Nova Scotian type Niemann-Pick disease
> Sea-blue histiocyte disease
> Sphingomyelin lipidosis
> Sphingomyelinase deficiency

Excludes:
> **Gaucher disease** (0406)
> **G(M1)-gangliosidosis, type 1** (0431)
> **G(M2)-gangliosidosis with hexosaminidase A deficiency** (0434)
> **Wolman disease** (1003)

Major Diagnostic Criteria: Enlargement of liver or spleen; presence of foam cells in bone marrow, liver, or spleen; demonstration of abnormal intracellular accumulation of sphingomyelin, and a negative search for other situations that may produce secondary formation of similar foam cells.

Clinical Findings: The term "Niemann-Pick disease" is applied to five phenotypes that have areas of clinical and genetic difference but a presumed biochemical relationship:
Group A: Acute neuronopathic form.
Group B: Chronic form without nervous system involvement.
Group C: Chronic neuronopathic form.
Group D: Nova Scotia variant.

Group E: Adult non-neuronopathic form.

Enlargement of the spleen and liver is common to all Groups and is usually quite notable, while lymphadenopathy is not prominent. The hematologic effects of the spenomegaly ("hypersplenism") are common, but are less intense than in **Gaucher disease**. Pulmonary infiltration is characteristic in the circumstances in which organomegaly is of high order and growth impairment is of varying degree. All forms except the remarkable "adult" type (Group B) have increasingly serious neurologic involvement, including developmental delay and arrest followed by general functional deterioration. Occasional patients have seizures, and the older children may show ataxia or other cerebellar signs. Cherry-red macular changes are noted in some of the patients, especially the younger ones. Occasional children develop small papular or nodular skin xanthomas, which are apparently not secondary to hyperlipidemia, the latter being seen only in Group A and B patients. It is usual to find vacuolization of some of the lymphocytes in the peripheral blood. The diagnosis can be made by recognition of a large foamy cell in the bone marrow. Electron microscopic studies show cytoplasmic lipid inclusions consisting of concentric laminar bodies.

A sixth form, sometimes called Group F, has been identified in populations of Spanish background. This group is distinguished, in part, by sea-blue or foamy histiocytes. At present, it is not clear if this is a unique form of Niemann-Pick, a specific condition sometimes called *Sea-blue histiocyte disease*, or a variation of Groups A, B, or C Niemann-Pick disease.

Complications: Chronic nutritional failure eventually ensues, as well as progressive debility and mental retardation (except in Group B patients). Bronchopneumonia occurs in the terminal patients, as does anemia and ascites. Hepatic failure has been described in Group B.

Associated Findings: Prolonged jaundice of moderate degree in the first 6 months of life is reported in about one-quarter of the patients and is of unknown significance.

Etiology: Autosomal recessive inheritance.

Pathogenesis: Specific sphingomyelinase deficiency has been identified in the tissues, cultured fibroblasts, and white blood cells of patients from Group A and B. In Group C the exact enzymatic defect is not known; recent works seem to demonstrate that the impairment of sphingomyelin metabolism is not the primary defect, the sphingomyelinase levels are normal in most of the tissues, and there is accumulation of cholesterol, which could be responsible for the inhibition of sphingomyelin degradation. Pentchev et al (1984) found Group C cell lines to differ from Group A and B in that Group C showed a major block in cholesterol esterification. Somatic cell hybridization experiments suggest that the defect in Group C is under separate genetic control from that in Groups A and B. Group D might represent an allelic form of the Group C gene.

It appears reasonable to assume that local tissue sphingomyelin accumulation can be adequately explained on the basis of the lysosomal enzyme insufficiency. An explanation is also needed, however, for the simultaneous cholesterol increase in tissues, unless, as Brady (1983) has suggested, a specific intermolecular complex (of cholesterol and sphingomyelin) is formed. The specific origin of the CNS defect is incompletely understood. Only in Group A patients is there a cortical increase in sphingomyelin, per se, and in Group B patients (with the same enzymopathy) the brain is normal.

MIM No.: *25720, *25722, *25725, 26960

POS No.: 3334

Sex Ratio: M1:F1

Occurrence: Several hundred cases reported. About 80% of Group A patients, which account for about 85% of all Niemann-Pick cases, are of Ashkenazi Jewish ancestry. The carrier rate among Jews is about 1:100. Group D is usually found among decendents of a 17th Century French Acadian couple from Yarmouth county, Nova Scotia.

Risk of Recurrence for Patient's Sib:

See Part I, *Mendelian Inheritance.*

Risk of Recurrence for Patient's Child:

See Part I, *Mendelian Inheritance.* A number of persons with Group B involvement are now known to have had normal children.

Age of Detectability: Prenatal diagnosis is possible for Groups A and B patients. Hepatosplenomegaly is detectable after age 2–3 months, and developmental delays are detectable shortly thereafter. Group C and D patients often have prolonged jaundice in the early months of life.

Gene Mapping and Linkage: SMPD1 (sphingomyelin phosphodiesterase 1, acid lysosomal) has been provisionally mapped to 17.

Prevention: None known. Genetic counseling indicated.

Treatment: No specific therapy is known. Supportive treatment is important for the child and family. This includes assistance in feeding, control of infection, anticonvulsants where needed, transfusion, or splenectomy.

Prognosis: Group A patients present the so-called classic picture, with onset of symptoms in early infancy, marked organomegaly, rapidly advancing CNS handicaps, and death by three years of age. Group B patients show the same massive sphingomyelin accumulation in the liver and spleen, and the pulmonary changes, as seen in the classically involved infants (Group A), but the nervous system is not affected. Although these patients survive into adulthood, they may not live a normal life span because of complications from visceral lipid storage. Group C patients show a pattern now being identified with reasonable frequency, characterized by developmental slowing beginning in late infancy, moderate chemical changes, enlargement of the liver and spleen, and gradual debilitation leading to death by 3 to 9 years of age. Group D involvement has been found most notably in persons of French-Canadian ancestry from Nova Scotia, with neurologic difficulties in mid-childhood (including cerebellar and athetoid symptoms), and survival until 12–20 years of age. Group E occurs in adults with moderate hepatosplenomegaly and no neurologic signs. Some of these could be a late onset variant of Group C.

Detection of Carrier: Parents and uninvolved sibs have no known clinical handicaps. The level of sphingomyelinase activity in the white blood cells and cultured fibroblasts from Group A and B is significantly reduced.

Special Considerations: A new classification system proposed by Spence and Callahan (1989) is expected to replace the old A-E classifications.

The author is indebted to Allen C. Crocker for his contributions to an earlier version of this article.

References:

Fried K, et al.: Biochemical, genetic and ultrastructural study of a family with sea-blue histiocyte syndrome: chronic and non-neuropathic Niemann-Pick disease. Europ J Clin Invest 1978; 8:249–253.

Walton DS, et al: Ocular manifestations of group A Niemann-Pick disease. Am J Ophthal 1978; 85:174–180. †

Winsor EJT, Welch JP: Genetic and demographic aspects of Nova Scotia Niemann-Pick disease (type D). Am J Hum Genet 1978; 30:530–538.

Wenger DA, et al.: Niemann-Pick disease type B: prenatal diagnosis and enzymatic and chemical studies on fetal brain and liver. Am J Hum Genet 1981; 33:337–344.

Pentchev PG, et al.: A genetic storage disorder in BALB/C mice with a metabolic block in esterification of exogenous cholesterol. J Biol Chem 1984; 259:5784–5791.

Palmer M, et al.: Niemann-Pick disease, type C: ocular, histopathologic and electron microscopic studies. Arch Ophthal 1985; 103:817–822. †

Levade T, Salvayre R, Douste-Blazy: Sphingomyelinases and Niemann-Pick disease. J Clin Chem Clin Biochem 1986; 24:205–220.

Maciejko D, Tylky-Szymanska A: Clinical and biochemical diagnostics of Niemann-Pick Disease. Klin Padiat 1986; 198:103–106.

Spence MW, Callahan JW: Sphingomyelin-cholesterol lipidosis: the Niemann-Pick group of diseases. In: Scriver CR, et al, eds: The metabolic basis of inherited disease, 6th ed. New York: McGraw-Hill, 1989:1655–1676.

TR008

Carlos J. Trujillo-Botero

Niemann-Pick disease with cholesterol esterification block
  See NIEMANN-PICK DISEASE
Nievergelt syndrome
  See MESOMELIC DYSPLASIA, NIEVERGELT TYPE
Nightblindness (congenital stationary) with normal fundus
  See NIGHTBLINDNESS, CONGENITAL STATIONARY, AUTOSOMAL DOMINANT

NIGHTBLINDNESS, CONGENITAL STATIONARY, AUTOSOMAL DOMINANT   3205

Includes:
  Hemeralopia
  Nightblindness (congenital stationary) with normal fundus
  Nougaret disease

Excludes:
  Nightblindness with myopia
  Nightblindness, congenital stationary, X-linked recessive (0718)
  Nightblindness, congenital stationary, autosomal recessive (3204)
  Nightblindness, Oguchi type (0740)

Major Diagnostic Criteria: Infantile onset, nonprogressive nightblindness with normal visual acuity, visual fields, and fundus. There is generally a positive family history. Electrophysiologic testing is diagnostic with a diminished ERG and an abnormal EOG. The ERG shows a very reduced photopic response without any scotopic increment.

Clinical Findings: Infantile onset nightblindness of a nonprogressive nature. Visual acuity is normal as are the visual fields and color vision. The paradoxical (Flynn-Barricks) pupil response may occur. Funduscopically the disc, macula, retinal vessels, and periphery are normal. The ERG shows a very reduced photopic response without scotopic increment. The initial 'a' wave is attenuated and there is an absence of the large 'b' wave response. In affected patients, the EOG is abnormal with a marked reduction in the EOG light rise.

Complications: Unknown.

Associated Findings: Syndactyly has been reported in one family member of a five generation pedigree.

Etiology: Autosomal dominant inheritance.

Pathogenesis: Apparently a result of a defect in neural transmission. The defect may lie at the level of the inner segment of the photoreceptors. Histology has been shown to be normal (except for slightly weak staining with Mac Mannus staining of the outer segments of the photorecptors.) Rhodopsin metabolism is normal.

MIM No.: *16350

Sex Ratio: M1:F1

Occurrence: Several hundred cases have been documented, including Blacks, since Cunier (1838) first identified the condition among decendants of Jean Nougaret, a French butcher.

Risk of Recurrence for Patient's Sib:
  See Part I, *Mendelian Inheritance.*

Risk of Recurrence for Patient's Child:
  See Part I, *Mendelian Inheritance.*

Age of Detectability: Correlation of history, clinical findings, and electrophysiologic testing allow early diagnosis.

Gene Mapping and Linkage: Unknown.

Prevention: None known. Genetic counseling indicated.

Treatment: Unknown.

Prognosis: This is a nonprogressive disorder. Visual acuity remains stable.

Detection of Carrier: Unknown.

Special Considerations: It must be noted that patients may have either of two types of ERG response and the response is not specific to a particular hereditary pattern, although a "Nougaret type" ERG response refers to one in which there is a reduced photopic response and no scotopic increment.

References:
Cunier F: Historie d'une hemeralopie hereditaire du puis deux siecles dans une famille de al commune de Vendemian pres Montpellier. Annales de la societe de medicin de Gaand 1838; 4:385–395.
Nettleship E: A history of congenital stationary nightblindness in nine consecutive generations. Trans Ophthalmol Soc U.K. 1907; 27:269–293.
Carr RE: Congenital stationary nightblindness. Trans Am Ophthalmol Soc 1974; 82:448–487.

AL031
MA054

Deborah Alcorn
Irene H. Maumenee

NIGHTBLINDNESS, CONGENITAL STATIONARY, AUTOSOMAL RECESSIVE   3204

Includes:
  Myopia (high-grade)-nightblindness
  Nightblindness-high-grade myopia
  Stationary nightblindness with normal fundus, congenital

Excludes:
  Nightblindness, congenital stationary, autosomal dominant (3205)
  Nightblindness, congenital stationary, X-linked recessive (0718)
  Nightblindness, Oguchi type (0740)
  Retina, amaurosis congenita, Leber type (0043)
  Retina, fundus albipunctatus (0399)

Major Diagnostic Criteria: Infantile onset, nonprogressive nightblindness. Most have normal visual acuity, but it may be diminished secondary to myopic changes. Most patients demonstrate a "negative" type ERG. Dark adaptation testing shows a bipartite curve with very slight adaptation of the rod system and the cone level is above the threshold.

Clinical Findings: Infantile onset nightblindness, nonprogressive. Visual acuity is normal as are the visual fields and color vision. The paradoxical (Flynn-Barricks) pupil always occurs. Funduscopically the disc, macula, retinal vessels, and periphery are normal unless there is associated myopia. ERG findings may be of two types. The first shows a reduced photopic response with any scotopic increment. In these patients the EOG is abnormal with a marked reduction in the light rise. The second type shows a "negative" ERG in which the 'a' wave is normal to increased in size and the positive 'b' wave is absent or markedly reduced. EOG in this second group shows a normal light rise.

Complications: Patients may be at increased risk of rhegmatogenous retinal detachments, associated with the myopia.

Associated Findings: None known.

Etiology: Autosomal recessive inheritance.

Pathogenesis: It has been shown that the rods have a normal density of pigment and that following bleaching, rod pigment regenerates normally, and manifest a normal 'a' wave on ERG testing. All of the above indicate that the rod outer segments are functioning. But the 'b' wave is markedly reduced and therefore it has been suggested that the defect may lie in the neural transmission from the photoreceptor terminals to bipolar cells.

MIM No.: *25727

Sex Ratio: M1:F1

Occurrence: Undetermined but presumably rare.

Risk of Recurrence for Patient's Sib:
  See Part I, *Mendelian Inheritance.*

Risk of Recurrence for Patient's Child:
  See Part I, *Mendelian Inheritance.*

Age of Detectability: Correlation of history, clinical findings, and electrophysiologic testing allows early diagnosis.

Gene Mapping and Linkage: Unknown.

Prevention: None known. Genetic counseling indicated.

Treatment: Unknown.

Prognosis: This is a stationary disease and visual acuity should remain stable.

Detection of Carrier: Unknown.

Special Considerations: In the cases of autosomal recessive CSNB with associated myopia, the patients may also have poor vision, strabismus, and nystagmus as seen in **Nightblindness, congenital stationary, X-linked recessive**. These patients are at increased risk of retinal detachments. They will also demonstrate a "negative" type ERG response and have a normal EOG.

References:

Gassler VJ: Ueber eine bis jetzt nicht bekannte recessive Verknuepfung von hochgradiger Myopie mit angeborener Hemaralopie. Arch Klaus Stift Vererbungoforsch 1925; 1:259–272.

Der Kaloustian VM, Baghdassarian SA: The autosomal recessive variety of congenital stationary night blindness with myopia. J Med Genet 1972; 9:67–69.

Carr RE: Congenital stationary nightblindness. Trans Am Ophthalmol Soc 1974; 72:448–487.

Weleber RG, Tongue AC: Congenital stationary night blindness presenting as Leber's congenital amaurosis. Arch Ophthal 1987; 105: 360–365.

AL031   **Deborah Alcorn**
MA054   **Irene H. Maumenee**

NIGHTBLINDNESS, CONGENITAL STATIONARY, X-LINKED RECESSIVE   0718

Includes:

Hemeralopia-myopia, X-linked
Myopia-nightblindness, X-linked
Stationary nightblindness with high myopia congenital

Excludes:

Forsius-Eriksson syndrome (3183)
Retina, fundus albipunctatus (0399)
Nightblindness, congenital stationary, autosomal dominant (3205)
Nightblindness, congenital stationary, autosomal recessive (3204)
Nightblindness, Oguchi type (0740)

Major Diagnostic Criteria: Infantile onset nonprogressive nyctalopia, nystagmus, and moderate to severe myopia. Corrected visual acuity is usually reduced and mild nystagmus may persist lifelong. The fundus is normal except for myopic changes. The ERG is characterized by small or absent oscillatory potentials and a "negative" ERG with a large "a" and a small "b" wave.

Clinical Findings: The nightblindness is congenital and stationary. Visual acuity is usually subnormal, and may vary from 20/20 to 3/200 among patients. The degree of myopia ranges from -2.00 D to -20.00 D. Patients with subnormal vision usually have associated horizontal nystagmus and strabismus is common. The visual fields are normal or reveal defects consistent with the degree of myopia. Color vision is usually normal, although slight abnormalities may be seen as a tritan axis on Farnsworth-Munsell 100 hue testing. The anterior segment examination is normal, although the paradoxical (Feynn-Barricks) pupil occurs in younger individuals. The fundus demonstrates myopic changes of the posterior pole of variable severity. This includes peripapillary choroidal atrophy, temporal disc pallor, or tilted disc. ERG testing after dark adaptation shows a large "a" wave with a distinctive squared-off appearance and a small "b" wave. This results in a "negative" ERG. There are identical peak times of the dark and light adapted responses. The oscillatory potentials under photopic testing are very small or absent. Dark adaptation testing reveals a delayed rod-cone break with an elevated cone and rod threshold. The EOG shows a normal light rise. The disease is stationary and visual acuity does not deteriorate. There may be an increase in the amount of myopia, particularly in those patients with a high degree of myopia at a young age.

It has been shown that the ERG pattern of congenital stationary nightblindness is not specific to any particular hereditary pattern.

Complications: Related to myopia, but without an increased frequency of retinal detachment compared to other patients with high myopia.

Associated Findings: None known.

Etiology: X-linked inheritance.

Pathogenesis: Because of the findings of a normal EOG and a normal "a" wave on ERG testing, the outer retinal layers are presumed to be normal. The abnormal "b" wave, originating from the bipolar cell regions suggests an abnormality in neural transmission. Both the rod and cone systems are affected. Rhodopsin kinetics are normal.

MIM No.: *31050

Sex Ratio: M1:F0

Occurrence: Undetermined but presumed rare.

Risk of Recurrence for Patient's Sib:
See Part I, *Mendelian Inheritance.*

Risk of Recurrence for Patient's Child:
See Part I, *Mendelian Inheritance.*

Age of Detectability: Congenital onset of nyctalopia with nonprogression of disease. Correlation of history, clinical findings, and electrophysiologic studies permits an early diagnosis.

Gene Mapping and Linkage: CSNB1 (congenital stationary night blindness 1) has been mapped to Xp21.1-p11.23.

Prevention: None known. Genetic counseling indicated.

Treatment: No effective treatment known except to accurately correct the refractive error (myopia).

Prognosis: Visual acuity usually remains stable, but with increasing degree of myopia with age, particularly those patients with high myopia at a young age. The visual function may actually improve with age. The nightblindness remains stationary.

Detection of Carrier: Carrier females have normal visual acuity, visual fields, and color vision. Their ERGs show a selective reduction in the amplitude of oscillatory potentials, but with peak time of each of the oscillatory potentials being normal.

References:

Morton AS: Two cases of hereditary congenital night blindness without visible fundus change. Trans Opthal Soc U.K. 1893;13:147–150.

Francois J, DeRouck A: Sex-linked myopic chorioretinal heredodegeneration. Am J Ophthal 1965;60:670–678.

Merin S, et al: Syndrome of congenital high myopia with nyctalopia. Am J Ophthalmol 1970;70:541–547.

Carr RE: Congenital stationary nightblindness. Trans Am Ophthalmol Soc 1974;72:448–487.

AL031   **Deborah Alcorn**
MA054   **Irene H. Maumenee**

NIGHTBLINDNESS, OGUCHI TYPE   0740

Includes: Oguchi disease types 1, 2A and 2B

Excludes:

Cone dystrophy, X-linked late onset
Nightblindness (other)
Retina, fundus albipunctatus (0399)

Major Diagnostic Criteria: Abnormal fundus discoloration in patient with nightblindness with characteristic disappearance of discoloration and occurrence of secondary dark-adaptation after prolonged period in the dark.

Clinical Findings: This form of stationary nightblindness is associated with a peculiar discoloration of the fundus, which, with prolonged dark-adaptation, will usually lead to a disappearance of the abnormal fundus coloration and marked improvement or normalization of subjective dark-adaptation. The coloration is described as grey or yellow and may be homogenous or streaky in appearance. The abnormal coloration may be found throughout the entire eyegrounds, only in the midperipheral area or mainly in the posterior eyegrounds. The abnormal zones of coloration are brilliant with more pronounced reflexes than normal. The underlying choroid is usually invisible under areas of abnormal coloration and it may be difficult to distinguish retinal veins from retinal arterioles in such areas.

Patients with Oguchi disease have been divided into two major types. Most patients fall into type 1 and are characterized by the occurrence of secondary or rod dark-adaptation after a sufficient period of time in the dark. The final threshold may be normal or elevated. With time in the dark, the abnormal fundus discoloration disappears. This latter event is known as Mizuo phenomenon. Patients with type 2 show no secondary or rod dark-adaptation. These patients have less striking abnormal fundus coloration than those classified as type 1. Some of these patients, type 2A, show Mizuo phenomenon, whereas others, type 2B, do not.

The disorder is stationary. Although some patients have been reported to have mild color defects and some visual field constriction, there is usually no other impairment of vision associated with the disease. The ERG shows a normal cone response. The rod response after several minutes of dark adaptation is grossly abnormal with mainly an A wave seen. Even after the patient is allowed to achieve a secondary dark adaptation and the Mizuo phenomenon, the ERG has been reported as abnormal by some investigators but a normal scotopic response to a single flash of light has been reported. The EOG is normal, reflection densitometry and rhodopsin kinetics are normal as is fluorescein angiography. The disorder is most likely one of neural transmission rather than a structural rod abnormality.

Complications: Unknown.

Associated Findings: None known.

Etiology: Autosomal recessive inheritance.

Pathogenesis: In two reports, light microscopy showed an abnormal number of cones, many of them larger than normal, in the posterior eyegrounds. Many of these cones were arranged in double rows and contained vesicular spaces between them. In addition there was an abnormal positioning of the cone nuclei, many lying outside of the external limiting membrane. Also, an extra layer with a syncytial structure and strongly pigmented was described between the photoreceptors and the true pigment epithelium. The pigment epithelium cells had dense and shrunken nuclei. However, in a recent histologic examination the extra layer was not detected. Although displaced cone nuclei were seen, the authors noted that in controls without Oguchi disease cone nuclei could sometimes be detected beyond the external limiting membrane. A nodular bulging of the inner side of the pigment epithelium was noted in some areas. This bulging was due to aggregates of fuchsin granules. These same granules were also seen to an abnormal degree among the rods and cones. In areas the pigment epithelium showed thinning and irregularities in cellular structure in many sites.

MIM No.: *25810

Sex Ratio: M1:F1

Occurrence: Undetermined. Has been reported in all races, but most patients were Japanese.

Risk of Recurrence for Patient's Sib:
See Part I, *Mendelian Inheritance.*

Risk of Recurrence for Patient's Child:
See Part I, *Mendelian Inheritance.*

Age of Detectability: When able to respond to necessary testing.

Gene Mapping and Linkage: Unknown.

Prevention: None known. Genetic counseling indicated.

Treatment: Unknown.

Prognosis: Normal life span.

Detection of Carrier: Unknown.

The authors are indebted to the late Alex E. Krill for his contributions to an earlier version of this article.

References:

Françis J, et al.: La maladie d'Oguchi. Ophthalmologica 1956; 131:1–40.

Carr RE, Gouras P: Oguchi's disease. Arch Ophthalmol 1965; 73:646–656.

Carr RE, Ripps H: Rhodopsin kinetics and rod adaptation in Oguchi's disease. Invest Ophthalmol 1967; 6:426–436.

Yamanaka M: Histologic study of Oquchi's disease: its relationship to pigmentary degeneration of the retina. Am J Ophthalmol 1969; 68:19–26.

Gouras P: Electroretinography: some basic principles. Invest Ophthalmol 1970; 9:557–569.

Gass JDM: Oguchi disease. Stereoscopic atlas of macular diseases. St. Louis: C.V. Mosby, 1987:270–271.

Remler B: New findings in Oguchi's disease. Klin Monatsbl Augenheilkd 1988; 192:239–243.

W0003
BE026
Mitchel L. Wolf
Donald R. Bergsma

Nightblindness-high-grade myopia
See *NIGHTBLINDNESS, CONGENITAL STATIONARY, AUTOSOMAL RECESSIVE*

Nigrospinodentatal degeneration with nuclear ophthalmoplegia
See *MACHADO-JOSEPH DISEASE*

Niikawa-Kuroki syndrome
See *KABUKI MAKE-UP SYNDROME*

Nijmegen chromosome breakage syndrome
See *CHROMOSOME INSTABILITY, NIJMEGEN TYPE*

Nipple, congenital absence
See *BREAST, AMASTIA*

Nipples, accessory
See *BREAST, POLYTHELIA*

Nipples, supernumerary nipples
See *BREAST, POLYTHELIA*

Noack syndrome
See *ACROCEPHALOSYNDACTYLY TYPE V*
also *ACROCEPHALOPOLYSYNDACTYLY*

Nodular erythema-digital changes
See *DIGITAL DEFECTS-NODULAR ERYTHEMA-EMACIATION, NAKAJO TYPE*

Non-African Burkitt lymphoma
See *LYMPHOMA, BURKITT TYPE*

Non-Hodgkin lymphoma of T-cell type
See *LEUKEMIA/LYMPHOMA, T-CELL*

Non-Hodgkin lymphoma of the B-cell type
See *LYMPHOMA, BURKITT TYPE*

Non-Hodgkin lymphoma of B-cell type
See *LEUKEMIA/LYMPHOMA, B-CELL*

Non-immune fetal hydrops
See *HYDROPS FETALIS, NON-IMMUNE*

Non-insulin dependent diabetes mellitus (NIDDM)
See *DIABETES MELLITUS, NON-INSULIN DEPENDENT TYPE*

Non-insulin-dependent diabetes of the young (NIDDY)
See *DIABETES MELLITUS, MATURITY ONSET OF THE YOUNG (MODY)*

Nondisjunction
See *CHROMOSOME 18, TRISOMY 18*

Nonketotic hyperglycinemia
See *HYPERGLYCINEMIA, NON-KETOTIC*

Nonne-Milroy type hereditary lymphedema
See *LYMPHEDEMA I*

Nonobstructive dilation of the intrahepatic biliary tree
See *LIVER, CONGENITAL CYSTIC DILATATION OF INTRAHEPATIC DUCTS*

Nonopalescent opalescent dentine
See *TEETH, DENTIN DYSPLASIA, RADICULAR*

Nonplasmatic thymic alymphoplasia or alymphocytosis
See *IMMUNODEFICIENCY, SEVERE COMBINED*

Nonpolyposis colerectal cancer, hereditary Lynch syndromes
See *CANCER, COLORECTAL*

Nonrotation of midgut
See *INTESTINAL ROTATION, INCOMPLETE*

Nonsteroidal synthetic estrogens, fetal effects
See *FETAL DIETHYLSTILBESTROL (DES) EFFECTS*

Nontropical sprue
See *GLUTEN-SENSITIVE ENTEROPATHY*

Nontumorous primary aldosteronism
See *HYPERALDOSTERONISM, FAMILIAL GLUCOCORTICOID SUPPRESSIBLE*

NOONAN SYNDROME   0720

Includes:

    Female pseudo-Turner syndrome
    Female Turner syndrome with normal XX karyotype
    Male Turner syndrome
    Neurofibromatosis-Noonan syndrome
    Noonan-neurofibromatosis syndrome
    Pterygium colli syndrome
    Status Bonnevie-Ullrich
    Turner phenotype with normal karyotype
    Turner syndrome, familial
    Ullrich-Noonan syndrome
    Ullrich syndrome
    XX-XY Turner phenotype

Excludes:

    Fetal primidone syndrome (2982)
    Klippel-Feil anomaly (2032)
    Lentigines syndrome, multiple (0586)
    Pterygium syndrome, multiple (2186)
    Pulmonic stenosis-cafe-au-lait spots, Watson type (2776)
    Turner syndrome (0977)

Major Diagnostic Criteria: The Noonan syndrome must be delineated at the clinical level. Cardinal features include congenital heart disease, particularly valvular pulmonary stenosis, mild mental retardation, short stature, broad or webbed neck, a peculiar chest deformity with pectus carinatum superiorly and pectus excavatum inferiorly, and characteristic facies that alter predictably with age to produce a discrete but changing phenotype.

Clinical Findings: Craniofacial dysmorphism is manifest in the newborn period, when the main features are hypertelorism with down-slanting palpebral fissures (95%), low-set posteriorly-rotated ears with a thick helix (90%), a deeply-grooved philtrum with high wide peaks of the vermilion border of the upper lip (95%), high-arched palate (45%), micrognathia (25%), and excess nuchal skin with a low posterior hairline (55%). There is a consistent predictable change in phenotype with age. In infancy, the head appears relatively large with turricephaly, prominent eyes with level palpebral fissures, hypertelorism, and thick-hooded eyelids or ptosis. The nose has a depressed root, wide base, and bulbous tip. In later childhood, the face often appears coarse or myopathic. With increasing age the contour of the face becomes more triangular. The neck lengthens, accentuating the webbing or prominent trapezius (90%). In the adolescent, the eyes are less prominent, the nose has a pinched root, thinner higher bridge, and wide base. In the older adult, there are prominent nasolabial folds, a high anterior hairline, and transparent wrinkled skin. Hair may be wispy in the infant, but often is curly or woolly in the older child and adolescent. Strikingly blue or blue-green irides, diamond-shaped arched eyebrows, and low-set posteriorly-rotated ears with a thick helix are frequently present.

Birth weight is generally normal (40%), but may be falsely elevated by the presence of subcutaneous edema. Failure to thrive in infancy is common (40%). Prepubertal growth often parallels the third percentile (60%), with a relatively normal growth velocity. The pubertal growth spurt may be reduced or absent. Bone age is delayed in up to 20% of cases. Cryptorchidism, commonly bilateral, occurs in 60% of affected males, and may lead to deficient spermatogenesis. However, normal virilization at puberty, with subsequent fertility, has been documented in males. In females, puberty may be normal or delayed, and fertility is generally unimpaired.

Congenital heart defects occur in approximately 66% of patients. Common lesions include **Pulmonary valve, stenosis** (50%), **Atrial septal defects** (10%), and asymmetric septal hypertrophy (10%). Electrocardiograph typically shows left axis deviation (33%) despite the fact that most cardiac lesions involve the right side of the heart.

A characteristic pectus deformity is seen (70%) with pectus carinatum superiorly and pectus excavatum inferiorly. Other skeletal anomalies include cubitus valgus (50%), clinobrachydactyly with blunt fingertips (30%), vertebral/sternal anomalies (25%), and dental malocclusion (35%).

IQ ranges between 64 and 127, with a median of 102. Mild mental retardation is seen in up to 33% of cases, and motor developmental delay is found in 25% of patients. Language delay (20%) may be secondary to perceptual motor disabilities (15%), mild hearing loss (12%), or articulation abnormalities (72%).

Various bleeding anomalies, including **Factor XI deficiency**, **Von Willebrand disease**, and platelet dysfunction, are documented (20%). Congenital lymphatic abnormalities (20%) may cause general or peripheral lymphedema, pulmonary or intestinal lymphangiectasia, hydrops fetalis, and cystic hygroma. Neonatal peripheral edema is common and may be associated with an increased total fingertip ridge count.

Wide intrafamilial variability in clinical expression is common. The phenotype, particularly in adults, may be extremely subtle. Careful examination of all first-degree relatives is essential, with a review of serial photographs, searching for the discrete change in phenotype.

Complications: In males, inadequate secondary sexual development and sterility may be associated with deficient spermatogenesis secondary to earlier cryptorchidism. Congestive heart failure or pulmonary complications resulting from the cardiac defect may occur.

Associated Findings: Various skin manifestations include café-au-lait patches (10%), pigmented nevi (25%), and lentigines (2%). Several patients with **Neurofibromatosis** and the Noonan phenotype are reported. Malignant hyperthermia is seen with the Noonan phenotype (see **King syndrome**).

Etiology: Autosomal dominant inheritance with variability in expression. Direct transmission from parent to child is documented in 30–75% of cases. "Sporadic" cases are thought to represent new dominant mutations. Maternal transmission of the gene is three times more common than paternal transmission.

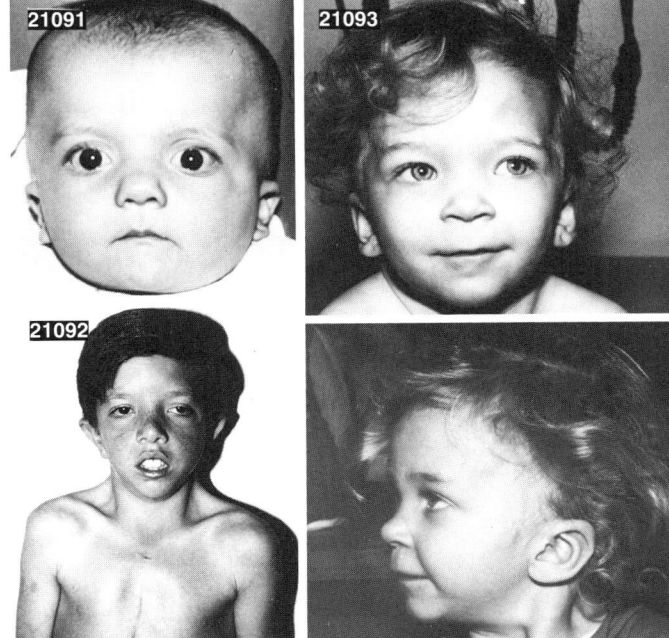

0720-21091: Infant with prominent eyes, hypertelorism, depressed nasal bridge and wide nasal base. **21092:** Adolescent male with triangular facies, coarse facial features, webbed neck and pectus deformity. **21093:** Face of a young child with Noonan syndrome; note the posteriorly angulated ears with a thickened helix.

This is probably attributable to the frequent occurrence of cryptorchidism and consequent male infertility.

Pathogenesis: One current hypothesis implicates lymphedema in the development of the Noonan phenotype. Disruption of normal tissue migration of organ placement by lymphedema may explain pterygium colli, cryptorchidism, wide-spaced nipples, low-set posteriorly-rotated ears, hypertelorism, abnormal dermatoglyphics, and congenital heart defects. The cause of lymphedema is unknown and is likely to be heterogeneous.

MIM No.: *16395, 16229

POS No.: 3335

CDC No.: 759.800

Sex Ratio: M1:F1

Occurrence: Incidence has been estimated to be between 1:1,000 and 1:2,500 live births.

Risk of Recurrence for Patient's Sib:
See Part I, *Mendelian Inheritance.*

Risk of Recurrence for Patient's Child:
See Part I, *Mendelian Inheritance.*

Age of Detectability: Clinically evident at birth. Prenatal detection of cystic hygroma and/or edema with ultrasound is possible in some cases.

Gene Mapping and Linkage: Unknown.

Prevention: None known. Genetic counseling indicated.

Treatment: Speech therapy is valuable for the child with language delay and/or articulation abnormalities. Cardiac surgery and orchidopexy may be indicated. Abnormal coagulation, when present, may require therapy.

Prognosis: Life expectancy is probably normal in those individuals without severe congenital heart disease or profound failure to thrive.

Detection of Carrier: Careful clinical examination of all first-degree relatives is essential to identify those who are minimally affected. Review of serial photographs will help to document the change in phenotype. Electrocardiogram and echocardiogram provide additional information when clinical examination is ambiguous.

Special Considerations: Preference for the term Noonan syndrome should avoid the confusing use of the *Turner* and *Ullrich* eponyms. While patients with Noonan syndrome, both male and female, share some phenotypic features with females with Turner syndrome, the absence of a detectable chromosome abnormality, the familial nature of Noonan syndrome, and careful clinical examination should allow differentiation of the two conditions.

No characteristic cytogenetic, biochemical, or metabolic abnormality has been detected. Several patients are reported with Noonan syndrome and trimethylaminuria or a fishy odor to the urine, in association with platelet dysfunction.

Lymphatic obstruction has been shown to cause left heart defects in a canine model. Lymphatic obstruction could similarly reduce right-sided cardiac blood flow and cause pulmonary stenosis.

The association between Noonan syndrome and **Neurofibromatosis** reported in several cases, remains controversial. Both neurofibromatosis and Noonan syndrome are common conditions with variable expression. The two conditions share some manifestations: short stature, learning disabilities or mild mental retardation, scoliosis or other skeletal abnormalities, and pulmonary stenosis. All cases of *neurofibromatosis-Noonan syndrome* until now appear to be sporadic. The presence of increased paternal age in some cases is suggestive of a new dominant mutation. Although occasional patients with neurofibromatosis may have a Noonan-like phenotype and although Noonan syndrome patients are predisposed to neural crest dysplasias (café-au-lait spots, multiple pigmented moles, tumors originating from neural tissue), it seems likely that the cases with neurofibromatosis-Noonan syndrome (or "*Noonan-neurofibromatosis*") have a separate "new" neurocristopathy.

References:
Noonan JA, Ehmke DA: Associated noncardiac malformations in children with congenital heart disease. J Pediatr 1963; 63:468–470.
Allanson JE, et al.: Noonan phenotype associated with neurofibromatosis. Am J Med Genet 1985; 21:457–462.
Allanson JE, et al.: Noonan syndrome: the changing phenotype. Am J Med Genet 1985; 21:507–514.†
Opitz JM, Weaver DD: The neurofibromatosis-Noonan syndrome. Am J Med Genet 1985; 21:477–490.
Mendez HMM, Opitz JM: Noonan syndrome: a review. Am J Med Genet 1985; 21:493–506. *
Allanson JE: Noonan syndrome. J Med Genet 1987; 24:9–13. * †
Witt DR, et al.: Lymphedema in Noonan syndrome: clues to pathogenesis and prenatal diagnosis and review of the literature. Am J Med Genet 1987; 27:841–856.
Witt DR, et al. Bleeding diathesis in Noonan syndrome. Am J Med Genet 1988; 31:305–317.

AL010   **Judith E. Allanson**

Noonan-like McDonough syndrome
See McDONOUGH SYNDROME
Noonan-like phenotype-malignant hyperthermia
See KING SYNDROME
Noonan-neurofibromatosis syndrome
See NOONAN SYNDROME
Norman-Roberts syndrome
See LISSENCEPHALY SYNDROME
Normokalemic periodic paralysis
See PARALYSIS, NORMOKALEMIC PERIODIC
Normopepsinogenemic I duodenal ulcer
See PEPTIC ULCER DISEASES, NON-SYNDROMIC
Norrbottnian Gaucher disease
See GAUCHER DISEASE

NORRIE DISEASE   0721

Includes:
Atrophia bulborum hereditaria
Episkopi blindness
Microcephaly-vitreoretinal dysplasia
Oculo-acoustic cerebral degeneration, congenital progressive
Pseudoglioma of the retina, congenital, bilateral, X-linked
Vitreoretinal dysplasia, X-linked

Excludes:
Chromosome 13, trisomy 13 (0168)
Encephaloretinal dysplasia
Retinal dysplasia (0866)
Eye, vitreous, persistent hyperplastic primary (0994)

Major Diagnostic Criteria: Recessive X-linked dysplasia of the retina existing bilaterally in boys blind from birth.

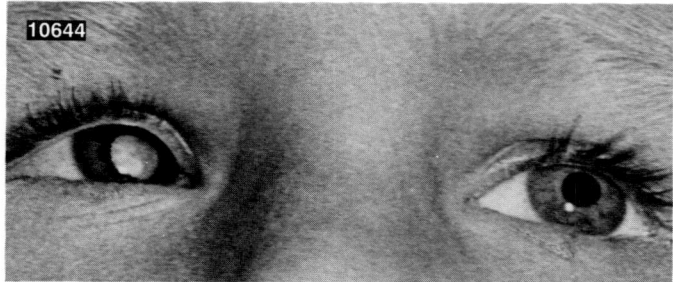

0721-10644: The right eye is deep-set. There is a white mass—not a cataract—behind the lens. This is the totally detached retina with hemorrhages and vascular hyperplasia. The left eye is artificial. This eye was removed due to suspicion of retinoblastoma.

Clinical Findings: The typical presenting sign is bilateral white pupillary reflexes (leukocoria) in micro-ophthalmic eyes evident at birth or shortly afterward. The anterior chamber is shallow, and the pupil is commonly dilated with no light reflex.

Posterior synechia, ectropion of the iris pigment fringe, and a hypoplastic iris usually are present. A gray membrane or gray-yellow opaque vascularized mass, which may be hemorrhagic, is apparent behind the lens. Elongated ciliary processes are often visible, and, in cases in which the fundus can be seen, retinal folds, retinal detachment, and pseudotumor formations may be observed. The affected patients are totally blind from birth. The lens and cornea are initially clear; however, both typically become opaque with time. Phthisis bulbi is the usual end result and typically occurs by age 10 years. Many of the observed patients become mentally retarded (25–40%) and severe deafness (25–35%) frequently develops later in life.

Complications: *Developmental:* mental retardation, sensorineural deafness.

Secondary: complicated cataract, retinal detachment, corneal opacities, secondary glaucoma, band keratopathy, phthisis bulbi.

Associated Findings: Microencephaly, cryptorchidism, hypogonadism, increased susceptibility to infection, growth disturbances.

Etiology: X-linked recessive inheritance.

Pathogenesis: Unknown.

MIM No.: *31060

POS No.: 3336

Sex Ratio: M1:F0. Homozygous affected females may occur.

Occurrence: About 100 cases from over a dozen kindreds have been reported in the literature, including a Greek family living in Episkopi, Cyprus.

Risk of Recurrence for Patient's Sib:
See Part I, *Mendelian Inheritance.*

Risk of Recurrence for Patient's Child:
See Part I, *Mendelian Inheritance.*

Age of Detectability: At birth. Prenatal diagnosis in utero by chorion villus biopsy is possible. Prenatal exclusion has also been accomplished using flanking DNA markers (Gal et al, 1988)

Gene Mapping and Linkage: NDP (Norrie disease (pseudoglioma)) has been mapped to Xp11.4-p11.3.

Prevention: None known. Genetic counseling indicated.

Treatment: Early surgical intervention consisting of cataract extraction, vitrectomy, and retinal detachment repair have been attempted. These procedures may prevent phthisis bulbi, but they will not improve vision.

Sound amplification and rehabilitation for hearing loss and appropriate treatment for each specific associated defect.

Prognosis: Irreversibly blind from birth.

Detection of Carrier: Chromosomal analysis; pedigree analysis to determine obligate heterozygotes.

Special Considerations: The ocular picture of Norrie disease is somewhat similar to the retinal dysplasia that occurs in **Chromosome 13, trisomy 13** and in other conditions. It is distinguished by the absence of other systemic abnormalities, by the concomitant mental retardation and deafness, and by the X-linked recessive mode of inheritance. *Pseudoglioma* is a clinical term describing a number of conditions that produce a white reflex or amaurotic "cat's eye reflex" in the pupil. Reese has grouped these conditions as "leukocoria" which may be produced by developmental abnormalities such as persistent hyperplastic primary vitreous, retinal dysplasia, congenital retinal folds, or by inflammatory conditions such as metastastic endophthalmitis, larval granulomatosis, and toxoplasmosis. Leukocoria may also be present in children with retinopathy of prematurity (retrolental fibroplasia and retinoblastoma.)

The psychiatric and otologic components of this syndrome are never congenital. If mental retardation begins early (age 3–4 years), the afflicted patient is more likely to be severely retarded.

Electrocochleography and brain stem-evoked responses reveal that the hearing loss is primarily of cochlear origin. A varient of Norrie disease with the typical stigmata and associated microcephaly has been well described (Moreira-Filho and Neustein, 1979).

References:
Warburg M: Norrie's disease: a congenital progressive oculo-acousti-cocerebral degeneration. Acta Ophthalmol 1966; 89:1–47.
Apple DJ, et al.: Ocular histopathology of Norrie's disease. Am J Ophthalmol 1974; 78:196–203.
Parving A, et al.: Electrophysiological study of Norrie's disease. Audiology 1978; 17:293–298.
Moreira-Filho CA, Neustein I: A presumptive new variant of Norrie's disease. J Med Genet 1979; 16:125–128.
de laChapelle A, et al.: Norrie disease caused by a gene deletion allowing carrier detection and prenatal diagnosis. Clin Genet 1985; 28:317–320.
Gal A, et al.: Submicroscopic interstitial deletion of the X chromosome explains a complex genetic syndrome dominated by Norrie disease. Cytogenet Cell Genet 1986; 42:219–224.
Gal A, et al.: Prenatal exclusion of Norrie disease with flanking DNA markers. Am J Med Genet 1988; 31:449–453.
Zhu D, et al.: Microdeletion in the X-chromosome and prenatal diagnosis in a family with Norrie Disease. Am J Med Genet 1989; 33:485–488.

EL007   **Robert M. Ellsworth**
HA068   **Barrett G. Haik**
WE038   **Robert A. Weiss**

North Carolina macular dystrophy (NCMD)
See EYE, MACULAR DYSTROPHY, NORTH CAROLINA TYPE
Norum disease
See ANEMIA, HEMOLYTIC, RED CELL MEMBRANE DEFECTS
also LECITHIN-CHOLESTEROL ACYL TRANSFERASE DEFICIENCY
Nose, absence of
See NOSE/NASAL SEPTUM DEFECTS
Nose, absence of half
See NOSE/NASAL SEPTUM DEFECTS

NOSE, ANTERIOR ATRESIA   **0723**

Includes:
    Anterior nasal atresia
    Atresia, nasal anterior
    Atresia of anterior nares
    Bony choanal atresia, anterior
    Choanal atresia, anterior
    Membranous choanal atresia, anterior
    Stenosis of anterior nares

Excludes:
    Nose and nasal septum defects
    Nose, nasopharyngeal stenosis (0707)
    Nose, posterior atresia (0727)

Major Diagnostic Criteria: Bony or membranous atresia of the anterior nares, with underdeveloped nostril. Anterior nasal atresia can be differentiated from half-nose by the presence of posterior choanae on examination of the nasopharynx, absence of purulent dacryocystitis, and presence of a partial nasal chamber and paranasal sinuses on X-ray examination.

Clinical Findings: A narrowing or stenosis of the anterior nares, usually unilateral, and either membranous or bony. The newborn may have respiratory distress when not crying if the lesion is bilateral. The nasolacrimal duct is present and normal, but X-ray examination may show lack of anterior ethmoid and maxillary sinuses. Computerized tomography will help to delineate the abnormality.

Complications: When bilateral, possible respiratory distress of the newborn.

Associated Findings: None known.

Etiology: Unknown.

Pathogenesis: The anterior nares are closed by epithelial plugs from the second to sixth month of intrauterine life. Failure of absorption of these plugs results in anterior atresia or stenosis of varying degrees.

CDC No.: 748.000

Sex Ratio: Presumably M1:F1

Occurrence: Undetermined but presumed rare.

Risk of Recurrence for Patient's Sib: Unknown.

Risk of Recurrence for Patient's Child: Unknown.

Age of Detectability: At birth.

Gene Mapping and Linkage: Unknown.

Prevention: None known. Genetic counseling indicated.

Treatment: Reconstructive surgery can be performed to provide an epithelial lined nasal cavity with cosmetically acceptable nostrils. This can be done through either a sublabial or a transnasal approach.

Prognosis: Good for life span, intelligence, and function, unless bilateral and associated with respiratory distress that is not recognized and not corrected.

Detection of Carrier: Unknown.

References:
Ballenger JJ: Diseases of the nose, throat and ear. Philadelphia: Lea & Febiger, 1969.
Maloney WH, ed: Otolaryngology, vol. 3. Hagerstown: Harper & Row, 1969.
Brown OE, et al.: Congenital piriform aperture stenosis in children. Larynoscope 1988; 99:86–91.

MY003   **Charles M. Myer III**

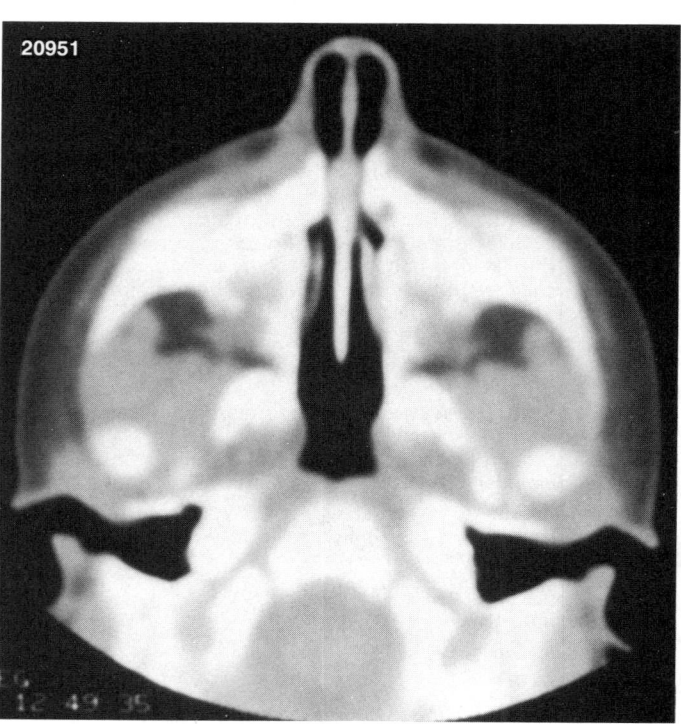

2718-20951: Anterior nasal stenosis as seen on CT scan.

NOSE, ANTERIOR STENOSIS   2718

Includes: Anterior nasal stenosis

Excludes:
    Choanal atresia
    Nose, anterior stenosis (2718)
    Nose, bifid (0724)
    Nose, dislocated nasal septum (2719)

Major Diagnostic Criteria: The affected infant presents with cyanosis and respiratory distress. On examination of the nose there is a hard bony mass presenting from the lateral nasal wall within the anterior nares, along with a narrowed nasal airway.

Clinical Findings: Infants with anterior nasal stenosis present with nasal airway obstruction, and may have a cyclic pattern of cyanosis relieved by crying (similar to infants with bilateral posterior choanal atresia or stenosis).

Nasal examination reveals a hard bony mass protruding medially at the area of the lumen vestibuli. The nasal airway is narrowed to 1–2 mm. It is frequently impossible to pass a small catheter through the nose.

Infants are obligate nasal breathers for a variable period of time; hence, a risk of nasal airway obstruction exists. Since the effects of this lesion are similar to those of bilateral posterior choanal atresia, sudden death due to an inadequate oral airway may result. Nasal airway obstruction may contribute to development of a "long face" syndrome.

Complications: Surgical complications include tooth bud damage, damage to nasolacrimal apparatus, maxillary sinus damage, and maldevelopment of the midface.

Associated Findings: None known.

Etiology: Unknown.

Pathogenesis: Unknown.

CDC No.: 748.000

Sex Ratio: Undetermined but presumably M1:F1.

Occurrence: Overall frequency < 1%.

Risk of Recurrence for Patient's Sib: Unknown.

Risk of Recurrence for Patient's Child: Unknown.

Age of Detectability: At birth.

Gene Mapping and Linkage: Unknown.

Prevention: None known.

Treatment: Sublateral resection of the bony stenosis.

Prognosis: Good.

Detection of Carrier: Unknown.

References:
Shetty R: Nasal pyramid surgery for correction of bony inlet stenosis. J Laryngol Otol 1977; 91:201–208.
Sprinkle PM, Sponck FT: Congenital malformations of the nose and paranasal sinuses. In: Bluestone CD, Stool SE, eds: Pediatric otolaryngology. Philadelphia: W.B. Saunders, 1983:769–779.

MY003   **Charles M. Myer III**
OR005   **Peter Orobello**

NOSE, BIFID   0724

Includes:
    Bifid nose
    "Doggennose"
    Nose, congenital median fissure of
    Nose, median cleft of

Excludes:
    Encephalocele (0343)
    Eye, hypertelorism (0504)
    Face, median cleft face syndrome (0635)
    Nose/nasal septum defects (0722)
    Nose, duplication (0725)

Major Diagnostic Criteria: Vertical midline cleft of the nose.

Clinical Findings: The tip and dorsum of the nose are divided by a vertical central sulcus of variable width, resulting in a broad and flat nose. The columella is broad and short, separating abnormally shaped nostrils. The septum may be duplicated, and the nasal bones may be normal or excessively broad. Computerized tomography is helpful in determining presence of the choanal atresia or associated abnormalities of the skull and sinuses.

Complications: Bifid nose is almost always found in association with hypertelorism, a real or illusory increase in interpupillary distance, and can be associated with other congenital midline defects of the face, such as cranium bifidum occultum (32%), median cleft lip (16%), and triad of bifid nose, cranium bifidum occultum, and cleft lip (12%). Incidence of severe mental retardation is 8%, and of borderline retardation, 12%.

Associated Findings: None known.

Etiology: Autosomal dominant and recessive inheritance has been reported in a few pedigrees. Three of 25 patients with bifid nose had ancestors with hypertelorism without bifid nose. One reported patient with a bifid nose had a normal twin.

Pathogenesis: In the five-week embryo the medial nasal processes are widely separated by the frontal process. Normally, the frontal process grows upward and away from the lower face, and the paired medial nasal processes grow toward the midline, over the frontal process to form the mesodermal structures of the midface. Failure of these processes to merge or failure of obliteration of ectodermal remnants may result in midline clefts of the nose.

MIM No.: 10974, 21040

CDC No.: 748.120

Sex Ratio: M1:F1

Occurrence: 1:1,000 congenital defects of the face. Over 140 cases have been reported in the literature.

Risk of Recurrence for Patient's Sib:
See Part I, *Mendelian Inheritance.*

Risk of Recurrence for Patient's Child:
See Part I, *Mendelian Inheritance.*

Age of Detectability: At birth.

Gene Mapping and Linkage: Unknown.

Prevention: None known. Genetic counseling indicated.

Treatment: Plastic surgical procedure to remove excess midline tissue and approximate nostrils. Use of flaps or skin grafts may be necessary to fill cleft defect.

Prognosis: Normal for life span, intelligence, and function if an isolated defect.

Detection of Carrier: Unknown.

References:
Boo-Chai K: The bifid nose; with a report of 3 cases in siblings. Plast Reconstr Surg 1965; 36:626–628.
Baibak G, Bromberg BE: Congenital midline defects of the midface. Cleft Palate J 1966; 3:392–401.
DeMyer W: The median cleft face syndrome: differential diagnosis of cranium bifidum occultum, hypertelorism, and median cleft nose, lip and palate. Neurology 1967; 17:961–971.
Kawamotod HK: The kaleidoscopic world of rare craniofacial clefts. Clinics in Plastic Surg 1976; 3:529–571, 533–534, 542–549.
Anyane-Yeboa K, et al.: Dominant inheritance of bifid nose. Am J Med Genet 1984; 17:561–563.
Miles JH, Smith V: Dominant bifid nose syndrome in four generations. (Abstract). Am J Hum Genet 1985; 37:A69.

BE028   **LaVonne Bergstrom**

NOSE, CHOANAL ATRESIA-LYMPHEDEMA   2597

Includes:
Atresia choanal posterior-lymphedema
Atresia of posterior nares-lymphedema
Bony choanal atresia, posterior-lymphedema
Choanal atresia, posterior-lymphedema
Lymphedema-choanal atresia
Nasal atresia, posterior-lymphedema

Excludes:
Brachydactyly (0114)
Charge association (2124)
Lymphedema I (0614)
Lymphedema II (0615)
Lymphedema, early onset
Lymphedema, other
Nose, anterior atresia (0723)
Nose, nasopharyngeal stenosis (0707)
Nose, posterior atresia (0727)

Major Diagnostic Criteria: Congenital bilateral posterior choanal atresia (PCA) detected soon after birth; onset of lymphedema of the lower extremities occurs after age two years.

Clinical Findings: Acute respiratory distress with cyanosis and struggling develops soon after birth due to atresia of the posterior nares, suspected by inability to pass a catheter in the oral pharynx and confirmed by lateral X-rays of the nasopharynx with radiopaque dye in the anterior portion of the nose. Infant is unable to nurse because of breathing difficulty.

Chronic, pitting edema is first noticed around the dorsal aspects of feet and ankles after the second birthday and progresses gradually upwards to involve the lower leg. The upper limb and thigh involvement may not be observed until ten years of age. The overlying skin appears shiny, but is otherwise normal. Older children have complained of tiredness during usual physical activities. The degree of involvement can be quite variable from individual to individual, and from side to side.

All causes of secondary lymphedema should be excluded. Lymphangiographic and Doppler studies may show aplasia, hypoplasia, or dilated lymph trunks. A history of PCA during the newborn period may be helpful in establishing the relationship between the two conditions. Physical growth is the normal range (height and weight between 5th and 45th percentiles); development and intelligence are normal.

Complications: Bilateral PCA causes serious breathing difficulty and may result in death unless an oral airway is established and surgical correction is carried out. Difficulties in nursing will result in failure to thrive. If the condition goes unrecognized and the infant suffers chronic hypoxia, intelligence and function may be affected. Although primarily a cosmetic and psychosocial handicap, the severe edema is likely to affect walking and movements.

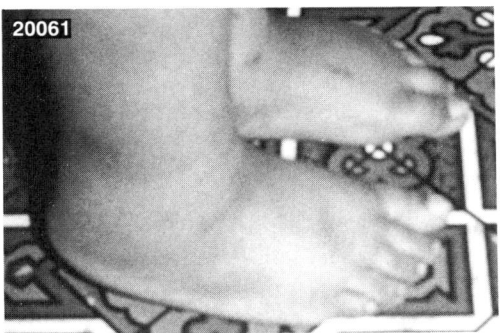

2597-20061: Note edema in both feet and lower legs. The edema is pitting type.

In addition, it may lead to recurrent episodes of lymphangitis or cellulitis, and to ulceration.

Associated Findings: Mild **Pectus excavatum** (5/5), highly arched palate (4/5), radial loop patterns on fourth fingertips (3/5), and relatively large head size (70–98th percentile) (4/5).

Etiology: Autosomal recessive inheritance.

Pathogenesis: The pathogenesis of PCA appears to be the failure of the bucconasal membrane to rupture between the 35th and 39th days of fetal life; persistent tissue is then carried posteriorly and vertically as the face develops. In 85% of the cases, the atresia is bony and is commonly located 1–2 mm anterior to the posterior edge of the hard palate.

Pathogenesis of lymphedema is largely unknown. The edema is likely due to a defect in the development of the lymphatic drainage associated with the congenital hypoplasia of the lymphatic system. The combined syndrome was observed in a large kindred in which several consanguinous marriages had taken place. The existence of tightly linked recessive genes for PCA and lymphedema in this an inbred kindred may explain concurrence of the two conditions. All children with PCA have already developed the edema.

POS No.: 4265

Sex Ratio: M1:F1

Occurrence: Observed in two generations of three sibships of one large kindred.

Risk of Recurrence for Patient's Sib:
See Part I, *Mendelian Inheritance.*

Risk of Recurrence for Patient's Child:
See Part I, *Mendelian Inheritance.*

Age of Detectability: Soon after birth because of respiratory difficulty and cyanosis. Lymphedema is detectable after the second birthday.

Gene Mapping and Linkage: Unknown.

Prevention: None known. Genetic counseling indicated.

Treatment: Early recognition of the PCA; establishing and maintaining an oral airway until surgery. Surgical correction can be performed intranasally during the newborn period, or transpalatally after the age of six months. Lymphedema is difficult to manage and treat. Partial and/or temporary response has been reported by administration of diuretics, bed rest, and use of a pararubber bandage or an elastic stocking. In severe and uncontrollable edema, resection of subcutaneous tissues with subsequent skin autografts may be performed. Supportive therapy for psychosocial problems may be needed.

Prognosis: Apparently normal for life span and intelligence once the PCA is surgically corrected. The prognosis for lymphedema is dictated by its severity and response to available treatment modalities.

Detection of Carrier: Unknown.

References:
Qazi QH, et al.: Inheritance of posterior choanal atresia. Am J Med Genet 1982; 13:413–416.
Sheikh TM, et al.: Posterior choanal atresia lymphedema association in a kindred. Pediatr Res 1986; 20:272A. *

QA000   **Qutub H. Qazi**

Nose, congenital median fissure of
See NOSE, BIFID

NOSE, DISLOCATED NASAL SEPTUM   2719

Includes:
Dislocation of the nasal septum
Nasal septum, subluxed or dislocated
Subluxed nasal septum, congenital

Excludes:
Choanal atresia
Nose, anterior stenosis (2718)
Turbinate defect

Major Diagnostic Criteria: Outward deviation of the nose to one side, accompanied by leaning of the columella and a loss of nasal tip stability.

Clinical Findings: Outward deviation of the nose to one side, leaning of the columella, loss of nasal tip stability, flattening of the nasal aperture on the side of dislocation, and diminished movement of the ala on the same side during inspiration.

Complications: Nasal obstruction, external deformity, risk of septal hematoma, and increased risk of upper and lower respiratory tract infections later in life.

Associated Findings: None known.

Etiology: Usually intrauterine pressure and strain, primarily during the first stage of labor in primipara.

Pathogenesis: The left occipitoanterior presentation results in a more frequent deviation to the right. Significant nasal trauma is possible any time after the fourth month of gestation and is subject to the pressure of intrauterine growths or fetal limbs.

CDC No.: 754.020

Sex Ratio: Undetermined but presumably M1:F1.

Occurrence: Overall frequency of < 1%.

Risk of Recurrence for Patient's Sib: Unknown.

Risk of Recurrence for Patient's Child: Unknown.

Age of Detectability: At birth.

Gene Mapping and Linkage: Unknown.

Prevention: None known.

Treatment: Manual reduction of septal cartilage into the septal groove within the first three days of life.

Prognosis: Once septal reduction has been performed, there is usually good stability.

Detection of Carrier: Unknown.

References:
Gray L: The deviated nasal septum. J Laryngol Otol 1965; 79:567–575.
Jazbi B: Subluxation of the nasal septum in the newborn: etiology, diagnosis and treatment. Otol Clin North Am 1977; 10:125–138.
Sprinkle PM, Sponck FT: Congenital malformations of the nose and paranasal sinuses. In: Bluestone CD, Stool SE, eds: Pediatric otolaryngology. Philadelphia: W.B. Saunders, 1983:769–779.

MY003   **Charles M. Myer III**
OR005   **Peter Orobello**

NOSE, DUPLICATION   0725

Includes: Nasal duplication

Excludes:
Amniotic bands syndrome (0874)
Nose/nasal septum defects (0722)
Nose, bifid (0724)
Supernumerary nostrils

Major Diagnostic Criteria: Two distinct and complete noses, each with two nostrils, two nasal cavities, a nasal septum, and alar cartilages.

Clinical Findings: In the newborn with nasal duplication, preliminary inspection reveals what appears to be a bifid nose with two well-developed nostrils; however, in addition, there exist between the nares two small sinus openings that, on careful examination, prove to be definite nostrils leading into separate nasal cavities. As the child grows, these openings develop into unmistakable nostrils with obvious alar cartilages. Finally, with further development, two separate and complete noses become distinctly evident. Although the small mesial nostrils usually open into definite nasal cavities separate from the lateral, larger nasal cavities, the former spaces may be nothing more than blind pouches without a posterior opening. However, the lateral nasal cavities may extend through choanae into the nasopharynx. X-rays are difficult to interpret but do reveal an indeterminate nasal defect.

Complications: Mild to moderate hypertelorism. The medially-placed nares and nasal chambers are smaller than the lateral ones, and may be patent or stenotic. Respiratory distress at birth, and excessive nasal discharge, may lead to exhaustion and interfere with sleeping and sucking.

Associated Findings: Muecke's (1923) patient had tiny, round depressions on the medial aspect of the root of each nose that Muecke speculated were lacrymal fissures. Ethmoid masses have been reported. One case was reported with a supplementary anterior cerebral lobe. A second complete nose, with or without duplication of the maxilla and/or orbits/eyes, is sometimes found in more severely affected cases of facial duplication.

Etiology: Possibly errors in cell duplication or reproduction.

Pathogenesis: From nasal embryology, one can assume that various forms of bifid nose, median clefts of the upper lip, notches in the nostrils, dermoid cysts, sinuses, and other ectodermal inclusions on the bridge of the nose are the result of arrested development of the frontonasal process (especially the globular processes) and the olfactory sacs.

Although it seems apparent that failure of the nasal laminae to consolidate into a single nasal septum is the cause of a bifid nose, it is most difficult to understand the faulty embryologic processes that initiate the formation of two noses with four nostrils and four nasal cavities. One can theorize that some irregularity in the evolution of the two olfactory placodes causes them to bring forth four olfactory pits, all in a horizontal plane, rather than two; such an anomaly would alter the developmental pattern of the medial nasal process. If such were the case, it would tend to explain why the lateral nostrils are larger and more normal in size than are the mesial nostrils, since the lateral nasal processes have not been involved in the developmental defect. Furthermore, it is possible that the two medial olfactory pits probably form olfactory sacs, which are interposed between the two nasal laminae. These sacs, which become medial nasal cavities, thus prevent the laminae from fusing into one nasal septum; instead, they stay divided and form two septa. With the presence of two septa, four nostrils, and four nasal cavities, the developmental anomaly goes on to form two separate noses.

CDC No.: 748.110

Sex Ratio: M1:F2 (observed).

Occurrence: About ten cases reported in the literature.

Risk of Recurrence for Patient's Sib: Unknown.

Risk of Recurrence for Patient's Child: Unknown.

Age of Detectability: At birth.

Gene Mapping and Linkage: Unknown.

Prevention: None known. Genetic counseling indicated.

Treatment: Surgical rectification of the deformity. The correction of nasal duplication requires three or four surgical procedures several years apart.

Prognosis: Normal for life span and intelligence.

Detection of Carrier: Unknown.

References:
Muecke FF, Souttar HS: Double nose. Proc R Soc Med 1924; 17:8–9.
Erich JB: Nasal duplication: report of case of patient with two noses. Plast Reconstr Surg 1962; 29:159–166.
Ghosh P, et al.: Double nose. J Laryngol Otolaryngol 1971; 85:963–969. †

Mazzola RF: Congenital malformations in the frontonasal area. Clin Plast Surg 1976; 3:573–609. * †
Barr M, Jr: Facial duplication: case review and embryogenesis. Teratology 1982; 25:152–159. *

ER001   **John B. Erich**
EV002   **Carla A. Evans**

Nose, ear, digital anomalies-gingival fibromatosis
    See GINGIVAL FIBROMATOSIS-DIGITAL ANOMALIES
Nose, flattened tip and depressed bridge (some)
    See CHONDRODYSPLASIA PUNCTATA, MILD SYMMETRIC TYPE

NOSE, GLIOMA   0726

Includes:
    Encephalochoristoma nasofrontalis
    Glioma, nasal
    Nasal glioma

Excludes:
    Neck/head, dermoid cyst or teratoma (0283)
    Encephalocele (0343)
    Hemangioma of nose
    Meningocele (0642)
    Nasal neurofibroma
    Nasal polyps

Major Diagnostic Criteria: A unilateral intra- or extranasal mass present at birth, producing a broad nasal bridge and wide-set eyes is the characteristic clinical picture. Sixty percent of nasal gliomas are extranasal, 30% are intranasal, and 10% are combined in location. Nasal gliomas have no fluid connection with the subarachnoid space. If, with straining or crying, the mass pulsates or increases in size, a spinal fluid communication may exist, and then a meningocele or an encephalocele must be ruled out. Biopsy of the mass with histopathologic study will help establish the diagnosis, but this should be delayed until appropriate X-ray studies have been performed and one is prepared definitively to excise the mass.

Clinical Findings: These congenital neurogenic tumors are often located externally at the nasal bridge; however, they can present as an intranasal or nasopharyngeal tumor. A combination of locations rarely will be evident. A nasal bridge that is broader in width and eyes that are more widely separated than normal suggest an intranasal tumor. The external tumor is raised and usually covered with intact skin. These tumors, ranging from 1 to 5 cm in diameter, are firm, mobile, round, and smooth. Color varies from pink to red.

Intranasal tumors are located high in the nasal cavity, but they may extend down to the anterior nares. These tumors appear to arise from above the middle turbinate or olfactory fissure; they should not be confused with nasal polyps. They are usually unilateral and cause airway obstruction.

Nasal gliomas are benign in clinical behavior. They rarely enlarge, and recurrence after complete excision is rare. Communication between the tumor and the anterior cranial fossa is not present in true nasal glioma, although a fibrous stalk is present about 20% of the time.

Complications: Nasal cosmetic deformities, rhinitis, meningitis, encephalitis, sinusitis, nasal obstruction, cerebrospinal fluid rhinorrhea, epistaxis, anosmia.

Associated Findings: Meningocele, encephalocele.

Etiology: Unknown.

Pathogenesis: Tumors probably arise from congenital malformations of the nose, the base of the skull, and CNS in the region of the foramen cecum. Glial tissue is separated from the CNS and remains outside the calvaria. These abnormalities result from developmental defects in the frontal, nasal, ethmoid, or sphenoid bones of the skull. Tumors composed of CNS tissues arise from such defects. Nasal gliomas contain glial tissues, are separated from the brain, and are occasionally connected to the base of the skull with a fibrous stalk. Nasal gliomas per se have no fluid connection with the CNS and hence contain no spinal fluid that circulates between the tumors and the subarachnoid space.

CDC No.: 748.180

Sex Ratio: M3:F1

Occurrence: Undetermined but presumed rare.

Risk of Recurrence for Patient's Sib: Unknown.

Risk of Recurrence for Patient's Child: Unknown.

Age of Detectability: At birth or soon after.

Gene Mapping and Linkage: Unknown.

Prevention: None known. Genetic counseling indicated.

Treatment: Complete surgical excision usually results in a cure. Intracranial communication must be ruled out before excising the tumor. If there is an intracranial connection, an intracranial excision should be performed before the external nasal mass is excised. Antibiotics for infections and rhinoplasty for nasal deformities may be necessary.

Prognosis: Good, when total excision is performed.

Detection of Carrier: Unknown.

Special Considerations: X-ray examination, including polytomography of the base of the skull and CT scans will often reveal a defect in the calvaria when a fluid communication does exist. The mass can be " tapped" with a needle to determine the presence of spinal fluid, but careful aseptic techniques must be used to avoid subsequent infections. When spinal fluid is present in the tumor, air or dye contrast studies of the CNS should be performed. The presence or absence of fluid communication must be determined before considering surgical therapy.

Encephaloceles may be difficult to differentiate from nasal gliomas, although they are quite different in structure. The encephalocele contains an ependyma-lined space filled with cerebrospinal fluid that communicates with the ventricles of the brain. Glial and fibrous tissues are present beneath the ependymal lining. A biopsy from the wall of such a tumor may not reveal the true nature of this tumor. A defect in the base of the skull on X-ray examination helps make this diagnosis. These tumors pulsate and increase in size when the infant strains or cries.

Meningoceles are rare and consist of meninges that herniate through a developmental defect in the cranium. They have clinical characteristics similar to those of the encephalocele. There are two types of meningocele that occur about the nose. The sphenopharyngeal dehiscence involves the sphenoid or ethmoid bones with a tumor presenting in the orbit, nasal cavity, nasopharynx, or medial to the ramus of the mandible. An intranasal (sincipital) dehiscence involves the cribriform plate, with a tumor either in the nasal cavity or externally at the medial canthus of the eye, or in the orbit.

References:
Black BK, Smith DE: Nasal glioma: two cases with recurrence. Arch Neurol Psychiatry 1950; 64:614–630.
Proctor B, Proctor C: Congenital lesions of the head and neck. Otolaryngol Clin North Am 1970; 3:221–248. *
Karma P, et al.: Nasal gliomas. A review and report of two cases. Laryngoscope 1977; 87:1169–1179.
Gorenstein A, et al.: Nasal gliomas. Arch Otolaryngol 1980; 106:536–540.
Hughes GB, et al.: Management of the congenital midline nasal mass: a review. Head Neck Surg 1980; 2:222–223.
Whitaker SR, et al.: Nasal glioma. Arch Otolaryngol 1981; 107:550–554. *
Bradley PJ, Singh SD: Nasal glioma. J Laryngol Otol 1985; 99:247–252.

EN002 **Gerald M. English**

Includes: Granulosis rubra nasi

Excludes:
　Acne rosacea
　Acne vulgaris
　Lupus erythematosis, systemic (2515)
　Lupus vulgaris
　Perioral dermatitis
　Other causes of erythema

Major Diagnostic Criteria: Hyperhidrosis of the nose. Erythema of the tip of the nose, which may extend to the rest of the nose.

Clinical Findings: Hyperhidrosis of the nose may be the first symptom. Erythema of the nasal tip, possibly the remainder of the nose, and sometimes migrating to involve the cheeks, upper lid and chin, is a reliable feature. Pinpoint to pinhead-sized dark red papules are scattered irregularly on the erythematous base associated with sweat droplets. Vesicles and small cystic lesions have been described. The nose feels cold to the touch, and there may be slight itching without other local symptoms. Volar hyperhidrosis and poor peripheral circulation are associated. Histopathologically, there is dilation of dermal blood and lymphatic vessels. There is perivascular infiltration, including mast cells and dilation of sweat ducts. The connective tissue, epidermis, and pilosebaceous elements are normal. Laboratory and X-ray findings are unremarkable.

The majority of patients are children, six months to 10 years of age. A few adult patients have been reported. The disease process commonly resolves at puberty.

Complications: Unknown.

Associated Findings: None known.

Etiology: Both autosomal recessive and dominant inheritance have been suggested.

Pathogenesis: Endocrinopathy, vasomotor disturbances in the form of sympathetic dysfunction, and a form of sweat retention are hypothesized causes.

MIM No.: 13900

CDC No.: 748.180

Sex Ratio: M1:F1

Occurrence: Unknown. At least one large kindred has been documented.

Risk of Recurrence for Patient's Sib:
　See Part I, *Mendelian Inheritance.*

Risk of Recurrence for Patient's Child:
　See Part I, *Mendelian Inheritance.*

Age of Detectability: Six months to 10 years.

Gene Mapping and Linkage: Unknown.

Prevention: None known. Genetic counseling indicated.

Treatment: No known effective therapy.

Prognosis: Excellent, with normal life span. Disease process usually resolves at puberty, but may persist indefinitely.

Detection of Carrier: Unknown.

References:
Binazzi M: Ulteriori relievi su di una osservazione di granulosis rubra nasi ereditaria. Rass Dermatol Sif 1958; 11:23–26.
Allen AC: The skin, ed 2, New York: Grune and Stratton, 1967.
Aram H, Mohagheghi AP: Granulosis rubra nasi. Cutis 1972; 10:463–464. *

HU015　　　　　　　　　　　　　　　　**Richard Hubbell**
MY003　　　　　　　　　　　　　**Charles M. Myer III**

NOSE, NASOPHARYNGEAL STENOSIS 0707

Includes:
> Nasopharyngeal atresia
> Nasopharyngeal stenosis

Excludes:
> **Nose, anterior atresia** (0723)
> **Nose, posterior atresia** (0727)

Major Diagnostic Criteria: Complete or incomplete attachment of the soft palate to the posterior nasopharynx. Nasopharyngeal stenosis should be considered in the newborn with obstruction of the nasal airway without choanal atresia.

Clinical Findings: The posterior soft palate and posterior nasopharynx are connected by a thin membrane. Although respiratory distress in the newborn with a complete membrane would be expected, it has not been reported. The patients do have excessive nasal discharge.

Complications: Reduced nasal airway proportional to the amount of obstruction produced by the membrane. Nasal discharge due to impaired flow of the nasal mucous into the pharynx.

Associated Findings: Shallow nasopharynx reported in about one-half of cases.

Etiology: Undetermined. One case of congenital syphilitic nasopharyngeal stenosis has been reported.

Pathogenesis: Undetermined. Incomplete rupture of buccopharyngeal membrane has been proposed; however, this is questionable since the buccopharyngeal membrane is thought to rupture prior to fusion of the lateral palatal processes to form the soft palate, and the buccopharyngeal membrane should not be attached to the posterior nasopharynx.

CDC No.: 748.180

Sex Ratio: Presumably M1:F1. Sex reported in only two cases, both of which were female.

Occurrence: Undetermined but presumed rare.

Risk of Recurrence for Patient's Sib: No known increase of risk.

Risk of Recurrence for Patient's Child: No known increase of risk.

Age of Detectability: At birth, by palpation between the soft palate and posterior pharyngeal wall.

Gene Mapping and Linkage: Unknown.

Prevention: None known.

Treatment: The cases of membranous connection between the palate and pharynx have responded to blunt penetration of the membrane followed by a digital dilation without recurrence of the stenosis. If a cicatricial stenosis or thick membrane is encountered, it can be treated with a seton suture or by mucosal flaps.

Although respiratory difficulties have not been reported, they would be expected in cases of complete or severe obstruction of the nasopharynx. This should be treated with an oral airway pending definitive treatment of the stenosis.

While membranous occlusion of the nasopharynx will respond to simple penetration and dilation of the stenotic segment, cicatricial stenosis will almost surely recur with this form of therapy.

Prognosis: *Treated:* Membranous stenosis: excellent prognosis for permanent establishment of a nasal airway. Cicatricial stenosis tends to recur; however, permanent establishment of a nasal airway has been accomplished with the seton procedure and with mucosal flaps.

Untreated: Death may result from complete or severe nasopharyngeal stenosis because the newborn does not breathe through his mouth except, when crying or gasping for air.

Detection of Carrier: Unknown.

References:
MacKenty JE: Nasopharyngeal atresia. Arch Otolaryngol 1927; 6:1–27.
Stevenson EW: Cicatricial stenosis of the nasopharynx. Laryngoscope 1969; 79:2035–2067.
Cotton RT: Nasopharyngeal stenosis. Arch Otolaryngol 1985; 111:146–148.

MY003   **Charles M. Myer III**

NOSE, POSTERIOR ATRESIA 0727

Includes:
> Atresia choanal posterior
> Atresia of posterior nares
> Bony choanal atresia, posterior
> Choanal atresia, posterior
> Membranous choanal atresia, posterior
> Posterior nasal atresia

Excludes:
> **Nose, nasopharyngeal stenosis** (0707)
> **Nose, anterior atresia** (0723)

Major Diagnostic Criteria: Obstruction to nasal breathing due to posterior choanal atresia. A lateral X-ray of the head will demonstrate radiopaque dye in the nasal cavities and air in the unoccluded nasopharynx behind the obstructing membrane. Computerized tomography and MRI scanning are helpful diagnostic procedures. The inability to pass nasal catheters through the nose a distance of 32 mm will confirm the diagnosis.

Clinical Findings: The newborn infant develops acute respiratory distress every time he or she attempts to breathe quietly with the mouth closed because most newborns are obligatory nasal breathers. Cyanosis, struggling, exhaustion, and death can occur

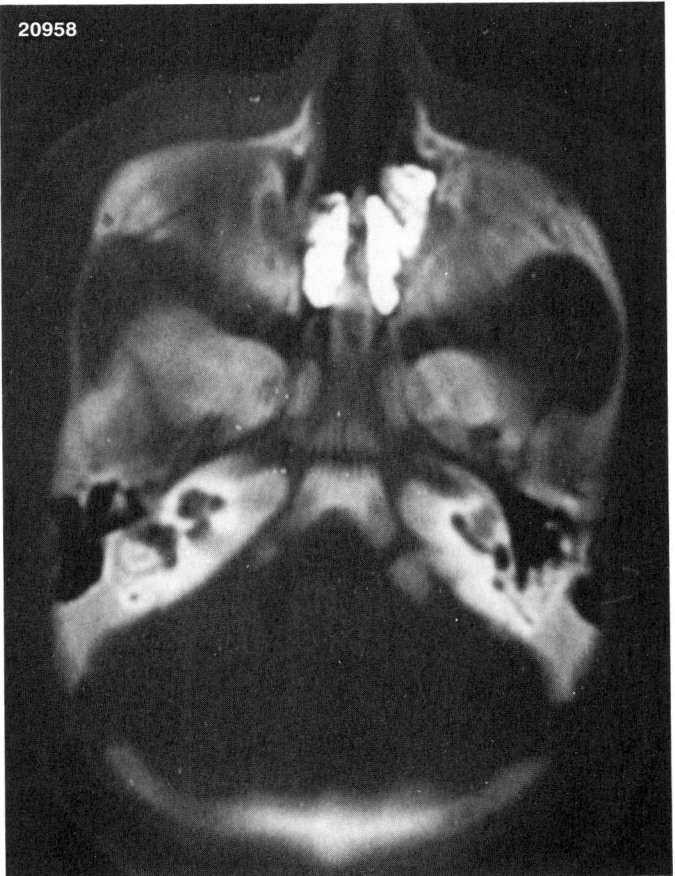

0727-20958: Choanal atresia.

unless an oral airway is obtained. When crying, the infant does well because the mouth is open. The newborn normally tends to breathe with the mouth closed. Nursing becomes a problem as the infant frequently has to stop feeding to gasp for breath.

A catheter cannot be passed into the oropharynx. If the airways are cleaned and decongested, an obstructing membrane may be seen in the depths of the nostril posteriorly, with a dimple in the center. Lateral X-rays of the head, with radiopaque dye injected into the nares, will demonstrate the soft tissue obstruction between the dye and the air in the nasopharynx. A computerized tomographic (CT) scan offers the most complete X-ray assessment of the problem.

Complications: Death may occur unless an oral airway is immediately placed and maintained.

Associated Findings: Cardiac defects (25%), branchial arch abnormalities (21%), abnormalities of pinna (15%), microcephaly (15%), micrognathia (15%), miscellaneous palatal abnormalities (15%), nasopharyngeal abnormalities (15%), mandibulofacial dysostosis (11%), cleft palate (10%), conductive or mixed hearing loss (3.5–7%), digital abnormalities (7%), miscellaneous tongue abnormalities (7%), cleft lip and palate (4%), tracheoesophageal fistula (3%), cervical meningocele, cleidocranial dysplasia, hiatus hernia, diaphragmatic hernia, oxycephaly, hypertelorism, facial cleft, absent nasal septum, imperforate anus, hydronephrosis, facial nerve paralysis, mental retardation, absent spleen, ileal atresia, cerebral agenesis, micropenis, coloboma. A feature of **Charge association**, it has also been observed in **Mandibulofacial dysostosis**.

Twenty-five percent of cases have a single minor associated abnormality; 25% have a single major associated abnormality, and 50% have multiple associated abnormalities. In unilateral choanal atresia, 45% have associated anomalies. In bilateral choanal atresia, 60% have associated anomalies. Sex incidence of associated anomalies: M2:F1.

Etiology: Presumably multifactorial.

Pathogenesis: Failure of complete excavation of the nasal cavities as they form (failure of rupture of buccopharyngeal membranes).

MIM No.: 21480

CDC No.: 748.000

Sex Ratio: M1:F2

Occurrence: Incidence 1:5,000 live births. Prevalence 1:4,000 to 1:8,000 in the general population.

Risk of Recurrence for Patient's Sib: Unknown.

Risk of Recurrence for Patient's Child: Unknown.

Age of Detectability: At birth by lack of a nasal airway causing acute respiratory distress with the mouth closed.

Gene Mapping and Linkage: Unknown.

Prevention: None known. Genetic counseling indicated.

Treatment: If the condition is bilateral, then an oral airway must be maintained until the bilateral choanal atresia is surgically corrected. The correction may be made immediately after birth by the intranasal or transpalatal route.

The application of modern otologic techniques, including micro instrumentation and the operating microscope, allow safe surgical correction with a relatively minor operative procedure in the first few days of life. Nonreactive silastic tubes maintain the patency of the corrected defect until re-epithelialization occurs and simultaneously allows for a patent airway.

Prognosis: Normal for life span, intelligence, and function if no life-threatening associated finding exists and if the infant survives the first few days or weeks of life when he or she tends to breathe entirely through the nose. Death occurring in the first days of life usually is from acute respiratory obstruction.

Detection of Carrier: Unknown.

References:
Baker MC: Congenital atresia of posterior nares. Arch Otolaryngol 1953; 58:431–434.

Singleton GT, Hardcastle B: Congenital choanal atresia. Arch Otolaryngol 1968; 87:620–625.
Evans JNG, MacLachlan RF: Choanal atresia. J Laryngol 1971; 85:903–929.
Feuerstein S, et al.: Transnasal correction of choanal atreasia. Head Neck Surg 1980; 3:97–104.
Maniglia AJ, Goodwin WJ: Congenital choanal atresia. Otolaryngol Clin North Am 1981; 14:167–173.
Qazi Q, et al.: Inheritance of posterior choanal atresia. Am J Med Genet 1982; 13:413–416.
Greenberg F: Choanal atresia and athelia: methimazole teratogenicity or a new syndrome? Am J Med Genet 1987; 28:931–934.

HA032 **B. Hardcastle**

NOSE, PROBOSCIS LATERALIS 0824

Includes:
  Proboscis lateral
  Lateral nasal proboscis
  Arrhinencephalia unilateralis
  Tubular nostril congenital

Excludes:
  Nose, bifid (0724)
  Nose/nasal septum defects (0722)

Major Diagnostic Criteria: A pendulous soft tissue tube resembling, as described in the literature, a "little elephant trunk" is attached at the medial orbit-nasal bridge area.

Clinical Findings: While usually a unilateral condition (90%), bilateral and midline cases have been reported. The unilateral cases are almost evenly divided between right and left sides of the face. A typical proboscis measures 20–40 mm in length and 10–15 mm in diameter. It may have a distal opening about 1 mm in size and is usually, but not always, blind. Heminasal aplasia commonly occurs on the side of the proboscis (90%). Eye defects, especially coloboma of the iris or eyelid, occur in nearly all individuals.

Complications: Abnormalities of the eye and its adnexa or the nasal wall are likely to cause disturbances in vision and handling of secretions.

Associated Findings: The adjacent nasal wall malformation may range from a soft tissue deficiency to absence of ipsilateral frontal and maxillary sinus, nasolacrimal apparatus, vomer, lateral nasal wall and nasal bone. Ophthalmic findings include coloboma of eyelid or iris, microphthalmia or anophthalmia, cystic degeneration of the optic nerve, cyclopean eye, and choroidal cleft.

Other associated findings are cleft lip/palate (20%); absence of the lateral incisor, vomer, premaxilla; and absence or diminution of the cribriform plate, olfactory bulb, and olfactory tract.

Etiology: Undetermined, but probably results from a defect in the anterior portion of the early neural crest and plate. Proboscis lateralis and microphthalmos has been produced in chicks with microlaser irratiation to anterior neural crest region.

Pathogenesis: Occurrence of proboscii may be related to facial clefting. The tube can be attached at various points along line of embryonic fusion between anterior maxillary process and frontonasal process. Imperfect mesodermal proliferation and epidermal breakdown produces a tube-like structure arising at frontonasal region.

CDC No.: 748.185

Sex Ratio: M2:F1

Occurrence: Approximately 40 cases reported.

Risk of Recurrence for Patient's Sib: Not increased.

Risk of Recurrence for Patient's Child: Not increased.

Age of Detectability: Proboscis lateralis has been detected in the fetus by sonography, but is usually noted at birth.

Gene Mapping and Linkage: Unknown.

Prevention: None known. Genetic counseling indicated.

Treatment: The nasal anomaly requires a surgical construction utilizing the proboscis when a tissue deficiency exists in the nasal wall. The plastic surgical procedure is usually staged. An early repair that improves esthetic appearance may promote more normal psychological development, but is more difficult to plan and execute due to the influences of growth on size and structure of the constructed nose.

Especially in heminasal aplasia, it is important to retain the proboscis so that adequate local tissue will be available for surgical procedures.

Prognosis: Unless severe cranial base and cerebral anomalies are present, a normal life span is expected.

Detection of Carrier: Unknown.

References:
Rontal M, et al: Proboscis lateralis: case report and embryologic analysis. Laryngoscope 1977; 87:996–1005. †
Lieuw Kie Song SH, et al.: Median faciocerebral anomalies in chick embryos resulting from local destruction of the anteriormost parts of the early neural plate and neural crest. Acta Morph Neerl Scand 1980; 18:231–252.
Wang S, et al.: Proboscis lateralis, microphthalmos, and cystic degeneration of the optic nerve. Ann Opthal 1983; 15:756–758.
Boo-Chai K: The proboscis lateralis-a 14-year follow-up. Plast Reconstr Surg 1985; 75:569–577.

EV002   **Carla A. Evans**

NOSE, TRANSVERSE GROOVE   0728

Includes:
    Nasal crease
    Nasal groove, familial transverse
    Nasal groove, transverse
    Nasal stripe, transverse

Excludes: Nose (other)

Major Diagnostic Criteria: A horizontal red depression or groove 1–3 mm wide and about 1 mm deep, located just caudad to the ala nasi.

Clinical Findings: A horizontal red depression or groove 1–3 mm wide and about 1 mm deep, located just caudad to the ala nasi has been observed in two affected families.

Complications: Unknown.

Associated Findings: Otosclerosis, hyperlaxity of the joints, severe dental caries.

Etiology: Autosomal dominant inheritance with variable penetrance.

Pathogenesis: Unknown.

MIM No.: *16150

CDC No.: 748.180

Sex Ratio: M1:F1

Occurrence: Documented in two kindreds.

Risk of Recurrence for Patient's Sib:
    See Part I, *Mendelian Inheritance.*

Risk of Recurrence for Patient's Child:
    See Part I, *Mendelian Inheritance.*

Age of Detectability: Becomes prominent in childhood, at which time it may have a rose color.

Gene Mapping and Linkage: Unknown.

Prevention: None known. Genetic counseling indicated.

Treatment: Not necessary.

Prognosis: Normal for life span, intelligence, and function; the groove disappears after puberty.

Detection of Carrier: Unknown.

References:
Anderson PC: Familial transverse nasal groove. Arch Dermatol 1961; 84:316–317.

Pierre ER, Teneyck FD: Hereditary hyperpigmentation anomalies in blacks. J Hered 1974; 65:157–159.

MY003   **Charles M. Myer III**

NOSE, TURBINATE DEFORMITY   2720

Includes:
    Nasal agenesis
    Turbinate deformity

Excludes:
    Choanal atresia
    Nose, anterior stenosis (2718)
    Nose, bifid (0724)
    Nose, dislocated nasal septum (2719)
    Nose/nasal septum defects (0722)

Major Diagnostic Criteria: The inferior or middle turbinate may acquire a rounded, bulbous appearance, causing airway obstruction.

Clinical Findings: There is extra space in one nasal cavity due to long standing septal deviation. Both bone and mucosal elements may be involved, and hypertrophy to fill the larger nasal cavity.

Complications: Nasal obstruction, and turbinate invasion by ethmoid air cells.

Associated Findings: None known.

Etiology: Unknown.

Pathogenesis: Whether the turbinate enlargement causes the septum to be deformed or the turbinate enlarges to fill the space created by the septal deformity is unknown.

CDC No.: 748.180

Sex Ratio: Undetermined but presumably M1:F1.

Occurrence: Ethmoid invasion of the middle turbinate is found in 12% of adults.

Risk of Recurrence for Patient's Sib: Unknown.

Risk of Recurrence for Patient's Child: Unknown.

Age of Detectability: During childhood.

Gene Mapping and Linkage: Unknown.

Prevention: It is undetermined whether repair of septal dislocation will prevent this deformity.

Treatment: It is controversial whether turbinate enlargement in children should be treated at all. Septal repair and surgical reduction procedure of turbinate (cautery vs. turbinectomy) is sometimes performed.

Prognosis: Good for function with treatment.

Detection of Carrier: Unknown.

References:
Sprinkle PM, Sponck FT: Congenital malformations of the nose and paranasal sinuses. In: Bluestone CD, Stool SE, eds: Pediatric otolaryngology. Philadelphia: W.B. Saunders, 1983:769–779.

MY003   **Charles M. Myer III**
OR005   **Peter Orobello**

NOSE/NASAL SEPTUM DEFECTS   0722

Includes:
    Dermoid cysts of nose of both skin and dural origin
    Nasal septum, absence of
    Nose, absence of
    Nose, absence of half
    Nose, half, plus proboscis
    Persistent frontonasal process
    "Potato" nose
    Triple nares

Excludes:
    Nasal deformities secondary to cleft lip or cleft palate

Nose, abnormalities of growth of the maxillary processes
Nose, anterior atresia (0723)
Nose, bifid (0724)
Nose, duplication (0725)

Major Diagnostic Criteria: Evidence of a nasal defect other than bifid nose or nasal duplication.

Clinical Findings: The degree of nasal deformity can vary from a small notch in one ala to total absence of the nose. The minor abnormalities are much more frequent.

Complications: Total nasal obstruction may be associated with asphyxia at birth. Intermediate degrees of nasal obstruction may also lead to a higher incidence of acquired ear disease. Speech defects are occasionally present. Psychologic problems occur due to the cosmetic deformity.

Associated Findings: Hypertelorism and abnormal location of the anterior fontanel are frequently seen with major deformities of the nose and are probably directly related to an abnormality of development of the frontonasal process.

Etiology: Some cases appear to be inherited.

Pathogenesis: The external nose and nasal septum are derived from a prolongation of the frontonasal process together with an infolding which produces the nasal septum. Unequal growth of the two sides of the nasal septum or excessive infolding of the septal portion without fusion of the 2 parts can account for the majority of the abnormalities of the nose and septum. The unusual inclusion dermoids of dural origin can be accounted for by dural extensions which have become included in the frontonasal process as it grows out from the anterior cranium.

MIM No.: 16400

Sex Ratio: M1:F1

Occurrence: Undetermined but presumed rare.

Risk of Recurrence for Patient's Sib: Unknown.

Risk of Recurrence for Patient's Child: Unknown.

Age of Detectability: At birth.

Gene Mapping and Linkage: Unknown.

Prevention: None known. Genetic counseling indicated.

Treatment: Operative repair of defect or reconstruction is indicated if either functional or cosmetic problems are present.

Prognosis: Generally good except for cases with total nasal obstruction occurring at birth when asphyxia may lead to death, or brain damage. Newborn infants are obligate nose breathers and temporary measures to keep the mouth open should be used until definitive surgery can be performed, including use of an oral airway.

Detection of Carrier: Unknown.

References:
Badrawy R: Mid-line congenital anomalies of the nose. J Laryngol Otol 1967; 81:419.
Toriello HV, et al.: Familial occurrence of a developmental defect of the medial nasal process. Am J Med Genet 1985; 21:131–135.

MY003   **Charles M. Myer III**

Nougaret disease
See NIGHTBLINDNESS, CONGENITAL STATIONARY, AUTOSOMAL DOMINANT
Nova Scotian type Niemann-Pick disease
See NIEMANN-PICK DISEASE
Nuchal lymphangioma
See NECK, CYSTIC HYGROMA, FETAL TYPE
Nuclear cataract
See CATARACT, AUTOSOMAL DOMINANT CONGENITAL
also CATARACT, COPPOCK
Nuclear facial palsy
See PALSY, CONGENITAL FACIAL
Nuclear hypoplasia congenital (6th and 7th cranial nerves)
See DIPLEGIA, CONGENITAL FACIAL
Nucleoside-phosphorylase deficiency
See IMMUNODEFICIENCY, NUCLEOSIDE-PHOSPHORYLASE DEFICIENCY

Nuidudui
See ANEMIA, SICKLE CELL
Nyssen-van Bogaert syndrome
See OPTICO-COCHLEO-DENTATE DEGENERATION
Nystagmus-brachydactyly-cerebellar ataxia syndrome
See BIEMOND I SYNDROME

Oast-house urine disease
    See *METHIONINE MALABSORPTION*
Obesity-hypotonia-prominent incisors
    See *COHEN SYNDROME*
Obstetric hepatosis
    See *INTRAHEPATIC CHOLESTASIS OF PREGNANCY (ICP)*
Obstructing muscular bands of the right ventricle
    See *VENTRICLE, DOUBLE CHAMBERED RIGHT*
Obstruction within the right ventricular body
    See *VENTRICLE, DOUBLE CHAMBERED RIGHT*
Obstructive hydrocephaly, extra- and intraventricular congenital
    See *HYDROCEPHALY*

OCCIPITAL HORN SYNDROME   3219

Includes:
    Cutis laxa, X-linked
    Ehlers-Danlos syndrome IX (obsolete)

Excludes:
    Ehlers-Danlos syndrome (0338)
    Menkes syndrome (0643)

Major Diagnostic Criteria: *Clinical:* Skin lax and mildly hyperextensible, hypermobile digits, and bony protuberances of the occiput.
    Biochemical: Moderate increase in serum copper and ceruloplasmin levels. Excess of copper and increased ^{64}Cu accumulation, attached to metallothionein, in cultured fibroblasts. Lysyl oxidase deficiency.
    The nosology of occipital horn syndrome (OHS) has been complicated; initially the condition was designated X-linked Cutis laxa and thereafter it was termed "Ehlers-Danlos syndrome type IX". Recently it has been established that OHS is due to a defect in copper metabolism and the OHS is now grouped with other disorders of copper transport.

Clinical Findings: The skin of the affected males is lax or mildly hyperextensible. Digits are hypermobile, while the elbows and knees have limitation of extension due to abnormalities of bone modelling. Bony protuberances of the occiput, known as occipital horns, which present as bony nubbins in the first decade are an important diagnostic indicator.
    Other skeletal stigmata include short clavicles, carpal bone coalescences and osteomalacia.
    Diverticulae of the bladder may rupture spontaneously. Chronic diarrhea and postural hypotension are inconsistent features.
    X-ray findings: occipital exostoses, clavicles short and thickened at horny distal ends. Micturating cystogram confirms bladder diverticulae. Other changes are variable.

Complications: Limitation of extension of knees and elbows; bladder rupture; **Hernia, inguinal**.

Associated Findings: None known.

Etiology: X-linked recessive inheritance.

Pathogenesis: Disorder of copper transport. Decreased activity of lysyl oxidase, the extracellular copper enzyme that initiates crosslinking of collagen and elastin. Corresponding to this decreased activity is a deficiency in the enzyme protein.

MIM No.: *30415

Sex Ratio: M1:F0

Occurrence: Undetermined but presumed rare, with no specific geographical grouping.

Risk of Recurrence for Patient's Sib:
    See Part I, *Mendelian Inheritance.*

Risk of Recurrence for Patient's Child:
    See Part I, *Mendelian Inheritance.*

Age of Detectability: In the first decade of life.

Gene Mapping and Linkage: LOX (lysyl oxidase; ?cutis laxa-X; ?Ehlers-Danlos V) has been provisionally mapped to X.

Prevention: None known. Genetic counseling indicated.

Treatment: Parenteral copper administration seems unlikely to remedy the low lysyl oxidase activity.

Prognosis: Life span is not significantly reduced.

Detection of Carrier: Unknown.

Special Considerations: The designation of this disorder as occipital horn syndrome, and the discontinuation of the use of the terms "EDS IX" or "XL Cutis Laxa", was formalized at the Workshop for the Nosology of Inherited Connective Tissue Disorders in Berlin in 1986 (Beighton et al, 1988).

References:
Byers PH, et al.: X-linked cutis laxa. New Engl J Med 1980; 303:61–65.
Sartons DJ, et al.: Type IX Ehlers-Danlos syndrome. Radiology 1984; 152:665–670.
Kuivaniemi H, et al.: Type IX Ehlers-Danlos syndrome and Menkes syndrome: the decrease in lysyl oxidase activity is associated with a corresponding deficiency in the enzyme protein. Am J Hum Genet 1985; 37:798–808.
Beighton P, et al.: International Nosology of Heritable Disorders of Connective Tissue, Berlin, 1986. Am J Med Genet 1988; 29:581–594.

WI055   **Ingrid M. Winship**

Occipito-facial-cervico-thoracic-abdomino-digital dysplasia
    See *SPONDYLOTHORACIC DYSPLASIA*
Ochoa syndrome
    See *UROFACIAL SYNDROME*
Ochronosis
    See *ALKAPTONURIA*
Ochronotic arthritis
    See *ALKAPTONURIA*
Octanoyl-CoA or general acyl-CoA dehydrogenase deficiency
    See *ACYL-CoA DEHYDROGENASE DEFICIENCY, MEDIUM CHAIN TYPE*
Ocular albinism
    See *ALBINISM*
    also *ALBINISM, OCULAR, AUTOSOMAL RECESSIVE TYPE*
    also *ALBINISM, OCULAR*

Ocular albinism, Forsius-Eriksson type
See FORSIUS-ERIKSSON SYNDROME
Ocular albinism-sensorineural deafness (OASD)
See ALBINISM, OCULAR-LATE-ONSET-SENSORINEURAL DEAFNESS, X-LINKED
Ocular and facial anomalies-proteinuria-deafness
See FACIO-OCULO-ACOUSTIC-RENAL SYNDROME (FOAR SYNDROME)
Ocular coloboma-imperforate anus-preauricular appendages
See CAT EYE SYNDROME

OCULAR DERMOIDS   0591

Includes:
   Conjunctival dermoid
   Dermoid of the cornea
   Epibulbar dermoid
   Eyelid tumor
   Limbal dermoid

Excludes:
   Eye, dermolipoma (0284)
   Orbital and periorbital dermoid cysts (0761)

Major Diagnostic Criteria: Congenital tumor composed of choristomatous tissues usually located at the limbus.

Clinical Findings: Solid or cystic, whitish mass located at the limbus, or upon the sclera, conjunctiva, or, rarely, the cornea. Usually single lesion involves one eye and remains stationary. Mattos, et al have reported five members of a three generation pedigree with bilateral annular limbal dermoids. Tumors are covered by stratified squamous epithelium with epidermal appendages, and may contain various well differentiated choristomatous tissues such as fat, smooth muscles or skeletal muscles, brain, teeth, cartilage, or bone.

Complications: If tumor encroaches upon cornea it may cause astigmatism, lipid deposits, or obstruct the visual axis. Extension into anterior chamber through a scleral defect may cause glaucoma.

Associated Findings: **Mandibulofacial dysostosis**, Goldenhar syndrome, **Proteus syndrome**, preauricular appendages, **Eyelid, coloboma**, and **Nevus, epidermal nevus syndrome**.

Etiology: Unknown.

Pathogenesis: Unknown.

Sex Ratio: Presumably M1:F1

Occurrence: Undetermined but presumably rare.

Risk of Recurrence for Patient's Sib: Unknown.

Risk of Recurrence for Patient's Child: Unknown.

Age of Detectability: At birth.

Gene Mapping and Linkage: Unknown.

Prevention: None known. Genetic counseling indicated.

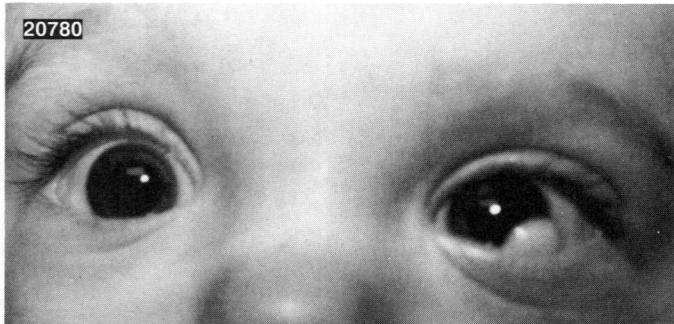

0591A-20780: Ocular dermoid OS.

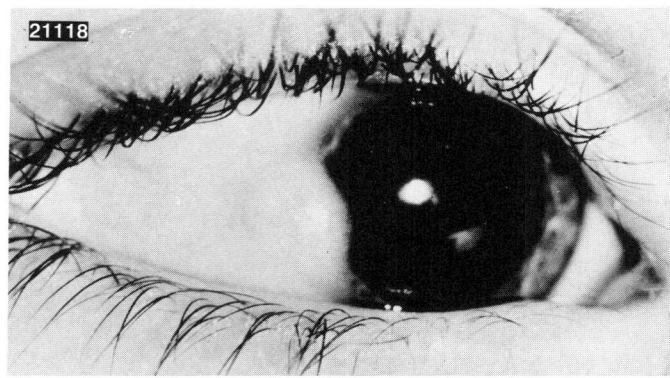

0591B-21118: Dermoid along the inferotemporal limbus.

Treatment: Excision. Caution is necessary during surgical excision since dermoid may be associated with area of thinned sclera (staphyloma).

Prognosis: Benign tumor. Unless dermoid involves cornea, visual function is normal.

Detection of Carrier: Unknown.

References:
Duke-Elder S: System of ophthalmology, vol. 3, Pt 2. Congenital deformities. St. Louis: CV Mosby, 1963:820–826.
Schultze RR: Limbal dermoid tumor with intraocular extension. Arch Ophthalmol 1966; 75:803–805.
Benjamin SJ, Allen HF: Classification for limbal dermoid, choristomatous and branchial arch anomalies. Arch Ophthalmol 1972; 87:305–314.
Hutchinson DS, et al.: Ectopic brain tissue in a limbal dermoid associated with a scleral staphyloma. Am J Ophthalmol 1973; 76:984–986.
Mattos J, et al.: Ring dermoid syndrome. Arch Ophthalmol 1980; 98:1059–1061.

WE035   **Avery H. Weiss**

OCULAR DRUSEN   0734

Includes:
   Colloid bodies, familial
   Doyne honeycombed retinal degeneration
   Drusen, ocular
   Drusen of Bruch membrane
   Hutchinson-Tay choroiditis
   Malattia levantinese

Excludes:
   Drusen secondary to disease of choroid
   Retina, fundus albipunctatus (0399)
   Retina, fundus flavimaculatus (0400)
   Giant drusen of optic disk

Major Diagnostic Criteria: Drusen beginning in the third or fourth decade with no evidence of other choroidal disease. Detection in more than one member of family helps to confirm the diagnosis.

Clinical Findings: The eyegrounds are characterized by deep yellowish lesions usually round or oval in configuration and varying in size from small, dot-like to larger foci about four times the caliber of the first order retinal arterioles. They may have pigment flecks in the center or around their borders, and frequently show secondary changes such as calcification. The lesions are usually of greatest concentration in the posterior polar region. They are frequently present in the periphery and are sometimes widespread over most of the retina. These lesions may become

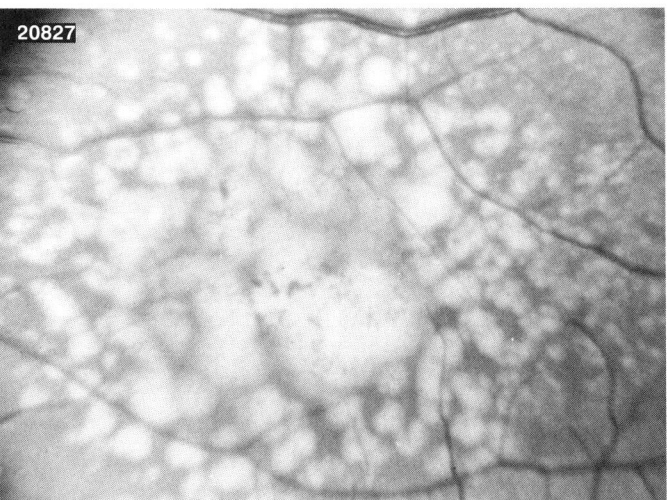

0734-20827: Retina, drusen.

confluent, particularly in or near the macular area into well-defined cloverleaf shapes or multilevel plaques. With fluorescein angiography, the lesions are well defined and overwhelmingly of distinct round shape with little tendency for confluence. These deposits are usually first seen in the third decade or first half of the fourth decade of life.

White or yellowish plaques may be seen in the macula and numerous clusters of drusen elsewhere. Secondary macular degeneration occurs frequently in the last stage. Not all cases follow the typical sequence. There is considerable variation in the ophthalmoscopic appearance even within the same family.

Visual acuity is affected when drusen appear in the fovea. The loss is often moderate with vision maintained at 20/30 to 20/60. However, widespread macular degeneration can occur either with extensive drusen or serous retinal detachment.

Peripheral vision remains good but central scotomas are present when macular degeneration supervenes. Dark adaptation may be mildly abnormal but the ERG is normal. The EOG was initially reported as severely affected but recent data do not support those claims and most patients have a normal EOG.

Complications: Macular degeneration.

Associated Findings: None known.

Etiology: Autosomal dominant inheritance, with occasional reports of autosomal recessive inheritance.

Pathogenesis: These deposits are hyaline excrescences in the cuticular portion of Bruch membrane--numerous discrete, round, fluorescent spots of varying size which far outnumber the drusen seen with the ophthalmoscope and are compatible with a diffuse pigment epithelium alteration. Pigment epithelium changes may be seen even in areas where there are no drusen, suggesting a widespread disturbance of the pigment epithelium in this condition. The drusen probably represent a secretion of the abnormal pigment epithelium.

MIM No.: *12660, 12670

Sex Ratio: M1:F1

Occurrence: More than a dozen kindreds have been well documented since Doyne (1899) first described the condition at the turn of the century, with many of them tracing their history back to the area around Oxford, England, and possibly to a common ancestor.

Risk of Recurrence for Patient's Sib:
  See Part I, *Mendelian Inheritance.*

Risk of Recurrence for Patient's Child:
  See Part I, *Mendelian Inheritance.*

Age of Detectability: Usually between 25–35 years of age.

Gene Mapping and Linkage: Unknown.

Prevention: None known. Genetic counseling indicated.

Treatment: Unknown.

Prognosis: Normal life span with frequent minimal reduction of vision in later life. Occasional moderate to severe reduction of vision.

Detection of Carrier: Clinical examination.

Special Considerations: Drusen may be secondary to numerous diseases of the choroid and are frequently noted in patients over 60 years of age on this basis. Melanoma of the choroid is a frequent cause of secondary drusen in younger patients.

  Retina, fundus flavimaculatus and **Retina, fundus albipunctatus** are both of autosomal recessive inheritance. Fluorescein characteristics particularly distinguish fundus flavimaculatus from drusen. The lesions of fundus albipunctatus are white or yellow-white, uniform, dot-like, discrete and are usually present over most of the fundus with greatest density in the midperiphery. Their size usually corresponds to a 2nd order arteriole. The early lesions of drusen may be confused with the typical lesions of fundus albipunctatus. Drusen, however, are eventually characterized by variability in size, shape, color and a tendency to confluence. The ERG and dark adaptation are always affected in fundus albipunctatus but these tests are normal in drusen.

References:

Doyne RW: A peculiar condition of choroiditis occuring in several members of the same family. Trans Ophthal Soc UK 1899; 19:71 only.

Krill AE, Klein BA: Flecked retina syndrome. Arch Ophthalmol 1965; 74:496–508.

Ernest JT, Krill AE: Fluorescein studies in flavimaculatus and drusen. Am J Ophthalmol 1966; 62:1–6.

Pearce WG: Doyne's honeycomb retinal degeneration: clinical and genetic features. Br J Ophthalmol 1968; 52:73–78.

Deutman AF, Janse LMAA: Dominantly inherited drusen of Bruch's membrane. Brit J Ophthal 1970; 54:373–382.

Fishman GA, et al.: The electrooculogram in diffuse (familial) drusen. Arch Ophthalmol 1971; 92:231–233.

W0003   **Mitchel L. Wolf**

Ocular fibrosis syndrome, congenital
  See EYE, FIBROSIS OF THE EXTRAOCULAR MUSCLES, GENERALIZED
Ocular hypertelorism
  See EYE, HYPERTELORISM
Ocular lens, dislocation of
  See LENS, ECTOPIC
Ocular lymphangioma
  See ORBITAL AND PERIORBITAL LYMPHANGIOMA
Ocular melanocytosis, congenital
  See EYE, MELANOSIS OCULI, CONGENITAL

OCULAR MOTOR APRAXIA, COGAN CONGENITAL TYPE   0191

Includes: Cogan ocular motor apraxia, congenital

Excludes: Ataxia-telangiectasia (0094)

Major Diagnostic Criteria: Failure of normal ocular fixation and head thrusting; retention of normal vertical eye movements. The possibility of blindness should be excluded by normal response on measurement of visual evoked response.

Clinical Findings: Congenital ocular motor apraxia is a defect in the horizontal eye movements involved in voluntary gaze and in the fast phase of both vestibular and optokinetic nystagmus. The pursuit movements are usually normal.

  Compensatory head thrusts on attempting to fixate an object to either side is the most obvious clinical sign. Being unable to initiate the eye movement readily, the infant or child rotates the head toward the object of regard. But, due to the associated defect in initiating the fast phase of the vestibular response, the eyes show a contraversive deviation during the rotation. This head thrust is highly characteristic of the clinical presentation. Also characteristic is the maintained deviation of the eyes when the patient is rotated about a vertical axis.

In contrast to the defect in voluntary eye movement, the patient makes normal random movements of the eyes when not alerted to make a voluntary fixation. Also, contrasting with the defect of horizontal gaze are the normal vertical movements for all parameters of gaze.

The head thrusts are usually noted at 3–4 months of age when the infant begins to hold his head erect. Prior to this, the failure to fixate an object may be misinterpreted as indicating blindness or cerebral palsy. General development is typically normal, but the child tends to be clumsy in sports and to be a poor reader in the first few years of school. The signs and symptoms progressively improve during childhood and are not known to cause any functional deficit in adult life.

Similar head thrusts and defects of the vestibular and optokinetic reflexes are seen with **ataxia telangiectasia** and possibly with other defects of the saccadic system, but, unlike congenital ocular motor apraxia, these involve the vertical as well as the horizontal eye movements.

Complications: Children are reported to be clumsy and are poor readers in the first few years of school.

Associated Findings: A similar ocular motor syndrome occurs frequently in **Gaucher disease** (type III), occasionally in patients with congenital defects of the midbrain, and rarely in infants with tumors of the pontocerebellar region (two cases). Two cases have been reported with brain tumors in the posterior fossa. Several cases have been reported with midline structural defects of the brain or with vermal aplasia of the cerebellum.

Etiology: Autosomal recessive inheritance. Several familial cases have been documented, including one family of apparent dominant transmission, and one occurrence in identical twins. Most cases occur sporadically unaccompanied by other abnormalities.

Pathogenesis: Unknown.

MIM No.: *21650

Sex Ratio: M2:F1

Occurrence: Some fifty cases documented.

Risk of Recurrence for Patient's Sib:
See Part I, *Mendelian Inheritance.*

Risk of Recurrence for Patient's Child:
See Part I, *Mendelian Inheritance.*

Age of Detectability: In infancy.

Gene Mapping and Linkage: Unknown.

Prevention: None known. Genetic counseling indicated.

Treatment: Unknown.

Prognosis: Symptoms progressively improve during the first two decades of life and are not known to cause any functional deficit in the adult.

Detection of Carrier: Unknown.

References:
Cogan DG: A type of congenital ocular motor apraxia presenting jerky head movements. Trans Am Acad Ophthalmol Otolaryngol 1952; 56:853–862.
Vassella F, et al.: Cogan's congenital ocular motor apraxia in two successive generations. Dev Med Child Neurol 1972; 14:788–796.
Zee DS, et al.: Congenital ocular motor apraxia. Brain 1977; 100:581–599.
Cogan DG, et al.: A long-term follow-up of congenital ocular motor apraxia. Neuro-ophthalmol 1980; 1:145–147.
Cogan DG, et al.: Notes on congenital ocular motor apraxia: associated anomalies. In: Glaser J, ed: Neuro-ophthalmology. St. Louis: C.V. Mosby, 1980:171–179.
Zaret CR, et al.: Congenital ocular motor apraxia and brain stem tumor. Arch Ophthalmol 1980; 98:328–330.
Gittinger JW, Sokol S: The visual-evoked potential in the diagnosis of congenital ocular motor apraxia. Am J Ophthalmol 1982; 93:700–703.

C0004

David G. Cogan

Ocular myopathy
See OPHTHALMOPLEGIA, PROGRESSIVE EXTERNAL
Ocular retraction syndrome
See EYE, DUANE RETRACTION SYNDROME
Ocular-scoliotic type Ehlers-Danlos syndrome
See EHLERS-DANLOS SYNDROME
Oculo-acoustic cerebral degeneration, congenital progressive
See NORRIE DISEASE

OCULO-AURICULO-VERTEBRAL ANOMALY 0735

Includes:
Facio-auriculo-vertebral spectrum
First and second branchial arch syndrome
Goldenhar syndrome
Goldenhar-Gorlin syndrome
Hemifacial microsomia

Excludes:
Acrofacial dysostosis, Nager type (2167)
Acrofacial dysostosis, postaxial type (2126)
Anus-hand-ear syndrome (0072)
Branchio-oto-renal dysplasia (2224)
Charge association (2124)

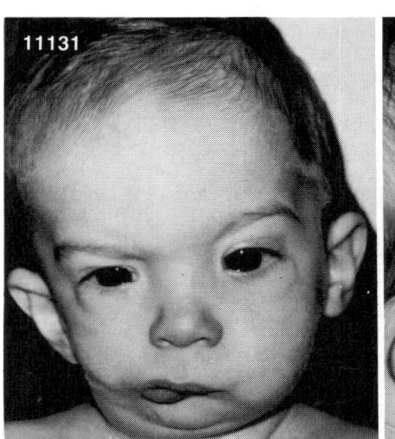
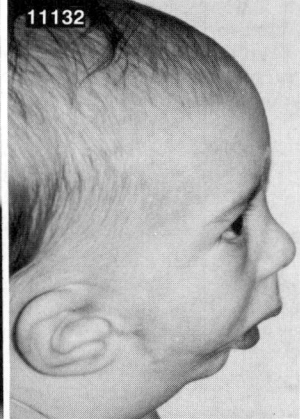
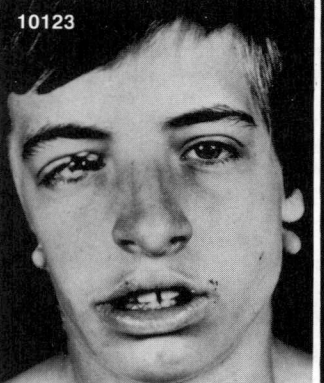
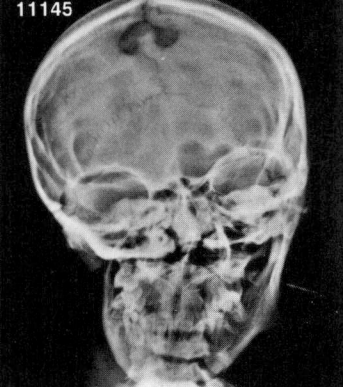

0735-11131–32: Facial asymmetry secondary to hemifacial microsomia. 10123: Coloboma of upper eyelid, abnormal auricles and unilateral facial hypoplasia. 11145: X-ray demonstrates right-sided hypoplasia of the face and right mandible.

Hemifacial atrophy, progressive (2615)
Mandibulofacial dysostosis (0627)
Mandibulo-facial dysostosis, Treacher-Collins type, recessive (2802)
MURCS association (2406)
Oro-facio-digital syndrome
Vater association (0987)

Major Diagnostic Criteria: External ear malformations with associated middle ear anomalies and conductive hearing loss, macrostomia, mandibular hypoplasia, epibulbar dermoids or lipodermoids, and/or anomalies of the cervical spine. X-ray may be required to detect vertebral anomalies and facial asymmetry. Microtia or preauricular tags may represent the most mild expression of the defect in some families.

Clinical Findings: Variability of expression is characteristic of oculo-auriculo-vertebral dysplasia (OAV). Ten to 33% of patients have bilateral facial involvement. The disorder is nearly always more severe on one side. The right side is involved more severely in over 60% of patients. Marked facial asymmetry is present in 20% of patients; some degree of asymmetry is evident in 65%. The asymmetry may not be apparent in the infant or young child but is usually evident by age four years.

The maxillary, temporal, and malar bones on the more severely involved side may be small and flattened. The mandibular ramus and condyle may be hypoplastic or absent. Reduced pneumatization of the mastoid region may be observed.

At least 35% of patients with agenesis of the mandibular ramus have associated macrostomia; i.e., lateral facial cleft, usually of a mild degree. The macrostomia is almost always unilateral and on the more severely affected side. There may be associated agenesis of the parotid gland. Intraorally, the palate and tongue muscles may be unilaterally hypoplastic.

Malformation of the external ear may vary from anotia to a mildly dysmorphic ear. Approximately one-third of cases show bilateral ear involvement. Preauricular tags of skin and cartilage are common and may occur anywhere from the tragus to the angle of the mouth. Preauricular sinuses may be present. Narrow or atretic external auditory canals may be observed. Small auricles with normal architecture may occasionally be seen. Conductive and, less frequently, sensorineural hearing loss occurs in the majority of patients because of hypoplasia or agenesis of ossicles, aberrant facial nerves, and abnormalities of the eustachian tube.

Blepharophimosis, or narrowing of the palpebral fissure, occurs in 10% of patients. Anophthalmia or microphthalmia has been described, as have retinal abnormalities. Epibulbar tumors (dermoids, lipodermoids) are found in 35% of patients; they appear as solid, yellow or pink ovoid masses up to 10mm in diameter. Bilateral lesions may occur. Vision may be impaired.

Cervical vertebral fusions occur in 20–25% of patients, and **Klippel-Feil anomaly** has occasionally been observed. Platybasia and occipitalization of the atlas is found in about 30% of patients.

Complications: Infants may be small for gestational age and may have feeding difficulties because of associated cleft lip and/or cleft palate or an anatomically narrow pharyngeal airway. Obstructive sleep apnea has been described.

Significant visual impairment may be present because of epibulbar tumors or anophthalmia/microphthalmia. Removal of epibulbar tumors can lead to scar formation with resultant leukoma.

Velopharyngeal insufficiency has been reported unassociated with cleft palate.

Associated Findings: Cranial defects consisting of plagiocephaly, microcephaly, skull defects, or intracranial dermoid cysts have been reported. Occipital encephalocele has been noted. Mental retardation occurs in 5–15% of the patients, and those with cranial defects are at higher risk. Unilateral or bilateral cleft lip and/or palate occurs in 7–15% of patients. Cleft palate is twice as common as cleft lip with or without cleft palate. Pulmonary anomalies, ranging in severity from incomplete lobulation to unilateral agenesis, have been reported. A variety of kidney abnormalities have been reported, including absent kidney, double ureter, ectopia, hydronephrosis, and hydroureter.

Congenital heart disease occurs with increased frequency; re-ported incidence figures range from 5 to 58%. Although no single cardiac lesion is characteristic, **Ventricular septal defect** and **Heart, tetralogy of Fallot** appear to be the most common.

A wide variety of skeletal abnormalities have been reported, affecting 30% of patients. Spina bifida, anomalous vertebrae, scoliosis, and anomalous ribs are relatively common. Talipes equinovarus has been reported in 20%. Limb anomalies may affect approximately 10% of patients. Radial limb anomalies may include aplasia of the radius and/or thumb or a bifid or digitalized thumb.

Etiology: There are multiple reports of familial cases, with widely varying expression between affected family members. Patterns of inheritance are consistent with autosomal dominant, autosomal recessive, and multifactorial inheritance. Several aberrant karyotypes have been reported.

Pathogenesis: May be related to abnormal neural crest cell morphology and subsequent malformation of the derivatives of the first and second visceral arches. Vascular abnormalities during embryogenesis have produced branchial arch anomalies in animals. Jongbloet (1987) suggested a theory of "overripeness ovopathy".

MIM No.: 14140, 16421, 25770

POS No.: 3339

CDC No.: 756.060

Sex Ratio: M3:F2

Occurrence: Grabb (1965) observed 1:5,600 births in the Midwest of the United States. Another study recorded 1:26,500 live births in a prospective study of United States newborns. No other population differences have been reported.

Risk of Recurrence for Patient's Sib: Empiric recurrence risk is 2–3%.

Risk of Recurrence for Patient's Child: Unknown.

Age of Detectability: At birth, based on clinical features. Mandibular hypoplasia may be masked by overlying soft tissue, but usually becomes apparent by age four years. Audiologic evaluation at an early age can detect hearing loss. High-resolution ultrasound may be used for prenatal detection of severe ear malformations, mandibular hypoplasia, facial clefts, and other skeletal abnormalities. Prenatal chromosome analysis may be helpful in some instances.

Gene Mapping and Linkage: Unknown.

Prevention: Avoidance of exposure to known teratogens.

Treatment: Detect and manage associated conductive hearing loss early in life. Repair facial clefts by age six months when possible. Speech therapy is often required. Orthodontic and dental care to correct malocclusion and other dental anomalies. Plastic surgery may improve the facial appearance. Surgical gastrostomy may be required for treatment of feeding problem. Other manifestations should be treated appropriately.

Prognosis: Varies with etiology and associated malformations. For those patients with no associated chromosomal anomalies or other severe associated malformations, life span is normal. Five to 15% have reduced intelligence. Some patients may develop emotional problems secondary to their facial defects.

Detection of Carrier: Careful evaluation of first degree relatives will help to identify individuals with mild facial manifestations of the condition and other extracranial anomalies.

Special Considerations: Originally, the term *hemifacial microsomia* was used do denote unilateral microtia, macrostomia, and failure of the formation of mandibular ramus and condyle. *Goldenhar syndrome* referred to a variant characterized by vertebral anomalies, most often hemivertebrae, and epibulbar dermoids. *First arch syndrome* and *First and second branchial arch syndrome* were also used, but implied that involvement was limited to facial structures.

As evidence emerged that each of these individual terms referred to variations within a single phenotypically variable and etiologically heterogeneous condition, which showed a wide range of clinical expression, Gorlin et al (1963) evolved the term *Oculo-auriculo-vertebral dysplasia* to describe the overall condition and its variants. Since forms of the condition may exists without "dysplasia" in the strict sense, the term "anomaly" has been substituted.

Within families, the spectrum of severity may range from severe microtia with significant mandibular involvement, to a unilateral ear tag. X-ray studies may be required to demonstrate a mildly hypoplastic mandible. Because of this wide range of expression, the numbers of alternative diagnoses with overlapping features becomes very extensive.

References:

Gorlin RJ, et al.: Oculoariculovertebral dysplasia. J Pediatr 1963; 63:991–999.

Grabb WC: The first and second branchial arch syndrome. Plast Reconstr Surg 1965; 36:485–508.

Rollnick BR, Kaye CI: Hemifacial microsomia and variants: pedigree data. Am J Med Genet 1983; 15:233–253.

Tenconi R, Hall BD: Hemifacial microsomia: phenotypic classification, clinical implications and genetic aspects. In: Harvold EP, ed: Treatment of hemifacial microsomia. New York: Alan R. Liss, 1983:39–49.

Mansour AM, et al.: Ocular findings in the facioauriculovertebral sequence (Goldenhar-Gorlin syndrome). Am J Ophthalmol 1985; 100:555–559.

Boles DJ, et al.: Goldenhar complex in discordant monozygotic twins: a case report and review of the literature. Am J Med Genet 1987; 28:103–109.

Jongbloet PH: Goldenhar syndrome and overlapping dysplasias, in vitro fertilization and ovopathy. J Med Genet 1987; 24:616–620.

Rollnick BR, et al.: Oculoauriculovertebral dysplasia and variants: phenotypic characteristics of 294 patients. Am J Med Genet 1987; 26:361–375.

Kay ED, Kay CN: Dysmorphogenesis of the mandible, zygoma, and middle ear ossicles in hemifacial microsomia and mandibulofacial dysostosis. Am J Med Genet 1989; 32:27–31.

R0016
KA029

Beverly R. Rollnick
Celia I. Kaye

OCULO-CEREBRO-CUTANEOUS SYNDROME 2752

Includes:

Delleman-Oorthuys syndrome
Orbital cyst-cerebral and focal dermal malformations

Excludes:

Dermal hypoplasia, focal (0281)
Oculo-auriculo-vertebral anomaly (0735)

Major Diagnostic Criteria: Orbital cysts in association with cerebral malformations, skin tags, and focal dermal regions of aplasia or hypoplasia. A computed tomographic scan or magnetic resonance image of the brain may be needed to document central nervous system malformations.

Clinical Findings: Clinical signs are recognized at birth. All patients exhibit orbital cysts, some of which (2/5) may be bilateral. Some of the orbital cysts may be filled with hamartomas containing distorted ocular structures including dysplastic rosettes of retinal neuroepithelium, as well as primitive tissue resembling brain. Other ophthalmic defects include eyelid colobomas (3/5), microphthalmos (4/5), and a persistent hyaloid artery (1/5).

Cerebral defects include multiple porencephalic cysts (4/4) and agenesis of the corpus callosum (3/4) which may been seen on X-ray. Mental retardation (4/5) and seizures (5/5) are common. These abnormalities may be unilateral or bilateral.

Skin tags are found in all infants in the periorbital and preauricular region. Multiple focal aplastic, hypoplastic, or punched-out skin lesions, also found in all children, are concentrated on the head and trunk but may be found anywhere on the body.

Other findings include skull defects and anomalies of the skeletal system, hands, feet, and genitalia. Generalized body asymmetry may occur (3/5) in association with both unilateral and bilateral orbital cysts.

Complications: Unknown.

Associated Findings: None known.

Etiology: Presumably sporadic, or possibly by autosomal dominant inheritance with variable expressivity or the result of an autosomal "dominant" lethal gene surviving by mosaicism (Happle, 1987).

Pathogenesis: The ocular involvement is possibly related to failure of the embryonic optic fissure and related structures to close during early development. There is no explanation for the systemic manifestations of the syndrome.

MIM No.: 16418

POS No.: 3506

Sex Ratio: M3:F2

Occurrence: Five cases have been reported in the literature; four of Dutch ancestry.

Risk of Recurrence for Patient's Sib: Unknown.

Risk of Recurrence for Patient's Child: Unknown.

Age of Detectability: At birth.

Gene Mapping and Linkage: Unknown.

Prevention: None known. Genetic counseling indicated.

Treatment: Surgical removal of the orbital cysts and hamartomas with cosmetic reconstruction is usually necessary. Anticonvulsant medication for seizures. Shunting procedures may be needed for **Hydrocephaly.**

Prognosis: Life span is undetermined. One child died at age two years from cerebral complications.

Detection of Carrier: Unknown.

References:

Delleman JW, et al: Orbital cyst in addition to congenital cerebral and focal dermal malformations: a new entity? Clin Genet 1981; 19:191–198. * †

Delleman JW, et al: Orbital cyst in addition of congenital cerebral and focal dermal malformations: a new entity. Clin Genet 1984; 25:470–472. †

Ferguson JW, et al: Ocular, cerebral, and cutaneous malformations: confirmation of an association. Clin Genet 1984; 25:464–469.

Wilson RD, et al: Oculocerebrocutaneous syndrome. Am J Ophthalmol 1985; 99:142–148. * †

Happle R: Lethal genes surviving by mosaicism: a possible explanation for sporadic birth defects involving the skin. J Am Acad Dermatol 1987; 16:899–906.

ST057
CH037

Gerald G. Striph
Fred C. Chu

OCULO-CEREBRO-FACIAL SYNDROME, KAUFMAN TYPE 2179

Includes:

Cerebro-oculo-facial syndrome
Facial-oculo-cerebro syndrome
Kaufman syndrome

Excludes:

Cerebro-oculo-facio-skeletal syndrome (0140)
Heart-Hand syndrome IV (3272)
Oculo-dento-osseous dysplasia (0737)
Oculo-mandibulo-facial syndrome (0738)

Major Diagnostic Criteria: The concomitant involvement of CNS (mental retardation, **Microcephaly**), eye (e.g., optic atrophy, microcornea), and mandibular arch (micrognathia, preauricular tags) is strongly suggestive of the diagnosis.

Clinical Findings: In three siblings on whom physical examinations were done and two other unrelated cases, the findings included: **Microcephaly** (5); sparse eyebrows (3); upslanting palpebral fissures (5); telecanthus (2); epicanthal folds (2); blepharophimosis or ptosis (2); microcornea (4); nystagmus (2); exotropia (1); amblyopia (1); strabismus (3); myopia (4); flat philtrum (2); highly arched palate (3); poorly formed teeth (4); micrognathia (4); preauricular tags (3); small, lowset ears (1); lordosis (2); large clitoris (1); joint contractures (2); edema of extremities (1); cutis

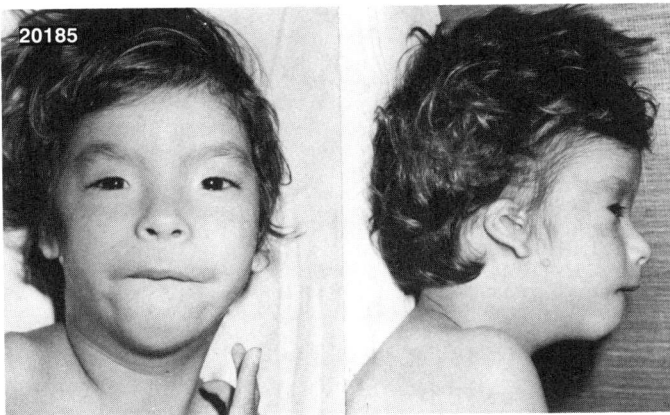

2179-20185: Note long narrow face, sparse eyebrows, mild blepharophimosis, epicanthal folds, telecanthus, large mouth with thin lips, poorly defined philtrum, bilateral skin tags, and micrognathia.

laxa (1); mental retardation (4); decreased muscle tone (3); respiratory difficulties in the newborn period (3); seizures (1); and choreiform movements (2).

Complications: Unknown.

Associated Findings: None known.

Etiology: Autosomal recessive inheritance.

Pathogenesis: Unknown.

MIM No.: *24445

POS No.: 3029

Sex Ratio: M2:F3 (observed in the five reported cases).

Occurrence: Four cases in one North American family of seven siblings, and two sporadic cases, have been reported.

Risk of Recurrence for Patient's Sib:
See Part I, *Mendelian Inheritance.*

Risk of Recurrence for Patient's Child:
See Part I, *Mendelian Inheritance.*

Age of Detectability: At birth, by physical examination.

Gene Mapping and Linkage: Unknown.

Prevention: None known. Genetic counseling indicated.

Treatment: Correction of ocular anomalies may be indicated.

Prognosis: Mental retardation is moderate to severe, lifespan is apparently not affected.

Detection of Carrier: Unknown.

References:
Kaufman RL, et al.: An oculocerebrofacial syndrome. BD:OAS VII(1). New York: March of Dimes Birth Defects Foundation, 1971:135–138.
Jurenka SB, Evans J: Kaufman oculocerebrofacial syndrome: case report. Am J Med Genet 1979; 3:15–19.
Garcia-Cruz D, et al.: Kaufman oculocerebrofacial syndrome: a corroborative report. Dysmorph Clin Genet 1988; 1:152–154.

Helga V. Toriello

OCULO-CEREBRO-RENAL SYNDROME   0736

Includes:
  Cerebro-oculo-renal syndrome
  Lowe syndrome
  Renal-oculo-cerebro syndrome

Excludes:
  Kidney, polycystic disease-cataract-blindness (3288)
  Renal tubular syndrome, Fanconi type (0864)

Major Diagnostic Criteria: Bilateral cataracts at birth, physical and mental retardation, and hypotonia in a male child are the clinical hallmarks. Evidence of renal tubular dysfunction includes some or all of the following: generalized renal hyperaminoaciduria; "tubular" proteinuria (soluble with heat after initial precipitation with 20% sulfosalicylic acid) comprising β-globulins; low T_m glucosuria; high renal clearance of inorganic phosphate with hypophosphatemia; renal tubular acidosis with impaired bicarbonate conservation; defect in H^+ secretion and ammonia production.

Clinical Findings: The complete phenotype is expressed uniformly in males only and is characterized by dense to mature cataracts (100%); glaucoma with or without buphthalmos, corneal scarring, or superficial granulations (50%); enophthalmos; growth failure; mental retardation; hypotonia at birth; reduced or absent deep tendon reflexes; metabolic acidosis; generalized hyperaminoaciduria; and tubular proteinuria after early infancy. Hypophosphatemic rickets appears as a later manifestation in about one-half the untreated patients. Bilateral cryptorchidism is common.

The tubular dysfunction increases in severity with age; its manifestations are thought to be minimal at birth, although only

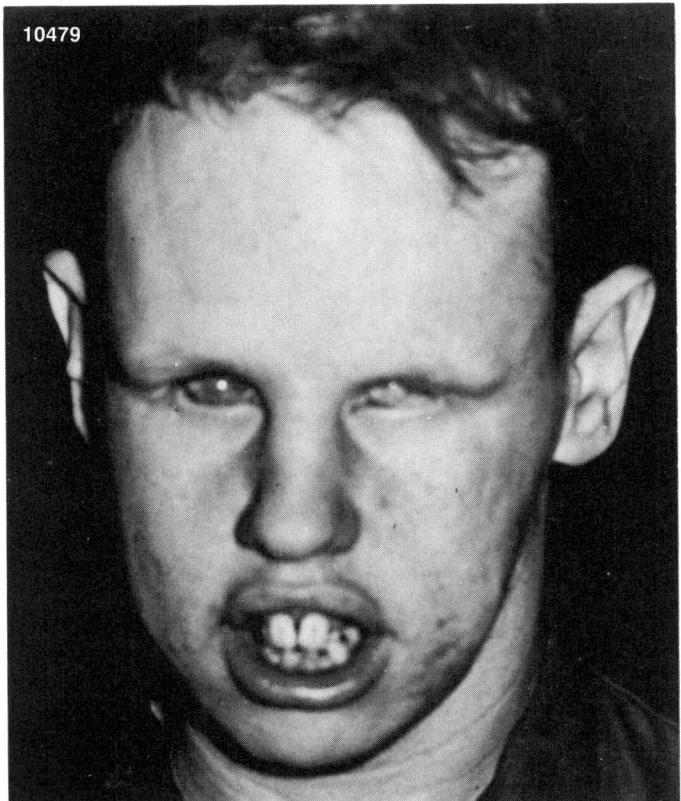

0736-10479: Cataracts, corneal scarring and enophthalmos are present in this 23-year-old mentally retarded male.

a few patients have yet been studied from birth onward. Rickets and/or osteomalacia are secondary to hypophosphatemia. Progresssive glomerular and interstitial fibrosis have been reported.

Histologic examination of eyes reveals warty excrescences and defects of the capsule of microphakic lenses. It has been postulated that the glaucoma is secondary to the small lens pulling on the ciliary body centrally, and thus preventing normal anterior chamber angle cleavage.

Complications: In untreated patients, renal tubular dysfunction appears during early infancy; failure to offset the latter is followed by predictable complications.

Associated Findings: Unknown.

Etiology: X-linked recessive inheritance.

Pathogenesis: It is presumed that all features are related to an undefined derangement of metabolism. The condition is expressed prenatally; a cataract-like lesion has been described in a male fetus (24th week) at risk; patients are born with cataracts. Deficient γ-glutamyl transpeptidase activity is not substantiated.

Reduced sulfation of glycosaminoglycans has been studied in several laboratories anticipating an abnormality in this condition. Recent studies of the synthesis of proteoglycans and glycosaminoglycans revealed marked variation in the rate of synthesis in normal and mutant cultures, but no significant difference in the two phenotypes. The authors (Harper et al, 1987) concluded that Lowe syndrome fibroblasts do not express a defect in sulfation of glycosaminoglycans or in the synthesis of proteoglycans.

MIM No.: *30900

POS No.: 3340

Sex Ratio: M1:F0

Occurrence: Undetermined. Established literature.

Risk of Recurrence for Patient's Sib:
See Part I, *Mendelian Inheritance.*

Risk of Recurrence for Patient's Child:
See Part I, *Mendelian Inheritance.*

Age of Detectability: At birth for cataracts; three to six months for tubular manifestations.

Gene Mapping and Linkage: OCRL (oculocerebrorenal syndrome of Lowe) has been mapped to Xq25-q26.1.

Prevention: None known. Genetic counseling indicated.

Treatment: Early treatment and good clinical home care reduce the phenotypic impact of the mutation; metabolic treatment includes correction of acidosis, hypophosphatemia, and other manifestations of tubulopathy. Care of ocular manifestations as indicated.

Prognosis: Poor for normal lifestyle, development, and longevity. All patients have loss of vision. Without treatment, the majority die in their first decade; a few survive into adolescence or beyond. Life span is increased by early diagnosis and symptomatic treatment.

Detection of Carrier: A study of the correlation between lecticular opacities and DNA haplotypes, using polymorphic markers in the region Xq24-q26, showed that carriers can be detected by slit lamp. Females at risk who have >100 opacities in the equatorial area of *both* lenses can be considered carriers (Wadelius et al., 1989).

Support Groups: IN; West Lafayette; Lowe's Syndrome Association

References:
Abbassi V, et al.: Oculo-cerebro-renal syndrome: a review. Am J Dis Child 1968; 115:145–168.
Witzleben CL, et al.: Progressive morphologic renal changes in the oculo-cerebro-renal syndrome of Lowe. Am J Med 1968; 44:319–324.
Gardner RJM, Brown N: Lowe's syndrome: identification of carriers by lens examination. J Med Genet 1976; 13:449–464.
Manz F, et al.: Renal transport of amino acids in children with oculocerebrorenal syndrome. Helv Paediatr Acta 1978; 33:37–44.
Hodgson SV, et al.: A balanced de novo X/autosome translocation in a girl with manifestations of Lowe syndrome. Am J Med Genet 1986; 23:837–847.
Tripathi R, et al.: Lowe's syndrome. BD:OAS XVIII(6). New York: March of Dimes Birth Defects Foundation, 1986:629–644.
Harper GS, et al.: Proteoglycan synthesis in normal and Lowe syndrome fibroblasts. J Biol Chem 1987; 262:5637–5643.
Wadelius C, et al.: Lowe-oculocerebral syndrome: DNA-based linkage of the gene Xq24-q26 using tightly linked flanking markers and the correlation to lens examination in carrier diagnosis. Am J Hum Genet 1989; 44:241–247.

SC050   **Charles R. Scriver**

Oculo-cervico-acoustic syndrome
See CERVICO-OCULO-ACOUSTIC SYNDROME
Oculo-cranio-somatic neuromuscular disease with ragged-red fibers
See OPHTHALMOPLEGIA, PROGRESSIVE EXTERNAL
Oculo-dento-digital dysplasia
See OCULO-DENTO-OSSEOUS DYSPLASIA

OCULO-DENTO-OSSEOUS DYSPLASIA   0737

Includes:
    Dento-oculo-osseous dysplasia
    Oculo-dento-digital dysplasia
    ODD syndrome
    Osseous-oculo-dento dysplasia

Excludes:
    Acrocephalosyndactyly type III (0229)
    Microcornea
    Oro-cranio-digital syndrome (0769)
    Teeth, amelogenesis imperfecta (0046)

Major Diagnostic Criteria: Characteristic facies, consisting of thin nose, hypoplastic alae and narrow nostrils, microcornea, and syndactyly of the fourth and fifth fingers.

Clinical Findings: Head circumference may be somewhat reduced. Characteristic facies exhibiting thin nose with hypoplastic alae and thin, anteverted nostrils, microcornea, soft tissue syndactyly, and camptodactyly of fourth and fifth fingers (rarely the third); less often second, third, and fourth toes are involved; hypoplasia of enamel and microdontia. The fifth fingers may only exhibit clinodactyly in some patients. There may be associated epicanthal folds, strabismus, short narrow palpebral fissures, and various other eye findings such as secondary glaucoma, persistence of pupillary membranes, and optic atrophy. The iris appears porous, and the frill may overide the pupillary rim. The lip and/or palate are cleft in a few cases. The hair may be dry and lusterless and grows very slowly. Frequent skeletal alterations include thickened mandible, metaphyseal widening of long bones, lack of formation of middle phalanges of toes, and hypoplasia of middle phalanx of fifth fingers.

There may be a less common autosomal recessive form of this condition. Affected patients are more severly affected; marked cranial hyperostosis, massive mandibular overgrowth, gross clavicular widening, blindness, microphthalmia, calcification of basal ganglia, cataracts, cleft lip-palate, spastic quadriplegia, and persistence of primary vitreous have been reported.

Complications: Blindness may result.

Associated Findings: None known.

Etiology: Autosomal dominant inheritance. New mutations represent about one-half of the new cases. Paternal age appears to be a factor in new mutations. Genetic heterogeneity has been suggested.

Pathogenesis: Unknown.

MIM No.: *16420

POS No.: 3341

Sex Ratio: M1:F1

Occurrence: About 85 cases have been documented in the literature.

Risk of Recurrence for Patient's Sib:
See Part I, *Mendelian Inheritance.*

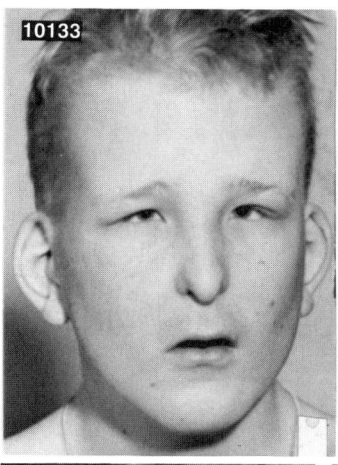
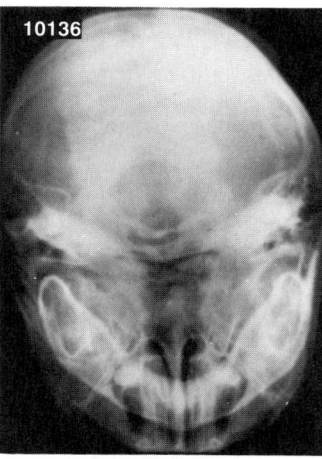
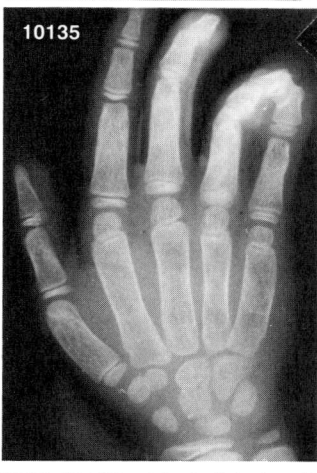
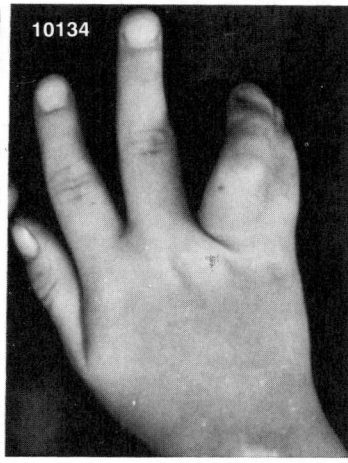

0737-10133: Typical facies characterized by pinched nose, small mouth, and overlapping upper lip. 10136: X-ray shows thickened mandible. 10134–35: Typical 4-5 syndactyly with ulnar deviation of the involved fingers. Note the lack of modeling; tiny, cube-shaped middle phalanges in the involved digits; and terminal bony syndactyly.

Risk of Recurrence for Patient's Child:
See Part I, *Mendelian Inheritance.*

Age of Detectability: At birth.

Gene Mapping and Linkage: Unknown.

Prevention: None known. Genetic counseling indicated.

Treatment: Surgical correction of syndactyly, crowning of teeth.

Prognosis: Good. No reduction in lifespan.

Detection of Carrier: Unknown.

References:
Reisner SH, et al.: Oculodentodigital dysplasia. Am J Dis Child 1969; 118:600–607.
Dudgeon J, Chisolm IA: Oculo-dento-digital dysplasia. Trans Ophthalmol Soc UK 1974; 94:203–210.
Fára M, et al.: Oculodentodigital dysplasia. Acta Clin Plast (Praha) 1977; 19:110–114.
Beighton P, et al.: Oculo-dento-osseous dysplasia: heterogeneity or variable expression? Clin Genet 1979; 16:169–177.
Judisch GF, et al.: Oculodentodigital dysplasia: four new reports and a literature review. Arch Ophthalmol 1979; 97:878–884.
Patton MA, Lawrence KM: Three new cases of oculodentodigital

(ODD) syndrome: development of the facial phenotype. J Med Genet 1985; 22:386–389.

G0038

Robert J. Gorlin

OCULO-ENCEPHALO-HEPATO-RENAL SYNDROME   3242

Includes:
   COACH syndrome
   Hepatic fibrosis-polycystic kidneys-colobomata
   Hunter oculo-encephalo-hepato-renal syndrome
   Thompson-Baraitser syndrome

Excludes:
   Joubert syndrome (2908)
   Meckel syndrome (0634)

Major Diagnostic Criteria: Congenital ataxia with cerebellar vermis hypo/aplasia, coloboma, and hepatic fibrosis.

Clinical Findings: Clinical delineation is based on seven known patients. At birth, coloboma of variable size (6/6), occipital encephalocele (1/7), and postaxial **Polydactyly** (1/7) may be present. Neurologic findings include marked hypotonia (3/4), and tachypnea (4/4) observed since the first weeks, and are related to vermis malformation in 4/4 cases who had CT scan. Ataxia (6/6) and psychomotor retardation (7/7) are obvious before one year of age. Mental retardation (6/6) and some degree of spasticity (3/6) are observed later. Hepatomegaly due to fibrocirrhosis occurs between 1–6 years of age (7/7). Kidney involvement includes small subcapsular or tubular cysts (2/3), interstitial fibrosis (1/3), proximal tubular acidosis, kidney hypoplasia, and slight functional impairment. Dysmorphic features include flat, round facies, **Eye, hypertelorism**, mild ptosis, upturned nose, macrostomia, and small chin, somewhat reminiscent of **Smith-Lemli-Opitz syndrome**.

Complications: Life-threatening esophageal bleeding of infantile onset.

Associated Findings: None known.

Etiology: Autosomal recessive inheritance. The condition has been reported in three pairs of sibs, one with consanguineous parents.

Pathogenesis: Unknown.

Sex Ratio: M1:F1

Occurrence: Seven cases have been reported from Europe and United States.

Risk of Recurrence for Patient's Sib:
See Part I, *Mendelian Inheritance.*

Risk of Recurrence for Patient's Child:
See Part I, *Mendelian Inheritance.*

Age of Detectability: During infancy.

Gene Mapping and Linkage: Unknown.

Prevention: None known. Genetic counseling indicated.

Treatment: Portal shunting may be required during childhood.

Prognosis: Survival beyond age 20 years is likely if portal hypertension is successfully managed.

Detection of Carrier: Unknown.

Special Considerations: The acronym COACH (Cerebellar vermis hypo/aplasia, Oligophrenia, congenital Ataxia, Coloboma, Hepatic fibrocirrhosis) has been proposed.
   Nosology of this syndrome is unclear. Clinical overlap does exist with syndromes such as **Smith-Lemli-Opitz syndrome, type II** and **Meckel syndrome**. The original patients with oculo-encephalo-hepato-renal syndrome (Hunter et al. 1974; Thompson et al. 1986) had slight differences (spasticity, lack of renal fibrosis) from the three children reported by Verloes & Lambotte (1989).

References:
Hunter AGW, et al.: Hepatic fibrosis, polycystic kydneys, colobomata and encephalopathy in siblings. Clin Genet 1974; 6:82–89.
Thompson E, Baraitser M: An autosomal recessive mental retardation syndrome. Am J Med Genet 1986; 24:151–158.

Verloes A, Lambotte C: Further delineation of a syndrome of cerebellar vermis hypo/aplasia, oligophrenia, congenital ataxia, coloboma and hepatic fibrosis. Am J Med Genet 1989; 32:227–232.

VE010   **A. Verloes**

OCULO-FACIAL SYNDROME, BENCZE TYPE   2364

Includes:
> Bencze syndrome
> Facial-oculo syndrome
> Hemifacial hyperplasia with strabismus (HFH)

Excludes:
> **Hemifacial atrophy, progressive** (2615)
> **Hemihypertrophy** (0458)
> **Oculo-auriculo-vertebral anomaly** (0735)

Major Diagnostic Criteria: Facial asymmetry, esotropia, and amblyopia with normal intelligence.

Clinical Findings: The most consistent finding is facial asymmetry, affecting soft tissue and bone, but not the eyeball. Teeth are often larger on the larger half of the face, although there is no evidence that they erupt sooner than those on the smaller half. Esotropia is a common finding; often, but not always, it affects the eye on the smaller side of the face. The palpebral fissure of the smaller side is often upslanting and narrow. Submucous cleft palate occurred in one-half of the members of one reported family. Intellectual development appears normal.

Complications: If strabismus is untreated, amblyopia may result. Malocclusion is a common complication of the asymmetry.

Associated Findings: One affected male had growth deficiency, mild mental retardation, primary telecanthus, mild thoracolumbar scoliosis, and hyperextensible knees; these were thought to be unrelated to the primary defect.

Etiology: Autosomal dominant inheritance.

Pathogenesis: Unknown.

MIM No.: *14135

POS No.: 3492

Sex Ratio: M1:F1

Occurrence: Two kinships have been reported.

Risk of Recurrence for Patient's Sib:
> See Part I, *Mendelian Inheritance.*

Risk of Recurrence for Patient's Child:
> See Part I, *Mendelian Inheritance.*

Age of Detectability: In early childhood.

Gene Mapping and Linkage: Unknown.

Prevention: None known. Genetic counseling indicated.

Treatment: Orthodontic and/or dental treatment may be indicated. Correction of strabismus is also indicated.

Prognosis: Life span and intelligence are normal.

Detection of Carrier: Unknown.

References:
Bencze J, et al.: Dominant inheritance of hemifacial hyperplasia associated with strabismus. Oral Surg 1973; 35:489–501.
Kurnit D, et al.: An autosomal dominantly inherited syndrome of facial asymmetry, esotropia, amblyopia, and submucous cleft palate (Bencze syndrome). Clin Genet 1979; 16:301–304. * †

T0007   **Helga V. Toriello**

Oculo-mandibulo dyscephaly
See OCULO-MANDIBULO-FACIAL SYNDROME

OCULO-MANDIBULO-FACIAL SYNDROME   0738

Includes:
> Dyscephaly with congenital cataract and hypotrichosis
> Facial-oculo-mandibulo syndrome
> Francois dyscephalic syndrome
> Hallermann-Streiff syndrome
> Mandibulo-facial-oculo syndrome
> Oculo-mandibulo dyscephaly

Excludes:
> **Chondroectodermal dysplasia** (0156)
> **Cleidocranial dysplasia** (0185)
> **Dermo-chondro-corneal dystrophy, Francois type** (0282)
> **Mandibulofacial dysostosis** (0627)
> **Oculo-dento-osseous dysplasia** (0737)
> **Progeria** (0825)
> **Pyknodysostosis** (0846)
> **Seckel syndrome** (0881)

Major Diagnostic Criteria: Proportionate dwarfism, normal mentation, congenital cataracts, microphthalmia, dyscephaly with mandibular and nasal cartilage hypoplasia, hypotrichosis, cutaneous atrophy limited to scalp and nose, and dental anomalies.

Clinical Findings: Dyscephaly is the most constant feature. Brachycephaly, microcephaly, frontal bossing, and disproportionately small face with a narrow nose are common features. Parietal and occipital bossing may be present. The rami of the mandible are hypoplastic, with their condylar heads being displaced anteriorly.

Dental anomalies, hypotrichosis, and cataracts are constant features. There may be natal teeth, hypodontia, malformed teeth, enamel dysplasia, or malocclusion. Other intraoral features include abnormally high palatal vault, microglossia or macroglossia, glossoptosis, and microstomia. The hypotrichosis is most common and most pronounced over the scalp, but also involves the eyelashes and eyebrows, beard, and axillary and public hair. Cataracts are always bilateral and complete. Micropthalmia is commonly reported. Other ocular defects include nystagmus, strabismus, blue sclerae, and in descending order of frequency, various defects of the fundus, conjunctiva, cornea, and iris.

Atrophy of the facial skin is common. The skin over the nose is thin, dry, smooth, and covered by telangiectasias. Other reported skin defects include vitiligo, nevi, and ichthyosis.

Feeding and respiratory difficulties are common during infancy, and can be fatal. Visual acuity is frequently decreased. Mentation is usually within normal limits.

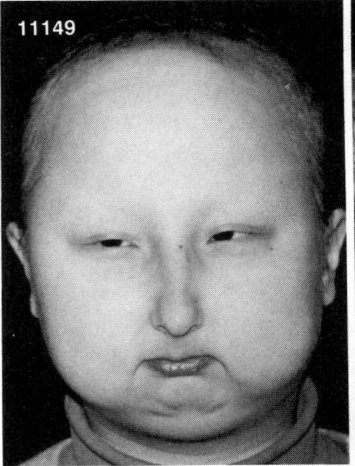 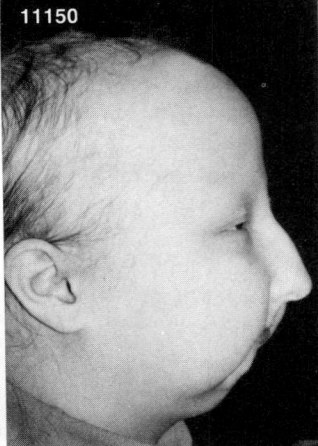

0738-11149–50: Hypotrichosis, narrow, beaked nose; small mandible and microphthalmia.

Complications: Vitiligo, respiratory and feeding difficulties in infancy, blindness, psychological disturbances, and deafness.

Associated Findings: A few instances of death in childhood from pulmonary infection have been recorded.

Etiology: The mode of transmission is unclear. Although most cases reported are sporadic, an equal sex ratio of affected persons, parental consanguinity (7% of cases), and several pairs of affected sibs suggest autosomal recessive inheritance. However, at least three multigenerational families, one with male-to-male transmission, have been reported.

Pathogenesis: Undetermined. Developmental defect early in embryonic life (perhaps as early as the fifth week). A defect of elastin has been reported, and glycoprotein metabolism has been suggested to be abnormal.

MIM No.: 23410

POS No.: 3342

CDC No.: 756.046

Sex Ratio: M1:F1

Occurrence: More than 150 cases reported.

Risk of Recurrence for Patient's Sib:
See Part I, *Mendelian Inheritance.*

Risk of Recurrence for Patient's Child:
See Part I, *Mendelian Inheritance.* Reproductive fitness is greatly reduced.

Age of Detectability: Within first year of life.

Gene Mapping and Linkage: Unknown.

Prevention: None known. Genetic counseling indicated.

Treatment: Tracheostomy in cases of severe respiratory distress.

Prognosis: Average life span is undetermined.

Detection of Carrier: Unknown.

References:
Franqis J: A new syndrome: dyscephalia with bird face and dental anomalies, nanism, hypotrichosis, cutaneous atrophy, microphthalmia, and congenital cataract. Arch Ophthalmol 1958; 60:842–862. *
Steele RW, Bass JW: Hallermann-Streiff syndrome: clinical and prognostic considerations. Am J Dis Child 1970; 120:462–465. * †
Imamura S, et al.: Hallermann-Streiff syndrome. Dermatologica 1980; 160:354–357.
Franqis J: Francois' dyscephalic syndrome. Birth Defects 1982; 18:595–619. *
Slootweg PJ, Huber J: Dento-alveolar abnormalities in oculomandibulodyscephaly (Hallermann-Streiff syndrome). J Oral Path 1984; 13:147–154. *

J0027   **Ronald J. Jorgenson**

OCULO-OSTEO-CUTANEOUS SYNDROME, TOUMAALA-HAAPANEN TYPE   2078

Includes:
Anodontia-hypotrichosis syndrome
Brachymetapody-anodontia-hypotrichosis-albinoidism
Toumaala-Haapanen syndrome

Excludes:
Brachydactyly (0114)
Ectodermal dysplasia, hidrotic (0334)
Parathormone resistance (0830)

Major Diagnostic Criteria: A combination of ocular, cutaneous and skeletal anomalies should be present to suspect the diagnosis. Ocular anomalies include convergent strabismus, myopia, nystagmus, lenticular opacities, foveal hypoplasia. Cutaneous anomalies include scanty hair and hypopigmentation. Skeletal anomalies include short stature, small maxilla and short metacarpals and metatarsals (3–5). Congenital edentia is also a consistent finding.

Clinical Findings: In three reported cases, short stature (3); light, relatively inelastic skin (3); hypotrichosis (3); short skull A-P diameter (3); antimongoloid slant of the palpebral fissures (3); hypoplastic tarsus (3); strabismus (3); nystagmus (3); lenticular opacities (3); foveal hypoplasia (3); high myopia (3); distichiasis (3); small maxilla (3); edentia (3); prominent mandible (3); hypoplastic genitalia (2); short fingers and toes (especially 3–5) (3); normal great toes and thumbs (3); congenital palmar hyperkeratosis (1).

Complications: Poor vision and possible blindness were the only complications noticed.

Associated Findings: None known.

Etiology: Possibly autosomal recessive inheritance.

Pathogenesis: Unknown. Although several findings are consistent with an ectodermal dysplasia, others are more likely attributable to a mesodermal defect. Skin biopsies were normal.

MIM No.: 21137

POS No.: 3044

Sex Ratio: M1:F2 (in the three observed siblings).

Occurrence: One family from northeast Finland has been documented.

Risk of Recurrence for Patient's Sib:
See Part I, *Mendelian Inheritance.*

Risk of Recurrence for Patient's Child:
See Part I, *Mendelian Inheritance.*

Age of Detectability: At birth, by physical examination.

Gene Mapping and Linkage: Unknown.

Prevention: None known. Genetic counseling indicated.

Treatment: Correction of vision problems, as indicated.

Prognosis: Life span is apparently normal; one affected individual was described as intellectually normal. Nothing is known about the intelligence of the other two affected individuals.

Detection of Carrier: Unknown.

References:
Tuomaala P, Haapanen E: Three siblings with similar anomalies in the eyes, bones and skin. Acta Ophthalmol 1968; 46:365–371.

T0007   **Helga V. Toriello**

OCULO-OTO-NASAL MALFORMATIONS WITH OSTEO-ONYCHO DYSPLASIA   2188

Includes: Osteo-onycho dysplasia and oculo-oto-nasal defects

Excludes: **Oculo-cerebro-facial syndrome, Kaufman type** (2179)

Major Diagnostic Criteria: Ptosis, prominent midface, large ears, large penis, dystrophic nails, large first and second toes.

Clinical Findings: Facial findings include ptosis, absence of medial eyebrows and eyelashes, hypertelorism, prominent midface, and receding chin. The ears are large, low-set, and have simply formed pinnae. The penis is large, with hypospadias. The nails are dystrophic with longitudinal ridges. Some are partially absent. The first and second toes are broad and large. X-rays show enlargement of the lateral part of the clavicle, resorption of some of the tufts of the terminal phalanges, broadened epiphyses of long bones, poorly formed acetabulum, and synostoses of the tarsals and metacarpals.

Complications: Unknown.

Associated Findings: None known.

Etiology: Possibly autosomal recessive inheritance.

Pathogenesis: Unknown.

Sex Ratio: The only reported case was male.

Occurrence: One case has been reported.

Risk of Recurrence for Patient's Sib: Unknown.

Risk of Recurrence for Patient's Child: Probably negligible.

Age of Detectability: At birth.

Gene Mapping and Linkage: Unknown.

Prevention: None known. Genetic counseling indicated.

Treatment: Unknown.

Prognosis: Unknown.

Detection of Carrier: Unknown.

References:
Leiba S, et al.: Oculootonasal malformations associated with osteoony-chodysplasia. BD:OAS XI(2). New York: March of Dimes Birth Defects Foundation, 1975:67–73.

TH017
UR001

T.F. Thurmon
S.A. Ursin

Oculo-oto-radial syndrome
  See IVIC SYNDROME
Oculo-palatal-cerebral dwarfism
  See DWARFISM, OCULO-PALATO-CEREBRAL TYPE

OCULO-RENO-CEREBELLAR SYNDROME   3050

Includes:
  Cerebellar-oculo-renal syndrome
  Renal-oculo-cerebellar syndrome

Excludes:
  Cerebellar granular layer, isolated absence of
  Oculo-cerebro-renal syndrome (0736)
  Nephritis
  Nephronophthisis, juvenile
  Retinopathy-hypotrichosis syndrome (2627)

Major Diagnostic Criteria: A progressive condition that leads to early dementia and choreoathetosis, accompanied by tapetoretinal degeneration, spastic diplegia, and a glomerulopathy. A single autopsied case had absence of the cerebellar granular layer.

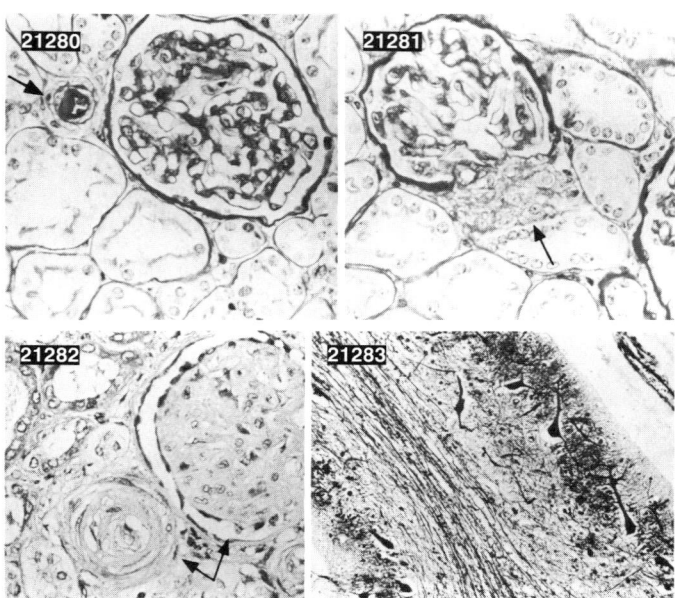

3050B-21280: Section from renal biopsy showing glomerulus in deep cortex with mild thickening of the basement membrane and PAS-positive material in an adjacent arteriole. **21281:** Juxtaglomerular prominence seen in renal biopsy section. **21282:** Completely sclerosed glomerulus and "onion skin" appearance in the adjacent arteriole. **21283:** Silver-stain preparation from cerebellum showing lack of granular layer, disorganization of the Purkinje cells; and normal orientation of underlying axons.

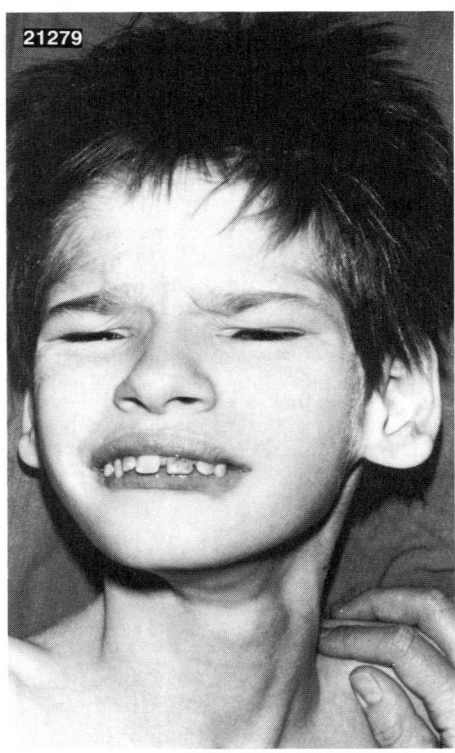

3050A-21279: Note large mouth and prominent ears; in profile the nose has a "ski-jump" shape.

Clinical Findings: By history, affected children had some very early development, but quickly (within 1–3 months) deteriorated to become profoundly demented. Choreoathetoid movement was an early sign, later accompanied by spastic diplegia, but with continued joint hyperextensibility. Death occurred within the first two decades from renal failure, which was due to a progressive glomerulopathy, with pathologic findings similar to segmental or focal hyalinosis. A severe progressive tapetoretinal degeneration was accompanied by dramatic hypoplasia of the retinal vasculature, which reached the point where retinal vessels were no longer clinically visible. There was hypoplasia of the cerebellum, which on light microscopy showed absence of granular cells in the internal granular layer, a reduced thickness of the molecular layer, and disoriented, displaced Purkinje cells with infrequent axons and occasional asteroid bodies.

Proteinuria was an early sign of the renal impairment, and the typical renal pathology of focal/segmental hyalinosis was seen in biopsy material. Periglomerular asteroids often contained a thick, PAS-positive basement membrane or hyaline deposits. Presumably imaging techniques now available would demonstrate the cerebellar hypoplasia.

Complications: Profound retardation, progressive visual impairment and blindness, progressive renal failure, and death.

Associated Findings: **Microcephaly**, strabismus, and cataracts were variable features. An unusual facial appearance that differed from other family members may simply have reflected poor muscle bulk and tone.

Etiology: Autosomal recessive inheritance.

Pathogenesis: Unknown. Some signs could result from progressive small vessel disease, as seen in the kidney and eye.

MIM No.: *25797

POS No.: 3995

Sex Ratio: M1:F1; M3:F2 observed.

Occurrence: Five members of one Mennonite family from Manitoba, Canada, have been reported.

Risk of Recurrence for Patient's Sib:

See Part I, *Mendelian Inheritance.*

Risk of Recurrence for Patient's Child:

See Part I, *Mendelian Inheritance.* Affected individuals are not expected to survive to reproduce.

Age of Detectability: Signs of delay are apparent within the first few months. The earliest age of appearance of renal and visual signs is unknown but is within the first decade (one child died at age seven years), and cerebellar pathology is probably also early (possibly during infancy).

Gene Mapping and Linkage: Unknown.

Prevention: None known. Genetic counseling indicated.

Treatment: Supportive care for child and family.

Prognosis: Profound dementia and early death from renal disease.

Detection of Carrier: Unknown.

References:

Hunter AGW, et al.: Absence of the cerebellar granular layer, mental retardation, tapetoretinal degeneration, and progressive glomerulopathy: an autosomal recessive oculo-renal-cerebellar syndrome. Am J Med Genet 1982; 11:383–395.

HU008   **Alasdair G.W. Hunter**

Oculocerebral syndrome with hypopigmentation
*See GINGIVAL FIBROMATOSIS-DEPIGMENTATION-
    MICROPHTHALMIA*
Oculocraniodental syndrome
See ACROCEPHALOSYNDACTYLY TYPE III
Oculocraniosomatic neuromuscular disease
See KEARNS-SAYRE DISEASE
Oculocraniosomatic syndrome
See OPHTHALMOPLEGIA, PROGRESSIVE EXTERNAL
Oculocutaneous albinism
See ALBINISM
Oculocutaneous albinoidism
See ALBINOIDISM
Oculocutaneous melanosis
See NEVUS OF OTA
Oculocutaneous pigmentation syndrome
See NEVUS OF OTA
Oculocutaneous tyrosinemia or tyrosinosis
See TYROSINEMIA II, OREGON TYPE
Oculodermal melanocytosis
See NEVUS OF OTA
Oculogastrointestinal muscular dystrophy
See MUSCULAR DYSTROPHY, OCULO-GASTROINTESTINAL
Oculoleptomeningeal type amyloidosis
See AMYLOIDOSIS, OHIO TYPE
Oculomotor apraxia-contractures-muscle atrophy
See CONTRACTURES-MUSCLE ATROPHY-OCULOMOTOR APRAXIA
Oculopharyngeal muscular dystrophy
See MUSCULAR DYSTROPHY, OCULOPHARYNGEAL
Oculopharyngeal myopathy
See MUSCULAR DYSTROPHY, OCULOPHARYNGEAL
Oculopupillary syndrome
See HORNER SYNDROME
Oculosympathetic syndrome
See HORNER SYNDROME
ODD syndrome
See OCULO-DENTO-OSSEOUS DYSPLASIA

ODONTO-ONYCHODERMAL DYSPLASIA   **2618**

Includes: Ectodermal dysplasia, odonto-onychodermal dysplasia type

Excludes: **Odonto-onychodysplasia-alopecia** (2890)

Major Diagnostic Criteria: Erythema, atrophy, and scalings on cheeks, nose, upper lip, chin, and forehead. Diffuse erythema and mild-to-moderate hyperkeratosis, fissuring, and hyperhidrosis of palms and soles. Dry and sometimes sparse scalp hair. Abnormal and missing teeth. Peg-shaped or conical maxillary central incisors. Thickening of toenails.

Clinical Findings: The disease is apparent early in childhood. There are ill-defined patches of erythema, atrophy, and scaliness on cheeks, nose, upper lip, and, to a lesser extent, on the chin and forehead. Cherry-red spots and telangiectases can be seen over the cheeks and nose. The skin is generally dry and scaly. Scalp hair is dry and may be sparse. The palms have diffuse erythema with mild-to-moderate hyperkeratosis and fissuring. The soles are similarly affected, but to a lesser extent. In addition, there is hyperhidrosis of the palms and soles and thickening of the nails of the big toes. The nipples and areolae are normal.

Oral examination may reveal a class I occlusion with severe overbite. Panorex film of the teeth may show peg-shaped or conical maxillary central incisors with a large diastema. The deciduous teeth have a marked erosion of their occlusal surfaces.

The X-ray survey of the axial skeleton shows no abnormalities. In particular, there is no fusion of the metacarpals and no evidence of **Polydactyly.**

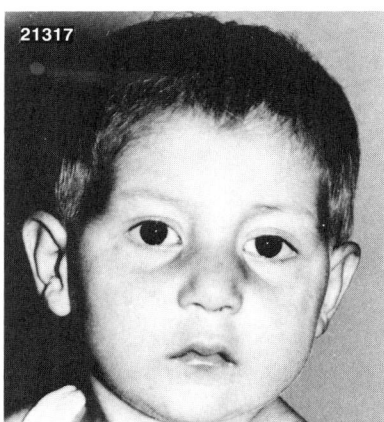

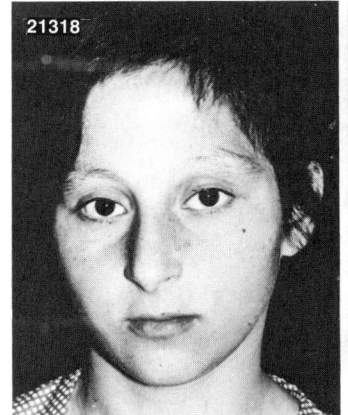 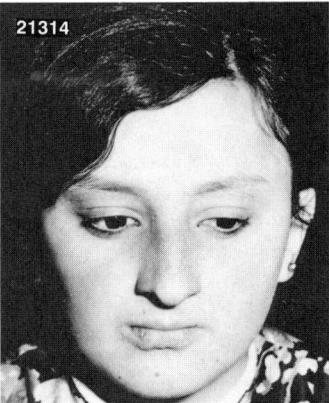

2618A-21317, 18, 14: Note facial erythema, sparse hair and eyebrows.

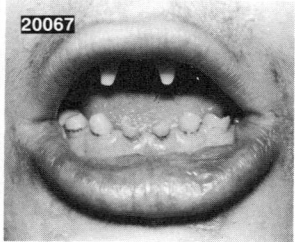

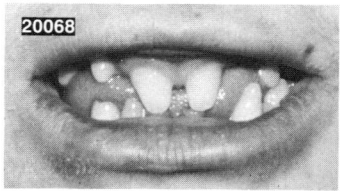

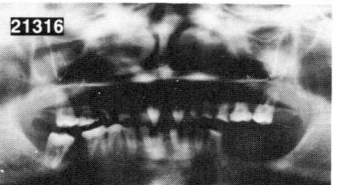

2618B-20066–68: Note the range of dental defects. 21316:
Panorex film of hypoplastic teeth.

The audiogram documents normal hearing.

Biopsy from the skin of the face may demonstrate basket-weave hyperkeratosis and spotty parakeratosis, irregular acanthosis alternating with atrophy, and effacement of the rete ridges. The basal cell layer is preserved. The dermis may show basophilic degeneration, compatible with solar-elastosis, and dilated blood

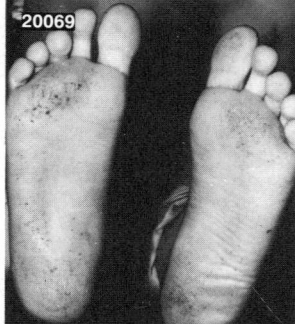

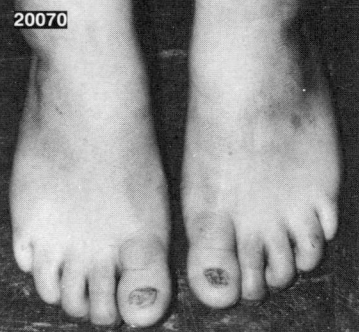

2618C-21323: Note the moderate hyperkeratosis and fissuring of the palms. 20069: Hyperkeratosis and fissuring of the soles. 20070: Irregular and thickened first toenails.

vessels. The sebaceous glands may be decreased in size and number, and the eccrine glands appear normal.

Biopsy from the sole shows hyperkeratosis, irregular hypergranulosis, and mild acanthosis in the epidermis. The dermis is unremarkable.

Complications: The abormalities of the teeth interfere with a comfortable chewing process.

Associated Findings: Recurrent ear discharges.

Etiology: Probably autosomal recessive inheritance. Parents of the affected individuals (five males and two females) are normal and first cousins, and the segregation ratio in the reported families is 7:24 (close to 0.25).

Pathogenesis: Freire-Maia (1971, 1977) suggested that in order to classify disorders as ectodermal dysplasias, they should have at least two of the following disturbances: 1) trichodysplasia, 2) dental defects, 3) onychodysplasia, and 4) dyshidrosis (group A) or at least one of the above plus at least one other ectodermal defect (group B). Odonto-onychodermal dysplasia belongs to the 1–2–3–4 subgroup of group A. Solomon and Keuer (1980) have reserved the term *ectodermal dysplasia* for conditions that 1) are congenital; 2) have diffuse involvement of the epidermis, and at least one of the following: hair, sebaceous glands, eccrine glands, nail, mucosa, or teeth; and 3) are not progressive. Odonto-onychodermal dysplasia is also an ectodermal dysplasia according to these criteria.

MIM No.: 25798

POS No.: 3609

Sex Ratio: M5:F2 (observed).

Occurrence: Seven cases from two Lebanese Moslem Shiite families have been observed.

Risk of Recurrence for Patient's Sib:
See Part I, *Mendelian Inheritance.*

Risk of Recurrence for Patient's Child:
See Part I, *Mendelian Inheritance.*

Age of Detectability: Usually clinically diagnosable by age 1.5 years, when the abnormalities of the teeth become evident.

Gene Mapping and Linkage: Unknown.

Prevention: None known. Genetic counseling indicated.

Treatment: Symptomatic care for the skin lesions and orthodontic treatment.

Prognosis: Normal life span.

Detection of Carrier: Unknown.

References:
Freire-Maia N: Ectodermal dysplasias. Hum Hered 1971; 21:309–312.
Freire-Maia N: Ectodermal dysplasias revisited. Acta Genet Med Gemellol 1977; 26:121–131.
Solomon LM, Keuer EJ: The ectodermal dysplasias: problems of classification and some newer syndromes. Arch Dermatol 1980; 116:1295–1299.
Pinheiro M, et al.: A previously undescribed condition, tricho-odonto-onycho-dermal syndrome: a review of the tricho-odonto-onychial subgroup of ectodermal dysplasias. Br J Dermatol 1981; 105:371–382.
Fadhil M, et al.: Odonto-onychodermal dysplasia: a previously apparently undescribed ectodermal dysplasia. Am J Med Genet 1983; 14:335–346.

DE030   **Vazken M. Der Kaloustian**

ODONTO-ONYCHODYSPLASIA-ALOPECIA   2890

Includes:
    Alopecia-odonto-onychodysplasia
    Ectodermal dysplasia, odonto-onychodysplasia-alopecia
       type

Excludes:
    Ectodermal dysplasia, Christ-Siemens-Touraine type (0333)
    Ectodermal dysplasia, hidrotic (0334)
    Odonto-onychodermal dysplasia (2618)
    Tricho-dermodysplasia-dental defects (2903)
    Tricho-odonto-onychial dysplasia (2889)

Major Diagnostic Criteria: Trichodysplasia, dental anomalies, and onychodysplasia.

Clinical Findings: Almost total alopecia; sparse, thin, brittle, and slow-growing hair at the occipital and temporal regions; scanty

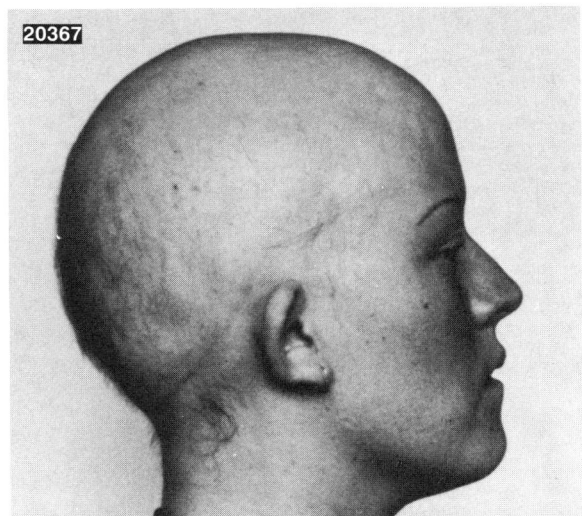

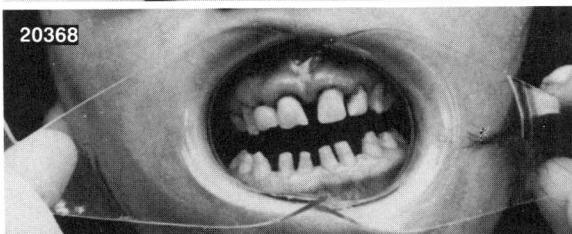

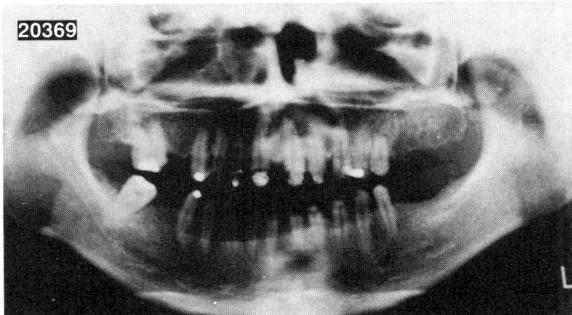

2890-20367: Odonto-onychodysplasia-alopecia; note anteverted auricles, absent eyebrows that are pencilled in, and alopecia with sparse hair at the base of the skull. **20368:** The apparently normal upper incisors are capped. **20369:** Orthopantomogram showing dental alterations.

eyebrows and lashes; absent axillary and pubic hair; hypodontia of both dentitions; enamel hypoplasia; microdontia; widely spaced and abnormally shaped teeth; dystrophic finger- and toenails with subungual corneal layer; sparse café-au-lait spots; irregular outlines of areolae; hypertrophied Montgomery glands; extranumerary nipples; palmoplantar keratosis; toe syndactyly; flat feet; anteverted auricles; recurrent atrophic rhinitis and external otitis; cysts of both ovaries; uterine fibroma; uterine retroversion; unilateral deviation of the lacrimal duct; dermatoglyphic changes; transpalmar creases.

Complications: Psychologic problems due to hair and dental alterations.

Associated Findings: None known.

Etiology: Probably autosomal recessive inheritance. Parental consanguinity is probable.

Pathogenesis: Defective formation of several derivatives of the embryonic ectoderm suggests that this condition must be classified as an ectodermal dysplasia.

Sex Ratio: Presumably M1:F1; M0:F2 observed.

Occurrence: Reported in two Caucasian Brazilian sisters; the only children of a probably consanguineous, normal couple.

Risk of Recurrence for Patient's Sib:
    See Part I, *Mendelian Inheritance.*

Risk of Recurrence for Patient's Child:
    See Part I, *Mendelian Inheritance.*

Age of Detectability: During childhood, by physical examination.

Gene Mapping and Linkage: Unknown.

Prevention: None known. Genetic counseling indicated.

Treatment: Prosthetic replacement and orthodontic treatment; wigs are cosmetically and psychologically helpful; surgery for uterine fibroma.

Prognosis: Normal for life span.

Detection of Carrier: Unknown.

References:
Pinheiro M, et al.: Odontoonychodysplasia with alopecia: a new pure ectodermal dysplasia with probable autosomal recessive inheritance. Am J Med Genet 1985; 20:197–202.

PI008   **Marta Pinheiro**

Odonto-onychohypohidrotic dysplasia with midline scalp defect
    See ECTODERMAL DYSPLASIA-ADRENAL CYST
Odonto-trichomelic hypohidrotic dysplasia
    See ODONTO-TRICHOMELIC SYNDROME

ODONTO-TRICHOMELIC SYNDROME   2887

Includes:
    Cleft lip-tetramelia-deformed ears-ectodermal dysplasia
    Ectodermal dysplasia, tetramelic
    Freire-Maia syndrome
    Odonto-trichomelic hypohidrotic dysplasia
    Tetramelic deficiencies-ectodermal dysplasia-deformed ears

Excludes: Ectrodactyly-ectodermal dysplasia-clefting syndrome (0337)

Major Diagnostic Criteria: Extensive tetramelic deficiencies, severe hypotrichosis, abnormal dentition, and deformed auricles.

Clinical Findings: Extensive deficiencies of the four limbs associated with dermatoglyphic abnormalities; hypotrichosis; small, conical, and widely spaced teeth; persistence of deciduous teeth; hypodontia; large, thin, protruding, and deformed auricles; hypoplastic areolae and nipples; thin, dry, and shiny skin; abnormalities of tyrosine and/or tryptophane metabolism; growth retardation; cleft lip; and EEG and EKG abnormalities.

Complications: Unknown.

Associated Findings: Hypoplastic nails.

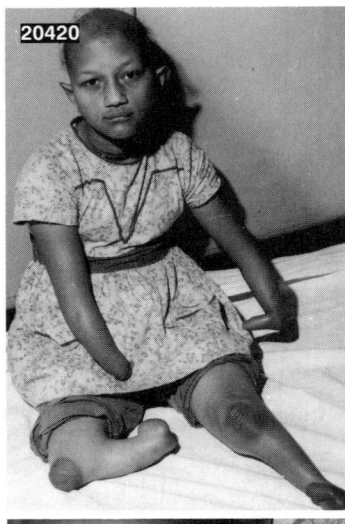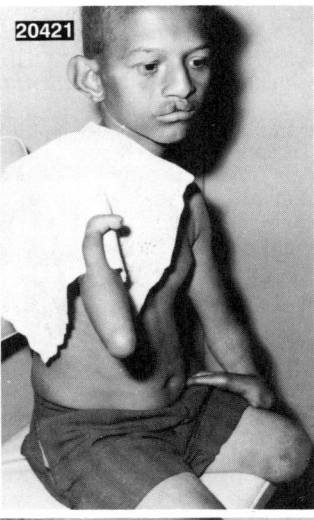
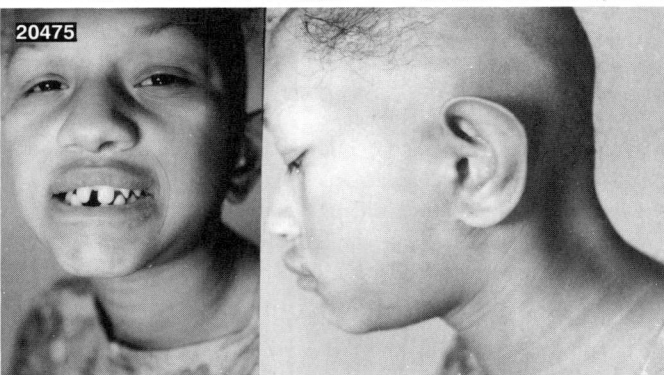

2887-20420: Affected girl at age 12 years; note hypotrichosis, abnormal auricles, and extensive tetramelic reductions. 20421: Affected boy at age 14 years, note hypotrichosis, abnormal auricle, incomplete left cleft lip and extensive tetramelic reductions. The reduction deformity of the left leg is identical to that of the right leg. 20475: Affected female at 12 years of age; note extensive hypotrichosis, abnormal auricle, dental alterations and unusual number of wrinkles.

Etiology: Probably autosomal recessive inheritance. The two sibships thus far investigated have normal parents. In one instance the parents were possibly consanguineous, while in the other they are first cousins.

Pathogenesis: Unknown.

MIM No.: 27340

POS No.: 3355

Sex Ratio: Presumably M1:F1; M3:F2 observed.

Occurrence: Four of eight siblings in one Caucasian Brazilian family, and one of three siblings in a Caucasian Italian family, have been reported in the literature.

Risk of Recurrence for Patient's Sib:
See Part I, *Mendelian Inheritance.*

Risk of Recurrence for Patient's Child:
See Part I, *Mendelian Inheritance.*

Age of Detectability: At birth, on the basis of physical findings.

Gene Mapping and Linkage: Unknown.

Prevention: None known. Genetic counseling indicated.

Treatment: Orthopedic services. Plastic surgery and use of wigs and dental prostheses are cosmetically and psychologically helpful.

Prognosis: Normal for life span.

Detection of Carrier: Unknown.

References:
Chautard EA, Freire-Maia N: Dermatoglyphic analysis in a highly mutilating syndrome. Acta Genet Med Gemellol 1970; 3:421–424. †
Freire-Maia N: A newly recognized genetic syndrome of tetramelic deficiencies, ectodermal dysplasia, deformed ears, and other abnormalities. Am J Hum Genet 1970; 22:370–377. * †
Freire-Maia N, et al.: A new malformation syndrome? Lancet 1970; I:840–841. †
Cat I, et al.: Odontotrichomelic hypohidrotic dysplasia: a clinical reappraisal. Hum Hered 1972; 22:91–95.
Pinheiro M, Freire-Maia N: EEC and odontotrichomelic syndromes. Clin Genet 1980; 17:363–364.
Pavone L, et al.: A case of the Freire-Maia odontotrichomelic syndrome: nosology with EEC syndrome. Am J Med Genet 1989; 33:190–193. †

FR033   **Newton Freire-Maia**

Odontoblastic dysplasia, focal
See TEETH, ODONTOBLASTIC DYSPLASIA, FOCAL
Odontodysplasia
See TEETH, ODONTODYSPLASIA
Odontogenesis imperfecta
See TEETH, ODONTODYSPLASIA
Odontogenic dysplasia
See TEETH, ODONTODYSPLASIA
Oguchi disease types 1, 2A and 2B
See NIGHTBLINDNESS, OGUCHI TYPE
Ohdo-Hirayama-Terawaki syndrome
See ECTODERMAL DYSPLASIA-ECTRODACTYLY-MACULAR DYSTROPHY
Ohdo-Madokoro-Hayakawa syndrome
See MENTAL RETARDATION-HEART DEFECTS-BLEPHAROPHIMOSIS
Ohio type amyloidosis
See AMYLOIDOSIS, OHIO TYPE
Oily ear wax
See EAR, CERUMEN VARIATIONS
Okihiro syndrome
See RADIAL-RENAL-OCULAR SYNDROME
also EYE, DUANE RETRACTION SYNDROME
Oldfield syndrome
See INTESTINAL POLYPOSIS, TYPE III
Olfaction loss, congenital
See ANOSMIA, CONGENITAL
Olfactogenital dysplasia
See KALLMANN SYNDROME
Oligoazoospermia, idiopathic
See ANDROGEN INSENSITIVITY (RESISTANCE), MINIMAL
Oligodactyly-hydronephrosis
See HAND, ULNAR AND FIBULAR RAY DEFICIENCY, WEYERS TYPE
Oligodontia, isolated
See TEETH, ANODONTIA, PARTIAL OR COMPLETE
Oligodontia-cleft lip/palate-syndactyly-hair defects
See CLEFT LIP/PALATE-OLIGODONTIA-SYNDACTYLY-HAIR DEFECTS
Oligohydramnios, fetal, with NSAID exposure
See FETAL EFFECTS OF NONSTEROIDAL ANTI-INFLAMMATORY DRUGS (NSAIDS)
Oligophrenia phenylpyruvica
See PHENYLKETONURIA
also FETAL EFFECTS FROM MATERNAL PKU
Oligophrenia-aniridia-cerebellar ataxia
See ANIRIDIA-CEREBELLAR ATAXIA-MENTAL DEFICIENCY
Oligophrenia-cochlear deafness-myopia
See DEAFNESS-MYOPIA
Oligophrenia-epilepsy-ichthyosis syndrome
See SEIZURES-ICHTHYOSIS-MENTAL RETARDATION
Oligophrenia-gingival fibromatosis-depigmentation-microphthalmia
See GINGIVAL FIBROMATOSIS-DEPIGMENTATION-MICROPHTHALMIA
Oligophrenia-ichthyosis-spasticity
See SJOGREN-LARSSON SYNDROME

Oligophrenic cerebello-lental degeneration
See *MARINESCO-SJOGREN SYNDROME*
Oliguria, neonatal, with NSAID exposure
See *FETAL EFFECTS OF NONSTEROIDAL ANTI-INFLAMMATORY DRUGS (NSAIDS)*
Oliver-MacFarlane syndrome
See *TRICHOMEGALY-RETARDATION-DWARFISM-RETINAL PIGMENTARY DEGENERATION*
Olivopontocerebellar atrophy I
See *OLIVOPONTOCEREBELLAR ATROPHY, DOMINANT MENZEL TYPE*
Olivopontocerebellar atrophy II
See *OLIVOPONTOCEREBELLAR ATROPHY, RECESSIVE FICKLER-WINKLER TYPE*
Olivopontocerebellar atrophy III (OPCA type III)
See *OLIVOPONTOCEREBELLAR ATROPHY, DOMINANT WITH RETINAL DEGENERATION*
Olivopontocerebellar atrophy IV
See *OLIVOPONTOCEREBELLAR ATROPHY, DOMINANT SCHUT-HAYMAKER TYPE*
Olivopontocerebellar atrophy V
See *OLIVOPONTOCEREBELLAR ATROPHY, DOMINANT WITH OPHTHALMOPLEGIA*

OLIVOPONTOCEREBELLAR ATROPHY, DOMINANT MENZEL TYPE   0742

Includes:
Olivopontocerebellar atrophy I
OPCA I

Excludes:
Olivopontocerebellar atrophy, dominant Schut-Haymaker type (0743)
Olivopontocerebellar atrophy (others)

Major Diagnostic Criteria: Adult life onset of progressive ataxia, computed tomography of the brain indicating olivopontocerebellar atrophy (OPCA), and evidence of autosomal dominant transmission.

Clinical Findings: Onset in the second to fifth decades of life, (usually about 30 years of age), of a slowly progressive unsteadiness of gait, and later of all limbs. There is progressive dysarthria with scanning speech, tremors, involuntary movements, often of choreiform type, and sensory impairment. Later, upper motor neuron signs with extensor plantar responses may develop.

There is moderate variability in some of the signs of this disease. Some cases may have no apparent sensory loss. Some patients may show weakness due to lower motor neuronal loss, while others have normal strength.

Complications: Patients become bedridden and debilitated.

Associated Findings: None known.

Etiology: Autosomal dominant inheritance. Penetrance appears complete, but age of onset is variable.

Pathogenesis: The brain shows the changes of OPCA with sparing of the cerebellar vermis, marked loss of cerebellar Purkinje cells, and less striking granule cell loss in the remainder of the cerebellum. The dentate nucleus is usually involved, and there is decreased size of the superior cerebellar peduncles and cerebellar white matter. The basis pontis is small, with loss of transverse fibers and fiber loss in the middle cerebellar peduncles. There is marked neuronal loss in the inferior olivary nuclei. The substantia nigra also frequently shows neuronal loss. In most cases the spinal cord shows loss of fibers in the posterior funiculus, spinocerebellar tracts, and, on occasion, in the pyramidal tracts. Sometimes neuronal loss is found in the posterior horns, Clarke column, or anterior horns. Clues to the biochemical origin of this disease are provided by studies in other inherited ataxias that demonstrate deficiencies in pyruvate dehydrogenase and mitochondrial enzymes.

MIM No.:   *16440

Sex Ratio: M1:F1

Occurrence: Although only a few families with this particular variant have been described in the United States, the combined

prevalence of the dominantly inherited forms of OPCA is estimated to be 1:31,250.

Risk of Recurrence for Patient's Sib:
See Part I, *Mendelian Inheritance.*

Risk of Recurrence for Patient's Child:
See Part I, *Mendelian Inheritance.*

Age of Detectability: At about age 30 years when onset of symptoms occurs.

Gene Mapping and Linkage: SCA1 (spinal cerebellar ataxia (olivopontocerebellar ataxia)) has been mapped to 6p24-p21.3.

Prevention: None known. Genetic counseling indicated.

Treatment: The evidence for pyruvic dehydrogenase deficiency has led to the use of cholinergic agonists (physostigmine and lecithin) with some efficacy. However, supportive personal and family therapy remain the mainstay of treatment.

Prognosis: Patients may die in their fourth to seventh decades of life, usually of debilitation and pneumonia.

Detection of Carrier: In some families, HLA typing may be helpful in carrier identification, but only after an index case has been discovered.

References:
Menzel P: Beitrag Zur Kenntniss der hereditaeren Ataxie und Kleinhirnatrophie. Arch Psychiatr Nervenkr 1890; 22:160–190.
Konigsmark BW, Weiner LP: The olivopontocerebellar atrophies: a review. Medicine 1970; 49:227–242. *
Skre H: Spino-cerebellar ataxia in western Norway. Clin Genet 1974; 6:265–288.
Jackson JF, et al: Spinocerebellar ataxia and HLA linkage: risk prediction by HLA typing. New Engl J Med 1977; 296:1138–1141. *
Rodriguez-Budelli M, et al.: Action of physostigmine on inherited ataxia. In: Kark RAP, et al, eds: The inherited ataxias. New York: Raven Press, 1978:195–202.
Gilman S, et al.: Disorders of the cerebellum. Philadelphia: F.A. Davis, 1981.
Stumpf DA, et al.: Mitochondrial malic enzyme deficiency in Friedreich's ataxia. Ann Neurol 1981; 10:283 only.
Sorbi S, et al.: Abnormal platelet glutamate dehydrogenase activity and activation in dominant and nondominant olivopontocerebellar atrophy. Ann Neurol 1986; 19:239–245.

CR011   **Carl J. Crosley**

OLIVOPONTOCEREBELLAR ATROPHY, DOMINANT SCHUT-HAYMAKER TYPE   0743

Includes:
Olivopontocerebellar atrophy IV
OPCA IV

Excludes:
Olivopontocerebellar atrophy, dominant Menzel type (0742)
Olivopontocerebellar atrophy (other)

Major Diagnostic Criteria: Adult life onset of cerebellar ataxia and variable upper motor neuron signs; computed tomography of the brain or autopsy findings of olivopontocerebellar atrophy (OPCA) with variable anterior horn cell and spinocerebellar tract loss, and loss of neurons in 9th, 10th and 12th cranial nerves. Evidence of autosomal dominant transmission helps to confirm the diagnosis.

Clinical Findings: Onset between about 17 and 35 years of age of a slowly progressive cerebellar ataxia. Tendon reflexes vary from completely absent to hyperactive. Plantar responses are flexor in most cases, but extensor in a few. Muscle tone varies from minimal to marked rigidity. Sensation varies from normal to moderate loss of position and pain sensation. Some cases may show clinical signs of **Ataxia, Friedreich type,** with absent deep tendon reflexes and mild coordination defect; others may show more prominent cerebellar ataxia, with variable deep tendon reflexes and moderate coordination disturbances, and some will show prominent pyramidal signs suggesting spastic quadriplegia.

Of all the olivopontocerebellar degenerations, this disease shows the greatest variation in clinical signs and pathologic changes. Schut and Haymaker (1951), who reported 42 affected persons in one kindred, divided the clinical types in this family into three groups: Friedreich ataxia type, cerebellar ataxia type, and spastic paraplegia type. The pathologic findings showed a similar variation, with a variable degree of severity of involvement of different structures.

Complications: Patients become incapacitated and bedridden.

Associated Findings: None known.

Etiology: Autosomal dominant inheritance with complete penetrance.

Pathogenesis: The brain shows the changes of OPCA with moderate-to-severe cerebellar atrophy and cerebellar cortical cell loss. Most severely affected in all cases are the inferior olivary nuclei, restiform bodies, brachium conjunctivum, cerebellum, and 12th nerves. There is marked neuronal and fiber loss in the inferior olivary nuclei. The basis pontis shows some variation from case to case with moderate atrophy in some cases and no changes in others. In the brainstem, neuronal loss varies in the 9th, 10th and 12th cranial nerves and substantia nigra. The white matter of the spinal cord varies from normal to severe fiber loss in the posterior funiculus and spinocerebellar tracts. The anterior motor horn cells may be normal or may show moderate loss. Clues to the biochemical origin of this disease are provided by studies in other inherited ataxias that demonstrate deficiencies in pyruvate dehydrogenase and mitochondrial malic enzyme.

MIM No.: *16460

Sex Ratio: M1:F1

Occurrence: In one western European population, 1:300,000.

Risk of Recurrence for Patient's Sib:
See Part I, *Mendelian Inheritance.*

Risk of Recurrence for Patient's Child:
See Part I, *Mendelian Inheritance.*

Age of Detectability: At about age 25 years.

Gene Mapping and Linkage: Unknown.

Prevention: None known. Genetic counseling indicated.

Treatment: The evidence for pyruvic dehydrogenase deficiency has led to the use of cholinergic agonists (physostigmine and lecithin) with some efficacy. However, supportive personal and family therapy remain the mainstay of treatment.

Prognosis: Patients die about 15 years after onset, usually of debilitation and infection.

Detection of Carrier: In some families, HLA typing may be helpful in carrier identification, but only after an index case has been discovered.

References:
Schut JW, Haymaker W: Hereditary ataxia: pathologic study of five cases of common ancestry. J Neuropathol Clin Neurol 1951; 1:183–213.
Konigsmark BW, Weiner LP: The olivopontocerebellar atrophies: a review. Medicine 1970; 49:227–242. *
Skre H: Spino-cerevellar ataxia in western Norway. Clin Genet 1974; 6:265–288.
Jackson JF, et al.: Spino-cerebellar ataxia and HLA linkage: risk prediction by HLA typing. New Engl J Med 1977; 296:1138–1141.
Rodriguez-Budelli M, et al.: Action of physostigmine on inherited ataxia. In: Kark RAP, et al, eds: The inherited ataxias. New York: Raven Press, 1978:195–202.
Gilman S, et al.: Disorders of the cerebellum. Philadelphia: F.A. Davis, 1981.
Stumpf DA, et al.: Mitochondrial malic enzyme deficiency in Friedreich's ataxia. Ann Neurol 1981; 10:283 only.

CR011   **Carl J. Crosley**

OLIVOPONTOCEREBELLAR ATROPHY, DOMINANT WITH OPHTHALMOPLEGIA   0744

Includes:
Cerebelloolivary degeneration-rigidity and dementia
Olivopontocerebellar atrophy V
Olivopontocerebellar atrophy-dementia-extrapyramidal signs
OPCA V

Excludes: Olivopontocerebellar atrophy (other)

Major Diagnostic Criteria: Adult life onset of progressive ataxia, tremor, rigidity, ophthalmoplegia, and severe mental deterioration. Computed tomography of the brain, or autopsy findings, of olivopontocerebellar atrophy (OPCA), and cerebral cortical atrophy. Evidence of autosomal dominant transmission helps to confirm the diagnosis.

Clinical Findings: Adult onset of progressive ataxia, dysarthria, rigidity, tremor, and mental deterioration. Patients may be diagnosed as having Parkinson disease when the rigidity and tremor are prominent. Walking, writing, and speech generally become difficult. Patients in their third decade of life show mental deterioration, with disorientation to time and place, and are only able to follow simple commands. Dysarthria is characterized by a high-pitched scanning voice. Eye movements become involved first with paresis of upward and lateral gaze and then complete external ophthalmoplegia. Marked rigidity and coarse resting and intention tremor become evident.

Complications: Patients become bedridden and debilitated.

Associated Findings: None known.

Etiology: Autosomal dominant inheritance with complete penetrance.

Pathogenesis: The gross brain is small, ranging from 700 to 1200g. There is OPCA, as well as cerebral cortical atrophy. There is a severe loss of neurons in the inferior olivary nuclei, the basis pontis, and the cerebellar cortex. In the spinal cord there is loss of posterior funiculus fibers. The substantia nigra shows marked neuronal loss, and there is a mild neuronal loss in the globus pallidus, caudate nuclei, and cerebral cortex. Clues to the biochemical origin of this disease are provided by studies in other inherited ataxias that demonstrated deficiencies in pyruvate dehydrogenase and mitochondrial malic enzyme.

MIM No.: *16470

Sex Ratio: M1:F1

Occurrence: While there are only a few kindreds reported in detail with this specific variant, the combined prevalence of the dominantly inherited forms of OPCA is estimated to be 1:31,250.

Risk of Recurrence for Patient's Sib:
See Part I, *Mendelian Inheritance.*

Risk of Recurrence for Patient's Child:
See Part I, *Mendelian Inheritance.*

Age of Detectability: At about age 20 years.

Gene Mapping and Linkage: Unknown. A single family has been described in whom HLA typing has accurately predicted the presence of ataxia. More tentative evidence is available in another family in which linkage between glyoxalase and spino-cerebellar degeneration is suggested.

Prevention: None known. Genetic counseling indicated.

Treatment: Supportive therapy for ataxia, and for the mental deterioration and disorientation.

Prognosis: Affected persons die about 10 years after onset of symptoms, usually from debility and infection.

Detection of Carrier: In some families, HLA typing may be helpful in carrier identification, but only after an index case has been discovered.

Special Considerations: This disease differs clinically from the other OPCAs because of the marked mental deterioration, and pathologically because of the marked brain atrophy with olivopontocerebellar degeneration and cerebral cortical neuronal loss.

Some patients have been diagnosed as having Parkinson disease because of prominent rigidity and tremor. Heterogeneity within and among reported families, both clinically and pathologically, has been observed.

References:
Konigsmark BW, Lipton HL: Dominant olivopontocerebellar atrophy with dementia and extrapyramidal signs: report of a family through three generations. BD:OAS VII(1). Baltimore: Williams & Wilkins for The National Foundation March of Dimes, 1971:178–202. *
Skre H: Spino-cerebellar ataxia in western Norway. Clin Genet 1974; 6:265–288.
Jackson JF, et al.: Spino-cerebellar ataxia and HLA linkage. N Engl J Med. 1977; 296:1138–1141.
Rodriguez-Budelli M, et al.: Action of physostigmine on inherited ataxia. In: Kark RAP, et al, eds: The inherited ataxias. New York: Raven Press, 1978:195–202. *
Gilman S, et al.: Disorders of the cerebellum. Philadelphia: F.A. Davis, 1981.
Stumpf DA, et al.: Mitochondrial malic enzyme deficiency in Friedreich's ataxia. Ann Neurol 1981; 10:283 only.

CR011   **Carl J. Crosley**

OLIVOPONTOCEREBELLAR ATROPHY, DOMINANT WITH RETINAL DEGENERATION   0745

Includes:
Cerebellar-macular abiotrophy
Infantile cerebellar atrophy with retinal degeneration
Olivopontocerebellar atrophy III (OPCA type III)
OPCA III
Retinal dystrophy associated with spinocerebellar ataxia

Excludes:
Cerebro-hepato-renal syndrome (0139)
Neuronal ceroid-lipofuscinoses (NCL) (0713)
Olivopontocerebellar atrophy (other)
Phytanic acid oxidase deficiency, infantile type (2278)

Major Diagnostic Criteria: Infancy or adult onset of ataxia, dysarthria and tremor; progressive visual loss, beginning about the same time as the ataxia and involving the macula and then remainder of the retina; evidence of autosomal dominant transmission, and computed tomography of the brain or neuropathologic findings of OPCA.

Clinical Findings: This disease is characterized by a remarkably variable age of onset of cerebellar ataxia and retinal dystrophy. The disease may show first signs from the age of one year to over 50 years of age; however, the usual age of onset is about 20 years. The syndrome is characterized by a progressive visual loss, ataxia and tremor. Clinically, eye signs are prominent with an unusual retinal pigmentary dystrophy and sometimes with ophthalmoplegia and nystagmus. When the disease begins in infancy, retinal involvement is diffuse with fine pigmentary changes in the macula and fundus periphery. When symptoms begin in adulthood, retinal changes typically remain restricted to the macula and take the form of a bull's eye lesion with mild pigmentary changes. Geographic atrophy of the retinal pigment epithelium and visual loss is much more severe and rapidly progressive when the disease has its onset in infancy. Cerebellar ataxia involving the limbs and speech begins about the same time as the retinal changes. The ataxia and rigidity progress leading to confinement in bed about 10 years after onset. The syndrome in infancy is characterized by tremor, ataxia, retinal dystrophy weakness, and early death.

Complications: Affected persons become bedridden, with death usually resulting from infection.

Associated Findings: None known.

Etiology: Autosomal dominant inheritance. Penetrance is complete, with variability in age of onset and rate of progression.

Pathogenesis: The changes of olivopontocerebellar (OPCA) atrophy are seen grossly and histologically. Cerebellar Purkinje cells are markedly decreased in numbers, particularly in the vermis, while granule cells are relatively preserved. There is also moderate loss of substantia nigra neurons. In early cases, the retina shows marked loss of rods and cones outer segments with preservation of bipolar cells and ganglion cells. The choriocapillaris is normal. The retinal pigment epithelium is variably pigmented. The pathology seems to start in the central retina and spreads to involve the periphery. With advanced disease, there is neuronal dropout in other retinal layers. The optic nerve is generally normal in appearance and color.

Clues to the biochemical origin of these diseases have been provided by studies demonstrating deficiencies in pyruvate dehydrogenase and by other studies recording mitochondrial malic enzyme deficiencies in patients with various inherited ataxias.

MIM No.: *16450

Sex Ratio: M1:F1

Occurrence: Only a few kindreds affected with this disease have been described in the United States. The prevalence of dominantly inherited OPCA is estimated to be 1:31,250.

Risk of Recurrence for Patient's Sib:
See Part I, *Mendelian Inheritance.*

Risk of Recurrence for Patient's Child:
See Part I, *Mendelian Inheritance.*

Age of Detectability: Highly variable, usually at about 20 years of age.

Gene Mapping and Linkage: Unknown.

Prevention: None known. Genetic counseling indicated.

Treatment: Supportive.

Prognosis: Affected persons generally die of debilitation and infection about 15 years after onset.

Detection of Carrier: There is no known method for the identification of asymptomatic carriers.

Special Considerations: In one family studied, two sibs died of this disease before the diagnosis was made in the affected father, who had only minimal retinal changes. Clinically this disease generally shows more rigidity than the other types of OPCA, and ophthalmoplegia is a prominent feature.

References:
Carpenter S, Schumacher GA: Familial infantile cerebellar atrophy associated with retinal degeneration. Arch Neurol 1966; 14:82–94.
Weiner LP, et al.: Herediatary olivopontocerebellar atrophy with retinal degeneration: report of a family through six generations. Arch Neurol 1967; 16:364–376.
Skre H: Spino-cerebellar ataxia in western Norway. Clin Genet 1974; 6:265.
Ryan SJ, et al.: Olivopontocerebellar degeneration: clinicopathologic correlation of the associated retinopathy. Arch Ophthalmol 1975; 93:169–172.
deJong PTVM, et al.: Olivopontocerebellar atrophy with visual disturbances: an ophthalmologic investigation into four generations. Ophthalmology 1980; 87:793–804.
Stumpf DA, et al.: Mitochondrial malic enzyme deficiency in Friedreich's ataxia. Ann Neurol 1981; 10:287.
Harding AE: The clinical features and classification of the late onset autosomal dominant cerebellar ataxia: a study of 11 families including descendants of the Drero family of Walworth. Brain 1982; 105:1–28.
Harding AE: Classification of the hereditary ataxias and paraplegia. Lancet 1983; 1:1151–1154.

CR011   **Carl J. Crosley**

OLIVOPONTOCEREBELLAR ATROPHY, LATE-ONSET   0746

Includes: N/A

Excludes:
Holmes cerebelloolivary atrophy
Marie ataxia
Olivopontocerebellar atrophy (other)

Major Diagnostic Criteria: Onset in adult life of progressive ataxia, tremor, and dysarthria with olivopontocerebellar atrophy (OPCA) as demonstrated by computed tomography of the brain or by autopsy.

Clinical Findings: Onset is in the fifth or sixth decades of life, with a progressive cerebellar ataxia of the limbs and trunk, slowness of voluntary movements, scanning speech, nystagmus, and tremor of the head and trunk. In some cases, Parkinsonian signs are prominent, with rigidity, tremor, bradykinesia, and immobile facies. Urinary incontinence and other frontal lobe signs will occur occasionally. Reflexes are usually normal, although there may be loss of knee and ankle jerks or an extensor plantar response.

Complications: Patients become incapacitated in 5–10 years.

Associated Findings: None known.

Etiology: Undetermined. May be **Olivopontocerebellar atrophy, recessive Fickler-Winkler type** with very late expressivity. Other etiologic possibilities include toxic factors or a specific deficiency.

Pathogenesis: There may be neuronal loss in the cerebellar dentate nuclei or substantia nigra. The spinal cord and cerebral cortex are minimally affected. Clues to the biochemical origin of this disorder are provided by studies in other inherited ataxias that demonstrate deficiencies in pyruvate dehydrogenase and mitochondrial malic enzyme.

Sex Ratio: M1:F1

Occurrence: The prevalence of **Olivopontocerebellar atrophy, recessive Fickler-Winkler type**, of which this may or may not be a subset, was determined to be 1.2:100,000 in one western European population.

Risk of Recurrence for Patient's Sib:
See Part I, *Mendelian Inheritance.*

Risk of Recurrence for Patient's Child:
See Part I, *Mendelian Inheritance.*

Age of Detectability: Onset of symptoms at about age 45 years.

Gene Mapping and Linkage: Unknown.

Prevention: None known. Genetic counseling indicated.

Treatment: Recognition that defects in pyruvate oxidation result in inhibition of the synthesis of acetylcholine has led to the use of cholinergic agonists (physostigmine and lecithin) with some efficacy. However, supportive personal and family therapy remain the mainstay of treatment.

Prognosis: Slow progression, with incapacitation in 5–10 years, and death due to debility and infection about five years later.

Detection of Carrier: In some families, HLA typing may be helpful in carrier identification, but only after an index case has been discovered.

References:
Jackson JF, et al.: Spino-cerebellar ataxia and HLA linkage. New Engl J Med 1977; 296:1138–1141. *
Rodriguez-Budelli M, et al.: Action of physostigmine on inherited ataxia. In: Kark RAP, et al, eds: The inherited ataxias. New York: Raven Press, 1978:195–202.
Skre H: Spino-cerebellar ataxia in western Norway. Clin Genet 1974; 6:265–288. *
Gilman S, et al.: Disorders of the cerebellum. Philadelphia: F.A. Davis, 1981.
Stumpf DA, et al.: Mitochondrial malic enzyme deficiency in Friedreich's ataxia. Ann Neurol 1981; 10:283 only.

CR011   **Carl J. Crosley**

OLIVOPONTOCEREBELLAR ATROPHY, RECESSIVE FICKLER-WINKLER TYPE   0747

Includes:
Fickler-Winkler olivopontocerebellar atrophy
Olivopontocerebellar atrophy II
OPCA II

Excludes: **Olivopontocerebellar atrophy** (other)

Major Diagnostic Criteria: Progressive cerebellar ataxia and dysarthria, computed tomography of the brain or autopsy findings of olivopontocerebellar atrophy, and evidence of autosomal recessive transmission.

Clinical Findings: Variable age of onset, between about seven and 50 years of age, of a slowly progressive cerebellar ataxia, head tremor, and dysarthria, with scanning speech. There are no choreiform movements; strength and sensation are normal.

The age of onset generally is younger than that of **Olivopontocerebellar atrophy, dominant Menzel type**, and there is no sensory loss or involuntary movements.

Complications: Patients gradually become bedridden and debilitated.

Associated Findings: None known.

Etiology: Autosomal recessive inheritance. Penetrance appears to be complete.

Pathogenesis: Clues to the biochemical origin of this disease are provided by studies in other inherited ataxias that demonstrate deficiencies in pyruvate dehydrogenase and mitochondrial malic enzyme.

MIM No.: *25830

Sex Ratio: M1:F1

Occurrence: Although Fickler and Winkler reported only two sibs with this condition, Skre (1974) has documented nine families with autosomal recessive OPCA. The prevalence of autosomal recessive OPCA has been reported to be 1.2:100,000 in a western European population.

Risk of Recurrence for Patient's Sib:
See Part I, *Mendelian Inheritance.*

Risk of Recurrence for Patient's Child:
See Part I, *Mendelian Inheritance.*

Age of Detectability: At onset of symptoms, from about age 7–50 years.

Gene Mapping and Linkage: Unknown.

Prevention: None known. Genetic counseling indicated.

Treatment: Recognition that defects in pyruvic oxidation result in inhibition of the synthesis of acetylcholine has led to the use of cholinergic agonists (physostigmine and lecithin) with some efficacy. However, supportive personal and family therapy remain the mainstay of treatment.

Prognosis: Affected persons die from 5–15 years after onset, usually of debilitation and infection.

Detection of Carrier: In some families, HLA typing may be helpful in carrier identification, but only after an index case has been discovered.

References:
Winkler C: A case of olivo-pontine cerebellar atrophy and our conceptions of neo and palaeocerebellum. Schweiz Arch Neurol Neurochir Psychiatr 1923; 13:684–702.
Konigsmark BW, Weiner LP: The olivopontocerebellar atrophies: a review. Medicine 1970; 49:227–240.
Skre H: Spino-cerebellar ataxia in western Norway. Clin Genet. 1974; 6:265–288.
Jackson JF, et al.: Spino-cerebellar ataxia and HLA linkage. New Engl J Med 1977; 296:1138–1141.
Rodriguez-Budelli M, et al.: Action of physostigmine on inherited ataxia. In: Kark RAP, et al, eds: The inherited ataxias. New York: Raven Press, 1978:195–202.
Gilman S, et al.: Disorders of the cerebellum. Philadelphia: F.A. Davis, 1981.

Stumpf DA, et al.: Mitochondrial malic enzyme deficiency in Friedreich's ataxia. Ann Neurol 1981; 10:283 only.

CR011 **Carl J. Crosley**

Olivopontocerebellar atrophy-dementia-extrapyramidal signs
See OLIVOPONTOCEREBELLAR ATROPHY, DOMINANT WITH OPHTHALMOPLEGIA
Ollier syndrome
See ENCHONDROMATOSIS
Omenn syndrome
See IMMUNODEFICIENCY, RETICULOENDOTHELIOSIS WITH EOSINOPHILIA

OMODYSPLASIA 3280

Includes:
Dwarfism, omodysplasia
Maroteaux rhizomelic dysplasia
Rhizomelic dysplasia, familial
Viljoen rhizomelic dysplasia
Excludes:
Humerus varus
Rhizomelic syndrome, Urbach type (2816)
Robinow syndrome (0876)

Major Diagnostic Criteria: Short humerus with a defect of growth of the distal end of the humerus and upper radio-ulnar diastasis.

Clinical Findings: Recognized at birth on the basis of shortened humeri; flexion and extension of the elbow are limited. Craniofacial morphology is characterized by a small but broadened nose, depressed nasal bridge, and a long philtrum. This upper limb anomaly can be isolated, but in some cases a severe micromelic dwarfism, with short and stubby femora and restricted motions of the hips and knees, is also present.

On X-ray, the diaphysis of the humerus is twisted, so that the distal end appears *en profil*. The condyle is hypoplastic and laterally everted. The radial head is dislocated anteriorly and laterally. There is a diastasis of the proximal end of the radius and ulna. If the lower limbs are involved, the diaphyses of the femora are short, broadened and twisted, and the tibiae and fibulae are short and thick.

Complications: In cases with severe micromelic dwarfism, patients may die shortly after birth.

Associated Findings: Congenital heart defects.

Etiology: Autosomal dominant inheritance has been observed in a family without shortness of the lower limbs. In the family reported by Viljoen et al (1987), recessive inheritance was suggested.

Pathogenesis: Unknown.

Sex Ratio: Presumably M1:F1.

Occurrence: Fewer than ten cases have been reported in the literature.

Risk of Recurrence for Patient's Sib:
See Part I, *Mendelian Inheritance*.

Risk of Recurrence for Patient's Child:
See Part I, *Mendelian Inheritance*.

Age of Detectability: At birth on the basis of shortened humeri, or possibly prenatally by fetal ultrasound.

Gene Mapping and Linkage: Unknown.

Prevention: None known. Genetic counseling indicated.

Treatment: Unknown.

Prognosis: The defect in the growth of the lower limbs may result in severe dwarfism. Intelligence is unaffected.

Detection of Carrier: Unknown.

References:
Vallee L, et al.: Syndrome de Robinow à transmission dominante. Arch Fr Pédiatr 1982; 39:447–448.

Viljoen D, et al.: Familial rhizomelic dysplasia: phenotype variation or heterogeneity. Am J Med Genet 1987; 26:941–947.
Maroteaux P, et al.: Omodysplasia. Am J Med Genet 1989; 32:371–375.

MA034 **Pierre Maroteaux**

OMPHALOCELE 0748

Includes:
Celosomia
Herniation into the umbilical cord
Umbilical cord hernia
Excludes:
Gastroschisis (0405)
Hernia, umbilical (2575)
Omphalomesenteric duct anomalies (2574)
Schisis association (2249)
Umbilical cord, large

Major Diagnostic Criteria: A transparent sac covering the umbilical ring, with the umbilical cord inserted onto the sac rather than the abdominal wall. Ultrasonography offers antenatal diagnosis of anterior abdominal wall defects, including omphalocele and gastroschisis.

Clinical Findings: Intra-abdominal viscera herniate the umbilical cord. The mass is not covered with peritoneum, fascia, muscles, or skin. The size of an omphalocele depends on the amount of the abdominal viscera herniated into the amniotic sac surrounding the umbilical cord.

Complications: Infection, dehydration, and trauma or vascular compromise to the herniated abdominal viscera may occur; prenatal as well as postnatal rupture of the covering sac.

Associated Findings: Associated anomalies occur in 67% of patients with omphalocele (Rickham et al, 1978). Such anomalies include those in the cardiovascular, genitourinary, and central nervous systems. Of special importance is the diagnosis of **Beckwith-Wiedemann syndrome** (omphalocele, macroglossia, and gigantism) because of the associated intractable hypoglycemia due to pancreatic hyperplasia.

Etiology: Unknown. Autosomal dominant and X-linked inheritance have been reported.

Pathogenesis: Failure of migration and fusion of the two lateral embryonic folds of the anterior abdominal wall. Central herniation of the contents of the abdomen through the umbilical ring into a transparent sac composed of amnion and peritoneum with Wharton's jelly between them.

MIM No.: 16475, 31098

CDC No.: 756.700

Sex Ratio: M1:F1

Occurrence: 1:4,000 births.

Risk of Recurrence for Patient's Sib: Unknown.

Risk of Recurrence for Patient's Child: Unknown.

Age of Detectability: At birth.

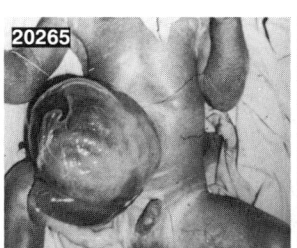
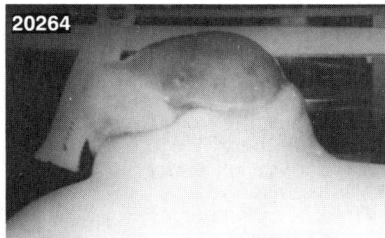

0748-20265–64: The transparent sac of the omphalocele covers the abdominal viscera.

Gene Mapping and Linkage: Unknown.

Prevention: None known. Genetic counseling indicated.

Treatment: Surgical closure, either primary or staged using silicone rubber parasthesis.

Prognosis: With early recognition and successful repair, survival in 50–60% of cases. Most deaths due to associated anomalies.

Detection of Carrier: Unknown.

References:
Rickham PP, et al.: Neonatal surgery. London: Butterworth & Co, 1978.
Seashore JH: Congenital abdominal wall defects. Clinics in Perinatology 1978; 5:61–78.
Havalad S, et al.: Familial occurrence of omphalocele suggesting sex-linked inheritance. Arch Dis Child 1979; 54:142–151.
DiLiberti JH: Familial omphalocele: analysis of risk factors and case report. Am J Med Genet 1982; 13:263–268.
Lurie IW, Ilyina HG: Familial omphalocele and recurrent risk. (Letter) Am J Med Genet 1984; 17:541–543.

SE006   **John H. Seashore**

Omphalocele with hypoplasia of pharynx and larynx
  See PHARYNX/LARYNX HYPOPLASIA-OMPHALOCELE, SHPRINTZEN-GOLDBERG TYPE
Omphalocele-cleft palate
  See CLEFT PALATE-OMPHALOCELE
Omphalocele-exstrophy-imperforate anus-spina bifida (OEIS)
  See EXSTROPHY OF CLOACA SEQUENCE
Omphalocele-pharynx/larynx hypoplasia, Shprintzen-Goldberg type
  See PHARYNX/LARYNX HYPOPLASIA-OMPHALOCELE, SHPRINTZEN-GOLDBERG TYPE
Omphalocele-visceromegaly-macroglossia syndrome
  See BECKWITH-WIEDEMANN SYNDROME
Omphalomesenteric duct
  See MECKEL DIVERTICULUM

OMPHALOMESENTERIC DUCT ANOMALIES   2574

Includes:
  Enteroumbilical fistula
  Meckel diverticulum
  Omphalomesenteric duct cyst
  Omphalomesenteric sinus
  Patent omphalomesenteric duct
  Umbilical polyp
  Vitelline cyst
  Vitelline duct anomalies

Excludes:
  Angiomyxomas
  Hemangiomas
  Teratomas (2919)
  Umbilical cord, large
  Umbilical cord, tumors
  Umbilical cysts
  Urachal anomalies (2573)

Major Diagnostic Criteria: A visible or palpable umbilical mass with or without a discharge. The type of lesion may be outlined by injecting contrast material into the sinus.

Clinical Findings: *Patent omphalomesenteric duct*: fecal discharge from the umbilicus or the umbilical stump coupled with visualiation of the fistulous tract following injection of a radio-opaque material.
Omphalomesenteric sinus: presents as a pouting mucous membrane projecting from the base of the umbilical wall and draining mucoid discharge.
Umbilical polyp: a bright red nodule with no demonstrable orifice or sinus tract.
Vitelline cyst: a palpable cystic mass buried superficially beneath the umbilicus.
Meckel diverticulum: the most common symptom is abdominal pain accompanied by sudden profuse rectal bleeding. Intussus-

ception occurs as the presenting problem in 25% of individuals with **Meckel diverticulum**.

Complications: Early and definitive diagnosis of the type of lesion is desirable because of the potential hazards of infection, injury, dehydration, and small bowel obstruction or perforation.

Associated Findings: None known.

Etiology: Aberrant development of the yolk sac coupled with an abnormal closure of the omphalomesenteric duct.

Pathogenesis: The wall in the nonobliterated vitelline duct may be lined by cuboidal or columnar epithelium with gastrointestinal differentiation with or without mucous production.

CDC No.: 751.000

Sex Ratio: M4:F1 for omphalomesenteric duct cyst
  M8:F1 for complete patency of the duct
  M6:F1 for cutaneous remnants of the duct

Occurrence: Varies according to the type of malformation. A completely patent omphalomesenteric duct is rare, occurring in 6.7:100,000 population.

Risk of Recurrence for Patient's Sib: Probably not increased.

Risk of Recurrence for Patient's Child: Probably not increased.

Age of Detectability: At birth or in the first year of life. Asymptomatic lesions may be discovered accidentally during abdominal operation or at autopsy.

Gene Mapping and Linkage: Unknown.

Prevention: None known. Genetic counseling indicated.

Treatment: Surgical excision of patent omphalomesenteric, omphalomesenteric duct cyst, or sinus and prompt treatment of symptomatic **Meckel diverticulum** is advisable. In the absence of a sinus tract, the treatment of choice of an umbilical polyp is cauterization.

Prognosis: Unknown.

Detection of Carrier: Unknown.

References:
Brown KL, Glover DM: Persistent omphalomesenteric duct. Am J Surg 1952; 83:680–685.

EL013   **Sami B. Elhassani**

Omphalomesenteric duct cyst
  See OMPHALOMESENTERIC DUCT ANOMALIES
Omphalomesenteric sinus
  See OMPHALOMESENTERIC DUCT ANOMALIES
Omphalopagus
  See TWINS, CONJOINED
Oncogene B-cell leukemia
  See LEUKEMIA/LYMPHOMA, B-CELL
Oncogene B-cell leukemia-2
  See LYMPHOMA, NON-HODGKIN
Ondine curse-Hirschprung disease
  See HYPOVENTILATION, CONGENITAL CENTRAL ALVEOLAR TYPE
Onion bulb neuropathy
  See DEJERINE-SOTTAS DISEASE
Onychial dysplasia, hereditary
  See NAILS, ANONYCHIA, HEREDITARY
Onycho-osteo dystrophy-deafness
  See DEAFNESS-TRIPHALANGEAL THUMBS-ONYCHODYSTROPHY

ONYCHO-TRICHODYSPLASIA-NEUTROPENIA   2331

Includes:
  Nails (hypoplastic)-neutropenia-onychorrhexis
  Neutropenia-onychotrichodysplasia
  Onychotrichodysplasia-chronic neutropenia-mild mental retardation
  Tricho-onycho-dysplasia-neutropenia

Excludes:
  Ectodermal dysplasia, Christ-Siemens-Touraine type (0333)
  Ectodermal dysplasia, hidrotic (0334)
  Ectodermal dysplasia (other)

Immunodeficiency, agranulocytosis, infantile Kostmann type (2197)
Nail dysplasia
Nails, hypoplastic
Nails, pachyonychia congenita (0789)
Nail-patella syndrome (0704)
Nails, koilonychia (0559)
Neutropenia, benign familial (2215)

Major Diagnostic Criteria: Neutropenia, trichorrhexis, hypoplastic nails.

Clinical Findings: The scalp and body hair is scanty, fine, dry, lusterless, short, curly, and sparse. Other characteristic findings are mild keratosis follicularis, hypoplastic nails, onychorrhexis, and koilonychia.

White blood cell counts show neutropenia (neutrophil counts range from 502 to 2,633/μl) and monocytosis (ranging from 1% to 6%). Immunoglobulin levels (IgA, IgG, and IgM), immune response to vaccination with common antigens, antistreptolysins, and C-reactive protein are normal. Responses to coccidioidin and histoplasmin are negative. Microscopic studies of the hair, eyebrows, and eyelashes show trichorrhexis.

Complications: Recurrent infections, i.e., conjunctivitis, tonsillitis, sinusitis, otitis, vaginitis, and cystitis.

Associated Findings: Verhage et al (1987) has suggested that the mild mental retardation (IQ ranges from 62 to normal), observed in most cases, may be a result of repeated infestions.

Etiology: Autosomal recessive inheritance.

Pathogenesis: Neutropenia is probably present from birth, leading to increased susceptibility to infections.

MIM No.: *25836

POS No.: 3490

Sex Ratio: M1:F3 (observed)

Occurrence: About a half-dozen cases have been reported.

Risk of Recurrence for Patient's Sib:
See Part I, *Mendelian Inheritance.*

Risk of Recurrence for Patient's Child:
See Part I, *Mendelian Inheritance.*

Age of Detectability: At birth.

Gene Mapping and Linkage: Unknown.

Prevention: None known. Genetic counseling indicated.

Treatment: Symptomatic.

Prognosis: One affected child died from acute meningitis. Two other affected individuals were alive beyond 20 years of age.

Detection of Carrier: Unknown.

References:
Cantú JM, et al.: Syndrome of onychotrichodysplasia with chronic neutropenia in an infant from consanguineous parents. BD:OAS XI(2). New York: March of Dimes Birth Defects Foundation, 1975: 63–66.
Hernández A, et al.: Autosomal recessive onychotrichodysplasia, chronic neutropenia and mild mental retardation: delineation of the syndrome. Clin Genet 1979; 15:147–152. *
Corona-Rivera E, et al.: Further delineation of the onycho-trichodysplasia, chronic neutropenia and mild retardation syndrome. (Abstract) Sixth Int Cong Hum Genet, Jerusalem 1981:267.
Verhage J, et al.: A patient with onychotrichodysplasia, neutropenia, and normal intelligence. Clin Genet 1987; 31:374–380.

HE039   **Alejandro Hernández**
CA011   **José María Cantú**

Onycho-trichodysplasia-xeroderma
See TRICHO-ONYCHODYSPLASIA-XERODERMA
Onychodystrophy-conical teeth-hearing loss
See ONYCHODYSTROPHY-CONIFORM TEETH-SENSORINEURAL HEARING LOSS

ONYCHODYSTROPHY-CONIFORM TEETH-SENSORINEURAL HEARING LOSS   2034

Includes:
   Deafness-onychodystrophy, dominant form
   Ectodermal dysplasia-hearing loss (sensorineural)-digital defects
   Onychodystrophy-conical teeth-hearing loss
   Robinson ectodermal dysplasia-deafness
   Teeth (coniform)-onychodystrophy-deafness

Excludes:
   Chondroectodermal dysplasia (0156)
   Deafness-onychodystrophy (0252)
   Ectodermal dysplasia, hidrotic (0334)

Major Diagnostic Criteria: The combination of nail dystrophy, missing and/or conical teeth, and sensorineural hearing loss and, in some cases, polydactyly and/or syndactyly.

Clinical Findings: This condition has only been reported in four individuals in a single family, and is considered a hidrotic ectodermal dysplasia. Affected individuals all have sensorineural hearing loss, which is more severe in the higher tones. The nails are small and dystrophic, with furrows and cracks. All individuals had delayed dentition, partial anodontia, and conical teeth, affecting both primary and secondary dentition. One individual had unilateral post-axial polydactyly of the hand, and another had unilateral syndactyly of toes 1 and 2, and 3 and 4. Laboratory investigations showed elevated sweat chloride and sodium.

Complications: Unknown.

Associated Findings: None known.

Etiology: Autosomal dominant inheritance, probably with a high degree of penetrance.

Pathogenesis: An ectodermal dysplasia seems most likely, although no specific defect has been identified.

MIM No.: *12448

Sex Ratio: M1:F1

Occurrence: Documented in a five members across three generations of one family.

Risk of Recurrence for Patient's Sib:
See Part I, *Mendelian Inheritance.*

Risk of Recurrence for Patient's Child:
See Part I, *Mendelian Inheritance.*

Age of Detectability: At birth, by the presence of polydactyly, syndactyly, or nail defects.

Gene Mapping and Linkage: Unknown.

Prevention: None known. Genetic counseling indicated.

Treatment: Orthodontic treatment for anodontia or hypodontia is indicated; appropriate schooling for deafness.

Prognosis: Life span and intellect appear normal.

Detection of Carrier: Unknown.

References:
Robinson GC, et al.: Familial ectodermal dysplasia with sensorineural deafness and other anomalies. Pediatrics 1962; 30:797–802. *

T0007   **Helga V. Toriello**

Onychodystrophy-deafness
See DEAFNESS-ONYCHODYSTROPHY
Onychodystrophy-digital malformation-deafness
See DEAFNESS-TRIPHALANGEAL THUMBS-ONYCHODYSTROPHY
Onycholysis-hypohidrosis-enamel hypocalcification
See AMELO-ONYCHO-HYPOHIDROTIC SYNDROME
Onychoosteodysplasia
See NAIL-PATELLA SYNDROME
Onychotrichodysplasia-chronic neutropenia-mild mental retardation
See ONYCHO-TRICHODYSPLASIA-NEUTROPENIA
Opalescent dentin
See TEETH, DENTINOGENESIS IMPERFECTA

OPCA I
  See OLIVOPONTOCEREBELLAR ATROPHY, DOMINANT MENZEL TYPE
OPCA IV
  See OLIVOPONTOCEREBELLAR ATROPHY, DOMINANT SCHUT-HAYMAKER TYPE
OPCA V
  See OLIVOPONTOCEREBELLAR ATROPHY, DOMINANT WITH OPHTHALMOPLEGIA
Ophiasis
  See HAIR, ALOPECIA AREATA
Ophthalmo-acromelic syndrome
  See ANOPHTHALMIA-LIMB ANOMALIES
Ophthalmo-mandibulo-melic dwarfism
  See DWARFISM (SHORT LIMBED)-PETERS ANOMALY OF THE EYE

OPHTHALMO-MANDIBULO-MELIC DWARFISM 3259

Includes:
  Dwarfism, ophthalmo-mandibulo-melic
  Mandibulo-melic dwarfism with corneal clouding
  Pillay syndrome

Excludes:
  Dwarfism (short limbed)-Peters anomaly of the eye (2812)
  Eye, anterior segment dysgenesis (0439)
  Fetal alcohol syndrome (0379)
  Walker-Warburg syndrome (2869)

Major Diagnostic Criteria: Mesomelic dwarfism with bowed radius and short ulna. Congenital corneal clouding. Micrognathia, obtuse jaw angle, temporomandibular joint fusion.

Clinical Findings: Bowed forearms due to radial bowing and marked shortening of ulna. Corneal clouding due to **Eye, anterior segment dysgenesis**. Relative shortening of tibia and fibula.

Complications: Visual loss from corneal opacities.

Associated Findings: Pupillary membrane.

Etiology: Autosomal dominant inheritance.

Pathogenesis: Unknown.

MIM No.: *16490

Sex Ratio: M1:F1

Occurrence: Pillay described a father with an affected daughter and son (1964). Another possible case in a female who underwent corneal transplantation has been observed. The histology revealed Peters anomaly (see **Eye, anterior segment dysgenesis**).

Risk of Recurrence for Patient's Sib:
  See Part I, *Mendelian Inheritance.*

Risk of Recurrence for Patient's Child:
  See Part I, *Mendelian Inheritance.*

Age of Detectability: At birth.

Gene Mapping and Linkage: Unknown.

Prevention: None known. Genetic counseling indicated.

Treatment: Early management of ocular conditions to promote normal visual development.

Prognosis: Guarded for vision. Severe short stature.

Detection of Carrier: Unknown.

References:
Pillay, VK: Ophthalmo-mandibulo-melic dysplasia: a hereditary syndrome. J Bone Joint Surg 1964; 46A:858–862.

KI021   **Jane D. Kivlin**

Ophthalmoarthropathy
  See ARTHRO-OPHTHALMOPATHY, HEREDITARY, PROGRESSIVE, STICKLER TYPE

OPHTHALMOPLEGIA EXTERNA-MYOPIA 0750

Includes:
  External ophthalmoplegia-myopia
  Myopia-external ophthalmoplegia

Excludes:
  Eyelid, ptosis, congenital (0834)
  Ocular myasthenia gravis
  Ophthalmoplegia, familial static (0751)
  Ophthalmoplegia, progressive external (0752)
  Ophthalmoplegia secondary to generalized myopathy or neuropathy

Major Diagnostic Criteria: Clinical diagnosis based upon limited mobility of extraocular muscles (external ophthalmoplegia) at birth and high myopia.

Clinical Findings: Although congenital, external ophthalmoplegia is difficult to detect in the newborn period; bilateral blepharoptosis is the most obvious sign. Ocular excursions are severely limited in all directions of gaze, vertical more than horizontal. High myopia is prevalent. The pupil is frequently eccentric. Examination of the fundi shows thinning of the choroid and retina, owing to high myopia.

Complications: The major ophthalmological complications are macular degeneration with visual loss and increased incidence of retinal detachment due to the high myopia. Some patients have strabismus. Moderate to severe blepharoptosis causes hyperextension of the neck which explains abnormal head posture and musculoskeletal strain.

Associated Findings: Systemic findings include absent knee and ankle jerks, spina bifida, scoliosis, dental malocclusion, cardiac defects, and hernia.

Etiology: X-linked recessive inheritance.

Pathogenesis: Thought to be due to dysgenesis of extraocular muscle, although mitochondrial cytopathies have not been excluded.

MIM No.: *31100

Sex Ratio: M1:F0

Occurrence: One pedigree from Argentina has been described (Salleras and Ortiz de Zarate, 1950) and reviewed again in a 15-year follow-up (Ortiz de Zarate, 1966).

Risk of Recurrence for Patient's Sib:
  See Part I, *Mendelian Inheritance.*

Risk of Recurrence for Patient's Child:
  See Part I, *Mendelian Inheritance.*

Age of Detectability: Soon after birth.

Gene Mapping and Linkage: OPEM (ophthalmoplegia, external, with myopia) has been provisionally mapped to X.

Prevention: None known. Genetic counseling indicated.

Treatment: Ptosis surgery is indicated for visual deprivation or chin-up head posture. Eye muscle surgery is not beneficial to those with their eyes aligned in primary position but, may be to those with strabismus or both eyes fixed in downgaze.

Prognosis: Life expectancy is dependent upon the severity of the associated findings.

Detection of Carrier: Female carriers have absent knee and ankle jerks.

References:
Salleras A, Ortiz de Zarate JC: Recessive sex-linked inheritance of external ophthalmoplegia and myopia coincident with other dysplasias. Br J Ophthalmol 1950; 34:662–667.
Ortiz de Zarate JC: Recessive sex-linked inheritance of congenital ophthalmoplegia and myopia coincident with other dysplasias: a reappraisal after 15 years. Br J Ophthalmol 1966; 50:606–607.

WE035   **Avery H. Weiss**

Ophthalmoplegia plus syndrome
See KEARNS-SAYRE DISEASE
also OPHTHALMOPLEGIA, PROGRESSIVE EXTERNAL
Ophthalmoplegia totalis
See OPHTHALMOPLEGIA, FAMILIAL STATIC
Ophthalmoplegia, chronic progressive external
See OPHTHALMOPLEGIA, PROGRESSIVE EXTERNAL
Ophthalmoplegia, congenital
See EYE, FIBROSIS OF THE EXTRAOCULAR MUSCLES,
GENERALIZED

OPHTHALMOPLEGIA, FAMILIAL STATIC   0751

Includes:
External ophthalmoplegia congenita
Ophthalmoplegia, hereditary congenital nonprogressive
Ophthalmoplegia totalis

Excludes:
Eye, fibrosis of the extraocular muscles, generalized (3185)
Ocular myasthenia gravis, congenital
Ophthalmoplegia externa-myopia (0750)
Ophthalmoplegia, progressive external (0752)
Ophthalmoplegia secondary to generalized myopathy or
neuropathy
Ophthalmoplegia, total with ptosis and miosis (0753)

Major Diagnostic Criteria: Clinical diagnosis based upon limited mobility of extraocular muscles (external ophthalmoplegia) from birth.

Clinical Findings: Congenital external ophthalmoplegia presents with bilateral ptosis and limitation of ocular excursions in all directions of gaze. Clinical variability is common. Ptosis is the only manifestation in some cases, while ptosis and complete external ophthalmoplegia are evident in others. Ocular alignment is usually normal in primary gaze due to the symmetrical involvement. Various abnormalities of the pupillary response are described; pupillary constriction to accomodative stimuli is sometimes decreased while the response to light stimuli is usually normal. Visual acuity is normal (except for those with strabismus amblyopia). Examination of the anterior and posterior segments is normal. Familial static ophthalmoplegia is one type of congenital external ophthalmoplegia, but there are other types with different associated manifestations and different patterns of inheritance. Also, the condition should be distinguished from *fibrosis of the extraocular muscles* (Harley, et al, 1978).

Complications: Bilateral ptosis, or hypodeviation of both eyes, causes compensatory hyperextension of the neck and musculoskeletal strain. Strabismus occurs in some cases. Amblyopia may complicate strabismus or severe ptosis in infancy.

Associated Findings: None known.

Etiology: Autosomal dominant inheritance with variable expression. Rarely, autosomal recessive inheritance.

Pathogenesis: A few histopathological studies have shown atrophy of muscle associated with variable amounts of fibrous tissue. Metabolic defects, such as mitochondrial cytopathies, have not been excluded.

MIM No.: *16500

Sex Ratio: M1:F1

Occurrence: Several kinships have been documented, including one Sicilian family.

Risk of Recurrence for Patient's Sib:
See Part I, *Mendelian Inheritance.*

Risk of Recurrence for Patient's Child:
See Part I, *Mendelian Inheritance.*

Age of Detectability: Soon after birth.

Gene Mapping and Linkage: Unknown.

Prevention: None known. Genetic counseling indicated.

Treatment: Surgical treatment of ptosis is indicated predominantly for abnormal head posture, and to prevent deprivation amblyopia in infant. Eye muscle surgery does not correct the limited ocular motility, and is recommended only for ocular misalignment (strabismus) or deviation of both eyes downwards in primary gaze.

Prognosis: Normal life span. Vision is usually normal.

Detection of Carrier: Examination of relatives for evidence of ptosis and external ophthalmoplegia.

References:
Holmes WJ: Hereditary congenital ophthalmoplegia. Am J Ophthalmol 1956; 28:23–30.
Lees F: Congenital static familial ophthalmoplegia. J Neurol Neurosurg Psych 1960; 23:46–51. *
Mace JW, et al.: Congenital hereditary nonprogressive external ophthalmoplegia. Am J Dis Child 1971; 122:261–263.
Harley RD, et al.: Congenital fibrosis of the extraocular muscles. J Pediat Ophthal 1978; 15:346–358.
Mollica F, et al.: Variabilite intrafamiliale de l'ophthalmologie externe congenitale: etude d'une famille sicilienne. J Hum Genet 1980; 28:23–30.

WE035   **Avery H. Weiss**

Ophthalmoplegia, hereditary congenital nonprogressive
See OPHTHALMOPLEGIA, FAMILIAL STATIC

OPHTHALMOPLEGIA, PROGRESSIVE EXTERNAL   0752

Includes:
Abiotrophic ophthalmoplegia externa
Extraocular muscular dystrophy, progressive
Mitochondrial cytopathy
Myopathic ophthalmoplegia externa
Oculo-cranio-somatic neuromuscular disease with ragged-red fibers
Ocular myopathy
Oculocraniosomatic syndrome
Ophthalmoplegia, chronic progressive external
Ophthalmoplegia-pigmentary dystrophy of retina-cardiomyopathy
Ophthalmoplegia plus syndrome
Ophthalmoplegia, progressive external, recessive
Ophthalmoplegia, progressive external, with ragged-red fibers

Excludes:
Abetalipoproteinemia (0002)
Diplegia, congenital facial (0376)
Eye, fibrosis of the extraocular muscles, generalized (3185)
Eyelid, ptosis, congenital (0834)
Kearns-Sayre disease (2070)
Muscular dystrophy, oculopharyngeal (0692)
Ocular myasthenia gravis
Ophthalmoplegia externa-myopia (0750)
Ophthalmoplegia, familial static (0751)
Ophthalmoplegia secondary to generalized myopathy or
neuropathy
Ophthalmoplegia secondary to thyroid disease
Ophthalmoplegia, total with ptosis and miosis (0753)
Phytanic acid storage disease (0810)

Major Diagnostic Criteria: Differentiation from other causes of ptosis and ophthalmoplegia is necessary. Myasthenia gravis is diagnosed by a characteristic response to anticholinesterases or the presence of antiacetylcholine receptor antibody. Ptosis also occurs with sympathetic lesions (see **Horner syndrome**), oculomotor nerve lesions, and after head trauma; but these causes are seldom confused with progressive external ophthalmoplegia.

Isolated ptosis does occur. Such cases are not considered *formes frustes* of progressive external ophthalmoplegia. **Muscular dystrophy, oculopharyngeal** presents with bilateral ptosis, which does not usually involve eye movement disorders, and swallowing difficulties; it is most prevalent among elderly French-Canadians. Rarely, ophthalmoplegia occurs with other neuromuscular diseases (Type I muscle fiber hypotrophy and central nuclei, myotonic atrophy, and even isolated case reports of polymyositis and **Spinal muscular atrophy**).

The presence of characteristic abnormalities on skeletal muscle biopsy strongly supports the diagnosis. These consist of accumulations of abnormal mitochondria subsarcolemmally, and lipids diffusely, in histochemical Type I muscle fibers. On light microscopy, after modified Masson trichrome staining, these are described as ragged-red fibers. By electron microscopy, the mitochondria have whorled lamellae, paracrystalline inclusions, and are of abnormal size. The mitochondrial abnormalities are also found in the liver, sweat glands, and brain. Ocular muscle biopsies are more difficult to interpret, since some ragged-red fibers are a normal constituent. Rarely, otherwise typical cases of progressive external ophthalmoplegia lacking ragged-red fibers on skeletal muscle biopsy are reported. Autopsied cases of progressive external ophthalmoplegia have shown both normal ocular motor nuclei and a spongiform encephalopathy.

Clinical Findings: A bilateral, often asymmetrical, ptosis presents at any age. This is followed by the insidious, usually asymptomatic, onset of ophthalmoplegia. Downward gaze may be relatively spared as compared to lateral and upward gaze. Before the ophthalmoplegia becomes complete, normally rapid eye movements are slowed. Orbicularis weakness is regularly associated; pupillary reactions remain normal in most cases.

Complications: Visual difficulties occur when the ptosis occludes the pupillary axis. Affected individuals often develop a chin elevation-backward head tilt in an attempt to compensate. The most serious complications of progressive external ophthalmoplegia arise from its associated disorders.

Associated Findings: Progressive external ophthalmoplegia has been reported with endocrine abnormalities (diabetes mellitus, hypoparathyroidism, thyroid disease, hyperaldosteronism, and hypogonadism), other neuromuscular abnormalities (small stature, weakness, intellectual deterioration, ataxia, spasticity, retinal degeneration, abnormal electroencephalogram, and increased cerebrospinal fluid protein), and cardiac defects (heart block, Wolff-Parkinson-White syndrome, cardiomyopathy).

Considerable debate has centered around whether particular combinations of these numerous associations represent separable nosological entities. The combination of heart block, retinal pigmentary degeneration and progressive external ophthalmoplegia is referred to as the **Kearns-Sayre disease**. A familial ophthalmoplegia with ataxia and amyotrophy is sometimes called the *Stephens syndrome* (see **Kearns-Sayre disease**). A variant of progressive external ophthalmoplegia occurs in **Abetalipoproteinemia** (*Bassen-Kornsweig*).

Etiology: Possibly autosomal dominant inheritance, or rarely autosomal recessive inheritance.

Pathogenesis: A history of meningitis-encephalitis in sporadically occurring cases of the **Kearns-Sayre disease** variant, and the similarity of the central nervous system pathology to the spongiform encephalopathy of *Creutzfeldt-Jacob disease* has led some authors to suggest the possibility of a slow virus infection, but this is unsupported by animal inoculations. Whitaker et al (1987), upon restudy of the pituitary from one of Kearns and Sayre's cases, concluded that the patient actually had **Laurence-Moon syndrome**.

There is a disagreement as to whether the ophthalmoplegia is primarily neurogenic or myogenic in origin. The regular association of neuropathological alterations argues for the former; the experimental production of morphological changes resembling ragged-red fibers in animal muscle perfused with metabolic poisons may support the latter.

MIM No.: 16510, 16513, 25845

Sex Ratio: M1:F1

Occurrence: About 30 kinships documented in the literature.

Risk of Recurrence for Patient's Sib:
See Part I, *Mendelian Inheritance*.

Risk of Recurrence for Patient's Child:
See Part I, *Mendelian Inheritance*.

Age of Detectability: Infancy to old age; most commonly in second decade of life.

Gene Mapping and Linkage: Unknown.

Prevention: None known. Genetic counseling indicated.

Treatment: Surgical treatment of strabismus is rarely indicated. Ptosis surgery should be approached with great caution because of the risk of exposure keratitis postoperatively. Ptosis crutch spectacles are occasionally tolerated.

Treatment of the associated disorders is important. Several cases of sudden death in patients with cardiac conduction defects are reported; pacemaker insertion is indicated when heart block is present. Death from hyperglycemic acidotic coma has been reported following administration of oral prednisone. Early studies of metabolic therapy with coenzyme Q_{10} have been promising, with improvement of EKG abnormalities and neurologic symptoms.

Prognosis: Progressive external ophthalmoplegia is compatible with a normal lifespan. In patients with retinal pigmentary degeneration, the visual prognosis is better than in the usual **Retinitis pigmentosa**. Children with the **Kearns-Sayre disease** variant have a poor prognosis, with progression of weakness, intellectual deterioration, visual loss, and death from cardiac complications or intercurrent infection.

Detection of Carrier: Unknown.

References:
Drachman DA: Ophthalmoplegia plus: the neurodegenerative disorders associated with progressive external ophthalmoplegia. Arch Neurol 1968; 18:654–674.
Daroff RB: Chronic progressive external ophthalmoplegia. Arch Ophthalmol 1969; 82:845–851.
Butler IJ, Gadoth N: Kearns-Sayre syndrome: a review of a multisystem disorder of children and young adults. Arch Intern Med 1976; 136:1290–1293.
Berenberg RA, et al.: Lumping or splitting? Ophthalmoplegia plus or Kearns-Sayre syndrome. Ann Neurol 1977; 1:37–54.
Ringel SP, et al.: Extraocular muscle biopsy in chronic progressive external ophthalmoplegia. Ann Neurol 1979; 6:326–341.
Eagle RC, Jr., et al.: The atypical pigmentary retinopathy of Kearns-Sayre: a light and electron microscope study. Ophthalmology 1982; 89:1433–1440.
Egger J, Wilson J: Mitochondrial inheritance in a mitochondrially mediated disease. New Engl J Med 1983; 309:142–146.
Mitsumoto H, et al.: Chronic progressive external ophthalmoplegia: clinical, morphologic, and biochemical studies. Neurology 1983; 33:452–461.
Ogasahara S, et al.: Improvement of abnormal pyruvate metabolism and cardiac conduction defect with coenzyme Q(10) in Kearns-Sayre syndrome. Neurology 1985; 35:372–377.
Whitaker MD, et al.: The pituitary gland in the Lawrence-Moon syndrome. Mayo Clin Proc 1987; 62:216–222.

DE034
BE026

Monte A. Del Monte
Donald R. Bergsma

Ophthalmoplegia, progressive external, recessive
See OPHTHALMOPLEGIA, PROGRESSIVE EXTERNAL
Ophthalmoplegia, progressive external, with ragged-red fibers
See OPHTHALMOPLEGIA, PROGRESSIVE EXTERNAL

OPHTHALMOPLEGIA, TOTAL WITH PTOSIS AND MIOSIS 0753

Includes: Ptosis and miosis with ophthalmoplegia totalis

Excludes:
Eyelid, ptosis, congenital (0834)
Ocular myasthenia gravis, congenital
Ophthalmoplegia externa-myopia (0750)
Ophthalmoplegia, familial static (0751)
Ophthalmoplegia, progressive external (0752)
Ophthalmoplegia secondary to generalized myopathy or neuropathy

Major Diagnostic Criteria: Clinical diagnosis based upon the presence of external and internal ophthalmoplegia (total ophthalmoplegia), blepharoptosis, and pupillary miosis.

Clinical Findings: Bilateral blepharoptosis and limitation of ocular movement in all directions of gaze (external ophthalmoplegia) are noted soon after birth. Pupillary miosis is present. Pupillary constriction in response to light and accomodative stimuli are decreased (internal ophthalmoplegia). Visual acuity and examination of the anterior and posterior segments are normal.

Complications: Blepharoptosis causes affected patients to hyperextend the neck, leading to abnormal head posture and musculoskeletal strain. Strabismus and deprivation amblyopia can occur in infants.

Associated Findings: None known.

Etiology: Autosomal recessive inheritance.

Pathogenesis: Congenital ophthalmoplegias are thought to be due to dysgenesis of extraocular muscle, although metabolic disorders, such as mitochondrial cytopathies, have not been excluded.

MIM No.: *25840

Sex Ratio: M1:F1

Occurrence: Two families have been described.

Risk of Recurrence for Patient's Sib:
See Part I, *Mendelian Inheritance.*

Risk of Recurrence for Patient's Child:
See Part I, *Mendelian Inheritance.*

Age of Detectability: Clinically evident in infancy.

Gene Mapping and Linkage: Unknown.

Prevention: None known. Genetic counseling indicated.

Treatment: Ptosis surgery is indicated when upper eyelid obstructs visual axis and induces chin-up head posture. Eye muscle surgery is not beneficial to those with eyes aligned in the primary position, but may be beneficial to those with strabismus, or those with both eyes fixed in downgaze.

Prognosis: Normal life span.

Detection of Carrier: Examination of relatives for evidence of the trait.

References:
Francois J: Heredity in ophthalmology. St Louis: C.V. Mosby, 1961:242 only.
Waardenberg PJ: Genetics and ophthalmology, vol 2. Springfield: Charles C Thomas, 1963:78 only.

WE035 **Avery H. Weiss**

Ophthalmoplegia-intestinal pseudo-obstruction
See MUSCULAR DYSTROPHY, OCULO-GASTROINTESTINAL
Ophthalmoplegia-pigmentary degeneration of retina-cardiomyopathy
See KEARNS-SAYRE DISEASE
Ophthalmoplegia-pigmentary dystrophy of retina-cardiomyopathy
See OPHTHALMOPLEGIA, PROGRESSIVE EXTERNAL
Ophthalmoplegic migraine
See MIGRAINE
Opitz G-syndrome
See G SYNDROME
Opitz oculo-genital-laryngeal syndrome
See HYPERTELORISM-HYPOSPADIAS SYNDROME
Opitz oculo-genito-laryngeal syndrome
See G SYNDROME
Opitz trigonocephaly syndrome
See C SYNDROME
Opitz-Frias syndrome
See G SYNDROME
Opitz-Kaveggia FG syndrome
See FG SYNDROME, OPITZ-KAVEGGIA TYPE
Opitz-Pallister-Herrmann syndrome
See HERRMANN-PALLISTER-OPITZ SYNDROME

OPSISMODYSPLASIA 2240

Includes:
Chondrodysplasia secondary to chondroosseous transformation defect
Skeletal dysplasia, opsismodysplasia

Excludes:
Achondroplasia (0010)
Asphyxiating thoracic dysplasia (0091)
Spondyloepiphyseal dysplasia congenita (0897)

Major Diagnostic Criteria: Micromelia, very retarded bone maturation, marked shortness of the bones of the hands and feet, concave metaphyses, and thin lamellar vertebral bodies.

Clinical Findings: Opsismodysplasia is recognized at birth on the basis of micromelia and facial abnormalities. Hands and feet are notably short and stocky with clubby fingers. Hypotonia is striking. The craniofacial morphology is characterized by frontal bossing, large fontanelles, and short nose, with a flattened root contrasting with the length of the upper lip. The upper part of the auricle deviates outward and the helix pattern is abnormal.

On X-ray, the retardation in ossification is very striking. The height of the vertebral bodies is very much reduced. The iliac bones have a square appearance. The diaphyses of the long bones are short, and the metaphyses are irregular and enlarged. The

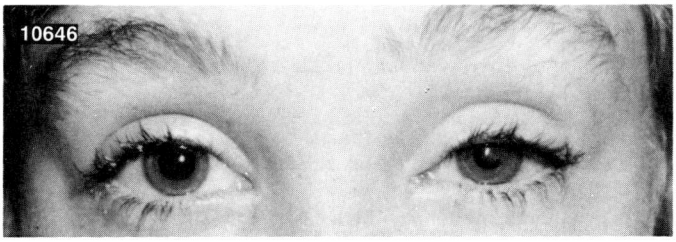

0753-10646: Ptosis and miosis OS; acute ulcer of the left cornea produces haziness.

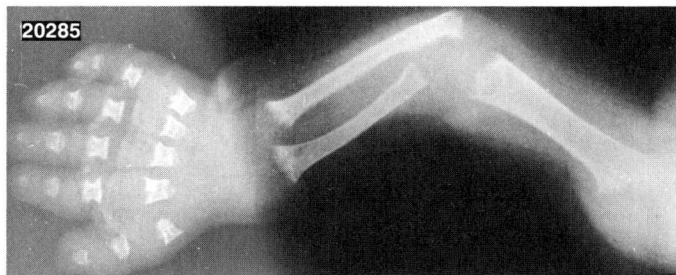

2240-20285: Opsismodysplasia, hand and arm X-ray of a 15-month-old male; note short hand bones with cup-shaped deformation of the metaphyses and retarded ossification.

appearance of the hand bones is typical and their extreme short-ness is associated with a cup-shaped deformation of the epiphy-seal and nonepiphyseal ends of the metaphyses.

Complications: Severe dwarfism and a particular susceptibility to respiratory infections. Most patients died in the first three years of life.

Associated Findings: None known.

Etiology: Autosomal recessive inheritance.

Pathogenesis: The most striking abnormality of the growth cartilage is the wide and irregular hypertrophic zone. This pro-vides a strong immunologic reaction for type I collagen, which is shown by gel electrophoresis analysis. It may be that the abnormal calcification and bone induction observed in these patients result because cells secreted predominantly type I collagen instead of type II.

MIM No.: 25848

POS No.: 3649

Sex Ratio: Presumably M1:F1.

Occurrence: Less than a dozen cases have been reported.

Risk of Recurrence for Patient's Sib:
See Part I, *Mendelian Inheritance.*

Risk of Recurrence for Patient's Child:
See Part I, *Mendelian Inheritance.* Few affected individuals sur-vive to reproduce.

Age of Detectability: In the newborn period, by X-ray study.

Gene Mapping and Linkage: Unknown.

Prevention: None known. Genetic counseling indicated.

Treatment: Treatment of respiratory infection or distress.

Prognosis: Usually fatal during infancy.

Detection of Carrier: Unknown.

References:
Zonana J, et al.: A unique chondrodysplasia secondary to a defect in chondroosseous transformation. BD:OAS XIII(3D). New York: March of Dimes Birth Defects Foundation, 1973:155–163.
Maroteaux P, et al.: Opsismodysplasia: a new type of chondrodyspla-sia with predominant involvement of the bones of the hand and the vertebrae. Am J Med Genet 1984; 19:171–182. *

MA034   **Pierre Maroteaux**

OPTIC ATROPHY, INFANTILE HEREDOFAMILIAL   0755

Includes:
Atrophy, optic
Behr syndrome (complicated optic atrophy)

Excludes:
Optic atrophy, Kjer type (3069)
Optic atrophy, Leber type (0579)
Optic atrophy of metabolic, degenerative, and demyelinating causes
Optic atrophy of inflammatory and toxic causes
Optic nerve anomalies, congenital

Major Diagnostic Criteria: Hereditary optic atrophy may occur with or without associated neurologic or systemic signs. Inheri-tance pattern and degree of visual impairment vary.

Clinical Findings: The recessive type of congenital optic atrophy is extremely rare. Profound visual loss, occurring early in life, causes nystagmus and allows detection during the first year of life. Visual loss is stationary without associated neurologic or systemic signs. Dominant optic atrophy is the most common hereditary form. Visual acuity ranges between 20/30 and 20/200, pallor is often limited to the temporal segment of the nerve, and the color defect is blue-yellow rather than red-green. Visual field defects are central or paracentral and nystagmus is typically absent. Usually presents between 1–8 years of age with no associated neurologic or systemic signs. Mental retardation and

sensorineural hearing loss can occur (see, also, **Optic atrophy, Kjer type**).

Because the normal newborn optic nerve is often pale, fundus examination is suboptimal, and it is difficult to diagnose optic atrophy within the first year of life. Anomalous optic nerve development, ocular albinism, and congenital cone-rod dysfunc-tion, are more common causes of visual loss and nystagmus in this age group and need to be carefully excluded by detailed ocular examination and visual electro-physiologic testing (electroretino-gram, visual evoked response).

Complications: Visual acuity reduction and loss of visual field. Neurologic and systemic complications vary with the associated conditions.

Associated Findings: Hereditary optic atrophy can be associated with a variety of neurologic or systemic signs, including congen-ital deafness, **Diabetes (insipidus/mellitus)-optic atrophy-deafness** (DIDMOAD), **Ataxia, Friedreich type**, Marie's ataxia, Charcot-Marie-Tooth disease, or various combinations of pyramidal tract signs, mental retardation, urinary incontinence, and pes cavus (Behr syndrome).

Etiology: Possibly autosomal recessive inheritance.

Pathogenesis: Undetermined. Muscle biopsy material has dis-closed extensive collections of "cylindrical spiral structures" like myelin figures or onion-skin lesions.

MIM No.: 21000

Sex Ratio: Presumably M1:F1

Occurrence: Several kinships documented in a literature which extends back to the turn of the century.

Risk of Recurrence for Patient's Sib:
See Part I, *Mendelian Inheritance.*

Risk of Recurrence for Patient's Child:
See Part I, *Mendelian Inheritance.*

Age of Detectability: At birth, or in the first decade of life.

Gene Mapping and Linkage: Unknown.

Prevention: None known. Genetic counseling indicated.

Treatment: Appropriate vision aids

Prognosis: Vision is in the range of 20/200.

Detection of Carrier: Clinical examination of first degree rela-tives.

References:
Glaser J: Heredofamilial disorders of the optic nerve. In: Goldberg M, ed: Genetic and metabolic eye disease. Boston: Little, Brown, 1974.
Hoyt CS: Autosomal dominant optic atrophy: a spectrum of disability. Ophthalmology 1980; 87:245–251.
Miller, et al.: Clinical neuro-ophthalmology, vol. 1: The hereditary optic neuropathies. Baltimore: Williams & Wilkins, 1982.
Thomas PK, et al.: Behr's syndrome: a family exhibiting pseudodom-inant inheritance. J Neurol Sc 1984; 64:137–148.

WE035   **Avery H. Weiss**

Optic atrophy, juvenile (infantile), dominant
See OPTIC ATROPHY, KJER TYPE

OPTIC ATROPHY, KJER TYPE   3069

Includes:
Kjer optic atrophy
Optic atrophy, juvenile (infantile), dominant

Excludes:
Deafness-optic nerve atrophy, progressive (0253)
Diabetes (insipidus/mellitus)-optic atrophy-deafness (0550)
Optic atrophy, infantile heredofamilial (0755)
Optic atrophy, Leber type (0579)

Major Diagnostic Criteria: Bilateral visual loss with insidious onset usually appears before ten years of age. Central or cecen-tral scotomata are present on visual field testing. Tritan dyschro-matopsia or severe generalized dyschromatopsia including blue-yellow axes is typical. Temporal optic disk pallor is evident in every patient. Visual evoked responses may be reduced in amplitude and have a prolonged latency even in the presence of good visual acuity.

Clinical Findings: Clinical onset is often undefinable and symptoms can be present as early as age two years; the majority of patients are affected by age twenty years. Visual loss is slowly progressive with visual acuities, even in adulthood, varying widely from 20/25 to less than 20/400. Visual loss is bilateral but may be asymmetric. Both interfamilial and intrafamilial variation in acuity and attendant dyschromatopsia have been reported.

A characteristic central or cecocentral scotoma of variable density is present on visual field testing. Other visual field abnormalities include paracentral scotomas, pericecal enlargement, and depression of isopters in the temporal field, simulating bitemporal hemianopsia, although generally the peripheral field is intact. A tritan color defect is characteristic, at times coexisting with a non-specific red-green dyschromatopsia. Neither the severity or the type of dyschromatopsia necessarily relate directly to either visual acuity or duration of disease. Ophthalmoscopically, temporal optic pallor is evident, with neuroretinal rim defects visible on monochromatic examination, which appear to be characteristic (although not unique) of this disease.

The nasal three-fourths of the optic nerve is either uninvolved, or diffusely pale, but invariably less severely affected than the papillomacular nerve fiber bundle insertion. Pupillary light reflexes may be slightly diminished with reduced visual acuity and paradoxical pupils (constriction to an "off" response) have been documented. Electroretinography and dark adaptation studies are normal. Nystagmus is only rarely present, eg, when acuity is extremely poor and early in life. Neurologic examinations are normal.

Complications: Reduced visual acuity to levels ranging from 20/25 to less or equal to 20/400. Various color vision defects, always including the tritan axis.

Associated Findings: None known.

Etiology: Autosomal dominant inheritance with almost complete penetrance but variable expressivity.

Pathogenesis: The optic atrophy in this disease appears to be due to a primary degeneration of the ganglion cell layer in the retina with ascending optic atrophy. Histopathology has shown atrophy of the retinal ganglion cell layer and gliosis of the optic nerve. The optic nerves, optic chiasm, and optic tracts show an increased content of collagen tissue and a decreased number of neurofibrils and myelin sheaths. In the lateral geniculate body, extensive loss of ganglion cells has been seen. There are no changes in the calcarine cortex.

MIM No.: *16550

Sex Ratio: M1:F1

Occurrence: Undetermined. Several large kindreds have been reported; some 200 cases examined by Kjer alone.

Risk of Recurrence for Patient's Sib:
See Part I, *Mendelian Inheritance.*

Risk of Recurrence for Patient's Child:
See Part I, *Mendelian Inheritance.*

Age of Detectability: During the first decade of life in severe cases. Some mildly expressed individual may escape detection until adulthood, when a severely affected sibling or offspring mandates complete family screening. No congenital case has been documented.

Gene Mapping and Linkage: OPA1 (optic atrophy (autosomal dominant)) is unassigned.

One gene for this disease may be located on chromosome 2 (linkage with Kidd blood group, lod score 2.0 at 0 = 0.18) (Kivlin et al., 1984).

Prevention: None known. Genetic counseling indicated.

Treatment: Unknown.

Prognosis: The overall prognosis is unpredictable with final visual acuity ranging from 20/25 to 20/400. None of the 200

individuals examined by Kjer had vision reduced to hand motions or light perception levels.

Detection of Carrier: Prolonged latency of visual evoked responses precedes visual loss and theoretically may be used to detect affected individuals. Careful ophthalmoscopy and standardized color screening is probably more efficient.

Special Considerations: The differential diagnosis of Kjer optic atrophy includes other entitites presenting with insidious reduction of visual acuity and central or cecocentral scotomas, such as nutritional amblyopia, toxic optic neuropathy, demyelinating disease, mistaken oversight of hereditary macular dystrophies, and other hereditary optic atrophies. The separation of Kjer optic atrophy from other hereditary atrophies should be based on detailed family history, careful examination of family members, clinical presentation and course, color-vision testing, and absence of neurosensory hearing impairment.

References:

Kjer P: Infantile optic atrophy with dominant mode of inheritance: a clinical and genetic study of 29 Danish families. Acta Ophthalmol (suppl) 1959; 54:1–146. *

Kline LB, Glaser JS: Dominant optic atrophy: the clinical profile. Arch Ophthalmol 1979; 97:1680–1686. *

Kjer et al.: Histopathology of eye, optic nerve and brain in a case of dominant optic atrophy. Acta Ophthalmol 1983; 61:300–312.

Kivlin JD, et al.: Optic atrophy possibly linked to the Kidd blood group locus. (Abstract) Cytogenet Cell Genet 1984; 37:512 only.

CH042   **Georgia A. Chrousos**
TR009   **Elias I. Traboulsi**

OPTIC ATROPHY, LEBER TYPE   0579

Includes:
Leber optic atrophy
Neuroretinopathy, optic Leber type

Excludes:
Optic atrophy, infantile heredofamilial (0755)
Retina, amaurosis congenita, Leber type (0043)

Major Diagnostic Criteria: Central visual loss, optic atrophy.

Clinical Findings: Sudden loss of central vision occurs in the second and third decades of life. The loss of central vision, which is usually bilateral, progresses rapidly. Elevation of the optic disk and swelling of nerve fiber bundles may be observed. Headaches may accompany the onset of visual loss. Progressive optic atrophy ensues, leaving a flat pale disk. The visual fields show large dense central scotomas.

Complications: Unknown.

Associated Findings: None known.

Etiology: The disorder, with male preponderance, has been considered X-linked recessive, but does not conform to rigid Mendelian rules. There is absence of transmission through males, and passage occurs from the female to most of her offspring.

Pathogenesis: Older theories included: an infective agent, especially a slow virus; failure to detoxify cyanide; and opticochiasmatic arachnoidal adhesions. Recently, however, Wallace et al. (1988) discovered a characteristic mitochondrial DNA mutation that encodes a histidine instead of an arginine in a respiratory protein.

MIM No.: 30890

Sex Ratio: Undetermined; 84.8% of European cases, but only 59.1% of Japanese cases, are male.

Occurrence: Undetermined; extensive literature.

Risk of Recurrence for Patient's Sib: Maternal transmission.

Risk of Recurrence for Patient's Child: Maternal transmission.

Age of Detectability: Typically in the late teens to middle 20s, but the range is from 5–65 years.

Gene Mapping and Linkage: Unknown.

Prevention: None known. Genetic counseling indicated.

Treatment: Unconfirmed approaches include the use of hydroxycobalamin, and lysis of opticochiasmatic arachnoidal adhesions. Metabolic therapies that increase cellular respiratory metabolism have been proposed.

Prognosis: Progressive visual loss.

Detection of Carrier: Neuro-ophthalmologic testing has revealed abnormalities of color discrimination in asymptomatic individuals thought to be at risk by pedigree analysis.

References:

Livingstone IR, et al.: Leber's optic neuropathy: clinical and visual evoked response studies in asymptomatic and symptomatic members of a 4-generation family. Br J Ophthalmol 1980; 64:751–757.

Nikoskelainen E, et al.: Ophthalmoscopic findings in Leber's hereditary optic neuropathy. Arch Ophthalmol 1983; 101:1059–1068.

Nikoskelainen E: New aspects of genetic etiology and the clinical puzzle of Leber's disease. Neurology 1984; 34:1482–1484.

Novotny EJ, Jr., et al.: Leber's disease and dystonia: a mitochondrial disease. Neurology 1986; 36:1053–1060.

Nikoskelainen EK, et al.: Leber's hereditary optic neuroretinopathy, a maternally inherited disease: a genealogic study in four pedigrees. Arch Ophthal 1987; 105:665–671.

Wallace DC, et al.: Mitochondrial DNA mutation associated with Leber's hereditary optic neuropathy. Science 1988; 242:1427–1430.

CH034

Philip F. Chance
Morton E. Smith

Optic atrophy-deafness, progressive
See DEAFNESS-OPTIC NERVE ATROPHY, PROGRESSIVE
Optic atrophy-juvenile diabetes-deafness
See DIABETES (INSIPIDUS/MELLITUS)-OPTIC ATROPHY-DEAFNESS
Optic atrophy-nerve deafness-distal neurogenic amyotrophy
See DEAFNESS-POLYNEUROPATHY-OPTIC ATROPHY

OPTIC DISK, MORNING GLORY ANOMALY 3158

Includes:
  Handmann disk anomaly
  Morning glory disk anomaly

Excludes:
  Optic disk pits (0756)
  Uveoretinal coloboma, typical

Major Diagnostic Criteria: An excavated, funnel-shaped but anomalously large optic nerve head with white glial elements at its center, surrounded by a variably pigmented and elevated annulus of subretinal tissues.

Clinical Findings: Strabismus, especially exotropia, is the presenting sign in 40–50% of cases, usually in the first two years of life. Poor vision in the affected eye leads to the detection of older patients. Occasionally a white or altered pupillary reflex from the enlarged optic nerve leads to eye examination and diagnosis.

Ophthalmoscopic findings vary with the degree of dysplasia, excavation, central glial proliferation, sheathing of retinal vessels, pigmentation of the surrounding annulus, and neuroretinal dysplasia. Visual acuity ranges from 20/100 to poor light perception, although rarely good visual acuity has been reported.

Complications: Poor visual acuity probably results from dysplasia of both the neural retina and the optic nerve. Strabismic amblyopia also contributes. Retinal detachment occurs in one-third of reported cases and is thought to be due to cerebrospinal fluid leakage into the subretinal space via a communication through either an anomalous nerve or its dural sheaths. Results of surgical repair of retinal detachment are poor.

Associated Findings: Common ocular findings in the same eye include retinal detachment, strabismus, hyaloid remnants, and **Retinal dysplasia**. Rare findings include **Cataracts**, epiretinal membranes, ciliary body cysts, vitreous cysts, pupillary membrane remnants, microphthalmos (see **Eye, microphthalmia/coloboma**), and rarely **Aniridia**.

Rare associations in the fellow eye are retinal vascular tortuos-

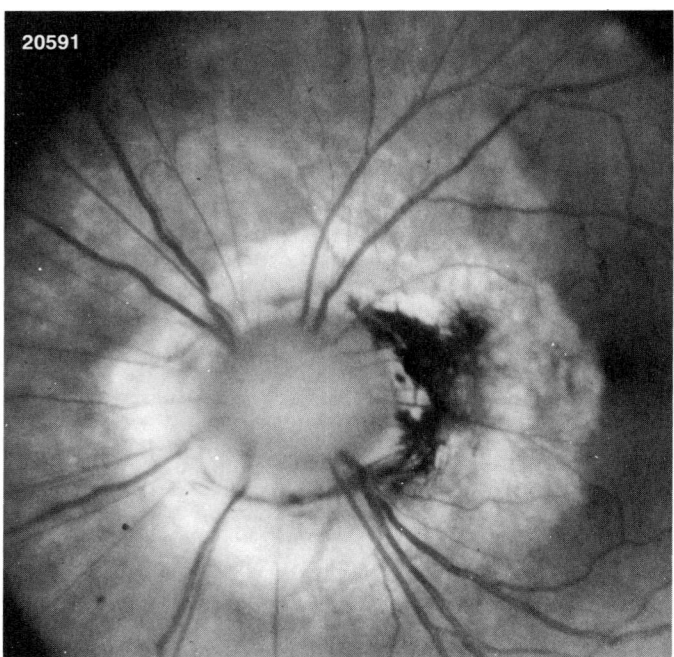

20591

3158-20591: Classical "morning glory" configuration of optic nerve head. Note enlarged excavated nerve head, central patch of gliotic tissue and peripapillary pigmented annulus. Retinal vessels, derived from central retinal artery, leave disk at its edge and run a straight course to the periphery of the fundus.

ity, **Optic disk pits**, microphthalmos, **Eye, anterior segment dysgenesis**, **Eye, Duane retraction syndrome**, and persistent pupillary membrane remnants. Various craniofacial anomalies include **Eye, hypertelorism**, basal (and other) **Encephalocele**, **Corpus callosum agenesis**, and **Cleft lip** and/or **Cleft palate** (occasionally occult).

Etiology: Unknown.

Pathogenesis: Defective formation of posterior sclera and lamina cribrosa with herniation of disk tissue and cone formation. Neuroectodermal layers in the area may be secondarily involved. Hyaloid system may fail to resolve completely resulting in presence of remnants at the center of the disk. The findings of an optic pit in the fellow eye of two unrelated patients in the literature, and the similar mechanism of retinal detachment in both anomalies suggest that these two malformations may share common pathogenetic mechanisms. The association with various midline brain and craniofacial defects suggests an early embryologic defect in fusion.

CDC No.: 743.520

Sex Ratio: M1:F1. Some authors have suggested a slight female predominance.

Occurrence: More than 70 cases have been reported in the literature.

Risk of Recurrence for Patient's Sib: Isolated defect; recurrence risk not increased.

Risk of Recurrence for Patient's Child: Presumbably not increased.

Age of Detectability: During infancy or early childhood. Occasionally cases may go undetected until adulthood.

Gene Mapping and Linkage: Unknown.

Prevention: None known. Genetic counseling indicated.

Treatment: Correction of strabismus for cosmesis. Amblyopia therapy is generally unrewarding. Surgical treatment of associated retinal detachment is usually unsatisfactory, however successful reattachment has been reported. Spontaneous reattachment has also occurred.

Prognosis: Most reported patients have had poor visual outcomes. This should not preclude all efforts toward amblyopia therapy and retinal reattachment surgery.

Detection of Carrier: Unknown.

Special Considerations: Consider this diagnosis in infants presenting with total retinal detachment. Midline cranial defects, especially basal encephaloceles should be sought with non-invasive scanning; nasal masses have been biopsied and found to contain brain tissue.

References:

Handman M: Erbliche, vermutlich angeborene zentrale gliose Entartunk des Sehnerven mit besonderer Beteilgung der Zentralgefasse. Klin Monatsbl Augenheilkd 1929; 83:145–152.

Kindler P: Morning glory syndrome: unusual congenital optic disk anomaly. Am J Ophthalmol 1970; 69:376–384.

Steinkuller PG: The morning glory disk anomaly: case report and literature review. J Pediatr Ophthalmol Strabismus 1980; 17:81–87.

Koenig SB, et al.: The morning glory syndrome associated with sphenoidal encephalocele. Ophthalmology 1982; 89:1368–1373.

Dempster AG, et al.: The "morning glory syndrome": a mesodermal defect? Ophthalmologica 1983; 187:222–230.

Chang S, et al.: Treatment of total retinal detachment in morning glory syndrome. Am J Ophthalmol 1984; 97:596–600.

Traboulsi EI, O'Neill JF: The spectrum in the morphology of the so-called "morning glory disc anomaly". J Pediatr Ophthalmol Strabism 1988; 25:93–98. †

TR009   **Elias I. Traboulsi**

Optic disk holes
See OPTIC DISK PITS

OPTIC DISK PITS   0756

Includes:
> Kranenburg syndrome
> Optic disk, crater-like cavities in
> Optic disk holes

Excludes:
> Ocular colobomas
> **Optic nerve hypoplasia** (0758)

Major Diagnostic Criteria: Sharp-edged pits in the optic disk.

Clinical Findings: The pits occur typically as oval depressions in the optic disk. They are usually one-eighth to one disk diameter in size, with sharp edges and of varying depth (approximately 1.5–20 diopters; average 2–7 diopters). They usually occur in the lower temporal quadrant of the disk; the floor may be covered with a soft gray tissue or may be heavily pigmented. The pits are single and unilateral in the majority (95%) of cases, but bilateral pits and multiple pits in the same disk do occur. The pit may have a partial or total overlying membrane, obscuring view of its true dimensions. The arrangement of the retinal vessels is usually not disturbed, but, in some cases, branches of the central retinal vessels or opticociliary veins descend into it and occasionally cilioretinal arteries emerge from it.

Symptoms may be absent, but frequently there is enlargement of the blind spot or sector defects in the visual field. If the maculopapillary bundle is involved, acuity may be diminished and a partial or complete paracentral or central scotoma may be present. In about 30% of these cases, associated fluid accumulation in the macula and serous detachment of the sensory retina is observed. The fluid appears to originate from either the cerebrospinal fluid or vitreous and passes from the nervehead to the macula.

Complications: *Developmental:* true colobomas of the optic disk, retina, or choroid; abnormalities of the retinal vasculature; peripapillary subretinal neovascularization.
Secondary: serous macular detachment, now believed to be due

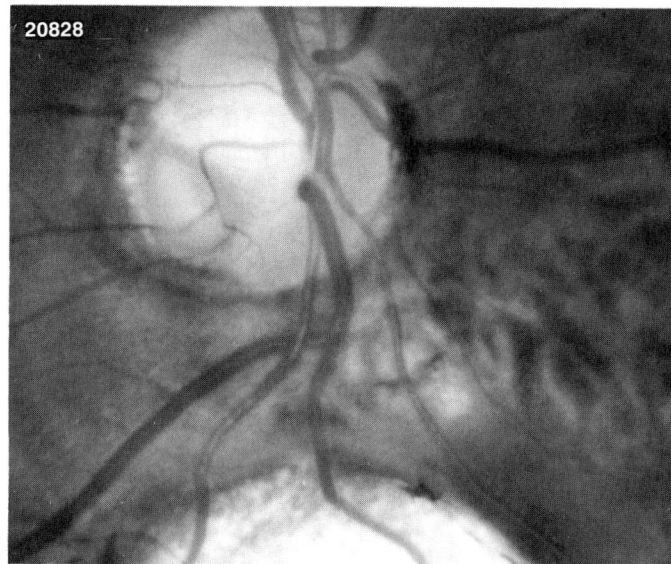

0756-20828: Optic disk pit with coloboma of retina and choroid.

---

to Schisis-like separation of the internal retinal layers and secondary macular detachment after formation of the outer layer macular hole (Lincoff et al, 1988).

Associated Findings: None known.

Etiology: Unknown.

Pathogenesis: A developmental defect of the optic nerve head. During differentiation of the primitive epithelial papilla, the pluripotential neuroepithelial cells of the walls of the optic vesicle may form atypical transparent retinal tissue instead of neuroglial supporting tissue at about the 15-mm stage. Some investigators believe that optic disk pits may represent atypical colobomas secondary to incomplete fusion of the embryonic fissure (the opening along the inferior aspect of the optic cup and optic stalk).

CDC No.: 743.520

Sex Ratio: M1:F1

Occurrence: Undetermined.

Risk of Recurrence for Patient's Sib: Unknown.

Risk of Recurrence for Patient's Child: Unknown.

Age of Detectability: The pit in the optic nerve is present at birth, but the related macular lesion occurs later, usually during the second or third decade of life.

Gene Mapping and Linkage: Unknown.

Prevention: None known. Genetic counseling indicated.

Treatment: The use of photocoagulation to the temporal margin of the optic disk adjacent to the pits remains controversial, but appears to speed resorption of subretinal fluid in some cases. This form of treatment may result in visual field defects and, therefore, is considered only after a significant delay, when there has been ample opportunity for spontaneous resorption.

Prognosis: Good, except in cases with secondary degenerative macular lesions, in which central acuity is lost. In a relatively large series of cases, the vision was good in 40% of cases, diminished but useful in 35%, and seriously diminished in 25%. Some investigators believe that photocoagulation can positively alter the long-term prognosis of this disease.

Detection of Carrier: Unknown.

Special Considerations: An acquired form may exist, and enlargement of pits has been noted; however, these observations are probably secondary to movement, thinning, or loss of an overlying glial veil that previously obscured visualization of the pit.

This condition has been confused with low-tension glaucoma and other causes of optic atrophy, especially when associated visual field defects exist. Careful stereoscopic ophthalmoscopy should allow this differentiation.

There is a rare association between optic pits and other optic nerve anomalies with midline defects, such as basal encephalocele and **Corpus callosum agenesis**. Therefore, it is appropriate to perform computed tomography (CT) or magnetic resonance imaging (MRI) studies, even if midline facial defects (hypertelorism, broad-based flat nose, cleft lip, cleft palate, or cleft face) are not present.

References:

Weithe T: Ein Fall von angeborener Difformitat der Sehnervenpapille. Arch Augenheilkd 1882; 11:14–19.
Kranenburg EW: Crater-like holes in the optic disc and central serous retinopathy. Arch Ophthalmol 1960; 64:912.
Sugar HS: Congenital pits in the optic disk. Am J Ophthalmol 1967; 63:298.
Gass JDM: Serous detachment of the macula secondary to pit of the optic nerve head. Am J Ophthalmol 1969; 67:821–841.
Brown GC, et al.: Congenital pits of the optic nerve-head: II: clinical studies in humans. Ophthalmology 1980; 87:51–65.
Alexander TA, Billson FA: Vitrectomy and photocoagulation in the management of serous detachment associated with optic nerve pits. Aust J Ophthalmol 1984; 12:139–142.
Borodic GE, et al.: Peripapillary subretinal neovascularization and serous macular detachment association with congenital optic nerve pits. Arch Ophthalmol 1984; 102:229–231.
Lincoff H, et al.: Retinoschisis associated with optic nerve pits. Arch Ophthalmol 1988; 106:61–67. *

EL007
HA068
WE038

Robert M. Ellsworth
Barrett G. Haik
Robert A. Weiss

Optic disk, crater-like cavities in
See OPTIC DISK PITS
Optic disk, crescent, congenital
See OPTIC DISK, TILTED
Optic disk, dysversion of
See OPTIC DISK, TILTED
Optic disk, melanocytoma
See OPTIC DISK, MELANOCYTOMA

OPTIC DISK, MELANOCYTOMA   0639

Includes:
Magnocellular nevus
Melanocytoma, optic disk
Melanoma, benign of optic nerve head
Optic disk, melanocytoma
Optic disk, pigmentation of, congenital

Excludes:
Eye, melanosis oculi, congenital (0640)
Melanosis oculi, acquired

Major Diagnostic Criteria: Grey, or more often jet-black, discolorations of the optic nerve head, rarely more than 1–2 mm in height.

Clinical Findings: Grey or black tumor of the optic disk usually less than two disk diameters in size with extension into the adjacent retina giving the lesion a feathered margin. More common in Negroes and other heavily pigmented non-Caucasians. Visual acuity is normal, and visual fields usually normal except for enlargement of blind spot. Most tumors remain stationary, but growth can occur, and histologic transformation to melanoma has presented (Zimmerman, 1975). Sometimes melanocytoma may appear in the uveal tract and rarely the conjunctiva or sclera.

Complications: Glaucoma can occur if there is extensive tumor in the posterior pole or when there is diffuse uveal involvement. Visual loss can occur if optic disk tumors cause optic atrophy or

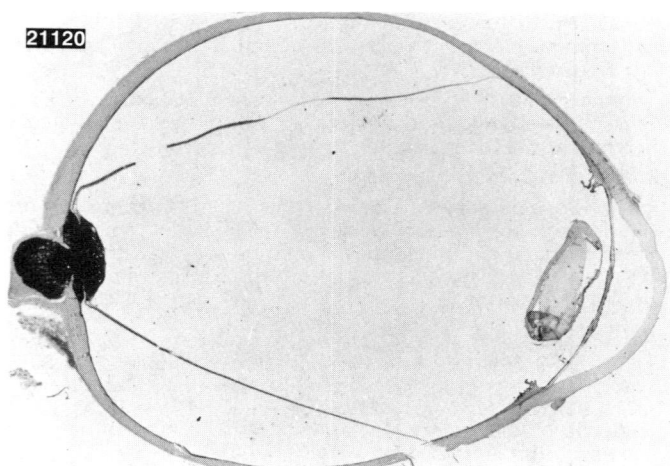

0639-21120: Histopathologic specimen shows whole globe with extensive optic disk melanocytoma.

associated choroidal involvement extends into the macula. Although these tumors can be locally invasive, there are no reports of orbital extension or metastases.

Associated Findings: Choroidal nevi, melanocytosis of the meninges, retinal pigment epithelial hypertrophy.

Etiology: Unknown.

Pathogenesis: This lesion is considered to be hamartomatous or progonomatous rather than neoplastic and can probably be regarded as atavistic, comparable with the tumor-like pigment formation in the optic nerve of certain subhuman species.

CDC No.: 743.520

Sex Ratio: M1:F>1

Occurrence: Undetermined but presumed rare

Risk of Recurrence for Patient's Sib: Unknown.

Risk of Recurrence for Patient's Child: Unknown.

Age of Detectability: At birth

Gene Mapping and Linkage: Unknown.

Prevention: None known.

Treatment: Unknown.

Prognosis: Excellent; visual impairment is unusual and no threat to life.

Detection of Carrier: Unknown.

Special Considerations: This lesion is a benign pigmented tumor involving the optic disk and needs to be distinguished from choroidal melanoma invading the nerve. Similarly, melanocytomas of uveal tract, sclera and conjunctiva need to be distinguished from malignant melanoma.

References:

Zimmerman LE, Garron LK: Melanocytoma of the optic disk. Int Ophthalmol Clinic 1962; 2:431–440.
Zimmerman LE, Spindle A: Melanoma emerging from a melanocytoma of the optic disc. Read before the Verhoeff Society Meeting, Washington, D.C., April 14–15, 1975.
Joffe L, Shields JA: Clinical and follow-up studies of melanocytoma of the optic disc. Ophthalmology 1979; 86:1067–1083.
Lee JS, Smith RE, Minckler DS: Scleral melanocytoma. Ophthalmology 1982; 89:178–182.
Croxatto JO, et al.: Angle closure glaucoma as initial manifestation of melanocytoma of the optic disc. Ophthalmology 1983; 90:830–834.
Frangieh GT, et al.: Melanocytoma of the ciliary body: presentation of

four cases and review of nineteen reports. Surv Ophthalmol 1985; 29:328–334. *

WE035   Avery H. Weiss

Optic disk, pigmentation of, congenital
See OPTIC DISK, MELANOCYTOMA
Optic disk, situs inversus of
See OPTIC DISK, TILTED

OPTIC DISK, TILTED   0757

Includes:
Conus, congenital
Fuch coloboma
Nasal fundus ectasia
Optic disk, crescent, congenital
Optic disk, dysversion of
Optic disk, situs inversus of

Excludes:
Coloboma of optic nerve
Optic nerve, congenital pit of

Major Diagnostic Criteria: Tilted appearance of disk with D-shaped scleral opening; congenital peripapillary crescent (conus); oblique direction of major retinal vessels; myopic astigmatism; inferonasal thinning of the choroid and retinal pigment epithelium; relative superotemporal field depression (or other field defects).

Clinical Findings: Normally the excavation in the optic disk is directed toward the lens or is tilted slightly temporally in the direction of the macula. In a "tilted disk," the disk is tilted in another direction, usually nasally or inferiorly. The disk appears abnormally D-shaped, and the central retinal vessels stream out in the direction of the tilt. The condition is bilateral in 80% of cases, and typical crescents appear in the direction of the tilt (nasally, 60%; infero-temporally, 28%; and inferiorly, 12%). Hypopigmentation and decreased nerve fiber density are noted in the inferonasal fundus of most patients. B-scan ultrasonography and histopathology may reveal a local ectasia in this area. An A-scan may demonstrate an increase in the dural diameter of the optic nerve. The condition is often associated with a major refractive error, usually (90%) myopia and astigmatism at an oblique axis. Temporal depression (usually superotemporal) of the visual field is most common; however, altitudinal defects, arcuate scotomas, and bizarre defects have been noted in the visual field. The field defect does not change with time and often slopes across the vertical meridian.

Complications: *Developmental:* refractive errors, usually myopic with oblique astigmatism.
Secondary: occasionally amblyopia in unilateral cases secondary to anisometropia.

Associated Findings: Oxycephaly, corneal opacities, ectopia of the macula, cilioretinal arteries, strabismus, and early open angle glaucoma are rarely associated.

Etiology: Unknown.

Pathogenesis: Developmental, possibly involving an anomalous insertion of the optic stalk into the optic vesicle, misdirection of retinal ganglion cell fibers, and anomalous closure of the embryonic fissure. Considered by some to be a form of optic nerve hypoplasia; however, none of the midline defects often associated with optic nerve hypoplasia are present. Mechanical compression of the optic nerve fibers or abnormalities in vascularization of the nerve during development may also contribute to the pathogenesis of this condition. Visual field defects may be related to ectasia of the posterior portion of the globe with or without hypoplasia of the optic nerve, retina, and choroid.

CDC No.: 743.520
Sex Ratio: M1:F1
Occurrence: Undetermined.
Risk of Recurrence for Patient's Sib: Unknown.

Risk of Recurrence for Patient's Child: Unknown.
Age of Detectability: At birth.
Gene Mapping and Linkage: Unknown.
Prevention: None known. Genetic counseling indicated.
Treatment: Unknown.
Prognosis: Field defects do not progress.
Detection of Carrier: Unknown.

Special Considerations: The often encountered bitemporal depression on visual field testing seen in this condition must be differentiated from that of a chiasmal lesion. In chiasmal lesions, the field defect tends to respect the midline and end in a sharp edge, which in the early stages does not cross into the nasal field. In contrast, with a tilted disk, rather than a distinct midline step, there is sloping of the temporal defect. In addition, patients with tilted optic disks do not demonstrate red hemianopsia (particularly when tested centrally) as is evident in chiasmal lesions. In some patients with tilted disks, the visual fields improve with refractive correction. The anatomic abnormalities of the tilted disk often are confused with papilledema, and may lead to unnecessary neurodiagnostic studies.

References:
Rucker CW: Bitemporal defects in visual fields resulting from developmental anomalies of optic discs. Arch Ophthalmol 1946; 35:546.
Graham M, Wakefield G: Bitemporal visual field defects associated with anomalies of the optic disc. Br J Ophthalmol 1973; 57:307.
Young SE, et al.: The tilted disc syndrome. Am J Ophthalmol 1976; 82:16.
Dorrel D: The tilted disc. Br J Ophthalmol 1978; 62:16.
Brown G, Tasman W: Congenital anomalies of the optic disc. New York: Grune & Stratton, 1983.
Guiffre G: Hypothesis on the pathogenesis of the papillary dysversion syndrome. J Fr Ophthalmol 1985; 8:565–572.
Singh J: Echographic features of tilted optic disc. Ann Ophthalmol 1985; 17:382–383.

EL007   Robert M. Ellsworth
HA068   Barrett G. Haik
WE038   Robert A. Weiss

Optic glioma, orbital
See ORBITAL NERVE GLIOMA

OPTIC NERVE HYPOPLASIA   0758

Includes:
Hypoplasia of optic nerve
Optic nerve, partial absence of
Quinine, fetal effects of
Sulfonamides, fetal effects of

Excludes: Optic nerve aplasia

Major Diagnostic Criteria: Ophthalmoscopic appearance in conjunction with reduced vision.

Clinical Findings: Hypoplasia of the optic nerve is not uncommon, and may be unilateral or bilateral in equal frequency. It is more often found with other anomalies than as an isolated entity. The optic nerve appears small, pale, and misshapen. It may have a greyish or brownish-black pigment crescent on the temporal side, a deep physiologic cup, a peripapillary cuff, or may appear mottled throughout. The foveolar reflex may be absent. The retinal vasculature is normal or tortuous. The visual acuity, if diminished in the affected eye, is proportionate to the severity of the hypoplastic disk with or without strabismus on the same side. Visual field defects, and on X-ray, a small optic foramen has been noted on the involved side.

Complications: Unknown.

Associated Findings: Microphthalmia, nystagmus, partial fourth or sixth nerve palsies, dacryostenosis, cyclopia, anencephaly, hydrocephaly, orbital encephalomeningocele, ptosis, blepharophimosis, hypopituitarism, and agenesis of the septum pellucidum (*DeMorsier syndrome*, see **Kallmann syndrome**); deafness, and anomalies of the urinary and skeletal systems. The majority of patients with unilateral or segmental optic nerve hypoplasia have no accompanying abnormalities.

Etiology: A familial tendency has been observed in bilateral cases, suggesting autosomal dominant inheritance. Maternal diabetes causing an adverse intrauterine environment may also be a cause.

Pathogenesis: Embryologic defect of differentiation in the ganglion cell layer. Some of the optic nerve fibers fail to develop and reach the disk, but mesoderm has invaginated the optic stalk, and retinal vessels exist. Teratogenic substances, for example drugs such as quinine and possibly sulfonamides, have been implicated if taken during the early weeks of gestation.

MIM No.: 16555

CDC No.: 743.520

Sex Ratio: Presumably M1:Fl

Occurrence: Undetermined but presumed rare. More common when found in association with hypopituitarism.

Risk of Recurrence for Patient's Sib:
See Part I, *Mendelian Inheritance.*

Risk of Recurrence for Patient's Child:
See Part I, *Mendelian Inheritance.*

Age of Detectability: In infancy, by ophthalmoscopic examination.

Gene Mapping and Linkage: Unknown.

Prevention: None known. Genetic counseling indicated.

Treatment: Unknown.

Prognosis: Visual prognosis dependent upon degree of severity of the hypoplasia and associated anomalies.

Detection of Carrier: Clinical examination of first degree relatives.

References:
Whinery RD, Blodi FC: Hypoplasia of the optic nerve: a clinical and histopathologic correlation. Trans Am Acad Ophthalmol Otolaryngol 1963; 67:733–738.
Helveston EM: Unilateral hypoplasia of the optic nerve. Arch Ophthalmol 1966; 76:195–196.
Ewald RA: Unilateral hypoplasia of the optic nerve. Am J Ophthalmol 1967; 63:763–767.
Hackenbrauch Y, et al.: Familial bilateral optic nerve hypoplasia. Am J Ophthalmol 1975; 79:314–320.
Patel H, et al.: Optic nerve hypoplasia with hypopituitarism. Am J Dis Child 1975; 129:175–180.
Petersen RA, Walton DS: Optic nerve hypoplasia with good visual acuity and visual field defects. Arch Ophthalmol 1977; 95:254–258.
Lambert SR, et al.: Optic nerve hypoplasia. Surv Ophthalmol 1987; 32:1–9.

RA004   **Elsa K. Rahn**

Optic nerve, partial absence of
See OPTIC NERVE HYPOPLASIA
Optic-septo dysplasia
See SEPTO-OPTIC DYSPLASIA

OPTICO-COCHLEO-DENTATE DEGENERATION   0759

Includes: Nyssen-van Bogaert syndrome

Excludes:
  Deafness-optic nerve atrophy, progressive (0253)
  Deafness-polyneuropathy-optic atrophy (0268)
  G(M2)-gangliosidosis
  Huntington disease (0478)
  Pelizaeus-Merzbacher syndrome (0803)

Major Diagnostic Criteria: Optic atrophy, sensorineural deafness, and spastic quadriplegia.

Clinical Findings: Most reported cases have presented before age one, and all by early childhood. The disorder presents with motor disturbances in early-onset cases; poor head control, decreased lower limb use, inability to sit or stand, flexion contractures of the legs, and kyphoscoliosis are seen. Spastic quadriplegia developed progressively with marked involvement of lower limbs in late-onset cases; ataxic gait, intention tremor with spasticity, and cerebellar myoclonus were present. Tendon stretch reflexes were hyperactive or absent. All patients have a thin, wasted appearance, with disuse atrophy. Progressive blindness caused by optic atrophy is frequent. In two cases, nystagmus was seen before age one year. All developed progressive sensorineural deafness caused by atrophy of the acoustic nerve nucleus, most within the first decade of life. Eight patients never developed speech. Neuropathologic lesions included atrophy and demyelination of the primary optic and cochlear pathways, atrophy of the nerve cells of dorsal and ventral cochlear nuclei, disseminated nerve cell loss of the dentate nucleus, degeneration of the medial lemnisci and, in some cases, of the pyramidal tracts. Nonspecific parenchymal losses (diffuse cortical nerve cell loss producing brain atrophy) and alteration of blood vessels may be seen. It appears that the severity of the disorder, head circumference, level of mental functioning, and degree of neuronal loss correlate with the age of onset.

Complications: Microcephaly, speech disturbances, mental retardation.

Associated Findings: In late-onset cases, deafness and blindness may cause psychologic isolation, which may give rise to affective disturbances. Intercurrent infections.

Etiology: Autosomal recessive inheritance with variability of expressivity. This syndrome represents a nosologic entity, but genetic heterogeneity is possible.

Pathogenesis: Unknown.

MIM No.: *25870

Sex Ratio: M7:F5 (observed).

Occurrence: Twelve cases have been recorded; two or more sibs have been involved in each family.

Risk of Recurrence for Patient's Sib:
See Part I, *Mendelian Inheritance.*

Risk of Recurrence for Patient's Child:
See Part I, *Mendelian Inheritance.*

Age of Detectability: Most often in early infancy.

Gene Mapping and Linkage: Unknown.

Prevention: None known. Genetic counseling indicated.

Treatment: Physical therapy, positioning to prevent decubitus ulcers.

Prognosis: Progression varies and may be very rapid or slow, 80% of deaths have occurred before puberty. Onset of vision loss usually precedes the onset of hearing loss.

Detection of Carrier: Unknown.

References:
Müller J, Zeman W: Dégénérescence systématisée optico-cochléo-dentelée. Acta Neuropathol (Berl) 1965; 5:26–39.
Zeman W: Dégénérescence systématisée optico-cochléo-dentelée. Handbook Clin Neurol 1975; 21:535 only.
Konigsmark BW, Gorlin RJ: Genetic and metabolic deafness. Philadelphia: W.B. Saunders, 1976.

MI029   **Joyce Mitchell**
                                              Cor W.R.J. Cremers

ORAL DERMOIDS 0760

Includes:
Cyst, developmental
Cyst, dysontogenetic
Cyst, epidermoid
Cyst, teratoid
Cystic teratoma
Dermoids, oral
Teratoma

Excludes:
Neck, Branchial cleft, cysts or sinuses (0117)
Cellulitis of the floor of the mouth
Cystic hygroma
Ranula
Thyroglossal duct remnant (0945)

Major Diagnostic Criteria: An elevation of the floor of the mouth, or a slight fullness in the submental area, usually eliciting the complaint of a "fullness" of the floor of the mouth which interferes with speaking or eating.

Clinical Findings: Dermoids present as sublingual masses and are located either above or below the mylohyoid muscle, usually in the midline. They may occasionally be on one side only. When below the mylohyoid muscle, they will present as pendulous, submental masses beneath the mandible.

Oral dermoids generally feel "dough-like," but may feel cystic, depending on the consistency of the contents, which may vary from a cheesy, sebaceous-like substance to a more liquefied material. They may contain hair, nails, and keratin, and may contain pus when secondarily infected.

These lesions vary in weight from 1 gram to several hundred grams, and may vary from a small pea-sized growth to the size of a grapefruit. Fistulous tracts may develop, opening either intraorally into the floor of the mouth, or extraorally into the skin beneath the chin.

Dermoids may undergo malignant degeneration and metastasize to lymph nodes.

A classification of dysontogenetic cysts of the floor of the mouth based upon embryology and histopathology has been presented by Meyer (1955) as follows:

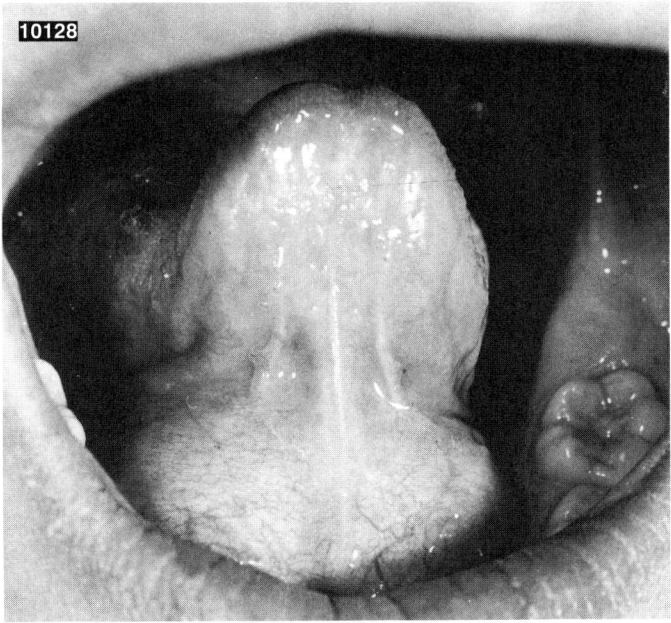

0760-10128: Sublingual oral dermoid.

Epidermoid: An epithelial-lined cavity surrounded by a capsule with no skin appendages; this is a simple-type lesion with embryologic ectodermal elements.

Dermoid: An epithelial-lined cavity with 1) skin appendages of hair, hair follicles, sebaceous glands, sweat glands, and 2) connective tissue, fat tissue, etc. This is a compound-type of cyst with ectodermal and mesodermal derivatives.

Teratoid: An epithelial-lined cavity with the following elements present in the capsule: 1) skin appendages including hair follicles, sebaceous glands, keratin, etc., 2) connective tissue derivatives such as fibers, bone, muscle, blood vessels, etc., and 3) respiratory and GI tissues. This is a complex cyst with derivatives of all three embryonic tissues of ectoderm, mesoderm and endoderm.

The term dermoid cyst is, unfortunately, frequently used as a synonym for benign cystic teratoma. That the same name is applied justifiably to unrelated sequestration cysts makes separation of the two types of lesions difficult.

Complications: Interference with speaking, eating or breathing; disfigurement; secondary infection with or without cellulitis; fistulae.

Associated Findings: None known.

Etiology: Unknown.

Pathogenesis: The majority of the oral dermoids are developmental cysts derived from epithelial rests enclaved during the midline closure of the bilateral mandibular (first) and hyoid (second) branchial arches. Some of these dermoid cysts may possibly be formed by remnants of the tuberculum impar of His, which together with the lateral processes from the inner surface of each mandibular arch form the body of the tongue and the floor of the mouth. These developments take place during the third and fourth weeks of embryonic life.

The growth of these cysts may be either gradual or sudden. It is suggested that the development of oral dermoids occurs during the period of increased activity of epithelial tissues, such as sweat glands or hair, which fill the lumen of the cyst. This increased growth activity coincides with the ages of 15–35 years, when most of these lesions become clinically evident.

Sex Ratio: M1:F1

Occurrence: Over 200 cases reported in the world literature. Of 1,495 dermoid cysts at Mayo Clinic (1910–1935), 103 (6.94%) were in the head and neck and of these only 24, or 0.6%, were in the floor of the mouth. There is no known predilection for race or ethnic group.

Risk of Recurrence for Patient's Sib: Unknown.

Risk of Recurrence for Patient's Child: Unknown.

Age of Detectability: Clinically, from birth on. Most come to clinical attention at age 15–35 years.

Gene Mapping and Linkage: Unknown.

Prevention: None known. Genetic counseling indicated.

Treatment: Either intraoral or extraoral surgical removal, depending on the position of the dermoid in relation to the mylohyoid muscle. Those lying between the mylohyoid muscle and oral mucous membrane (sublingual) are best removed by an intraoral approach, while those lying between the mylohyoid muscle and platysma muscle are approached through an extraoral or skin incision.

Prognosis: Excellent, if the tumor is surgically removed in its entirety. If the lesion is incompletely removed, the remaining epithelial cells may proliferate to form a new lesion. Dermoids may undergo malignant degeneration and may even metastasize to lymph nodes, and, therefore, should be completely removed when first diagnosed.

Detection of Carrier: Unknown.

References:
New GB, Erich JB: Dermoid cysts of the head and neck. Surg Gynecol Obstet 1937; 65:48–55.
Meyer I: Dermoid cysts (dermoids) of the floor of the mouth. Oral Surg 1955; 8:1149–1164.

Howell CJ: The sublingual dermoid cyst: report of five cases and a review of the literature. Oral Surg Med Oral Pathol 1985; 59:578–580.

ME028   **Irving Meyer**

Oral-facial-digital syndrome
See ORO-FACIO-DIGITAL SYNDROME I
Oral-facial-digital syndrome II
See ORO-FACIO-DIGITAL SYNDROME, MOHR TYPE
Oral-facial-digital syndrome IV
See ORO-FACIO-DIGITAL SYNDROME, BARAITSER-BURN TYPE
Oral-facial-digital syndrome V
See ORO-FACIO-DIGITAL SYNDROME, THURSTON TYPE

ORBITAL AND PERIORBITAL DERMOID CYSTS   0761

Includes: Dermoid cysts, orbital and periorbital

Excludes:
    Corneal dermoid
    Eye, dermolipoma (0284)
    Limbal dermoid
    Orbital cyst-microphthalmia, congenital

Major Diagnostic Criteria: Periorbital dermoids are diagnosed clinically on the basis of circumscribed subcutaneous tumors located near the orbital rim and present since birth. Orbital dermoids present as expanding masses within the orbit that displace the globe. CT scan shows their cystic nature. Histopathological examination shows an encapsulated tumor with stratified squamous epithelium and skin appendages in its wall and desquamated keratin and hair shafts within its lumen.

Clinical Findings: Although congenital, periorbital dermoids become clinically apparent as they enlarge between one and three years of age. They appear as firm circumscribed masses, ranging from 0.5 to 1.5cm, located usually along the superotemporal rim of the orbit and less frequently along the nasal rim. In general, they are attached to the underlying bone but not the overlying skin. Skull X-rays show a concave depression of bone underlying the tumor. Orbital dermoids are less frequent and often go undetected until adulthood. As they enlarge, dermoids displace the globe or restrict its movement. Orbital CT scan is necessary to delineate its size, and position. The cystic appearance of dermoids on CT scan helps to distinguish it from other orbital tumors.

Complications: Spontaneous rupture or incomplete excision of the tumor incites acute and sometimes chronic inflammation in or around the orbit. As dermoids enlarge, they can cause significant displacement of the globe.

Associated Findings: None known.

Etiology: Sporadic.

Pathogenesis: Recent evidence indicates that most of the mesenchymal tissues of the eye and the orbit are derived from neural crest cells. As a consequence of abnormal cellular interactions with the overlying ectoderm, these ectodermal tumors develop beneath the skin.

Sex Ratio: Presumably M1:F1.

Occurrence: Comprise nearly 40% of orbital tumors of childhood.

Risk of Recurrence for Patient's Sib: Probably not increased.

Risk of Recurrence for Patient's Child: Probably not increased.

Age of Detectability: Although present at birth, periorbital dermoids usually manifest between one and three years of age as they enlarge, while orbital dermoids usually manifest in adulthood.

Gene Mapping and Linkage: Unknown.

Prevention: None known. Genetic counseling indicated.

Treatment: Surgical excision. The tumor should be excised intact to avoid release of cystic contents which leads to inflammation within surrounding tissues. Orbital CT scan is necessary in orbital dermoids, and some periorbital dermoids, to delineate their extent of involvement.

Prognosis: Dermoids are benign with no malignant potential.

Detection of Carrier: Unknown.

Special Considerations: In adults, so called "giant" dermoid cysts can be equal to or greater in size than the globe. Such lesions can be mistaken for lacrimal gland tumors. Excision of these is technically difficult.

References:
Duke-Elder S: System of ophthalmology, vol 3, part 2, Congenital deformities. London: Henry Kimptom, 1964:956–963.
Reese AB: Hamartomas, progonomas, choristomas, miscellaneous tumors and tumefactions. In: Reese AB, ed: Tumors of the eye. New York: Harper and Row, 1976:15:416–417.
Iliff WJ, Green WR: Orbital tumors in children. In: Jakobiec FA, ed: Ocular and adnexal tumors. Birmingham: Aesculapius 1978:47:673–675.
Nevares RL, et al.: Ocular dermoids. Plast Reconstr Surg 1989; 82:959–964.

WE035   **Avery H. Weiss**

ORBITAL AND PERIORBITAL LYMPHANGIOMA   0765

Includes:
    Capillary lymphangiomas of orbit
    Cavernous lymphangiomas of orbit
    Cystic lymphangiomas of orbit
    Ocular lymphangioma

Excludes:
    Arteriovenous malformations
    Capillary hemangioma, orbital
    Cavernous hemangioma, orbital
    Venous varix of the orbit

Major Diagnostic Criteria: The tumor appears as a cystic mass of the eyelid, conjunctiva, or orbit. On histopathological examination, lymphangiomas are comprised of flattened endothelial cells without surrounding smooth muscle or pericytes, which distinguishes them from hemangiomas and venous varices.

Clinical Findings: These tumors may occur in the eyelid, conjunctiva, or orbit. Jones (1978) reported the following distributions for location of 61 lymphangiomas: lid, conjunctiva, and face (18%); conjunctiva only (35%); and orbit only (47%). When visible, they appear as a bluish cystic mass. Orbital tumors cause progressive proptosis that increases with an upper respiratory infection or Valsalva maneuver. Spontaneous hemorrhage into a lymphangioma, so-called "chocolate cyst", may cause subconjunctival hemorrhage or increasing proptosis. Orbital echography shows multiple irregular echos intermixed with cystic spaces. Orbital CT scan shows nonenhancing diffusely infiltrating mass with expansion of the orbit in some cases.

Complications: Expansion of orbital lymphangioma may displace the globe, restrict ocular motility, and cause optic atrophy.
    Acute hemorrhage into such tumors can be an emergency if vascular perfusion to the optic nerve or retina is compromised. Cellulitis within a facial lymphangioma can spread to the orbit.

Associated Findings: Occasionally associated with similar tumors elsewhere: face, oropharynx, and paranasal sinuses.

Etiology: Unknown.

Pathogenesis: Since the orbit, unlike the eyelid and conjunctiva, does not normally contain lymphatic tissue, the origin of lymphangiomas is not established. Lymphangiomas may arise from primordial cells destined to become endothelial cells that remain isolated and fail to interconnect with arteries or veins.

Sex Ratio: M1:F1

Occurrence: Lymphangiomas were found in 2.8% of 358 children with orbital tumors.

Risk of Recurrence for Patient's Sib: Unknown.

Risk of Recurrence for Patient's Child: Unknown.

Age of Detectability: Lymphangiomas of the eyelid and conjunctiva can present at any time in the child or adult.

Gene Mapping and Linkage: Unknown.

Prevention: None known. Genetic counseling indicated.

Treatment: Surgical excision of symptomatic tumors is treatment of choice. As they diffusely infiltrate surrounding tissues, excision from the eyelid and orbit are seldom complete. There is no proven role for radiation therapy or use of sclerosing agents.

Prognosis: In the absence of complications, there is no impairment of visual function.

Detection of Carrier: Unknown.

References:

Jones IS, Desjardins L: Management of orbital neurofibromatosis and lymphangiomas. In: Jakobiec FA, ed: Ocular and adnexal tumors. Birmingham: Aesculapius, 1978:50:735–740.

Iliff WJ, et al.: Orbital lymphangiomas. Ophthalmology 1979; 86:914–929.

Jakobiec FA, Jones IS: Vascular tumors, malformations and degenerations. In: Duane TD, ed: Clinical ophthalmology. Philadelphia: Harper and Row, 1986.

Rootman J, et al.: Orbital-adnexal lymphangiomas: a spectrum of hemodynamically isolated vascular hamartomas. Ophthalmology 1986; 93:1558–1570.

WE035   **Avery H. Weiss**

ORBITAL CEPHALOCELES   0762

Includes:

    Encephalocele, orbital
    Orbital encephalocele
    Orbital hydrocephalocele
    Orbital meningocele

Excludes:

    Basal encephaloceles to nasal or nasopharyngeal passageways
    Encephaloceles, nonsphenoidal, nonethmoidal
    Posttraumatic pseudomeningocele

Major Diagnostic Criteria: True cephaloceles have specific constituents derived from remnant protrusions of encephalic tissues from within the cranial vault. They may contain meningeal or cerebral tissues or both. There may or may not be any identifiable connecting remnant through the optic foreamen or at fusion lines of facial or orbital bones.

    Orbital cephaloceles are one of three types of basal encephalo-

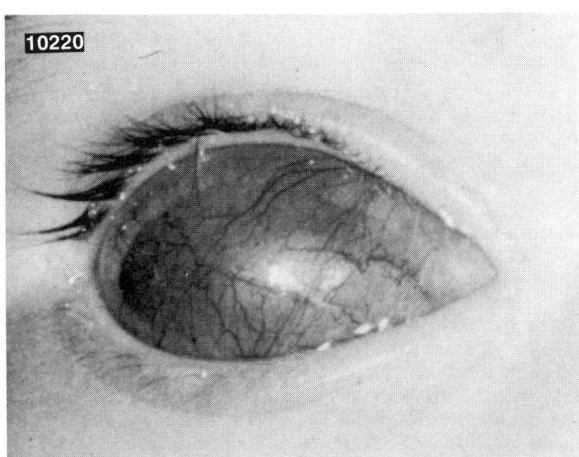

0762-10220: Encephalocele in orbit.

celes in which the meninges and brain substance in varied amounts protrude through the sphenoid and sometimes the ethmoid bones: 1) sphenopharyngeal (seen in the nasopharynx), 2) transethmoidal and sphenoethmoidal (seen in the nose), and 3) sphenorbital (seen in the orbit). The literature uses the term *encephalocele* to cover all varieties of tissue components, but the protrusion should be named according to the tissues within. If only meningeal membranes are present, then the term *orbital meningocele* is used; if neural tissue is present, then *orbital encephalocele* is used; and if cerebrospinal fluid is included, it is an *orbital hydrocephalocele*.

Clinical Findings: The orbit is distorted, most often by a protrusion of the eye, usually with displacement downward and outward. The mass appears cystic and may be fluctuant or pulsatile. Pressure may produce an oculocardiac reflex. Proptosis is often progressive and may increase transiently upon straining, sneezing, or coughing. Bony defects may show on X-ray or computed tomography (CT) scan. Orbital echography will demonstrate the density and complexity of the lesion.

    There are two types by location and site of origin of orbital cephaloceles: 1) an *anterior* group arising from the nasofrontal or anterior part of the orbit, and 2) a less frequent *posterior* group arising from the middle cerebral fossa with protrusion through the optic foramen or the sphenoid bone. Clinically, the differential diagnosis includes other swellings of the orbit, such as specific tumors, pseudotumors, and other anomalies. Pulsatile exophthalmos may result from defects in the bony orbit without encephalocele. The pathological differential diagnosis includes hemangioma and teratoma. Hemangiomas are farily common in brain, meningeal, and cephalic tissues, and their hypervascularity and connective tissue patterns can be confused with cephalocele. Spontaneous regression of hemangioma has been noted, but this is unlikely in cephalocele. Teratoma is less common, perhaps 10–20% as frequent, and is harder to distinguish, in part because some cephaloceles have solid areas and some teratomas are cystic and would be indistinguishable from cephaloceles, were it not for tissues of other germ layers. Nasofrontal glioma is a known entity, possibly different from encephalocele, but since some cases have a transcranial connection (Younun and Coode, 1986) these lesions may well be simply points along a developmental spectrum. The connecting pathway between the orbit and the intracranial space has great potential for complex lesions, including cephalocele. This is shown by a unique case of combined orbital-intracranial teratoma (Garden and McManis, 1986).

Complications: Papilledema, compressive optic atrophy, oculomotor palsies, pits, colobomas and other dysplasias of the optic disk, and megalopapilla.

Associated Findings: Acrocephaly, microphthalmos, anophthalmia, uveoretinal colobomas, **Optic disk, morning glory anomaly**, and atresia of the lacrimal passages. **Corpus callosum agenesis** is occasionally associated. May be a feature of other complex malformation syndromes.

Etiology: Undetermined. Familial and ethnic patterns have been noted.

Pathogenesis: Unknown.

Sex Ratio: From M5:F7 to M1:F3.

Occurrence: Estimated at 1:80,000 to 1:400,000 births.

Risk of Recurrence for Patient's Sib: Unknown.

Risk of Recurrence for Patient's Child: Unknown.

Age of Detectability: Early life; may be present *in utero*, allowing possible detection by prenatal ultrasound.

Gene Mapping and Linkage: Unknown.

Prevention: None known. Genetic counseling indicated.

Treatment: Surgical removal of the tumefaction with effort at salvage of the eye is the only useful treatment, and may require sealing of the deep orbital bony defect(s). Decompression rather than removal has the risk of leaving behind teratomatous tissues with malignant potential (Garden and McManis, 1986).

Prognosis: Moderately good in isolated cases; poor when part of multiple malformations of the brain and head. Salvage of functional vision is possible only rarely.

Detection of Carrier: Unknown.

References:

Cook GR, Knobloch WH: Autosomal recessive vitreoretinopathy and encephaloceles. Am J Ophthalmol 1982; 94:18–25.

Koenig SB, et al.: The morning glory syndrome associated with sphenoidal encephalocelle. Ophthalmology 1982; 89:1368–1373.

van Nouhuys E: Autosomal recessive vitreoretinopathy and encephaloceles. Am J Ophthalmol 1982; 94:820.

Ferguson JW, et al.: Ocular, cerebral and cutaneous malformations: confirmation of an association. Clin Genet 1984; 25:464–469.

Shields JA, et al.: Classification and incidence of space-occupying lesions of the orbit. Arch Ophthalmol 1984; 102:1606–1611.

Grossniklaus HE, et al.: Childhood orbital pseudotumor. Ann Ophthalmol 1985; 17:372–377.

Mamalis N, et al.: Congenital orbital teratoma: a review and report of two cases. Surv Ophthalmol 1985; 30:41–46.

Garden JW, McManis J: Congenital orbital-intracranial teratoma with subsequent malignancy: case report. Br J Ophthalmol 1986; 70:111–113.

Younus M, Coode PE: Nasal glioma and encephalocele: two separate entities. J Neurosurg 1986; 64:516–519.

ES003
SH054

John R. Esterly
Douglas R. Shanklin

Orbital cyst-cerebral and focal dermal malformations
See OCULO-CEREBRO-CUTANEOUS SYNDROME
Orbital encephalocele
See ORBITAL CEPHALOCELES

ORBITAL HEMANGIOMA   0764

Includes:
Cellular hemangioma of infancy
Hemangioma of eye lids and orbit
Infantile hemangioendothelioma

Excludes: Orbital lymphangioma

Major Diagnostic Criteria: Hemangioma of the ocular adnexae.

Clinical Findings: These are the most common orbital tumors in children. Any portion of the ocular adnexae may be involved. They present as a soft compressible purplish mass often palpable through the lids or conjunctiva and may produce unilateral exophthalmos. There might be an increase in tumor volume or depth of bluish discoloration when the child cries. Around 25% have coexisting nonophthalmic strawberry marks. Visual acuity may be unaltered or the tumor might press on the optic nerve, leading to papilledema and optic atrophy.

Complications: Visual defects secondary to papilledema. Occlusion of the eye by the tumor, or induced refractive errors due to its impingement on the eye, can cause amblyopia. Occasionally they cause strabismus by interfering with muscle action. Thrombocytopenia due to entrapment of platelets within the capillary hemangioma can lead to bleeding. The tumor may also ulcerate and become necrosed.

Associated Findings: Occasionally there are hemangiomas elsewhere in the body. Typically there are no associated retinal or intraocular malformations.

Etiology: Unknown.

Pathogenesis: The lesion is considered to be a congenital hamartoma.

Sex Ratio: M1:F2

Occurrence: In 1% to 2% of newborn children.

Risk of Recurrence for Patient's Sib: Unknown.

Risk of Recurrence for Patient's Child: Unknown.

Age of Detectability: About one-third of lid and orbital hemangiomas are evident at birth, and 95% are recognized by six months of age.

Gene Mapping and Linkage: Unknown.

Prevention: None known. Genetic counseling indicated.

Treatment: The overwhelming majority of these lesions will spontaneously subside within the first few years of life. The mainstay of management is directed primarily toward correction of associated refractive errors, and vigorous treatment of amblyopia if tumor causes eyelid to occlude pupillary axis. If a lesion is so extensive as to threaten vision, a trial of therapy with systemic corticosteroids should be considered. Direct injections of corticosteroids into the lesion have also been effective in provoking involution of the hemangioma. Low doses of radiotherapy might also be beneficial. Surgery is sometimes necessary.

Prognosis: Normal for life and intelligence; vision might be decreased due to amblyopia.

Detection of Carrier: Unknown.

Special Considerations: It is important to distinguish the orbital hemangiomas from the port wine stain or **Nevus flammeus**. This is a flat vascular malformation that represents telangiectasia, not a true angioma. When this lesion occurs on the eyelids it may be part of the **Sturge-Weber syndrome**.

References:

de Venecia G, Lobeck CC: Successful treatment of eyelid hemangioma with prednisone. Arch Ophthalmol 1970; 84:98.

Jakobiec FA: Ocular and adnexal tumors. Birmingham: Aesculapius, 1978.

Kushner BJ: Local steroid therapy in adnexal hemangioma. Ann Ophthalmol 1979; 11:1005.

Nicholson DH, Green RW: Pediatric ocular tumors. Masson, 1981.

Crawford JS, Morin JD: The eye in childhood. Grune & Stratton, 1983.

MU026

Michelle Munoz
Morton E. Smith

Orbital hydrocephalocele
See ORBITAL CEPHALOCELES
Orbital meningocele
See ORBITAL CEPHALOCELES

ORBITAL NERVE GLIOMA   0763

Includes:
Glioma, of optic nerve
Optic glioma, orbital

Excludes: Meningioma of the optic nerve

Major Diagnostic Criteria: Optic nerve glioma is diagnosed clinically on the basis of visual loss, proptosis, or optic atrophy associated with X-ray evidence of optic nerve tumor. Disk swelling is rarely observed. Histopathologically, optic nerve glioma is a pilocytic astrocytoma of the juvenile type. In most cases, the astrocytomas belong to grade I group due to absence of histologic features indicative of infiltration or spread.

Clinical Findings: Tumors of the optic nerve are uncommon. Optic glioma is the most prevalent tumor arising in the optic nerve. Approximately 85% are present in childhood before 15 years of age. Patients present with visual loss, proptosis, and disk atrophy and swelling. With chronic compression, optic atrophy, and rarely optociliary shunt veins may occur. Visual fields show constriction of peripheral field with depression or scotoma of central field. Some tumors are confined to the orbital segment of the nerve but a substantial proportion extend intracranially. Thin-section computed tomography (CT) scan of the orbit, or magnetic resonance imaging (MRI), shows fusiform swelling of the nerve. CT scan or MRI studies of the brain with detailed views of optic canal, chiasm, optic tracts, and surrounding structures are necessary to define intracranial extension. Adults with optic gliomas may present with visual loss that is rapidly progressive and disk swelling with superimposed vascular occlusion. In this group, the tumor is very aggressive and frequently invades the CNS leading to death.

Complications: Progressive enlargement of the orbital segment of the nerve causes increasing visual loss, proptosis, restricted ocular motility, and pressure on the posterior aspect of the globe. Primary involvement or extension into the chiasmal region can disturb hypothalamic and pituitary function, raise intracranial pressure, induce seizures, and invade surrounding structures causing variable neurological impairment and even death.

Associated Findings: Among all individuals with **Neurofibromatosis**, gliomas of the anterior visual pathways occur in the CT and MRI studies of 15%.

Etiology: Usually sporadic, except when associated with **Neurofibromatosis**.

Pathogenesis: Unknown.

Sex Ratio: M1:F>1

Occurrence: In large series of orbital tumors not biased by neurosurgical or pathological referral basis, optic nerve glioma comprises 1.6 to 5.6% of orbital tumors in childhood.

Risk of Recurrence for Patient's Sib:
See Part I, *Mendelian Inheritance.*

Risk of Recurrence for Patient's Child:
See Part I, *Mendelian Inheritance.*

Age of Detectability: Usually by the second decade of life.

Gene Mapping and Linkage: Unknown.

Prevention: None known. Genetic counseling indicated.

Treatment: Treatment is controversial. Some authors view glioma as a benign tumor with self-limited pattern of growth. Surgical excision is recommended only if tumor growth and severe visual loss is documented. Others view optic nerve glioma as a malignant astrocytoma with invasive potential; thus aggressive surgical excision is advised to prevent intracranial extension.

Prognosis: Gliomas which remain confined to the optic nerve have a good prognosis whether excised or not. Gliomas which extend into the chiasm or other intracranial structures may respond to chemotherapy or irradiation, but some tumors continue to grow resulting in death. Visual morbidity varies with the severity of optic nerve involvement.

Detection of Carrier: Clinical examination of first degree relatives.

Special Considerations: The presence of nystagmus strongly suggests chiasmal involvement and less likely optic nerve involvement bilaterally. Numerous reports have noted spasmus nutans, an acquired benign condition, is frequently confused with chiasmal glioma in young children. Since there are no other ocular or CNS abnormalities in spasmus nutans, the distinction is made on clinical grounds or by brain CT or MRI scan.

References:
Hoyt W, Baghdassarian S: Optic glioma of childhood: natural history and rationale for conservative treatment. Br J Ophthalmol 1969; 53:793–798.
Hoyt WF, et al.: Malignant optic glioma of adulthood. Brain 1973; 96:121–132.
Yanoff M, et al.: Juvenile pilocytic astrocytoma ("Glioma") of optic nerve: clinicopathologic study of sixty-three cases. In: Jakobiec FA, ed: Ocular and adnexal tumors. Birmingham: Aesculapius 1978:685–707.
Riccardi VM: von Recklinghausen neurofibromatosis. New Engl J Med 1981; 305:1617–1627.
Rush JA, et al.: Optic glioma: long-term follow-up of 85 histopathologically verified cases. Ophthalmology 1982; 89:1213–1219.
Imes RK, Hoyt WF: Childhood chiasmal gliomas: update on the fate of patients in the 1969 San Francisco Study. Br J Ophthalmol 1986; 70:179–182.
Alvord EC, Lofton S: Gliomas of the optic nerve or chiasm: outcome by patient's age, tumor, site and treatment. J Neurosurg 1988; 68:85–98.

WE035   **Avery H. Weiss**

Orbital teratoma
See EYE, ORBITAL TERATOMA, CONGENITAL

Orbitopagus parasiticus
See EYE, ORBITAL TERATOMA, CONGENITAL
'Oregon type' tyrosinosis
See TYROSINEMIA II, OREGON TYPE
Orengua
See ANEMIA, SICKLE CELL
Organoid nevus syndrome
See PROTEUS SYNDROME
Organomercurials (phenyl and alkylmercury), fetal effects
See FETAL METHYLMERCURY EFFECTS
Ornithine carbamoyl transferase deficiency
See ORNITHINE TRANSCARBAMYLASE DEFICIENCY
Ornithine ketoacid aminotransferase deficiency
See GYRATE ATROPHY OF THE CHOROID AND RETINA

ORNITHINE TRANSCARBAMYLASE DEFICIENCY   3023

Includes:
Hyperammonemia due to ornithine transcarbamylase deficiency
Ornithine carbamoyl transferase deficiency
Valproate sensitivity

Excludes:
Aciduria, argininosuccinic (0087)
Argininemia (0086)
Carbamoyl phosphate synthetase deficiency (3022)
Citrullinemia (0174)
Hyperdibasic aminoaciduria (0491)
Hyperornithinemia-hyperammonemia-homocitrullinuria (3169)
Lactic acidosis, congenital
N-acetylglutamate synthetase deficiency (3170)
Organic acidemias
Reye syndrome
Transient hyperammonemia of the newborn
Transient hyperammonemia of the newborn

Major Diagnostic Criteria: In most hemizygous affected males, coma associated with hyperammonemia (plasma ammonium >500 μM, normal <50 μM) occurs in the first three days of life. However, some males have first developed symptoms in later childhood and may have clinical findings similar to symptomatic female heterozygotes. Some ten percent of heterozygous females are symptomatic. In symptomatic heterozygotes, recurrent episodes of ataxia, migraine-like headaches, vomiting, lethargy, and coma with elevated plasma ammonium levels (>100 μM) and low serum urea nitrogen levels occur. Plasma amino acids show low levels of citrulline (absent or trace levels in the neonatal onset form of the disorder) distinguishing it from citrullinemia and argininosuccinic aciduria, in which citrulline levels are high. Plasma arginine level is low, in contrast to that in argininemia, in which arginine level is elevated. Plasma glutamine and alanine levels are elevated. Urinary orotic acid excretion is high, distinguishing this disorder from carbamyl phosphate synthetase deficiency, in which urinary orotic acid excretion is low. Organic acids and dibasic amino acids are not found in the urine. A definitive diagnosis can be made by measuring activity of ornithine transcarbamylase in liver, duodenal, or rectal tissue. The enzyme is not expressed in fibroblasts or leukocytes.

Clinical Findings: Hemizygous males generally present with respiratory distress, poor feeding, hypotonia, progressive lethargy, and coma within the first three days of life. Untreated, there is universal mortality. Approximately one-half survive following treatment with hemodialysis/peritoneal dialysis. Pulmonary and gastrointestinal hemorrhages have been reported. Girls with partial deficiencies have recurrent episodes of vomiting, hyperactivity, lethargy, and coma, occurring from early childhood and often associated with protein loads or intercurrent illnesses.

Complications: In children with neonatal-onset hyperammonemic coma lasting longer than 48 hours, there is a high incidence of cortical atrophy associated with mental retardation and other developmental disabilities. Despite treatment, affected children are at risk for future episodes of coma, which may cause further brain damage or death.

Associated Findings: Chronic anorexia, food avoidance.

Etiology: X-linked dominant inheritance.

Pathogenesis: Ornithine transcarbamylase deficiency is caused by a deficiency of the mitochondrial urea cycle enzyme ornithine transcarbamylase. Ornithine transcarbamylase is the second enzyme in the urea cycle. Deficient activity leads to an accumulation of ammonium in blood and brain, especially following a protein load or an intercurrent infection. Ammonia is a neurotoxin. Additionally, there may be alterations in brain energy and neurotransmitter metabolism induced by prolonged hyperammonemic coma that result in brain damage. Alzheimer type II cells have been found in the brain.

MIM No.: *31125

Sex Ratio: M1:F1 (manifestations vary by sex).

Occurrence: About 1:30,000. More than 100 cases have been reported.

Risk of Recurrence for Patient's Sib:
See Part I, *Mendelian Inheritance.*

Risk of Recurrence for Patient's Child:
See Part I, *Mendelian Inheritance.*

Age of Detectability: In the neonatal period for affected males and later in childhood, generally ages 2–4 years, in females. Prenatal detection by RFLP is possible in about 85% of affected families. Prospective treatment is possible for at-risk infants from birth.

Gene Mapping and Linkage: OTC (ornithine carbamoyltransferase) has been mapped to Xp21.1.

Prevention: None known. Genetic counseling indicated.

Treatment: Treatment involves combining protein restriction with the induction of alternate pathways of nitrogen waste excretion. This is accomplished using a protein-restricted diet supplemented with essential amino acids (including citrulline) and providing sodium benzoate and sodium phenylacetate. Liver transplant has been performed in two affected males.

Prognosis: The few affected children who have been treated prospectively from birth, because of a previously affected sib, have done better developmentally than those rescued from hyperammonemic coma. The majority of children who have suffered neonatal hyperammonemic coma are mentally retarded. Symptomatic female heterozygotes have a better prognosis, depending on maintaining adequate control of plasma ammonium levels. Life span is uncertain because of the risk of intercurrent hyperammonemic episodes.

Detection of Carrier: Carrier detection has been done using protein tolerance tests or allopurinol tests and then measuring urinary excretion of orotic acid or other pyrimidines. RFLP has also been useful in carrier detection of informed families.

References:
Hokanson JT, et al.: Carrier detection in ornithine transcarbamylase deficiency. J Pediatr 1978; 93:75–78.
Bachmann C, Colombo JP: Diagnostic value of orotic acid excretion in heritable disorders of the urea cycle and in hyperammonemia due to organic aciduria. Eur J Pediatr 1980; 134:109–113.
Zimmermann A, et al.: Ultrastructural pathology in congenital defects of the urea cycle: ornithine transcarbamylase and carbamyl phosphate synthetase deficiency. Virchows Arch Pathol 1981; 393:321.
Batshaw ML, et al.: Treatment of inborn errors of urea synthesis: activation of alternative pathways of waste nitrogen synthesis and excretion. New Engl J Med 1982; 306:1387–1392. *
Batshaw ML: Hyperammonemia. Curr Prob Pediatr 1984; 16:1–69. *
Msall M, et al.: Neurologic outcome of children with inborn errors of urea synthesis. New Engl J Med 1984; 310:1500–1505. *
Fox J, et al.: Prenatal diagnosis of ornithine transcarbamylase deficiency with use of DNA polymorphisms. New Engl J Med 1986; 315:1205–1208.
Rowe PC, et al.: Natural history of symptomatic partial ornithine transcarbamylase deficiency. New Engl J Med 1986; 314:541–547.
Schwartz M, et al.: Detection and exclusion of carriers of ornithine transcarbamylase deficiency by RFLP analysis. Clin Genet 1986; 29:449–452.
Brusilow SW: Urea cycle disorders and other hereditary hyperammonemic syndromes. In: Scriver CR, et al, eds: The metabolic basis of inherited disease, 6th ed. New York: McGraw-Hill, 1989:629–664. *
Spence JE, et al.: Prenatal diagnosis and heterozygote detection by DNA analysis in ornithine transcarbamylase deficiency. J Pediatr 1989; 114:582–588.

BA066   **Mark L. Batshaw**

Ornithine-delta-aminotransferase deficiency
See GYRATE ATROPHY OF THE CHOROID AND RETINA
Ornithinemia with gyrate atrophy of the choroid & retina
See GYRATE ATROPHY OF THE CHOROID AND RETINA

ORO-CRANIO-DIGITAL SYNDROME 0769

Includes:
Cleft lip/palate-abnormal thumbs-microcephaly
Cranio-oro-digital syndrome
Digital-oro-cranio syndrome
Juberg-Hayward syndrome

Excludes:
Acrocephalosyndactyly type III (0229)
Oculo-dento-osseous dysplasia (0737)
Oro-facio-digital syndrome (see all)
Oto-palato-digital syndrome (see all)

Major Diagnostic Criteria: For an isolated case: bilateral or unilateral cleft lip, cleft palate, or occult cleft of the lip; microcephaly; anomaly of the thumbs such as hypoplasia, distal placement, or inflexibility; anomaly of the toes such as mediodorsal curvature or syndactyly. Fewer criteria apparently are needed, once the syndrome is recognized in a sibship.

Clinical Findings: Mediodorsal curvature of the fourth toes (4/5); minimal syndactyly of the second and third toes (4/5); growth

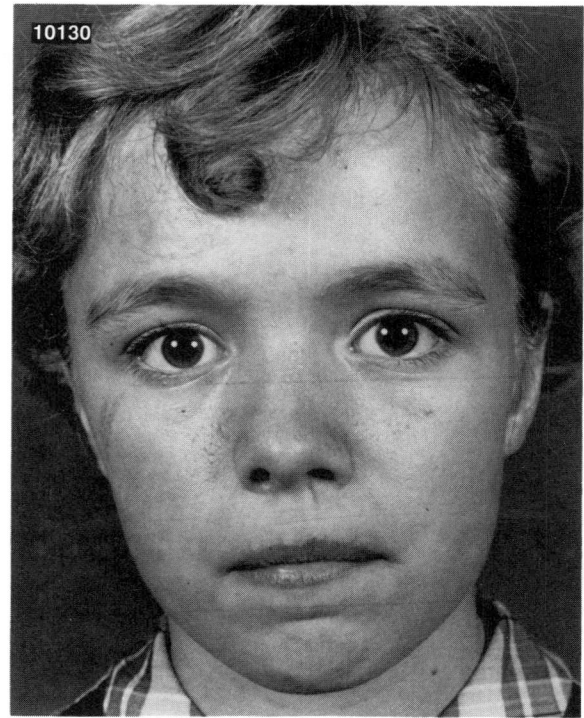

0769A-10130: Occult cleft lip, left edge of philtrum, and wide nasal septum.

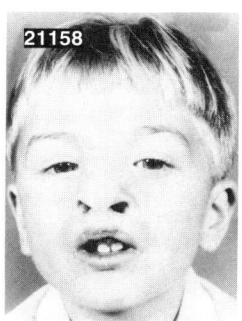
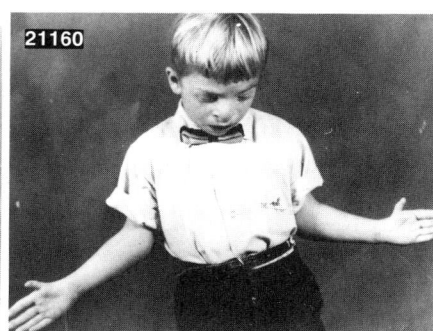
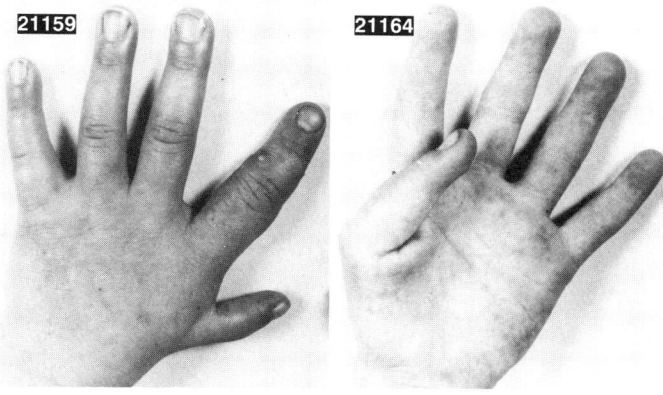

0769B-21158: Propositus at age five years; note repaired cleft lip and ptosis. **21160:** Incomplete extension at both elbows. **21159:** Hypoplasia and distal displacement of the thumb. **21164:** Interphalangeal inflexibility of the thumb is bilateral in this affected sib.

retardation (3/5); microcephaly (3/5); hypoplasia and inflexibility of thumbs (3/5); low birthweight (3/5); dislocation and shortening of radii (2/5); cleft lip or palate (2/5); mental retardation (1/5); and occult cleft lip (1/5).

Complications: Speech defect will accompany cleft palate defect. Difficulty in upper extremity range of motion occurs with dislocation and shortening of the radii.

Associated Findings: Absence of pituitary fossa (reported in one isolated female).

Etiology: Possibly autosomal recessive inheritance.

Pathogenesis: Unknown.

MIM No.: 21610

POS No.: 3138

Sex Ratio: M2:F3 (observed in one sibship).

Occurrence: One sibship of five, and two isolated cases, have been reported.

Risk of Recurrence for Patient's Sib:
See Part I, *Mendelian Inheritance.*

Risk of Recurrence for Patient's Child:
See Part I, *Mendelian Inheritance.*

Age of Detectability: During neonatal period, by clinical examination.

Gene Mapping and Linkage: Unknown.

Prevention: None known. Genetic counseling indicated.

Treatment: Plastic and orthopedic operative procedures, speech correction, physical therapy.

Prognosis: Probably normal life expectancy.

Detection of Carrier: Undetermined. Parents of the one reported sibship were phenotypically normal.

References:
Juberg, RC, Hayward JR: A new familial syndrome of oral, cranial, and digital anomalies. J Pediatr 1969; 74:755–762. * †
Nevin NC, et al.: A case of orocraniodigital (Juberg-Hayward) syndrome. J Med Genet 1981; 18:478–480.
Kingston HM, et al.: Orocraniodigital (Juberg-Hayward) syndrome with growth hormone deficiency. Arch Dis Child 1982; 57:790–792.

JU000   **Richard C. Juberg**

Oro-digito-facial dysostosis
See ORO-FACIO-DIGITAL SYNDROME I

ORO-FACIO-DIGITAL SYNDROME I	**0770**

Includes:
Gorlin-Psaume syndrome
Oral-facial-digital syndrome
Oro-facio-digital syndrome I (OFD I)
Oro-digito-facial dysostosis
Papillon-Leage syndrome
Psaume syndrome

Excludes: **Oro-facio-digital syndrome** (all others)

Major Diagnostic Criteria: Patients are all females (except in the case of **Klinefelter syndrome**) with multiple hyperplastic frenula, multilobulated tongue, broad nasal root, evanescent facial milia, and digital anomalies (brachydactyly, clinodactyly).

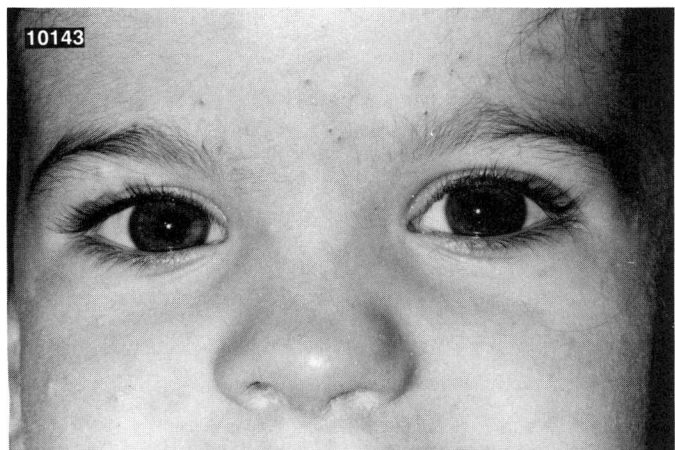
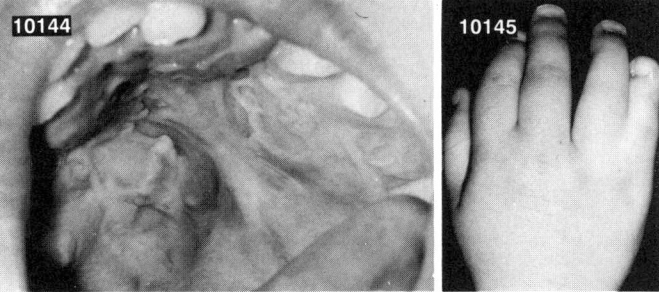

0770-10143: Milia, dystopia canthorum and asymmetric alar cartilages. **10144:** Bizarre clefting of the palate. **10145:** Brachydactyly and partial soft-tissue syndactyly of the 4th and 5th digits.

Clinical Findings: Hyperplastic frenula (ca. 75%); tongue cleft into two or more lobes (ca. 80%); hamartoma of tongue (40%); cleft palate (35%); median cleft of upper lip (35%); dystopia canthorum (30%); hypoplasia of malar bone (25%); clinodactyly, brachydactyly or syndactyly (60%); duplicated hallux (unilateral) (25%); mental retardation (40%); hypoplastic alar cartilages (35%); alopecia (30%); and evanescent facial milia (35%).

Complications: Unknown.

Associated Findings: Various cerebral abnormalities (10%); coarse dry hair (15%); polycystic kidney (15%); agenesis of lower lateral incisor teeth (20%); supernumerary teeth (20%); ankyloglossia (10%); grooved anterior alveolar process of mandible (10%); and lateral grooving of maxillary alveolar process (10%).

Etiology: X-linked dominant inheritance, lethal in male. Segregation analysis has shown some female lethality in lyonized heterozygotes.

Pathogenesis: Unknown.

MIM No.: *31120

POS No.: 3347

CDC No.: 759.800

Sex Ratio: M0:F1

Occurrence: Possibly 1:50,000 live births. Over 200 cases reported.

Risk of Recurrence for Patient's Sib:
See Part I, *Mendelian Inheritance.* If male receives mutant gene from mother, the pregnancy is not completed.

Risk of Recurrence for Patient's Child:
See Part I, *Mendelian Inheritance.* Fifty percent if a daughter; zero if a son. Hence there is a M1:F2 ratio in all offspring of affected females. The overall ratio of affected to unaffected offspring of affected mothers is 1:2.

Age of Detectability: At birth.

Gene Mapping and Linkage: OFD1 (oral-facial-digital syndrome I) is X.

Prevention: None known. Genetic counseling indicated.

Treatment: Plastic surgery for correctible defects.

Prognosis: Normal life span, with average IQ about 70. Functional limitations primarily due to mental retardation.

Detection of Carrier: Clinical examination of first degree relatives.

References:
Gorlin RJ, Psaume J: Orodigitofacial dysostosis: a new syndrome, a study of 22 cases. J Pediatr 1962; 61:520–530.
Fuhrmann W, et al.: Das oro-facio-digitale Syndrom: zugleich eine Diskussion der Erbgänge mit geschlechtsbegrenztem Letaleffekt. Humangenetik 1966; 2:133–164.
Gorlin RJ: The oral-facial-digital (OFD) syndrome. Cutis 1968; 4:1345–1349.
Melnick M, Shields ED: Orofaciodigital syndrome, type I: a phenotype and genetic analysis. Oral Surg 1975; 40:599–610.
Wood BP, et al.: Cerebral abnormalities in the oral-facial-digital syndrome. Pediatr Radiol 1975; 3:130–136.
Townes PL, et al.: Further heterogeneity of the oral-facial-digital syndrome. Am J Dis Child 1976; 130:548–554.
Towfighi J, et al.: Neuropathology of oro-facial-digital syndrome. Arch Path Lab Med 1985; 109:642–646.
Donnai D, et al.: Familial orofaciodigital syndrome type I presenting as adult polycystic disease. J Med Genet 1987; 24:84–87.

G0038   **Robert J. Gorlin**

Oro-facio-digital syndrome I (OFD I)
  See ORO-FACIO-DIGITAL SYNDROME I
Oro-facio-digital syndrome II (OFD II)
  See ORO-FACIO-DIGITAL SYNDROME, MOHR TYPE
Oro-facio-digital syndrome III
  See ORO-FACIO-DIGITAL SYNDROME, SUGARMAN TYPE
Oro-facio-digital syndrome IV
  See ORO-FACIO-DIGITAL SYNDROME, BARAITSER-BURN TYPE

Oro-facio-digital syndrome V
  See ORO-FACIO-DIGITAL SYNDROME, THURSTON TYPE
Oro-facio-digital syndrome VI
  See ORO-PALATAL-DIGITAL SYNDROME, VARADI TYPE
Oro-facio-digital syndrome VII
  See ORO-FACIO-DIGITAL SYNDROME, WHELAN TYPE

ORO-FACIO-DIGITAL SYNDROME, BARAITSER-BURN TYPE   **2585**

Includes:
  Digital-oro-facio syndrome
  Facio-digital-oro syndrome
  Oral-facial-digital syndrome IV
  Oro-facio-digital syndrome IV

Excludes:
  Chondroectodermal dysplasia (0156)
  Oro-facio-digital syndrome, Mohr type (0771)
  Oro-facio-digital syndrome (others)
  Short rib-polydactyly syndrome, type II (0883)

Major Diagnostic Criteria: The combination of tibial defects with oral, facial, and digital anomalies.

Clinical Findings: Facial anomalies include broad nasal root and/or tip, hypertelorism or telecanthus, micrognathia, and low-set ears. Oral anomalies are similar to those reported for other oro-facio-digital syndromes, and include midline cleft lip, cleft or highly arched palate, bifid uvula, oral frenulae, and lingual hamartoma. Absent or supernumerary teeth are occasionally found. Pre- and/or post-axial **Polydactyly** is found in most, but not all cases. **Syndactyly**, clinodactyly, and brachydactyly are sometimes present. However, all cases (and thus the reason for inclusion in this category) have had some degree of tibial dysplasia, ranging from pseudoarthrosis to metaphyseal flaring on X-ray. Short stature, conductive deafness, **Pectus carinatum** or **Pectus excavatum** and clubfoot occasionally occur. Mental retardation can be present, but is not a consistent finding.

Complications: Unknown.

Associated Findings: None known.

Etiology: Possibly autosomal recessive inheritance.

Pathogenesis: Unknown.

MIM No.: 25886

POS No.: 3147

CDC No.: 759.800

Sex Ratio: M1:F1

Occurrence: Undetermined but presumed rare. Many cases were originally described as **Oro-facio-digital syndrome, Mohr type** or a Mohr-Majewski compound (see **Short rib-polydactyly syndrome, type II**). Cases from different parts of the world have been described.

Risk of Recurrence for Patient's Sib:
See Part I, *Mendelian Inheritance.*

Risk of Recurrence for Patient's Child:
See Part I, *Mendelian Inheritance.*

Age of Detectability: At birth, although prenatal ultrasound may detect severe tibial defects.

Gene Mapping and Linkage: Unknown.

Prevention: None known. Genetic counseling indicated.

Treatment: Orthopedic treatment may be indicated.

Prognosis: Life span appears unimpaired; mental retardation, when present, can be mild to severe.

Detection of Carrier: Unknown.

Special Considerations: Further heterogeneity within this category may be possible, in that some individuals have rather severe limb defects and mental retardation, whereas others have short long bones and normal intellect. There appears to be consistency within families regarding the severity of the condition.

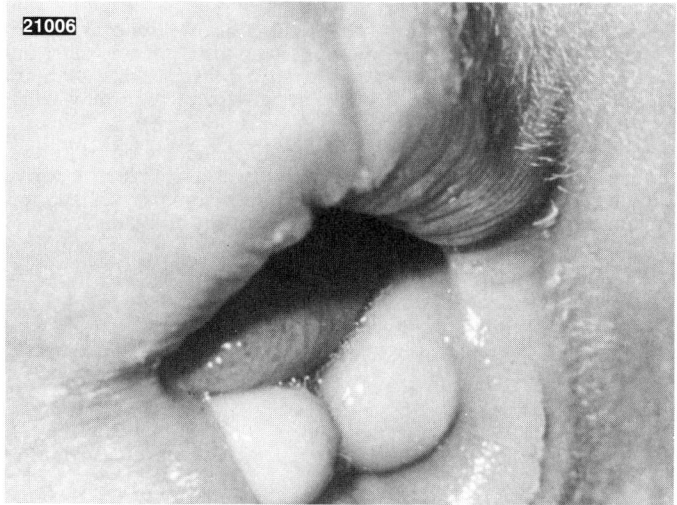

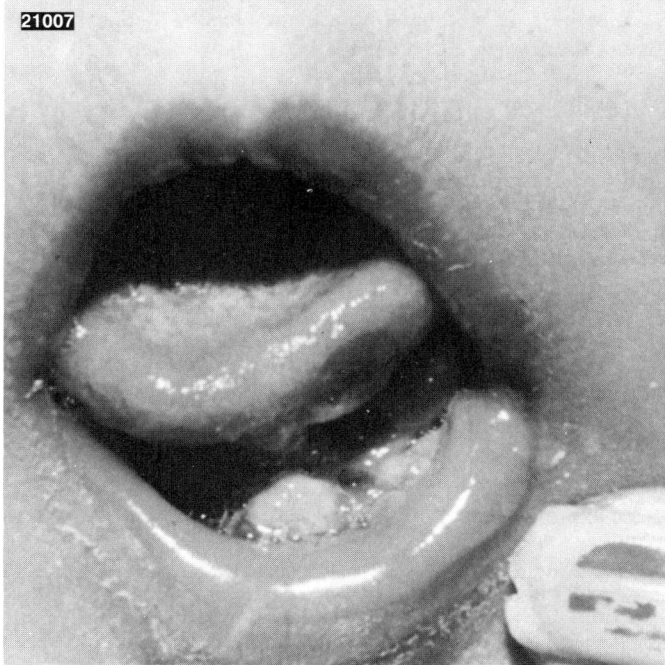

2585A-21006–07: Sublingual hamartomas.

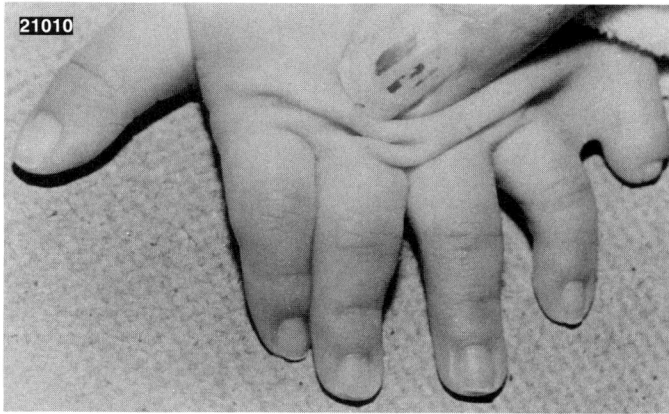

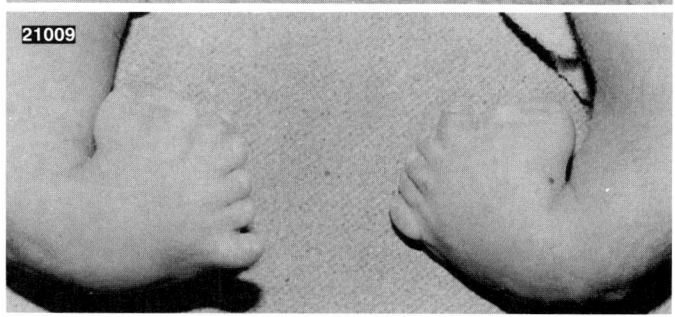

2585B-21010: Post-axial polydactyly. 21009: Pre- and post-axial polydactyly.

ORO-FACIO-DIGITAL SYNDROME, MOHR TYPE   0771

Includes:
    Mohr syndrome
    Oral-facial-digital syndrome II
    Oro-facio-digital syndrome II (OFD II)

Excludes:
    Acrocallosal syndrome, Schinzel type (2263)
    Asphyxiating thoracic dysplasia (0091)
    Chondroectodermal dysplasia (0156)
    Oro-facio-digital syndrome (type I and others)
    Short rib-polydactyly syndrome, type II (0883)

Major Diagnostic Criteria: Oral manifestations include lingual or sublingual hamartomatous nodules with or without a lobate tongue, hypodontia, hyperplastic frenula, pseudocleft of the upper lip, broad nasal bridge, broad or bifid nasal tip, zygomatic hypoplasia and hypoplasia of the body of the mandible, and polysyndactyly.

Clinical Findings: The cleft upper lip may be severe or so mild as to be considered a "pseudocleft." The upper lip may appear to be tethered by the hypertrophied midline frenula. Multiple lateral frenula are present less frequently. A midline cleft of the lower alveolar ridge may also be present and may be severe enough to require bone grafting. Hypodontia involving the central lower incisors is common. Other dental abnormalities may include absence of other teeth, small malformed teeth, and dental malocclusion related to the mandibular defects.

On X-ray, there is hypoplasia of the body of the mandible, and clinically there is often micrognathia. Less frequently there is prognathism because of marked midface hypoplasia. The nasal root and tip are broad, and the tip may be bifid but without a true cleft. True hypertelorism occurs rarely if at all, but dystopia canthorum may be present.

The most characteristic digital abnormality is duplication of the

References:
Baraitser M, et al.: A female infant with features of Mohr and Majewski syndromes: variable expression, a genetic compound, or a distinct entity? J Med Genet 1983; 20:65–67.
Burn J, et al.: Orofacial digital syndrome with mesomelic limb shortening. J Med Genet 1984; 21:189–192. * †
Fenton OM, Watt-Smith SR: The spectrum of the oro-facial digital syndrome. Br J Plast Surg 1985; 38:532–539.
Baraitser M: The orofaciodigital (OFD) syndromes. J Med Genet 1986; 23:116–119.
Nevin NC, Thomas PS: Orofaciodigital syndrome type IV: report of a patient. Am J Med Genet 1989; 32:151–154. †

     Helga V. Toriello

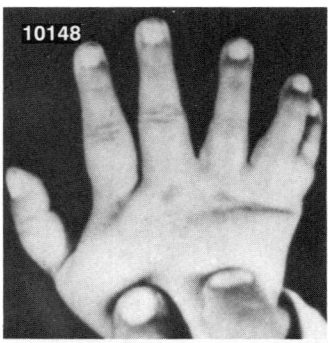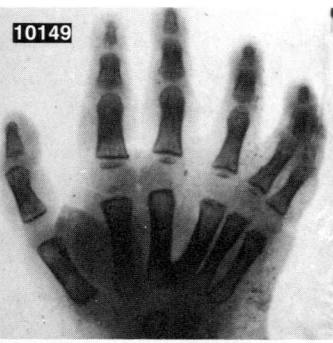

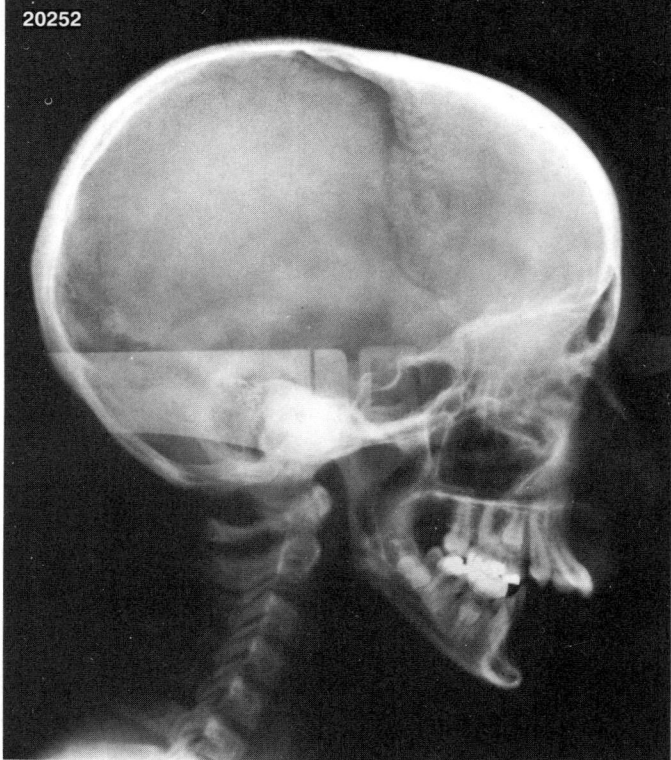

0771-10148–49: Postaxial polydactyly. 20252: Lateral skull X-ray shows hypoplasia of the body of the mandible.

hallux; almost always bilateral. Although usually clinically obvious, hallucal defects may be demonstrated in other cases on X-ray as broad first metatarsals and notching of the distal phalanx. Duplication of the medial cuneiform and navicular bones may be present. Polydactyly and syndactyly of other digits are frequently present; the average number of fingers per hand in one selected series of patients was 5.8 (post-axial polydactyly was more common than pre-axial) and of toes was 6.0 (pre-axial more common than post-axial). Up to seven digits may be present on each hand or foot. Syndactyly may involve the extra digits, fingers 3–4 or 4–5, or toes 2–3 or 1–7. In addition, fifth finger clinodactyly and brachydactyly may be present. Mild short stature and mesomelic shortening of extremities, especially of the tibia, may be present. X-rays may show metaphyseal flaring and irregularity of the tibia. Metaphyseal and sometimes epiphyseal abnormalities of the radius are less frequently observed. Some patients have equinovarus deformities.

Moderately severe conductive hearing loss may be present, and in one case it was related to a malformed incus that did not articulate with the stapes. No patient has had complete hearing loss. Intellect ranges from normal to significant subnormality. In several families, intellect seems to be similar in affected sibs, but severity in general cannot be predicted because stillbirths, infant deaths, and prolonged survival with good outcome may occur within a single sibship.

Complications: There is an increased frequency of stillbirths. Infant deaths related to respiratory problems and failure to thrive may occur, but other infants thrive. In survivors, mental subnormality and hearing loss are the major medical problems.

The lobate tongue and hamartomatous nodules infrequently interfere with speech development, but usually do not impair speech, respirations or feeding.

Associated Findings: None known.

Etiology: Autosomal recessive inheritance.

Pathogenesis: Unknown.

MIM No.: *25210

POS No.: 3348

CDC No.: 759.800

Sex Ratio: M1:F1

Occurrence: About 25 cases have been documented.

Risk of Recurrence for Patient's Sib:
See Part I, *Mendelian Inheritance.*

Risk of Recurrence for Patient's Child:
See Part I, *Mendelian Inheritance.*

Age of Detectability: At birth. Prenatal diagnosis has not been reported, but an affected fetus could potentially be detected by ultrasound on the basis of polydactyly.

Gene Mapping and Linkage: Unknown.

Prevention: None known. Genetic counseling indicated.

Treatment: Surgical correction of cleft lip and palate, polysyndactyly, and, if warranted, lingual abnormalities. Hearing aids are helpful for patients with conductive hearing deficits. Mandibular and dental procedures may alleviate dental malocclusion and improve cosmetic appearance. Clubfoot deformity may respond to casting.

Prognosis: An increased frequency of stillbirths and infant deaths. In survivors, outcome is mainly determined by intellectual status.

Detection of Carrier: By clinical examination, and X-rays of mandible and feet.

Special Considerations: Misdiagnosis may account for some of the clinical heterogenity with regard to presence or absence of structural central nervous system malformations, severe limb defects, and renal abnormalities. Alternatively, these features may represent a more severe clinical spectrum of this condition.

Although many patients with this condition have mild mesomelic shortening of the tibia, some researchers have designated patients with more severe limb defects as having **Oro-facio-digital syndrome, Baraitser-Burn type**. Others maintain that these patients simply have a more severe form of **Oro-facio-digital syndrome, Mohr type**, and also classify patients with tibial pseudoarthroses as having the Mohr type. It has even been suggested that **Short rib-polydactyly syndrome, type II** ("Majewski") represents a severe spectrum of the Mohr type, but it is nevertheless reasonable to maintain for the moment that this uniformly severe and lethal disorder is a distinct clinical entity. Whether or not some of these disorders are allelic is undetermined.

Some consider patients with central nervous system abnormalities such as Dandy-Walker malformation, porencephalic cysts and agenesis of the corpus callosum to have Mohr type OFD. However, some of these patients may have **Joubert syndrome** or some other distinct condition. It is difficult to definitely categorize some of these patients because of overlapping clinical features. Similarly, some patients with renal hypoplasia or aplasia have overlapping features with Mohr OFD, and it is not clear if these patients have a separate disorder.

Finally, some have suggested that **Acrocallosal syndrome, Schin-**

zel type is a related genetic entity with an additional loss of the corpus callosum.

References:
Mohr O: A hereditary sublethal syndrome in man. Avh Norske Videnskad Oslo 1941; 14:1–18.
Rimoin DL, Edgerton MT: Genetic and clinical heterogeneity in the oral-facial-digital syndromes. J Pediatr 1967; 71:94–102. *
Haumont D, Pelc S: The Mohr syndrome: are there two variants? Clin Genet 1983; 24:41–46.
Anneren G, et al.: Oro-facio-digital syndromes I and II: radiological methods for diagnosis and the clinical variations. Clin Genet 1984; 26:178–182.
Michels VV, et al.: Polysyndactyly in the orofacial digital syndrome, Type II. J Clin Dysmorphol 1985; 3:2–9.
Baraitser M: The orofacial digital (OFD) syndromes. J Med Genet 1986; 23:116–119. *
Silengo MC, et al.: Oro-facial-digital syndrome II: transition type between the Mohr and the Majewski syndromes: report of 2 new cases. Clin Genet 1987; 31:331–336.

MI002   **Virginia V. Michels**

ORO-FACIO-DIGITAL SYNDROME, SUGARMAN TYPE   3058

Includes:
Digital-oro-facio syndrome III
Facio-oro-digital syndrome III
Oro-facio-digital syndrome III
Sugarman syndrome

Excludes:
Bardet-Biedl syndrome (2363)
Oro-facio-digital syndrome (other)

Major Diagnostic Criteria: The combination of oral, facial, and digital anomalies with see-saw winking or myoclonic jerks affecting the ocular area is necessary to make the diagnosis.

Clinical Findings: Phenotypic features include lobed tongue with hamartomas, malocclusion and supernumerary teeth, bifid uvula, postaxial **Polydactyly** of hands and feet, **Pectus excavatum**, short sternum, kyphosis, and mental retardation. One child had see-saw winking of the eyelids, one had blepharospasm, and three had myoclonic jerks of the eyelids and extraocular muscles.

Complications: Unknown.

Associated Findings: None known.

Etiology: Autosomal recessive inheritance.

Pathogenesis: Unknown.

MIM No.: *25885

POS No.: 3098

Sex Ratio: M1:F1

Occurrence: Five patients in two families have been reported, both from the United States.

Risk of Recurrence for Patient's Sib:
See Part I, *Mendelian Inheritance.*

Risk of Recurrence for Patient's Child:
See Part I, *Mendelian Inheritance.*

Age of Detectability: At birth, although prenatal diagnosis using ultrasound may also be useful.

Gene Mapping and Linkage: Unknown.

Prevention: None known. Genetic counseling indicated.

Treatment: Unknown.

Prognosis: Mental retardation has been severe in all cases; life span is unknown.

Detection of Carrier: Unknown.

Special Considerations: Three of the five cited cases of this condition consist of two brothers and a sister observed (unpublished) by Victor McKusick, for whom other diagnoses have been suggested.

References:
Sugarman GI, et al.: See-saw winking in a familial oral-facial-digital syndrome. Clin Genet 1971; 2:248–254.

T0007   **Helga V. Toriello**

ORO-FACIO-DIGITAL SYNDROME, THURSTON TYPE   2592

Includes:
Cleft lip-polydactyly
Oral-facial-digital syndrome V
Oro-facio-digital syndrome V
Polydactyly, postaxial-median cleft of upper lip
Thurston syndrome

Excludes:
Cleft lip (0178)
Oro-facio-digital syndrome (others)
Polydactyly (0814)

Major Diagnostic Criteria: The combination of median **Cleft lip** and **Polydactyly** without other anomalies confirms the diagnosis.

Clinical Findings: The only anomalies consist of median **Cleft lip** and **Polydactyly** of hands and/or feet, which can be unilateral or bilateral. Polydactyly is usually post-axial, and six or seven digits may be present.

Complications: Unknown.

Associated Findings: None known.

Etiology: Possibly autosomal recessive inheritance.

Pathogenesis: Unknown.

MIM No.: 17430

POS No.: 3870

CDC No.: 759.800

Sex Ratio: M1:F1

Occurrence: Undetermined but presumed rare. All cases have been of Indian ethnic origin.

Risk of Recurrence for Patient's Sib:
See Part I, *Mendelian Inheritance.*

Risk of Recurrence for Patient's Child:
See Part I, *Mendelian Inheritance.*

Age of Detectability: At birth by the presence of the cleft lip and/or polydactyly.

Gene Mapping and Linkage: Unknown.

Prevention: None known. Genetic counseling indicated.

Treatment: Repair of the cleft lip. Removal of the extra digits for cosmetic reasons may also be considered.

Prognosis: Life span and intelligence are normal.

Detection of Carrier: Unknown.

References:
Thurston EO: A case of median hare-lip associated with other malformations. Lancet 1909; II:996–997.
Chowdhury J: A study of five siblings with median cleft lips and polydactyly. Trans 6th Cong Plast Reconstr Surg Paris, 1975:208–211.
Khoo CT, Saad MN: Median cleft of the upper lip in association with bilateral hexadactyly and accessory toes. Plast Reconstr Surg 1980; 33:407–409.
Gopalakrishna A, Thatte RL: Median cleft lip associated with bimanual hexadactyly and bilateral accessory toes: another case. Br J Plast Surg 1982; 35:354–355. †

T0007   **Helga V. Toriello**

ORO-FACIO-DIGITAL SYNDROME, WHELAN TYPE   2586

Includes:
Digital-facio-oro syndrome
Facio-oro-digital syndrome
Oro-facio-digital syndrome VII
Whelan syndrome

Excludes:
Oculo-auriculo-vertebral anomaly (0735)
Oro-facio-digital syndrome (other)

Major Diagnostic Criteria: Facial asymmetry, unilateral pseudo-cleft lip, and hydronephrosis, in addition to oral anomalies and clinodactyly.

Clinical Findings: In a reported mother and daughter; apparent hypertelorism, pseudocleft upper lip, highly arched palate, lobed tongue, and facial asymmetry. The daughter also had unilateral preauricular tags and low-set ears. Both had clinodactyly, but no other digital anomalies, and hydronephrosis.

Complications: Renal complications secondary to hydronephrosis.

Associated Findings: None known.

Etiology: Possibly X-linked or autosomal dominant inheritance.

Pathogenesis: Unknown.

CDC No.: 759.800

Sex Ratio: M0:F2 (observed).

Occurrence: Reported in a mother and daughter.

Risk of Recurrence for Patient's Sib:
See Part I, *Mendelian Inheritance.*

Risk of Recurrence for Patient's Child:
See Part I, *Mendelian Inheritance.*

Age of Detectability: At birth.

Gene Mapping and Linkage: Unknown.

Prevention: None known. Genetic counseling indicated.

Treatment: Appropriate treatment for hydronephrosis is indicated.

Prognosis: Mental retardation is mild to minimal; life span appears unimpaired.

Detection of Carrier: Unknown.

Special Considerations: This case was reported as an example of **Oro-facio-digital syndrome I**; however, the presence of some findings in both mother and daughter, but not in other cases of OFD I syndrome, suggests, albeit tentatively, that this may be a distinct condition.

References:
Whelan DT, et al.: The oro-facial-digital syndrome. Clin Genet 1975; 8:205–212.

T0007   **Helga V. Toriello**

Oro-ocular cleft
See FACIAL CLEFT, OBLIQUE

ORO-PALATAL-DIGITAL SYNDROME, VARADI TYPE   2368

Includes:
Digital-oro-palatal syndrome
Joubert syndrome with polydactyly
Oro-facio-digital syndrome VI
Palatal-digital-oro syndrome
Polydactyly-cleft lip/palate/lingual lump-psychomotor retardation
Varadi-Papp syndrome

Excludes:
Joubert syndrome (2908)
Oro-facio-digital syndrome, Mohr type (0771)
Oro-facio-digital syndrome (others)

Major Diagnostic Criteria: Oral, facial, digital (OFD) and cerebellar anomalies.

Clinical Findings: Facial features consist of hypertelorism, epicanthal folds, broad nasal tip, **Cleft palate**, and posteriorly rotated, low-set ears. Oral frenulae, lingual nodules, cleft or highly arched palate are the oral findings. Postaxial polydactyly, clinodactyly, and syndactyly affect the hands; on X-ray, a bifid metacarpal has been noted in all cases. The feet can have pre- or postaxial polydactyly. Cerebellar defects range from features of the Dandy-Walker malformation to hypoplasia of the vermis. Severe mental retardation is a constant finding; growth delay, hypotonia, and deafness also occur.

Complications: Motor incoordination and speech delay are likely secondary to the cerebellar defects.

Associated Findings: Findings reported in one case only include arhinencephaly, **Aortic valve stenosis**, **Aorta, coarctation**, and **Renal agenesis, unilateral.**

Etiology: Possibly autosomal recessive inheritance.

Pathogenesis: Unknown.

MIM No.: 27717

Sex Ratio: M1:F1

Occurrence: Undetermined but presumed rare. Cases have been reported from different areas of the world.

Risk of Recurrence for Patient's Sib:
See Part I, *Mendelian Inheritance.*

Risk of Recurrence for Patient's Child:
See Part I, *Mendelian Inheritance.*

Age of Detectability: At birth, although prenatal diagnosis by ultrasound may be possible.

Gene Mapping and Linkage: Unknown.

Prevention: None known. Genetic counseling indicated.

Treatment: Supportive.

Prognosis: Mental retardation is severe; life span is unknown. Some cases have died in infancy.

Detection of Carrier: Unknown.

References:
Varadi V, et al.: Syndrome of polydactyly, cleft lip/palate or lingual lump, and psychomotor retardation in endogamic gypsies. J Med Genet 1980; 17:119–122. †
Haumont D, Pelc SC: The Mohr syndrome: are there two variants? Clin Genet 1983; 24:41–46.
Mattei JF, Ayme S: Syndrome of polydactyly, cleft lip, lingual hamartomas, renal hypoplasia, hearing loss, and psychomotor retardation: variant of the Mohr syndrome or a new syndrome? J Med Genet 1983; 20:433–435. * †

T0007   **Helga V. Toriello**

Oromandibular limb hypoplasia
See HYPOGLOSSIA-HYPODACTYLIA
Oromandibular-limb hypogenesis syndrome
See DIPLEGIA, CONGENITAL FACIAL
Orotate phosphoribosyltransferase-omp decarboxylase deficiency
See ACIDEMIA, OROTIC
Orotic acidemia
See ACIDEMIA, OROTIC
Orotic aciduria
See ACIDEMIA, OROTIC
Orotidylic decarboxylase deficiency
See ACIDEMIA, OROTIC
Orotidylic pyrophosphorylase-orotidylic decarboxylase deficiency
See ACIDEMIA, OROTIC
Orthochromatic leukodystrophy
See ADRENOLEUKODYSTROPHY, X-LINKED
Osgood-Schlatter disease (tibial tubercle)
See JOINTS, OSTEOCHONDRITIS DISSECANS
Osler disease
See TELANGIECTASIA, OSLER HEMORRHAGIC
Osler-Weber-Rendu disease
See TELANGIECTASIA, OSLER HEMORRHAGIC

Osseous-oculo-dento dysplasia
  See *OCULO-DENTO-OSSEOUS DYSPLASIA*
Ossicle malformations
  See *EAR, OSSICLE AND MIDDLE EAR MALFORMATIONS*
Ossicles, malformed and conductive hearing loss
  See *EAR, MICROTIA-ATRESIA*
Ossifying fibroma of the long bones
  See *OSTEOFIBROUS DYSPLASIA OF TIBIA AND FIBULA*
Osteitis deformans
  See *BONE, PAGET DISEASE*
Osteo-onycho dysplasia and oculo-oto-nasal defects
  See *OCULO-OTO-NASAL MALFORMATIONS WITH OSTEO-ONYCHO DYSPLASIA*
Osteoarthropathy, hypertrophic
  See *PACHYDERMOPERIOSTOSIS*
Osteochondritis deformans juvenilis
  See *HIP, OSTEONECROSIS, CAPITAL FEMORAL EPIPHYSIS*

OSTEOCHONDRODYSPLASIA WITH HYPERTRICHOSIS   2332

Includes: Hypertrichotic osteochondrodysplasia

Excludes:
  Gingival fibromatosis-hypertrichosis (0410)
  Hair, hypertrichosis, lanuginosa (0507)
  Hair, hypertrichosis, X-linked (2314)
  Hypertrichosis, acquired
  Hypertrichosis, other forms of familial localized
  Localized hypertrichosis, sporadic or associated with spina bifida

Major Diagnostic Criteria: Excessive generalized hairiness at birth with macrosomy, typical facial appearance, and X-ray findings that include narrow thorax, cardiomegaly, wide ribs, platyspondyly, hypoplastic ischiopubic branches, bilateral coxa valga, "Erlenmeyer flask" long-bone appearance, wide distal phalanx of the first toes, and generalized osteopenia.

Clinical Findings: Excessive hairiness occurs practically all over the body, except the palms, soles, and mucous membranes. Coarse facial features; abundant and curly eyelashes; epicanthal folds; flattened, broad nasal bridge; small nose with hypoplastic alae nasi (in younger patients); anteverted nostrils; long philtrum; prominent mouth; short neck; narrow shoulders and thorax; cardiomegaly; some patients with confirmed cardiopathy (**Ductus arteriosus, patent**, **Aortic valve stenosis**); **Hernia, umbilical**; short hands; clinodactyly of the fifth fingers; and short, wide thumbs and first toes.

Typical X-ray findings: narrow thorax, global cardiomegaly, wide ribs, platyspondyly, irregularities on the articular surfaces of the vertebral bodies (in oldest patients), vertebral bodies with an ovoid shape (in youngest patients), hypoplastic ischiopubic branches, small obturator foramen, bilateral coxa valga, enlarged medullary canal, long bones with an "Erlenmeyer flask" appearance, thick and bright cortical margins, generalized osteopenia, bands of growth arrest, shortness of the distal phalanx of the first fingers, short and wide distal phalanx of the first toe and delayed bone age.

This is a distinct osteochondrodysplasia with congenital hypertrichosis. The physical appearance in some patients during early infancy may erroneously suggest hypothyroidism. The typical abnormal skeletal findings are easily distinguishable from other skeletal dysplasias.

Complications: Psychosocial impact from the physical appearance.

Associated Findings: Some patients may have dental anomalies and, rarely, gingival hyperplasia. Hepatomegaly of unknown cause was observed in one patient, and mild mental deficiency in another.

Etiology: Although no parental consanguinity can be found in any family, the presence of affected males and females from healthy parents and its occurrence in sibs suggest autosomal recessive inheritance.

Pathogenesis: Unknown.

MIM No.: 23985

POS No.: 3941

CDC No.: 756.580

Sex Ratio: M1:F1

Occurrence: Seven cases have been observed from three families.

Risk of Recurrence for Patient's Sib:
  See Part I, *Mendelian Inheritance.*

Risk of Recurrence for Patient's Child:
  See Part I, *Mendelian Inheritance.*

Age of Detectability: At birth.

Gene Mapping and Linkage: Unknown.

Prevention: None known. Genetic counseling indicated.

Treatment: Cosmetic treatment of the hair by depilatory applications, shaving, diathermy, radiation, or bleaching.

Prognosis: Normal life span, no functional impairment, and normal intelligence.

Detection of Carrier: Unknown.

References:
Cantú JM, et al.: A distinct osteochondrodysplasia with hypertrichosis: individualization of a probable autosomal recessive entity. Hum Genet 1982; 60:36–41. * †

CA011
CR023

José María Cantú
Diana García-Cruz

Osteochondroma of the distal femoral epiphysis
  See *DYSPLASIA EPIPHYSEALIS HEMIMELICA*
Osteochondroma, intra-articular of the astragalus
  See *DYSPLASIA EPIPHYSEALIS HEMIMELICA*
Osteochondromatosis
  See *ENCHONDROMATOSIS*
Osteodermatopoikilosis
  See *OSTEOPOIKILOSIS*
Osteodysgenesis, multisynostotic, with fractures
  See *ANTLEY-BIXLER SYNDROME*
Osteodysplasia enostotica
  See *OSTEOPOIKILOSIS*
Osteodysplasia with acro-osteolysis, hereditary
  See *HAJDU-CHENEY SYNDROME*
Osteodysplasia, auricular
  See *AURICULO-OSTEODYSPLASIA*

OSTEODYSPLASIA, LIPOMEMBRANOUS POLYCYSTIC-DEMENTIA   2227

Includes:
  Brain-bone-fat disease
  Dementia (progressive)-lipomembranous polycystic osteodysplasia
  Lipomembranous osteodystrophy
  Membranous lipodystrophy
  Nasu-Hakola disease
  Polycystic lipomembranous osteodysplasia-leukoencephalopathy

Excludes:
  Alzheimer disease, familial (2354)
  Fibrous dysplasia, monostotic (0390)
  Fibrous dysplasia, polyostotic (0391)
  Gaucher disease (0406)
  Hallervorden-Spatz disease (2526)
  Wolman disease (1003)

Major Diagnostic Criteria: Pain and tenderness in wrists, ankles or knees of a young adult with X-ray evidence of pathologic fractures; with onset in the fourth or fifth decade of dementia, neurologic defects and seizures.

Clinical Findings: Infancy and childhood are usually unremarkable but the young adult has onset of pain and tenderness in ankles, wrists or knees with X-ray evidence of pathologic fractures. Bone biopsy shows yellow gelatinous substance with markedly abnormal fat cell histology. Also, in adulthood, there is onset of slowly progressive dementia typically beginning in the fourth or fifth decade. Dementia is often accompanied by frontal lobe signs, confabulation, euphoria, upper motor neuron signs, and there is also adult onset of generalized seizures. CT brain scan shows evidence of cerebral cortical atrophy and calcification in the basal ganglia. Pathologic fractures, progressive dementia and generalized seizures occur in almost every patient. Death occurs in a vegetative state with poorly controlled seizures and aspiration pneumonia, typically in the fifth decade. The EEG may show typical symmetrical, synchronous, episodic 6–8 Hz activity with diffuse slow wave activity.

Complications: Severe dementia; vegetative state.

Associated Findings: Two patients have been described with associated megacolon and paralytic ileus. One patient also had chronic myelogenous leukemia. Senile plaques and neurofibrillary tangles were found in the cortex of a single 48-year-old-man, but have not been found in other patients. Myoclonic twitches have been reported in some cases.

Etiology: Autosomal recessive inheritance, with affected siblings and unaffected parents.

Pathogenesis: No specific metabolic or chemical abnormality has been found. Histologic changes have been noted in fat cells throughout the body, including tissue from the bone cysts and subcutaneous fat. Fat cell membranes are markedly convoluted, and lipid vesicles may accumulate in the extracellular space. The jelly-like material in the bone cysts is PAS positive, suggesting a glycoprotein structure. Arteries, including those in the basal ganglia, have been abnormal with poorly developed tunica media, abnormal elastica exterma, and interna with thickened intima. Arterioles may be completely blocked and calcified. The brain shows generally normal gray matter with atrophy and marked gliosis of subcortical white matter, compatible with a leukodystrophy. One autopsied Japanese case demonstrated a sudanophilic leukodystrophy with an increase in brain free fatty acids and a decrease in unsaturated fatty acids.

MIM No.: *22177

POS No.: 4262

Sex Ratio: M1:F1

Occurrence: At least 55 cases from 16 kinships have been reported. Most cases have been reported from Finland, Sweden, and Japan.

Risk of Recurrence for Patient's Sib:
See Part I, *Mendelian Inheritance.*

Risk of Recurrence for Patient's Child:
See Part I, *Mendelian Inheritance.*

Age of Detectability: No specific test, but earliest abnormality may be bone cysts noted on careful X-ray examination in adolescence or young adulthood.

Gene Mapping and Linkage: Unknown.

Prevention: None known. Genetic counseling indicated.

Treatment: Symptomatic as needed. Seizures should be treated with long-term anticonvulsant therapy.

Prognosis: Poor. Death typically in the fifth decade following a five to 20 year course of increasing pathologic fractures, initially mild psychiatric symptoms progressing to a severe dementia, poorly controlled seizures, and end-stage vegetative neurologic state.

Detection of Carrier: Unknown.

Special Considerations: The slowly progressive presenile dementia can be confused with **Alzheimer disease, familial**, but can be distinguished from Alzheimer's by the presence of polycystic bone disease, calcification of the basal ganglia on CT scan, and sometimes, a history of affected sibs. The cystic bone lesions must be distinguished from the nonspecific and more common X-ray diagnosis of fibrous dysplasia. X-rays of wrists and ankles should probably be obtained in all cases of unexplained presenile dementia. Biopsy of bone cysts in suspicious cases may provide valuable diagnostic information.

References:
Hakola HPA: Neuropsychiatric and genetic aspects of a new hereditary disease characterized by progressive dementia and lipomembranous polycystic osteodysplasia. Acta Psychiatry Scand (Suppl) 1972; 232:1–171. *
Hakola HPA, Iivanainen M: A new hereditary disease with progressive dementia and polycystic osteodysplasia: neuroradiological analysis of seven cases. Neuroradiology 1973; 6:162–168.
Nasu T, et al.: A lipid metabolic disease: 'membranous lipodystrophy' an autopsy case demoonstrating peculiar membrane-structures composed of lipid in bone and bone marrow and various adipose tissues. Acta Pathol Jpn 1973; 23:539–558.
Tanaka J: Leukoencephalopathic alteration in membranous lipodystrophy. Acta Neuropathol (Berl) 1980; 50:193–197.
Matsushita M, et al.: Nasu-Hakola's disease (membraneous lipodystrophy). Acta Neuropathol (Berl) 1981; 54:89–93.
Bird TD, et al.: Lipomembranous polycystic osteodysplasia (brain, bone, and fat disease): a genetic cause of presenile dementia. Neurology 1983; 33:81–86. *

BI019   **Thomas D. Bird**

Osteodysplasias
See DWARFISM
Osteodysplastic primordial dwarfism, type II
See DWARFISM, OSTEODYSPLASTIC PRIMORDIAL, MAJEWSKI-RANKE TYPE
Osteodysplastic primordial dwarfism, type IV
See DWARFISM, MICROCEPHALIC PRIMORDIAL WITH CATARACTS
Osteodysplastic primordial dwarfism, types I and III
See DWARFISM, OSTEODYSPLASTIC PRIMORDIAL, MAJEWSKI-WINTER TYPE

OSTEODYSPLASTICA GERODERMIA, BAMATTER TYPE   2099

Includes:
Bamatter syndrome
Geroderma osteodysplastica hereditaria (GOH)
Gerodermia osteodysplastica
Walt Disney dwarfism

Excludes:
Cockayne syndrome (0189)
Cutis laxa (0233)
Cutis laxa-growth defect, De Barsy type (2138)
Ehlers-Danlos syndrome (0338)
Werner syndrome (0998)

Major Diagnostic Criteria: A combination of lax, wrinkled skin; aged appearance; osteoporosis; and joint laxity.

Clinical Findings: In 17 affected individuals, the findings have included lax, wrinkled skin from birth (17); joint hyperextensibility (17); short stature (8); brachycephaly (7); prominent forehead (10); ptosis of upper eyelids (7); microcornea (3); malar flushing (5); malar flattening (8); down-turned corners of the mouth (7); narrow and/or highly arched palate (13); dental malocclusion (12); mandibular hypoplasia (9); narrow chest (4); kyphosis plus scoliosis (11); winged scapulae (10); **Hernia, inguinal** (4); dislocated hips (14); minor hand anomalies (8); flat feet (14); increased lambdoid wormian bones (6); vertebral compression (14); osteoporosis (16).
The skin shows lack of normal recoil, although there is no abnormality with scar formation, nor is skin fragility or bruisability increased. Laboratory studies which have been done, and found to be normal, include blood and urine metabolic studies, creatinine phosphokinase levels, thyroxine levels, electromyography, nerve conduction studies, EEG, EKG, and chromosome studies. In some patients skin biopsies have been interpreted as normal. However, in others excessive fragmentation of collagen fibers was noted, and in one, elastic fibers were found to be underdeveloped as well. On X-ray, osteoporosis is most marked in the vertebrae. Bone age has been normal.

Complications: Fractures following minimal trauma are common.

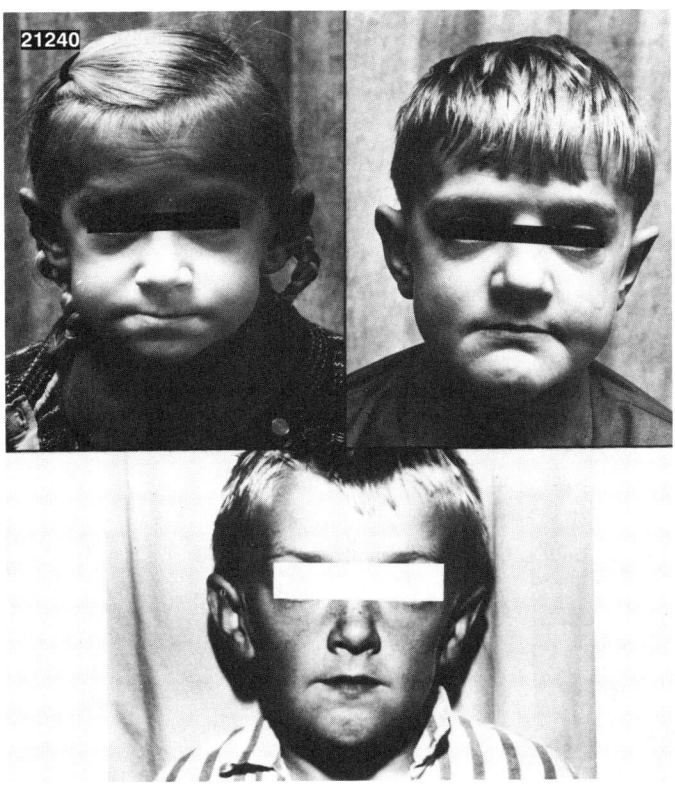

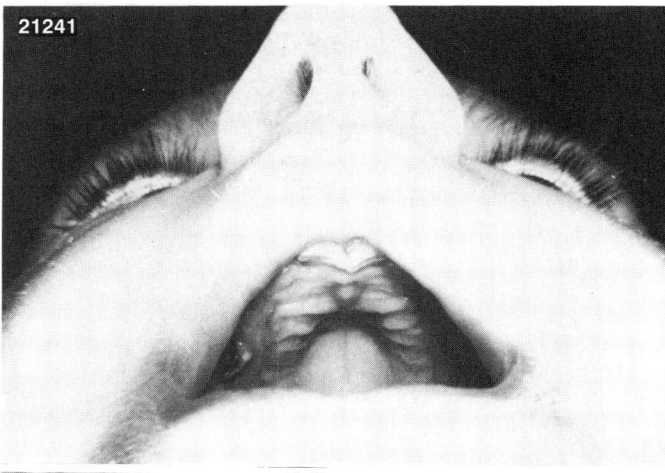

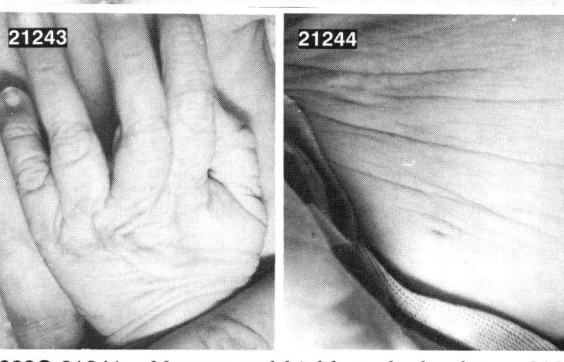

2099A-21240: Note prominent forehead, ptosis, malar flush and flattening, downturned corners of the mouth and small chin.

2099C-21241: Narrow and highly arched palate. 21243: Lax and wrinkled skin is seen in this child's hand. 21244: Lax and wrinkled abdominal skin.

Associated Findings: Reported in only one or two affected individuals were exophthalmos, iris heterochromia, premature arcus senilis, strabismus, **Tongue, geographic**, inverted nipples, cryptorchidism, simian crease, hyperconvex nails, small sella turcica, and absent left pisiform bone.

Etiology: Autosomal recessive inheritance.

Pathogenesis: Unknown. Both ectodermal and mesodermal derivatives are involved.

MIM No.: *23107

POS No.: 3243

Sex Ratio: M1:F1

Occurrence: Reported in four kinships plus isolated cases.

Risk of Recurrence for Patient's Sib:
See Part I, *Mendelian Inheritance*.

Risk of Recurrence for Patient's Child:
See Part I, *Mendelian Inheritance*.

Age of Detectability: At birth, by physical examination.

Gene Mapping and Linkage: Unknown.

Prevention: None known. Genetic counseling indicated.

Treatment: If indicated, treatment for hip dislocation, and prevention of excessive trauma to minimize fracture incidence.

Prognosis: Life span appears normal, and intelligence is usually not impaired, although one patient had an IQ of 68.

Detection of Carrier: Unknown.

References:
Bamatter F, et al.: Gerodermie osteodysplastique hereditaire. Ann Pediatr 1950; 174:126–127
Boreux G: La gerodermie osteodysplastie. J Genet Hum 1969; 17:137–178
Hunter AGW, et al.: Geroderma osteodysplastica: a report of two affeted families. Hum Genet 1978; 40:311–325.
Lisker R, et al.: Geroderma osteodysplastica hereditaria: report of three affected brothers and a literature review. Am J Med Genet 1979; 3:389–395
Suter H, et al.: Geroderma osteodysplastica hereditaria (GOH) in a girl. In: Papadatos CT, Bartsocas CS, eds: Skeletal dysplasias. New York: Alan R. Liss, 1982:327–329.
Hall BD: Geroderma osteodysplastica: a rare autosomal recessive

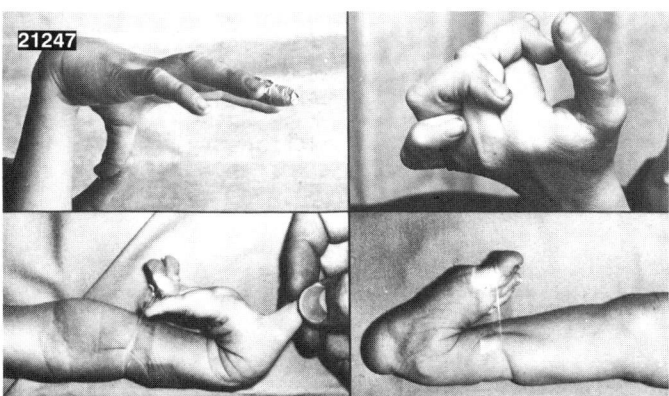

2099B-21247: Note joint hyperextensibility.

connective tissue disorder with either variability or heterogeneity or both. Proc Greenwood Genet Center 1983; 2:101–102.

T0007 **Helga V. Toriello**

OSTEODYSPLASTY 0775

Includes:
Melnick-Needles osteodysplasty
Osteodysplasty, precocious, of Danks-Mayne-Kozlowski

Excludes: N/A

Major Diagnostic Criteria: Generalized bone dysplasia characterized primarily by cortical irregularity, shortening, bowing, and metaphyseal flaring of the long bones.

Clinical Findings: In addition to the unusual cortical irregularity of the long bones, this rare skeletal dysplasia is identified by a ribbon-like appearance of the ribs, an increase in height with anterior concavity of the vertebral bodies, pelvic contracture, sternal abnormalities, delayed closure of the anterior fontanel, sclerosis at the base of the skull, and scoliosis. Facial dysmorphia consisting of exophthalmos, hypertelorism, micrognathia, dental malocclusion, and full cheeks are prominent features. Adults have only mildly reduced stature, normal intelligence, no increase in bone fragility, normal serum chemistries, and a normal life expectancy. At least four cases of affected males born to mothers with osteodysplasty have been reported, but all died in utero or immediately after birth. In addition to micrognathia, exophthalmos, thin calvaria, and severe long bone, rib, and clavicular irregularity and bowing, these males were growth retarded, had hypoplastic thoraces, abdominal wall defects, and abnormalities in their renal collecting systems.

Complications: Gait disturbances, osteoarthritis of the hips, predisposition to urinary tract infections, and difficulty in childbirth secondary to contracted pelvis.

Associated Findings: Vesico-ureteral reflux, congenital heart disease.

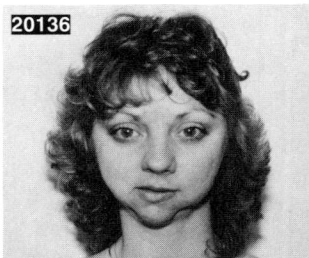
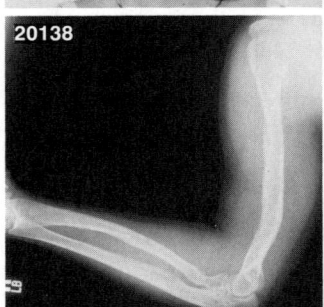
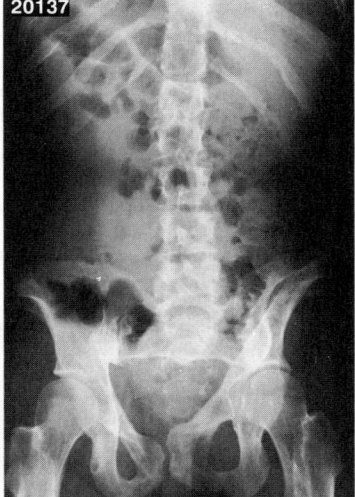

0775-20136: Note hypertelorism, micrognathia and full cheeks. 20137: Ribbon-like ribs, increased height of vertebral bodies and contracted pelvis. 20138: Unusual cortical irregularity of the long bones.

Etiology: Usually X-linked dominant inheritance with lethality in hemizygous males. Autosomal dominant and autosomal recessive (ter Haar et al, 1982) inheritance have also been suggested.

Pathogenesis: Unknown.

MIM No.: *30935, 24942, 25927

POS No.: 3354

CDC No.: 756.580

Sex Ratio: M0:F1. All viable individuals are female. Males usually die *in-utero* or immediately after birth.

Occurrence: Unknown. At least 30 viable individuals have been reported, all female. Four males with malformations incompatible with life have been identified.

Risk of Recurrence for Patient's Sib:
See Part I, *Mendelian Inheritance.*

Risk of Recurrence for Patient's Child:
See Part I, *Mendelian Inheritance.*

Age of Detectability: At birth, by physical and X-ray examination. Affected males have been recognized *in utero* by ultrasound in the early second trimester.

Gene Mapping and Linkage: Unknown.

Prevention: None known. Genetic counseling indicated.

Treatment: Appropriate dental and orthopedic management.

Prognosis: Females have normal life span in most cases, and normal intelligence. Affected males have malformations incompatible with life.

Detection of Carrier: Unknown.

Special Considerations: This condition is very similar to *Osteodysplasty, precocious, of Dank-Mayne-Kozlowski* (1974). Three patients with this condition, two being siblings of Albanian extraction, were reported with a generalized disturbance of modeling of the long and tubular bones and pelvis, with severe hypoplasia of the bones of the fingers and toes. All three died before reaching their first birthday.

References:
Melnick JC, Needles CF: An undiagnosed bone dysplasia: a two family study of four generations and three generations. Am J Roentgen 1966; 98:39–48.
Maroteaux P, et al.: L'osteodysplastie (syndrome de Melnick et de Needles). Presse Med 1968; 76:715–718.
Danks DM, et al.: Precocious autosomal recessive type of osteodysplasty. BD:OAS X(12). New York: March of Dimes Birth Defects Foundation, 1974:124–127.
Gorlin RJ, Knier J: X-linked or autosomal dominant lethal in the male inheritance of the Melnick-Needles (osteodysplasty) syndrome? a reappraisal. Am J Med Genet 1982; 13:465–467. *
ter Haar B, et al.: Melnick-Needles syndrome: indication for an autosomal recessive form. Am J Med Genet 1982; 13:469–477.
von Oeyen P, et al.: Omphalocele and multiple severe congenital anomalies associated with osteodysplasty (Melnick-Needles syndrome). Am J Med Genet 1982; 13:453–463.
Donnenfeld AE, et al.: Melnick-Needles syndrome in males: a lethal multiple congenital anomalies syndrome. Am J Med Genet 1987; 27:159–173.

D0025 **Alan E. Donnenfeld**
ZA000 **Elaine H. Zackai**

Osteodysplasty, precocious, of Danks-Mayne-Kozlowski
See *OSTEODYSPLASTY*
Osteodystrophy-mental retardation
See *OSTEODYSTROPHY-MENTAL RETARDATION, RUVALCABA TYPE*

OSTEODYSTROPHY-MENTAL RETARDATION, RUVALCABA TYPE   2076

Includes:
Mental retardation-osteodystrophy, Ruvalcaba type
Osteodystrophy-mental retardation
Ruvalcaba syndrome

Excludes:
Oculo-mandibulo-facial syndrome (0738)
Tricho-rhino-phalangeal syndrome, type I (0966)
Tricho-rhino-phalangeal syndrome, type II (0967)

Major Diagnostic Criteria: The combination of mental retardation, postnatal growth failure, characteristic facies, hypoplastic skin lesions, and skeletal anomalies.

Clinical Findings: Prenatal growth is normal, whereas postnatal growth failure occurs. Clinical findings in 11 evaluated individuals include mental retardation (6); short stature (8); delayed adolescence (5); **Microcephaly** (3); down-slanting palpebral fissures (5); narrow, small nose (9); down-turned mouth (5); narrow maxilla (9); low-set ears (1); **Pectus carinatum** (5); narrow trunk (6); scoliosis (6); kyphosis (5); abnormal kidney position (2); **Hernia, inguinal** (2); undescended testes (2); hypoplastic genitalia (5); joint limitation (3); prominent elbows (2); short limbs (6); short hands (9); proximal thumbs (4) clinodactyly (6); small feet (7); small toes (7); enlarged areola (2); and hypoplastic skin lesions (3).

X-ray findings include spine osteochondritis (4); fusion of scaphoid and lunate (2); short metacarpals (6); short phalanges (4); short metatarsals (6); cone-shaped epiphyses (2).

Complications: Unknown.

Associated Findings: One individual had low frontal hairline with a white forelock, and broad great toe with valgus defect. Craniosynostosis and cardiac defects were reported in three generations of a family by Hunter et al (1977). Another boy had an apparently balanced 13;14 translocation which he inherited from his apparently unaffected father.

Etiology: Probably autosomal dominant inheritance with reduced penetrance and variable expressivity.

Pathogenesis: Unknown. Growth hormone levels, thyroid studies, metabolic studies, calcium, phosphorus, alkaline phosphatase, immunoglobulins, cortisol, uric acid, and banded karyotype have all been normal.

MIM No.: 18087

POS No.: 3131

Sex Ratio: M1:F1

Occurrence: Sixteen cases have been reported from Europe, Japan, and North America.

Risk of Recurrence for Patient's Sib:
See Part I, *Mendelian Inheritance.*

Risk of Recurrence for Patient's Child:
See Part I, *Mendelian Inheritance.*

Age of Detectability: At birth by physical examination.

Gene Mapping and Linkage: Unknown.

Prevention: None known. Genetic counseling indicated.

Treatment: Unknown.

Prognosis: Mental retardation can occur as part of the phenotype; life span is normal.

Detection of Carrier: Unknown.

References:
Ruvalcaba RHA, et al.: A new familial syndrome with osseous dysplasia and mental deficiency. J Pediatr 1971; 79:450–455.
Hunter AGW, et al.: A "new" syndrome of mental retardation with characteristic facies and brachyphalangy. J Med Genet 1977; 14:430–437
Geormaneanu M, et al.: Veberein "neus syndrome" in verbindung mit familiaerer translokation 13/14. Klin Paediat 1978; 190:500–506.
Sugio Y, Kajii T: Ruvalcaba syndrome: autosomal dominant inheritance. Am J Med Genet 1984; 19:741–753. * †

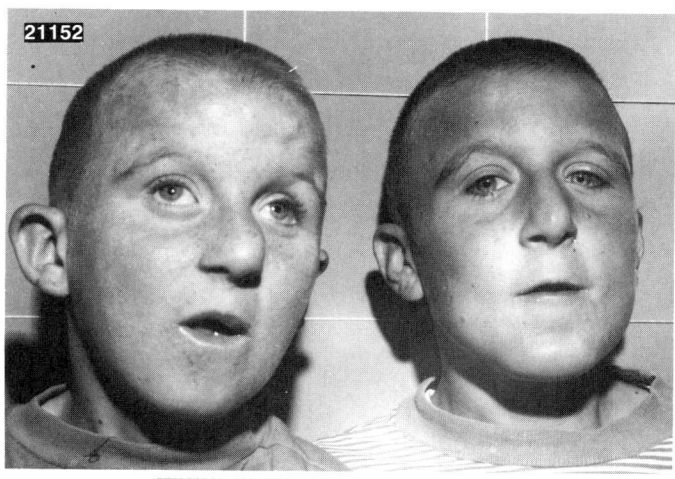

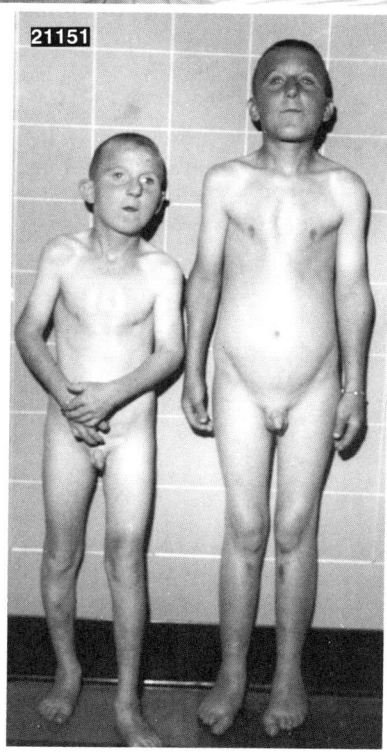

2076-21152: Two brothers with microcephaly, downslanting palpebral fissures, small alae nasi, small mouth, thin lips with downturned corners, and low-set ears. **21151:** Short stature, microcephaly, unusual facies, narrow trunk, pectus carinatum, small genitalia, and prominent elbows.

Bianchi E, et al.: Ruvalcaba syndrome: a case report. Europ J Pediatr 1984; 142:301–303.
Hunter A: Ruvalcaba syndrome. (Letter) Am J Med Genet 1985; 21:785–786.

T0007   **Helga V. Toriello**

OSTEOECTASIA 0776

Includes:
Bone, excessive turnover
Chronic osteopathy with hyperphosphatasia
Hyperostosis corticalis deformans juvenilis
Hyperphosphatasemia, chronic congenital idiopathic
Osteoectasia with macrocranium (with hyperphosphatasia)
Paget disease, juvenile

Excludes:
Cortical hyperostosis, infantile (0221)
Hyperostosis, Worth type (2691)

Major Diagnostic Criteria: Calvarial thickening; demineralization and expansion of the tubular bones; and elevated alkaline phosphatase.

Clinical Findings: Small stature; large skull, progressive bowing of the legs and arms with pain, tenderness, and muscular weakness; tendency to bone fractures. X-rays show a thickened calvaria, with loss of normal bone structure and changes reminiscent of Paget disease; generalized demineralization; expansion and bowing of the long bones, and widening of the short tubular bones. In some patients and some sites, there is dissolution of the normal cortical architecture of the tubular bones.

Laboratory findings include an elevated activity of serum alkaline and acid phosphatase, and of serum aminopeptidase. Uric acid levels are increased in serum and urine. There is an elevation of the urinary peptide-bound hydroxyproline.

Complications: Angioid streaks of the retina, macular atrophy, vascular hypertension. Hearing deficit and optic atrophy due to continued new bone formation at the skull base.

Associated Findings: None known.

Etiology: Autosomal recessive inheritance with considerable variability of expression.

Pathogenesis: Excessive bone turnover, which leads to decreased amounts of mature lamellar bone. The defect is possibly related to a defective production or action of calcitonin.

MIM No.: *23900

CDC No.: 756.580

Sex Ratio: M1:F1

Occurrence: Over thirty cases have been documented.

Risk of Recurrence for Patient's Sib:
See Part I, *Mendelian Inheritance.*

Risk of Recurrence for Patient's Child:
See Part I, *Mendelian Inheritance.*

Age of Detectability: Between the third and eighteenth month of life.

Gene Mapping and Linkage: Unknown.

Prevention: None known. Genetic counseling indicated.

Treatment: Long-term treatment with calcitonin seems to be highly effective. Surgical correction of bone deformities; removal of excessive bone compressing the optic nerves, if necessary.

Prognosis: Untreated, most patients are severely deformed and incapacitated by the age of 14 years. Vascular hypertension may lead to cerebrovascular accidents and death.

Detection of Carrier: Undetermined. Possibly through serum phosphatases.

References:
Caffey J: Familial hyperphosphatasemia with ateliosis and hypermetabolism of growing membranous bone. Progr Pediatr Radiol 1973; 4:438–468.
Iancu TC, et al.: Chronic familial hyperphosphatasemia. Radiology 1978; 129:669–676.
Dunn V, et al.: Familial hyperphosphatasemia: diagnosis in early infancy and response to human calcitonin therapy. Am J Roentgen 1979; 132:541–545.

Jürgen W. Spranger

Osteoectasia with macrocranium (with hyperphosphatasia)
See OSTEOECTASIA

OSTEOFIBROUS DYSPLASIA OF TIBIA AND FIBULA 2502

Includes:
Monostotic cortical fibrous dysplasia
Ossifying fibroma of the long bones
Osteogenic fibroma

Excludes:
Fibrous dysplasia, monostotic (0390)
Fibrous dysplasia, polyostotic (0391)
Neurofibromatosis (0712)

Major Diagnostic Criteria: *Clinical:* isolated, unilateral bowing of the leg associated with a painless mass. *Radiologic:* localized diaphyseal enlargement; intracortical radiolucence, with thinning of the external cortex and sclerosis of the medullary surface; and narrowing of the medullary canal. *Histopathologic:* fibrous tissue surrounding bone trabeculae lined by osteoblasts; "zonal" architecture.

Clinical Findings: Isolated bowing of the leg, usually in its middle one-third, but occasionally in the distal one-third; the bowing is usually anterior. A painless mass is generally apparent. A pathologic fracture may occur, and rarely pseudoarthrosis may develop. A lesion may heal spontaneously or be slowly progressive. Relapse after surgical treatment is frequent. The presence of other findings, particularly patchy skin hyperpigmentation anywhere on the body or additional sites of osseous abnormalities, should suggest an alternative diagnosis.

Complications: Relapse after surgical treatment; permanent bowing deformity; and, rarely, pseudoarthrosis.

Associated Findings: Possibly the histologic presence of an adamantinoma.

Etiology: Unknown.

Pathogenesis: Unknown.

CDC No.: 756.580

Sex Ratio: M1:F<1

Occurrence: About 100 cases have been reported.

Risk of Recurrence for Patient's Sib: Presumably very low.

Risk of Recurrence for Patient's Child: Unknown.

Age of Detectability: During the first decade of life.

Gene Mapping and Linkage: Unknown.

Prevention: None known. Genetic counseling indicated.

Treatment: If minor, close observation. Otherwise, curettage or other surgical techniques to limit or remove the lesion, although relapse is frequent after curettage. In general, surgery is restricted to patients more than five years of age who have extensive lesions.

Prognosis: Generally good, but variable, depending on the presence of complications as noted above.

Detection of Carrier: Unknown.

References:
Campanacci M: Osteofibrous dysplasia of long bones: a new clinical entity. Ital J Orthop Traumatol 1976; 2:221–237.
Capusten BM, et al.: Osteofibrous dysplasia. J Can Assoc Radiol 1980; 31:50–53.
Campanacci M, Laus M: Osteofibrous dysplasia of the tibia and fibula. J Bone Joint Surg 1981; 63:367.
Campbell CJ, Hawk T: A variant of fibrous dysplasia (osteofibrous dysplasia). J Bone Joint Surg 1982; 64:231–236.
Nakashima Y, et al.: Osteofibrous dysplasia (ossifying fibroma of long bones): A study of 12 cases. Cancer 1983; 52:909–914.
Sissons HA, et al.: Ossifying fibroma of bone: report of two cases. Bull Hosp Joint Dis Orthop Inst 1983; 43:1–14.
Alguacil-Garcia A, et al.: Osteofibrous dysplasia (ossifying fibroma) of the tibia and fibula and adamantinoma: a case report. Am J Clin Pathol 1984; 82:470–474.

Kerr R: Radiologic case study: osteofibrous dysplasia. Orthopedics 1987; 10:1085–1089.

RI000   **Vincent M. Riccardi**

OSTEOGENESIS IMPERFECTA   0777

Includes:

Lobstein syndrome
Osteogenesis imperfecta congenita, neonatal lethal
Osteogenesis imperfecta congenita-microcephaly-cataracts
Osteogenesis imperfecta, lethal preinatal
Osteogenesis imperfecta, progressively deforming, normal sclerae
Osteogenesis imperfecta tarda
Osteogenesis imperfecta-blue sclerae
Osteogenesis imperfecta-normal sclerae
Osteogenesis imperfecta-opalescent teeth
Osteogenesis imperfecta-opalescent teeth-Wormian bones
Vrolik disease

Excludes:

Hypophosphatasia (0516)
Osteoporosis, juvenile idiopathic (0782)
Osteoporosis-pseudoglioma syndrome (0783)

Major Diagnostic Criteria: Skeletal fractures with minimal trauma and/or evidence of osteopenia and/or blue sclerae; typical X-ray changes or otosclerosis. Considerable heterogeneity exists in phenotype and in genetic transmission.

Clinical Findings: Osteogenesis imperfecta (OI) is a descriptive term applied to a group of multisystem diseases involving the skeletal, ocular, cutaneous, otologic, dental and vascular tissues, with the greatest morbidity arising from the skeletal manifestations. The spectrum of severity varies considerably. Patients range from those with severe neonatal onset characterized by multiple intrauterine fractures of the limbs and ribs, soft membranous cranium, and usually neonatal death from intracranial hemorrhage or respiratory distress; to those manifesting only a slight tendency toward, or no history at all of bone fractures, but with blue sclerae or mild deafness. The current nomenclature divides OI into four major types (Beighton 1988) with type I and IV subdivided according to presence or absence of opalescent dentin (see **Teeth, dentinogenesis imperfecta**) (Sillence 1988) and type II

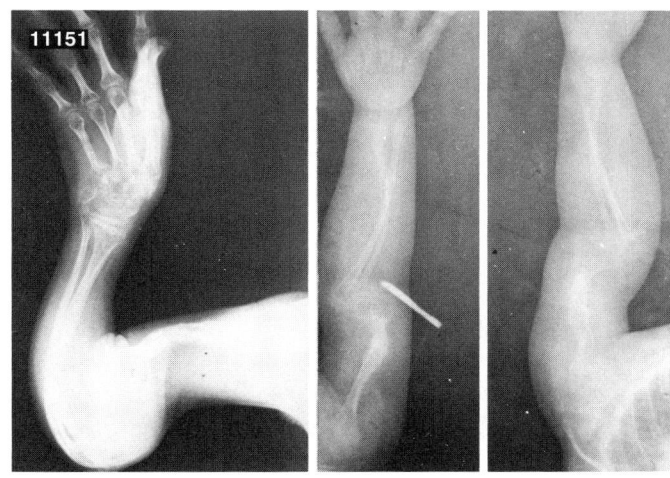

0777B-11151: Note thin, severely bowed long bones.

subdivided into 3 sub-groups on the basis of X-ray findings in the long bones and ribs (Thompson et al. 1987). The majority of cases can be encompassed by one of these eight types.

OI type I: The classic syndrome of dominantly inherited OI with distinctly blue-gray sclerae. It is further subdivided into families with normal teeth (OI type I, group A), and families with opalescent dentin (OI type I, group B). The dental involvement

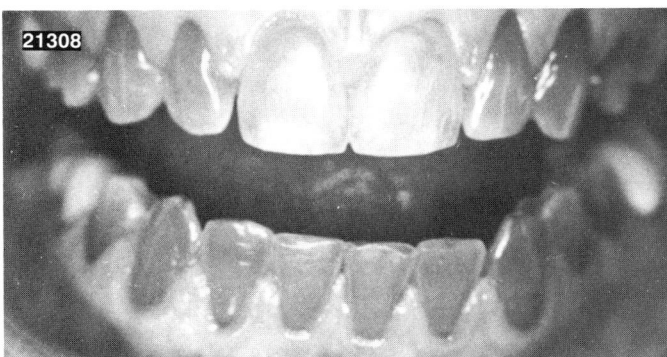

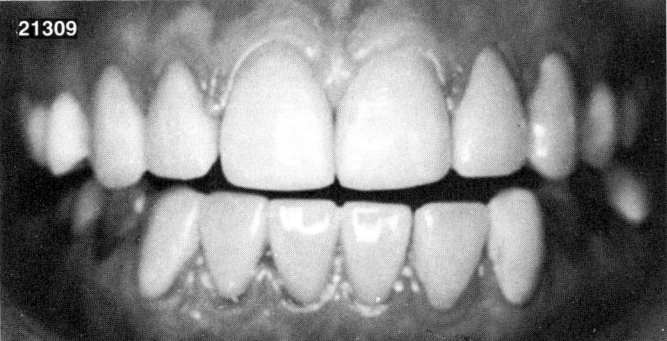

0777C-21308: Teeth of a woman with type IB osteogenesis imperfecta; note the good formation of the teeth despite the hypoplasia of the dentin with translucency of the teeth.   21309: Same woman as shown in **21308** after dental lamination of all teeth; note the untreated mandibular premolars.

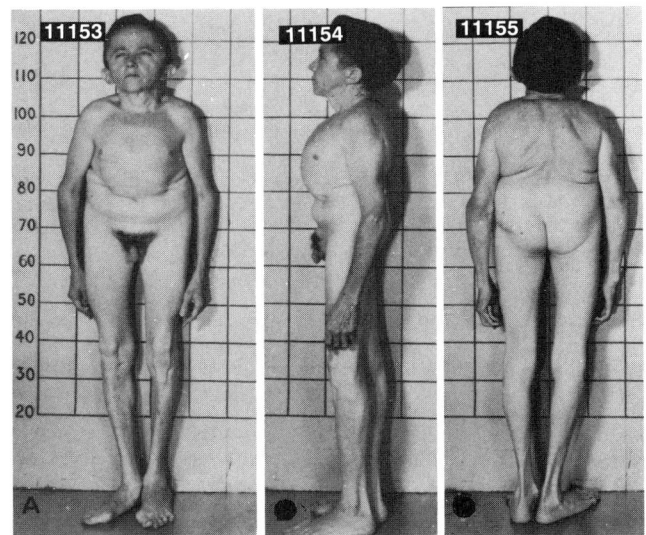

0777A-11153–55: Note short barrel-shaped chest and short neck.

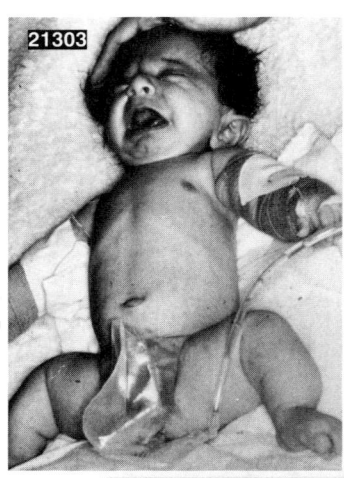

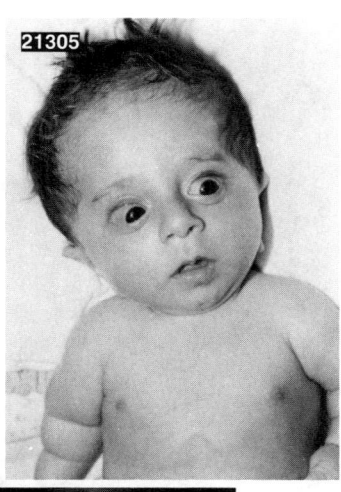

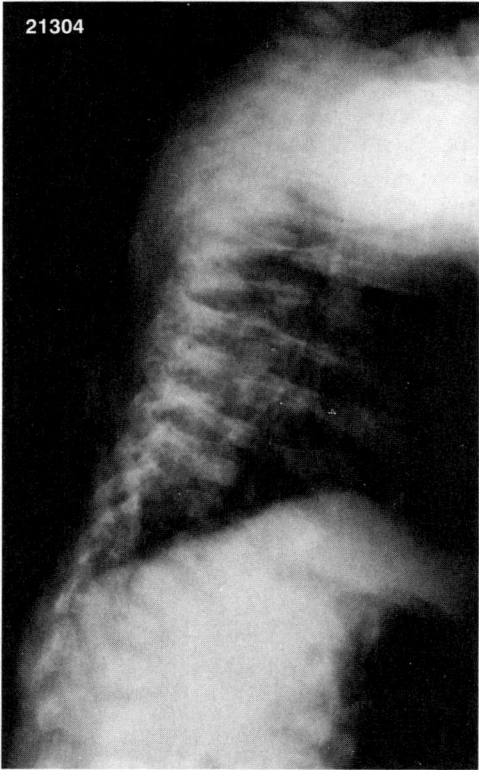

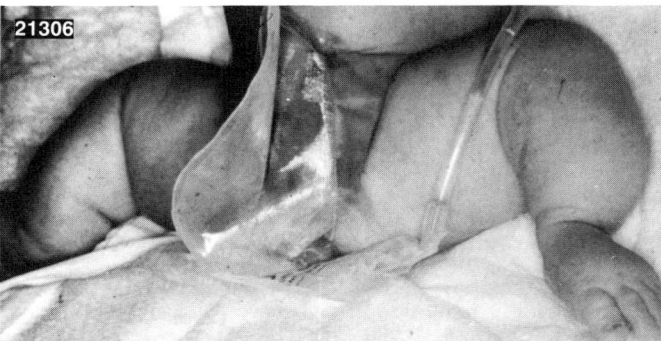

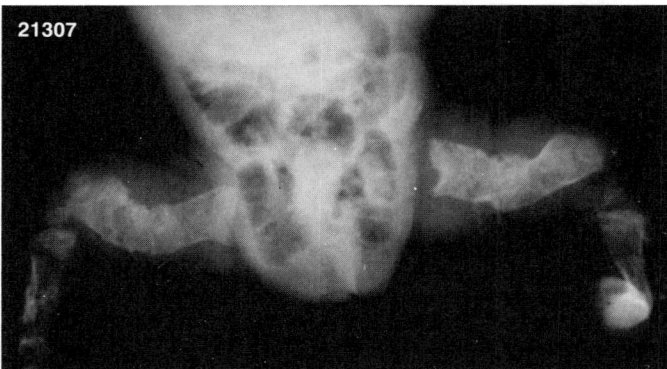

0777E-21306: Neonate with phenotypic OI type II with short and bowed lower limbs. 21307: X-ray shows multiple fractures and crumpled appearance of the long bones, which are shortened and deformed. Note also the poorly ossified callus and deformed, heart-shaped pelvis.

0777D-21303: Male infant with osteogenesis type II; note short and deformed limbs from congenital fractures. 21305: Round facies with prominent eyes and blue sclerae; note the short limbs with excessive skin folds secondary to multiple healed fractures. 21304: Lateral spine of a neonate with OI type II shows osteoporotic platyspondyly with vertebrae resembling those of a fish (fish spine) and thin ribs.

can be highly variable, and these sub-categories are not always clear-cut. Some 10% of individuals in these families present with fractures at birth. The majority of affected persons have their first fractures before five years of age; other persons may have no fractures during childhood or adult life. In all affected persons the sclerae are distinctly blue-gray and remain so throughout life. The hearing impairment is predominantly conductive and is due to sclerosis and deformity of the ossicles, but in some cases mixed conductive and sensory hearing impairment occurs, with high frequency loss. While these patients have a high fracture frequency, bowing and curvature deformity of long bones and spine are usually mild. Although kyphosis and loss of skeletal height with age are frequent findings, only a few affected adults develop severe scoliosis. In families with opalescent dentin (group B), the teeth appear yellow-brown in color; they are easily cracked or worn. X-rays of these teeth show constricted corono-radicular junctions. X-rays also indicate that the predominant feature throughout the skeleton is osteopenia, with deformity of the spine and long bones in some cases. Wormian bones are seen in the skull of the majority of individuals with OI type I. Biochemical studies show a quantitative defect in the production of type I procollagen. Linkage has been demonstrated to COL I A1 by RFLP analysis.

OI type II: This syndrome, characterized by extreme bone fragility, leads to intrauterine fractures and either stillbirth or neonatal death. Considerable clinical heterogeneity exists. Three subgroups can be defined by X-ray (Sillence et al. 1984, Thompson et al. 1987). Type II group A shows broad crumpled femora with continuous rib beading on, X-ray; group B has broad crumpled femora but minimal or no rib fractures; and group C has thin femora with fractures and thin ribs with extensive fracturing. Biochemical studies in group A patients show a marked reduction in type I collagen synthesis. Collagen protein and gene studies show defects which for the most part are heterozygous deletions:

(a) COL I A1 glycine 988 → cysteine (Steinmann et al. 1988)
(b) COL I A1 glycine 664 → arginine (Bateman et al. 1988)

A few patients with type II OI have demonstrated a marked diversity of specific defects; however, all lead to a decrease in type I collagen or a structurally abnormal type I collagen. The nature of the defects often suggest new dominant mutations, thus genetic heterogeneity is likely.

OI type III: This group is probably heterogeneous, but in each case inheritance is autosomal recessive (by definition). These individuals frequently survive the newborn period, i.e. in these cases the disease is not generally lethal; their X-rays lack the continuously beading ribs and crumpled long bones that are seen in the OI type II cases in the newborn period. However, in some instances there is overlap of OI type III cases with OI type II. Survivors have severe short stature and with age develop progressive deformities of long bones and spine. The sclerae, although bluish at birth, become progressively less blue with age, and are usually white by late childhood. In the third and fourth decades there is a high mortality from cardiorespiratory failure. Biochemical studies in one instance show decreased collagen synthesis due to mutation affecting transcription of the alpha 2 chain of type I collagen (Nicholls et al. 1984).

OI type IV: The major characteristic of this dominantly inherited form of OI is normal sclerae. Although at birth the sclerae of affected individuals are bluish, they become progressively less blue with age; by adolescence, they have a normal hue. This group can be further subdivided into families with normal teeth (OI type IV group A) and families with opalescent dentin (OI type IV group B). The onset of fractures frequently occurs in the newborn period although some affected persons show only the congenital bowing of the long bones and have no subsequent fractures; they appear to improve with age. As in OI type III progressive kyphoscoliosis may occur in adult life. Available biochemical data suggest that structural alterations in the alpha 2(I) chain of type I collagen may be the underlying mechanism in some affected families.

Complications: In addition to those mentioned above, other complications include tendon sprains, tendon avulsion, increased capillary fragility, subcutaneous hemorrhage, peri-operative malignant hyperthermia, and neurologic dysfunction due to platybasia.

Associated Findings: Elastosis perforans (rarely).

Etiology: Osteogenesis imperfecta appears to be clinically and genetically very heterogeneous. The classic syndrome (OI type I) is by far the most prevalent form of OI in most populations.

The vast majority of sporadic cases appear to be inherited in an autosomal dominant manner from the previous generation, or represent new dominant mutations. When parents are consanguineous and clinically normal, autosomal recessive inheritance should be suspected.

Pathogenesis: In view of the clinical and genetic heterogeneity, it is clear that OI must be pathogenetically heterogeneous. As the manifestations include abnormality of the skeleton, eye, and skin, the OI disorders must represent generalized defects in connective tissue.

Available data indicates marked heterogeneity at the biochemical level in OI type II. However, the defects appear to reduce the amount of type I collagen or to produce a structurally abnormal type I collagen. Fewer patients with the other types of OI have been studied, but structural or functional defects of the constituent chains of type I collagen are suspected.

An absence of secretion of the alpha 2(I) collagen by cultured fibroblasts in one patient with an autosomal recessive non-lethal form of OI (OI type III) has been reported. In this patient α_2 (I) collagen is not recoverable from tissues, and structural collagen presumably consists of α_1 (I) trimers.

MIM No.: *16620, *16621, *16622, 16623, 16624, *25940, 25941, *25942, *12015, *12016

POS No.: 3349

CDC No.: 756.500

Sex Ratio: M1:F1

Occurrence: Based on an Australian study, the incidence of OI type I is 3.5:100,000 live births; and of type II is 1.6:100,000 live births. Prevalence of OI type I was calculated at 3.4:100,000 population. OI type III is common in the black population of South Africa, where more than 80 cases have been documented.

Risk of Recurrence for Patient's Sib:
See Part I, *Mendelian Inheritance.* If there is no consanguinity, and neither parent has evidence of the disorder (i.e. blue sclerae and excessive fractures), then the risk is generally small unless the patient has the severe perinatal lethal OI type II group B or OI type II group C.

Where X-ray changes are of OI type II group B, a recurrence risk of 8% can be given. Similarly with OI type II group C a risk of 25%. When X-ray studies are not available in severe lethal OI, a British study suggests a recurrence risk of 6%. (Thompson et al, 1987).

Risk of Recurrence for Patient's Child:
See Part I, *Mendelian Inheritance.*

Age of Detectability: Because of clinical variability, detection may range from birth through adulthood. Prenatal diagnosis of OI type II has been accomplished using ultrasonography. In addition, biochemical studies on cultured amniotic cells have been employed to confirm a decreased type I collagen secretion in recurrence of OI type II. Chorion villus specimens can be investigated for over-modification of lysine residues in pregnancies at risk for OI type II where study of fibroblasts from a previous affected have shown this abnormality. Ultrasound studies may be used in conjunction with X-ray studies to screen pregnancies at risk for severe forms of OI type III. However, no measure of reliability can yet be placed on such studies.

Gene Mapping and Linkage: OI4 (osteogenesis imperfecta type IV) has been provisionally mapped to 7q21.3-q22.1.

COL1A1 (collagen, type I, alpha 1) has been mapped to 17q21.3-q22.

COL1A2 (collagen, type I, alpha 2) has been mapped to 7q21.3-q22.1.

Prevention: None known. Genetic counseling indicated.

Treatment: Oral magnesium oxide, calcitonin, sodium fluoride, and vitamin C have been suggested to be potentially useful therapeutic agents; however, definite improvement of clinical symptoms with any of these treatments is yet to be documented. Immobilization should be avoided. Careful alignment of fractures may reduce residual deformity. Multiple fragmentation and intramedullary rodding may be useful in some patients in stabilizing a long bone subject to recurrent fractures and in correcting the deformity. Selective spinal fusion has been reported to be useful in stabilizing spinal curvature (scoliosis).

Because of hormonal effects, pregnancy may be deleterious to severely affected females. An increase in fracture frequency may occur, and hearing may deteriorate. Cesarean section is usually indicated.

Prognosis: Dependent upon type of OI. Ranges from death in perinatal period to normal life span with little if any morbidity.

Detection of Carrier: There is a wide range of expressivity within families showing autosomal dominant inheritance. An affected member may demonstrate only blue sclerae, while sibs or offspring may demonstrate the full manifestations of the disorder. At present no biochemical test is available to routinely distinguish carriers; however if a specific collagen biochemical defect is known in a patient, carrier testing may be possible.

Support Groups:
DC; Washington; Osteogenesis Imperfecta National Capital Area

PA; West Chester; American Brittle Bone Society (ABBS)

NH; Manchester; Osteogenesis Imperfecta Foundation (OIF)

References:
Paterson CR, et al.: Heterogeneity in osteogenesis imperfecta type I. J Med Genet 1983; 20:203–205.
Paterson CR, et al.: Osteogenesis imperfecta with dominant inheritance and normal sclerae. J Bone Joint Surg 1983; 65B:35–39.
Nicholls et al.: The clinical features of homozygous α_2(I) collagen deficient Osteogenesis Imperfecta. J Med Genet 1984; 21:257–262.
Sillence DO, et al.: Osteogenesis imperfecta type II: delineation of the phenotype with reference to genetic heterogeneity. Am J Med Genet 1984; 17:407–423.
Beighton P, Versfeld GA: On the paradoxically high relative preva-

lence of osteogenesis imperfects type III in the Black population of South Africa. Clin Genet 1985; 27:398–404.

Byers PH, Bonadio JF: The molecular basis of clinical heterogeneity in osteogenesis imperfecta: mutations in type I collagen genes have different effects on collagen processing. In: Lloyd JK, Scriver CR, eds: Genetics and metabolic disease in pediatrics. London: Butterworths, 1985:56–90.

Sillence DO, et al: Osteogenesis imperfecta type III: delineation of the phenotype with special reference to genetic heterogeneity. Am J Med Genet 1986; 23:821–832.

Thompson EM, et al.: Recurrence risks and prognosis in severe sporadic osteogenesis imperfecta. J Med Genet 1987; 24:390–405.

Tsipouras P, et al.: Prenatal prediction of osteogenesis imperfecta type IV: exclusion of inheritance using a collagen gene probe. J Med Genet 1987; 24:406–409.

Bateman JF, et al.: Biochemical heterogeneity of type I collagen mutations in Osteogenesis Imperfecta. Ann New York Acad Sci 1988; 543:95–105.

Beighton P, et al.: International nosology of heritable disorders of connective tissue. Am J Med Genet 1988; 29:581–594.

Sillence DO: Osteogenesis imperfecta: nosology and genetics. Ann New York Acad Sci 1988; 543:1–15.

Steinmann B, et al.: Imperfecta collagenesis in Osteogenesis Imperfecta. Ann New York Acad Sci 1988; 543;47–61.

SI009
BA021
David Sillence
Kristine K. Barlow

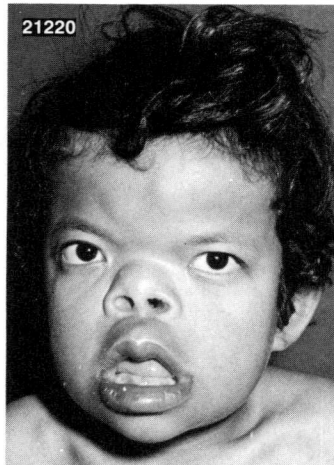 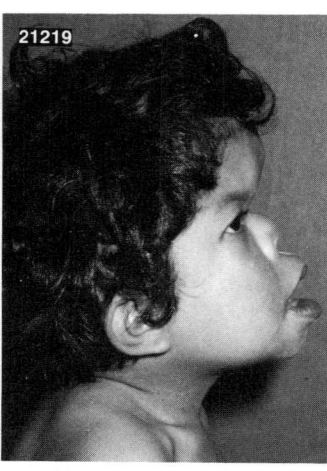

2571A-21219–20: Affected 12-year-old girl with hypertelorism, mandibular prognathism, depressed nasal bridge and bossing of the forehead.

Osteogenesis imperfecta congenita, neonatal lethal
  See OSTEOGENESIS IMPERFECTA
Osteogenesis imperfecta congenita-microcephaly-cataracts
  See OSTEOGENESIS IMPERFECTA
Osteogenesis imperfecta tarda
  See OSTEOGENESIS IMPERFECTA
Osteogenesis imperfecta, lethal preinatal
  See OSTEOGENESIS IMPERFECTA
Osteogenesis imperfecta, ocular form
  See OSTEOPOROSIS-PSEUDOGLIOMA SYNDROME
Osteogenesis imperfecta, possible variant
  See SHORT STATURE-WORMIAN BONES-JOINT DISLOCATIONS
Osteogenesis imperfecta, progressively deforming, normal sclerae
  See OSTEOGENESIS IMPERFECTA
Osteogenesis imperfecta-blue sclerae
  See OSTEOGENESIS IMPERFECTA
Osteogenesis imperfecta-normal sclerae
  See OSTEOGENESIS IMPERFECTA
Osteogenesis imperfecta-opalescent teeth
  See OSTEOGENESIS IMPERFECTA
Osteogenesis imperfecta-opalescent teeth-Wormian bones
  See OSTEOGENESIS IMPERFECTA
Osteogenic fibroma
  See OSTEOFIBROUS DYSPLASIA OF TIBIA AND FIBULA
Osteogenic sarcoma
  See OSTEOSARCOMA
Osteoglophonic dwarfism
  See OSTEOGLOPHONIC DYSPLASIA

OSTEOGLOPHONIC DYSPLASIA 2571

Includes: Osteoglophonic dwarfism

Excludes:
  Craniofacial dysostosis (0225)
  Craniometaphyseal dysplasia (0228)
  Hypophosphatasia (0516)
  Skeletal dysplasia (others)

Major Diagnostic Criteria: Dwarfism, gross craniofacial abnormalities and characteristic metaphyseal lucencies on X-ray.

Clinical Findings: Rhizomelic dwarfism and limb malalignment are associated with frontal prominence, hypertelorism and massive mandibular prognathism. The palate is high, the teeth are maldeveloped and the nostrils are anteverted. Developmental milestones are delayed, due to the skeletal problems, but intelligence is normal. There are no visceral ramifications.

On X-ray the skull is scaphocephalic, due to sagittal stenosis, with gross frontal bossing. Cystic changes are present in the mandibular ramus, and the teeth may remain unerupted. In the spine, platyspondyly with anterior projection of the vertebral bodies is a striking feature. The ribs and clavicles are normal, but the pelvis is distorted, with radiolucent areas in the ilia. The long bones show gross undermodeling, with generalized osteoporosis, cortical thinning and loss of the normal trabecular pattern. Lucent patches throughout the metaphyses, especially in the distal femora and proximal tibiae, produce a hollowed out appearance. The tubular bones of the extremities are short and broad, with dysplastic epiphyseal ossification centers.

Complications: Craniosynostosis may produce severe facial abnormalities. Dental maleruption may be troublesome. The narrow nasal passages predispose to recurrent upper respiratory infections. Gait is impaired due to the skeletal abnormalities.

Associated Findings: None known.

Etiology: Possibly autosomal dominant inheritance, although most cases have been sporadic.

Pathogenesis: Unknown.

MIM No.: 16625

POS No.: 4004

CDC No.: 756.580

Sex Ratio: M1:F1

Occurrence: Six patients have been reported in the United Kingdom and United States, and another affected female infant is known in Portugal.

Risk of Recurrence for Patient's Sib:
  See Part I, *Mendelian Inheritance.*

Risk of Recurrence for Patient's Child:
  See Part I, *Mendelian Inheritance.*

Age of Detectability: At birth.

Gene Mapping and Linkage: Unknown.

Prevention: None known. Genetic counseling indicated.

Treatment: Craniotomy in infancy may diminish craniofacial distortion. Orthodontic measures may be necessary for dental maldevelopment.

Prognosis: Intelligence and general health are normal. Dwarfism is severe, and the facial appearance is grotesque.

Detection of Carrier: Unknown.

References:
Fairbank T: An atlas of general affections of the skeleton. Edinburgh: Livingstone, 1959.

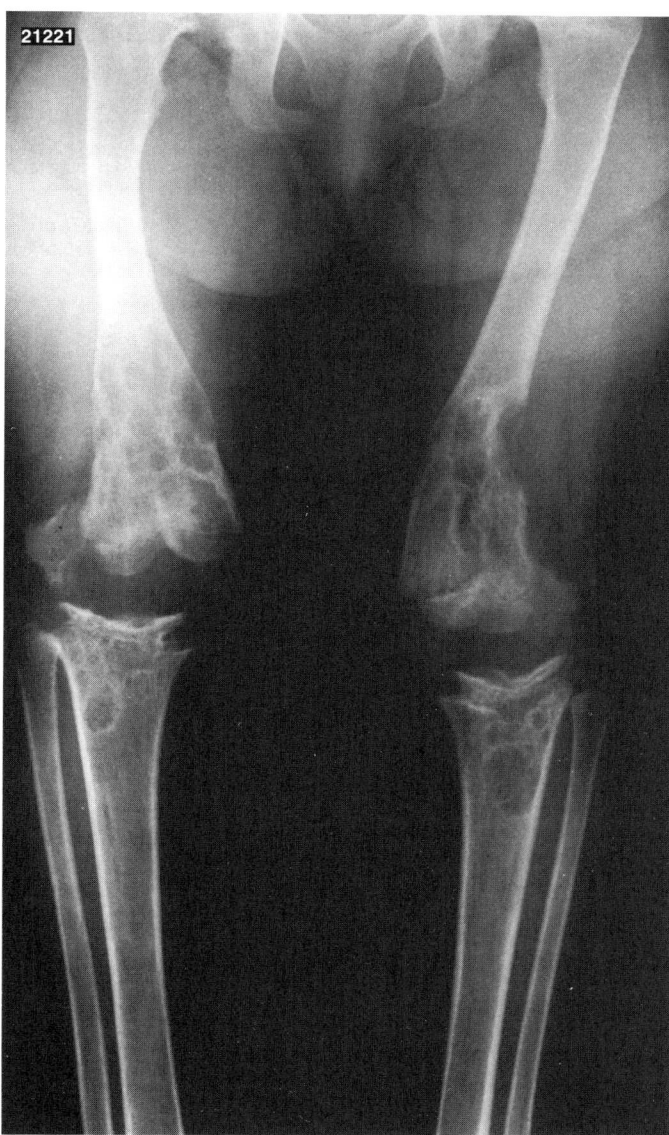

2571B-21221: A-P view of the legs of an affected girl aged 12 years; note multiple irregular lucent areas in the metaphyses.

Keats TE, et al.: Craniofacial dysostosis with fibrous metaphyseal defects. Am J. Roentgenol 1975; 124:271–275.
Beighton P, et al.: Osteoglophonic dwarfism. Pediatr Radiol 1980; 10:46–50. * †
Kelley RI, et al.: Osteoglophonic dwarfism in two generations. J Med Genet 1983; 20:436–440.

BE008   **Peter Beighton**

OSTEOLYSIS   **1521**

Osteolysis is a general term referring to the appearance on X-ray of intense, focal resorption of bone. The resorption may be either focal and segmental or focal and generalized. The term osteolysis is used to distinguish focal bone resorption from generalized osteopenia, and it should be used to express an X-ray finding rather than a specific disease process.

Osteolysis can be caused by a myriad of disorders such as osteomyelitis, tuberculosis, granulomatous bone disease, stress fractures, benign or malignant primary bone tumors, multiple myeloma, leukemia, mast cell disease, histiocytosis, metastatic carcinoma, metabolic disorders (such as brown tumors of hyperthyroidism or the lytic phase of **Bone, Paget disease**), extreme pressure on bone, periarticular inflammation, inflammatory arthropathies, reflex sympathetic dystrophy, transient regional osteoporosis, migratory osteolysis, the lytic phase of osteonecrosis, focal denervation (pseudomyelomatous osteopenia), or several specific and extremely rare genetic conditions such as **Osteopoikilosis; Fibromatosis, juvenile hyaline; Pyknodysostosis; Winchester syndrome**; or **Osteolysis, carpal-tarsal and chronic progressive glomerulopathy**.

In light of the myriad causes of osteolysis, the age of onset can vary widely from prenatal to beyond the tenth decade of life, and it has no sex predilection. Depending on the cause, the condition may be either painless or painful. The treatment of the condition is essentially the treatment of the underlying condition, if known.

KA033   **Frederick S. Kaplan**

OSTEOLYSIS, CARPAL-TARSAL AND CHRONIC PROGRESSIVE GLOMERULOPATHY   **0128**

Includes:
    Carpal-tarsal osteolysis-chronic progressive glomerulopathy
    Essential osteolysis-nephropathy
    Gorham osteolysis
    Osteolysis, essential hereditary, of carpal bones-nephropathy
    Osteolysis-proteinuria
    Proteinuria-osteolysis

Excludes:
    Acro-osteolysis, dominant type (0021)
    Arthritis, rheumatoid (2517)
    Conorenal syndrome
    Hajdu-Cheney syndrome (2022)
    Osteoarthropathy of Schinz and Furtwaengler
    Osteolysis, essential (2596)
    Osteolysis, recessive carpal-tarsal (0129)
    Various aseptic necrosis syndromes

Major Diagnostic Criteria: Osteolysis of carpal and tarsal bones associated with moderate-to-marked involvement of adjacent tubular bones, proteinuria, and microscopic hematuria.

Clinical Findings: Osteolysis of carpal and tarsal bones begins in the first decade, usually before age 5 years. It may occur without symptoms or may be accompanied by tenderness, swelling, and painful limitation of motion of ankle or wrist. As a rule, osteolysis is bilaterally symmetric and progresses slowly to complete dissolution of carpal and tarsal bones. Adjacent tubular bones are shortened with marked tapering, resembling a "sucked-candy" appearance on X-ray. Progressive shortening of the forearms is noted, and lytic involvement of the elbow leads to loss of mobility and function. Cortical thinning of the nonaxial tubular bones also becomes evident. Other nonprogressive skeletal defects have been associated with this syndrome.

Progressive proteinuria with onset at about the end of the first decade, associated with microscopic hematuria, is found. Azotemia is usually manifested by the late second early third decade; nonoliguric renal insufficiency (with the nephrotic syndrome) rapidly progresses to frank renal failure and death.

Pathologic examination of affected wrists has revealed replacement of bone and cartilage by fibrofatty tissue, and a notable lack of inflammatory response or vascular or hemangiomatous changes. Arrest of endochondral bone formation and areas of fibrocartilaginous metaplasia have been observed. Both percutaneous biopsy and autopsy specimens of kidney have demonstrated a proliferative glomerulopathy with epithelial crescent formation and numerous hyalinized glomeruli. Unusual neovascularization of glomeruli by capillary ingrowths from the Bowman capsule have been observed. Immunopathologic studies show some IgM in unsclerosed segments of glomeruli.

Laboratory evaluations early in the course of this syndrome are normal; erythrocyte sedimentation rate, latex fixation, and LE preparations are normal. Somewhat later, proteinuria and hematuria are found; and, finally, the chemical finding of uremia and massive proteinuria becomes manifest.

Complications: Painful limitation of motion of affected areas with progressive dysfunction due to loss of bone and resultant deformity (volar subluxation of hands, flexion contractures of elbows and pes cavum). Marked muscle atrophy without neurologic deficit is presumably due to loss of bony insertions. Progressive chronic renal insufficiency results in death in the late second to third decade.

Associated Findings: None known.

Etiology: Autosomal dominant inheritance. Monocentric massive osteolysis (Gorham and Stout, 1955) appears to be non-Mendelian.

Pathogenesis: Unknown.

MIM No.: *16630

POS No.: 3053

CDC No.: 756.580

Sex Ratio: Presumably M1:F1

Occurrence: Undetermined. Extensive literature.

Risk of Recurrence for Patient's Sib:
See Part I, *Mendelian Inheritance.*

Risk of Recurrence for Patient's Child:
See Part I, *Mendelian Inheritance.*

Age of Detectability: First decade of life.

Gene Mapping and Linkage: Unknown.

Prevention: None known. Genetic counseling indicated.

Treatment: Symptomatic treatment with mild analgesics for wrist and ankle pain. Supportive therapy for chronic renal failure. There is no reported experience with immunosuppressive agents.

Prognosis: Death from uremia in late second to early third decades. Function is variable depending on degree and extent of osteolysis.

Detection of Carrier: Unknown.

Special Considerations: Whether carpal-tarsal osteolysis without glomerulopathy and with extensive lytic involvement of adjacent tubular bones and elbow joints is a separate entity is not clear. This syndrome is easily distinguished from **Osteolysis, recessive carpal-tarpal** by the above criteria and by the notable osteoporosis, cortical thinning, and especially increased caliber of phalanges and metacarpals found in the recessive syndrome. The syndrome is easily distinguished from the various acro-osteolysis syndromes and aseptic necrosis syndromes by distribution of the lesions. The lack of acute phase reactants, systemic illness, and inflammatory reaction in biopsy material distinguishes this syndrome from rheumatoid arthritis. The lack of generalized joint stiffness and other skeletal disorders separates this syndrome from the osteoarthropathy of Schinz and Furtwaengler.

References:
Gorham LW, Stout AP: Massive osteolysis. J Bone Joint Surg 1955; 37A:985–1004.
Marie J, et al.: Acro-osteolyse essentielle compliquée d'insuffisance renal d'evolution fatale. Presse Med 1963; 71:249–252.
Shurtleff DB, et al.: Hereditary osteolysis with hypertension and nephropathy. JAMA 1964; 188:363–368.

Lagier R, Rutishauser E: Osteoarticular changes in a case of essential osteolysis. J Bone Joint Surg 1965; 47B:339–353. *
Torg JS, Steel HH: Essential osteolysis with nephropathy. J Bone Joint Surg 1968; 50A:1629–1638.
Counahan, R et al.: Multifocal osteolysis with nephropathy. Arch Dis Child 1976; 51:717–719. *
Hardegger F, et al.: The syndrome of idiopathic osteolysis: classification, review, and case report. J Bone Joint Surg 1985; 67B:89–93. *

B0025

Zvi Borochowitz
David L. Rimoin

Osteolysis, distal-short stature-characteristic facies
See OSTEOLYSIS, ESSENTIAL

OSTEOLYSIS, ESSENTIAL   2596

Includes:
Acroosteolysis
Acroosteolysis-osteoporosis-skull and mandible changes
Arthrodentoosteodysplasia
Cheney syndrome
Essential carpotarsal osteolysis
Multicentric osteolysis
Osteolysis, distal-short stature-characteristic facies
Osteolysis, idiopathic
Osteolysis, idiopathic multicentric
Osteolysis, idiopathic phalangeal

Excludes:
Acroosteolysis, secondary
Acroosteolysis-neurologic deficit
Hajdu-Cheney syndrome (2022)
Osteolysis, carpal-tarsal and chronic progressive glomerulopathy (0128)
Osteolysis, recessive carpal-tarsal (0129)

Major Diagnostic Criteria: X-ray demonstration of osteolytic destruction of clinically affected bones.

Clinical Findings: In all types of idiopathic osteolyses, osteolytic bone changes result in variable degrees of disability. The osteolytic process starts in early infancy and is characterized by arthritis-like episodes with pain and swellings of the affected bones. Concomitant atrophy of the muscles and flexion contractures progressively become evident in most patients. In all of the subtypes of essential osteolyses, the osteolytic destruction is more or less diffuse and not exclusively restricted to one or another bone segment. All patients have characteristc facial changes

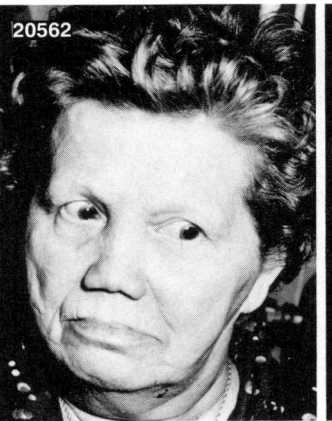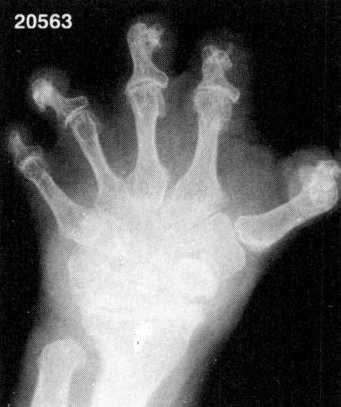

2596-20562: Characteristic facial changes: maxillary hypoplasia, relative exophthalmos, and broad nasal tip. **20563:** Note destruction of the distal phalanges of all fingers.

consisting of maxillary hypoplasia, relative exophthalmos, and broad nasal tip.

Complications: Unknown.

Associated Findings: Associated renal abnormalities and hypertension have been documented. Whereas in most patients the renal symptoms are limited to a fluctuating proteinuria and an abnormal cell count, in a few patients death occurred about the age of 20 years from renal failure with histologic lesions resembling chronic glomerulonephritis. Corneal opacities were reported in at least four patients.

Etiology: Different forms of idiopathic osteolysis have been differentiated on the basis of clinical, X-ray, and genetic criteria. *Idiopathic multicentric osteolysis* has been reported as an autosomal dominant condition. At least three apparently distinct types of acro-osteolysis have been delineated, each with autosomal dominant inheritance: *essential carpotarsal osteolysis*, **Hajdu-Cheney syndrome**, and *idiopathic acroosteolysis* of the phalanges. A few examples of probable autosomal recessive types of essential osteolysis have been reported. For all types of essential osteolysis, the etiology remains obscure.

Pathogenesis: Vascular and immunological disturbances have been considered, but biopsy and necropsy studies have failed to provide definite clue as to the nature of the disorder.

MIM No.: *10250, 25961

CDC No.: 756.580

Sex Ratio: M1:F1

Occurrence: Undetermined but presumed rare.

Risk of Recurrence for Patient's Sib:
See Part I, *Mendelian Inheritance.*

Risk of Recurrence for Patient's Child:
See Part I, *Mendelian Inheritance.*

Age of Detectability: The osteolytic process usually starts in early childhood and is slowly progressive. Facial changes become evident after puberty.

Gene Mapping and Linkage: Unknown.

Prevention: None known. Genetic counseling indicated.

Treatment: In addition to supportive treatment, sympathectomy has been performed in some patients, with inconsistent results. Treatment of hypertension and renal insufficiency, if present.

Prognosis: The osteolytic changes start in early childhood and are slowly progressive, resulting in functional disability, muscular atrophy, and joint contractures. Life span prognosis is generally good, except in patients with renal involvement.

Detection of Carrier: Unknown.

References:
Joseph R, et al.: Acro-ostéolyse idiopathique familiale. Ann Pediatr 1959; 35:622–629.
Spranger J, et al.: Bone dysplasias: an atlas of constitutional disorders of skeletal development. Stuttgart: Gustav Fischer Verlag 1974: 209–218. *
Beals RK, Bird CB: Carpal and tarsal osteolysis. J Bone Joint Surg 1975; 57A:681–686.
Bennett WM, et al.: Nephropathy of idiopathic multicentric osteolysis. Nephron 1980; 25:134–138.
Petit P, Fryns JP: Distal osteolysis, short stature, mental retardation, and characteristic facial appearance: delineation of an autosomal recessive subtype of essential osteolysis. Am J Med Genet 1986; 25:537–541. †
Osterberg PH, et al.: Familial expansile osteolysis: a new dysplasia. J Bone Joint Surg 1988; 70:255–260.
Barr RJ, et al.: Idiopathic multicentric osteolysis: report of two new cases and a review of the literature. Am J Med Genet 1989; 32:556 only.

FR030 **Jean-Pierre Fryns**

Osteolysis, idiopathic multicentric
See OSTEOPOIKILOSIS
Osteolysis, idiopathic
See OSTEOLYSIS, ESSENTIAL

Osteolysis, idiopathic multicentric
See OSTEOLYSIS, ESSENTIAL
Osteolysis, idiopathic phalangeal
See OSTEOLYSIS, ESSENTIAL

OSTEOLYSIS, RECESSIVE CARPAL-TARSAL 0129

Includes:
Carpal-tarsal osteolysis, recessive
Multicentric osteolysis with recessive transmission

Excludes:
Acro-osteolysis (all forms)
Arthritis, rheumatoid (2517)
Aseptic necrosis in other syndromes
Gorham disease
Hajdu-Cheney syndrome (2022)
Osteoarthropathy of Schinz and Furtwaengler
Osteolysis, carpal-tarsal and chronic progressive glomerulopathy (0128)
Osteolysis, essential (2596)
Osteolysis with dominant transmission, idiopathic hereditary
Winchester syndrome (1000)

Major Diagnostic Criteria: Flexion contractures of the knees, hips, and elbows; fusiform enlargement of the digits; and the absence of systemic renal and neurological defects. X-rays show collapse and resorption of carpal and tarsal bones, and appendicular osteopenia, cortical thinning, and an increased diameter of long and tubular bones. Evidence of autosomal recessive inheritance is helpful.

Clinical Findings: A single pedigree with three young affected members has been described. Beginning in early childhood, onset of a progressive osteolysis of the carpal and tarsal bones occurs, usually accompanied by swelling, tenderness, and painful limitation of motion of the affected area. Fusiform swelling of the fingers may be observed, with deformity of the proximal interphalangeal joints. In at least one patient, nontender subcutaneous nodules on knees, feet, elbows, and fingers were observed, and "hyperpigmented and erythematous" skin lesions were noted.

X-rays prior to the onset of osteolysis demonstrate decreased mineralization of the hand bones and increased caliber of phalanges, metacarpals, and long tubular bones of the upper limbs with thinning of cortical bone. Osteolysis of carpal and tarsal bones is usually bilaterally symmetric but may be unilateral. In the most advanced case (age 10 years), complete loss of all carpal bones and extensive lysis of tarsal bones was found with increased caliber, osteoporosis, and cortical thinning of nonaxial tubular bones. The phalanges demonstrated focal areas of resorption. There was a notable lack of metacarpal erosion or resorption of long tubular bone with the exception of the distal epiphyses of the radius and ulna.

Length discrepancies of a limb may develop, apparently secondary to involvement of epiphyses of long tubular bones. In addition to the deformities due to bony loss at the wrist and ankle, flexion contractures of elbows and knees and deformities of metacarpophalangeal and interphalangeal joints gradually develop.

Biopsy of a metacarpal bone demonstrated only osteopenia; the subcutaneous nodules showed only normal fibrofatty tissue, and the hyperpigmented skin lesions demonstrated normal histology.

Laboratory studies in a 7-year-old boy revealed increased erythrocyte sedimentation rate (ESR) and +1 latex fixation; all other blood and urine studies were normal.

The original family as described by Torg and Steel (1968) is thought to demonstrate an autosomal recessively transmitted trait as there was consanguinity and expression in one generation only with 3/6 children affected.

Complications: Limb length discrepancies and contractures at multiple small and large joints may occur. Painful joint limitation may compromise function as does deformity secondary to bony loss (volar subluxation of the hand and pes cavum).

Associated Findings: None known.

Etiology: The pattern is consistent with either autosomal recessive or X-linked recessive inheritance.

Pathogenesis: Unknown.

MIM No.: 25960

CDC No.: 756.580

Sex Ratio: M3:F0 Observed.

Occurrence: One family reported.

Risk of Recurrence for Patient's Sib:
See Part I, *Mendelian Inheritance.*

Risk of Recurrence for Patient's Child:
See Part I, *Mendelian Inheritance.*

Age of Detectability: Two to six years by clinical and X-ray examinations.

Gene Mapping and Linkage: Unknown.

Prevention: None known. Genetic counseling indicated.

Treatment: Orthopedic care may be appropriate for specific developmental deformities, but the lifelong natural history of the untreated condition is not known, and the potential benefits of orthopedic modalities such as casting, bracing, physical therapy medication, and/or surgery can only be surmized.

Prognosis: Unknown for life span (oldest reported patient reached at least early teens), apparently normal for intelligence, variable for function, but probably poor for hand and foot function depending on degree and extent of osteolysis.

Detection of Carrier: Unknown.

Special Considerations: The various aseptic necrosis syndromes and acro-osteolysis syndromes are distinguished by the distribution and extent of the lesions. Subcutaneous nodules, elevated ESR, swelling and tenderness, and a positive latex fixation may suggest **Arthritis, rheumatoid,** but biopsy materials fail to reveal the characteristic pathologic changes. The lack of generalized joint stiffness and other skeletal disorders separates this syndrome from the osteoarthropathy of Schinz and Furtwaengler. Lack of corneal opacity, coarse face, and generalized osteoporosis distinguish this from **Winchester syndrome.**

Several other conditions involving idiopathic osteolysis are known. These include Gorham disease (massive osteolysis or disappearing bone disease) in which generalized intraosseous hemangiomatosis has been described; essential multifocal osteolysis with nephropathy, a progressive nonfamilial disorder characterized by carpo-tarsal osteolysis and progressive nephropathy; and idiopathic hereditary osteolysis with dominant transmission but without nephropathy, a disorder in which an inherent vascular abnormality has been hypothesized.

Advances in the cellular biology of bone modeling and remodeling, along with specific noncollagenous protein markers of bone metabolism and undercalcified processing of bone biopsy specimens following dynamic tetracycline labeling hold promise of bringing a more basic understanding to these complex but related disorders.

References:
Abell JM, Badgley CE: Disappearing bone disease. JAMA 1961; 177: 771.
Halliday DR, et al.: Massive osteolysis and angiomatosis. Radiology 1964; 82:637.
Shurtleff DB, et al.: Hereditary osteolysis with hypertension and nephropathy JAMA 1964; 188:363.
Torg JS, Steel HH: Essential osteolysis with nephropathy: case report of an unusual syndrome. J Bone Joint Surg 1968; 50A:1629.
Torg JS, et al.: Hereditary multicentric osteolysis with recessive transmission: a new syndrome. J Pediatr 1969; 75:243–252.
Kohler E, et al.: Hereditary osteolysis. Radiology 1973; 108:99.

KA033
B0025

Frederick S. Kaplan
Zvi Borochowitz
David L. Rimoin

Osteolysis-proteinuria
See OSTEOLYSIS, CARPAL-TARSAL AND CHRONIC PROGRESSIVE GLOMERULOPATHY
Osteolysis. essential hereditary, of carpal bones-nephropathy
See OSTEOLYSIS, CARPAL-TARSAL AND CHRONIC PROGRESSIVE GLOMERULOPATHY
Osteomata, multiple compact
See EAR, EXOSTOSES
Osteomesopycnose
See OSTEOMESOPYKNOSIS

OSTEOMESOPYKNOSIS 2695

Includes:
Axial osteosclerosis
Osteomesopycnose

Excludes:
Craniometaphyseal dysplasia (0228)
Dysosteosclerosis (0310)
Osteomalacia, atypical axial
Osteopetrosis, benign dominant (0779)
Pyknodysostosis (0846)

Major Diagnostic Criteria: X-rays show osteosclerosis localized to the axial spine, the pelvis, and the proximal part of the long bones.

Clinical Findings: Osteomesopycnosis is usually discovered because of chronic lower back pain. Sometimes, the patient is asymptomatic and is diagnosed on incidental X-rays or because of a genetic analysis of his family. Physical examination is normal, except for tenderness in the back or moderate dorsal kyphosis.

X-ray examination reveals the increased bone density in the vertebral bodies, the pelvis, and the proximal part of the femora. Sclerosis does not involve the skull, clavicles, ribs, hands, feet, or tubular bones other than the proximal part of the femora. Inconstantly the height of the vertebral bodies may be slightly reduced with an ovalar form. A "sandwich" appearance can develop with the densification of the upper and lower plates or more in homogenous patches of osteosclerosis. A radiolucent defect has been described in the proximal part of the femur in three patients.

Complications: The severe complications of osteopetrosis are absent.

Associated Findings: Tubular acidosis and abnormal aminoaciduria were reported in one case.

Etiology: Probably autosomal dominant inheritance.

Pathogenesis: Unknown.

MIM No.: 16645

POS No.: 4457

CDC No.: 756.580

Sex Ratio: M1:F1

Occurrence: At least six kinships have been reported.

Risk of Recurrence for Patient's Sib:
See Part I, *Mendelian Inheritance.*

Risk of Recurrence for Patient's Child:
See Part I, *Mendelian Inheritance.*

Age of Detectability: During adolescence or in the young adult for chronic lower back pain.

Gene Mapping and Linkage: Unknown.

Prevention: None known. Genetic counseling indicated.

Treatment: Physiotherapy.

Prognosis: Functional impairment is possible. Should be clearly distinguished from **Osteopetrosis, benign dominant** because of their different prognoses.

Detection of Carrier: Examination of relatives for evidence of vertebral anomalies.

References:
Simon D, et al.: Une ostéosclérose axiale de transmission dominante autosomique: une nouvelle entité? Rev Rhum 1979; 46:375–382.

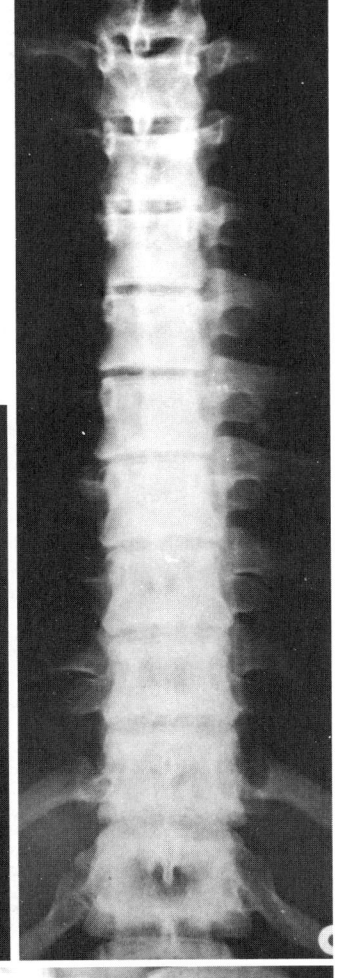

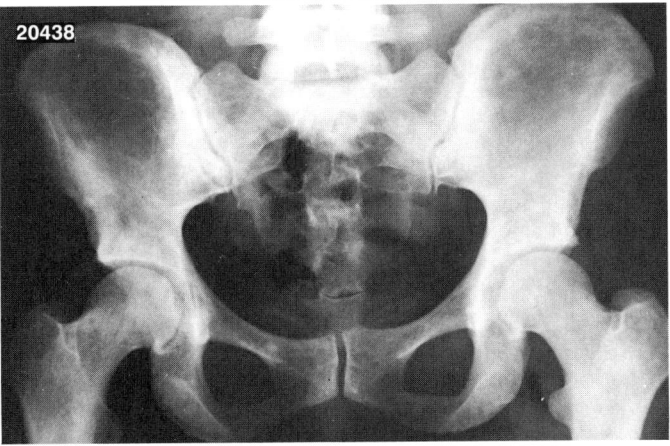

2695-20284: Sclerosis of vertebral bodies. 20435: Increased density of the upper and lower vertebral plates; these changes are similar to those seen in osteopetrosis except in osteomesopycnosis the long bones are normal except for the proximal femur. 20438: Sclerosis in the pelvis.

Maroteaux P: L'ostéomésopycnose: une nouvelle affection conden-
sante de transmission dominante autosomique. Arch Fr Pédiatr
1980; 37:153–157. *

Stoll CG, et al.: Osteomesopyknosis: an autosomal dominant osteosclerosis. Am J Med Genet 1981; 8:349–353.

Maroteaux P, et al.: Four recently described osteochondrodysplasias.
In: Papadatos CJ, Bartsocas CS, eds: Skeletal dysplasias. New York:
Alan R. Liss, 1982:345–350.

Proschek R, et al.: Osteomesopyknosis: case report. J Bone Joint Surg
1985; 67A:652–653.

Griffith TM, et al.: Osteomesopyknosis benign axial osteosclerosis. Br
J Radiol 1988; 61:951–953.

Delcambre B, et al.: Osteomesopyknosis: report of two new cases.
Skeletal Radiol 1989; 18:21–24.

MA034   **Pierre Maroteaux**

Osteopathia hyperostotica scleroticans multiplex infantilis
See DIAPHYSEAL DYSPLASIA

OSTEOPATHIA STRIATA   0778

Includes:
Osteopathia striata with pigmentary dermopathy-white
forelock
Voorhoeve disease

Excludes:
Osteopathia striata-cranial sclerosis (2237)
Osteopoikilosis (0781)

Major Diagnostic Criteria: The typical X-ray appearance of longitudinal striations of osteosclerosis in the long bones.

Clinical Findings: Patients with striated bony lesions have been
reported with dermatofibrosis lenticularis, and in families with
osteopoikilosis.

X-rays show longitudinal striations in the long bones, beginning
at the epiphyseal line and most prominently in the metaphyses.
Irregular fan-like striations are seen in the ilium. Increased bone
density has been reported in the skull and ribs. Thickening of the
cranial vault, with projection of dense bone from the inner table,
and obliteration of the sinuses has been observed, but this
condition may be a separate entity. No abnormal laboratory
results have been reported. Unilateral involvement has been
reported.

Complications: Conductive deafness has been reported in two
cases, probably resulting from the narrow auditory canals, fixation
of the ossicular chain, and loss of mastoid air cells.

Associated Findings: Reduced intelligence has been reported in
two patients, cleft palate in two cases, and premature cortical
cataracts have been reported in one patient. Dermatofibrosis
lenticularis has also been reported. Osteopathis striata is frequently seen in **Dermal hypoplasia, focal**. Associated X-ray findings
include small areas of translucency in the metaphysis, localized
thinning of the cortex, and small exostoses.

Etiology: Undetermined. An X-linked variant with dermopathy
and white forelock has been described.

Pathogenesis: Pathology has been reported to be similar to
Osteopetrosis in involved areas, with loss of lamellar structure due
to the obliteration of canaliculi. The pathogenesis is unknown,
although similar lesions have been produced in mice by inhibition
of resorption of metaphyseal spongiosa with estrogens.

MIM No.: 31128

POS No.: 3795

CDC No.: 756.580

Sex Ratio: Presumably M1:F1, except in X-linked instances.

Occurrence: Over a dozen cases documented, plus three sisters
reported with X-linked variant.

Risk of Recurrence for Patient's Sib: Unknown.

Risk of Recurrence for Patient's Child: Unknown.

Age of Detectability: Usually detected in adults as an incidental X-ray finding, although it is probably detectable in childhood, and severe cases may be detected prenatally.

Gene Mapping and Linkage: Unknown.

Prevention: None known. Genetic counseling indicated.

Treatment: Hearing aid and surgical mobilization of the ossicles may be necessary for accompanying deafness.

Prognosis: Normal for life span, probably normal for intelligence and function, except for possible loss of hearing or sight.

Detection of Carrier: Unknown.

References:

Hurt RL: Osteopathia striata-Voorhoeve's disease; report of a case presenting the features of osteopathia striata and osteopetrosis. J Bone Joint Surg 1953; 35B:89.

Walker BA: Osteopathia striata with cataracts and deafness. BD:OAS V(4). White Plains: The National Foundation-March of Dimes, 1969:295–297.

Larregue M, et al.: L'osteopathie striee, symptome radiologique de l'hypoplasie dermique en aires. Ann Radiol 1972; 15:287–295.

Horan FT, Beighton PH: Osteopathia striata with cranial sclerosis: an autosomal dominant entity. Clin Genet 1978; 13:201–206.

Whyte MP, Murphy WA: Osteopathia striata associated with familial dermopathy and white forelock: evidence for postnatal development of osteopathia striata. Am J Med Genet 1980; 5:227–234.

Coutina H, et al.: Familial osteopathia striata with cranial condensation. Pediatr Radiol 1981; 11:87–90.

LA006   Ralph S. Lachman

Osteopathia striata with pigmentary dermopathy-white forelock
See OSTEOPATHIA STRIATA

OSTEOPATHIA STRIATA-CRANIAL SCLEROSIS-MEGALENCEPHALY   2237

Includes:
Cranial sclerosis-osteopathia striata-macrocephaly
Hyperostosis generalisata with striations
Megalencephaly-cranial sclerosis-osteopathia striata

Excludes:
Cranial sclerosis (others)
Dermal hypoplasia, focal (0281)
Osteopathia striata (0778)

Major Diagnostic Criteria: **Osteopathia striata**, non-progressive **Megalencephaly** (head circumference paralleling the normal curve), and progressive cranial sclerosis.

Clinical Findings: **Megalencephaly** with prominant forehead, hypoplastic orbital ridges, and moderate **Eye, hypertelorism**.

X-ray features: longitudinal striations of tubular bones and pelvis, progressive sclerosis of cranial bones, gradual development of generalized hyperostosis.

Complications: Neurosensory deafness, facial nerve palsy.

Associated Findings: **Cleft palate**, mental retardation.

Etiology: Autosomal dominant inheritance with high penetrance but variable expressivity.

Pathogenesis: Osteopathia striata has been attributed to persistence of the fetal pattern of bone trabeculation.

MIM No.: *16650

POS No.: 4249

CDC No.: 756.580

Sex Ratio: Presumably M1:F1, but current observed M1:F2.

Occurrence: About 25 cases have been reported.

Risk of Recurrence for Patient's Sib:
See Part I, *Mendelian Inheritance.*

Risk of Recurrence for Patient's Child:
See Part I, *Mendelian Inheritance.*

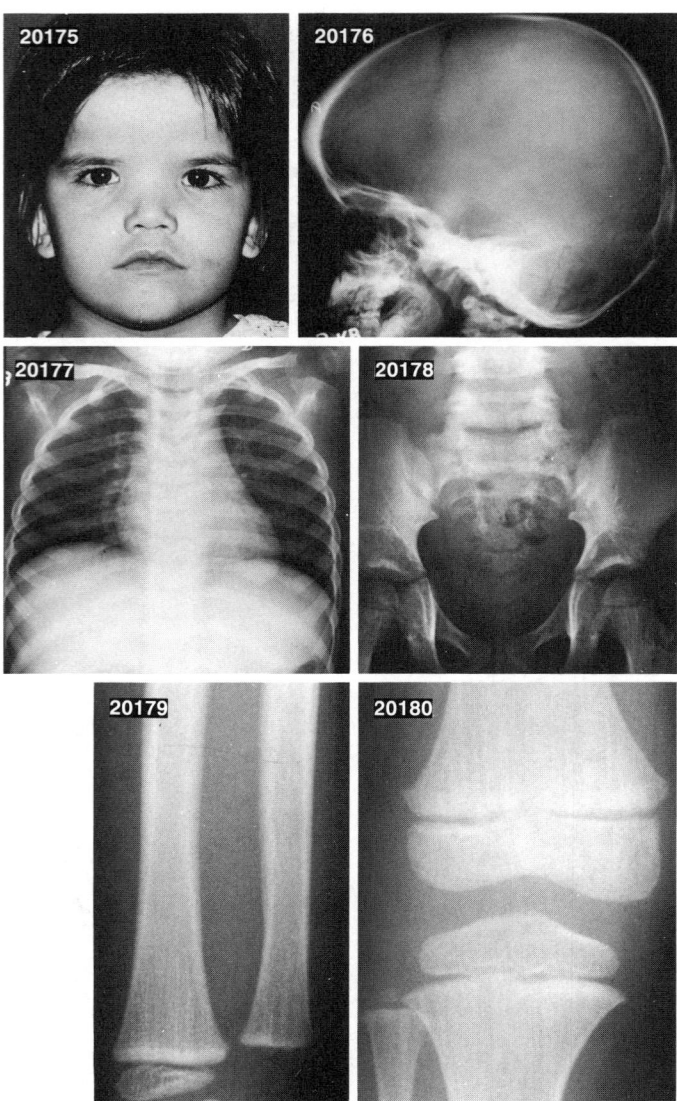

2237-20175: Note prominent forehead, hypertelorism, telecanthus and hypoplastic orbital ridges. **20176:** Lateral skull X-ray shows craniomegaly, thickened frontal bone, sclerosis of the skull base, poor mastoid pneumatization and lack of sinus aeration. **20177:** Chest X-ray shows generalized hyperostosis with widening of the ribs. **20178:** Longitudinal striations appear in the proximal femora and central ilia. **20179:** Striations appear in the distal ulna and radius. **20180:** Striations in distal femora and proximal tibia. There is no cortical thickening, periosteal new bone formation or defective tubular modeling.

Age of Detectability: Usually in infancy or childhood. One familial case was diagnosed prenatally by ultrasonography.

Gene Mapping and Linkage: Unknown.

Prevention: None known. Genetic counseling indicated.

Treatment: Unknown.

Prognosis: Hyperostosis, usually progressive, is in some cases stationary. Life span is normal. No functional impairment except for rare cases with facial palsy or neurosensory deafness.

Detection of Carrier: Skeletal X-rays may detect previously unsuspected heterozygotes.

Special Considerations: The triad of osteopathia striata, macrocephaly, and cranial sclerosis was first delineated in 1978 by Horan and Beighton. Classification of several earlier published cases of osteopathia striata combined with **Osteopoikilosis** or with generalized osteosclerosis and medullary expansion remains uncertain.

References:
Horan FT, Beighton PH: Osteopathia striata with cranial sclerosis: an autosomal dominant entity. Clin Genet 1978; 13:201–206. * †
Winter RM, et al.: Osteopathia striata with cranial sclerosis: highly variable expression within a family including cleft palate in two neonatal cases. Clin Genet 1980; 18:462–474.
Robinow M, Unger F: Syndrome of osteopathia striata, macrocephaly, and cranial sclerosis. Am J Dis Child 1984; 138:821–823. * †

R0004 **Meinhard Robinow**

Osteopathic childhood osteoporosis
See OSTEOPOROSIS, JUVENILE IDIOPATHIC
Osteoperiostosis, secondary hypertrophic with pernio
See DIGITAL DEFECTS-NODULAR ERYTHEMA-EMACIATION, NAKAJO TYPE
Osteopetrosis tardia
See OSTEOPETROSIS, BENIGN DOMINANT
Osteopetrosis with late manifestation
See OSTEOPETROSIS, BENIGN DOMINANT
Osteopetrosis, benign adult form of
See OSTEOPETROSIS, BENIGN DOMINANT

OSTEOPETROSIS, BENIGN DOMINANT 0779

Includes:
Albers-Schonberg disease
Marble bone disease
Osteopetrosis, benign adult form of
Osteopetrosis, dominant
Osteopetrosis tardia
Osteopetrosis with late manifestation
Osteosclerosis fragilis generalisata

Excludes:
Craniometaphyseal dysplasia (0228)
Diaphyseal dysplasia (0290)
Dysosteosclerosis (0310)
Hyperostosis generalisata
Leontiasis ossea
Osteopetrosis (other)
Osteopoikilosis (0781)
Pyknodysostosis (0846)

Major Diagnostic Criteria: The clinical features are variable. X-rays shows pathologic fractures, dental abscesses, and cranial hyperostosis later in life. Serum chemistry shows elevated acid phosphatase levels in some cases.

Clinical Findings: Clinically the disorder is detected later in life, usually in adolescence, and sometimes upon routine X-ray of the chest. It is characterized by a generalized sclerosis of the bone, with marked variability in its clinical manifestations.

Close to 50% of patients are asymptomatic and are diagnosed on incidental X-rays or because of genetic analysis of their family due to a more severely affected relative. The most common problem in this disorder is pathologic fractures; 40% of reported cases had a history of fractures. About 10% have osteomyelitis of the mandible. Dental abscesses are frequent.

Bone pain, primarily of the lumbar spine, occurs in 20% of patients. The cranial hyperostosis may result in cranial nerve palsies which have been described in 16% of cases. The nerves most commonly affected are the 2nd, 3rd, and 7th cranial nerves, resulting in optic atrophy, extraocular muscle palsies, and facial palsy. Frontal bossing, exophthalmos, or facial palsies may result in a peculiar facial appearance. There is marked intrafamilial variability in the clinical features of this disorder, and nonpenetrance has been described. Hepatosplenomegaly and severe anemia are usually not features of the dominant form of osteopetro-

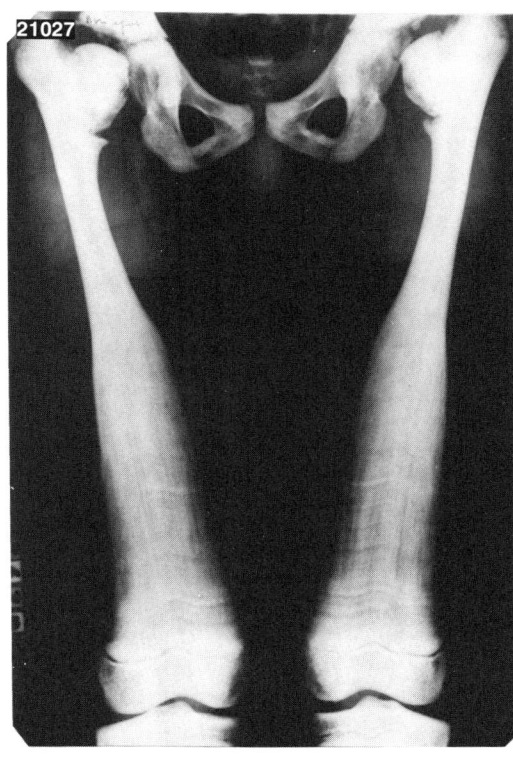

0779A-21027: Osteopetrosis, autosomal dominant; note generalized sclerosis and parallel radiolucent striations in the metaphyseal region.

sis. Elevated serum acid phosphatase levels have been found in almost all reported cases, but other serum chemistries and calcium balance studies have been normal.

Skeletal X-rays reveal a generalized sclerotic process. The earliest features are an increase in the density of the diaphyseal regions of the growing bone, with parallel radiolucent striations in the metaphyseal regions. The vertebral bodies may develop a "sandwich" appearance, with sclerosis of the upper and lower plates and an intervening less dense appearance. The tubular bones, especially the metacarpals, may show a "bone within a bone" appearance. The skull is thickened and dense, especially at the base. The sinuses decrease in size and even disappear.

Histologic examination of the affected bones shows absence of a true medullary cavity with noncalcified hyaline cartilage remnants scattered diffusely within the bone. The bone itself is made up primarily of Haversian systems with scanty fibrillar composition. Foci of osteoblastic and osteoclastic activity can be seen.

Complications: Teeth are affected by dental abscesses and osteomyelitis. Pathologic fractures occur following minor trauma.

Associated Findings: Cranial nerve palsy, strabismus.

Etiology: Autosomal dominant inheritance with variable expressivity. Could be non-penetrant.

Pathogenesis: Of several hypotheses, the most favored is defective resorption of primary spongiosa by abnormal osteoclasts, which results in increased osseous density.

MIM No.: *16660
CDC No.: 756.540
Sex Ratio: M1:F1
Occurrence: About 1:100,000, based on data from Brazil.
Risk of Recurrence for Patient's Sib:
See Part I, *Mendelian Inheritance.*

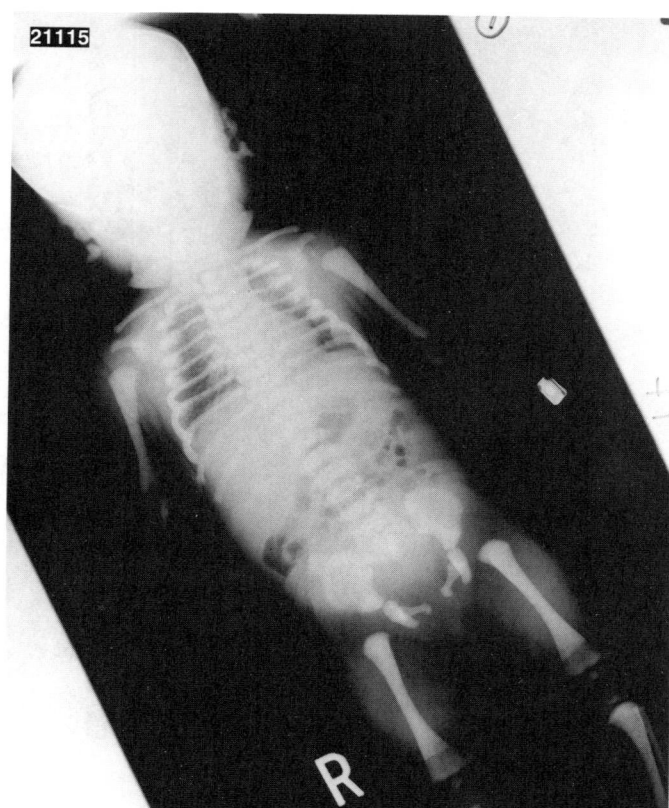

0779B-21115: X-ray of an infant shows increased bone density.

Risk of Recurrence for Patient's Child:
See Part I, *Mendelian Inheritance.*

Age of Detectability: Clinically not remarkable within the first several years of life, but could be detected early by skeletal X-rays. It is often not diagnosed until adolescence or adulthood.

Gene Mapping and Linkage: Unknown.

Prevention: None known. Genetic counseling indicated.

Treatment: Successful use of calcitriol has been reported. Calcitriol is a metabolite of vitamin D with a bone-resorbing effect.

Prognosis: Life span is not affected.

Detection of Carrier: Unknown.

Special Considerations: This disorder is distinct from the congenital malignant form of the disease, both clinically and genetically. Severe anemia and hepatosplenomegaly are not features of this dominant disorder. Any adolescent or adult with the X-ray features of osteopetrosis will almost certainly have the dominant form of the disease. This disease must be differentiated from the other forms of skeletal sclerosis such as fluorosis, heavy metal intoxication, **Craniometaphyseal dysplasia**, **Osteopoikilosis**, Camurati-Engelmann disease, **Cranio-diaphyseal dysplasia**, Schwarz-Lélek syndrome, **Endosteal hyperostosis**, **Sclerosteosis**, and **Pyknodysostosis**.

Support Groups: PA; West Chester; American Brittle Bone Society (ABBS)

References:
Ghormley RK: A case of congenital osteosclerosis. Bull Johns Hopkins Hosp 1922; 33:444–446.
Welford NP: Facial paralysis associated with osteopetrosis (marble bones). J Pediatr 1959; 55:67–72.
Salzano FM: Osteopetrosis: review of dominant cases and frequency in a Brazilian state. Acta Genet Med Gemellol (Roma) 1961; 10:353–358.
Johnston CC Jr, et al.: Osteopetrosis. Medicine 1968; 47:149–167. *
Beighton P, et al.: A review of the osteopetroses. Postgrad Med J 1977; 53:507–515.
Key L, et al.: Treatment of congenital osteopetrosis with high dose calcitrol. New Engl J Med 1984; 310:409–415.

CE003

Jaroslav Červenka
David L. Rimoin
David W. Hollister

Osteopetrosis, dominant
See OSTEOPETROSIS, BENIGN DOMINANT
Osteopetrosis, intermediate type
See OSTEOPETROSIS, MILD RECESSIVE

OSTEOPETROSIS, MALIGNANT RECESSIVE   0780

Includes:
   Albers-Schonberg disease
   Carbonic anhydrase II deficiency
   Guibaud-Vainsel syndrome
   Infantile malignant osteopetrosis
   Lethal osteopetrosis
   Malignant congenital osteopetrosis
   Marble bone disease
   Marble brain disease
   Osteopetrosis-renal tubular acidosis

Excludes:
   Craniometaphyseal dysplasia (0228)
   Diaphyseal dysplasia (0290)
   Dysosteosclerosis (0310)
   Osteopetrosis (other)
   Osteopoikilosis (0781)

Major Diagnostic Criteria: Skeletal X-rays show sclerosis of all bones. Serum chemistry sometimes shows hypocalcemia and hyperphosphatemia. Clinically, early onset of deafness, blindness, severe anemia, hepatosplenomegaly, facial paralysis, and macrocephaly is observed.

Clinical Findings: Dense brittle bones, macrocephaly, progressive deafness and blindness, hepatosplenomegaly, and severe anemia beginning in early infancy or in utero. Affected children may be stillborn or exhibit failure to thrive; they may die in infancy

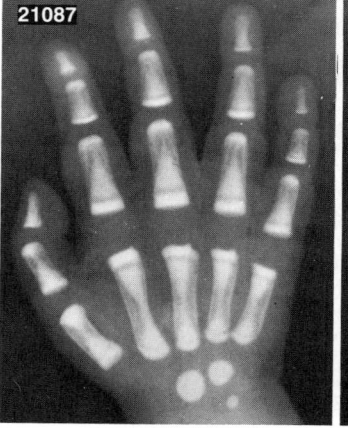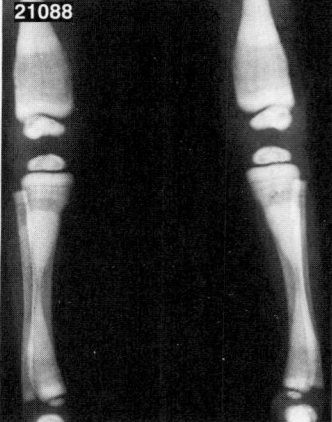

0780-21087: Hand X-ray shows the "bone within a bone" appearance in the tubular bones. **21088:** The long bones are undermodelled and the lower femoral metaphyses have a club-shaped configuration. The bones show regions of lucency and increased density.

or early childhood. The osteosclerotic process impinges on the marrow cavity, resulting in severe anemia and pancytopenia with extramedullary hematopoiesis producing hepatosplenomegaly and lymphadenopathy, often with nucleated red blood cells in the peripheral blood (myeloid metaplasia). Cranial sclerosis may result in macrocephaly and hydrocephaly, as well as impingement on the cranial nerve foramina, leading to blindness with optic or retinal atrophy, deafness, facial palsies, and strabismus. Dentition may be delayed and severe dental caries has been reported. Growth and developmental retardation are common, but intelligence is normal in over 75% of cases. The sclerotic skeletal system predisposes to pathologic fractures and osteomyelitis. Serum chemistry is usually normal, although hypocalcemia and hyperphosphatemia may be detected and tetany has been described.

Skeletal X-rays reveal uniformly dense sclerotic bones, with associated metaphyseal splaying and clubbing. The medullary canals and trabecular patterns are obliterated. Radiolucent streaks appear in the long bone metaphyses, while the epiphyses are sclerotic but of normal contour. The skull is thickened, particularly at the base, with narrowing of the cranial foramina. The mastoids and paranasal sinuses are poorly aerated. The metacarpals and metatarsals may appear block-shaped, with a "bone in bone" appearance, and there may be partial aplasia of the distal phalanges. The vertebrae are of normal shape, but the ribs appear flared.

Histologic examination of bone reveals obliteration of the medullary cavity by a lattice-like network of hyaline cartilage surrounded by thick bone that exhibits a paucity of fibrils. Foci of osteoblastic and osteoclastic activity can be seen.

Complications: Cranial nerve palsies and facial paralysis, deafness, strabismus, nystagmus, blindness, anemia, failure to thrive, and short life span.

Associated Findings: A possible form in which osteoclasts are markedly reduced was reported by El Khazen et al (1986) and designated *lethal osteopetrosis.*

Etiology: Autosomal recessive inheritance.

Pathogenesis: Several hypotheses have been proposed. It appears likely that the abnormality of osteoclasts leads to the disease. Dysfunctioning osteoclasts then fail in resorption of primary spongiosa.

MIM No.: *25970, *25973, 25972

POS No.: 3374

CDC No.: 756.540

Sex Ratio: M1:F1

Occurrence: Less than 100 cases have been reported. A high frequency has been observed in Costa Rica.

Risk of Recurrence for Patient's Sib:
See Part I, *Mendelian Inheritance.*

Risk of Recurrence for Patient's Child:
See Part I, *Mendelian Inheritance.* Affected individuals are not expected to survive to reproduce.

Age of Detectability: Usually at birth. Prenatal diagnosis is made by X-ray, revealing a generalized sclerotic skeletal system.

Gene Mapping and Linkage: Unknown.

Prevention: None known. Genetic counseling indicated.

Treatment: Steroid therapy has been reported to be of some value, and an increasing experience with bone marrow transplantation has demonstrated that the disease can be greatly ameliorated.

Prognosis: Survival past the age of 20 years is rare. Death in infancy or childhood is usually due to anemia or secondary infection.

Detection of Carrier: Unknown.

Special Considerations: The eponym *Albers-Schonberg disease* is usually reserved for the benign dominant form of this disorder (see **Osteopetrosis, benign dominant**).

Autosomal recessive osteopetrosis with renal tubular acidosis, also known as *carbonic anhydrase II deficiency*, *Guibaud-Vainsel syndrome* and *marble brain disease* (Sly et al, 1985) is a separate

entity. Affected individuals have reduced intelligence, short stature, pancytopenia, basal ganglion calcification, renal tubular acidosis, and deficiency of carbonic anhydrase II in erythrocytes. This is a severe form of osteopetrosis, with early onset.

Support Groups: PA; West Chester; American Brittle Bone Society (ABBS)

References:
Moe PJ, Skjaeveland A: Therapeutic studies in osteopetrosis. Acta Paediatr Scand 1969; 58:593–600.
Loria-Cortés R, et al.: Osteopetrosis in children: a report of 26 cases. J Pediatr 1977; 91:43–47. *
Beighton P, Cremin BJ: Sclerosing bone dysplasias. New York: Springer Verlag, 1980. *
Coccia PF, et al.: Successful bone-marrow transplantation for infantile malignant osteopetrosis. New Engl J Med 1980; 302:701–708.
Sorrel M, et al.: Marrow transplantation for juvenile osteopetrosis. Am J Med 1981; 70:1280–1287.
Sieff CA, et al.: Allogeneic bone-marrow transplantation in infantile malignant osteopetrosis. Lancet 1983; I:437–441.
Sly WS, et al.: Carbonic anhydrase II deficiency in 12 families with the autsomal recessive syndrome of osteopetrosis with renal tubular acidosis and cerebral calcification. New Engl J Med 1985; 313:139–145.
El Khazen N, et al.: Lethal osteopetrosis with multiple fractures in utero. Am J Med Genet 1986; 23:811–819.
Fischer A, et al.: Bone-marrow transplantation for immunodeficiencies and osteopetrosis: European survey 1968–1985. Lancet 1986; II:1080–1084.
Bollerslev J: Osteopetrosis: a genetic and epidemiologic study. Clin Genet 1987; 31:86–90.

CE003

Jaroslav Červenka
David L. Rimoin
David W. Hollister

OSTEOPETROSIS, MILD RECESSIVE   2253

Includes: Osteopetrosis, intermediate type

Excludes:
   Osteopetrosis, benign dominant (0779)
   Osteopetrosis, malignant recessive (0780)
   Renal tubular acidosis-osteopetrosis syndrome (3086)

Major Diagnostic Criteria: Characteristic X-ray changes, including sclerosis of the cranial base, generally increased bone density, sclerosis of the vertebral end plates, and transverse bands and poor diaphyseal modeling of the long bones. Pedigree consistent with autosomal recessive inheritance.

Clinical Findings: Physical findings include relative or absolute short stature, with increased upper/lower segment ratio and decreased arm span. Mandibular prognathism may also be a feature, along with dental abnormalities. Patients have often been asymptomatic in childhood, except for increased susceptibility to fractures or mandibular osteomyelitis. The X-ray changes are probably present from early childhood. Clinical manifestations are much milder than in **Osteopetrosis, malignant recessive**.

Complications: Osteomyelitis, especially mandibular actinomycosis; mild anemia due to marrow encroachment, with compensatory extramedullary hematopoiesis; impacted teeth; fractures.

Associated Findings: Midface hypoplasia was thought to be part of the syndrome in one family. Acid or alkaline phosphatase was elevated in some patients.

Etiology: Autosomal recessive inheritance.

Pathogenesis: Unknown.

MIM No.: 25971

CDC No.: 756.540

Sex Ratio: M12:F6 (observed).

Occurrence: About 20 cases have been documented.

Risk of Recurrence for Patient's Sib:
See Part I, *Mendelian Inheritance.*

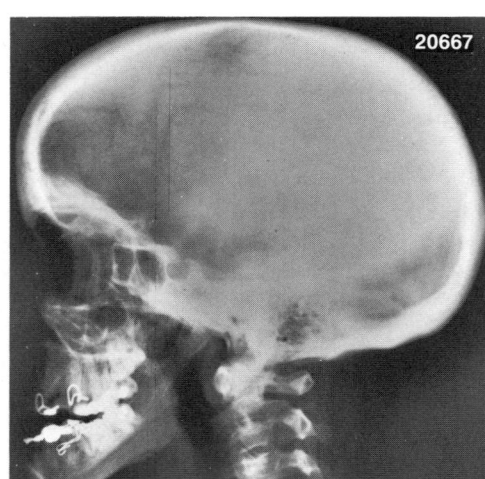

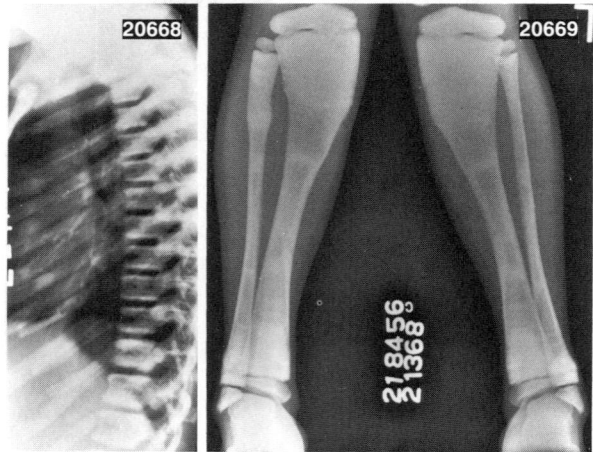

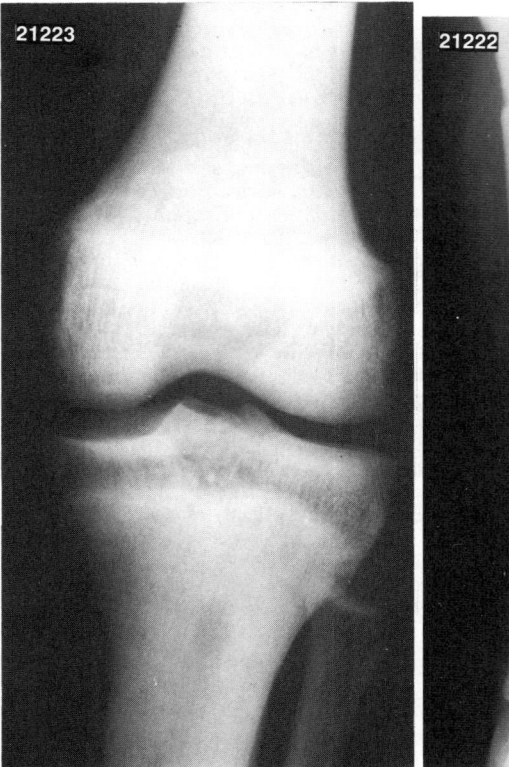

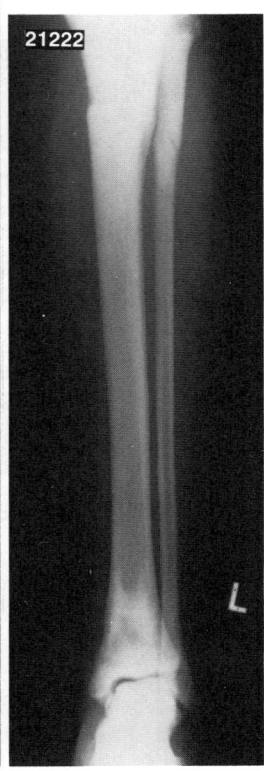

2253B-21223: The bones are brittle with a propensity to fracture. 21222: The tubular bones are sclerotic but their external contours are undisturbed. Note the transverse fracture of the tibia and fibula.

2253A-20667: Osteoporosis, mild autosomal recessive type; note lateral view of the skull shows marked thickening of the base. The cranium also shows increased bone density and there is mid-face hypoplasia. 20668: Lateral view of the spine shows increased density at the ends of the vertebral bodies ("rugger-jersey" appearance), and widening and increased density of the ribs. 20669: AP view of the lower legs shows generalized increased density of bone with horizontal areas of greater and lesser density, widening of the metaphyses, and deformation of the shaft of the long bones.

Support Groups: PA; West Chester; American Brittle Bone Society (ABBS)

References:

Trias A, Fery A: Osteopetrosis in adults. Rev Chir Orthop 1974; 60:593–606.
Beighton P, et al.: Osteopetrosis in South Africa. S Afr Med J 1979; 55:659–665.
Horton WA, et al.: Osteopetrosis: further heterogeneity. J Pediatr 1980; 97:580–585.
Kahler SG, et al.: A mild autosomal recessive form of osteopetrosis. Am J Med Genet 1984; 17:451–464. * †

KA002   **Stephen G. Kahler**

Osteopetrosis-renal tubular acidosis
See OSTEOPETROSIS, MALIGNANT RECESSIVE
Osteopetrosis-renal tubular acidosis-cerebral calcification
See RENAL TUBULAR ACIDOSIS-OSTEOPETROSIS SYNDROME

Risk of Recurrence for Patient's Child:
See Part I, *Mendelian Inheritance.*

Age of Detectability: In childhood.

Gene Mapping and Linkage: Unknown.

Prevention: None known. Genetic counseling indicated.

Treatment: No specific treatment known. Osteomyelitis must be treated early and vigorously. Mandibular actinomycosis may be fatal, but it has been treated successfully with long-term penicillin augmented with hyperbaric oxygen. Dental abnormalities, fractures, and cranial nerve compression (optic, facial, and acoustic) may occur and require treatment.

Prognosis: Good for health and life span.

Detection of Carrier: Unknown.

OSTEOPOIKILOSIS   **0781**

Includes:
    Buscke-Ollendorf syndrome
    Dermatoosteopoikilosis
    Disseminated dermatofibrosis-osteopoikilosis
    Osteodermatopoikilosis
    Osteodysplasia enostotica
    Osteolysis, idiopathic multicentric
    "Spotted bones"

Excludes:
    Chondrodysplasia punctata, X-linked dominant type (2730)

Osteoblastic metastases
Osteopetrosis, benign dominant (0779)
Osteosclerosis of other etiologies

Major Diagnostic Criteria: Typical grain-to-pea size densities on X-rays.

Clinical Findings: This disorder is usually discovered accidently, by X-ray. The typical appearance is oval or round densities, oriented in longitudinal directions, and most abundant in the pelvis and shoulder girdles and in the epiphyses and metaphyses of the long bones. The skull is rarely involved. Although the round densities are rarely seen in the diaphyses, the distinct parallel lines of density extending from the epiphyseal line down into the diaphyses, as seen in osteopathia striata, may be found in patients with osteopoikilosis or in their relatives. This has led some observers to consider them as the same process. Dermatofibrosis lenticularis is the skin manifestation of the disorder, occurring in over 50% of patients with X-ray changes. These are raised, yellowish lesions, which may coalesce and form stripes. The common locations are the buttocks, thighs, back, and abdominal skin, but not the face. The skin lesions have been reported without the X-ray changes in families with osteopoikilosis. The eponym "Buscke-Ollendorf" is applied to the syndromic association of the bone and skin abnormalities.

Complications: Keloids.

Associated Findings: Fibrous nodules of the peritoneal lining. Associations that have been reported but may not be real are short stature, diabetes, cleft lip, scleroderma, palmar and plantar keratosis, subcutaneous fibrous nodules, and hyperostosis frontalis interna. Osteopoikilosis is usually innocuous, but a single report of the development of osteosarcoma may have serious implications. Spinal canal stenosis and basal cell nevus syndrome have also been recognized in persons with osteopoikilosis. The significance of these inter-relationships is undetermined.

Etiology: Autosomal dominant inheritance with incomplete penetrance. Skipped generations are common. The skin lesions and bony lesions may occur separately in the same family.

Pathogenesis: Appears to be a spotty hyperplasia of collagen in the corium and bone matrix. The bony lesions are due to a thickening of the trabecular spongiosa.

MIM No.: *16670

CDC No.: 756.560

Sex Ratio: Presumably M1:F1, although males are more frequently detected because they more frequently have X-rays for trauma, etc.

Occurrence: 1:20,000 X-rays in a German survey (Jonaseh, 1955).

Risk of Recurrence for Patient's Sib:
See Part I, *Mendelian Inheritance.*

Risk of Recurrence for Patient's Child:
See Part I, *Mendelian Inheritance.*

Age of Detectability: At birth, but has been detected prenatally.

Gene Mapping and Linkage: Unknown.

Prevention: None known. Genetic counseling indicated.

Treatment: Unknown.

Prognosis: Normal for life span, intelligence, and function.

Detection of Carrier: Unknown.

References:
Busch KFB: Familial disseminated osteosclerosis. Acta Radiol (Stockh) 1937; 18:693–714.
Danielsen L, et al.: Osteopoikilosis associated with dermatofibrosis lenticularis disseminata. Arch Dermatol 1969; 100:465–470.
Mindell ER, et al.: Osteosarcoma associated with osteopoikilosis: case report. J Bone Joint Surg (Am) 1978; 60:406 only.
Weisz GM: Lumbar spinal canal stenosis in osteopoikilosis. Clin Orthopaed 1982; 166:89–92.
Blinder G, et al.: Widespread osteolytic lesions of the long bones in the basal cell nevus syndrome. Skel Radiol 1984; 12:196–198.
Lagier R, et al.: Osteopoikilosis: a radiological and pathological study. Skel Radiol 1984; 11:161–168.
Verbov J, et al.: Disseminated dermatofibrosis osteopoikilosis. Clin Exper Derm 1986; 11:17–26.
Carnevale A, et al.: Idiopathic multicentric osteolysis with facial anomalies and nephropathy. Am J Med Genet 1987; 26:877–886.

BE008   **Peter Beighton**

OSTEOPOROSIS, JUVENILE IDIOPATHIC   **0782**

Includes:
Juvenile osteoporosis
Osteopathic childhood osteoporosis

Excludes:
Osteogenesis imperfecta (0777)
Osteoporosis secondary to any identifiable cause

Major Diagnostic Criteria: Fractures follow minor trauma in a previously normal child or adolescent who has no signs or family history of osteogenesis imperfecta. X-rays show diminished bone density in the absence of any defined underlying disease.

Clinical Findings: Juvenile osteoporosis is a disease of childhood and adolescence exhibiting marked clinical variability. The disease usually begins in the peripubertal period (age 8–13 years), but several younger cases (age 3–8 years) have been reported, and the disorder has been documented in at least one adult. The affected individuals are clinically normal, as are their X-rays, until the onset of fractures following minor trauma. The fractures usually occur in the vertebrae, but long bone fractures are also common. Metabolic studies indicate negative calcium balance, but serum calcium, phosphorus, and alkaline-phosphatases are often normal. Calcitriol (1,25 dihydroxycholecalciferol) deficiency has been documented in one case. X-rays typically show marked diminution in bone density. The disease can persist for many years, but usually remits, or markedly improves, within five years. Even after remission, severe sequelae due to spinal cord compression, malaligned long bones, and pseudoarthroses can persist. It has not been determined if these patients have an increased propensity for senile osteoporosis.

Complications: Bony deformities secondary to fractures lead to decreased height, kyphosis, protuberant sternum and malalignment of long bones, and pseudoarthroses.

Associated Findings: None known.

Etiology: Possibly autosomal recessive inheritance, but a clear inheritance pattern has not been established. This condition might not represent a single entity, but rather a heterogeneous group of disorders with a common clinical appearance. Dent (1969) has emphasized that the younger onset group (3–8 years) may comprise a distinct entity called *osteopathic childhood osteoporosis.*

Pathogenesis: Undetermined. Calcitriol deficiency and negative calcium balance have been documented.

MIM No.: 25975

CDC No.: 756.580

Sex Ratio: M1:F1

Occurrence: About 50 cases reported. Mild cases may go unrecognized.

Risk of Recurrence for Patient's Sib:
See Part I, *Mendelian Inheritance.*

Risk of Recurrence for Patient's Child:
See Part I, *Mendelian Inheritance.*

Age of Detectability: Early childhood to adulthood.

Gene Mapping and Linkage: Unknown.

Prevention: None known. Genetic counseling indicated.

Treatment: Avoidance of any activity that might cause fractures or exacerbate old fractures is recommended. Calcitriol was reported as helpful in one patient.

Prognosis: Normal life span and intelligence. Spontaneous remission is usual, but long standing cases have had severe residual damage.

Detection of Carrier: Unknown.

Support Groups: PA; Marshallton; American Brittle Bone Society

References:
Dent CE, Friedman M: Idiopathic juvenile osteoporosis. Q J Med 1965; 34:177–210. *
Dent CE: Idiopathic juvenile osteoporosis. BD:OAS V(4). New York: The National Foundation-March of Dimes, 1969:134–147. *
Marder HK, et al.: Calcitriol deficiency in idiopathic juvenile osteoporosis. Am J Dis Child 1982; 136:914–917.

AL006   **Kirk Aleck**

Osteoporosis-ocular pseudoglioma
See OSTEOPOROSIS-PSEUDOGLIOMA SYNDROME

OSTEOPOROSIS-PSEUDOGLIOMA SYNDROME   0783

Includes:
Blindness (pseudogliomatous)-osteoporosis-mild mental retardation
Osteogenesis imperfecta, ocular form
Osteoporosis-ocular pseudoglioma

Excludes:
Osteogenesis imperfecta (0777)
Osteoporosis (all other forms)

Major Diagnostic Criteria: Blindness from "pseudogliomatous" retinal detachment causing phthisis bulbi; osteoporosis; fractures from minor accidents and deformities; and mild mental retardation.

Clinical Findings: Blindness in infancy is probably due to "pseudogliomatous" retinal detachment or from fetal uveitis, resulting in microphthalmia, phthisis bulbi, corneal opacity, and cataracts; calcification of the lens may occur. Osteoporosis of variable severity is manifested at age 2–3 years, sometimes resulting in incapacitating deformities secondary to multiple fractures from minor trauma. Vertebral deformities result in a short trunk. Ligaments are lax. Microcephaly and macular hypotonia are present in some. Mental retardation when present usually is of mild-to-borderline degree (special verbal abilities are occasionally seen, e.g. idiot savant). Hearing is usually normal. X-ray findings include osteoporosis, thin cortex, and coarse trabecular structure of long bones; spontaneous fractures, bowing of limbs, metaphyseal cysts, codfish vertebrae, and wormian bones.

Complications: Blindness, deformities, physical handicap, and mental deficiency.

Associated Findings: Ventricular septal defect.

Etiology: Autosomal recessive inheritance.

Pathogenesis: Unknown.

MIM No.: *25977

POS No.: 3711

CDC No.: 756.580

Sex Ratio: M1:F1

Occurrence: About a dozen families have been documented. May be more frequent in Mediterranean countries.

Risk of Recurrence for Patient's Sib:
See Part I, *Mendelian Inheritance.*

Risk of Recurrence for Patient's Child:
See Part I, *Mendelian Inheritance.*

Age of Detectability: Infancy (blindness) and early childhood (fractures and osteoporosis).

Gene Mapping and Linkage: Unknown.

Prevention: None known. Genetic counseling indicated.

Treatment: Treatment of osteoporosis; care for fractures and deformities. Prevention of retinal detachment in patients at risk.

Prognosis: Osteoporosis may progress during childhood; stabilization usually occurs after childhood.

Detection of Carrier: Incomplete manifestation of the syndrome may be seen in heterozygotes.

Special Considerations: "Pseudoglioma" is a nonspecific term; usually retinal detachment is the cause of blindness. The syndrome is probably a connective tissue dysplasia primarily involving eyes, bones, and ligaments. Biochemical findings reported from some cases include hypercalcinuria and hydroxyprolinuria as nonspecific secondary manifestations of osteoporosis. A decreased rate of bone formation and an increased rate of bone resorption have been shown by microautoradiographic studies.

Support Groups: PA; Marshallton; American Brittle Bone Society

References:
Bianchine JW, Murdoch JL: Juvenile osteoporosis (?) in a boy with bilateral enucleation of the eyes for pseudoglioma. BD:OAS V(4). New York: The National Foundation-March of Dimes, 1969:225–226.
Neuhäuser G, et al.: Autosomal recessive syndrome of pseudogliomatous blindness, osteoporosis and mild mental retardation. Clin Genet 1976; 9:324–332.
Bartsocas CS, et al.: Syndrome of osteoporosis with pseudoglioma. Ann Genet 1982; 25:61–62.
Frontali M, et al.: Osteoporosis-pseudoglioma syndrome: report of three affected siblings and a review. Am J Med Genet 1985; 22:35–47.
Beighton P, et al.: The ocular form of osteogenesis imperfecta. Clin Genet 1986; 28:69–75.
Teebi AS, et al.: Osteoporosis-pseudoglioma syndrome with congenital heart disease. J Med Genet 1988; 25:32–36.

NE012   **Gerhard Neuhäuser**

OSTEOSARCOMA   3101

Includes:
Cancer, osteosarcoma
Multicentric osteosarcoma
Osteogenic sarcoma
Periosteal osteosarcoma
Telangiectatic osteosarcoma

Excludes:
Bone, Paget disease (3081)
Dedifferentiated chondrosarcoma
Low-grade osteosarcoma
Malignant fibrous-histiocytoma
Parosteal osteosarcoma

Major Diagnostic Criteria: Pain and a tender mass are present usually at the metaphyseal end of a long bone. X-rays reveal a destructive lesion of bone and a soft tissue mass, often mineralized. Alkaline phosphatase level may be elevated. Histology

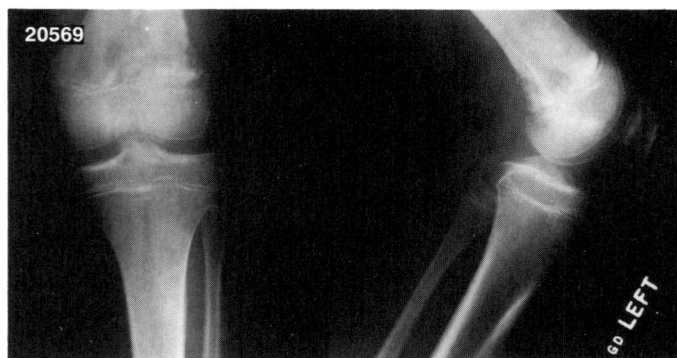

3101-20569: AP and lateral views of a typical osteosarcoma of the distal femur showing a poorly defined destructive lesion in the metaphysis. The cortex has been transgressed and there is a soft tissue mass which is partially mineralized. A Codman's triangle is evident.

shows a highly pleomorphic sarcoma with tumor bone production.

Clinical Findings: Osteosarcoma is a rare malignant neoplasm of bone occurring most frequently in the second decade of life. It usually presents as a painful mass of one or several months duration, located most commonly about the knee or shoulder. There is often a history of trauma that is not considered etiologic. The symptoms are progressive and the soft tissue mass may grow to large proportions, or a pathological fracture of the involved bone may occur if treatment is not instituted. Without treatment, patients would die of metastatic disease (most commonly pulmonary), and even with local treatment (amputation or radiation) of the primary disease, 80–90% will develop metastatic disease, suggesting that micrometastases are present in most patients at presentation.

The metaphyses of the long bones are the sites most frequently involved, but any bone may be affected. The distal femur is the most common site, followed by the proximal tibia (approximately 50% occur about the knee), proximal humerus, and femur. X-rays show a poorly defined destructive lesion of bone, which may be purely lytic or extremely blastic, but is usually a combination of both. The lesion is not marginated and usually transgresses the cortex of the bone to involve the adjacent soft tissues. The soft tissue component is variably mineralized, sometimes producing vertical striations: the so-called starburst appearance. An incomplete periosteal reaction (Codman triangle) is seen at the periphery of the lesion, but this is not specific for osteosarcoma. Computed tomograms and magnetic resonance images show the intramedullary and soft tissue extent more precisely than do plane X-rays and are useful in planning surgical approaches. Radionuclide bone scans show uptake in the area of involvement and are needed to exclude bony metastases.

There are no laboratory blood tests specific for osteosarcoma, although the alkaline phosphatase may be elevated, and patients with serum lactic dehydrogenase elevations were shown in one study to have a less favorable prognosis.

The diagnosis is made by biopsy of the lesion. Histologic findings are variable and may contain areas of fibrosarcomatous and chondrosarcomatous change, but the presence of a highly pleomorphic stroma producing tumor osteoid or bone is diagnostic.

Complications: Metastases, primarily to the lung, occur within two years in patients receiving local treatment only. Other bones are the second most common site for metastatic disease, and other organs, such as the brain, heart, and liver, are involved as a late, terminal event. Locally, if untreated, the large soft tissue mass may fungate through the skin, and a pathologic fracture may develop in the involved bone.

Associated Findings: Adults with **Bone, Paget disease** have a 5–10% incidence of osteosarcoma. Osteosarcoma has been reported in association with other congenital diseases and bone dysplasias such as **Enchondromatosis, Enchondromatosis and hemangiomas, Exostoses, multiple cartilaginous,** and **Osteogenesis imperfecta.** Some patients with osteosarcoma have been found to have abnormal glucose metabolism.

Etiology: There is no established inheritance of classic osteosarcoma; however, autosomal recessive inheritance has been suggested in several families with multiple cases of osteosarcomas, and sets of sibs with osteosarcoma have been reported. Among patients with **Retinoblastoma,** the incidence of osteosarcoma is increased 500 times above the incidence in other groups.

Pathogenesis: An association with growth is presumed because the peak incidence is during the adolescent growth spurt, and the most frequent locations are in the skeletal areas of most rapid growth. Similarly, in dogs, osteosarcoma occurs predominantly in large breeds (Great Danes, Saint Bernards, and German shepherds). Ionizing radiation to bone and thorium derivative administration is associated with the subsequent development of osteosarcoma. Viruses have been shown to cause osteosarcoma in some experimental animal systems, but not in humans.

MIM No.: 25950

Sex Ratio: During preadolescent years, M1:F1; overall, M1.6:F1.

Occurrence: Among patients <20 years old in the United States: 3.36:1,000,000 whites; 2.88:1,000,000 Blacks. Higher incidence in United Kingdom due to Paget disease. There is an initial peak incidence of occurrence during the adolescent years, followed by a second peak later in life (fifth and sixth decades) due to osteosarcomas in **Bone, Paget disease** and radiation-associated sarcomas.

Risk of Recurrence for Patient's Sib:
See Part I, *Mendelian Inheritance.* At least 16 sets of sibs with osteosarcoma have been reported.

Risk of Recurrence for Patient's Child: Unknown.

Age of Detectability: Rare under age five years, but case reports of patients as young as age two years have been reported.

Gene Mapping and Linkage: OSRC (osteosarcoma) has been DISCONTINUED.

Prevention: None known. Genetic counseling indicated. Avoidance of irradiation and thorium derivatives is encouraged.

Treatment: Wide or radical resection of the primary tumor is necessary to achieve local control. Traditionally this has been accomplished by amputation, but recent efforts at limb-preserving resection and reconstruction seem to provide equivalent disase control and adequate function. Recent randomized studies confirm the benefit of multiagent chemotherapy in improving the disease-free survival in patients without detectable metastases at diagnosis.

Prognosis: With adequate surgical control of the primary and adjuvant chemotherapy, disease-free survival figures of 50–70% at five years and an overall survival of 70–80% have been reported from several cancer centers.

Detection of Carrier: Unknown.

Special Considerations: Osteosarcoma, although rare, has a considerable impact because of its highly malignant nature and occurrence during the adolescent years. Great strides have been made in treatment with adjuvant chemotherapy, but controversy exists regarding the timing of surgery and chemotherapy. Preliminary evidence suggests that preoperative administration ("neo-adjuvant chemotherapy") may be beneficial because it treats micrometastatic disease earlier, identifies "responders" (those who demonstrate nearly complete necrosis of the tumor after treatment), allows for the possibility of tailoring postoperative therapy for those who do not respond, and may make surgical resection easier and safer.

Other efforts are being directed toward identifying markers to predict prognosis and response to therapy, such as DNA aneuploidy and labeling index. Further informations regarding genetic markers (such as the deletion of the Rb locus) will add to the understanding of the disease and hopefully to improved treatment outcomes. Finally, much effort is being directed toward means of reconstruction following limb-sparing procedures and in evaluating the functional results of these procedures relative to amputation.

Support Groups: New York; American Cancer Society

References:
Colyer RA: Osteogenic sarcoma in siblings. Johns Hopkins Med J 1979; 145:131–135.
Bode U, Levine AS: The biology and management of osteosarcoma. In: Levine A, ed: Cancer in the young. New York: Masson, 1982:575–602.
Goorin AM, et al.: Osteosarcoma: fifteen years later. New Engl J Med 1985; 313:1637–1643.
Friend, SH, et al.: A human DNA segment with properties of the gene that predisposes to retinoblastoma and osteosarcoma. Nature 1986; 323:643–646.
Link MP et al.: The effect of adjuvant chemotherapy on relapse-free survival in patients with osteosarcoma of the extremity. New Engl J Med 1986; 314:1600–1606.
Dahlin DC: Osteosarcoma. In: Dahlin DC, ed: Bone tumors. Springfield, II: Charles C. Thomas, 1987:226–260.

Mark C. Gebhardt

Osteosarcoma, retinoblastoma-related
  See RETINOBLASTOMA
Osteosclerosis fragilis generalisata
  See OSTEOPETROSIS, BENIGN DOMINANT
Osteosclerosis, autosomal dominant
  See HYPEROSTOSIS, WORTH TYPE
Osteosclerosis-ichthyosis-fractures
  See SKELETAL BOWING-CORTICAL THICKENING-BONE FRAGILITY-ICTHYOSIS
Osteosclerosis-platyspondyly
  See DYSOSTEOSCLEROSIS
Osteosis eburnisans monomelica
  See MELORHEOSTOSIS
Ostertag type amyloidosis, familial
  See AMYLOIDOSIS, FAMILIAL VISCERAL
Ostium primum atrial septal defect, persistent ostium primum
  See HEART, ENDOCARDIAL CUSHION DEFECTS
'Ostrich-footed' tribe
  See ECTRODACTYLY
Oto-branchio-renal dysplasia
  See BRANCHIO-OTO-RENAL DYSPLASIA
Oto-branchio-ureteral syndrome
  See BRANCHIO-OTO-URETERAL SYNDROME

OTO-DENTAL DYSPLASIA   0784

Includes:
   Dental-oto dysplasia
   Globodontia-high frequency hearing loss
   Otodental syndrome

Excludes:
   Teeth, macrodontia (0617)
   Molarization of premolar teeth

Major Diagnostic Criteria: Large, globe-shaped molar teeth occur with sensorineural hearing loss.

Clinical Findings: Large, globe-shaped tooth crowns occur in both dentitions affecting the canine teeth and teeth posterior to the canines. Some affected persons have only the molar teeth involved. The incisor teeth are spared and are of normal size and shape. Over one-half have one or more congenitally missing premolars, or the premolars may be small. Age of onset of hearing loss varies from birth to third and fourth decade. The sensorineural hearing loss is high frequency and moderate to profound (50 db or greater hearing loss). Persons with only isolated hearing loss have transmitted the full syndrome. Data from one kindred show 30/37 had the full syndrome, 3/37 had globodontia only and 4/37 had only hearing loss. The last two had offspring affected with both defects. Local spots of yellow hypomature enamel have been noted in those with large teeth. Duplication of pulp chambers in molar teeth is seen on X-ray.

Complications: Malocclusion, full-face appearance, long philtrum, delayed eruption of teeth, and impacted teeth.

Associated Findings: Some families have shown thin enamel with large interrod spaces.

Etiology: Autosomal dominant inheritance. Patients within affected kindreds with isolated hearing loss have had offspring with the complete syndrome. High frequency hearing loss is common and can be due to a number of other genetic and environmental causes. Thus within kindreds, isolated hearing loss may indicate incomplete expression of the gene, but also may not indicate those bearing the gene.

Pathogenesis: Abnormal tooth form appears to be result of massive development of each tooth mamelon, or twinning-fusion of tooth germ.

MIM No.: *16675

Sex Ratio: M1:F1

Occurrence: At least eight kindreds with 62 affected members have been reported.

Risk of Recurrence for Patient's Sib:
  See Part I, *Mendelian Inheritance.*

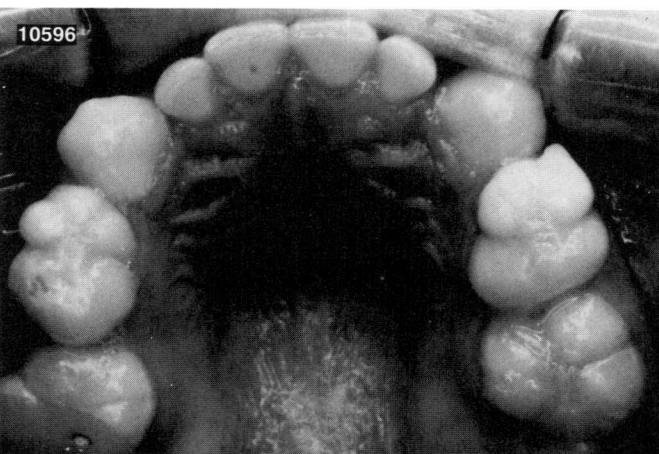
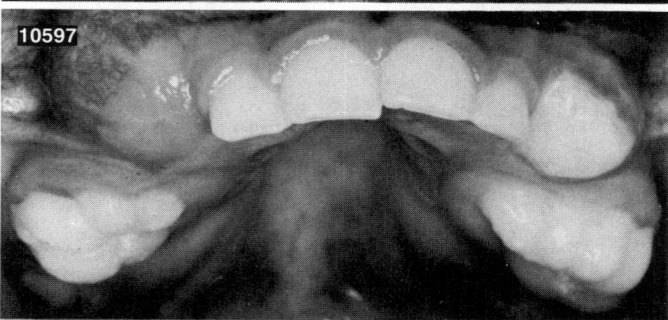

0784-10596–97: Abnormally large and globular-shaped molars.

Risk of Recurrence for Patient's Child:
  See Part I, *Mendelian Inheritance.*

Age of Detectability: At time of eruption of posterior primary teeth, 18 months-2 years of age.

Gene Mapping and Linkage: Unknown.

Prevention: None known. Genetic counseling indicated.

Treatment: Orthodontic treatment with selected tooth extraction. Hearing aids.

Prognosis: Does not appear to affect longevity. Hearing loss may be progressive, and eventually involve conversational frequencies.

Detection of Carrier: Examination of first degree relatives.

References:
Levin LS, et al.: Otodental dysplasia: a new ectodermal dysplasia. Clin Genet 1975; 8:136–144. *
Witkop CJ Jr, et al.: Globodontia in the otodental syndrome. Oral Surg 1976; 41:472–483. †
Cook RA, et al.: Otodental dysplasia: a five year study. Ear Head 1981; 2:90–94.

WI043   Carl J. Witkop, Jr.
LE028   L. Stefan Levin

Oto-facio-cervical syndrome
  See BRANCHIO-OTO-RENAL DYSPLASIA
Oto-limb-cardiac syndrome
  See LIMB-OTO-CARDIAC SYNDROME

OTO-OCULO-MUSCULO-SKELETAL SYNDROME 0785

Includes:
Cataract-deafness-musculo-skeletal defects
Deafness-cataract-muscular atrophy-skeletal defects
Musculo-skeletal-oto-oculo syndrome
Nathalie syndrome

Excludes: Deafness and cataract in other syndromes

Major Diagnostic Criteria: Early childhood deafness, cataract, muscular atrophy, EKG abnormalities.

Clinical Findings: This syndrome was reported in four of seven sibs (Cremers, 1975), one of which was named Nathalie. Early childhood (2–10 years) deafness was present in 4/4, cataract in 4/4, spinal muscular atrophy in 3/4, skeletal defects (osteochondrosis) in 3/4, retardation of growth in 3/4, EKG abnormalities in 4/4 and underdeveloped sexual characteristics in 2/4. The proposita suffered intermittently from regular and very frequent palpitations of the heart. The EKG showed ventricular extrasystoles, possibly multifocal in origin, or supraventricular extrasystoles with an aberrant intraventricular conduction. The proposita died during an attack of these palpitations.
Sensorineural hearing loss (slopes from a 25–60 dB loss at 250 Hz to a 100 dB loss at 4000 Hz - nonprogressive in 3/4 cases) was diagnosed at the age of 5 in 3/4 and by the age of 4 in 1/4. X-rays of the temporal bones in the proposita were normal. Vestibular function examined in 2/4 was normal.

Complications: Death secondary to extrasystoles.

Associated Findings: Enuresis, nocturia in some cases and some family members, albuminuria in one case.

Etiology: Presumably autosomal recessive inheritance.

Pathogenesis: Unknown.

MIM No.: 25599

POS No.: 3351

Sex Ratio: Presumably M1:F1 (M1:F3 observed)

Occurrence: Four affected sibs reported.

Risk of Recurrence for Patient's Sib:
See Part I, *Mendelian Inheritance.*

Risk of Recurrence for Patient's Child:
See Part I, *Mendelian Inheritance.*

Age of Detectability: In the first years of life.

Gene Mapping and Linkage: Unknown.

Prevention: None known. Genetic counseling indicated.

Treatment: Special education for deafness. Lens discission for cataract, and orthopedic treatment of skeletal defects. Medication for extrasystoles.

Prognosis: Possibly diminished life span due to cardiac rhythm disturbances.

Detection of Carrier: Unknown.

References:
Cremers CWRJ, et al.: The Nathalie syndrome: a new hereditary syndrome. Clin Genet 1975; 8:330–340.

MI029

Joyce Mitchell
Cor W.R.J. Cremers

OTO-ONYCHO-PERONEAL SYNDROME 2810

Includes:
Anonychia-fibular dysplasia
Fibula dysplasia-anonychia-abnormal ears

Excludes:
Craniosynostosis-fibular aplasia, lowry type (2184)
Fibula, congenital absence of (2229)
Nails, anonychia, hereditary (0066)
Pterygium syndrome, popliteal (0818)
Skeletal dysplasia, Fuhrmann type (2696)

Major Diagnostic Criteria: Dysplasia of the fibula associated with anonychia of several medial fingers and toes. Abnormally shaped ears with missing lobules are also possibly characteristic.

Clinical Findings: Craniofacial dysmorphy with dolichocephaly; flared temporal areas; depressed nose; epicanthal folds; strabismus; large, floppy, peculiarly shaped ears; and hypoplastic lobules. Nails are missing on the first and second fingers and toes, partially absent and replaced by a cutaneous fold on the third, and hypoplastic folds on the other digits. The fibulae are either hypoplastic or absent. There are contractures of the hips, knees, and ankle joints with pes calcaneovalgus position. Mental retardation is moderate. One child died unexpectedly after an attack of respiratory asphyxia. Similar episodes and rare general fits have been noted in the surviving child in whom optic atrophy has also been noted.

Complications: Episodic asphyxia.

Associated Findings: Difficulty walking, even with orthopedic aid.

Etiology: Autosomal recessive inheritance has been proposed on the basis of possibly remote consanguinity.

Pathogenesis: Unknown.

MIM No.: 25978

POS No.: 3582

Sex Ratio: Presumably M1:F1; M2:F0 observed.

Occurrence: The condition has been documented in two brothers.

Risk of Recurrence for Patient's Sib:
See Part I, *Mendelian Inheritance.*

Risk of Recurrence for Patient's Child:
See Part I, *Mendelian Inheritance.*

Age of Detectability: Prenatally by ultrasound of the fibulae, or at birth.

Gene Mapping and Linkage: Unknown.

Prevention: None known. Genetic counseling indicated.

Treatment: Orthopedic treatment as necessary, but has proven of limited benefit.

Prognosis: Probably poor because of attacks of asphyxia, motor handicap, and mental retardation.

Detection of Carrier: Unknown.

References:
Pfeiffer RA: The oto-onycho-peroneal syndrome: a probably new genetic entity. Eur J Pediatr 1982; 138:317–320.

PF001

Rudolf A. Pfeiffer

OTO-PALATO-DIGITAL SYNDROME, I 0786

Includes:
> Digito-oto-palatal syndrome
> Palato-oto-digital syndrome

Excludes:
> Cleft palate-flattened facies-multiple congenital dislocations
> **Larsen syndrome** (0570)
> **Oro-cranio-digital syndrome** (0769)
> **Oto-palato-digital syndrome, II** (2258)

Major Diagnostic Criteria: Cleft palate, downward slant of palpebral fissures, severe conductive hearing loss, and shortness of the terminal phalanges.

Clinical Findings: Cleft palate, downward slant of palpebral fissures, conductive hearing loss, short halluces, clinodactyly and variable syndactyly of other toes, flattened and short terminal phalanges, subluxation of head of radius, and broad nasal bridge giving pugilistic facial appearance.

X-ray findings include frontal and occipital bossing and thickening giving, the skull a mushroom-like appearance. The base of the skull is thick; the facial bones are hypoplastic, and the paranasal sinuses and mastoids are poorly pneumatized. The mandibular plane angle is increased, and the clivus or base sphenoid tends to be more vertical. There is lack of normal flare of ilia, mild coxa valga, secondary ossification centers of proximal second metacarpal, and second and third metatarsals, which fuse with the cuneiform bones, producing paddle-shaped structures. Intertarsal fusion is common.

Abnormalities of the ossicles and chronic serous otitis media are frequently noted.

Complications: Speech development is slow; this may be related to bilateral conductive hearing loss.

Associated Findings: Scoliosis.

Etiology: X-linked recessive inheritance, with variable expression in females.

Pathogenesis: Unknown.

MIM No.: *31130

POS No.: 3352

Sex Ratio: M1:F0

Occurrence: About 30 cases documented in the literature.

Risk of Recurrence for Patient's Sib:
> See Part I, *Mendelian Inheritance.*

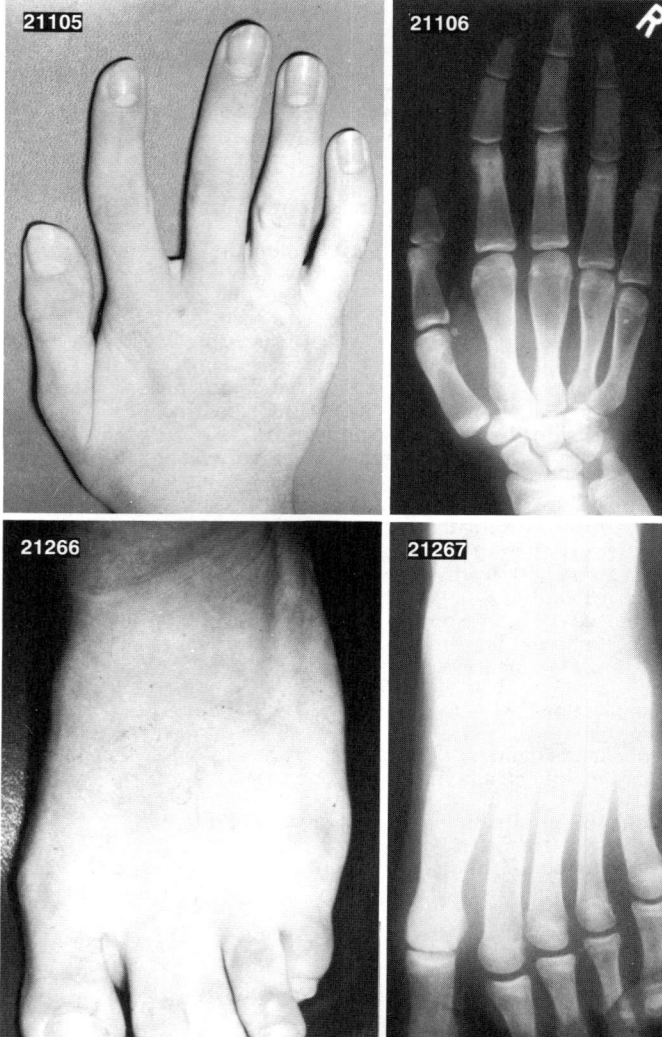

0786B-21105–06: Short distal phalanges and characteristic flask-shaped metacarpals in an affected female. 21266–67: Tree frog toes, shortened great toe and distal phalanges in the toes of an affected female.

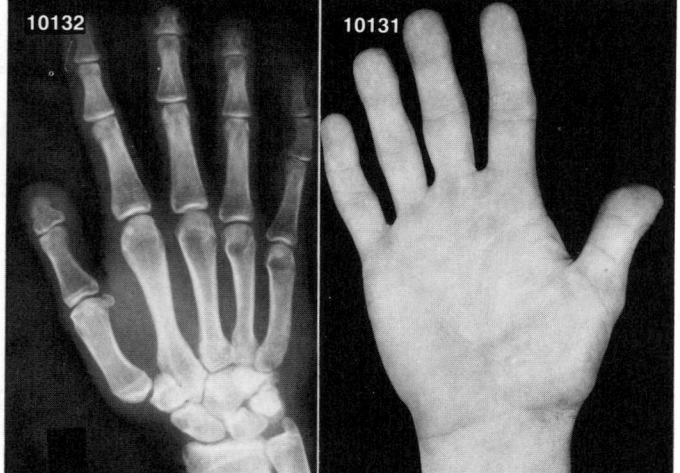

0786A-10132–31: Short distal phalanges of thumb and digits 3 and 4, and fusion of hamate and capitate bones.

Risk of Recurrence for Patient's Child:
> See Part I, *Mendelian Inheritance.*

Age of Detectability: At birth.

Gene Mapping and Linkage: OPD (otopalatodigital syndrome) has been provisionally mapped to X.

Prevention: None known. Genetic counseling indicated.

Treatment: Repair of cleft palate. Treatment of hearing loss has been limited, with variable improvement. No therapy is needed for the abnormalities of hands or feet.

Prognosis: Good, except for deafness.

Detection of Carrier: Facial features in the female heterozygote are variable. Most constant is overhanging brow with prominent supraorbital ridges, depressed nasal bridge, and flat midface.

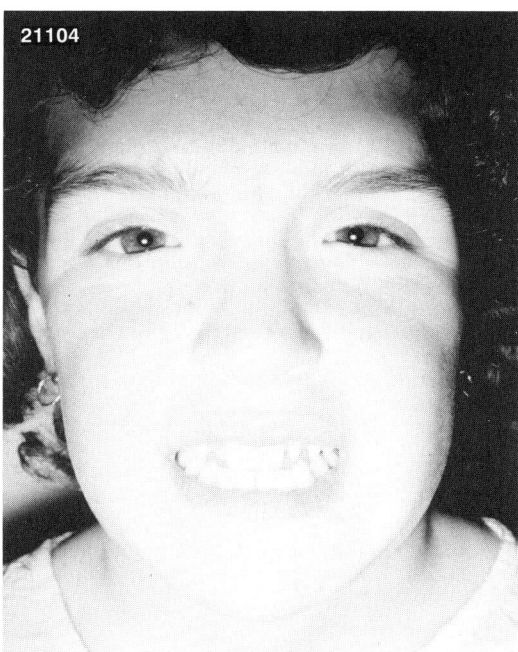

0786C-21104: Note hypertelorism and telecanthus, and down-slanting palpebral fissures in an affected female.

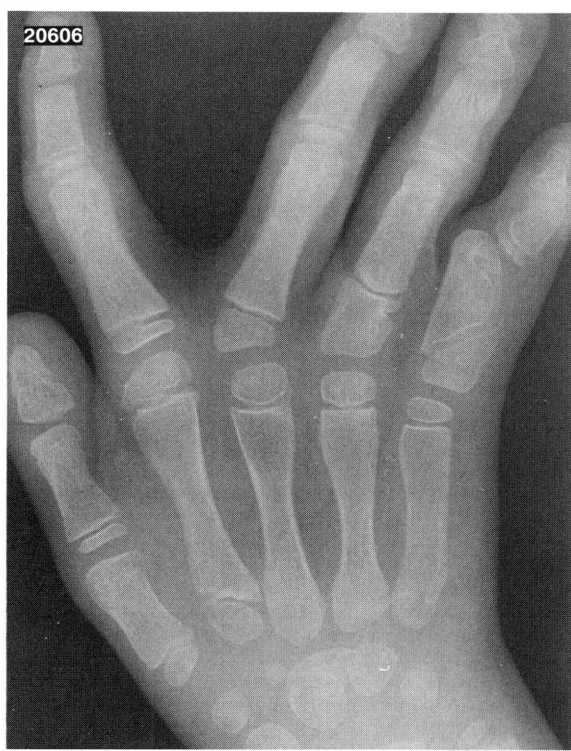

2258-20606: Oto-palato-digital syndrome, type II; note transverse capitate bone and extra bone in the capitate-hamate complex in this 5-year-old subject. The first metacarpal is short and there is digital deviation.

Other skeletal alterations are variable. Females have a higher frequency of greater multangular-navicular fusion.

References:

Dudding B, et al.: The otopalato-digital syndrome: a new symptom-complex consisting of deafness, dwarfism, cleft palate, characteristic facies, and a generalized bone dysplasia. Am J Dis Child 1967; 113:214–221.

Gall JC Jr, et al.: Oto-palato-digital syndrome. Comparison of clinical and radiographic manifestations in males and females. Am J Hum Genet 1972; 24:24–36.

Gorlin RJ, et al.: The oto-palato-digital syndrome in females: hetero-zygous expression of an X-linked trait. Oral Surg 1973; 35:218–224.

Poznanski AK, et al.: The hand in the oto-palato-digital syndrome. Ann Radiol 1973; 16:203–206.

Kozlowski K, et al.: Oto-palato-digital syndrome with severe x-ray changes in two half brothers. Pediatr Radiol 1977; 6:97–103.

Pazzaglia UE, Beluffi G: Oto-palato-digital syndrome in four generations of a large family. Clin Genet 1986; 30:338–344.

G0038   **Robert J. Gorlin**

OTO-PALATO-DIGITAL SYNDROME, II   **2258**

Includes:
    Andre syndrome
    Cranio-oro-digital syndrome
    Digital-oto-palato syndrome
    Facio-palato-osseous syndrome
    Palato-digital-oto syndrome

Excludes:
    Frontometaphyseal dysplasia (0394)
    Oto-palato-digital syndrome, I (0786)
    Cleft palate-dysmorphic facies-digital defects, Martsolf type
    (2579)

Major Diagnostic Criteria: Typical facies with broad forehead, hypertelorism, apparently low-set ears, downward obliquity of palpebral fissures, flattened nose bridge, microstomia, microg-

nathia and **Cleft palate**, fingers overlapping and flexed, short thumbs and short big toes, curved long bones in forearm and legs at birth, short first metacarpal, wide proximal phalanges 2–4 in the hand and clinodactyly of fingers 2 and 4, short or absent metatar-sal, proximal phalanx and distal phalanx in big toe. Other meta-tarsals and middle toe phalanges may be short or absent.

Clinical Findings: The newborn infant usually has a large ante-rior fontanelle, wide sutures, low-set ears, prominent forehead, antimongoloid slant, flattened bridge of nose, micrognathia, cleft palate, flexed overlapping fingers, and short thumbs and big toes.
X-ray findings include small facial bones, small mandible with obtuse angle, dense long bones at birth, and curved long bones in arms and legs. The fibula may be small or absent, elbow and sometimes the wrist dislocated or subluxated, and ribs may be short and wavy. The vertebral bodies and acetabula are flat. The first metacarpal is short; the proximal phalanges 2–4 in the hand are wide and there is clinodactyly of fingers 2 and 4. Foot abnormalities include short or absent metatarsal 1, short or absent metatarsals 2 and 5, and short or absent proximal phalanges 1 and 5. The distal phalanx of the big toe is short or absent.
The neonatal period is usually complicated by respiratory and feeding difficulties, and six of the nine known patients died in infancy. Those who survived had bilateral conductive hearing loss. One was severely mentally retarded, and one had normal intelligence; there is no information on the mental status of the third case. The capitate bone is transverse, and an extra bone in the capitate-hamate complex may be present. The osteosclerosis, with the exception of the skull, tends to disappear, as does the long bone curvature.

Complications: Unknown.

Associated Findings: None known.

Etiology: X-linked semidominant inheritance.

Pathogenesis: Undetermined. Chondro-osseous histopathology is normal.

MIM No.: 30412

POS No.: 3710

Sex Ratio: M9:F0 (observed).

Occurrence: Nine cases, all male, have been described.

Risk of Recurrence for Patient's Sib:
See Part I, *Mendelian Inheritance*.

Risk of Recurrence for Patient's Child:
See Part I, *Mendelian Inheritance*.

Age of Detectability: In the newborn period.

Gene Mapping and Linkage: OPD (otopalatodigital syndrome) has been provisionally mapped to X.

Prevention: None known. Genetic counseling indicated.

Treatment: Repair of cleft palate.

Prognosis: May be mentally retarded.

Detection of Carrier: The mothers of two of the patients described by André et al. (1981) had broad facies, midline frontal bossing, downward slant of palpebral fissures, flattened noses, hypertelorism, and low-set ears. Both had hyperostosis frontalis interna, hypoplastic mandibles, and a narrow pelvis. The mother of patient 3 had a normal face, but the same X-ray anomalies. In addition, she had had an operation for conductive deafness when it was noticed that the stapes was ankylosed and crudely formed, there was a knuckle in the descending branch of the incus, and the right stapedial arch was completely closed. The sister of patient 2 had the same dysmorphic face and a cleft palate. The mother of the boys described by Fitch et al. (1976) had a highly arched palate, bifid uvula, and clinodactyly fingers 3–5. Her mother had a cleft palate. The mother of the infant described by Kaplan and Maroteaux (1984) had polydactyly of the hands and feet, and the mother of the infants described by Brewster et al. (1985) had mild frontal bossing and downslanting palpebral fissures.

References:
Fitch N, et al.: A familial syndrome of cranial, facial, oral and limb anomalies. Clin Genet 1976; 10:226–231.
Kozlowski K, et al: Oto-palato-digital syndrome with severe X-ray changes in two half brothers. Pediatr Radiol 1977; 6:97–102. *
André M, et al.: Abnormal facies, cleft palate and generalized dysostosis: a lethal X-linked syndrome. J Pediatr 1981; 98:747–752. †
Fitch N, et al.: The oto-palato-digital syndrome, proposed type II. Am J Med Genet 1983; 15:655–664. *
Kaplan J, Maroteaux P: Syndrome oto-palato-digital de Type II. Ann Gent 1984; 27:79–82.
Brewster TG, et al.: Oto-palato-digital type II: an X-linked skeletal dysplasia. Am J Med Gent 1985; 20:249–254.

FI020   **Naomi Fitch**

Oto-spondylo-megaepiphyseal dysplasia
See CHONDRODYSTROPHY-SENSORINEURAL DEAFNESS, NANCE-INSLEY TYPE

OTO-SPONDYLO-MEGAEPIPHYSEAL DYSPLASIA   2304

Includes:
Chondrodystrophy-sensorineural deafness
Megaepiphyseal dwarfism
Nance-Insley syndrome

Excludes:
Arthro-ophthalmopathy, hereditary, progressive, Stickler type (0090)
Arthro-ophthalmopathy, Weissenbacher-Zweymuller variant (2424)
Deafness-myopia-cataract-saddle nose, Marshall type (0261)
Kniest dysplasia (0557)
Metatropic dysplasia (0656)
Oto-palato-digital syndrome, I (0786)
Oto-palato-digital syndrome, II (2258)

Major Diagnostic Criteria: Short-limbed skeletal dysplasia with large epiphyses, sensorineural hearing loss, and platyspondyly.

Clinical Findings: Most patients have shown prenatal onset of short-limbed disproportionate short stature, although some demonstrate the disproportion with overall height remaining in the normal range. The facies are distinctive, with severely depressed nasal bridge and an upturned "snubbed" nose, retrognathia, **Cleft palate**, and malar hypoplasia. Some patients have had epicanthal folds. Sensorineural hearing loss is accompanied in some patients by a conductive hearing loss due to recurrent otitis media. No severe visual defects have been seen. Mild **Camptodactyly** of the hands is present. Kyphosis and hyperlordosis are common. During the second decade there is onset of progressive contractures of the major joints. Intelligence has been normal in all except one patient who also had homocystinuria.

On X-ray, the long bones are short and broad with flaring of the metaphyses. The femora are described as "dumb-bell shaped" in some cases. The vertebrae show platyspondyly, coronal clefts in the lumbar vertebrae, and molding deformities. Large epiphyses at the knees, ankles, elbows, and first interphalangeal joints are the hallmark of the disease. Progressive fusion of the carpal bones has been noted.

Complications: Progressive joint limitation and pain are seen in the second decade. Some patients have had osteophytic changes in the spine or deformities of the femoral heads.

Associated Findings: None known.

Etiology: Autosomal recessive inheritance.

Pathogenesis: Unknown.

MIM No.: *21515

POS No.: 3630

Sex Ratio: M1:F1

Occurrence: Two or three kindreds have been reported.

Risk of Recurrence for Patient's Sib:
See Part I, *Mendelian Inheritance*.

Risk of Recurrence for Patient's Child:
See Part I, *Mendelian Inheritance*.

Age of Detectability: At birth.

Gene Mapping and Linkage: Unknown.

Prevention: None known. Genetic counseling indicated.

Treatment: Orthopedic surgery as indicated.

Prognosis: Normal life span.

Detection of Carrier: Unknown.

Special Considerations: The patients described appear to have the same clinical entity. Without a defined etiology, however, genetic heterogeneity cannot be excluded.

Support Groups:
MA; Quincy; Prescription Parents, Inc.
CANADA: Ontario; Toronto; Canadian Cleft Lip and Palate Family Association

References:
Nance WE, Sweeney A: A recessively inherited chondrodystrophy. BD:OAS VI(4). New York: March of Dimes Birth Defects Foundation, 1970:25–27.
Gorlin RJ, et al.: Megaepiphyseal dwarfism. J Pediatr 1973; 83:633–635.
Insley J, Astley R: A bone dysplasia with deafness. Br J Radiol 1974; 47:244–251.
Giedion A, et al.: Oto-spondylo-megaepiphyseal dysplasia (OSMED). Helv Paediatr Acta 1982; 37:361–380.
Miny P, Lenz W: Autosomal recessive deafness with skeletal dysplasia and facial appearance of Marshall syndrome. Am J Med Genet 1985; 21:317–324.
Salinas C, et al.: Bone dysplasia, deafness and cleft palate syndrome. (Abstract) 7th Int Cong Hum Genet, Berlin, 1986; 1:259 only.

H0025   **O.J. Hood**
H0033   **William A. Horton**

Otocephaly
See AGNATHIA-MICROSTOMIA-SYNOTIA
Otodental syndrome
See OTO-DENTAL DYSPLASIA

OTOSCLEROSIS 0787

Includes:
Labyrinthine otosclerosis
Labyrinthine otosclerosis-fixed stapes footplate

Excludes:
Hearing loss, postinflammatory conductive
Ossicular fixation, congenital
Osteogenesis imperfecta (0777)
Stapes fixation due to Paget osteitis deformans
Tympanosclerosis

Major Diagnostic Criteria: Progressive conductive or mixed hearing loss in a young or middle-aged adult without evidence of other middle ear disease. Clinical onset prior to age six years has rarely been reported.

Clinical Findings: With otosclerosis there is a slowly progressive conductive or mixed hearing loss of insidious onset unrelated to inflammatory middle ear findings. Approximately 75% of cases are bilateral. The patient may describe a history of hearing better in noisy situations ("paracusis Willisiani"). Tinnitus is a frequent complaint and is usually a low-frequency type sometimes accompanied by an audible pulse. Vertigo is found in about 5–8% of patients with otosclerosis.

The tympanic membranes are normal at inspection, and their mobility is unaltered. There may be a pink flush seen through the eardrum caused by increased vascularity of the mucosa over the otosclerotic focus on the promontory of the middle ear ("Schwartze sign"). This sign is believed to be correlated with increased vascularity in the mucosa of the promontory overlying the focus, and is believed to signify an "active" focus. An "inactive" focus is thought to be a healed area of otosclerosis and grossly appears whiter than the surrounding normal area. Audiometry reveals a conductive hearing loss of varying severity, which is initially more marked in the lower frequencies, but as the lesion progresses with increased stapes fixation, all frequencies are affected. Middle ear impedance is increased as measured by an acoustic bridge. Labyrinthine or cochlear otosclerosis results in a sensorineural hearing loss. This may or may not be accompanied by a conductive component. The pathology is not clear but seems to be related to destruction of the endosteal membrane of the cochlea adjacent to the spiral ligament. X-ray examination by high-resolution computerized tomography is generally not necessary clinically, but may be helpful in distinguishing otosclerotic stapes fixation from other acquired ossicular fixation or in identifying otosclerotic invasion of the cochlea in a patient with an associated sensorineural loss.

At surgery the stapes footplate is found to be partially or completely fixed to the otic capsule by an otosclerotic focus. This most commonly occurs at the anterior footplate, but it can be at any other location; it may be circumscribed, or the lesion may obliterate the oval window niche.

Complications: Labyrinthine or cochlear otosclerosis has been suspected to be a cause of severe sensorineural hearing loss. There has been evidence that sensorineural hearing losses are not increased in otosclerosis compared to the normal population, but there is a small percentage of these patients who show a severe progressive sensorineural hearing loss long before presbycusis could be assumed to be an explanation.

Associated Findings: Vestibular disturbances are more common in patients with otosclerosis than in the general population. There is a statistically significant correlation with the ability to taste phenylthiocarbamide, but the significance of this is unknown.

Etiology: Autosomal dominant inheritance with incomplete penetrance, estimated at between 25 to 40%, depending on the series studied.

Pathogenesis: Otosclerosis is a focal, progressive replacement of the endochondral bone of the otic capsule with abnormal bone, which has the microscopic appearance of healing fibrous bone, but which is normally calcified. The site of predilection is the otic capsule anterior to the stapes footplate, and the process progresses to involve the stapes footplate and fix it to the surrounding bone. The pathogenesis of the sensorineural hearing loss is not yet completely understood.

MIM No.: *16680

Sex Ratio: M1:F1

Occurrence: Clinical otosclerosis is 1:330 in the White population, about 1:3,300 in the Black population, and estimated to be 1:33,000 in the Oriental. Series of temporal bone specimens which show histologic otosclerosis, not necessarily with hearing loss, have shown the histologic changes to be present in 1:14 to 1:10 of white subjects studied in the United States, and approximately 1:100 in Blacks.

Risk of Recurrence for Patient's Sib:
See Part I, *Mendelian Inheritance*. If only one parent is affected, 1:5 to 1:8 depending on expressivity.

Risk of Recurrence for Patient's Child:
See Part I, *Mendelian Inheritance*. If mate is not affected, 1:5 to 1:8.

Age of Detectability: A conductive hearing loss is first seen at age 11–15 years in 10% of cases, progressing to 50% at age 21–25 years, and reaching 100% at age 40 years. Earlier detectability could possibly be achieved with temporal bone tomograms in the absence of clinical findings, but the significance of this in terms of morbidity is unclear.

Gene Mapping and Linkage: Unknown.

Prevention: None known. Genetic counseling indicated.

Treatment: Stapedectomy to restore hearing in those with a conductive loss secondary to otosclerosis has been highly developed and is generally very successful. The most common procedure is removal of the fixed stapes from the oval window and replacement with a wire or Teflon prosthesis. The oval window is cleaned of otosclerotic bone and covered with Gelfoam^, fat, or vein and the prosthesis is placed between the incus and this new membrane. Improvement in hearing occurs in approximately 90+%, with an incidence of surgical complications of about 3%. Sodium fluoride has been used orally to treat cochlear otosclerosis, but the treatment is controversial.

Prognosis: Normal for life span and intelligence.

Detection of Carrier: Unknown.

References:
Kelemen G, Linthicum FH Jr: Labyrinthine otosclerosis. Acta Otolaryngol [suppl] (Stockh) 1969; 253:1–12.
Morrison AW, Bundey SE: The inheritance of otosclerosis. J Laryngol Otol 1970; 84:921–932.
Johnsson LG, et al.: Cochlear and vestibular lesions in capsular otosclerosis as seen in microdissection. Ann Otol Rhinol Laryngol (Suppl) 1978; 87:48:1–40.
Schaap T, Gapany-Gapanavicius B: The genetics of otosclerosis. I. Distorted sex ratio. Am J Hum Genet 1978; 30:59–64. *
Schuknecht HF, Jones DD: Stapedectomy postmortem findings. Ann Otol Rhinol Laryngol (Suppl 88) 1979; 55:1–43.
Vollrath M, Schreiner C: Influence of argon laser stapedectomy on cochlear potentials. Acta Oto Laryngologica (suppl) 1982; 385:1–31.

BE028   **LaVonne Bergstrom**

Oudtshoorn skin
See SKIN, ERYTHROKERATOLYSIS HIEMALIS
Ovalocytoses, Malaysian-Melanesian type
See ELLIPTOCYTOSIS
Ovalocytosis, hereditary
See ELLIPTOCYTOSIS
Ovarian dysgenesis, familial
See GONADAL DYSGENESIS, XX TYPE
Ovarian dysgenesis-sensorineural deafness
See PERRAULT SYNDROME
Overgrowth disorder, hemihypertrophy
See HEMIHYPERTROPHY

OVERGROWTH, BANNAYAN TYPE　　　2381

Includes:

Bannayan-Zonana syndrome
Lipomatosis-angiomatosis-macrencephalia
Macrocephaly-diffuse hamartomas
Macrocephaly-multiple lipomas-hemangiomata
Protean gigantism, Bannayan type
Zonana syndrome

Excludes:

Angio-osteohypertrophy syndrome (0055)
Chromosome abnormalities
Cutis marmorata (2296)
Disseminated hemangiomatosis
Neurofibromatosis (0712)
Overgrowth, macrocephaly-hemangioma, Riley-Smith type
(2192)
Overgrowth, Ruvalcaba-Myhre-Smith type (2120)
Proteus syndrome (2382)

Major Diagnostic Criteria: The diagnosis is based on **Megalencephaly** with normal ventricles and mesodermal multiple hamartomas. Motor, speech, and coordination delays are common and transient. Intelligence is usually within the average range. Computerized tomographic (CT) head scan is necessary to confirm the normal size of the ventricles. Familial occurrence is also of help to the diagnosis.

Clinical Findings: The **Megalencephaly** is present at birth, with head circumference at least 2 SD above the mean. Hamartomas may be apparent at that time; these usually manifest in infancy or early childhood. The majority of the tumors are subcutaneous lipomas. Some may show elements of lymphangioma and/or hemangioma. Spontaneous regression of these tumors may occur. Congenital macrosomia may be present. Periods of decelerated growth and occasional transient failure to thrive have been reported. Ultimate height is within normal range. Other nonspecific signs delineate further the phenotype.

In the fewer than 20 reported patients, the approximate frequency of the clinical features is: **Megalencephaly** (18/18), accelerated fetal growth (5/9), decelerated postnatal growth (10/10), lipomas (14/18), hemangiomas (8/18), lymphangioma (2/18), other tumors (3/18), motor delay (9/12), speech delay (10/18), adult motor dysfunction (4/5), mental retardation (3/18), seizures (3/18), strabismus/amblyopia (3/18), obliquity of palpebral fissures (7/13), high palate (6/10), joint hyperextensibility (5/10), **Pectus excavatum** (2/10), hypotonia (2/10) and drooling (4/10). Clinical variability appears to exist. First degree relatives should have genetic evaluation to detect minimally affected individuals.

Complications: Localization, size, and structure of the hamartomas may lead to space occupying symptomatology particularly within the central nervous system. Manifestations of the infrequent arteriovenous malformations may also complicate the clinical picture.

Associated Findings: Follicular cell carcinoma of the thyroid was found in one patient; it is not clear whether or not the carcinoma was causally related to the syndrome. Meningoepithelial meningioma has also been reported in one patient and angioleiomyoma in another. One patient with *de novo* translocation, t(Y;19), had a similar phenotype to that of Bannayan syndrome.

Etiology: Autosomal dominant inheritance with variable expressivity.

Pathogenesis: One of the mesodermal phakomatoses. The pathogenesis probably represents a genetically determined interference with the differentiation, migration, and interaction of the mesodermal cells within the affected organs. Dysregulated paracrine growth factor may play a critical role in pathogenesis.

MIM No.: *15348

POS No.: 3556

Sex Ratio: M4:F1

Occurrence: Reported in about 15 kinships, including an American Black family. As with most other hamartoses, the syndrome is most likely underdiagnosed.

Risk of Recurrence for Patient's Sib:
See Part I, *Mendelian Inheritance.*

Risk of Recurrence for Patient's Child:
See Part I, *Mendelian Inheritance.*

Age of Detectability: **Megalencephaly** is present at birth. Prenatal diagnosis is theoretically possible. The hamartomas become apparent in infancy or later.

Gene Mapping and Linkage: Unknown.

Prevention: None known. Genetic counseling indicated.

Treatment: The usually noninvasive hamartomas are amenable to surgery.

Prognosis: Normal life span is presumed.

Detection of Carrier: Detailed diagnostic evaluation of the first degree relatives may detect minimally affected individuals.

Special Considerations: Bannayan syndrome appears to be the same as Zonana syndrome. However, other proposals to unify various overgrowth syndromes into a single entity are considered premature at this time.

References:
Bannayan GA: Lipomatosis, angiomatosis and macrencephalia. Arch Pathol 1971; 92:1–5.
Zonana J, et al.: Macrocephaly with multiple lipomas and hemangiomas. J Pediatr 1976; 89:600–603.
Higginbottom MC, Schultz C: The Bannayan syndrome: an autosomal dominant disorder consisting of macrocephaly, lipomas, hemangiomas, and risk of intracranial tumors. Pediatrics 1982; 69:632–634.
Miles JH, et al.: Macrocephaly with hamartomas: Bannayan-Zonana syndrome. Am J Med Genet 1984; 19:225–234.
Israel JN: 19/Y translocation in a patient with features of Zonana syndrome. Am J Hum Genet 1985; 37:A60.
Saul RA, Stevenson RE: Bannayan syndrome and Ruvalcaba-Myhre-Smith syndrome discrete entities? Proc Greenwood Genet Center 1986; 5:3–7.
Kousseff BG, Madan S: The phakomatoses - an hypothesis: paracrine growth regulation disorders? Dysmorph Clin Genet 1988; 2:76–90.

K0018　　　　　　　　　　　　　　**Boris G. Kousseff**

Overgrowth, encephalo-cranio-cutaneous lipomatosis type
See PROTEUS SYNDROME
Overgrowth, Golabi-Rosen type
See SIMPSON-GOLABI-BEHMEL SYNDROME

OVERGROWTH, MACROCEPHALY-HEMANGIOMA, RILEY-SMITH TYPE　　　2192

Includes:

Bannayan-Riley-Ruvalcaba syndrome
Macrocephaly-hemangioma
Macrocephaly-pseudopapilledema-multiple hemangiomata
Multiple hemangiomata-macrocephaly-pseudopapilledema
Pseudopapilledema-macrocephaly-multiple hemangiomata
Riley-Smith syndrome

Excludes:

Enchondromatosis and hemangiomas (0346)
Hemangioma-thrombocytopenia syndrome (0456)
Macrocephaly, benign familial
Overgrowth, Bannayan type (2381)
Sturge-Weber syndrome (0915)
Von Hippel-Lindau syndrome (0995)

Major Diagnostic Criteria: The combination of **Microcephaly**, pseudopapilledema, and multiple hemangiomata are strongly suggestive of the diagnosis. If the family history is positive, then one of the above features is sufficient to make the diagnosis.

Clinical Findings: In the five reported and two subsequently identified affected individuals, the following clinical features were observed: congenital macrocephaly (7); pseudopapilledema (6);

cutaneous and/or subcutaneous hemangiomata (4); and frequent respiratory infections (4).

The only significant X-ray finding has been increased thickness of the cranial bones. Chest X-rays have revealed minimal pulmonary fibrosis in three affected individuals. Histologic studies of nodules have been characteristic for hemangiomata. Ophthalmologic findings have been consistent with pseudopapilledema (blurred disk margins). Metabolic and hematologic studies, pneumoencephalograms, electroencephalograms, and electrocardiograms have all been normal.

Complications: Posttraumatic bleeding of the hemangiomata and bronchopneumonia have been reported.

Associated Findings: One affected individual also had a **Tracheoesophageal fistula.**

Etiology: The presence of the syndrome in four generations of a single family is strongly suggestive of autosomal dominant inheritance.

Pathogenesis: Unknown.

MIM No.: 15350

Sex Ratio: M3:F4 (in the seven known cases).

Occurrence: A mother and sibs in one family have been reported.

Risk of Recurrence for Patient's Sib:
See Part I, *Mendelian Inheritance.*

Risk of Recurrence for Patient's Child:
See Part I, *Mendelian Inheritance.*

Age of Detectability: Macrocephaly is present at birth, whereas the hemangiomata were congenital in two cases and appeared after the age of three years in two cases.

Gene Mapping and Linkage: Unknown.

Prevention: None known. Genetic counseling indicated.

Treatment: Unknown.

Prognosis: Vision and intellect are unimpaired. Life span appears to be normal.

Detection of Carrier: A large head size may be the only obvious finding. A funduscopic exam is necessary to detect pseudopapilledema.

Special Considerations: Although Cohen suggested that this condition is the same as the **Overgrowth, Bannayan type** and **Overgrowth, Ruvalcaba-Myhre-Smith type** syndromes, based on a paper published by Dvir et al in 1988, Di Liberti suggested that, in a companion letter, that appropriate research needs to be done before these conditions be "lumped" into a *Bannayan-Riley-Ruvalcaba syndrome.* It is possible that the condition Dvir et al is describing, which included macrocephaly, hamartomas, pseudopapilledema and macropenia as phenotypic features, could be a distinct, albeit pathogenetically related, syndrome.

References:
Riley HD, et al.: Macrocephaly, pseudopapilledema and multiple hemangiomata. Pediatrics 1960; 26:293–300.
Dvir M, et al.: Heredofamilial syndrome of mesodermal hamartomas, macrocephaly, and pseudopapilledema. Pediatrics 1988; 81:287–290.
Cohen MM Jr.: Bannayan-Riley-Ruvalcaba syndrome: renaming three formerly recognized syndromes as one etiologic entity. (Letter) Am J Med Genet 1990; 35:291.
Di Liberti JH: Comments on Dr. Cohen's letter. (Letter) Am J Med Genet 1990; 35:292.

T0007
RI018

Helga V. Toriello
Harris D. Riley

Overgrowth, Proteus type
See PROTEUS SYNDROME

OVERGROWTH, RUVALCABA-MYHRE-SMITH TYPE   2120

Includes:
   Genitalia, pigmentary changes-megalencephaly-intestinal polyposis
   Intestinal polyposis-pigmentary changes of genitalia-megalencephaly
   Megalencephaly-intestinal polyposis-pigmentary changes of genitalia
   Myopathy, lipid storage (one form)
   Ruvalcaba-Myhre-Smith syndrome

Excludes:
   Overgrowth, Bannayan type (2381)
   Cebebral gigantism (0137)
   Overgrowth, macrocephaly-hemangioma, Riley-Smith type (2192)

Major Diagnostic Criteria: Clinical findings include megalencephaly, hypotonia or developmental delay, normal stature, pigmented macules on the penis, prominent Schwalbe's lines and corneal nerves, hamartomatous intestinal polyps, lipid storage myopathy, and lipomas or angiolipomas.

Clinical Findings: **Megalencephaly** is often present at birth, and the head circumference remains large (≥97th percentile) throughout life. The CT scan is always normal except for the increased head size. Hypotonia (90%) is a common problem in childhood but appears to improve with age. Signs of proximal muscle weakness may be present in the pre-school child. Mental retardation is found in some affected patients but normal intellect has been observed in several. Pigmented macules on the glans and shaft of the penis (80%) are first noted between infancy and adulthood. Similar lesions may be found on other parts of the body. Hamartomatous intestinal polyps (<20%) may produce intestinal bleeding or intussusception and have been found in early childhood through adulthood. Prominent Schwalbe's lines and corneal nerves (50%) do not appear to cause clinical problems.

An unusual lipid storage myopathy is often present (≥50% in children), even in asymptomatic patients. The EMG may be abnormal without clinical signs of myopathy, and no signs of deterioration have been observed. Serum CPK activity is normal. In spite of a high mean birth weight (4,120 g), growth rates are normal and adult stature is average.

Complications: Anemia, intestinal bleeding, and intussusception occur secondary to hamartomatous polyps.

Associated Findings: Acanthosis nigricans, mucoepidermoid carcinoma of the parotid, lipoma, **Pectus excavatum**, accessory nipples, diabetes mellitus, epilepsy.

Etiology: Possibly autosomal dominant inheritance.

Pathogenesis: Unknown.

MIM No.: 18089

POS No.: 3526

Sex Ratio: Presumably M1:F1, although a disproportionate number of males have been observed.

Occurrence: A dozen or so cases have been reported in the literature.

Risk of Recurrence for Patient's Sib:
See Part I, *Mendelian Inheritance.*

Risk of Recurrence for Patient's Child:
See Part I, *Mendelian Inheritance.*

Age of Detectability: At birth.

Gene Mapping and Linkage: Unknown.

Prevention: None known. Genetic counseling indicated.

Treatment: Unknown.

Prognosis: Variable. One patient was severely retarded, but intellectual performance in others has varied through the normal range, at least in childhood. Most known patients have done well in follow-up, although the lipomas may grow quite large and cause cosmetic problems. The myopathy does not appear to be progressive and has not caused problems beyond mid-childhood.

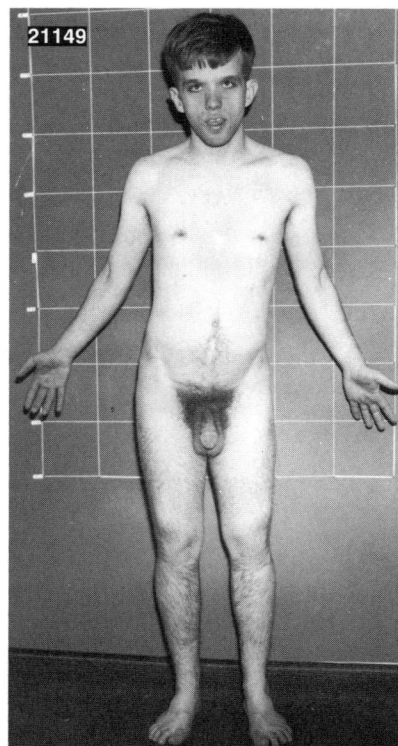

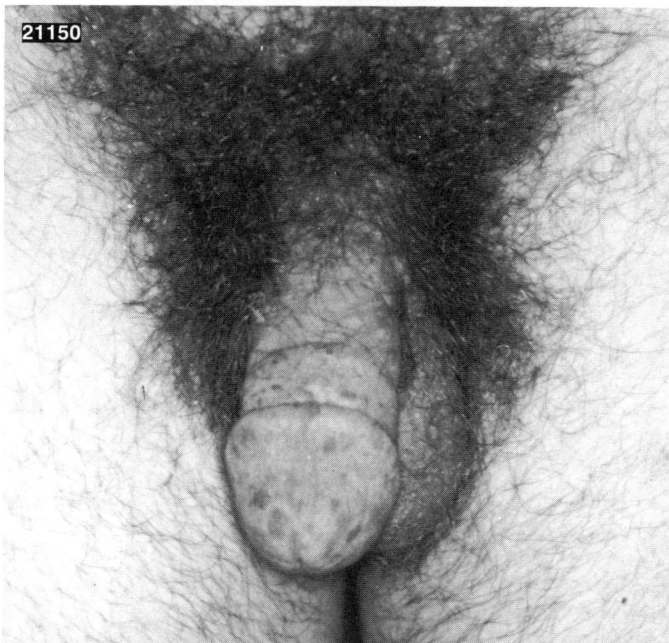

2120-21149: Macrocephaly, supernumerary nipple, and scar from early colectomy. 21150: Tan macular lesions on the glans and shaft of the penis.

One adult patient continues to have difficulties caused by intestinal polyps. Life span appears to be normal.

Detection of Carrier: Megalencephaly or prominent Schwalbe's lines may be the only manifestations in some individuals.

Special Considerations: This disorder has similarities to **Overgrowth, Bannayan type** and other reported conditions which feature macrocephaly and hamartoma. Available data do not permit differentiation between a single allele-variable expression model or multiple genotypes (see **Overgrowth, macrocephaly-hemangioma, Riley-Smith type**).

References:

Ruvalcaba RHA, et al.: Sotos syndrome with intestinal polyposis and pigmentary changes of the genitalia. Clin Genet 1980; 18:413–416. * †
Di Liberti JH, et al.: The Ruvalcaba-Myhre-Smith syndrome: a case with probable dominant inheritance and additional manifestations. Am J Med Genet 1983; 15:491–496. * †
Di Liberti JH, et al.: A new lipid storage myopathy in the the Ruvalcaba-Myhre-Smith syndrome. Am J Med Genet 1984; 18:163–167. †
Gretzula JC, et al.: Ruvalcaba-Myhre-Smith syndrome. Pediatr Dermatol 1988; 5:28–32. †
Halal F, Silver K: Slowly progressive macrocephaly with hamartomas: a new syndrome? Am J Med Genet 1989; 33:182–185. †

DI001   **John H. Di Liberti**

Overgrowth-congenital edema-positional defects of the feet
See NEVO SYNDROME
Overgrowth-mental retardation syndrome, X-linked
See SIMPSON-GOLABI-BEHMEL SYNDROME

OVERGROWTH-RENAL HAMARTOMA, PERLMAN TYPE   2241

Includes:
     Fetal ascites-macrosomia-Wilms tumor
     Hamartoma and nephroblastomatosis
     Perlman syndrome
     Renal hamartoma syndrome
     Renal hamartomas-nephroblastomatosis-fetal gigantism

Excludes:
     Beckwith-Wiedemann syndrome (0104)
     Hemihypertrophy (0458)

Major Diagnostic Criteria: Macrosomia at birth; unusual facial appearance; distended abdomen; hypoglycemia.

Clinical Findings: Macrosomia at birth; unusual facial appearance characterized by upsweep of anterior hairline, apparent enophthalmos, hypoplastic bridge of nose, inverted "V" shape of the upper lip, micrognathia; prominent, bifid xiphisternum; distended abdomen; cryptorchidism in males; and hypoglycemia.

Complications: **Cancer, Wilms tumor**; hypoglycemic coma; developmental delay.

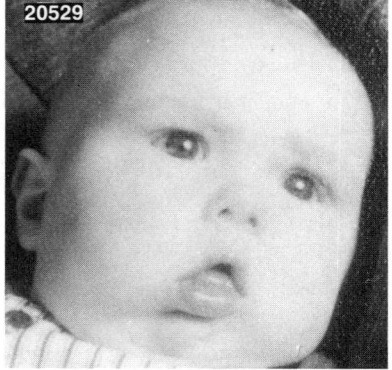 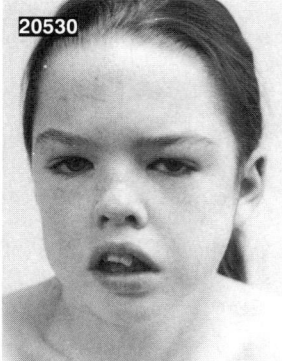

2241-20529–30: Perlman syndrome; note these 2 affected sibs at ages 6 months and 12 years respectively. The inverted "v" shaped upper lip is characteristic.

Associated Findings: Polyhydramnios; fetal ascites.

Etiology: Autosomal recessive inheritance.

Pathogenesis: It has been suggested that a defect in a gene regulating cell proliferation during embryonic and fetal life causes macrosomia with minor anomalies, hyperplasia of the endocrine pancreas and renal dysplasia with nephroblastomatosis. Macrosomia regresses during postnatal life, with ensuing developmental delay and so probably does the pancreatic hyperplasia, although hypoglycemia can be a persistent complication and hypoglycemic coma a possible cause of death. The kidney dysplasia, on the other hand, has a strong tendency to develop into a Wilms tumor.

MIM No.: *26700

POS No.: 3648

Sex Ratio: M1:F1

Occurrence: Ten patients, of both sexes, have been described from three families, one of Jewish Yemenite origin (six affected sibs) and another Caucasian (two affected sibs). Origin of the third family (two patients) was not stated. Parents were healthy, and consanguineous in the Jewish family.

Risk of Recurrence for Patient's Sib:
See Part I, *Mendelian Inheritance.*

Risk of Recurrence for Patient's Child:
See Part I, *Mendelian Inheritance.* There are no reports of an affected individual having reproduced.

Age of Detectability: At birth. Prenatal diagnosis may be possible.

Gene Mapping and Linkage: Dao et al (1987) studied chromosome 11 p markers in a bilateral Wilms tumor from a patient with this condition and found the same loss of 11p DNA sequences found in non-syndromal cases of **Cancer, Wilms tumor.** Genetic differences between the two tumors indicated that they developed independently, and were the results of different genetic events.

Prevention: None known. Genetic counseling indicated.

Treatment: Surgical excision of Wilms tumor, followed by chemo- and radiotherapy as indicated.

Prognosis: Most affected individuals so far described died in the neonatal period. At least one survivor was reported at age 14 years, with some psychomotor retardation. Early diagnosis may lead to effective treatment of the kidney dysplasia through appropriate chemotherapy, and of the developmental delay through adequate correction of the hypoglycemia.

Detection of Carrier: Unknown.

References:
Liban E, Kozenitsky I: Metanephric hamartomas and nephroblastomatosis in siblings. Cancer 1970; 25:885–888.
Perlman M, et al.: Renal hamartomas and nephroblastomatosis with fetal gigantism: a familial syndrome. J Pediatr 1973; 83:414–418.
Perlman M, et al.: Syndrome of fetal gigantism, renal hamartomas, and nephroblastomatosis with Wilms tumor. Cancer 1975; 35:1212–1217.
Neri G, et al.: The Perlman syndrome: familial renal dysplasia with Wilms tumor, fetal gigantism and multiple congenital anomalies. Am J Med Genet 1984; 19:195–207. †
Greenberg F, et al.: The Perlman familial nephroblastomatosis syndrome. Am J Med Genet 1986; 24:101–110. †
Perlman M: Perlman syndrome: familial renal dysplasia with Wilms tumor, fetal gigantism, and multiple congenital anomalies. Am J Med Genet 1986; 25:793–795. †
Dao DD, et al.: Genetic mechanisms of tumor-specific loss in 11p DNA sequences in Wilms tumor. Am J Hum Genet 1987; 41:202–217.
Greenberg F, et al.: Expanding the spectrum of the Perlman syndrome. Am J Med Genet 1988; 29:773–776.

NE019   **Giovanni Neri**

Oviducts in males, persistence of
See MULLERIAN DERIVATIVES IN MALES, PERSISTENT

OVULATION INDUCTION TRISOMY — 2993

Includes:
 Chlomaphen, ovulation induction trisomy
 Chromosome, ovulation induction trisomy
 Clomid△, ovulation induction trisomy
 Clomiphene ovulation induction trisomy
 Menotropin, ovulation induction trisomy
 Trisomy, ovulation induction

Excludes:
 Chromosome (other)
 Fetal effects (other)

Major Diagnostic Criteria: Trisomy with ovulation induction.

Clinical Findings: Oakley and Flynt (1972) reported six **Chromosome 21, trisomy 21** cases among 2,239 infants in the new drug investigations for ovulation-inducing agents (five following clomiphene, one following menotropin administration). This was 2.5 times the expected number. A further suggestion of association between trisomy and ovulation induction was found in the data of Boue et al (1975) on karyotyped spontaneous abortions. The ratio of trisomies to normal karyotypes was 3.5 times as high in spontaneous abortions following ovulation-inducing agent administration as in controls.

A total of 30 trisomy births following clomiphene ovulation induction are known to the Food and Drug Administration (FDA). Twenty of the cases were **Chromosome 21, trisomy 21**; two were **Chromosome 18, trisomy 18** (or trisomy 17); four were **Chromosome 13, trisomy 13** (or trisomy 14 or 15); two were **Chromosome 8, trisomy 8**; and two were unspecified trisomies. Five cases occurred among 2,082 investigational patients (included in Oakley and Flynt's data). Ten cases occurred among 3,815 exposed pregnancies in other cohorts in the scientific literature. Both the numerator and the denominator in the latter data may be undercounted: the numerator because some cases were not followed-up long enough to identify trisomy cases and the exposure denominator because some of the numerous small cohorts not having abnormalities were unpublished. Although maternal age is not given in some of these reports, available information indicates that the age of ovulation induction is not sufficiently elevated to be a substantial confounding factor. Fifteen other isolated case reports of trisomy births with maternal clomiphene exposure submitted to the FDA include 12 from the United States and three from other countries.

The possible association has also been examined in case control studies because of adequate maternal recall for ovulation induction and good definition of cases. However, the case control data available to date, limited to about 400 cases of **Chromosome 21, trisomy 21**, do not show an association. This discrepancy between the cohort and case control data could be due to mothers avoiding trisomy births on the basis of antenatal testing.

Complications: Unknown.

Associated Findings: None known.

Etiology: Maternal nondisjunction associated either with fertility problems for which ovulation-inducing agents are given, or with the agents themselves.

Pathogenesis: Unknown. Infertility problems in the mother could be a factor.

Sex Ratio: Presumably M1:F1.

Occurrence: Unlikely to exceed one trisomy birth in 300 exposures.

Risk of Recurrence for Patient's Sib: Unknown.

Risk of Recurrence for Patient's Child: Unknown.

Age of Detectability: At birth, or by amniocentesis.

Gene Mapping and Linkage: Unknown.

Prevention: An association, if present, does not mean the agent caused the defect. However, a practical clinical question, regardless of cause, is whether risk is sufficiently high to justify the hazard of amniocentesis in subfertile women strongly desiring a child.

Treatment: Unknown.

Prognosis: Unknown.

Detection of Carrier: Unknown.

References:

Oakley GP, Flynt GO: Increased prevalence of Down's syndrome (mongolism) among offspring of women treated with ovulation-inducing agents. (Abstract) Teratology 1972; 5:264 only.

Boue J, et al.: Retrospective and prospective studies of 1,500 karyotyped spontaneous human abortions. Teratology 1975; 14:11–26.

Merrill National Laboratories: Pregnancy outcome of humans following Clomid (clomiphene citrate USP) with summary of information of reported possible neural related anomalies of offspring. NDA 15–131, October 14, 1980.

Rosa FW: Ovulation induction trisomy. Food and Drug Administration ADR Highlight, 1981, No. 20.

Kurachi K, et al.: Congenital malformation of newborn infants after clomipene induced ovulation. Fertil Steril 1983; 40:187–189.

Wramsby H, et al.: Chromosome analysis of human oocytes recovered from preovulatory follicles in stimulated cycles. New Engl J Med 1987; 316:121–124.

R0018   **Franz W. Rosa**

Owren parahemophilia
  See FACTOR V DEFICIENCY
'Ox eye' (buphthalmos)
  See GLAUCOMA, CONGENITAL
Oxazepam, fetal effects of
  See FETAL BENZODIAZEPINE EFFECTS
Oxycephally
  See CRANIOSYNOSTOSIS

❖ P ❖

P450 side-chain cleavage enzyme, deficiency of
See STEROID 20-22 DESMOLASE DEFICIENCY
P450C11B1, deficiency of
See STEROID 11 BETA-HYDROXYLASE DEFICIENCY

PACHYDERMOPERIOSTOSIS   0788

Includes:
Hypertrophic osteoarthropathy, primary or idiopathic
Osteoarthropathy, hypertrophic
Rosenfeld-Kloepfer syndrome
Touraine-Solente-Gole syndrome

Excludes:
Pulmonary hypertrophic osteoarthropathy
Thyroid acropachy

Major Diagnostic Criteria: The presence of at least two of the three major abnormalities; clubbing, periostosis, cutis gyrata; in an individual with a negative family history and no sign of a predisposing lesion (e.g. bronchogenic carcinoma), or the presence of one of these major lesions in a close relative of a typical case.

Clinical Findings: Clubbing of the fingers and toes; periosteal new bone formation, especially over the distal ends of the long bones; coarse facial features with thickening, furrowing, and excessive oiliness of the skin of the face and forehead; cutis verticis gyrata (often appearing in the early teenage years); hyperhidrosis of the hands and feet and occasional intermittent swelling or pain in the large joints. X-rays reveal irregular subperiosteal ossification over the long bones, primarily at the distal ends and most pronounced at the insertion of tendons and ligaments. There is marked variability in expressivity, the disorder being more severe in males than in females.

A combination of pubertal onset, male predominance, feminine hair distribution, increased estrogen excretion, and decreased serum sodium with increased aldosterone excretion suggests an endocrinologic disturbance.

Complications: Ptosis due to hypertrophy of the eyelids, skeletal pain secondary to periostosis, and seborrheic dermatitis and secondary folliculitis associated with large and open skin pores.

Associated Findings: A severe duodenal ulcer presented in an affected individual at the third decade of life.

Etiology: Presumably autosomal dominant inheritance with marked variability in expression. Usually more severe in males.

Pathogenesis: This syndrome usually appears around puberty, slowly progresses for about 10 years, and is self-limited thereafter. Periostosis and clubbing may be related to an autonomic nervous system defect, since there is a decrease in peripheral blood flow, and vagal resection has been reported to improve joint swelling.

MIM No.: 16710

POS No.: 3369

Sex Ratio: M7:F1 observed among reported cases, but possibly related to increased severity of the disease in males.

Occurrence: Undetermined but presumed rare.

Risk of Recurrence for Patient's Sib:
See Part I, *Mendelian Inheritance.*

Risk of Recurrence for Patient's Child:
See Part I, *Mendelian Inheritance.*

Age of Detectability: In childhood or adolescence, by clinical features.

Gene Mapping and Linkage: Unknown.

Prevention: None known. Genetic counseling indicated.

Treatment: Plastic surgery to improve facial appearance. Vagotomy is reported to relieve skeletal pain and swelling.

Prognosis: Normal life span.

Detection of Carrier: Skeletal X-rays may detect periosteal new bone formation in otherwise unaffected female relatives.

Special Considerations: It is important to distinguish this disorder from secondary hypertrophic osteoarthropathy, as the latter condition may be associated with a treatable primary lesion (e.g. bronchogenic carcinoma, bronchiectasis, ulcerative colitis). A full clinical examination for a primary lesion must be performed on all sporadic cases of pachydermoperiostosis, as the diagnosis of this genetic disorder in isolated cases can only be made by exclusion.

0788-11181: Diffuse enlargement of fingers with clubbing producing drumstick appearance.

The unequal sex ratio is probably due to the variable expression of this dominant trait, which is much more severe in males. The phenotypic expression of this trait in females may be limited to asymptomatic periosteal new bone formation, and these individuals would go undetected unless skeletal X-rays were obtained.

The *Rosenfeld-Kloepfer syndrome* (Rosenthal & Kloepfer, 1962) is usually considered to be a variant of pachydermoperiostosis. This autosomal dominant condition is characterized by acromegaloid features, prominence of the frontal bone, cutis verticus gyrata, and corneal leukoma.

The authors are indebted to Sonja A. Rasmussen and Jaime L. Frias for their contributions to this article.

References:
Rosenthal JW, Kloepfer HW: An acromegaloid, cutis verticis gyrata, corneal leukoma syndrome. Arch Ophthalmol 1962; 68:722–726.
Vogl A, Goldfischer S: Pachydermoperiostosis: primary or idiopathic hypertrophic osteoarthropathy. Am J Med 1962; 33:166–187.
Rimoin DL: Pachydermoperiostosis (idiopathic clubbing and periostosis): genetic and physiologic considerations. New Engl J Med 1965; 272:923–931.
Hambrick GW Jr, Carter BM: Pachydermoperiostosis: Touraine-Solente-Golé syndrome. Arch Dermtol 1966; 94:594–608.
Hedayati H, et al.: Acrolysis in pachydermoperiostosis (primary or idiopathic hypertrophic osteoarthropothy). Arch Intern Med 1980; 140:1087–1088.
Shiu Kum Lana, et al.: Pachydermoperiostosis, hypertrophic gastropathy, and peptic ulcer. Gastroenterology 1983; 84:834–839.

B0025

Zvi Borochowitz
David L. Rimoin

Pachyonychia congenita
See NAILS, PACHYONYCHIA CONGENITA
Pachyonychia congenita, Jackson-Lawler type
See PACHYONYCHIA CONGENITA-STEATOCYSTOMA MULTIPLEX

PACHYONYCHIA CONGENITA-STEATOCYSTOMA MULTIPLEX   2905

Includes:
Nails, pachyonychia congenita, Jackson-Lawler type
Pachyonychia congenita, Jackson-Lawler type
Steatocystoma-pachyonychia congenita

Excludes:
Dyskeratosis congenita (2024)
Keratoderma of palms and soles
Nails, pachyonychia congenita (0789)
Steatocystoma multiplex, isolated

Major Diagnostic Criteria: Milia in infancy, supernumerary teeth, subcutaneous cysts, and thickened nails that are almost impossible to cut.

Clinical Findings: The disease affects the nails and skin. Clinical signs, especially milia and neonatal teeth, may be present at birth. The former disappears in childhood. Deformed nails appear shortly after birth. The free edge of the nail is raised in a thick, horny mass, while the base is normal. Finger- and toenails may have to be cut with a hacksaw. Subcutaneous cysts that are painful, enlarge, become infected, and discharge pus are common. Other skin manifestations include hyperhidrosis, bullae, follicular keratoses, ichthyosis, and acne conglobata. Skin lesions may be scattered to almost confluent. The soles of the feet are hyperkeratotic and painful, and there is hyperhidrosis of both palms and soles. Corneal dystrophy may be present. Pachyonychia congenita may occur as an isolated condition or with various skin and oral lesions. There is obviously much heterogeneity.

Complications: Infection of the cysts. Psychologic problems due to the cosmetic effects.

Associated Findings: None known.

Etiology: Autosomal dominant inheritance.

Pathogenesis: The cysts appear to be hamartomas.

MIM No.: 16721

Sex Ratio: Presumably M1:F1.

Occurrence: About 20 cases have been documented in the literature.

Risk of Recurrence for Patient's Sib:
See Part I, *Mendelian Inheritance.*

Risk of Recurrence for Patient's Child:
See Part I, *Mendelian Inheritance.*

Age of Detectability: At birth.

Gene Mapping and Linkage: Unknown.

Prevention: None known. Genetic counseling indicated.

Treatment: Symptomatic. Antibiotics as needed for infection.

Prognosis: Apparently consistent with normal life span. Scarring after spontaneous evacuation of skin lesions.

Detection of Carrier: By clinical examination.

Special Considerations: Gorlin et al (1976) discuss the distinction between this Jackson-Lawler form of pachyonychia congenita and the Jadassohn-Lewandowsky form (see **Nails, pachyonychia congenita**).

References:
Jackson ADM, Lawler SD: Pachyonychia congenita: a report of six cases in one family, with a note on linkage data. Ann Eugen 1951; 16:142–146.
Vineyard WR, Scott RA: Steatocystoma multiplex with pachyonychia congenita: eight cases in four generations. Arch Dermatol 1961; 84:824–827.
Gorlin RJ, et al.: Syndromes of the head and neck, ed 2. New York: McGraw-Hill, 1976:600–603.
Hodes ME, Norins AL: Pachyonychia congenita and steatocystoma multiplex. Clin Genet 1977; 11:359–364.
Hurwitz S: Clinical pediatric dermatology. Philadelphia: W.B. Saunders, 1981:183.

H0003
N0008

M.E. Hodes
A.L. Norins

Pachyonychia ichthyosiforme
See NAILS, PACHYONYCHIA CONGENITA
Pachyonychia neonatorum
See NAILS, PACHYONYCHIA CONGENITA
Paget disease
See BONE, PAGET DISEASE
Paget disease, juvenile
See OSTEOECTASIA
Pagon syndrome
See WALKER-WARBURG SYNDROME
Pain, insensitivity to, with anhidrosis of Swanson (congenital)
See NEUROPATHY, CONGENITAL SENSORY WITH ANHIDROSIS
Palatal incompetence, congenital
See PALATOPHARYNGEAL INCOMPETENCE
Palatal-digital-oro syndrome
See ORO-PALATAL-DIGITAL SYNDROME, VARADI TYPE
Palate enlargement
See PALATE, TORUS PALATINUS
Palate, cleft, occult submucous
See PALATOPHARYNGEAL INCOMPETENCE
Palate, cleft, submucous with a bifid uvula
See CLEFT PALATE
Palate, congenital short
See PALATOPHARYNGEAL INCOMPETENCE

PALATE, FISTULA 0790

Includes: Fistula of palate

Excludes:
Median palatal fistula and cyst
Nasoalveolar fistula and cyst

Major Diagnostic Criteria: Small openings in anterior pillars at the junction of the soft palate and pharynx.

Clinical Findings: Bilateral or unilateral fistulas at junction of soft palate and pharynx in the anterior pillars without cicatrization.

Complications: Unknown.

Associated Findings: Absence or hypoplasia of one or both palatine tonsils, preauricular fistulas, deafness and strabismus.

Etiology: Unknown.

Pathogenesis: Maldevelopment of the second branchial pouch occurs with failure of complete obliteration of the pouch. The resultant fistulas are lined by stratified squamous epithelium, with lymphoid tissue adjacent.

Sex Ratio: Presumably M1:F1.

Occurrence: Undetermined but presumed rare.

Risk of Recurrence for Patient's Sib: Unknown.

Risk of Recurrence for Patient's Child: Unknown.

Age of Detectability: At birth, by visual examination.

Gene Mapping and Linkage: Unknown.

Prevention: None known. Genetic counseling indicated.

Treatment: Unknown.

Prognosis: Excellent.

Detection of Carrier: Unknown.

References:

Claiborne JH Jr: Hiatus in the anterior pillar of the fauces of the right side with congenital absence of tonsil on either side. Am J Med Sci 1885; 89:490–491.

Miller AS, et al.: Lateral soft palate fistula. Arch Otolaryngol 1970; 91:200.

Gorlin RJ, et al.: Syndromes of the head and neck. 2nd ed. New York: McGraw-Hill, 1976.

Saito T: Congenital fistulas of the cleft and palate. J Jap Cleft Palate Asso 1982; 7:189–193.

JI001 **Jan E. Jirásek**

PALATE, TORUS PALATINUS 0959

Includes:
Palate enlargement
Torus palatinus

Excludes: N/A

Major Diagnostic Criteria: A rounded elevation in the midline of the palate, with a smooth edge.

Clinical Findings: A slowly growing enlargement of bone on the hard palate at the junction of the midpalatal suture usually covered with normal appearing mucosa. These can be single or lobulated, and show remarkable variation in morphology (flat, spindle, nodular).

Complications: Complications occur only if the palatal elevations grow so large as to interfere with mastication, speech, or the fitting of a denture.

Associated Findings: None known.

Etiology: Probably autosomal dominant inheritance with variable expressivity and penetrance close to 85%, although X-linked dominant inheritance has also been proposed, and there is also evidence also for multifactorial inheritance. There is no evidence of sporadic cases. Suzuki and Sakai (1960) have suggested this condition is due to the same gene as that responsible for **Mandible, torus mandibularis**.

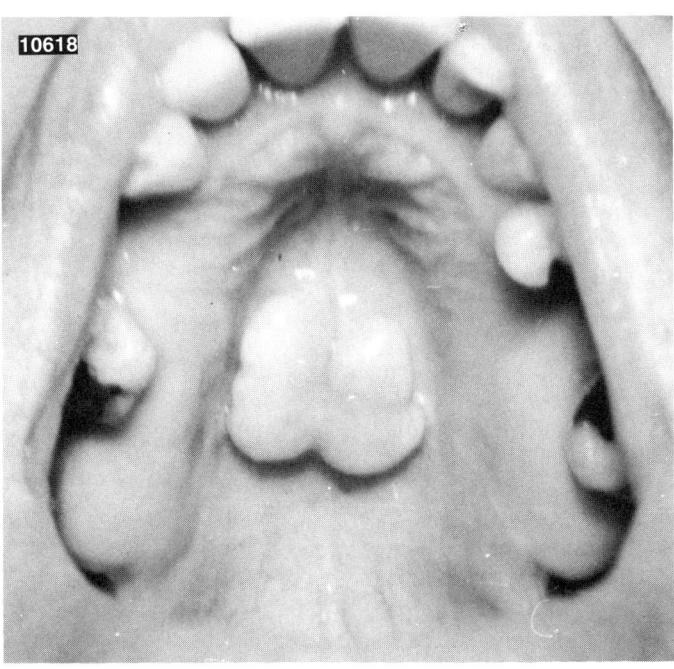

0959-10618: Torus palatinus.

Pathogenesis: Gradual enlargement of bone in the region of the midpalatal suture.

MIM No.: *18970

Sex Ratio: Estimated M1:F2 in Caucasians; M3:F1 American Indians.

Occurrence: Incidence 1:5 in a midwestern United States Caucasian population. Prevalence 1:50 children.

Risk of Recurrence for Patient's Sib:
See Part I, *Mendelian Inheritance.*

Risk of Recurrence for Patient's Child:
See Part I, *Mendelian Inheritance.*

Age of Detectability: Occasionally seen in children, but usually apparent by puberty.

Gene Mapping and Linkage: Unknown.

Prevention: None known. Genetic counseling indicated.

Treatment: Surgical removal, if interfering with oral function or placement of denture.

Prognosis: Excellent.

Detection of Carrier: By clinical examination of first degree relatives.

References:

Kolos S, et al.: The occurrence of torus palatinus and torus mandibularis in 2,478 dental patients. Oral Surg 1953; 6:1134.

Suzuki M, Sakai T: A familial study of torus palatinus and torus mandibularis. Am J Phys Anthrop 1960; 18:263–272.

Gould AW: An investigation of the inheritance of torus palatinus and torus mandibularis. J Dent Res 1964; 43:159.

Gorlin RJ: Developmental anomalies of the face and oral structures. In: Gorlin RJ, Goldman HM, eds: Thoma's oral pathology, ed 6. vol. 1. St. Louis: C.V. Mosby, 1970:21.

King DR, Moore GE: The prevalence of torus palatinus. J Oral Med 1971; 26:113.

Barbujani G, et al.: Torus palatinus: a segregation analysis. Hum Hered 1986; 36:317–325.

J0011 **Clinton C. Johnson**

Palato-digital-oto syndrome
See OTO-PALATO-DIGITAL SYNDROME, II
Palato-oto-digital syndrome
See OTO-PALATO-DIGITAL SYNDROME, I

PALATOPHARYNGEAL INCOMPETENCE 2118

Includes:
    Cleft palate, occult submucous
    Palatal incompetence, congenital
    Palate, congenital short
    Palate, cleft, occult submucous
    Rhinolalia
    Speech, hypernasal
    Velopharyngeal incompetence
    Velopharyngeal insufficiency

Excludes: **Cleft palate** (0180)

Major Diagnostic Criteria: An abnormal resonance of speech in the nasal cavity as a result of a failure of closure of the palato-pharyngeal (velopharyngeal) orifice during phonation. The nasal resonance is variable from person to person depending partly upon the size of the palato-pharyngeal opening during speech as well as other vocal tract dynamics. Occasionally, abnormal speech may be accompanied by nasal regurgitation of food or fluids during deglutition, but this is a relatively rare occurrence. Frequently, nasal resonance is accompanied by audible nasal air flow (nasal turbulence, or "snorting").

Clinical Findings: Palatal-pharyngeal gaps are most easily diagnosed and recognized by motion picture fluoroscopic studies of the palato-pharyngeal orifice during speech, or by direct nasal endoscopy. A variety of other procedures, such as nasal airflow studies, may be helpful in confirming the presence of abnormal nasal resonance, but the final determination of the degree of abnormality of the speech symptom depends most heavily upon a thorough speech evaluation. Palato-pharyngeal incompetence may be related to any disorder of the palate, pharynx, or nervous system (central or peripheral), including structural anomalies, neuromuscular disease, and anomalies of the CNS. Palato-pharyngeal incompetence is a nonspecific finding symptomatic of a broad range of disorders; it is not characterized by any particular set of physical findings (such as short stature, reduced head size, etc.). The relative frequency of palato-pharyngeal incompetence rank-ordered by pathogenesis is probably as follows:
    1. cleft palate, submucous cleft palate, occult submucous cleft palate.
    2. trauma or degenerative disease of the CNS.
    3. CNS malformations.
    4. neuromuscular disease or peripheral nerve damage.
    5. iatrogenic (usually a complication of adenotonsillectomy).

Complications: Developmental problems occur because proper functioning of the palato-pharyngeal valve is necessary for the acquisition of normal speech and articulation. Many individuals with palato-pharyngeal incompetence develop compensatory errors in their speech patterns. This often makes their speech entirely unintelligible and may give the appearance of significant language delay at ages one to two years due to the inability to decode their utterances. Patients with palato-pharyngeal incompetence also often develop facial grimaces in their efforts to constrict the abnormal nasal air flow at the nostrils.

Some patients may tend to avoid speech or speaking situations because of the secondary psychological complications of poor intelligiblity.

Associated Findings: Bifid uvula, highly arched palate, dental anomalies (especially in the area of the lateral incisors, cuspids, and bicuspids), notching of the maxillary alveolus, conductive hearing loss with recurrent middle ear effusions, **Microcephaly**, small stature, congenital heart disease, auricular anomalies, and orbital hypertelorism. Such associated findings may be related to the large number of malformation syndromes with palato-pharyngeal incompetence as a feature.

Etiology: Unknown.

Pathogenesis: Occurs in association with multiple types of anomalies and syndromes. Etiologically, three types of anomalies can cause palato-pharyngeal incompetence: structural anomalies of the palate and pharynx, neuromuscular disorders, and CNS anomalies.

Structural anomalies of the palate and pharynx may include abnormal insertions of the palatal muscles, missing muscle groups in the palate, excessively large pharynx, asymmetry of the palate and/or pharynx, and abnormal structural relationships between the palate and pharynx. As such, palato-pharyngeal incompetence can occur in a variety of disorders with multiple pathogeneses, such as **Mandibulofacial dysostosis, Acrofacial dysostosis, Nager type, Oto-palato-digital syndrome, I,** and **Chromosome 21, trisomy 21.**

Neuromuscular disorders are frequently first expressed by speech abnormalities such as hypernasality indicative of palato-pharyngeal incompetence. Many of the muscular dystrophies have associated palato-pharyngeal incompetence, most particularly **Myotonic dystrophy.** Palato-pharyngeal incompetence is also a frequent finding in **Neurofibromatosis.**

CNS anomalies, both malformations and deformations, frequently result in palato-pharyngeal incompetence. Hypernasality is associated with the Arnold-Chiari deformation, among others. Any disorder with involvement of the motor cortex and upper pyramidal tracts may result in palato-pharyngeal incompetence.

MIM No.: 16750

CDC No.: 750.210

Sex Ratio: M1:F1

Occurrence: Prevalence more than 1:1,000.

Risk of Recurrence for Patient's Sib:
See Part I, *Mendelian Inheritance.* If an isolated trait, the risk may be as high as 50%. Otherwise the risk is that of the condition with which the palato-pharyngeal incompetence is associated.

Risk of Recurrence for Patient's Child:
See Part I, *Mendelian Inheritance.*

Age of Detectability: With the onset of speech (approximately 10–18 months of age).

Gene Mapping and Linkage: Unknown.

Prevention: None known. Genetic counseling indicated.

Treatment: Depending on etiology, may be surgical reconstruction of the palate and/or pharynx, prosthetic augmentation of the palato-pharyngeal orifice, or speech therapy.

Prognosis: With treatment, prognosis for normal speech is excellent.

Detection of Carrier: Unknown.

Special Considerations: Because of the multiple etiologies of palato-pharyngeal incompetence, some potentially serious, it is extremely important to determine the reason for this common disorder in each individual case. For example, surgical correction of palato-pharyngeal incompetence is usually performed without complication in most instances. However, such surgery could prove to be hazardous in patients with **Myotonic dystrophy** because of the risk of malignant hyperthermia under anesthesia, or in patients with **Mandibulofacial dysostosis** because of the risk of obstructive apnea postoperatively. Furthermore, because this disorder may be the first noticeable symptom of a variety of syndromes, its source must be delineated to provide appropriate counseling (both genetic and treatment). The first clinically evident symptom of **Cleft lip/palate-lip pits or mounds**, for example, is often palato-pharyngeal incompetence. This is also true for such conditions as **Velo-cardio-facial syndrome** and **Neurofibromatosis.** Therefore, this disorder must be regarded in a broader context than simply speech impairment.

References:
Peterson-Falzone S, Pruzansky S: Cleft palate and congenital palatopharyngeal incompetency in mandibulofacial dysostosis: frequency and problems in treatment. Cleft Palate J 1976; 13:354–360.
Luce EA, et al.: Velopharyngeal insufficiency in hemifacial microsomia. Plast Reconstr Surg 1977; 60:602–606.

Pollack MA, et al.: Velopharyngeal insufficiency: the neurologic perspective. Dev Med Child Neurol 1979; 21:194–201. *
Lewin ML, et al.: Velopharyngeal insufficiency due to hypoplasia of the musculus uvulae and occult submucous cleft palate. Plast Reconstr Surg 1980; 65:585–591. * †
Andres R, et al.: Dominant inheritance of velopharyngeal incompetence. Clin Genet 1981; 19:443–447.
Pollack MA, Shprintzen RJ: Velopharyngeal insufficiency in neurofibromatosis. Int J Pediatr Otorhinolaryngol 1981; 3:257–262.
Williams MA, et al.: Adenoid hypopladia in the velo-cardio-facial syndrome. J Craniofac Genet Devel Biol 1987; 7:23–26.

SH040   **Robert J. Shprintzen**

Pallister mosaic syndrome
See PALLISTER-KILLIAN MOSAIC SYNDROME
Pallister syndrome
See ULNAR-MAMMARY SYNDROME
Pallister-Hall syndrome
See HYPOTHALAMIC HAMARTOBLASTOMA SYNDROME, CONGENITAL
Pallister-Herrmann-Opitz syndrome
See HERRMANN-PALLISTER-OPITZ SYNDROME

PALLISTER-KILLIAN MOSAIC SYNDROME   2189

Includes:
> Chromosome 12, isochromosome 12p mosaicism
> Killian syndrome
> Pallister mosaic syndrome
> Teschler-Nicola/Killian syndrome

Excludes:
> **Chromosome 12, partial trisomy 12p** (2130)
> Chromosome 21, mosaic tetrasomy 21
> **Hypomelanosis of Ito** (2264)

Major Diagnostic Criteria: Affected newborn infants are profoundly hypotonic with sparsity of scalp hair, especially bitemporally, and a prominent forehead. There is coarsening of facial features over time. Blood chromosomes are usually normal. Analysis of fibroblast chromosomes shows mosaicism for an isochromosome of 12p.

Clinical Findings: Clinical signs are evident at birth with profound hypotonia, distinct facial appearance, and sparsity of scalp hair, especially bitemporally. Birth weight is within the normal range. Craniofacial manifestations include "coarse" face with prominent high forehead, normal head circumference, hypertelorism, epicanthal folds, flat bridge of nose, highly arched palate, and abnormal ears. Most affected individuals have a generalized pigmentary dysplasia, which may vary from sparse hypopigmented macules to an incontinentia pigmenti-like pattern. Pigmentary changes may be evident only with a Woods lamp in some individuals. Many have accessory nipples.

In infancy the facial appearance becomes more "coarse," hypotonia persists, cognitive delays are obvious, and seizures may occur. Contractures may also develop, and strabismus is common. Cranial CT scan abnormalities were found in 10/15 tested, with cerebral atrophy being the most common finding.

Of the three adult patients, two are severely retarded, bedridden, have seizures and severe contractures of limbs, and lack speech and all self-help skills. The third adult is healthy, ambulatory, and has no contractures but is profoundly retarded, nonverbal, has seizures, and lacks self-help skills.

Complications: **Laryngomalacia** may cause respiratory problems in the newborn period. Gastroesophageal reflux and poor feeding may be secondary to hypotonia. Contractures (2/3) and cataracts (2/3) may develop in adulthood.

Associated Findings: Congenital heart defects (3/33), **Diaphragmatic hernia** (3/33), sensorineural hearing loss (3/33), imperforate anus (2/33).

Etiology: Tetrasomy for chromosome 12p. All cases have been sporadic. There is no significant pattern of advanced parental age, and there is no history of recurrent fetal wastage in their families.

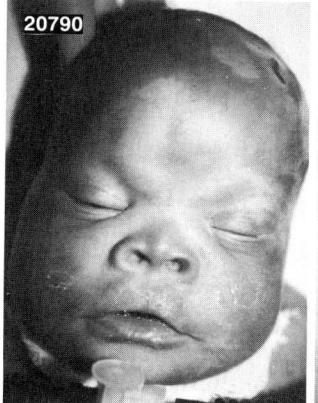
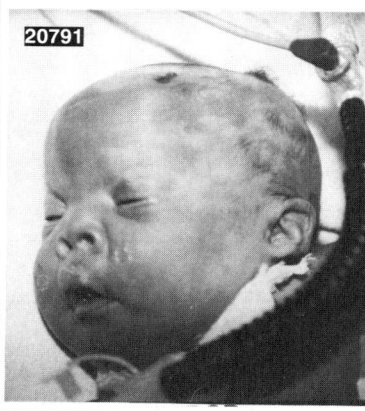
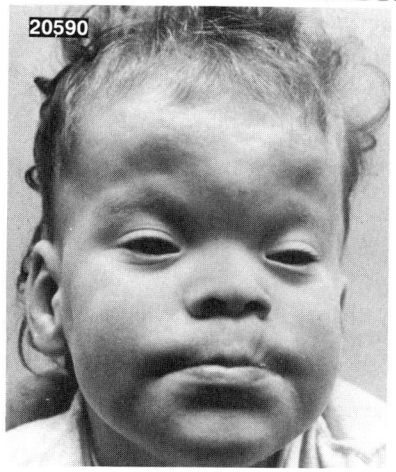

2189-20790–91: Pallister-Killian mosaic syndrome in an infant; note epicanthal folds, upward slanted palpebral fissures, anteverted nares, flat nasal bridge and prominent cheeks. **20590:** Facial coarsening, high forehead and flat nasal bridge. There is now hair in the area where frontal balding occurs in infancy.

Pathogenesis: Unknown.

POS No.: 3800

Sex Ratio: M1:F1

Occurrence: More than 30 cases have been reported.

Risk of Recurrence for Patient's Sib: Low. All cases are sporadic.

Risk of Recurrence for Patient's Child: Unknown. No affected individuals are known to have reproduced.

Age of Detectability: At birth. Has been detected prenatally in amniocytes.

Gene Mapping and Linkage: See *Gene Map.*

Prevention: None known. Genetic counseling indicated.

Treatment: Unknown.

Prognosis: Athough early death does occur, oldest patients are in their 40s. Severe mental retardation is common, but some children are attending special education classes. Contractures may develop with time.

Detection of Carrier: Unknown.

References:
Pallister PD, et al.: The Pallister mosaic syndrome. BD:OAS XIII(3B). New York: March of Dimes Birth Defects Foundation, 1977:103–110.
Teschler-Nicola M, Killian W: Case report 72. Synd Ident 1981; 7:6–7.
Reynolds JF, et al.: Isochromosome 12p mosaicism (Pallister mosaic

aneuploidy or Pallister-Killian syndrome): report of 11 cases. Am J Med Genet 1987; 27:257–274. * †

Warburton D, et al.: Mosaic tetrasomy 12p: four new cases, and confirmation of the chromosomal origin of the supernumerary chromosome in one of the original Pallister-mosaic syndrome cases. Am J Med Genet 1987; 27:275–283.

RE029   **James F. Reynolds**

PALLISTER-W SYNDROME   0791

Includes: W Syndrome

Excludes: Oto-palato-digital syndrome

Major Diagnostic Criteria: Mental retardation, some manifestations of a median oral cleft, the characteristic facial appearance, and mild skeletal abnormalities of the upper limbs. Patients present very much like the **Oto-palato-digital syndrome**, but without the characteristic hand and foot manifestations.

Clinical Findings: Presently the syndrome is defined on the basis of two male sibs having a malformation-mental retardation syndrome with the following features: moderate mental retardation, grand mal seizures, tremor, mild spasticity, an incomplete median cleft in the palate and upper lip, broad tip of nose, broad and flat maxilla, telecanthus, alternating esotropia, and high forehead. Skeletal abnormalities in the upper limbs included cubitus valgus, shortness of the ulnae, bowing of the radii, and clinocamptodactyly. One patient had pes cavus; the other had metatarsus varus and pes planus.

Complications: Broad uvula, absent incisors, and nasal speech secondary to oral cleft; antimongoloid slant of palpebral fissures secondary to hypoplastic maxillae; anterior cowlick secondary to high forehead. Injury secondary to seizures and mental retardation.

Associated Findings: Prematurity.

Etiology: Probably X-linked recessive inheritance (with some expression in female heterozygotes), or possibly autosomal dominant inheritance (with manifestations expressed more severely in males than in females).

Pathogenesis: A number of the facial manifestations can be related to incomplete median clefting.

MIM No.: 31145

POS No.: 3357

Sex Ratio: Presumably M1:F1 (2 brothers had severe symptoms, their mother and sister had mild manifestations).

Occurrence: One family consisting of two brothers, their mother, and a sister has been documented. The sister has since produced a severely affected son.

Risk of Recurrence for Patient's Sib:
See Part I, *Mendelian Inheritance.*

Risk of Recurrence for Patient's Child:
See Part I, *Mendelian Inheritance.*

Age of Detectability: At birth.

Gene Mapping and Linkage: Unknown.

Prevention: None known. Genetic counseling indicated.

Treatment: Cleft palate care and repair, correction of strabismus, orthopedic surgery. Special education, speech therapy, seizure control.

Prognosis: Survival into adulthood.

Detection of Carrier: Carrier females may show mild craniofacial manifestations.

References:
Pallister PD, et al.: The W syndrome. BD:OAS X(7). Miami: Symposia Specialists for The National Foundation-March of Dimes. 1974:51–60.

PA010   **Philip D. Pallister**
HE023   **Jürgen Herrmann**

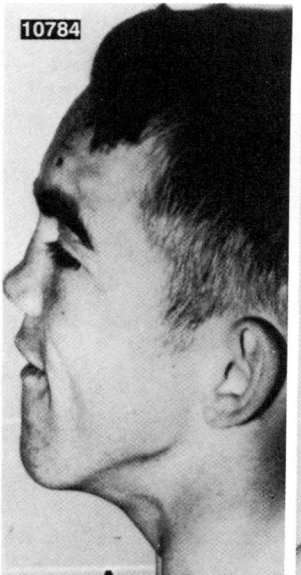
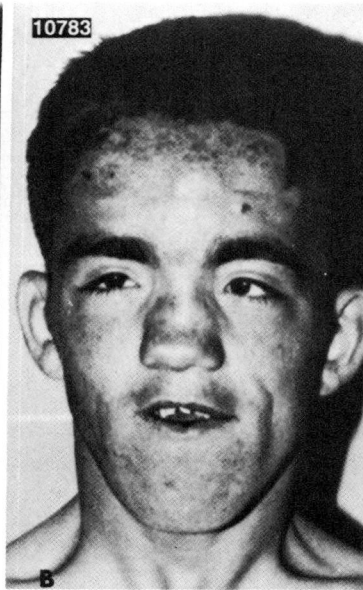
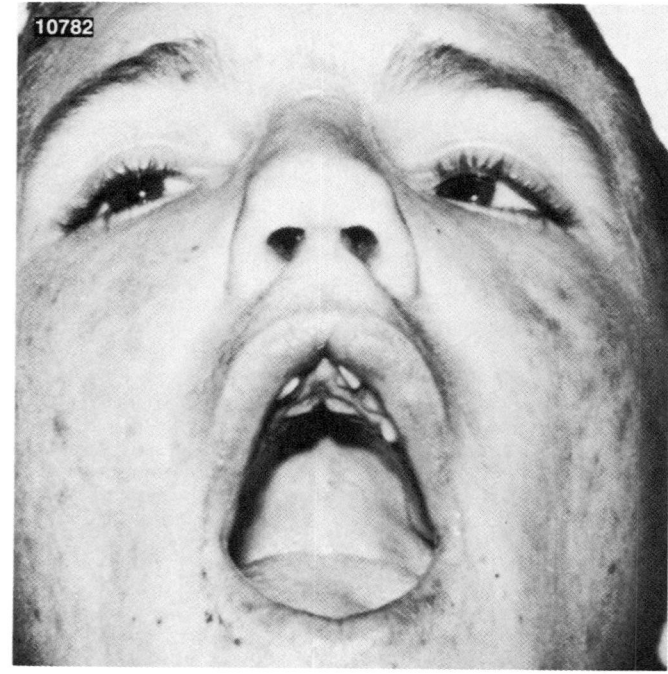

0791-10784–83: Characteristic facies shows broad nasal tip, broad maxilla, telecanthus, broad forehead and long chin. 10782: Incomplete median cleft of the palate and upper lip.

Palm, single line
See SKIN CREASE, SINGLE PALMAR
Palmar clinodactyly
See CAMPTODACTYLY
Palmar crease, single transverse
See SKIN CREASE, SINGLE PALMAR
Palmar fibromatosis
See CONTRACTURE, DUPUYTREN
Palmityl-CoA dehydrogenase deficiency
See ACYL-CoA DEHYDROGENASE DEFICIENCY, LONG CHAIN TYPE

Palmo-plantar erythema
    See *SKIN, PALMO-PLANTAR ERYTHEMA*
Palmo-plantar keratoderma, hereditary epidermolytic
    See *KERATOSIS PALMARIS ET PLANTARIS OF UNNA-THOST*
Palmo-plantar keratodermas
    See *ICHTHYOSIS*
Palmo-plantar keratodermia with carcinoma of esophagus
    See *HOWEL EVANS SYNDROME*
Palmo-plantar keratodermia, diffuse hereditary
    See *KERATOSIS PALMARIS ET PLANTARIS OF UNNA-THOST*
Palmoplantar hyperkeratosis-gingival hyperkeratosis
    See *SKIN, HYPERKERATOSIS, FOCAL PALMOPLANTAR AND GINGIVAL*
Palmoplantar hyperkeratosis-reticular pigmentation
    See *ECTODERMAL DYSPLASIA, NAEGELI TYPE*
Palmoplantar hyperkeratosis-spastic paraplegia-retardation
    See *HYPERKERATOSIS PALMOPLANTARIS-SPASTIC PARAPLEGIA-RETARDATION*
Palpebral coloboma-lipoma syndrome
    See *NASOPALPEBRAL LIPOMA-COLOBOMA SYNDROME*
Palpebromaxillary synergy, hereditary
    See *JAW-WINKING SYNDROME*

PALSY, CONGENITAL FACIAL   0377

Includes:
    Facial palsy, congenital partial
    Facial palsy, congenital unilateral or bilateral
    Facial paralysis, familial congenital peripheral
    Nuclear facial palsy

Excludes:
    Agenesis of facial musculature
    Bell palsy, sporadic cases of
    Facial palsy as part of a complex malformation syndrome
    Facial palsy due to birth trauma or application of forceps
    Palsy, late-onset facial, familial (0378)

Major Diagnostic Criteria: Bilateral (occasionally unilateral) peripheral palsy present from birth and not caused by trauma. Electrodiagnostic tests will show denervation as differentiated from muscular agenesis. Petrous pyramid polytomography may show middle ear anomalies or an aberrant course of the facial nerve canal.

Clinical Findings: Peripheral facial palsy is present at birth and is usually bilateral. Some pedigrees have been described in which each affected member was involved unilaterally and on the same side. History and physical findings are negative for birth trauma and, unlike most cases due to obstetric forceps pressure, no degree of recovery has been reported. In most instances no other neurologic deficits can be found, although in some families scattered members have shown associated homolateral ptosis or nystagmus or strabismus. In some instances associated congenital conductive hearing loss due to middle ear malformations has been reported, but these appeared to be sporadic. Various laboratory tests may be helpful in differential diagnosis, prognosis and in determining whether therapy might be beneficial in some instances. However, for therapy to have optimum results, evaluation should be carried out at about 7–14 days of age. Four tests have been found useful: the facial nerve excitability test, the strength-duration or intensity-duration test (recorded graphically), electromyography, and facial muscle biopsy in selected cases. Acoustic middle ear reflex (stapedius reflex) testing may help establish the site of lesion but needs to be combined with audiologic evaluation, probably including brainstem auditory evoked response testing, so that the level of hearing and type of hearing loss (if one exists) may be documented. The facial nerve-excitability test is most useful in unilateral cases where the response between the normal and abnormal side can be compared. In neurapraxia (physiologic or conductive block), there will be no difference in excitability between the normal and abnormal nerve. In partial denervation, the involved nerve will require more intensity of stimulation to evoke a response. In both of these instances, recovery can be anticipated and a good prognosis given but confirmation should be obtained using strength-duration testing. This test is of no value if performed before the 14th day

after onset of paralysis. However, the time of onset of paralysis in congenital cases is unknown. Therefore, it might be worthwhile trying the test before the 14th day of life. In total denervation no response to facial nerve-excitability stimulation is seen. Accordingly, this test is useful for both unilateral and bilateral facial weakness. Strength-duration curves are confirmatory. Facial nerve-excitability and strength-duration tests are best carried out in the infant under light general anesthesia which can then be deepened for definitive surgery, should this prove advisable. Electromyography and stapedius reflex testing should be done without anesthetic, although sedation may be required. In the absence of muscle potentials of any kind, specific muscle biopsy might be advisable in some instances to rule out absence of muscle fibers. The stapedius reflex will be absent in lesions proximal to the takeoff of the main trunk of the facial nerve as it descends through the mastoid. If hearing loss is also present, it is important to measure acoustic impedance to see if an associated anomaly of the middle ear ossicles may exist. Instances of partial facial palsy have been reported in which only the lower half of the face was paralyzed. The stapedius reflex was also impaired but taste and lacrimation were unimpaired. This was believed to be a partial nuclear lesion, not cortical. Petrous pyramid computerized tomography may delineate the anatomy of the facial nerve canal in the temporal bone and is a useful adjunct to diagnosis and therapy. It should be remembered, however, that the facial nerve may not be in the fallopian canal.

Complications: Corneal drying and ulceration could occur if the eye is unable to be closed sufficiently. Most patients, however, have an adequate eye closure. Eventually, denervated muscles undergo atrophy and fibrosis, and if the defect is unilateral, pulling of the opposite facial muscles will make the asymmetry even more noticeable. Bilateral involvement of the buccinator muscles may make feeding of the newborn infant very difficult but children and adults compensate for this.

Associated Findings: Middle ear anomalies, usually of second branchial arch origin but sometimes involving first arch structures, may be associated without mandibulofacial anomalies. Associated deficits of other cranial nerves have been reported in a few patients. Isolated absence or abnormality of the ramus mandibularus of the facial nerve associated with cardiac defects has been reported but this appears to be a separate entity. Congenital facial palsy may be found in a variety of syndromes.

Etiology: Autosomal dominant inheritance with high penetrance. It is possible that idiopathic, sporadic cases of congenital facial palsy are representative of autosomal dominance with variable penetrance. In congenital unilateral facial palsy, partial agenesis of the motor nucleus of the seventh cranial nerve has been found at autopsy. If hypoplasia of the facial nerve is found combined with middle ear anomalies, a nongenetic cause for branchial arch malformation may exist. Thalidomide ingestion by the mother during pregnancy may cause facial nerve agenesis.

Pathogenesis: The pathogenesis is unknown except that in instances of bony compression of the facial nerve within the temporal bone, it is believed the blood supply to the nerve is compromised. Wide variations in the anatomy of the facial nerve and the fallopian canal are known to occur. Hypoplasia and ''hyperplasia'' of the nerve have been reported. The facial nerve lies encased in a bony canal which may be abnormally narrow and compress the nerve. Narrowing at the stylomastoid foramen has been reported. Secondary edema may cause further decrease of the blood supply with death of the nerve fibers. There is some experimental evidence that ischemia of the facial nerve causes paralysis.

MIM No.: 13410

Sex Ratio: M1:F1

Occurrence: Several kindreds have been documented.

Risk of Recurrence for Patient's Sib:
    See Part I, *Mendelian Inheritance.*

Risk of Recurrence for Patient's Child:
    See Part I, *Mendelian Inheritance.*

Age of Detectability: At birth. In unilateral cases the facial asymmetry is obvious. Bilateral cases may go unrecognized for a prolonged time. Detection is by physical examination and confirmation is by electrodiagnostic testing.

Gene Mapping and Linkage: Unknown.

Prevention: None known. Genetic counseling indicated.

Treatment: Surgical decompression of the facial nerve in the temporal bone may be useful in early cases. This technique has been used so seldom in such ideal cases that its success cannot be assessed. Later, plastic and reconstructive procedures, such as fascial slings and reinnervation of the facial musculature using other nearby motor nerves, might be done. Reinnervation of already atrophic or fibrotic muscles is hopeless, and electromyography should be done before attempting any such procedure. If the patient has inadequate eye closure, tarsorrhaphy should be performed and the patient given safety glasses as additional protection. Tube feeding, gavage, or feeding with a syringe may be necessary in the bilaterally affected infant who cannot suck. Gastrostomy may be indicated in extreme cases. Surgical correction of associated middle ear anomalies that have caused conductive hearing loss may be feasible. In inoperable cases a hearing aid should be prescribed if the hearing loss is bilateral.

Prognosis: Normal for life span and intelligence. For function, no recovery can be anticipated without therapy. With therapy, variable degrees of recovery may be possible.

Detection of Carrier: Unknown.

Special Considerations: Physicians caring for these infants need to be aware that a more sophisticated approach to the problem than mere observation is now available. Facial paralysis is a major disability, and every attempt should be made to diagnose and, if possible, treat it early. Middle ear anomalies may be present in some instances, causing maximum conductive hearing loss. Audiometry should be done early to rule out this possibility, and appropriate habilitation should be begun. In many cases the etiology or pathogenesis remain unknown because either a "wait-and-see" or a hopeless attitude is taken by parents or physician. Very few patients have electrodiagnostic studies made shortly after birth, and even fewer patients have surgical exploration and decompression of the facial nerve as it courses through the temporal bone.

References:

Skyberg D, Van der Hagen CB: Congenital hereditary unilateral facial palsy in four generations. Acta Paediatr Scand 1965; 159(suppl):77–79.

Rubin A: Handbook of congenital malformations. Philadelphia: WB Saunders, 1967.

Cayler CG: Cardiofacial syndrome: congenital heart disease and facial weakness. Arch Dis Child 1969; 44:69–75.

McHugh HE, et al.: Facial paralysis and muscle agenesis in the newborn. Arch Otolaryngol 1969; 89:131–143.

Bergstrom L, Baker B: Syndromes associated with congenital facial paralysis. Otolaryngol Head Neck Surg 1981; 89:336–342.

BE028   **LaVonne Bergstrom**

Palsy, double elevator
See EYELID, PTOSIS, CONGENITAL

PALSY, LATE-ONSET FACIAL, FAMILIAL   **0378**

Includes:
   Bell palsy, single or recurrent episodes of
   Facial palsy, familial recurrent peripheral
   Facial palsy, late-onset

Excludes:
   Bell palsy, sporadic cases of
   Cheilitis granulomatosa, Melkersson-Rosenthal type (2083)
   Fetal effects from Lyme disease (3212)
   Palsy, congenital facial (0377)

Major Diagnostic Criteria: Typical peripheral facial palsy not present at birth, often recurrent; occurring in a family or kindred.

Clinical Findings: Inability to move the ipsilateral muscles of the face or close the eye. Decreased salivary secretion of the submaxillary gland, decreased tearing of the eye, diminished or absent stapedius reflex, impaired taste sensation on the ipsilateral side may be present.

Affected persons may show one or repeated episodes of peripheral facial palsy. Family history for more than one generation reveals an increased incidence of Bell palsy among family members. One survey found such an incidence to be nine times greater in the families of patients with Bell palsy as compared to the families of control patients. The same study showed that the episodes of Bell palsy in families could not be associated with exogenous factors, such as viral outbreaks. Although in one family several members had repeated episodes of facial palsy associated with upper respiratory and ear infections. Disorders such as diabetes or hypertension do not seem to be associated with an increased incidence of familial facial palsy.

There is a tendency for episodes of recurrent Bell palsy to recur on the same side, suggesting an anatomic variation as a factor in etiology. Usually the palsy clears spontaneously. However, in some instances nerve excitability may be lost; and in those instances the nerve would not be expected to recover without treatment. Pain, when it occurs, is a poor prognostic sign and also suggests the need for urgent surgical intervention. Jepson reported the following findings for facial nerve lesions at different levels:

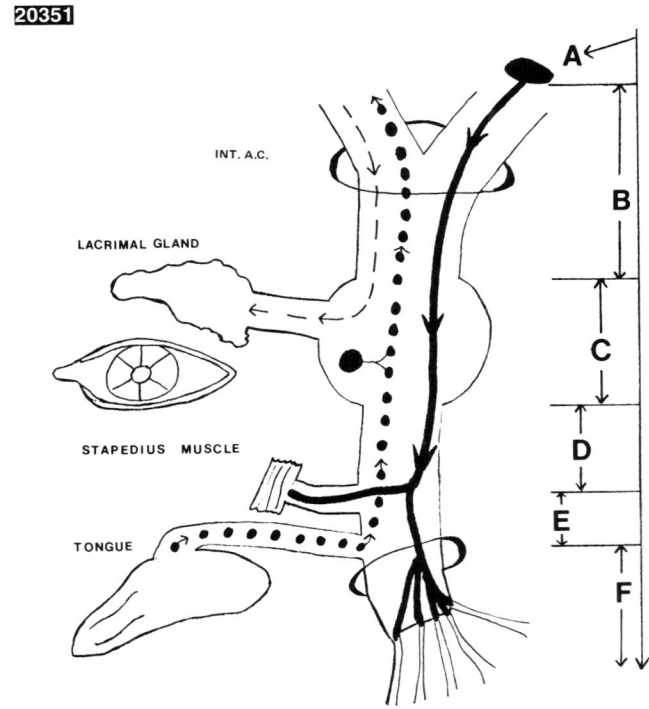

0378-20351: Schematic drawing of the facial nerve restricted to motor, gustatory (via chorda tympani nerve), and lacrimal (via greater superficial petrosal nerve) branches. INT. A. C. = internal auditory canal. A, seventh (facial) nerve nucleus; B, suprageniculate; C, geniculate ganglion; D, suprastapedial; E, infrastapedial; F, infrachordal.

Facial Nerve Lesions by Level

Regional Diagnosis	Taste	Lacrimation	Stapedius Reflex
Nuclear	+	+	-
Suprageniculate	+/-	-	-
Transgeniculate	-	-	-
Suprastapedial	-	+	-
Infrastapedial	-	+	+
Infrachordal	+	+	+

Complications: The nerve may fail to recover causing permanent paralysis. This may occur in 10–25% of cases. There is some evidence that recovery is less after repeated episodes of facial palsy. Corneal drying and ulceration may occur if there is inadequate eye closure.

Associated Findings: None known.

Etiology: Autosomal dominant inheritance with reduced penetrance. There may also be instances of autosomal recessive inheritance. Hypersensitivity to cold or to horse serum has been associated with increased susceptibility to facial paralysis in experimental animals.

Pathogenesis: Unknown.

MIM No.: *13420

Sex Ratio: M1:F1

Occurrence: Undetermined. At least a dozen kindreds have been documented.

Risk of Recurrence for Patient's Sib:
See Part I, *Mendelian Inheritance*.

Risk of Recurrence for Patient's Child:
See Part I, *Mendelian Inheritance*.

Age of Detectability: When it first occurs, usually in adults.

Gene Mapping and Linkage: Unknown.

Prevention: None known. Genetic counseling indicated.

Treatment: If nerve excitability remains equal to that of the normal side, a conduction block exists. Nerve conduction should be tested twice daily for up to two weeks to be certain denervation is not occurring. Probably no therapy is needed in these cases but if the palsy persists more than a few weeks, massage, local heat and electrical stimulation of the facial muscles to minimize atrophy and fibrosis may be beneficial.

If denervation occurs and if other neurologic deficits or a systemic cause are not present, immediate surgical decompression of the nerve throughout its course in the temporal bone seems to be of benefit. This should be done as soon as denervation becomes apparent. However, it may be of some benefit even after a prolonged period of denervation. In late cases, anastomosis of the facial nerve with another nerve, excision of an involved segment and grafting have been proposed. To minimize deformity, facial slings may be created to support the sagging paralyzed side of the face.

If coverage of the eye is inadequate, temporary or permanent tarsorrhaphy should be done.

Other medical treatments have been proposed. These include the administration of steroids, vasodilating drugs and stellate ganglion block. However, their efficacy seems to approximate the spontaneous recovery rate.

Prognosis: Normal for life span and intelligence. Spontaneous recovery of nerve function occurs in 75–90% of cases. In some cases recovery is partial, resulting in synkinesis or only partial movement.

Detection of Carrier: Unknown.

Special Considerations: Careful electrodiagnostic testing and neurologic examination of patients are essential for accurate diagnosis and rational therapy.

References:
Danforth HB. Familial Bell's palsy. Ann Otol Rhinol Laryng. 1964; 73:179–183.

McGovern FH. A review of the experimental aspects of Bell's palsy. Laryngoscope. 1968; 78:324.

DeSanto LW, Schubert HA. Bell's palsy: ten cases in a family. Arch Otolaryngol. 1969; 89:700–702.

Sullivan JA, et al. Management of Bell's palsy. Arch Otolaryngol. 1969; 89:144.

Auerbach SH, Depiero TJ, Mejlszenkier J. Familial recurrent peripheral facial palsy: observations of the pediatric population. Arch Neurol. 1981; 38:463–464.

Markby DP: Lyme disease facial palsy: differentiation from Bell's palsy. Br Med J 1989; 299:605–606.

BE028   **LaVonne Bergstrom**

PALSY, PROGRESSIVE BULBAR OF CHILDHOOD   2045

Includes:
> Brown-Vialetto-Van Leare syndrome
> Bulbopontine paralysis, chronic-deafness
> Fazio-Londe disease
> Progressive bulbar palsy associated with neural deafness (PBPND)
> Progressive bulbar palsy of childhood (PBPC)

Excludes:
> **Amyotrophic lateral sclerosis, familial adult and juvenile types** (2069)
> Amyotrophy in multisystem disease
> **Arthrogryposes** (0088)
> **G(M2)-gangliosidosis with hexosaminidase A deficiency** (0434)
> Motor neuron disorders due to other causes
> Poliomyelitis and other viral encephalitides
> **Spinal muscular atrophy** (0895)

Major Diagnostic Criteria: Progressive paralysis of cranial nerve innervated muscles with or without upper motor neuron signs. EMG evidence of a diffuse neuropathic process in the absence of neuromuscular junction defect and exclusion of an infectious or neoplastic lesion helps to make the diagnosis of PBPC.

Clinical Findings: PBPC is probably not a single entity, and its symptomatology of progressive paralysis of cranial nerve innervated muscles is a common signature of different etiologic agents. Less than 20 cases of Fazio-Londe disease have been published. PBPC most frequently manifests as unilateral facial paralysis, followed in frequency by dysarthria associated with facial weakness, dysphagia and difficulty with chewing, palpebral ptosis, and palatal weakness. Progression to involve other cranial nerve innervated muscle occurs over a period of months or years. The facial nerve is affected in all cases, followed in frequency by the hypoglossal, vagus, trigeminal, spinal accessory, abducens, oculomotor, cochlear, and glossopharyngeal. Corticospinal tract involvement has been reported but may be rare. The disease may progress relentlessly to the patient's death in as short as nine months, or it may have a slower evolution with plateaus and the patient may live for more than eight years.

There are 20 cases of Brown-Vialetto-Van Leare (PBPND) disease (chronic bulbopontine paralysis with deafness) described in the world literature. Four autopsy reports are available. Clinical PBPND resembles Fazio-Londe disease except for sensorineural deafness (eighth nerve involvement) and usually, though not always, a more indolent course and a much more variable age of onset. Corticospinal tract involvement may be present.

PBPC must be diagnosed after the common causes of bulbar palsy in childhood are excluded. These include astrocytomas of the brain stem or extramedullary tumors, progressive myopathies, vascular malformations and congenital anomalies, cranial polyneuritis, brain stem encephalitis, myasthenia gravis or pseudobulbar palsy associated with perinatal hypoxia. Neuroimaging techniques, together with EMG examination, CSF examination, and antiacetylcholine receptor antibody titers usually help to differentiate these entities.

Complications: Muscle weakness interferes with basic functions of life, such as sucking of milk, breathing, and speaking. Motor milestones gained may be lost. Scoliosis develops in the more chronic cases. Hearing loss poses a problem in appropriate communication.

Associated Findings: **Retinitis pigmentosa** has been reported.

Etiology: Usually autosomal recessive inheritance. Patients with giant axonal neuropathy have been reported to have findings of PBPC. Nosologically, some cases with upper motor neuron findings and without extraocular muscle weakness may be diagnosed as juvenile-onset **Amyotrophic lateral sclerosis**, and others may be form-frustes of **Spinal muscular atrophy**. Dominant, recessive, and sporadic patterns of inheritance have been described in PBPC.

Pathogenesis: Degeneration of motor neurons of cranial nerve nuclei and sometimes spinal motor neurons. Corticospinal and spinocerebellar tracts may also be involved. The ventral portion of the cochlear nuclei shows severe neuronal loss in PBPND.

MIM No.: *21150

Sex Ratio: M1:F1

Occurrence: About 40 cases have been described in the literature.

Risk of Recurrence for Patient's Sib:
See Part I, *Mendelian Inheritance.*

Risk of Recurrence for Patient's Child:
See Part I, *Mendelian Inheritance.*

Age of Detectability: In Fazio-Londe disease, age of detectability may vary from one to 12 years, and in juvenile-onset disorder it may be even later. In PBPND, age of onset of sensorineural hearing defect may occur simultaneously with other bulbar and spinal symptoms or it may be separated from them by as many as three years. Sensorineural deafness may be present as early as the first year of life or as late as three years. In PBPND patients onset is before the age of 10 years.

Gene Mapping and Linkage: Unknown.

Prevention: None known. Genetic counseling indicated.

Treatment: Appropriate measures to ensure feeding. Respiration may have to be supported depending on the severity of involvement. A tracheostomy may help breathing in patients with vocal cord paralysis. Physical therapy measures for range of motion exercises to prevent contractions is indicated.

Prognosis: Some patients die within a year of onset of symptoms. Others may live longer, with long plateaus in the progression of illness.

Detection of Carrier: Unknown.

References:
Gomez MR: Progressive bulbar paralysis of childhood. In: Vinken PJ, Bruyn GW, eds: Handbook of clinical neurology. Amsterdam: North-Holland, 1975:103–109.
Latbrisseau A, et al.: Generalized giant axonal neuropathy: a case with features of Fazio-Londe disease. Neuropaediatrie 1979; 1:76–86.
Gallai V, et al.: Ponto-bulbar palsy with deafness (Brown-Vialetto-Van Leare syndrome). J Neurol Sci 1981; 50:259–275.
Albers JW, et al.: Juvenile progressive bulbar palsy: clinical and electrodiagnostic findings. Arch Neurol 1983; 40:351–353.

SI032   **Teepu Siddique**

PANCREAS, ANNULAR   0062

Includes:
Annular pancreas
Pancreas, malrotation of

Excludes: **Duodenum, atresia or stenosis** (0300)

Major Diagnostic Criteria: Intestinal obstruction with a "double bubble" gas pattern by X-ray, and demonstration of a collar of pancreas surrounding the duodenum at laparotomy.

Clinical Findings: All grades of obstruction ranging from complete duodenal obstruction in the neonate, associated with maternal hydramnios and with bile-stained vomiting, to intermittent

vomiting and failure to thrive. Nonobstructing forms may be found at operation or autopsy without symptoms.

Complications: Defective pancreatic drainage with pancreatitis later in life; occasional stasis ulcer of the duodenum with perforation into the annular pancreas; failure to thrive, secondary to occasional vomiting.

Associated Findings: **Chromosome 21, trisomy 21** occurs in 20–30% of patients with annular pancrease; anomalies in other organs in 40–50% of cases (Merrill and Raffensperger, 1976).

Etiology: Possibly autosomal dominant inheritance.

Pathogenesis: There are several versions of basic incomplete rotation of the dorsal and ventral anlagen of the pancreas so that portions of the pancreas remain on both sides of the second portion of the duodenum. The exact mode of formation of the defect is not known; perhaps several different variations in rotation may result in annular rings of the pancreas and various grades of obstruction. Several investigators believe that the obstruction when present is due to a stenosis of the duodenum and that there is no true constriction by the surrounding pancreas.

MIM No.: 16775

CDC No.: 751.720

Sex Ratio: Presumably M1:F1

Occurrence: 1:10,000 live births.

Risk of Recurrence for Patient's Sib:
See Part I, *Mendelian Inheritance.*

Risk of Recurrence for Patient's Child:
See Part I, *Mendelian Inheritance.*

Age of Detectability: At birth.

Gene Mapping and Linkage: Unknown.

Prevention: None known. Genetic counseling indicated.

Treatment: Duodenojejunostomy or duodenoduodenostomy should be performed. Cutting into pancreatic substance is dangerous, since it may produce a pancreatic fistula.

Prognosis: Excellent for relief of obstruction. There is normal life expectancy. Rarely, pancreatitis or biliary tract disease may occur in later life. Mortality is usually due to associated anomalies.

Detection of Carrier: Unknown.

References:
Merrill JR, Raffensperger JG: Pediatric annular pancreas: twenty year's experience. J Pediatr Surg 1976; 11:921–925.
Jackson LG, Apostolides P: Autosomal dominant inheritance of annular pancreas. Am J Med Genet 1978; 1:319–321.
MacFadyen UM, Young ID: Annular pancreas in mother and son (letter). Am J Med Genet 1987; 27:987–988.

SE006   **John H. Seashore**

PANCREATITIS, HEREDITARY   0793

Includes: Pancreatitis, familial

Excludes:
> Cystic fibrosis (0237)
> Pancreatitis, acute idiopathic
> Pancreatitis associated with hyperlipidemia or
> hyperparathyroidism

Major Diagnostic Criteria: Increased serum amylase and lipase during the acute phase of illness are diagnostic features of pancreatitis. Increased urinary amylase-to-creatinine clearance ratio helps confirm serum values, and should be performed when possible. Some patients will not have elevated enzyme tests, particularly those with advanced disease.

Calcifications distributed throughout the pancreas, especially if apparent in childhood, strongly suggest hereditary pancreatitis.

The diagnosis can be made if there is documentation of repeated episodes of acute pancreatitis and a family history of similar illness. Analysis of serum lipoproteins and evaluation of parathyroid function are necessary to exclude familial hyperlipidemia and hyperparathyroidism.

Clinical Findings: Hereditary pancreatitis presents with episodes of recurrent epigastric or abdominal pain that may radiate through to the back and subscapular area. The pain is often initiated by a large fatty or spicy meal. The attack progresses to maximal intensity in 24–48 hours and abates in four days to several weeks. Nausea and vomiting frequently accompany the pain and may result in serum electrolyte disturbances. Serum and urinary amylase and lipase will be elevated during the active phase. The attacks of acute pancreatitis are separated by symptom-free periods of days to years in duration. During the symptom-free periods there will be no disturbance in serum amylase and lipase.

In time, the repeated episodes of pancreatitis result in pancreatic fibrosis, with exocrine insufficiency (30–50%) or glucose intolerance (30%). Pancreatic exocrine insufficiency produces steatorrhea in most instances, but subclinical disease may be diagnosed by measurement of the pancreatic peptidases or lipase obtained at duodenal intubation. Secretin stimulation may provide another degree of discrimination of exocrine function.

Pancreatic calcifications observed on abdominal X-ray are of diagnostic importance. Some patients (50%) will exhibit coarse, rounded calcifications in the head of the pancreas. Linear distribution is consistent with the anatomic finding of calcifications in the major pancreatic ducts. CT scanning improves the sensitivity for detecting pancreatic calcifications.

Involvement of multiple family members has been documented in all series.

Complications: Acute dehydration and serum electrolyte disturbances (common in acute attacks); pancreatic exocrine insufficiency (often with steatorrhea); pancreatic endocrine insufficiency (glucose intolerance); pancreatic carcinoma (25%); portal or splenic vein thrombosis (rare); acute hemorrhagic pancreatitis (with or without hemorrhagic pleural and peritoneal effusions) (rare); and pancreatic pseudocyst.

Associated Findings: Aminoaciduria (cystine and lysine) has been documented in two families. Abnormal sweat electrolytes have been found in one family.

Etiology: Autosomal dominant inheritance with variable expressivity.

Pathogenesis: Unknown.

MIM No.: *16780

CDC No.: 751.780

Sex Ratio: M1:F1

Occurrence: About 400 known or suspected cases have been reported.

Risk of Recurrence for Patient's Sib:
See Part I, *Mendelian Inheritance.*

Risk of Recurrence for Patient's Child:
See Part I, *Mendelian Inheritance.*

Age of Detectability: The majority of cases have their onset in childhood, often in infancy.

Gene Mapping and Linkage: Unknown.

Prevention: None known. Genetic counseling indicated.

Treatment: Supportive measures during acute attacks include restorative and maintenance intravenous fluids and electrolytes, nothing orally, nasogastric suction; and narcotic pain medication. Enzyme replacement and a low-fat diet for pancreatic exocrine insufficiency. Appropriate measures for control of glucose intolerance.

Prognosis: Life expectancy is generally normal, if acute attacks are managed appropriately and if pancreatic carcinoma is not a complicating factor.

Detection of Carrier: Asymptomatic parents of affected individuals have been shown to have abnormalities in pancreatic exocrine function.

References:
Gross JB, et al.: Hereditary pancreatitis: description of a fifth kindred and summary of clinical features. Am J Med 1962; 33:358–364.
Kattwinkel J, et al.: Hereditary pancreatitis: three new kindreds and a critical review of the literature. Pediatrics 1973; 51:55–69.
Girard RM, et al.: Hereditary pancreatitis: report of an affected Canadian kindred and review of the disease. Can Med Asso J 1981; 125:576–580.
Dalton-Clark HJ, et al.: Familial chronic calcific pancreatitis: a family study. Br J Surg 1985; 72:307–308.

WH007   **Peter F. Whitington**

PANCYTOPENIA SYNDROME, FANCONI TYPE   2029

Includes:
> Estren-Dameshek variant of Fanconi anemia
> Fanconi anemia, I
> Fanconi pancytopenia, type I

Excludes:
> Anemia, hypoplastic congenital (0051)
> Anemia, hypoplastic-triphalangeal thumbs, Aase-Smith type (2028)
> Bloom syndrome (0112)
> Dyskeratosis congenita (2024)
> Thrombocytopenia-absent radius (0941)
> Thrombocytopenia-multiple malformations-neurologic dysfunction
> WT syndrome (3145)

Major Diagnostic Criteria: Progressive pancytopenia and spontaneous chromosome breakage, which worsens after exposure to bifunctional alkylating agents. Multiple congenital anomalies may occur, including low birth weight, abnormal skin pigmentation, skeletal deformities, kidney malformations, and hypogonadism. Variation in number and severity of anomalies precludes diagnosis on clinical grounds alone. Clinical diagnosis must be confirmed cytogenetically.

Clinical Findings: The usual symptoms relate to anemia or thrombocytopenia. Most affected children present with pallor, fatigue, bleeding, or easy bruisability. The history reveals that the child was small for gestational age and had congenital anomalies. Review of 155 patients with Fanconi anemia showed that 76% of probands had hyperpigmentation, café-au-lait spots, or both; 65% were of small stature for age; 40% had thumb anomalies (aplasia, hypoplasia, supernumerary); 30% were microcephalic, 31% had renal anomalies (including absent kidney, duplication of the kidney or collecting system, renal ectopia, or a horseshoe kidney); 28% had other skeletal malformations (most commonly of the skull, spine, and extremities), 23% had strabismus; 20% hyperreflexia; 19% microophthalmia; 18% mental retardation; 12% ear anomalies or deafness; and 7% congenital heart disease. Absence of congenital anomalies, however, does not rule out a diagnosis of Fanconi anemia. In a study of 44 affected siblings of probands,

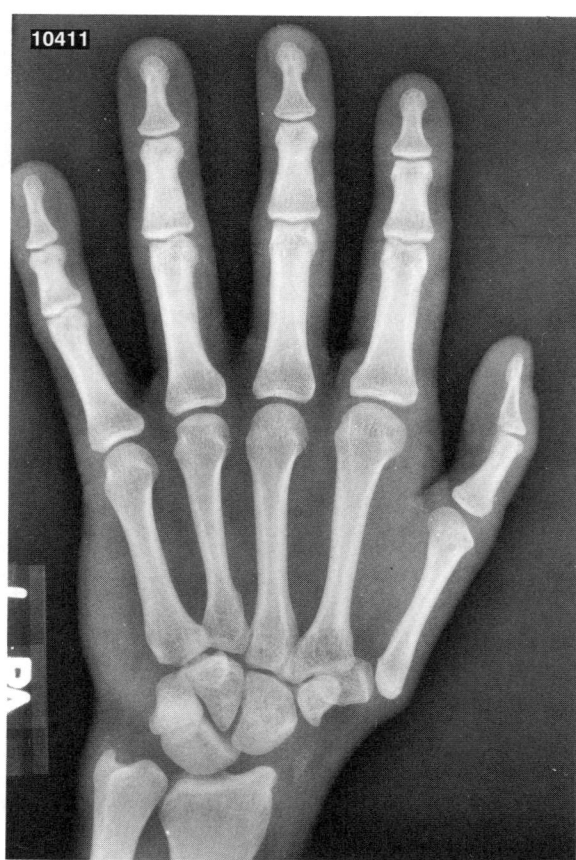

2029-10411: Hypoplastic 1st metacarpal and phalanges of thumb; absent navicular.

25% had no dysmorphic features. There may be wide clinical variability, even within families.

Anemia characteristically develops in early to mid-childhood. Laboratory findings may include macrocytosis, mild poikilocytosis, mild anisocytosis, leukopenia, thrombocytopenia, and reticulocytopenia. The stressed hypocellular bone marrow will produce erythrocytes with fetal-like qualities (expressing i surface antigen and containing fetal hemoglobin).

The most specific laboratory finding for Fanconi anemia is in the metaphase chromosomes of affected individuals. Typical abnormalities include chromatid breaks, gaps, chromosome rearrangements, endoreduplication, or formation of triradials or quadriradials. In an affected patient, the number of abnormalities will dramatically increase after cells have been exposed to the difunctional alkylating agents mitomycin C or diepoxybutane. Because of the low mitotic index often seen in cells from patients with Fanconi anemia, additional methods of diagnosis have been developed using flow cytometry and DNA histograms. After exposure to mitomycin C, Fanconi cells will characteristically accumulate in the G_2 phase of the cell cycle.

Complications: Recurrent infections, growth hormone deficiency, cryptorchidism, primary testicular failure, hepatomas (may be reversible), peliosis hepatis, unusual sensitivity to chemotherapeutic agents used to prepare for bone marrow transplantation, and severe graft-vs-host disease following bone marrow transplantation.

Associated Findings: Acute nonlymphatic leukemia, hepatocellular carcinoma, squamous cell carcinomas. Leukemia is the terminal event in 5–10% of patients with Fanconi anemia. It was formerly thought that Fanconi anemia heterozygotes were at increased risk for developing malignancies. This has now been disproved.

Etiology: Autosomal recessive inheritance. Heterogeneity is postulated.

Pathogenesis: Fanconi anemia is the most common heritable aplastic anemia. If all cases of childhood aplastic anemia are taken together, approximately one-fifth will be diagnosed as Fanconi anemia. The association between the bone marrow failure and the congenital anomalies is not understood but is presumed to be related to simultaneous developmental events occurring at 25–34 days gestation. Fanconi anemia is possibly a hematopoietic stem cell disorder. Cultures of bone marrow cells from Fanconi patients reveal markedly decreased or absent progenitor cells (CFU-C, CFU-E, BFU-E). The biochemical basis for the enhanced sensitivity to DNA cross-linking agents is unknown, but it is hypothesized to be due to abnormal DNA repair mechanisms. Recent experiments have shown that the subcellular distribution of topoisomerase (a DNA-related enzyme) is different in Fanconi placental cells when compared with normals. In Fanconi patients, the DNA topoisomerase activity is high in the cytoplasm, where it is produced, but low in the nucleus, where it is utilized for DNA repair. Other experiments have shown that mitomycin-C-treated Fanconi cells, when fused with normal fibroblasts, have a decreased number of chromosome abnormalities. This implies production of a clastogenic factor by the Fanconi cells.

MIM No.: *22765

POS No.: 3234

Sex Ratio: M1.9:F1

Occurrence: Heterozygote frequency has been estimated at between 1:300 and 1:600. Most of the reported cases have been in whites, although Black, Oriental, Turkish, Arab, and Indian patients have been described. The incidence among white Afrikaans-speaking South Africans is particularly high, with the heterozygote prevalence calculated at about 1:77, and a birth incidence of 1:22,000.

Risk of Recurrence for Patient's Sib:
See Part I, *Mendelian Inheritance.*

Risk of Recurrence for Patient's Child:
See Part I, *Mendelian Inheritance.* If an affected patient marries a Fanconi heterozygote, half of the offspring will be affected. Risk = 1/300 x 1/2 = 0.16%.

Age of Detectability: Rarely present at birth. The onset of pancytopenia is slightly earlier in males than in females. Median age for clinical diagnosis in a male is six years; median age in a female is 7 1/2 years. For males, 90% are diagnosed by age 12 years; in females, 90% are diagnosed by age 14 years. Ultrasound may be helpful in detecting skeletal, renal, or cardiac anomalies.

Diagnosis is available at birth or prenatally. Amniotic fluid cells, fetal blood lymphocytes, and chorionic villus cells, when treated with diepoxybutane, reveal increased chromosome breakage and rearrangements as compared with controls. First trimester prenatal diagnosis based on clastogen-induced chromosomal breakage is now available (Auerbach et al, 1986).

Gene Mapping and Linkage: FA (Fanconi anemia) is unassigned.

Prevention: None known. Genetic counseling indicated.

Treatment: Support with specific transfusions of red cells, white cells, and platelets. Splenectomy is not indicated. Androgen therapy causes definite improvement in blood counts but will have masculinizing side effects. Bone marrow transplantation is a potential form of treatment, although studies have indicated that Fanconi patients are unusually sensitive to chemotherapeutic agents and have a severe problem with graft-vs-host disease.

Prognosis: In older studies, an overall 80% mortality by age 12 years. Survival is prolonged with androgen therapy. An association between androgen therapy and the subsequent development of hepatocellular carcinoma has not been proved. Fanconi anemia patients usually die of bleeding, intercurrent infection, or malignancy.

Detection of Carrier: In one study, lymphocytes from parents and siblings exhibited a significantly increased diepoxybutane-induced chromosome breakage compared with normal subjects.

Special Considerations: This condition should be distinguished from *Thrombocytopenia-multiple malformations-neurologic dysfunction* (Gardner et al, 1983).

Support Groups: OR; Eugene; Fanconi Anemia Support Group

References:

Fanconi G: Familial constitutional panmyelocytopathy, Fanconi's anemia. I. Clinical aspects. Seminars in Hematology 1967; 4:233–240.

Schroeder TM, et al.: Formal genetics of Fanconi's anemia. Hum Genet 1976; 32:257–288.

Glanz A, Fraser FC: Spectrum of anomalies in Fanconi anemia. J Med Genet 1982; 19:412–416. *

Latts A, et al.: Cytogenetic and flow cytometric studies of cells from patients with Fanconi's anemia. Cytogenet Cell Genet 1982; 33:133–138.

Alter BP, Potter NU: Long-term outcome in Fanconi's anemia: description of 26 cases and review of the literature. In: German J, ed: Chromosome mutation and neoplasia. New York: Alan R. Liss, 1983:43–62. *

Deeg HJ, et al.: Fanconi's anemia treated by allogeneic marrow transplantation. Blood 1983; 61:954–959.

Gardner RJM, et al.: A syndrome of congenital thrombocytopenia with multiple malformations and neurologic dysfunction. J Pediatr 1983; 102:600–603.

Duckworth-Rysiecki G, et al.: Clinical and cytogenetic diversity in Fanconi's anemia. J Med Genet 1984; 21:197–203.

Auerbach AD, et al.: Clastogen-induced chromosomal breakage as a marker for first trimester prenatal diagnosis of Fanconi anemia. Hum Genet 1986; 73:86–88.

Rosendorff J, et al.: Fanconi anemia: another disease of unusually high prevalence in the Afrikaans population of South Africa. Am J Med Genet 1987; 27:793–797.

Schweiger M, et al.: DNA repair in human cells: biochemistry of the hereditary diseases Fanconi's anemia and Cockayne syndrome. Eur J Biochem 1987; 165:235–242.

BIOO1   **Diana W. Bianchi**

PAPILLOMA VIRUS, CONGENITAL INFECTION   2965

Includes:
   Anogenital warts, congenital
   Condylomata acuminata, congenital
   Fetal effects from papilloma virus
   Laryngeal papillomatosis, juvenile
   Papilloma virus infection, congenital susceptibility
   Recurrent respiratory papillomatosis
   Respiratory papillomatosis, juvenile

Excludes:
   Common warts (verruca vulgaris)
   Condylomata lata
   Plane warts (verruca plana)
   Plantar warts (verruca plantaris)

Major Diagnostic Criteria: Multiple respiratory papillomas or anogenital condylomata that are either present at birth or detected during infancy or early childhood. Histopathologic examination of excised tissues can confirm the clinical diagnosis. The specific human papillomavirus (HPV) involved can be determined by DNA hybridization studies.

Clinical Findings: All areas of the respiratory tract are susceptible to HPV infection. The larynx is the most commonly involved site, but as many as 15% of patients with recurrent respiratory papillomatosis have no apparent laryngeal lesions. Suggestive symptoms may be present from birth, but the diagnosis is not usually made until later. About 15% of patients have onset of their disease during the first year of life, about 30–50% by age five years, but over one third of all patients initially present after age 20 years (adult onset). Presenting symptoms of recurrent respiratory papillomatosis may include hoarseness, abnormal cry, aphonia, stridor or dyspnea. A history of maternal genital warts can be elicited in at least one half of all patients with juvenile-onset disease.

Laryngeal papillomas are usually multiple. They typically regrow after surgical removal, and recurrences may occur within periods as short as 2–3 weeks or as long as several years. DNA hybridization studies have also demonstrated that clinically uninvolved laryngeal sites may harbor a latent HPV infection. Distal extension of papillomas into the trachea has been noted in as many as one third of all patients, but pulmonary involvement is uncommon. Spontaneous remissions of laryngeal papillomas occur in most patients, but their durations are variable.

Laryngeal papillomas can be visualized at endoscopy and the diagnosis confirmed by pathologic examination of excised tissues. Histologically, the lesions are benign squamous papillomas. The presence of koilocytes is indicative of HPV infection. In some patients, HPV particles can be visualized by electron microscopy or detected by immunoperoxidase staining of tissues using antibodies against a genus-specific antigen. DNA hybridization studies are needed to determine the specific HPV type involved.

The moist mucosal surfaces of the anogenital area are also susceptible to HPV infection. The characteristic abnormalities, or condylomata acuminata, are clusters of soft cauliflower-like lesions involving the vulva, perianal area, and, less commonly, the vagina, urethral meatus, or rectum. They may also involve the conjunctiva, mouth, axilla, or umbilicus. A latent HPV infection in clinically and histologically normal sites that are in close proximity to condylomatous lesions may also be present. Condylomata acuminata are uncommon in children and when encountered should arouse the suspicion of sexual abuse. However, several cases with disease onset in the newborn period or early infancy are documented in the literature, suggesting intrauterine or intrapartum transmission. A history of maternal genital warts during pregnancy is commonly elicited. Many condylomata acuminata regress spontaneously.

The diagnosis of condyloma acuminatum is usually based on its typical gross morphology. Cervical lesions are often flat growths and require colposcopy for visualization. The diagnosis is based on characteristic histologic and cytologic features. DNA hybridization is required to establish a specific HPV type as the etiologic agent.

Complications: The most feared complication of recurrent respiratory papillomatosis is life-threatening airway obstruction. Malignant transformation of respiratory papillomas is uncommon, but the risk appears higher for patients with prolonged and widespread disease. Although malignant changes are more likely in patients receiving radiation therapy for their disease, this complication also occurs in those not receiving this treatment. Psychosocial complications may include communication difficulties and poor school performance.

Complications of condylomata acuminata may include ulceration, secondary infection, and bleeding. A more serious complication is that of malignant transformation, but the magnitude of this risk is unknown. HPVs have been associated with a variety of genital tract malignancies, including cervical, vulvar, and anorectal carcinomas. Condylomata acuminata may also enlarge during pregnancy to an extent that hampers vaginal delivery. These lesions typically regress after delivery.

Associated Findings: None known.

Etiology: Both juvenile- and adult-onset respiratory papillomas are associated with infection by HPV types 6 or 11. On the other hand, carcinoma of the larynx may be rarely associated with infection by HPV types 11, 16 or 30.

Condylomata acuminata are most commonly caused by HPV types 6 or 11. HPV types 16, 18, or 31 are found almost exclusively in patients with genital carcinoma.

Recurrent conjunctival papillomatosis has been associated with HPV types 6, 11, and 16.

Associations between chromosome 12 and HPV 18 integration sites have been reported.

Pathogenesis: Intrauterine transmission of HPV may occur, since some patients with recurrent respiratory papillomatosis have disease symptoms at birth and at least one newborn with congenital condylomata acuminata has been described in the literature. Viremia is not known to occur with HPV infection, thereby favoring the idea of an ascending route of transmission for these patients. Intrapartum acquisition of HPV appears to be a more significant pathway of infection because over one-half of the patients with juvenile-onset recurrent respiratory papillomatosis have a history of maternal genital warts but only very rarely a history of cesarean delivery. Postnatal transmission of HPV is theoretically possible but unlikely for patients with juvenile-onset respiratory disease. The pathogenesis of adult-onset disease is not understood at the present time. Comparable information for condylomata acuminata presenting in the neonatal period or early infancy is not available.

MIM No.: 16796

Sex Ratio: Presumably M1:F1, although there appears to be a slight preponderance of males among reported cases.

Occurrence: Condylomata acuminata may be found in 0.2% of pregnant women in the United States. However, clinically inapparent cervical HPV infection has been found in as many as 29% of pregnant women in Germany. Foreskins from 70 unselected newborns analyzed by dot blot hybridization revealed that at least 4% contained HPV DNA. About 1,500 new cases of recurrent respiratory papillomatosis are diagnosed each year in the United States.

Risk of Recurrence for Patient's Sib: Unknown.

Risk of Recurrence for Patient's Child: Unknown.

Age of Detectability: Recurrent respiratory papillomatosis may occur at any age, but about one-half of the patients have disease onset by age five years. Condylomata acuminata may be present at birth or first manifest during infancy. Lesions appearing later in childhood or adolescence are due to postnatal acquisition of HPV.

Gene Mapping and Linkage: Unknown.

Prevention: Delivery by cesarean section for mothers with genital HPV infection would theoretically be helpful, but this has not been studied to date. This method would not prevent cases resulting from intrauterine or postnatal infection by HPV.

Treatment: Surgical excision of respiratory papillomas using the carbon dioxide laser. Tracheostomy is sometimes needed to maintain an open airway. Data suggest that the beneficial effect of alpha-interferon in inducing clinical remission is not sustained.

The preferred treatment of condylomata acuminata varies with the age of the patient and extent of the lesions. Carbon dioxide laser therapy, cryosurgery, electrodesiccation and curettage, surgical excision, and podophyllin are commonly used therapeutic modalities. The local injection of interferon alpha-2b or autogenous vaccine has been reported to be beneficial in adults.

Prognosis: Respiratory papillomas typically recur after variable periods of time following their removal, thereby necessitating repeated surgical procedures. About one-half of the patients suffer management-related complications such as the development of mucosal webs, hemorrhage, and vocal cord scarring. Extension of disease into the lung parenchyma is rare and carries a poor prognosis, with a mortality rate of about 40%. Spontaneous remissions for variable periods of time are seen in many patients. Malignant transformation is rare but may worsen the prognosis.

The frequency of either spontaneous regression or malignant transformation of anogenital warts is not known.

Detection of Carrier: Visual inspection, colposcopy, cytology, and histopathologic examination of biopsy specimens can all be used to detect women with genital HPV infection. DNA hybridization can also detect clinically and histologically inapparent HPV infection in biopsied tissues. Preliminary data indicate that the polymerase chain reaction can be used to increase the frequency of HPV detection in biopsied tissues, swab specimens, and urine from infected individuals.

Special Considerations: An accurate estimate of the risk of HPV infection for an infant delivered through an infected birth canal is not available. When one considers the high prevalence of genital HPV infection in pregnant women and the low incidence of clinically apparent recurrent respiratory papillomatosis, the risk appears small. DNA hybridization studies are revolutionizing the understanding of the epidemiology, pathogenesis, and natural history of HPV infection and will undoubtedly resolve many of the currently unanswered questions.

References:

Tang C-K, et al.: Congenital condylomata acuminata. Am J Obstet Gynecol 1978; 131:912–913.

De Jong AR, et al.: Condyloma acuminata in children. Am J Dis Child 1982; 136:704–706.

Mounts P, Shah KV: Respiratory papillomatosis: etiological relation to genital tract papillomaviruses. Prog Med Virol 1984; 29:90–114. *

Roman A, Fife K: Human papillomavirus DNA associated with foreskins of normal newborns. J Infect Dis 1986; 153:855–861.

Shah K, et al.: Rarity of cesarean delivery in cases of juvenile-onset respiratory papillomatosis. Obstet Gynecol 1986; 68:795–799.

Byrne JC, et al.: Human papillomavirus-11 DNA in a patient with chronic laryngotracheobronchial papillomatosis and metastatic squamous-cell carcinoma of the lung. New Engl J Med 1987; 317:873–878.

Popescu NC, et al.: Human papillomavirus type 18 DNA is integrated at a single chromosome site in cervical carcinoma cell line SW756. J Virol 1987; 61:1682–1685.

Healy GB, et al.: Treatment of recurrent respiratory papillomatosis with human leukocyte interferon: results of a multicenter randomized clinical trial. New Engl J Med 1988; 319:401–407.

Davis AJ, Emans SJ: Human papilloma virus infection in the pediatric and adolescent patient. J Pediatr 1989; 115:1–9. *

Young LS, et al.: The polymerase chain reaction: a new epidemiological tool for investigating cervical human papillomavirus infection. Br Med J 1989; 298:14–18.

FR039
SE021

Bishara J. Freij
John L. Sever

PARALYSIS, HYPERKALEMIC PERIODIC 0794

Includes:
Adynamia episodica hereditaria
Hyperkalemic periodic paralysis
Periodic paralysis, II
Periodic paralysis, hyperpotassemic

Excludes:
Paralysis, hypokalemic periodic (0795)
Paralysis, normokalemic periodic (2050)
Paramyotonia congenita (0796)

Major Diagnostic Criteria: Attacks of paralysis associated with elevated serum potassium. Positive family history.

Clinical Findings: The condition is usually first detected by the parents in infancy or in childhood. Affected children have episodes during which they become unusually floppy and move poorly. Onset may be delayed till adulthood, and onset up to 31 years of age has been reported. The frequency of attacks varies between once a week to several mild attacks a day. Most attacks have a short duration, 30–60 minutes. Weakness is usually noticed first in the lower back, thighs, and calves, then spreads to arms and neck. Rarely, there may be difficulty in swallowing and coughing. Clinical myotonia, especially eyelid myotonia, may be a diagnostic clue for the condition. This is characterized by slow opening of the eyelids after forced active closure of the eyes. Myotonic symptoms are not present in all patients.

The paralytic attacks are usually provoked by rest after exercise, but unlike the hypokalemic form, the weakness develops in a shorter period of time (average duration is 30 minutes). One patient became weak when resting after swimming. Sometimes the patients may be able to "walk off" the symptoms early in an attack. This postponement of an attack seems to be only temporary, and the maneuver is sometimes associated with the development of muscle cramps. Factors other than exercise that can precipitate clinical attacks include emotion, cold, hunger, infection, and general anesthesia. This condition may also worsen during pregnancy.

Physical evaluation during the attacks shows variable weakness, usually more prominent in the proximal muscles. Severe flaccid quadriplegia is less frequently seen than in the hypokalemic type. Deep tendon reflexes are diminished or absent in severe attacks.

Physical evaluation between attacks usually shows no abnormality early in life. However, a proximal myopathy with permanent weakness develops later in many patients. The weakness affects pelvic muscles and then spreads to shoulder muscles. Occasionally a wheelchair is needed. Potentially fatal cardiac dysrhythmia with sudden death was described in several families with hyperkalemic periodic paralysis.

Laboratory findings include a rise in serum potassium during attacks. Affected persons appear to be hypersensitive to changes in serum potassium concentration, because weakness develops at lower levels than in normal individuals. Between attacks the serum potassium is normal. An abnormally high serum potassium level between attacks suggests secondary rather than primary hyperkalemic periodic paralysis. The electrocardiogram shows an increase in amplitude of precordial T waves during the attacks, consistent with hyperkalemia. Permanent bidirectional ventricular tachydysrythmia was reported in two patients. Electromyography may show myotonic discharges. During an attack, the muscle is inexcitable. The serum creatine kinase may be elevated. Muscle biopsy shows myopathic changes, particularly in advanced cases. Variability in the size of muscle fibers, increased numbers of internal nuclei, vacuoles, and tubular aggregates were described. Decreased potassium levels in the muscle and an increase in the sodium, water, and chloride contents were reported.

Oral administration of potassium chloride (0.10 g per kg body weight) under electrocardiographic monitoring induces a paralytic attack within 90–180 minutes and supports the clinical diagnosis.

Complications: Dysphagia with aspiration pneumonitis, and occasionally marked hypoventilation during attacks.

Associated Findings: Progressive myopathy with severe weakness may develop late in life.

Etiology: Autosomal dominant inheritance with high penetrance in both sexes.

Pathogenesis: Undetermined, but may involve an alteration of sodium-potassium ion transport mechanisms across the defective muscle cell membrane. Recent electrophysiologic studies in myotonic and nonmyotonic hyperkalemic periodic paralysis suggest that the failure of propagation of action potentials in the paralytic attacks may be related to the abnormality of the sodium-potassium pump.

MIM No.: *17050

Sex Ratio: Presumably M1:F1.

Occurrence: The hyperkalemic type is the second most frequent of the periodic paralyses. The incidence in Sweden is 0.2: 1,000,000. Two Swedish kinships alone accounted for 138 patients in five generations.

Risk of Recurrence for Patient's Sib:
See Part I, *Mendelian Inheritance.*

Risk of Recurrence for Patient's Child:
See Part I, *Mendelian Inheritance.*

Age of Detectability: Usually in infancy or early childhood.

Gene Mapping and Linkage: Unknown.

Prevention: None known. Genetic counseling indicated.

Treatment: The acute attack can be treated with calcium gluconate (0.5–2 g given intravenously), glucose by mouth (2 g per kg of body weight), insulin (15–20 units subcutaneously), or beta-adrenergic agents (1.3 mg metaproterenol inhalation).

Preventive therapy consists of frequent meals of high carbohydrate content; avoidance of fasting, exposure to cold or overexertion, and diuretic agents such as acetazolamide or thiazides. The lowest dose of diuretic required to prevent attack should be used, and the dose should not lower the serum potassium below 3.7 mEq/liter.

Prognosis: Generally good for life span, although a very small percentage (less than 1%) of patients may die during a paralytic attack. Myopathic patients with permanent weakness may have a severe motor handicap.

Detection of Carrier: By inducing attacks with potassium chloride loading test or by demonstration of myotonia.

Special Considerations: Heterogeneity may exist within the clinical entities corresponding to myotonic and nonmyotonic types of hyperkalemic periodic paralysis.

References:
Gamstorp I: Adynamia episodica hereditaria. Acta Paediatr Scand 1956; 45(suppl 108):1–126. *
Lehmann-Horn F, et al.: Two cases of adynamia episodica hereditaria: in vitro investigation of muscle cell membrane and contraction parameters. Muscle Nerve 1983; 6:113–120.
Bendheim PE, et al.: Beta-adrenergic treatment of hyperkalemic periodic paralysis. Neurology 1985; 35:746–749.
Gould RJ, et al.: Potentially fatal cardiac dysrhythmia and hyperkalemic periodic paralysis. Neurology 1985; 35:1208–1212.
Lehmann-Horn F, et al.: Adynamia episodica hereditaria with myotonia: a non-inactivating sodium current and the effect of extracellular pH. Muscle Nerve 1987; 10:363–374.

I0000

Victor V. Ionasescu

PARALYSIS, HYPOKALEMIC PERIODIC　　0795

Includes:
> Hypokalemic periodic paralysis
> Periodic paralysis, II
> Periodic paralysis, familial
> Periodic paralysis, hypopotassemic

Excludes:
> **Paralysis, hyperkalemic periodic** (0794)
> **Paralysis, normokalemic periodic** (2050)
> **Paramyotonia congenita** (0796)

Major Diagnostic Criteria: Attacks of paralysis in conjunction with lowered serum potassium levels. Positive family history.

Clinical Findings: This disorder is characterized by attacks of flaccid quadriplegia lasting usually several hours and frequently occurring in the early morning. The muscles of speech, deglutition, and respiration are usually spared. The attacks begin in the second decade of life and are most frequent between the ages of 20 and 35 years, after which they tend to decrease in number and severity, and may completely disappear. The weakness can vary in severity from mild to almost complete paralysis of the neck, trunk, and extremities. Most moderate attacks last 6–24 hours, but severe paralysis may last for 2–3 days or longer. It is characteristic for the lower limbs to be affected first, then the arms, the trunk, and finally the neck. The proximal muscles of the limbs are the first to be affected, while the distal muscles (hands, feet) can move slightly even in severe attacks. The most important predisposing factors are prolonged rest after vigorous exercise and large carbohydrate meals. The plasma potassium falls coincidentally with the development of an attack. Administration of glucose or glucose and insulin leads to hypopotassemia and induces a paralytic attack. Death occurs rarely in an attack.

Examination during an attack shows flaccid paralysis, predominantly in the proximal muscles. The paralyzed muscles fail to respond to direct mechanical or electrical stimulation. The EKG shows bradycardia, prominent U waves, and flattening of the T waves in conjunction with the lowered serum potassium to the level of 2.0 to 2.5 mEq/liter. Muscle biopsy performed during paralytic attack shows multiple vacuoles of the muscle fibers and alterations of the sarcoplasmic reticulum.

Between attacks, patient's strength and serum potassium are within the normal range. Older patients frequently show some degree of proximal limb weakness and atrophy, with nonvacuolar myopathy at biopsy.

Complications: During attacks, severe dysphagia with aspiration pneumonitis and respiratory failure from intercostal weakness may occur.

Associated Findings: A slowly progressive myopathy with proximal weakness may develop late in life after the paralytic attacks have almost completely disappeared.

Etiology: Autosomal dominant inheritance with complete penetrance in males. Cases have been reported in up to six consecutive generations. There is a sex limitation, with frequent failure of manifestation in females in whom the disease, when it occurs, tends to be milder. Less than 10% female patients were reported in several kindreds. For this reason, X-linked recessive inheritance has been discussed in some families in which only male patients were noticed. Hypokalemic periodic paralysis occurs also as a rare, probably genetically determined, complication of thyrotoxicosis.

Pathogenesis: A shift of potassium, sodium, chloride and phosphate ions, and water into muscle has been documented during hypopotassemic attacks. Most likely, the fluid and electrolyte movements are caused by a defect in the muscle membrane with increased sodium permeability. Both the surface membrane of muscle and the T tubules, which represent an inward extension of the surface membrane, fail to conduct an action potential during attacks. The abnormal electrolyte shifts and the electrical inexcitability of the muscle fiber may influence the development of the permanent late myopathy.

MIM No.: *17040

Sex Ratio: M1:F<1

Occurrence: The hypokalemic is the most frequent type of periodic paralysis. The incidence in Denmark is 0.8:1,000,000. The association of hypokalemic variant and hyperthyroidism is higher in Japanese and Chinese patients.

Risk of Recurrence for Patient's Sib:
> See Part I, *Mendelian Inheritance*. Risk 1:2 to 1:10 for female.

Risk of Recurrence for Patient's Child:
> See Part I, *Mendelian Inheritance*. Risk 1:2 to 1:10 for female.

Age of Detectability: Usually by the second decade of life.

Gene Mapping and Linkage: Unknown.

Prevention: None known. Genetic counseling indicated.

Treatment: Paralysis is reversible during an attack by oral administration of 10 g potassium chloride for an adult. If the patient shows no signs of recovery after 3 to 4 hours, the dose may be repeated. Preventive therapy consists of a relatively low-sodium (2–3 g per day) and low-carbohydrate (60 to 80 g per day) diet and supplemental oral doses of potassium chloride, 2.5 g per day as 10% aqueous solution. Acetazolamide (up to 1 g per day) is the drug of choice in preventing paralytic attacks. Spironolactone and diazoxide are also used prophylactically.

Prognosis: Generally good for life span, but about 2–5% of the patients may die in a severe attack. Permanent late onset myopathy with physical handicap due to weakness and muscle atrophy is relatively common in older patients.

Detection of Carrier: Oral administration of glucose (2 g per kg of body weight) combined with 10 to 20 units of crystalline insulin given subcutaneously may precipitate an attack of weakness within 2 to 3 hours in an otherwise asymptomatic carrier.

References:
Johnsen T: Familial periodic paralysis with hypokalaemia: experimental and clinical investigations. Dan Med Bull 1981; 28:1–27. *
Rudel R, et al.: Hypokalemic periodic paralysis: in vitro investigation of muscle fiber membrane parameters. Muscle Nerve 1984; 7:110–120.
Buruma OJS, et al.: Familial hypokalemic periodic paralysis: 50 year follow-up of a large family. Arch Neurol 1985; 42:28–31.

I0000　　　　　　　　　　　　　　　**Victor V. Ionasescu**

PARALYSIS, NORMOKALEMIC PERIODIC　　2050

Includes:
> Normokalemic periodic paralysis
> Periodic paralysis, normopotassemic
> Periodic paralysis, III

Excludes:
> **Paralysis, hyperkalemic periodic** (0794)
> **Paralysis, hypokalemic periodic** (0795)
> **Paramyotonia congenita** (0796)

Major Diagnostic Criteria: Attacks of paralysis with normal serum potassium levels. Positive family history.

Clinical Findings: Twenty-one of 45 members were affected in the kinship originally described. The paralytic attacks began in the first decade and were provoked by rest after exercise, exposure to cold, alcohol in excess and potassium loading. The episodes of weakness occurred at intervals of one to three months lasting from two days to three weeks, often of a severe degree, including quadriplegia and weakness of the muscles of mastication but excluding facial expression, bladder and bowel function, and respiration. Large doses of sodium chloride improved the weakness. The urinary potassium retention, lack of a beneficial effect of glucose, and failure of the serum potassium to increase in attacks distinguished this disease from primary hyperkalemic periodic paralysis.

The diagnosis of normokalemic periodic paralysis was also well documented in another kinship in which a mother and her son were affected. In that family, paralysis was not provoked by lowering the serum potassium to 2 mEq/liter by glucose and insulin or by raising the serum potassium level to 6.6 mEq/liter by oral potassium loading. The resistance to the potassium loading test distinguished this kinship from the previous one.

Physical examination between attacks was normal in all patients. There was no evidence of weakness, myotonia, or changes of reflexes. Weakness during the attacks sometimes involved selective muscles, such as calf muscles and arm extensors. Reflexes were reduced or absent.

Electromyography during a paralytic attack in one patient showed mostly a myopathic pattern (full interference with greatly reduced amplitude). There were several large motor units, which raised the possibility of an associated neurogenic lesion. Motor nerve conduction velocities were normal. Muscle biopsy obtained at the height of an episode of paralysis demonstrated vacuolation of muscle fibers and focal areas of muscle degeneration. Some patients also showed tubular aggregates by electron microscopy, suggesting proliferation of the reticular system of the muscle. Serum creatine kinase was elevated during the paretic attacks in several cases.

There were doubts in the literature about the distinctness of the normokalemic and hyperkalemic types, because some patients with normokalemic periodic paralysis had positive potassium loading test.

Complications: Unknown.

Associated Findings: None known.

Etiology: Autosomal dominant inheritance with complete penetrance.

Pathogenesis: A defect in the membrane of the sarcoplasmic reticulum has been postulated.

MIM No.: *17060

Sex Ratio: Presumably M1:F1.

Occurrence: The incidence is 1:100,000 population in the area of Newcastle upon Tyne, England. Undetermined elsewhere, but presumed rare.

Risk of Recurrence for Patient's Sib:
See Part I, *Mendelian Inheritance.*

Risk of Recurrence for Patient's Child:
See Part I, *Mendelian Inheritance.*

Age of Detectability: In the first decade of life.

Gene Mapping and Linkage: Unknown.

Prevention: None known. Genetic counseling indicated.

Treatment: Sodium chloride taken at the onset of an attack will reduce its severity or shorten it. Severe attacks when fully developed may no longer be responsive to this form of therapy. Combination of 9-alpha-fluoro-hydrocortisone and acetazolamide has proved effective in preventing attacks in several cases.

Prognosis: Generally good for life span. There were no reports of patients dying during a paralytic attack. The episodic weakness becomes milder and occurs less frequently with age.

Detection of Carrier: In families with weakness triggered by potassium chloride, attacks can be induced with the potassium chloride loading test.

References:
Poskanzer DC, Kerr DNS: A third type of periodic paralysis with normokalemia and favorable response to sodium chloride. Am J Med 1961; 31:328–342. *
Meyers KR, et al.: Periodic muscle weakness, normokalemia and tubular aggregates. Neurology 1972; 22:269–279. *
Danowski TS, et al.: Clinical and ultrastructural observations in a kindred with normo-hyperkalemic periodic paralysis. J Med Genet 1975; 12:20–28.
Rudel R: The pathophysiologic basis of the myotonias and of the periodic paralyses. In: Engel AG, Banker BQ, eds: Myology. New York: McGraw-Hill, 1986:1297–1319.

I0000   **Victor V. Ionasescu**

Paralysis, periodica hypokaliemica
See PARALYSIS, HYPOKALEMIC PERIODIC

Parana hard skin syndrome
See SKIN, PARANA HARD SKIN SYNDROME
Paramedian lower lip pits-popliteal pterygium
See PTERYGIUM SYNDROME, POPLITEAL
Paramedian pits of lower lip (isolated trait)
See LIP, PITS OR MOUNDS
Paramethadione, fetal effects of
See FETAL TRIMETHADIONE SYNDROME
Paramolar
See TEETH, SUPERNUMERARY

PARAMYOTONIA CONGENITA   0796

Includes:
Eulenburg disease
Myotonia congenita intermittens
Paralysis periodica paramyotonica
von Eulenburg paramyotonia congenita

Excludes:
Myotonia in other syndromes or conditions
Myotonic dystrophy (0702)
Nephrosis, familial type (0710)
Paralysis, hyperkalemic periodic (0794)

Major Diagnostic Criteria: Myotonia is induced or aggravated by cold. Positive family history.

Clinical Findings: This condition is manifested mainly by myotonia worsened after exposure to cold. There is predilection of the myotonia for facial, lingual, and hand muscles. Myotonia is also aggravated by repeated muscle contraction (paradoxical myotonia). In addition, some of the patients experience attacks of flaccid weakness after exercise or after cold exposure, accompanied by increased serum potassium. The condition is usually evident in infancy, is not progressive, does not affect life expectancy and does not interfere with a reasonably normal social and economic life. Dystrophic features are not present.

Paramyotonia is distinguished from myotonia congenita by the attacks of muscular weakness. The paralytic attacks are quite similar to those that occur in hyperkalemic periodic paralysis. Several authors suggested that the two conditions are identical. However, other authors report cases in which myotonia and weakness were induced in the cold and not accompanied by significant changes in the serum potassium. Therefore, the diagnosis of paramyotonia congenita should be limited only to patients in whom myotonia and paralysis are induced or aggravated by cold with normal serum potassium.

Neurologic evaluation shows myotonic signs and intermittent flaccid weakness with decreased or absent deep tendon reflexes. Patients of three families with paramyotonia congenita had no myotonia in a warm environment.

Electromyography in a cold environment (20°C) showed a significant fall in the amplitude of the compound muscle action potentials (CMAP) obtained from patients with paramyotonia congenita. Cold also induced or worsened a significant decremental response to 2-Hz nerve stimulation and virtually abolished voluntary recruitment of motor unit potentials. None of these changes occurred in patients with myotonia congenita.

Complications: Unknown.

Associated Findings: Muscle hypertrophy and persistent weakness (myopathy) were reported in older patients.

Etiology: Autosomal dominant inheritance with high penetrance in both sexes.

Pathogenesis: A muscle membrane defect different from myotonic and nonmyotonic hyperkalemic periodic paralysis has been postulated based on in vitro electrophysiologic studies. In paramyotonia congenita depolarization and paralysis are caused by an abnormal temperature dependence of the Na^+ channel kinetics.

MIM No.: *16830

Sex Ratio: M1:F1

Occurrence: Undetermined but presumed rare. Two large families alone account for 17 and 30 affected members across five and six generations respectively.

Risk of Recurrence for Patient's Sib:
See Part I, *Mendelian Inheritance.*

Risk of Recurrence for Patient's Child:
See Part I, *Mendelian Inheritance.*

Age of Detectability: In early childhood, based on clinical and EMG signs of myotonia.

Gene Mapping and Linkage: Unknown.

Prevention: None known. Genetic counseling indicated.

Treatment: Regulation of serum potassium levels by acetazolamide or thiazide diuretics has proved helpful in some families with paramyotonia congenita and hyperkalemia by decreasing the number of paralytic attacks, but it did not change the myotonic findings. Treatment with tocainide (400–1200 mg/day) has been successful in seven patients with paramyotonia congenita.

Prognosis: Generally good for life span and function.

Detection of Carrier: Demonstration of myotonia, clinically and electromyographically, often at room temperature and always upon exposure to cold.

Special Considerations: Heterogeneity of this condition is suggested by the variability of the clinical picture. The molecular genetic basis of the heterogeneity remains unknown.

References:
Thrush DC, et al.: Paramyotonia congenita: a clinical, histochemical and pathological study. Brain 1972; 95:537–552. *
Haas A, et al.: Clinical study of paramyotonia congenita with and without myotonia in a warm environment. Muscle Nerve 1981; 4:388–395.
Lehmann-Horn F, et al.: Membrane defects in paramyotonia congenita with and without myotonia in a warm environment. Muscle Nerve 1981; 4:396–406.
Subramony SH, et al.: Distinguishing paramyotonia congenita and myotonia congenita by electromyography. Muscle Nerve 1983; 6:374–379.
Streib EW: Paramyotonia congenita: successful treatment with tocainide: clinical and electrophysiologic findings in seven patients. Muscle Nerve 1987; 10:155–162.

I0000   **Victor V. Ionasescu**

Paranasal sinuses, absent
See SINUS, ABSENT PARANASAL

PARAPLEGIA, FAMILIAL SPASTIC   0295

Includes:
Spastic paraplegia, hereditary
Spastic paraplegia, pure hereditary
Spastic paraplegia, X-linked, complicated
Strumpell familial spastic paraplegia
Strumpell-Lorrain syndrome

Excludes:
Ataxia, Friedreich type (2714)
Ataxia, hereditary
Adrenomyeloneuropathy
Cerebellar ataxia
Cerebral palsy (2931)
Charcot-Marie-Tooth disease
Lison syndrome
Parasagittal intracranial mass
Sjogren syndrome (2101)
Spastic paraplegia, familial, in other syndromes
Spastic paraplegia of perinatal onset
Thoracic spinal cord lesion

Major Diagnostic Criteria: Progressive spasticity of the lower extremities with exaggerated deep tendon reflexes and Babinski signs. A positive family history in the autosomal dominant pedigrees is a helpful but not necessary criterion.

Clinical Findings: The age of onset is usually in the first decade in the autosomal recessive families. In the autosomal dominant families, there are two groups: type I with age of onset at 13.49 ± 12.25 years and type II with age of onset at 44.9 ± 13.9 years. Intellect is preserved. Dragging of one leg is often the first symptom to be noted. Leg cramps follow, and within 2 to 3 years a scissoring spastic gait emerges. Urinary frequency and urgency occur in 50% of cases. In the older-onset male patients, 60% develop secondary impotence. Their inability to have erections is presumably based on spinal cord pathology, and does not affect biologic reproductive fitness. Increased tone and flexion spasms are frequently reported. Ultimately, one-third of the older patients require wheelchair assistance. Increased deep tendon reflexes and Babinski signs are found in all those affected. Motor weakness occurs late in the illness, and sensory findings are limited to mildly diminished vibratory response below the ankles in 60% of patients. There may be abnormal release of H-reflexes from the small muscle of the foot on tibial nerve stimulation; otherwise, neurophysiologic and X-ray studies are normal. Expressivity of the disease is variable, and mildly affected individuals may be unaware of their problem unless examined by a neurologist. This may be important for counseling issues.

Complications: Pes cavus; kyphoscoliosis; hip, knee, and joint contractures, with late-onset entrapment neuropathies.

Associated Findings: Late-onset distal wasting of the muscles and urinary tract infections. Patients with the X-linked form frequently have signs of cerebellar dysfunction.

Etiology: The majority of reported families show autosomal dominant inheritance. Thirty percent of reported cases are autosomal recessive. Few pedigrees are reported with X-linked inheritance.

Pathogenesis: The underlying mechanism is unknown. The predominant neuropathologic lesion is a loss of myelin and axons in the lateral corticospinal tract. The fasciculus gracilis and, to a minor extent, the fasciculus cuneatus are involved at the thoracic and lower cervical levels. Rarely is there involvement of the spinocerebellar and anterior corticospinal tracts.

MIM No.: *18260, *27080, *31290

Sex Ratio: Probably M1:F1 in non-X-linked cases. M1:F1, M60:F40, and M1:F2 have been reported.

Occurrence: Over 200 cases have been reported in the literature.

Risk of Recurrence for Patient's Sib:
See Part I, *Mendelian Inheritance.*

Risk of Recurrence for Patient's Child:
See Part I, *Mendelian Inheritance.*

Age of Detectability: The autosomal recessive form can usually be detected in the first decade. Dominant familial spastic paraplegia is of two forms, one that presents before age 35 years (type I) and one that presents after age 35 years (type II). Spasticity of the lower limbs is more severe in type I families. However, progression is more rapid in the type II families. The few cases described with X-linked recessive inheritance were diagnosed in the first or second decade.

Gene Mapping and Linkage: SPG1 (spastic paraplegia, complicated) has been provisionally mapped to Xq27-q28.

Prevention: None known. Genetic counseling indicated.

Treatment: Dantrolene sodium and baclofen (Lioresal) have been tried with variable success for marked spasticity. Treatment is supportive, with attention to bladder care in those prone to infections.

Prognosis: Most patients continue to be gainfully employed and productive in life in spite of their difficulty walking. Life span is not affected.

Detection of Carrier: Twenty percent of affected individuals are asymptomatic, but have increased tone and exaggerated reflexes on physical examination. Parents should be examined carefully in all instances.

Special Considerations: The variable expressivity of this disease necessitates careful neurologic examination of all family members once a case has been identified. Treatable causes of lower extremity spasticity need to be ruled out, particularly parasagittal masses, thoracic spinal cord tumors, and adrenomyeloneuropathy, which may benefit from dietary therapy.

References:

Strümpell A: Über eine bestimmte Form der primaren combinierten Systemerkrankung des Rückenmarks. Arch Psychiatr Nervenkr 1886; 17:217–238.

Behan WMH, Maia M: Strümpell's familial spastic paraplegia: genetics and neuropathology. J Neurol Neurosurg Psychiatry 1974; 37:8–20.

Harding AE: Hereditary "pure" spastic paraplegia: a clinical and genetic study of 22 families. J Neurol Neurosurg Psychiatry 1981; 44:871–888. *

Harding AE: Classification of the hereditary ataxias and paraplegias. Lancet 1983; I:1151–1155.

Kenwrick S, et al.: Linkage analysis of several cloned DNA sequences with the locus of X-linked recessive spastic paraplegia. Am J Hum Genet 1985; 37:A160.

Boustany R-MN, et al.: The autosomal dominant form of "pure" familial spastic paraplegia: clinical findings and linkage analysis of a large pedigree. Neurology 1987; 37(6):910–915. *

B0053   **Rose-Mary N. Boustany**

Parasternal hernia
See DIAPHRAGMATIC HERNIA
Parastremmatic dwarfism
See PARASTREMMATIC DYSPLASIA

PARASTREMMATIC DYSPLASIA   0798

Includes:
Dwarfism, parastremmatic
Parastremmatic dwarfism

Excludes:
Diastrophic dysplasia (0293)
Metatropic dysplasia (0656)
Osteogenesis imperfecta (0777)

Major Diagnostic Criteria: Severe dwarfism with progressive spinal malalignment, short limbs, and rigid joints. On X-ray, the skeleton has a pathognomonic "flocky" appearance due to patchy undermineralization.

Clinical Findings: The features are evident at birth, and become progressively more severe. The forehead is high, with brachycephaly and a temporal bulge. The extremities are short, with bilateral genu valgum, bowing of the shins, osseous enlargement of the knees, and contractures of the hip joints. Scoliosis appears in early infancy. Intelligence is normal and there are no visceral ramifications.

On X-ray, the skeleton is grossly undermineralized, coarsely trabeculated, and contains areas of irregular stippling which produces a "flocky" appearance. The vertebral bodies are flattened and irregular, and the pelvic bones are dysplastic. The metaphyses and epiphyses of the tubular bones are severely malformed.

Complications: Articular rigidity causes severe handicap, which is accentuated by the effects of spinal cord compression due to progressive spinal malalignment. Cardio-respiratory failure may develop.

Associated Findings: None known.

Etiology: Presumably autosomal dominant inheritance, with sporadic cases representing new mutations. Neither affected sibs nor parental consanguinity have been recorded. The only report of generation to generation transmission concerns an affected father and daughter. The mother had **Osteogenesis imperfecta**, and the daughter was thought to have inherited both conditions.

Pathogenesis: Unknown.

MIM No.: 16840

POS No.: 3358

Sex Ratio: M1:F5 (Observed).

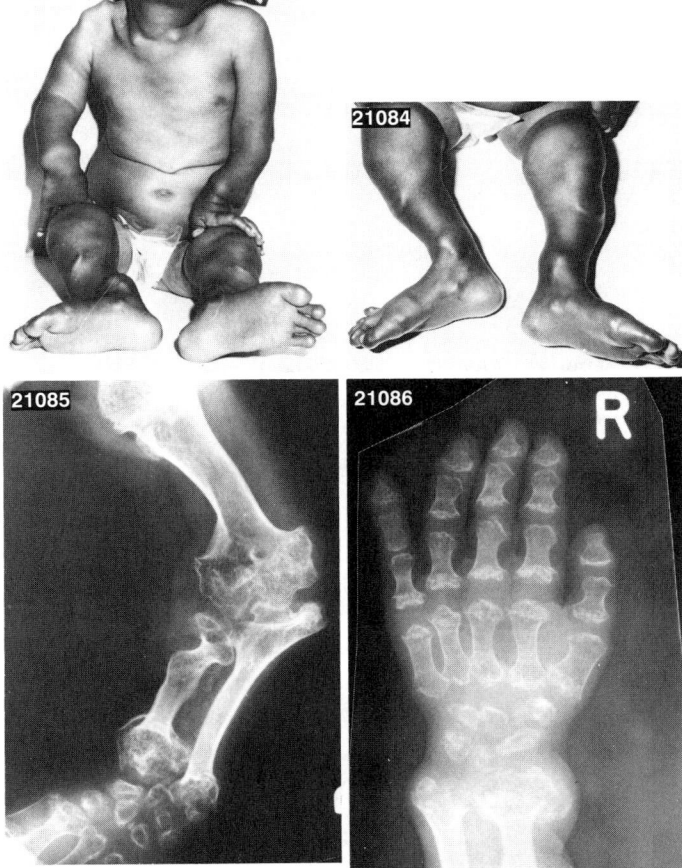

0798-21083: An affected girl with dwarfism and malformation of the limbs and trunk. 21084: The legs of the affected girl show irregular expansion of the shins and ankles. 21085: X-ray of the arm shows very dysplastic bones with a characteristic "flocky" appearance. 21086: Hand X-ray shows short tubular bones that are dysplastic with irregular expansion of the metaphyses.

Occurrence: Six cases have been reported, including four unrelated females, and a father and daughter.

Risk of Recurrence for Patient's Sib:
See Part I, *Mendelian Inheritance.*

Risk of Recurrence for Patient's Child:
See Part I, *Mendelian Inheritance.*

Age of Detectability: At birth.

Gene Mapping and Linkage: Unknown.

Prevention: None known. Genetic counseling indicated.

Treatment: Orthopedic correction of limb and spinal malalignment.

Prognosis: Progressive physical handicap. Eventual spinal cord compression and cardio-respiratory failure. Intelligence remains unimpaired.

Detection of Carrier: Unknown.

References:
Rask MR: Morquio-Brailsford osteochondrodystrophy and osteogenesis imperfecta: report of a patient with both conditions. J Bone Joint Surg 1963; 45A:561–570.
Langer LO, et al.: An unusual bone dysplasia: parastremmatic dwarfism. Am J Roentgenol Rad Ther Nuc Med 1970; 110:550–560. *
Horan F, Beighton P: Parastremmatic dwarfism. J Bone Joint Surg 1976; 58B:343–346. * †

BE008   **Peter Beighton**

Parathormone resistance
See PARATHYROID HORMONE RESISTANCE

| **PARATHYROID HORMONE RESISTANCE** | **0830** |

Includes:
Albright hereditary osteodystrophy
Hypoparathyroidism, resistant (ineffective) hormone
Parathormone resistance
Pseudohypoparathyroidism, type 1a or 1b (PHP-1a or b)
Pseudohypoparathyroidism, type 2 (PHP-2)
Pseudo-pseudohypoparathyroidism

Excludes:
Brachydactyly (0114)
Hypoparathyroidism, idiopathic

Major Diagnostic Criteria: Either the presence of a characteristic clinical somatotype, referred to as Albright Hereditary Osteodystrophy (AHO), or the demonstration of renal unresponsiveness to parathyroid hormone (PTH) has been considered a sufficient criterion for the diagnosis of pseudohypoparathyroidism (PHP), but the classical description includes both features. At least two biochemical phenotypes (PHP-1 and PHP-2) have been recognized. The major findings are as follows:

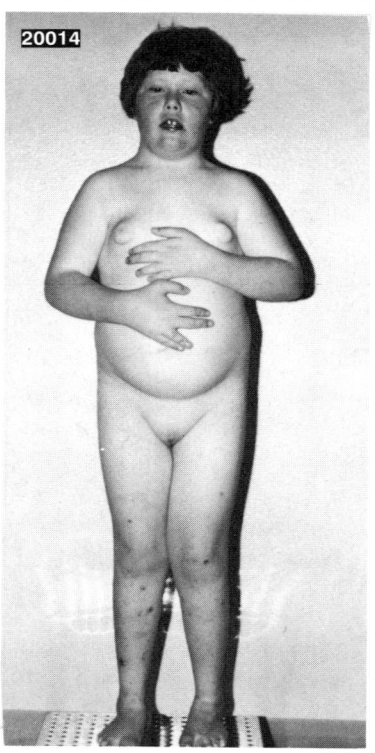

0830A-20014: Note characteristic body habitus with truncal obesity, brachydactyly and dysmorphic facies.

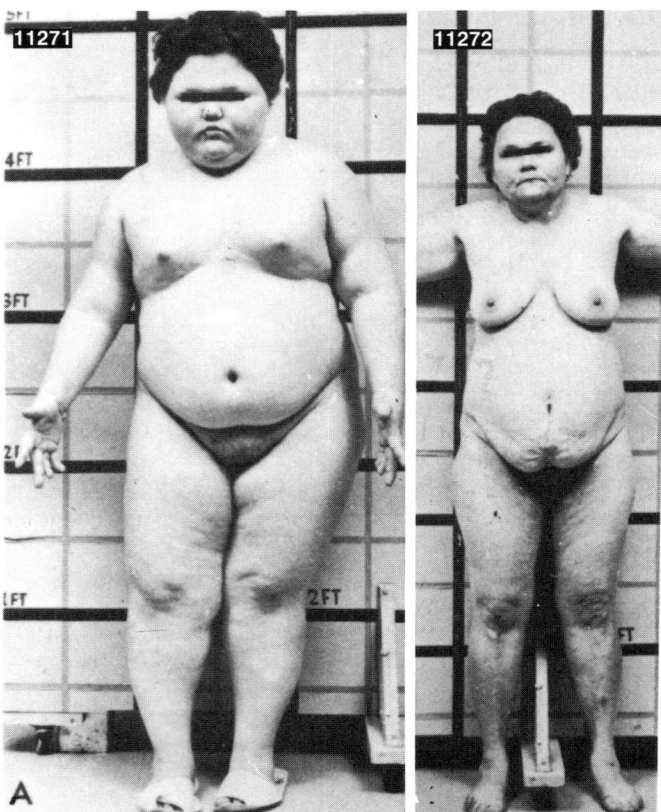

0830B-11271: Thirteen-year-old girl with pseudohypoparathyroidism who was the daughter of woman shown in 11272. 11272: Woman with pseudo-pseudohypoparathyroidism.

Feature	PHP-1	PHP-2
Serum		
-calcium	low	low
-phosphate	high	normal or high
-immunoreactive PTH (iPTH)	high	high
Renal response to PTH challenge		
-phosphate excretion	decreased	decreased
-3', 5' cyclic AMP (cAMP) excretion	decreased	normal
-1,25 $(OH)_2D_3$ synthesis	decreased	? normal
Stimulatory guanine nucleotide nucleotide-binding protein (G_s) activity	decreased in some	normal
AHO somatotype	present in most	usually absent

Patients with reduced activity of the G_s (or N_s) protein, which is a component of the hormone-sensitive adenylcyclase complex, are subclassified as PHP-1a. Those with normal G_s activity are designated PHP-1b. Normocalcemic individuals with PHP-2 or 2 may be said to have pseudo-pseudohypoparathyroidism (PPHP). They may still show target organ resistance to PTH with or without the G_s protein defect or the AHO somatotype.

Clinical Findings: Clinical features of AHO are variable but include short stature, obesity, round face, brachydactyly (particularly the fourth and fifth metacarpals and the distal first phalanx), and mild-to-moderate mental retardation. Other signs of abnormal mineral metabolism include ectopic calcifications in brain (particularly the choroid plexus) and skin, delayed tooth

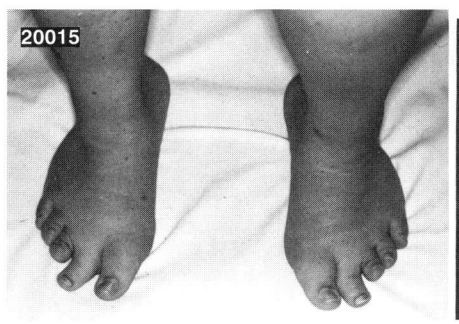 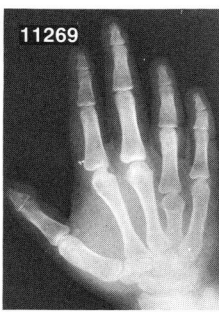

0830C-20015: Note brachydactyly; the third, fourth and fifth metatarsals are short. **11269:** Shortened fourth metacarpal.

eruption, enamel hypoplasia, and X-ray features in keeping with hypoparathyroidism. In some patients, isolated skeletal responsiveness to PTH may be inferred from radiographically demonstrable features of hyperparathyroidism (osteitis fibrosa).

Complications: Patients may present with hypocalcemic tetany and convulsions. Cataracts and corneal opacities have been described. Moderate to severe hypertension may be found in more than one-half of the adult patients.

Associated Findings: In PHP-1a patients, the G_s protein defect is is widespread, and therefore other physiologic functions mediated by the hormone-sensitive adenyl cyclase may also be affected. Thyroid dysfunction may only be evidenced by an exaggerated thyroid-stimulating hormone (TSH) response to thyrotropin-releasing hormone (TRH), but infants with PHP have presented with hypothyroidism. Other hormonal abnormalities include hypergonadotrophic hypogonadism and decreased cAMP responses to glucagon and isoproterenol. Patients with the G_s deficit have anosmia, presumably because a hormone-sensitive adenylcyclase system is required in the transduction of the receptor signal (generated by binding of odiferous molecules) to an electrical impulse in the olfactory neuroepithelial membrane.

Etiology: Although considered to be X-linked, many authorities suggest that autosomal dominant inheritance is more compatible with most pedigrees. In PHP-1a, the decrease in Gs activity has been related to an alpha subunit (Gs) deficiency, which is transmitted in an autosomal dominant fashion. In different kindreds, levels of Gs mRNA may be decreased or normal, suggesting further genetic heterogeneity.

Pathogenesis: Because there is incomplete concordance between the G_s protein defect and the AHO somatotype or any of the biochemical findings associated with disturbed mineral metabolism, it is suggested that at least one other gene must be involved in the full expression of the PHP phenotype. It has been suggested that the Gs protein defect in the parathyroid gland itself may interfere with synthesis and secretion of PTH, thereby accounting for altered bioactivity of the circulating hormone found in some PHP patients. Multiple forms of the PTH molecule, with agonist or inhibitory activity, may account for some of the temporal and intrafamilial variability that is characteristic of this disorder.

In PHP-1b and PHP-2 individuals, defects in the PTH molecule itself, the PTH receptor, or in the intracellular transduction of the cAMP signal to distal cellular events (e.g. increased 25-hydroxyvitamin D, 1 α hydroxylase activity) have been postulated, but definitive evidence is lacking. The origin of the increased prevalence in females is unknown.

MIM No.: *10358, 20333, 30080

Sex Ratio: M1:F2.3 (PHP-1 with AHO).

Occurrence: Over 50 kindreds documented in the literature.

Risk of Recurrence for Patient's Sib:
See Part I, *Mendelian Inheritance.*

Risk of Recurrence for Patient's Child:
See Part I, *Mendelian Inheritance.*

Age of Detectability: Elevated serum iPTH or decreased RBC G_s activity can be determined shortly after birth. Clinical features (AHO, hypocalcemia, etc.) may not be manifest until later childhood or adulthood.

Gene Mapping and Linkage: Unknown.

Prevention: None known. Genetic counseling indicated.

Treatment: Hypocalcemia associated with decreased circulating 1,25(OH)D levels can be effectively treated with vitamin D or its analogs--dihydrotachysterol, calcitriol [1,25(OH)$_2$D$_3$] or alphacalcidol [1 α (OH)D$_3$]. Adjunctive therapy may include supplemental oral calcium to help normalize serum calcium and thiazides or acetazolamide to reduce calcium excretion. Whether or not very early detection and treatment of associated hypothyroidism will reduce the extent of the mental deficit is not known.

Prognosis: Normal life span.

Detection of Carrier: Formal testing for G_s activity and delineation of biochemical phenotype may be useful in identifying asymptomatic, clinically normal adults.

Special Considerations: Because of the significant clinical, biochemical, and genetic heterogeneity, caution should be exercised in counselling with regard to risks of recurrence or ultimate outcome.

References:
Chase LR, et al.: Pseudohypoparathyroidism: defective excretion of 3'–5' CAMP in response to parathyroid hormone. J Clin Invest 1969; 48:1832–1844.
Fitch N: Albright's hereditary osteodystrophy: a review. Am J Med Genet 1982; 11:11–29.
Okano K, et al.: Comparative efficacy of various vitamin D metabolites in the treatment of various types of hypoparathyroidism. J Clin Endocrinol Metab 1982; 55:238–243.
Goltzman DA, et al.: Studies of the multiple molecular forms of bioactive parathyroid hormone and parathyroid hormone-like substances. Recent Prog Horm Res 1986; 42:665–703.
Levine MA, et al.: Activity of the stimulatory guanine nucleotide-binding protein is reduced in erythrocytes from patients with pseudohypoparathyroidism and pseudopseudohypoparathyroidism: biochemical, endocrine, and genetic analysis of Albright's hereditary osteodystrophy in six kindreds. J Clin Endocrinol Metab 1986; 62:497–502.
Radeke HH, et al.: Multiple pre- and postreceptor defects in pseudohypoparathyroidism (a multicenter study with twenty four patients). J Clin Endocrinol Metab 1986; 62:393–402.
Weinstock RS, et al.: Olfactory dysfunction in humans with deficient guamine nucleotide-binding protein. Nature 1986; 322:635–636.
Brickman AS, et al.: Hypertension in pseudohypoparathyroidism type 1. Am J Med 1988; 85:785–792.
Levine MA, et al.: Genetic deficiency of the alpha subunit of the guanine nucleotide-binding protein G(s) as a molecular basis for Albright hereditary osteodystrophy. Proc Nat Acad Sci 1988; 85:617–621.
Spiegel AM: Pseudohypoparathyroidism. In: Scriver CR, et al, eds: The metabolic basis of inherited disease, 6th ed. New York: McGraw-Hill, 1989:2013–2028.

C0016   **David Cole**

Parathyroid hyperplasia, hereditary
See HYPERPARATHYROIDISM, FAMILIAL
Parchment right ventricle
See VENTRICLE, RIGHT, UHL ANOMALY

PARIETAL FORAMINA-CLAVICULAR HYPOPLASIA 2769

Includes: Cleidocranial dysplasia-parietal foramina

Excludes: **Cleidocranial dysplasia** (0185)

Major Diagnostic Criteria: The combination of parietal foramina and clavicular hypoplasia.

Clinical Findings: Eckstein and Hoare (1963) described a mother and son with bilateral clavicular hypoplasia and parietal foramina (oval defects in the parietal bone which are covered by skin). Golabi et al (1984) expanded on the phenotype, and described a three generation pedigree with five affected family members. **Megalencephaly** was present in all five. Occipital dermoid with a hair tuft was present in 4/5. Other findings included prominent forehead (2/5), prominent eyes (2/5), midfacial hypoplasia (2/5), short nasal septum (2/5), long philtrum (2/5), thin upper lip (2/5), and small ears or microtia (2/5).

Complications: Unknown.

Associated Findings: One affected individual also had lacrimal stenosis and epicanthal folds.

Etiology: Presumably autosomal dominant inheritance.

Pathogenesis: Unknown.

MIM No.: 16855

POS No.: 3643

CDC No.: 755.555

Sex Ratio: M1:F1

Occurrence: Two families have been reported.

Risk of Recurrence for Patient's Sib:
See Part I, *Mendelian Inheritance.*

Risk of Recurrence for Patient's Child:
See Part I, *Mendelian Inheritance.*

Age of Detectability: At birth, by physical examination.

Gene Mapping and Linkage: Unknown.

Prevention: None known. Genetic counseling indicated.

Treatment: Undetermined, although removal of the hair tuft for cosmetic reasons may be desirable.

Prognosis: Excellent. Life span and intellect are not affected.

Detection of Carrier: Unknown.

References:
Eckstein HB, Hoare RD: Congenital parietal "foramina" associated with faulty ossification of clavicles. Br J Radiol 1963;36:220–221.
Golabi M, et al: Parietal foramina-clavicular hypoplasia. Am J Dis Child 1984; 138:596–599.

T0007 **Helga V. Toriello**

Parkes-Weber syndrome
See ANGIO-OSTEOHYPERTROPHY SYNDROME
Parkinson disease, early onset-mental retardation
See X-LINKED MENTAL RETARDATION-BASAL GANGLION DISORDER
Parodontopathia acroectodermalis
See HYPERKERATOSIS PALMOPLANTARIS-PERIODONTOCLASIA
Parotid aplasia or hypoplasia
See ALACRIMA-APTYALISM
Parotid gland, swelling of
See BRANCHIAL CLEFT CYSTS
Parotitis associated with Sjogren syndrome
See PAROTITIS, PUNCTATE
Parotitis of childhood, chronic recurrent
See PAROTITIS, PUNCTATE

PAROTITIS, PUNCTATE 0799

Includes:
Parotitis of childhood, chronic recurrent
Sialangiectasis
Sialectasis
Mikulicz disease
Parotitis associated with Sjogren syndrome

Excludes:
Parotid infection, other forms (e.g. viral, sarcoid, bacterial)
Sjogren syndrome (2101)

Major Diagnostic Criteria: Evidence of punctate sialectasis on sialography. If possible, a tissue examination of the gland should be done to confirm the pathology.

Clinical Findings: A unique pathologic process that appears to occur in three different clinical forms:
Chronic recurrent parotitis of childhood: Usually misdiagnosed as "recurrent mumps." It is usually not infectious or contagious. Attacks subside about the time of puberty in about 90% of cases.
Mikulicz disease: Occurs in adults who have no evidence of systemic disease. In most cases, only the parotid gland is involved. There may be recurrent attacks of parotid swelling or there may be a chronic diffuse enlargement or a discrete mass. Involvement may be unilateral or bilateral.
Punctate parotitis: A very frequent, if not a constant, component of **Sjogren syndrome**. The parotitis may be recurrent or may be chronic, diffuse enlargement. Clinically only one gland may be involved, but on X-ray and pathologically, both are affected.
Pathologic and X-ray findings in the parotid gland are similar in all three clinical types. There appear to be three primary histopathologic lesions: hyperplasia of the epithelial and myoepithelial cells of the intralobular ducts, disappearance of acinar structures, and replacement of the glandular parenchyma by a diffuse infiltration of lymphoid cells.
Involvement of larger ducts and gross glandular destruction, with increased fibrosis, is thought to be associated with secondary infection. Occasionally cystic lesions develop from the hyperplastic ducts. In longstanding cases the pathology may undergo involution and fatty replacement.
The classic X-ray findings are demonstrated by sialography in which terminal or punctate sialectasis is seen. Some workers have reported that the lesion then progresses through globular, cavitary, and destructive stages. These may be caused by bacterial infection secondary to reduced salivary flow. Although there is no unanimity of opinion, many feel that the punctate areas are an artifact due to extravasation of contrast material, but nevertheless are a valuable diagnostic sign.

Complications: Secondary bacterial infection due to diminution of salivary flow from acinar destruction.

Associated Findings: Other manifestations of **Sjogren syndrome**, i.e., xerophthalmia, connective tissue disorders, and lymphoepithelial malignancy.

Etiology: This is an inflammatory lesion but not a bacteriologic disease. A chronic viral infection is possible, but this has not been adequately evaluated. Evidence for a genetic etiology in at least some cases is as follows: definite familial incidence, occurrence in very young children, and preliminary studies indicating hereditary factors in **Sjogren syndrome** with which punctate parotitis is usually associated.

Pathogenesis: Unknown.

Sex Ratio: Varies by clinical type. Chronic recurrent parotitis of childhood, M>1:F1. Mikulicz disease, M1:F>1. See also **Sjogren syndrome**.

Occurrence: Undetermined but presumed rare. Seen most frequently during childhood.

Risk of Recurrence for Patient's Sib: Unknown.

Risk of Recurrence for Patient's Child: Unknown.

Age of Detectability: Whenever clinical involvement of the parotid occurs.

Gene Mapping and Linkage: Unknown.

Prevention: None known. Genetic counseling indicated.

Treatment: The type of treatment depends on the gross pathology and severity of clinical symptoms. Mild cases may require only observation and management of secondary infection. Among available treatments are massage of the gland, stimulation of salivary flow by chewing gum or wax, treating infections of the teeth or tonsils, antibiotics for the acute attack, sialography (because the iodides it contains may be beneficial), injection of antibiotics into the duct system, and small doses (800–1,800r) of X-ray therapy, with or without duct ligation. Surgical treatment includes tympanic neurectomy to eliminate the parasympathetic nerve supply to the gland, and either subtotal or total parotidectomy, sparing the facial nerve. The latter treatment is preferred.

Prognosis: Chronic recurrent parotitis of childhood subsides around the age of puberty in about 90% of cases. The parotitis of Mikulicz disease and Sjögren syndrome seems to subside spontaneously after a variable length of time.

Detection of Carrier: Unknown.

References:

Blatt IM. On sialectasis and benign lymphosialadenopathy (the pyogenic parotitis, Goujerot-Sjögren's syndrome, Mikulicz's disease complex), a 10-year study. Laryngoscope 1964; 74:1684–1746.
Bunim JJ. A broader spectrum of Sjögren's syndrome and its pathogenic implications. Ann Rheum Dis 1961; 20:1–10.
Hemenway WG. Chronic punctate parotitis. Laryngoscope 1971; 81:485–509.
Konno A: A study on the pathogenesis of recurrent parotitis in childhood. Ann Otol Rhinol Laryngol 1979; 88(Suppl)63:1–20. *

BE028   **LaVonne Bergstrom**

PECTUS CARINATUM   0801

Includes:
    Chicken breast
    Chondrosternal prominence, congenital
    Pigeon breast
    Pyramidal chest
    Sternogladiolar prominence
    Thorax cuneiforme

Excludes: Pectus excavatum (0802)

Major Diagnostic Criteria: Prominence of sternum with lateral depression of ribs.

Clinical Findings: There are three types. *Type I:* "Keel" chest, most common of the three, consists of symmetrical protrusion of the sternum and the costal cartilages. *Type II:* Pouter breast consists of protrusion of the manubrium and the first two sternal cartilages, with depression of the body of the sternum and protrusion of the tip of the xiphoid process. It is the least common of the three. *Type III:* Lateral pectus carinatum consists of asymmetric unilateral protrusion of the anterior chest wall.

The condition is present at birth but may not become obvious until recession of the prominent abdomen in later childhood. There is usually no associated significant limitation of cardiorespiratory function.

Complications: Possible psychological effects. Occasionally fatigue, nondescript chest pain, and possibly dyspnea from decreased respiratory excursion of the thorax.

Associated Findings: Marfan syndrome, Homocystinuria, Mucopolysaccharidosis, rickets, and various malformation syndromes.

Etiology: Unknown.

Pathogenesis: Several theories have been proposed. Brodkin believes that the various sternal deformities are the result of failure of the development of muscle in the ventral segment of the diaphragm, and that these portions of the muscle exert a pull on the attached chest wall as a result of the unopposed action of muscles on the other side. Robicsek et al (1979) believe this deformity is due to an overgrowth of the costal cartilages and thus, if the sternum is pushed inward, **Pectus excavatum** results. But, if the sternum is outward, pectus carinatum develops.

CDC No.: 754.800

Sex Ratio: Presumably M1:F1.

Occurrence: Reported as 1:1,660 in the school population of Newark, New Jersey.

Risk of Recurrence for Patient's Sib: Unknown.

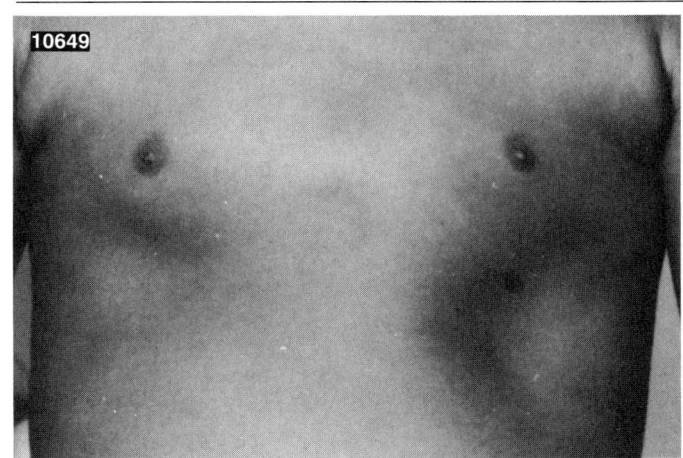

0801-10649:   Asymmetric pectus carinatum.

Risk of Recurrence for Patient's Child: Unknown.

Age of Detectability: At birth, by physical examination.

Gene Mapping and Linkage: Unknown.

Prevention: None known. Genetic counseling indicated.

Treatment: Surgery is usually for cosmetic effect and because of the variety of defects, individuality of approach is required. Although it appears that pectus carinatum does not interfere with normal activity, there have been no good reported studies of intrathoracic gas volumes or mechanics of breathing. The deformity is not caused by or related to airway obstruction. It is generally agreed by surgeons that surgical correction should be deferred until the chest wall is stable.

Prognosis: Normal for life span and intelligence. Function may depend on severity.

Detection of Carrier: Unknown.

References:

Ravitch MM: Congenital deformities of the chest wall. In: Benson CD, et al., eds: Pediatric surgery, vol. 1. Chicago: Year Book Medical Publishers, 1962:227.

Pickard LR, et al.: Pectus carinatum: results of surgical therapy. J Ped Surg 1979; 14:228–230.

Robicsek F, et al.: Pectus carinatum. J Thorac Cardiovas Surg 1979; 78:52–61.

Wesselhoeft CW, DeLuca FG: A simplified approach to the repair of pediatric pectus deformities. Ann Thorac Surg 1982; 34:640–646.

J0010   **Virginia P. Johnson**

PECTUS EXCAVATUM   0802

Includes:

> Chest, funnel
> Chonechondrosternon
> Funnel chest
> Pectum recurvatum
> Schusterbrust
> Trichterbrust

Excludes: Pectus carinatum (0801)

Major Diagnostic Criteria: Central depression of the chest at the level of the sternum.

Clinical Findings: The anteroposterior diameter of the lower thorax is decreased by the posterior dislocation of the lower sternum, the costal cartilages, and the anterior part of the ribs. The affected portion of the sternum is concavely deformed. The manubrium is generally normal, whereas the xiphoid may extend so far posteriorly as to impinge on the vertebral bodies or the paravertebral gutters. The left side of the chest bulges slightly because the heart underlies it very close to the surface.

Children with this anomaly are usually asymptomatic, unless they have primary lung or heart disease. Only occasionally are vague complaints heard about decreased exercise tolerance and chest discomfort. Auscultatory findings may simulate mild pulmonary stenosis and small atrial septal defects. Scalar electrocardiographic and X-ray features may resemble mild right ventricular overload. These are not specific enough to suggest cardiac malformation and are explainable on the basis of heart displacement. Thus cardiac catheterization is often not needed. However, pectus excavatum can reduce the pumping capacity of the heart during upright exercise, and hemodynamic improvement may be achieved with surgery.

Complications: Psychologic effects are noted. In the presence of chronic lung disease, congenital or acquired heart conditions, or calcification of cartilages with advanced age, a severe chest deformity can further impair the function of the intrathoracic organs, by dislocation, distortion, compression, or restriction of mobility.

Associated Findings: Occurs in association with various syndromes (e.g. **Marfan syndrome**, **Noonan syndrome**), and chronic airway obstruction in infants.

Etiology: Possibly autosomal dominant inheritance. There are many sporadic cases.

Pathogenesis: Disputed, but the most probable mechanism is an intrinsic failure of osteogenesis. Other theories include a partial weakness of the diaphragm, with the stronger portions causing an asymmetric pull on the chest wall; an abnormally short tendon or fibrous central portion of the diaphragm; and either persistent obstructive respiratory disease causing an increased transpulmonary pressure gradient during respiration, or secondary displacement of the sternum from overgrowth of the costal cartilages, or both.

MIM No.: 16930

CDC No.: 754.810

Sex Ratio: M3:F2 observed.

Occurrence: 13–40:10,000.

Risk of Recurrence for Patient's Sib:
See Part I, *Mendelian Inheritance.*

Risk of Recurrence for Patient's Child:
See Part I, *Mendelian Inheritance.*

Age of Detectability: Usually present at birth, often undetected until some months later.

Gene Mapping and Linkage: Unknown.

Prevention: None known. Genetic counseling indicated.

Treatment: Surgical repair of deformity by mobilization and repositioning of the body of the sternum after a subperichondrial resection or morcellation of costal cartilages, or by replacing deformed portions or correcting contours with bone grafts or with prosthetic materials. Temporary internal support with a malleable strut passed transternally is often necessary. The approach to surgical repair depends on individual assessment of the relative significance of physiologic and psychologic indications, and on the balance between operative risks and expectable results. In cases of independent heart or lung diseases, the same factors must be weighed with particular care, and in some cases a more radical approach may be indicated.

Prognosis: Probably normal life span. May be progressive or stationary; recurrence after operation not uncommon unless internal strut is used.

Detection of Carrier: Unknown.

References:

Beiser GD, et al.: Impairment of cardiac function in patients with pectus excavatum with improvement after operative correction. New Engl J Med 1972; 287:267–272.

Haller JA Jr., Turner CS: Diagnosis and operative management of

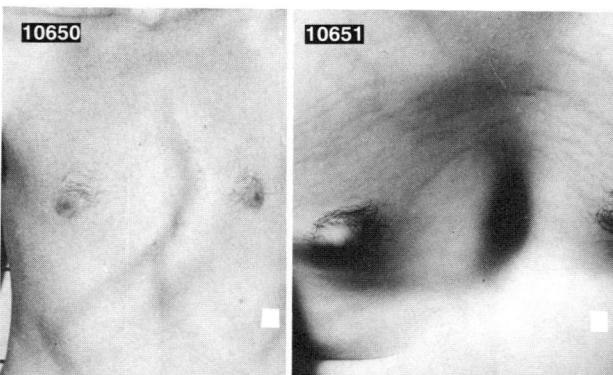

0802-10650: Asymmetric pectus excavatum. **10651:** Asymmetric pectus excavatum with striae cutis distensae.

chest wall deformities in children. Surg Clin North Am 1981; 61:1199–1207.

Castile R, et al.: Symptomatic pectus deformities of the chest. Am Rev Respir Dis 1982; 126:564–568.

Wesselhoeft CW, DeLuca FG: A simplified approach to the repair of pediatric pectus deformities. Ann Thorac Surg 1982; 34:640–646.

Cahill JL, et al.: A summary of preoperative and postoperative cardiorespiratory performance in patients undergoing pectus excavatum and carinatum repair. J Ped Surg 1984; 19:430–433.

Leung AKC, Hoo JJ: Familail congenital funnel chest. Am J Med Genet 1987; 26:887–890.

J0010   **Virginia P. Johnson**

Pedersen hypothesis
  See FETAL EFFECTS FROM MATERNAL DIABETES
Pee deficiency
  See BIOPTERIN SYNTHESIS DEFICIENCY
Peg-shaped lateral incisor
  See TEETH, ENAMEL HYPOPLASIA
Pelizaeus-Merzbacher disease (PMD), connatal type
  See PELIZAEUS-MERZBACHER SYNDROME

PELIZAEUS-MERZBACHER SYNDROME   0803

Includes:
  Cerebral sclerosis, diffuse chronic infantile
  Pelizaeus-Merzbacher disease (PMD), connatal type
  Proteolipid protein, myelin
  Leukodystrophy, sudanophilic
  Seitelberg variant, Pelizaeus-Merzbacher syndrome

Excludes:
  Adrenoleukodystrophy, X-linked (2533)
  Brain, spongy degeneration (0115)
  Cockayne syndrome (0189)
  Leukodystrophy, adult onset progressive dominant type (2975)
  Leukodystrophy, globoid cell type (0415)
  Leukodystrophies of nervous system, other
  Metachromatic leukodystrophies (0651)
  Nervous system, other degenerative diseases of

Major Diagnostic Criteria: A pattern of involvement of males, with onset around age 4–6 months, and with peculiar pendular nystagmus followed by delay in motor development should strongly suggest the diagnosis. A family history compatible with a pattern of X-linked recessive inheritance is also suggestive.

Clinical Findings: The disease is slowly progressive, with onset usually at 4–6 months of age. The distinctive clinical features are that of a chaotic, pendular nystagmus, often accompanied by shaking movements of the head, combined with hypotonia. Later, choreoathetoid movements develop, and optic atrophy is common. The patients are delayed in early motor milestones and, in the later stage of disease, they often develop contractures and spasticity of the lower limbs. Movements of the arms, particularly fine motor movements, are jerky and clumsy. Speech development may be slightly delayed, but is often within the normal range. Mentation, early in the course of the disease, seems to be relatively normal. Progression is gradual, with increasing involvement of the lower and upper limbs. The nystagmus persists and ataxia becomes a prominent symptom. There is slow progression, and death usually occurs in the third decade.

Renier et al (1981) delineated three variants: the classic type discussed above; a connatal or Seitelberg variant, in which onset is in the neonatal period, the course of the disease is more rapid and severe, and death usually occurs before five years of age; and an intermediate transitional form.

Complications: Progressive neurologic disease. Terminal pneumonia is frequent.

Associated Findings: None known.

Etiology: X-linked recessive inheritance.

Pathogenesis: Probably a defect in the lipophilin constituent of myelin. The pathology is distinctive, with a marked loss of myelin except for relatively well-preserved areas or islands of normal myelin (Tigroid patten). In the severe form (Seitelberg variant), there is more extensive and complete loss of myelin. A similar disorder in the jimpy mouse is due to abnormal synthesis of proteolipid protein associated with an abnormality of the PLP gene resulting in abnormal splicing of the mRNA.

MIM No.: *31208

Sex Ratio: M1:F0

Occurrence: Undetermined but presumed rare. Extensive literature.

Risk of Recurrence for Patient's Sib:
  See Part I, *Mendelian Inheritance*.

Risk of Recurrence for Patient's Child:
  See Part I, *Mendelian Inheritance*. Affected individuals are not expected to survive to reproduce.

Age of Detectability: Usually by 4–18 months of age. The condition can be diagnosed by magnetic resonance imaging (MRI).

Gene Mapping and Linkage: PLP (proteolipid protein (Pelizaeus-Merzbacher disease)) has been mapped to Xq21.3-q22.

Prevention: None known. Genetic counseling indicated.

Treatment: Unknown.

Prognosis: A slowly progressive leukodystrophy, with few patients surviving the third decade of life.

Detection of Carrier: Unknown.

Special Considerations: This condition was first reported in the German literature prior to the turn of the century.

Closely related processes, with sporadic appearance and without nystagmus as a prominent early sign, but which also have a slowly progressive course compatible with a leukodystrophy, have been observed. Pathologically, these cases do have islands of normal myelin adjacent to areas of marked demyelination.

References:
Renier WO, et al.: Connatal Pelizaeus-Merzbacher disease with congenital stridor in two maternal cousins. Acta Neuropath 1981; 54:11–17.

Boulloche J, Aicardi J: Pelizaeus-Merzbacher disease: clinical and nosological study. J Child Neurol 1986; 1:233–239. *

Dautigny A, et al.: The structural gene coding for myelin-associated proteolipid protein is mutated in jimpy mice. Nature 1986; 321:867–869.

Koeppen AH, et al.: Defective biosynthesis of proteolipid protein in Pelizaeus-Merzbacher disease. Ann Neurol 1987; 21:159–170.

GI010   **Herbert Gilmore**

Pelvofemoral muscular dystrophy
  See MUSCULAR DYSTROPHY, LIMB-GIRDLE
Pelvospondylitis ossificans
  See ANKYLOSING SPONDYLITIS

PEMPHIGUS, BENIGN FAMILIAL   3255

Includes:
  Hailey-Hailey disease
  Skin, pemphigus, benign familial

Excludes:
  Darier disease (2865)
  Pemphigus vulgaris

Major Diagnostic Criteria: A rash of the intertriginous areas, occurring in early adulthood, and typical histological findings on skin biopsy. These include suprabasal lacunae or fully developed blisters, with acantholysis showing a dilapidated brick wall appearance. Dyskeratotic cells (corps ronds) may be present in the granular layer.

Clinical Findings: A chronic recurrent eruption occurring in the intertriginous areas, especially the axillae and groins. Consists of vesicles on an erythematous base that coalesce to form circinate well defined plaques, sometimes with crusting and exudation. Mucosal lesions appear rarely. Healing occurs spontaneously without scarring. These patients often experience exacerbations during warm weather, associated with sweating and friction. Seventy percent of patients report a positive family history.

Complications: Bacterial or candidal contamination are often found. It is felt that these organisms may precipitate exacerbations, although it is possible that they are a secondary phenomenon.

Associated Findings: None known.

Etiology: Autosomal dominant inheritance.

Pathogenesis: The basic defect as seen by electron microscopy is a defect in cellular cohesion. This is thought to arise either due to a defect in the tonofilament-desmosome complex or due to a defect in the synthesis of intercellular substance.

MIM No.: *16960

Sex Ratio: M1:F1

Occurrence: Undetermined but presumed rare.

Risk of Recurrence for Patient's Sib:
See Part I, *Mendelian Inheritance.*

Risk of Recurrence for Patient's Child:
See Part I, *Mendelian Inheritance.*

Age of Detectability: Usually at adolescence or early adulthood.

Gene Mapping and Linkage: Unknown.

Prevention: None known. Genetic counseling indicated.

Treatment: Unknown.

Prognosis: Unknown.

Detection of Carrier: Unknown.

References:
Hailey J, Hailey H: Familial benign chronic pemphigus. Arch Dermatol Syphilol 1939; 39:679–685.
Lever WF: Familial benign pemphigus. In: Dermatology in general medicine. New York: McGraw-Hill, 1987.

GH001   **Ruby Ghadially**

Pena-Shokeir II syndrome
See CEREBRO-OCULO-FACIO-SKELETAL SYNDROME

PENA-SHOKEIR SYNDROME   2080

Includes:
Arthrogryposis multiplex congenita-pulmonary hypoplasia
Fetal akinesia deformation sequence, Pena-Shokeir I phenotype

Excludes:
Cerebro-oculo-facio-skeletal syndrome (0140)
Hutterite syndrome, Bowen-Conradi type (2422)
Neu-laxova syndrome (2092)
Pterygium syndrome, multiple lethal (2274)

Major Diagnostic Criteria: The combination of multiple joint contractures, facial anomalies, and pulmonary hypoplasia. However, these features are really a phenotype that can be produced by decreased fetal movement. The cases which have been reported in the literature represent a heterogeneous group of disorders, on the basis of neuropathic and myopathic evaluations. Nevertheless, as pointed out by Moessing (1983), a typical phenotype is produced with decreased early fetal movement. These same anomalies can be produced by curarizing rats.

Clinical Findings: Based on more than 30 cases, the major findings include pulmonary hypoplasia; low-set appearing malformed ears; multiple joint contractures; **Camptodactyly**; clubfeet; **Eye, hypertelorism**; depressed nasal tip; micrognathia; intrauterine growth retardation; and polyhydramnios. Cryptorchidism was seen in all males evaluated. Relatively common features included abnormal placentas, epicanthal folds, highly arched or cleft palate, hypoplastic dermal ridges, webbing across joints, and a short neck.

Complications: Most infants have severe respiratory distress at birth because of underdeveloped lungs. Some catch-up growth

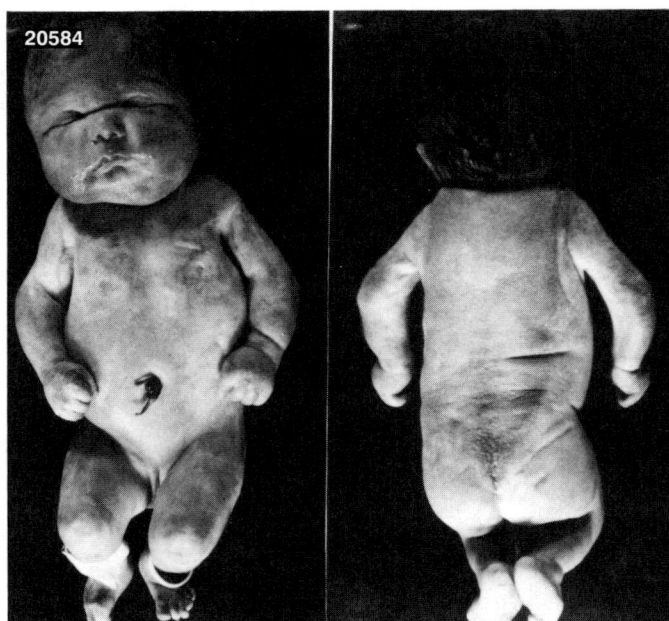

20584

2080-20584: Pena-Shokier syndrome; note multiple joint contractures, and dysmorphic facies. There is also pulmonary hypoplasia.

does appear to be possible. One child survived to 20 months of age.

Associated Findings: A few affected infants have had cardiac defects (including hypoplasia, **Aorta, coarctation, Ductus arteriosus, patent**, right ventricular hypertrophy, **Heart, transposition of great vessels**, and cor pulmononale), genitourinary defects (renal microcysts, megaloureter, persistent or cystic urachus, **Hypospadias**, or micropenis), **Cleft palate**, choanal atresia, laryngeal stenosis, microphthalmia, **Optic atrophy, Torticollis**, abnormal lung lobation, pulmonary hemangiomata, thymic hyperplasia, **Adrenal hypoplasia**, islet cell hyperplasia, gastroschisis, intestinal malrotation, **Meckel diverticulum**, anorectal atresia, preaxial **Polydactyly**, absent lower limb, and multiple skin nevi.

Etiology: Cases diagnosed as Pena-Shokeir are clearly a heterogeneous group of disorders secondary to several causes, including neurogenic atrophy, anterior horn cell changes, abnormal skeletal musculature, congenital myopathy, and maternal myasthenia gravis. All of these reflect decreased intrauterine movement which produces the common phenotype described in Pena-Shokeir; pulmonary hypoplasia, congenital contractures, depressed nasal tip, micrognathia, and hypertelorism. Many of the specific entities are inherited on an autosomal recessive basis.

Pathogenesis: Most, if not all the phenotypic features seen in Pena-Shokeir can be attributed to fetal akinesia or hypokinesia, e.g., lack of in utero movement. Moessinger's (1983) work with rats has shown that the polyhydramnios is associated with decreased or absent swallowing; that the congenital contractures are seen with decreased or absent fetal movement; that the lack of normal fetal respiratory activity is associated with pulmonary hypoplasia; and that the facial anomalies present in these cases are likely to be secondary to decreased facial and jaw movement in utero.

MIM No.: *20815

POS No.: 3135

Sex Ratio: M1:F1

Occurrence: Several dozen cases have been reported in the literature.

Risk of Recurrence for Patient's Sib:
See Part I, *Mendelian Inheritance.*

Risk of Recurrence for Patient's Child:
See Part I, *Mendelian Inheritance.* Affected individuals are not expected to survive to reproduce.

Age of Detectability: Prenatal diagnosis with real-time ultrasound is possible, but there may be a risk of missing a case early in the second trimester. Most cases are detected at birth by physical examination.

Gene Mapping and Linkage: Unknown.

Prevention: None known. Genetic counseling indicated.

Treatment: Vigorous physical therapy and pulmonary support during the newborn period give a chance for catch-up growth and survival.

Prognosis: Survival depends on the degree of pulmonary hypoplasia. Most affected infants have died soon after birth. Although a few have survived several months, all survivors have had delayed motor development. Mental development has ranged from severly retarded to normal.

Detection of Carrier: Unknown.

Special Considerations: It bears repeating that Pena-Shokeir is actually a phenotype and represents a heterogeneous group of disorders. Even those cases with decreased numbers of anterior horn cells may be heterogeneous. Within a specific family, however, there is usually a fairly consistent picture, and in all cases there has been decreased intrauterine movement prior to 24 weeks. Herva et al (1985) have reported 16 cases with the Pena-Shokeir phenotype and anterior horn call atrophy, but with severe edema and stillbirth prior to the 35th week of gestation; concluding that this represented a distinct syndrome.

References:
Moessinger AC: Fetal akinesia deformation sequence: an animal model. Pediatrics 1983; 72:857–863.
Herva R, et al: A lethal autosomal recessive syndrome of multiple congenital contractures. Am J Med Genet 1985; 20:431–439.
Lindhout D, et al.: The Pena-Shokeir syndrome: report of nine Dutch cases. Am J Med Genet 1985; 21:655–668.
Hall JG: Analysis of the Pena-Shokeir phenotype. Am J Med Genet 1986; 25:99–117. *
Hageman G, et al.: The heterogeneity of the Pena-Shokeir syndrome. Neuropediatrics 1987; 18:45–50.
Davis JE, Kalousek DK: Fetal akinesia deformation sequence in previable fetuses. Am J Med Genet 1988; 29:77–87.
Katzenstein M, Goodman RM: Pre- and postnatal findings in Pena Shokeir I syndrome: case report and a review of the literature. J Craniofac Genet Devel Biol 1988; 8:111–126.
Ohlsson A, et al.: Prenatal sonographic diagnosis of Pena-Shokeir syndrome. Am J Med Genet 1988; 29:59–65.

HA014
T0007

Judith G. Hall
Helga V. Toriello

PENTALOGY OF CANTRELL 3121

Includes:
Cantrell-Haller-Ravitch syndrome
Cantrell pentalogy
Pentalogy syndrome
Peritoneopericardial diaphragmatic hernia
Thoracoabdominal ectopia cordis

Excludes:
Diaphragmatic hernia (0289)
Heart, cordis ectopia (0335)
Heart, pericardium agenesis (0805)
Pectus excavatum (0802)

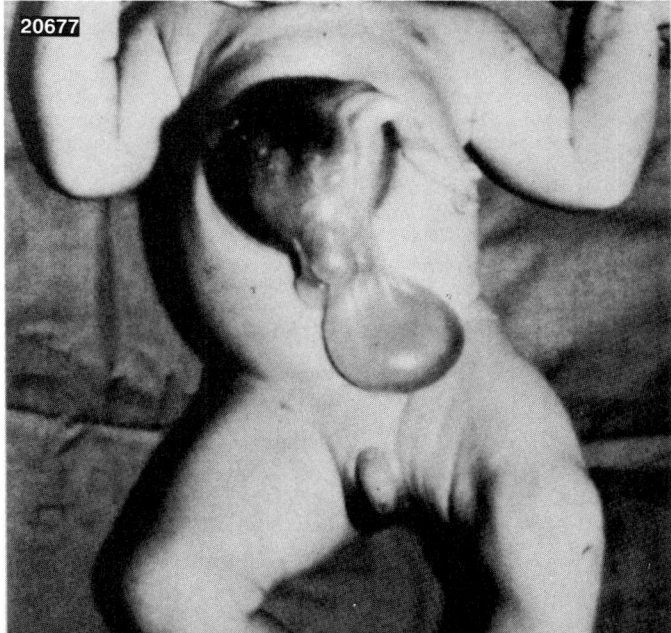
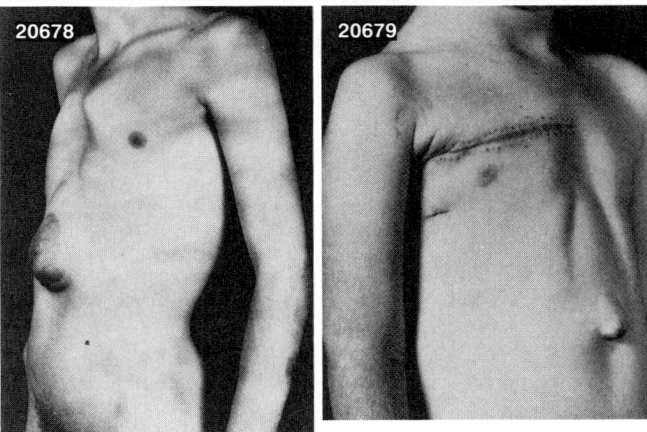

3121-20677: Newborn infant with a supraumbilical omphalocele with heart contour visible beneath the skin of the unusually high epigastrium. The child subsequently proved to have tetralogy of Fallot. **20678:** Twenty-year-old male who has tetralogy of Fallot, a broad sternal cleft, diastasis recti, and a supraumbilical hernia covered by thin hyperpigmented skin. **20679:** Two-year-old boy with distal sternal cleft and diastasis recti, shortly after Blalock shunt for tetralogy of Fallot.

Major Diagnostic Criteria: Midline, supraumbilical abdominal wall defect; defect of the lower sternum; deficiency of the anterior diaphragm; a defect in the diaphragmatic pericardium; and congenital intracardiac defects. Although a definite diagnosis is made by the presence of all five components, a probable diagnosis is suggested by any four features, and three should prompt consideration of this condition.

Clinical Findings: In the full syndrome, there is a distal sternal cleft, an omphalocele-like ventral abdominal defect with diastasis recti, a crescentic midline anterior diaphragmatic defect, a free pericardioperitoneal communication, and an internal cardiac malformation, suggesting a field defect.

The *sternal* defect may range from inconspicuous absence of the xyphoid or shortening to complete clefting or absence. The *abdominal wall* defect may be wide rectus muscle diastasis with the heart often palpable beneath loose hyperpigmented overlying skin. At the other extreme, a huge omphalocele may be present that contains bowel, liver, and the cardiac apex, covered by a translucent membrane. The semilunar *diaphragmatic* defect is unrelated to the more common diaphragmatic defects and is usually relatively small. Occasionally bowel gains entry into the pericardial cavity via the pericardioperitoneal communication. Defects in the *pericardium* typically involve its diaphragmatic aspect. A significant number of patients have a vermiform diverticulum of the left ventricle that may protrude through this communication. Congenital *intracardiac* defects are almost invariably present in the pentalogy and usually include **Atrial septal defects** or **Ventricular septal defect**; tetralogy of Fallot is very common.

Except for some degree of dextrorotation, which is often present, the heart usually lies in normal relationship to the other thoracic viscera. The appearance of ectopia is created by the concomitant defects of the sternum, diaphragm, and abdominal wall, which occasionally leave the heart abnormally exposed. The presence and full extent of the pentalogy may not be readily apparent on initial examination of an infant with a supraumbilical hernia. Several patients have undergone repair of what was assumed to be a simple omphalocele and were only later found to have the pentalogy at the time their cardiac defects were discovered and repaired.

Complications: Depend on the severity of the defects and may include rupture of abdominal viscera during delivery, sepsis from peritonitis, cyanosis, congestive heart failure, cardiorespiratory difficulty from visceral herniation into the thorax, and cardiac compression. Most of these complications are currently remediable with surgical therapy. A number of patients have succumbed to respiratory insufficiency secondary to pulmonary hypoplasia. The major morbidity after the newborn period is related to the congenital heart disease. Intelligence is usually normal.

Associated Findings: Intestinal malrotation and **Hernia, umbilical** are common. Rarely, severe malformations such as **Exstrophy of cloaca sequence** and neural tube defects may accompany the pentalogy.

Etiology: Unknown. Pentalogy of Cantrell is unlikely to be the result of a single gene defect, since, other than one pair of monozygotic twins both with the pentalogy, no cases of affected sibs have been reported. The presence of the pentalogy in only one twin of four reported cases of presumed dizygotic twins suggests that a transmitted maternal infection or toxin is also unlikely.

Pathogenesis: A proposed theory postulates that an abnormality must occur prior to or immediately after differentiation of the intraembryonic mesoderm into its splanchnic and somatic layers at about 14–18 days after conception. The diaphragmatic defect results from total or partial failure of the septum transversum to develop from a segment of somatic mesoderm. The pericardium arises from somatic mesoderm immediately adjacent to that from which the septum transversum is derived. The sternum and abdominal wall defects appear to arise from faulty migration of paired mesodermal structures. Since the normal elements of the sternum and abdominal wall are usually present but not fused in affected individuals it is thought that perhaps there is a deficiency

of the ventral paramidline mesoderm into which the migrating premordia of these structures grow.

POS No.: 3248

CDC No.: 754.820

Sex Ratio: M1:F1

Occurrence: About 50 cases have been reported in the literature.

Risk of Recurrence for Patient's Sib: Unknown. Probably low, since, except for one pair of concordant twins with the pentalogy, no affected sibs have been reported.

Risk of Recurrence for Patient's Child: Unknown.

Age of Detectability: At birth, or prenatally by ultrasound examination if defects are severe.

Gene Mapping and Linkage: Unknown.

Prevention: None known. Genetic counseling indicated.

Treatment: In most cases in which an **Omphalocele** is present, immediate surgical intervention is mandatory. Repair of sternal, diaphragmatic, and pericardial anomalies are secondary to the problems involved in satisfactory closure of a large omphalocele; however, they are usually most easily corrected at the time of the initial surgery. Recognition and management of the intracardiac lesion is important in infancy. Palliative surgery may be needed early, although a definitive procedure to correct the heart defect is often performed when the child is older.

Prognosis: Is primarily determined by the extent of the ventral wall and cardiac defects. May be lethal during the neonatal period. Reports in the literature describe patients with less extensive defects who survived into adulthood without surgical corrective procedures.

Detection of Carrier: Unknown.

Special Considerations: This specific combination of five anomalies has in the past occasionally been classified as an example of *thoracoabdominal ectopia cordis*. Since the heart defect only appears superficial secondary to the thoracoabdominal defects and is not actually ectopic, this association of birth defects should be classified as a separate entity.

Since the pentalogy has been found in two unrelated cases of **Chromosome 18, trisomy 18** and in one case of 45,X/46,XX mosaicism, chromosome studies should be considered when evaluating patients with this field defect.

References:
Cantrell JR, et al.: A syndrome of congenital defects involving the abdominal wall, sternum, diaphragm, pericardium, and heart. Surg Gynecol Obstet 1958; 107:602–614. * †
Toyama WM: Combined congenital defects of the anterior abdominal wall, sternum, diaphragm, pericardium, and heart: a case report and review of the syndrome. Pediatrics 1972; 50:778–792.
Ravitch MM: Cantrell's pentalogy and notes on diverticulum of the left ventricle. In: Ravitch MM: Congenital deformities of the chest wall and their operative correction. Philadelphia: W.B. Saunders, 1977: 53–77. * †

BR041
BR007

Christine R. Bryke
W. Roy Breg

Pentalogy syndrome
See PENTALOGY OF CANTRELL
Pentazocine induced scleroderma
See SCLERODERMA, FAMILIAL PROGRESSIVE

PENTOSURIA   0804

Includes:
L-xylulose reductase deficiency
L-xylulosuria
Xylitol dehydrogenase deficiency

Excludes: Alimentary pentosuria

Major Diagnostic Criteria: Pentosuric individuals excrete 1–4 gm of L-xylulose per day. Unlike glucose or galactose, xylulose (as well as ketoses such as fructose) reduces Benedict's solution at low temperatures. Consequently, the Lasker and Enklewitz Benedict's test (55° C, 10 minutes) should be used as the first and most convenient diagnostic test. Paper chromatography will provide direct evidence that the urinary sugar is xylulose.

Clinical Findings: Pentosuria is not accompanied by any functional disturbances or symptoms other than the daily excretion of gram quantities of the pentose, L-xylulose. The pentose is present in only trace quantities in normal urine. However, presumably as a result of a defect in the liver enzyme system, which acts on this ketopentose, the sugar is poorly metabolized and is largely excreted in the urine. The condition is usually discovered when patients with high levels of urinary sugar are found to be without diabetic symptoms. Analysis of the urine discloses that the reducing sugar is not glucose.

Complications: None. Early reports of unusual psychologic manifestations were probably a consequence of the uncertainty of diagnosis and of unnecessary or ineffective attempts at treatment.

Associated Findings: **Diabetes mellitus** is occasionally found in pentosuric individuals, but as yet there are no valid data on whether the coincidence of the two conditions is other than rare and random.

Etiology: Autosomal recessive inheritance of the enzyme NADP-xylitol (L-xylulose) dehydrogenase. The exception was one study suggesting that in a particular Lebanese family the mechanism of inheritance appeared to be that of a dominant gene with reduced penetrance; subsequent restudy of this family with an improved enzyme assay (Lane and Jenkins, 1985) indicated pseudodominance.

Pathogenesis: No specific pathology has been demonstrated. Although it has been stated that the pentosuric condition persists relatively unchanged throughout life, members of one Lebanese family were reported to show pentosuria after earlier urine tests for pentose had been negative. The urinary level of xylulose is not markedly influenced by ordinary variations in diet. A direct test of pentosuric liver has not as yet been possible. Although there is no well-established relationship between pentosuria and diabetes mellitus, there is suggestive evidence that the latter disease may be accompanied by a disturbance in the glucuronate-xylulose pathway. Further work on this possible interrelationship is required. Wang and van Eys (1970) have shown a decrease of NADP-linked xylitol dehydrogenase in red cells of patients with pentosuria.

MIM No.: *26080

Sex Ratio: M1:F1

Occurrence: 1:2,500 births among Ashkenazim. The condition has been encountered almost exclusively in Ashkenazi Jews of Polish-Russian extraction and, occasionally, in individuals of Lebanese descent.

Risk of Recurrence for Patient's Sib:
See Part I, *Mendelian Inheritance.*

Risk of Recurrence for Patient's Child:
See Part I, *Mendelian Inheritance.*

Age of Detectability: In infants, as early as two weeks of age.

Gene Mapping and Linkage: Unknown.

Prevention: None known. Genetic counseling indicated.

Treatment: Unknown.

Prognosis: Normal life span.

Detection of Carrier: Carriers appear to be capable of handling the normal load of L-xylulose produced in normal metabolism. However, by stressing the glucuronic acid-xylulose metabolic pathway by the administration of a large test dose of D-glucuronolactone, it has been found that the heterozygous carrier of the pentosuric gene is less able than homozygous normal individuals to metabolize the L-xylulose produced from the glucuronolactone.

Special Considerations: It is unnecessary to demonstrate that the xylulose is of the L form, since D-xylulosuria has never been reported. However, when desired, the osazone of L-xylulose can be prepared and characterized by its melting point behavior when mixed with D-xylosazone. The derivative mixture melts approximately 40 ° C higher than the separate isomers.

References:
Touster O: Pentose metabolism and pentosuria. Am J Med 1959; 26:724–735.
Touster O: Essential pentosuria and the glucuronate-xylulose pathway. Fed Proc 1960; 19:977.
Politzer WM, Fleischmann H: L-xylulosuria in a Lebanese family. Am J Hum Genet 1962; 14:256–260.
Hollmann S, Touster O: Non-glycolytic pathways of metabolism of glucose. New York: Academic Press, 1964:95.
Wang YM, van Eyes JO: The enzymatic defect in essential pentosuria. New Engl J Med 1970; 282:892–896.
Lane AB, Jenkins T: Human L-xylulose reductase variation: familial and population studies. Ann Hum Genet 1985; 49:227–235.
Hiatt HH: Pentosuria. In: Scriver CR, et al, eds: The metabolic basis of inherited disease, 6th ed. New York: McGraw-Hill, 1989:481–493.

T0010   **Oscar Touster**

Pepper syndrome
See COHEN SYNDROME

PEPTIC ULCER DISEASES, NON-SYNDROMIC   2233

Includes:
Antral G-cell hyperfunction DU
Combined duodenal and gastric ulcer
Duodenal ulcer (DU)
Gastric ulcer
Hyperpepsinogenemic I duodenal ulcer
Normopepsinogenemic I duodenal ulcer
Rapid gastric emptying duodenal ulcer
Ulcer, duodenal
Ulcer, gastric
Ulcer, peptic

Excludes:
Amyloidoses
Endocrine neoplasia, multiple type I (0350)
Histamine excess (mastocytosis) associated peptic ulcer
Tremor-duodenal ulcer syndrome (0963)
Ulcer-leukonychia-gallstones (2234)

Major Diagnostic Criteria: Endoscopically or X-ray barium study proven ulcer crater, or characteristic scarring of the duodenal bulb.

Clinical Findings: The patient usually presents with abdominal pain and is diagnosed by endoscopy or barium X-ray studies, or presents with perforation or upper gastrointestinal bleeding. The pain commonly follows a chronic course with exacerbations and recurrences. There is strong evidence that this disease is a collection of multiple diseases each having distinct underlying mechanisms, but resulting in a similar clinical picture; at least as currently delineated.

Complications: Perforation, bleeding, and obstruction.

Associated Findings: None known.

Etiology: It is clear from family studies demonstrating increased family aggregation, and from twin studies demonstrating increased concordance of disease in monozygotic versus dizygotic twins, that there is a major genetic component or susceptibility to the peptic ulcer diseases.

The etiology appears to be extensively heterogeneous, with dominant inheritance of some specific disorders that predispose to the ulcer diathesis.

Gastric and duodenal ulcers have been found to be distinct disorders by studies that have shown that the increased familial risk for ulcer is site specific. Combined ulcer, i.e., gastric and duodenal, has also been delineated as a distinct entity, through epidemiologic studies showing that the incidence of duodenal and gastric ulcers in the same patient is about twenty times that expected from the relative frequencies of the two disorders in the population.

Heterogeneity of duodenal ulcer disease itself has been shown by family studies. Specific and different pathophysiologic markers that cosegregate with the ulcer disease, some of which have a dominant pattern of inheritance, have been identified.

The most extensive studies have indicated that approximately one-half of the duodenal ulcer population in the Western world have elevated serum pepsinogen I (and total serum pepsinogen as well) and that this hyperpepsinogenemia I is often inherited in a dominant pattern with variable penetrance of the clinical ulcer disease. This physiologically related serum marker appears to identify those who are genetically predisposed to duodenal ulcer disease on the basis of increased pepsin and acid secretion, secondary to an increased mass of chief and parietal cells in the mucosal lining of the body of the stomach.

A subgroup of duodenal ulcer patients with hyperpepsinogenemia I may have it associated with, and possibly due to antral G-cell hyperfunction. These patients have an exaggerated serum gastrin response to feeding and some have an elevated basal acid level.

The remaining one-half of duodenal ulcer patients are normopepsinogenemic I on a familial basis. Rapid gastric emptying has been found to cosegregate with duodenal ulcer in one large family with normopepsinogenemia I duodenal ulcer. This suggests that altered motility leading to an increased acid load to the duodenum is the abnormality resulting in the duodenal ulcer in this family.

Other predisposing familial/inherited factors that have been identified are immunologic associations and gastritis/duodenitis. These suggest autoimmune mechanisms in some subtypes of duodenal ulcer.

Thus duodenal ulcers can have many different predisposing pathophysiological conditions, and the etiology in a given patient can be one or a combination of these abnormalities.

Pathogenesis: Multiple distinct factors have been identified. These appear to differ from patient to patient and family to family, and may be multiple in some patients. Excess acid and pepsin secretion, altered gastric motility, and increased gastrin response to a meal are three documented mechanisms. Immunologic derangements and decreased mucosal protection are likely additional mechanisms. Environmental factors include smoking, nonsteroidal inflammatory agents, and possibly the bacterium *campylobacter pyloridis* recently isolated from the stomach and associated with peptic ulcers in some studies.

MIM No.: *12685

Sex Ratio: M2:F1 in the United States.

Occurrence: Estimated at a lifetime prevalence of up to 5% in the United States.

Risk of Recurrence for Patient's Sib: Estimated at 10–20%

Risk of Recurrence for Patient's Child: Estimated at 10–20%

Age of Detectability: Most commonly third to fourth decade of life. Earlier presentations do exist, even in childhood, and may be associated with specific genetic syndromes. Variability of age of onset exists between cultures, suggesting even further heterogeneity.

Gene Mapping and Linkage: Unknown.

Prevention: None known. Genetic counseling indicated. Recurrence can be prevented by anti-ulcer therapy.

Treatment: Treatment is usually symptomatic and empiric but is still very effective. The specific underlying mechanisms for the peptic ulcer diathesis in a given patient often goes unrecognized. Agents are used that either affect acid secretion or its neutralization: antacids, H_2 receptor antagonists; or agents that affect mucosal protection, e.g. sucralfate (a sulfated disaccharide), all have all been shown to be effective in promoting the rate of ulcer healing.

A variety of surgeries (highly selective vagotomy, vagotomy and pyloroplasty, vagotomy and antrectomy) are used for selected patients. We urge that appropriate caution be used before such therapy is performed. It will become increasingly important that attempts are made to identify preoperatively the cause of duodenal ulcer. Specific etiologies might in some cases, e.g. rapid gastric emptying, preclude surgery. Others, such as antral G-cell hyperfunction, might lead to the suggestion of a specific surgery, e.g., antrectomy.

It is likely that identifying the specific components contributing to the ulcer diathesis in a given patient will lead to more specific and efficacious therapy; though at this time this is only true for specific limited subgroups. An example may be prostaglandin agents for non-steroidal anti-inflamatory drug-induced ulcer.

Prognosis: Good, especially with recent advances in medical therapy.

Detection of Carrier: Hyperpepsinogenemia I can be assayed in serum. This would identify some high-risk individuals in specific families. Antral G-cell hyperfunction can be identified as a predisposing factor in a family member of a patient with this syndrome by demonstrating a markedly enhanced gastric response to a meal. Gastric motility studies can be performed in relatives of those patients found to have rapid gastric emptying. These are markers for specific underlying mechanisms and while they identify individuals at increased risk for disease, these individuals will not necessarily develop the disease, as a wide degree of penetrance exists.

Special Considerations: Those families with one clear abnormality, such as hyperplasia of the chief and parietal cells, ascertained by an elevated pepsinogen I or altered gastric motility, allow us to identify the inheritance patterns of peptic ulcer disease susceptibility and are increasing our knowledge regarding specific mechanisms of ulcer development. This will allow us to be more precise in our therapeutic intervention and counseling for prevention. It is clear that the genetic basis is heterogeneous, but this does not preclude the hypothesis of a multifactorial component in expression of some forms of the disease, and the involvement of environmental factors as well.

References:

Rotter JI, et al.: Genetic heterogeneity of hyperpepsinogenemic I and normopepsinogenemic I duodenal ulcer disease. Ann Intern Med 1979; 91:372–377. *

Rotter JI: The genetics of peptic ulcer: more than one gene, more than one disease. Progress in Medical Genetics, Vol. IV: Genetics of Gastrointestinal Disease. Philadelphia: W.B. Saunders, 1980:1–58.

Taylor IL, et al.: Family Studies of hypergastrinemic, hyperpepsinogenemic I duodenal ulcer. Ann Intern Med 1981; 95:421–425.

Rotter JI: Peptic Ulcer. In: Emery AE, Rimoin DL: Principles and practice of medical genetics. New York: Churchill Livingstone, 1983:863–878.

Rotter JI, et al.: Pepsinogens and other physiologic markers in genetic studies of peptic ulcer and related disorders. In: Kreuning J, et al, eds: Pepsinogens in man: clinical and genetic advances. New York: Alan R. Liss, 1985:227–244.

Sumii K, et al.: Familial aggregation of duodenal ulcer and an autosomal dominant inheritance of hyperpepsinogenemia I. Hiroshima J Med Sci 1986; 35:171–175.

Andersen LP, et al.: Gastric and duodenal infection caused by C. pyloridis: histopathologic and microbiologic findings. Scand J Gastroenterol 1987; 22:219–224.

Eliakim R, et al.: Duodenal ulcer mucosal injury with nonsteroidal anti-inflammatory drugs. J Clin Gastroenterol 1987; 9:395–399.

ES005

Theresa J. Escalante
Jerome I. Rotter

Peptidase D deficiency
See PROLIDASE DEFICIENCY
Perceptive deafness-corneal dystrophy
See CORNEAL DYSTROPHY-SENSORINEURAL DEAFNESS
Perceptive hearing loss
See DEAFNESS
Pericardial constriction-arthritis-camptodactyly
See PERICARDITIS-ARTHRITIS-CAMPTODACTYLY
Pericardial constriction-growth failure
See DWARFISM, MULIBREY TYPE
Pericardial defects, congenital
See HEART, PERICARDIUM AGENESIS

PERICARDITIS-ARTHRITIS-CAMPTODACTYLY 2811

Includes:
Arthritis-pericarditis-camptodactyly
Camptodactyly-pericarditis-arthritis
Pericardial constriction-arthritis-camptodactyly

Excludes:
Arthritis, rheumatoid (2517)
Dwarfism, Mulibrey type (2081)
Lupus erythematosus, systemic (2515)
Synovitis, familial hypertrophic (2155)

Major Diagnostic Criteria: The combination of constrictive pericarditis, arthritis, and flexion contractures of the fingers.

Clinical Findings: In all known cases, **Camptodactyly** affecting thumbs and/or fingers and arthritis with or without synovitis affecting the large joints where present. The arthritis is reportedly not painful. Eight of ten affected children also had restrictive pericarditis. Histologically the pericardium showed fibrosis, which was also noted on synovial biopsy.

In some affected children, elbow, knee, and hip joints had limited movement as well, not always secondary to arthritis or synovitis. Coxa vara was also described in one family.

Complications: In some children with restrictive pericarditis, hepatomegaly and jugular vein distension also occurred. These findings disappeared after treatment of the pericarditis.

Associated Findings: None known.

Etiology: Autosomal recessive inheritance.

Pathogenesis: Unknown.

MIM No.: *20825

POS No.: 4071

Sex Ratio: M1:F1

Occurrence: One family from Mexico with five affected sibs, one family from Turkey with four affected sibs, and one isolated case from Canada have been reported.

Risk of Recurrence for Patient's Sib:
See Part I, *Mendelian Inheritance.*

Risk of Recurrence for Patient's Child:
See Part I, *Mendelian Inheritance.*

Age of Detectability: In some children, joint limitation was present at birth. In others it occurred in early childhood. Joint enlargement occurred between ages one and eight years; restrictive pericarditis was usually diagnosed within the following two years.

Gene Mapping and Linkage: Unknown.

Prevention: None known. Genetic counseling indicated.

Treatment: Pericardiectomy is indicated. The arthritis was resistant to treatment with corticosteroids or aspirin.

Prognosis: Appears to be normal for life span and intelligence.

Detection of Carrier: Unknown.

References:
Martinez-Lavin M, et al.: A familial syndrome of pericarditis, arthritis, and camptodactyly. New Engl J Med 1983; 309:224–225.
Bulutlar G, et al.: A familial syndrome of pericarditis, arthritis, camptodactyly, and coxa vara. Arthritis Rheum 1986; 29:436–438.
Laxer RM, et al.: The camptodactyly-arthropathy-pericarditis syndrome: case report and literature review. Arthritis Rheum 1986; 29:439–444.

T0007 **Helga V. Toriello**

Pericarditis-arthropathy-camptodactyly (CAP) syndrome
See SYNOVITIS, FAMILIAL HYPERTROPHIC
Pericardium agenesis
See HEART, PERICARDIUM AGENESIS
Pericardium, congenital partial or complete absence of
See HEART, PERICARDIUM AGENESIS
Peridens
See TEETH, SUPERNUMERARY
Perilymphatic gusher during stapes surgery
See DEAFNESS WITH PERILYMPHATIC GUSHER
Perinatal conduction system defects
See ARRHYTHMIA, CARDIAC CONDUCTION DEFECTS, NEONATAL
Perinatal effects of nonsteroidal anti-inflammatory drugs (NSAIDS)
See FETAL EFFECTS OF NONSTEROIDAL ANTI-INFLAMMATORY DRUGS (NSAIDS)
Perinatal transmission of hepatitis B infection
See FETAL EFFECT FROM HEPATITIS B INFECTION
Perinatal/neonatal cardiac conduction system defects-arrhythmia
See ARRHYTHMIA, CARDIAC CONDUCTION DEFECTS, NEONATAL
Perineal anus
See ANORECTAL MALFORMATIONS
Perinuclear cataract
See CATARACT, AUTOSOMAL DOMINANT CONGENITAL
Periodic disease
See FEVER, FAMILIAL MEDITERRANEAN (FMF)
Periodic fever
See FEVER, FAMILIAL MEDITERRANEAN (FMF)
Periodic neutropenia
See NEUTROPENIA, CYCLIC
Periodic paralysis, familial
See PARALYSIS, HYPOKALEMIC PERIODIC
Periodic paralysis, hyperpotassemic
See PARALYSIS, HYPERKALEMIC PERIODIC
Periodic paralysis, hypopotassemic
See PARALYSIS, HYPOKALEMIC PERIODIC
Periodic paralysis, II
See PARALYSIS, HYPERKALEMIC PERIODIC
also PARALYSIS, HYPOKALEMIC PERIODIC
Periodic paralysis, III
See PARALYSIS, NORMOKALEMIC PERIODIC
Periodic paralysis, normopotassemic
See PARALYSIS, NORMOKALEMIC PERIODIC
Periodic peritonitis
See FEVER, FAMILIAL MEDITERRANEAN (FMF)
Periodontitis, generalized juvenile
See TEETH, PERIODONTITIS, JUVENILE
Periodontitis, localized juvenile
See TEETH, PERIODONTITIS, JUVENILE
Periodontoclasia-hyperkeratosis palmoplantaris
See HYPERKERATOSIS PALMOPLANTARIS-PERIODONTOCLASIA
Periodontosis (misnomer)
See TEETH, PERIODONTITIS, JUVENILE
Periodontosis type Ehlers-Danlos syndrome
See EHLERS-DANLOS SYNDROME
Periosteal osteosarcoma
See OSTEOSARCOMA
Peripartum cardiomyopathy (some cases)
See CARDIOMYOPATHY, FAMILIAL DILATED
Peripheral neuroblastoma
See CANCER, EWING SARCOMA
Peritoneopericardial diaphragmatic hernia
See PENTALOGY OF CANTRELL
Perlman syndrome
See OVERGROWTH-RENAL HAMARTOMA, PERLMAN TYPE
Pernicious anemia, due to defect in intrinsic factor
See ANEMIA, PERNICIOUS CONGENITAL
Pernicious anemia, juvenile-proteinuria
See VITAMIN B(12) MALABSORPTION
Peromelia-micrognathia
See HYPOGLOSSIA-HYPODACTYLIA
Peroneal muscular atrophy, axonal type
See NEUROPATHY, HEREDITARY MOTOR AND SENSORY, TYPE I
Peroneal muscular atrophy, hypertrophic
See NEUROPATHY, HEREDITARY MOTOR AND SENSORY, TYPE I
Peroneal muscular atrophy, neuronal
See NEUROPATHY, HEREDITARY MOTOR AND SENSORY, TYPE II

Peroutka sneeze
  See ACHOO SYNDROME
Peroxisomal biogenesis, disorders of
  See CEREBRO-HEPATO-RENAL SYNDROME
Peroxisomal disorder (one form)
  See CHONDRODYSPLASIA PUNCTATA, RHIZOMELIC TYPE
Peroxisome deficiency
  See CEREBRO-HEPATO-RENAL SYNDROME

PERRAULT SYNDROME   2350

Includes:

    Deafness-gonadal dysgenesis
    Gonadal dysgenesis, XX type, with deafness
    Ovarian dysgenesis-sensorineural deafness

Excludes:

    Gonadal dysgenesis, XX type (0436)
    Gonadal dysgenesis, XY type (0437)
    Turner syndrome (0977)

Major Diagnostic Criteria: 46,XX individuals with infantile female phenotype; streak gonads demonstrated by direct visualization or elevated gonadotropin levels; and sensorineural deafness. Males (46,XY) with normal gonadal function and sensorineural deafness and females (46,XX) with isolated gonadal dysgenesis and normal hearing may be included if they have a positive family history.

Clinical Findings: Female individuals with Perrault syndrome have gonadal dysgenesis with an apparently normal (46,XX) chromosomal complement. Both the internal and external genitalia are female, but remain infantile. External genitalia, streak gonads, and endocrine function are indistinguishable from individuals with other types of gonadal dysgenesis, such as 45,X and gonadal dysgenesis, XX type. Hearing loss is usually moderate-to-severe sensorineural deafness and has been documented as early as one year of age. However, one individual had onset of significant hearing loss at age 31 years. Normal hearing has been documented in one female sib who also had gonadal dysgenesis; thus, hearing loss does not appear to be an obligatory manifestation in homozygous females. Male individuals (46,XY) who are sibs of affected females and apparently possess the same genotype have sensorineural hearing loss. However, they appear to have normal gonadal function with normal sexual development. Pallister and Opitz (1979) suggested that the low male-to-female ratio may indicate that hearing loss is not an obligate manifestation in male homozygotes, and thus these individuals have not been detected.

The majority of individuals with Perrault syndrome do not have additional anomalies. However, nine individuals had short stature (height at or below the third centile). Four females had at least one of the following features of **Turner syndrome**: cubitus valgus, congenital lymphedema, short neck, and short fourth and fifth metacarpals. Mental retardation was reported in three affected sibs, one of whom also had a right bundle branch block. Two affected females had lower limb weakness. One of these females was also mentally retarded and had spastic diplegia but also had a history of significant birth trauma. The other individual had ataxia. Both females had limited extraocular eye movements.

Laboratory evaluation of females with Perrault syndrome reveals decreased estrogen levels and increased follicle-stimulating hormone (FSH) and luteinizing hormone (LH) levels. One female also had partial growth hormone deficiency. Streak gonadal biopsy in one patient showed cortical fibrous tissue with absence of primordial follicles. Audiograms in seven patients suggested a pattern of mid-frequency depression and severe loss of high frequencies. Dermatoglyphics were normal in three patients but were mildly abnormal in two patients due to increased ridge count and alteration of main line termination. Bone age was retarded in seven of eight patients studied.

Complications: Hypogonadism and infertility in females. Severe speech deficits are common secondary to hearing loss.

Associated Findings: Possibly mental retardation, short stature.

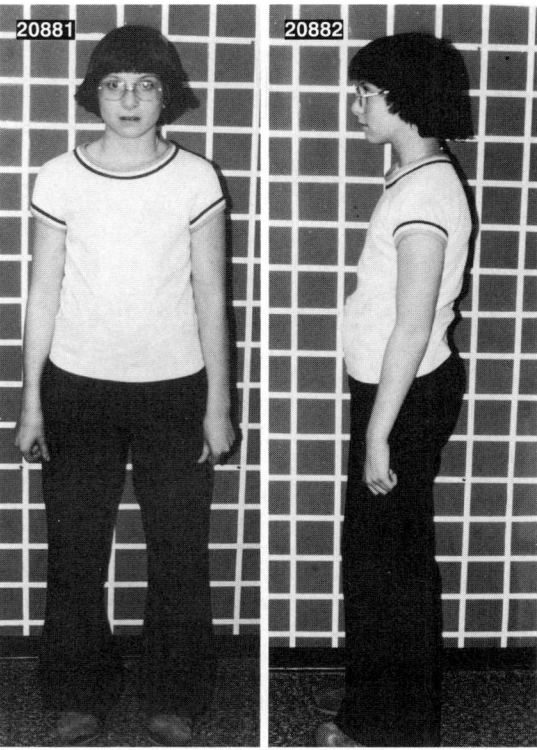

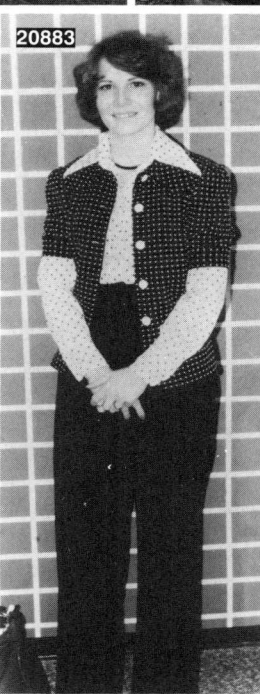

2350-20881–83: Perrault syndrome; two sisters who are affected; note the body habitus.

Etiology: Autosomal recessive inheritance. Parental consanguinity was reported in two families.

Pathogenesis: Gonadal dysgenesis and sensorineural deafness appear to be pleiotropic manifestations of the same gene. It has not been established whether the deafness and the streak gonads are due to a congenital developmental defect or arrest, or to a degenerative process.

MIM No.: *23340

POS No.: 3764

Sex Ratio: Presumably M1:F1; however, in the 21 reported cases the ratio was M1:F6, or M1:F3 if probands are excluded.

Occurrence: Nineteen additional individuals in seven families have been reported since Perrault's initial description of two affected sisters in 1951. Two sibships were from western Montana.

Risk of Recurrence for Patient's Sib:
See Part I, *Mendelian Inheritance.*

Risk of Recurrence for Patient's Child:
See Part I, *Mendelian Inheritance.* 46,XX patients are infertile. 46,XY patients probably have a less than 1% risk in the absence of consanguinity.

Age of Detectability: Sensorineural hearing loss can be detected in the first year of life. Diagnosis of Perrault syndrome is usually determined at puberty due to primary amenorrhea and lack of development of secondary sexual characteristics.

Gene Mapping and Linkage: Unknown.

Prevention: None known. Genetic counseling indicated.

Treatment: Estrogen replacement for hypogonadism; specialized educational programs for hearing impairment.

Prognosis: Probable normal for life span. Infertility in homozygous females. Varying degrees of hearing and speech deficits. The risk for mental retardation is uncertain.

Detection of Carrier: Unknown.

References:

Perrault M, et al.: Deux cas de syndrome de Turner avec surdi-multité dans une même fratrie. Bull Mém Soc Méd Hôp Paris 1951; 16:79–84.

Pallister PD, Opitz JM: The Perrault syndrome: autosomal recessive ovarian dysgenesis with facultative, non-sex-limited sensorineural deafness. Am J Med Genet 1979; 4:239–246. *

Bosze P, et al.: Perrault's syndrome in two sisters. Am J Med Genet 1983; 16:237–241.

McCarthy DJ, Opitz JM: Perrault syndrome in sisters. Am J Med Genet 1985; 22:629–631.

Nishi Y, et al.: The Perrault syndrome: clinical report and review. Am J Med Genet 1988; 31:623–629.

MO039 **Cynthia A. Moore**
WE005 **David D. Weaver**

Persistent ductus arteriosus
See DUCTUS ARTERIOSUS, PATENT
Persistent frontonasal process
See NOSE/NASAL SEPTUM DEFECTS
Persistent hypertrophic primary vitreous in OPC dwarfism
See DWARFISM, OCULO-PALATO-CEREBRAL TYPE
Persistent oviduct syndrome
See MULLERIAN DERIVATIVES IN MALES, PERSISTENT
Perthes disease
See JOINTS, OSTEOCHONDRITIS DISSECANS
also HIP, OSTEONECROSIS, CAPITAL FEMORAL EPIPHYSIS
Peters anomaly
See EYE, ANTERIOR SEGMENT DYSGENESIS
Peters anomaly-aortic stenosis-growth and mental retardation
See AORTC STENOSIS-CORNEAL CLOUDING-GROWTH AND MENTAL RETARDATION
Peters anomaly-short limbed dwarfism
See DWARFISM (SHORT LIMBED)-PETERS ANOMALY OF THE EYE
Peters plus
See DWARFISM (SHORT LIMBED)-PETERS ANOMALY OF THE EYE
also EYE, ANTERIOR SEGMENT DYSGENESIS
Petit mal automatism
See SEIZURES, CENTRALOPATHIC
Petit mal lapse ("absence")
See SEIZURES, CENTRALOPATHIC
Petit mal seizures
See SEIZURES, CENTRALOPATHIC
Petrous pyramid cholesteatoma
See EAR, CHOLESTEATOMA OF TEMPORAL BONE
Peutz-Jeghers syndrome
See INTESTINAL POLYPOSIS, TYPE II
Pfeiffer acrocephalopolysyndactyly
See ACROCEPHALOPOLYSYNDACTYLY
Pfeiffer syndrome
See ACROCEPHALOSYNDACTYLY TYPE V
PFK, liver type
See GLYCOGENOSIS, TYPE VII
Phagocytosis, plasma-related defect in
See IMMUNODEFICIENCY, PLASMA-ASSOCIATED DEFECT OF PHAGOCYTOSIS
Phalangeal hypoplasia-gingival fibromatosis
See GINGIVAL FIBROMATOSIS-DIGITAL ANOMALIES
Pharyngeal cyst or fistula
See NECK, BRANCHIAL CLEFT, CYSTS OR SINUSES
Pharyngeal muscular dystrophy
See MUSCULAR DYSTROPHY, OCULOPHARYNGEAL
Pharyngeal pouch syndrome
See IMMUNODEFICIENCY, THYMIC AGENESIS
Pharyngoesophageal diverticulum
See ESOPHAGUS, DIVERTICULUM
Pharynx cancer
See CANCER, LUNG, FAMILIAL

PHARYNX/LARYNX HYPOPLASIA-OMPHALOCELE, SHPRINTZEN-GOLDBERG TYPE — 2774

Includes:
Omphalocele-pharynx/larynx hypoplasia, Shprintzen-Goldberg type
Omphalocele with hypoplasia of pharynx and larynx
Shprintzen-Goldberg syndrome

Excludes: **Beckwith-Wiedemann syndrome** (0104)

Major Diagnostic Criteria: **Omphalocele** was found in two of the three cases examined. All known cases have learning disabilities, orbital hypertelorism or telecanthus, downturned oral commisures, hypotonia, scoliosis or kyphosis, reduced pharyngeal circumference, and a hypoplastic larynx.

Clinical Findings: **Omphalocele** and respiratory distress are present at birth. Hypotonia is also present at birth and persists into adult life. The face becomes increasingly dysmorphic with age. Orbital hypertelorism or telecanthus is relatively mild. The lower eye lids are S-shaped. The columella is slightly short, and there is bimaxillary protrusion, giving the nose a broad-based appearance. The oral commisures are downturned. Learning disabilities become apparent at school age. The voice is high pitched, which is secondary to a hypoplastic larynx. The epiglottis is similarly small and immature in configuration. The pharynx is very small, resulting in infantile apnea and frequent respiratory illness. The severity of learning disabilities and neurologic impairment has been variable, but intellectual testing has been within normal limits in all cases.

Complications: The constriction of the pharynx and larynx causes severe respiratory distress, especially in the newborn period, often requiring hospitalization and resulting in death in one patient at age four months. Learning disabilities and persistent hypotonia may limit certain activities in school, but cognitive development is not severely impaired. The small larynx causes vocal pitch to be high throughout life. Spinal abnormalities (i.e., scoliosis and lordosis) are probably secondary to hypotonia.

Associated Findings: Chronic serious otitis with subsequent mild conductive hearing loss.

Etiology: Presumably autosomal dominant inheritance, though there has not been an instance of male-to-male transmission.

Pathogenesis: Unknown.

MIM No.: 18221

POS No.: 4022

Sex Ratio: Presumably M1:F1.

Occurrence: Reported in a father and three daughters.

Risk of Recurrence for Patient's Sib:
See Part I, *Mendelian Inheritance.*

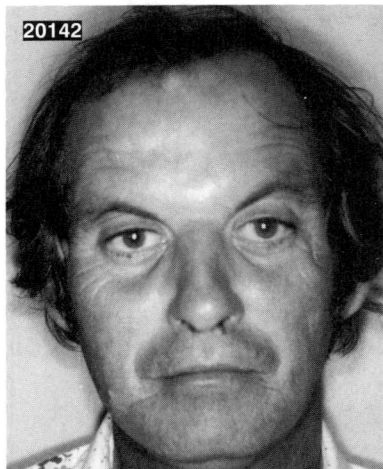

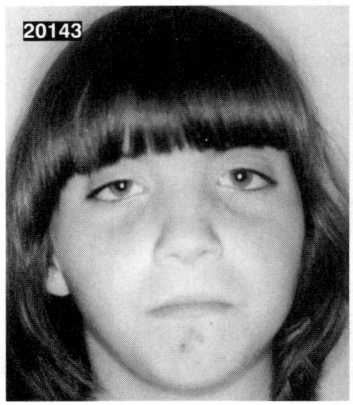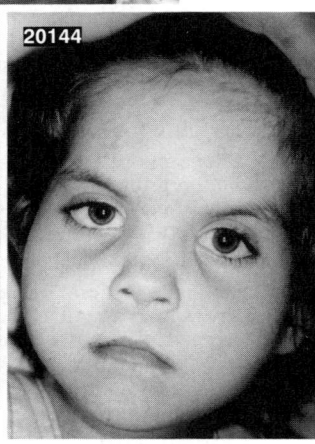

2774-20142–44: Subject with his two affected daughters; note epicanthal folds, broad nasal base, short columella, downturned lips and bimaxillary protrusion.

Risk of Recurrence for Patient's Child:
See Part I, *Mendelian Inheritance.*

Age of Detectability: If **Omphalocele** is present, diagnosis with prenatal ultrasound or fetoscope is possible. If omphalocele is not present, the detection may not occur until laryngeal abnormalities or learning disabilities become apparent during childhood.

Gene Mapping and Linkage: Unknown.

Prevention: None known. Genetic counseling indicated.

Treatment: Surgery for omphalocele as indicated. Laryngeal anomalies do not require intervention. Learning disabilities respond well to educational regimens. Physical therapy for hypotonia is indicated.

Prognosis: Normal life span. Hypotonia, high-pitched voice, and appearance are not severe enough to cause major problems, though they may limit certain choices of occupation, as may the learning disabilities.

Detection of Carrier: Fiber optic endoscopy of the upper airway is indicated for direct view of pharyngeal dimensions and laryngeal morphology. Testing of peripheral strength and cognitive testing for learning disabilities are possible. Presence of omphalocele should prompt further examination for other features.

References:
Shprintzen RJ, Goldberg RB: Dysmorphic facies, omphalocele, laryngeal and pharyngeal hypoplasia, spinal anomalies, and learning disabilities in a new dominant malformation syndrome. BD:OAS XV(5B). New York: March of Dimes Birth Defects Foundation, 1979:347–353.

SH040
G0008

Robert J. Shprintzen
Rosalie B. Goldberg

Phencyclidine, fetal effects
See FETAL EFFECTS FROM ANGEL DUST (PHENCYCLIDINE OR PCP)

Phenylalanine hydroxylase deficiency
See FETAL EFFECTS FROM MATERNAL PKU
also PHENYLKETONURIA

Phenylketonuria
See FETAL EFFECTS FROM MATERNAL PKU

PHENYLKETONURIA   0808

Includes:
Folling disease
Hyperphenylalaninemia
Oligophrenia phenylpyruvica
Phenylalanine hydroxylase deficiency
PKU1

Excludes:
Biopterin synthesis deficiency (2002)
Dihydropteridine reductase deficiency (2001)
Hyperphenylalanemia, transient

Major Diagnostic Criteria: Persistent elevation of blood phenylalanine concentrations above 6 mg/dl with normal or reduced blood tyrosine.

Clinical Findings: The major problem in untreated phenylketonuria, and sometimes the only problem, is mental retardation. During the first few weeks of life, there may be severe vomiting and epileptic seizures. Irritability may be seen in infancy. Some children have an eczematoid eruption; others have dry skin. Children may have a "mousy" smell due to phenylacetic acid in the urine and sweat. Although there are exceptions, phenylketonuric individuals tend to have blue eyes, blond hair, and fair skin.

Approximately two-thirds of those with concentrations of phenylalanine in serum above 6 mg/dl will develop moderate-to-severe mental retardation. Neurologic examination in these children may reveal **Microcephaly**, hand posturing with purposeless movements, and increased deep tendon reflexes. Many have abnormal EEG patterns. Some have seizures.

Biochemical characteristics are elevated blood phenylalanine (mean 20 mg/dl with a range of 10–60 mg/dl), urinary excretion of o-hydroxyphenylacetic acid (mean 1.6 μM/g creatinine), and excretion of urinary phenylpyruvic acid, phenyllacticacid and phenylacetylglutamine.

Complications: Mental retardation, seizures.

Associated Findings: None known.

Etiology: Autosomal recessive inheritance.

Pathogenesis: Deficiency of liver phenylalanine hydroxylase (PAH) reduces ability to form tyrosine. The accumulation of phenylalanine, phenylpyruvic acid, and other metabolites leads in some way to mental retardation, since prevention of accumulation through dietary restriction of phenylalanine prevents mental retardation.

MIM No.: *26160

POS No.: 3533

CDC No.: 270.100

Sex Ratio: M1:F1

Occurrence: 1:15,000 live births in the United States. Lower in Blacks and Ashkenazi Jews.

Risk of Recurrence for Patient's Sib:
See Part I, *Mendelian Inheritance.*

Risk of Recurrence for Patient's Child:
See Part I, *Mendelian Inheritance.* Heterozygous offspring of a

homozygous mother can be mentally retarded (see **Fetal effects from maternal PKU**).

Age of Detectability: At 48 hours, by measurement of blood phenylalanine if protein intake is normal. By the sixth day, the diagnosis should virtually always be clear. The gene for phenylalanine hydroxylase has been cloned, and while the cDNA probe does not recognize the patient with PKU as different from control individuals, there are a number of linked restriction fragment length polymorphisms (RFLPs).

Gene Mapping and Linkage: PAH (phenylalanine hydroxylase) has been mapped to 12q22-q24.2.

Prevention: None known. Genetic counseling indicated.

Treatment: The low-phenylalanine diet is effective in preventing mental retardation. Treatment must be started during the early weeks of life, but this is the logical consequence of the availability of programs of routine neonatal screening in most of the developed countries of the world.

Prognosis: In the untreated patient with mental retardation and seizures, there may be reduced life span. With treatment, the prognosis for life span and intelligence should be excellent.

Detection of Carrier: The cDNA probe and assessment of RFLPs is successful in identifying heterozygotes in an informative family known to be at risk.

Special Considerations: In a collaborative study of newborn screening programs of patients with high concentrations of phenylalanine and normal tyrosine, it was found that about one fourth have had persistent phenylalaninemia between 6 and 19.9 mg/dl, and the remainder have had phenylalaninemia greater than 20 mg/dl. Among untreated patients, normal mental development has been found in almost all of those with phenylalanine concentrations less than 19.9 mg/dl. In treated patients, a diet low in phenylalanine was effective in preventing mental deficiency, particularly if started at less than 30 days of age. A number of terms have been employed in hyperphenylalaninemic patients including phenylketonuria, hyperphenylalanemia, persistent hyperphenylalanemia, phenylalanemia, and atypical phenylketonuria. These patients may represent heterogeneity in the phenylalanine hydroxylase enzyme.

Support Groups:
CA; Los Altos; PKU Parents Group
ENGLAND: Kent; Bexley; National Society for Phenylketonuria

References:

Lyman FL, ed. Phenylketonuria. Springfield, CC Thomas, 1963.
Berman JL, et al.: Causes for high phenylalanine with normal tyrosine in newborn screening programs. Am J Dis Child 1969; 117:54.
Koch R, et al.: Phenylalaninemia and phenylketonuria. In: Nyhan WL, ed: Heritable disorders of amino acid metabolism. New York: John Wiley & Sons, 1974:109–140.
Shear CS, et al.: Phenylketonuria: experience with diagnosis and management. In: Nyhan WL, ed: Heritable disorders of amino acid metabolism. New York: John Wiley & Sons, 1974:141–159.
Koch R, et al.: Preliminary report on the effects of diet discontinuation in PKU. J Pediatr 1982; 100:870–875.
Güttler F, et al.: Prenatal diagnosis and carrier detection by gene analysis. In: Inherited diseases of amino acid metabolism. Recent progress in the understanding, recognition and management, international symposium in Heidelberg, 1984, Bickel H and Wachtel U, eds., Stuttgart/New York: Georg Thiem Verlag Thieme, 1985:18–36.
Nyhan WL: Diagnostic recognition of genetic disease. Philadelphia, Lea & Febiger, 1987:100–106.

NY000   **William L. Nyhan**

Phenylketonuria II
See DIHYDROPTERIDINE REDUCTASE DEFICIENCY
Phenylketonuria III
See BIOPTERIN SYNTHESIS DEFICIENCY
Phenylketonuria VI
See BIOPTERIN SYNTHESIS DEFICIENCY
Phenylthiocarbamide tasting
See TASTING DEFECT, PHENYLTHIOCARBAMIDE
Phenylthiourea insensitivity
See TASTING DEFECT, PHENYLTHIOCARBAMIDE

Phenytoin, fetal effects of
See FETAL HYDANTOIN SYNDROME
also HOLOPROSENCEPHALY
Phenytoin-type embryopathy
See FETAL PRIMIDONE EMBRYOPATHY
Pheochromocytoma and amyloid-producing medullary thyroid carcinoma
See ENDOCRINE NEOPLASIA, MULTIPLE TYPE II
Pheochromocytoma-medullary thyroid carcinoma-multiple neuroma
See ENDOCRINE NEOPLASIA, MULTIPLE TYPE III
Phocomelia
See LIMB REDUCTION DEFECTS
Phocomelia, deficiency of
See HAND, RADIAL CLUB HAND
Phocomelia-ectrodactyly-oto-sinus arrhythmia syndrome
See LIMB-OTO-CARDIAC SYNDROME
Phosphatase, liver alkaline
See HYPOPHOSPHATASIA
Phosphate-eliminating enzyme, deficiency of
See BIOPTERIN SYNTHESIS DEFICIENCY
Phosphate-pyrophosphate translocase
See GLYCOGENOSIS, TYPE Ic
Phosphatidylcholine red cell membrane disorder
See ANEMIA, HEMOLYTIC, RED CELL MEMBRANE DEFECTS
Phosphoethanolaminuria
See HYPOPHOSPHATASIA
Phosphofructokinase (PFK) deficiency
See GLYCOGENOSIS, TYPE VII
Phosphofructokinase, muscle type
See GLYCOGENOSIS, TYPE VIII
Phosphoglucomutase
See GLYCOGENOSES
Phosphoglucose isomerase
See GLYCOGENOSES
Phosphoglucose isomerase inhibitor
See GLYCOGENOSIS, TYPE VIII
Phosphoglucose isomerase, deficiency of
See ANEMIA, GLUCOSE PHOSPHATE ISOMERASE DEFICIENCY
Phosphoglucose isomerase, Homberg type
See GLYCOGENOSES
Phosphoglycerate kinase (PGK) deficiency, erythrocyte
See ANEMIA, HEMOLYTIC, ERYTHROCYTE PHOSPHOGLYCERATE KINASE DEFICIENCY
Phosphoglycerate kinase, M isozyme
See GLYCOGENOSES
Phosphoglycerate mutase, M isozyme
See GLYCOGENOSES
Phosphohexose isomerase, deficiency of
See ANEMIA, GLUCOSE PHOSPHATE ISOMERASE DEFICIENCY

**PHOSPHORIBOSYL PYROPHOSPHATE (PRPP)
SYNTHETASE ABNORMALITY**   **0508**

Includes:
Ataxia-deafness (sensorineural)-hyperuricemia
Deafness-hyperuricemia-ataxia
Hyperuricemia-deafness (sensorineural)-ataxia
Phosphoribosylpyrophosphate synthetase

Excludes:
Gout (0441)
Lesch-Nyhan syndrome (0588)
Lipodystrophy and neurologic defects

Major Diagnostic Criteria: Progressive spinocerebellar ataxia and sensorineural hearing loss with hyperuricemia. Abnormal hyperactivity of PRPP synthetase.

Clinical Findings: Onset of elevated blood uric acid is in infancy, but may not be recognized until late childhood or at puberty. Similarly, sensorineural hearing loss may be congenital, or it may first be recognized in adolescence or early adult life. Progressive spinocerebellar ataxia, when present, begins later, along with slurred speech. Renal disease and any of the manifestations of **Gout** may occur in the absence of effective treatment. Two adult females with the syndrome have also developed cervicodorsal fat pad ("buffalo hump") without Cushing syndrome and with normal steroid levels. Muscle wasting and weakness are inconstant features. One member of a family studied has developed cardiomyopathy. There is no mental retardation or self-mutilation as in the **Lesch-Nyhan syndrome**.

Audiograms usually show a high-frequency sensorineural loss in the younger affected members, and a sloping sensorineural loss in early adult life. The most severely affected individuals have virtually complete loss of hearing, and this may be congenital. A highly positive SISI (short increment sensitivity index) is found on special testing, indicating cochlear involvement rather than neural or central involvement. Electronystagmography shows changes consistent with a vestibular lesion central to the labyrinth. Petrous pyramid tomography is normal.

Standard renal function tests are normal in the younger affected members. Erythrocyte hypoxanthine-guanine phosphoribosyltransferase levels are normal. Muscle biopsies of affected members with muscle weakness are consistent with a neurogenic myopathy.

Complications: Nephrolithiasis, nephropathy, gouty arthritis, tophi.

Associated Findings: Congestive heart failure secondary to cardiomyopathy. One patient was reported with limited intelligence and absent lacrimal glands.

Etiology: X-linked inheritance.

Pathogenesis: Defect of phosphoribosyl pyrophosphate (PRPP) synthetase. This is an unusual defect in that the enzyme is superactive rather than hypoactive. Nevertheless, it may be unstable and short lived. Activities in erythrocytes may accordingly be normal or low. Studies in fibroblasts are usually required. Hyperuricemia results in renal dysfunction and associated symptoms.

MIM No.: *31185

POS No.: 4266

Sex Ratio: M1:F<1

Occurrence: Undetermined. Described in a large Mexican-American kindred living in Pueblo, Colorado.

Risk of Recurrence for Patient's Sib:
See Part I, *Mendelian Inheritance*.

Risk of Recurrence for Patient's Child:
See Part I, *Mendelian Inheritance*.

Age of Detectability: Prenatally by enzyme analysis. In infancy by blood uric acid. In childhood by audiometry. Often in adolescence by clinical evaluation.

Gene Mapping and Linkage: PRPS1 (phosphoribosyl pyrophosphate synthetase 1) has been mapped to Xq21-q27.

Prevention: None known. Genetic counseling indicated.

Treatment: Allopurinol will reduce blood uric acid levels and should prevent gout, nephropathy, and nephrolithiasis. However, it has had no retarding or beneficial effects on the deafness, ataxia, muscle weakness, or wasting. Hearing aids and speech training. Treatment for congestive heart failure secondary to cardiomyopathy.

Prognosis: Progression of hearing loss, ataxia, and muscle weakness.

Detection of Carrier: By PRPP synthetase in cultured fibroblasts.

References:
Kelley WN, et al.: A specific enzyme defect in gout assoicated with overproduction of uric acid. Proc Natl Acad Sci USA 1967; 57:1735.
Rosenberg AL, Bartholomew B: Gout and uric acid. Bull Rheum Dis 1969; 19:543.
Rosenberg AL, et al.: Hyperuricemia and neurologic deficits: a family study. New Engl J Med 1970; 282:992–997.
Simmond HA, et al.: An X-linked syndrome characterised by hyperuricaemia, deafness, and neurodevelopmental abnormalities. Lancet 1982; II:68–70.
Becker MA, et al.: Phosphoribosylpyrophosphate synthetase superactivity. Arthritis Rheum 1986; 29:880–888.

BE028
NY000

LaVonne Bergstrom
William L. Nyhan

Phosphoribosylpyrophosphate synthetase
See *PHOSPHORIBOSYL PYROPHOSPHATE (PRPP) SYNTHETASE ABNORMALITY*
Phosphorylase deficiency glycogen-storage disease of liver
See *GLYCOGENOSIS, TYPE VI*
Phosphorylase kinase deficiency of liver
See *GLYCOGENOSIS, TYPE IXa*
also *GLYCOGEN STORAGE DISEASE, X-LINKED WITH NORMAL HEPATIC ENZYMES*
Phosphorylase kinase deficiency, generalized
See *GLYCOGENOSIS, TYPE IXb*
Photic sneeze reflex
See *ACHOO SYNDROME*
Photogenic epilepsy
See *EPILEPSY, REFLEX*
Photomyoclonus-deafness-diabetes-nephropathy
See *DEAFNESS-DIABETES-PHOTOMYOCLONUS-NEPHROPATHY*
Photosensitivity with defective DNA synthesis
See *XERODERMA PIGMENTOSUM*
Photosensitivity, from protoporphyria
See *PORPHYRIA, PROTOPORPHYRIA*
Phytanic acid oxidase deficiency
See *PHYTANIC ACID STORAGE DISEASE*

PHYTANIC ACID OXIDASE DEFICIENCY, INFANTILE TYPE   2278

Includes:
Adrenoleukodystrophy, neonatal (some forms)
Infantile phytanic acid storage disease
Pipecolic acidemia (some forms)
Refsum disease, infantile form

Excludes:
Adrenoleukodystrophy, X-linked (2533)
Cerebro-hepato-renal syndrome (0139)
Phytanic acid storage disease (0810)

Major Diagnostic Criteria: Retinitis pigmentosa, severe neurosensory deafness, severe developmental delay, peripheral neuropathy, hepatomegaly, facial dysmorphism, simian creases, minor elevation in serum phytanic acid. Serum pipecolic acid and very long chain (C_{24} and C_{26}) fatty acids are elevated. Plasmalogen synthesis is impaired. Activities of several enzymes, including phytanic acid oxidase, Acyl-CoA:dihydroxyacetone phosphate acyltransferase and other enzymes now known to be peroxisomal are deficient in several tissues including cultured skin fibroblasts.

Clinical Findings: The condition is apparent in infancy, when hepatomegaly (2–5 cm below the costal margin) is noted; several cases have had steatorrhea with a marked bleeding diathesis responsive to Vitamin K. The steatorrhea has resolved spontaneously after some months or years. Most cases have not been

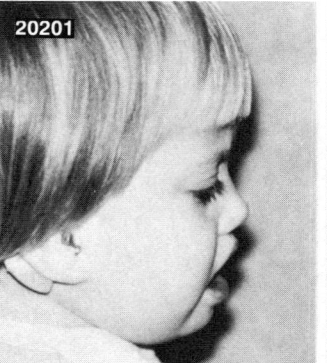
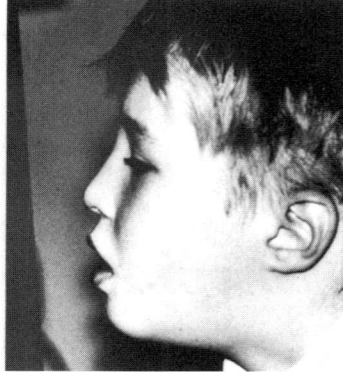

2278-20201: Note flattened facies in these two subjects with phytanic oxidase deficiency, infantile type.

investigated in early infancy, so the frequency of the steatorrhea is unclear.

Severe sensorineural hearing loss becomes evident (100%) within the first year, and a severe devlopmental delay is apparent before the first birthday. **Retinitis pigmentosa** has developed within the first two years of life in all cases studied to date. This includes a prominent macular dystrophic component, and is similar to that seen in advanced **Phytanic acid storage disease**. Electroretinography shows severely subnormal rod- and cone-mediated responses. The characteristic facies are considered by some to be reminiscent of **Chromosome 21, trisomy 21**. From the side view, the face is flattened with the nose being rather less prominent than normal. A **Skin crease, single palmer** has been noted in at least five cases. The children are hypotonic, and the tendon reflexes are diminished or absent, consistent with a peripheral neuropathy.

Standard liver function tests are not consistently abnormal, but the liver biopsy is definitely abnormal. On regular microscopy, the architecture of the lobules and hepatocytes is preserved but there is interlobular bridging by bands of fibrous tissue which emanate from the portal triads. On electron microscopy, at least two groups have reported characteristic long, linear, trilaminar membrane bound inclusions within the hepatocytes and probably the Kupffer cells. The composition of these materials is unknown.

Laboratory Findings: the level of phytanic acid in the serum is usually elevated (0.5–20mg/dl; normal <0.2 mg/dl) but may occasionally be normal. Pipecolic acid (0.3–3 mg/dl; normal <0.05 mg/dl) has been elevated in all patients in whom it has been measured. The plasma very long chain fatty acids are also elevated, resulting in an increased ratio of hexacosanoate:docosanoate (C_{26}:C_{22}) and tetracosanoate:docosanoate (C_{24}:C_{22}). Plasmalogen levels are lower than normal; plasma bile acid intermediates may be elevated in some patients.

Multiple enzyme defects are known, including phytanic acid oxidase, dihydroxyacetone phosphate acyltransferase, alkyldihydroxyacetone phosphate synthase, peroxisomal acyl-CoA oxidase, bifunctional protein, and thiolase.

Complications: Hemorrhagic episodes, such as cerebral hemorrhage, in the early months due to the bleeding diathesis caused by the malabsorption and steatorrhea. The retinal dystrophy can be severe enough for the patients to be classified as legally blind.

Associated Findings: Plasma cholestrol tends to be low, with reduced levels of alpha- and sometimes also beta-lipoproteins in the plasma.

Etiology: Presumably autosomal recessive inheritance.

Pathogenesis: Early reports emphasized the abnormal levels of phytanic acid in plasma, and it was presumed that the phytanic acid somehow caused the symptoms by a mechanism similar to that in **Phytanic acid storage disease** (Refsum disease). The recent discovery of many other biochemical abnormalities such as elevated pipecolic acid, which is a metabolite of lysine, and the biochemical findings outlined above, all indicate a major defect in peroxisomal function. Not all peroxisomal enzymes are compromised. For example, catalase activity, at least in fibroblasts, is normal, although less than 5% of it is particle bound. There is some debate over whether peroxisomes are absent as in **Cerebro-hepato-renal syndrome** (Zellweger syndrome), or present but diminished in number and metabolic function.

Complementation studies of cell lines from **Cerebro-hepato-renal syndrome**, hyperpipecolicacidemia, and infantile Refsum patients indicate no complementation. Whether this reflects total absence of peroxisomes or allelic mutations is not clear. Conversely, complementation appears to occur with cell fusions of lines from **Cerebro-hepato-renal syndrome** and neonatal adrenoleukodystrophy patients.

The obvious relationship of this disorder to **Cerebro-hepato-renal syndrome** in which serum phytanic acid, pipecolic acid, and very long chain fatty acids are also elevated, and liver peroxisomes are severely deficient, suggests that infantile phytanic acid oxidase deficiency may represent another disorder of peroxisomal function. The cause of the steatorrhea may be from low levels of lipoprotein in the plasma, similar to what is seen in **Abetalipopro-**

teinemia. The facial dysmorphism associated with this syndrome implies that the damage is of prenatal onset.

Sex Ratio: Presumably M1:F1.

Occurrence: A few dozen cases have been documented.

Risk of Recurrence for Patient's Sib:
See Part I, *Mendelian Inheritance.*

Risk of Recurrence for Patient's Child:
See Part I, *Mendelian Inheritance.*

Age of Detectability: In the neonatal period. Prenatal diagnosis is possible.

Gene Mapping and Linkage: Unknown.

Prevention: None known. Genetic counseling indicated.

Treatment: A phytanic acid restricted diet has been tried in one patient. The diet lowered the phytanic acid level in the plasma and improved the patient's behavior, but did nothing to improve the other symptoms. Therapy for steatorrhea in the early months includes a low lipid diet, probably with medium chain triglycerides and supplements of the fat soluble vitamins. No other specific therapy is currently available.

Prognosis: The patients reported to date have all presented similar symptoms in early infancy, and have survived into adolescence with severe and stable developmental delay. It is not known whether there are milder or more severe cases in whom the prognosis may be different.

Detection of Carrier: In four obligate heterozygotes, serum phytanic acid was normal, as was the ratio of C_{26}:C_{22} and C_{24}:C_{22} very long chain fatty acids. Thus, carrier detection for infantile phytanic acid oxidase deficiency is not yet possible.

References:
Scotto, JM, et al.: Infantile phytanic acid storage disease, a possible variant of Refsum's disease: three cases, including ultrastructural studies of the liver. J Inherit Metab Dis 1982; 5:83–90.

Poulos A, et al.: Infantile Refsum's disease (phytanic acid storage disease): a variant of Zellweger's syndrome? Clin Genet 1984; 26:579–586.

Budden SS, et al.: Dysmorphic syndrome with phytanic acid oxidase deficiency, abnormal very long chain fatty acids, and pipecolic acidemia: studies in four children. J Pediatr 1986; 108:33–39.

Kelley RI, et al.: Neonatal adrenoleukodystrophy: new cases, biochemical studies and differentiation from Zellweger and related peroxisomal polydystrophy syndromes. Am J Med Genet 1986; 23:869–901.

Wanders RJA, et al.: Infantile Refsum disease: deficiency of catalase-containing particles (peroxisomes), alkyldihydroxyacetone phosphate synthase and peroxisomal β-oxidation enzyme proteins. Eur J Pediatr 1986; 145:172–175.

Schutgens RBH, et al.: Peroxisomal disorders: a newly recognized group of genetic diseases. Eur J Pediatr 1986; 144:430–440.

Lazarow PB, Moser HW: Disorders of peroxisome biogenesis. In: Scriver CR, et al, eds: The metabolic basis of inherited disease, 6th ed. New York: McGraw-Hill, 1989:1479–1510.

KE022   **Nancy G. Kennaway**
BU009   **Neil R. M. Buist**

PHYTANIC ACID STORAGE DISEASE   **0810**

Includes:
Heredopathia atactica polyneuritiformis
Phytanic acid oxidase deficiency
Refsum disease

Excludes:
Adrenoleukodystrophy, X-linked (2533)
Cerebro-hepato-renal syndrome (0139)
Elevated pipecolic acid, other syndromes with
Phytanic acid oxidase deficiency, infantile type (2278)
Retinal pigmentation without accumulation of phytanic acid
Retinal pigmentation without deficiency in phytanic acid oxidation
Very long chain fatty acids, other syndromes with

Major Diagnostic Criteria: Demonstration should be made of abnormal concentrations of phytanic acid in plasma or tissues. The major "clinical triad" consists of retinitis pigmentosa, peripheral neuropathy, and cerebellar ataxia. Cerebrospinal fluid protein level is increased without cells present.

Clinical Findings: The clinical features found at the time of reporting are listed here for patients in whom the actual biochemical defect was confirmed. Onset of symptoms is usually before adulthood. Retinal degeneration, with nightblindness, concentric narrowing of visual fields, and an atypical retinal pigmentation are virtually always found. There is peripheral neuropathy in 90% of the patients, with motor weakness, muscular atrophy, loss of deep tendon reflexes, electromyographic evidence of denervation, and loss of superficial sensation to pain, touch, or temperature. Muscle pain, or paresthesias, are infrequent. Other neurologic features include cerebellar signs (75%), nerve deafness (50%), pupillary abnormalities (40%), anosmia (35%), and nystagmus (25%). Cardiac involvement can sometimes be shown, with nonspecific ST-T changes in the precordial EKG or left ventricular enlargement. Cataracts were seen in 40% of the patients, and 60% have some skeletal malformations (shortening of the metatarsals, osteochondritis dissecans, pes cavus, etc). Some patients have ichthyotic skin changes, occasionally florid (trunk, palms, soles). Spinal fluid protein levels are increased in 85% of the patients (55–730 mg/dl, mean: 275), without increased cells present.

Complications: Four patients have died suddenly, possibly from cardiac arrhythmias, and two have died with respiratory paralysis. Renal function has been impaired in four patients, and increased urine lipid was noted in one (with severe fatty infiltration of the kidneys).

Associated Findings: Aminoaciduria has been reported in two patients, of uncertain relationship to the primary defect.

Etiology: Autosomal recessive inheritance, with high consanguinity, and a partial defect in heterozygotes.

Pathogenesis: Phytanic acid accumulation has been shown to be secondary to deletion of a phytanic acid oxidizing system, with the specific metabolic block involving the initial α-oxidation. This probably involves specifically an α-hydroxylating system that converts phytanic acid to α-hydroxyphytanic acid.

It is likely that the accumulation of phytanic acid in itself leads to the clinical manifestations of the disease. Animal feeding experiments have been negative, however, and rare instances of moderately elevated plasma phytanic acid levels have been found in parents of patients without clinical signs. It is pertinent that in some patients the course of the illness has been favorably influenced by dietary restriction of phytanic acid.

It is of interest that the nervous system is a natural site of high concentrations of α-hydroxy fatty acids, but skin and nerve tissue from patients analyzed to date have not shown alteration in concentration or composition of these acids.

MIM No.: *26650

POS No.: 3463

Sex Ratio: M1:F1

Occurrence: About 100 cases have been documented.

Risk of Recurrence for Patient's Sib:
See Part I, *Mendelian Inheritance.*

Risk of Recurrence for Patient's Child:
See Part I, *Mendelian Inheritance.*

Age of Detectability: The earliest clinical manifestations (e.g. nightblindness) usually occur within the first two decades of life.

Gene Mapping and Linkage: Unknown.

Prevention: None known. Genetic counseling indicated.

Treatment: It is possible to limit the accumulation of phytanic acid and to decrease body stores by a diet from which phytanic acid and its precursors have been removed. Dairy products (butter, milk, cheese) and ruminant fats (beef and sheep) are the major sources, but phytanic acid is widely distributed in foodstuffs, including lipids of marine animals. Phytol in its unesterified form is a precursor for phytanic acid, but when esterified in

the chlorophyll molecule it is apparently minimally absorbed. Plasma phytanate levels have dropped in all patients who have adhered to the special diet, and in none of those adhering has there been a clinical relapse. In four patients follow-up data are now available for up to 10 years; some improvement in symptomatology occurs over the first 6–12 months (excluding cranial nerve manifestations), after which the clinical picture seems to stabilize. Obviously one would anticipate that institution of the diet in childhood would be most advantageous. Repeated plasmapheresis or plasma exchange may also be helpful in depleting body stores of phytanic acid.

Supportive measures for consequences of neuropathy (physiotherapy, orthopedic devices); cataract extraction when indicated.

Prognosis: The course of the untreated disease is slowly progressive, with frequent exacerbations and remissions of symptoms (occasionally correlated with intercurrent viral infection). Life expectancy is shortened, but the age at death varies greatly. Expiration in childhood is rare, but death before age 40 years occurred in six of the 33 chemically-established cases. Cardiac and respiratory problems appear to be the major threat to survival.

Detection of Carrier: Parents, sibs, and children of known patients are clinically unaffected, and their plasma phytanic acid levels have been normal except in two instances (mothers of patients). Cell cultures from skin biopsies of patients show oxidation of phytanic acid at 1–2% of the normal rate. Cultures from heterozygote individuals have a partial defect, and hence this technique could be used in the detection of heterozygosity.

References:
Refsum S: Heredopathia atactica polyneuritiformis; familial syndrome not hitherto described: contribution to clinical study of hereditary diseases of nervous system. Acta Psychiatr Scand 1946; 38 (Suppl.):1.
Steinberg D, et al.: Refsum's disease: a recently characterized lipidosis involving the nervous system. Ann Intern Med 1967; 66:365–395.
Steinberg D, et al.: Refsum's disease: nature of the enzyme defect. Science 1967; 156:1740–1742.
Poulos A, et al.: Patterns of Rufsum's disease: phytanic acid oxidase deficiency. Arch Dis Child 1984; 59:222–229.
Steinberg D: Refsum disease. In: Scriver CR, et al, eds: The metabolic basis of inherited disease, 6th ed. New York: McGraw-Hill, 1989: 1533–1550.

ST012   **Daniel Steinberg**
BU009   **Neil R. M. Buist**
KE022   **Nancy G. Kennaway**

Pi phenotype ZZ, SZ, Z- and --
See ALPHA(1)-ANTITRYPSIN DEFICIENCY

PICK DISEASE OF THE BRAIN 3243

Includes:
Brain, lobar atrophy of
Dementia-lobar atrophy and neuronal cytoplasmic inclusions
Lobar atrophy

Excludes:
Alzheimer disease
Creutzfeldt-Jakob disease (3244)
Multi-infarct dementia
Subcortical atherosclerotic encephalopathy

Major Diagnostic Criteria: A rare degenerative disease of the central nervous system characterized by the insidious onset and slow progression of dementia, frequently with prominent behavioral symptoms and language impairment. It is relentlessly progressive over 2–12 years, leading to death. Brain computerized tomography (CT) or magnetic resonance imaging (MRI) may show characteristic focal or lobar atrophy. There is considerable overlap in clinical symptoms with **Alzheimer disease**, which frequently leads to diagnostic uncertainty. Presumptive clinical diagnosis is confirmed by post-mortem examination of the brain. This demonstrates prominent atrophy in a lobar distribution involving the frontal and/or temporal lobes and distinctive histologic changes of argyrophilic cytoplasmic inclusions (Pick bodies) within neurons and "ballooned" or "inflated" neurons (Pick cells), in the absence of neuritic plaques and neurofibrillary tangles characteristic of Alzheimer disease.

Clinical Findings: Symptoms usually begin in the fifth or sixth decade (average age of onset is 54 years), but may occur as early as the third or as late as the ninth decades. The disease is characterized by progressive cognitive deterioration, with specific clinical features reflecting the distribution of the pathologic changes, usually predominantly frontal or temporal lobe involvement. Eighty percent of cases of Pick disease appear to be sporadic while 20% are thought to be familial. There are no consistent differences between the apparently sporadic and familial cases. There is no evidence of differences between maternal and paternal rates of transmission.

The disease can be divided into three stages. The initial stage (usually lasting 1–3 years) is characterized by prominent personality, behavioral, and emotional changes. Judgement is impaired early, insight is lacking and social behavior deteriorates. A wide variety of personality changes can be seen (such as depression, apathy, euphoria and irritability); behavioral changes frequently seen include inappropriate or disinhibited actions, particularly sexual indiscretions. Perhaps the most striking behavioral manifestation is the development of symptoms resembling the Kluver-Bucy syndrome, including emotional blunting, hypersexuality, hyperorality, markedly increased eating, hypermetamorphosis, and visual or auditory agnosia. Language alterations may be noted early but become particularly prominent as the disease progresses.

In the second stage (lasting 3–6 years) cognitive deterioration becomes evident and language disturbance (anomia, verbal stereotypias, impaired comprehension and aphasia) become a dominant feature. It is interesting that memory, calculations, and visuospatial skills remain relatively unimpaired during this phase, which is in contrast to Alzheimer disease where early impairment in these areas is quite characteristic.

In the final stage of Pick disease (lasting 6–12 years), diffuse cognitive deterioration with profound dementia occurs, the person becomes mute or incomprehensible, and a progressive extrapyramidal syndrome usually develops. There is a marked lack of focal motor, sensory or visual signs, such as hemiplegia or visual field deficits. Myoclonus sometimes occurs, but generalized motor seizures are uncommon.

Routine laboratory studies of blood, serum, urine, and cerebrospinal fluid are normal. Vitamin B12 and folate deficiency, neurosyphillis and hypothyroidism should be excluded since they represent potentially treatable causes of dementia. Some investigators have found increased levels of urinary zinc. Neuroimaging studies (brain CT or MRI) may show focal lobar atrophy and provide supportive evidence for the clinical diagnosis as well as serve to exclude other causes of dementia such as multiple infarcts, tumors, and normal pressure **Hydrocephaly**. Positron emission tomography (PET scan) shows hypometabolism of cortical glucose in the anterior frontal and temporal association cortices and is perhaps the best current imaging technique to reliably distinguish Pick disease from Alzheimer disease. The EEG typically remains normal, but may show diffuse, or rarely focal, slowing of the background. Formal neuropsychological evaluation is useful for characterizing the cognitive deficits and quantifying changes as the disease progresses. This may also disclose an anatomical pattern of functional impairment that supports the diagnosis of Pick disease and assists in differentiating it from Alzheimer disease.

Complications: Progressive behavioral and cognitive deterioration frequently lead to loss of employment as well as disruption of familial and interpersonal relationships. In the terminal stage of the disease, common complications of the bedridden state such as aspiration pneumonia, urinary tract infections, decubitus ulcers and progressive inanition are seen.

Associated Findings: Although it has not been widely investigated, increased urinary excretion of zinc has been found in some patients. An increase in psychiatric symptoms in first degree relatives has been reported.

Etiology: Autosomal dominant inheritance with age-dependent penetrance is found in familial cases, which accounts for approximately 20% of the reported cases.

Pathogenesis: Unknown. A variety of theories have been proposed, including an axonal disorder with secondary changes in the cell body, a defect in zinc transport by plasma proteins leading to elevated intracortical zinc levels and selective disruption of glutamate function, viral infection, and primary degeneration of the neuronal cell body.

MIM No.: 17270

Sex Ratio: Probably M1:F1. However, most epidemiologic studies have found a higher overall prevalence and age-specific incidence rates for females (approximately M1:F2).

Occurrence: Prevalence is estimated to be less than 1%. The precise incidence and prevalence are unknown since the accurate diagnosis requires pathologic confirmation and the disease is clinically likely to be misdiagnosed as Alzheimer disease.

Risk of Recurrence for Patient's Sib:
See Part I, *Mendelian Inheritance*.

Risk of Recurrence for Patient's Child:
See Part I, *Mendelian Inheritance*. This risk has not been adequately studied.

Age of Detectability: Symptoms may begin as early as the third decade, although the average age of onset is in the fifth or sixth. Pick disease appears to increase in frequency until about age 58; then its frequency decreases until after age 70 its onset becomes rare.

Gene Mapping and Linkage: Unknown.

Prevention: None known. Genetic counseling indicated.

Treatment: There is no effective treatment or cure. Treatment is symptomatic and may include minor and major tranquilizers for control of behavioral symptoms. Supportive medical care, educational and supportive interventions for the family, and symptomatic treatment of complications (e.g. infections, seizures, feeding problems) are provided as indicated. Constantinidis has reported symptomatic improvement in a small number of patients with heavy-metal chelation.

Prognosis: The disease progresses over 2–12 years, from the onset of clinical symptoms to the time of death. Decreased life expectancy is observed, with approximately 80% of patients dying within ten years after the onset of the disease.

Detection of Carrier: Careful pedigree analysis may allow detection of families and individuals at high risk. There is no laboratory or other test to identify asymptomatic carriers. Groen and Endtz (1982) investigated persons at risk from a large, well-documented family with EEGs and CT scans and found frontal atrophy in four cases out of 12. In one of these cases, clinical signs of Pick disease became manifest a year after the investigation. Formal neuropsychological assessment may detect individuals early in the course of the disease.

References:
Malamud N, Waggoner RW: Genealogic and clinicopathologic study of Pick disease. Arch Neurol and Psychiat 1943; 50:288–303.
Sjogren T, et al.: Morbus Alzheimer and morbus Pick: a genetic, clinical, and patho-anatomical study. Acta Psychiat Scand 1952; 82:9–66.
Schenk VWD: Re-examination of a family with Pick's disease. Ann Hum Genet 1959; 23:325–333.
Heston LL: The clinical genetics of Pick's disease. Acta Psychiat Scand 1978; 57:202–206.
Groen JJ, Endtz LJ: Hereditary Pick's disease: second re-examination of a large family and discussion of other hereditary cases, with particular reference to electroencephalography and computerized tomography. Brain 1982; 105:443–459.
Cummings JL, Benson DF: Dementia: a clinical approach. Stoneham, MA: Butterworth Publishing, 1983.
Morris JC, et al.: Hereditary dysphasic dementia and the Pick-Alzheimer spectrum. Ann Neurol 1984; 16:455–466.

Constantinidis J: Heredity and dementia. Gerontol 1986; 32:73–79.
Heston LL, et al.: Pick's disease: clinical genetics and natural history. Arch Gen Psych 1987; 44:409–411.

EA005   **Nancy Lorraine Earl**

PILI TORTI-CLEFT LIP/PALATE-SYNDACTYLY   3126

Includes:
  Cleft lip/palate-syndactyly-pili torti
  Syndactyly-cleft lip/palate-pili torti
  Zlotogora-Zilberman-Tenenbaum syndrome
Excludes:
  Cleft lip/palate-ectodermal dysplasia-syndactyly (0179)
  Cleft lip/palate-oligodontia-syndactyly-hair defects (2898)
  Ectodermal dysplasia, Rapp-Hodgkin type (3056)
  Ectrodactyly-ectodermal dysplasia-clefting syndrome (0337)

Major Diagnostic Criteria: The combination of pili torti, **Cleft lip** with or without **Cleft palate**, **Syndactyly**, and mental retardation should help to distinguish this syndrome from others.

Clinical Findings: Sparse scalp hair, pili torti, downslanting palpebral fissures, malformed protruding ears, cleft lip with or without cleft palate, micrognathia, partial **Syndactyly** of fingers and toes 3–4, single transverse palmar crease (either simian or Sydney line), and severe head lag in infancy. Additional features noted in the older of two reported sib include widely spaced teeth, widely spaced nipples (>97th percentile), and hypoplastic scrotum with cryptorchidism.

This condition has been reported in sibs from one family. A similar condition, **Cleft lip/palate-oligodontia-syndactyly-hair defects**, was also reported in 1987, although the presence of the condition in a mother and daughter, and other clinical differences, suggest that these may be distinct conditions.

Complications: Unknown.

Associated Findings: None known.

Etiology: The presence of this syndrome in sibs of each sex, whose parents are consanguineous, is strongly suggestive of autosomal recessive inheritance.

Pathogenesis: Unknown. This condition could be considered an ectodermal dysplasia.

POS No.: 4480

Sex Ratio: Presumably M1:F1.

Occurrence: Two siblings from Israel has been documented.

Risk of Recurrence for Patient's Sib:
  See Part I, *Mendelian Inheritance.*

Risk of Recurrence for Patient's Child:
  See Part I, *Mendelian Inheritance.*

Age of Detectability: At birth, by physical examination.

Gene Mapping and Linkage: Unknown.

Prevention: None known. Genetic counseling indicated.

Treatment: Supportive, with repair of the cleft lip and palate indicated.

Prognosis: Mental retardation is part of the syndrome. Life span is unknown; the younger sib died at age eight months from an illness.

Detection of Carrier: Unknown.

References:
Zlotogora J, et al.: Cleft lip and palate, pili torti, malformed ears, partial syndactly of fingers and toes, and mental retardation: a new syndrome? J Med Genet 1987; 24:291–293.

T0007   **Helga V. Toriello**

PILO-DENTO-UNGULAR DYSPLASIA WITH MICROCEPHALY   2636

Includes: Ectodermal dysplasia, pilo-dento-ungular type
Excludes:
  Ectodermal dysplasia, Christ-Siemens-Touraine type (0333)
  Ectodermal dysplasia, Passarge type (3120)
  Ectodermal dysplasia, hidrotic (0334)
  Tricho-odonto-onychial dysplasia (2889)

Major Diagnostic Criteria: **Microcephaly**, trichodysplasia, onychodysplasia, dental alterations, and gastroesophageal disturbances.

Clinical Findings: Thin and sparse scalp hair, synophrys, hypodontia of permanent dentition, dystrophic finger- and toenails, **Microcephaly**, mental retardation, increased deep tendon reflexes, spasticity, scoliosis, advanced bone age, retrognathism, blue sclerae, strabismus, high-arched palate, clinodactyly, dermatoglyphic alterations, nocturnal enuresis, intestinal and respiratory infections, gastroesophageal reflux, esophagus hypotonia, compression of the anterior wall of the upper one-third of the esophagus, and anterior deviation of the trachea.

Complications: May gag on solid food and tolerate only liquids.

Associated Findings: None known.

Etiology: Possibly autosomal recessive inheritance. Parental consanguinity has been reported.

Pathogenesis: Unknown.

POS No.: 4391

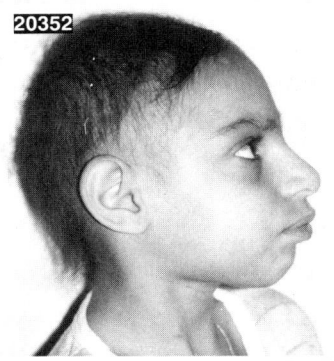
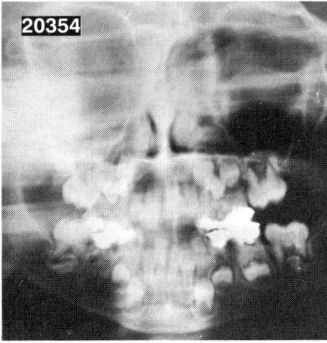
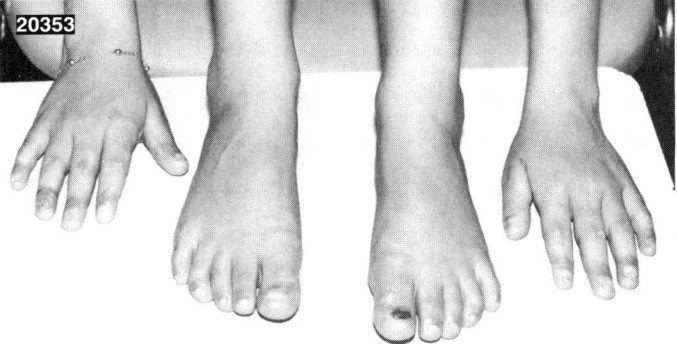

2636-20352: Note microcephaly, thin and sparse hair, synophrys, and retrognathism in this affected 6-year-old girl. 20353: Note dystrophic nails. 20354: Orthopantomogram at age 6 years; note dental defects.

Sex Ratio: Presumably M1:F1.

Occurrence: One Brazilian Caucasian girl in a sibship of two, from normal first cousin parents, has been reported.

Risk of Recurrence for Patient's Sib:
See Part I, *Mendelian Inheritance.*

Risk of Recurrence for Patient's Child:
See Part I, *Mendelian Inheritance.*

Age of Detectability: At birth, by physical examination.

Gene Mapping and Linkage: Unknown.

Prevention: None known. Genetic counseling indicated.

Treatment: Use of wigs and dental prosthesis may be cosmetically and psychologically helpful.

Prognosis: The only affected person known died at age seven years due to a combination of bone-marrow aplasia (possibly produced by drugs), multiple infections, hemorrhages, and acute anemia.

Detection of Carrier: Unknown.

References:
Tajara EH, et al.: Displasia pilodentoungular, uma nova sindrome de displasia e malformação. Ciênc Cult (suppl) 1986; 38:894 only.
Tajara EH, et al.: Pilodentoungulardysplasia with microcephaly: a new ectodermal dysplasia/malformation syndrome. Am J Med Genet 1987; 26:153–156.

FR033   **Newton Freire-Maia**

Pilomatricoma
See PILOMATRIXOMA

PILOMATRIXOMA   2589

Includes:
   Calcifying epithelioma of Malherbe
   Cancer, trichomatrical
   Pilomatricoma
   Trichoepithelioma

Excludes:
   Calcified hamartomas
   Calcified lymph nodes
   Calcinosis cutis
   Dermoid cysts
   Hemangiomas
   Parotid gland tumors
   Sebaceous adenoma or carcinoma
   Skin and subcutaneous cysts
   Squamous cell carcinomas
   Xanthogranuloma, juvenile

Major Diagnostic Criteria: Cytologic evaluation following biopsy, excision, or fine-needle aspiration. Cytologic criteria include 1) presence of cells with large, vesicular nuclei with distinct nucleoli that form clusters or occur singly; and 2) presence of numerous naked nuclei with well-preserved chromatin structure and distinct nucleoli.

Clinical Findings: Small, mobile nodules occur in the dermis or subcutaneous tissue, and are usually located in the head and neck. Consistency of the nodules is variable, ranging from cystic, to firm, to stony hard. A reddish-blue mass with areas of yellow-white patches is seen through the overlying layer of skin. Telangiectatic vessels are sometimes present on the overlying skin. Occasionally, overlying skin ruptures, with extrusion of friable granulation or calcified material. Pilomatrixomas are usually well-circumscribed and solitary lesions, but up to 6% are multiple. Average size is 1–3 cm in diameter, but "giant" pilomatrixomas of 15 cm diameter have been reported.

Pilomatrixomas are often preceded by a history of trauma. Growth is slow and usually asymptomatic. Pain may result from pressure or pinching of the lesion or from secondary infection with bleeding and ulceration. The majority (50–70%) occur in the head and neck region, most frequently on the brow, eyelid, or cheek. No cases have been reported on the palms or soles.

Modified mammographic techniques have been used to show fine speckled calcification in the lesions. Routine X-ray rarely shows calcifications.

Histologic appearance is distinctive and allows differentiation from other possible skin lesions. The tumor is made up of irregularly shaped islands of epithelial cells surrounded by a dense fibrous tissue. There are two distinctive cell types: basophilic, and "shadow" or "ghost" cells. The basophilic cells represent immature hair matrix cells and are usually at the periphery. Moving toward the center, there is a transition zone where the cells gradually lose their nuclei. In the center of this area one sees "shadow" or "ghost" cells. These cells have distinct borders but are devoid of their nuclei and display cellular dystrophy and degeneration. The stroma surrounding these cells is made up of granulation tissue with foreign body giant cells. Calcification is present in 75–80% of lesions. Ossification is found in 15–20%. Occasionally, melanin is seen. Aspirates contain only scant cellular granulomatous tissue which is more prevalent on histologic examination. Also, "ghost" or "shadow" cells are more frequently seen singly on cytologic examinations, as opposed to large groups seen on tissue section.

Complications: Recurrence is likely if the lesion is not totally excised. There are at least five reported cases of malignant transformation with invasion of local structures.

Associated Findings: Multiple pilomatrixomas may be associated with **Intestinal polyposis, type III** and **Myotonic dystrophy**. This association may represent a pleiotropic effect of the myotonic dystrophy gene.

Etiology: A benign tumor of hair cell origin.

Pathogenesis: First described by Malherbe and Chenantais (1880), who thought the condition originated from sebaceous glands. However, electron microscopy and histochemical studies show that the outer root sheath of the hair follicle is the cell of origin. The calcium deposits that occur in 80% of these lesions are felt to be the result of a dystrophic process. No abnormality in calcium metabolism is present.

Sex Ratio: M2:F3

Occurrence: The second most common superficial "lump" excised on a child; 1:824 dermatologic pathologic specimens and 1:2,200 surgical pathologic specimens. Most (97%) of the reported cases were Caucasians.

Risk of Recurrence for Patient's Sib: Unknown. A familial incidence has been noted in only six cases.

Risk of Recurrence for Patient's Child: Unknown.

Age of Detectability: While the condition has been identified in neonates, 40% occur in patients less than 10 years of age, and 60% occur in patients less than 20 years of age. The peak incidence is 8–13 years of age.

Gene Mapping and Linkage: Unknown.

Prevention: None known. Genetic counseling indicated.

Treatment: Total excision is needed; and this may need to include overlying skin. Incision and curettage are also advocated.

Prognosis: Recurrence is unlikely after adequate surgical excision. Lesions are felt to be benign, but there are reported cases of malignant transformation to a "giant" pilomatrixoma with locally aggressive and invasive behavior. Wide excision is needed in these cases.

Detection of Carrier: Unknown.

Special Considerations: *Trichoepithelioma* is a tumor similar to the pilomatrixoma. In these tumors, the hair matrix or basophilic cells do not develop into "shadow" cells. Instead, they develop into keratinized areas of "horn cysts." Eosinophils often surround these horn cysts, shown by electron microscope studies to represent immature hair structures. The malignant variant is the *trichomatrical carcinoma*.

References:

Malherbe A, Chenantais J: Note sur l'epitheliome calcifie des glands sebaces. Progr Med (Paris) 1880; 8:826–828.

Harper PS: Calcifying epithelioma of Malherbe-Association with myotonic muscular dystrophy. Arch Dermatol 1972; 106:41–44.

Moehlenbeck FW: Pilomatrixoma (calcifying epithelioma). Arch Dermatol 1973; 108:532–534.

Hernandez-Perez E, Cestoni-Parducci RF: Pilomatricoma (calcifying epithelioma): a study of 100 cases in El Salvador. Int J Dermatol 1981; 9:491–494.

Woyke S, et al.: Pilomatrixoma: a pitfall in the aspiration cytology of skin tumors. Acta Cytol 1982; 26:189–194.

Van der Walt JD: Carcinomatous transformation in a pilomatrixoma. Am J Dermatopathol 1984; 6:63–69.

Hawkins DB, Chen WT: Pilomatrixoma of the head and neck in children. Int J Pediatr Otorhinolaryngol 1985; 8:215–223.

MY003
SH050

Charles M. Myer III
Sally Shott

Pineal teratomas
See TERATOMAS
Pinealomas, ectopic
See CNS NEOPLASMS
Pinna, ectopic placement of pinna
See EAR, ECTOPIC PINNA
Pinna, hypogenesis of, with associated atresia of external ear
See EAR, MICROTIA-ATRESIA
Pipecolic acidemia
See CEREBRO-HEPATO-RENAL SYNDROME
Pipecolic acidemia (some forms)
See PHYTANIC ACID OXIDASE DEFICIENCY, INFANTILE TYPE
Pits of upper lip
See LIP, PITS OR MOUNDS
Pitt syndrome
See DWARFISM-DYSMORPHIC FACIES-RETARDATION, PITT TYPE

Pitt-Rogers-Danks syndrome
See DWARFISM-DYSMORPHIC FACIES-RETARDATION, PITT TYPE
Pituitary cretinism
See THYROTROPIN DEFICIENCY, ISOLATED
Pituitary dwarfism II
See DWARFISM, LARON
Pituitary dwarfism III
See DWARFISM, PANHYPOPITUITARY
Pituitary dwarfism IV
See DWARFISM, PANHYPOPITUITARY
Pituitary dwarfism-sella turcica defect
See DWARFISM, PITUITARY WITH ABNORMAL SELLA TURCICA
Pituitary gland hypoplasia-adrenal hypoplasia, congenital
See ADRENAL HYPOPLASIA, CONGENITAL
Pityriasis pilaris
See SKIN, PITYRIASIS RUBRA PILARIS
Pityriasis rubra pilaris
See SKIN, PITYRIASIS RUBRA PILARIS
PKU
See FETAL EFFECTS FROM MATERNAL PKU
PKU, atypical
See DIHYDROPTERIDINE REDUCTASE DEFICIENCY
PKU1
See PHENYLKETONURIA
Placenta, circumvallate
See CIRCUMVALLATE PLACENTA SYNDROME
Placental hypoperfusion fetal developmental retardation
See FETAL DEVELOPMENTAL RETARDATION WITH MATERNAL HYPERTENSION
Placental steroid sulfatase deficiency
See ICHTHYOSIS, X-LINKED WITH STEROID SULFATASE DEFICIENCY
Plagiocephaly
See CRANIOSYNOSTOSIS

PLAGIOCEPHALY 2939

Includes:
> Head, rhomboid-shaped
> Positional plagiocephaly
> Postural plagiocephaly

Excludes:
> **Oculo-auriculo-vertebral anomaly** (0735)
> Craniosynostosis, unilateral coronal
> Craniosynostosis, unilateral lambdoidal

Major Diagnostic Criteria: The term *plagiocephaly* is used by some authors to include any asymmetric head shape of any cause. The term is used more specifically here to mean a rhomboid-shaped head with a shift of the cranial base. One side of the face and the contralateral occipital parietal region are flattened, while the opposite sides of the skull seem to bulge. X-rays of the cranial sutures show them to be patent, while CT or MRI scans of the brain demonstrate normal anatomy.

Clinical Findings: Generally the infant's head has a normal shape at birth and becomes progressively distorted over the next four months of life as the infant maintains a consistent head posture against his or her mattress and other flat head supports. Then, as the infant develops improved head control, the distortion begins to resolve spontaneously. The head shape usually achieves its maximal resolution by ages 6–8 months. The distinction between positional plagiocephaly from structural facial asymmetry (hemifacial microsomia) may be difficult at times, since the flattened side of the face may be distorted and appear to feature a smaller jaw, abnormal auricle, and decreased unilateral facial movement. The correct diagnosis can be made by noting the overall head shape of plagiocephaly, which is rare in conditions featuring hemifacial microsomia, and then through X-ray assessment of the face.

Complications: Plagiocephaly is solely a cosmetic distortion of the skull. The only complication is its failure to resolve spontaneously.

Associated Findings: Plagiocephaly is generally associated with congenital muscular torticollis. Presumably the limited neck movement forces the head to remain in limited posture against the mattress. Cervical hemivertebrae or other structural anomalies of

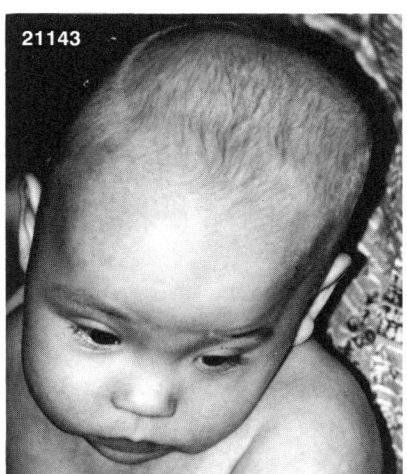

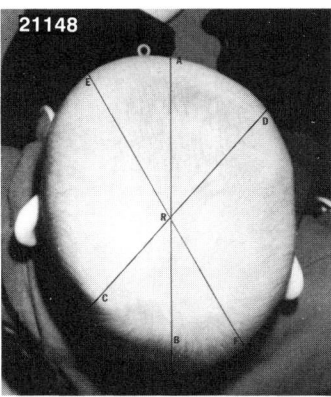

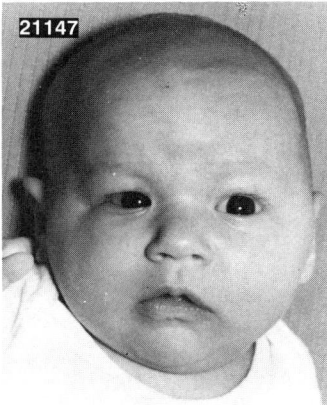

2939-21143: An infant with typical positional plagiocephaly. 21148: Positional plagiocephaly is best appreciated from the superior view of the head. The cranium takes on a rhomboid shape with frontal and contralateral occipital flattening (CD) and apparent bulging in the reverse direction (EF). 21147: Characteristic asymmetry of the entire face is seen in full facial view.

---

neck bones or muscles may also occasionally result in abnormal head shape. Some infants with hypotonia will prefer a single head position and produce a plagiocephalic skull in spite of full passive range in neck movement.

Etiology: Postnatal deformation.

Pathogenesis: Unknown.

CDC No.: 754.050

Sex Ratio: M1:F1

Occurrence: It is estimated that 8–10:10,000 newborns have some evidence of deformational plagiocephaly.

Risk of Recurrence for Patient's Sib: Dependent on the risk of recurrence for the underlying cause of limited head movement.

Risk of Recurrence for Patient's Child: Not increased.

Age of Detectability: Generally, cosmetically important plagiocephaly is noted by ages 6–8 weeks and progresses to a maximum distortion by age four months.

Gene Mapping and Linkage: N/A

Prevention: Attempts at increasing neck movement to minimize consistent head positioning is extremely difficult prior to ages 4–6 months. Placing the small infant in a swing, a front- or back-pack, or in other ways maintaining the head in space without any

---

surface pressure for as many hours a day as is practicable may be a more successful preventive approach.

Treatment: The facial asymmetry of deformational plagiocephaly will generally continue to improve for several years and rarely pose a permanent cosmetic problem. The calvarial asymmetry that remains at ages 6–8 months is permanent. If the distortion cannot be easily disguised with hair, corrective treatment can be taken. Lightweight helmets can be fashioned to fit tightly where the head is prominent and allow for brain growth in the areas of normal flattening. Such helmets should be placed between ages 6–8 months to assure that maximum spontaneous recovery occurs while utilizing all remaining brain growth potential to restore head shape. Surgical corrections are possible through calvarectomy, but are rarely needed.

Prognosis: Restoration of symmetric head shape can be expected if helmets are employed when spontaneous resolution fails.

Detection of Carrier: N/A

References:
Dingwall EJ: Artificial cranial deformation. London: John Bale & Sones & Danielsson, 1931.
Clarren SK: Plagiocephaly and torticollis: etiology, natural history, and helmet treatment in 43 patients. J Pediatr 1981; 98:92–95. *
Clarren SK, et al.: Malformations of the cranium. In: Kelley V, ed: Practice of pediatrics. Philadelphia: J.B. Lippincott, 1986. †
Cohen MM, Jr., ed: Craniosynostosis: diagnosis, evaluation and management. New York: Raven, 1986.
Dunne KB, Clarren SK: The origin of prenatal and postnatal deformities. Pediatr Clin North Am 1986; 33:1277–1297.

CL006 **Sterling K. Clarren**

Plantar callosities, autosomal dominant painful
  See SKIN, PAINFUL PLANTAR CALLOSITIES
Plasma cell myeloma
  See CANCER, MULTIPLE MYELOMA
Plasma cholesteryl ester deficiency, familial
  See LECITHIN-CHOLESTEROL ACYL TRANSFERASE DEFICIENCY
Plasma cholinesterase, atypical
  See CHOLINESTERASE, ATYPICAL
Plasma protein S deficiency
  See PROTEIN S DEFICIENCY
Plasma thromboplastin antecedent (PTA) deficiency
  See FACTOR XI DEFICIENCY
Plasma thromboplastin component deficiency
  See HEMOPHILIA B
Plasma transglutaminase
  See FACTOR XIII (FIBRIN STABILIZING FACTOR)

PLASMA, GROUP-SPECIFIC COMPONENT **0446**

Includes:
  Gc plasma protein component
  Group-specific protein
  Protein Gc
  Vitamin D binding protein (VDBP)

Excludes: N/A

Major Diagnostic Criteria: The group-specific component is the vitamin D binding protein of human plasma.

Clinical Findings: The so-called group-specific component (Gc) is the vitamin D binding protein (VDBP) in the plasma of humans and other mammals. It serves as the transport protein for vitamin D_3 and the natural derivatives 25-hydroxy-vitamin D, 1,25-dihydroxy-vitamin D, and 24,25-dihydroxy-vitamin D. It has a single common binding site for these ligands with the greatest affinity for 25-OH-D and $24,25(OH)_2$-D. Thus far, a deficiency of this protein has not been identified. In the various genetic types of vitamin D resistant rickets, as well as in osteogenesis imperfecta, the plasma levels and the vitamin D binding function of this protein are normal. The serum concentration in healthy individuals is approximately 40 mg/dl. There are slight but significant differences in the concentrations among the different genetic Gc types: persons with

Gc 1–1 have on the average higher levels than individuals with Gc 2–1; persons with Gc 2–1 have higher concentrations than individuals with Gc 2–2. Gc is increased in sera of pregnant women. The group-specific component is synthesized in the liver; patients with severe liver diseases tend to have very low Gc serum levels. Gc is also present in cerebrospinal fluid (CSF), ascites fluid, and normal urine.

The vitamin D binding protein Gc is an $\alpha(2)$-globulin. It has a molecular weight of 50,000 daltons and a sedimentation rate of 4.1 S. It is devoid of lipids. Only the Gc 1 protein has a glycan moiety of 1%. Gc 2 contains no carbohydrate. It consists of a single polypeptide chain. The amino acid sequence and nucleotide sequence of the cDNA has been determined.

Genetic variations were demonstrated first by Hirschfeld in 1959. Three common Gc types were identified by electrophoresis: Gc 1–1, Gc 2–1, and Gc 2–2. They were determined by a pair of autosomal alleles, Gc[1] and Gc[2]. Gc 1–1 has the electrophoertic mobility of a $\alpha(2)$-globulin; it is electrophoretically heterogeneous and consists of two separable proteins. Gc 2–2 migrates as a slow $\alpha(2)$-globulin and is homogeneous. Individuals heterozygous for this trait (Gc 2–1) have the products of both alleles in their serum; by electrophoretic procedures three components can be disclosed. For the classification of Gc types, starch-, agarose- and polyacrylamide-gel electrophoresis have also been employed. Recently, isoelectric focusing on polyacrylamide gels followed by immunofixation has been applied for Gc typing. Six common Gc subtypes are designated as 1F-1F, 1F-1S, 1S-1S, 2–1F, 2–1S, and 2–2. They are controlled by three alleles, named Gc[1F], Gc[1S], and Gc[2].

The practical application of the Gc system is at present restricted to its use as a genetic marker in studies of human populations, in twin studies, and in cases of disputed paternity.

Complications: Unknown.

Associated Findings: None known.

Etiology: Autosomal co-dominant inheritance.

Pathogenesis: Unknown.

MIM No.: *13920

Sex Ratio: M1:F1

Occurrence: Gc[1] and Gc[2] appear to have a worldwide distribution; both alleles have been disclosed in every population examined. In most populations, Gc[1] is more common than Gc[2]; the frequency of the latter varies from 0.011 in an Australian aborigine tribe from Cundeelee in the Western Desert to 0.385 in a population of Finns from the island of Kokar. In some South American Indian tribes, however, Gc[2] is more common than Gc[1]. Most Caucasian and Asian populations have Gc[2] frequencies between 0.20 and 0.30, Black populations have lower Gc[2] frequencies between 0.03 and 0.11.

The distribution of the suballeles Gc [1F] and Gc [1S] also shows significant differences between human populations: Europeans tend to have high frequencies for Gc [1S] and low frequencies for Gc [1F], in African populations the opposite is found, whereas Asian populations have similar frequencies for Gc [1F] and Gc [1S]. Useful for anthropological studies is the consideration of the frequencies for Gc [1F] and Gc [2] which permits grouping of populations according to their geographic and/or ethnic origin. The allelic distribution is possibly related to variations in skin pigmentation: small differences in vitamin D-binding have been demonstrated for the different allelic products. It is, therefore, conceivable that differences in the vitamin D transport function of Gc are related to variations in skin pigmentation which in turn are associated with differences in sun shine exposure.

More than 100 genetic variants have, in addition, been identified in the Gc system. These are classified into phenotypes with a double banded and a single banded pattern. The former are mutants of Gc [1], the latter are variants of Gc [2]. Their isoelectric points are either shifted toward the anode or toward the cathode. Some of these variants have been observed only in single families. Others occur in certain populations in appreciable frequencies as, for instance, Gc [1A1] which is found in Australian aborigines and in Melanesians.

Risk of Recurrence for Patient's Sib:
See Part I, *Mendelian Inheritance.*

Risk of Recurrence for Patient's Child:
See Part I, *Mendelian Inheritance.*

Age of Detectability: In infancy.

Gene Mapping and Linkage: GC (group-specific component (vitamin D binding protein)) has been mapped to 4q12-q13.

Prevention: None known. Genetic counseling indicated.

Treatment: None required.

Prognosis: A recent debate centered on a possible relationship between Gc genotype and genetic susceptibility to acquired immunodeficiency syndrome, concluding that no such association existed (see *New Engl J Med* 1987; 317:630–632).

Detection of Carrier: Unknown.

References:

Daiger SP, et al.: Group-specific component (Gc) proteins bind vitamin D and 25-hydroxy-vitamin D. Proc Natl Acad Sci 1975; 72:2076–2080.

Mourant AE, et al.: Sunshine and the geographical distribution of the alleles of the Gc system of plasma proteins. Hum Genet 1976; 33:307–314.

Constans J, et al.: Group-specific component. Report on the First International Workshop. Hum Genet 1979; 48:143–149.

Constans J, et al.: The polymorphism of the vitamin D-binding protein (Gc); isoelectric focusing in 3M urea as additional method for identification of genetic variants. Hum Genet 1983; 65:176–180. *

Yang F, et al.: Human group-specific component (Gc) is a member of the albumin family. Proc Nat Acad Sci 1985; 82:7994–7998. *

CL014   **Hartwig Cleve**

Plasma, plasminogen defects
See PLASMINOGEN DEFECTS

PLASMINOGEN DEFECTS   3083

Includes:
> Microplasmin
> Plasma, plasminogen defects
> Plasminogen Tochigi

Excludes: N/A

Major Diagnostic Criteria: The plasminogen system is highly polymorphic, with many variant forms having been identified. Variant forms of the proenzyme may be identified by isoelectric focusing, immunoelectrophoresis, and measurements of functional activity in relation to enzyme protein. Most of the known plasminogen variants have no clinical significance; however, several of them have been shown to produce hypercoagulability with thromboembolic complications. Affected individuals in most cases exhibit approximately 50% of normal plasmin activity in their plasma.

Clinical Findings: Reported individuals having the apparently rare variant forms of plasminogen with deficient function have in some cases had severe and recurrent thromboembolic disease. In some families, however, other individuals with the enzyme deficiency have not experienced thrombotic complications, suggesting that other factors may also play a role in the clinical expression of these abnormalities.

Complications: Unknown.

Associated Findings: None known.

Etiology: Autosomal dominant inheritance.

Pathogenesis: Plasminogen is a single-chain protein that circulates in the plasma as an inactive zymogen. Its activation, by cleavage of an Arg-Val bond, converts the molecule to a protease (plasmin) with trypsin-like activity. The principal physiologic role of plasmin is as a fibrinolytic agent. Plasminogen in the blood has been shown to bind to fibrin during its polymerization in the formation of a blood clot. Endothelial cells contain plasminogen activator, which is released in association with thrombus formation. The fibrinolytic action of plasmin is believed to be essential for clot resolution and the re-establishment of the patency of the blood vessels. Diminished plasmin activity resulting from function-deficient mutations presumably interferes with this process and predisposes the affected individuals to thrombotic complications.

MIM No.: *17335

Sex Ratio: M1:F1

Occurrence: All of the function-deficient variants appear to be of rare occurrence.

Risk of Recurrence for Patient's Sib:
See Part I, *Mendelian Inheritance.*

Risk of Recurrence for Patient's Child:
See Part I, *Mendelian Inheritance.*

Age of Detectability: At birth.

Gene Mapping and Linkage: PLG (plasminogen) has been mapped to 6q26-q27.

Prevention: None known. Genetic counseling indicated.

Treatment: Plasma infusions might be anticipated to replenish deficient plasminogen; however, the efficacy of this form of treatment is as yet unknown. Efforts to manage deficient patients with anticoagulants have in general not been successful.

Prognosis: Most forms are compatible with good health and normal life span. Affected individuals may, however, be at risk for serious thromboembolic complications.

Detection of Carrier: As affected individuals are apparently heterozygous for the abnormality, the disorder is fully expressed in the carrier. Studies of some families, however, have shown the abnormality to be present in some family members who do not exhibit thromboembolic disease.

References:

Aoki N, et al.: Abnormal plasminogen: a hereditary molecular abnormality found in a patient with recurrent thrombosis. J Clin Invest 1978; 78:1186–1195.
Wohl RC, et al.: Physiological activation of the human fibrinolytic system. Isolation and characterization of human plasminogen variants Chicago I and Chicago II. J Biol Chem 1979; 254:9063–9069.
Soria J, et al.: Plasminogen Paris I: congenital abnormal plasminogen and its incidence in thrombosis. Thromb Res 1983; 32:229–238.
Miyata T, et al.: Plasminogens Tochigi II and Nagoya: two additional molecular defects with Ala-600→Thr replacement found in plasmin light chain variants. J Biochem 1984; 96:277–287.
Towne JB, et al.: Abnormal plasminogen: a genetically determined cause of hypercoagulability. J Vasc Surg 1984; 1:896–902.
Scharrer IM, et al.: Investigation of a congenital abnormal plasminogen, Frankfurt I, and its relationship to thrombosis. Thromb Haemost 1986; 55:396–401.
Skoda U, et al.: Proposal for the nomenclature of human plasminogen (PLG) polymorphism. Vox Sang 1986; 51:244–248.

H0024   **George R. Honig**

Plasminogen Tochigi
See PLASMINOGEN DEFECTS
Plasmodium vivax malaria
See MALARIA, VIVAX, SUSCEPTIBILITY TO
Platelet fibinogen receptor deficiency
See THROMBASTHENIA, GLANZMANN-NAEGELI TYPE
Platelet glycoprotein IIb-IIIa deficiency
See THROMBASTHENIA, GLANZMANN-NAEGELI TYPE
Platelet, May-Hegglin anomaly
See LEUKOCYTE, MAY-HEGGLIN ANOMALY
Platelet/fibronectin abnormality-Ehlers-Danlos syndrome
See EHLERS-DANLOS SYNDROME
Platyspondyly-osteosclerosis
See DYSOSTEOSCLEROSIS
Pleonosteosis
See LERI PLEONOSTEOSIS SYNDROME
Pleura and peritoneum, muscle deficiency between
See DIAPHRAGM, EVENTRATION

Plott syndrome
See VOCAL CORD PARALYSIS
also LARYNGEAL PARALYSIS
also LARYNGEAL ABDUCTOR PARALYSIS-MENTAL RETARDATION
Poikiloderma atrophicans-cataract
See ROTHMUND-THOMSON SYNDROME
Poikiloderma with bullae, Weary type
See POIKILODERMA, HEREDITARY ACROKERATOTIC, KINDLER-WEARY TYPE

POIKILODERMA, HEREDITARY ACROKERATOTIC, KINDLER-WEARY TYPE   3038

Includes:
Acrokeratotic poikiloderma, hereditary
Bullous acrokeratotic poikiloderma of Kindler and Weary
Kindler-Weary syndrome
Poikiloderma with bullae, Weary type

Excludes:
Dyskeratosis congenita (2024)
Epidermolysis bullosum, type I (2560)
Poikiloderma, congenital
Poikiloderma, sclerosing, hereditary (3262)
Rothmund-Thomson syndrome (2037)
Urticaria pigmentosa (UP) (3263)
Xeroderma pigmentosum (1005)

Major Diagnostic Criteria: Pigmentary anomaly; vesicopustules in infancy followed by gradually increasing diffuse poikiloderma with striate and reticulate atrophy.

Clinical Findings: The lesions vary with age. During *infancy* vesicopustules or bullae on hands and feet and occasionally the trunk beginning at ages 1–3 months. These lesions resolve in later childhood. From *infancy to five years* transient eczematous eruption in flexural areas with or without pruritus. This lesion resolves by about age five years. *Poikiloderma*: persistent diffuse poikiloderma, especially in the flexural areas and sparing the face, scalp, and ears. This lesions is progressive with striate and reticulate atrophy. Telangiectasia is not a feature. *Acrokeratosis*: keratotic "warty" papules on the hands, feet, knees, and elbows, which persist into adulthood. Families with the putative autosomal accessive type exhibit photosensitivity and intraoral anomalies.

Expression may be incomplete, or more than one gene may be responsible for the complete syndrome: one family in the group reported by Weary et al (1971) had acral blistering and acrokeratoses without eczema and poikiloderma. Photosensitivity and intraoral anomalies exist in the putative autosomal recessive type.

Histology: 1) *Vesicles*: in the epidermis, focal spongiosis and microvesicles and areas of hydropic degeneration of the basal cell layer of epidermis and hair follicles; in the dermis, focal lymphohistiocytic inflammatory infiltrates subepidermally, periappendageal, and perivascular and edema. 2) *Poikilodermatous lesions*: epidermal atrophy, pigmentary irregularity, pigmentary incontinence, and mild perivascular infiltration. 3) *Acrokeratotic lesions*: marked localized hyperkeratosis and hypergranulosis; irregular acanthosis; and prominent vessels in upper dermis without inflammatory response.

Immunology: elevated IgG levels in affected individuals. Rheumatoid factor was positive in the two oldest patients in the absence of rheumatoid arthritis. Antinuclear factor is of dubious significance.

Complications: Unknown.

Associated Findings: None known.

Etiology: Autosomal dominant inheritance, except in putative type, in which autosomal recessive inheritance in two related Kurdish Jewish sibs has been reported.

Pathogenesis: Unknown.

MIM No.: *17365

POS No.: 3382

Sex Ratio: M1:F1

Occurrence: About 60 cases have been documented in the literature, including ten persons in one family by Weary et al (1971), 41 persons in six families by Larregue et al (1981), and four cases by Hacham-Zadeh and Garfunkel (1985).

Risk of Recurrence for Patient's Sib:
See Part I, *Mendelian Inheritance.*

Risk of Recurrence for Patient's Child:
See Part I, *Mendelian Inheritance.*

Age of Detectability: During infancy, from ages five weeks to as late as six months.

Gene Mapping and Linkage: Unknown.

Prevention: None known. Genetic counseling indicated.

Treatment: Symptomatic as indicated.

Prognosis: Life span does not appear to be reduced; normal intelligence.

Detection of Carrier: Unknown.

Special Considerations: Genetic heterogeneity may exist, as evidenced by one family within the kindred reported by Weary et al (1971) who had acral blistering and acrokeratosis in the absence of eczema or poikiloderma. Some researchers consider this condition to be a variant of **Epidermolysis bullosum, type I** with mottled pigmentation. Photosensitivity in the putative autosomal recessive disorder may differentiate it as an entity separate from the dominant disorder.

References:
Kindler T: Congenital poikiloderma with traumatic bulla formation and progressive cutaneous atrophy. Br J Dermatol 1954; 66:104–111.
Weary PE, et al.: Hereditary acrokeratotic poikiloderma. Arch Dermatol 1971; 103:409–422.
Der Kaloustian VM: Genetic diseases of the skin. Berlin: Springer-Verlag, 1979:122–123.
Larregue M, et al.: Acrokeratose poikilodermique bulleuse et hereditaire de Weary-Kindler. Ann Dermatol Venereol 1981; 103:69–76.
Hacham-Zadeh S, Garfunkel AA: Kindler syndrome in two related Kurdish families. Am J Med Genet 1985; 20:43–48.

WI055   **Ingrid M. Winship**

POIKILODERMA, SCLEROSING, HEREDITARY   3262

Includes: Sclerosing poikiloderma, hereditary

Excludes:
Poikiloderma, congenital
Poikiloderma, hereditary acrokeratotic, Kindler-Weary type (3038)
Rothmund-Thomson syndrome (2037)
Xeroderma pigmentosum (1005)

Major Diagnostic Criteria: *Clinical:* Generalised poikiloderma of the skin, sclerosis of the palms and soles, hyperkeratotic and sclerotic bands in flexures, and clubbing of the fingers.
Laboratory: Histology of the skin from antecubital fossae and axillae reveals focal homogenisation of collagen, with a reduction in elastic tissue.

Clinical Findings: *Poikiloderma:* A generalised poikiloderma of the skin is accentuated in a flexural distribution, viz. axillae, antecubital and popliteal fossae, as well as the extensor surfaces of the knees, elbows and over the joints of the bands. True poikiloderma, ie hypo-and hyper-pigmentation with telangectasia and atrophy is interspersed with mottled pigmentary change alone.
Sclerosis: In addition to poikiloderma, sclerotic changes occur to the skin of the palms and soles; these differ from the changes of scleroderma.
Hyperkeratotic and sclerotic bands in either a reticulate or linear pattern occur in the flexural areas, viz. axillary vault and antecubital and popliteal fossae.
Clubbing: Clubbing of the fingers is a consistent feature of this syndrome.

Complications: Calcinosis of the tissues in older patients.

Associated Findings: Soft systolic murmurs are audible in different areas of the precordium in more than half of affected persons reported.

Etiology: Autosomal dominant inheritance.

Pathogenesis: A probable heritable disorder of connective tissue.

MIM No.: 17370

Sex Ratio: M1:F1

Occurrence: Rare; Seven affected persons in two unrelated Black families have been reported.

Risk of Recurrence for Patient's Sib:
See Part I, *Mendelian Inheritance.*

Risk of Recurrence for Patient's Child:
See Part I, *Mendelian Inheritance.*

Age of Detectability: Early signs in childhood (±4 years of age).

Gene Mapping and Linkage: Unknown.

Prevention: None known. Genetic counseling indicated.

Treatment: Symptomatic, using keratolytic agents.

Prognosis: Life span not affected.

Detection of Carrier: Unknown.

Special Considerations: This is an extremely rare genodermatosis; however, it would appear that it is indeed an autonomous syndrome.

References:
Weary PE, et al.: Hereditary sclerosing poikiloderma. Arch Derm 1969; 100:413–422.
Der Kaloustiaan VM, Kurban AK: Genetic diseases of the skin. Berlin: Springer-Verlag, 1979:122.

WI055   **Ingrid M. Winship**

Poland anomaly
See POLAND SYNDROME
Poland syndactyly
See POLAND SYNDROME

POLAND SYNDROME   0813

Includes:
Pectoralis muscle, absence of
Poland anomaly
Poland syndactyly
Poland-Moebius syndrome
Subclavian artery supply disruption sequence (SASDS)
Symbrachydactyly-ipsilateral aplasia of head of pectoralis muscle

Excludes:
Symbrachydactyly without associated muscle defect
Syndactyly (0923)
Syndactyly as a part of the acrocephalosyndactylies

Major Diagnostic Criteria: The association of symbrachydactyly with ipsilateral aplasia of the sternal head of the pectoralis major is diagnostic. The muscle defect is observed clinically as absence of the normal well-developed curved anterior axillary fold.

Clinical Findings: The two main components of the syndrome are symbrachydactyly and pectoral muscle defect. Symbrachydactyly is a specific hand malformation, always unilateral, characterized by the association of short digits and syndactyly. The phalanges are short or absent. The middle phalanges are affected more frequently, and in severe cases they are absent or fused with the distal phalanges (terminal symphalangism and assimilation hypoplasia). The distal phalanges are minimally affected and are rarely absent. The thumb is usually least affected. Syndactyly is either partial or complete, usually involving the soft tissues, and is not associated with bone synostosis. Syndactyly frequently involves the index and middle fingers.
The associated muscle defect is ipsilateral aplasia of the sternal

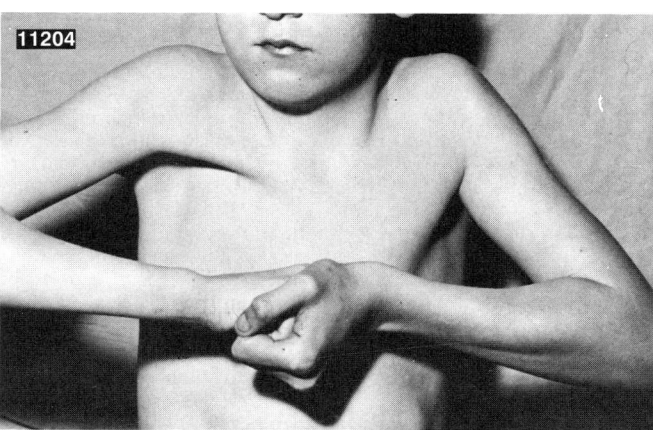

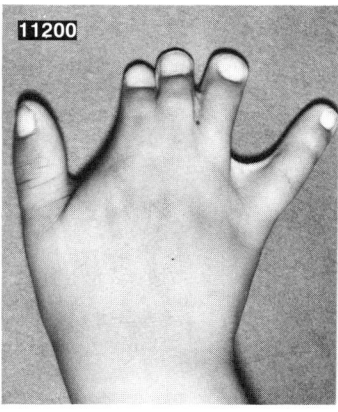 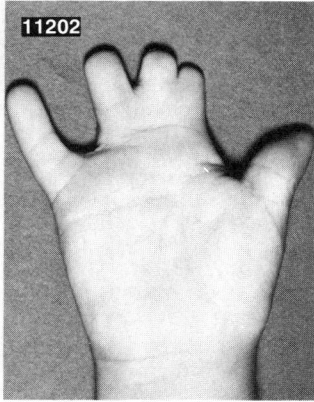

0813-11204: Absence of the sternal head of the right pectoral major muscle. 11200–02: Unilateral digital hypoplasia, brachydactyly and syndactyly.

head of the pectoralis major, while its clavicular head is always present and is sometimes hypertrophied.

Asymmetry of breast development, and ipsilateral absence of the breast and subcutaneous tissue, as well as ipsilateral webbing of the axilla, are sometimes noted.

Complications: Defects in pectoralis minor, rectus abdominis, latissimus dorsi, serratus anterior, and intercostal muscles have been reported. Associated bone defects have also been noted; examples are hypoplasia of upper ribs, Sprengel deformity of the scapulae, and shortening of arm and forearm bones.

Associated Findings: Ipsilateral hypoplasia of the kidney was noted once. An association with **Diplegia, congenital facial** (Moebius syndrome) has also been suggested.

Etiology: Practically all reported cases are sporadic. Some familial patterns have been reported (David and Winter, 1985).

Pathogenesis: Bavinck and Winter (1986) have suggested that this and related conditions result from interruption of the early embryonic blood supply in the subclavian arteries, the vertebral arteries and/or their branches. They have suggested the term *subclavian artery supply disruption sequence (SASDS)* for this group of birth defects.

MIM No.: 17380, 17375

POS No.: 3359

CDC No.: 756.800

Sex Ratio: M1:F1

Occurrence: Among 33 cases with symbrachydactyly, Pol in 1921 found 21 cases with ipsilateral aplasia of the sternal head of

the pectoralis major. Among 102 cases with absent sternal head of the pectoralis major, Bing in 1902 found 14 cases with associated symbrachydactyly. Sigiura et al (1962) found one boy with Poland syndactyly among 6,297 Japanese primary school children. In British Columbia, McGillivray and Lowry (1977) found an incidence of 1:32,000 live births. In Brazil, Castilla et al (1980) found 11 cases in 599,109 consecutive newborn infants.

Risk of Recurrence for Patient's Sib: Probably not increased.

Risk of Recurrence for Patient's Child: Probably not increased.

Age of Detectability: At birth, by clinical examination.

Gene Mapping and Linkage: Unknown.

Prevention: None known. Genetic counseling indicated.

Treatment: Surgical correction.

Prognosis: Normal life span.

Detection of Carrier: Unknown.

Special Considerations: At least a dozen instances of the association of the Poland and Moebius syndromes (*Polant-Moebius syndrome*) have been documented (see Stevenson, 1982).

References:
Clarkson P: Poland's syndactyly. Guys Hosp Rep 1962; 111:335–346.
McGivillray BC, Lowry RB: Poland syndrome in British Columbia: incidence and reproductive experience of affected persons. Am J Med Genet 1977; 1:65–74.
Temtamy SA, McKusick VA: The genetics of hand malformations. New York: Alan R Liss, for The National Foundation-March of Dimes, 1978.
Castilla EE, et al.: Syndactyly: frequency of specific types. Am J Med Genet 1980; 5:357.
Hegde HR, Shokeir MHK: Posterior shoulder girdle abnormalities with absence of pectoralis major muscle. Am J Med Genet 1982; 13:285–293.
Hester TR, Bostwick J: Poland's syndrome: correction with latissimus muscle transposition. Plast Reconstr Surg 1982; 69:226–233.
Stevenson RE: The Poland-Moebius syndrome. Proc Greenwood Genet Center 1982; 1:26–28.
Suzuki T, et al.: Computed tomography of the pectoralis muscles in Poland's syndrome. Hand 1982; 15:35–41.
David TJ, Winter RM: Familial absence of the pectoralis major, serratus anterior, and latissimus dorsi muscles. J Med Genet 1985; 22:390–392.
Bavinck JNB, Weaver DD: Subclavian artery supply disruption sequence: hypothesis of a vascular etiology for Poland, Klippel-Feil, and Moebius anomalies. Am J Med Genet 1986; 23:903–918.

TE004   **Samia A. Temtamy**

Poland-Moebius syndrome
  See POLAND SYNDROME
Polar and capsular cataracts
  See CATARACT, POLAR AND CAPSULAR
Polar cataract
  See CATARACT, AUTOSOMAL DOMINANT CONGENITAL
Polio, sensitivity to
  See POLIO, SUSCEPTIBILITY TO

POLIO, SUSCEPTIBILITY TO   **3109**

Includes:
  Acute anterior poliomyelitis
  Heine-Medin disease
  Infantile paralysis
  Polio, sensitivity to
  Poliomyelitis
  Poliovirus receptor
  Post-polio syndrome

Excludes:
  Amyotrophic lateral sclerosis
  Guillain-Barre syndrome
  Infectious meningo-encephalitides
  Lyme disease
  Motor neuron diseases

Porphyria
Sensitivity to other enteroviruses, such as Coxsackie and ECHO
Tick paralysis

Major Diagnostic Criteria: *Minor illness*: Polio virus usually causes an asymptomatic infection, but can present as a minor, non-specific systemic illness. Diagnosis at this stage can be made by culturing virus from stool.
Major illness: Poliomyelitis begins with upper respiratory and/or GI symptoms, with fever and signs of aseptic meningitis followed by usually asymmetrical paralysis of voluntary muscles. Definitive diagnosis is made by culturing one of the three serotypes of poliovirus from the patient's stool.

Clinical Findings: In an epidemic, 90–95% of all poliovirus-infected people are asymptomatic (inapparent). Four to eight percent may suffer a non-specific, abortive illness (minor illness), whereas 1–2% of infections result in neurologic symptoms or signs (major illness).
Minor illness: Most patients are asymptomatic, while others have sore throat, abdominal discomfort, vomiting accompanied by minor constitutional symptoms such as low-grade fever, malaise and mild headache. These symptoms last 1–4 days and recede (abortive infection). The incubation period is between 1–5 days.
Major Illness: The incubation period for the major illness is usually 4–10 days, rarely 3–35 days. A biphasic course is seen in one-third of 2–10 year-old patients, but is unusual in adults. The symptoms of aseptic meningitis begin with headache, vomiting, irritability and drowsiness. The neck and back may be stiff. The illness may abort at this stage. Paralysis usually develops on the second to fifth day after onset of headache. It may be delayed in children, or conversely, present as one of the initial symptoms. The pre-paralytic phase in adults is more severe than in children. Before onset of paralysis fasiculations may be present and the deep tendon reflexes may be hyperactive.
Spinal poliomyelitis primarily affects muscles of the extremities; the involvement is typically typically asymmetrical and the proximal muscles are more affected than distal. Lower extremities are more frequently involved then upper extremities. Affected muscles are flaccid and the deep tendon reflexes are absent. Atrophy is apparent as early as 5–7 days. When motor neurons of the brainstem are involved (bulbar poliomyelitis), paralysis of pharyngeal and laryngeal muscles is most common; facial muscles may also be involved. Less common is weakness of the muscles of the tongue and of mastication. External oculomotor weakness is rare. Brainstem reticular formation may also be involved, leading to disturbances of breathing, swallowing and cardiovascular control. A few adult patients may develop an encephalitic picture due to extensive involvement of neurons from the hypothalamus to the spinal cord. Such patients often die within 24–72 hours.

Complications: Complications of acute paralysis include respiratory failure, decubitus ulcers, and other systemic problems associated with decreased voluntary activity. Chronic complications of paralysis are contractures and weakness of limbs, scoliosis, reduced size or length of a limb, and sometimes persistent respiratory dependence.
A well-documented late complication of poliomyelitis is the occurrence of progressive motor complaints years or decades after the initial infection (*post-polio syndrome*). In some patients the complaints may be limited to joint pain and increased fatiguability, while in others, progressive weakness, atrophy and fasciculations are noted (*post-polio muscular atrophy PPMA*). Mulder's series (see Price and Plum, 1978) of 34 patients had a preponderance of men (M25:F9). Average age of onset of new symptoms was 34 years after recovery from acute poliomyelitis. Onset and involvement of weakness was not limited to limbs originally affected by poliomyelitis. Babinski signs were noted in some patients. The relationship of post-polio muscular atrophy (PPMA) to **Amyotrophic lateral sclerosis** (ALS) is unclear. Norris et al (see Price and Plum 1978) reported 2–8% of patients of adult motor neuron disease to have suffered from previous paralytic poliomyelitis. Poliomyelitis is 200 to 800-fold more common in the adult motor neuron disease group as compared to the general population.
Inflammatory changes in the muscle of patients with PPMA have been described. No evidence of antipolio antibodies has been noted in the CSF of these individuals, though oligoclonal bands may be seen. There is no evidence of persistence of poliovirus infection in these individuals. The speculated mechanisms of PPMA include: 1) Motor neuron damage induced by anti-idiotype antibodies. 2) Progressive decrease in the number of motor neurons as a result of normal aging or shortened lifespan of motor neurons originally damaged by polio infection. 3) A genetic susceptibility to motor neuron damage by poliovirus infection and aging processes, perhaps residing in the poliovirus receptor.

Associated Findings: Genetic polymorphisms of the poliovirus receptor have been postulated but not established. Physical signs and symptoms collectively referred to as the poliomyelitic constitution have been reported but never critically verified. Most patients with poliomyelitis have varying degrees of autonomic and sensory symptoms.

Etiology: Poliovirus sensitivity is an autosomal dominant trait. Poliomyelitis is transmittted by the three serotypes of the polio virus. Polio virus is an Enterovirus of the family Picornaviridae. It is transmitted by the oral-fecal route. Rarely it has been transmitted iatrogenically by the parenteral route. Family clusters of poliomyelitis have been described. Whether genetic predisposition plays a part in these clusters is unclear. Past studies have claimed that a hereditary factor or an autosomal recessive gene is responsible for paralytic polio. However, scientific documentation is lacking. An initial study reported an increased frequency of HLA-A3 and HLA-A7 histocompatibility antigens in patients with previous poliomyelitis, but a second study could not confirm an association between paralytic polio and HLA-A type. Pregnancy, trauma, increased age, and increased physical activity predispose to paralytic poliomyelitis.

Pathogenesis: Lytic poliovirus infection of neurons and the accompanying inflammatory response are the most likely mechanisms of central nervous system damage. Sensitivity to polio virus infection is mediated by a dominant gene localized to the proximal long arm of chromosome 19. The sensitivity is primarily a cell-surface characteristic which is thought to be receptor mediated. Binding studies have shown that the poliovirus receptor is widely present in the central nervous system, and may lie on axon terminals of motor neurons. The virus reaches neurons by hematogenous as well as axonal spread. The worsened severity of paralysis in exercised limbs may be explained by the postulated availability of poliovirus receptors at the neuromuscular junction, leading to axonal spread. Another explanation may be that exercise results in an increase in the number of poliovirus receptors on the motor neurons innervating the exercised limbs. Differences in susceptibility due to age may also be explained in terms of differences in type or number of receptors. However, no differences in the receptor types between different cells or between adult and children have been described, nor has the receptor been isolated or its gene cloned.
The mechanism for the post-polio syndrome or for PPMA is unclear. Persistent poliovirus infection has not been demonstrated in these individuals. Some investigators favor an "overuse" theory. Inflammatory cells have been noted in muscle of these individuals, and in one case, in the spinal cord. It is possible that the mechanism of this syndrome is through antibody directed against the poliovirus receptor on the motor neuron. If the receptor is bound to the antibody and deprived of its natural ligand, the receptor may no longer be able to fulfill its biological role, thereby resulting in motor neuron dysfunction. This theory can be tested by demonstrating receptor-binding antibodies in the sera or CSF of patients with PPMA.

MIM No.: *17385

Sex Ratio: M1:F1 for poliomyelitis. For PPMA, it has been reported as M2.7:F1 as well as M1:F1.

Occurrence: The incidence of poliomyelitis varies with the immune status of the population. In non-immunized populations, it is estimated to be about 1:10,000. Since the introduction of effective programs of vaccination, paralytic poliomyelitis occurs primarily in non-immunized individuals, children with immune deficiency, and susceptible individuals exposed to the vaccine virus, either directly or after fecal passage. Some data suggest attenuated-live virus can revert to a more virulent form in the GI tracts of immunized children; this process has been documented with Poliovirus III. In 1984 there were eight cases of poliomyelitis in the United States, most vaccine-related. In some underdeveloped countries, poliomyelitis continues to be epidemic, mainly due to inadequate immunization programs. Recurrence with a serotype of poliovirus different from the initial infection has occurred.

Risk of Recurrence for Patient's Sib: There is no evidence of increased risk of poliomyelitis in siblings, except in non-immunized or immune deficient populations.

Risk of Recurrence for Patient's Child: Little risk except in non-immunized or immune deficient populations. A greater risk is to non-immunized adults who come in contact with a child who has recently received the oral vaccine, since the attenuated virus may mutate into a virulent form after passage through the GI tract. Poliovirus sensitivity is an autosomal dominant trait, it is undetermined if receptors resistant to polio virus exist among the human population.

Age of Detectability: Poliomyelitis can occur at any age. The incidence and severity is age dependent. The ratio of inapparent to paralytic disease in children is 1000:1, while in adults it is 75:1. No case of *in-utero* poliomyelitis has been convincingly documented.

Gene Mapping and Linkage: PVS (poliovirus sensitivity) has been mapped to 19q12-q13.2.

Prevention: Paralytic poliomyelitis is preventable by either inactivated (Salk) or live-attenuated (Sabin) poliovirus vaccines. The use of these vaccines has brought about a dramatic decline in the number of paralytic cases in the United States from an average of 21,000 cases per year to just eight in 1984. Problems associated with inactivated vaccine have been generally overcome. The major complication of live-attenuated polio virus is the development of paralytic polio in vaccine recipients and contacts. This risk is low, but vaccine-related cases outnumber naturally occurring ones in immunized populations like the United States.

Treatment: Treatment for poliomyelitis is symptomatic. In an epidemic, during the preparalytic period, the patient should remain quiet and rest. Analgesics and hot packs are applied for comfort. In the paralyzed patient, intensive nursing care and positional measures are used to prevent complications. Respiratory support may be needed in case of respiratory failure. Orthopedic and physical therapy measures are instituted for rehabilitation.

There is no treatment for PPMA, although a trial of plasmapheresis for these patients has been proposed, based on the autoantibody theory.

Prognosis: Death in poliomyelitis is usually due to respiratory failure. Mortality varies with epidemics and has been reduced due to advanced treatment of complications. In 1916 the mortality was 26.9% in the United States. Patients who survive usually recover considerable motor function. Sixty percent of the eventual recovery occurs in the first three months, 80% in six months and the rest during the next two years. It is likely that improvement occurs due to recovery of sick neurons and due to collateral sprouting of healthy axons, which then innervate the denervated muscle fibers. Muscle fibers may hypertrophy with physical activity and further improve strength.

PPMA, when compared to **Amyotrophic lateral sclerosis**, is a relatively benign disease. In one series, 34 patients were observed for an average of 8.7 years. In only one did the clinical illness cause death.

Detection of Carrier: Poliovirus can be excreted for 4–8 weeks after immunization with live-attenuated virus. Some individuals may excrete virus for a prolonged period of time. The virus can be detected by stool culture.

Special Considerations: The genetic susceptibility of paralytic poliomyelitis remains unproven. The cause of PPMA as a remote complication of paralytic poliomyelitis remains enigmatic. Persistence of polio virus has not been demonstrated in PPMA or in other motor neuron diseases. What part, if any, the poliovirus receptor plays in inherited motor neuron diseases such as **Amyotrophic lateral sclerosis** and the spinal muscular atrophies is under investigation. As the genes for the poliovirus (sensitivity) receptor and myotonic dystrophy are linked to the same region of chromosome 19, the gene for the poliovirus receptor can be tested as a candidate gene for myotonic dystrophy once it has been cloned.

References:
Kovacs E: The biochemistry of poliomyelitis viruses. New York: Macmillan, 1964.
Price RW, Plum F: Handbook of clinical neurology, vol 34. Amsterdam: North Holland Publishing Co., 1978:93–132.
Dalakas MC, et al: A long term follow-up study of patients with post-poliomyelitis neuromuscular symptoms. New Engl J Med 1986; 313:959–963.
Mendelsohn C, et al: Transformation of a human poliovirus receptor gene into mouse cells. Proc Natl Acad Sci 1986; 83:7845–7849.
Siddique T, et al: The poliovirus sensitivity (PVS) gene is on chromosome 19q12-q13.2. Genomics 1988; 3:156–160.

SI032   **Teepu Siddique**
MC039   **Ross McKinney**

Poliodystrophica cerebri dystrophica
See ALPERS DISEASE
Poliomyelitis
See POLIO, SUSCEPTIBILITY TO
Poliovirus receptor
See POLIO, SUSCEPTIBILITY TO
Polish hereditary amyloidosis
See AMYLOIDOSIS, ASHKENAZI TYPE
Pollex varus
See THUMB, CLASPED
Pollitt syndrome
See TRICHOTHIODYSTROPHY
Polychlorinated biphenyl (PCB), fetal effects of
See FETAL EFFECTS OF POLYCHLORINATED BIPHENYL (PCB)
Polycystic disease of infancy and childhood
See KIDNEY, POLYCYSTIC DISEASE, RECESSIVE
Polycystic disease of the newborn
See KIDNEY, POLYCYSTIC DISEASE, RECESSIVE
Polycystic kidney disease, medullary type
See KIDNEY, NEPHRONOPHTHISIS-MEDULLARY CYSTIC DESEASE
Polycystic lipomembranous osteodysplasia-leukoencephalopathy
See OSTEODYSPLASIA, LIPOMEMBRANOUS POLYCYSTIC-DEMENTIA
Polycystic ovary disease due to 17-KSR deficiency
See STEROID 17-KETOSTEROID REDUCTASE DEFICIENCY
Polycystic renal disease, adult type (Potter type III)
See KIDNEY, POLYCYSTIC DISEASE, DOMINANT

POLYDACTYLY   0814

Includes:
Fromont anomaly
Index finger polydactyly
Preaxial polydactyly I, II, and III
Polydactyly of index finger
Postaxial polydactyly, types A and B
Thenar hypoplasia
Thumb polydactyly
Triphalangeal thumb, opposable

Excludes:
Chondroectodermal dysplasia (0156)
Chromosome 13, trisomy 13 (0168)
Laurence-Moon syndrome (0578)
Polydactyly, pre- or postaxial, in complex malformation syndromes
Polysyndactyly (0817)
Syndactyly (0923)

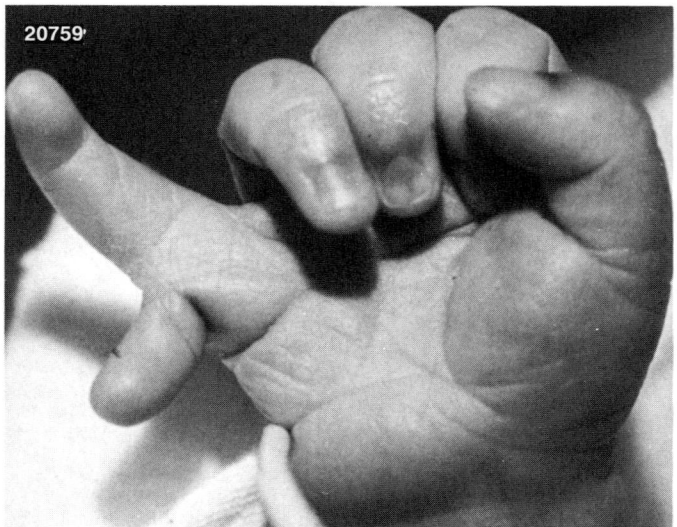
20759

0814-20759: Polydactyly, post-axial.

Major Diagnostic Criteria: An extra digital triradius is found at the base of the extra digit. When it is a pedunculated postminimus that was surgically removed or fell out spontaneously, the extra triradius in the dermatoglyphics may be the only evidence of postaxial polydactyly.

Clinical Findings: In *preaxial polydactyly* the extra digit is on the radial side of the hand. The deformity in polydactyly of the thumb is duplication of all or part of the components of a thumb. In polydactyly of a triphalangeal thumb, the thumb has three phalanges, with duplication of all or part of its components. In polydactyly of the index finger, the thumb is present and the index finger is duplicated. Dermatoglyphic findings in this case are diagnostic, since an extra A triradius and an A line are present, corresponding to the extra index finger. In polysyndactyly, preaxial polydactyly of the toes is associated with variable degrees of syndactyly of the toes and fingers.

In *postaxial polydactyly*, the extra digit is on the ulnar side in the upper limb and the fibular side in the lower limb. Two phenotypic and possibly genetically different varieties exist. In one of them, postaxial polydactyly type A, the extra digit is rather well formed and articulates with the fifty or extra metacarpal. In postaxial polydactyly type B, or pedunculated postminimus, the extra digit is not well formed and is frequently in the form of a skin tag.

Complications: Unknown.

Associated Findings: None known.

Etiology: Usually autosomal dominant inheritance with variable expressivity. Thumb polydactyly is frequently unilateral, and most cases are sporadic with no evidence of inheritance.

Pathogenesis: Unknown.

MIM No.: *17450, *17460, *17420, 17440

CDC No.: 755.0

Sex Ratio: M1:F1

Occurrence: Postaxial polydactyly is about ten times more frequent in Blacks than in Caucasians. In American whites, incidence figures vary from 1:3,300 to 1:630 live births, and in American Blacks figures vary from 1:300 to 1:100 live births.

Risk of Recurrence for Patient's Sib:
See Part I, *Mendelian Inheritance*.

Risk of Recurrence for Patient's Child:
See Part I, *Mendelian Inheritance*.

Age of Detectability: In utero by fetoscopy (polydactyly), and at birth.

Gene Mapping and Linkage: Unknown.

Prevention: None known. Genetic counseling indicated.

Treatment: Surgical removal of the extra digit.

Prognosis: Polydactyly as an isolated malformation does not affect life span.

Detection of Carrier: Unknown.

References:

Atasu M: Hereditary index finger polysyndactyly: phenotypic, radiological, dermatoglyphic, and genetic findings in a large family. J Med Genet 1976; 13:469–476.

Temtamy SA, McKusick VA: The genetics of hand malformations. New York: Alan R. Liss, for The National Foundation-March of Dimes, 1978.

Ventruto V, et al.: Postaxial polydactyly in two members of the same family. Clin Genet 1980; 18:342–347.

Kucheria K, et al.: An Indian family with postaxial polydactyly in four generations. Clin Genet 1981; 20:36–39.

Graham JM, Jr., et al.: Thumb polydactyly as part of the range of genetic expression for thenar hypoplasia. (Abstract) Am J Hum Genet 1985; 37:A132.

Merlob P, et al.: Familial opposable thriphalangeal thumbs associated with duplication of the big toes. J Med Genet 1985; 22:78–80.

TE004   **Samia A. Temtamy**

Polydactyly (postaxial)-cortical blindness-growth retardation
See BLINDNESS (CORTICAL)-RETARDATION-POSTAXIAL POLYDACTYLY
Polydactyly of index finger
See POLYDACTYLY
Polydactyly of thumbs/hallux-extra phalanges in the thumbs
See THUMB, TRIPHALANGEAL-DUPLICATED GREAT TOES
Polydactyly, postaxial type A-scalp defects
See SCALP DEFECTS-POSTAXIAL POLYDACTYLY
Polydactyly, postaxial-median cleft of upper lip
See ORO-FACIO-DIGITAL SYNDROME, THURSTON TYPE
Polydactyly, preaxial II
See THUMB, TRIPHALANGEAL-DUPLICATED GREAT TOES
Polydactyly-chondrodystrophy
See CHONDROECTODERMAL DYSPLASIA
Polydactyly-cleft lip/palate/lingual lump-psychomotor retardation
See ORO-PALATAL-DIGITAL SYNDROME, VARADI TYPE
Polydactyly-conical teeth-nail dysplasia-short limbs
See ACROFACIAL SYNDROME, CURRY-HALL TYPE

POLYDACTYLY-DISTAL OBSTRUCTIVE UROPATHY   2644

Includes:
Postaxial polydactyly-distal obstructive uropathy
Urethral valve, posterior-polydactyly

Excludes:
Meckel syndrome (0634)
Postaxial polydactyly as a part of other syndromes

Major Diagnostic Criteria: Postaxial polydactyly with or without **Syndactyly** in one or more limbs; posterior urethral valve.

Clinical Findings: The association of postaxial polydactyly with distal obstructive uropathy was described in two unrelated stillborn male babies of 36 and 36 1/2 weeks of age respectively. Patient one had Potter sequence involvement (see **Renal agenesis, bilateral** of the face, left postaxial synpolydactyly of the hand, and posterior urethral valve. Patient two had postaxial polydactyly of the left hand and right foot and probable posterior urethral valve.

Complications: Patient one had dilation of the proximal portion of the urethra, dilation of the bladder with thickening and a few trabeculations of its wall, bilateral hydroureters, marked bilateral hydronephrosis with renal cystic dysplasia type II-B of Potter, undescended testes, and hypospadias grade I. He also had congestion and complete atelectasis of the lungs. In patient two, catheterization of the urethra was possible for a distance of only 0.5 cm. The bladder was extremely dilated with a smooth wall. Hydroureters were bilateral with no evidence of ureteral stenosis. The kidneys showed marked bilateral hydronephrosis. There was bilateral cryptorchidism. Microscopic examination of the entire penile portion of the urethra failed to show any stenosis. It is likely that the obstruction was caused either by a posterior urethral valve (the abdominal portion of the urethra was not examined) or, less likely, by an anterior urethral stenosis in the region of the glans.

Associated Findings: Patient one had patent foramen ovale.

Etiology: Unknown.

Pathogenesis: Associated anomalies of the genitourinary tract are actually manifestations of the primary defect, namely, posterior urethral valve. Bona fide renal parenchymal malformations with polydactyly suggest the presence of an acrorenal developmental defect (DFD), in and of itself a causally nonspecific malformation. However, since the renal dysplasia in patient one and hydronephrosis in both patients were secondary to distal obstructive uropathy, the association probably does not represent an acrorenal DFD.

Sex Ratio: M1:F0. Only males are affected, since a posterior urethral valve is present only in males.

Occurrence: Two infants were seen in the months of December 1980 and December 1984 (from a total of approximately 7,502 births).

Risk of Recurrence for Patient's Sib: Unknown. Kidney echogram of patient one's brother showed a prominent cystic structure (4.5 ;ts 5 cm) involving the superior aspect of the left kidney. Urologic investigation showed bilateral duplication of the collecting system and ectopic ureterocele with megaureter and hydronephrosis of the left upper pole collecting system. A paternal cousin of the patient had bilateral hydroureters, right more than left.

Risk of Recurrence for Patient's Child: Unknown.

Age of Detectability: At birth. Prenatal diagnosis is probably possible by routine ultrasonography.

Gene Mapping and Linkage: Unknown.

Prevention: Prenatal treatment of hydronephrosis may be possible.

Treatment: Prenatal treatment of hydronephrosis may be possible.

Prognosis: Both known patients were stillborn.

Detection of Carrier: Careful clinical and urologic examinations of first degree relatives will help to clarify the spectrum of manifestations.

Special Considerations: Because advanced autolysis did not permit good examination of the central nervous system, associated anomalies of the brain could not be definitely excluded.

References:
Halal F: Distal obstructive uropathy with polydactyly: a new syndrome? (Letter) Am J Med Genet 1986; 24:753–757.

HA074   **Fahed Halal**

Polydactyly-ectrodactyly
  See ECTRODACTYLY-POLYDACTYLY
Polydactyly-imperforate anus
  See VATER ASSOCIATION
Polydactyly-Joubert syndrome
  See JOUBERT SYNDROME
Polydactyly-neonatal chondrodystrophy, type I
  See SHORT RIB-POLYDACTYLY SYNDROME, TYPE I
Polydactyly-neonatal chondrodystrophy, type II
  See SHORT RIB-POLYDACTYLY SYNDROME, TYPE II
Polydactyly-neonatal chondrodystrophy, type III
  See SHORT RIB-POLYDACTYLY SYNDROME, VERMA-NAUMOFF TYPE
Polydactyly-obesity-hypogenitalism-iris coloboma
  See BIEMOND II SYNDROME
Polydactyly-Robin anomaly-skeletal dysplasia
  See CLEFT PALATE-DYSMORPHIC FACIES-DIGITAL DEFECTS, MARTSOLF TYPE
Polydactyly-sex reversal-renal hypoplasia-unilobular lung
  See SMITH-LEMLI-OPITZ SYNDROME, TYPE II

Polydactyly-syndactyly-ear lobe syndrome
  See SYNDACTYLY-POLYDACTYLY-EAR LOBE SYNDROME
Polydontia
  See TEETH, SUPERNUMERARY
Polydysspondyly
  See SPONDYLOCOSTAL DYSPLASIA
Polydystrophia oligophrenia
  See MUCOPOLYSACCHARIDOSIS III

POLYGLANDULAR AUTOIMMUNE SYNDROME   2623

Includes:
  Autoimmune polyendocrinopathy-candidiasis-ectodermal dystrophy
  Candidiasis-endocrinopathy syndrome
  Hypoadrenocorticism-hypoparathyroidism-superficial moniliasis
  Moniliasis, familial
  Whitaker syndrome

Excludes: Candidiasis, familial chronic mucocutaneous (2117)

Major Diagnostic Criteria: Familial occurrence of chronic candidal infection of mucous membranes, skin, and nails. Polyendocrinopathy occurs in roughly one-half of the cases.

Clinical Findings: Chronic candidal infection of the oral mucous membranes is almost always evident and usually develops in early childhood, often before age two years. Chronic candidal infection of fingernails and toenails is also frequently present and may result in severe dystrophic changes. Cutaneous disease is somewhat less common and affects primarily the face, hands, and feet. Those severely affected may develop candidal granuloma (thick, hyperkeratotic plaques of the face or nails). Systemic candidiasis is uncommon. In those with endocrinopathy, symptoms and signs of deficient hormone production by the parathyroid, adrenal, and, less commonly, the thyroid, pancreas, stomach, and ovary usually become manifest in the second decade. In rare cases, endocrine abnormalities precede candidiasis by 5–10 years. Endocrinopathy is associated with autoimmunity to the involved gland. Chronic active hepatitis and cirrhosis occur in some patients. Alopecia and tooth hypoplasia are common. Chronic pulmonary disease occasionally develops.

Complications: Chronic hoarseness may result from candidal laryngitis. Disfiguring skin lesions may result in psychologic disturbances. Adrenal failure may result in sudden death. Tetany, seizures, cataracts, keratoconjunctivitis, and band keratopathy may occur as a result of hypoparathyroidism. Pancreatic insufficiency can result in steatorrhea and diabetes mellitus. Pernicious anemia and iron deficiency anemia are common.

Associated Findings: Thymoma, thymic dysplasia, and splenic agenesis.

Etiology: Autosomal recessive inheritance. Multifactorial etiology involving infectious and autoimmune components has also been suggested.

Pathogenesis: The frequent occurrence of abnormalities of the cellular immune system, including anergy, hypergammaglobulinemia, selective IgA deficiency, defective in vitro nonspecific T suppressor cell activity, impaired in vitro production of migration inhibition factor, and autoantibodies to endocrine tissue, have led to the theory that this condition results from an inherited abnormality of the immune system that primarily affects the T lymphocyte, which results in 1) abnormalities of immunoregulation leading to autoimmunity and 2) impaired host resistance to candidal infection.

MIM No.: *24030

Sex Ratio: M1:F1

Occurrence: About 150 cases have been reported, almost one-third from Finland.

Risk of Recurrence for Patient's Sib:
  See Part I, *Mendelian Inheritance.*

Risk of Recurrence for Patient's Child:
  See Part I, *Mendelian Inheritance.*

Age of Detectability: Usually clinically evident in early childhood.

Gene Mapping and Linkage: Unknown.

Prevention: None known. Genetic counseling indicated.

Treatment: Continuous antifungal therapy is usually required. Topical therapy with gentian violet, Mycostatin, and other similar agents is not curative but can prevent progression. Intravenous amphotericin B results in more marked improvement and clearing of lesions, but relapse is invariable. Renal toxicity limits its use. Surgical removal is the only definitive treatment for affected nails. Administration of transfer factor, thymosin, and levamisole have been used with only partial and inconsistent results. Bone marrow transplantation has been used successfully in a single case, but is not recommended because of the risk of graft-versus-host disease. In one study intravenous iron therapy provided a beneficial effect in 8:11 patients. Endocrinopathies must be treated as appropriate to each condition.

Prognosis: The outcome depends on the severity of such associated conditions as adrenal insufficiency, hypoparathyroidism, diabetes mellitus, and chronic liver disease. Normal life span is possible.

Detection of Carrier: Unknown.

References:

Wuepper KD, Fudenberg HH: Moniliasis, "autoimmune" polyendocrinopathy, and immunologic family study. Clin Exp Immunol 1967; 2:71–82.

Blizzard RM, Gibbs JH: Candidiasis: studies pertaining to its association with endocrinopathies and pernicious anemia. Pediatrics 1968; 42:231–237.

Wells RS, et al.: Familial chronic muco-cutaneous candidiasis. J Med Genet 1972; 9:302–310.

Arulanantham K, et al.: Evidence for defective immunoregulation in the syndrome of familial candidiasis endocrinopathy. New Engl J Med 1978; 300:164–168.

Stiehm ER, Fulginiti VA: Immunologic disorders in infants and children, ed 2. Philadelphia: W.B. Saunders, 1980. * †

Ahonen P: Autoimmune polyendocrinopathy-candidiasis-ectodermal dystrophy (APECED): autosomal recessive inheritance. Clin Genet 1985; 27:535–542.

Maclaren NK, Riley WJ: Inherited susceptibility to autoimmune Addison's disease is linked to human leukocyte antigens-DR3 and/or DR4, except when associated with type I autoimmune polyglandular syndrome. J Clin Endocr Metab 1986; 62:455–459.

KA038   **Joseph Kaplan**

POLYPOSIS-ALOPECIA-PIGMENTATION-NAIL DEFECTS   3040

Includes:
  Alopecia-polyposis-pigmentation-nail defects
  Cronkhite-Canada syndrome
  Gastrointestinal polyposis-ectodermal defects
  Pigmentation-alopecia-polyposis-nail defects

Excludes:
  Intestinal polyposis, type II (2344)
  Intestinal polyposis, type III (0536)

Major Diagnostic Criteria: Gastrointestinal symptoms (weight loss, vomiting, and diarrhea) associated with hair loss, nail atrophy, and skin hyperpigmentation should suggest the diagnosis.

Clinical Findings: Individuals with this condition present with diarrhea, vomiting, anorexia, and sometimes with abdominal pains. Alopecia, nail changes (in the form of loss or dystrophy), and hyperpigmentation of skin or mucosa accompany the gastrointestinal symptoms. X-ray evaluation of the GI tract demonstrates generalized polyposis of the stomach and colon, with occasional involvement of duodenum, rectum, and esophagus. Death usually occurs after a duration of 6–18 months. Onset is at 30–80 years of age. Early descriptions of the polyps have classified them as adenomas, histologically; more recently thay have been characterized as hamartomatous polyps of the juvenile type.

Complications: Weight loss, muscle weakness, anemia, and edema all occurred as complications.

Associated Findings: Six patients had numbness and tingling, four developed cataracts, two had seizures, and one each had syncope and transient ischemia.

Etiology: The cause of this condition is obscure, although it is not thought to be genetic. All reported cases have been sporadic occurrences in otherwise normal families.

Pathogenesis: It has been suggested that the ectodermal changes are secondary to an as yet unidentified nutritional deficiency caused by the diffuse polyposis. However, in one patient, the nail changes occurred years before onset of gastrointestinal symptoms, so the ectodermal changes may be concomitant, rather than secondary, findings.

MIM No.: 17550

POS No.: 3844

Sex Ratio: M1:F1

Occurrence: More than 50 cases, from all parts of the world, have been reported.

Risk of Recurrence for Patient's Sib: Probably not increased.

Risk of Recurrence for Patient's Child: Probably not increased.

Age of Detectability: Onset of the disorder has been between the ages of 40 and 70 years.

Gene Mapping and Linkage: Unknown.

Prevention: None known. Genetic counseling indicated.

Treatment: Aggressive supportive therapy is recommended over surgical intervention. However, hemicolectomy in one case and partial gastrectomy in another led to apparent recovery.

Prognosis: Death usually occurs 6–18 months from the onset of symptoms; however, some patients have survived for 15 years. Death usually occurs in severely symptomatic patients who fail to respond to therapeutic measurers.

Detection of Carrier: Unknown.

Special Considerations: This condition must be distinguished from the genetic polyposes so that accurate genetic counseling can be provided to relatives.

References:

Cronkhite LW, Jr., Canada WJ: Generalized gastrointestinal polyposis: an unusual syndrome of polyposis, pigmentation, alopecia and onychotrophia. New Engl J Med 1955; 252:1011–1015.

Jarnum S, Jensen H: Diffuse gastrointestinal polyposis with ectodermal changes: a case with severe malabsorption and enteric loss of plasma proteins and electrolytes. Gastroenterology 1966; 50:107–118.

Dacruz GMG: Generalized gastrointestinal polyposis: an unusual syndrome of adenomatous polyposis, alopecia, onychorotrophia. Am J Gastroenterol 1967; 47:504–510.

Daniel ES, et al.: The Cronkhite-Canada syndrome: an analysis of clinical and pathologic features and therapy in 55 patients. Medicine 1982; 61:293–309. *

T0007   Helga V. Toriello

Polysaccharide storage cardioskeletal myopathy
  See MYOPATHY-METABOLIC, GLYCOPROTEIN-GLYCOSAMINOGLYCANS STORAGE TYPE
Polyserositis, benign paroxysmal
  See FEVER, FAMILIAL MEDITERRANEAN (FMF)
Polyserositis, recurrent
  See FEVER, FAMILIAL MEDITERRANEAN (FMF)
Polysplenia syndrome
  See ASPLENIA SYNDROME

POLYSYNDACTYLY   0817

Includes:
  Preaxial polydactyly IV
  Preaxial polydactyly of toes associated with syndactyly

Excludes:
  Acrocephalosyndactyly
  Polysyndactyly-dysmorphic craniofacies, Greig type (2925)
  Syndactyly (0923)

Major Diagnostic Criteria: An extra or duplicated digit occurs with syndactyly (webbing between digits).

Clinical Findings: In the feet, preaxial polydactyly or duplication of the first or second toes is associated with syndactyly of various degrees. In the hands, the most common malformation is syndactyly of the third and fourth fingers; the terminal phalanx of the thumb is usually malformed, broad and short, or bifid, and sometimes radially deviated. Pedunculated postminimi is a feature in some families. While the hand malformation is mild and variable, malformation of the feet is constant and nearly uniform.

Complications: Unknown.

Associated Findings: None known.

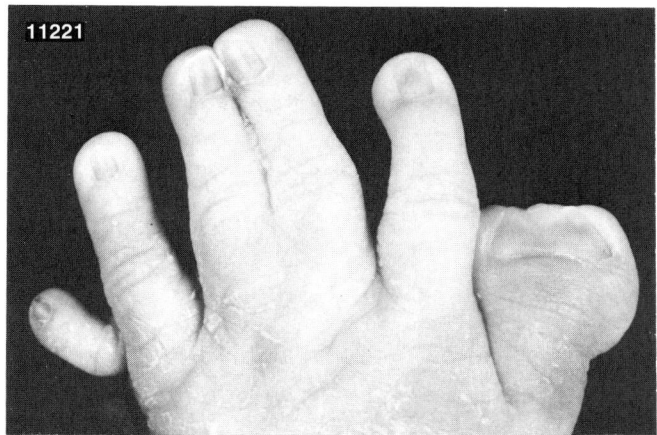

0817-11221:   Combined pre- and post-axial polysyndactyly.

Etiology: Autosomal dominant inheritance with variable expression and complete penetrance.

Pathogenesis: Unknown.

MIM No.: *17470

Sex Ratio: M1:F1

Occurrence: Undetermined. Several large kindreds have been reported.

Risk of Recurrence for Patient's Sib:
  See Part I, *Mendelian Inheritance.*

Risk of Recurrence for Patient's Child:
  See Part I, *Mendelian Inheritance.*

Age of Detectability: At birth.

Gene Mapping and Linkage: Unknown.

Prevention: None known. Genetic counseling indicated.

Treatment: Surgical correction of malformation.

Prognosis: Normal life span.

Detection of Carrier: Unknown.

Special Considerations: Recent research (Baraitser et al, 1983) has pointed out a similarity between polysyndactyly and **Polysyndactyly-dysmorphic craniofacies, Greig type**. The delineation of polysyndactyly as a distinct entity (Temtamy and McKusick, 1978) is, therefore, no longer certain.

References:

Goodman RM: A family with polysyndactyly and other anomalies. J Hered 1965; 56:37–38.

Temtamy SA, Loutfy AH: Polysyndactyly in an Egyptian family. BD:OAS X(5). New York: March of Dimes Birth Defects Foundation, 1974:207.

Temtamy SA, McKusick VA: The genetics of hand malformations. New York: Alan R. Liss, 1978.

Baraitser M, et al.: Greig cephalopolysyndactyly: report of 13 affected individuals in three families. Clin Genet 1983; 24:257–265.

Reynolds JF, et al.: Preaxial polydactyly type 4: variability in a large kindred. Clin Genet 1984; 25:267–272.

TE004   Samia A. Temtamy

Polysyndactyly, postaxial-frontonasal dysostosis-cleft lip/palate
  See ACRO-FRONTO-FACIO-NASAL DYSOSTOSIS

POLYSYNDACTYLY-CARDIAC MALFORMATIONS   2815

Includes: Heart defects-polysyndactyly

Excludes:
  Chondroectodermal dysplasia (0156)
  Oro-facio-digital syndrome, Mohr type (0771)
  Polysyndactyly-dysmorphic craniofacies, Greig type (2925)

Major Diagnostic Criteria: The combination of mild facial anomalies, **Syndactyly** of the fingers, duplicated great toes, and cardiac malformations.

Clinical Findings: The gestations of all affected individuals were complicated by polyhydramnios; two of the children were stillborn. Facial anomalies in the surviving child included **Eye, hypertelorism** with epicanthal folds, short nose with anteverted nares, long and poorly defined philtrum, micrognathia, posteriorly rotated ears, and creased earlobes. Hirsutism was present on the face and upper trunk. Limb defects were present in all three, and consisted of duplicated great toes (3/3) and **Syndactyly** of fingers 2–5 (2/3). The liveborn child had **Atrial septal defects** and **Ventricular septal defect**; the stillborn children had a single ventricle with a common atrioventricular valve.

Complications: Unknown.

Associated Findings: A **Urofacial syndrome** was present in one child but may have been a coincidental finding.

Etiology: Possibly autosomal recessive inheritance.

Pathogenesis: Unknown.

MIM No.: 26363

POS No.: 3814

Sex Ratio: Presumably M1:F1.

Occurrence: One sibship of three affected individuals has been reported from France.

Risk of Recurrence for Patient's Sib:
See Part I, *Mendelian Inheritance.*

Risk of Recurrence for Patient's Child:
See Part I, *Mendelian Inheritance.*

Age of Detectability: At birth, although prenatal diagnosis by ultrasound may be possible.

Gene Mapping and Linkage: Unknown.

Prevention: None known. Genetic counseling indicated.

Treatment: Supportive; surgical correction of the cardiac defect may be indicated.

Prognosis: Of three reported cases, two were stillborn, and the third died at age 5 1/2 months. Intellectual development is undetermined.

Detection of Carrier: Unknown.

References:
Bonneau JC, et al.: Polysyndactylie avec cardiopathie complexe a propos de trois cas dans une meme fratrie. J Genet Hum 1983; 31:93–105.

T0007   **Helga V. Toriello**

POLYSYNDACTYLY-DYSMORPHIC CRANIOFACIES, GREIG TYPE   2925

Includes:
Cephalopolysyndactyly syndrome, Greig type
Craniofacial anomalies-polysyndactyly
Frontodigital syndrome
Greig cephalopolysyndactyly syndrome
Skull, peculiar shape-polysyndactyly

Excludes:
Acrocallosal syndrome, Schinzel type (2263)
Cephalopolysyndactyly syndromes, other
Eye, hypertelorism (0504)

Major Diagnostic Criteria: Pronounced cutaneous **Syndactyly** of toes and fingers, postaxial **Polydactyly** of toes and fingers, complete or partial duplication of the halluces, and scaphocephaly.

Clinical Findings: Craniofacial features include **Megalencephaly,** scaphocephaly, prominent forehead (frontal bossing), and **Eye, hypertelorism** but no overt craniostenosis. Plagiocephaly may occasionally be seen. The most common features of the hands are syndactyly and pedunculated postminimi polydactyly. The syndactyly varies from mild cutaneous webbing to bony fusion. Occasionally, the thumbs may be duplicated or have broad tips. In the feet, the syndactyly is variable and the polydactyly is commonly preaxial, although postaxial polydactyly may be seen. Intelligence is normal in affected individuals, and CT scans show only mild-to-moderate enlargement of the lateral ventricles, basal cisterns, and sylvian fissures.

Complications: Palsy of fifth cranial nerve, divergent strabismus, and **Camptodactyly**.

Associated Findings: **Hernia, inguinal**. While mental development is usually normal, mental retardation and absence of corpus callosum has been documented in a small number of patients. Other rare occasional findings include growth retardation and genital hypoplasia. It is undetermined if **Acrocallosal syndrome, Schinzel type** is a distinct entity or a variable expression of the same condition.

Etiology: Autosomal dominant inheritance with wide variation in expression. Various chromosomal anomalies have also been suggested.

Pathogenesis: The skull congfiguration has led to the suggestion that the cranial features result from basal hypoplasia with compensatory calvarial expansion and retention of an infantile forehead.

MIM No.: *17570

POS No.: 3489

Sex Ratio: M1:F1

Occurrence: Unknown. A few dozen cases have been reported, but the features may be so mild that many affected individuals escape notice.

Risk of Recurrence for Patient's Sib:
See Part I, *Mendelian Inheritance.*

Risk of Recurrence for Patient's Child:
See Part I, *Mendelian Inheritance.*

Age of Detectability: Prenatal, by ultrasound observation of polydactyly and macrocephaly.

Gene Mapping and Linkage: GCPS (Greig cephalopolysyndactyly syndrome) has been mapped to 7p13.

Prevention: None known. Genetic counseling indicated.

Treatment: Surgical release of syndactyly and removal of supernumerary digits.

Prognosis: Good for life span and general health in the absence of major internal malformations.

Detection of Carrier: Unknown.

References:
Greig DM: Oxycephaly. Edinb Med J 1928; 33:189–218.
Marshall RE, Smith DW: Frontodigital syndrome: a dominantly inherited disorder with normal intelligence. J Pediatr 1970; 77:129–133. *
Hootnick D, Holmes LB: Familial polysyndactyly and craniofacial anomalies. Clin Genet 1972; 3:128–134. * †
Baraitser M, et al.: Greig cephalopolysyndactyly: report of 13 affected individuals in three families. Clin Genet 1983; 24:257–265. †
Fryns JP, et al.: The Greig polysyndactyly-craniofacial dysmorphism syndrome. Eur J Pediatr 1977; 126:283–287. †
Gallop TR, Fontes LR: The Greig cephalopolysyndactyly syndrome: report of a family and review of the literature. Am J Med Genet 1985; 22:59–68. †
Kruger G, et al.: Greig syndrome in a large kindred due to reciprocal chromosome translocation t(6;7)(q27;p13). Am J Med Genet 1989; 32:411–416.

J0027   **Ronald J. Jorgenson**
FR030   **Jean-Pierre Fryns**

Pompe disease
See GLYCOGENOSIS, TYPE IIa
Ponstel^, fetal effects
See FETAL EFFECTS OF NONSTEROIDAL ANTI-INFLAMMATORY DRUGS (NSAIDS)
Popliteal pterygium syndrome
See PTERYGIUM SYNDROME, POPLITEAL
Popliteal pterygium syndrome, lethal type
See PTERYGIUM SYNDROME, POPLITEAL, LETHAL

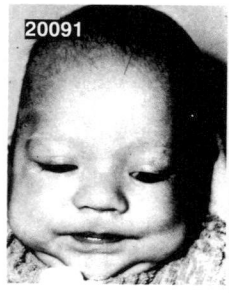 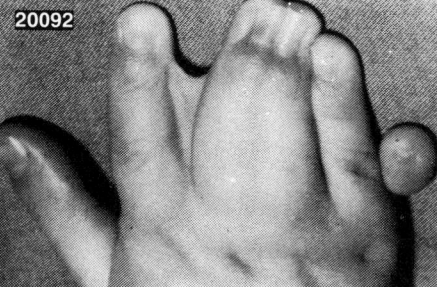

2925-20091: Typical craniofacies with high, broad forehead, hypertelorism and broad nasal base.   **20092:** Polysyndactyly of the hand.

Porcupine man
  See NEVUS, EPIDERMAL NEVUS SYNDROME
Porencephaly, prenatal
  See BRAIN, PORENCEPHALY
Porokeratosis of Mibelli
  See SKIN, POROKERATOSIS
Porokeratosis, linear
  See SKIN, POROKERATOSIS
Porokeratosis, plantaris
  See SKIN, POROKERATOSIS
Porphobilinogen deaminase deficiency
  See PORPHYRIA, ACUTE INTERMITTENT
Porphobilinogen synthase partial deficiency
  See DELTA-AMINOLEVULINIC ACID DEHYDRASE DEFICIENCY

PORPHYRIA CUTANEA TARDA   3064

Includes:
  Cutaneous porphyria
  Hepatoerythropoietic porphyria
  Porphyria, hepatocutaneous type
  Porphyria, hepatoerythropoietic
  Uroporphyrinogen decarboxylase deficiency

Excludes:
  Porphyria cutanea tarda, sporadic
  Porphyria (other)

Major Diagnostic Criteria: Characteristic bullous lesions on sun-exposed skin. Laboratory diagnosis requires measurement of porphyrins in both urine and stool. Traditional solvent partition methods demonstrate that uroporphyrin exceeds coproporphyrin in the urine, and coproporphyrin exceeds protoporphyrin in the stool. Chromatographic methods show mainly 8- and 7-carboxylate porphyrins in the urine and an increase of isocoproporphyrin in the stool.

Clinical Findings: Blisters form on the sun-exposed areas of the skin, particularly the dorsum of the hands and face. The involved skin is mechanically fragile. Subsequent ulceration and scarring may lead to a scleroderma-like thickening of the skin. Hyperpigmentation and hypertrichosis may also occur. Most patients have evidence of liver disease, with biopsy materials revealing hemosiderosis and lobular inflammatory cellular aggregates. Patients do not have acute photosensitivity and do not have acute porphyric attacks with neurovisceral symptoms.

Complications: Increased incidence of hepatocellular carcinoma.

Associated Findings: **Lupus erythematosus, systemic** and other autoimmune diseases.

Etiology: Autosomal dominant inheritance with variability in expression (the more common sporadic type appears to be the result of environmental injury without any evidence of a genetic component). *Hepatoerythropoietic porphyria* (Toback et al, 1987) is an autosomal recessive disease with less than 10% of normal activity of uroporphyriogen decarboxylase and might represent the homozygous form.

Pathogenesis: Fifty percent of normal activity of uroporphyrinogen decarboxylase (E.C. 4.1.1.37) in erythrocytes, liver, and other tissues. Additional agents, especially ethanol or estrogens, are required for overproduction of hepatic porphyrins. Hepatic iron plays a synergistic role in this toxic process by an unknown mechanism. The increased blood porphyrins cause the cutaneous manifestations, perhaps by activating the complement system.

MIM No.: *17610

Sex Ratio: M1:F1

Occurrence: Unknown. The most common porphyria. However, the vast majority of cases are believed to be sporadic, and only a small minority are familial.

Risk of Recurrence for Patient's Sib:
  See Part I, *Mendelian Inheritance.*

Risk of Recurrence for Patient's Child:
  See Part I, *Mendelian Inheritance.*

Age of Detectability: Rarely clinically evident before age 20 years and usually evident after age 40 years. The deficiency in the activity of uroporphyrinogen decarboxylase is detectable throughout life.

Gene Mapping and Linkage: UROD (uroporphyrinogen decarboxylase) has been mapped to 1p34.

Prevention: None known. Genetic counseling indicated.

Treatment: Elimination of potentially precipitating agents, including ethanol, oral iron supplements, oral estrogens, and halogenated aromatic hydrocarbons. Reduction of iron stores by phlebotomy or by subcutaneous desferoxamine infusion. Low-dose chloroquine or hydroxychloroquine is a secondary therapy.

Prognosis: Complete remission of symptoms occurs in the majority of patients with therapy. Compatible with a normal life span.

Detection of Carrier: Carriers have a 50% deficiency in the activity of uroporphyrinogen decarboxylase in the erythrocytes and liver.

References:
Lefkowitch JH, Grossman ME: Hepatic pathology in porphyria cutanea tarda. Liver 1983; 3:19–29.
de Verneuil H, et al.: Enzymatic and immunological studies of uroporphyrinogen decarboxylase in familial porphyria cutanea tarda and hepatoerythropoietic porphyria. Am J Hum Genet 1984; 36:613–622.
Dubart A, et al.: Assignment of human uroporphyrinogen decarboxylase (URO-D) to the p34 band of chromosome 1. Hum Genet 1986; 73(3):277–279.
Rocchi E, et al.: Serum ferritin in the assessment of liver iron overload and iron removal therapy in porphyria cutanea tarda. J Lab Clin Med 1986; 107:36–42.
Sweeney GD: Porphyria cutanea tarda, or the uroporphyrinogen decarboxylase deficiency diseases. Clin Biochem 1986; 19:3–15.
Toback AC, et al.: Hepatoerythropoietic porphyria: clinical, biochemical, and enzymatic studies in a three-generation family lineage. New Engl J Med 1987; 316:645–650.

BR038   **David A. Brenner**

Porphyria, acute hepatic
  See DELTA-AMINOLEVULINIC ACID DEHYDRASE DEFICIENCY

PORPHYRIA, ACUTE INTERMITTENT   0820

Includes:
  PBGD deficiency
  Porphobilinogen deaminase deficiency
  Pyrroloporphyria
  Swedish genetic porphyria
  UPS deficiency

Excludes:
  Delta-aminolevulinic acid dehydrase deficiency (3091)
  Porphyria, coproporphyria (0203)
  Porphyria, variegate (0822)

Major Diagnostic Criteria: Demonstration of significantly increased porphobilinogen excretion (Watson-Schwartz test), tachycardia, and abdominal pain.

Clinical Findings: This condition may exist in a latent form for a lifetime or may be manifest by attacks of neurologic dysfunction. Four known groups of precipitating causes are drugs (barbiturates, sulfonamides, griseofulvin, diphenylhydantoin, and so forth); estrogen and possibly progesterone, oral contraceptives in certain cases; infections; and starvation. Some attacks occur without obvious precipitating factors. In about 10–20% of women with this disease attacks occur in a cyclic pattern, usually beginning about 3 days before menstrual periods.
  The acute attack results from damage in any portion of the nervous system. Signs and symptoms of the acute attack, which are all attributable to autonomic neuropathy, include abdominal pain, constipation (occasionally diarrhea), tachycardia, sweating, labile hypertension, postural hypotension, retinal artery spasm,

and vascular spasm in the skin of the limbs. Peripheral neuropathy may be sensory or motor. There may be pain in the back or limbs (more commonly in the legs), which may persist for long periods without motor involvement or may precede motor paralysis. There may be paresthesias, but objective sensory findings are usually absent unless the sensory neuropathy is of long duration. Motor involvement is variable in terms of symmetry, severity, and rate of progress of the process. All peripheral nerves, including cranial, are subject to the neuropathy. CNS manifestations include bulbar paralysis, cerebellar and basal ganglion manifestations, hypothalamic dysfunction, seizures, acute and chronic psychoses, hallucinations, and coma.

Medullary and phrenic nerve involvement may cause respiratory paralysis, which is the most common cause of death. Hyponatremia, sometimes of severe degree, may result from excessive sodium loss from the GI tract or may be associated with the classic findings of the syndrome of inappropriate release of antidiuretic hormone (SIADH). Hypomagnesemia, occasionally sufficient to produce tetany, may accompany the hyponatremia.

The two most significant psychiatric syndromes associated with this disease are organic brain syndrome (irritability, restlessness, confusion, disorientation, hallucinations) and depression. BSP excretion may be normal or decreased during asymptomatic periods, but it is usually impaired during activity of the disease. Other frequent laboratory findings include hypercholesterolemia (40–50% of patients), increased serum PBI and thyroxin-binding globulin (TBG), and hyper-β-lipoproteinemia. During acute attacks, a diabetic glucose tolerance test is often demonstrable.

Complications: Chronic pain syndrome (peripheral or abdominal), motor paralysis (including respiratory paralysis), seizures, organic brain syndrome, depression.

Associated Findings: None known.

Etiology: Autosomal dominant inheritance.

Pathogenesis: An increase of delta-aminolevulinic acid synthase and rate-controlling enzyme of the heme biosynthetic pathway has been demonstrated in the livers of patients with this disease. The inherited defect is a decreased level of porphobilinogen deaminase (uroporphyrinogen I synthase). However, it is not clear how these findings relate to the acute attacks of neurologic dysfunction.

MIM No.: *17600

Sex Ratio: M1:F1.5

Occurrence: About 1:66,000 in the British Isles, but in certain areas such as Lapland it is much higher. Probably exceeds 1:66,000 worldwide.

Risk of Recurrence for Patient's Sib:
See Part I, *Mendelian Inheritance.*

Risk of Recurrence for Patient's Child:
See Part I, *Mendelian Inheritance.*

Age of Detectability: The disease is usually not manifest clinically, and is sometimes not evident biochemically before puberty.

Gene Mapping and Linkage: PBGD (porphobilinogen deaminase) has been mapped to 11q23.2-qter.

Prevention: None known. Genetic counseling indicated.

Treatment: Abdominal pain may be relieved by chlorpromazine. Demerol may be useful if chlorpromazine does not completely alleviate pain. The cause of hyponatremia must be determined before it is treated. If caused by primary salt loss from the GI tract, salt replacement is essential. If associated with the findings of the syndrome of inappropriate release of ADH, water restriction has been successful in raising serum sodium levels. The problem has been complicated by the frequent finding of hypovolemia, which, if sufficiently pronounced in the presence of hyponatremia, is an indication for hypertonic saline adminstration. Some patients have responded well to a high-carbohydrate intake-as high as possible (up to 400 g/day or more). Since the response is not uniform or predictable, a high-carbohydrate intake should be attempted in all patients experiencing an attack of an inducible porphyria.

Hematin infusions have been repeatedly shown to curtail an acute attack and have improved the prognosis for all "inducible" porphyrias. It is given at a dose of 2–4 mg/kg for three days (Pierach, 1982).

Supportive care during acute attacks is of great importance. When there is peripheral neuropathy, respiratory paralysis, dysphagia, or coma, careful attention to nursing care, avoidance of aspiration, assisted respiration, early recognition of pneumonia, and physiotherapy are of great importance. Splints and sandbags should be used for wrist- and footdrop.

In those women who experience regularly recurrent attacks in relation to menstrual cycles, administration of oral contraceptive preparations have been useful in preventing attacks. The schedule used is similar to that used for contraception, but the dosage required may or may not be higher. This approach should be used with caution, since experience with it in this type of patient is limited and oral contraceptives sometimes precipitate attacks in women who do not experience the regularly recurring cyclic attacks. A luteinizing hormone-releasing hormone analogue has been shown experimentally to suppress these premenstrual attacks (Anderson et al., 1984).

Prophylaxis is of great importance and involves warning patients and members of their families about avoiding the known precipitating factors.

Prognosis: A mortality rate of 24% over a five-year observation period has been reported. In the patient with known disease who has been warned about the precipitating factors, the prognosis is now much improved.

Detection of Carrier: In approximately 90% of patients with acute intermittent porphyria, porphobilinogen deaminase (the deficient enzyme) can be found to be decreased in their erythrocytes, thus lending itself very well to carrier detection (Pierach et al., 1987).

The author wishes to thank Donald P. Tschudy for his contribution to an earlier version of this article.

References:
Wetterberg L: A neuropsychiatric and genetical investigation of acute intermittent porphyria. Stockholm: Bokforlaget, 1968.
Tschudy DP, Lamon JL: Porphyrin metabolism and the porphyrias. In: Bondy PK, Rosenberg LE, ed: Metabolic control and disease. Philadelphia: W.B. Saunders, 1980:939–1008.
Pierach CA: Hematin therapy for the porphyric attack. Semin Liver Disease 1982; 2:125–131.
Anderson KE, et al.: Prevention of cyclical attacks of acute intermittent porphyria with a long-acting agonist of luteinizing hormone-releasing hormone. New Engl J Med 1984; 311:643–645.
Pierach CA, et al.: Red cell porphobilinogen deaminase in the evaluation of acute intermittent porphyria. JAMA 1987; 257:60–61.

PI009   **Claus A. Pierach**

PORPHYRIA, COPROPORPHYRIA   0203

Includes:
   Coproporphyrinogen oxidase deficiency
   Harderoporphyria

Excludes: Hepatic porphyria (other forms)

Major Diagnostic Criteria: Increased fecal and urine coproporphyrin with little increase of fecal protoporphyrin. Urinary delta-aminolevulinic acid and porphobilinogen are increased during acute attacks of neurovisceral symptoms.

Clinical Findings: Patients present with acute attacks of neurovisceral symptoms similar to those in acute intermittent porphyria. The manifestations of an acute attack may include abdominal pain, neurologic deficits, psychiatric symptoms (hallucinations, depression), and constipation. A minority of patients have photosensitivity, consisting of blistering of the sun-exposed skin. The majority of patients with the inherited defect and biochemical abnormalities are clinically asymptomatic.

Complications: Paralysis (rarely progressing to respiratory muscle paralysis), seizures, depression, psychosis, photosensitivity, hypertension.

Associated Findings: None known.

Etiology: Autosomal dominant inheritance of enzymatic defect. Homozygous cases with more severe clinical manifestations have been reported.

Pathogenesis: Enzymatic defect in coproporphyrinogen oxidase (E.C.1.3.3.3). Heterozygotic patients have 50% of the enzymatic activity of controls.

MIM No.: *12130

Sex Ratio: All patients, M1:F1; symptomatic, M1:F2.5

Occurrence: Rarest of the three types of acute hepatic porphyrias. No ethnic predisposition.

Risk of Recurrence for Patient's Sib:
See Part I, *Mendelian Inheritance*.

Risk of Recurrence for Patient's Child:
See Part I, *Mendelian Inheritance*.

Age of Detectability: Decreased activity of coproporphyrinogen oxidase is present at birth; biochemical abnormalities appear postpubescent.

Gene Mapping and Linkage: CPO (coproporphyrinogen oxidase) has been mapped to 9.

Prevention: Avoidance of precipitating drugs (most commonly phenobarbital, ethanol). Fasting should be avoided. Genetic counseling is indicated.

Treatment: Specific treatment of acute attacks includes high-carbohydrate diet and intravenous hematin. Most acute attacks resolve after discontinuing the precipitating drug(s). Specific therapy is the same for all acute hepatic porphyrias and consists of high carbohydrate diet and intravenous hematin.

Prognosis: Acute attacks are generally less severe than in acute intermittent porphyria. By avoiding precipitating agents, the disease is compatible with longevity.

Detection of Carrier: Decreased activity of coproporphyrinogen oxidase is detectable in cultured fibroblasts, peripheral lymphocytes, and buffy coat preparations. The enzyme activity assay is not widely available. Fecal coproporphyrin levels are elevated in nearly all carriers of the mutant gene.

References:
Elder GH, et al.: The primary enzyme defect in hereditary coproporphyria. Lancet 1976; II:1217–1219.
Brodie MJ, et al.: Hereditary coproporphyria: demonstration of the abnormalities in haem biosynthesis in peripheral blood. Q J Med 1977; 46:229–241.
Grandchamp B, et al.: Homozygous case of hereditary coproporphyria. Lancet 1977; II: 1348–1349.
Grandchamp B, et al.: Assignment of the human coproporphyrinogen oxidase to chromosome 9. Hum Genet 1983; 64:180–183.
Nordmann Y, et al.: Harderoporphyria: a variant hereditary coproporphyria. J Clin Invest 1983; 72:1139–1149.
Andrews J, et al.: Hereditary coproporphyria: incidence in a large English family. J Med Genet 1984; 21:341–349.

BR038   **David A. Brenner**

PORPHYRIA, ERYTHROPOIETIC   0821

Includes:
  Enamel and dentin staining from erythropoietic porphyria
  Erythrodontia
  Erythropoietic porphyria, congenital
  Gunther disease
  Hematoporphyria congenita
  Uroporphyrinogen III cosynthase deficiency
  UROS deficiency

Excludes:
  Nonporphyric photodermatoses such as xeroderma
    pigmentosum
  Photosensitizing porphyrias

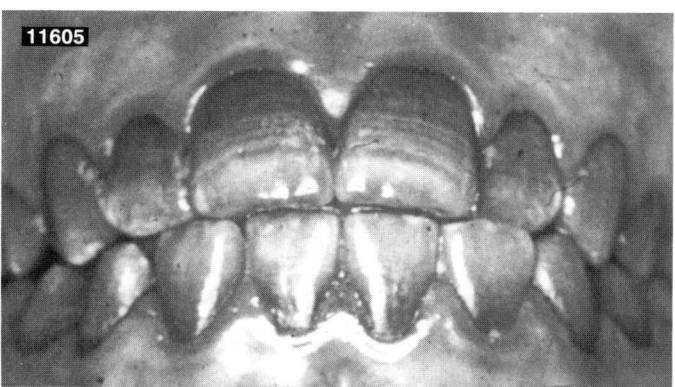

0821-11605: Red staining of the teeth.

Porphyria (others)
Teeth, enamel and dentin defects from erythroblastosis fetalis
(0340)

Major Diagnostic Criteria: Pink urine, photosensitivity, and hemolysis are the major findings. Demonstration by quantitative methods of greatly increased uroporphyrin I in the urine and fluorescence of red cells and marrow normoblasts. In addition, it is desirable to demonstrate increased erythrocyte uroporphyrin levels by direct analysis. Fluorescence of the teeth should be sought when erythrodontia is not obvious. Clinical pigmentation of teeth may be minimal in some cases, but an extract of ground tooth structure with 0.5 N HCl will normally exhibit brilliant red fluorescence.

Clinical Findings: The two organ systems mainly affected are the skin and bone marrow. The onset of symptoms is usually between birth and age 5 years. Pink or red urine may be the first obvious sign. Photosensitivity may manifest in infancy and may cause the child to cry when exposed to sunlight. The vesicles or bullae that appear on the exposed portions of the body often ulcerate and heal, with scarring. Secondary infections in the skin lesions and repeated episodes of ulceration and scarring lead to severe deformities of the nose, ears, eyes, and fingers. Conjunctivitis, keratitis, ectropion, and loss of fingernails and phalanges may occur. Hypertrichosis is often seen on the face and limbs, but areas of alopecia may occur on the scalp. Areas of pigmentation and depigmentation develop in exposed areas.
  Hemolysis occurs in the majority of patients with this disease, some of whom can increase red cell production sufficiently to prevent the normochromic anemia seen in others. The more active periods of hemolysis are accompanied by increased fecal urobilinogen, normoblastic hyperplasia of the marrow, and circulating normoblasts. Splenomegaly is present in about 75% of the patients with this disease. Thrombocytopenia, presumably secondary to hypersplenism, and clinically evident jaundice occur rarely.
  Bones are red-brown in color and fluoresce red in UV light.
  Teeth vary in color from yellow-brown to red-brown to violet. Teeth fluoresce distinctly red in Wood's (UV) light. Both enamel and dentin contain porphyrins. However, higher concentrations are found in dentin.

Complications: Varying degrees of deformity of nose, ears, eyes, and fingers. Areas of pigmentation and depigmentation occur on exposed areas. Ectropion, and the loss of nails and terminal phalanges may occur. Areas of alopecia in the scalp and hypertrichosis of the face and limbs. Hemolytic anemia and occasionally hypersplenism.

Associated Findings: None known.

Etiology: Autosomal recessive inheritance.

Pathogenesis: Deficiency of uroporphyrinogen III cosynthetase, which ranges from one-tenth to one-third of normal levels of activity.

Insufficient production or utilization of uroporphyrinogen isomerase resulting in the production of the unusable isomer uroporphyrinogen I. This isomer and its oxidized or decarboxylated products (uroporphyrin I, coproporphyrin I) have a high degree of physical affinity for calcium phosphate and are, therefore, incorporated into the bones and teeth during osteogenesis and odontogenesis. The pigmentation of the teeth is thus dependent primarily upon the level of circulating abnormal porphyrins at the time of initial calcification. In one reported case, a female with proven erythropoietic porphyria gave birth to a basically unaffected infant whose primary teeth, which formed and calcified in utero, were pigmented reddish-brown.

MIM No.: *26370

Sex Ratio: M1:F1

Occurrence: Over 100 cases reported in the literature.

Risk of Recurrence for Patient's Sib:
See Part I, *Mendelian Inheritance.*

Risk of Recurrence for Patient's Child:
See Part I, *Mendelian Inheritance.*

Age of Detectability: Uroporphyrinogen III cosynthetase is expressed in cultured amniotic cells, so prenatal diagnosis is possible. Clinical signs are evident from as early as birth up to age five years at the latest. Probably urinary porphyrin analysis will detect the disease within the first year of life in most cases.

Gene Mapping and Linkage: Unknown.

Prevention: None known. Genetic counseling indicated.

Treatment: Avoidance of light with a wavelength around 4,000 A as much as possible. Use of protective clothing and other protective measures. A sunscreen filter chemically induced in the skin may be useful (see Fusaro et al, 1966 for details). Splenectomy for severe hemolytic anemia has sometimes been useful. Porcelain or acrylic crowns may be useful. Transfusion to suppress erythropoiesis has been reported to be effective.

Prognosis: Death usually occurs before middle age.

Detection of Carrier: The level of uroporphyrinogen III cosynthetase of carriers is intermediate between normal and homozygotic levels.

The authors wish to thank Donald P. Tschudy for his contributions to a previous version of this article.

References:
Townes PL: Transplacentally acquired erythrodontia. J Pediatr 1965; 67:600–602.
Fusaro RM, et al.: Sunlight protection in normal skin. Arch Dermatol 1966; 93:106–111.
Deybach JC, et al.: Prenatal exclusion of congenital erythropoietic porphyria (Gunther's disease) in a fetus at risk. Hum Genet 1980; 53:217–221.
Piomelli S, et al.: Complete suppression of the symptoms of congenital erythropoietic porphyria by long-term treatment with high-level transfusions. New Engl J Med 1986; 314:1029–1031.
Pimstone NR, et al.; Therapeutic efficacy of oral charcoal in congenital erythropoietic porphyria. New Engl J Med 1987; 316:390–393.
Tsai SF, et al.: Coupled-enzyme and direct assays for uroporphrinogen III synthase activity in human erythrocytes and cultured lymphoblasts. Anal Biochem 1987; 166:120–133.
Kappas A, et al.: The porphyrias. In: Scriver CR, et al, eds: The metabolic basis of inherited disease, 6th ed. New York: McGraw-Hill, 1989:1305–1366.

BR038
TR003

David A. Brenner
John N. Trodahl

Porphyria, hepatocutaneous type
See PORPHYRIA CUTANEA TARDA
Porphyria, hepatoerythropoietic
See PORPHYRIA CUTANEA TARDA

PORPHYRIA, PROTOPORPHYRIA　　0362

Includes:
　　Erythrohepatic protoporphyria
　　Erythropoietic protoporphyria (EPP)
　　Ferrochelatase deficiency
　　Heme synthase deficiency
　　Light, sensitivity to
　　Liver disease-erythrohepatic protoporphyria
　　Photosensitivity, from protoporphyria
　　Protoporphyria, erythropoietic
　　Protoporphyria, porphyria

Excludes:
　　Porphyria cutanea tarda (3064)
　　Porphyria (others)

Major Diagnostic Criteria: The diagnosis of protoporphyria is made by demonstrating an increased level of protoporphyrin in erythrocytes, plasma, and stool. In contrast to lead poisoning and iron deficiency anemia, the increased protoporphyrin in erythrocytes occurs as free protoporphyrin and not the zinc chelate.

Clinical Findings: The major clinical manifestation of protoporphyria is photosensitivity. This is usually present from infancy, although patients occasionally have not had symptoms until adolescence or adulthood. They complain of burning, itching, or pain of the skin on exposure to sunlight, sometimes within a few minutes. This is followed by erythema and edema. Vesicles seldom develop unless sun exposure is prolonged. Small, shallow, pitted scars are characteristic. These occur mainly over the nose, cheeks, and backs of the hands. There is also thickening and lichenification of the skin in these areas.

The degree of photosensitivity is variable among patients, even among those in the same family. There is poor correlation between the severity of photosensitivity and the erythrocyte protoporphyrin level.

The other major clinical manifestation of protoporphyria is liver disease. Although the incidence is uncertain, it probably occurs in less than 10% of patients. Jaundice has frequently been the first manifestation of liver disease. This has been followed by a progressive downhill course, leading to death during hepatic failure. Only an occasional patient has recovered after the onset of jaundice. The livers of patients who have died during hepatic failure have been nodular due to cirrhosis and black due to massive deposits of protoporphyrin pigment in hepatobiliary structures. When liver biopsy specimens are examined by polarization microscopy the pigment deposits are birefringent, and by electron microscopy they are seen to contain crystals.

Complications: Unknown.

Associated Findings: Approximately 20–30% of patients have mild anemia, with hypochromic microcytic indices. There is an increased frequency of cholelithiasis, and some patients require cholecystectomy. Chemical analysis of gallstones has demonstrated the presence of protoporphyrin.

Etiology: Autosomal dominant inheritance with variable expression. Some individuals have no clinical manifestations of protoporphyria, but have increased levels of erythrocyte protoporphyrin. They are considered to be clinically unaffected carriers of the gene defect. However, more complex mechanisms of inheritance, in particular a three-allele system, have been postulated on the basis of multiple family studies.

Pathogenesis: A reduction in activity of ferrochelatase (also termed *heme synthase* or *protoheme ferrolyase*), which catalyzes the insertion of iron into protoporphyrin to form heme. The enzyme defect is present in all heme-forming tissues. The nature of the abnormality in ferrochelatase has not yet been determined.

As a result of the deficient ferrochelatase activity, protoporphyrin accumulates in excessive amounts. The bone marrow is the major source of the excess protoporphyrin, with a variable contribution from the liver and perhaps other heme-forming tissues.

MIM No.: *17700

Sex Ratio: M1:F1

Occurrence: Protoporphyria occurs in all ethnic groups. The incidence and prevalence have not been precisely determined for any group. It appears to be a relatively common type of porphyria, perhaps second only to porphyria cutanea tarda in frequency. Thus, a reasonable estimate of its prevalence is 1:5,000–10,000 individuals.

Risk of Recurrence for Patient's Sib:
See Part I, *Mendelian Inheritance.*

Risk of Recurrence for Patient's Child:
See Part I, *Mendelian Inheritance.*

Age of Detectability: Usually during infancy due to the photosensitivity, with the average age being approximately 4 years. Occasionally symptoms have not occurred until adolescence or adulthood.

Gene Mapping and Linkage: Unknown.

Prevention: None known. Genetic counseling indicated.

Treatment: Topical sunscreens are ineffective as protective agents against photosensitivity in patients with protoporphyria. However, oral administration of beta-carotene (Solatene) in a dose of 60–180 mg/day reduces photosensitivity in over 80% of patients.

Various therapeutic modalities have been proposed for treatment of hepatobiliary disease in protoporphyria. These include red cell transfusions or the intravenous administration of hematin to suppress erythropoiesis, oral iron therapy (particularly when there is iron deficiency), oral administration of chenodeoxycholic acid to enhance hepatic disposal of protoporphyrin, and oral administration of cholestyramine or activated charcoal to interrupt the enterohepatic circulation of protoporphyrin. None of these therapeutic modalities has been shown in a large group of patients to be the optimal form of therapy. Liver transplantation should be considered for patients with advanced liver disease.

Prognosis: Most patients with protoporphyria are expected to have normal life spans. However, patients with progressive liver damage have a poor prognosis.

Detection of Carrier: The asymptomatic carrier of the gene defect may be detected by demonstrating an increased level of erythrocyte protoporphyrin. Asymptomatic carriers may also be shown to have diminished ferrochelatase activity in cultured skin fibroblasts and lymphocytes isolated from the blood.

Special Considerations: Although serious liver disease appears to occur in less than 10% of patients with protoporphyria, the clinician must be vigilant in observing patients for this complication because of the ominous prognosis. Unfortunately, there is no precise means by which to identify patients who are at risk for this complication. Routine tests of liver function do not provide much information regarding the degree of liver damage since livers can remain mildly abnormal until hepatic decompensation occurs. Any patient with an unexplained abnormality should therefore be observed closely. Patients with high erythrocyte (greater than 1,500 μg/dl) and plasma (greater than 50 μg/dl) protoporphyrin levels must also be observed closely. Liver biopsy should be done to assess histology in such patients. Those with hepatocellular necrosis and fibrosis, even if mild, should be considered for therapeutic options outlined above.

An animal model of protoporphyria has been found in cattle. The disease differs from that in humans in that there is a homozygous deficiency of ferrochelatase activity. Cattle manifest photosensitivity but do not develop hepatobiliary disease, limiting their usefulness in studying the pathogenesis and treatment of clinical manifestations of protoporphyria.

References:
Magnus IA, et al.: Erythropoietic protoporphyria. A new porphyria syndrome with solar urticaria due to protoporphyrinemia. Lancet 1961; II:448–451.
Bonkowsky HL, et al.: Heme synthetase deficiency in human protoporphyria. Demonstration of the defect in liver and cultured skin fibroblasts. J Clin Invest 1975; 56:1139–1148.
DeLeo VA, et al.: Erythropoietic protoporphyria: 10 years experience. Am J Med 1976; 60:8–22. * †
Bloomer JR: Pathogenesis and therapy of liver disease in protoporphyria. Yale J Biol Med 1979; 52:39–48. †
Went LN, Klasen EC: Genetic aspects of erythropoietic protoporphyria. Ann Hum Genet 1984; 48:105–117.
Bloomer JR, Straka JG: Porphyrin metabolism. In: Arias IM, et al., eds: The liver: biology and pathobiology. New York: Raven, 1988. *

BL023   **Joseph R. Bloomer**

PORPHYRIA, VARIEGATE   0822

Includes:
Mixed porphyria
Protocoproporphyria
Protoporphyrinogen oxidase deficiency
South African porphyria

Excludes:
Porphyria, acute intermittent (0820)
Porphyria, coproporphyria (0203)

Major Diagnostic Criteria: Increased urinary excretion of porphobilinogen during an acute attack. Increased fecal coproporphyrin and protoporphyrin with normal red cell protoporphyrin.

Clinical Findings: This disease may present either cutaneous manifestations of photosensitivity or neurologic aspects identical to those described for acute intermittent porphyria or both.

The skin lesions may be vesicles, bullae, or erosion, with variable degrees of scarring and pigmentation of the skin exposed to sunlight. There may be increased skin fragility. Hypertrichosis on the face or chronic thickening of skin may occur with diffuse yellowish papules. Azotemia and electrolyte abnormalities are frequent and often result from the GI manifestations of the acute attack.

Complications: Chronic skin lesions, chronic pain syndrome (peripheral or abdominal), motor paralysis (including respiratory paralysis), seizures, organic brain syndrome, depression.

Associated Findings: None known.

Etiology: Autosomal dominant inheritance.

Pathogenesis: Increased levels of hepatic δ-aminolevulinic acid synthase have been demonstrated, but the relationship of this finding to the attacks of neurologic dysfunction is unknown. The basic genetic defect is probably a protoporphyrinogen oxidase deficiency (Brenner and Bloomer, 1980).

MIM No.: *17620

Sex Ratio: M1:F1.3 in one series of 66 cases.

Occurrence: In the total white population of South Africa it has been estimated as 1:330. Its incidence is probably somewhat less than 1:66,000 in most parts of the world.

Risk of Recurrence for Patient's Sib:
See Part I, *Mendelian Inheritance.*

Risk of Recurrence for Patient's Child:
See Part I, *Mendelian Inheritance.*

Age of Detectability: Usually after puberty.

Gene Mapping and Linkage: VP (variegate porphyria (protoporphyrinogen oxidase)) has been provisionally mapped to 14q.

Prevention: None known. Genetic counseling indicated.

Treatment: Avoidance of sunlight.

Hematin infusions have been repeatedly shown to curtail an acute attack and have improved the prognosis for all "inducible" porphyrias. It is given at a dose of 2–4 mg/kg for three days (Pierach, 1982).

Supportive care during acute attacks is of great importance. When there is peripheral neuropathy, respiratory paralysis, dysphagia, or coma, careful attention to nursing care, avoidance of aspiration, assisted respiration, early recognition of pneumonia, and physiotherapy are of great importance. Splints and sandbags should be used for wrist- and footdrop.

In those women who experience regularly recurrent attacks in relation to menstrual cycles, administration of oral contraceptive preparations have been useful in preventing attacks. The schedule used is similar to that used for contraception, but the dosage required may or may not be higher. This approach should be used with caution, since experience with it in this type of patient is limited and oral contraceptives sometimes precipitate attacks in women who do not experience the regularly recurring cyclic attacks. A luteinizing hormone-releasing hormone analogue has been shown experimentally to suppress these premenstrual attacks (Anderson et al., 1984).

Prophylaxis is of great importance and involves warning patients and members of their families about avoiding the known precipitating factors.

Prognosis: Unknown.

Detection of Carrier: Increased fecal protoporphyrin was demonstrated in members of one family with the disease (Fromke et al., 1978).

The author wishes to thank Donald P. Tschudy for his contribution to earlier versions of this article.

References:
Eales L: Porphyria as seen in Cape Town: a survey of 250 patients and some recent studies. S Afr J Lab Clin Med 1963; 9:151–162.
Waldenstrom J, Haeger-Aronsen B: The porphyrias: a genetic problem. Prog Med Genet 1967; 5:58–101.
Fromke VL, et al.: Porphyria variegata: study of a large kindred in the United States. Am J Med 1978; 65:80–88.
Brenner DA, Bloomer JR: The enzymatic defect in variegate porphyria: studies with human cultured skin fibroblasts. New Engl J Med 1980; 302:765–769.
Kushner JP, et al.: Congenital erythropoietic porphyria, diminished activity of uroporphyrinogen decarboxylase and dyserythropoiesis. Blood 1982; 59:725–737.
Mustajoki P, et al.: Homozygous variegate porphyria: a severe skin disease of infancy. Clin Genet 1987; 32:300–305.

PI009   **Claus A. Pierach**

Port-wine stain
  See NEVUS FLAMMEUS
Portal vein atresia
  See LIVER, VENOUS ANOMALIES
Portuguese (Andrade)-type hereditary amyloidosis
  See AMYLOIDOSIS, TRANSTHYRETIN METHIONINE-30 TYPE
Positional plagiocephaly
  See PLAGIOCEPHALY
Post-anesthesia apnea
  See CHOLINESTERASE, ATYPICAL
Post-polio syndrome
  See POLIO, SUSCEPTIBILITY TO
Postaxial acrofacial dysostosis syndrome (POADS)
  See ACROFACIAL DYSOSTOSIS, POSTAXIAL TYPE
Postaxial polydactyly, types A and B
  See POLYDACTYLY
Postaxial polydactyly-dental-vertebral syndrome
  See HEART-HAND SYNDROME IV
Postaxial polydactyly-distal obstructive uropathy
  See POLYDACTYLY-DISTAL OBSTRUCTIVE UROPATHY
Posterior embryotoxon
  See EYE, ANTERIOR SEGMENT DYSGENESIS
Posterior marginal dysplasia of cornea
  See EYE, ANTERIOR SEGMENT DYSGENESIS
Posterior nasal atresia
  See NOSE, POSTERIOR ATRESIA
Posterior polar
  See CATARACT, AUTOSOMAL DOMINANT CONGENITAL
Posterolateral diaphragmatic hernia
  See DIAPHRAGMATIC HERNIA
Postmortem dermatolysis, multiple cysts
  See FETAL MULTIPLE CYSTS ANOMALY
Postural plagiocephaly
  See PLAGIOCEPHALY
Postural torticollis
  See TORTICOLLIS
Potassium-losing nephropathy with low aldosterone
  See LIDDLE SYNDROME
Potassium-sodium disorder of erythrocyte
  See ANEMIA, HEMOLYTIC, RED CELL MEMBRANE DEFECTS

'Potato' nose
  See NOSE/NASAL SEPTUM DEFECTS
Potter syndrome
  See RENAL AGENESIS, BILATERAL
Potter type I infantile polycystic kidney disease
  See KIDNEY, POLYCYSTIC DISEASE, RECESSIVE
Potter type II renal dysplasia
  See KIDNEY, RENAL DYSPLASIA, POTTER TYPE II
Potter type III polycystic kidney disease
  See KIDNEY, POLYCYSTIC DISEASE, DOMINANT
Prader-Labhart-Willi syndrome
  See PRADER-WILLI SYNDROME

PRADER-WILLI SYNDROME   0823

Includes:
  Hypogenital dystrophy with diabetic tendency
  Hypotonia-hypomentia-hypogonadism-obesity (HHHO)
  Prader-Labhart-Willi syndrome
Excludes:
  Adiposogenital dystrophy
  Alstrom syndrome (0041)
  Angelman syndrome (2086)
  Atonic diplegia and other severe supranuclear hypotonias
  Cohen syndrome (2023)
  Hypotonia, other forms of infantile
  Laurence-Moon syndrome (0578)
  Myopathy (see others)

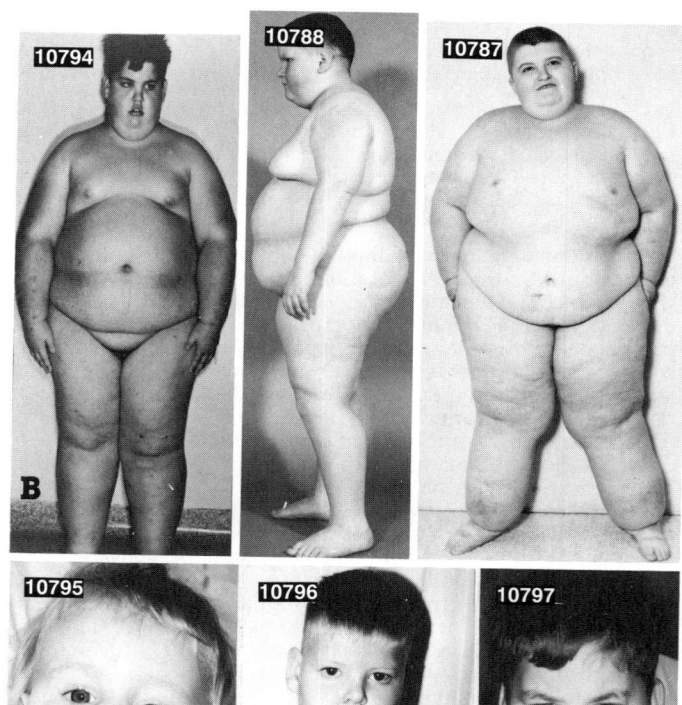

0823A-10794, 10788, 10787:   Moderate to severe obesity particularly in the trunkal region.   10795–97:   Characteristic facies include upslanted palpebral fissures, almond-shaped eyes and full cheeks.

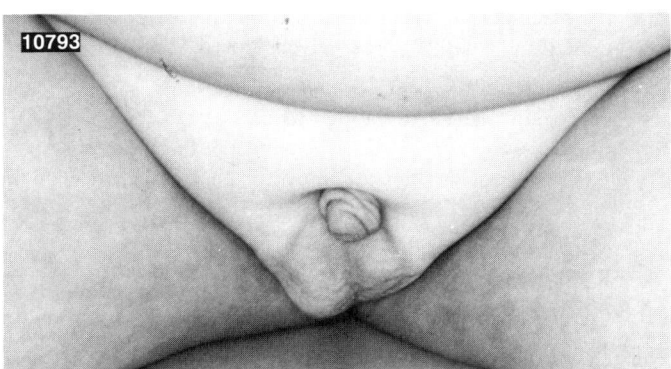

0823B-10793:   Genital hypoplasia in male with Prader-Willi.

Myotonic dystrophy (0702)
Spinal muscular atrophy (0895)
Williams syndrome (0999)
X-linked mental retardation, Fragile X syndrome (2073)
X-linked mental retardation-short stature-obesity-hypogonadism (3147)

Major Diagnostic Criteria: Severe muscular hypo- or atonia, are-flexia, feeding difficulties, and hypothermia characterize the first phase. Micropenis, hypoplastic scrotum, and cryptorchidism are present. Diagnosis of first phase is more difficult for Prader-Willi syndrome (PW) girls, though small or hypoplastic labia minora and clitoris may suggest PW if associated with the above criteria. The second phase is characterized by polyphagia or decreased perception of satiety, delayed psychomotor development, mental subnormality (90% of cases), obesity, short stature, hypogonadism, and behavioral peculiarities.

Clinical Findings: A decrease of fetal movements in the last months of pregnancy is sometimes noticed. Breech deliveries occur in 10–40% of the cases. The mean birthweight is several hundred grams less than the average birthweight of term babies. Mean duration of gestation is within the normal range. Some PW

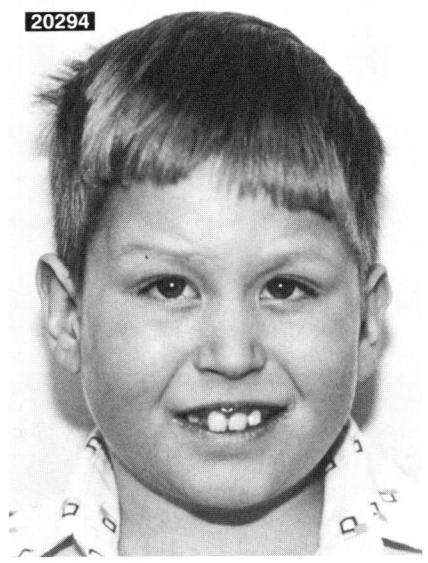

0823C-20294:   Prader-Willi syndrome; note almond-shaped eyes and full cheeks.

babies are born with dislocated hips and/or talipes valgoplanus. There may also be acromicria (small hands and feet).

The clinical course can be divided into two phases. The first phase is characterized by severe hypotonia or even atonia. There is evidence of facial diplegia with a flat face, a triangular mouth (tented upper lip), and narrow bifrontal diameter. Young infants with PW are almost motionless; Moro response, withdrawal reflex, and tendon reflexes are decreased or absent. Sucking and swallowing reflexes are very poorly developed and usually neces-sitate feeding by gavage, dropper, spoon, or premature nipple for weeks or even months. There is a tendency to hypothermia in early infancy. Penis and scrotum are hypoplastic; the latter often consists of not more than an area of corrugated skin in the anterior perineum. Testes may be cryptorchid or very small. Female external genitalia may show small or hypoplastic labia minora and clitoris.

Usually after a few months, the PW infants enter the second phase. They become more lively and responsive, and feeding difficulties subside; they become hungry and cry for food. Some PW children have a constant hunger, starting at age 1–6 years (usually age two) forcing them to incessantly seek food. Other PW patients may not seek food, but are unable to recognize satiety and eat as long as food is in sight. As a result, PW children become extremely obese, particularly in the trunk and proximal limbs. In some children forearms and lower legs become obese as well, but hands and feet remain disproportionately small. Longitudinal growth is impaired. Height is almost always below the 50th percentile. The prepubertal growth spurt does not occur, thus growth retardation becomes even more conspicuous at that age.

Psychomotor development is delayed, particularly with motor dependent skills; e.g. sitting and walking. Psychometric tests yield IQs between 20 and 90. A normal IQ is found in 10% of the cases. Some PW adults are able to function at a trainable level, but impaired speech clarity and emotional lability are common prob-lems. PW children show times of exuberant joy, yet they also have excessive outbursts of anger, and temper tantrums that become more severe in the second decade of life to the point where they become unbearable for other family members. Affected children may have mannerisms such as trichotillomania and constant plucking on sores, insect bites, and the like. The muscular hypotonia tends to improve with age. Episodes of incoercible sleep are sometimes observed and may be precipitated by small doses of anorexic drugs such as dexedrine sulfate. Periods of constitutional hyperthermia lasting for days and even weeks are noticed.

Other manifestations are microdontia, dental caries, enamel defects (notably in the first dentition), abnormal saliva (bubbly, viscous, decreased in volume), strabismus, high-arched palate, dry oral mucosa, mesobrachyphalangy, and simian creases. Poorly modeled ears and narrow external ear canals are occasion-ally encountered. Scoliosis is frequent. Hypopigmentation (fair coloring for their family) occurs in one-half of affected individuals. Osteoporosis, evidenced by radial bone mineral measurement, appears to be a fairly consistent finding. Most PW patients show hypogonadotropic hypogonadism, although hypergonadotropic hypogonadism has been observed. Male PW patients are infertile; the testes are extremely small and show immature and partially hyalinized seminiferous tubules, with decreased or absent sper-matogenesis. However, restoration of normal spermatogenesis was noted in at least one patient after he was treated for several months with clomiphene citrate. Leydig cells are present in normal or subnormal number; their maturation is at times inade-quate. Plasma testosterone levels are below normal and remain subnormal after clomiphene treatment. Anorchia is found in some cases. The development of secondary sex characteristics in PW males is delayed and incomplete; the voice remains high-pitched.

Female PW patients show either primary or secondary amenor-rhea, but are infertile. Menarche, if it occurs, is delayed, though precocious pubarche has been reported. Some females have anovulatory cycles. Estrogenization of the vaginal mucosa varies between moderately decreased and normal. Some cases of hypog-onadotropic hypogonadism show normal or more often subnor-mal responses to clomiphene and luteinizing hormone-releasing hormone. The clomiphene-induced maturation effect may subside after medication is stopped. Secondary sex characteristics of female PW patients vary between incomplete and normal.

Endocrine studies of the pituitary-adrenal and the pituitary-thyroid axes are normal, although mild and inconsistent abnormalities have been reported by some observers. A low somatomedin-C level, and linear growth rate, which respond to growth hormone treatment has been reported. Glucose metabolism disturbance is often found. Normal glucose tolerance is found in young PW patients, while glucose intolerance and insulin hypersensitivity often develop in obese patients. Normal laboratory findings include serum electrolytes, urinalysis, and blood morphology. EEGs are sometimes normal, but nonspecific abnormalities and even paroxysmal discharges such as spike-waves are reported. Muscles show signs of disuse atrophy in some cases.

Recent studies revealed anomalies of chromosome 15 in more than one-half of PW patients. *De novo* deletions of proximal parts of the long arm (del 15q11-q13) are most frequent, at times due to an unbalanced translocation in that region. Less frequently, a 15;15 translocation or an isodicentric chromosome 15 is found. Some of the later may be tetrasomic for 15pter-q11. Thus most chromosomally abnormal PW cases have a common deletion of the "critical" 15q11-q13 region, which may be due to unstable DNA sequences in that region. While there are no clinical differences between PW patients with and without chromosomal anomalies, molecular-genetic studies have isolated more than 10 DNA markers in this same region, including those associated with other variants of mental retardation such as **Angelman syndrome** which also show chromosomal abnormalities, although they may differ with respect to parental origin. A Prader-Willi-like phenotype has also been described in some instances of **X-linked mental retardation, Fragile X syndrome** (Fryns et al, 1988).

The chromosomal deletion has been shown to be paternally derived in almost every case. When the same or similar deletion is in the maternally derived chromosome it has been associated with the **Angelman syndrome** phenotype. Among those patients with Prader-Willi syndrome who do not have a cytogenetically detectable deletion, some have submicroscopic deletions (molecular deletions), others have no detectable paternal contribution and both maternal contributions in the 15q11-q13 region (maternal heterodisomy). These unique findings suggest that genes arising from different sex parents are modified differently prior to conception, and are expressed differently in their offspring (genetic imprinting).

Complications: Development of a Pickwickian, or obesity-hypoventilation syndrome, treatable with progesterone. Diabetes mellitus, adult type without tendency to ketosis, appears during second decade or later. Early development of atherosclerosis and glomerulosclerosis occurs. Gastric perforation may occur as a consequence of overeating.

Associated Findings: Rumination occurs in 10% to 17% of cases. Seizures (rarely).

Etiology: Heterogeneity of PW has been established. Sporadic cases with normal chromosomes may represent apparent autosomal dominant mutations. Recently, a few families with autosomal recessive inheritance have been reported.

Pathogenesis: A disturbance within the hypothalamic-pituitary pathway is debated. The few postmortem studies available show no evidence of a microscopic lesion in this area. However, destruction of the ventromedial hypothalamus produces a PW-like picture, with polyphagia and obesity in experimental animals.

MIM No.: *17627

POS No.: 3361

CDC No.: 759.870

Sex Ratio: M1:F1

Occurrence: About 1:15,000.

Risk of Recurrence for Patient's Sib: Estimated at 1:1,000, since most cases are sporadic.

Risk of Recurrence for Patient's Child: No PW patient is known to have reproduced.

Age of Detectability: At birth or shortly thereafter in male infants. Accurate diagnosis of PW in females is possible in the second phase only.

Gene Mapping and Linkage: PWCR (Prader-Willi syndrome chromosome region) has been mapped to 15q11-q12.

Prevention: None known. Genetic counseling indicated.

Treatment: 1. Passive physiotherapy can prevent disuse atrophy of muscle during the first phase. Active physiotherapy can be initiated as soon as the child reaches the second phase and before activity-limiting obesity develops.

2. Appetite depressants may be tried during the second phase. PW children are hypersensitive to dexedrine sulfate; therefore drug treatment should begin with very small doses. The growth-limiting effect of these drugs only occurs if the dose is higher than 30 mg/day.

3. Gastroplasty has proven to be successful in some cases when other attempts to regulate food intake fail.

4. Patients whose food intake cannot be controlled in the realm of the family, and patients who display severe and disruptive behavioral disorders, may benefit from institutionalization in group homes specializing in PW treatment.

5. To be effective, nutritional behavior modification must begin during the first phase when the child is on a normal caloric intake. The outcome, however, is still uncertain. Support of the family during periods of feeding difficulties and careful communication to them of the expected course of these difficulties should help early acceptance of behavior modification. A low-calorie formula, enough to guarantee adequate but not excessive weight increase, must be designed. Regular feeding hours and habits, such as feeding in the same location and with the same table mat and bib, and an acoustic signal indicating the time of feeding, may allow the regulating of feeding habits and possibly prevent overeating. Early nutritional behavior modification is still experimental, though it appears to be promising.

6. Jaw wiring is not recommended because of possible complications such as aspiration.

7. The greatest problem besides obesity are severe behavior disorders. Residential facilities with specific PW regimens have shown success in dealing with this problem.

8. Depo-Testosterone has been used to treat the microphallus of small boys (25mg IM every three weeks for a total of five injections). Cryptorchidism may respond to hormone therapy, specifically HCG, and should be corrected when the patient is 2–5 years of age, but it is not always possible to bring the testes to the scrotum.

9. Depo-Testosterone given to male adolescents and adults does not remedy the infertility, but may have a beneficial effect on behavior and in the development of secondary sex characteristic.

10. Growth hormone can be used to increase height in some individuals who have documented stimulated or neurosecretory growth hormone secretion.

Prognosis: Life expectancy is shortened. Sudden death may occur during the intercurrent infections due to the complicating obesity-hypoventilation syndrome. Early development of diabetic glomerulosclerosis has also been reported. However, some PW patients may reach 50 years of age or more, provided their obesity can be controlled.

Detection of Carrier: Unknown.

Special Considerations: This condition was first described in 1887 by Langdon-Down, the person who also described Down syndrome, who termed PW "polysarcia". The Prader-Willi Syndrome Association maintains a registry of United States and Canadian patients which currently contains about 1,600 entries.

Support Groups: MN; St. Louis Park (6490 Excelsior Blvd., E-102, 55426); Prader-Willi Syndrome Association (PWSA)

References:

Niikawa N, Ishikiriyama S: Clinical and cytogenetic studies of the Prader-Willi syndrome: evidence of phenotype-karyotype correlation. Hum Genet 1985; 69:22–27.

Butler M, et al.: Clinical and cytogenetic survey of 39 individuals with Prader-Labhart-Willi syndrome. Am J Med Genet 1986; 23:793–809.

Greenswag LR: Adults with Prader-Willi syndrome. Devel Med Child Neurol 1987; 29:145–152.

Lubinsky M, et al.: Familial Prader-Willi syndrome with normal chromosomes. Am J Med Genet 1987; 28:37–43.

Wiesner GL, et al.: Hypopigmentation in the Prader-Willi syndrome. Am J Hum Genet 1987; 40:431–442.

Fryns JP, et al.: A peculiar subphenotype in the fra(X) syndrome: extreme obesity - short stature - stubby hands and feet - diffuse hyperpigmentation. Clin Genet 1988; 32:388–392.

Greenswag LR, Alexander RC: Management of Prader-Willi syndrome. New York: Springer-Verlag, 1988.

Ledbetter DH, Cassidy SB: The etiology of Prader-Willi syndrome: clinical implications of the chromosome 15 abnormalities. In: Caldwell ML, Taylor RL, eds: Prader-Willi syndrome. New York: Springer-Verlag, 1988.

Knoll JHM, et al.: Angelman and Prader-Willi syndromes share a common chromosome 15 deletion but differ in parental origin of the deletion. Am J Med Genet 1989; 32:285–290.

Nicholls RD, et al.: Restriction fragment length polymorphisms within proximal 15q and their use in molecular cytogenetics and the Prader-Willi syndrome. Am J Med Genet 1989; 33:66–77.

Tantravahi U, et al.: Quantitative calibration and use of DNA probes for investigating chromosome abnormalities in the Prader-Willi syndrome. Am J Med Genet 1989; 33:78–87.

ZE001   **Hans Zellweger**

Prealbumin (TTR) Ala-60 amyloidosis
  See *AMYLOIDOSIS, APPALACHIAN TYPE*
Prealbumin (TTR) Ile-33 and/or Gly-49
  See *AMYLOIDOSIS, ASHKENAZI TYPE*
Prealbumin defect
  See *AMYLOIDOSIS, TRANSTHYRETIN METHIONINE-30 TYPE*
Prealbumin met-111 amyloidosis
  See *AMYLOIDOSIS, DANISH CARDIAC TYPE*
Prealbumin Tyr-77 amyloidosis
  See *AMYLOIDOSIS, ILLINOIS TYPE*
Prealbumin-84 isoleucine-to-serine
  See *AMYLOIDOSIS, INDIANA TYPE*
Preauricular appendages and deafness
  See *DEAFNESS-EAR PITS*
Preauricular fistulae
  See *EAR, PITS*
Preauricular pit-cervical fistula-hearing loss syndrome
  See *BRANCHIO-OTO-RENAL DYSPLASIA*
Preaxial polydactyly I, II, and III
  See *POLYDACTYLY*
Preaxial polydactyly IV
  See *POLYSYNDACTYLY*
Preaxial polydactyly of toes associated with syndactyly
  See *POLYSYNDACTYLY*
Preaxial upper limb deficiency
  See *HAND, RADIAL CLUB HAND*
Precalyceal canalicular ectasia
  See *KIDNEY, MEDULLARY SPONGE KIDNEY*
Precocious dentition
  See *TEETH, NATAL OR NEONATAL*
Precocious periodontitis
  See *TEETH, PERIODONTITIS, JUVENILE*
Preductal aortic coarctation
  See *AORTA, COARCTATION, INFANTILE TYPE*
Preduodenal portal vein
  See *LIVER, VENOUS ANOMALIES*
Preeclampsia, and fetal developmental retardation
  See *FETAL DEVELOPMENTAL RETARDATION WITH MATERNAL HYPERTENSION*
Pre-excitation syndromes
  See *ARRHYTHMIA, WOLFF-PARKINSON-WHITE TYPE*
Pregnancy-related cholestasis
  See *INTRAHEPATIC CHOLESTASIS OF PREGNANCY (ICP)*
Premature alopecia
  See *HAIR, BALDNESS, COMMON*
Premaxillary agenesis
  See *HOLOPROSENCEPHALY*
Premolar aplasia-hyperhidrosis-canities
  See *HYPERHIDROSIS-PREMATURE GREYING-PREMOLAR APLASIA*
Prepyloric membrane
  See *STOMACH, PYLORIC ATRESIA*
Presenile dementia, familial
  See *ALZHEIMER DISEASE, FAMILIAL*

'Pressure marks' (obsolete)
  See *NEVUS FLAMMEUS*
Pressure palsies (hereditary) and neuropathy
  See *NEUROPATHY, HEREDITARY WITH PRESSURE PALSIES*
Prieto mental retardation
  See *X-LINKED MENTAL RETARDATION-SUBCORTICAL ATROPHY-PATELLAR LUXATION*
Primaquine sensitive anemia
  See *GLUCOSE-6-PHOSPHATE DEHYDROGENASE DEFICIENCY*
Primary basilar impression
  See *BASILAR IMPRESSION, PRIMARY*
Primary diphallia
  See *DIPHALLIA*
Primary hypobetalipoproteinemia
  See *HYPOBETALIPOPROTEINEMIA*
Primary hypogonadism
  See *KLINEFELTER SYNDROME*
Primary Raynaud phenomenon
  See *RAYNAUD DISEASE*
Primary retinal telangiectasia
  See *RETINA, COATS DISEASE*
Primidone, fetal effects of
  See *FETAL PRIMIDONE EMBRYOPATHY*
Primitive renal tubule syndrome
  See *RENAL TUBULAR DYSGENESIS*
Primordial dwarfism
  See *GROWTH HORMONE DEFICIENCY, ISOLATED*
Pringle disease
  See *TUBEROUS SCLEROSIS*
Prinivil△, possible fetal effects
  See *FETAL ANGIOTENSIN CONVERTING ENZYME (ACE) INHIBITION RENAL FAILURE*
Proaccelerin deficiency
  See *FACTOR V DEFICIENCY*
Proalbumin Christchurch
  See *ANALBUMINEMIA*
Proboscis lateral
  See *NOSE, PROBOSCIS LATERALIS*
ProC deficiency
  See *PROTEIN C DEFICIENCY*
Procollagen peptidase deficiency
  See *EHLERS-DANLOS SYNDROME*
Procollagen protease deficiency
  See *EHLERS-DANLOS SYNDROME*
Progenie
  See *MANDIBULAR PROGNATHISM*

PROGERIA   **0825**

Includes:
  Acrogeria
  Aging, accelerated
  Hutchinson-Gilford progeria syndrome
  Progeronanism
  Senile nanism

Excludes:
  Cleidocranial dysplasia (0185)
  Cockayne syndrome (0189)
  Cutis laxa (0233)
  "Gerodermata" (various)
  Leprechaunism (0587)
  Mandibuloacral dysplasia (2082)
  Oculo-mandibulo-facial syndrome (0738)
  Pyknodysostosis (0846)
  Seckel syndrome (0881)
  Werner syndrome (0998)

Major Diagnostic Criteria: Appearance of accelerated aging, onset of growth failure in the first year of life, weight decreased for height, alopecia, loss of peripheral subcutaneous fat, prominent scalp veins, delayed and abnormal dentition, craniofacial disproportion with small face, micrognathia, prominent eyes, midfacial cyanosis, coxa valga, and normal intelligence.

Clinical Findings: The development of an extremely aged appearance is the most striking feature of the syndrome. At birth affected infants may already have suspicious findings ("sclerodermatous skin," midfacial cyanosis, sculptured nose) but are usually

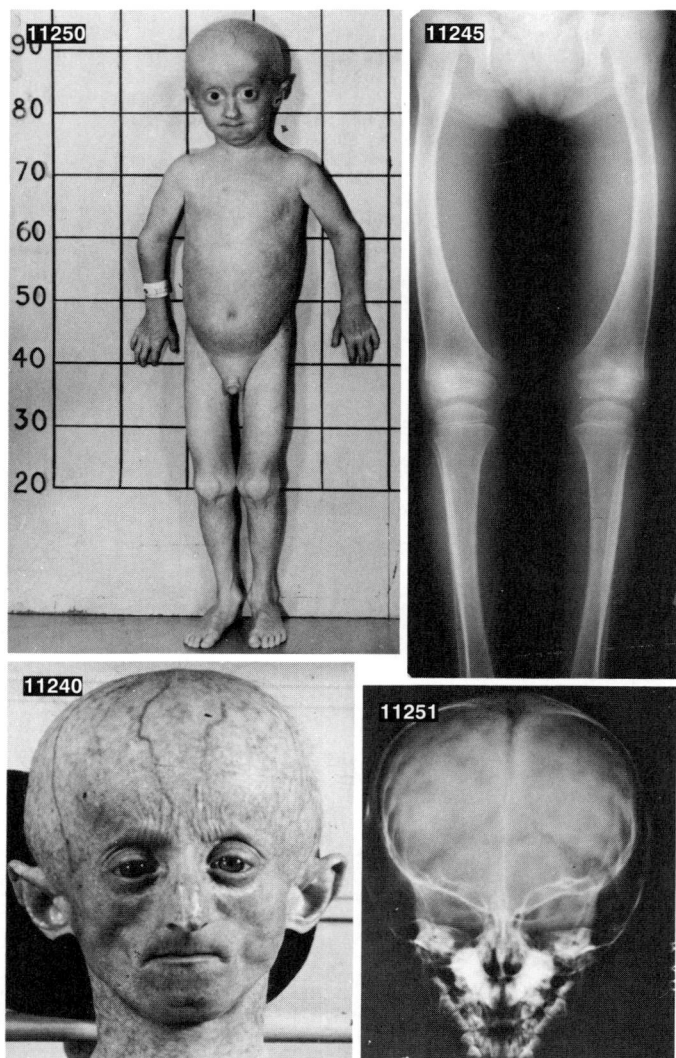

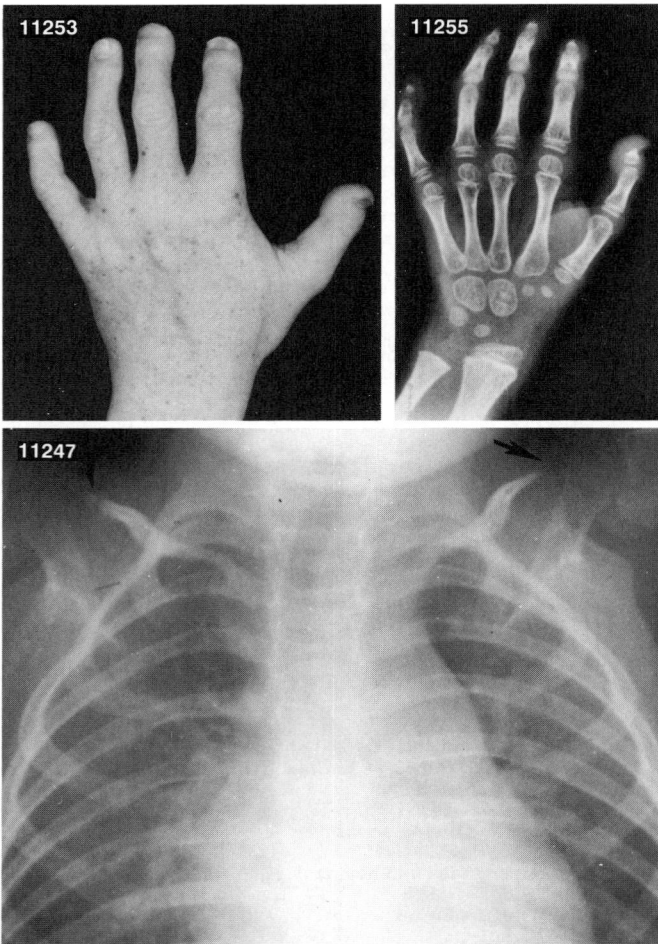

0825B-11253: Inability to extend fingers fully, knobby interphalangeal joints, and stubby terminal phalanges of several digits. **11255:** Retarded bone age and hypoplastic terminal phalanges. **11247:** X-ray of the chest shows osteolysis of the distal clavicles.

0825A-11250: Short stature, hairlessness and prominent scalp veins. **11245:** Delicate long bones and coxa valga. **11240:** Increased prominence of scalp veins and aged appearance in this affected 14-year-old. **11251:** X-ray of skull shows open fontanels and small facial bones relative to the calvarium.

considered to be normal appearing infants. During the second six months of life a profound and progressive retardation in weight gain and growth becomes apparent. Growth of the facial bones and mandible also fail, but the cranium remains relatively large. The eyes become prominent. The nose stays small, perhaps beaked, with nasal cartilage contours visible under the thin skin. The mandible continues to grow slowly, resulting in true micrognathia. At about the same time the scalp hair becomes sparse, and the scalp veins become prominent. Eyebrows and eyelashes may disappear during the first and second years of life. The result is total alopecia from the early years on, apart from a few downy, small, white or blond hairs, which may persist throughout life. The effect is to produce what has been called a "plucked-bird appearance."

Concurrent with the failure to gain weight and grow is the gradual disappearance of almost all subcutaneous fat. This absence of subcutaneous fat, along with failure of long bones to

grow in girth and in length, results in spindly limbs. The joints, especially the knees, become prominent. Stiffness of joints and limitation of motion develop. This and the invariable coxa valga are the basis for the wide-based "horse-riding stance," usually evident by age two or three years, which adds to the striking appearance. The voice is thin and high-pitched. The clavicles are usually short and thin; the distal one-third frequently becomes radiolucent. The anterior fontanelle remains patent, and there are occasional Wormian bones. The short clavicles are associated with narrow shoulders and pyriform thorax. Abnormalities of nails may become apparent by age two or three years. Nails may be dystrophic, small, and short. The terminal phalanges frequently develop acro-osteolysis and may become radiolucent. The skin develops an aged appearance, being thin, shiny, taut, and dry in some areas and dry, dull, and wrinkled in others. Small, blotchy, brownish pigmentations tend to develop with increasing age. There is a marked delay in dentition, with crowded maloccluded teeth that may be rotated, displaced, or overlapping. There are no ocular abnormalities as in oculomandibulofacial syndrome. Widespread atherosclerosis usually develops. Early death by myocardial infarction or cerebral vascular accident is common. Intelligence is normal or above average.

Excess urinary excretion of hyaluronic acid has been noted. No endocrine or metabolic abnormality has been documented other than an increase in metabolic rate without hyperthyroidism. Growth hormone responses are normal, but insulin tolerance may be increased. Collagen fiber bundles may be disorganized, thickened, and "hyalinized." Extracted collagen has been reported to show decreased solubility and abnormal thermal shrinkage. Chromosomal studies have been normal. There are no consistent abnormalities of serum lipids. Decreased growth capacity of fibroblasts has been variably noted. Abnormalities of DNA repair, HLA antigen expression, and thermolability of enzymes have not been consistently demonstrated.

The condition should be distinguished from *Acrogeria*, a rare condition in which the skin of the hands and feet show signs of premature aging, but there is no alopecia or atherosclerosis (De Groot et al, 1980).

Complications: Myocardial infarcts, congestive heart failure, limitation of motion of large and small joints.

Associated Findings: Cerebrovascular occlusions secondary to atherosclerosis; hip dislocations; aseptic femoral head necrosis; cephalohematomas; headaches; parathesias.

Etiology: In most instances, a sporadic autosomal dominant mutation. In support of this conclusion, there is a significant increase in the average paternal age. Maciel (1988), however, has made a case for autosomal recessive inheritance. A lack of affected sibs is the general rule. Occasional sibships may suggest somatic mosaicism, or stem cell mutation of ovary or testes. Several sets of identical twins have been noted.

Pathogenesis: An abnormality of glycosaminoglycan metabolism is suggested by elevated hyaluronic acid excretion. Such an abnormality could alter normal development.

MIM No.: 17667, 20120

POS No.: 3362

Sex Ratio: M1:F1

Occurrence: Since it was first described in 1886, approximately 100 cases of progeria have been reported. In the United States, the reported incidence over the past 60 years is about 1:8,000,000, although, since about one-half of cases go unreported, the true incidence may reach 1:4,000,000. In the United States, about 10–15 patients are living at any one time. Cases have been reported from all continents. Several cases have been reported in Black and Oriental populations.

Risk of Recurrence for Patient's Sib:
See Part I, *Mendelian Inheritance*. Probably around 1:500 because of the possible somatic mosaicism.

Risk of Recurrence for Patient's Child:
See Part I, *Mendelian Inheritance*. No affected individuals are known to have reproduced.

Age of Detectability: Generally first to second year of life, but possibly at birth if sclerodermatous skin, glyphic nose, and midfacial cyanosis are present.

Gene Mapping and Linkage: Unknown.

Prevention: None known. Genetic counseling indicated.

Treatment: No specific therapy; small dose aspirin is suggested.

Prognosis: General health usually good, with few infections. Physical handicaps due to size are usual. Joint problems are common with increasing age. Psychologic problems related to appearance and self-image are common. The age of nontraumatic death was reported for 18 cases to range from 7 to 27 years, with a median age of 12 years and a mean of 13.4 years. Death was usually due to heart failure.

Detection of Carrier: Unknown.

Special Considerations: Progeria has been considered a model of apparent accelerated aging, although dementia, cataracts, and tumors, which may be associated with normal aging, are not usually seen. Hyaluronic acid elevation in urine, also seen in **Werner syndrome**, may reflect a basic defect in metabolism.

Support Groups: NY; Manhasset (Tel. 516–562–4612); Progeria International Registry

References:
DeBusk FL: The Hutchinson-Gilford progeria syndrome. J Pediatr 1972; 80:697–724.
DeGroot WP, et al.: Familial acrogeria (Gottron). Btit J Derm 1980; 103:213–223.
Brown WT, et al.: Progeria, a model disease for the study of accelerated aging In: Woodhead AD, et al., eds: Molecular Biology of Aging. New York: Plenum, 1986:375–396.
Zebrower M, et al.: Urinary hyaluronic acid elevation in Hutchinson-Gilford progeria syndrome. Mech Ageing Dev 1986; 35:39–46.
Dyck JD, et al.: Management of coronary artery disease in Hutchinson-Gilford syndrome. J Pediat 1987; 111:407–410.

BR024   **W. Ted Brown**

Progeria adultorum
See WERNER SYNDROME

PROGERIA, NEONATAL RAUTENSTRAUCH-WIEDEMANN TYPE   2593

Includes:
> Progeroid syndrome, neonatal
> Rautenstrauch-Wiedemann syndrome
> Wiedemann-Rautenstrauch syndrome

Excludes:
> **Cockayne syndrome** (0189)
> **Cutis laxa-growth defect, De Barsy type** (2138)
> **Lipodystrophy syndrome, Berardinelli type** (2038)
> **Oculo-mandibulo-facial syndrome** (0738)
> **Progeria** (0825)

Major Diagnostic Criteria: Neonatal progeroid appearance, lipoatrophy, and slow growth.

Clinical Findings: Affected children are all small for gestational age and subsequently grow at a slower than average rate. A progeroid appearance is present at birth and consists of macrocephalic appearance, entropion, malar hypoplasia, sparse hair, prominent veins, widened anterior fontanelle, and absence of subcutaneous fat. In all cases, 2–4 incisors were present at birth. These teeth were eventually lost, and subsequent dentition was

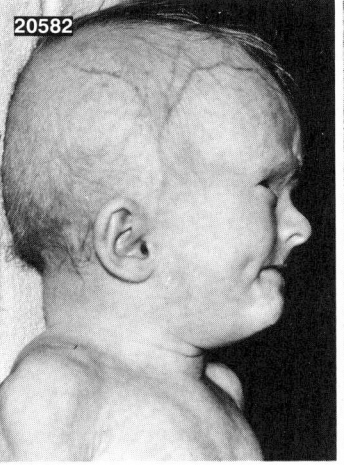
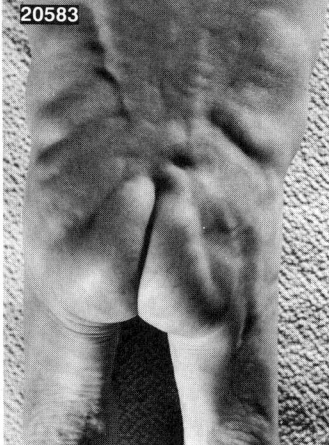

2593-20582: Progeria, neonatal Rautenstrauch-Wiedemann type; note hydrocephaloid cranium, prominent venous markings, sparse hair, prominent nose and low-set ears. **20583:** Paradoxical fat accumulation at the buttocks.

delayed. As the children aged, the nose appeared beak-shaped, and paradoxical caudal fat accumulation occurred. Mental retardation is mild to severe. Eyes and digits are normal, although the digits appear long.

Complications: May be more prone to feeding difficulties and recurrent respiratory infections.

Associated Findings: None known.

Etiology: Autosomal recessive inheritance.

Pathogenesis: A congenital hypotrophy of subcutaneous fat and mesenchymal tissues. Neuropathologic findings are those of pure sudanophilic leukodystrophy (Martin et al, 1984).

MIM No.: *26409

POS No.: 3721

Sex Ratio: M1:F1

Occurrence: Undetermined but presumed rare. All five reported cases have been from Europe.

Risk of Recurrence for Patient's Sib:
See Part I, *Mendelian Inheritance.*

Risk of Recurrence for Patient's Child:
See Part I, *Mendelian Inheritance.*

Age of Detectability: At birth by physical examination.

Gene Mapping and Linkage: Unknown.

Prevention: None known. Genetic counseling indicated.

Treatment: Unknown.

Prognosis: Mental retardation is usually present, and ranges from mild to severe. Longevity is unknown; the oldest patient was four years at the time of the last report.

Detection of Carrier: Unknown.

Special Considerations: One of the patients studied by Rautenstrauch (1977) showed decreased proliferative capacity of the fibroblasts, whereas this was not found in one of Wiedemann's patients (1979). This may indicate that heterogeneity exists, or that decreased proliferation is an inconstant finding, and therefore not of diagnostic value.

Support Groups: NY; Staten Island; Progeria International Registry

References:
Rautenstrauch T, Snigula F: Progeria: a cell culture study and clinical report of familial incidence. Eur J Pediatr 1977; 124:101–111.
Wiedemann HR: An unidentified neonatal progeroid syndrome: follow-up report. Eur J Pediatr 1979; 130:65–70.
Devos EA, et al.: The Wiedemann-Rautenstrauch or neonatal progeroid syndrome. Eur J Pediatr 1981; 136:245–248. * †
Martin JJ, et al.: The Wiedemann-Rautenstrauch or neonatal progeroid syndrome: neuropathological study of a case. Neuropediatrics 1984; 15:43–48.

T0007   **Helga V. Toriello**

Progeroid syndrome of De Barsy
See CUTIS LAXA-GROWTH DEFECT, DE BARSY TYPE

PROGEROID SYNDROME WITH EHLERS-DANLOS FEATURES   **3012**

Includes: Ehlers-Danlos features with progeroid facies

Excludes:
Ehlers-Danlos syndrome (0338)
Noonan syndrome (0720)

Major Diagnostic Criteria: Progeroid facies; curly hair; scanty eyebrows and eyelashes; multiple nevi, skin hyperextensibility, bruisability, and fragility; joint hypermobility in digits.

Clinical Findings: Mild mental retardation (mean IQ, 60), wrinkled facies, curly and fine hair, scanty eyebrows and eyelashes, telecanthus, periodontitis and multiple caries, low-set and prominent ears, **Pectus excavatum**, winged scapulae, pes planus, skin hyperextensibility and fragility, bruisability, dermatorrhesis, papiraceous scars, multiple nevi, joint hypermobility in digits,

varicose veins, **Hernia, inguinal**, bilateral cryptorchidism. Electron microscopy detects no abnormalities of the skin with exception of a slight distention of intracellular spaces; in the spinous layer the epidermal cells and the collagen bundles are normal.

Complications: Unknown.

Associated Findings: Mild aortic or pulmonary stenosis, **Brachydactyly** type E, variable stature, hypospadias.

Etiology: A *de novo* autosomal dominant mutation has been postulated since all patients were sporadic cases and the paternal age was increased.

This is a distinct nosologic entity that shows variable expression, principally in stature and psychomotor development. In one affected young boy no major handicap was noticed. However, he received psychiatric treatment because of abnormal behavior.

Pathogenesis: Probably a primary defect in the synthesis or structure of one of the components of the connective tissue. In one case only half of the amount of a mature proteoglycan was synthesized, and that glycosaminoglycan-free core protein was secreted in fibroblasts (Kreese et al, 1987).

MIM No.: 13007

Sex Ratio: Presumably M1:F1.

Occurrence: About a half-dozen cases have been reported in the literature.

Risk of Recurrence for Patient's Sib:
See Part I, *Mendelian Inheritance.*

Risk of Recurrence for Patient's Child:
See Part I, *Mendelian Inheritance.*

Age of Detectability: During early infancy.

Gene Mapping and Linkage: Unknown.

Prevention: None known. Genetic counseling indicated.

Treatment: Early stimulation; special education.

Prognosis: Good for life span; poor for intellectual development.

Detection of Carrier: Unknown.

References:
Hernández A, et al.: A distinct variant of the Ehlers-Danlos syndrome. Clin Genet 1979; 16:335–339.
Hernández A, et al.: Third case of a distinct variant of the Ehlers-Danlos syndrome. Clin Genet 1981; 20:222–224.
Hernández A, et al.: Ehlers-Danlos features with progeroid facies and mild mental retardation: further delineation of the syndrome. Clin Genet 1986; 30:456–461.
Krusius T, Ruoslahti E: Primary structure of an extracellular matrix proteoglycan core protein deduced from cloned cDNA. Proc Nat Acad Sci 1986; 83:7683–7687.
Kresse H, et al.: Glycosaminoglycan-free small proteoglycan core protein is secreted by fibroblasts from a patient with a syndrome resembling progeroid. Am J Hum Genet 1987; 41:436–453.

HE039   **Alejandro Hernández**
CA011   **José María Cantú**

Progressive chorea
  See HUNTINGTON DISEASE
Progressive diaphyseal dysplasia
  See DIAPHYSEAL DYSPLASIA
Progressive familial cholestasis
  See JAUNDICE, INTRAHEPATIC CHOLESTATIC, BYLER TYPE
Progressive hypertrophic interstitial neuritis of childhood
  See DEJERINE-SOTTAS DISEASE
Progressive lenticular degeneration
  See HEPATOLENTICULAR DEGENERATION
Progressive muscular dystrophy of childhood
  *See MUSCULAR DYSTROPHY, CHILDHOOD
    PSEUDOHYPERTROPHIC*
Progressive myoclonus epilepsy without Lafora bodies
  *See SEIZURES, PROGRESSIVE MYOCLONIC, UNVERRICHT-
    LUNDBORG TYPE*
Progressive systemic sclerosis (PSS)
  See SCLERODERMA, FAMILIAL PROGRESSIVE
Prolapse of laryngeal ventricle
  See LARYNX, VENTRICLE PROLAPSE

PROLIDASE DEFICIENCY   2616

Includes:
  Hyperimidodipeptiduria
  Imidodipeptidase deficiency
  Peptidase D deficiency

Excludes: Hyperamidodipeptiduria

Major Diagnostic Criteria: Cutaneous ulcers involving the extremities, mostly the legs and feet. Mental retardation is found in a significant percentage of patients. Large quantities of imidodipeptides are excreted in the urine, especially glycylproline. Prolidase activity in erythrocytes, leukocytes, or skin fibroblasts is absent or markedly diminished.

Clinical Findings: Skin pathology has been described in about 90% of reported patients, the most prominent lesions being multiple, recurrent ulcers of the lower extremities. Ulcers initially develop in childhood or adolescence and have been reported to appear as early as age 19 months. These scars may be atrophic or sclerotic and can be pigmented or depigmented. Ulcers have been described in two-thirds of reported cases, but their true frequency is probably lower since the diagnosis of prolidase deficiency may not be considered in the absence of these lesions.

Prolidase-deficient individuals may have a variety of other dermatologic lesions, including telangiectasias of the face, shoulders, and hands (40%); scaly erythematous maculopapular lesions (25%); and premature graying of the hair (25%). Few patients had photosensitivity, dry skin, hyperkeratosis of elbows and knees, purpura without underlying hematologic abnormalities, and lymphedema.

Involvement of other organ systems is common. Mild mental retardation is present in more than one-half of the patients. Dysmorphic features, though common, have no specific pattern. Eye examination may disclose hypertelorism, mild ptosis, optic atrophy, or keratitis. A history of recurrent infections such as otitis media or sinusitis has been noted in about 50% of the cases.

Urinary excretion of significant quantities of imidodipeptides, especially glycylproline, is characteristic of this condition. Absence of hyperimidodipeptiduria is strong evidence against the diagnosis of prolidase deficiency. Prolidase activity in erythrocytes, leukocytes, or skin fibroblasts is absent or less than 5% of that of normal controls.

Complications: Secondary bacterial infection of ulcerated skin areas.

Associated Findings: Obesity, a protuberant abdomen, splenomegaly, joint laxity, deafness, and short stature are present in some patients.

Etiology: Autosomal recessive inheritance.

Pathogenesis: Prolidase deficiency is the underlying biochemical defect. Prolidase (imidodipeptidase, - EC 3.4.13.9) is an enzyme that splits dipeptides with proline or hydroxyproline at the carboxyl terminal (e.g., glycylproline). Prolidase activity has been

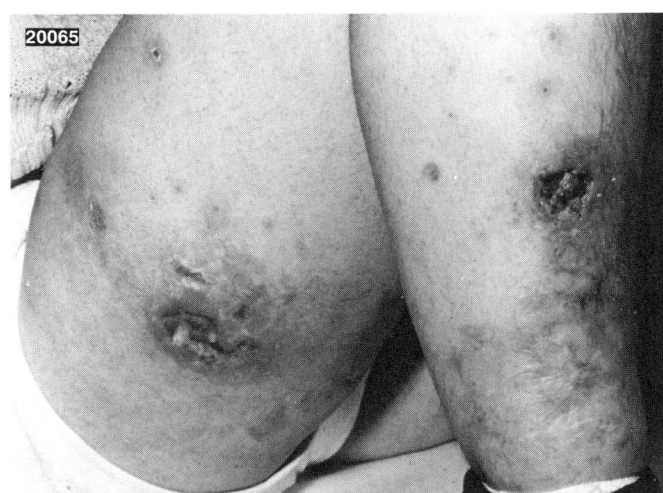

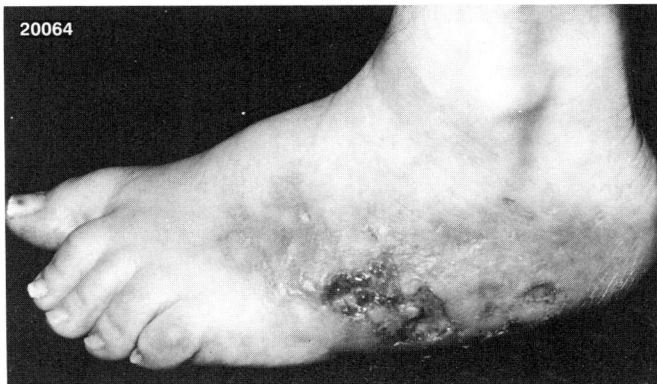

2616-20064–65: Note recurrent ulcerations of the leg and foot from prolidase deficiency.

detected in all tissues tested in normal individuals. The pathophysiology of the biochemical and clinical abnormalities in prolidase deficiency has not been delineated to date.

MIM No.: 26413

POS No.: 3767

Sex Ratio: M1:F1

Occurrence: More than 20 individuals with this condition have been described in the world literature. The patients are from ten different countries: Australia, Belgium, Canada, Denmark, France, Germany, Japan, Lebanon, the United Kingdom, and the United States. One thousand dried blood specimens from Japanese neonates assayed for prolidase activity revealed that about 2% of the samples had intermediate activity consistent with a heterozygote state.

Risk of Recurrence for Patient's Sib:
  See Part I, *Mendelian Inheritance.*

Risk of Recurrence for Patient's Child:
  See Part I, *Mendelian Inheritance.*

Age of Detectability: Prolidase deficiency can be detected in the newborn period by urine screening for imidodipeptide excretion followed by a confirmatory enzyme assay, long before signs or symptoms appear. Ulcers may develop during childhood or adolescence and have been reported to manifest as early as age 19 months. Prenatal diagnosis by amniocentesis or chorionic villus sampling is theoretically possible.

Gene Mapping and Linkage: PEPD (peptidase D) has been mapped to 19q12-q13.2.

PEPD has also been mapped to 19p13.2 by in situ hybridization. The gene has been cloned and sequenced. There is a close linkage between PEPD and apolipoprotein C 2 (apo-C2). The condition is linked to **Myotonic dystrophy** and probably linked to the C3-Le-DM-Se-Lu linkage group.

Prevention: None known. Genetic counseling indicated.

Treatment: Symptomatic treatment of the ulcers. An excellent response to the application of a 5% glycine-5% proline ointment on leg ulcers has been noted in the one patient treated with this modality.

Prognosis: Variable. Some patients become bedridden during the second decade of their life because of the severely disabling leg ulcers.

Detection of Carrier: Heterozygotes are asymptomatic, do not have imidodipeptiduria, but have reduced erythrocyte prolidase activity compared with normal controls.

Special Considerations: There are two main hypotheses for the pathogenesis of the leg ulcers and other manifestations in this condition. One of these attributes the clinical findings to the toxic effects of the imidodipeptides that are not broken down into individual amino acids. The other considers that the skin lesions may be due, to a great extent, to the losses of amino acids in the urine in the form of dipeptides. However, to date both hypotheses lack dependable supportive evidence.

The occurrence of prolidase-like activity about 5% of normal in amount but with a preference for substrate different from normal, in cells homozygous (or compound) for CRM-negative mutations, identified an alternative cleavage activity not encoded at the prolidase locus. Allelic heterogeneity at the major locus, and the amount of alternative peptidase activity encoded elsewhere, appear to be determinants of the associated and heterogeneous clinical phenotype.

References:
Der Kaloustian VM, et al.: Prolidase deficiency: an inborn error of metabolism with major dermatological manifestations. Dermatologica 1982; 164:293–304. * †
Freij BJ, et al.: Clinical and biochemical characteristics of prolidase deficiency in siblings. Am J Med Genet 1984; 19:561–571. * †
Arata J, et al.: Effect of topical application of glycine and proline on recalcitrant leg ulcers of prolidase deficiency. Arch Dermatol 1986; 122:626–627.
Freij BJ, Der Kaloustian VM: Prolidase deficiency: a metabolic disorder presenting with dermatologic signs. Int J Dermatol 1986; 25:431–433.
Boright AP, et al.: Prolidase deficiency: biochemical classification of alleles. Am J Med Genet 1989; 44:731–740.
Endo F, et al.: Primary structure and gene localization of human prolidase. J Biol Chem 1989; 264:4476–4481.
Phang JM, Scriver CR: Disorders of proline and hydroxyproline metabolism. In: Scriver CR, et al, eds: The metabolic basis of inherited disease, 6th ed. New York: McGraw-Hill, 1989:577–598.

DE030
FR039

Vazken M. Der Kaloustian
Bishara J. Freij

Proline oxidase deficiency
See HYPERPROLINEMIA
Prominent umbilicus
See HERNIA, UMBILICAL
Pronation, congenital
See RADIAL-ULNAR SYNOSTOSIS
Propionic acidemia
See ACIDEMIA, PROPIONIC
Propionicacidemia I
See ACIDEMIA, PROPIONIC
Propionyl-CoA-carboxylase deficiency, type I
See ACIDEMIA, PROPIONIC
Propylthiouracil (PTU) goiter
See GOITER, GOITROGEN INDUCED
Prostaglandin synthesis inhibition, fetal effects
See FETAL EFFECTS OF NONSTEROIDAL ANTI-INFLAMMATORY DRUGS (NSAIDS)
Prostatic male urethra, obstruction
See URETHRAL VALVES, POSTERIOR
Protanopia
See COLOR BLINDNESS, RED-GREEN PROTAN SERIES

Protean gigantism, Bannayan type
See OVERGROWTH, BANNAYAN TYPE
Protean gigantism, encephalo-cranio-cutaneous lipomatosis type
See PROTEUS SYNDROME
Protease inhibitor
See ALPHA(1)-ANTITRYPSIN DEFICIENCY

PROTEIN C DEFICIENCY 2918

Includes:
Heterozygous protein C deficiency
Homozygous protein C deficiency
Plasma protein C deficiency
ProC deficiency
Purpura fulminans, neonatal
Thrombophilia, inherited
Thromboses, and Protein C deficiency
Thrombotic disease, congenital

Excludes:
Antithrombin III deficiency (3066)
Fibrinogens, abnormal congenital (0004)
Plasminogen defects (3083)
Protein S deficiency (2950)
Vascular plasminogen activator deficiency

Major Diagnostic Criteria: Heterozygous protein C deficiency is a familial disorder in which there is an increased risk of thrombosis associated with isolated deficiency of protein C, with levels approximately 50% of normal. Other causes of acquired protein C deficiency, such as vitamin K deficiency, liver disease, or consumptive coagulopathy, must be excluded. Homozygous protein C deficiency is a severe disorder occurring in newborns in whom very low levels (1% of normal or less) of protein C are associated with a purpura fulminans-like syndrome or massive venous thrombosis.

Clinical Findings: In families with heterozygous protein C deficiency, levels of approximately 50% of normal protein C may lead to an increased risk of thromboembolic complications. Symptoms usually appear during adolescence or in the young adult and include recurrent thrombophlebitis or pulmonary emboli. In family studies, approximately 75% of protein C-deficient individuals experienced at least one thromboembolic episode. The most frequent site of thrombosis was the deep veins of the lower extremities, occurring in 75% of symptomatic persons. In 40% pulmonary embolism also occurred. Superficial thrombophlebitis was observed in 50%. Mesenteric and cerebral vein thromboses have also been reported. The mean age at which thrombotic events began was 29 years, ranging from 14 to 82 years. Pregnancy, surgery, trauma, parenteral injections, and contraceptive hormones were coexisting risk factors.

Complete (homozygous) deficiency of protein C is associated with purpura fulminans or massive venous thrombosis during the neonatal period. Thus far, there have been a dozen confirmed cases. Usually infants were born to asymptomatic, heterozygous, protein C-deficient parents. Pregnancies were full-term and uncomplicated. The major clinical symptoms included widely distributed purpuric lesions progressing to skin necrosis with bullae formation. Skin biopsy of the hemorrhagic lesions revealed microthrombi and fibrin deposition in capillaries and small vessels. A consumptive coagulopathy was associated with mucosal bleeding, intestinal hemorrhage, hematuria, and intracerebral hemorrhage. Widespread thrombosis included bilateral renal vein, hepatic venous, and inferior vena cava thromboses. Pulmonary emboli and hemorrhagic infarction of the lungs were common findings on autopsy. Cerebral thrombosis and hemorrhage lead to cortical necrosis, hydrocephalus, and seizures. Vitreous hemorrhage leading to cataracts and blindness was seen. The age of onset of lesions varied from 1 to 2 hours to 5 days after birth. Laboratory results were consistent with disseminated intravascular coagulation, including microangiopathic hemolysis, thrombocytopenia, hypofibrinogenemia, increased fibrin split products, and prolonged prothrombin and partial thromboplastin clotting times. Protein C antigen was undetectable or less than one percent in all but three patients. These three infants were reported to have 16–23% antigen, but undetectable protein C activity.

Protein C levels can be measured by assays for antigen or functional activity. Antigen assays include Laurell immunoelectrophoresis, enzyme-linked immunosorbent assay, or radioimmunoassay using either polyclonal rabbit or goat antibodies or monoclonal antibodies. Protein C function can be measured by a variety of methods, depending on its ability to act as an anticoagulant or to act upon a chromogenic substrate. For functional measurement, protein C must first be activated by thrombin (with or without the addition of thrombomodulin) or by a snake venom. Functional assays for protein C are technically more difficult to perform and are not as readily available as the antigenic assay. Normal adult levels of protein C antigen are approximately 65–165% of normal pooled plasma. In normal term infants, protein C antigen, like the other vitamin K proteins, may be reduced to 30% of normal. Protein C may also be secondarily reduced in the postoperative state and in massively obese individuals. Protein C may be elevated during pregnancy. To diagnose hereditary protein C deficiency, liver disease and a vitamin K deficiency must be ruled out. Normal levels of the vitamin K-dependent coagulation factors (Factors VII, IX, and X and prothrombin) should be present.

Plasma levels of protein C may be moderately decreased, secondarily, in persons with consumptive coagulopathy. This diagnosis should be excluded by the presence of normal levels of fibrinogen and platelets with normal fibrin split products in persons with suspected heterozygous protein C deficiency. Although disseminated intravascular coagulation is a feature of the severe homozygous form of protein C deficiency, the marked depression of the protein C level (less than two percent of normal) in association with appropriate family studies will confirm the diagnosis of primary, rather than secondary, protein C deficiency. Other causes of familial thrombosis should be excluded, including abnormalities of fibrinogen or deficiencies of antithrombin III, protein S, plasminogen, or vascular plasminogen activator. The definitive diagnosis of hereditary heterozygous protein C deficiency can only be made with certainty if at least one additional family member is affected. In homozygous protein C deficiency both parents should have reduced levels of protein C antigen or function.

Complications: Primarily the sequelae of venous thrombosis. Chronic venous insufficiency may result. Coumarin-induced skin necrosis has also been reported to develop in patients with protein C deficiency within a few days of initiating oral anticoagulant therapy. The lesions usually occur on the lower extremity, the abdominal wall, the breast, or the penis. Lesions progress rapidly to formation of hemorrhagic bullae and full-thickness skin infarction. The cause of coumarin necrosis is explained as resulting from a severe hypercoagulable state following initiation of coumarin therapy due to a rapid fall in protein C levels compared with the clotting factors II, IX, and X because of their different biologic half-lives. Coumarin necrosis may not be avoidable by simultaneous heparin therapy. Complications of homozygous protein C deficiency include sequelae of multiple organ infarct. Renal vein thrombosis has been associated with hypertension and uremia. Cerebral thrombosis or hemorrhage has resulted in developmental retardation, deafness, blindness, and death.

Associated Findings: None known.

Etiology: Heterozygous protein C deficiency by autosomal dominant inheritance with incomplete penetrance at the clinical level. In most families, the deficient family members show a severe thrombotic tendency in adult life. In homozygous protein C deficiency, both parents would be expected to have a deficiency of protein C. The thrombotic tendency of heterozygotes found by family studies of homozygous newborns is far less severe than in families with heterozygous protein C deficiency. Only six percent have been reported to have experienced venous thrombosis. It has been proposed that, on the basis of clinical manifestations, hereditary protein C deficiency may be divided into two distinct phenotypes: autosomal recessive and autosomal dominant. In the autosomal dominant phenotype, the heterozygotes have recur-

rent thrombosis during adult life. In the recessive phenotype, heterozygotes have no symptoms and the homozygotes are severely affected with purpura fulminans or massive thrombosis during the neonatal period. There is no clear explanation for the difference between these two apparent phenotypes.

Pathogenesis: Protein C is a vitamin K-dependent serine protease zymogen produced in the liver. Upon activation by thrombin, protein C exhibits anticoagulant activity by way of its ability to inactivate clotting factors Va and VIIIa in the presence of protein S, another vitamin K-dependent protein. In addition to this anticoagulant action, activated protein C promotes fibrinolysis probably by inhibiting the inactivator of plasminogen activator. The activation of protein C by thrombin is greatly accelerated if thrombin is first complexed with the endothelial-bound cofactor thrombomodulin. At present two types of protein C deficiency have been described. Type I, in which protein C activity and antigen are equally reduced, probably reflects decreased synthesis of protein C. Type II, in which the biologic activities of protein C are reduced whereas the antigen level is within the normal range, probably reflects production of a dysfunctional protein. Subtypes of type II deficiency may be defined according to the results of a chromogenic functional assay versus the anticoagulant assay. From a clinical standpoint, there appears to be no difference in the two types. In some cases of type II protein C deficiency, an abnormal electrophoretic migration of protein C has been demonstrated.

MIM No.: *17686

Sex Ratio: M1:F1

Occurrence: Prevalence of the autosomal dominant form has been estimated at 1:16,000. Prevalence of the autosomal recessive form in which heterozygotes have no symptoms has been estimated at 1:200–300.

Risk of Recurrence for Patient's Sib:
See Part I, *Mendelian Inheritance.*

Risk of Recurrence for Patient's Child:
See Part I, *Mendelian Inheritance.*

Age of Detectability: Homozygous protein C deficiency can be detected at birth. The diagnosis of heterozygous protein C deficiency should be made cautiously in the young child because of normal low levels of protein C under age six months. Prenatal diagnosis has not been reported.

Gene Mapping and Linkage: PROC (protein C (inactivator of coagulation factors Va and VIIIa)) has been mapped to 2q13-q21.

Isolation and characterization of the cDNA coding for human protein C has demonstrated the gene to span 11 kilobases of DNA. The coding and 3' noncoding portion of the gene consists of eight exons and seven introns. There is considerable similarity between the locations of the introns in the genes for protein C and Factor IX. Genotype studies in 14 families with hereditary protein C deficiency revealed a complete deletion of the protein C gene in three families. In two families, changes in Southern blot analysis were produced by either a deletion or insertion of new sequences. Nine families showed no detectable abnormality of the gene. It is likely that most families with protein C deficiency result from a point mutation in the protein C gene. Closely linked Pvu restriction enzyme polymorphism has been demonstrated in two related patients with type I protein C deficiency.

Prevention: None known. Genetic counseling indicated.

Treatment: In heterozygotes, heparin is effective for treatment of thrombosis. Coumarin therapy is effective in the long-term prevention of venous thromboembolism. Initiation of coumarin therapy has to be monitored carefully because of the risk of coumarin necrosis. Low initial loading doses are recommended to prevent marked and rapid decrease of protein C. Replacement of protein C with fresh-frozen plasma during life-threatening thromboembolism or coumarin necrosis has been reported. Anabolic steroids have been shown to raise protein C levels in heterozygous deficiency. Clinical usefulness of these agents would be expected in type I protein C deficiency only. In the purpura fulminans-like syndrome in homozygous protein C deficiency, infusions of fresh-frozen plasma and prothrombin complex concentrates have been life-saving. Protein C survival in the plasma of these infants has been biphasic, with a first-phase half-life of six hours and a second phase of 10–11 hours. Oral anticoagulant therapy has also been used with success.

Prognosis: Heterozygous protein C deficiency is compatible with a long life. Due to the risk of spontaneous recurrence of thrombosis after oral anticoagulation therapy is discontinued, prolonged therapy (possibly for life) is indicated. The ultimate prognosis of homozygous protein C deficiency is extremely guarded. Reported infants who have been maintained on protein C replacement therapy or oral anticoagulant therapy to prevent the catastrophic symptoms of homozygous protein C deficiency. The long-term effects of vitamin K antagonists in children on growth and development are undetermined.

Detection of Carrier: In type I heterozygous protein C deficiency, protein C antigen and function would be moderately and proportionately reduced to approximately 50% of normal. In type II protein C heterozygous deficiency, protein C function is reduced to approximately 50% of normal and is associated with normal protein C antigen. In patients on oral anticoagulant therapy, the diagnosis of protein C deficiency may be difficult. Simultaneous measurement of protein C and coagulation factors II and X have been used. If both the ratios of protein C: factor II antigen and protein C: factor X antigen are below 0.5, protein C deficiency may be presumed. This diagnostic determination should be made only after equilibrium of all clotting factors has been reached on oral anticoagulant therapy.

References:
Griffin JH, et al.: Deficiency of protein C in congenital thrombotic disease. J Clin Invest 1981; 68:1370–1373.
Crabtree GR, et al.: The range of genotypes underlying human protein C deficiency. Thromb Haemost 1985; 54:56.
Foster DC, et al.: The nucleotide sequence of the gene for human protein C. Proc Natl Acad Sci USA 1985; 82:4673–4677.
Marlar RA: Protein C in thromboembolic disease. Semin Thromb Hemostas 1985; 11:387–393.
Rocchi M, et al.: Mapping of coagulation factors protein C and factor X on chromosome 2 and 13 respectively. Cytogenet Cell Genet 1985; 40:734.
Clouse LH, Comp PC: The regulation of hemostasis: the protein C system. New Engl J Med 1986; 314:1298–1304.
Long GL: Structure and evaluation of the human genes encoding protein C and coagulation factors VII, IX and X. Cold Spring Harbor Symp Quant Biol 1986; 51:525–529.
Pabinger I: Clinical relevance of protein C. Blut 1986; 53:63–75.
Miletich J, et al.: Absence of thrombosis in subjects with heterozygous protein C deficiency. New Engl J Med 1987; 317:991–996.
Marlar RA, et al.: Diagnosis and treatment of homozygous protein C deficiency. J Pediatr 1989; 114:528–534.

GR036 **Ralph A. Gruppo**

Protein C inhibitor deficiency
See COAGULATION DEFECT, FAMILIAL MULTIPLE FACTORS
Protein Gc
See PLASMA, GROUP-SPECIFIC COMPONENT

PROTEIN S DEFICIENCY 2950

Includes:
Plasma protein S deficiency
Thromboses, and protein S deficiency

Excludes:
Antithrombin III deficiency (3066)
Protein C deficiency (2918)
Protein S deficiency, acquired

Major Diagnostic Criteria: Deep venous thrombosis, which can be recurrent; reduced plasma level of functional protein S.

Clinical Findings: Congenital deficiency of functional protein S with associated venous thrombosis. Pulmonary embolism occurs in over half of all patients, and are recurrent in 77% of these. There is no apparent relationship between the level of protein S and the frequency of thrombosis. Patients have been reported who have had severe deficiency of protein S and no history of thrombosis, and there are patients with moderate deficiency who have had recurrent thromboses.

Complications: Pulmonary embolism; death from thromboembolic disease.

Associated Findings: None known.

Etiology: Autosomal dominant inheritance.

Pathogenesis: Protein S exists in two forms, as free protein S and as a complex with C4b binding protein (a complement inhibitor protein). The free protein S is the functional protein. This protein S serves as a cofactor for activated protein C. Activated protein C functions as an inhibitor to activated Factors VIII and V.

MIM No.: *17688

Sex Ratio: M1.6:F1 (estimated).

Occurrence: Over a hundred cases have been documented in the literature. Occurrence is estimated to be higher than the number of reported cases would suggest.

Risk of Recurrence for Patient's Sib:
See Part I, *Mendelian Inheritance.*

Risk of Recurrence for Patient's Child:
See Part I, *Mendelian Inheritance.*

Age of Detectability: During adolescence.

Gene Mapping and Linkage: PROS1 (protein S, alpha) has been mapped to 3p11-q11.2.

Prevention: None known. Genetic counseling indicated.

Treatment: Coumarin anticoagulants (such as warfarin).

Prognosis: Unknown.

Detection of Carrier: By protein S levels of about 50% of normal.

References:
Comp PC, Esmon CT: Familial protein S deficiency is associated with recurrent thrombosis. J Clin Invest 1984; 74:2082–2088.
Comp PC, Esmon CT: Recurrent venous thromboembolism in patients with a partial deficiency of protein S. New Engl J Med 1984; 311:1525–1528.
Kamiya T, et al.: Inherited deficiency of protein S in a Japanese family with recurrent venous thrombosis: a study of three generations. Blood 1986; 67:406–410.
Engesser L, et al.: Hereditary protein S deficiency: clinical manifestations. Ann Intern Med 1987; 106:677–682.

C0068 **James J. Corrigan**

Protein-losing enteropathy with dilated intestinal lymphatics
See INTESTINAL LYMPHANGIECTASIA
Proteinuria-ocular and facial anomalies-deafness
See FACIO-OCULO-ACOUSTIC-RENAL SYNDROME (FOAR SYNDROME)
Proteinuria-osteolysis
See OSTEOLYSIS, CARPAL-TARSAL AND CHRONIC PROGRESSIVE GLOMERULOPATHY
Proteodermatan sulfate, defective biosynthesis of
See EHLERS-DANLOS SYNDROME
Proteolipid protein, myelin
See PELIZAEUS-MERZBACHER SYNDROME

PROTEUS SYNDROME 2382

Includes:
"Elephant man" (possible diagnosis)
Encephalo-cranio-cutaneous lipomatosis
Gigantism, hands and feet-nevi-hemihypertrophy-megalencephaly
Linear sebaceous nevus-mental retardation-seizures
Organoid nevus syndrome
Overgrowth, encephalo-cranio-cutaneous lipomatosis type
Overgrowth, Proteus type
Protean gigantism, encephalo-cranio-cutaneous lipomatosis type

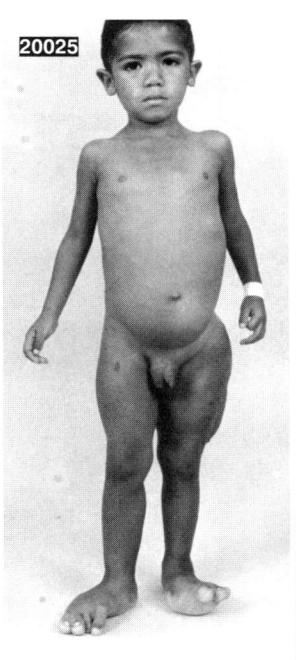
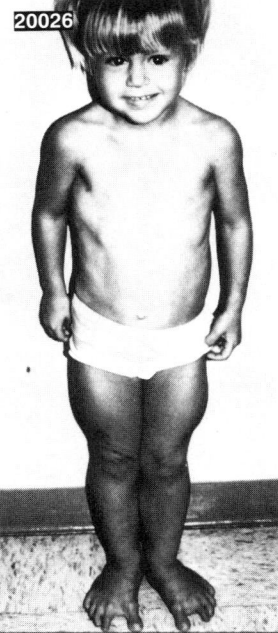
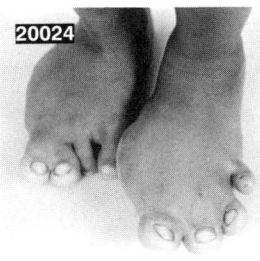
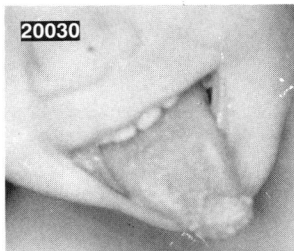
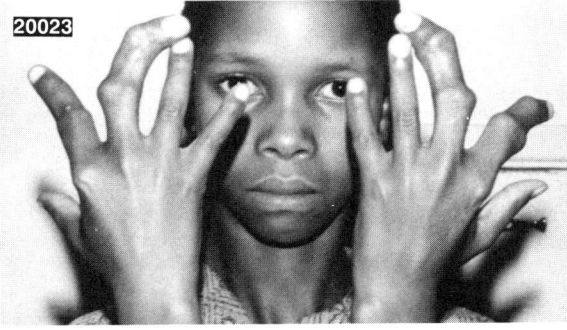

2382-20025: Six-year-old boy with asymmetric overgrowth, hypertrophy and syndactyly of the feet, right-sided hypertrophy, lymphangioma of the left thigh, and a right inguinal hernia. **20026:** Five-year-old girl with hemihypertrophy and partial gigantism of the feet. **20024:** Asymmetric hypertrophy of feet with syndactyly; both hallucès were surgically removed to improve ambulation. **20030:** Hypertrophy of the tip of the tongue. **20023:** Digital hypertrophy and bizarre angulation.

Schimmelpenning-Feuerstein-Mims syndrome

Excludes:
Angiomatosis, cutaneomedullar
Angiomatosis, retinomesencephalic
Angio-osteohypertrophy syndrome (0055)
Enchondromatosis and hemangiomas (0346)
Fibrous dysplasia, polyostotic (0391)

Gingival multiple hamartoma syndrome (0412)
Lipomatosis, diffuse
Neurofibromatosis (0712)
Nevus, blue rubber bleb nevus syndrome (0113)
Nevus of Ota (0716)
Overgrowth, Bannayan type (2381)
Overgrowth, macrocephaly-hemangioma, Riley-Smith type (2192)
Sturge-Weber syndrome (0915)
Telangiectasia, Osler hemorrhagic (2021)
Tuberous sclerosis (0975)
Von Hippel-Lindau syndrome (0995)

Major Diagnostic Criteria: Congenital lipomas, occasionally with elements of lymphangioma and/or hemangioma, predominately subcutaneous, on the cranium and/or intracranially, are essential for the diagnosis. Central nervous system (ectodermal) structural malformations represent a spectrum with frequent eye involvement. **Megalencephaly**, mental retardation, seizures, choristomas, and a variety of other hamartomas further delineate the phenotype, and confirm the diagnosis.

Clinical Findings: When present, the **Megalencephaly** is congenital; the head circumference is usually around 2 SD above the mean. Congenital cutaneous hamartomas frequently lead to asymmetry. Partial gigantism secondary to hypertrophy of soft and osseous tissues of the anterior feet and hands in several patients led to the emergence of the Proteus syndrome. Large hamartomas of the soles, predominately lipomatous, were another differentiating sign between Proteus syndrome and the encephalocraniocutaneous lipomatosis.

Until recently, seizures and mental retardation were considered characteristic of encephalocraniocutaneous lipomatosis and not of Proteus syndrome. Additional reported patients, however, seem to bridge the gap between those syndromes. Pigmented intradermal nevi, hyper- and hypopigmented cutaneous streaks, linear verrucose epidermoid nevi, as well as occasional linear subaceous nevi, further delineate the combined phenotype.

On the other hand, the latter clinical features raise the question of whether or not some patients described years ago represent separate entities. The clinical variability of encephalocraniocutaneous lipomatosis appears to be extraordinary, and challenges the current classification of phakomatoses. The symmetric or asymmetric hypertrophy of Proteus syndrome also does not appear to be an unique; i.e., diagnostic clinical feature of the condition.

Ophthalmologic features occasionally noted in patients are anisocoria, heterochromia irides, unilateral microphthalmos, scleral tumor, severe myopia, retinal detachment, cataract, strabismus, and chorioretinitis. Cyst-like alterations of the lungs were observed in two patients. Intelligence is usually normal.

X-ray features include osseous protruberances of the skull, hyperostoses in the external auditory canals and alveolar ridges, irregularly shaped vertebrae, dystrophic intervertebral disks, elongated cervical spine, and kyphoscoliosis.

Complications: Excessive localized growth may require surgery to improve function and appearance. The central nervous system malformations frequently lead to the inability to maintain an independent life style. Blindness can complicate the ophthalmologic findings.

Associated Findings: Macroorchidism, penile hypertrophy, goiter, early breast development, and congenital dislocation of the hip have been reported in single individuals.

Etiology: Unknown. Usually sporadic.

Pathogenesis: Possibly faulty embryonic differentiation in the induction, cell migration, and interaction of the cells of the ecto-, meso-, and entoderm. Paracrine growth factors dysregulation appears to play a role in pathogenesis. A somatic cell genetic disorder has also been suggested.

MIM No.: 17692

POS No.: 3515, 3655

Sex Ratio: M1:F1

Occurrence: Undetermined. Several dozen cases have been evaluated as possibly having this condition. There appears to be no ethnic predilection.

Risk of Recurrence for Patient's Sib: Unknown.

Risk of Recurrence for Patient's Child: Unknown.

Age of Detectability: At birth for the hamartomas. Several years may be necessary for the emergence of the complete phenotype. Prenatal diagnosis by ultrasound may be possible on the basis of asymmetric hypertrophy of limbs.

Gene Mapping and Linkage: Unknown.

Prevention: None known. Genetic counseling indicated.

Treatment: Orthopedic management of kyphoscoliosis and surgical excision of hamartomas may be performed when clinically indicated.

Prognosis: Unknown. A possible malignant potential exists as with other hamartomas.

Detection of Carrier: Unknown. First degree relatives should be examined for hamartomas and **Neurofibromatosis**.

References:

Gorlin RJ: Proteus syndrome. J Clin Dysmorphol 1984; 2:8–9.
Kousseff BG: Proteus syndrome or another hamartosis. J Clin Dysmorph 1984; 2:23–26.
Lezama DB, Buyse ML: The Proteus syndrome: the emergence of an entity. J Clin Dysmorphol 1984; 2:10–13.
Kousseff BG: Pleiotropy vs heterogeneity in Proteus syndrome. Pediatrics 1986; 78:544–546.
Wiedemann H-R, Burgio GR: Encephalocraniocutaneous lipomatosis and Proteus syndrome. Am J Med Genet 1986; 25:403–404.
Clark RD, et al.: Proteus syndrome: an expanded phenotype. Am J Med Genet 1987; 27:99–117.
Malamitsi-Puchner A, et al.: Severe Proteus syndrome in an 18-month-old boy. Am J Med Genet 1987; 27:119–125.
Viljoen DL, et al.: Proteus syndrome in Southern Africa: natural history and clinical manifestations in six individuals. Am J Med Genet 1987; 27:87–98. †
Cohen MM, Jr: Further diagnostic thoughts about the Elephant Man. Am J Med Genet 1988; 29:777–782.
Kousseff BG, Madan S: The phakomatoses - an hypothesis: paracrine growth regulation disorders? Dysmorph Clin Genet 1988; 2:76–90 †

K0018
VI005

Boris G. Kousseff
Denis L. Viljöen

Prothrombin
See HYPOPROTHROMBINEMIA
Proto-collagen lysyl hydroxylase deficiency
See EHLERS-DANLOS SYNDROME
Protocoproporphyria
See PORPHYRIA, VARIEGATE
Proto-oncogene homologous to myelocytomatosis virus
See LYMPHOMA, BURKITT TYPE
Protoporphyria, erythropoietic
See PORPHYRIA, PROTOPORPHYRIA
Protoporphyria, porphyria
See PORPHYRIA, PROTOPORPHYRIA
Protoporphyrinogen oxidase deficiency
See PORPHYRIA, VARIEGATE
Proximal femoral focal deficiency
See FIBULA, CONGENITAL ABSENCE OF

PRUNE-BELLY SYNDROME	**2007**

Includes:
　　Abdominal muscles, absence-urinary tract anomaly-
　　　　cryptorchidism
　　Abdominal musculature, agenesis, congenital
　　Eagle-Barrett syndrome

Excludes:
　　Bladder exstrophy (3015)
　　Ventral hernia

Major Diagnostic Criteria: Partial or complete absence of abdominal musculature, urinary tract malformations, and bilateral cryp-

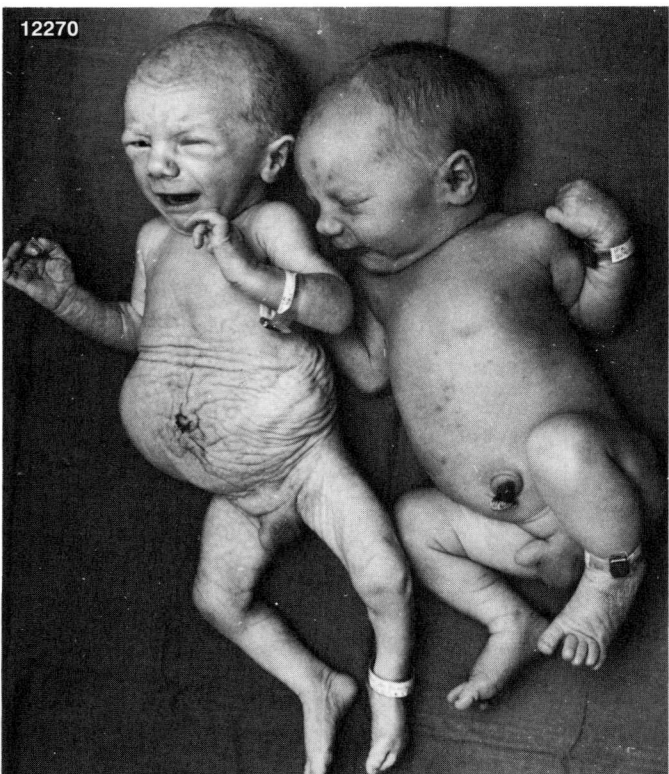

2007-12270: Three-day-old monozygotic twins discordant for the abdominal muscle triad. Note the wrinkled and distended abdomen of the affected twin on the left.

---

torchidism. Confirmation depends on intravenous pyelography (IVP), renal scan and voiding cystourethrogram. Retrograde studies may be necessary in some cases. Urine cultures, renal function tests and biochemical profiles play an important part in the diagnosis and management of the patient.

Clinical Findings: This syndrome is recognized at birth, since deficiency of lower and medial parts of the abdominal musculature give the skin the wrinkled appearance of a prune. The fully developed syndrome occurs almost exclusively in males. The defect is quite variable and often asymmetrical, ranging from hypoplasia to complete absence of the abdominal muscles. The lower rectus and oblique muscles are usually intact, pulling the umbilicus cephalad. Ribs are usually flared; Harrison's groove is present.

In the fully developed syndrome the entire genitourinary tract is affected. The kidneys may be dysplastic, cystic, hypoplastic or grossly hydronephrotic. These findings are frequently asymmetric in distribution and kidney function is usually good and does not deteriorate rapidly. Progressive renal failure is the result of chronic urinary tract infection and obstruction uropathy. The dilated and elongated ureters are quite striking on X-ray.

Hydro-ureter or megalo-ureter with poor contractility power are observed by cineradiography. In some cases the ureters are atretic: vesico-urethral reflux is present in most.

The bladder has an enlarged capacity and is trabeculated or megacystic. The apex is attached to the umbilicus; at times the urachus is patent. Although bladder neck obstruction or atresia is rarely reported, this is not a usual finding.

When posterior urethral valves are present, the penile urethra balloons out, often with distention of the prostatic utricle and thickening of the bladder neck. Urachus may be patent allowing leakage of urine through the umbilicus in infants surviving to term. Twenty percent of infants are stillborn; these manifest Potter facies (see **Kidney, polycystic disease, recessive**) and anuria due to renal agenesis. If oliguria is present in the newborn, the survival is poor. Most infants with prune belly syndrome can void normally at birth, but urinary tract infections, and impending chronic renal failure makes early intervention appropriate.

There are milder cases with good renal function in whom surgery can be delayed.

Complications: With passage of time the wrinkles flatten out, and the lower abdominal wall bulges in a "pot belly" appearance; this makes it difficult for the child to rise from the supine position. Chronic urinary tract infections eventually lead to uremia.

The time of end stage renal failure depends on the extent of malformations and infection.

When the urinary tract anomaly is severe, such as with complete atresia of the urethra or bilateral renal agenesis oligohydramnios occurs, resulting in multiple compression deformities of the limbs.

Talipes equinovarus and bilateral dislocated hips are the two most common physical abnormalities. Similarly, the hypoplasia of the lungs due to the embarrassment of intrauterine respiratory movements may cause respiratory distress soon after birth. Older children have a tendency to increased respiratory infections.

Associated Findings: *Musculoskeletal malformations*: (20–50% of cases): club foot is common. Congenital hip dislocation, skin dimples of elbows, knees, scoliosis, arthrogryposis, **Pectus excavatum** or **Pectus carinatum** hemimelia, myelomeningocele, **Polydactyly**, **Torticollis**, flaired iliac wings, and diastasis of pubis have all been reported.

Intestinal tract: imperforate anus is common in the severely affected neonate. Universal mesentery with unattached cecum may cause malrotation of intestines in later life.

Respiratory tract: pulmonary hypoplasia with association of oligohydramnios, spontaneous pneumothorax in neonatal period.

Cardiovascular system: congenital heart disease is reported in some cases, including **Ductus arteriosus, patent** and septal defects.

CNS: craniostenosis and **Microcephaly** have been reported rarely. This may be related to oligohydramnios.

Etiology: Undetermined. Discordance was reported seven times, concordance once, in monozygotic twins. One patient was reported to be one of a set of homozygous triplets. The condition has been reported in association with diverse chromosomal anomalies, but most patients have had normal karyotypes.

Pathogenesis: The most commonly affected abdominal muscles are the derivatives of the first lumbar myotome, which differentiates between the sixth and tenth week of gestation. Microscopic studies of the muscles show profound alteration, degeneration, and fibrosis.

Two major hypotheses in the pathogenesis of prune belly syndrome exist: one suggests primary distal obstruction in the urinary tract leading to bladder distention and lower abdominal muscular atrophy by duct pressure in early fetal life. The second hypothesis suggests a primary somatic defect in the abdominal musculature. Recent evidence implies that the primary pathogenetic event in the observed pattern of anomalies is overdistension of the fetal abdomen. In some instances, in males particularly, this early distension is associated with urethral obstruction and bladder distension. In the majority of cases, anatomic obstructive lesions could not be identified. In some cases, prune belly results from fetal ascites secondary to various causes.

MIM No.: 10010

POS No.: 3003

CDC No.: 756.720

Sex Ratio: M20:F1. Only males have the fully developed syndrome.

Occurrence: Over 300 cases have been reported in the English literature.

Risk of Recurrence for Patient's Sib: Unknown.

Risk of Recurrence for Patient's Child: Unknown. There is no reported case of a prune belly syndrome patient fathering a child.

Age of Detectability: At birth. Prenatal diagnosis may be accomplished by ultrasonography after the 20th week of gestation.

Gene Mapping and Linkage: Unknown.

Prevention: None known. Genetic counseling indicated.

Treatment: The primary goal of treatment is the preservation of renal function. This should be directed towards the control of infection and relief of obstruction when present. Surgical management consists of high tubeless urinary diversion, usually pyelostomy, with total reconstruction at the later stage when feasible.

One stage surgery consists of shortening, tapering and reimplantation of ureters, reduction cytoplasty, orchiopexy and plication of abdominal wall. Complete reconstruction of the drainage system and abdominal wall leads to a better prognosis.

Prognosis: Survival is related to the level of kidney function. In severe bilateral renal dysplasia, the prognosis is guarded.

Excellent results in children with good renal function and early surgical intervention have been reported.

Detection of Carrier: Unknown.

Special Considerations: There are only ten reported cases of prune belly syndrome in females. The characteristic urinary tract anomalies are usually missing. Whether these cases represent true prune belly syndrome or are lateral ventral hernias is still debatable.

References:

Moine IW, Moine BJ: Prune belly syndrome and fetal ascites. Teratology 1979; 19:111–118.
Pagon RA, et al.: Urethral obstruction malformation complex: a cause of abdominal muscle deficiency and the "prune belly". J Pediatr 1979; 94:900–906.
Woodhouse CRJ, et al.: Prune belly syndrome: report of 47 cases. Arch Dis Child 1982; 57:856–859.
Frydman M, et al.: Chromosome abnormalities in infants with prune belly anomaly. Am J Med Genet 1983; 15:127–135.
Burton BK, Dillard RG: Prune belly syndrome: observations supporting the hypothesis of abdominal overdistension. Am J Med Genet 1984; 17:669–475.
Moerman P, et al.: Pathogenesis of the prune belly syndrome: a functional urethral obstruction caused by prostatic hypoplasia. Pediatrics 1984; 73:470–475.

BIO12
SA008

Nesrin Bingol
Inge Sagel

Prurigo Besnier
See SKIN, ATOPY, FAMILIAL
Pruritus gravidarum
See INTRAHEPATIC CHOLESTASIS OF PREGNANCY (ICP)

PRURITUS, HEREDITARY LOCALIZED   0827

Includes: Itching, hereditary localized

Excludes: Pruritus, non-hereditary

Major Diagnostic Criteria: A localized, familial pruritus unassociated with other causes and without significant skin changes.

Clinical Findings: Hereditary localized area of pruritus unassociated with any significant skin changes. In the two families reported to date, it occurred on the back. The age of onset is usually in the third decade, but ranges from age four to 41 years.

Complications: Unknown.

Associated Findings: None known.

Etiology: Possibly autosomal dominant or X-linked dominant inheritance.

Pathogenesis: Unknown.

MIM No.: 17710

Sex Ratio: M1:F7 in the reported family. This family also had one male carrier without symptoms who had five affected daughters and two unaffected sons.

Occurrence: One kinship reported.

Risk of Recurrence for Patient's Sib:
See Part I, *Mendelian Inheritance.*

Risk of Recurrence for Patient's Child:
See Part I, *Mendelian Inheritance.*

Age of Detectability: Generally in the second to third decade of life.

Gene Mapping and Linkage: Unknown.

Prevention: None known. Genetic counseling indicated.

Treatment: Symptomatic.

Prognosis: Normal life span.

Detection of Carrier: Unknown.

References:
Comings DE, Comings SN: Hereditary localized pruritus. Arch Dermatol 1965; 92:236–237.

C0030   **David E. Comings**

Psaume syndrome
  See ORO-FACIO-DIGITAL SYNDROME I
Pseudo (platelet-type) von Willebrand disease
  See VON WILLEBRAND DISEASE
Pseudo-arylsulfatase A deficiency
  See METACHROMATIC LEUKODYSTROPHIES
Pseudo-Crouzon disease
  See CRANIOFACIAL DYSOSTOSIS
Pseudo-Hurler disease
  See G(M1)-GANGLIOSIDOSIS, TYPE 1
Pseudo-Hurler polydystrophia
  See MUCOLIPIDOSIS III
Pseudo-pseudohypoparathyroidism
  See PARATHYROID HORMONE RESISTANCE

PSEUDOACHONDROPLASTIC DYSPLASIA   0828

Includes:
  Gonadal mosaicism in pseudoachondroplasia
  Pseudoachondroplastic spondyloepiphyseal dysplasia
  Spondyloepiphyseal dysplasia, pseudoachondroplastic type

Excludes:
  Achondroplasia (0010)
  Epiphyseal dysplasia, multiple (0358)
  Hypochondroplasia (0510)
  Spondyloepiphyseal dysplasia congenita (0897)
  Spondyloepiphyseal dysplasia, late (0898)

Major Diagnostic Criteria: Normal at birth. Normal skull, disproportionate short stature, with long trunk and short limbs, and typical vertebral and epiphyseal dysplasia during growth.

Clinical Findings: Disproportionate dwarfism with relatively long trunk, short arms and legs, and normal skull and facies; normal-appearing at birth (X-rays taken at birth have been normal); growth retardation and disproportion usually present by two years of age. Growth curve falls off during childhood. Limbs generally shortened; particularly hands and feet. Joint laxity except at elbows. The patient may be knock-kneed or have bowed knees. Trunk relatively long; may be absolutely normal or mildly shortened, with marked lumbar lordosis and mild-to-moderate scoliosis in some individuals. Moderate-to-severe short stature (91.5–137.2 cm adult height). Growth falls off during late childhood and adolescence. X-rays in childhood show oval shape, then moderate flattening of the vertebral bodies, irregularity, and tongue-like projections of central portion of vertebral body; during adolescence, markedly irregular calcification of vertebrae occurs, with partial restoration of normal vertebral form by adulthood. Generalized epiphyseal dysplasia and delay in ossification, particularly in weight bearing joints; capital femoral epiphyses, knees, wrists, and short tubular bones with small, irregular, flat epiphyses, as well as mildly irregular metaphyses during childhood leading to flattening and irregularity of the joint when epiphyses fuse. Faces of affected individuals are similar.

There are no clear differences between the postulated sub-types (I,II,III and IV), although they do differ in apparent inheritance

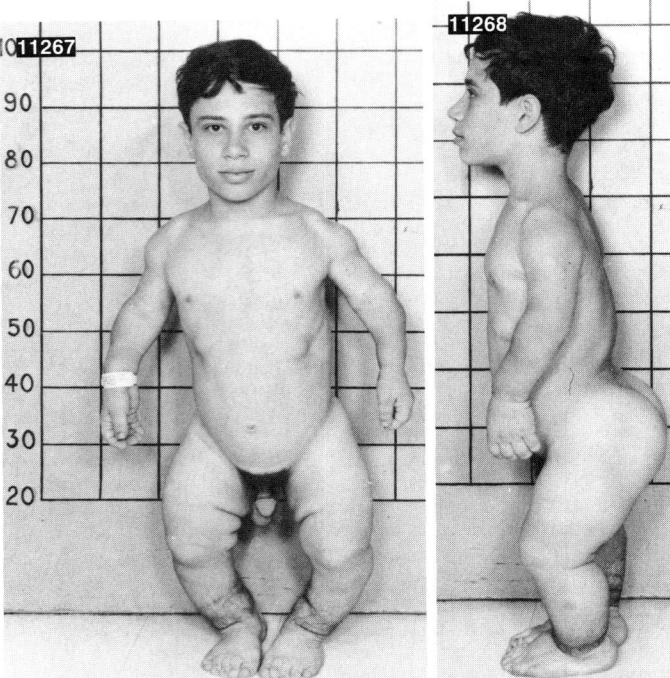

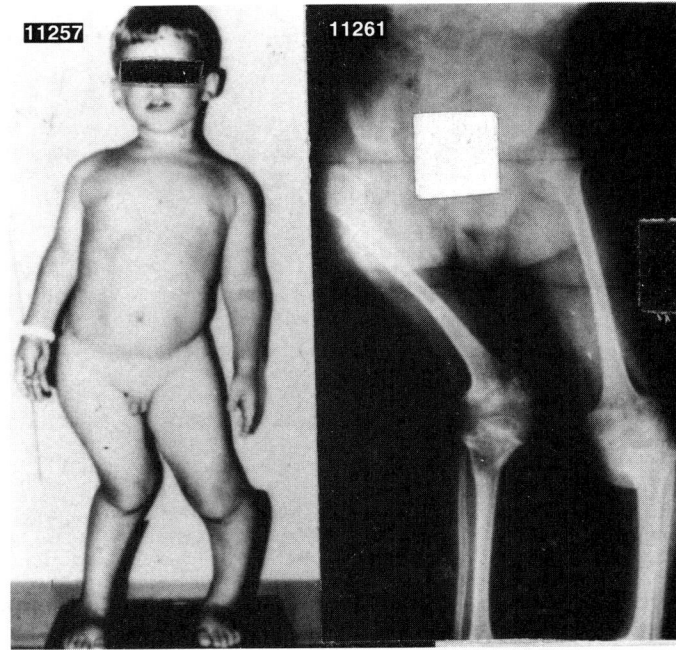

0828A-11267: Short stature with short limbs, relatively long trunk and normal skull. **11268:** Lateral view shows short limbs and exaggerated lumbar lordosis. **11257–61:** Windswept appearance with knock-knees on right and bow-leg on the left.

---

patterns and severity. Skeletal, X-ray, and pathologic changes of each sub-type show similar patterns.

Complications: Arthritis, particularly hip and knee; scoliosis; ulnar deviation of hand, and joint laxity making functional fixa-

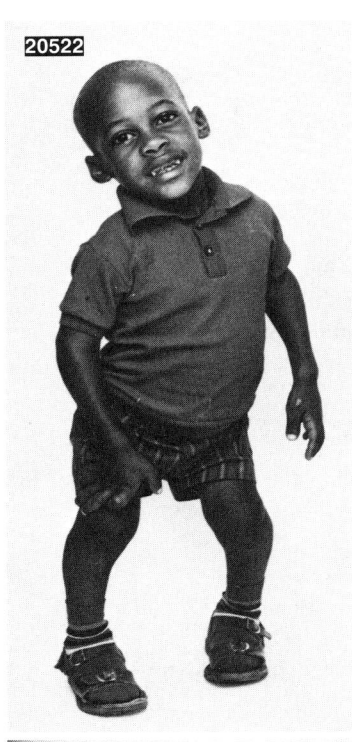

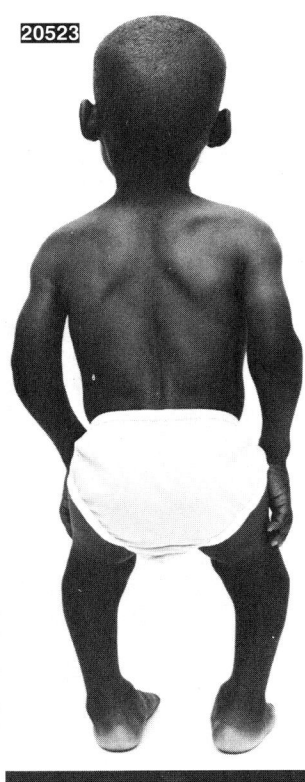

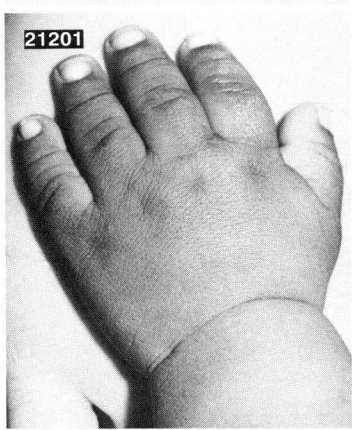

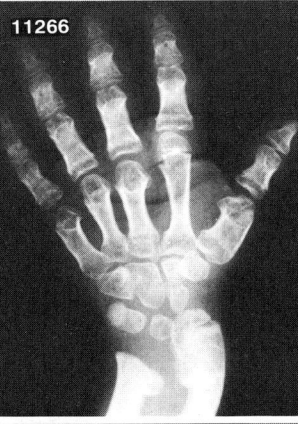

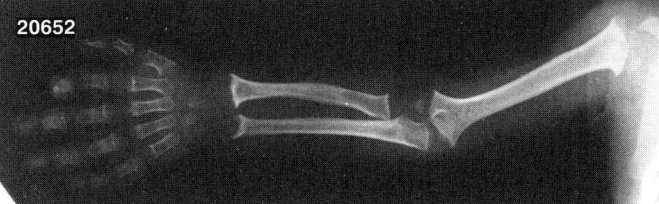

0828B-20522–23: Disproportionate short stature with bowed legs and limb deformities. **21201:** Short hand with short digits. **11266:** X-ray of the hand shows abnormality in epiphyseal formation of the distal ulna resulting in relative overgrowth of the radius and ulnar deviation of the hand. The metacarpals and phalanges are all short and stubby. **20652:** X-ray of an affected 4-year-old shows short tubular bones and irregular mushroomed epiphyses.

tion of joints difficult; slow developmental landmarks or waddling gait; social and psychologic adjustments to short stature.

Associated Findings: Cord compression has been described.

Etiology: Almost all cases have autosomal dominant inheritance or represent new dominant mutations. While penetrance is 100%, fairly marked intrafamilial variability does occur. Some cases previously reported as autosomal recessive inheritance represented parental gonadal mosaicism. A rare condition with autosomal recessive inheritance may, however, exist.

Pathogenesis: Accumulation of non-collagenous protein material in the rough endoplasmic reticulum of chondrocytes, and the absence of a specific proteoglycan in cartilage (i.e. not transferred to the Golgi system), appears to be the basic defect.

MIM No.: *17715, *17717, *26415, 26416

POS No.: 3363

Sex Ratio: M1:F1

Occurrence: Undetermined, but presumably one-quarter to one-fiftieth as common as **Achondroplasia**.

Risk of Recurrence for Patient's Sib:
See Part I, *Mendelian Inheritance.*

Risk of Recurrence for Patient's Child:
See Part I, *Mendelian Inheritance.*

Age of Detectability: Usually 2–4 years of age. If the parents have a previously affected child, they may suspect the diagnosis at about one year because of short fingers, short arms, or inability to straighten elbow completely.

Gene Mapping and Linkage: Unknown.

Prevention: None known. Genetic counseling indicated.

Treatment: Avoid vigorous athletics, since trauma to joints seems to hasten arthritis. Symptomatic orthopedics for arthritis and bowing. Splinting of wrists and ankles for loose jointedness.

Prognosis: Normal for life span and intelligence; fairly severe degenerative arthritis; social, emotional, and vocational problems.

Detection of Carrier: Unknown.

References:
Maroteaux P, Lamy M: Les formes pseudo-achondroplastiques des dysplasias spondylo-epiphysaires. Presse Med 1959; 67:383–386.
Hall JG: Pseudoachondroplasia. BD:OAS XI(6). Miami: Symposia specialists for The National Foundation-March of Dimes, 1975:187–202. *
Horton WA, et al.: Growth curves for height for diastrophic dysplasia, spondyloepiphyseal dysplasia congenita, and pseudoachondroplasia. Am J Dis Child 1982; 136:316–319.
Stanescu V, et al.: The pathogenetic mechanism in osteochondroplasias. J Bone Joint Surg 1984; 66A:817–836.
Young ID, Moore JR: Severe pseudoachondroplasia with parental consanguinity. J Med Genet 1985; 22:150–153.
Wynne-Davies R, et al.: Pseudoachondroplasia: clinical diagnosis at different ages and comparison of autosomal dominant and recessive types: a review of 32 patients (26 kindreds). J Med Genet 1986; 23:425–434.
Hall JG, et al.: Gonadal mosaicism in pseudoachondroplasia. Am J Med Genet 1987; 28:143–151.

HA014   **Judith G. Hall**

Pseudoachondroplastic spondyloepiphyseal dysplasia
See PSEUDOACHONDROPLASTIC DYSPLASIA
Pseudoaldosteronism
See LIDDLE SYNDROME

PSEUDOAMINOPTERIN SYNDROME   2628

Includes: Aminopterin syndrome without aminopterin (ASSA)

Excludes: Fetal aminopterin syndrome (0380)

Major Diagnostic Criteria: Ocular hypertelorism, ossification defects of cranium, upswept frontal hair pattern, flared eyebrows, and short stature.

Clinical Findings: Dysmorphic signs strongly resembling those described in children who were exposed to aminopterin or to methotrexate in early pregnancy (see **Fetal aminopterin syndrome**). Signs include ocular hypertelorism (4/4); bitemporal flattening (3/4); widow's peak with temporal hairline recession and upswept pattern (4/4); arched eyebrows with medial flaring, thinning, and perhaps hypopigmentation laterally (4/4); hypoplastic supraorbital ridges (4/4) with prominent eyeballs (3/4); small palpebral fissures (3/4); prominent nose root (4/4); highly arched or cleft palate (4/4); micrognathia (3/4); and low-set, posteriorly rotated ears (4/4).

The skull is brachycephalic, with incomplete ossification of cranial bones (4/4), delayed fontanelle closure, and synostosis of lambdoid or coronal sutures. Skeletal findings include short stature (4/4), limitation of elbow movement (3/4) with subluxation of radial heads, stenosis of tubular bones, and digital anomalies (3/4). There is mild-to-moderate mental retardation (3/4) and cryptorchidism (3/3).

Complications: Unknown.

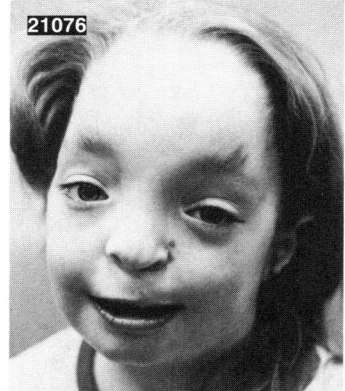

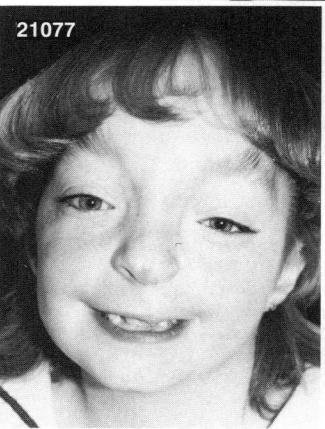
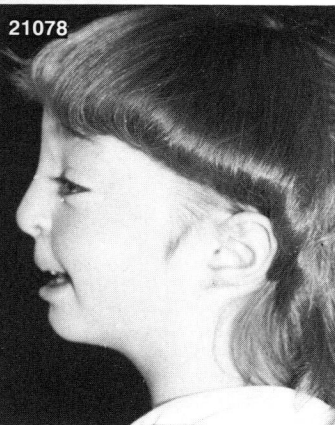

2628-21076–77: Note similarity of facial features to those of fetal aminopterin syndrome including ocular hypertelorism, widow's peak, temporal hair recession and upswept pattern, arched eyebrows with medial flaring. **21078:** Lateral view demonstrates the prominent nasal root, micrognathia and low-set ear.

Associated Findings: Findings in only one of four patients include **Cleft lip**, **Hydrocephaly**, distal shortening of limbs, and thin long bones with constricted narrow cavities (as in the aminopterin syndrome).

Etiology: Possibly autosomal recessive inheritance, if sibs reported by Crane and Heise (1981) represent this condition. One case was found to be mosaic for an apparently symmetrical translocation involving 5q35 and 10q22.

Pathogenesis: Unknown.

Sex Ratio: Undetermined but presumably M1:F1.

Occurrence: Four cases have been reported in the literature.

Risk of Recurrence for Patient's Sib: Unknown.

Risk of Recurrence for Patient's Child: Unknown.

Age of Detectability: At birth. Prenatal detection of some signs may be possible by ultrasound.

Gene Mapping and Linkage: Unknown.

Prevention: None known. Genetic counseling indicated.

Treatment: Surgical management of craniosynostosis, hydrocephalus, possibly hypertelorism, and digital anomalies when indicated.

Prognosis: Unknown.

Detection of Carrier: Unknown.

References:

Shaw EB, Rees EL: Fetal damage due to aminopterin ingestion: follow-up at 17 1/2 years of age. Am J Dis Child 1980; 134:1172–1173.

Crane JP, Heise RL: New syndrome in three affected siblings. Pediatrics 1981; 68:235–237.

Fraser FC, et al.: An aminopterin-like syndrome without aminopterin (ASSAS). Clin Genet 1987; 32:28–34. * †

FR009   **F. Clarke Fraser**

Pseudoleprechaunism
See PSEUDOLEPRECHAUNISM, PATTERSON TYPE

PSEUDOLEPRECHAUNISM, PATTERSON TYPE   2626

Includes:
    Patterson pseudoleprechaunism
    Pseudoleprechaunism

Excludes: Leprechaunism

Major Diagnostic Criteria: The combination of normal birth weight, bronzed hyperpigmentation, cutis laxa of large hands and feet, hirsutism, and skeletal dysplasia.

Clinical Findings: Findings reported in two affected individuals include normal birth weight (2/2), congenital redundant skin folds (2/2), bronze hyperpigmentation (2/2), hirsutism (2/2), large and beaked nose (2/2), large ears (2/2), large hands and feet with cutis gyrata (2/2), endocrine anomaly (premature adrenarche in one, hyperadrenocorticism in one), severe mental retardation (2/2), seizures (1/2), and skeletal anomalies that include severely delayed bone age (1/2), kyphoscoliosis (1/2), swelling of distal ends of long bones (1/2), genu valgum (1/2), and thickened cranial vault and abnormal metaphyses and diaphyses of the long bones on X-ray (1/2). Abnormal urinary glycosaminoglycan excretion was noted in one patient.

Complications: Unknown.

Associated Findings: None known.

Etiology: Possibly autosomal dominant inheritance.

Pathogenesis: Unknown.

MIM No.: 16917

POS No.: 3494

Sex Ratio: M1:F1

Occurrence: Two unrelated cases have been reported in the literature.

Risk of Recurrence for Patient's Sib:
    See Part I, *Mendelian Inheritance.*

Risk of Recurrence for Patient's Child:
    See Part I, *Mendelian Inheritance.*

Age of Detectability: At birth by physical examination.

Gene Mapping and Linkage: Unknown.

Prevention: None known. Genetic counseling indicated.

Treatment: Unknown.

Prognosis: One patient died at age seven years. The other patient was age 12 years at the time of the report. Both were severely mentally retarded.

Detection of Carrier: Unknown.

References:
Patterson JH: Presentation of a patient with leprechaunism. BD:OAS V(4). New York: March of Dimes Birth Defects Foundation, 1969: 117–121.
David TJ, et al.: The Patterson syndrome, leprechaunism, and pseudoleprechaunism. J Med Genet 1981; 18:294–298.

T0007   **Helga V. Toriello**

Pseudometatropic dwarfism
See KNIEST DYSPLASIA
Pseudoobstruction, chronic idiopathic intestinal, neuronal type
See INTESTINAL PSEUDO-OBSTRUCTION SYNDROMES
Pseudopapilledema-macrocephaly-multiple hemangiomata
See OVERGROWTH, MACROCEPHALY-HEMANGIOMA, RILEY-SMITH TYPE
Pseudopolysystrophy
See MUCOLIPIDOSIS III
Pseudothalidomide syndrome
See ROBERTS SYNDROME
Pseudothalidomide-SC syndrome
See ROBERTS SYNDROME
Pseudotoxoplasmosis syndrome
See MICROCEPHALY WITH CHORIORETINOPATHY

Pseudovaginal perineoscrotal hypospadias
See STEROID 5 ALPHA-REDUCTASE DEFICIENCY
Pseudovitamin D-deficiency rickets (PDR)
See RESISTANCE TO 1,25 DIHYDROXY VITAMIN D
Pseudovitamin D-deficiency rickets (PDR), hereditary
See RICKETS, VITAMIN D-DEPENDENT, TYPE I

PSEUDOXANTHOMA ELASTICUM   0832

Includes:
    Angioid streaks with skin changes
    Elastosis dystrophica
    Groenblad-Strandberg syndrome
    PXE
    Systemic elastorrhexis

Excludes: Senile elastosis

Major Diagnostic Criteria: Angioid streaks and typical pseudoxanthoma elasticum (PXE) skin changes in the absence of **Bone, Paget disease**. Angioid streaks also occur with Paget disease of bone and with **Anemia, sickle cell**. Encrustation of a normal Bruch membrane by calcium and iron, respectively, may be responsible.

Clinical Findings: Changes occur in the skin, eyes, and arteries. The name used for this condition refers to the skin changes which superficially resemble xanthoma and histologically show degeneration of elastic fibers. The skin lesions are usually discernible by the second decade at the latest and are most striking around the neck and in the axilla. The skin of the antecubital area, groin, penis, and periumbilical area may be affected also. The changes consist of yellowish nodular or reticular thickening. The skin about the mouth and chin and in the areas of the nasolabial folds is loose and thickened. The mucosa on the inside of the lower lip may be thickened and yellow, with a superficial vascular network. Not all patients show the chracteristic skin lesions, and scar biopsy may be helpful in establishing the diagnosis in such cases.

    In the eyes, the hallmark is angioid streaks: irregular streaking radiating from the disk and lying behind the retinal vessels; so called because of their superficial resemblance to vessels. They are likely to disappear when pressure is applied to the globe. Histologically they can be shown to result from breaks in the Bruch membrane. Hemorrhages also occur in the fundus and threaten vision, especially when they are located in the region of the macula.

    Degeneration in the elastic fibers of arteries is accompanied by rupture (especially in the submucosa of the alimentary tract, so that GI bleeding is a major complication in terms of frequency and clinical significance) or occlusion (e.g. in coronary arteries, cerebral arteries, or arteries of limbs).

Complications: Blindness, rarely complete. Occlusion of cerebral, coronary, or peripheral arteries with expected clinical results. In pregnant women; deceleration of fetal growth.

Associated Findings: None known.

Etiology: Autosomal recessive or autosomal dominant inheritance. The autosomal recessive form may be less prone to vascular complications than the autosomal dominant form. Indeed, two distinct autosomal dominant forms may exist. One has severe vascular and ocular changes. The second is accompanied by mild ocular changes, blue sclerae, high palate, and loose jointedness.

Pathogenesis: Earliest discernible change in elastic fibers of corium is accretion of calcium salts. Since the fibers, as well as the Bruch membrane, seem to become brittle and fracture, this is presumably a primary disorder of elastic tissue. An inborn error of metabolism with secondary damage to the connective tissue elements (as in **Alkaptonuria** and **Homocystinuria**) is theoretically plausible, but none has been demonstrated.

MIM No.: *17785, *26480

POS No.: 3346

Sex Ratio: Presumably M1:F1 (More females come to medical attention).

Occurrence: Several hundred cases have been documented in the literature.

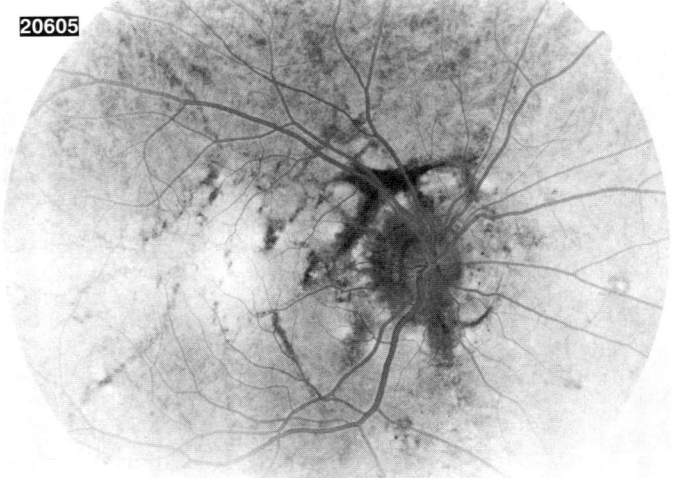

0832A-11278: Note excess and moderately loose skin of neck.

Risk of Recurrence for Patient's Sib:
See Part I, *Mendelian Inheritance.*

Risk of Recurrence for Patient's Child:
See Part I, *Mendelian Inheritance.*

Age of Detectability: Varies; from birth to third or fourth decade.

Gene Mapping and Linkage: Unknown.

Prevention: None known. Genetic counseling indicated.

Treatment: Both vitamin E and vitamin C have been recommended, but there is no evidence of benefit and little rationale for their use. Restriction of calcium intake may be advisable.

Prognosis: Normal for intelligence and early function, but life span is significantly reduced by GI bleeding and arterial occlusion.

Detection of Carrier: Unknown.

0832B-20605: Pseudoxanthoma elasticum; note angioid streaks in the fundus.

References:
McKusick VA: Heritable disorders of connective tissue, 4th ed. St. Louis: C.V. Mosby, 1972.
Pope FM: Autosomal dominant pseudoxanthoma elasticum. J Med Genet 1974; 11:152–157.
Elejalde BR, et al.: Manifestations of pseudoxanthoma elasticum during pregnancy: a case report and review of the literature. Am J Med Genet 1984; 18:755–762.
Remie WA, et al.: Pseudoxanthoma elasticum: high calcium intake in early life correlates with severity. Am J Med Genet 1984; 19:235–244.
Lebwohl M, et al.: Diagnosis of pseudoxanthoma elasticum by scar biopsy in patients without chracteristic skin lesions. New Engl J Med 1987; 317:347–350.
Beighton P, et al.: International nosology of heritable disorders of connective, Berlin, 1986. Am J Med Genet 1988; 29:581–594.

MC023   **Victor A. McKusick**

Psoriasis
See SKIN, PSORIASIS VULGARIS
Psoriasis-mental retardation, X-linked
See X-LINKED MENTAL RETARDATION-PSORIASIS
Psoriatic arthritis
See ANKYLOSING SPONDYLITIS
Psychosine lipidosis
See LEUKODYSTROPHY, GLOBOID CELL TYPE
PTA deficiency
See FACTOR XI DEFICIENCY
PTC syndrome
See ENDOCRINE NEOPLASIA, MULTIPLE TYPE II
PTC taster defect
See TASTING DEFECT, PHENYLTHIOCARBAMIDE

PTERYGIA-DYSMORPHIC FACIES-SHORT STATURE-MENTAL RETARDATION   **2770**

Includes:
Face, dysmorphic-pterygia-short stature-mental retardation
Pterygia-mental retardation-distinctive craniofacial features
Short stature-pterygia-dysmophic facies-mental retardation

Excludes:
Arthrogryposes (0088)
Arthrogryposis, distal types (2280)
Pterygium syndrome

Major Diagnostic Criteria: Shortness, unusual combination of craniofacial anomalies (trigonocephaly; bulging forehead; flat face; posteriorly angulated, low-set ears; and microretrognathia), genital hypoplasia, and multiple pterygia.

Clinical Findings: The three known patients presented with severe mental retardation and multiple congenital anomalies. The full clinical expression was present in one female: multiple pterygia (see **Pterygium syndrome, multiple**), **Cleft palate**, and genital hypoplasia. The absence of evident pterygia in the other two known patients precludes classification of this condition as a separate **Pterygium syndrome.**

Complications: Unknown.

Associated Findings: Hypothyroidism was documented in two of the three patients.

Etiology: Possibly autosomal dominant inheritance. The presence of similar facial findings in two grandmothers suggests variable expression and penetrance.

Pathogenesis: Unknown.

MIM No.: 17798

POS No.: 3843

Sex Ratio: Three females have been reported.

Occurrence: Reported cases consist of three related females who were detected in a survey of 2,000 institutionalized moderately and severely mentally retarded persons.

Risk of Recurrence for Patient's Sib:
See Part I, *Mendelian Inheritance.*

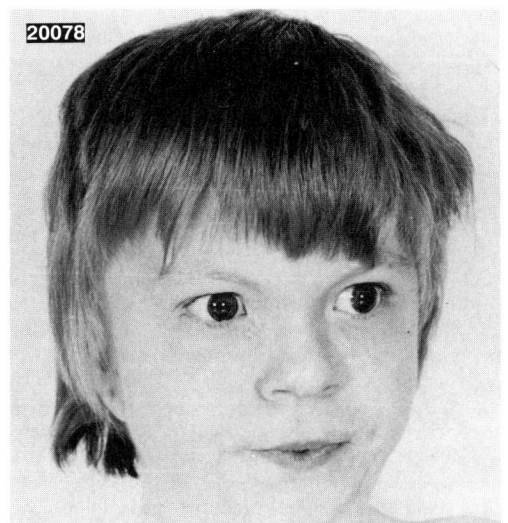

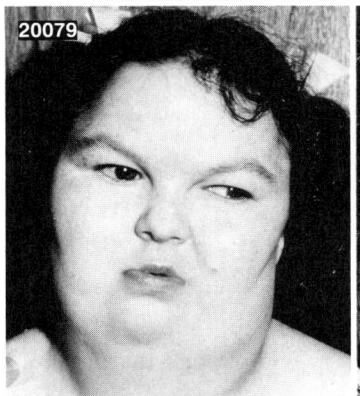 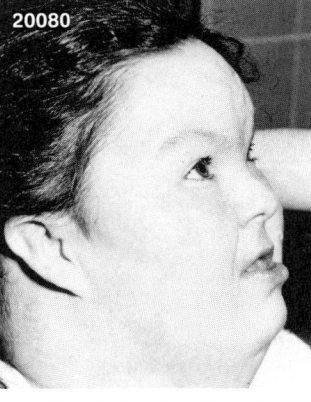

2770-20078: Note facies with prominent forehead and flat facies. 20079: Note prominent forehead and micrognathia. 20080: Lateral view of face shows prominent forehead, low-set posteriorly rotated ears and microretrognathia.

Pterygium colli
 See NECK, CYSTIC HYGROMA, FETAL TYPE
Pterygium colli syndrome
 See PTERYGIUM SYNDROME, MULTIPLE
 also NOONAN SYNDROME

PTERYGIUM SYNDROME, MULTIPLE   2186

Includes:
 Escobar syndrome
 Pterygium colli syndrome

Excludes:
 Arthrogryposes (0088)
 Pterygium syndrome, multiple lethal (2274)
 Pterygium syndrome, popliteal (0818)
 Pterygium syndrome, popliteal, lethal (3233)

Major Diagnostic Criteria: Pterygia of the neck, axillae, antecubital fossae, popliteal fossae, intercrural areas, and fingers in combination with multiple joint flexion contractures and crouched stance.

Clinical Findings: The most consistent malformations present in the multiple pterygium syndrome include growth retardation (100%), webbing of the neck (100%), antecubital fossae (90%), popliteal fossae (90%), and intercrural area (63%) all of which prevent full extension of arms and legs. Syndactyly (74%) and camptodactyly (84%) of the fingers as well as foot deformities (74%) are common findings. Multiple joint flexion contractures are common (74%) as are epicanthal folds (68%), which give the impression of hypertelorism.

Other findings reported in over 40% of the patients include long philtrum, antimongoloid slanting of the palpebral fissures, low-set ears, micrognathia, eyelid ptosis, cleft palate, down-turned corners of the mouth, rib and vertebral anomalies, scoliosis with or without lordosis, talipes equinovarus and rocker-bottomed feet. Genital anomalies in the male consist of small penis and cryptorchidism, and in the female one may see hypoplastic or absent labia majora.

Malformations less often reported are **Hernia, umbilical** (26%), **Hernia, inguinal** (26%), congenital hip dislocation (21%), and hypoplastic nipples (11%). Rare abnormalities reported in isolated cases include spina bifida occulta, **Cutis laxa**, **Hydrocephaly**, platy-

Risk of Recurrence for Patient's Child:
 See Part I, *Mendelian Inheritance.* No affected individuals are known to have reproduced.

Age of Detectability: At birth.

Gene Mapping and Linkage: Unknown.

Prevention: None known. Genetic counseling indicated.

Treatment: Thyroid substitution in patients with associated hypothyroidism. Severe mental retardation and poor motoric prognosis make institutionalization of most patients necessary.

Prognosis: Life span does not appear to be affected.

Detection of Carrier: Unknown.

References:
Hall JG, et al.: The distal arthrogryposes: delineation of new entities - review and nosologic discussion. Am J Med Genet 1982; 11:185–239.
Haspeslagh M, et al.: Mental retardation with pterygia, shortness and distinct facial appearance: a new MCA/MR syndrome. Clin Genet 1985; 28:550–555.

FR030   **Jean-Pierre Fryns**

Pterygia-mental retardation-distinctive craniofacial features
 See PTERYGIA-DYSMORPHIC FACIES-SHORT STATURE-MENTAL RETARDATION

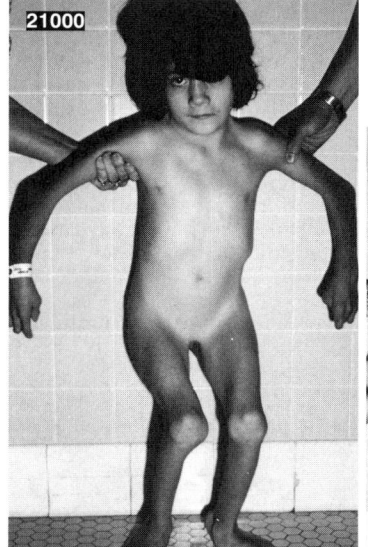 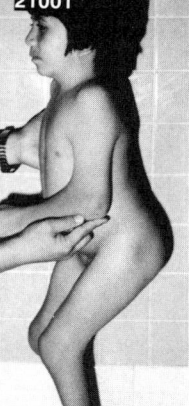

2186A-21000–01: Pterygium syndrome, multiple; note restricting pterygia and rocker-bottom feet.

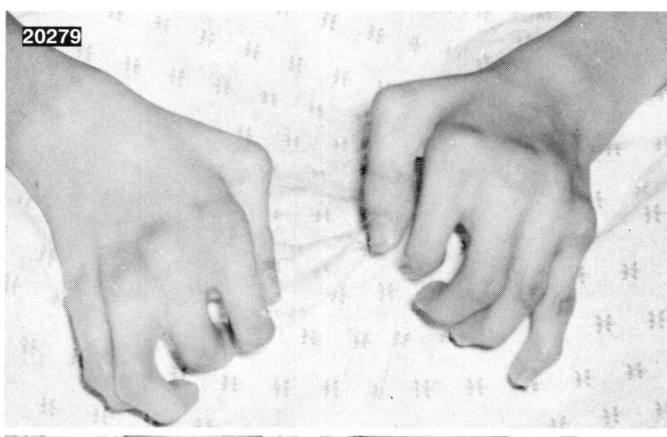

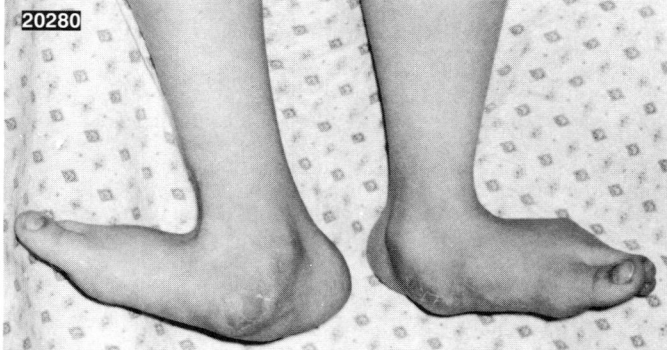

2186B-20279: Digital camptodactyly. 20280: Rocker-bottom feet.

spondyly, clitoromegaly, **Ventricular septal defect, Pectus excavatum**, bilateral pulmonary hypoplasia, small heart, absent appendix, and attenuated ascending and transverse colon.

Complications: Inability to ambulate independently because of limited extension of the legs. Lack of neck movement due to cervical vertebral fusion.

Associated Findings: Progressive joint contractures with fixation and fusion due to lack of movement. Speech difficulties. Psychologic abnormalities may develop due to crippling by the disease in the presence of an otherwise normal IQ.

Etiology: Although most cases have been sporadic, occurrences of affected sibs have been reported, lending support to an autosomal recessive pattern of inheritance.

The question of genetic heterogeneity has been raised by reports of a lethal form of multiple pterygium syndrome (see **Pterygium syndrome, multiple lethal**). Gillin and Pryse-Davies (1976) and by Hall (1984) have suggested that two other forms of the syndrome may occur: one with spinal fusion and one with congenital bone fusions.

With the exception of the patient reported by Pashayan et al. (1973) who had 47,XXY/48,XXXY mosaicism, no other chromosomal abnormalities have been reported.

Pathogenesis: The origins of the various pterygia are unknown, but biopsy specimens show the presence of muscle degeneration and disorganization of the myofibrils, a finding compatible with muscles not in use.

MIM No.: *26500

POS No.: 3472

Sex Ratio: M1:F1

Occurrence: About 50 cases reported in the French, German, and English literature.

Risk of Recurrence for Patient's Sib: See Part I, *Mendelian Inheritance*.

Risk of Recurrence for Patient's Child: See Part I, *Mendelian Inheritance*.

Age of Detectability: At birth, with affected individuals showing multiple pterygia and joint flexion contractures. Prenatal diagnosis by ultrasound may be possible.

Gene Mapping and Linkage: Unknown.

Prevention: None known. Genetic counseling indicated.

Treatment: Plastic reconstructive surgery for the cleft palate, popliteal and antecubital fossae pterygia, and the syndactyly. Physical therapy helps to prevent joint fixation.

Prognosis: After surgery and with the help of physical therapy, walking and body movements will improve. Life span appears to be normal.

Detection of Carrier: Because of phenotypic variation, a careful clinical examination and history of all relatives of an affected patient will help to identify those who are minimally affected.

Special Considerations: Major nerves and blood vessels lie free within the pterygia and may be too short for full extension of the extremity. Also, if plastic surgery of the pterygium is attempted and these facts are unrecognized, sectioning of major motor nerves may occur.

References:

Pashayan H, et al.: Bilateral aniridia, multiple webs and severe mental retardation in a 47 XXY/48 XXXY mosaic. Clin Genet 1973; 4:126–129.
Gillin ME, Pryse-Davies J: Pterygium syndrome. J Med Genet 1976; 13:249–251.
Escobar V, et al.: Multiple pterygium syndrome. Am J Dis Child 1978; 132:609–611.
Chen H, et al.: Multiple pterygium syndrome. Am J Med Genet 1980; 7:91–102.
Stoll C, et al.: Familial pterygium syndrome. Clin Genet 1980; 18:317–320.
Hall JG, et al.: Limb pterygium syndromes: a review and report of eleven patients. Am J Med Genet 1982; 12:377–409.
Hall JG: The lethal multiple pterygium syndromes.(Editorial) Am J Med Genet 1984; 17:803–807.
Thompson EM, et al.: Multiple pterygium syndrome: evolution of the phenotype. J Med Genet 1987; 24:733–749. *

ES000   **Victor Escobar**

PTERYGIUM SYNDROME, MULTIPLE LETHAL   **2274**

Includes: Lethal multiple pterygium syndrome

Excludes:

    Pena-Shokeir syndrome (2080)

    Pterygium syndrome, multiple (2186)

    Pterygium syndrome, popliteal, lethal (3233)

Major Diagnostic Criteria: Multiple pterygia with flexion contractures, intrauterine growth retardation, cystic hygroma and/or fetal hydrops, and uniform lethality (12 cases: mean gestational age, 29 menstrual weeks).

Clinical Findings: Early in the second trimester some fetuses have appeared normal but subcutaneous edema and cystic hygroma of the neck have been seen, and the ultrasonic measurements have frequently suggested intrauterine growth retardation. Later in gestation, nuchal cystic hygroma and/or fetal hydrops, absent limb movements in the fetus, or polyhydramnios in the mother may be visualized by ultrasound.

Clinically, the multiple pterygia are seen in the chin-to-sternum, cervical, axillary, antecubital, crural, and popliteal regions in association with prominent flexion contractures of the limbs. Nuchal cystic hygroma, generalized fetal hydrops, and loose edematous skin are also observed. Facial dysmorphology has included epicanthal folds, flattened nose, apparently low-set ears, hypertelorism, micrognathia and, occasionally, cleft lip and/or palate.

X-ray studies have revealed microbrachydactyly, a flattened

mandibular angle, absence of the normal cervicothoracic curvature, thiness of the ribs and other bones (some associated with fractures and dislocations), and fusions of the posterior vertebral spinous processes and elbows in the older fetuses.

At autopsy, hypoplastic lungs and heart, and atrophic musculature have been consistently present, and in the fetuses studied, degeneration and paucity of anterior horn motor neurons were observed. One of 46,XY monozygotic twins had female genitalia similar to the sex reversal seen in **Smith-Lemli-Opitz syndrome, type II**.

Complications: Malignant hyperthermia was reported in one case (Robinson et al, 1987).

Associated Findings: There appear to be several subtypes which are consistent within a family but quite variable between families. One subtype is associated with spinal fusion (Chen et al, 1984), and another with bone fusions (Chen et al, 1984; Van Regemorter, 1984).

Etiology: Usually autosomal recessive inheritance, although a few families have shown apparent X-linked inheritance. Sporadic cases have been reported.

Pathogenesis: Unknown.

MIM No.: 25329, 31215

POS No.: 4255

Sex Ratio: M1:F1

Occurrence: About 200 cases have been observed.

Risk of Recurrence for Patient's Sib:
See Part I, *Mendelian Inheritance.*

Risk of Recurrence for Patient's Child:
See Part I, *Mendelian Inheritance.* Affected individuals are not expected to survive to reproduce.

Age of Detectability: Ultrasound examination has detected affected sibs in families at risk on the basis of **Hydrops fetalis, non-immune**, cystic hygroma on the back of the head and neck, diminished fetal activity, short or fixed limbs, intrauterine growth retardation, and/or by maternal polyhydramnios. Real-time ultrasound will probably detect decreased fetal movement by 10–12 weeks; however, in one of the first families reported, a normal ultrasound examination at 22 menstrual weeks failed to detect an affected fetus.

Gene Mapping and Linkage: Unknown.

Prevention: None known. Genetic counseling indicated.

Treatment: Unknown.

Prognosis: Uniformly lethal.

Detection of Carrier: Unknown.

References:

Hall JG, et al.: Limb pterygium syndromes: a review and report of eleven patients. Am J Med Genet 1982; 12:377–409.
Hall JG: The lethal multiple pterygium syndromes. Am J Med Genet 1984; 17:803–807.
Chen H, et al.: Syndrome of multiple pterygia, camptodactyly, facial anomalies, hypoplastic lungs and heart, cystic hygroma, and skeletal anomalies; delineation of a new entity and review of lethal forms of multiple pterygium syndrome. Am J Med Genet 1984; 17:809–826.
Van Regemorter N, et al.: Lethal multiple pterygium syndrome. Am J Med Genet 1984; 17:827–834.
Herva R, et al.: A lethal autosomal recessive syndrome of multiple congenital contractures. Am J Med Genet 1985; 20:431–439.
Hogge WA, et al.: The lethal multiple pterygium syndromes: is prenatal detection possible? (Letter) Am J Med Genet 1985; 20:441–442.
Martin NJ, et al.: Lethal multiple pterygium syndrome: three consecutive cases in one family. Am J Med Genet 1986; 24:295–304.
Robinson LK, et al.: Lethal multiple pterygium syndrome. Clin Genet 1987; 32:5–9.

DU003   **Peter A. Duncan**
SH009   **Lawrence R. Shapiro**

PTERYGIUM SYNDROME, POPLITEAL   **0818**

Includes:
>   Cleft lip/palate-popliteal pterygium-digital and genital anomalies
>   Facio-genito-popliteal syndrome
>   Paramedian lower lip pits-popliteal pterygium
>   Popliteal pterygium syndrome
>   Webbing, popliteal

Excludes:
>   **Arthrogryposes** (0088)
>   **Cleft lip/palate-lip pits or mounds** (0177)
>   **Noonan syndrome** (0720)
>   **Pterygium syndrome, multiple** (2186)
>   **Pterygium syndrome, popliteal, lethal** (3233)
>   **Sirenomelia sequence** (3191)

Major Diagnostic Criteria: Popliteal webbing (pterygium); pits of lower lip; cleft lip-palate or cleft palate; and genital anomalies.

Clinical Findings: Bilateral, rarely unilateral, popliteal pterygium extending from the heel to the ischial tuberosity; intercrural pterygia; cleft lip-palate; and pits or fistulas of the lower lip. Genital anomalies in the male include cryptorchidism and absent or cleft scrotum, and in the female include absence of labia majora and enlarged clitoris. **Syndactyly** of hands or feet, filiform adhesions between the upper and lower lids, and hypoplasia or agenesis of digits may also be present.

Complications: Walking difficulties due to limited extension, rotation and abduction of the legs; speech impairment, hearing impairment, and frequent otitis media with conductive hearing loss in patients with cleft palate.

Associated Findings: None known.

Etiology: Autosomal dominant inheritance with variable expressivity.

2274-20585: Pterygium syndrome, multiple lethal; note skin webbing at the neck, axillae, antecubital, crural and popliteal areas along with marked edema of the skin and maceration. The nasal bridge was flattened with hypoplastic nasal alae; the ears were low-set and the mouth small.

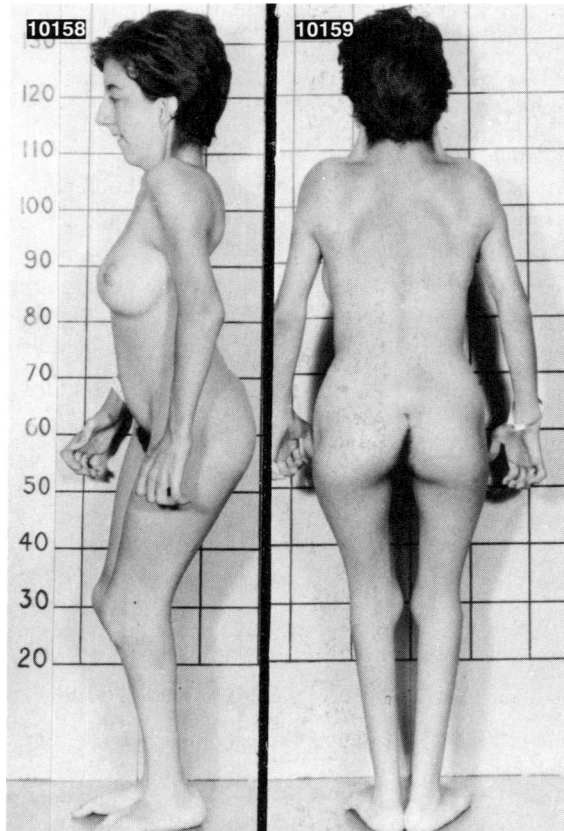

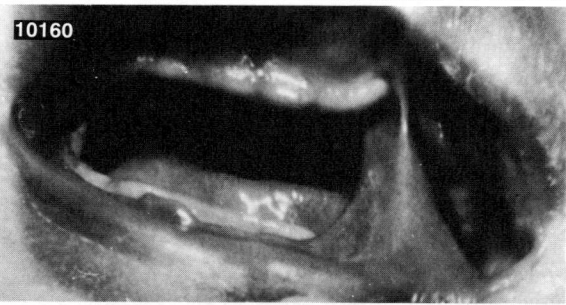

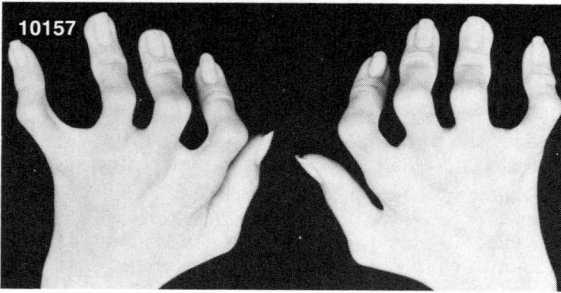

0818A-10158–59: Short stature, marked webbed neck, low posterior hairline, flexion contractures of the fingers and knees and foot deformities. 10160: Soft tissue bands extending from the lower lip to maxillary alveolus at site of incomplete cleft palate. 10157: Maximal extension of fingers with flexion contractures.

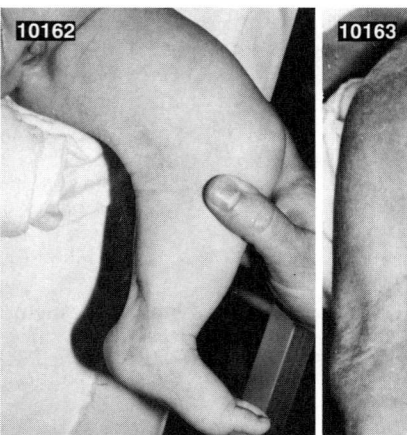

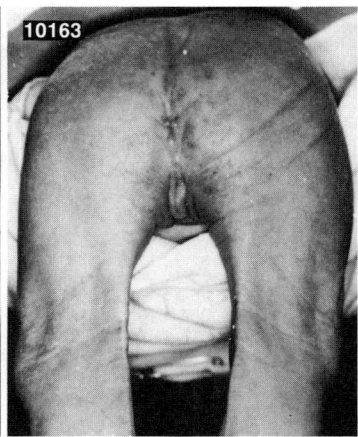

0818B-10162: Popliteal ptyergium extending over the popliteal space to the intercrural area with hypoplasia of the labia minora. 10163: Posterior view of popliteal ptyergium and hypoplasia of the labia minora.

Pathogenesis: Unknown.

MIM No.: *11950

POS No.: 3360

Sex Ratio: M1:F1

Occurrence: Undetermined. Some 60 cases reported in the literature.

Risk of Recurrence for Patient's Sib:
See Part I, *Mendelian Inheritance.*

Risk of Recurrence for Patient's Child:
See Part I, *Mendelian Inheritance.*

Age of Detectability: At birth.

Gene Mapping and Linkage: Unknown.

Prevention: None known. Genetic counseling indicated.

Treatment: Plastic reparative surgery for cleft lip-palate, lip pits, popliteal pterygium (the sciatic nerve lies free within the pterygium; if plastic surgery of the webbing is attempted and this is not recognized, sectioning of the nerve may occur), ankyloblepharon, and syndactyly; speech therapy. Myringotomy and placement of ventilation tubes if middle ear fluid persists.

Prognosis: After surgery, walking will improve as well as speech. General health is not impaired, but disability may be extensive.

Detection of Carrier: Unknown.

References:
Gorlin RJ, et al.: Popliteal pterygium syndrome: syndrome comprising cleft lip-palate, popliteal and intercrural pterygia, digital and genital anomalies. Pediatrics 1968; 41:503–509.
Bixler D, et al.: Phenotypic variation in the popliteal pterygium syndrome. Clin Genet 1973; 4:220–228.
Escobar V, Weaver, DD: The facio-genito-popliteal syndrome. BD: OAS XIV(6B). New York: March of Dimes Birth Defects Foundation, 1978:185–192.
Pashayan HM, Lewis MB: A family with the popliteal pterygium syndrome. Cleft Palate J 1980; 17:48–51.
Hall J, et al.: Limit pterygium syndromes: a review and report of eleven patients. Am J Med Genet 1982; 12:377–409.
Audino G, et al.: Popliteal pterygium syndrome present with orofacial abnormalities. J Maxellofac Surg 1984; 12:174–177.
Steinberg B, Saunders V: Popliteal pterygium syndrome. Oral Surg 1987; 63:17–20.

Heddie O. Sedano

PTERYGIUM SYNDROME, POPLITEAL, LETHAL 3233

Includes:
Bartsocas-Papas syndrome
Popliteal pterygium syndrome, lethal type

Excludes:
Pena-Shokeir syndrome (2080)
Pterygium syndrome, multiple (2186)
Pterygium syndrome, multiple lethal (2274)
Pterygium syndrome, popliteal (0818)

Major Diagnostic Criteria: Marked popliteal pterygium with cord containing nerve and vessels, synostosis of hand and foot bones, digital hypoplasia, and **Syndactyly.**

Clinical Findings: Marked popliteal pterygium with cord containing nerve and vessels, synostosis of hand and foot bones, digital hypoplasia, and **Syndactyly** of the hands and feet. Facial clefts, ectropion, **Eyelid, ankyloblepharon,** hypoplastic nasal tip, filiform bands between the jaws, and corneal anomalies have also been reported.

Complications: Unknown.

Associated Findings: Supernumerary nipples, hypoplastic external genitalia, and lanugo hair.

Etiology: Autosomal recessive inheritance.

Pathogenesis: Unknown.

MIM No.: *26365

Sex Ratio: M1:F1

Occurrence: About a half-dozen cases have been reported.

Risk of Recurrence for Patient's Sib:
See Part I, *Mendelian Inheritance.*

Risk of Recurrence for Patient's Child:
See Part I, *Mendelian Inheritance.*

Age of Detectability: At birth. Prenatal diagnosis may be possible by ultrasound.

Gene Mapping and Linkage: Unknown.

Prevention: None known. Genetic counseling indicated.

Treatment: Unknown.

Prognosis: Lethal.

Detection of Carrier: Unknown.

References:
Bartsocas CS, Papas CV: Popliteal pterygium syndrome: evidence for a severe autosomal recessive form. J Med Genet 1972; 9:222–226.
DiStefano G, Romeo MG: La sindrome dello pterigio popliteo. Riv Ped Sic 1974; 29:54–75.
Hall JG, et al.: Limb pterygium syndromes: a review and report of eleven patients. Am J Med Genet 1982; 12:377–409.
Hall JG: The lethal multiple pterygium syndromes. Am J Med Genet 1984; 17:803–807.
Papadia F, et al.: The Bartsocas-Papas syndrome: autosomal recessive form of popliteal pterygium syndrome in a male infant. Am J Med Genet 1984; 17:841–847. * †

DU003
SH009

Peter A. Duncan
Lawrence R. Shapiro

Pterygoid-levator synkinesis
See JAW-WINKING SYNDROME
Ptosis and miosis with ophthalmoplegia totalis
See OPHTHALMOPLEGIA, TOTAL WITH PTOSIS AND MIOSIS
Ptosis, congenital
See EYELID, PTOSIS, CONGENITAL
Ptosis-epicanthus
See EYELID, PTOSIS, CONGENITAL
Ptosis-inferior rectus fibrosis, congenital hereditary
See EYE, FIBROSIS OF THE EXTRAOCULAR MUSCLES, GENERALIZED
Ptosis-superior rectus weakness
See EYELID, PTOSIS, CONGENITAL
Puberty, incoordinate pattern of in adult male
See ANDROGEN INSENSITIVITY (RESISTANCE), MINIMAL

Pulmonary arterial stenosis-neonatal liver disease
See ARTERIO-HEPATIC DYSPLASIA
Pulmonary artery absent, blood supplied by ductus arteriosus
See PULMONARY ARTERY, ORIGIN FROM DUCTUS ARTERIOSUS
Pulmonary artery origin from contralateral ductus arteriosus
See PULMONARY ARTERY, ORIGIN FROM DUCTUS ARTERIOSUS
Pulmonary artery origin from ipsilateral ductus arteriosus
See PULMONARY ARTERY, ORIGIN FROM DUCTUS ARTERIOSUS
Pulmonary artery ring
See PULMONARY ARTERY, ORIGIN OF THE LEFT FROM RIGHT PULMONARY ARTERY
Pulmonary artery stenosis
See PULMONARY ARTERY, COARCTATION
Pulmonary artery subclavian steal
See AORTA, ISOLATION OF SUBCLAVIAN ARTERY FROM AORTA
Pulmonary artery, aberrant left
See PULMONARY ARTERY, ORIGIN OF THE LEFT FROM RIGHT PULMONARY ARTERY

PULMONARY ARTERY, COARCTATION 0835

Includes:
Pulmonary artery stenosis
Pulmonary branch stenosis
Supravalvular pulmonary stenosis

Excludes:
Pulmonary artery atresia
Pulmonary hypertension, primary or secondary
Pulmonary stenosis, infundibular
Pulmonary valve, stenosis (0839)
Pulmonary vascular disease, occlusive

Major Diagnostic Criteria: The characteristic systolic murmurs, heard equally well in both axillae and back as over the base, should suggest the diagnosis, particularly when the patient has **Fetal rubella syndrome, Williams syndrome, Noonan syndrome,** or biliary dysgenesis. Pulmonary artery angiocardiography demonstrates the anatomic constrictions. Differentiation between transient, anatomic, hemodynamic, and syndrome categories is advisable.

Clinical Findings: The murmurs of pulmonary artery coarctations are the most common murmurs encountered in the newborn nursery (5% of newborns in one series). In the great majority of cases, these murmurs represent a transient benign condition which disappears with the normal growth and maturation of the pulmonary vascular bed. In a small percentage of cases, the murmurs are produced by the high pulmonary flow of a left-to-right shunt or true anatomic constriction of the pulmonary arteries. In the case of true coarctation the pathologic anatomy varies from a discrete, abrupt narrowing (often at a bifurcation) to a diffuse elongation. Generalized hypoplasia is rarely present in 1 or both main branches. Stenoses often are multiple, but in most cases are only mildly obstructive. Histologically there is intimal thickening and fibrosis with fragmentation of the internal elastic laminae at the site of the obstruction with vein-like dilatation of the distal artery. There may be calcification of the intima in later stages. Four anatomic groups have been described: Type I: in which the stenosis is in the main pulmonary trunk or near its point of bifurcation into the main pulmonary arteries; Type II: stenosis at the bifurcation extending into the left or right branch, or both; Type III: multiple peripheral stenoses; and Type IV: stenosis of the main pulmonary trunk plus peripheral stenoses. Associated cardiac anomalies are common, particularly **Pulmonary valve, stenosis, Ductus arteriosus, patent, Ventricular septal defect, Atrial septal defects,** and **Heart, tetralogy of Fallot.** The likelihood that the coarctations are anatomically significant is greatly increased if the patient has any one of the following syndromes: **Fetal rubella syndrome, Williams syndrome,** or **Noonan syndrome.** In fact, most patients who have severe pulmonary artery coarctations have one of these three syndromes.

The hemodynamic alterations, and consequently the clinical picture, will vary with the degree of obstruction of the pulmonary artery coarctation(s). The presence of an associated lesion will influence the clinical picture. The presence of branch stenosis may be masked by pulmonary valvar or infundibular stenosis, or accentuated by increased pulmonary flow.

The pathophysiology resembles that of pulmonary valve stenosis. With increasing degrees of obstruction there is increased right ventricular hypertension and, consequently, hypertrophy. Certain cases may be progressive and eventually lead to severe and extensive stenosis. Cardiac failure may then occur, resulting in cardiomegaly and right atrial hypertension. A right-to-left shunt across a patent foramen ovale then causes cyanosis.

Continuous murmurs are rarely heard. The usual murmur in pulmonary artery coarctation consists of high-pitched ejection murmur(s) heard in the right axilla, left axilla and back, as well as over the base. There is usually no ejection click and the second heart sound is normal in most cases. The murmurs resemble the peripheral lung murmurs caused by very large atrial level left-to-right shunts. It should be emphasized that, although the great majority of newborns who have murmurs of peripheral pulmonary artery coarctation have a benign, transient condition, these newborns should be followed through sequential visits until the murmurs disappear. If the murmurs are present for more than 3 months, anatomic coarctation or increased pulmonary flow from a shunt should be suspected. Atrial septal defect is not infrequently misdiagnosed as benign pulmonary artery coarctation (until congestive heart failure becomes manifest).

The EKG may be normal in the presence of very mild obstruction. Usually right ventricular hypertrophy of the pressure overload type is present (the degree depending on the severity of the obstruction).

The X-ray findings in isolated pulmonary artery stenosis are not characteristic. With severe bilateral stenosis, the pulmonary arterial vascular workings are diminished. The cardiac silhouette may assume a right ventricular contour, but the pulmonary artery segment is not enlarged.

At cardiac catheterization, a consistent peak systolic pressure gradient within the pulmonary arterial bed of 10mm Hg is consistent with anatomic pulmonary artery coarctation (but may also be found in high pulmonary flow from left-to-right shunts). With severe bilateral stenoses, the morphology of the proximal main pulmonary artery pressure pulse often exhibits a wide pulse pressure characterized by a fast upstroke, a depressed dicrotic notch and a slow diastolic runoff. Indeed, it may show "ventricularization," ie resemble the right ventricular pressure tracing, very similar to that of massive pulmonic valve regurgitation. The degree of right ventricular and right atrial hypertension depends on the severity of the obstruction. In the presence of an associated lesion, the above findings will be changed. For example, an increase in the pressure difference across the coarctation is seen with a large left-to-right shunt.

Complications: Right heart failure, right-to-left shunt at atrial level with desaturation and elevated hematocrit, progressive stenosis of coarctations with increasing right ventricular hypertension, pulmonary artery thrombosis, rupture of distal dilated arteries with hemoptysis, and persistent right ventricular hypertension after total correction of the associated cardiac defect (such as tetralogy of Fallot).

Associated Findings: Pulmonary artery coarctations are particularly common in certain syndromes. These include **Fetal rubella syndrome, Williams syndrome, Noonan syndrome** and biliary dysgenesis (with or without peculiar facies).

Etiology: Multifactorial inheritance is postulated in **Williams syndrome** and in sporadic cases. The condition is found in the autosomal dominant **Noonan syndrome**, following profound teratogenic maternal exposure to rubella virus. and in the biliary dysgenesis syndrome, which may have a teratogenic basis.

Pathogenesis: A teratogenic insult (e.g. rubella) may cause a defect in the internal elastic laminae of the artery, producing a localized weakness in the wall in response to pulsatile pressure at systemic levels in utero. Resultant medial damage will then cause intimal hyperplasia and fibrosis.

Other theories include: an inflammatory lesion in an area of turbulent flow (arterial branch) may cause intimal fibrosis, or a

teratogenic insult may cause slowing of the maturation and development of certain segments of the pulmonary vascular bed.

MIM No.: *18550

CDC No.: 747.380

Sex Ratio: M1:F1

Occurrence: The occurrence of hemodynamically significant branch stenosis is small: of the order of 1:20,000. The frequency of transient benign disease in the newborn is about 5%. Prevalence varies from higher rates during the rubella pandemic of 1964–65, to lower rates at present.

Risk of Recurrence for Patient's Sib:
See Part I, *Mendelian Inheritance*. Varies depending on etiology.

Risk of Recurrence for Patient's Child:
See Part I, *Mendelian Inheritance*. Varies depending on etiology.

Age of Detectability: In infancy.

Gene Mapping and Linkage: Unknown.

Prevention: Rubella vaccination for non-pregnant females. Genetic counseling is indicated.

Treatment: Arterial reconstruction if stenosis is severe enough and repair is anatomically feasible; lobectomy if multiple peripheral stenoses are localized to one area of the lung. Symptomatic therapy for relief of congestive heart failure.

Prognosis: The severity, location, and extent of the stenoses, and the presence or absence of associated syndromes and cardiac defects, determine the prognosis.

Detection of Carrier: Varies depending upon etiology.

References:
Dunkle LM, Rowe RD: Transient murmur simulating pulmonary artery stenosis in premature infants. Am J Dis Child 1972; 124:666.
Nora JJ, et al.: The Ullrich-Noonan syndrome (Turner phenotype). Am J Dis Child 1974; 127:48. *
Toews WH, et al.: Presentation of atrial septal defect in infancy. JAMA 1975; 234:1250.
Nora JJ, Nora AH. Genetics and counseling in cardiovascular diseases. Springfield: Charles C. Thomas, 1978:105–108.
O'Connor WN, et al.: Supravalvular aortic stenosis: clinical and pathologic observations in six patients. Arch Path Lab Med 1985; 109:179–185.

N0003   **James J. Nora**
N0004   **Audrey H. Nora**

PULMONARY ARTERY, ORIGIN FROM ASCENDING AORTA   0767

Includes: Ascending aorta, origin of pulmonary artery

Excludes: Pulmonary artery, origin from ductus arteriosus (0768)

Major Diagnostic Criteria: Cases of congenital origin of either the right or left pulmonary artery in which the affected lung in actual fact is supplied by a vessel arising from the ascending aorta proximal to the take-off of the first (brachio) cephalic vessel, with or without other cardiac defects.

Diagnosis must be established by cardiac catheterization with angiography in the aortic root, showing a pulmonary artery arising from the ascending aorta.

Clinical Findings: Origin of a pulmonary artery from the ascending aorta may occur either on the right or left side. Those on the right tend to be posterior in origin and those on the left anterior. Abnormal origin of one of the pulmonary arteries is usually, not always, contralateral to the aortic arch. The branching pattern of the other aortic arch vessels is usually normal for the situs of the arch. Most commonly the right pulmonary artery is anomalous. With **Heart, tetralogy of Fallot**, the left pulmonary artery is more commonly anomalous, regardless of the sites of the aortic arch.

Symptoms are similar to those of a large left-to-right shunt, and occur in early infancy. Heart failure is common while pulmonary resistances allow a large flow. Elevated pressures in both pulmonary arteries are generally found. If pulmonary resistances increase, as is usual in untreated cases, pulmonary flow will decrease, and eventually cyanosis and hemoptysis will occur, with pulmonary vascular obstructive disease.

The EKG will usually reveal biventricular hypertrophy in early cases, evolving to right ventricular hypertrophy if pulmonary vascular obstructive disease develops. X-ray of the chest may show increased vascularity and cardiomegaly in cases with large left-to-right shunts. Progressive pulmonary vascular obstruction results in decreased heart size and vascularity. Pulmonary function studies may show that the involved lung contributes very little, if any, to gas exchange, although ventilation is normal.

Radioactive isotopes injected intravenously will result in no uptake in the affected side.

Complications: Congestive heart failure occurs with large pulmonary blood flow. Hypoxia and hemoptysis result from pulmonary vascular obstructive disease.

Associated Findings: If the defect is associated with **Heart, tetralogy of Fallot, Ventricular septal defect**, or **Ductus arteriosus, patent**, complications of those defects may be present.

Etiology: Unknown.

Pathogenesis: *Anterior type*: In these cases the anomalous pulmonary artery is made up of the left 4th arch (in cases with a right aortic arch), a segment of the dorsal aorta, the distal portion of the left 6th arch, and the left embryonic pulmonary artery. Presumably, in such cases, the segment of the left dorsal aorta between the 6th arch and the 7th intersegmental artery is interrupted, resulting in a left subclavian artery arising anomalously from the descending aorta.

Posterior type: The artery is made up of the proximal portion of the 6th arch and the embryonic pulmonary artery. Apparently, at the time of partitioning of the truncus and truncoaortic sac, it was left "stranded." It may therefore be expected to be located always on the right side in situs solitus individuals with either a right or left aortic arch.

MIM No.: 12100

CDC No.: 747.380

Sex Ratio: M1:F1

Occurrence: Undetermined but presumed rare.

Risk of Recurrence for Patient's Sib: Predicted risk < 1:100. Empiric risk undetermined.

Risk of Recurrence for Patient's Child: Predicted risk < 1:100. Empiric risk undetermined.

Age of Detectability: In infancy.

Gene Mapping and Linkage: Unknown.

Prevention: None known. Genetic counseling indicated.

Treatment: Surgical anastomosis of the anomalous artery to the main pulmonary trunk, either primarily or with a prosthetic graft, has been successful, and must be undertaken early to avoid pulmonary vascular obstructive disease. Ligation and division of an associated patent ductus arteriosus on the unaffected side is recommended. If associated with tetralogy of Fallot, repair of this defect must also be undertaken.

Prognosis: If diagnosis and surgical correction are undertaken early, prognosis is good.

Detection of Carrier: Unknown.

References:
Netter FH: The Ciba collection of medical illustrations, vol. 5. The heart. New Jersey: Ciba Publications Dept, 1969:162 only.
Cissman NJ: Anomalies of the aortic arch complex. In: Adams FH, Emmanoulides GC, eds: Heart disease in infants, children and adolescents, 3rd ed. Baltimore: Williams & Wilkins, 1983:199–215.

James J. Nora

PULMONARY ARTERY, ORIGIN FROM DUCTUS ARTERIOSUS   0768

Includes:
>   Pulmonary artery absent, blood supplied by ductus arteriosus
>   Pulmonary artery origin from contralateral ductus arteriosus
>   Pulmonary artery origin from ipsilateral ductus arteriosus

Excludes:
>   Pulmonary artery, absence of, blood not via ductus arteriosus
>   **Pulmonary artery, origin from ascending aorta** (0767)

Major Diagnostic Criteria: Discrepancy in the vascular pattern between the two lungs may suggest the diagnosis, particularly in patients in whom the symptoms and signs suggest presence of **Heart, tetralogy of Fallot**. Aortic angiography is the procedure of choice in establishing the diagnosis.

Clinical Findings: The distal pulmonary artery receives its blood supply not from the pulmonary trunk, but from a ductus arteriosus. Such a ductus arteriosus originates from the aortic arch, if the arch is on the same side, or from the innominate artery if the aortic arch is on the opposite side. There is a tendency for the ductus arteriosus to close at least partially, and thus, as a rule, a large left-to-right shunt is not present. The anomaly is uncommon as an isolated lesion. The clinical findings are largely determined by other cardiovascular anomalies, usually some form of tetralogy of Fallot. Although it most commonly occurs on the left, there have been cases reported on the right side. Recently a case was reported of both pulmonary arteries arising from a normally septated truncus, the right originating from the aorta and the left pulmonary artery from a ductus arteriosus.

If no associated lesions are present, symptoms and signs depend on the magnitude of the left-to-right shunt. If the shunt is small, or if the blood supply to the affected lung is actually decreased, patients are asymptomatic. X-rays of the chest may show discrepancy in the vascularity of the lung fields. If so, the affected lung generally shows a reduced vascular pattern. The unaffected side may show hypervascularity if no significant intracardiac right-to-left shunt is present, such as is seen in cases associated with various forms of tetralogy of Fallot. The lung on the affected side may be smaller than normal. EKG findings are usually determined by associated cardiovascular defects, and may be normal if the anomaly occurs as an isolated lesion.

Pulmonary function tests may show that the involved lung participates very little, if any, in oxygen exchange, although ventilation is normal.

Complications: In the unusual case where the lesion is isolated and the ductus arteriosus remains widely patent causing a large left-to-right shunt, congestive heart failure and respiratory infections may occur.

Associated Findings: Signs and symptoms of additional lesions such as tetralogy of Fallot may be present.

Etiology: Presumably multifactorial inheritance.

Pathogenesis: In both forms, the anomaly appears to be due to early obliteration and disappearance of the proximal portion of one or the other sixth arch. The corresponding embryonic pulmonary artery, therefore, will be supplied instead by the distal sixth arch segment, i.e. the ductus arteriosus. In some cases it may be difficult to distinguish the precise origin of the anomalous vessel, i.e. cases of origin of the pulmonary artery from the ascending aorta may occur so close to the innominate artery that a ductal origin is implicated, especially if the origin of the vessel has a narrow caliber.

MIM No.: 12100

CDC No.: 747.380

Sex Ratio: M1:F1

Occurrence: Undetermined but presumed rare.

Risk of Recurrence for Patient's Sib: Unknown.

Risk of Recurrence for Patient's Child: Unknown.

Age of Detectability: Depends largely on associated lesions. Can be detected at birth.

Gene Mapping and Linkage: Unknown.

Prevention: None known. Genetic counseling indicated.

Treatment: Surgery might be considered in those cases where the lesion is isolated, and a large left-to-right shunt is present. Anastomosis of the anomalous vessel to the pulmonary trunk may be attempted. In patients who in addition, however, have tetralogy of Fallot, the anomalous vessel may represent the main pulmonary blood supply. Then no such surgical procedure is indicated until complete correction of the tetralogy is accomplished.

Prognosis: Depends largely on associated cardiovascular anomalies. If the anomaly is the sole cardiovascular defect, prognosis depends on the magnitude of any left-to-right shunt, and on the pulmonary arteriolar resistance in the affected lung.

Detection of Carrier: Unknown.

References:
Netter FH: The Ciba collection of medical illustrations, vol. 5. The heart. New Jersey: Ciba Publications Dept, 1969:162 only.
Cissman NJ: Anomalies of the aortic arch complex. In: Adams FH, Emmanoulides GC, eds: Heart disease in infants, children and adolescents, 3rd ed. Baltimore: Williams & Wilkins, 1983:199–215.

N0003   **James J. Nora**

PULMONARY ARTERY, ORIGIN OF THE LEFT FROM RIGHT PULMONARY ARTERY   0766

Includes:
Pulmonary artery, aberrant left
Pulmonary artery ring
Pulmonary vascular ring
Vascular ring from aberrant left pulmonary artery

Excludes: Vascular rings, other

Major Diagnostic Criteria: This anomaly is characterized by the presence of a normal main pulmonary artery which courses undivided toward the right lung. The left pulmonary artery arises from the right pulmonary artery at a point just anterior and to the right of the carina of the trachea. The left pulmonary artery passes toward the left lung, posterior to the right mainstem bronchus, then posteriorly to the trachea and anteriorly to the esophagus. This is the only vascular anomaly which results in a major vessel coming between the trachea and esophagus.

Clinical Findings: Respiratory symptoms, which are usually severe, develop in early infancy. Stridor, wheezing, cyanosis, dyspnea, and recurrent respiratory infections may be present. Inspiratory stridor and chest retraction with inspiration are more prominent in this anomaly than in other types of vascular rings with expiratory stridor. Rarely, onset of respiratory symptoms have presented after the second year of life. A few children and adults with this defect have also been reported without respiratory symptoms. Clinical features are due to associated intracardiac defects or associated noncardiac congenital defects.

Chest X-ray may show hyperinflation, atelectasis, or segmental atelectasis of either lung, although the right lung is more often affected. The trachial air column above the carina may appear narrow. Tracheal indentation, anterior bowing of the right mainstem bronchus, and a downward displacement of the carina may be noticed. An anterior and leftward indentation of the barium-filled esophagus near the level of the carina is diagnostic. This finding requires lateral views. Bronchoscopy, although not diagnostic, may reveal extrinsic compression. 2-dimensional echocardiography from the suprasternal notch, computerized axial tomography, and digitally enhanced angiography may aid in the diagnosis. Pulmonary artery angiography is confirmatory. Cardiac catheterization may be required in the evaluation of associated intracardiac defects.

Complications: Pulmonary complications are characteristic because a portion of the lung is supplied by a compressed bronchus. Neurologic abnormalities or death may occur as a sequela of hypoxia. Esophageal complications do not occur in this anomaly because the esophagus is not compressed by a ring.

Associated Findings: Intracardiac defects are found in about half of the cases. Patent ductus arteriosus (25%), persistent left superior vena cava (20%), **Atrial septal defects** (20%), **Ventricular septal defect** (10%), **aortic valve stenosis, Heart, tetralogy of Fallot, Aorta, coarctation** and aberrant right subclavian artery, persistent atrioventricular canal, single ventricle, and isolation of the left subclavian artery are among the associated defects.

Associated tracheobronchial abnormalities are also found in approximately half of the cases. Complete tracheal rings ("napkin ring cartilage") occur in about 10% of cases. Direct attachment of the right upper lobe bronchus to the trachea (bronchus suus), left epiarterial bronchus, unilateral single-lobed lung, tracheomalacia, and hypoplasia of the distal trachea or bronchus may occur.

Other reported association findings are imperforate anus, **Diaphragmatic hernia**, absent gallbladder, **Biliary atresia**, partial intestinal malrotation, asplenia, **Colon, aganglionosis**, cleft lip and palate, absent left lobe of the thyroid, thymic rests, hemivertebrae, **Aorta, isolation of subclavian artery from aorta**, forearm anomalies, and **Chromosome 21, trisomy 21**.

Etiology: Unknown.

Pathogenesis: An artery from the pulmonary plexus of the embryonic lung bud normally joins a projection from the ventral part of the aortic sac to form the left pulmonary artery. These vessels and the ventral portion of the aortic arch eventually form the left pulmonary artery. The dorsal left 6th arch persists as the patent ductus arteriosus. If connection of the pulmonary plexus with the right 6th arch caudal to the lung bud across the midline occurs, the developing left pulmonary artery courses behind the developing tracheobronchial tree.

MIM No.: 12100

CDC No.: 747.380

Sex Ratio: M1:F1

Occurrence: More than 75 cases have been reported. This defect was found in approximately 1.6% of vascular rings in one large series.

Risk of Recurrence for Patient's Sib: Unknown. No affected siblings reported.

Risk of Recurrence for Patient's Child: Unknown. No affected offspring reported.

Age of Detectability: From birth. Death from airway obstruction has occurred as early as the second day of life.

Gene Mapping and Linkage: Unknown.

Prevention: None known. Genetic counseling indicated.

Treatment: Selected cases with mild symptoms may not require surgical intervention. In severe cases, surgical treatment may be effective, although the operative mortality is quite high. Division of the aberrant vessel and reanastomosis to the main pulmonary artery is required in these cases. Aggressive nonoperative management of the patient's pulmonary status is required in the mildly symptomatic patient, as well as in the preoperative stabilization of the severely symptomatic individual.

Prognosis: Severely symptomatic individuals have over 90% mortality without operative intervention. Mortality with surgical intervention is also high (38%). Persistent airway symptoms and lack of patency of the repaired left pulmonary artery are commonly found in patients surviving operation.

Detection of Carrier: Unknown.

References:
Clarkson PM, et al.: Aberrant left pulmonary artery. Am J Dis Child 1967; 113:373–377.
Nora JJ, McNamara DG: Vascular rings and related anomalies. In: Watson H, ed: Pediatric cardiology. St. Louis: C.V. Mosby, 1968: 233–241.

Tan PM, et al.: Aberrant left pulmonary artery. Br Heart J 1968; 30:110–114.
Gumbiner CH, et al.: Pulmonary artery sling. Am J Cardiol 1980; 45:311–315. * †

BR014   **J. Timothy Bricker**
MC028   **Dan G. McNamara**

Pulmonary atresia with hypoplastic right ventricle
    See PULMONARY VALVE, ATRESIA
Pulmonary atresia with normal aortic root
    See PULMONARY VALVE, ATRESIA
Pulmonary branch stenosis
    See PULMONARY ARTERY, COARCTATION
Pulmonary hypertension, familial
    See PULMONARY HYPERTENSION, PRIMARY

PULMONARY HYPERTENSION, PRIMARY   2116

Includes:
    Aminorex, effects of
    Pulmonary hypertension, familial

Excludes: Pulmonary hypertension, secondary

Major Diagnostic Criteria: Characteristic clinical findings without evidence of underlying anomalies that produce secondary pulmonary hypertension.

Clinical Findings: Accentuated pulmonary closure sound with split S2. No significant murmurs or non-specific murmurs. Severe RVH on electrocardiogram, cardiomegaly in advanced cases and increased hilar markings on chest films. Cyanosis in advanced cases. At heart catheterization the pulmonary artery and right ventricular pressures are elevated, often to systemic level, with no evidence of gradients and no findings of structural anomalies of the heart or great vessels.

Complications: Congestive heart failure, cyanosis, sudden death.

Associated Findings: Has occasionally been found associated with **Raynaud disease**.

Etiology: Some families show autosomal dominant inheritance. Certain environmental agents have been implicated, such as in the epidemic of pulmonary hypertension associated with aminorex.

Pathogenesis: Progressive occlusive changes with intimal proliferation and medial hypertrophy culminating in the characteristic plexiform lesion of the pulmonary arteries.

MIM No.: *17860

CDC No.: 747.680

Sex Ratio: M1:F1 in childhood. Females predominate among adults.

Occurrence: More than 1,000 cases have been reported. This entity represented 1–2% of adults coming to cardiac catheterization at one laboratory.

Risk of Recurrence for Patient's Sib:
    See Part I, *Mendelian Inheritance.*

Risk of Recurrence for Patient's Child:
    See Part I, *Mendelian Inheritance.* Some familial cases occur among sibs without an affected parent.

Age of Detectability: Childhood or early adult age.

Gene Mapping and Linkage: Unknown.

Prevention: Genetic counseling. Removal of environmental hazards such as animorex.

Treatment: No consistently effective program is yet available. Oxygen and vasodilators may be used in some selected cases and situations.

Prognosis: Guarded to grave.

Detection of Carrier: Unknown.

Support Groups: Dallas; American Heart Association

References:
Kingdon HS, et al.: Familial occurrence of primary pulmonary hypertension. Ann Intern Med 1966; 118:422–426.
Rogge JD, et al.: The familial occurrence of primary pulmonary hypertension. Ann Intern Med 1966; 65:672–684.
Thompson P, McRae C: Familial pulmonary hypertension: evidence of autosomal dominant inheritance. Br Heart J 1970; 32:758–760.
Lloyd JE, et al.: Familial primary pulmonary hypertension: clinical patterns. Am Rev Respir Dis 1984; 129:194–197. *

N0003   **James J. Nora**
N0004   **Audrey H. Nora**

Pulmonary regurgitation due to abnormality of pulmonary valve
    See PULMONARY VALVE, INCOMPETENCE
Pulmonary sequestration, extralobar
    See LUNG, LOBE SEQUESTRATION
Pulmonary sequestration, intralobar
    See LUNG, LOBE SEQUESTRATION
Pulmonary stenoses (peripheral)-brachytelephalangy-deafness
    See KEUTEL SYNDROME
Pulmonary stenosis, isolated infundibular
    See VENTRICLE, OBSTRUCTION WITHIN RIGHT VENTRICLE OR ITS OUTFLOW TRACT
Pulmonary stenosis-cafe-au-lait spots-mental retardation
    See PULMONIC STENOSIS-CAFE-AU-LAIT SPOTS, WATSON TYPE
Pulmonary valve atresia with intact ventricular septum
    See PULMONARY VALVE, ATRESIA
Pulmonary valve dysplasia
    See PULMONARY VALVE, STENOSIS
Pulmonary valve stenosis with intact ventricular septum
    See PULMONARY VALVE, STENOSIS
Pulmonary valve stenosis with normal aortic root
    See PULMONARY VALVE, STENOSIS

PULMONARY VALVE, ABSENT   0836

Includes:
    Tetralogy of Fallot with absent pulmonary valve
    Ventricular septal defect with absent pulmonary valve

Excludes: Pulmonary valve, atresia (0837)

Major Diagnostic Criteria: A diastolic murmur in the second and third left intercostal space at the sternal border, with enlarged pulmonary artery on X-ray and normal pulmonary vascularity, and a normal EKG, or one showing right ventricular hypertrophy, suggests the diagnosis.
    Selective pulmonary artery angiocardiography is confirmatory as it will show absence of pulmonary valve tissue or a thickened ridge of tissue with massive reflux of contrast media from the large pulmonary artery into the right ventricle.

Clinical Findings: At the site of the pulmonary valve, a ring of nodular tissue is present which has no structural characteristics of a pulmonary valve. Histologically, this tissue is composed of large pale-staining, myxomatous appearing cells. The pulmonary valvar annulus is frequently hypoplastic and therefore stenotic. Because of the pulmonic regurgitation, the right ventricle is enlarged. In addition, the pulmonary trunk and major pulmonary arterial branches are dilated, often appearing aneurysmal. The pulmonary trunk has been studied histologically and found in some cases to present a mosaic of fibers, rather than normal lamellar configuration. In the majority of patients with absent pulmonary valve a **Ventricular septal defect** coexists, usually as part of a **Heart, tetralogy of Fallot** malformation.
    The clinical findings vary depending upon the type of associated cardiac malformation. In patients with absent pulmonary valve coexisting with ventricular septal defect, the signs and symptoms of congestive cardiac failure occur in infancy. The predominant shunt in infancy is left to right with minimal cyanosis. Pulmonary insufficiency due to isolated absent pulmonary valve usually results in severe congestive heart failure early in infancy or even in utero. Patients with isolated absence of the pulmonary valve are generally asymptomatic until adulthood. The major bronchi may be partially compressed by the aneurysmally

dilated pulmonary arteries which may lead to obstructive emphysema.

Cardiac findings are those of pulmonary stenosis and pulmonary insufficiency. A to-and-fro murmur is present along the left upper sternal border. The systolic portion of the murmur is of the ejection type and may be harsh and loud, especially in those with coexistent cardiac anomalies, whereas it is softer in patients with the isolated anomaly. A diastolic murmur of pulmonary insufficiency is present and its intensity is related to the degree of reflux. The second heart sound is single. A pulmonic systolic ejection click may be present. EKG may be normal if pressures are normal, regurgitation is not gross, and there are no complicating conditions. The EKG of infants with isolated symptomatic absence of the pulmonary valve reveals right ventricular hypertrophy. Among those with coexistent ventricular septal defect, biventricular hypertrophy is observed; and in those with tetralogy of Fallot, right ventricular hypertrophy of pressure overload type. In patients with ventricular septal defect and absent pulmonary valve, generalized cardiomegaly is present on the roentgenogram. The pulmonary trunk and pulmonary vessels, especially the right pulmonary artery, are greatly enlarged and may be misinterpreted as a tumor mass. Tetralogy of Fallot with absent pulmonary valve reveals enlarged pulmonary trunk, but near normal sized cardiac silhouette. With minimal or moderate isolated pulmonary valve anomaly the cardiac size is usually normal, but in symptomatic neonates it is greatly enlarged. The pulmonary trunk is dilated.

A major echocardiographic finding is the inability to image the pulmonary valve. However, a failure to find this structure is relatively weak evidence for diagnosis. Additionally, the right pulmonary artery and right ventricle are usually dilated. Paradoxical septal motion may be present. The tricuspid valve may flutter. The remainder of the echocardiographic examination is normal. Doppler interrogation of the right vantricular outflow area shows the regurgitant flow and the data used to estimate the level of pulmonary artery pressure.

For patients with a ventricular septal defect, additional findings specific for that condition may be present. See **Ventricular septal defect**.

In patients with absent pulmonary valve associated with tetralogy of Fallot, the catheterization data are similar to those of patients with tetralogy of Fallot. Whether the shunt is right to left or left to right depends entirely upon the degree of right ventricular obstruction. In isolated absent pulmonary valve, the right ventricular systolic pressure may be normal or slightly elevated with a small systolic pressure difference across the valve related to increased pulmonary flow. In all cases, the pulmonary arterial pulse pressure contour is characteristic, showing a wide pulse pressure, low diastolic pressure (similar to the right ventricular end diastolic pressure) and a low dicrotic notch. Angiography assists in identifying the presence of associated cardiac malformations. The pulmonary trunk and major pulmonary vessels are greatly dilated and pulsatile. The right ventricular chamber is enlarged and may remain opacified for a prolonged period. The pulmonary valve is not distinct and the pulmonary annulus is narrowed. Pulmonary arteriography reveals reflux of opaque material into the right ventricle.

Complications: Congestive cardiac failure, obstructive emphysema.

Associated Findings: None known.

Etiology: Unknown.

Pathogenesis: Unknown.

Sex Ratio: M1:F1

Occurrence: 2:1,000 in one large series of operated or catherized patients.

Risk of Recurrence for Patient's Sib: Unknown.

Risk of Recurrence for Patient's Child: Unknown.

Age of Detectability: At birth.

Gene Mapping and Linkage: Unknown.

Prevention: None known. Genetic counseling indicated.

Treatment: Congestive cardiac failure and the pulmonary complications must be vigorously treated. Patients with isolated absence of pulmonary valve or with coexistent malformations who are asymptomatic do not require operation. In patients with coexistent congenital cardiac anomalies, particularly ventricular septal defect, management is more difficult and controversial. Several options have been used. Pulmonary arterial banding is a palliative procedure used in some infants with cardiac failure to reduce the left to right shunt, while others would have the ventricular septal defect closed. It may be necessary to simultaneously perform pulmonary angioplasties to reduce the size of the enlarged central pulmonary arteries. Occasionally, the pulmonary valve is replaced.

Prognosis: Poor in patients with coexistent defects, with many dying in infancy from congestive cardiac failure complicated by pulmonary disorders. Patients with tetralogy of Fallot may survive relatively symptom free into teens and 20s. Patients with isolated absent pulmonary valve survive until their 70s, although there is increasing evidence that this is not always as benign a condition as once believed. Particularly, in adults who develop unrelated pulmonary diseases resulting in pulmonary hypertension, symptoms may develop because of the increased right ventricular pressure and volume work.

Detection of Carrier: Unknown.

References:

Miller RA, et al.: Congenital absence of the pulmonary valve: the clinical syndrome of tetralogy of fallot with pulmonary regurgitation. Circulation 1962; 26:266–278.

Venables AW: Absence of the pulmonary valve with ventricular septal defect. Br Heart J 1962; 24:293–296.

Goldberg SJ, et al.: Pediatric and adolescent echocardiography: a handbook. Chicago: Year Book Medical Publishers, 1975.

M0005   **James H. Moller**

PULMONARY VALVE, ATRESIA   0837

Includes:

Atresia of pulmonary valve
Pulmonary atresia with hypoplastic right ventricle
Pulmonary atresia with normal aortic root
Pulmonary valve atresia with intact ventricular septum

Excludes:

Pulmonary valve, stenosis (0839)
Tetralogy of Fallot with pulmonary valve atresia

Major Diagnostic Criteria: Selective right ventricular angiocardiography is needed to establish the pathologic anatomy of pulmonary atresia.

Clinical Findings: The pulmonary valve is an imperforate membrane, with two or three small raphae. Right ventricular size in pulmonary atresia with intact ventricular septum is variable, the size corresponding with the size of the tricuspid valve. Small and stenotic tricuspid valves are associated with hypoplastic right ventricle while marked tricuspid insufficiency or Ebstein anomaly of the tricuspid valve occurs with an enlarged right ventricle.

Although the right ventricular infundibulum may be patent to the level of the atretic pulmonary valve, the infundibulum is markedly hypoplastic and may be separated from the atretic pulmonary valve by muscular tissue.

The right ventricle is hypertrophied and endocardial fibroelastosis may coexist. Enlarged myocardial sinusoids may connect to the coronary arterial branches. During systole blood leaves the right ventricle through the sinusoids and flows into the coronary arterial system. An atrial communication is present, usually a patent foramen ovale, or less frequently, an ostium secundum atrial septal defect.

In neonates the patent ductus arteriosus provides the sole source of pulmonary blood flow but it usually closes in the neonatal period. The diameter of the pulmonary trunk varies from normal to hypoplastic and the size does not correlate with the size of the underlying right ventricle. The pulmonary trunk is usually patent to the level of the atretic pulmonary valve and is usually hypoplastic.

Ventricular size has been broadly classified as either hypoplastic or normal. Regardless of the size of the right ventricular cavity, the clinical manifestations are similar. Cyanosis is present at birth or shortly thereafter. If the ductus remains patent, however, only mild cyanosis is present. Cyanosis increases quickly as the ductus closes. The other prominent finding is dyspnea. The signs of cardiac failure are prominent only in patients with tricuspid regurgitation. Physical examination reveals a cyanotic, dyspneic infant with cardiomegaly. The second heart sound is single. In more than half the patients, there is a systolic murmur which is usually soft, and may be related to either the ductus arteriosus or tricuspid regurgitation. The pulmonary vascularity is decreased with markedly ischemic lung fields. There is a tendency for the cardiac silhouette to be larger in patients with an enlarged right ventricle, especially in those with tricuspid insufficiency. The pulmonary arterial segment is concave and the right atrium is greatly enlarged. The upper mediastinum often is narrow and the aortic knob inapparent.

The EKG reveals normal or right axis deviation. This serves to distinguish this condition from tricuspid atresia in which left axis deviation is the rule. Furthermore, a qR pattern in lead aVF suggests pulmonary atresia, whereas such a qR pattern is seen in lead AVL in tricuspid atresia. Right atrial enlargement is present although not always in the first week of life. A few older cases show left atrial enlargement. The precordial leads are useful in distinguishing the 2 types of pulmonary valvar atresia. With a hypoplastic right ventricle, a pattern of "absence of right ventricular forces" is present with an rS in lead V1 and an R in V6. Normal or enlarged right ventricles are associated with classic patterns of right ventricular hypertrophy.

The pulmonary valve can be imaged on echocardiography, but absence of Doppler detected pulmonary flow is inconclusive since the same may exist in cases of pulmonary hypertension in the presence of a patent pulmonary valve. The right ventricular outflow tract usually appears narrowed. In most instances, the aorta will be larger than normal. Right ventricular cavity size depends upon the exact anatomy of a particular patient. Right ventricular hypertrophy almost always is present. If pulmonary blood flow is low, left atrial size is small. If the right pulmonary artery is present, it can be imaged and measured via the suprasternal notch approach.

Cardiac catheterization is useful in establishing the diagnosis. It is not always possible to advance the catheter tip into a hypoplastic right ventricle. The right ventricular pressure is elevated with the peak systolic pressure exceeding the systemic arterial pressure, unless there is marked tricuspid insufficiency, when the right ventricular systolic pressure may be as low as 40 mmHg. Right atrial pressure is elevated and shows large "a" waves. Oxygen saturations on the right side of the heart are low and blood from the left atrium is desaturated. Indicator dilution curves performed from either atrium are practically identical, showing a common pathway of circulation.

Angiocardiography confirms the diagnosis and yields information regarding right ventricular size. The angiocardiogram reveals no passage of contrast material from the right ventricle into the pulmonary artery. Contrast may be seen escaping from the right ventricle either through an insufficient tricuspid valve or through myocardial sinusoids with retrograde filling of coronary arteries. In some cases, opacification of the aortic root occurs as well. Right atrial injections show contrast material flowing from right-to-left atrium, but frequently fail to distinguish this condition from **Tricuspid valve, atresia**. The pulmonary arteries fill by way of a patent ductus arteriosus or enlarged bronchial arteries.

Complications: Acidosis secondary to hypoxia, cardiac failure.

Associated Findings: None known.

Etiology: Undetermined but presumably multifactorial inheritance.

Pathogenesis: Probably due to early fusion of the pulmonary valvar primordia.

CDC No.: 746.000

Sex Ratio: M1:F1

Occurrence: Approximately 1:10,000 live births. Prevalence diminishes to only the rare survivors of palliative surgery.

Risk of Recurrence for Patient's Sib: Predicted risk: 1:100; Empiric risk: undetermined.

Risk of Recurrence for Patient's Child: Affected individuals are not expected to survive to reproduce.

Age of Detectability: At birth.

Gene Mapping and Linkage: Unknown.

Prevention: None known. Genetic counseling indicated.

Treatment: Following cardiac catheterization, operation is mandatory. If the right ventricle is of normal size and the infundibulum patent to the level of the pulmonary valve, pulmonary valvotomy can be performed. This may be combined with placement of an outflow tract patch across the pulmonary annulus. When the right ventricle is either hypoplastic and associated with a very stenotic infundibulum or greatly enlarged and associated with massive tricuspid insufficiency, an aortopulmonary shunt should be created and an atrial septostomy performed. Subsequently, in patients with a hypoplastic right ventricle a pulmonary valvotomy should be performed at an early age to reduce the elevated right ventricular systolic pressure.

Prognosis: Perioperative use of prostaglandin E1 has dramatically improved the surgical outcome for neonates with pulmonary atresia and intact ventricular septum. The long-term prognosis of these operative survivors has not been determined.

Detection of Carrier: Unknown.

References:
Zuberbuhler JR, et al.: Morphological variations in pulmonary atresia with intact ventricular septum. Br Heart J 1979; 41:281–288.
Patel RG, et al.: Right ventricular volume determinations in 18 patients with pulmonary atresia and intact ventricular septum. Analysis of factors influencing right ventricular growth. Circulation 1980; 61: 428–440.
Brunlin EA, et al.: Angio-pathological appearances of pulmonary valve in pulmonary atresia with intact ventricular septum. Br Heart J 1982; 47:281–289.
Freedom RM: The morphologic variations of pulmonary atresia with intact ventricular septum: guidelines for surgical intervention. Pediatr Cardiol 1983; 4:183–188.
Freedom RM, et al.: Pulmonary atresia and intact ventricular septum. Scand J Thorac Cardiovasc Surg 1983; 17:1–28.
Smallhorn JF, et al.: Noninvasive recognition of functional pulmonary atresia by echocardiography. Am J Cardiol 1984; 54:925–926.

M0005   **James H. Moller**
BR040   **Elizabeth A. Braunlin**

PULMONARY VALVE, BICUSPID   0109

Includes: Bicuspid pulmonary valve with or without a raphe

Excludes:
   Pulmonary valve, atresia (0837)
   Pulmonary valve, atresia (0837)

Major Diagnostic Criteria: Soft or moderately loud systolic pulmonic ejection murmur unassociated with electrocardiographic or vectorcardiographic abnormalities of any kind may suggest a pulmonary valve lesion.

Clinical Findings: Two functional pulmonary valve cusps are present rather than 3. The 2 cusps may be approximately equal in size in which case there usually is no raphe in either sinus of Valsalva. Both sinuses of Valsalva, while larger than normal, are well-formed. More commonly, however, one of the cusps is somewhat larger than the other and contains a raphe which partially divides the sinus of Valsalva into more or less equal sized shallow components. Since by definition neither stenosis nor incompetence is present, the lesion is asymptomatic. Even in nonstenotic bicuspid valves, however, turbulence is usually produced which is responsible for the soft or moderately loud systolic ejection type murmur usually present in these patients. A suprasternal systolic thrill may be present.

The EKG and vectorcardiogram are normal in uncomplicated simple bicuspid pulmonary valve. X-rays of the chest may show minimal "poststenotic" dilatation of the pulmonary trunk. Cross-sectional echocardiography in some instances can show the bicuspid nature of the valve. At cardiac catheterization, no pressure difference is found across the valve and the physiologic findings are normal. A pulmonary arterial angiogram or right ventriculogram may demonstrate the true nature of the anomaly.

Complications: Calcification of the bicuspid pulmonary valve is unusual, as is bacterial endocarditis.

Associated Findings: A bicuspid pulmonary valve is commonly associated with **Heart, tetralogy of Fallot**, in which case it does not have to be stenotic but may be hypoplastic. Other cardiovascular lesions may be present. Also commonly associated with **Chromosome 18, trisomy 18.**

Etiology: Presumably multifactorial inheritance.

Pathogenesis: True bicuspid pulmonary valve without a raphe is probably due to absence of one of the pulmonary valve cusp anlagen. This may be the intercalated valve swelling of either of the anlagen derived from the truncus septum. In a bicuspid pulmonary valve with a raphe, all 3 anlagen are present, 2 of these have fused to form a functionally single cusp with 2 poorly developed sinuses of Valsalva separated by a raphe.

CDC No.: 746.080

Sex Ratio: M1:F1

Occurrence: Unknown.

Risk of Recurrence for Patient's Sib: Unknown.

Risk of Recurrence for Patient's Child: Unknown.

Age of Detectability: Probably in early childhood, if all soft pulmonic murmurs are investigated.

Gene Mapping and Linkage: Unknown.

Prevention: None known. Genetic counseling indicated.

Treatment: None if lesion is an isolated one.

Prognosis: The prognosis of bicuspid pulmonary valve is excellent, if it occurs as an isolated lesion. If other congenital cardiac defects are present, the prognosis is determined by the associated lesion.

Detection of Carrier: Unknown.

References:
Koletsky S: Congenital bicuspid pulmonary valve. Arch Pathol 1941; 31:338–353. *
Ford AB, et al.: Isolated congenital bicuspid pulmonary valve: clinical and pathologic study. Am J Med 1956; 20:474–486.
Pierpont MEM, et al.: Chromosomal anomalies. In Pierpont MEM, Moller, JH eds: Genetics of cardiovascular disease. Boston: Martinus Nijhoff, 1987:83–84.

M0005   **James H. Moller**

PULMONARY VALVE, INCOMPETENCE   **0838**

Includes: Pulmonary regurgitation due to abnormality of pulmonary valve

Excludes:
    Pulmonary valve, absent (0836)
    Pulmonary valve, secondary incompetence

Major Diagnostic Criteria: An early diastolic murmur along the left sternal border with EKG evidence of right ventricular hypertrophy suggests the diagnosis. Pulmonary artery angiocardiography confirms the diagnosis.

Clinical Findings: Incompetence of the pulmonary valve results from a structural abnormality of the valve which may be bicuspid, tricuspid or quadricuspid. Functional pulmonary incompetence may also be present in patients with idiopathic dilatation of the

pulmonary artery or other lesions which cause dilatation of the pulmonary artery.

Because of incompetence of the pulmonary valve, the right ventricular stroke volume is increased. As a result, the main pulmonary artery, its major branches and the right ventricular chamber are dilated. The degree of dilatation of the right side of the heart is dependent not only upon the degree of pulmonary incompetence but also on the level of pulmonary arterial pressure. If sufficient regurgitation occurs and marked right ventricular dilatation develops, congestive cardiac failure may occur.

The clinical findings are related primarily to the degree of incompetence and the level of pulmonary arterial pressure. Patients with minor degrees of incompetence are asymptomatic. The elevated pulmonary vascular resistance that is normally present in the neonatal period, or that may develop secondarily later in life, tends to augment the degree of regurgitation, thereby imposing an excessive pressure load upon the right ventricle and leading to congestive cardiac failure. Newborn infants with pulmonary insufficiency can thus present with signs of severe cardiac failure. A systolic ejection type murmur is present, which is related to increased right ventricular stroke volume. This murmur is followed by a medium to low-pitched diastolic regurgitant murmur along the left sternal border. The pulmonary component of the second heart sound may be absent if the valve is rudimentary. If both components of the second sound are present, the degree of splitting may be increased because of the increased right ventricular stroke volume. When pulmonary arterial hypertension is present, the pulmonic component is accentuated. A pulmonary ejection click may be present.

Thoracic X-rays in most children show a normal-sized cardiac silhouette with prominent pulmonary trunk and major arterial branches. With severe incompetence or pulmonary hypertension, the right-sided cardiac chambers are enlarged. Cardiac fluoroscopy shows increased pulsations of the pulmonary trunk and main arteries.

The EKG findings may reflect the volume overload on the right ventricle. It may either be normal or reveal mild right ventricular hypertrophy. The latter is manifested as an rSR' pattern in lead V_1, a larger than normal S wave in lead V_6, and terminal slowing of the QRS electrical forces.

The pulmonary valvular abnormality cannot be visualized by echocardiography. If the insufficiency is of moderate or greater degree, the right ventricular cavity is dilated. In more advanced instances, paradoxical septal motion may be present. Tricuspid flutter has been reported but it is relatively rare. Thickness of the right ventricular wall depends on the level of right ventricular systolic pressure. The right pulmonary artery is usually dilated.

In the presence of significant pulmonary valve incompetence, cardiac catheterization characteristically reveals a wide pulmonary arterial pulse pressure with the diastolic pressure similar to that of right ventricular end diastolic pressure. The dicrotic notch is low. Small systolic pressure gradients may be present between the right ventricle and the pulmonary artery secondary to the increased forward flow.

Angiocardiography shows an enlarged right ventricle especially the infundibulum. The pulmonary trunk is dilated. In severe cases, the main pulmonary arteries may show considerable dilatation as well. Pulmonary arteriography shows retrograde opacification of the right ventricle.

Complications: Congestive cardiac failure.

Associated Findings: None known.

Etiology: Unknown.

Pathogenesis: Unknown.

CDC No.: 746.020

Sex Ratio: M1:F1

Occurrence: Less than 1% of all cases of congenital heart defects.

Risk of Recurrence for Patient's Sib: Unknown.

Risk of Recurrence for Patient's Child: Unknown.

Age of Detectability: At birth.

Gene Mapping and Linkage: Unknown.

Prevention: None known. Genetic counseling indicated.

Treatment: If cardiac failure occurs, medical treatment is possible. Surgical therapy is rarely indicated. It could, however, be accomplished by homograft replacement of the pulmonary valve, or other type of valvar prosthesis.

Prognosis: Pulmonary valve incompetence has been generally considered a benign condition, but reports of death in the neonatal period and in later life have been reported. Short-term animal studies of surgically induced insufficiency have indicated its benign nature. Longer periods of observation are needed to determine the future course of the child or younger adult with symptom-free isolated pulmonary valvar incompetence.

Detection of Carrier: Unknown.

References:
Collins NP, et al.: Isolated congenital pulmonic valvular regurgitation; diagnosis by cardiac catheterization and angiocardiography. Am J Med 1960; 28:159–164.
Vlad P, et al.: Congenital pulmonary regurgitation: a report of six autopsied cases. Am J Dis Child 1960; 100:640–641.
Gasul BM, et al.: Congenital isolated pulmonary valvular insufficiency. In: Heart disease in children: diagnosis and treatment. Philadelphia: J.B. Lippincott, 1966:807.
Goldberg SJ, et al.: Pediatric and adolescent echocardiography: a handbook. Chicago: Year Book Medical Publishers, 1975.
Buendia A, et al.: Congenital absence of pulmonary valve leaflets. Br Heart J 1983; 50:31–41. *
Hiraishi S, et al.: Ventricular and pulmonary artery volumes in patients with absent pulmonary valve: factors affecting the natural course. Circulation 1983; 67:183–190.

M0005   **James H. Moller**

Pulmonary valve, quadricuspid
See PULMONARY VALVE, TETRACUSPID

PULMONARY VALVE, STENOSIS   0839

Includes:
> Pulmonary valve dysplasia
> Pulmonary valve stenosis with intact ventricular septum
> Pulmonary valve stenosis with normal aortic root
> Pulmonic stenosis

Excludes:
> **Heart, tetralogy of Fallot** (0938)
> Infundibular pulmonic stenosis
> **Pulmonary artery, coarctation** (0835)

Major Diagnostic Criteria: A harsh systolic murmur, maximal in the second left intercostal space, with an enlarged main pulmonary artery on X-ray with normal pulmonary vascularity, plus right ventricular hypertrophy on the EKG, indicate the diagnosis. Echocardiography is confirmatory.

Clinical Findings: In the majority of patients with pulmonary valvar stenosis, the pulmonary valve is dome-shaped, with partial commissural fusion, resulting in a central circular orifice of variable size. Less frequently, the valve shows no commissural fusion. In the latter form, called pulmonary valvar dysplasia, three distinct cusps and commissures are present, the valvar tissue being greatly thickened and redundant. The sinuses of Valsalva are partly obliterated by tissue composed of large, pale-staining myxomatous-like cells. In this form, pulmonary stenosis results from the mass of valvar tissue encroaching on the pulmonary orifice. Secondary anatomic features of pulmonary valve stenosis include poststenotic dilatation of both the pulmonary trunk and usually also the left pulmonary artery. The right ventricle is hypertrophied in proportion to the severity of the stenosis. With time, two alterations occur in the right ventricle which significantly alter right ventricular function. One of these is the development of myocardial fibrosis and the other is the development of infundibular stenosis. Right atrial enlargement and hypertrophy are present in the more severe cases, and this may be of sufficient degree to open a previously competent patent foramen ovale.

The clinical and laboratory findings are dependent in part upon the severity of the stenosis. The majority of patients with pulmonary valve stenosis are asymptomatic and show normal growth and development. With moderate stenosis, easy fatigability may be present. Congestive cardiac failure and cyanosis (related to a right-to-left atrial shunt) may develop but usually only in patients with severe pulmonary valvar stenosis. These findings may be present in the infant with severe stenosis or may develop gradually in the adult with significant pulmonary valve stenosis. The prominent physical finding is a loud pulmonary systolic ejection murmur, which is usually associated with a thrill along the upper left sternal border and in the suprasternal notch. The murmur is usually introduced by a pulmonic systolic ejection click, but this may be absent in severe cases. Other auscultatory features may be indicative of the severity of the stenosis. With significant pulmonary stenosis, the murmur becomes longer and the peak intensity of the murmur is delayed further into systole. The development or presence of a murmur of tricuspid insufficiency is indicative of severe pulmonary stenosis. The components of the second heart sound are normal in mild stenosis, but with increasing degrees of severity, the pulmonic component becomes delayed and softer, or even inaudible.

Attention must be directed to the general appearance and physical characteristics of the child. They may indicate the etiology of the pulmonary valve stenosis, as in post-rubella syndrome. Children with a dysplastic pulmonary valve are generally small in stature, retarded in sexual development, and have a rather typical triangular shaped face with ptosis, hypertelorism and low-set ears. Pulmonic systolic ejection clicks are rarely heard among these patients. Usually the heart size is normal as is the pulmonary vasculature. There is prominence of the pulmonary trunk and left pulmonary artery. In patients with severe stenosis, the pulmonary artery segment is usually inapparent. With severe or long-standing moderate pulmonary stenosis, the overall cardiac size may be slightly enlarged, representing primarily right ventricular and right atrial enlargement. In patients with cyanosis related to right-to-left atrial shunt, the pulmonary vasculature is diminished, but left atrial enlargement is then present. Combination of decreased pulmonary vascularity and left atrial enlargement should suggest a large right-to-left shunt at atrial level.

In mild pulmonary valvar stenosis, the EKG is normal, or shows only minimal evidence of right ventricular hypertrophy (T wave positive in V_1). With more severe stenosis, there is progressively more right axis deviation and right ventricular hypertrophy. Right atrial enlargement may be observed. There is a rough correlation between the height of the R wave in right precordial leads and the severity of the stenosis. In children with dysplastic pulmonary valves, Noonan syndrome with pulmonary stenosis, and rubella patients with stenotic pulmonary valves, the EKG findings of severe right axis deviation (more than $+210°$) and rS deflections in all precordial leads suggest a degree of right ventricular hypertrophy which is not actually present.

In most instances, the echocardiographic "a" wave amplitude of the pulmonary valve is excessive in some beats; in other beats, the "a" wave appears normal. In some children with pulmonary valvular stenosis, the "a" wave appears normal. Right ventricular anterior wall thickness is related to the severity of the disease. Right ventricular cavity size may vary from small to dilated. If the right ventricular cavity is dilated, paradoxical septal motion may be present even in the absence of a right ventricular volume overload. The right pulmonary artery is usually dilated. Doppler interrogation of the transvacuar jet allows estimation of the gradient.

Cardiac catheterization reveals a systolic pressure difference across the pulmonary valve and there may be a right-to-left shunt at the atrial level. Simultaneous measurement of the cardiac output and the gradient across the pulmonary valve permit calculation of the size of the stenotic pulmonary valvar orifice. Measurement of hemodynamic parameters during exercise permits assessment of right ventricular function. Right ventricular angiography demonstrates a dome-shaped pulmonary valve with a jet of contrast passing through the small central orifice. The angiocardiogram reveals hypertrophy of the right ventricle, especially the crista supraventricularis, which forms the posterior wall of the right ventricular infundibulum. Generally, the infundibulum narrows during systole, but widens significantly during diastole. In patients with a dysplastic pulmonary valve, the valve cusps do not dome and there is no jet. The thickened cusps maintain a fixed position in both diastole and systole; the sinuses of Valsalva are nearly occluded.

Complications: Congestive cardiac failure, **Tricuspid valve, insufficiency**, development of myocardial fibrosis, increased hematocrit.

Associated Findings: May be seen as part of the **Fetal rubella syndrome, Noonan syndrome**, and **Lentigines syndrome, multiple**.

Etiology: Multifactorial inheritance in the majority of cases. May be seen as part of the **Fetal rubella syndrome** and the **Lentigines syndrome, multiple**. Variable expressivity is seen in autosomal dominant **Noonan syndrome**.

Pathogenesis: Dome-shaped pulmonary valve probably results from fusion of the embryonic valvar cusps. Dysplastic pulmonary valve probably results from failure of reabsorption of the embryonic cusp tissue that normally occurs in the formation of the sinuses of Valsalva.

MIM No.: 26550

CDC No.: 746.010

Sex Ratio: M1:F1

Occurrence: Prevalence is approximately 1:1,250 of the general population. About 10% of congenital heart disease.

Risk of Recurrence for Patient's Sib: About 2%.

Risk of Recurrence for Patient's Child: If mother is affected, empiric risk is about 6.5%. If father is affected, empiric risk is about 1.8%.

Age of Detectability: From birth, by clinical examination and cardiac catheterization.

Gene Mapping and Linkage: Unknown.

Prevention: Genetic counseling is indicated as is rubella vacciniation. Special attention must be paid to a possible association with **Noonan syndrome**.

Treatment: Medical, symptomatic treatment of congestive cardiac failure, when this is present. The valvar obstruction should be relieved when the calculated pulmonary valve area is less than 0.5 cm²/meter² of body surface area. With a normal cardiac output, this valve area is usually associated with a right ventricular systolic pressure in the range of 75 mm Hg. The traditional approach of operative pulmonary valvotomy has been replaced by an interventional catheter technic -- balloon valve dilatation. This procedure is extremely safe, and leads to excellent relief of the valvar stenosis, except in individuals with a dysplastic pulmonary valve. In patients with significant infundibular stenosis, it may be necessary to resect a portion of the obstructing muscle as well as open the pulmonary valve. In patients with a dysplastic pulmonary valve, the operation involves excision of the valvar tissue or the placement of an outflow patch across the pulmonary annulus.

Infants with severe pulmonary stenosis and cardiomegaly represent surgical emergencies. Prompt performance of diagnostic procedures and pulmonary valvotomy may be lifesaving.

Prognosis: Serial cardiac catheterization studies have indicated that beyond infancy patients with mild-to-moderate pulmonary valvar stenosis show no increase in the level of right ventricular pressure. There are suggestions, however, that the incidence of coexistent infundibular pulmonary stenosis increases in each decade of life. As a result, the infundibular stenosis may result in increased levels of right ventricular systolic pressure and complicate operation. With time, right ventricular myocardial fibrosis develops which may significantly alter the compliance and function of the right ventricle. The results of operation in children are excellent and pulmonary valvotomy can be performed successfully at low risk. In adults, particularly those with poor right ventricular function, the operative risk is higher, and the postoperative catheterization data frequently reveal continued poor right ventricular myocardial performance.

Detection of Carrier: Unknown.

References:

Klinge T, Laursen HB: Familial pulmonary stenosis with underdeveloped or normal right ventricle. Br Heart J 1975; 37:60–64.

Kan JS, et al.: Percutaneous balloon valvuloplasty: a new method for treating congenital pulmonary valve stenosis. New Engl J Med 1982; 307:540–542.

Johnson GL, et al.; Accuracy of combined two-dimensional echocardiography and continuous wave Doppler recordings in the estimation of pressure gradient in right ventricular obstruction. J Am Coll Cardiol 1984; 3:1013–1018.

Trowitzsch E, et al.: Two-dimensional echocardiographic evaluation of right ventricular size function in newborns with severe right ventricular outflow tract obstruction. J Am Coll Cardiol 1985; 6:388–393.

Radtke W: Percutaneous balloon valvotomy of congenital pulmonary stenosis using oversized balloons. J Am Coll Cardiol 1986; 8:909–915.

Nora JJ, Nora AH: Maternal transmission of congenital heart disease. Am J Cardiol 1987; 59:459–463. *

Emmanouilides GC, Baylen BG: Obstructive lesions of the right ventricle and pulmonary arterial tree. In: Adams FH, Emmanouilides GC, eds: Heart disease in infants, children, and adolescents. Baltimore: Williams & Wilkins, 1989.

M0005   **James H. Moller**

PULMONARY VALVE, TETRACUSPID   0840

Includes: Pulmonary valve, quadricuspid

Excludes: **Pulmonary valve** (other defects)

Major Diagnostic Criteria: Selective pulmonary artery angiocardiography is necessary to establish the diagnosis. Even then, exact delineation of a tetracuspid pulmonary valve is difficult. Thus, necropsy is required to definitively document the diagnosis.

Clinical Findings: The pulmonary valve has four valve cusps. The cusps may each be of equal size, or one may be smaller. Often it is the supernumerary cusp that is deformed, imperfect, or smaller. When present as an isolated anomaly, the right-sided cardiac chambers are normal. If the valve is insufficient, the pulmonary artery and right ventricle may be dilated. Symptoms and signs are only present if the pulmonary valve is incompetent or stenotic.

Complications: Pulmonary valve insufficiency, bacterial endocarditis.

Associated Findings: None known.

Etiology: Unknown.

Pathogenesis: Probably results from the formation of an additional intercalated pulmonary valve swelling.

CDC No.: 746.080

Sex Ratio: M1:F1

Occurrence: About 50 autopsy cases reported.

Risk of Recurrence for Patient's Sib: Unknown.

Risk of Recurrence for Patient's Child: Unknown.

Age of Detectability: At birth.

Gene Mapping and Linkage: Unknown.

Prevention: None known.

Treatment: Unknown.

Prognosis: Good; the anomaly usually being an incidental finding at necropsy.

Detection of Carrier: Unknown.

References:

Kissin M: Pulmonary insufficiency with a supernumerary cusp in the pulmonary valve: report of a case with review of the literature. Am Heart J 1936; 12:206–227.

Hurwitz LE, Roberts WC: Quadricuspid semilunar valve. Am J Cardiol 1973; 31:623–626.

Davia JE, et al.: Quardicuspid semilunar valves. Chest 1977; 72:186–189.

M0005   **James H. Moller**

Pulmonary vascular ring
See PULMONARY ARTERY, ORIGIN OF THE LEFT FROM RIGHT PULMONARY ARTERY
Pulmonary vein, stenosis of the common
See HEART, COR TRIATRIATUM
Pulmonary venous connection, anomalous (partial)
See PULMONARY VENOUS CONNECTION, PARTIAL ANOMALOUS

PULMONARY VENOUS CONNECTION, PARTIAL ANOMALOUS — 0841

Includes:
Great veins, transposition of (partial)
Pulmonary venous connection, anomalous (partial)
Venous return, anomalous (partial)

Excludes: **Pulmonary venous connection, total anomalous** (0842)

Major Diagnostic Criteria: Typical physical examination, electrocardiographic features, and X-ray features of **Atrial septal defects**. Although cardiac catheterization, including selective pulmonary arteriogram, confirms the diagnosis, two-dimensional echocardiography with imaging of pulmonary veins can be diagnostic as well. Computerized tomography also may provide positive identification of partial anomalous pulmonary venous connection (PAPVC).

Clinical Findings: *Anatomy:* Partial anomalous pulmonary venous connection occurs when one or more, but not all, of the pulmonary veins connect to the systemic venous circulation instead of the left atrium. Almost every conceivable connection between the pulmonary veins and the proximal systemic veins has been reported. The abnormally draining veins may be either from the entire right or left lung or from only several segments. Right-sided anomalous pulmonary veins usually empty into the superior vena cava, right atrium, or occasionally into the inferior vena cava and other sites. Anomalous left pulmonary veins usually drain into a left superior vena cava, and occasionally left innominate vein, left subclavian veins, or coronary sinus.

Partial anomalous pulmonary venous connection (PAPVC) is usually associated with an atrial septal defect of the sinus venosus type. Occasionally PAPVC is seen with **Mitral valve stenosis**. Other major associated cardiac anomalies are present in approximately 20% of the cases.

Physiology: The fundamental hemodynamic alteration is similar to an atrial septal defect. Increased pulmonary blood flow occurs as a consequence of recirculation through the lungs. The magnitude of the recirculation is determined by: 1) the number of anomalous pulmonary veins, 2) the presence and the size of the atrial septal defect, 3) the pulmonary vascular resistance, and (4) ssociated anomalies. When the atrial septum is intact, the number of anomalously connected veins and the state of the parenchyma determine the amount of blood which drains anomalously. When a single pulmonary vein is anomalously connected, the anomalously draining blood approximates 20% of total pulmonary blood flow. This amount is clinically inapparent. With anomalous drainage of several lobes of the lungs or when PAPVC and atrial septal defect coexist, the hemodynamic picture is similar to that of an uncomplicated atrial septal defect. The left-to-right shunt is usually large.

Clinical features: The anomalous connection of one pulmonary vein is inapparent clinically. If all but one of the veins connect anomalously, the clinical features mimic those of total anomalous pulmonary venous connection. Children with PAPVC are usually asymptomatic but may have dyspnea on exertion. Patients presenting with cyanosis in their third and fourth decades occur due to elevated pulmonary vascular resistance.

Physical findings are similar to those of **Atrial septal defects**. These include 1) right ventricular lift, 2) when associated with ASD, the S_2 is split widely and fixed. When the atrial septum is intact, the S_2 is normal, 3) a grade II-III/VI systolic ejection murmur at the upper left sternal border, and 4) a mid-diastolic rumble, due to increased flow across the tricuspid valve. Electrocardiographic findings are similar to those seen in uncomplicated atrial septal defects.

The chest X-ray reflects the increased pulmonary blood flow and right ventricular dilatation. Occasionally, a dilated superior vena cava, a crescent-shaped vertical shadow in the right lower lung, or a distended vertical vein may suggest the site of anomalous drainage.

Complications: As a consequence of increased pulmonary blood flow, pulmonary vascular hypertension rarely occurs in the third and fourth decade. Pulmonary infections are common in patients with anomalous drainage of the right pulmonary veins to the inferior vena cava associated with pulmonary sequestration (see **Scimitar syndrome**).

Associated Findings: Partial anomalous pulmonary venous connection of the right lung is typically a connection of one or more veins from the upper and middle lobes to the superior vena cava and the right atrium near the cavo-atrial junction, usually in association with a sinus venosus type of atrial septal defect. Atrial defects of the fossa ovalis type may also be seen with PAPVC. Partial anomalous pulmonary venous connection occurs in approximately 15% - 25 of cases of cor triatriatum.

Other associated findings include **Mitral valve stenosis**, polysplenia, and **Asplenia syndrome**. Major additional cardiac anomalies are present in approximately 20% of cases of PAPVC. **Turner syndrome** has been reported in association with PAPVC.

Etiology: Presumably multifactorial inheritance.

Pathogenesis: The lungs arise from a portion of the foregut. Initially pulmonary veins draining the splanchnic plexus and empty into the systemic venous system. If one or more of these pulmonary veins fail to connect with the left atrium, the original drainage into the systemic venous system will persist.

MIM No.: 12100

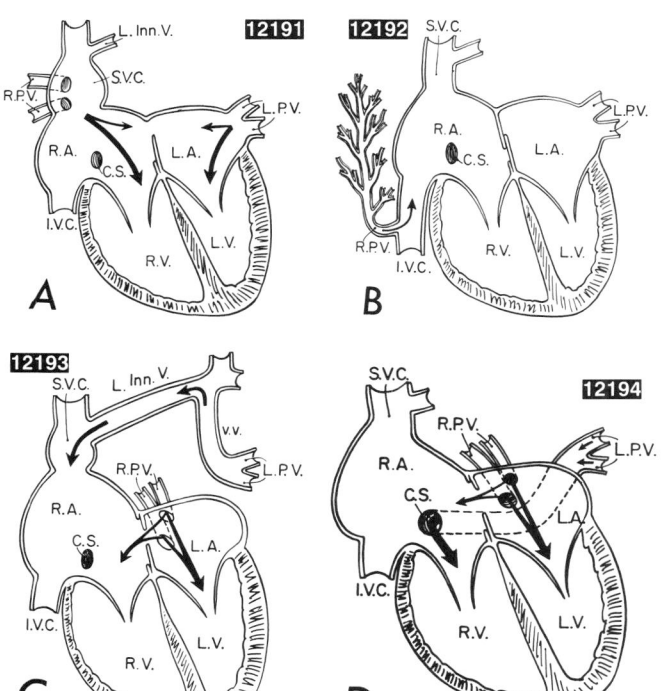

0841-12191–94: Common forms of partial anomalous pulmonary venous connection.

Sex Ratio: M1:F1

Occurrence: 7:1,000 in the general population; authorities have quoted figures from 6–600:100,000 in the general population. The higher prevalence figure is not compatible with general clinical experience.

Risk of Recurrence for Patient's Sib: Unknown.

Risk of Recurrence for Patient's Child: Unknown.

Age of Detectability: At birth, by echocardiogram or angiography.

Gene Mapping and Linkage: Unknown.

Prevention: None known. Genetic counseling indicated.

Treatment: Exercise restriction is generally not required. Bacterial endocarditis prophylaxis is probably not indicated. Medical therapy may be required. Surgical correction is carried out under cardiopulmonary bypass. The specific procedure to be performed depends on the site of anomalous drainage. An isolated single lobe anomaly is not ordinarily corrected surgically. Timing of surgery is usually at 4–5 years of age, if clinically indicated. Mortality for surgical repair is less than 1%. Most common complications of surgery are superior vena caval obstruction, supraventricular arrhythmias and symptomatic sinus node dysfunction ("sick sinus syndrome").

Prognosis: Pathologic studies indicate that patients with one pulmonary vein connected anomalously and with an intact septum have an excelent prognosis with normal life expectancy. The natural history in symptomatic patients seems comparable to those with uncomplicated atrial septal defects. The prognosis is determined by severity of associated anomalies in patients with complicated anatomy.

Detection of Carrier: Unknown.

References:

Alpert JS, et al.: Anomalous pulmonary venous return with intact atrial septum: diagnosis and pathophysiology. Circulation 1977; 56:870–875.

Price WH, Willey RF: Partial anomalous pulmonary venous drainage in two patients with Turner's syndrome. J Med Genet 1980; 17:133–134.

Whittemore R, et al.: Pregnancy and its outcome in women with and without surgical treatment of congenital heart disease. Am J Cardiol 1982; 50:641–651.

Lucas RV Jr: Anomalous venous connections, pulmonary and systemic. In: Adams FM, Emmanoulides GC, eds: Moss's heart disease in infants, children and adolescents. 3rd ed. Baltimore: Williams & Wilkins, 1983:458–491. *

Rose V, et al.: A possible increase in the incidence of congenital heart defects among the offspring of affected parents. J Am Coll Cardiol 1985; 6:376–382.

Wolf WJ: Diagnostic features and pitfalls in the two-dimensional echocardiographic evaluation of a child with cor triatriatum. Pediatr Cardiol 1986; 6:211–213.

PE019
BR014

Angel Perez
J. Timothy Bricker

PULMONARY VENOUS CONNECTION, TOTAL ANOMALOUS   0842

Includes:
  Great veins, transposition of (complete)
  Pulmonary venous, anomalous return (total)

Excludes:
  Pulmonary valve, atresia (0837)
  Pulmonary valve, stenosis (0839)
  Pulmonary venous connection, partial anomalous (0841)
  Pulmonary venous connection, subtotal
  Scimitar syndrome (0879)

Major Diagnostic Criteria: Total anomalous pulmonary venous connection (TAPVC) with obstruction: Neonate with intense cyanosis and respiratory distress, X-ray signs of pulmonary venous congestion, and a normal heart size.

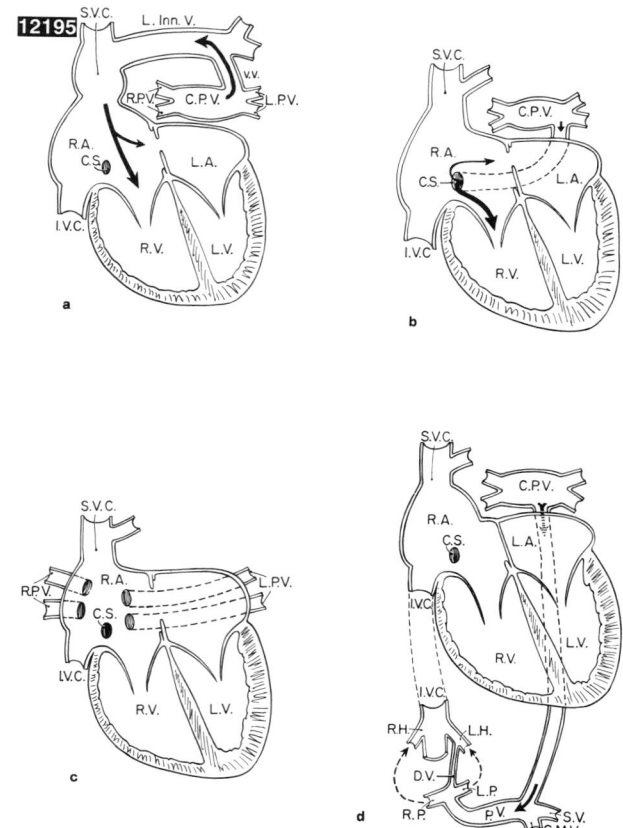

0842-12195: Common forms of total anomalous pulmonary venous connection.

TAPVC without obstruction: Infant with cyanosis and signs of congestive heart failure, EKG evidence of right atrial enlargement and right ventricular hypertrophy, and X-ray signs of increased pulmonary blood flow and enlarged right heart structures.

In both forms of TAPVC, selective pulmonary angiography will demonstrate the route of anomalous connection, but in TAPVC with obstruction, pulmonary blood flow may be slowed, and the sites of connection and obstruction not seen until late in levophase. Echocardiography may be diagnostic and angiography is not always required.

Clinical Findings: All pulmonary veins drain by abnormal routes directly or indirectly to the right atrium. Interatrial communication, either by atrial septal defect or patent foramen ovale, is therefore an essential component of TAPVC. Approximately 40% of patients with TAPVC have other associated cardiac anomalies. The site of anomalous connection may be classified as (I) supracardiac: to a left vertical vein, left superior vena cava, right superior vena cava or azygous vein, (II) intracardiac: to the coronary sinus or right atrium, (III) infracardiac: to the portal vein, ductus venosus, inferior vena cava or hepatic veins, (IV) mixed: one or more of the above.

The presence or absence of obstruction to pulmonary venous drainage dictates the hemodynamic consequences and therefore the clinical features of TAPVC. Obstruction can occur secondary to a narrow anomalous channel, extrinsic compression of an anomalous channel, interposition of the hepatic sinusoids in infracardiac TAPVC, or a restrictive interatrial communication.

TAPVC with obstruction to pulmonary venous drainage: Pulmonary venous obstruction occurs most often with infracardiac connections but may be secondary to other etiologies as above.

Prenatal changes consisting of increased pulmonary vein and capillary wall thickness may contribute to both pre- and postoperative pulmonary hypertension. Elevated pulmonary resistance and a thickened, non-compliant right ventricle lead to diminished pulmonary blood flow and increased right-to-left atrial shunting. Physical exam therefore reveals cyanosis and respiratory distress at or soon after birth. There are generally no murmurs heard, the pulmonary closure sound is accentuated and the heart is not enlarged. There are rales secondary to pulmonary edema and the liver is enlarged.

X-ray findings are those of pulmonary venous obstruction and pulmonary edema without cardiomegaly. The diffuse reticular pattern of pulmonary vascular markings may resemble those of hyaline membrane disease, but differ in that air bronchograms are absent. Kerley B lines may be seen.

The electrocardiogram usually shows right ventricular hypertrophy, but the QRS axis, atrial and ventricular forces may also be within normal limits for age.

Echocardiograms: two-dimensional echocardiography is a reliable means of diagnosing both the presence and routes of abnormal pulmonary venous connection. In the presence of pulmonary venous obstruction, however, pulmonary blood flow is diminished and the site of connection is more difficult to visualize. Two-dimensional directed Doppler echocardiograms, and more recently, color Doppler flow studies, help identify patterns of blood flow and sites of obstruction. An echo-free space posterior to the left atrium (common pulmonary vein) is a characteristic finding in TAPVC, but may be lacking in some patients with right atrial or mixed connections.

Cardiac catheterization: systemic saturations may be very low secondary to diminished pulmonary blood flow. Streaming of highly saturated renal vein blood can cause confusion in interpretation of inferior vena caval oxygen saturations. Right ventricular pressure is systemic or greater. Right atrial pressure is higher and systemic saturations lower in patients with a restrictive interatrial communication and these patients benefit from balloon atrial septostomy. Pulmonary arteriograms generally require longer film duration (10–15 sec) to allow opacification of pulmonary venous return because of low pulmonary blood flow.

TAPVC without obstruction to pulmonary venous drainage: Age of presentation can vary considerably. With postnatal decrease in pulmonary vascular resistance, pulmonary blood flow increases to exceed systemic flow. Patients therefore may be asymptomatic at birth, then develop congestive heart failure, grow poorly and have frequent respiratory infections. Physical exam reveals a variable degree of cyanosis with cardiovascular findings resembling atrial septal defect. An infant may be irritable and poorly nourished. Tachypnea and tachycardia are found as well as a right ventricular heave. The second heart sound is well split with little or no change with respiration and the pulmonary closure sound is accentuated, reflecting pulmonary hypertension. Gallop rhythms are frequent. A grade II-III/VI blowing systolic murmur is audible at the mid-to-upper left sternal border and a diastolic murmur secondary to increased blood flow across the tricuspid valve is present at the lower left sternal border. With anomalous venous connection to the left innominate vein, a venous hum may be present at either upper sternal border. Hepatomegaly is present.

X-ray findings all show increased pulmonary arterial markings and cardiomegaly secondary to right atrial and right ventricular enlargement. The left atrium handles a normal volume of blood and is not enlarged. Occasionally, the chest radiograph allows definition of the route of anomalous drainage. In connection to a left superior vena cava, the "snowman" or "figure of eight" silhouette may be seen, the lower portion formed by the heart and the upper portion formed by the enlarged left SVC-innominate vein - right SVC system. This appearance may be obscured by or confused with a neonatal thymic shadow. Connection to the right SVC may cause dilatation and blurring of the SVC-right atrial junction and connection to the coronary sinus may cause an indentation anteriorly on barium-swallow just below the left atrial shadow.

The EKG invariably shows right atrial enlargement and right ventricular hypertrophy. Approximately half show a qR pattern in the right precordial leads, while the other half show an rR' or rsR'. These findings occur independent of the degree of pulmonary flow or pulmonary arterial pressure.

Echocardiograms: as mentioned previously, two-dimensional Doppler echocardiography is a reliable means of diagnosing TAPVC. Difficulties arise in patients with right atrial isomerism, mixed-type TAPVC and complex cardiac anatomy. The finding of a dilated coronary sinus should lead to searches for anomalous drainage through that structure.

Cardiac catheterization: high oxygen saturations in a systemic vein may allow identification of the site of anomalous connections. Saturations are generally the same in right atrium, right ventricle, pulmonary artery and aorta. Due to the degree of pulmonary to systemic shunting, systemic saturations may be near normal. There may be mild to moderate elevations of both right ventricular and pulmonary artery pressures. Pulmonary arteriograms require large volumes of contrast injected rapidly because of high pulmonary flow. Pulmonary venous opacification is thereby adequate, allowing visualization of the site of connection.

Complications: With obstruction, death usually occurs from the first day to the second month. Without obstruction, symptoms of congestive heart failure may begin in infancy. The minority surviving the first year of life generally do not have pulmonary hypertension but are at risk for developing pulmonary vascular disease. Unoperated, overall mortality for TAPVC is 80% in the first year of life.

Associated Findings: Other major cardiac defects (excluding interatrial communications) are seen in 5–40%; including transposition of the great arteries, **Ventricular septal defect**, mitral atresia-hypoplastic left heart syndrome, **Tricuspid valve, atresia, Heart, tetralogy of Fallot**, truncus arteriosus, the association of right atrial isomerism with dextrocardia, common AV valve, single ventricle and pulmonary stenosis/atresia.

A low frequency of occurrence of TAPVC has been reported in association with **Heart-hand syndrome**, **Noonan syndrome**, **Klippel-Feil anomaly**, **Cat eye syndrome**, conjoined twins, and agenesis of the right lung and phocomelia. A higher incidence is seen in **Asplenia syndrome**.

Etiology: Presumably multifactorial inheritance, although both sporadic geographic clusters in non-related patients and familial recurrences have been reported.

Pathogenesis: Embryologically, the inital route of pulmonary venous drainage is through the cardinal veins and the umbilico-vitelline system. Normally, these channels involute after successful anastomosis of pulmonary veins to an outpouching of the sinoatrial portion of the heart. Failure of development of this communication between the common pulmonary vein and left atrium results in TAPVC with persistence of either the cardinal or umbilicovitelline system or both.

MIM No.: 10670

CDC No.: 747.420

Sex Ratio: Reported M3.6:F1 for TAPVC to portal vein. Other sites of connection felt to be M1:F1, but reports show slight male predominance.

Occurrence: 1:5,000 live births. 25:1,000 of infants under one year old referred to New England Regional Infant Cardiac Program (NERICP).

Risk of Recurrence for Patient's Sib: Unknown.

Risk of Recurrence for Patient's Child: Unknown.

Age of Detectability: At birth. Fetal echocardiography probably difficult secondary to low pulmonary blood flow in utero.

Gene Mapping and Linkage: Unknown.

Prevention: None known. Genetic counseling indicated.

Treatment: Balloon and blade atrial septostomy improves atrial shunting in TAPVC without obstruction and those with TAPVC and obstruction secondary to a restrictive interatrial communication. This may improve hemodynamics and systemic saturation prior to surgery. Use of prostaglandin E1 is not helpful and in patients with low blood flow secondary to pulmonary venous obstruction could worsen pulmonary edema and exacerbate systemic desaturation.

Some patients without obstruction present later in infancy or childhood and can be managed medically to allow later surgical intervention. Most patients require early surgical correction using hypothermic circulatory arrest.

Prognosis: Eighty percent of all unoperated children with TAPVC are dead within the first year of life. Nearly half die in the first three months of life. In TAPVC with obstruction and/or restrictive interatrial communication, death usually occurs in the first weeks of life. In the presence of a large ASD and unobstructed TAPVC, some patients may not present until late childhood or early adulthood. Surgical mortality for the child under one year of age approximates 25–30%, with a mortality closer to 50% for those under one month of age. This is, in part, due to extremely ill neonates with obstruction who present with acidosis and shock. Overall, surgical mortality in the patient over one year of age is less than 5%.

Detection of Carrier: Unknown.

References:

Nora JJ, Nora AH: Genetics and counseling in cardiovascular diseases. Springfield, IL: Thomas Books, 1978.
Norwood WI, et al.: Total anomalous pulmonary venous connection: surgical considerations. In: Engle ME, ed: Pediatric cardiovascular disease, cardiovascular clinics, 1980:353–364.
Whittemore R, et al.: Pregnancy and its outcome in women with and without surgical treatment of congenital heart disease. Am J Cardiol 1982; 50:641–651.
Lucas RV Jr: Anomalous venous connections, pulmonary and systemic. In: Adams FH, Emmanouilides GS, eds: Heart disease in infants, children and adolescents, 3rd ed. Baltimore: Williams & Wilkins, 1983:458–491. *
Huhta JC, et al.: Cross-sectional echocardiographic diagnosis of total anomalous pulmonary venous connection. Brit Heart J 1985; 53:525–534.
Rose V, et al.: A possible increase in the incidence of congenital heart defects among the offspring of affected parents. J Am Coll Cardiol 1985; 6:376–382.
Solymar L, et al.: Total anomalous pulmonary venous connection in siblings. Acta Paediat Scand 1987; 76:124–127.

PE020
BR014

James C. Perry
J. Timothy Bricker

Pulmonary venous return, partial anomalous
See SCIMITAR SYNDROME
Pulmonary venous, anomalous return (total)
See PULMONARY VENOUS CONNECTION, TOTAL ANOMALOUS
Pulmonic stenosis
See PULMONARY VALVE, STENOSIS

PULMONIC STENOSIS-CAFE-AU-LAIT SPOTS, WATSON TYPE 2776

Includes:
Cafe-au-lait spots-pulmonary stenosis
Pulmonary stenosis-café-au-lait spots-mental retardation
Watson syndrome

Excludes:
Lentigines syndrome, multiple (0586)
Neurofibromatosis (0712)
Noonan syndrome (0720)

Major Diagnostic Criteria: Pulmonic stenosis, cafe-au-lait spots, and limited intelligence inherited in an autosomal dominant fashion.

Clinical Findings: Based on 18 patients in four families, pulmonic stenosis occurs in 60%; it may present with exertional dyspnea in childhood or may be a symptomless, incidental finding. Cafe-au-lait spots are found in 100%, but may vary from a few large (more than 5 cm in diameter) spots to about 100 smaller spots. Freckles are common, and axillary freckling occurs. Intelligence has usually

been described as low normal or dull (11/18), but three boys have mild and one girl severe mental retardation. All affected members (3/3) of one family had short adult stature.

Complications: Pulmonic stenosis may cause significant exertional dyspnea and cyanosis with right-to-left shunting at the atrial level. One 57-year-old man with pulmonic stenosis and coronary ectasia presented with angina when exerting effort.

Associated Findings: One girl has severe soft tissue limitation of movement of her ankles and knees.

Etiology: Autosomal dominant inheritance.

Pathogenesis: Unknown. The only vascular lesion found clinically, at operation or at autopsy, has been valvular pulmonic stenosis except for the one adult with associated coronary ectasia.

MIM No.: *19352

Sex Ratio: M1:F1

Occurrence: Three families have been described from England, one probable family from France, and one from Canada.

Risk of Recurrence for Patient's Sib:
See Part I, *Mendelian Inheritance.*

Risk of Recurrence for Patient's Child:
See Part I, *Mendelian Inheritance.*

Age of Detectability: At birth, if there are other affected members of the family. Otherwise diagnosis has usually been in mid-childhood.

Gene Mapping and Linkage: NF1 (neurofibromatosis 1 (von Recklinghausen disease, Watson disease)) has been mapped to 17q11.2.

Prevention: None known. Genetic counseling indicated.

Treatment: Pulmonic stenosis is treatable surgically. However, most patients do well without surgical treatment, and two out of three patients have died postoperatively following valvotomy.

Prognosis: Unknown. At least two males, one with and one without pulmonic stenosis, have lived into the sixth decade.

Detection of Carrier: Clinical examination and cardiac investigation.

Special Considerations: Until recently, Watson syndrome has been confused with **Lentigines syndrome, multiple** on the one hand and **Neurofibromatosis** on the other. However, the clinical picture seems sufficiently consistent and different from these two conditions to warrant consideration as a separate disorder.

References:

Watson GH: Pulmonary stenosis, cafe-au-lait spots and dull intelligence. Arch of Dis in Child 1967; 42:303–307. * †
Partington MW, et al.: Pulmonary stenosis, cafe au lait spots and dull intelligence: the Watson syndrome revisited. Proc Greenwood Genet Center 1985; 4:105 only.
Allanson JE, Watson GH: Watson syndrome: nineteen years on. Proc Greenwood Genet Center 1987; 6:173 only.

PA026

M.W. Partington

Pulmonic stenosis-congenital nephrosis
See NEPHROSIS, CONGENITAL
Pulp stones
See TEETH, DENTIN DYSPLASIA, CORONAL
Pulverulent nuclear cataract
See CATARACT, COPPOCK
Pulverulent zonular cataract
See CATARACT, COPPOCK
also CATARACT, AUTOSOMAL DOMINANT CONGENITAL
Pupil and lens, ectopic
See LENS AND PUPIL, ECTOPIC
Pupil shape abnormalities
See PUPIL, DYSCORIA
Pupil size unequal
See PUPIL, ANISOCORIA

PUPIL, ANISOCORIA   0058

Includes:
    Anisocoria
    Eye, anisocoria
    Pupil size unequal

Excludes:
    Acquired anisocoria
    Horner syndrome (0475)
    Rieger syndrome (2139)

Major Diagnostic Criteria: Unequal pupil size greater than 20%.

Clinical Findings: Defining the upper limit of normal pupillary inequality at 20%, then 2% of the population have anisocoria ranging from 0.5 to 2.0 mm.

Complications: Unknown.

Associated Findings: None known.

Etiology: Possibly autosomal dominant inheritance. Heterogeneity exists. Other disorders such as iris atrophy and stromal hypoplasia must be excluded as causes.

Pathogenesis: Unknown.

MIM No.: 10624

Sex Ratio: M1:Fl

Occurrence: 1:50 live births.

Risk of Recurrence for Patient's Sib:
    See Part I, *Mendelian Inheritance.*

Risk of Recurrence for Patient's Child:
    See Part I, *Mendelian Inheritance.*

Age of Detectability: In childhood.

Gene Mapping and Linkage: Unknown.

Prevention: None known. Genetic counseling indicated.

Treatment: Unknown.

Prognosis: Normal for life span and intelligence. Visual prognosis good.

Detection of Carrier: Unknown.

References:
Duke-Elder S: System of ophthalmology, vol. 3, part 2. congenital deformities. London: Henry Kimpton, 1964: 592.
Lam BL, et al.: The prevalence of simple anisocoria. Am J Ophthal 1987; 104:69–73.

CR012   **Harold E. Cross**

PUPIL, DYSCORIA   0309

Includes:
    Dyscoria
    Pupil shape abnormalities

Excludes:
    Corectopia
    Eye, anterior segment dysgenesis (0439)
    Eye, microphthalmia/coloboma (0661)
    Eye, pupillary membrane persistence (0845)
    Polycoria
    Pupil, anisocoria (0058)

Major Diagnostic Criteria: Abnormality in the shape of the pupil, in the absence of neoplasia or inflammatory processes with synechiae.

Clinical Findings: Abnormally shaped pupils may take the form of a slit (most commonly), hourglass, rectangle or pear. White and Fulton (1937) reported a woman of Russian-Jewish extraction and her daughters with "egg-shaped" pupils. In the absence of malformations of the globe, vision is usually good.

Complications: Unknown.

Associated Findings: Anterior chamber cleavage syndromes.

Etiology: Usually autosomal dominant inheritance. May also occur sporadically.

Pathogenesis: Probably related to abnormal "cleavage" of the anterior chamber during embryonic life.

MIM No.: 17880

Sex Ratio: M1:F1

Occurrence: Unknown.

Risk of Recurrence for Patient's Sib:
    See Part I, *Mendelian Inheritance.*

Risk of Recurrence for Patient's Child:
    See Part I, *Mendelian Inheritance.*

Age of Detectability: At birth.

Gene Mapping and Linkage: Unknown.

Prevention: None known. Genetic counseling indicated.

Treatment: None indicated in the absence of associated ocular malformations.

Prognosis: Normal for life and intelligence. Good for vision, if independent of associated ocular malformations.

Detection of Carrier: Unknown.

References:
White BV Jr., Fulton MN: A rare pupillary defect inherited by identical twins. J Hered 1937; 28:177–179.
Duke-Elder S: System of ophthalmology. vol. 3, part 2. Congenital deformities. London: Henry Kimpton, 1964.
Henkind P, et al.: Mesodermal dysgenesis of the anterior segment: Rieger's anomaly. Arch Ophthalmol 1965; 73:810–817.
Reese AB, Ellsworth RM: The anterior chamber cleavage syndrome. Arch Ophthalmol 1966; 75:307–318.

SU001   **Joel Sugar**
G0006   **Morton F. Goldberg**

Pupillary membrane persistence
    See EYE, PUPILLARY MEMBRANE PERSISTENCE
Pupils, fixed, dilated
    See EYE, IRIDOPLEGIA, FAMILIAL
Pure testicular dysgenesis
    See GONADAL DYSGENESIS, XY TYPE
Puretic syndrome
    See FIBROMATOSIS, JUVENILE HYALINE
Purine autism
    See ADENYLOSUCCINATE MONOPHOSPHATE LYASE DEFICIENCY
Purine-nucleoside: orthophosphate ribosyltransferase
    See IMMUNODEFICIENCY, NUCLEOSIDE-PHOSPHORYLASE DEFICIENCY
Purpura fulminans, neonatal
    See PROTEIN C DEFICIENCY
Purtilo syndrome
    See IMMUNODEFICIENCY, X-LINKED LYMPHOPROLIFERATIVE DISEASE
Pustular psoriasis
    See SKIN, PSORIASIS VULGARIS
PXE
    See PSEUDOXANTHOMA ELASTICUM
Pycnodysostosis
    See PYKNODYSOSTOSIS
Pygopagus
    See TWINS, CONJOINED

PYKNODYSOSTOSIS   0846

Includes:
    Pycnodysostosis
    Toulouse-Lautrec (possible diagnosis)

Excludes:
    Cleidocranial dysplasia (0185)
    Osteopetrosis (see all)

Major Diagnostic Criteria: Short stature with craniofacial dysmorphism and pathologic fractures. On X-rays, generalized increased density of the skeleton, delayed closure of the cranial sutures, mandibular hypoplasia, narrowness, partial amputation, or osteolysis of the distal phalanges.

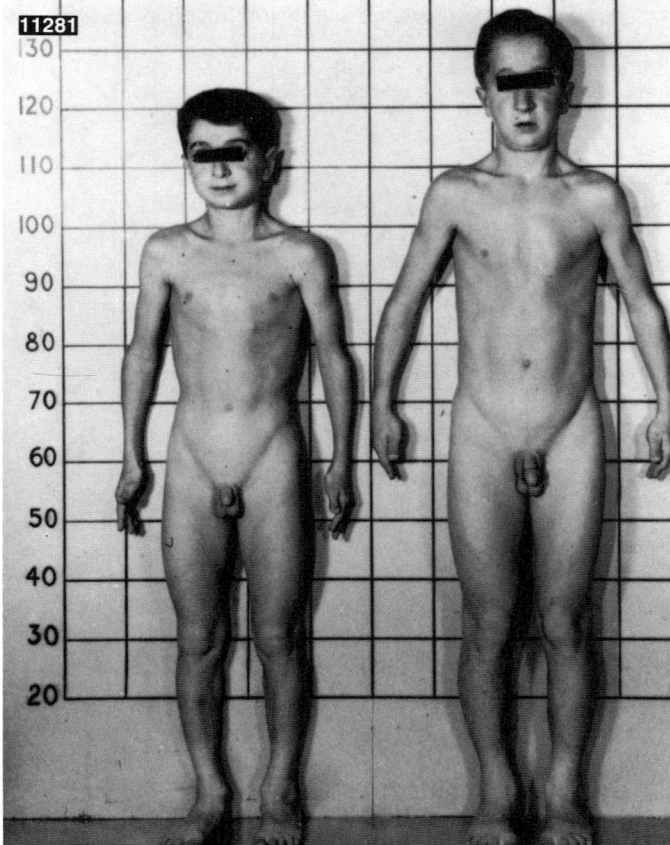

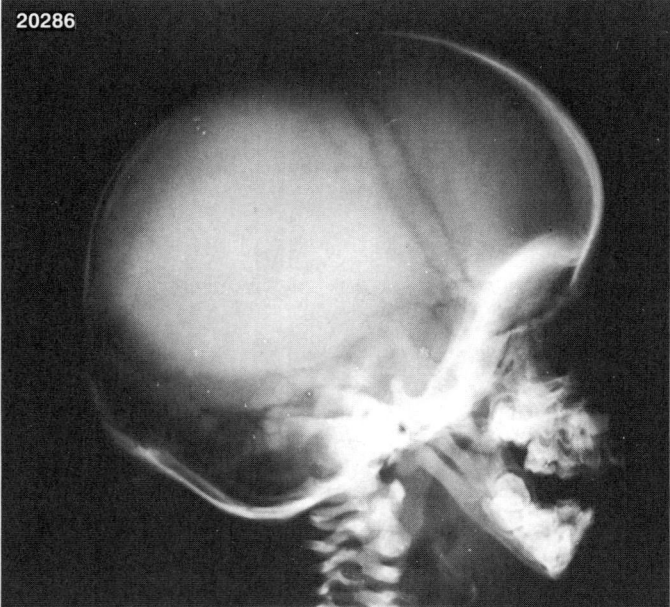

0846-11281: Pyknodysostosis in cousins; note short stature and craniofacial disproportion. **20286:** Skull X-ray of a 30-month-old male; note lack of closure of the anterior fontanel, marked enlargement of the lamboid suture, and hypoplasia of the mandible, which is almost rectilinear.

Clinical Findings: Patients are of short stature, with a final height of 1.35 to 1.50 m. The head is large with protrusion of the frontal bone; the anterior fontanelle remains largely open, and the chin is small and receding. Usually the sclerae have a bluish color, and dental anomalies with malplacements are frequent. The extremities are short, with a square aspect of the distal phalanges. Abnormal but moderate fragility of bones is usually present.

X-rays show the generally increased density of the skeleton without defective metaphyseal modeling of the long bones. On the hands, the terminal phalanges are narrow, and their distal portion disappears or is replaced by irregular bony fragments (an aspect comparable to that of a local osteolysis). The lack of closure of the anterior fontanelle, marked enlargement of the lambdoid suture, and mandibular hypoplasia are the most striking features. The angle of the mandible is wide so that the entire bone appears to be almost rectilinear. Teeth are irregularly aligned and in the adult total edentia is possible.

Complications: The risk of fracture is increased, but the complications of osteopetrosis (nervous compression, anemia) are absent.

Associated Findings: In one patient, dyspneic spells occurred as a consequence of mandibular hypoplasia. Spondylolisthesis is also possible.

Etiology: Autosomal recessive inheritance.

Pathogenesis: Ultrastructural study of growth cartilage reveals the presence of abnormal inclusions in the chondrocytes. These inclusions contain granular material and irregularly interwoven lamellar structure and can be excreted in the cell lacunae. The histochemical characteristics (coloration with Nile blue), and the ultrastructure probably indicate the phospholipid content of the vacuoles (Stanescu et al., 1984).

MIM No.: *26580

POS No.: 3365

Sex Ratio: M1:F1

Occurrence: About 30 cases have been documented.

Risk of Recurrence for Patient's Sib:
See Part I, *Mendelian Inheritance.*

Risk of Recurrence for Patient's Child:
See Part I, *Mendelian Inheritance.*

Age of Detectability: Usually during the first five years of life, on the basis of short stature, delayed closure of the anterior fontanelle, or fracture.

Gene Mapping and Linkage: Unknown.

Prevention: None known. Genetic counseling indicated.

Treatment: Orthopedic management of fracture; fixation with expanding intramedullary rods if repetition of tibial fractures.

Prognosis: Normal life span. The dwarfism is moderate.

Detection of Carrier: Unknown.

Special Considerations: There are good reasons to believe that the painter Henri de Toulouse Lautrec suffered from pyknodysostosis.

References:
Maroteaux P, Lamy M: La pycnodysostose. Presse Med 1962; 70:999–1002.
Maroteaux P, Lamy M: The malady of Toulouse-Lautrec. J Am Med Assoc 1965; 191:715–717.
Elmore SM, et al.: Pycnodysostosis, with a familial chromosome anomaly. Am J Med 1966; 40:273–282.
Maroteaux P, Fauré C: Pycnodysostosis. Prog Pediatr Radiol 1973; 4:403–413. *
Meredith SC, et al.: Pycnodysostosis: a clinical, pathological and ultramicroscopic study of a case. J Bone Joint Surg 1978; 60A:1122–1128.
Stanescu V, et al.: Pathogenic mechanisms in osteochondrodysplasias. J Bone Joint Surg 1984; 66A:817–836.

Pierre Maroteaux

PYLE DISEASE
0847

Includes: Metaphyseal dysplasia

Excludes: Craniometaphyseal dysplasia (0228)

Major Diagnostic Criteria: Gross metaphyseal expansion associated with few, if any, clinical manifestations.

Clinical Findings: Valgus deformity of the knees may be the only obvious abnormality, but muscular weakness, scoliosis, and bone fragility are sometimes present. In contrast to the mild clinical signs, the X-ray changes are striking. The tubular bones of the legs show gross "Erlenmeyer flask" flaring, particularly in the distal portions of the femora. The long bones of the arms are also undermodeled, and the cortices are generally thin. The skull is virtually normal, apart from a supraorbital prominence. The bones of the pelvis and thoracic cage are expanded.

Complications: There may be a mild tendency to fracturing.

Associated Findings: None known.

Etiology: Autosomal recessive inheritance.

Pathogenesis: Unknown.

MIM No.: *26590

POS No.: 3367

Sex Ratio: M1:F1

Occurrence: About 20 cases have been documented. The wide geographic distribution includes the United States, Germany, France, South Africa, India, and Saudi Arabia.

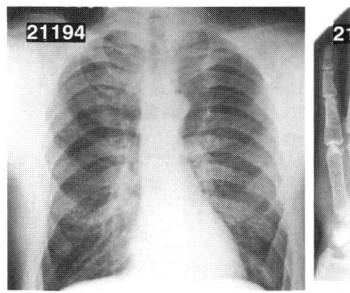
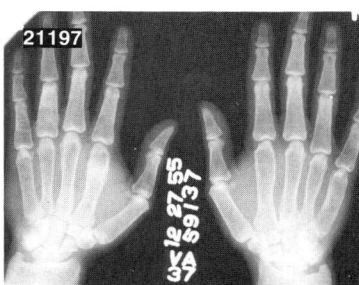
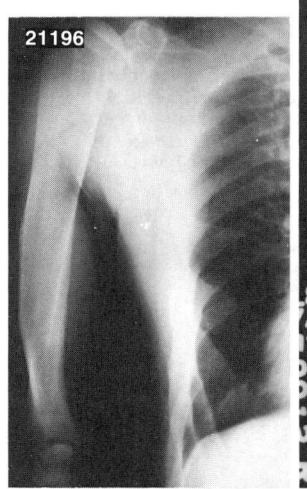
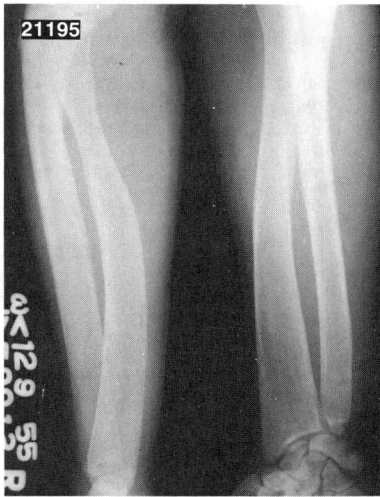
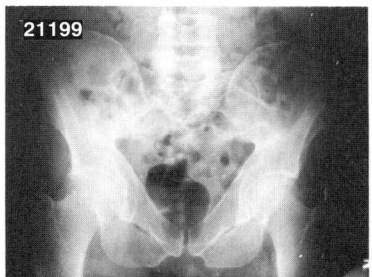
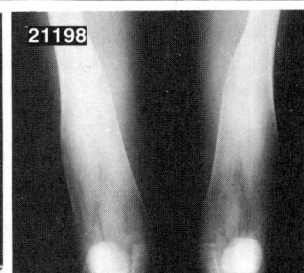

0847B-21194: Ribs and clavicles are markedly thickened. **21197:** Tubular bones of the hands show marked distal flaring of the metacarpals and proximal flaring of the phalanges. **21196:** Humerus is undermodeled in the proximal two-thirds. **21195:** Radius and ulna are undermodeled in the distal two-thirds. **21199:** Pelvis and ischial bones are thickened. **21198:** Femora exhibit most marked "Erlenmeyer flask"-like flare which extends far up the diaphysis.

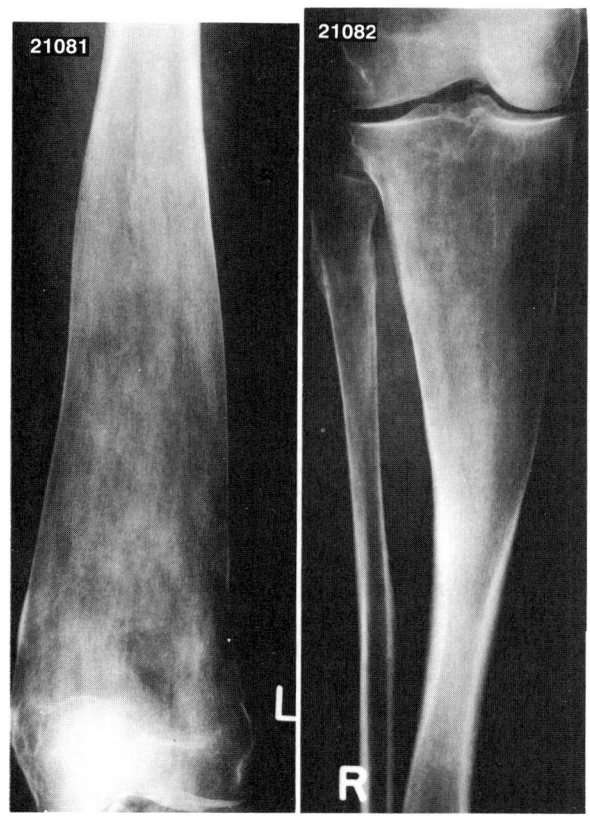

0847A-21081: X-ray of the femur of an affected male showing gross Erlenmeyer flask appearance and marked cortical thinning. **21082:** The proximal regions of the tibia and fibula are flared and the cortices are thin.

Risk of Recurrence for Patient's Sib:
See Part I, *Mendelian Inheritance.*

Risk of Recurrence for Patient's Child:
See Part I, *Mendelian Inheritance.*

Age of Detectability: In early childhood, by X-ray.

Gene Mapping and Linkage: Unknown.

Prevention: None known. Genetic counseling indicated.

Treatment: Unknown.

Prognosis: Intelligence and lifespan are normal. General health is good.

Detection of Carrier: Heterozygotes have minor disturbances of modelling in the metaphyses of the tubular bones, especially the distal femora.

Special Considerations: This condition is named after Edwin Pyle (1891–1961), an orthopedic surgeon from Waterbury, Connecticut, who published the first case in 1931.

There has been nosologic confusion between Pyle disease and the autosomal recessive form of **Craniometaphyseal dysplasia.** It must be emphasized that these conditions are distinct and separate entities.

References:
Pyle E: Case of unusual bone development. J Bone Joint Surg 1931; 13:874–876.
Gorlin RJ, et al.: Pyle's disease (familial metaphyseal dysplasia). J Bone Joint Surg 1970; 52A:345–354.
Raad MS, Beighton P: Autosomal recessive inheritance of metaphyseal dysplasia (Pyle's disease). Clin Genet 1978; 14:251–256. * †
Heselson NG, et al.: The radiological manifestations of metaphyseal dysplasia (Pyle's disease). Brit J Radiol 1979; 52/618:431–440. * †
Beighton P: Pyle disease (metaphyseal dysplasia). J Med Genet 1987; 24:321–324.

BE008   **Peter Beighton**

Pyloric atresia
  See STOMACH, PYLORIC ATRESIA
Pyloric atresia, hereditary
  See PYLORODUODENAL ATRESIA, HEREDITARY
Pyloric diaphragm, incomplete
  See STOMACH, PYLORIC ATRESIA

PYLORIC STENOSIS   0848

Includes: Hypertrophic pyloric stenosis, congenital

Excludes: Pylorospasm

Major Diagnostic Criteria: Nonbilious vomiting and pyloric hypertrophy identified by palpation of a pyloric "tumor." Sonography or upper GI series may be diagnostic when "tumor" cannot be palpated.

Clinical Findings: Nonbilious projectile vomiting, characteristically beginning at 2–3 weeks of age, which progresses to almost complete gastric outlet obstruction associated with constipation, weight loss, dehydration, and electrolyte imbalance (hypokalemic alkalosis). Eagerness to nurse after vomiting is common. Visible gastric peristaltic waves proceed from left to right after feeding. The thickened, hypertrophied, muscular pylorus can be palpated in the epigastrium as an olive-sized and olive-shaped movable mass or "tumor." Contrast X-ray studies (using a barium-water mixture) identify an elongated, curved, pyloric channel, with proximal and distal protrusion of the hypertrophied pyloric musculature into the duodenal and gastric lumen to cause the so-called "shoulder" sign. Delayed gastric emptying is not a valid specific diagnostic sign.

Complications: Starvation, dehydration, and severe electrolyte imbalance. Jaundice (unusual, less than 3%), with predominance of indirect bilirubin. Hematemesis.

Associated Findings: Jaundice (< 3%), gastric ulcer.

Etiology: Probably polygenic and sex modified. It is improbable that just one gene makes a major contribution to its genetic liability.

Pathogenesis: The hypertrophy of the circular (and some longitudinal) musculature of the pylorus is progressive, to some extent. Variations in mucosal edema account for changes in the degree of obstruction.

MIM No.: 17901

CDC No.: 750.510

Sex Ratio: M4:F1

Occurrence: 1:250 births (1:200 males; 1:1,000 females). Most frequent in Caucasians; uncommon in non-Caucasians, rare in Asiatics (especially Chinese). The most common problem requiring abdominal surgery in infancy.

Risk of Recurrence for Patient's Sib: If mother was affected, 1:5 (20%) for brothers, and 1:14 (7%) for sisters. If father was affected, 1:20 (5%) for brothers, and 1:40 (21/2 %) for sisters.

Risk of Recurrence for Patient's Child: If patient is female, 1:5 (20%) for sons, and 1:14 (7%) for daughters. If patient is male, 1:20 (5%) for sons, and 1:40 (21/2 %) for daughters.

Age of Detectability: Usually at 2–4 weeks of age.

Gene Mapping and Linkage: Unknown.

Prevention: None known. Genetic counseling indicated.

Treatment: Laparotomy and Ramstedt pyloromyotomy are curative. Nonsurgical treatment with antispasmodics is generally unsatisfactory.

Prognosis: Excellent. Following pyloromyotomy symptoms vanish, and the pyloric hypertrophy disappears. Some evidence suggests a higher incidence of peptic ulcer in later life.

Detection of Carrier: Unknown.

References:
Carter CO, Evans KA: Inheritance of congenital pyloric stenosis. J Med Genet 1969; 6:233.
Rickham PP, et al., eds: Congenital hypertrophic pyloric stenosis. In: Rickham PP, et al., eds: Neonatal surgery. New York: Appleton-Century-Crofts, 1969:271.
Fried K, et al.: Probable autosomal dominant infantile pyloric stenosis in a large kindred. Clin Genet 1981; 20:328–330.
Spicer RD: Infantile hypertrophic pyloric stenosis: a review. Br J Surg 1982; 69:128–135. *
Tunell WP, Wilson DA: Diagnosis by real time sonograph. J Pediatr Surg 1984; 19:795–199. *

SI004   **William K. Sieber**

PYLORODUODENAL ATRESIA, HEREDITARY   2617

Includes:
  Duodenal atresia of the first segment, hereditary
  Pyloric atresia, hereditary

Excludes:
  Intestinal atresia, multiple (2933)
  Jejunal atresia (2934)

Major Diagnostic Criteria: The pylorus and the first part of the duodenum are reduced to a fibrous band or are obstructed by a diaphragm.

Clinical Findings: The pregnancy is complicated by polyhydramnios in about 90% of the cases. The newborn presents with low birth weight in 60% of the cases, and continuous projectile, nonbileous vomiting in 95% of patients. On physical examination, the epigastric region may be distended (in 85%). X-ray studies reveal complete obstruction of the pylorus.

At exploratory laparotomy, there is complete diaphragmatic obstruction (in the majority) or a fibrous band blocking the lumen of the pylorus and the first portion of the duodenum.

Complications: If untreated, the patient may die of starvation or perforation of the stomach.

Associated Findings: Epidermolysis bullosum associated with complete pyloric atresia was reported in four cases.

Etiology: Autosomal recessive inheritance.

Pathogenesis: Possibly derangement in the vacuolization of the "solid" stage of the embryonic pylorus.

MIM No.: 22340, *26595

CDC No.: 751.100

Sex Ratio: M1:F1

Occurrence: Fewer than 50 patients with the hereditary type have been reported.

Risk of Recurrence for Patient's Sib:
  See Part I, *Mendelian Inheritance.*

Risk of Recurrence for Patient's Child:
See Part I, *Mendelian Inheritance.* The gene frequency of this disorder is very low.

Age of Detectability: During the neonatal period.

Gene Mapping and Linkage: Unknown.

Prevention: None known. Genetic counseling indicated.

Treatment: Preferably gastroduodenostomy. Gastrojejunostomy only if gastroduodenostomy is not possible.

Prognosis: Excellent with proper surgical intervention.

Detection of Carrier: Unknown.

Special Considerations: In all cases of pyloroduodenal atresia, it is very important to keep the possibility of the hereditary type in mind for proper counseling of the family. Thus, fetal sonography or postdelivery investigations can be done on time for early surgical intervention, if necessary. This may be life-saving.

References:
Mishalany HG, et al.: Familial congenital duodenal atresia. Pediatrics 1970; 46:629–632. *
Bronsther B, et al.: Congenital pyloric atresia: a report of three cases and review of the literature. Surgery 1971; 69:130–136.
Mishalany HG, et al.: Familial congenital duodenal atresia. (Letter) Pediatrics 1971; 47:633–634.
Bar-Maor JA, et al.: Pyloric atresia: a hereditary congenital anomaly with autosomal recessive transmission. J Med Genet 1972; 9:70–72.
Tan KL, Murugasu JJ: Congenital pyloric atresia in siblings. Arch Surg 1973; 106:100–102.
Der Kaloustian VM, et al.: Familial congenital duodenal atresia (cont.). (Letter) Pediatrics 1974; 54:118 only.
Rosenbloom MS, Ratner M: Congenital pyloric atresia and epidermolysis bullosa letalis in premature siblings. J Pediat Surg 1987; 22:374–375.

DE030   **Vazken M. Der Kaloustian**
MI039   **Henry G. Mishalany**

Pyorrhea-epilepsy-alopecia-mental retardation
See ALOPECIA-SEIZURES-MENTAL RETARDATION, SHOKEIR TYPE
Pyramidal chest
See PECTUS CARINATUM
Pyridoxine deficiency induced by isoniazid therapy
See NEUROPATHY, HERITABLE ISONIAZIDE TYPE (INH)
Pyridoxine dependency
See SEIZURES, VITAMIN B(6) DEPENDENCY
Pyridoxine-responsive homocystinuria
See HOMOCYSTINURIA
Pyroglutamic acidemia
See ACIDEMIA, PYROGLUTAMIC
Pyroglutamic aciduria
See ANEMIA, HEMOLYTIC, GLUTATHIONE SYNTHETASE DEFICIENCY
Pyropoikilocytosis
See ELLIPTOCYTOSIS
Pyropoikilocytosis, hereditary
See ANEMIA, HEMOLYTIC, RED CELL MEMBRANE DEFECTS
Pyrroloporphyria
See PORPHYRIA, ACUTE INTERMITTENT

PYRUVATE CARBOXYLASE DEFICIENCY WITH LACTIC ACIDEMIA   0850

Includes:
Ataxia with lactic acidosis II
Lactic acidemia without hypoxemia
Leigh necrotizing encephalopathy (some cases)

Excludes:
Carboxylase deficiency, multiple
Fructose-1-phosphate aldolase deficiency (0395)
Fructose-1,6-diphosphatase deficiency (0396)
Lactate elevation secondary to other causes
Myopathy, mitochondrial
Pyruvate dehydrogenase deficiency (0851)

Major Diagnostic Criteria: Neurologic deterioration with lactic and pyruvic acidemia. Demonstration of decreased pyruvate carboxylase activity in cultured skin fibroblasts, leukocytes, or liver confirms the diagnosis.

Clinical Findings: Pyruvate carboxylase deficiency has been found in patients who develop severe neonatal lactic acidosis, and those whose clinical disease has a later onset. In the later case, the patient may appear normal at birth and during infancy, but whose development tends to be slow. More serious difficulties become apparent by one year of age. Abnormalities have included "failure to thrive", vomiting, irritability, apathy, inactivity, hypotonia, areflexia, spasticity, cerebellar ataxia, abnormal eye movements, and seizures. The course is usually progressive, with neurologic and intellectual deterioration, and death has occurred within several years. Some children have been diagnosed as having **Encephalopathy, necrotizing** (subacute).

Lactate, pyruvate, and alanine are elevated on most occasions, and the lactate-to-pyruvate ratio is usually in the normal range. In the acute form, the lactate levels may be catastrophically high, and in some instances ammonia, citrulline, proline, and lysine have been described as elevated. Those patients with later onset of obvious symptoms may have lactate levels in the range of 20–40 mg/dl (2–4 mMol/L); levels which do not obviously distort the acid base balance. EEG abnormalities have occurred in some patients. Pyruvate carboxylase activity has been decreased or absent in liver biopsy specimens.

Complications: Neurologic and intellectual deterioration. Death, in most instances.

Associated Findings: None known.

Etiology: Autosomal recessive inheritance.

Pathogenesis: Pyruvate carboxylase is important both in gluconeogenesis and in maintaining adequate levels of oxaloacetate to support full activity of the tricarboxylic acid cycle. Hypoglycemia has not been a prominent part of the clinical picture in most patients.

MIM No.: *26615

Sex Ratio: M1:F1

Occurrence: Undetermined but presumed rare. Established literature.

Risk of Recurrence for Patient's Sib:
See Part I, *Mendelian Inheritance.*

Risk of Recurrence for Patient's Child:
See Part I, *Mendelian Inheritance.* Affected individuals are not expected to survive to reproduce.

Age of Detectability: Earliest diagnoses were made within the first several days for the neonatal form, and the first several months for less severely affected patients. Lactate and pyruvate theoretically should be elevated within the first week of life in all patients. Diagnosis is confirmed by liver biopsy or study of cultured skin fibroblasts, and should be positive at birth.

Gene Mapping and Linkage: PC (pyruvate carboxylase) has been provisionally mapped to 11q.

Prevention: None known. Genetic counseling indicated.

Treatment: Thiamine, lipoic acid, glutamine, and aspartic acid in pharmacologic doses have all been reported to be helpful in reducing lactate and pyruvate levels, and in mitigating the symptoms and their rate of progression.

Prognosis: Poor. Death usually occurs within several years.

Detection of Carrier: Unknown.

Special Considerations: The signs and symptoms of this disorder are nonspecific and inconsistent. Primary suspicion is caused by elevated lactate, pyruvate, or alanine, and the diagnosis must be confirmed by liver biopsy. It cannot be readily distinguished from **Pyruvate dehydrogenase deficiency** on clinical or biochemical grounds alone. The assay for pyruvate carboxylase is reported to be difficult and is best performed in a laboratory with experience in the methodology.

Biotin-responsive multiple carboxylase deficiency may present as lactic acidemia due to a predominant deficiency of pyruvate carboxylase. Diagnosis can be confirmed by urinary organic acid analysis.

Lactic acidemia is defined by the presence of a blood lactate in excess of 15 mg/dl and becomes lactic acidosis when compensatory mechanisms are no longer able to maintain the arterial pH in the normal range. Lactate exists in equilibrium with pyruvate and with alanine. The NADH/NAD ratio reflects the ratio of lactate (L) to pyruvate (P). In some instances, the L/P ratio provides a clue to the nature of the primary metabolic error.

Elevation of blood lactate is a laboratory abnormality that may be due to a variety of inherited and acquired conditions. Within each entity, the severity may vary with the nature and degree of the enzyme deficiency. Seizure activity may raise blood and cerebrospinal fluid lactate levels. It is prudent to wait 12–24 hours after the control of electrical seizure activity before assessing lactate and pyruvate.

Because lactate and pyruvate are readily measured in most clinical laboratories, elevations in these compounds may be detected in cases of acidosis, even though the primary cause of the acidosis may be an entirely different disorder. Conversely, significant elevations in both lactate and pyruvate may cause no obvious alteration in plasma bicarbonate and thus be overlooked entirely.

The assessment of patients with elevations of lactate must include measurement of the lactate/pyruvate ratio, urinary lactate excretion, association between lactate and pyruvate levels and meals, plasma and urinary ketone body levels, blood sugar measurement in the fasting and post-prandial state, plasma amino acids, urinary amino and organic acids, and a history for sensitivity to dietary factors or other minor environmental stress. High levels of pyruvate may cause an apparent false-positive test for ketones when using a commercial nitroprusside reagent (Acetest, Ames).

In a decreasing but still significant number of patients with an apparently primary elevation of lactate and pyruvate, no definite enzymatic diagnosis is made. In these instances, some people use empiric dietary therapy or pharmacologic doses of thiamine, biotin, or lipoic acid. False-positive and nonspecific chemical responses to thiamine have been reported.

In most cases in which no enzymatic diagnosis is made, it is most prudent to assume that the inheritance is autosomal recessive. Exceptions include those instances of a similar disease in a parent or those cases of primary myopathy in which autosomal dominant or other inheritance mechanisms may be operating.

References:
Saudubray JM, et al.: Neonatal congenital lactic acidosis with pyruvate carboxylase deficiency in two siblings. Acta Pediatr Scand 1976; 65:717–724.
Robinson BH, et al.: The genetic heterogeneity of lactic acidosis: occurrence of recognizable inborn errors of metabolism in a pediatric population with lactic acidosis. Pediatr Res 1980; 14:956–962.
Freytag SO, Collier KJ: Molecular cloning of a cDNA for human pyruvate carboxylase. J Biol Chem 1984; 259:12831–12837.
Robinson BH, et al.: The French and North American phenotypes of pyruvate carboxylase deficiency. Am J Hum Genet 1987; 40:50–59.
Robinson BH: Lactic acidemia. In: Scriver CR, et al, eds: The metabolic basis of inherited disease, 6th ed. New York: McGraw-Hill, 1989: 869–888. *

CE001

Stephen D. Cederbaum
John P. Blass

PYRUVATE DEHYDROGENASE DEFICIENCY   0851

Includes:
Alaninuria
Ataxia, intermittent-pyruvate dehydrogenase deficiency
Ataxia, intermittent-pyruvate decarboxylase deficiency
Ataxia with lactic acidosis I
Lactic and pyruvic acidemia with carbohydrate sensitivity
Lactic and pyruvic acidemia with episodic ataxia and weakness

Excludes:
Fructose-1,6-diphosphatase deficiency (0396)
Lactic acidosis-persistently increased lactate: pyruvate ratio
Lactic and pyruvic acidemia due to other causes

Major Diagnostic Criteria: Persistent or recurrent pyruvic and usually lactic acidemia. Enzyme deficiency must be confirmed using skin fibroblasts or other tissue.

Clinical Findings: Findings may vary from severe acidosis appearing in the first few days of life to recurrent episodes of ataxia and weakness following upper respiratory infection or other minor stress. Growth retardation has been frequent. Varying permanent neurologic deficits and mental retardation have been seen in most patients. Near-normal resting levels of lactate and pyruvate have been associated with severe neurologic damage in several patients.

Biochemical findings vary from severe lactic acidosis appearing shortly after birth to minimal pyruvic acidemia (1.5–1.8 mg/dl; normally <1.2) 2 hours following a meal high in carbohydrates. In some instances elevation of blood pyruvate levels is seen only during the acute episodes of ataxia and weakness. The blood lactate:pyruvate ratio has almost always been normal (< 20). Alanine excretion of greater than 100 mg/g creatinine is a variable finding and often is present only during acute episodes. Blood alanine has been elevated above 6 mg/dl only with pyruvate values persistently greater than 2.0 mg/dl. Cerebrospinal fluid pyruvate and lactate also have been elevated. Increased lactate in the urine (> 0.7 mg/mg creatine) is seen when blood lactate is 2–4 times normal or more.

Complications: Mental retardation and neurologic damage; in some instances, early death from lactic acidosis.

Associated Findings: None known.

Etiology: Autosomal recessive inheritance.

Pathogenesis: Defective oxidation of pyruvate and deficiency of pyruvate dehydrogenase have been demonstrated in cultured skin fibroblasts, peripheral lymphocytes, muscle, and other visceral tissues. Increased dietary carbohydrates typically precipitate lactic acidosis in the more severely affected patients.

MIM No.: *20880

Sex Ratio: Presumably M1:F1, but males predominate in reported cases.

Occurrence: Over 100 cases have been documented.

Risk of Recurrence for Patient's Sib:
See Part I, *Mendelian Inheritance.*

Risk of Recurrence for Patient's Child:
See Part I, *Mendelian Inheritance.*

Age of Detectability: Shortly after birth, by skin fibroblast assay or other tissue assay. Age at which pyruvate and lactate elevation is detected will probably depend on the nature and severity of the biochemical defect.

Gene Mapping and Linkage: One subunit of the complex has been mapped to the X chromosome; the others are autosomal.

Prevention: None known. Genetic counseling indicated.

Treatment: The disorder is exacerbated by increased carbohydrate intake and improved by increased dietary fat. Avoidance of infection and undue stress is desirable. High doses of thiamine have not yet proven beneficial. Corticosteroid therapy has been reported to abort the acute episodes of ataxia and weakness in several instances.

Prognosis: In most instances irreversible neurologic damage and mental retardation have occurred by the time of diagnosis. The impact of a high-fat diet instituted at an early age has not been assessed. The ultimate risk of permanent neurologic handicap to those patients with only episodic symptoms is unknown.

Detection of Carrier: By analysis of skin fibroblasts. Discrimination incomplete.

Special Considerations: Blood pyruvate levels have always been abnormal following a meal high in carbohydrate. The long-term impact of a high-fat diet has not been determined. Dietary trial for pyruvic and lactic acidemia should be undertaken with care, since other causes of pyruvic acidemia may lead to carbohydrate dependence.

Pyruvate dehydrogenase is a complex of three catalytic and two regulatory enzymes. Deficiency of all three catalytic enzymes, and of the activating enzyme, have been reported. Ultimately, the disorders caused by each defect may be distinguishable clinically and prognostically.

References:

Falk RE, et al.: Ketogenic diet in the treatment of pyruvate dehydrogenase deficiency. Pediatrics 1976; 58:713–721.

Robinson BH, et al.: The genetic heterogeneity of lactic acidosis: occurrence of recognizable inborn errors of metabolism in a pediatric population with lactic acidosis. Pediat Res 1980; 14:956–962. *

Prick M, et al.: Pyruvate dehydrogenase deficiency restricted to brain. Neurology 1981; 31:398–404.

McKay N, et al.: Lacticacidemia due to pyruvate dehydrogenase deficiency, with evidence of protein polymorphism in the α-subunit of the enzyme. Eur J Pediat 1986; 144:445–450.

Patel M, Roche T, eds: Alpha ketoacid dehydrogenase complexes: organization, regulation and biochemical aspects. New York: New York Academy of Sciences, 1989.

Robinson BH: Lactic acidemia. In: Scriver CR, et al, eds: The metabolic basis of inherited disease, 6th ed. New York: McGraw-Hill, 1989: 869–888. *

CE001

Stephen D. Cederbaum
John P. Blass

PYRUVATE KINASE DEFICIENCY   0852

Includes:

  Anemia, hemolytic pyruvate kinase type
  Pyruvate kinase deficiency of erythrocyte

Excludes:

  Nonspherocytic hemolytic anemias from other enzyme deficiencies
  Nonspherocytic hemolytic anemias from unstable hemoglobin

Major Diagnostic Criteria: Pallor due to hemolytic anemia with reticulocytosis. There is no specific abnormality of erythrocyte morphology. Increased autohemolysis of affected erythrocytes in vitro is usually demonstrable, usually uncorrected by glucose but corrected by adenosine triphosphate (ATP). Erythrocyte 2, 3DPG levels are unusually high, in severely anemic patients reaching levels greater than 3 times normal. Erythrocyte pyruvate kinase activity is reduced, usually to 5–20% of normal. Occasionally, maximal pyruvate kinase activity is normal but the enzyme exhibits unfavorable kinetic properties at low substrate (phospho-enol-pyruvate) concentrations. International standards for biochemical characterization of pyruvate kinase mutants have been developed.

Clinical Findings: Signs of excessive hemolysis of varying grades of severity and changing from time to time; chronic hemolytic anemia, hyperbilirubinemia, splenomegaly, reticulocytosis.

Complications: Gallstones are secondary to chronic hyperbilirubinemia. Exacerbations of anemia, resulting from transient marrow erythroid hypoplasia, are usually associated with infections. Leg ulcers rarely occur.

Associated Findings: Leukocyte pyruvate kinase is normal, but liver pyruvate kinase activity may be reduced.

Etiology: Autosomal recessive inheritance.

Pathogenesis: The sequence of events preceding hemolysis of pyruvate kinase deficient erythrocytes is poorly understood. Deficient erythrocytes usually have low glycolytic rates in vitro (particularly when compared to control erythrocytes of similar age) and are unable to maintain intracellular ATP levels. However, in vivo erythrocyte ATP levels may be normal. Nevertheless, ATP depletion as a result of inadequate glycolysis is thought to be the central event resulting in premature hemolysis. The almost immediate destruction of a portion of newly formed reticulocytes

in the spleen or elsewhere in the reticuloendothelial system contributes importantly to the observed hemolysis. Molecular variants of erythrocyte pyruvate kinase have been characterized by their abnormal substrate kinetics, but no detailed studies of molecular structure are as yet available.

MIM No.: *26620

Sex Ratio: M1:F1

Occurrence: Undetermined but presumed rare. Most affected individuals thus far described have been of European or Amish origin. Extensive literature. An estimated 2.4:1,000 heterozygotes for enzyme deficiency variants.

Risk of Recurrence for Patient's Sib:
  See Part I, *Mendelian Inheritance.*

Risk of Recurrence for Patient's Child:
  See Part I, *Mendelian Inheritance.*

Age of Detectability: At birth, by assay of erythrocyte pyruvate kinase.

Gene Mapping and Linkage: PKLR (pyruvate kinase, liver and RBC) has been provisionally mapped to 1q21.

Prevention: None known. Genetic counseling indicated.

Treatment: Splenectomy reduces or eliminates the need for blood transfusions in severely anemic patients but is not curative. Anemia persists, but usually a higher hemoglobin level can be maintained. Postsplenectomy reticulocyte counts usually rise rather than fall and may occasionally exceed 90%. Supportive blood transfusions should be given when indicated. Cholecystectomy is indicated if gallstones form.

Prognosis: Varies with severity of anemia (e.g. high mortality in early childhood described in unsplenectomized Amish kindred). Most patients survive to adulthood, and mildly anemic patients may expect to have a near-normal life span unless complications (e.g. gallstones) supervene.

Detection of Carrier: Carriers are clinically and hematologically normal, but their erythrocyte pyruvate kinase activity is usually one-half the normal level. Alternatively, carriers may have normal enzyme activity, but abnormal substrate kinetics (altered Km of PEP).

Special Considerations: Pyruvate kinase deficient reticulocytes are protected from the consequences of their glycolytic defect by the availability of alternate metabolic pathways (oxidative phosphorylation).

Oxidative phosphorylation in such reticulocytes may be inhibited during sequestration in hypoxic, acidic regions of the spleen whereupon glycolysis alone is inadequate to support their increased ATP requirements. The result is ATP depletion which induces a membrane lesion characterized by massive prelytic loss of intracellular potassium and water, cell shrinkage, and increased cell rigidity. The shrunken rigid cell produced is presumed to be susceptible to further sequestration because of difficulty in traversing the 3 micron pores separating splenic cords from sinuses. Eventually, cell lysis occurs. Splenectomy, by removal of a stagnant, hypoxic trap, allows reticulocytes to survive, and partially alleviates the anemia.

References:

Keitt AS, Bennett DC: Pyruvate kinase deficiency and related disorders of red cell glycolysis. Am J Med 1966; 41:762–785.

Miwa S: Recommended methods for the characterization of red cell pyruvate kinase variants. Br J Haematol 1979; 43:275–286.

Mentzer WC Jr.: Pyruvate kinase deficiency and disorders of glycolysis. In: Nathan DG, Oski FA, eds: Hematology of infancy and childhood, 3rd ed. Philadelphia: W.B. Saunders, 1987:545–582.

Valentine WN, et al.: Pyruvate kinase and other enzyme deficiency disorders of the erythrocyte. In: Scriver CR, et al, eds: The metabolic basis of inherited disease, 6th ed. New York: McGraw-Hill, 1989: 2341–2366.

ME019

William C. Mentzer, Jr.

Pyruvate kinase deficiency of erythrocyte
See PYRUVATE KINASE DEFICIENCY

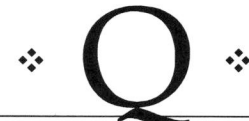

Quinine, fetal effects of
  See OPTIC NERVE HYPOPLASIA
Quinoform induced subacute myelo-optico neuropathy (SMON)
  See NEUROPATHY, MYELO-OPTICO, SUBACUTE TYPE
Quinoid dihydropteridine reductase deficiency
  See DIHYDROPTERIDINE REDUCTASE DEFICIENCY
Quivering of chin, hereditary
  See CHIN, TREMBLING

❖ R ❖

Rabenhorst syndrome
  See VENTRICULAR SEPTAL DEFECT
Rabson-Mendenhall syndrome
  See LIPODYSTROPHY-COARSE FACIES-ACANTHOSIS NIGRICANS,
    MIESCHER TYPE
Rachipagus
  See TWINS, CONJOINED
Racial lactase deficiency
  See LACTASE DEFICIENCY, PRIMARY
Radial aplasia-cleft lip/palate
  See RADIAL DEFECTS
Radial aplasia-craniosynostosis
  See CRANIOSYNOSTOSIS-RADIAL APLASIA SYNDROME

RADIAL DEFECTS   0853

Includes:
    Deficiency of radial rays and radius and phocomelia
    Phocomelia and radial ray defects
    Radial aplasia-cleft lip/palate
    Radial dysplasia
    Thumb defects

Excludes:
    Craniosynostosis (0230)
    Fetal thalidomide syndrome (0386)
    Heart-hand syndrome (0455)
    Pancytopenia syndrome, Fanconi type (2029)
    Thrombocytopenia-absent radius (0941)
    Vater association (0987)
    Ventriculoradial dysplasia

Major Diagnostic Criteria: Hypoplasia of the thumb or first metacarpal in the absence of other malformations.

Clinical Findings: Several degrees of severity occur. In the mildest form, there is hypoplasia of the first metacarpal often combined with hypoplasia of the thumb. With increasing severity, there is complete loss of the first metacarpal producing a small flail thumb attached to the index finger by soft tissue. The next level of severity is characterized by hypoplasia or aplasia of the radius associated with varying degrees of thumb and first metacarpal hypoplasia (see **Hand, radial club hand**). Both the radius and ulna are absent in the most severe form which is associated with variable radial ray abnormalities and often hypoplasia of the humerus. Approximately 20% of all affected individuals have radial defects alone, of which about two-thirds are unilateral.

A possible variant, *radial aplasia-cleft lip/palate*, has been reported in at least 18 cases (Immeyer, 1967).

Complications: Dysfunction of upper limbs related to severity of malformation.

Associated Findings: Possibly cleft lip/palate, or this association may constitute a distinct condition.

Etiology: If all cases of radial defects with associated anomalies are excluded, most cases are sporadic.

Pathogenesis: Suppression of developing limb structures.

MIM No.: 17910, 17940

CDC No.: 755.280

Sex Ratio: M1:F1

Occurrence: Undetermined but presumed rare.

Risk of Recurrence for Patient's Sib: Undetermined, but probably low.

Risk of Recurrence for Patient's Child: Undetermined, but probably low.

Age of Detectability: At birth.

Gene Mapping and Linkage: Unknown.

Prevention: None known. Genetic counseling indicated.

Treatment: Surgery may improve function in certain cases.

Prognosis: Normal intelligence and life span. Dysfunction is related to severity of deformity.

Detection of Carrier: Unknown.

Special Considerations: For accurate genetic counseling, as well as proper treatment, it is important to exclude the many complex syndromes in which radial defects occur. In particular, the cardiovascular, GU, and hematologic systems should be carefully examined. Although families have been reported showing autosomal dominant inheritance of isolated radial defects, it is very difficult to completely rule out the more complex syndromes; e.g. **Heart-hand syndrome** with no or only minor heart manifestations.

References:
Immeyer F: Lippen-Kiefer-Gaumenspalten bei thalidomidgeschaedigten Kindern. Acta Genet Med Gemellol 1967; 16:244–274.
Carroll RE, Louis DS: Anomalies associated with radial dysplasia. J Pediatr 1974; 84:409–411.
Temtamy SA: On anomalies associated with radial dysplasia. J Pediatr 1974; 85:585 only.

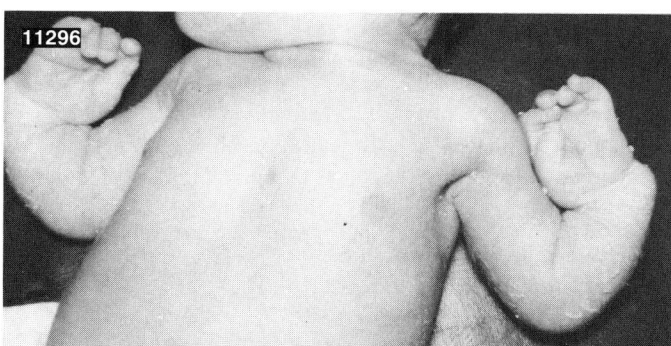

0853-11296:   Radial aplasia.

Temtamy SA, McKusick VA: The genetics of hand malformation. New York: Alan R. Liss, 1978.

H0033   **William A. Horton**
H0025   **O.J. Hood**

Radial deficiency or defect
See HAND, RADIAL CLUB HAND
Radial dysplasia
See HAND, RADIAL CLUB HAND
also RADIAL DEFECTS
Radial hemimelia
See HAND, RADIAL CLUB HAND
Radial hypoplasia-deafness-ophthalmoplegia-thrombocytopenia
See IVIC SYNDROME

RADIAL HYPOPLASIA-TRIPHALANGEAL THUMBS-HYPOSPADIAS-DIASTEMA   2772

Includes:
  Diastema-radial hypoplasia-triphalangeal thumbs-
    hypospadias
  Hypospadias-radial hypoplasia-triphalangeal thumbs-
    diastema
  Schmitt syndrome
  Thumbs, triphalangeal-radial hypoplasia-diastema-
    hypospadias

Excludes:
  Heart-hand syndrome (0455)
  Pancytopenia syndrome, Fanconi type (2029)
  Roberts syndrome (0875)
  Thrombocytopenia-absent radius (0941)

Major Diagnostic Criteria: In the single described family, all indicated features were present (except hypospadias in the females). The diagnosis should not be entertained in a family unless all the features are present in at least one member or collectively in several family members.

Clinical Findings: The hands demonstrate triphalangeal, nonopposable thumbs without flexion creases. Flexion creases are hypoplastic on the second digits. The hands are radially deviated and the forearms are markedly shortened, with limitation in pronation, supination, and extension. Despite the deformities, adults have good manual dexterity and hand-writing skills. In males, the hypospadias consists of a pinpoint meatus on the distal ventral shaft of the penis. A 1–2-mm gap between the upper central incisors (maxillary diastema) is present in all affected individuals; no other dental anomalies were noted.

Complications: As with any case of hypospadias, other urinary tract anomalies or obstruction should be investigated, but no urinary complications were noted in the family studied.

Associated Findings: None known.

Etiology: Autosomal dominant inheritance with complete penetrance and little variability.

Pathogenesis: Unknown.

MIM No.:   17925

POS No.:   3551

Sex Ratio: M1:F1

Occurrence: One kinship has been reported.

Risk of Recurrence for Patient's Sib:
  See Part I, *Mendelian Inheritance.*

Risk of Recurrence for Patient's Child:
  See Part I, *Mendelian Inheritance.*

Age of Detectability: During the newborn period.

Gene Mapping and Linkage: Unknown.

Prevention: None known. Genetic counseling indicated.

Treatment: Surgical repair of hypospadias. The triphalangeal thumb can be rendered opposable and the radially deviated hand supported by a brace if functionally indicated.

Prognosis: Normal life span. Minimal associated disability.

Detection of Carrier: By clinical examination.

References:
Schmitt E, et al.: An autosomal dominant syndrome of radial hypoplasia, triphalangeal thumbs, hypospadias and maxillary diastema. J Med Genet 1982; 13:63–69.

KE012   **Thaddeus E. Kelly**

Radial ray hypoplasia syndrome
See RADIAL-RENAL-OCULAR SYNDROME
Radial rays, deficiency of
See HAND, RADIAL CLUB HAND

RADIAL-RENAL SYNDROME   2771

Includes:
  Acro-renal syndrome, Sofer type
  Renal-radial syndrome
  Siegler syndrome
  Sofer syndrome

Excludes:
  Lacrimo-auriculo-dento-digital syndrome (2180)
  Pancytopenia syndrome, Fanconi type (2029)
  Thrombocytopenia-absent radius (0941)
  Vater association (0987)

Major Diagnostic Criteria: Radial aplasia, renal anomalies, and short stature.

Clinical Findings: All affected individuals have had bilateral absence or hypoplasia of the radius and absence of the thumbs. In one case the humerus was hypoplastic and the index fingers were absent. Renal anomalies were consistent and included crossed-fused ectopia and unilateral renal agenesis. Vesicoureteral reflux occurred in two cases. The ear was described as malformed in two cases. All affected individuals were below the third percentile for stature. Intellectual development was normal.

Complications: Renal failure secondary to reflux nephropathy.

Associated Findings: One affected individual has a **Tracheoesophageal fistula** and **Ventricular septal defect**.

Etiology: One report was of an affected father and son; the other was of sibs. Therefore, this condition could be heterogeneous and exist in both recessive and dominant forms. Conversely, reduced penetrance or germinal mosaicism could also be the case in one of the parents of the affected sibs.

Pathogenesis: Unknown.

MIM No.:   17928

POS No.:   3633

Sex Ratio: M4:F0 (observed).

Occurrence: Two families have been reported in the literature. A father and son were reported in Israel, brothers in Utah.

Risk of Recurrence for Patient's Sib:
  See Part I, *Mendelian Inheritance.*

Risk of Recurrence for Patient's Child:
  See Part I, *Mendelian Inheritance.*

Age of Detectability: At birth, although it is likely that prenatal diagnosis by ultrasound is possible.

Gene Mapping and Linkage: Unknown.

Prevention: None known. Genetic counseling indicated.

Treatment: Supportive. Ureteral reimplantation may be indicated.

Prognosis: Life span may be affected by the renal anomaly; intellectual development is normal.

Detection of Carrier: Unknown.

References:
Siegler RL, et al.: Upper limb anomalies and renal disease. Clin Genet 1980; 17:117–119. †

Sofer S, et al.: Radial ray aplasia and renal anomalies in father and son: a new syndrome. Am J Med Genet 1983; 14:151–157. †

T0007   **Helga V. Toriello**

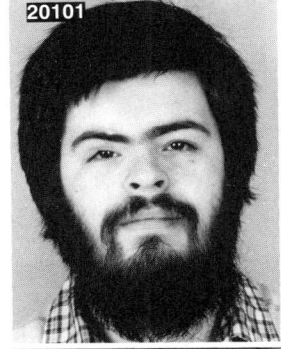
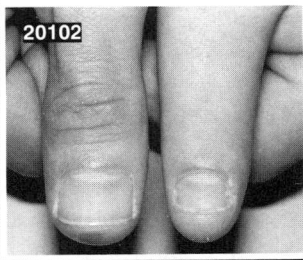

RADIAL-RENAL-OCULAR SYNDROME   2643

Includes:
> Acro-renal-ocular syndrome
> DR syndrome
> Duane syndrome-radial defects
> Ferrell-Okihiro-Halal syndrome
> Okihiro syndrome
> Radial ray hypoplasia syndrome
> Thumb-renal-ocular syndrome

Excludes:
> **Acro-renal-mandibular syndrome** (2778)
> **Anus-hand-ear syndrome** (0072)
> **Cervico-oculo-acoustic syndrome** (0142)
> **Eye, Duane retraction syndrome** (3180)
> **Heart-hand syndrome** (0455)
> **IVIC syndrome** (3043)
> **Macular coloboma-brachydactyly** (0621)

Major Diagnostic Criteria: Thumb anomalies include mild (limited motion at the IP joint) to severe hypoplasia or absent thumb and first metacarpal, with **Syndactyly** between digits I-II, or preaxial **Polydactyly**. Renal anomalies include ectopia, fusion, vesicoureteral reflux, bladder diverticulum, recurrent urinary tract infections, hypertension, and mild malrotation. Ocular features consist of **Eye, Duane retraction syndrome**, lid ptosis, uveal coloboma, microcornea, optic nerve coloboma, or choroid atrophy.

Clinical Findings: Seven individuals from three generations of a French-Canadian family had various combinations of acral, renal, and ocular defects (Halal et al, 1984). Three of the seven affected individuals had the complete triad. An eye defect was absent in four individuals. When present, it consisted of bilateral **Eye, Duane retraction syndrome** with unilateral palpebral ptosis (1/7), or bilateral uveal coloboma with unilateral microcornea (1/7), or unilateral coloboma of optic nerve (1/7). Acral anomalies were present in all affected individuals, varying from mild hypoplasia of the tip of the thumbs (but on X-ray, normal distal phalanx) with limited active motion of IP joints (4/7) to moderately severe bilateral hypoplasia of the thumb (1/7), unilateral severe hypoplasia (nonfunctional) of the thumb with hypoplastic first metacarpal (1/7), and preaxial **Polydactyly** type 1 (1/7). Urinary tract anomaly was present in all affected individuals; varying from mild vesicoureteral reflux (1/7) to bladder diverticulum (1/7), renal ectopia (crossed without fusion, 2/7; sacral, 1/7), and mild malrotation (2/7).

In addition, the family history of an additional adopted boy with the condition indicates no other affected family members; however, the parents were first cousins. The boy had hypoplastic thumbs, **Eye, Duane retraction syndrome** (Duane anomaly), ureteral reflux with posterior urethral valves, hypospadias, membranous imperforate anus, bilateral choanal atresia, small larynx, vocal cord fibrosis, cholesteatoma, a jugular bulb which prolapsed into the middle ear cavity, congenital ossicular chain abnormality, slightly malformed auricles, severe low frequency hearing loss, and moderate hearing loss for the higher frequencies. Average non-verbal intelligence was noted. His WISC-R verbal score showed a pattern consistent with his hearing impairment.

Complications: Functional vision impairment and hearing loss, recurrent urinary tract infections, hypertension, impaired fine motor abilities, and school performance problems.

Associated Findings: Onychodystrophy of toenails (4/7), gastroduodenal ulcer, **Hernia, hiatal**, **Cancer, colorectal**, spina bifida occulta, pulmonic stenosis, preauricular tag, choanal atresia, hearing loss, hypospadias, small larynx, vocal cord fibrosis, jugular bulb prolapse into the middle ear cavity, malformed auricles, cholesteatoma, membranous imperforate anus, and conjunctival dermolipoma.

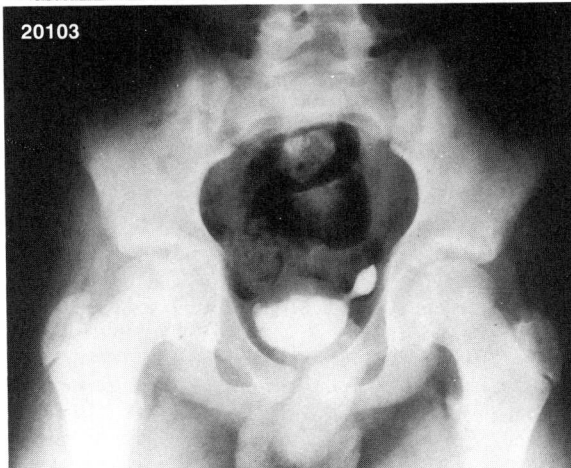
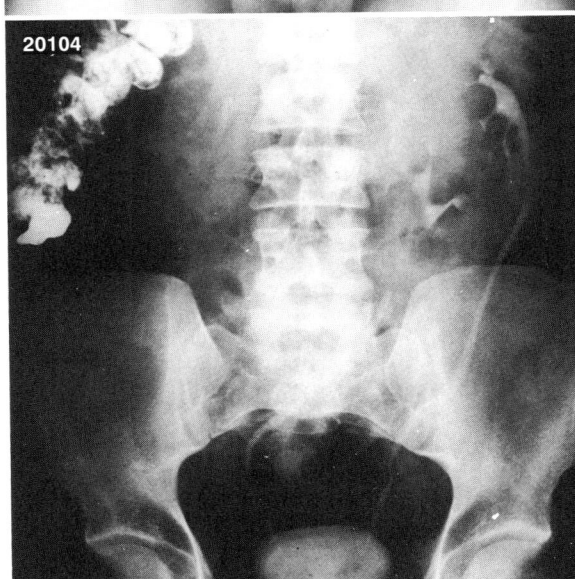

2643-20101: Note right palpebral ptosis. 20102: Left, hypoplastic distal portion of the thumb with absent flexion creases; right, normal thumb. 20103: Cystogram showing left paraureteral bladder. 20104: IVP showing crossed renal ectopia without fusion; right, absent kidney.

Etiology: Possibly autosomal dominant inheritance with variable expressivity.

Pathogenesis: Possibly an incompletely delineated heritable developmental field defect.

MIM No.: 10249

Sex Ratio: M1:F1

Occurrence: Undetermined but presumed rare.

Risk of Recurrence for Patient's Sib:
See Part I, *Mendelian Inheritance*.

Risk of Recurrence for Patient's Child:
See Part I, *Mendelian Inheritance*.

Age of Detectability: Clinically evident at birth. Prenatal diagnosis by ultrasonography appears to be possible.

Gene Mapping and Linkage: Unknown.

Prevention: None known. Genetic counseling indicated.

Treatment: Hand surgery to improve function; early recognition of vision and hearing problems with use of appropriate aids; monitoring for urinary tract infections; surgical management of urinary tract anomalies when appropriate; regular monitoring of blood pressure; and appropriate special education services when needed.

Prognosis: Life span appears to be normal. Intelligence is normal; special education may be needed if functional vision or hearing problems are present.

Detection of Carrier: Careful clinical thumb examination, since mild hypoplasia of the distal portion of the thumb could be the only apparent manifestation of the syndrome.

Special Considerations: The association of **Eye, Duane retraction syndrome** (Duane anomaly) with radial defects was reported previously in two families (Ferrell et al, 1966; Temtamy and McKusick, 1978). In the family reported by Ferrell et al (1966), a father and three of his five children had radial defects that varied in expression from mild hypoplasia of the thenar muscles to absence of the thumb and first metacarpal. The father had radial defects and the Duane anomaly, and the proposita had radial defects and **Atrial septal defects** but did not have the Duane anomaly. A paternal aunt had radial defects and the Duane anomaly, and a paternal uncle had radial malformations only. There was no mention of intravenous pyelogram studies on affected members of the family.

In the family (father and son) reported by Temtamy and McKusick (1978), the father had Duane anomaly with radial defects (bilateral thenar and thumb hypoplasia, with syndactyly of the index finger and unilateral clubhand deformity) and malrotation of both kidneys with partial horseshoe anomaly; his son had apparently normal eyes, bilateral clubhand with absent thumbs, and renal anomalies (absent right kidney, malrotation of left kidney). Associated anomalies were malformed pinnas, pectoral and upper limb hypoplasia, and congenital deafness and facial nerve weakness. Dermatoglyphics in the father showed abnormal flexion creases, absent axial triradius on the left, and distal axial triradius on the right. Temtamy and McKusick (1978) proposed the acronym *DR syndrome* (Duane/radial dysplasia).

More recently, Hayes et al (1985) reported on a child with Duane anomaly, deafness, cervical spine, and radial ray abnormalities. A sister of the proposita had **Oculo-auriculo-vertebral anomaly**, cervical abnormalities, and hypoplasia of the thenar eminence. Four relatives had hypoplasia of the thenar eminence. A fifth had preaxial polydactyly. Duane anomaly was present in two sixth-degree relatives. There was no mention of renal anomaly in any of the affected members. The authors suggested that the disorder be designated the *Okihiro syndrome*, since Okihiro et al (1977) were the first to recognize the constellation of non-ocular abnormalities in a single pedigree.

McDermot and Winter (1987) have also reported a family in which radial defects and Duane anomaly occurred in an autosomal dominant pattern. Anal stenosis was present in one affected individual but no urogenital anomalies were found. Goldblatt and Viljoen (1987) described a father and two daughters with radial ray hypoplasia, esotropia, and choanal atresia with normal hematologic and renal studies.

Although the constellation of radial, renal and ocular anomalies probably represents a distinct autosomal dominant trait of variable expressivity, the possibility that it may also comprise part of the spectrum of the previously reported syndrome of Duane anomaly with radial defects cannot be excluded.

References:
Ferrell RL, et al.: Simultaneous occurrence of the Holt-Oram and the Duane syndrome. J Pediatr 1966; 69:630–634.
Okihiro MM, et al.: Duane syndrome and congenital upper-limb anomalies. Arch Neurol 1977; 34:174–179.
Temtamy S, McKusick VA: The genetics of hand malformations. New York: Alan R. Liss, 1978.
Halal F, et al.: Acro-renal-ocular syndrome: autosomal dominant thumb hypoplasia, renal ectopia, and eye defect. Am J Med Genet 1984; 17:753–762. * †
Hayes A, et al.: The Okihiro syndrome of Duane anomaly, radial ray abnormalities, and deafness. Am J Med Genet 1985; 22:273–280.
Temtamy SA: The DR syndrome or the Okihiro syndrome? (Letter) Am J Med Genet 1986; 25:173–174.
MacDermot K, Winter RM: Radial ray defect and Duane anomaly: report of a family with autosomal dominant trasmission. Am J Med Genet 1987; 27:313–319.
Goldblatt J, Viljoen D: New autosomal dominant radial ray hypoplasia syndrome. Am J Med Genet 1987; 28:647–654.

HA074   **Fahed Halal**
M0000   **John B. Moeschler**
GR000   **John M. Graham, Jr.**

RADIAL-ULNAR SYNOSTOSIS   0854

Includes:
　　Pronation, congenital
　　Synostosis, radial cubital

Excludes:
　　Acrocephalosyndactyly type V (2284)
　　Fetal thalidomide syndrome (0386)
　　Humero-radial synostosis (0477)
　　Mandibulofacial dysostosis (0627)
　　Mesomelic dysplasia, Nievergelt type (0647)
　　Poland syndrome (0813)
　　Radio-ulnar synostosis as a component of a syndrome
　　Radio-ulnar synostosis secondary to trauma
　　Roberts syndrome (0875)
　　Synostosis, multiple synostosis syndrome (2312)

Major Diagnostic Criteria: Restriction of pronation-supination at the elbow with X-ray evidence of fusion of the proximal radius and ulna.

Clinical Findings: Pronation-supination is restricted or absent, and the elbow is often fixed in pronation. Some patients show mild limitation of extension and flexion at the elbow. Sporadic cases may be unilateral or bilateral, whereas familial cases are usually bilateral.

Complications: Restriction of pronation-supination.

Associated Findings: Other skeletal malformations, including **Craniosynostosis** and congenital hyperthyroidism.

Etiology: Most cases are sporadic; about 10% autosomal dominant inheritance (variable expressivity and may occasionally be nonpenetrant, especially in females); occasionally secondary to sex chromosome aneuploidy, notably 48,XXXY and 49,XXXXY.

Pathogenesis: Unknown.

MIM No.: *17930

CDC No.: 755.536

Sex Ratio: M2:F1

Occurrence: Undetermined. Davenport et al (1924) documented an extensive kindred, and Hansen and Andersen (1970) reported 37 cases.

Risk of Recurrence for Patient's Sib:
See Part I, *Mendelian Inheritance*.

Risk of Recurrence for Patient's Child:
See Part I, *Mendelian Inheritance*.

Age of Detectability: At birth, by clinical examination, and by X-ray when the intervening cartilage has ossified.

Gene Mapping and Linkage: Unknown.

Prevention: None known. Genetic counseling indicated.

Treatment: Rarely surgery may be required to improve the functional position of the forearm.

Prognosis: Normal life span.

Detection of Carrier: Unknown.

References:

Abbott FC: Hereditary congenital dislocations of the radius. Trans Pathol Soc (Lond) 1892; 43:129–139.

Davenport CB, et al.: Radio-ulnar synostosis. Arch Surg 1924; 8:705–762.

Hansen OH, Andersen NO: Congenital radio-ulnar synostosis: report of 37 cases. Acta Orthop Scand 1970; 41:225–230.

Jancu J: Radioulnar synostosis. a common occurrence in sex chromosomal abnormalities. Am J Dis Child 1971; 122:10–11.

Spritz RA: Familial radioulnar synostosis. J Med Genet 1978; 15:160–162.

Cleary JE, Omer GE: Congenital proximal radio-ulnar synostosis: natural history and functional assessment. J Bone Joint Surg 1985; 67A:539–545.

C0066

J. Michael Connor

Radiation embryopathy
See FETAL RADIATION SYNDROME
Radiation teratogenesis
See FETAL RADIATION SYNDROME
Radiation, fetal effects of
See FETAL RADIATION SYNDROME
Radicular dentin dysplasia
See TEETH, DENTIN DYSPLASIA, RADICULAR
Radius absent-thrombocytopenia
See THROMBOCYTOPENIA-ABSENT RADIUS
Radius, congenital absence of the
See HAND, RADIAL CLUB HAND
Radius, deficiency of
See HAND, RADIAL CLUB HAND
Radix in radice
See TEETH, DENS INVAGINATUS
Radon gas, fetal effects of
See FETAL RADIATION SYNDROME

RAG SYNDROME   2578

Includes:
Aniridia-Robin sequence-growth delay
Robin sequence-aniridia-growth delay (RAG)

Excludes:
Chromosome 11, partial monosomy 11p (2245)
Chromosome 13, monosomy 13q (0167)
Progeria (0825)

Major Diagnostic Criteria: Robin sequence with micrognathia and U-shaped cleft palate, absence of the iris bilaterally, and severe growth retardation. Characteristic elfin-like features. The hands are small, with long, pointed fingers and abnormal palmar creases.

Clinical Findings: Severe prenatal developmental and growth delay, with reduced amniotic fluid volume and no obvious prenatal fetal movements. The infant has a birth weight of below 1,000 g, but is otherwise strong and healthy. Clinically, characteristic elfin-like facies with aniridia and the Robin anomaly with cleft palate are evident at birth. Weight gain is very slow (less than eight pounds at age two years), and length is short; both parameters being well below the normal percentiles. Chromosomes have been normal. Endocrine findings are normal with normal growth hormone levels.

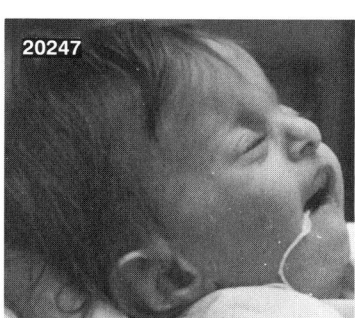
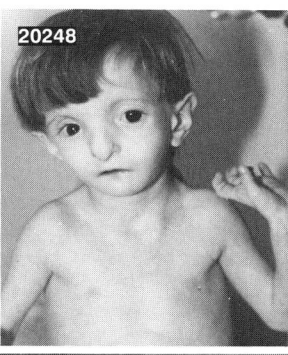
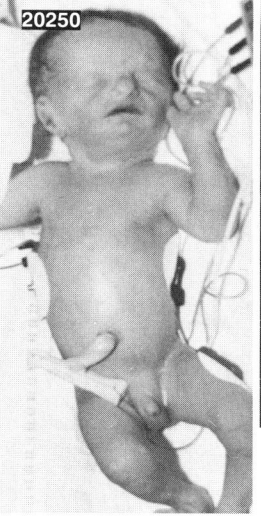
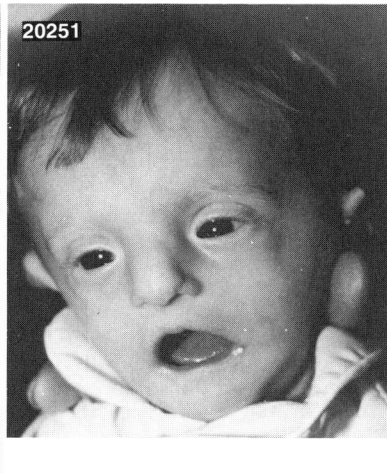

2578-20247: Lateral view of proposita with RAG syndrome at age 2 months; note micrognathia. **20248:** Proposita at age 3 years; note unusual triangular facies. **20250:** Younger brother of the proposita at birth. **20251:** Proposita's brother at age 1 year; note the facies are similar to his sister's.

Development is very delayed. By age four years, there is no speech; motor skills included standing with support. Only two teeth had erupted in the reported case, although all the dentition appeared to be present. The head circumference was well below normal. Cranial bones were infantile with domes in the center and open sutures. The child was reportedly irritable.

Complications: Unknown.

Associated Findings: None known.

Etiology: Possibly autosomal recessive inheritance.

Pathogenesis: Unknown.

Sex Ratio: M1:F1

Occurrence: One family with two sibs has been described.

Risk of Recurrence for Patient's Sib:
See Part I, *Mendelian Inheritance*.

Risk of Recurrence for Patient's Child:
See Part I, *Mendelian Inheritance*.

Age of Detectability: At birth, or prenatally by ultrasound detection of severe intrauterine growth retardation early in the second trimester.

Gene Mapping and Linkage: Unknown.

Prevention: None known. Genetic counseling indicated.

Treatment: Unknown.

Prognosis: Unknown.

Detection of Carrier: Unknown.

References:
Saal HM, et al.: The RAG syndrome: a new autosomal recessive syndrome with the Robin sequence, aniridia and profound growth retardation and developmental delays. Am J Hum Genet (suppl) 1986; 39:78A.

P0007   **Andrew E. Poole**
SA001   **Howard M. Saal**

Ragged red fibers-myoclonic epilepsy
See MYOCLONIC EPILEPSY-RAGGED RED FIBERS
Ragin' Cajun
See JUMPING FRENCHMAN OF MAINE

RAGWEED POLLEN SENSITIVITY   3082

Includes:
Asthma, ragweed pollen-induced
Hayfever
HLA-A histocompatibility type
Ragweed sensitivity, asymptomatic
Rhinitis, ragweed pollen-induced

Excludes:
Skin, atopy, familial (3150)
Ragweed oleoresin contact dermatitis

Major Diagnostic Criteria: Demonstrable presence of IgE antibody to ragweed pollen components, based on environmental exposure, constitutes ragweed pollen sensitivity. This condition may remain asymptomatic despite annual dispersion of the sensitizer(s) or may manifest as allergic rhinitis or reactive airways disease. Wheal and flare reactions in skin, peaking 15 minutes after intradermal testing with ragweed pollen extracts, indicate allergen-specific, tissue-fixed IgE. Additional, *in vitro* studies, (viz., RAST, ELISA, and other solid-phase immunosorbent tests, as well as leukocyte histamine release) allow assay of specific IgE in serum and tissue fluids. Aerosol challenge, with pollen extracts, of the upper and lower airways can confirm the potential for specific reactivity using patency or secretion-based response parameters. However, a certain clinical diagnosis rests on confirmation of characteristic respiratory symptoms during natural exposure periods.

Clinical Findings: Like other atopic individuals (i.e., those prone to synthesize significant IgE following mucosal allergen contact), ragweed-sensitive persons commonly display multiple IgE-based sensitivities, and at least 50% have at least one atopic first-degree relative. Histories of childhood atopic dermatitis with or without gastrointestinal allergy are abnormally frequent. Allergic rhinitis presents as variable nasal obstruction; repetitive sneezing; thin, copious rhinorrhea; and pruritus of eyes, nose, and pharynx. Lacrimation, periorbital swelling, and conjunctival injection often coexist. Symptoms tend to peak shortly after arising, but persist diurnally, often disturbing sleep and contributing to a more or less prominent lassitude. The nasal mucosa commonly reflects prominent edema and venostasis, appearing pale and bluish-gray, and stained mucus often reveals numerous eosinophils. Heightened nasal reactivity is characteristically evident, obstruction and other symptoms readily following chilling, recumbency, and exposure to volatile and particulate irritants. A minority of sensitive persons manifest asthma (bouts of potentially reversible bronchial obstruction and general airway lability) in response to ragweed allergens. In most, sensitivity to additional factors with or without resulting factors, with or without resulting respiratory allergy, is demonstrable. Where ragweed pollen is annually prevalent, symptoms most commonly appear after three to five seasons of exposure. As a result, an onset of pollinosis in childhood is frequent. Spontaneous attenuation of symptoms may occur with advancing age in endemic areas or may continue lifelong.

Complications: Because isolated ragweed pollinois lasts, at most, 2–3 months annually, infectious and structural complications are less than in those with perennial symptoms due to diverse sensitivities. However, purulent rhinitis, bronchitis, and sinusitis often complicate pollinosis. In children especially, purulent otitis media or, less commonly, serous otitis reflect accompanying eustachian tube dysfunction. Bouts of intractable, irresistible, repetitive sneezing can pose hazards for operation of vehicles and other machinery requiring constant hand-eye coordination. As in responses to other allergens, ragweed pollinosis confers upper and lower airway hyperreactivity to additional allergens and irritant factors.

Associated Findings: A significant minority of ragweed-sensitive persons have experienced skin or gastrointestinal allergy. Most have additional sensitivities with or without resulting respiratory conditions.

Etiology: Possibly autosomal dominant inheritance of differential sensitivity. A series of smaller proteins and polypeptides are the sensitizing agents. Of these, antigens E (MW ca. 38,700) constitute 6% of the pollen protein of short (dwarf) ragweed and appears to be its single most important allergen. IgE-reactive materials are eluted at mucous surfaces from intact grains. Additional small micronic and submicronic aerosols carrying pollen allergens occur in nature and may augment exposure.

Genetic associations of several immune response determinants of ragweed pollinosis have been examined. Associations between HLA haplotypes and IgE-mediated skin reactivity to Amb a I (antigen E) of short ragweed in multiple generations of selected kindreds have been reported (Blumenthal and Amos, 1987). However, others (Bias & Marsh, 1975, Marsh et al, 1987) have questioned these conclusions which center on a relatively complex (M.W. 37,800) protein antigen having multiple epitopes. Polygenic factors, or failure of certain family members to express reactivity when studied, has been postulated. More recently, responses to a smaller ragweed pollen component, Amb a V (antigen Ra5); a single chain polypeptide with M.W. *ca* 5,000; have been found strongly associated with Dw 2 and DR2 typing by Marsh et al (1987). Both IgE and IgG reactivity have showed this correlation. Similarly, in persons responding with IgE and IgG to Amb t V of giant ragweed pollen, associations with Dw2 have been described. Most recently Marsh et al (1987) have shown a concordance of response of Amb a VI, (an 11,500 dalton ragweed pollen allergen) and HLA-DR5+ status.

Total IgE level, while not regarded as HLA-assocaited, is a trait for which genetic control is strongly suggested, and high responders appear more prone to pollinosis. The heritability of high and low IgE status has been well supported by twin studies (especially in childhood) by Bazaral et al (1974). In addition, families studied by Gerrard et al (1978) have confirmed the genetic control of IgE, suggesting that high response acts as a recessive trait, although polygenic control seems to be exerted.

Pathogenesis: Pollenosis essentially reflects tissue effects of mast cell and basophil secretion following bridging, by allergen, of specific IgE molecules on cell surface receptors. Laboratory-based allergen challenges have confirmed the appearance of proinflammatory mediators, including histamine, prostaglandin D_2, sulfidopeptide leukotrienes, and various esterases in nasal washings. Similar events appear to follow bronchial provocation with allergen. Heightened vascular permeability results with tissue edema and hypersecretion by organized glands and goblet cells. In subglottic airways, an intense spasm of mural smooth muscle is associated. Both permeability factors and agents chemotactic for eosinophils and neutrophils follow allergen challenge with immediate (0–90-minute) and late (3–6-hour) appearance peaks. In lower airways, late reactions with neutrophil influx appear to foster bronchial hyperresponsiveness. Nasal hyperreactivity may reflect demonstrated factors including increased mucosal permeability, influxes of mast cells and basophils, and changes in the density of receptors for autonomic neurotransmitters. Additional determinants of symptom severity, including circadian, reflex, and endocrine influences, are suspected.

MIM No.: *14280, 17945

Sex Ratio: Presumably M1:F1, although an earlier childhood onset in males has been suggested.

Occurrence: Rates of sensitization approach or exceed 25% in endemic areas. Symptomatic pollenosis affecting up to 25% of exposed young adults has been observed. Familial clustering of respiratory allergy (including ragweed pollinosis) is prominent, at least 50% of affected persons having one or more first degree relatives with IgE-mediated conditions. However, no simple pattern of inheritance is discernible. Family studies have suggested genetic control(s) of high (vs. normally low) total serum IgE levels. Reported linkage disequilibrium between IgE responsiveness to specific ragweed pollen allergens (E, Ra3, Ra5) and one or more HLA haplotypes also implies a role for immune response genes. In addition, independent transmission of bronchial hyperresponsiveness, a trait promoting asthma, is strongly suggested.

Risk of Recurrence for Patient's Sib:
See Part I, *Mendelian Inheritance.*

Risk of Recurrence for Patient's Child:
See Part I, *Mendelian Inheritance.*

Age of Detectability: Usually during pre-school years in suitably exposed individuals, but may appear later.

Gene Mapping and Linkage: HLA-A (major histocompatibility complex, class I) has been mapped to 6p21.3.

Prevention: None known. Genetic counseling indicated. While seldom feasible, (geographic) removal of patients from seasonal exposure effectively terminates clinical pollinosis, although asymptomatic sensitivity remains. Patients with severe ragweed-induced rhinitis may have their risk of subsequent asthma diminished by specific (injection) immunotherapy.

Treatment: Symptom amelioration by agents that block the release and tissue effects of mast cell-derived mediators has been increasingly successful. H1 antihistamines and topical cromolyn sodium or corticosteroids are mainstays for relief of rhinitis. Asthma often is benefitted by inhaled cromolyn and corticosteroids, as well as by aerosolized and oral bronchodilators; systemic steroids may be required. Immunotherapy with ragweed pollen extracts has proven valuable in hayfever and remains to be critically evaluated in asthma.

Prognosis: The proportion of ragweed pollen-sensitive persons who will develop specific symptoms is undefined, but appears large. Determinants of the clinical illness in this risk group remain controversial. However, once pollinosis is established, it tends to recur annually with seasonal exposure. Rhinitis severity seems to augment the small increased risk of de novo asthma in those (initially) with ragweed hayfever alone. A fraction of sensitive persons manifest only asthma over extended periods in response to ragweed pollen.

Detection of Carrier: Unknown.

Special Considerations: Patients with pollen sensitivity have little, if any, increased risk of adverse reactivity to drugs, radiocontrast media, and hymenoptera (insect) stings when compared with comparable exposed, nonsensitive subjects.

References:
Bazaral M, et al.: Genetics of IgE and allergy: serum IgE levels in twins. J Allergy Clin Immunol 1974; 54:288–304.
Blumenthal MN, et al.: Genetic mapping of Ir locus in man: linkage to second locus of HL-A. Science 1974; 184:1301–1303.
Bias WB, Marsh DG: HLA linked antigen E immune response genes: an unproved hypothesis. Science 1975; 188:375–377.
Gerrard JW, et al.: A genetic study of immunoglobulin E. Am J Hum Genet 1978; 30:46–58.
Marsh DG, et al.: HLA-Dw2: a genetic marker for human immune response to short ragweed pollen allergen Ra5. I. Response resulting primarily from natural antigenic exposure. J Exper Med 1982; 155:1439–1451.
Mygind N, Weeke B: Allergic and non-allergic rhinitis. In: Middleton E Jr., et al., eds: Allergy: principles and practice, ed 2. St. Louis: C.V. Mosby, 1983:1101–1117.
Roebber M, et al.: Immunochemical and genetic studies of Amb .t. v (Ra5G), an Ra5G homologue from giant ragweed pollen. J Immunol 1985; 134:3062–3069.
Blumenthal MN, Amos DB: Genetic and immunologic basis of atopic responses. Chest 1987; 91S:176S.
Marsh DG, et al.: Immune responsiveness to Ambrosia artemisiifolia (short ragweed) pollen allergen Amb a VI (Ra6) is associated with HLA-DR5 in allergic humans. Immunogenetics 1987; 26:230–236.
Meyers DA, et al.: Inheritance of total serum IgE (basal levels) in man. Am J Hum Genet 1987; 41:51–62.

S0015   **William R. Solomon**

Ragweed sensitivity, asymptomatic
See RAGWEED POLLEN SENSITIVITY
Ramon syndrome
See GINGIVAL FIBROMATOSIS-CHERUBISM-SEIZURES, RAMON TYPE
Ramon syndrome-juvenile rheumatoid arthritis
See GINGIVAL FIBROMATOSIS-CHERUBISM-SEIZURES, RAMON TYPE
Ramsay-Hunt syndrome (some cases)
See SEIZURES, PROGRESSIVE MYOCLONIC, UNVERRICHT-LUNDBORG TYPE
Ranula congenita
See CYSTIC HYGROMA
Raphe, supraumbilical midline-cavernous facial hemangiomas
See HEMANGIOMAS OF THE HEAD AND NECK
Rapid gastric emptying-duodenal ulcer
See PEPTIC ULCER DISEASES, NON-SYNDROMIC
Rapid isoniazid (INH) inactivation
See ACETYLATOR POLYMORPHISM
Rapp-Hodgkin ectodermal dysplasia
See ECTODERMAL DYSPLASIA, RAPP-HODGKIN TYPE
Rautenstrauch-Wiedemann syndrome
See PROGERIA, NEONATAL RAUTENSTRAUCH-WIEDEMANN TYPE

RAYNAUD DISEASE   **2115**

Includes:
Fingers, cold, hereditary
Primary Raynaud phenomenon
Raynaud phenomenon

Excludes:
Raynaud phenomenon, secondary
Scleroderma, familial progressive (2154)

Major Diagnostic Criteria: Bilateral clinical findings in absence of demonstrable cause of secondary Raynaud phenomenon; duration of symptoms for at least two years.

Clinical Findings: Changes in skin color (pallor) and temperature (coolness) mainly involving the hands and feet; excited by cold temperatures and emotional stress.

Complications: Raynaud disease, unlike secondary Raynaud phenomenon, is not accompanied by extensive gangrene. Major amputations are never necessary.

Associated Findings: Numbness, livido reticulares; rarely, acrocyanosis

Etiology: Autosomal dominant and multifactorial inheritance.

Pathogenesis: Arteriospasm of unkown cause. Affected individuals have decreased capillary blood flow as compared to unaffected persons.

MIM No.: *17960

Sex Ratio: M1:F1 in the autosomal dominant form. M1:F>1 in the idiopathic, presumably multifactorial form.

Occurrence: Undetermined. Lewis and Pickering (1933) reported 23 cases in two working-class British families.

Risk of Recurrence for Patient's Sib:
See Part I, *Mendelian Inheritance.*

Risk of Recurrence for Patient's Child:
See Part I, *Mendelian Inheritance.*

Age of Detectability: Late childhood or early adulthood.

Gene Mapping and Linkage: Unknown.

Prevention: None known. Genetic counseling indicated.

Treatment: Avoidance of cold temperatures and emotional stress. Nifedipine and ketanserin have been used with success.

Prognosis: Good.

Detection of Carrier: Unknown.

Special Considerations: As the nature of this condition has become clearer, there is an emerging consensus that the name should be changed to *Raynaud phenomenon*.

Support Groups: Dallas; American Heart Association

References:
Allen EV, Brown GE: Raynaud's disease a critical review of minimal requisites for diagnosis. Am J Med Sci 1932; 183:187–200. *
Lewis T, Pickering GW: Observations upon maladies in which the blood supply to digits ceases intermittently or permanently, and upon bilateral gangrene of digits, observations relevant to so-called "Raynauds disease". Clin Sci 1933; 1:327–366. *
Gifford RW Jr, Hines EA Jr: Raynaud's disease among women and girls. Circulation 1957; 16:1012.
White CJ, et al.: Objective benefit of nifedipine in the treatment of Raynauds phenomenon. Am J Med 1986; 80:623–625.
Coffman JD, et al.: International study of ketanserin in Raynaud's phenomenon. Am J Med 1989; 87:264–268.

N0004   **Audery H. Nora**
N0003   **James J. Nora**

Raynaud phenomenon
  See RAYNAUD DISEASE
Reactive arthritis
  See ANKYLOSING SPONDYLITIS
Reading disorder, developmental
  See DYSLEXIA
Reading disorder, specific
  See DYSLEXIA
Reading epilepsy
  See EPILEPSY, REFLEX
REAR syndrome
  See ANUS-HAND-EAR SYNDROME
Recessive dystrophic epidermolysis bullosa (RDEB)
  See EPIDERMOLYSIS BULLOSUM, TYPE III
Recessive optic atrophy-hearing loss-juvenile diabetes
  See DIABETES (INSIPIDUS/MELLITUS)-OPTIC ATROPHY-DEAFNESS
Rectal aganglionosis
  See COLON, AGANGLIONOSIS
Rectal atresia or stenosis
  See COLON, ATRESIA OR STENOSIS
Rectal duplication
  See COLON, DUPLICATION
Rectoperineal fistula
  See ANORECTAL MALFORMATIONS
Rectus muscle, congenital fibrosis of the inferior
  See EYE, FIBROSIS OF THE EXTRAOCULAR MUSCLES, GENERALIZED
Recurrent erosive corneal dystrophy
  See CORNEAL DYSTROPHY, RECURRENT EROSIVE
Recurrent intrahepatic cholestasis of pregnancy (RICP)
  See INTRAHEPATIC CHOLESTASIS OF PREGNANCY (ICP)
Recurrent respiratory papillomatosis
  See PAPILLOMA VIRUS, CONGENITAL INFECTION
Red cell aregenerative anemia, congenital
  See ANEMIA, HYPOPLASTIC CONGENITAL
Red cell membrane defects
  See ANEMIA, HEMOLYTIC, RED CELL MEMBRANE DEFECTS
Red cell membrane phosphatidylcholine hemolytic anemia
  See ANEMIA, HEMOLYTIC, ERYTHROCYTE PHOSPHOLIPID DEFECT
Red cell permeability defect
  See ANEMIA, HEMOLYTIC, RED CELL MEMBRANE DEFECTS
Red cell phospholipid defect-hemolysis
  See ANEMIA, HEMOLYTIC, RED CELL MEMBRANE DEFECTS
Red palms
  See SKIN, PALMO-PLANTAR ERYTHEMA
Red-fleck retina
  See RETINA, FLECKED KANDORI TYPE
Red-green deutan series color blindness
  See COLOR BLINDNESS, RED-GREEN DEUTAN SERIES
Red-green protan series color blindness
  See COLOR BLINDNESS, RED-GREEN PROTAN SERIES
Reducing body myopathy
  See MYOPATHY, REDUCING BODY
Reduction defects of limb
  See LIMB REDUCTION DEFECTS

Refetoff syndrome
  See THYROID, HORMONE RESISTANCE
Reflux, esophageal
  See ESOPHAGUS, CHALASIA
Refsum disease
  See PHYTANIC ACID STORAGE DISEASE
Refsum disease (some neonatal or infantile forms)
  See CEREBRO-HEPATO-RENAL SYNDROME
Refsum disease, infantile form
  See PHYTANIC ACID OXIDASE DEFICIENCY, INFANTILE TYPE
Regional enteritis/ileitis
  See INFLAMMATORY BOWEL DISEASE
Regional odontodysplasia
  See TEETH, ODONTODYSPLASIA
Reifenstein syndrome
  See ANDROGEN INSENSITIVITY SYNDROME, INCOMPLETE
Reiger anomaly-growth retardation
  See SHORT SYNDROME
Reinclusion of permanent molars, familial
  See TEETH, MOLAR REINCLUSION
Reinhardt-Pfeiffer mesomelic dysostosis
  See MESOMELIC DYSPLASIA, REINHARDT-PFEIFFER TYPE
Reis-Bucklers corneal dystrophy
  See CORNEAL DYSTROPHY, REIS-BUCKLERS TYPE
Reiter syndrome
  See ANKYLOSING SPONDYLITIS
Renal (hyper)uricosuria, isolated
  See RENAL HYPOURICEMIA
Renal 25-hydroxyvitamin D1-hydroxylase deficiency
  See RICKETS, VITAMIN D-DEPENDENT, TYPE I
Renal adysplasia
  See RENAL AGENESIS, BILATERAL

RENAL AGENESIS, BILATERAL   0856

Includes:
  Kidneys, absence of
  Kidneys, congenital bilateral absence of
  Potter syndrome
  Renal adysplasia
  Urogenital adysplasia

Excludes:
  Potter syndrome associated with infantile polycystic kidney
  Potter syndrome associated with renal dysplasia

Major Diagnostic Criteria: Lack of kidneys.

Clinical Findings: At birth, infants may show the following features: Potter facies (an appearance of redundant and dehydrated skin, wide-set eyes, prominent fold arising at inner canthus of each eye, "parrot-beak" nose, receding chin, facial expression of an older infant); large, low-set ears with deficient auricular cartilages; no urine output; no kidneys palpable. About 40% of these infants are stillborn, and the majority of those born alive die within four hours. Rarely an infant may survive more than two days, since the condition is incompatible with life.

Complications: Death shortly after birth is attributed to asphyxia secondary to pulmonary hypoplasia due to compression of chest from lack of amniotic fluid. Renal failure is usually the other cause of death.

Associated Findings: History of oligohydramnios or total absence of amniotic fluid or amnion nodosum. Often premature onset of labor, breech delivery, and birth weight disproportionately low. The patient may have multiple malformations including bilateral pulmonary hypoplasia; genital organ abnormalities such as absence of vas deferens and seminal vesicles or absence of uterus and upper vagina; GI malformations such as anal atresia, absent sigmoid and rectum, and esophageal and duodenal atresia; single umbilical artery; major deformities of lower part of body (sirenomelia) or lower limbs such as clubfoot.

Etiology: Bilateral renal agenesis may represent the severe expression of autosomal dominant inheritance of a gene that in its milder expression causes unilateral renal agenesis, double ureter, renal cyst, or hydronephrosis (Roodhooft et al, 1984).

Pathogenesis: Unknown.

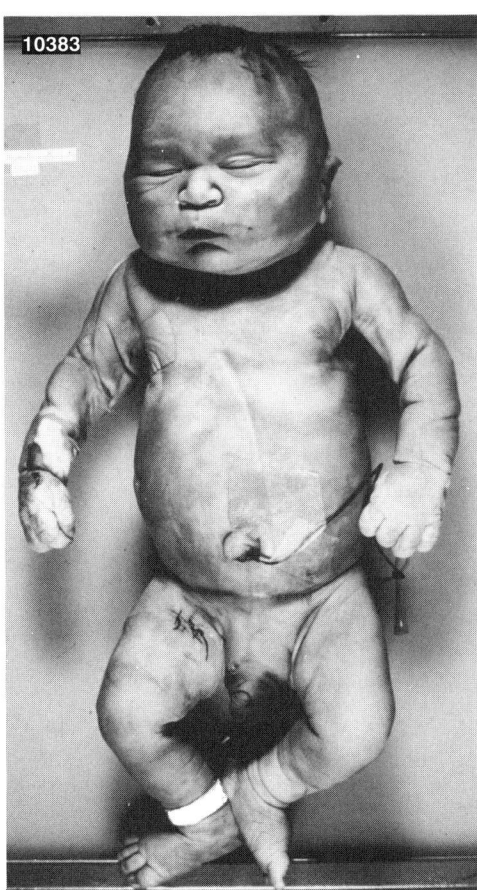

0856-10383: Potter facies, redundant skin and pulmonary hypoplasia secondary to oligohydramnios from bilateral renal agenesis.

MIM No.: *19183

POS No.: 3368

CDC No.: 753.000

Sex Ratio: M2.5:F1

Occurrence: Estimated at 12:100,000 total births (Carter et al, 1979).

Risk of Recurrence for Patient's Sib:
See Part I, *Mendelian Inheritance*. The proportion of sibs affected with bilateral renal agenesis was 6:199 (3.0%) in one study in England (Carter et al, 1979).

Risk of Recurrence for Patient's Child:
See Part I, *Mendelian Inheritance*. Affected individuals are not expected to survive to reproduce.

Age of Detectability: Prenatal exam by ultrasound can detect some cases; all others are evident in the neonate.

Gene Mapping and Linkage: Unknown.

Prevention: None known. Genetic counseling indicated.

Treatment: Unknown. Dialysis/renal transplantation is usually not considered because of the pulmonary hypoplasia.

Prognosis: Inevitably fatal.

Detection of Carrier: Unknown.

Special Considerations: Parents and unaffected children have increased risk of having silent genitourinary malformations; especially unilateral renal agenesis (Roodhooft et al, 1984). Parents and sibs should be screened by ultrasound for asymptomatic malformations.

Support Groups: New York; National Kidney Foundation

References:
Potter EL: Bilateral absence of ureters and kidneys: a report of 50 cases. Obstet Gynecol 1965; 25:3–12.

Cain DR, et al.: Familial renal agenesis and total dysplasia. Am J Dis Child 1974; 128:377–380.

Carter CO, et al.: A family study of renal agenesis. J Med Genetics 1979; 16:176–188.

Roodhooft AM, et al.: Familial nature of congenital absence and severe dysgenesis of both kidneys. New Engl J Med 1984; 310:1341–1345. *

Bankier A, et al.: A pedigree study of perinatal lethal renal disease. J Med Genet 1985; 22:104–111.

McPherson E, et al.: Dominantly inherited renal adysplasia. Am J Med Genet 1987; 26:863–872.

Morse RP et al.: Bilateral renal agenesis in three consecutive siblings. Prenatal Diag 1987; 7:573–579.

M0035   **Donald I. Moel**

RENAL AGENESIS, UNILATERAL   0857

Includes:
    Kidney, congenital solitary
    Renal aplasia, unilateral

Excludes:
    Renal agenesis, bilateral (0856)
    Renal atrophy, unilateral
    Renal dysgenesis, unilateral
    Renal hypoplasia, unilateral

Major Diagnostic Criteria: Unilateral renal agenesis is discovered incidentally on X-ray or other examination.

Clinical Findings: The affected infant usually appears normal at birth. Most frequently clinical recognition of unilateral renal agenesis results from an incidental examination during an illness.

Absence of one renal outline, most commonly on the left side; enlarged renal shadow on the opposite side; asymmetry of the outlines of the psoas muscles; renal pelvis of moderate size that does not parallel the degree of parenchymal hypertrophy; ectopy or malrotation of the single kidney in 5–10% of cases. Cystoscopy reveals absence of a ureteral orifice on one side and often absence or deformity of the corresponding half of the interureteral ridge of the trigone. Ultrasonography shows the presence of only one kidney.

Complications: Unless the solitary kidney becomes infected, obstructed, or exposed to toxins, the condition is not clinically significant. Sterility has been noted.

Associated Findings: Usually the ipsilateral ureter is absent or poorly developed; the adrenal gland on the side of anomaly may be absent. Absence or agenesis of the vagina (Mayer-Rokitansky syndrome) is associated with a high rate of urologic abnormalities including renal agenesis, ectopia, fusion anomalies, horseshoe kidneys, duplication anomalies, and ureteroceles. In the male, there may be ipsilateral absence of the testis, vas deferens and/or the seminal vesicles.

A defect in mesodermal development at the primitive streak level is called by the acronym VATER (see **VATER association**). Renal anomalies are also observed in 50% of patients and include renal agenesis, dysplasia or hypoplasia).

Etiology: Possibly autosomal dominant inheritance with variable expressivity and penetrance. In some families, unilateral renal agenesis may be considered a mild expression of a more severe abnormality (i.e. bilateral renal agenesis or dysgenesis).

Pathogenesis: Unknown.

MIM No.: *19183

CDC No.: 753.010

Sex Ratio: Presumably M1:F1. Autopsy studies indicate solitary kidney to be more common among males; however, clinical studies indicate it to be more common among females. This apparent difference in sex incidence is attributable to fact that associated complications and other anomalies are more frequently recognized in females.

Occurrence: About 1:1,000 infants.

Risk of Recurrence for Patient's Sib:
See Part I, *Mendelian Inheritance.*

Risk of Recurrence for Patient's Child:
See Part I, *Mendelian Inheritance.*

Age of Detectability: During investigation of kidney disease, or as a chance finding.

Gene Mapping and Linkage: Unknown.

Prevention: None known. Genetic counseling indicated.

Treatment: Treatment of infection and/or obstruction in the remaining kidney to preserve renal function. If severely diseased, renal transplantation.

Prognosis: Generally good, but depends on remaining kidney function and other associated anomalies.

Detection of Carrier: Unknown.

Support Groups: New York; National Kidney Foundation

References:
Thompson DP, Lynn HB: Genital anomalies associated with solitary kidney. Mayo Clin Proc 1966; 41:538–548.
Emanuel B, et al.: Congenital solitary kidney: a review of 74 cases. Am J Dis Child 1974; 127:17–19.
Carter CO, et al.: A family study of renal agenesis. J Med Genet 1979; 16:176–188.
Uehling DT, et al.: Urologic implications of the VATER association. J Urol 1983; 129:352–354.
Roodhooft AM, et al.: Familial nature of congenital absence and severe dysgenesis of both kidneys. New Engl J Med 1984; 310:1341–1345. *

M0035 **Donald I Moel**

Renal and X-ray anomalies-midface retraction-hypertrichosis
See SCHINZEL-GIEDION SYNDROME
Renal aplasia, unilateral
See RENAL AGENESIS, UNILATERAL
Renal artery stenosis, congenital
See ARTERY, RENAL FIBROMUSCULAR DYSPLASIA

RENAL BICARBONATE REABSORPTIVE DEFECT   0858

Includes:
Bicarbonate-wasting renal tubular acidosis
Renal tubular acidosis, proximal
Renal tubular acidosis, rate type
Renal tubular acidosis, type II

Excludes:
Renal tubular acidosis (0862)
Renal tubular acidosis, type IV
Renal tubular syndrome, Fanconi type (0864)

Major Diagnostic Criteria: Hyperchloremic acidosis with reduced renal threshold for bicarbonate-producing bicarbonaturia in the range of 15–25% of the filtered load. Before acidosis is treated, urine pH is less than 6.0. Evidence of a more generalized dysfunction of the proximal tubule (renal Fanconi syndrome) such as amino aciduria, glucosuria, and phosphaturia are absent.

Clinical Findings: A small number of children have been reported who exhibit an isolated defect in proximal tubular bicarbonate reabsorption in infancy associated with hyperchloremic metabolic acidosis and failure to thrive. Most cases have been males without a family history of the problem. It is notable that nephrocalcinosis, hypokalemia, hypocitraturia, and metabolic bone disease are absent. These patients have done well on high-dose bicarbonate therapy (15–25 mEq/kg/day), with resolution of acidosis and growth failure.

Complications: Failure to thrive, episodes of fever and dehydration.

Associated Findings: None reported except in one Norwegian family in which mental retardation, developmental delay, corneal opacities, glaucoma, and hypothyroidism were found in two brothers with pure proximal renal tubular acidosis. It is likely that this family represents a form of the disease different from the sporadic cases.

Etiology: Possibly X-linked inheritance. Many cases are sporadic.

Pathogenesis: Defective reabsorption of bicarbonate in the proximal tubule leads to bicarbonate loss, sodium wasting, volume contraction, and acidosis.
There is controversy as to whether proximal tubular carbonic anhydrase activity is normal. Some have speculated that a defect in proximal hydrogen ion secretion or pyruvate carboxylase activity might produce the syndrome. More than one type is likely.

MIM No.: 31240

Sex Ratio: M1:F0. Nearly all cases have been males.

Occurrence: Undetermined but presumed rare.

Risk of Recurrence for Patient's Sib:
See Part I, *Mendelian Inheritance.*

Risk of Recurrence for Patient's Child:
See Part I, *Mendelian Inheritance.*

Age of Detectability: In infancy.

Gene Mapping and Linkage: Unknown.

Prevention: None known. Genetic counseling indicated.

Treatment: Administration of large amounts of sodium bicarbonate (15–25 mEq/kg/day) in divided doses is required to correct acidosis. Polyuria persists.

Prognosis: Good with treatment. In most of the sporadic cases, the requirement for bicarbonate therapy has slowly resolved.

Detection of Carrier: Unknown.

Support Groups: New York; National Kidney Foundation

References:
Soriano JR, et al.: Proximal renal tubular acidosis: a defect in bicarbonate reabsorption with normal urinary acidification. Pediatr Res 1967; 1:81–98.
Donckerwolcke RA, et al.: A case of bicarbonate-losing renal tubular acidosis and defective carbonic anhydrase activity. Arch Dis Child 1970; 45:769–773.
Brenes LG, et al.: Familial proximal renal tubular acidosis: a distinct clinical entity. Am J Med 1977; 63:244–252.
Winsnes A, et al.: Congenital, persistent proximal type renal tubular acidosis in two brothers. Acta Paediatr Scand 1979; 68:861–868.
DuBose TD, Jr., Alpern RF: Renal tubular acidosis. In: Scriver CR, et al, eds: The metabolic basis of inherited disease, 6th ed. New York: McGraw-Hill, 1989:2539–2568.

G0052 **Paul Goodyer**

Renal blastema, nodular or persistent
See CANCER, WILMS TUMOR
Renal calculi-ulcer-leukonychia
See ULCER-LEUKONYCHIA-GALLSTONES
Renal cell carcinoma
See CANCER, RENAL CELL CARCINOMA
Renal disease, polycystic adult type
See KIDNEY, POLYCYSTIC DISEASE, DOMINANT
Renal disease-deafness-ichthyosis
See DEAFNESS-HYPERPROLINURIA-ICHTHYOSIS
Renal duplication-hearing loss-external ear anomalies
See BRANCHIO-OTO-URETERAL SYNDROME
Renal dysplasia, Elejalde type
See ACROCEPHALOPOLYDACTYLOUS DYSPLASIA
Renal dysplasia-blindness, hereditary
See RENAL DYSPLASIA-RETINAL APLASIA, LOKEN-SENIOR TYPE
Renal dysplasia-primitive renal tubules
See RENAL TUBULAR DYSGENESIS

RENAL DYSPLASIA-RETINAL APLASIA, LOKEN-SENIOR TYPE 2687

Includes:

Loken-Senior syndrome
Nephronophthisis-associated ocular anomalies, familial
   juvenile
Renal-retinal dystrophy, familial
Renal-retinal syndrome
Renal dysplasia-blindness, hereditary
Senior-Loken syndrome

Excludes:

Kidney, nephronophthisis-medullary cystic desease (3018)
Kidney, polycystic disease-cataract-blindness (3288)
Retina, amaurosis congenita, Leber type (0043)
Retinitis pigmentosa (0869)
Saldino-Mainzer syndrome

Major Diagnostic Criteria: Nephronophthisis (with or without medullary cystic renal disease) and a progressive pigmentary retinal dystrophy, with onset typically in the first year of life.

Clinical Findings: In some cases, the progressive pigmentary retinal dystrophy is like those of **Retina, amaurosis congenita, Leber type** and children present with visual impairment in the first year of life. In other cases, the tapetoretinal dystrophy resembles **Retinitis pigmentosa** and develops later. Renal involvement is always insidious in onset. There is a progressive renal insufficiency secondary to abiotrophy of the distal part of the renal tubules, which results in a chronic interstitial nephritis and uremia.

Complications: Severely impaired visual acuity secondary to retinal dystrophy and renal failure.

Associated Findings: None known.

Etiology: Autosomal recessive inheritance. Concordance is observed in monozygotic twins. Consanguinity of the parents is frequent. It has been reported that, in one affected sibship, one child may show only the tapetoretinal dystrophy and another only the nephronophthisis; thus the disease is either due to a gene with pleiotrophic effects and variable expressivity or two closely linked genes, one acting on the renal tubule and the other on the retina.

Pathogenesis: May be due to a genetic enzymatic disorder which involves vitamin A metabolism in the retina and changes the metabolism of the retinal tubules. There has been one report of an associated lipidosis.

MIM No.: *26690

POS No.: 3455

Sex Ratio: M1:F1

Occurrence: About 150 cases have been documented in the literature.

Risk of Recurrence for Patient's Sib:
See Part I, *Mendelian Inheritance.*

Risk of Recurrence for Patient's Child:
See Part I, *Mendelian Inheritance.*

Age of Detectability: If the tapetoretinal dystrophy resembles **Retina, amaurosis congenita, Leber type** with nystagmus, it is detected early in infancy and the electroretinogram is abnormal. Renal function should be followed sequentially to note the abnormality that may not present until later on in the first decade of life.

Gene Mapping and Linkage: Unknown.

Prevention: None known. Genetic counseling indicated.

Treatment: None for the eye; appropriate management of renal failure and its complications. Renal transplant has been performed.

Prognosis: The ocular prognosis is poor. Prognosis for renal function is also poor.

Detection of Carrier: Scotopic impairment of the ERG in healthy heterozygoes parents has been reported.

References:
Senior B: Familial renal-retinal dystrophy. Am J Dis Child 1973;125: 442–447.
François J, et al: Familial juvenile nephronophthisis and associated ocular anomalies (Senior's syndrome): a study of three families. Ophthalmic Paed Genet 1982; 1:97–105.

ME032   **Marilyn B. Mets**

Renal glucosuria-hyperglycinuria
See GLUCOGLYCINURIA

RENAL GLYCOSURIA 0861

Includes:

Benign mellituria
Glucosuria
Glycosuria, renal
Renal glycosuria, A and B types
Renal glycosuria, 0 type

Excludes:

Diabetes mellitus (see all)
Glucose-galactose malabsorption (0419)
Renal tubular syndrome, Fanconi type (0864)

Major Diagnostic Criteria: The reducing substance in urine is glucose; glycosuria during an otherwise normal oral glucose tolerance test; excretion of > 300 mg glucose per 24 hours on standard carbohydrate diet; and demonstration of reduced renal threshold for glucose by renal titration techniques. Type A renal glycosuria is characterized by reduced threshold and reduced tubular maximum for glucose reabsorption (T_mG). Type B renal glycosuria demonstrates reduced threshold, exaggerated "splay", and normal T_mG. Type 0 has no threshold or T_mG (tubular glucose reabsorption is completely absent). All three forms have no other proximal or distal tubular abnormalities.

Clinical Findings: Asymptomatic glucosuria is not associated with any presenting complaints other than rare episodes of hypoglycemia reported during pregnancy. The condition is usually detected on routine urinalysis.

Complications: Iatrogenically induced hypoglycemia in patients misdiagnosed as diabetics and treated with insulin.

Associated Findings: None known.

Etiology: Autosomal recessive inheritance. Several distinct autosomal mutations are likely.

Pathogenesis: Transport defect leads to reduced threshold or reduced T_m for glucose.

MIM No.: *23310

Sex Ratio: M1:F1

Occurrence: Undetermined. Established literature.

Risk of Recurrence for Patient's Sib:
See Part I, *Mendelian Inheritance.*

Risk of Recurrence for Patient's Child:
See Part I, *Mendelian Inheritance.*

Age of Detectability: During neonatal period.

Gene Mapping and Linkage: Unknown.

Prevention: None known. Genetic counseling indicated.

Treatment: Unknown.

Prognosis: No apparent effect on longevity or health.

Detection of Carrier: No reliable means; some carriers do demonstrate mild renal glycosuria.

Special Considerations: Early studies using glucose tolerance tests suggested that renal glycosuria is inherited as a dominant trait; recent pedigree analyses using glucose titration techniques indicate that the disorder is inherited in an autosomal recessive fashion and that types A and B renal glycosuria may be found in a single sibship; thus several different mutations affecting one or more glucose transport systems in the kidney may be responsible.

Gut transport system for glucose is not affected in pedigrees studied so far.

Support Groups: New York; National Kidney Foundation

References:

Elsas LJ, Rosenberg LE: Familial renal glycosuria: a genetic reappraisal of hexose transport by kidney and intestine. J Clin Invest 1969; 48:1845–1854.

Elsas LJ, et al.: Autosomal recessive inheritance of renal glycosuria. Metabolism 1971; 20:968–975.

Oemar BS, et al.: Complete absence of tubular glucose reabsorption: a new type of renal glucosuria (type 0). Clin Nephrol 1987; 27:156–160.

Desjeux, J-F: Congenital selective Na+, D-glucose cotransport defects leading to renal glycosuria and congenital selective intestinal malabsorption of glucose and galactose. In: Scriver CR, et al, eds: The metabolic basis of inherited disease, 6th ed. New York: McGraw-Hill, 1989:2463–2478.

SC050   **Charles R. Scriver**

Renal glycosuria, 0 type
 See RENAL GLYCOSURIA
Renal glycosuria, A and B types
 See RENAL GLYCOSURIA
Renal hamartoma syndrome
 See OVERGROWTH-RENAL HAMARTOMA, PERLMAN TYPE
Renal hamartomas-nephroblastomatosis-fetal gigantism
 See OVERGROWTH-RENAL HAMARTOMA, PERLMAN TYPE
Renal histidinura
 See HISTIDINURIA
Renal hypoplasia-unilobular lung-polydactyly-sex reversal
 See SMITH-LEMLI-OPITZ SYNDROME, TYPE II

RENAL HYPOURICEMIA   2005

Includes:

 Dalmatian hypouricemia
 Hypouricemia-hypercalciuria-decreased bone density
 Renal (hyper)uricosuria, isolated
 Uric acid urolithiasis

Excludes:

 Hypouricemia secondary to antidiuretic hormone, drugs or neoplasm
 Renal tubular syndrome, Fanconi type (0864)
 Transport, renal, defects of (1501)
 Xanthine oxidase deficiency (2411)

Major Diagnostic Criteria: 1) serum urate <2 mg/dl (<120 μmol/liter); 2) normal renal excretion of xanthine and absence of other renal tubular abnormalities; 3) increased renal clearance of uric acid (urate/creatinine clearance ratio >0.2).

Clinical Findings: There are no characteristic somatic features associated with this condition.

Complications: Urolithiasis (calcium urate stones).

Associated Findings: Hypercalciuria is not uncommon and may be causally related to increased urate excretion. Other associated conditions include osteoporosis, **Osteopetrosis** (without renal tubular acidosis (RTA)), and infections.

The combination of *hypouricemia, hypercalciuria, and decreased bone density* has been reported in a kindred by Sperling et al (1974).

Etiology: Autosomal recessive inheritance. Genetic heterogeneity appears likely, since several different transport defects have been identified.

Pathogenesis: Renal handling of urate involves filtration, presecretory reabsorption, secretion, and postsecretory reabsorption. Tests with specific inhibitors of urate secretion (pyrazinamide) and postsecretory reabsorption (probenecid) have been used to show isolated defects in each of these transport pathways. In some cases, a combined defect appears likely.

MIM No.: *22015, 24205

Sex Ratio: M1:F1

Occurrence: Hypouricemia is seen in less than 1% of the population. Two-thirds of these cases are secondary hypouricemia; of the remainder, some may be due to xanthuria or decreased urate synthesis. Published reports suggest an increased frequency in non-Ashkenazi Jewish populations.

Risk of Recurrence for Patient's Sib:
 See Part I, *Mendelian Inheritance.*

Risk of Recurrence for Patient's Child:
 See Part I, *Mendelian Inheritance.*

Age of Detectability: Infants of two to four years of age have been described.

Gene Mapping and Linkage: Unknown.

Prevention: None known. Genetic counseling indicated.

Treatment: Urolithiasis can be avoided with standard regimens, including hydration and alkalinization to increase volume and pH of the urine, and with use of xanthine oxidase inhibitors (allopurinol).

Prognosis: A benign disorder, apart from the increased risk of urolithiasis.

Detection of Carrier: Urate clearances measured in some obligate heterozygotes are elevated and appear to be intermediate between normals and affected individuals.

Special Considerations: The human phenotype is analogous to the well-described autosomal recessive renal hyperuricosuria found in the Dalmatian coachhound. Studies in the latter indicate that transport is also abnormal in erythrocytes.

Support Groups: New York; National Kidney Foundation

References:

Greene ML, et al.: Hypouricemia due to isolated renal tubular defect: dalmatian dog mutation in man. Am J Med 1972; 53:361–367.

Sperling O, et al.: Hypouricemia, hypercalcinuria, and decreased bone density: a hereditary syndrome. Ann Intern Med 1974; 80:482–487.

Fujiwara Y, et al.: Hypouricemia due to an isolated defect in renal tubular urate reabsorption. Clin Nephrol 1980; 13:44–48.

Takeda E, et al.: Hereditary hypouricemia in children. J Pediatr 1985; 107:71–74.

Sperling O: Hereditary renal hypouricemia. In: Scriver CR, et al, eds: The metabolic basis of inherited disease, 6th ed. New York: McGraw-Hill, 1989:2605–2618.

C0016   **David Cole**

Renal iminoglycinuria
 See IMINOGLYCINURIA
Renal medulla, familial disease
 See KIDNEY, NEPHRONOPHTHISIS-MEDULLARY CYSTIC DESEASE

RENAL MESANGIAL SCLEROSIS-EYE DEFECTS   2805

Includes:
 Eye defects-diffuse renal mesangial sclerosis
 Mesangial sclerosis, diffuse renal-ocular abnormalities

Excludes:
 Cataract-renal tubular necrosis-encephalopathy, Crome type (2162)
 Oculo-cerebro-renal syndrome (0736)
 Oculo-reno-cerebellar syndrome (3050)
 Renal dysplasia-retinal aplasia, Loken-Senior type (2687)
 Wilms tumor-pseudohermaphroditism-glomerulopathy, Denys-Drash type (3139)

Major Diagnostic Criteria: Nephrotic syndrome secondary to diffuse mesangial sclerosis, eye abnormalities, chronic renal failure, and death in early childhood.

Clinical Findings: The condition presents in the first year of life with nephrotic syndrome secondary to diffuse mesangial sclerosis and eye abnormalities consisting of nystagmus, optic atrophy, narrowing of retinal arterioles, and abnormal macular areas. Renal failure occurs in early childhood.

Complications: Chronic renal failure.

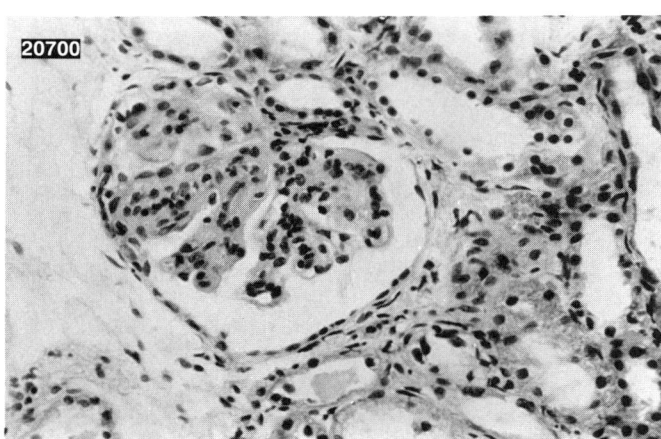

2805-20700: Renal mesangial sclerosis-eye defects; renal histology of glomeruli showing diffuse mesangial sclerosis.

Associated Findings: Diffuse mesangial sclerosis may be associated with male pseudohermaphroditism, **Cancer, Wilms tumor,** hypertension, and psychomotor retardation. May also be seen in **Wilms tumor-pseudohermaphroditism-glomerulopathy, Denys-Drash type.**

Etiology: Possibly autosomal recessive inheritance.

Pathogenesis: Possibly an antenatal dysgenetic process.

MIM No.: 24966

Sex Ratio: Presumably M1:F1

Occurrence: This association has been observed in two siblings.

Risk of Recurrence for Patient's Sib:
See Part I, *Mendelian Inheritance.*

Risk of Recurrence for Patient's Child:
See Part I, *Mendelian Inheritance.*

Age of Detectability: Early in the first year of life.

Gene Mapping and Linkage: Unknown.

Prevention: None known. Genetic counseling indicated.

Treatment: Renal transplantation has been performed successfully in patients with diffuse mesangial sclerosis.

Prognosis: Chronic renal failure occurs in early childhood.

Detection of Carrier: Unknown.

Support Groups: New York; National Kidney Foundation

References:
Barakat AY, et al.: Diffuse mesangial sclerosis and ocular abnormalities in two siblings. Int J Pediatr Nephrol 1982; 3:33–35. †

BA065
NA009

Amin Y. Barakat
Samir S. Najjar

Renal reabsorption of carnitine, defect in
See MYOPATHY-METABOLIC, CARNITINE DEFICIENCY, PRIMARY AND SECONDARY
Renal transport defects
See TRANSPORT, RENAL, DEFECTS OF

RENAL TUBULAR ACIDOSIS | 0862

Includes:
Deafness (sensorineural)-renal tubular acidosis
Distal renal tubular acidosis
Gradient type renal tubular acidosis
Renal tubular acidosis, classic type
Renal tubular acidosis, type I

Excludes:
Renal bicarbonate reabsorptive defect (0858)
Renal tubular acidosis (0862)
Renal tubular acidosis (incomplete distal), type IV
Renal tubular acidosis-osteopetrosis syndrome (3086)
Renal tubular acidosis-sensorineural deafness (0863)

Major Diagnostic Criteria: Persistent elevation of urinary pH (usually > 6.0) despite acidosis; abnormal distal hydrogen ion secretory capacity reflected by abnormally low urine-to-blood CO_2 gradient (pCO_2 < 35 mm Hg) despite bicarbonate, sulfate, or phosphate loading or furosemide administration.

Clinical Findings: Usually presents in infancy as failure to thrive, hyperchloremic acidosis, hypokalemia, and episodes of vomiting and dehydration. Twenty-five percent may develop a metabolic emergency. In infants, bicarbonaturia may be profound and is the major determinant of the therapeutic sodium bicarbonate requirement; this aspect gradually improves so that, in adults, acidosis is limited to the magnitude of endogenous acid production.

Complications: Untreated or partially treated acidosis leads to growth failure, hypercalciuria, hypocitraturia, and nephrocalcinosis by 2–4 years. Hypokalemia and acidosis produce a proximal myopathy and listlessness. Moderate nephrocalcinosis causes interstitial nephritis and sterile pyuria; advanced nephrocalcinosis predisposes to urinary tract infection and occasionally to chronic renal failure.

Associated Findings: Ehlers-Danlos syndrome, Elliptocytosis. A recessive form associated with progressive nerve deafness has also been identified.

Etiology: Autosomal dominant inheritance.

Pathogenesis: The distal hydrogen ion secretory defect is independent of transepithelial voltage and availability of urinary buffers. There is some controversy as to whether hypercalciuria is secondary to acidosis or is a direct consequence of the mutation.

MIM No.: *17980

Sex Ratio: M1:F1

Occurrence: Undetermined. Established literature.

Risk of Recurrence for Patient's Sib:
See Part I, *Mendelian Inheritance.*

Risk of Recurrence for Patient's Child:
See Part I, *Mendelian Inheritance.*

Age of Detectability: Usually during the neonatal period; becomes clinically overt by two years of age.

Gene Mapping and Linkage: Unknown.

Prevention: None known. Genetic counseling indicated.

Treatment: Oral sodium bicarbonate 5–15 mEq/kg/day in divided doses is believed to normalize growth, repair hyperkalemia and myopathy, and prevent nephrocalcinosis. Potassium supplementation may be required to avoid hypokalemia and episodes of muscle weakness.

Prognosis: Apparently good if compliant with high-dose sodium bicarbonate therapy.

Detection of Carrier: Unknown.

Support Groups: New York; National Kidney Foundation

References:
Rodriquez-Soriano J: The renal regulation of acid-base balance and the disturbances noted in renal tubular acidosis. Pediatr Clin North Am 1971; 18:529–545.
McSherry E, Morris RC, Jr.: Attainment and maintenance of normal

stature with alkali therapy in infants and children with classical renal tubular acidosis. J Clin Invest 1978; 61:509–527.

McSherry E: Renal tubular acidosis in childhood. Kidney Int 1981; 20:799–809.

DuBose TD, Jr., Alpern RF: Renal tubular acidosis. In: Scriver CR, et al, eds: The metabolic basis of inherited disease, 6th ed. New York: McGraw-Hill, 1989:2539–2568.

G0052   **Paul Goodyer**

Renal tubular acidosis, classic type
   See RENAL TUBULAR ACIDOSIS
Renal tubular acidosis, proximal
   See RENAL BICARBONATE REABSORPTIVE DEFECT
Renal tubular acidosis, rate type
   See RENAL BICARBONATE REABSORPTIVE DEFECT
Renal tubular acidosis, type I
   See RENAL TUBULAR ACIDOSIS
Renal tubular acidosis, type II
   See RENAL BICARBONATE REABSORPTIVE DEFECT

RENAL TUBULAR ACIDOSIS-OSTEOPETROSIS SYNDROME   3086

Includes:
   Carbonic anhydrase B
   Carbonic anhydrase II deficiency
   Carbonic anhydrase II, erythrocyte, electrophoretic variant
   Guibaud-Vainsel syndrome
   Marble brain disease
   Osteopetrosis-renal tubular acidosis-cerebral calcification

Excludes:
   Osteopetrosis, benign dominant (0779)
   Osteopetrosis, malignant recessive (0780)
   Renal bicarbonate reabsorptive defect (0858)
   Renal tubular acidosis (0862)

Major Diagnostic Criteria: Metabolic acidosis of varying severity secondary to impaired urinary acidification is present from birth. Osteopetrosis, evident on X-rays, develops by one year of age. Cerebral calcification, most evident on CT scan, appears during the first decade. Additional features are mental retardation, growth failure, abnormal dentition, and bone fractures. Anemia, if present, is usually mild. Diagnosis is established by demonstration of absence of carbonic anhydrase II in erythrocyte lysates. This enzyme deficiency has been demonstrated in every known patient with **Osteopetrosis** and **Renal tubular acidosis**.

Clinical Findings: Skeletal X-ray findings include increased bone density, abnormal modeling, transverse banding of metaphyses, fractures, and "bone in bone" appearance. Distal renal tubular acidosis is suggested by metabolic acidosis with hyperchloremia, normal anion gap, and inappropriately alkaline urine pH (over 6.0) without reduction in glomerular filtration rate or elevated urea nitrogen. Bicarbonaturia when plasma HCO_3- is raised to normal levels indicates the presence of a proximal tubular component also. Growth retardation begins after birth, and improves with treatment of the acidosis. Mental retardation is common, and may be severe. Intercranial calcifications are detected by 18 months by CT scan, and later by X-ray. Nephrocalcinosis is absent.

Complications: Multiple bone fractures in the first two decades. Episodes of severe hypokalemia may occur. Optic nerve atrophy and other cranial nerve compressions occur.

Associated Findings: Restrictive lung disease has been reported.

Etiology: Autosomal recessive inheritance.

Pathogenesis: Carbonic anhydrase II isozyme (CA II) is absent in erythrocytes. Although not demonstrated in humans, the absence of CAII in renal parenchyma, osteoclasts, and oligodendrial cells is inferred, and presumed to be the basis for the mixed (proximal and distal) renal tubular acidosis, the defect in bone resorption leading to osteopetrosis, and the cerebral calcification.

MIM No.: *25973, 11481

POS No.: 4170

Sex Ratio: M1:F1

Occurrence: About 15 kindreds are known, nearly half of which are from Saudi Arabia, Kuwait, and North Africa.

Risk of Recurrence for Patient's Sib:
   See Part I, *Mendelian Inheritance.*

Risk of Recurrence for Patient's Child:
   See Part I, *Mendelian Inheritance.*

Age of Detectability: At birth.

Gene Mapping and Linkage: CA2 (carbonic anhydrase II) has been mapped to 8q22.

Prevention: None known. Genetic counseling indicated.

Treatment: Treatment of renal tubular acidosis with alkali and symptomatic treatment of bone fractures and skeletal deformities.

Prognosis: Multiple fractures in childhood, but X-rays and clinical course improve in adolescents. Learning disabilities are usually substantial. Treatment of acidosis improves growth.

Detection of Carrier: Possible by demonstrating one-half normal CA II level with normal CA I level in erythrocyte lysate.

Special Considerations: Since this disorder may present in infancy, it can be confused with **Osteopetrosis, malignant recessive**. Diagnosis is important because of the much better prognosis in CA II deficiency.

Support Groups: New York; National Kidney Foundation

References:
Sly WS, et al: Carbonic anhydrase II deficiency identified as the primary defect in the autosomal recessive syndrome of osteopetrosis with renal tubular acidosis and cerebral calcification. Proc Natl Acad Sci USA 1983; 80:2752–2756.

Sly WS, et al: Carbonic anhydrase II deficiency in 12 families with the autosomal recessive syndrome of osteopetrosis with renal tubular acidosis and cerebral calcification. New Engl J Med 1985; 313:139–145.

Ohlsson A, et al: Carbonic anhydrase II deficiency syndrome: recessive osteopetrosis with renal tubular acidosis and cerebral calcification. Pediatrics 1986; 77:371–381.

Sundaram V, et al: Carbonic anhydrase II deficiency: diagnosis and carrier detection using differential enzyme inhibition and inactivation. Am J Hum Genet 1986; 38:125–136.

SL001   **William S. Sly**

RENAL TUBULAR ACIDOSIS-SENSORINEURAL DEAFNESS   0863

Includes:
   Carbonic anhydrase B deficiency
   Deafness, sensorineural-renal tubular acidosis

Excludes:
   Oculo-cerebro-renal syndrome (0736)
   Renal tubular acidosis (0862)
   Renal tubular acidosis with other associated defects

Major Diagnostic Criteria: Renal tubular acidosis with a defect in tubular HCO_3-resorption and sensorineural hearing loss or deafness.

Clinical Findings: At birth or soon thereafter, vomiting, dehydration, polydipsia, polyuria, hyposthenuria, and failure to thrive. Nephrocalcinosis was observed in some cases.

Renal tubular acidosis is a clinical syndrome of disordered renal acidification which is out of proportion to the impairment of glomerular filtration and in which metabolic acidosis results from abnormalities of renal tubular function. This type of renal tubular acidosis is associated with a defect in tubular HCO_3-resorption. Deficient carbonic anhydrase B (CA-B) activity in the affected individuals of one family has been suggested; however, repeat evaluations of one of these patients showed normal red cell carbonic anhydrase.

Deafness is variable. In most cases, a sensorineural deafness is present in early childhood. In two sibs the onset of hearing loss was during late childhood, and in two other sibs there was a striking difference in the degree of hearing loss.

Complications: Nephrocalcinosis.

Associated Findings: Mild mental retardation.

Etiology: Autosomal recessive inheritance.

Pathogenesis: Unknown.

MIM No.: *26730

POS No.: 4463

Sex Ratio: M5:F4

Occurrence: More than 20 cases have been documented in the literature.

Risk of Recurrence for Patient's Sib:
See Part I, *Mendelian Inheritance.*

Risk of Recurrence for Patient's Child:
See Part I, *Mendelian Inheritance.*

Age of Detectability: Early childhood.

Gene Mapping and Linkage: CA2 (carbonic anhydrase II) has been mapped to 8q22.

Prevention: None known. Genetic counseling indicated.

Treatment: Treatment with alkalinizing solutions and high fluid intake. Hearing aid; special training if the hearing loss is severe.

Prognosis: Probably normal life span, assuming good medical care.

Detection of Carrier: Unknown.

Support Groups: New York; National Kidney Foundation

References:
Simon H, et al.: The acidification defect in the syndrome of renal tubular acidosis with nerve deafness. Acta Pediatr Scand 1979; 68:291–295.
Cremers CWRJ, et al.: Renal tubular acidosis and sensorineural deafness: an autosomal recessive syndrome. Arch Otolaryngol 1980; 106:287–289.
Dunger DB, et al.: Renal tubular acidosis and nerve deafness. Arch Dis Child 1980; 55:221–225.
Tashian RE, et al.: Inherited variants of human red cell carbonic anhydrase. Hemoglobin 1980; 4:635–651.
Anai T, et al.: Siblings with renal tubular acidosis and nerve deafness: the first family in Japan. Hum Genet 1984; 66:282–285. *

BA033   **James A. Bartley**
                                         Cor W.R.J. Cremers

RENAL TUBULAR DYSGENESIS   2608

Includes:
Primitive renal tubule syndrome
Renal dysplasia-primitive renal tubules
Renal tubular immaturity
Renotubular dysgenesis

Excludes:
Kidney, polycystic disease, recessive (2003)
Kidney, renal dysplasia, Potter type II (3028)
Renal agenesis, unilateral (0857)

Major Diagnostic Criteria: Diagnosis is made by histological findings only. The proximal convoluted tubules are lined with poorly differentiated, crowded cuboidal and columnar epithelial cells which appear abnormally primitive. Normal proximal tubule brush borders are not demonstrated by periodic acid-Schiff stain or by peroxidase-labeled winged pea (Tetragonolobus lotus) lectin, which is a selective marker for proximal tubules. Electron microscopy demonstrates only rare rudimentary brush borders. Glomeruli are normal in appearance, but appear crowded due to a reduced number of tubular cross-sections. The corticomedullary margin is well demarcated, however, the medullary rays are poorly delineated. Renal size may be normal or enlarged.

Clinical Findings: Anuria in the neonatal period or prenatal diagnosis of oligohydramnios and inability to demonstrate fetal bladder are often the presenting clinical signs. All published cases have been preterm deliveries.

Complications: The neonatal course is complicated by pulmonary hypoplasia. Clinical findings may include Potter facies (see **Renal agenesis, bilateral**), compression deformity of the cranium, and joint contractures.

Associated Findings: **Eye, hypertelorism** (one case), **Heart, tetralogy of Fallot** (one case), **Microcephaly** (two cases), and open cranial sutures (three cases), rocker-bottom feet (two cases) and abnormal body proportions (one case).

Etiology: Autosomal recessive inheritance.

Pathogenesis: The cause of oligohydramnios in these patients is unclear, but the presence of short and undifferentiated tubules might be expected to result in decreased fluid resorption and increased fluid output. Therefore, it seems likely that abnormal glomerular filtration plays a role. No anatomic basis for decreased filtration has been identified, as the glomeruli appear to be histologically normal and well vascularized.

MIM No.: *26743

Sex Ratio: M8:F4 (observed).

Occurrence: Five families have been identified as follows: 1) a nonconsanguineous Chinese mating; 2) first cousin once-removed Sicilian mating; 3) first cousin Egyptian mating; 4) nonconsanguineous American mating of parents of Northern European background; and 5) nonconsanguineous American mating, ethnicity unspecified.

Risk of Recurrence for Patient's Sib:
See Part I, *Mendelian Inheritance.*

Risk of Recurrence for Patient's Child:
See Part I, *Mendelian Inheritance.* Affected individuals are not expected to survive to reproduce.

Age of Detectability: Due to the late onset of oligohydramnios, reliable prenatal diagnosis may not be possible. There have been two cases with amniotic fluid volume at the lower limit of normal at 22 weeks gestation, which progressed to oligohydramnios at 32 weeks gestation. One case presented with oligohydramnios at 26 weeks gestation.

Gene Mapping and Linkage: Unknown.

Prevention: None known. Genetic counseling indicated.

Treatment: Unknown.

Prognosis: Lethal.

Detection of Carrier: Unknown.

Support Groups: New York; National Kidney Foundation

References:
Allanson JE, et al.: Possible new autosomal recessive syndrome with unusual renal histopathological changes. Am J Med Genet 1983; 16:57–60.
Voland JR, et al.: Congenital hypernephrotic nephromegaly with tubular dysgenesis: a distinctive inherited renal anomaly. Pediatr Pathol 1985; 4:231–245.
Schwartz BR, et al.: Isolated congenital renal tubular immaturity in siblings. Hum Pathol 1986; 17:1259–1263.
Bernstein J: Congenital malformations of the kidney. In Tisher CC and Brenner BM, (eds): Renal Pathology, vol 2. Philadelphia: J.B. Lipincott, 1989:1278–1304.
Swinford AE, et al.: Renal tubular dysgenesis: delayed onset of oligohydramnios. Am J Med Genet 1989; 32:127–132.

SW007   **Ann E. Swinford**
HI004   **James V. Higgins**

Renal tubular immaturity
See RENAL TUBULAR DYSGENESIS
Renal tubular insufficiency-biliary malformation
See BILIARY ATRESIA
Renal tubular necrosis-cataract-encephalopathy
See CATARACT-RENAL TUBULAR NECROSIS-ENCEPHALOPATHY, CROME TYPE

RENAL TUBULAR SYNDROME, FANCONI TYPE 0864

Includes:

Adult Fanconi syndrome
Fanconi-like syndrome
Fanconi renotubular syndrome I, childhood and infantile
forms
Fanconi renotubular syndrome II, adult form
Fanconi syndrome-intestinal malabsorption-galactose
intolerance
Luder-Sheldon syndrome

Excludes: Pancytopenia syndrome, Fanconi type (2029)

Major Diagnostic Criteria: All aspects of this syndrome reflect impaired renal tubular transport. These include generalized hyperaminoaciduria resembling plasma ultrafiltrate, hypophosphatemia and hyperphosphaturia, low tubular maximum (T_m) glucosuria, type II (proximal) renal tubular acidosis with bicarbonate loss, high free water clearance, and high renal clearance of other filtered solutes (e.g., uric acid, potassium). An analogous impairment of intestinal transport may also exist.

The morphologic lesion that affects the proximal tubule, often called a "swan neck lesion," is probably secondary to the functional deficit; it represents atrophy of epithelial cells and loss of volume of proximal tubular mass.

Progressive nephron failure and decreased glomerular filtration can abate phenotypic expression of the Fanconi syndrome in its later stages in some traits (e.g., **Cystinosis**).

Clinical Findings: This is a syndrome of many causes, some of which are inherited, yet often unidentified. The clinical manifestations are, in essence, peripheral, being dependent either on the condition causing the syndrome, or on the sequelae of the syndrome itself. The fully expressed syndrome comprises a generalized disturbance of proximal renal tubular transport. The most frequent clinical consequences include hypophosphatemic rickets (phosphate loss), acidosis (bicarbonate loss), weakness (potassium loss), and dehydration (water loss). Growth failure or weight loss may also occur in the uncompensated syndrome.

Time of onset of the trait depends on its cause. Exposure to toxic agents directly precedes most acquired causes, which must be

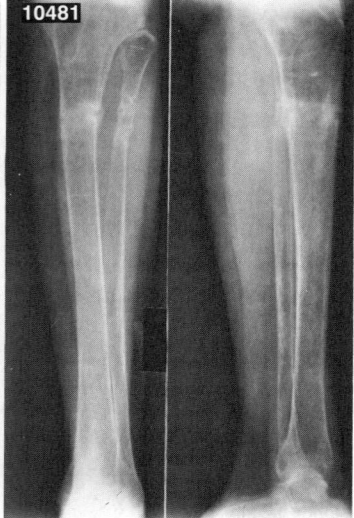

0864-10480: Skeletal changes of hypophosphatemia; note grossly deformed chest, foreshortened limbs, limb and joint defects. **10481:** X-ray shows hypophosphatemic rickets with severe nonmineralization with "looser zones" of healing fractures in proximal tibia and fibula.

eliminated before attributing the syndrome to an inherited cause. Inherited traits may produce the Fanconi syndrome either early or late in life; galactosemia and fructosemia produce the syndrome rapidly after the metabolite accumulates in the blood, while prolonged copper accumulation is required in **Hepatolenticular degeneration** before the syndrome is noticed. The recessively inherited Fanconi syndrome associated with **Cystinosis** appears in the first six months of life. The noncystinotic adult idiopathic syndrome may not appear until the fourth decade.

A possible variant, *Luder-Sheldon syndrome* (autosomal dominant), has also been described (Sheldon et al, 1961). A *Fanconi-like* syndrome (Abels and Reed, 1973) also has similarities to yet differences from the recognized Fanconi variants, including multiple cutaneous malignancies.

Complications: All clinical manifestions (e.g., rickets or osteomalacia, renal tubular acidosis and dehydration) can be considered as "complications" of the transport defect. Death secondary to uncorrected hypokalemia or dehydration can occur in infants.

Associated Findings: Those of the primary trait (e.g., **Cystinosis**, "tyrosinosis," **Hepatolenticular degeneration**) should be considered in their own terms. Death may be the end stage of a number of primary traits associated with the syndrome.

Fanconi syndrome-intestinal malabsorption-galactose intolerance has been reported in a brother and sister of Turkish-Assyrian extraction (Aperia et al, 1981).

Etiology: This condition may be acquired or inherited. While autosomal dominant inheritance has been reported, autosomal recessive inheritance of many mutant alleles at numerous autosomal loci determine most of the various forms of the syndrome. Some mutant alleles are easily recognized as primary traits, such as hereditary tyrosinemia, infantile nephropathic cystinosis, galactosemia, fructosemia, and **Hepatolenticular degeneration**. In these, the syndrome is clearly secondary to the expression of the primary trait. Other mutant genes are identifiable only through the presence of the Fanconi syndrome itself, as in the adult idiopathic Fanconi syndrome.

Pathogenesis: Impaired *net reabsorption* ability for solute and water across the tubular cell seems to be the fundamental lesion of the syndrome; *affinity* of the solutes for their binding site is apparently not altered. The inhibition of membrane transport is probably linked to specific forms of impaired availability or transduction of metabolic energy for transport.

MIM No.: *13460, 22770, 22780, 22781, 22785

Sex Ratio: M1:F1

Occurrence: Varies with primary cause.

Risk of Recurrence for Patient's Sib:
See Part I, *Mendelian Inheritance.*

Risk of Recurrence for Patient's Child:
See Part I, *Mendelian Inheritance.*

Age of Detectability: Varies with primary cause. Prenatal diagnosis is feasible in certain forms (causes), e.g., in cystinosis, hereditary tyrosinemia, and galactosinemia.

Gene Mapping and Linkage: Unknown.

Prevention: Elimination of etiologic factor in acquired forms. Genetic counseling is indicated.

Treatment: Offset phenotypic effects of trait; e.g., phosphate supplementation of diet to prevent hypophosphatemia; potassium and bicarbonate replacement to prevent hypokalemia and renal tubular acidosis; high fluid intake to prevent dehydration.

Prognosis: Depends upon the cause. Some forms respond better to treatment than do others.

Detection of Carrier: This depends on the cause. The syndrome is usually never expressed in carriers, except in unusual pedigrees, such as that described by Ben-Ishay et al. (1961), or by Sheldon et al (1961) where a dominantly inherited trait was identified. Carrier detection is feasible in cases of **Cystinosis** by measurement of cellular lysosomal cystine content, but each cause of Fanconi syndrome must be considered on its own terms (e.g., possible galactosemia; not possible yet, in hereditary tyrosinemia or idiopathic forms).

Support Groups: New York; National Kidney Foundation

References:
Ben-Ishay D, et al.: Fanconi syndrome with hypouricemia in an adult: family study. Am J Med 1961; 31:793–800.
Sheldon W, et al.: A familial tubular absorption defect of glucose and amino acids. Arch Dis Child 1961; 36:90–95.
Abeles D, Reed WB: Fanconi-like syndrome: immunologic deficiency, pancytopenia, and cutaneous malignancies. Arch Derm 1973; 107: 419–423.
Friedman AL, et al.: Autosomal dominant Fanconi syndrome with early renal failure. Am J Med Genet 1978; 2:225–232.
Aperia A, et al.: Familial Fanconi syndrome with malabsorption and galactose intolerance, normal kinase and transferase activity. Acta Paediat Scand 1981; 70:527–533.
Brenton DP, et al.: The adult presenting idiopathic Fanconi syndrome. J Inherit Metab Dis 1981; 4:211–215.
Patrick A, et al.: A family with a dominant form of idiopathic Fanconi syndrome leading to renal failure in adult life. Clin Nephrol 1981; 16:289–292.
Bergeron M, Gougoux A: The renal Fanconi syndrome. In: Scriver CR, et al, eds: The metabolic basis of inherited disease, 6th ed. New York: McGraw-Hill, 1989:2569–2580.

SC050   **Charles R. Scriver**

Renal type amyloidosis
  See AMYLOIDOSIS, FAMILIAL VISCERAL
Renal-acro-mandibular syndrome
  See ACRO-RENAL-MANDIBULAR SYNDROME
Renal-branchio-oto dysplasia
  See BRANCHIO-OTO-RENAL DYSPLASIA
Renal-facio-oculo-acoustic syndrome
  See FACIO-OCULO-ACOUSTIC-RENAL SYNDROME (FOAR SYNDROME)

RENAL-GENITAL-MIDDLE EAR ANOMALIES   0860

Includes:
  Genital-renal-middle ear anomalies
  Ear, middle-genitourinary anomalies
  Winter syndrome
Excludes:
  Deafness-renal-digital anomalies
  Nephritis-deafness (sensorineural), hereditary type (0708)
  Renal agenesis, bilateral (0856)
  Renal agenesis, unilateral (0857)

Major Diagnostic Criteria: Conductive hearing loss, variable renal anomalies, and vaginal atresia.

Clinical Findings: Renal abnormalities vary from unilateral hypoplasia to unilateral or bilateral renal agenesis. Vaginal atresia may be associated with normal external genitalia, uterus, fallopian tubes, and ovaries or with extensive internal genital anomalies. Hearing loss is conductive and associated with stenotic external auditory canals. Audiogram shows a conductive loss with a normal bone line. An absent or malformed incus has been described in two patients who had middle ear explorations. Variable features include a beaked nose, micrognathia, low-set small ears, clinodactyly, and mild mental retardation. One sib 47XX +c is presumed **Chromosome X, triplo-X.**

Complications: Delayed development of language secondary to the hearing loss. If renal anomalies are extensive enough, they may be incompatible with life. Undiagnosed vaginal atresia can lead to hydrometrocolpos at menarche.

Associated Findings: Mild mental retardation, beaked nose, micrognathia, low-set small ears, congenital heart disease, pulmonary hypoplasia.

Etiology: Possibly autosomal recessive inheritance with variable expressivity, and possibly sex-influenced. It is not known if there is a form of this syndrome in males.

Pathogenesis: Unknown.

MIM No.: 26740

POS No.: 3376

Sex Ratio: M0:F1 (observed).

Occurrence: Four, possibly five cases reported, all female.

Risk of Recurrence for Patient's Sib:
  See Part I, *Mendelian Inheritance.* Expression of this defect in males is undetermined.

Risk of Recurrence for Patient's Child:
  See Part I, *Mendelian Inheritance.* Reproductive fitness undetermined, although those with more severe abnormalities are probably infertile.

Age of Detectability: At birth, by clinical examination, although the vaginal atresia and conductive hearing loss may be difficult to detect until later.

Gene Mapping and Linkage: Unknown.

Prevention: None known. Genetic counseling indicated.

Treatment: Middle ear surgery may improve the hearing, although amplification and special training may be necessary prior to middle ear surgery. A vagina may be created by plastic surgery. Other therapy may be required for secondary renal complications.

Prognosis: Death may occur in infancy if renal abnormalities are severe, or if associated abnormalities are present. Milder forms are probably compatible with a normal life span.

Detection of Carrier: Unknown.

Special Considerations: Turner (1970) reported a patient with a narrow external auditory meatus with mild deafness, vaginal atresia, and an absent left kidney. In addition, this patient had crowded dentition, lacrimal duct stenosis, and an anteriorly placed rectum with mild rectal stenosis. This patient may represent an additional example of this syndrome. One affected female is reported to have 47XX+c karyotype that may represent a third X chromosome.

Support Groups: New York; National Kidney Foundation

References:
Winter JS, et al.: A familial syndrome of renal, genital and middle ear anomalies. J Pediatr 1968; 72:88–93.
Turner G: A second family with renal, vaginal and middle ear anomalies. J Pediatr 1970; 76:641 only.
Franek A: Ein oto-uro-genitales Syndrom Mit Mindervuchs. Monatsschr Kinderheizkd 1982; 130:730–731.
King LA, et al.: Syndrome of genital, renal and middle ear anomalies: a third family and report of a pregnancy. Obstet Gynec 1987; 69:491–493.

Janet M. Stewart

Renal-hepatic-pancreatic dysplasia (one form)
  See KIDNEY, POLYCYSTIC DISEASE, RECESSIVE
Renal-oculo-cerebellar syndrome
  See OCULO-RENO-CEREBELLAR SYNDROME
Renal-oculo-cerebro syndrome
  See OCULO-CEREBRO-RENAL SYNDROME
Renal-radial syndrome
  See RADIAL-RENAL SYNDROME
Renal-retinal dystrophy, familial
  See RENAL DYSPLASIA-RETINAL APLASIA, LOKEN-SENIOR TYPE
Renal-retinal syndrome
  See RENAL DYSPLASIA-RETINAL APLASIA, LOKEN-SENIOR TYPE
Rendu-Osler disease
  See TELANGIECTASIA, OSLER HEMORRHAGIC
Rendu-Osler-Weber disease
  See TELANGIECTASIA, OSLER HEMORRHAGIC
Reno-digito-cerebral syndrome
  See DIGITO-RENO-CEREBRAL SYNDROME
Renotubular dysgenesis
  See RENAL TUBULAR DYSGENESIS
Renpenning syndrome
  See X-LINKED MENTAL RETARDATION, RENPENNING TYPE
Reproductive tract injuries in DES daughters
  See FETAL DIETHYLSTILBESTROL (DES) EFFECTS

RESISTANCE TO 1,25 DIHYDROXY VITAMIN D 2953

Includes:

Alopecia-rickets syndrome
Autosomal recessive vitamin D dependency (ARVD)
End-organ unresponsiveness to 1,25
    dihydroxycholecalciferol
End-organ unresponsiveness to vitamin D
Hair, development in utero
Hypocalcemic, hypophosphatemic rickets with
    aminoaciduria
Hypocalcemic rickets, type IIa
Pseudovitamin D-deficiency rickets (PDR)
Rickets-alopecia syndrome
Rickets, hereditary hypocalcemic type IIa
Rickets, vitamin D-dependent, type II
Vitamin D dependency IIa
Vitamin D-dependent rickets, type IIa
Vitamin D-dependent rickets, type IIb

Excludes:

Hypophosphatasia (0516)
Hypophosphatemia, non X-linked (2040)
Hypophosphatemia, X-linked (0517)
Pseudohypoparathyroidism
Rickets, vitamin D-dependent, type I (0873)

Major Diagnostic Criteria: The general features of patients with this defect are rickets or osteomalacia, alopecia, hypocalcemia, secondary hyperparathyroidism, and high serum concentrations of 1,25-dihydroxyvitamin D (1,25[OH]$_2$D), the biologically active form of vitamin D, before or during treatment with calciferols.

Clinical Findings: *Resistance to 1,25(OH)$_2$D* is a term applied to a hereditary (and sometimes sporadic) form of hypocalcemic rickets in which there is diminished or absent target tissue responsiveness to the actions of the active form of vitamin D, 1,25(OH)$_2$D. Affected infants appear normal at birth, since fetal mineral homeostasis is determined primarily by maternal calcium and phosphate concentrations. However, serum 1,25(OH)$_2$D levels are probably abnormally high early in life (within the first few weeks). Rickets usually presents prior to age three years; however, some patients presented with osteomalacia as late as age 45 years. All cases with late onset have been eucalcemic. Approximately one-half of the reported cases have total alopecia or sparse hair. Although sometimes present at birth, alopecia is not usually obvious until ages 3–6 months. Alopecia correlates well with the severity of the resistance to 1,25(OH)$_2$D. It is always associated with early age of presentation and is always present in those patients who cannot become normocalcemic with high doses of exogenous calciferols.

Although some patients with alopecia have become normocalcemic with calciferol therapy, none have shown improvement in hair growth. Parental consanguinity has been noted in many of the reported cases, especially those with alopecia. For unknown reasons, there is a striking clustering of cases close to the Mediterranean, even though different cellular defects have been implicated in these cases. Except for patients with alopecia, rickets is the usual presenting complaint.

Clinical manifestations are similar to those of vitamin D-deficiency rickets. Symptoms usually appear before age one year and may occur as early as the first months of life. These include hypotonia, weakness, and growth failure. Motor retardation may be apparent or real. Enamel defects are seen in teeth that calcify postnatally. Pathologic fractures may occur. Later, bony deformities develop. Convulsions or tetany may be the presenting clinical feature. Rickets with a reliable history of adequate intake of vitamin D may be a clue to the diagnosis.

Prominent physical findings are shortness of stature, hypotonia, and the characteristic features of rickets, including thickening of the wrists and ankles, frontal bowing of lower limbs, and positive Trousseau and Chvostek signs.

The X-ray findings are not distinguishable from those associated with other forms of rickets. The diagnosis is documented in the laboratory with hypocalcemia, hypophosphatemia, elevated urinary cyclic AMP, and elevated serum levels of parathyroid hormone, alkaline phosphatase, and 1,25(OH)$_2$D. Serum levels of 25-(OH)D are normal. Pretreatment concentrations of 1,25(OH)$_2$D have ranged from 54 to 966 pg/ml, and from 189 to 4,800 pg/ml during calciferol therapy. Confirmation of the diagnosis requires failure to respond to an adequate trial of supplemental calcium and normal replacement doses of calciferols for three months. Although recent studies have shown an important role for 1,25(OH)$_2$D in regulating immune function, it is not known if resistance to 1,25(OH)$_2$D *per se* in these subjects leads to increased morbidity or mortality from infectious diseases or immune abnormalities. Finally, endocrine studies in several affected patients have indicated that secretion of insulin, TSH, prolactin, growth hormone, and testosterone were either normal or correctable by restoration of eucalcemia with calcium infusions. One affected woman, who was successfully treated with high doses of 1,25(OH)$_2$D, has been reported to become pregnant and bear a normal child.

Complications: Bony deformities related to severity of unresponsiveness to calciferol therapy and delay in making diagnosis and initiating treatment.

Associated Findings: Alopecia, aminoaciduria, hypotonia, tetany, enamel hypoplasia of teeth that form post-natally.

Etiology: Although about one-half of the cases have been sporadic, several kindreds with parental consanguinity and multiple affected children suggests autosomal recessive inheritance.

Pathogenesis: This syndrome can be explained on the basis of end-organ resistance to the actions of 1,25(OH)$_2$D. The resistance is due to an abnormality in the receptor for 1,25(OH)$_2$D, or in a post-receptor process. All tissues appear to be affected, although the classic vitamin D target tissues (intestine, bone, and kidney) seem to be the ones primarily responsible for the clinical manifestations of rickets, hypocalcemia, and secondary hyperparathyroidism.

Based on studies in skin fibroblasts cultured from many of the reported kindreds, the lack of tissue responsiveness results from a heterogeneity of at least five defects: 1) Hormone-binding negative. Radioligand binding studies *in vitro* document total lack of functional receptor in about one-half of all the cases, although immunochemical assays demonstrate that a receptor polypeptide is synthesized. 2) Diminished quantity of receptor. Only 10% normal binding capacity with normal receptor affinity has been documented in two kindreds. 3) Reduced affinity of receptor for 1,25(OH)$_2$D. Two kindreds have shown a 20- to 30-fold reduction in the affinity constant for the hormone, but normal receptor binding capacity. 4) Failure of nuclear localization. Cells from two kindreds contained an apparently normal 1,25(OH)$_2$D receptor in soluble extracts, but studies with radioligand in intact cells show no detectable hormone localization to the nucleus as occurs with normal cells. 5) Nuclear uptake-positive resistance.

In three of the four kindreds with the pattern five, receptor elution from DNA-cellulose *in vitro* was abnormal, suggesting that the mutation involved the DNA binding domain of the receptor. Following successful cloning of the vitamin D receptor gene, two kindreds with this pattern have been found to have point mutations in the "zinc finger" loops in the DNA binding region of the receptor gene. Bioassay of fibroblasts from affected patients using induction of an enzyme, 25 hydroxy D-24-hydroxylase or inhibition of cell proliferation by 1,25(OH)$_2$D, has generally correlated well with clinical responsiveness to large doses of calciferols. In the one kindred where osteoblast-like cells were cultured from bone at the time of a surgical procedure, an identical cellular defect was found in the bone cells as was found with fibroblasts, confirming the validity of the fibroblast model system. Finally, lymphocytes, obtained by phlebotomy and activated in culture have also been found to be useful for 1,25(OH)$_2$D receptor and responsiveness studies, recapitulating observations made earlier with fibroblasts.

The frequency of alopecia in the more severely resistant patients suggests a key role for 1,25(OH)$_2$D and its receptor in hair follicle development and/or metabolism *in utero*.

MIM No.: 27742, *27744

Sex Ratio: Presumably M1:F1.

Occurrence: Several kindreds have been reported.

Risk of Recurrence for Patient's Sib:
See Part I, *Mendelian Inheritance.*

Risk of Recurrence for Patient's Child:
See Part I, *Mendelian Inheritance.*

Age of Detectability: Usually the condition is detected in the first 2–3 years of life. Amniotic fluid cells have receptors and a bioresponse to 1,25(OH)₂D, thus allowing for the possibility of prenatal diagnosis.

Gene Mapping and Linkage: VDR (vitamin D receptor) has been tentatively mapped to 12.

Prevention: None known. Genetic counseling indicated.

Treatment: In many cases, supplemental $1,25(OH)_2D$, up to 20 μg daily, along with calcium replacement corrects the hypocalcemia, secondary hyperparathyroidism, and rickets. However, some patients are completely refractory to all forms of calciferol therapy. One unusual patient responded permanently to a short course of treatment with $24,25(OH)_2D$. One totally resistant patient was treated successfully with prolonged intravenous calcium infusion over several months in the hospital; another was treated with long-term nocturnal calcium infusions.

Prognosis: With correction of rickets and hypocalcemia in patients who respond to therapy, the prognosis appears to be good for growth, development, and reproduction. However, the prognosis for totally resistant patients is uncertain.

Detection of Carrier: Unknown. Screening of sibs' or parents' fibroblasts *in vitro* has thus far failed to distinguish heterozygotes from normal persons.

References:
Marx SJ, et al.: A familial syndrome of decrease in sensitivity to 1,25-dihydroxyvitamin D. J Clin Endocrinol Metab 1978; 47:1303–1310.
Rosen JF, et al.: Rickets with alopecia: an inborn error of vitamin D metabolism. J Pediatrics 1979; 94:729–735. †
Eil C, et al.: A cellular defect in hereditary vitamin-D-dependent rickets type II: defective nuclear uptake of 1,25-dihydroxyvitamin D in cultured skin fibroblasts. New Engl J Med 1981; 304:1588–1591.
Marx SJ, et al.: Hereditary resistance to 1,25-dihydroxyvitamin D. Rec Prog Horm Res 1984; 40:589–615.
Gamblin GT, et al.: Vitamin D-dependent rickets type II: defective induction of 25-hydroxyvitamin D(3)-24-hydroxylase by 1,25-dihydroxyvitamin D₃ in cultured skin fibroblasts. J Clin Invest 1985; 75:954–960.
Hirst M, et al.: Vitamin D resistance and alopecia: a kindred with normal 1,25-dihydroxyvitamin D binding, but decreased receptor affinity for deoxyribonucleic acid. J Clin Endocrinol Metab 1985; 60:490–495.
Hochberg L, et al.: Does 1,25-dihydroxyvitamin D participate in the regulation of hormone release from endocrine glands. J Clin Endocrinol Metab 1985; 60:57–61.
Koren R, et al.: Defective binding and function of 1,25-dihydroxyvitamin D3 receptors in peripheral mononuclear cells of patients with end-organ resistance to 1,25-dihydroxyvitamin D. J Clin Invest 1985; 76:2012–2015.
Balsan S, et al.: Long-term nocturnal calcium infusions can cure rickets and promote normal mineralization in hereditary resistance to 1,25-dihydroxyvitamin D. J Clin Invest 1986; 77:1661–1667.
Delvin EE, et al.: Specific 1,25-hydroxycholecalciferol receptors and stimulation of 25-hydroxycholecalciferol-24R hydroxylase in human amniotic cells. Pediatr Res 1987; 21:432–435.
Hughes MR, et al.: Point mutation in the human vitamin D receptor gene associated with hypocalcemic rickets. Science 1988; 242:1702–1705.

EI002   **Charles Eil**

Respiratory papillomatosis, juvenile
See PAPILLOMA VIRUS, CONGENITAL INFECTION
Restoril^, fetal effects
See FETAL BENZODIAZEPINE EFFECTS

RESTRICTIVE DERMATOPATHY   2757

Includes:
    Contractures-hyperkeratosis
    Hyperkeratosis-contracture syndrome
    Late fetal epidermal dysplasia, type II
    Skin, tight
    Tight skin contracture syndrome

Excludes:
    Ichthyosis
    Skin, localized absence of (0608)

Major Diagnostic Criteria: The combination of congenital contractures, hyperkeratosis, and characteristic facial appearance distinguishes this condition from other lethal skin defects.

Clinical Findings: All affected infants were born prematurely (31–33 weeks), with the majority of pregnancies complicated by polyhydramnios. Umbilical cords are often short. At birth, all skin had an abnormal appearance, ranging from a hard, shell-like structure, to a translucent, thin skin with prominent vasculature and diffuse erythema. Joint contractures were present in all cases, with knees, elbows, wrists, and ankles generally held in flexion. Fontanelles were wide in almost all cases. Facial anomalies consistently present included apparent hypertelorism; small nose; small, open mouth; micrognathia; and low-set, anomalous ears.

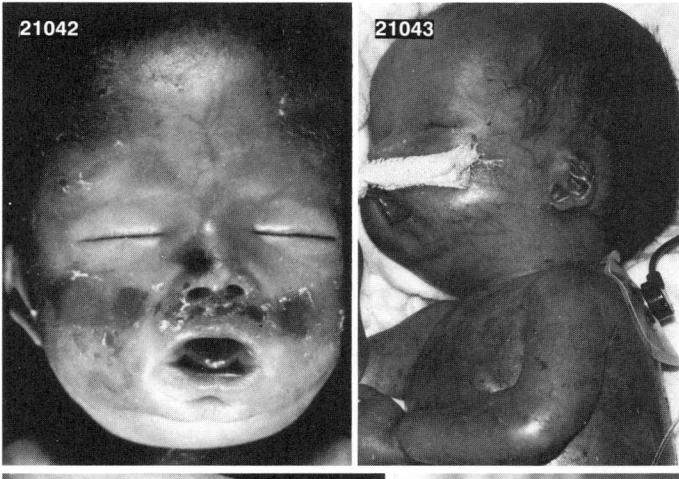

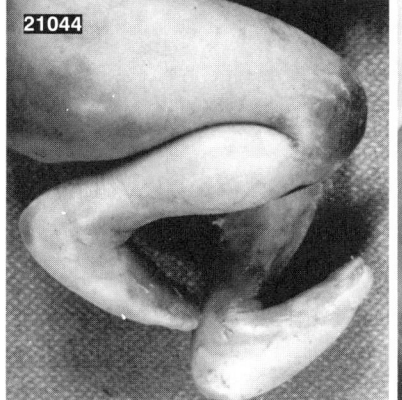
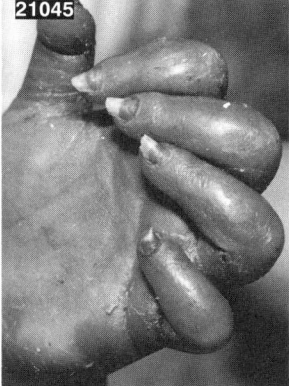

2757-21042–44: Restrictive dermatopathy: note small jaw and mouth; pinched, narrow nose; thick, dysplastic ears; relatively large head. All major joints are in a fixed, flexed position with tense, stiff skin which is sloughing in places. **21045:** Camptodactyly of fingers with long, thickened nails.

Occasional anomalies included ectropion and skeletal anomalies, including hypoplastic clavicles, scapulae, and/or long bones.

Histologically, the epidermis is thickened, with hyperkeratosis of the stratum corneum. The pilosebaceous structures and eccrine sweat glands were hypoplastic. The dermis was thinner than normal, with abnormal connective tissue. In cases of Hutterite ethnic origin, muscle immaturity was also noted.

Complications: Sepsis was frequently noted. Most of the facial features and contractures are thought to be secondary to fetal hypokinesia, which in turn may be caused by the tight skin.

Associated Findings: Present in only one case each were gyral immaturity, choanal atresia, submucous cleft palate, **Ductus arteriosus, patent** with patent foramen ovale, absent adrenal cortex, left ureter duplication, and **Hypospadias.**

Etiology: Autosomal recessive inheritance is suggested by the presence of the condition in sibs of both sexes.

Pathogenesis: Thought to be a biochemical defect leading to abnormal keratin formation and failure of differentiation.

MIM No.: 27521

POS No.: 3799

Sex Ratio: M1:F1

Occurrence: Several sibships have been reported, including two from a Mennonite kindred.

Risk of Recurrence for Patient's Sib:
See Part I, *Mendelian Inheritance.*

Risk of Recurrence for Patient's Child:
See Part I, *Mendelian Inheritance.*

Age of Detectability: At birth, although prenatal diagnosis by amniocentesis or fetoscopy with skin biopsy may be possible.

Gene Mapping and Linkage: Unknown.

Prevention: None known. Genetic counseling indicated.

Treatment: Unknown.

Prognosis: All affected infants died soon after birth.

Detection of Carrier: Unknown.

Special Considerations: There are slight differences in cases of Hutterite origin, e.g., intrauterine growth retardation in Hutterite cases, which may indicate heterogeneity. Furthermore, Stevenson et al (1987) reported a case with virtually identical histologic skin abnormalities, yet a phenotype that was quite different; in their case, the skin seemed to form a cocoon around the fetus, and the facial appearance was different. It is unknown whether this case represents a phenotypic continuum of the same defect, or a distinct condition with similar histology, but different biochemistry.

References:
Lowry RB, et al.: Congenital contractures, edema, hyperkeratosis, and intrauterine growth retardation. Am J Med Genet 1985; 22:531–543.
Schuur RE, et al.: A lethal ichthyosis variant with arthrogryposis. Am J Hum Genet 1985; A76.
Toriello HV: Restrictive dermopathy and report of another case. Am J Med Genet 1986; 24:625–629.
Witt DR, et al.: Restrictive dermopathy: a newly recognized autosomal recessive skin dysplasia. Am J Med Genet 1986; 24:631–648.
Stevenson RE, et al.: Cocoon fetus-fetal encasement secondary to ectodermal dysplasia. Proc Greenwood Genet Center 1987; 6:10–15.

T0007   **Helga V. Toriello**

Rethore syndrome
See CHROMOSOME 9, TRISOMY 9p
Reticular dysgenesis
See IMMUNODEFICIENCY, SEVERE COMBINED
Reticular pigmented anomaly of flexures
See SKIN CREASES, RETICULATE PIGMENTED FLEXURES, DOWLING-DEGOS TYPE
Reticular pigmented dermatosis
See ECTODERMAL DYSPLASIA, NAEGELI TYPE
Reticuloendotheliosis, nonlipoid
See LETTERER-SIWE DISEASE

Reticulosis, familial histiocytic
*See LETTERER-SIWE DISEASE
also IMMUNODEFICIENCY, RETICULOENDOTHELIOSIS WITH EOSINOPHILIA*
Reticulosis, familial histiocytic
See LYMPHOHISTIOCYTOSIS, FAMILIAL ERYTHROPHAGOCYTIC

RETINA, AMAUROSIS CONGENITA, LEBER TYPE   0043

Includes:
Amaurosis congenita of Leber, types I and II
Amaurosis of retinal origin, congenital
Dysgenesis neuroepithelialis retinae
Pigmentary retinitis-congenital amaurosis
Retinal aplasia, hereditary
Retinal blindness, congenital
Retinal degeneration, congenital
Retinitis pigmentosa, congenital

Excludes:
Albinism, ocular (0032)
Color blindness, total (0198)
Nightblindness, congenital stationary, autosomal dominant (3205)
Nightblindness, congenital stationary, autosomal recessive (3204)
Nightblindness, congenital stationary, X-linked recessive (0718)
Renal dysplasia-retinal aplasia, Loken-Senior type (2687)
Retinitis pigmentosa (0869)

Major Diagnostic Criteria: Congenital nystagmus and severely impaired visual function are detected in infancy. The ocular fundi are normal or show optic atrophy with pigmentary disturbances. The photopic and scotopic electroretinograms (ERGs) are severely decreased or extinguished.

Clinical Findings: Amaurosis congenita of Leber is a devastating visual disorder of infants first suspected on the basis of severely impaired visual function and congenital nystagmus. Visual acuity usually ranges from "counting fingers" at a few feet to "no light perception" with severe constriction of the visual field. A few patients show 20/100 vision or better and preserved visual fields. At birth, the fundi could appear normal or show optic atrophy, retinal vascular attenuation and pigmentary disturbances. With advancing age, some fundi remain normal while others show progressive changes with "bone spicule" formation, similar to that noted in retinitis pigmentosa. On ERG the photopic and scotopic responses are severely decreased or extinguished. High hyperopia has been suggested as a diagnostic criteria. A small percentage of patients develop cataracts and keratoconus in the second decade. The pleiotropy of the ocular manifestations suggests heterogeneity for isolated amaurosis congenita.

Amaurosis congenita is sometimes a part of a systemic disease associated with a variety of neurological, renal or skeletal abnormalities. The frequency of the association with neurological disorders is controversial. Alstrom found no neurological involvement in 175 patients. In a recent series, Nickel and Hoyt, found one of 31 with psychomotor retardation and 3 with cerebellar hypoplasia. On the other hand, Schappert-Kimmijser et al found 25% of 227 patients and Vaizey found 52% of 21 with significant psychomotor retardation and muscular hypotonia. In a recent series of 43 cases, 10 had mental retardation and other associated systemic findings were noted. Moore and Taylor (1984) have described 3 boys, including 2 brothers, with palsy of saccadic eye movements, suggestive of oculomotor apraxia.

Complications: Psychomotor retardation and muscular hypotonia are complications of visual deprivation during childhood development.

Associated Findings: *Ocular:* Enophthalmos is frequently present due to repetitive self digital stimulation of the globe causing atrophy of orbital fat. Documentation of decreased total axial length of the globe in a few cases and high hyperopia as a frequent finding suggest that microphthalmia is common. On occasion, macular colobomas and optic disc edema are found.

Neurologic: Psychomotor retardation, muscular hypotonia, enlargement of ventricles and cisterns, with widening of cerebral sulci. Cigarette paper scars and increased hyperextensability of skin suggestive of **Ehlers-Danlos syndrome** has been described in one pedigree.

Etiology: Autosomal recessive inheritance in some cases, but most are sporadic.

Pathogenesis: Undetermined. Some histopathological studies have shown a marked decrease or absence of rod and cone photoreceptors in the retina. Others show immature development or degeneration of photoreceptors.

MIM No.: *20400, *20410

Sex Ratio: M1:F1

Occurrence: Amaurosis congenita of Leber is the diagnosis in 10 to 18% of children in some institutions for the blind in the Netherlands.

Risk of Recurrence for Patient's Sib:
See Part I, *Mendelian Inheritance.*

Risk of Recurrence for Patient's Child:
See Part I, *Mendelian Inheritance.*

Age of Detectability: In infancy.

Gene Mapping and Linkage: Unknown.

Prevention: None known. Genetic counseling indicated.

Treatment: Referral to services for visually impaired to learn non-visual means of communication, and to maximize educational, vocational and social skills.

Prognosis: Normal life expectancy. Intelligence is usually normal. Visual handicap leads to a major change in lifestyle.

Detection of Carrier: Examination of relatives for evidence of the trait.

Special Considerations: Amaurosis congenita has been reported with various congenital renal abnormalities. The ophthalmological manifestations vary: some have congenital blindness with fundus findings consistent with amaurosis congenita while others have acquired visual disturbances with findings more consistent with retinitis pigmentosa. Some authors consider amaurosis congenita associated with renal disease as a separate condition (See **Renal dysplasia-retinal aplasia, Loken-Senior type**).

References:
Schappert-Kimmijser J, et al.: Amaurosis congenita (Leber). Arch Ophthalmol 1959; 61:211–218.
Vaizey MJ, et al.: Neurological abnormalities in congenital amaurosis of Leber. Arch Dis Child 1977; 52:399–402.
Nickel B, Hoyt CS: Leber's congenital amaurosis: is mental retardation a frequent associated defect. Arch Ophthalmol 1982; 100:1089–1092.
Foxman SG, et al.: Leber's congenital amaurosis and high hyperopia: a discrete entity. In: Henkind P, ed: Acta 25th International Congress of Ophthalmology. Philadelphia: Lippincott, 1983:85–88.
Moore AT, Taylor SI: A syndrome of congenital retinal dystrophy and saccade palsy - a subset of Leber's amaurosis. Br J Ophthalmol 1984; 68:421–431.
Carr RC, Heckenlively JR: Hereditary pigmentary degenerations of the retina. In: Duane TD, ed: Clinical ophthalmology. vol. 3. Philadelphia: Harper and Row, 1986:9–11.
Schroeder R, et al.: Leber's congenital amaurosis: retrospective review of 43 cases and a new fundus finding in two cases. Arch Ophthal 1987; 105:356–359.

Avery H. Weiss

RETINA, CAVERNOUS HEMANGIOMA   3176

Includes:
Angiomas (cavernous) of CNS and retina
Cavernoma multiplex
Familial cavernous malformations of the CNS and retina (FCMCR)
Gass syndrome
Vascular formations, familial

Excludes:
Retinal capillary hemangioma
Retina, Coats disease (3135)
Retinal telangiectasia-hypogammaglobulinemia (0868)
Sturge-Weber syndrome (0915)
Von Hippel-Lindau syndrome (0995)

Major Diagnostic Criteria: Cavernous hemangiomas of the retina and/or central nervous system. The retinal lesions are best detected by indirect ophthalmoscopy and their diagnosis confirmed by retinal fluorescein angiography. The central nervous system lesions are seen on magnetic resonnance imaging (MRI) and computed tomographic (CT) scanning. These findings may be accompanied by cutaneous angiomas as well as by a family history of other affected individuals.

Clinical Findings: In 1940, Weskamp and Cotlier described a neuro-oculo-cutaneous syndrome that consists of cavernous angioma of the central nervous system, cavernous hemangioma of the retina or optic nerve head, and cutaneous angiomas. An affected individual may have either the intracranial or retinal hemangioma, or both. Cutaneous angiomas are a less consistent finding.

Cavernous hemangiomas of the retina rarely cause a decrease in vision and therefore are most often discovered on routine ophthalmoscopic exam. The lesion is usually unilateral and best detected with indirect ophthalmoscopy of the retinal periphery. It has the appearance of a sessile tumor composed of saccular aneurysms filled with dark venous blood looking like a group of grapes projecting from the inner retinal surface. These aneurysms rarely leak and therefore there is no surrounding exudate. Occasionally a lesion will be covered by a gray-white substance suggestive of fibrous tissue or an epiretinal membrane. Spontaneous vitreous hemorrhage can occur particularly from larger lesions. Fluorescein angiography typically shows delayed and incomplete filling of the lesion. Fluorescein caps are highly characteristic and result from sedimentation of the erythrocytes in the dependent portion of the aneurysms. Filling of the angioma is incomplete as a result of thrombosis of some of the aneurysms. The surrounding retinal vasculature appears normal.

The long-term course is believed to be nonprogressive, although some of these lesions clinically appear to have an increase in the size of their associated fibrovascular or epiretinal membranes. The visual acuity is usually unaffected; however, there is a visual field defect corresponding to the location of the retinal lesion.

Cavernous malformations of the central nervous system may be associated with headaches, seizures, or intracranial hemorrhage. There is a high risk of symptomatic disease. One study reporting on 54 patients with FCMCR found that 24 patients (44%) had seizures, while 26 patients (48%) had recognized intracranial hemorrhages of which nine died. These lesions are demonstratable on CT scanning, and may show calcification.

Cutaneous vascular anomalies have been described in association with this syndrome, although it is an inconsistent finding and may be absent in certain pedigrees. Cutaneous hemangiomas are the most typical lesion but a variety of vascular anomalies have been seen in patients with FCMCR.

Complications: Headaches, seizures, and strokes are seen in association with the intracranial hemangioma. The retinal lesion does not usually affect vision.

Associated Findings: Congenital malformation of the heart and great vessels, and **Nevus, blue rubber bleb nevus syndrome**.

Etiology: Autosomal dominant inheritance with high penetrance and variable expressivity.

Pathogenesis: This syndrome is considered by some to be a phakomatoses or hamartosis affecting the retina, central nervous system, and skin.

MIM No.: *14080

Sex Ratio: M1:F1

Occurrence: At least 54 patients have been reported from 17 families.

Risk of Recurrence for Patient's Sib:
See Part I, *Mendelian Inheritance.*

Risk of Recurrence for Patient's Child:
See Part I, *Mendelian Inheritance.*

Age of Detectability: These vascular tumors are felt to be congenital and therefore should be present at birth. A retinal cavernous hemangioma was discovered on ophthalmoscopic exam of a full-term baby who had subconjunctival hemorrhages after a prolonged delivery.

Gene Mapping and Linkage: Unknown.

Prevention: None known. Genetic counseling indicated.

Treatment: No treatment required for the retinal lesion.

Prognosis: Risk of intracranial hemorrhage or seizures; otherwise life span and lifestyle is unaffected.

Detection of Carrier: By fundus and dermatologic exam, as well as neuro-radiologic evaluation.

Special Considerations: All first degree relatives of the affected individual are at risk for harboring an intracranial cavernous malformation and should be evaluated. Presymptomatic diagnosis in affected relatives would allow genetic counseling and close monitoring so that prompt treatment can be instituted if symptoms occur.

References:
Weskamp C, Cotlier E: Angioma del cerebro y de la retina con malformaciones capilares de la piel. Arch Oftal Buenos Aires, 1940; 15:1–10.
Gass JD: Cavernous Hemangioma of the Retina. Am J Ophthalmol 1971; 71:779–814.
Lewis RA, et al: Cavernous haemangioma of the retina and optic disc: a report of three cases and a review of the literature. Br J Ophthalmol 1975; 59:422–434.
Goldberg RE, et al: Cavernous hemangioma of the retina. Arch Ophthalmology 1979; 97:2321–2324. †
Messmer E, et al: Cavernous hemangioma of the retina: immunohistochemical and ultrastructura observations. Arch Ophthalmol 1984; 102:413–418.
Schwartz AC, et al: Cavernous hemangioma of the retina, cutaneous angiomas, and intracranial vascular lesion by computed tomography and nuclear magnetic resonance imaging. Am J Ophthalmol 1984; 98:483–487.
Dobyns WB, et al: Familial cavernous malformations of the central nervous system and retina. Ann Neurol 1987; 21:578–583. *

SC067
JA016

Bruce M. Schnall
Mohammad S. Jaafar

RETINA, COATS DISEASE   3135

Includes:
Coats disease
Leber miliary aneurysms
Primary retinal telangiectasia
Telangiectasia, congenital retinal

Excludes:
Neovascularization, diseases associated with peripheral
Telangiectasia, Osler hemorrhagic (2021)
White pupillary reflex (leukocoria), all causes

Major Diagnostic Criteria: A predominantly unilateral exudative retinopathy caused by a developmental anomaly (telangiectasia) of retinal vessels. Involved vessels show anomalous capillary branching and connections, capillary enlargement, wider than normal perivascular capillary-free zone, small caliber arterio-venous shunts, and balloon-shaped structures resembling macroaneurysms on arterioles and even venules, typically in a non-anatomic field of the retina. In the early stages of the disease, the telangiectatic vessels may be invisible on ophthalmoscopy; in later stages, and after intraretinal edema and exudation, the telangiectatic vessels may be visible only using flurescein angiography.

Clinical Findings: Coats disease presents in a bimodal age distribution depending on the extent, severity, and size of blood vessels involved. About two-thirds of patients are diagnosed between 18 months and 18 years of age. Up to one-third of patients are 30 years or older before the disease is discovered. Some patients present in the first two years of life, and the disease tends to be more severe in patients younger than four years of age at diagnosis. The peak presentation of diagnosis occurs towards the end of the first decade of life. About three-quarters of patients are males. Approximately one-fourth of cases are discovered on routine ophthalmoscopic examination. Leukocoria (white pupil) is the presenting sign in about one-third of patients, especially infants, and strabismus in about one-sixth of patients.

Disease progression, with subretinal exudation and secondary retinal detachment, correlates with the size of the vessels in the involved vascular bed and the number of retinal quadrants involved. In two-thirds of patients the telangiectasias involve only one quadrant, and in the other third they involve two quadrants; three and four quadrant involvement is rare and associated with poor visual prognosis. The temporal retina is affected preferentially. Subretinal exudation from peripheral lesions tends to pool into the macular area as an elevated mound of yellow material and has been confused with a choroidal tumor or infection or with retinoblastoma. Accurate diagnosis requires thought to the source of the exudation and indirect ophthalmoscopy with 360 degree scleral depression. Cystoid macular edema may develop in patients with either posterior or peripheral telangiectasia and cause decreased visual acuity. Spontaneous regression of the telangiectasia is rare except in advanced stages of the disease.

Complications: Serous and exudative retinal detachment; periretinal fibroproliferation; neovascular glaucoma (with total retinal detachment) and cataracts in long-standing disease.

Associated Findings: Isolated cases have been reported with a variety of non-specific and inconsistent findings including facial angioma, progressive facial hemiatrophy, **Nephritis-deafness (sensorineural), hereditary type** and **Nevus, epidermal nevus syndrome**. Peripheral retinal vasculopathy similar to Coats disease has been reported in association with **Retinitis pigmentosa** and in a single patient with **De Lange syndrome**. Bilateral Coats-like reaction has been reported in multiple members of a family with muscular dystrophy, deafness, and mental retardation (Small, 1968). Adults with Coats disease have been reported to have elevated serum cholesterol levels.

Etiology: An isolated embryologic malformation.

Pathogenesis: Unknown. The formation of incompetent and leaky retinal telangiectatic vessels causes the clinical manifestations of the disease.

MIM No.: 21635

Sex Ratio: In children probably M9:F1; in older patients close to M3:F1.

Occurrence: Probably less than 1:5,000.

Risk of Recurrence for Patient's Sib: Usually not increased.

Risk of Recurrence for Patient's Child: Usually not increased.

Age of Detectability: The majority of patients are seen in the first two decades of life, but the disease may be seen at birth or as late as the seventh decade of life.

Gene Mapping and Linkage: Unknown.

Prevention: None known. Genetic counseling indicated.

Treatment: Early treatment of the abnormal vessels by cryotherapy or photocoagulation (argon laser or xenon arc) as soon as the diagnosis is made, in order to prevent the inexorable development of subretinal exudation, macular edema, and exudative retinal detachment. Retinal reattachment surgery is indicated in cases with total exudative retinal detachment. In cases with vitreoretinal traction, vitrectomy, including retinotomy and drainage of sub-retinal fluid, may be indicated.

Prognosis: Good in cases with limited involvement and early treatment, as long as the foveal vasculature is not involved.

Detection of Carrier: Affected individuals are detected by indirect ophthalmoscopy and/or fluorescein angiography.

References:
Small RG: Coats' disease and muscular dystrophy. Trans Am Acad Ophthalmol Otolaryngol 1968; 72:225–231.
Folk JC, et al: Coats' disease in a patient with Cornelia de Lange syndrome. Am J Ophthalmol 1981; 91:607.
Ridley ME, et al: Coats' disease: evaluation of management. Ophthalmology 1982; 89:1381–1387.
Siegelman S: Coats' disease. In: Retinal diseases: pathogenesis, laser therapy and surgery. Boston: Little Brown, 1984:332–349. *
Gass RDM: Primary or congenital retinal telangiectasis (Leber's miliary aneurysm, Coats' syndrome). In: Stereoscopic Atlas of Macular Diseases. St. Louis: C. V. Mosby, 1987:384–389. *

KA045 **Hassan M. Kattan**
TR009 **Elias I. Traboulsi**

Retina, coloboma
See EYE, MICROPHTHALMIA/COLOBOMA

RETINA, COMBINED CONE-ROD DEGENERATION   **0201**

Includes:
> Cone-rod degeneration, progressive
> Cone-rod dystrophy (degeneration)
> Retinitis pigmentosa, atypical (some forms)

Excludes:
> **Choroideremia** (0925)
> **Color blindness, blue monocone-monochromatic** (0195)
> **Color blindness, total** (0198)
> Cone dystrophies (pure)
> Drug-induced retinopathies (e.g., thioridazine, chloroquine)
> Hyperornithinemia-gyrate atrophy
> **Nightblindness, congenital stationary**
> **Retina, fundus albipunctatus** (0399)
> **Retina, fundus flavimaculatus** (0400)
> **Retinitis pigmentosa** (0869)
> Retinitis punctata albescens

Major Diagnostic Criteria: A heterogeneous group of genetic retinal disorders characterized by a history of progressive loss of the psychophysiologic functions associated with cones to an earlier or more severe degree than rods. Thus, losses of central visual acuity, of color vision, and of tolerance to bright daylight (evidenced as photodysphoria or hemeralopia) are proportionately more obvious than difficulty with night (dim-light) or peripheral vision. Color vision under standard illumination, central and peripheral perimetry, dark adaptometry, and electroretinogram (ERG) may be needed if anamnesis is equivocal. Pigmentary changes in the ocular fundus are not mandatory, for or exclusive of, the diagnosis.

Clinical Findings: The term *cone-rod dystrophy* may be confusing, because currently there is no standard nomenclature for genetic disorders of the retina. One usage of the linear order of these attributive nouns emphasizes the clinician's history that the patient loses central or color vision earlier than night or peripheral vision; the other derives from responses to electroretinography. The cone system is tested by light-adapting the retina so that rods are light-saturated and thus will not respond to the flash stimulus, resulting in a characteristic waveform. After the retina has been dark adapted for at least 25 minutes, a dim (blue or white) flash below the cone threshold elicits rod-mediated function. When both the cone and the rod components of these elicited waves are abnormal, the more severely affected is listed first: combined cone-rod dystrophy.

Diminished central vision is usually associated with retinal pigment epithelial alterations within the central 30 degrees of the ocular fundi. Evidence of diffuse cone involvement includes sensitivity/discomfort in daylight (photodysphoria), altered color vision, abnormal contrast sensitivity and central visual field sensitivity, elevated thresholds or altered regeneration times on cone dark adaptation, and reduced amplitudes and prolonged implicit times on ERG. Evidence of diffuse rod involvement is often more subtle and includes peripheral visual losses, abnormally elevated rod thresholds on dark adaptation, and reduced amplitudes and altered implicit times on the rod phases of the ERG.

Combined cone-rod dystrophies must be differentiated from congenital and historically stationary disorders affecting either the cone systems alone (e.g., the cone monochromacies and rod monochromacy) or apparently both the photoreceptors and the neuroepithelial integration (e.g., the congenital stationary night blindnesses and fundus albipunctatus), since both groups may also appear to alter acuity, color, and night visual functions. In addition, they must be distinguished from progressive degenerations of both photoreceptor systems in which the rods are more severely afflicted (rod-cone dystrophies), one subset of which has characteristic ophthalmoscopic retinal changes (the **Retinitis pigmentosa**).

The onset may appear from childhood to late adulthood, with reasonable symmetry of the age of onset among affected members of the same family, especially in recessive variants. The rate of progression and the ultimate severity, as monitored by threshold visual fields or by ERG, are more variable among families with autosomal dominant transmission.

Individuals with autosomal recessive cone-rod dystrophy usually have a decrease in visual acuity during the first two decades of life and may have characteristic "bull's-eye" foveal lesions, which should be differentiated from drug toxicities (e.g., chloroquine), other lipofuscin-storage disorders, or late-onset neuronal ceroid lipofuscinoses.

Complications: Unknown.

Associated Findings: *Ocular*: posterior cortical cataracts among older individuals; rarely, vitreous syneresis and cells.
Extraocular: may occur as part of **Bardet-Biedl syndrome**.

Etiology: Autosomal dominant or autosomal recessive inheritance. Numerous sporadic cases have been reported.

Pathogenesis: Unknown.

MIM No.: *12097

Sex Ratio: M1:F1

Occurrence: Undetermined. Probably less than one-tenth as common as **Retinitis pigmentosa**.

Risk of Recurrence for Patient's Sib:
> See Part I, *Mendelian Inheritance.*

Risk of Recurrence for Patient's Child:
> See Part I, *Mendelian Inheritance.*

Age of Detectability: Usually during the second or third decades; later onset does occur.

Gene Mapping and Linkage: CORD (cone rod dystrophy (autosomal dominant)) is unassigned.

Prevention: None known. Genetic counseling indicated.

Treatment: Primary intervention is unavailable. Low-vision aids and visual rehabilitation are appropriate.

Prognosis: Visual impairment varies from moderate to considerably less than legal blindness. Most affected individuals cannot maintain a driver's license and do require magnification for reading.

Detection of Carrier: At-risk relatives may be examined for minor manifestations or early onset of disease.

References:
Krill AE, et al.: The cone degenerations. Doc Ophthalmol 1973; 35:1–80.
Francois J, et al.: Progressive cone dystrophies. Ophthalmologica 1976; 173:81–101.
Grey RHB, et al.: Bull's eye maculopathy with early cone degeneration. Br J Ophthalmol 1977; 61:702–718.

Ferrell RE, et al.: Autosomal dominant cone-rod dystrophy: a linkage study with 17 biochemical and serological markers. Am J Med Genet 1981; 8:363–369.

Marmor MF, et al.: Retinitis pigmentosa: a symposium on terminology and methods of examination. Ophthalmology 1983; 80:126–131.

Rabb MF, et al.: Cone-rod dystrophy: a clinical and histopathologic report. Ophthalmology 1986; 93:1443–1451.

Ripps H, et al.: Progressive cone dystrophy. Ophthalmology 1987; 94:1401–1409.

LE039   **Richard Alan Lewis**

RETINA, CONE DYSTROPHY, X-LINKED   3228

Includes: Cone dystrophy, X-linked with tapetal-like sheen

Excludes:
   Color blindness, blue monocone-monochromatic (0195)
   Nightblindness, Oguchi type (0740)

Major Diagnostic Criteria: Evidence of major cone dysfunction on electroretinogram (ERG) with normal or only mildly subnormal rod mediated responses.

Clinical Findings: Young patients may not be symptomatic. Patients usually present within the first to third decades of life with decreased visual acuity, defective color vision, and myopia. Vision loss may begin in childhood but is not congenital as is the case in **Color blindness, blue monocone-monochromatic.** The visual acuity may be initially as good as 20/25, but in later years may drop to counting fingers or hand motion as macular changes occur. Patients may complain of photophobia or glare sensitivity and may say their vision is best at twilight. Color vision may show either red-green or blue-yellow defects and eventually scotopization on anomaloscope testing similar to that seen in achromatopsia. Nystagmus is not a reported feature.

In all cases the ERG at the earliest age tested has shown generalized loss of cone mediated responses with normal or mildly subnormal rod responses. The EOG light-to-dark ratio may be supernormal early in the disorder but becomes subnormal later in life. Dark adaptometry demonstrates elevation of the cone portion of the curve. Pinckers (1987) believes that the disorder begins as a peripheral cone disorder (abnormal cone ERG with relative preservation of central cone function, including visual acuity) that progresses to a diffuse cone disease (including loss of central cone function). As disease progresses the macular regions develop atrophy of the pigment epithelium and choriocapillaris. At least one form demonstrates a golden-yellow tapetal-like sheen throughout the retina. This sheen appeared to fade somewhat after dark adaptation (the Mizuo-Nakamura phenomenon).

Complications: Central or pericentral scotomas develop and enlarge with passing decades. Eventually patients become legally blind, usually from loss of central visual acuity to 20/200 or worse in the better seeing eye. Rod ERG function may be normal or subnormal. It is likely that rod function loss is progressive.

Associated Findings: None known.

Etiology: X-linked recessive inheritance.

Pathogenesis: Unknown.

MIM No.: 30402, 30403

Sex Ratio: Theoretically M1:F0. Because of carrier manifestations, some women have had significant but usually mild features of the disorder.

Occurrence: One of the rarest forms of cone dystrophy, although Pinckers (1987) believes that, because of lack of recognition, X-linked cone dystrophy may be more common than previously realized.

Risk of Recurrence for Patient's Sib:
   See Part I, *Mendelian Inheritance.*

Risk of Recurrence for Patient's Child:
   See Part I, *Mendelian Inheritance.*

Age of Detectability: The electroretinogram has been shown to be abnormal by the end of the first decade of life. The ERG may show abnormality earlier.

Gene Mapping and Linkage: COD1 (cone dystrophy 1 (X-linked)) has been provisionally mapped to Xp21.1-p11.3.

Prevention: None known. Genetic counseling indicated.

Treatment: Routine ophthalmological care, with consideration of low vision aids to regain ability to read as visual acuity decreases. Consider special glasses, such as Corning 550 CPF, which protect rods from excessive light adaptation, and for many patients provide comfort. However, such glasses have not been shown to alter course of the disease.

Prognosis: Legal blindness by mid-life. Intelligence, life span, and health are otherwise normal.

Detection of Carrier: Carriers usually have normal visual acuity (20/30 or better) but may have subnormal cone ERG responses and abnormal color vision.

Special Considerations: Heterogeneity probably exists for X-linked cone dystrophy. It is uncertain whether the disorder described by Heckenlively and Weleber (1986) is the same as that described by Pinckers et al (1981). Heckenlively and Weleber's patients demonstrated a striking tapetal-like sheen. Jacobson et al (1989) reported nine affected males, three of whom showed a bronze-green tapetal-like sheen, and six female carriers from a large four generation family with X-linked cone dystrophy. Fleischman and O'Donnell (1981), described a black kindred with what they call X-linked incomplete achromatopsia. Pinckers believes that Fleischman and O'Donnell's family instead probably represents X-linked cone dystrophy, but that family had gross pathology of the macula not present in Heckenlively's family.

References:
Fleischman JA, O'Donnell FE: Congenital X-linked incomplete achromatopsia: evidence for slow progression, carrier fundus findings, and possible genetic linkage with glucose-6-phosphate dehydrogenase locus. Arch Ophthalmol 1981; 99:468–472.

Pinckers A, Timmerman GJMEN: Sex-difference in progressive cone dystrophy I. Ophthalmic Paediatr Genet 1981; 1:17–24.

Pinckers A, et al.: Sex-difference in progressive cone dystrophy II. Ophthalmic Paediatr Genet 1981; 1:25–36. * †

Heckenlively JR, Weleber RG: X-linked recessive cone dystrophy with tapetal-like sheen. Arch Ophthalmol 1986; 104:1322–1328. * †

Pinckers A, Deutman AF: X-linked cone dystrophy: an overlooked diagnosis? Internat Ophthalmol 1987; 10:241–243.

Weleber RG, Eisner A: Cone degeneration ("bull's-eye dystrophies") and color vision defects. In: Newsome DA, ed: Retinal dystrophies and degenerations. New York: Raven Press, 1988:233–256.

Jacobson DM, et al.: X-linked progressive cone dystrophy: clinical characteristics of affected male and female carriers. Ophthalmol 1989; 96:885–895.

WE042   **Richard G. Weleber**

Retina, congenital detachment of
See RETINAL DYSPLASIA

RETINA, CONGENITAL HYPERTROPHY OF RETINAL
PIGMENT EPITHELIUM   3134

Includes:
   CHRPE, isolated
   CHRPE in adenomatous polyposis (Intestinal polyposis, type III)
   Congenital hypertrophy of the retinal pigment epithelium (CHRPE)
   Retina, pigmentation of, congenital grouped

Excludes:
   Adenoma of the retinal pigment epithelium
   Choroidal nevus
   Intestinal polyposis, type III (0536)
   Melanocytoma of choroid

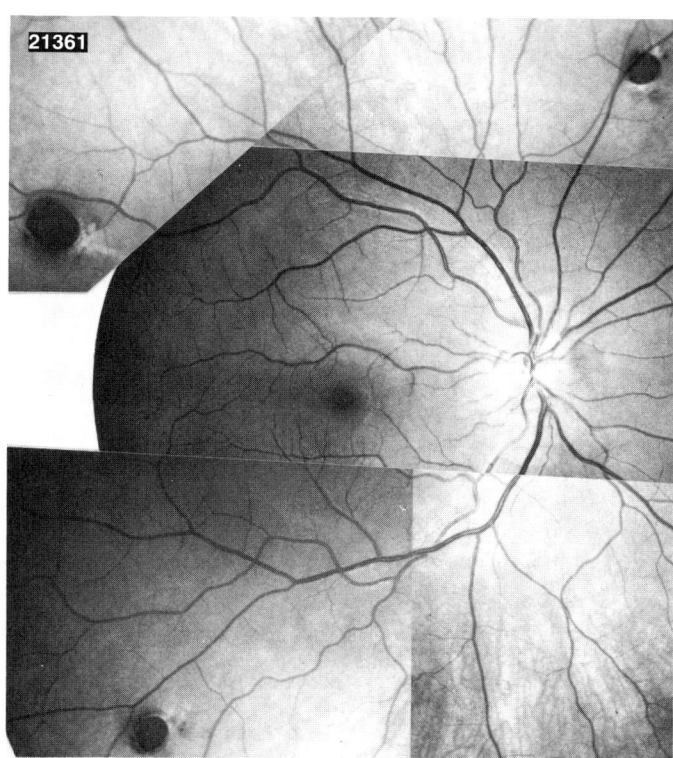

3134-21361: Retina, congenital hypertrophy of the retinal pigment epithelium.

Retina, grouped hypertrophy of retinal pigment epithelium (3203)

Major Diagnostic Criteria: Brown to black, flat, usually solitary, round to oval, sharply demarcated lesions of the ocular fundus at the level of the retinal pigment epithelium.

Clinical Findings: Isolated patches of congenital hypertrophy of retinal pigment epithelium (CHRPE) range from isolated dots less than 100 microns up to several disc diameters in size and are densely hyperpigmented (brown to black); they have smooth, sharp margins, and are usually surrounded by a subtle, but sharply defined depigmented halo. These are typically located in the peripheral fundus. With age, small and/or multiple lacunae may develop within the pigmented portion and may enlarge to become confluent and leave a sharp scleral patch in older adults. The frequency of a solitary lesion of any size in one eye in the general population is probably between 1:10 and 1:5. Congenital grouped pigmentation of the retina or "beartracks" (because they resemble animal tracks) are usually unilateral, typically sectoral, pigmented oval patches of CHRPE occurring as clumps of three or four, larger lesions occurring more peripheral to smaller clusters.

The histopathology of both isolated CHRPE and of congenital grouped pigmentation of the retina consists of hypertrophic retinal pigment epithelial cells with agenesis or atrophy of the overlying outer retina.

Complications: CHRPE does not affect vision unless it involves the fovea.

Associated Findings: Bilateral multiple but isolated and unclustered patches of CHRPE of various sizes and configurations have been found recently to be specific and sensitive markers of adenomatous polyposis in families with familial adenomatous polyposis (see **Intestinal polyposis, type III**). A total of more than three lesions in one or both eyes of an individual at risk indicates probable inheritance of the disease. The pigmented lesions have been observed as early as three months of age (presumably present at birth) and are due apparently to the pleiotropic effects of one gene responsible for familial adenomatous polyposis. These retinal pigment epithelial lesions have not been observed in hereditary colon cancer.

Etiology: Undetermined in isolated CHRPE and in congenital grouped pigmentation of the retina.

Pathogenesis: Unknown.

MIM No.: *17530

Sex Ratio: M1:F1

Occurrence: Small, solitary, and isolated patches of CHRPE are estimated to occur in 1:10 to 1:5 normal individuals.

Risk of Recurrence for Patient's Sib: Unknown.

Risk of Recurrence for Patient's Child: Unknown.

Age of Detectability: At birth.

Gene Mapping and Linkage: Unknown.

Prevention: None known. Genetic counseling indicated.

Treatment: None necessary.

Prognosis: Excellent for vision.

Detection of Carrier: Retinal examination with indirect ophthalmoscope.

Special Considerations: Because multiple patches of CHRPE are an excellent clinical marker in families with familial adenomatous polyposis, ocular examination with dilated indirect ophthalmoscopy is indicated in families of patients with adenomatous polyposis. If the lesions are present, close monitoring for the development of intestinal polyps and later colon cancer is imperative.

References:
Kurz GH, Zimmerman LE: Vagaries of the retinal pigment epithelium. Int Ophthalmol Clin 1962; 2:441–464.
Buettner H: Congenital hypertrophy of the retinal pigment epithelium. Am J Ophthalmol 1975; 79:177–189.
Shields JA, Tso MOM: Congenital grouped pigmentation of the retina: a histopathologic description and report of a case. Arch Ophthalmol 1975; 93:1153–1155.
Blair NP, Trempe CL: Hypertrophy of the retinal pigment epithelium associated with Gardner's syndrome. Am J Ophthalmol 1980; 90: 661–667.
Lewis RA, et al.: The Gardner syndrome: significance of ocular features. Ophthalmology 1984; 91:916–925.
Traboulsi EI, Krush AJ, Gardner EJ, et al.: Prevalence and importance of pigmented ocular fundus lesions in Gardner's syndrome. New Engl J Med 1987; 316:661–667.
Baker RH, et al.: Hyperpigmented lesions of the retinal pigment epithelium in familial adenomatous polyposis. Am J Med Genet 1988; 31:427–435.
Lyons LA, et al.: A genetic study of Gardner syndrome and congenital hypertrophy of the retinal pigment epithelium. Am J Hum Genet 1988; 42:290–296.

TR009

Elias I. Traboulsi

RETINA, FLECKED KANDORI TYPE   2110

Includes:
Fleck retina of Kandori
Kandori fleck retina
Red-fleck retina

Excludes:
Ocular drusen (0734)
Retina, fundus albipunctatus (0399)
Retina, fundus flavimaculatus (0400)

Major Diagnostic Criteria: Typical fundus changes, mild delays in reaching normal dark adaptation final threshold, and normal electrophysiologic testing.

Clinical Findings: Characteristic lesions are noted in the equatorial regions of the fundus. These are sharply defined flecks of varying size and shape ranging from the diameter of a retinal vessel to 1.5 times the size of the optic disc. The color has been described by Kandori as "dirty yellow". There are none of the dark pigment spicules seen in primary retinal pigmentary diseases. The disc, macula, vessels and posterior are normal. Fluorescein angiography has shown the flecks to act like pigment epithelial defects, with fluorescence appearing early in the arterial phase, remaining constant in size without leakage into the surrounding retina. Patients followed since 1958 have had no changes in their lesions. This differs from **Retina, fundus flavimaculatus** in which lesions change with time, originally blocking fluorescein and later with destruction of pigment epithelium transmitting fluorescein.

Complications: Unknown.

Associated Findings: None known.

Etiology: One patient was the product of a consanguinous marriage, but the total number of patients is too small to be certain if this is an autosomal recessive disorder.

Pathogenesis: No pathologic specimens have been studied but this appears to be a disorder of the retinal pigment epithelium.

MIM No.: 22899

Sex Ratio: M1:F1

Occurrence: Undetermined but presumably rare.

Risk of Recurrence for Patient's Sib:
See Part I, *Mendelian Inheritance.*

Risk of Recurrence for Patient's Child:
See Part I, *Mendelian Inheritance.*

Age of Detectability: In the second decade of life.

Gene Mapping and Linkage: Unknown.

Prevention: None known. Genetic counseling indicated.

Treatment: Night vision aids.

Prognosis: Non-progressive or minimally progressive.

Detection of Carrier: Unknown.

References:
Kandori F: Very rare cases of congenital non-progressive night blindness with fleck retina. Jpn J Ophthalmol 1959; 13:384–386.
Krill AE, Klien BA: Flecked retina syndrome. Arch Ophthalmol 1965; 74:496–508.
Duke-Elder S: System of ophthalmology, vol. 10. St. Louis: C.V. Mosby, 1967:629 only.
Kandori F, et al.: Fleck retina. Am J Ophthalmol 1972; 73:673–685.

W0003   **Mitchel L. Wolf**

RETINA, FUNDUS ALBIPUNCTATUS   0399

Includes:
　　Fleck retina disease (one form)
　　Fundus albipunctatus

Excludes:
　　Basal laminar drusen
　　Canthaxanthine retinopathy
　　Cystimers
　　Oxalate retinopathy
　　Progressive albipunctate dystrophy
　　Retina, flecked Kandori type (2110)
　　Retinitis punctata albescens
　　Uyemura syndrome
　　Vitamin A deficiency

Major Diagnostic Criteria: Typical fundus findings with nightblindness that becomes normal with time and a normal ERG after appropriate adaptation.

Clinical Findings: Multiple yellow-white dots, sparing the macula, are seen deep in the retina and are associated with congenital stationary nightblindness. The dots are most dense in the posterior pole and are more scattered towards the periphery. The size of the spots has been described as that of a second order arteriole,

and they are fairly uniform. The retinal vessels and the optic disk remain normal. The dots may fade as the patient advances in age.

Visual functions are well preserved; acuity is normal, color vision is normal and visual fields are full.

Dark adaptometry shows a marked delay in both cone and rod function so that the normal cone threshold, usually achieved at 10 minutes after a standard bleach, is delayed for up to 1 hour and the final rod threshold may not be achieved for 3 hours with a normal of 30 minutes. Electroretinography parallels the course of adaptation so that a normal ERG is recordable after appropriate adaptation but only a cone-dominated ERG is seen if done in a routine fashion. The EOG has a reduced light rise but this, too, becomes normal after prolonged dark adaptation. Kinetic studies of pigment regeneration show marked delays in both rods and cones.

A variant form with faster, but delayed, regeneration has also been reported.

Complications: Unknown.

Associated Findings: None known.

Etiology: While most fleck retina disease is autosomal recessive, this specific form may follow a pattern of autosomal dominant inheritance (Krill, 1977).

Pathogenesis: All evidence points to a defect in rate of pigment regeneration with a disturbance in the receptor outer segment-pigment epithelial complex. No histologic examinations have yet been reported.

MIM No.: 13688

Sex Ratio: M1:F1

Occurrence: Undetermined but presumed rare.

Risk of Recurrence for Patient's Sib:
See Part I, *Mendelian Inheritance.*

Risk of Recurrence for Patient's Child:
See Part I, *Mendelian Inheritance.*

Age of Detectability: First decade of life.

Gene Mapping and Linkage: Unknown.

Prevention: None known. Genetic counseling indicated.

Treatment: Night vision pocketscope.

Prognosis: Normal life span.

Detection of Carrier: Unknown.

Special Considerations: The appearance of white dots in the fundus has been reported in vitamin A deficiency and generalized oxalosis. However, these abnormalities have not been seen in fundus albipunctatus patients.

References:
Carr RE, et al.: Visual pigment kinetics and adaptation in fundus albipunctatus. Doc Ophthol Proc Ser 1974; 4:193–204.
Franceschetti A, et al.: Chorioretinal heredodegenerations. Springfield: Charles C Thomas, 1974.
Carr RE, et al.: Fluorescein angiography and vitamin A and oxalate levels in fundus albipunctatus. Am J Ophthalmol 1976; 82:549–558.
Krill AE: Hereditary retinal and choroidal diseases: flecked retina diseases; vol 2. Hagerstown, MD: Harper & Row, 1977:739–819.
Marmor MF: Fundus albipunctatus: a clinical study of the fundus lesions, the physiologic defect and the vitamin A metabolism. Doc Ophthal 1977; 43:277–302.
Margolis S, et al.: Variable expressivity in fundus albipunctatus. Ophthalmol 1987; 94:1416–1422.

W0003   **Mitchel L. Wolf**

RETINA, FUNDUS FLAVIMACULATUS 0400

Includes:

Fundus flavimaculatus with macular degeneration
Juvenile macular degeneration, hereditary
Macular degeneration and fundus flavimaculatus
Stargardt disease

Excludes:

Ocular drusen (0734)
Retina, flecked Kandori type (2110)
Retina, fundus albipunctatus (0399)

Major Diagnostic Criteria: Characteristic ophthalmoscopic appearance. Fluorescein angiographic finding may be helpful in diagnosis.

Clinical Findings: This is a group of retinal diseases that include yellow flecks at the level of the pigmented epithelium. Stargardt originally described patients with macular disease in 1909. Even though he included both patients with extensive retinal involvement and patients with little involvement outside the macula, the term "Stargardt disease" is generally used for the more limited macular disease. Franceschetti, in describing his fundus flavimaculatus patients, included another subgroup that had only widespread flecks and no macular involvement; thus, visual acuity was good. His patients with macular involvement and widespread flecks appears to be identical to those described by Stargardt.

Patients are subdivided according to age of onset, retinal involvement and electro-physiological findings:

Group I is the pure form of fundus flavimaculatus. It is found in adults, often on routine examination. Despite widespread flecks, these patients initially have good visual acuity and color vision, and normal electro-physiological findings. some patients later develop macular involvement and poor vision.

Group IIa patients have a childhood onset of the disease, which remains limited to within the retinal arcades. The ERG and EOG remain normal.

Group IIb patients also have an early onset of disease, but have widely scattered flecks. There is early depression of the EOG and photopic ERG. Extensive progressive chorioretinal atrophy involving the macula causes these patients to be more disabled than Group IIa patients.

There have been two families in which Group I disease occurred in the first generation, and severe Group IIb disease occurred in the second generation. This suggests that the Group I disease is the heterozygous form of a subgroup of Group IIb disease.

Complications: Macular degeneration; severe progressive visual loss in some cases.

Associated Findings: None known.

Etiology: Autosomal recessive inheritance is most common for Groups IIa and IIb. Several dominant pedigrees have been reported for Groups I and IIb. Segregation of severe and mild forms of the disease by generation suggests that Group I may be a heterozygous form of a subgroup of Group IIb. Many Group IIb patients have children and parents with normal retinas. In one series 10/27 cases were classified as familial, so sporadic occurrences likely account for the majority of cases.

Pathogenesis: Histologic studies of eyes from three Group IIb patients have shown accumulation of a lipofuscin-like substance in the pigmented epithelial cells. One Group I patient has shown enlarged RPE cells, but no lipofuscin.

MIM No.: 23010

Sex Ratio: M1:F1

Occurrence: At least 50 cases have been documented.

Risk of Recurrence for Patient's Sib:

See Part I, *Mendelian Inheritance.*

Risk of Recurrence for Patient's Child:

See Part I, *Mendelian Inheritance.* Autosomal dominant pedigrees have been quite rare.

Age of Detectability: Group I: Uncertain, since usually found on routine exams; visual loss can occur as late as age 65.

Groups IIa and IIb: Visual loss usually occurs between 8 and 30 years of age.

Gene Mapping and Linkage: Unknown.

Prevention: None known. Genetic counseling indicated.

Treatment: Unknown.

Prognosis: Normal life span; variable vision loss according to subgroup.

Detection of Carrier: By fundus exam.

References:

Klein BA, Krill AE: Fundus flavimaculatus, clinical, functional and histopathologic observations. Am J Ophthalmol 1967; 64:3–23.
Merin S, Landau J: Abnormal findings in relatives of patients with juvenile hereditary macular degeneration (Stargardt's disease). Ophthalmologica 1970; 161:1–10.
Krill AE: Krill's hereditary retinal and choroidal diseases. Clinical characteristics. vol. 2. Hagerstown: Harper & Row, 1972. †
Cibis GW, et al.: Dominantly inherited macular dystrophy with flecks (Stargardt). Arch Ophthalmol 1980; 98:1785–1789.
Moloney JBM, et al.: Retinal function in Stargardt's disease and fundus flavimaculatus. Am J Ophthalmol 1983; 96:57–65. *
McDonnel PJ, et al.: Fundus flavimaculatus without maculopathy: a clinicopathologic study. Ophthalmology 1986; 93:116–119.

KI021   **Jane D. Kivlin**

Retina, giant cyst of
See RETINOSCHISIS

RETINA, GROUPED HYPERTROPHY OF RETINAL PIGMENT EPITHELIUM 3203

Includes:

Bear tracks
Melanosis retinae
Melanosis retinae, congenital grouped
Nevoid pigmentation of the retina

Excludes:

Choroidal nevus
Fetal rubella syndrome (0384)
Malignant melanoma
Pigment proliferation secondary to trauma or hemorrhage
Retina, congenital hypertrophy of retinal pigment epithelium (3134)
Sector retinitis pigmentosa

Major Diagnostic Criteria: An asymptomatic congenital disorder occurring most frequently unilaterally. Diagnosis of the condition is usually made during a routine ophthalmoscopic exam.

Characteristically, the lesion consists of several well defined flat, gray to black colored areas, more often confined to one sector of the fundus. Each pigmented lesion may range in size from 0.1 to 3.0 mm in diameter occurring in groups of 3 to 30 foci. The

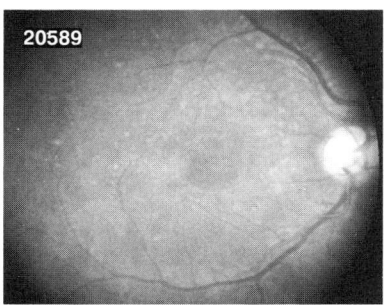
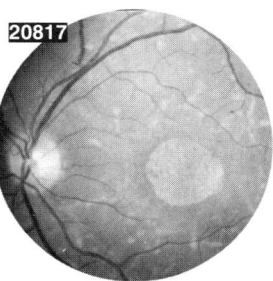

0400-20589: Multiple hypopigmented areas of varying shape; visual acuity is 20/100. **20817:** Fundus flavimaculatus with macular degeneration (Stargardt disease).

lesion is commonly larger in the retinal periphery with the surrounding retina being normal. The similarity of grouped hypertrophy of the retinal pigment epithelium to animal footprings has caused them to be termed "bear tracks."

Clinical Findings: Grouped hypertrophy of the retinal pigment epithelium should not be confused with **Retina, congenital hypertrophy of retinal pigment epithelium**. In the latter condition, a singular lesion, often surrounded by a thin hypopigmented ring, occurs frequently with depigmented lacunae within the pigmented lesion. The histologic appearance of the two conditions is similar; one being multifocal and the other unifocal.

It is important to note that grouped hypertrophy of the retinal pigment epithelium is a benign lesion. The lesions are nonprogressive and not associated with decrease in vision, visual field defects or electroretinogram change. In addition, no definite associated systemic conditions have been reported.

Complications: Unknown.

Associated Findings: None known.

Etiology: Unknown.

Pathogenesis: Unknown.

Sex Ratio: M1:F1

Occurrence: Undetermined but presumably very uncommon.

Risk of Recurrence for Patient's Sib: Presumably low.

Risk of Recurrence for Patient's Child: Presumably low.

Age of Detectability: At birth.

Gene Mapping and Linkage: Unknown.

Prevention: None known. Genetic counseling indicated.

Treatment: None needed.

Prognosis: No association with visual loss. Lesions are nonprogressive.

Detection of Carrier: Unknown.

References:

Tower P: Congenital grouped pigmentation of the retina. Arch Ophthalmol 1948; 39:536.
Purcell JJ, Shields JA: Hypertrophy with hyperpigmentation of the retinal pigment epithelium. Arch Ophthalmol 1975; 93:1122.
Shields JA, Tso MO: Congenital grouped pigmentation of the retina. Arch Ophthalmol 1975; 93:1153.
Deutman AF: Focal retinal pigment epithelial dystrophies. In: Krill AE, Archer DB, eds.: Krill's hereditary retinal and choroidal diseases, vol 2. Hagerstown: Harper and Row, 1977.
Newsome DA: Pigment epithelial dystrophies. In: Newsome DA, ed.: Retinal dystrophies and degenerations. New York: Raven Press, 1988.

P0025
BE026

Scott L. Portnoy
Donald R. Bergsma

Retina, gyrate atrophy
See GYRATE ATROPHY OF THE CHOROID AND RETINA

RETINA, HYALOIDEORETINAL DEGENERATION OF WAGNER 0479

Includes:
Hyaloideoretinal degeneration of Wagner
Wagner syndrome

Excludes:
Arthro-ophthalmopathy, hereditary, progressive, Stickler type (0090)
Arthro-ophthalmopathy, Weissenbacher-Zweymuller variant (2424)
Clefting syndromes
Retina, vitreoretinopathy, familial exudative (3133)
Retinal detachments, familial
Vitreoretinopathy, familial exudative

Major Diagnostic Criteria: Mild to moderate myopia, retinal dystrophy, presenile cataracts, vitreous veils, in the absence of retinal detachments.

Clinical Findings: Mild nightblindness has its onset in early childhood and is slowly progressive. A mild myopic prescription may be required during early school years, but the visual status will remain stable until the age of 30 to 40 years, when posterior cortical and subcapsular cataracts develop, which in recent years have been successfully removed in the presence of fluid vitreous, vitreous strands and peripheral circumferential vitreous bands. Complications in previous generations included vitreous loss, postoperative hypotony and glaucoma, but not retinal detachments. Only recently has the focus shifted to the progressive retinal dystrophic changes seen in these patients with the development of ring scotomata and night blindness and ultimate blindness in their sixties. On slit lamp examination there is obvious vitreous liquefaction in early life. On fundus examination one observes an at times contiguous, at others interrupted circumferential vitreous band and, emanating from this ring are avascular strands floating freely in the vitreous cavaty. Large areas of chorioretinal dystrophy originating from the disc in a helicoidal pattern are obvious in the older patient.

Complications: Large angle kappa with temporal dragging of the macula in some patients, presenile cataracts, glaucoma, retinal dystrophy.

Associated Findings: None known.

Etiology: Autosomal dominant inheritance.

Pathogenesis: The absence of normal vitreous structures suggests an abnormality of type IV collagen. These are, however, not pathognomonic for the condition.

MIM No.: *14320

Sex Ratio: M1:F1

Occurrence: Unknown.

Risk of Recurrence for Patient's Sib:
See Part I, *Mendelian Inheritance.*

Risk of Recurrence for Patient's Child:
See Part I, *Mendelian Inheritance.*

Age of Detectability: Usually not clinically evident until nightblindness is noted in childhood. Mild myopia becomes evident during the early school years, vitreous changes are present during those early years, but not diagnosed unless searched for.

Gene Mapping and Linkage: Unknown.

Prevention: None known. Genetic counseling indicated.

Treatment: Cataract extraction and glaucoma management as indicated. While results have been good, the ultimate vision loss from retinal dystrophic changes cannot be prevented.

Prognosis: Life expectancy is normal and there are no extraocular complications. The visual prognosis is guarded.

Detection of Carrier: The diagnosis is obvious in all affected if slit lamp and fundus examinations are performed. There have been no skipped generations.

Special Considerations: This disease should not be confused with **Arthro-ophthalmopathy, hereditary, progressive, Stickler type**. The patients in Wagner's original family do not have extraocular features and retinal detachments have not occured in any of the affected members. X-ray examinations for epiphyseal changes were normal in five personally examined members, who also had no systemic findings of clefting of the hard or soft palate, nor deafness or subjective joint disease.

This condition has generated an extensive literature and considerable debate, and there is, in fact, no concensus that true Wagner syndrome has ever existed beyond the members of Wagner's original family. A good overview of the debate appears in McKusick's *Mendelian inheritance in Man.*

References:

Wagner H: Ein bisher unbekanntes Erbleiden des Auges (Degeneratio hyaloideo-retinalis hereditaria), beobachtet im Kanton Zurich. Klin Monatsbl Augenheilkd 1938; 100:840–857.

Maumenee IH, et al: The Wagner syndrome versus hereditary arthroophthalmopathy. Tr Am Ophth Soc 1982; 80:349–365.

MA054   **Irene H. Maumenee**

RETINA, MACULAR DEGENERATION, VITELLIRUPTIVE   0622

Includes:
> Best disease
> Central cystoid dystrophy
> Exudative detachment of retina, central
> Macular degeneration, polymorphic vitelliruptive
> Macular dystrophy, atypical vitelliform
> Macular pseudocysts
> Vitelliform cysts of macula, congenital
> Vitelliform macular dystrophy
> Vitelliruptive macular degeneration, hereditary

Excludes:
> Central serous retinopathy
> Foveomacular vitelliruptive dystrophy, adult type (GASS)
> Progressive foveal dystrophy
> Pseudovitelliform macular degeneration

Major Diagnostic Criteria: Typical appearing lesion in younger members of a family with macular degeneration of autosomal dominant inheritance. Abnormal electrooculogram with normal electroretinogram.

Clinical Findings: The age of onset of the macular lesion is usually between 5–15 years, but it has been seen as early as one week of age. The typical features of the lesion are seen in early cases. It has been described as looking like "an egg with sunny-side up," at a somewhat later stage like a "scrambled egg," or like a "cystic lesion filled with exudates and precipitates, sometimes with a definite level, resembling a hypopyon." The early lesion is usually yellow or orange in color, elevated, has sharp borders and is frequently almost circular in outline. However, it eventually loses its cystic appearance and the exudate-like material disappears. Rarely, there may be multiple vitelliform lesions in the posterior pole areas. A macular degeneration may then follow which is indistinguishable from other types of macular degenerations. Visual acuity, particularly in the early stages of the disease, is usually better than anticipated from the appearance of the macula. However, deep retinal hemorrhage may occur, probably from the choriocapillaris, with eventual hypertrophic scar formation so that vision can be reduced early in life.

Visual acuity typically remains good until the 4th decade when a secondary macular degeneration frequently occurs. On the other hand, secondary intraretinal macular changes may be minimal and fairly good visual acuity may be maintained throughout life. Visual fields are normal except for central scotoma when acuity is abnormal. Dark adaptation and ERG are usually normal but minimal abnormality has been noted. The electrooculogram is always abnormal.

Complications: Intraretinal macular degeneration, macular hemorrhage.

Associated Findings: Hyperopia, esotropia, amblyopia (strabismus). Best disease has co-existed with so-called pattern dystrophies of the retinal epithelium in the same families

Etiology: Autosomal dominant inheritance with many examples of reduced penetrance and expressivity.

Pathogenesis: Three early pathologic reports were from patients who were elderly with extensive choroidal and retinal changes. A recent report from a 29-year-old in the scrambled egg stage showed generalized retinal pigment epithelial (RPE) abnormalities with accumulation of lipofuscin not only in the RPE but also in subretinal macrophages and free in the choroid. Frangieh et al (1982) described the histopathology of the eyes of an 80-year-old lady and postulated that the disease starts in the neurosensory retina, and that the RPE changes are secondary. The electrooculogram is markedly abnormal in all cases tested, even in younger members with early stages of the disease. This finding suggests that a diffuse abnormality of the pigment epithelium exists in this

disease even though only the macular area shows ophthalmoscopic changes. With red light, which penetrates the retinal pigment epithelium, the typical lesion of younger subjects is observed. On the other hand, blue light, which does not penetrate beyond the retinal receptors, does not show the typical lesion. Therefore early lesions are probably external to the pigment epithelium. Blue light shows the typical features of the secondary macular degeneration in older subjects indicating its intraretinal location. Fluorescence is not observed with very early lesions; however, after an uncertain period of time, fluorescence characteristic of defective pigment epithelium is seen in the macula and is dependent on the size and position of the original lesion.

MIM No.: *15370, *15384

Sex Ratio: M1:F1

Occurrence: Several large kindreds have been reported, and one study in Sweden traced 250 cases to a single 17th Century source.

Risk of Recurrence for Patient's Sib:
> See Part I, *Mendelian Inheritance.*

Risk of Recurrence for Patient's Child:
> See Part I, *Mendelian Inheritance.*

Age of Detectability: Usually detected between 5–15 years of age, but occasionally may not be noted until the third or even beginning of the fourth decade of life.

Gene Mapping and Linkage: Best disease itself has not been mapped, although 6q25 has been suggested as the possible locus (Rivas et al, 1986).

VMD1 (vitelliform macular dystrophy, atypical) has been provisionally mapped to 8q.

Prevention: None known. Genetic counseling indicated.

Treatment: Unknown.

Prognosis: Life span normal, guarded for vision.

Detection of Carrier: A carrier with no macular abnormality can be identified by an abnormal EOG.

Special Considerations: Patients with typical vitelliform fusions have been recently reported who have normal EOGs. These patients are not part of a familial disease, have visual loss associated with the lesions, and represent a different entity which has been called "pseudovitelliform degeneration." A late onset dominant disease with small lesions and a mildly abnormal EOG has also been described.

Macular dystrophy, atypical vitelliform (Ferrell et al, 1983) has a similar phenotype, and may be simply an allelic mutation.

References:

Braley AE, Spivey BE: Hereditary vitelline macular degeneration: a clinical and functional evaluation of a new pedigree with variable expressivity and dominant inheritance. Arch Ophthalmol 1964; 72:743–762.

Krill AE, et al.: Hereditary vitelliruptive macular degeneration. Am J Ophthalmol 1966; 61:1405–1415.

Deutman AF: Electro-oculography in families with vitelliform dystrophy of the fovea: detection of the carrier state. Arch Ophthalmol 1969; 81:305–316.

Frangieh GT, et al.: A histopathologic study of Best's macular dystrophy. Arch Ophthalmol 1982; 100:1115–1121.

Weingeist TA, et al.: Hystopathology of Best's macular dystrophy. Arch Ophthalmol 1982; 100:1108–1114.

Ferrell RE, et al.: Linkage of atypical vitelliform macular dystrophy (VMD-1) to the soluble glutamate pyruvate transaminase (GPT1) locus. Am J Hum Genet 1983; 35:78–84.

Godel V, et al.: Best's vitelliform macular dystrophy. Acta Ophthalmolgica 1986; 175(suppl):1–31. *

Grieffre G, Lodato G: Vitelline dystrophy and pattern dystrophy of the retinal pigment epithelium: concomitant presence in a family. Br J Ophthalmol 1986; 70:526–532.

Rivas FE, et al.: De novo del(6)(q25) associated with macular degeneration. Ann Genet 1986; 29:42–44.

Yoder FE, et al.: Linkage studies of Best's macular dystrophy. Clin Genet 1988; 34:26–30.

W0003   **Mitchel L. Wolf**

Retina, pigmentation of, congenital grouped
See RETINA, CONGENITAL HYPERTROPHY OF RETINAL PIGMENT EPITHELIUM
Retina, tapetochoroidal dystrophy
See CHOROIDEREMIA

RETINA, VITREORETINOPATHY, FAMILIAL EXUDATIVE   3133

Includes:
Criswick-Schepens syndrome
Exudative vitreoretinopathy

Excludes:
Arthro-ophthalmopathy, hereditary, progressive, Stickler type (0090)
Eales disease
Retina, Coats disease (3135)
Retina, hyaloideoretinal degeneration of Wagner (0479)
Retinopathy of prematurity (0872)
Retinoschisis (0871)

Major Diagnostic Criteria: In the later stages of this ocular disease: organized vitreous membranes and prominent vitreoretinal adhesions, temporal dragging and heterotopia of the macula, peripheral subretinal and intraretinal exudates, and localized retinal detachment. Fluorescein angiography shows disorganization of the architecture and abrupt cessation of the retinal capillary network in the temporal periphery. Fluorescein angiography is essential in establishing the diagnosis of mild cases and asymptomatic family members.

Clinical Findings: The fundus changes in advanced familial exudative vitreoretinopathy (FEVR) are most similar to those of **Retinopathy of prematurity** (ROP), with vitreoretinal adhesions, abnormalities of the retinal vasculature, and temporal dragging of the macula. The differentiating features include normal birth weight, absence of a history of prematurity and oxygen administration in FEVR, and the familial (dominant) occurrence of FEVR. Myopia is present in 80% of patients with ROP but is infrequent in FEVR. The severity of the vitreoretinal changes is extremely variable in FEVR and a majority of patients may have normal visual acuity and ocular examination and may only be detected by abnormalities of the peripheral retinal vasculature on wide-field (60–90 degrees) fluorescein angiography; other patients, sometimes in the same family, will have severe bilateral disease with retinal detachment, macular dragging, and poor vision. Both eyes are affected, sometimes with marked asymmetry of the retinal pathology. The disease is generally stable or slowly progressive and may manifest as early as three months of age or be diagnosed as late as 57 years. The severity of the disease does not correlate with advancing patient age. Subretinal exudates are seen in about 15–20% of patients.

Complications: Late complications include rubeosis irides, secondary glaucoma, secondary cataract, and band keratopathy. A peripheral "mass-like" appearance has sometimes led to unnecessary enucleation in the mistake diagnosis of **Retinoblastoma**.

Associated Findings: Platelet aggregation defects have been detected in all affected members of two families reported by Chaudhuri et al (1983).

Etiology: Autosomal dominant inheritance with variability in expression. X-linked inheritance postulated (though unlikely) to be possible in the original report by Criswick and Schepens (1969).

Pathogenesis: A defect in peripheral maturation of retinal capillaries has been postulated.

MIM No.: *13378, 22723.

Sex Ratio: M1:F1

Occurrence: About 140 cases have been reported in the world literature; from the United States, Japan, South America, Europe, and (unpublished reports) from the Middle East.

Risk of Recurrence for Patient's Sib:
See Part I, *Mendelian Inheritance.*

Risk of Recurrence for Patient's Child:
See Part I, *Mendelian Inheritance.*

Age of Detectability: Depends on severity of retinal changes. May be as early as three months or as late as the fifth decade. Mean age at diagnosis in one series was ten years.

Gene Mapping and Linkage: Unknown.

Prevention: None known. Genetic counseling indicated.

Treatment: Value of prophylactic cryotherapy is questionable. Vitrectomy and peeling of epiretinal membranes may be performed in very selected cases.

Prognosis: Generally good if retinal involvement is mild at initial diagnosis, because of the slowly progressive nature of the disease process.

Detection of Carrier: Fluorescein angiography of peripheral fundus should be performed in parents and sibs of affected individuals, and detects silent carriers of the disease.

References:
Criswick VG, Schepens CL: Familial exudative vitreoretinopathy. Am J Ophthalmol 1969; 68:578–594.
Gow CLB, Oliver GL: Familial exudative vitreoretinopathy: an expanded view. Arch Ophthalmol 1971; 86:150–155.
Laqua H: Familial exudative vitreoretinopathy. Graefe's Arch Clin Exp Ophthalmol 1980; 213:121–133.
Ober RR, et al.: Autosomal dominant exudative vitreoretinopathy. Br J Ophthalmol 1980; 64:112–120.
Tasman W, et al.: Familial exudative vitreoretinopathy. Trans Am Ophthalmol Soc 1981; 79:211–226. *
Miyakubo H, et al.: Retinal involvement in familial exudative vitreoretinopathy. Ophthalmologica 1982; 185:125–135.
Van Nauhuys CE: Dominant exudative vitreoretinopathy and other vascular developmental disorders of the peripheral retina. The Hague: W Junk Publishers, 1982.
Chaudhuri PR, et al.: Familial exudative vitreoretinopathy associated with familial thrombocytopathy. Br J Ophthalmol 1983; 67:755–758.

TR009   **Elias I. Traboulsi**

Retinal anlage tumor
See JAW, NEUROECTODERMAL PIGMENTED TUMOR
Retinal anomalies-corneal hypesthesia-deafness-unusual facies
See CORNEAL ANESTHESIA-RETINAL DEFECTS-UNUSUAL FACIES-HEART DEFECT
Retinal aplasia, hereditary
See RETINA, AMAUROSIS CONGENITA, LEBER TYPE
Retinal aplasia-cystic kidneys-Joubert syndrome
See JOUBERT SYNDROME
Retinal blindness, congenital
See RETINA, AMAUROSIS CONGENITA, LEBER TYPE
Retinal choristoma
See JAW, NEUROECTODERMAL PIGMENTED TUMOR
Retinal cyst, congenital
See RETINOSCHISIS
Retinal degeneration, congenital
See RETINA, AMAUROSIS CONGENITA, LEBER TYPE

RETINAL DYSPLASIA   0866

Includes:
Falciform retinal fold
Retina, congenital detachment of
Retinal dysplasia, Reese type
Retinal nonattachment and falciform detachment

Excludes:
Eye, vitreous, persistent hyperplastic primary (0994)
Retina, Coats disease (3135)
Retina, vitreoretinopathy, familial exudative (3133)
Retinoblastoma (0870)
Retinopathy of prematurity (0872)

Major Diagnostic Criteria: Retinal dysplasia is a pathologic term referring to the abnormal differentiation of retinal elements, as a result of either genetic or environmental factors. The major histopathologic feature of this disorder is the formation of rosettes by the immature photoreceptor segments. Neural cells forming the rosettes are variably differentiated and are arranged in palisading or radiating formations about a central lumen or space. The retina may appear ophthalmoscopically normal, or may show a variety of topographic abnormalities. The electroretinogram is abnormal and parallels the severity of retinal involvement.

Clinical Findings: Retinal dysplasia may be unilateral or bilateral and may appear as an isolated finding or in association with other ocular or systemic abnormalities. The clinical findings are determined primarily by the extent of retinal involvement and usually become evident by early childhood. There is a manifest disturbance of visual function in one or both eyes; nystagmus, strabismus, and abnormal head postures may develop. The retinal findings vary from an isolated fold to total disruption of the retinal structures. The folds generally extend from the optic nerve temporally to the retinal periphery, thus usually involving the macula, and resulting in loss of central vision. In more severe cases, there is marked retinal disruption and cicatrization, with a white mass protruding into the vitreous cavity. Such instances must be differentiated from other conditions causing a white retinal mass.

Visual loss is usually marked but nonprogressive, since retinal damage occur *in utero* and appears not to progress after birth. Visual function and prognosis may, however, be affected by associated ocular abnormalities (*vide infra*).

In genetically determined cases, there may be a positive family history of early visual loss.

Complications: The most common complication is visual loss or blindness. Nystagmus and strabismus may occur as a result of visual impairment and macular heterotopia.

Associated Findings: Associated ocular abnormalities may include microphthalmos, megalocornea, **Eye, anterior segment dysgenesis**, anterior chamber angle abnormalities with secondary glaucoma, cataract, colobomas of the optic disc or choroid, and optic nerve hypoplasia.

Retinal dysplasia may also occur in association with multiple systemic abnormalities as **Chromosome 13, trisomy 13**, **Chromosome 18, trisomy 18**, **Walker-Warburg syndrome**, and **Norrie disease**. There is no correlation between the severity of systemic abnormalities and the extent of retinal dysplasia.

Etiology: Retinal dysplasia may occur as an isolated defect, or as a part of many malformation syndromes or chromosomal associated diseases. Autosomal dominant, autosomal recessive, and X-linked recessive inheritance has been reported. Retinal dysplasia has been reported with maternal use of LSD, and has been induced experimentally *in utero* in animal models by radiation, viral infection, and vitamin A deficiency.

Pathogenesis: Retinal dysplasia is felt to be a non-specific response of the retina to a variety of noxious influences during various, perhaps critical, periods of its development. Since the retinal pigment epithelium (RPE) is a major organizing factor in the development of normal retinal architecture, any detachment of the sensory retina from the underlying RPE during development results in its disorganization and in dysplasia. Such dysplastic changes do not occur with disruption of the normal sensory retina-pigment epithelium interface after maturation is complete.

MIM No.: 18007, *22190, 26640, 31255

Sex Ratio: Presumably M1:F1, except in cases of X-linked inheritance.

Occurrence: Undetermined.

Risk of Recurrence for Patient's Sib:
See Part I, *Mendelian Inheritance.*

Risk of Recurrence for Patient's Child:
See Part I, *Mendelian Inheritance.*

Age of Detectability: Usually present at birth, but often not clinically evident until several months or years later.

Gene Mapping and Linkage: Unknown.

Prevention: Avoidance of fetal exposure to LSD, irradiation, and other teratogens. Genetic counseling is indicated.

Treatment: Unknown.

Prognosis: Poor for vision. Life expectancy and general development depends on associated systemic findings.

Detection of Carrier: Visually insignificant mild retinal fold changes have been observed in female carriers of the X-linked recessive form. Iris stromal changes (decreased pigmentation and lack of normal surface markings) were also reported in female carriers, but the significance of these anterior segment changes is unclear as they have not been observed in affected males.

Special Considerations: The term retinal dysplasia was once used to designate a specific syndrome of multiple congenital anomalies involving the brain, heart, limbs, mouth and eye, in which the dysplastic retina was one of the most consistent findings. It has since become evident that most of the affected children, including those reported by Reese and diagnosed as having "Reese retinal dysplasia", probably had **Chromosome 13, trisomy 13** or **Walker-Warburg syndrome**. Retinal dysplasia is a pathologic term which is now generally used to refer to the retinal lesion rather than to a specific syndrome, except when inherited as an isolated condition.

The authors wish to thank Lorenz E. Zimmerman for his suggestions in the preparation of this article.

References:

Reese AB, Straatsma BR: Retinal dysplasia. Am J Ophthalmol 1958; 45:199–211.
Silverstein AM, et al.: The pathogenesis of retinal dysplasia. Am J Ophthalmol 1971; 72:13–21. * †
Lahav M, Albert DM: Clinical and histopathologic classification of retinal dysplasia. Am J Ophthalmol 1973; 75:648–667. * †
Fulton AB, et al.: Human retinal dysplasia. Am J Ophthalmol 1978; 85:690–698. †
Godel V, Goodman RM: X-linked recessive primary retinal dysplasia: clinical findings in affected males and carrier females. Clin Genet 1981; 20:260–266.
Pagon RA, et al.: Autosomal recessive eye and brain anomalies: Warburg syndrome. J Pediatr 1983; 102:542–546.

F0013   **David J. Forster**
TR009   **Elias I. Traboulsi**
P0024   **Robert C. Polomeno**

Retinal dysplasia, Reese type
See RETINAL DYSPLASIA
Retinal dystrophy associated with spinocerebellar ataxia
See OLIVOPONTOCEREBELLAR ATROPHY, DOMINANT WITH RETINAL DEGENERATION
Retinal dystrophy, posterior pole-congenital total hypotrichosis
See RETINOPATHY-HYPOTRICHOSIS SYNDROME

RETINAL FOLD   **0867**

Includes:
Falciform detachment, congenital
Hydrocephaly-retinal nonattachment-falciform fold
Microcephaly-microphthalmia-falciform retinal folds
Retinal septum, congenital

Excludes:
Acquired retinal folds secondary to iatrogenic etiologies
Acquired retinal folds secondary to inflammatory disease
Acquired retinal folds secondary to intraocular foreign bodies
Chromosome 13, trisomy 13 (0168)
Retina, vitreoretinopathy, familial exudative (3133)
Retinopathy of prematurity (0872)
Rhegmatogenous retinal detachments
Walker-Warburg syndrome (2869)

Major Diagnostic Criteria: Tractional retinal fold running from the disk to the periphery.

Clinical Findings: The folds occur in otherwise normal eyes and are occasionally bilateral. Ophthalmoscopically, they are seen as elevated gray folds or ridges, running from the optic nervehead

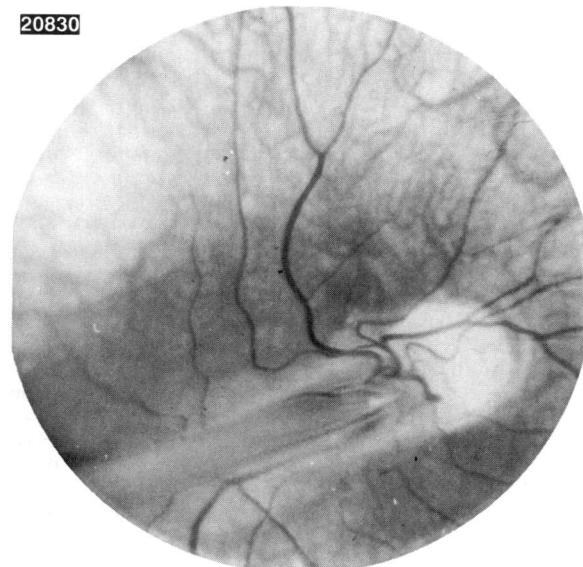

0867-20830: Retinal fold.

into the retinal periphery where they commonly expand in a gray fan over the peripheral retina and the pars plana. These folds occur most commonly in the lower temporal quadrant of the retina and, occasionally, send strands forward to the posterior capsule of the lens. Often, there is considerable disturbance in the retinal pigment epithelium along the borders of the fold, and there may be traction or detachment at various places along its course. Remnants of the hyaloid arterial system may be adherent to the surface of the fold. The normal retinal blood vessels appear to be pulled up into this fold, and vessels may be absent from other areas of the retina. Visual acuity is minimal from birth, and the first signs of the condition are strabismus, nystagmus, or, if the folds are bilateral, poor vision.

Complications: Cataract formation, traction retinal detachments, and phthisis bulbi have been reported to occur rarely.

Associated Findings: Hydrocephaly, microphthalmia, congenital dislocation of the hip, mental retardation, **Microcephaly**, hypogenitalism, cryptorchidism.

Etiology: May represent a persistence of the posterior primary vitreous, and although this condition may be associated with persistence of the anterior hyperplastic vitreous, it is distinctly different. Pseudogliomas, congenital retinal nonattachment, and retinal dysplasia, have been reported in the second eye of some patients.

In complex syndromes with congenital falciform folds, there are many associated congenital defects in addition to the retinal fold. **Retina, Coats disease** is characterized by retinal telangiectasia and more widespread retinal detachment without a discrete isolated fold. Any inflammatory disease, especially toxoplasmosis and toxocariasis, can cause a retinal fold. In this case, however, the folds run from the area of the granuloma to the retinal periphery and usually do not insert at the disk unless the granuloma is in the peripapillary region.

Retinal falciform folds are characteristic of grade III **Retinopathy of prematurity** (retrolental fibroplasia). Although controversial, some investigators believe that falciform folds may occasionally represent a form of retinopathy of prematurity that occurs without a history of oxygen exposure, prematurity, or low birth weight.

Retinal folds may be the result of retinal detachment surgery secondary to scleral buckling or intraocular gas. Falciform retinal folds may also be a sign of **Retina, vitreoretinopathy, familial exudative**.

Many cases are sporadic, but autosomal dominant, autosomal recessive, and X-linked recessive inheritance has been reported. A syndrome consisting of congenital hydrocephalus, microophthalmia, retinal detachment, or retinal falciform fold, which may or may not be distinct from **Walker-Warburg syndrome**, appears to exist and to be transmitted as an autosomal recessive trait (Warburg, 1978).

Pathogenesis: The folds may be caused by a localized persistence of the primary vitreous with adherence of the retina. Other possibilities include an overgrowth of a localized area of the retina, or a difference in the growth rate of the two layers of the optic cup.

MIM No.: 18006

Sex Ratio: M1:F1

Occurrence: Undetermined.

Risk of Recurrence for Patient's Sib: Unknown.

Risk of Recurrence for Patient's Child: Unknown.

Age of Detectability: At birth.

Gene Mapping and Linkage: Unknown.

Prevention: None known. Genetic counseling indicated.

Treatment: Unknown.

Prognosis: The condition is static and generally shows no progression. Vision in the involved eye remains static unless the rare complications of detachment or phthisis bulbi occur.

Detection of Carrier: Unknown.

References:
Mann I: Developmental abnormalities of the eye. Philadelphia: J.B. Lippincott, 1957:200.
Godel V, et al.: Primary retinal dysplasia transmitted as a chromosome-linked recessive disorder. Am J Ophthalmol 1978; 86:221–227.
Warburg M: Hydrocephaly, congenital retinal nonattachment, and congenital falciform fold. Am J Ophthalmol 1978; 85:88–94.
Godel V, et al.: Falciform form of the retina. Can J Ophthalmol 1979; 14:192–194.
Jarmas AL, et al.: Microcephaly, microphthalmia, falciform retinal folds and blindness. Am J Dis Child 1981; 135:930–933.
Young ID, et al.: Microcephaly, microphthalmos, and retinal folds: report of a family. J Med Genet 1987; 24:172–184.

EL007   **Robert M. Ellsworth**
HA068   **Barrett G. Haik**
WE038   **Robert A. Weiss**

Retinal nonattachment and falciform detachment
See RETINAL DYSPLASIA
Retinal pigmentary degeneration-microcephaly-mental retardation
See RETINOPATHY-MICROCEPHALY-MENTAL RETARDATION
Retinal septum, congenital
See RETINAL FOLD

RETINAL TELANGIECTASIA-HYPOGAMMAGLOBULINEMIA   0868

Includes: Hypogammaglobulinemia-retinal telangiectasia

Excludes:
  Ataxia-telangiectasia (0094)
  Retina, Coats disease (3135)
  Waldenstrom macroglobulinemia

Major Diagnostic Criteria: Retinal telangiectasia plus hypogammaglobulinemia.

Clinical Findings: Frenkel and Russe (1967) reported two sibs with retinal telangiectasia. The male had absence of IgA and IgM immunoglobulins, and reduction of IgG immunoglobulin. The female had normal immunoglobulin levels but had a deficiency in delayed hypersensitivity. Both individuals had normal karyotypes. Six other unrelated individuals with hypogammaglobulinemia were found to have normal retinal vasculature.

Complications: Recurrent infections.

Associated Findings: None known.

Etiology: Possibly a variant anomaly in segmentation of retinal capillaries.

Pathogenesis: Unknown.

POS No.: 3913

Sex Ratio: Presumably M1:F1.

Occurrence: Two siblings reported.

Risk of Recurrence for Patient's Sib: Unknown.

Risk of Recurrence for Patient's Child: Unknown.

Age of Detectability: In infancy.

Gene Mapping and Linkage: Unknown.

Prevention: None known. Genetic counseling indicated.

Treatment: Avoidance of pathogens, treatment of infections as indicated.

Prognosis: Unknown.

Detection of Carrier: Unknown.

References:
Frenkel N, Russe HP: Retinal telangiectasia associated with hypogammaglobulinemia. Am J Ophthalmol 1967; 63:215–220.

G0006   **Morton F. Goldberg**
SU001   **Joel Sugar**

RETINITIS PIGMENTOSA   0869

Includes:
    Pigmentary retinal degeneration
    Rod-cone dystrophy

Excludes:
    Choroideremia (0925)
    Cone-rod degeneration
    Gyrate atrophy of the choroid and retina (0449)
    Myopia, malignant
    Nightblindness, congenital stationary (see all)
    Retina, fundus albipunctatus (0399)
    Retinitis punctata albescens
    Usher syndrome (0983)

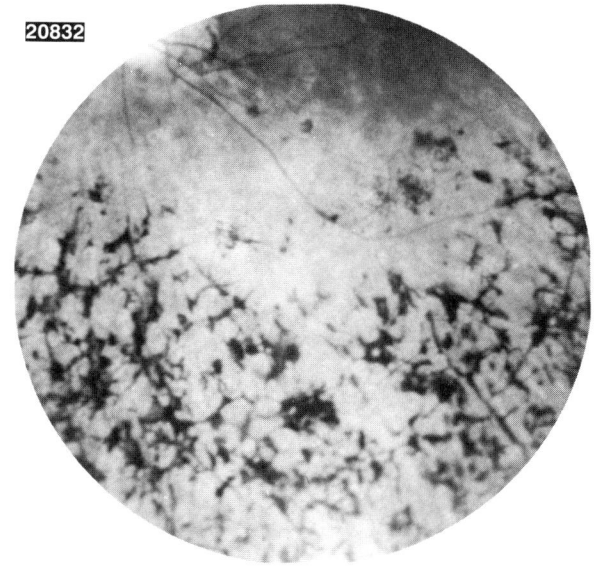

0869-20832: Retinitis pigmentosa.

Major Diagnostic Criteria: Characteristic impaired rod and cone (photoreceptor) function, and evidence of retinal and pigment epithelial disease by ERG, in the presence or absence of morphologic retinal changes.

Clinical Findings: Decreased dim light vision and constricted visual fields are the earliest signs of retinitis pigmentosa (RP), and these may occur prior to the onset of morphologic retinal changes. The common ocular complications which add to the severity of the disease are posterior cortical cataracts and macular involvement, often with cystoid macular edema.

Retinitis pigmentosa may be inherited as a dominant, recessive, or X-linked trait, but 40–50% of affected individuals are isolated cases within their families. *Autosomal recessive* is the most common form, comprising 30–40% of all cases. There is no proof that isolated and recessive forms are the same. Onset is during the first two decades of life, and usually progresses to severe visual loss by the fifth decade.

A slowly progressive adult onset form has been noted with a recordable ERG. This type, although uncommon, is compatible with good visual function. In the more usual cases, the ERG has typically been reported as unrecordable. With the use of a computer-averaged ERG, signals of less than 10μ can be measured easily, and the truly unrecordable ERG is rare.

Some *autosomal dominant* forms also have an onset in the first or second decade, but some may not begin until the fourth or fifth decade. The initial findings are mild, progression is slow, and although night vision and peripheral vision end up severely affected, central vision may be maintained into the sixth or seventh decade. Although complete penetrance is common, some families with variable penetrance have been described, with characteristic changes in the temporal aspects of the ERG. A sectoral form of RP has been documented in some dominant pedigrees, progresses slowly, and is compatible with good function in the normal patches of retina. The sectoral form can masquerade as a nerve fiber bundle defect, or other neurologic visual field deficit, if corresponding pigmentary changes are not noted in the fundus. Dominant cases have been subdivided by their ERG characteristics and these are highly predictive of visual outcome.

The *X-linked* forms are the least common type of RP (8–10%) but tend to be the most severe, with profound visual loss by the fourth decade. The female carriers will often show signs of retinal involvement and may even be symptomatic. Two carrier states are recognized, each unique to a given family, which suggest that there are at least two, not necessarily allelic, genotypes for X-linked RP. Some female carriers show a congenital golden-metallic sheen, which may progress to pigmentary changes in mid-life. In other families, the carriers have normal fundi but develop islands or sectors of pigmentary RP-like degeneration in their mid-30s and 40s.

The typical retinal changes are clumps of pigment resembling bone spicules in the equatorial region, attenuated arterioles, and a waxy somewhat pale disk. The pigment epithelium often develops white dots or diffuse depigmentation easily seen on fluorescein angiography. The pigment dispersion in the retina may take the form of round clumps and, rarely, no pigment clumping is seen. The initial changes are often fine pigment granularity with accumulations over the retinal vessels. Fine salt-and-pepper changes characterized by tiny pigment clumps surrounded by rings of depigmentation help to distinguish the pathologic fundus of early RP from normal blond fundi.

Dark adaptometry invariably shows elevated thresholds in areas of abnormal retina. However, mild and atypical cases may possibly demonstrate normal dark adaptation in some areas of the retina with elevated thresholds elsewhere. The visual field is often first affected in the equatorial region producing an encircling ring-type scotoma which widens toward the periphery and the center with resulting tubular vision. Arcuate or sector defects are also possible. Color vision may be affected. The early changes are tritanopic, and all color perception may be lost in advanced disease. Electrophysiologic studies are abnormal early in the course of the disease. A reduced ERG is the rule, and the early receptor potential (ERP) is also abnormal. Although the rate of progression varies greatly, recent research has carefully examined the natural history in a quantitative fashion. Psychophysical studies comparing rod and cone function across the retina have allowed further subclassification.

Complications: Unknown.

Associated Findings: *Ocular:* Myopia, macular involvement, cataracts, drusen of the optic nerve, achromatopsia, ophthalmoplegia.

Extraocular: The combination of RP and congenital hearing loss is known as **Usher syndrome**. There are a host of genetic disorders with associated RP including **Abetalipoproteinemia, Phytanic acid storage disease, Neuronal ceroid-lipofuscinoses (NCL), Mucopolysaccharidosis** types I-H, I-S, II and III, **Bardet-Biedl syndrome, Olivopontocerebellar atrophy, dominant with retinal degeneration, Renal dysplasia-retinal aplasia, Loken-Senior type**, and **Asphyxiating thoracic dysplasia.**

Etiology: Autosomal recessive, autosomal dominant, and X-linked recessive inheritance. The mothers of all males presenting with apparently isolated disease should be examined for X-linked carrier states.

Pathogenesis: There is a progressive degeneration of the receptors with associated neuroepithelial atrophy, and glial overgrowth, and an eventual narrowing of the retinal vessels. Depigmentation of the retinal epithelium, with a migration of its pigment into the retina, is characteristic.

The initial site of tissue abnormality is unknown. Both the neuroepithelium, with progressive loss of rods and cones, and the pigment epithelium are abnormal. Degenerated receptors may become partly replaced by neuroglia. The ganglion cells and the nerve fiber layer remain relatively unchanged. The retinal vessels, arterioles, and veins alike, always show marked changes, generally atrophic.

Electron microscopic studies in RP emphasize the relationship between the pigment epithelium and the neural retina. Specimens have been obtained in increasing numbers, and careful studies have been performed on eyes of all genetic subtypes. The question of whether the disease is primary to the receptors or the pigment epithelium has not been conclusively answered.

MIM No.: *18010, *26800, 26801, 26802, 26803, *31260, 30320, *31261

CDC No.: 362.700

Sex Ratio: M1:F1 for all but X-linked forms.

Occurrence: Prevalence varies from 1:2,000 to 1:7,000, with an estimated carrier rate of 1:80 to 1:100. An unique form may exist among the Navajo (Heckenlively et al, 1981).

Risk of Recurrence for Patient's Sib:
See Part I, *Mendelian Inheritance.*

Risk of Recurrence for Patient's Child:
See Part I, *Mendelian Inheritance.*

Age of Detectability: Depends on the mode of transmission, with the most frequent onset at the end of the first decade or the beginning of second decade of life.

Gene Mapping and Linkage: RP1 (retinitis pigmentosa 1) has been tentatively mapped to 1.
RP2 (retinitis pigmentosa 2) has been mapped to Xp11.4-p11.2.
RP3 (retinitis pigmentosa 3) has been mapped to Xp21.1-p11.4.
CRD (choroidoretinal degeneration) has been mapped to X.

Prevention: None known. Genetic counseling indicated.

Treatment: Night vision aids and optical field wideners may help some symptoms. Protecting the retina from bright light by sunglasses or occlusion has been advocated, but remains with no substantive proof of benefit. Appropriate therapy for hearing loss may be needed. Vitamin therapy has been associated with slower progression than normal, and treatment trials are being actively investigated.

Prognosis: Normal life span unless influenced by an associated systemic problem. There is always impairment of visual fields and night vision, but acuity may be normal.

Detection of Carrier: In the X-linked form, the carrier may show a golden glistening "spotty" or "streaky" reflex in the post-equatonal retina area or throughout most of the eyegrounds. This change has been called a "tapetal" reflex. A few carriers will show some of the changes seen in males, but usually, in general, only minimal functional disturbances are noted. Occasionally a mild abnormality, particularly of dark adaptation, is found. Rarely the female carrier will show marked symptoms. The full field ERG and vitreous fluorophotometry have been able to detect a high percentage of carriers. The ERP has also been used to identify carriers. Carriers generally cannot be detected in the autosomal recessive form. Pedigree analysis may reveal obligate carriers.

Support Groups:
MD; Baltimore; RP Foundation Fighting Blindness
CANADA: Ontario; Toronto; National Retinitis Pigmentosa Foundation of Canada

References:
Merin S, Auerbach E: Retinitis pigmentosa. Surv Ophthalmol 1976; 20:303–346.
Heckenlively J, et al.: Retinitis pigmentosa in the Navajo. Metab Pediat Ophthal 1981; 5:201–206.
Hu D-N: Genetic aspects of retinitis pigmentosa in China. Am J Med Genet 1982; 12:51–56.
Marmor MF, et al.: Retinitis pigmentosa: a symposium on terminology and methods of examination. Ophthalmology 1983; 90:126–131.
Bhattacharya SS, et al.: Close genetic linkage between X-linked RP and a restriction fragment length polymorphism identified by recombinant DNA probe LI.28. Nature 1984; 309:253–255.
Bunker CH, et al.: Prevalence of retinitis pigmentosa in Maine. Am J Ophthalmol 1984; 97:357–365.
Berson EL, et al.: Natural course of RP over a three year interval. Am J Ophthal 1985; 99:240–251.
Fishman GA, et al.: Autosomal dominant retinitus pigmentosa: a method of classification. Arch Ophthal 1985; 103:366–374.
Grohdahl J: Estimation of prognosis and prevalence of retinitus pigmentosa and Usher syndrome in Norway. Clin Genet 1987; 31:255–264.
Heckenlively JR, et al.: Clinical findings and common symptoms in retinitis pigmentosa. Am J Ophthalmol 1988; 105:504–511.
Heckenlively JR: Retinitis pigmentosa. Philadelphia: J.B. Lippincott, 1988.
Pagon RA: Retinitis pigmentosa. Survey of Ophthalmology 1988; 33:137–177.

W0003   **Mitchel L. Wolf**

Retinitis pigmentosa, atypical (some forms)
See RETINA, COMBINED CONE-ROD DEGENERATION
Retinitis pigmentosa, congenital
See RETINA, AMAUROSIS CONGENITA, LEBER TYPE
Retinitis pigmentosa-hearing loss (sensorineural)
See USHER SYNDROME

RETINOBLASTOMA   **0870**

Includes:
Cancer, retinoblastoma
Endophytum type retinoblastoma
Exophytum type retinoblastoma
Osteosarcoma, retinoblastoma-related
Trilateral retinoblastoma

Excludes:
CNS neoplasms (0188)
Diktyoma
Pupil, other causes of white (leukocoria)

Major Diagnostic Criteria: Characteristic ophthalmoscopic appearance of a tumor arising in the retina of one or both eyes, usually occurring in an infant less than three years of age. When the tumor is obscured by overlying detachment or inflammatory reaction in the vitreous, neuro-imaging and ultrasonography are useful.

P-32 uptake studies may be useful in special situations, although the injection of P-32 into infants must be regarded with

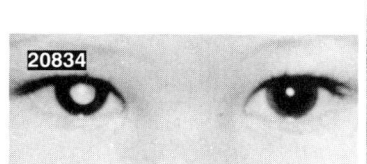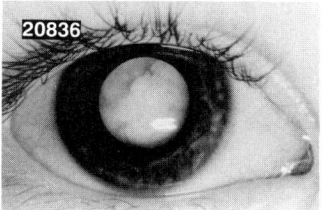

0870-20834–36: Typical white "cat's eye" reflex in the affected eye.

great circumspection. Computed axial tomography has been of great value, both in detecting a mass lesion within the eye, and appreciating calcific densities that cannot be demonstrated by other techniques. CT scanning may be useful in detecting extension of tumor into the optic nerve, into the orbit, and into the middle cranial fossa.

Increased levels of lactic acid dehydrogenase have been found in almost all patients with retinoblastoma. The absolute level of this enzyme is increased in the aqueous humor. The aqueous: serum LDH ratio is always greater than one, and there is a fairly characteristic isoenzyme pattern. Aqueous gamma enolase levels may prove to be a more specific marker for cells of neural crest origin.

Clinical Findings: The average age at the time of tumor diagnosis is 12 months. The most common presenting sign is a white "cat's eye reflex" in the pupil, and the second most common sign is strabismus. Occasionally, spontaneous necrosis in the tumor will lead to a red, painful eye, with or without secondary glaucoma. In older children, poor vision or vitreous floaters are rarely presenting complaints. Because of a family history, younger sibs should be examined early in life. Consequently about 3% of tumors are identified on routine examination.

In hereditary cases, the tumor arises multifocally in the retina, and at least one-half of all cases have more than one tumor in an involved eye. The tumor arises bilaterally in one-third of all cases. Retinoblastoma occurs in eyes of normal size, and cataract is never seen except as a rare, late complication. The tumor may grow from the retina forward into the vitreous space, the endophytum type, when it can be clearly seen with an ophthalmoscope during the early stages. These tumors usually have a very characteristic creamy-pink color with numerous blood vessels on the surface. The exophytum type, however, grows beneath the retina, in the subretinal potential space. This lesion may be obscured by an overlying detachment, and the borders and surface characteristics cannot be clearly seen.

Two clinical findings are more or less pathognomonic of retinoblastoma. The first is calcification within the tumor which may be seen either with the ophthalmoscope or by X-ray. Approximately 75% of retinoblastomas will show intraocular calcification if the X-rays or CT are properly exposed. When the tumor has achieved a relatively large size, the stroma breaks down and portions of the tumor seeds into the vitreous and may go to the anterior chamber where they may implant on the iris or present as a hypopyon.

Complications: *Ocular*: Retinal detachment. Inflammatory reaction due to spontaneous necrosis. Rubeosis iridis. Secondary glaucoma. Phthisis bulbi.

Systemic complications: This tumor may spread directly by the optic nerve into the subarachnoid space, and the base of the brain may be seeded with tumor which then produces central nervous system (CNS) symptoms and death. It may also metastasize hematogenously following extension into the choroid. The bone marrow is probably the tissue first invaded, but multiple viscera may be involved later. It is curious that lung parenchyma is rarely involved. If the tumor extends out of the eye into the orbit, it may then spread lympatically to the regional nodes.

Associated Findings: The clinical phenotype is usually limited to the retinal tumors, but infants with a detectable defect in the long arm of chromosome 13 have psychomotor retardation and a variety of skeletal defects. About 5% of patients with retinoblastoma have mental retardation, but the vast majority of patients have normal intellectual development.

Patients with the germinal mutation for retinoblastoma seem to have both increased susceptibility to radiation-induced tumors at relatively low dosage levels, and a high incidence (>50%) of second primary neoplasms later in life unrelated to retinoblastoma or the treatment thereof. Osteogenic sarcoma is the most common second tumor, although a variety of other neoplasms have been reported, such as soft tissue sarcomas, and cutaneous malignant melanomas.

Some patients with retinoblastoma have associated ectopic retinoblastoma in the pineal gland or in the parasellar location and are said to have *trilateral retinoblastoma*. When such tumors are considered, a computed tomogram of the head is obtained for a patient with retinoblastoma.

Etiology: Autosomal dominant inheritance in 8–10% of cases. About 5–7% of patients demonstrate deletion of the q14 band on the long arm of chromosome 13 in fresh tumor preparations. These may be unilateral or bilateral cases. Only 8% of patients present with a family history at time of diagnosis.

All patients with a family history, all patients with bilateral disease, and all patients with multicentric tumor (even if unilateral) are assumed to have germinal mutations. Approximately 15% of unilateral isolated cases are found to have germinal mutations, but the remainder are not transmitted as would be expected of an autosomal dominant disease. These latter may represent somatic mutations and have one tumor in one eye. Recent information suggests, however, that the molecular defect requires simultaneous alterations at each chromosome 13 locus, this behaving as a "recessive" molecular disease.

Pathogenesis: Tumors arise in one or both eyes, probably as photoreceptor precursor cells, and then grow at variable rates, until the globe is entirely filled with tumor. Loss of or mutation of both alleles of the normally present retinoblastoma suppressor oncogene on the long arm of chromosome 13 are needed for a tumor to develop.

MIM No.: *18020

CDC No.: 190.500

Sex Ratio: M1:Fl

Occurrence: The tumor now appears to arise in 1:20,000 births. Approximately 200 new cases are seen in the United States each year. Some populations (e.g. Saudi Arabia) appear to have higher prevalence. As more patients with germinal mutations live to reproductive age, an increase in incidence may be expected.

Risk of Recurrence for Patient's Sib: With no family history: 1%. With a positive family history: 40%.

Risk of Recurrence for Patient's Child: 8–25% if parent had unilateral involvement; almost 40% if parent had bilateral or multicentric retinoblastoma.

Age of Detectability: The vast majority of patients are detected before the age of two years. It is extremely unlikely to see the appearance of a new tumor beyond the age of three years. At least two cases with metastatic retinoblastoma at birth are known, and an occasional patient with spontaneous regression has been identified up to the age of 62 years.

Gene Mapping and Linkage: RB1 (retinoblastoma 1 (including osteosarcoma)) has been mapped to 13q14.2.

Prevention: None known. Genetic counseling indicated.

Treatment: Even in isolated cases, *both* parents must have complete medical eye examinations to identify possible spontaneous regression of tumor, which would indicate that the case is "genetic" rather than isolated.

In families with a positive history, all possible effort must be made to examine all children within one week of birth. Supervoltage radiation is the most effective form of treatment, as this tumor is radiocurable. The average tumor dose is 3500–4000r delivered over 3–4 weeks. Radioactive cobalt applicators, light coagulation, diathermy, and cryotherapy are valuable adjunctive measures. Eyes with large tumors, filling more than one-half of the globe, are usually enucleated.

The tumor is sensitive to various chemotherapeutic agents including nitrogen mustard, TEM, thio-TEPA, methotrexate, Cytoxan, actinomycin-D, and vincristine. These agents are not curative, however, and should be used only in conjunction with radiation or in the treatment of as-yet incurable metastatic disease.

Prognosis: Overall mortality in the United States is 20%; much higher in less-developed countries. The stage of the disease at the time that diagnosis is made is the most significant factor in the eventual outcome.

For practical purposes, all fatal cases have one or both eyes in group 5 of the Reese-Ellsworth classification. If cases are detected at any earlier stage, and adequate treatment is undertaken, there is virtually no mortality from the primary tumor.

Prognosis appears to be correlate better with size and extent of tumor than with cytologic differentiation.

Several articles have claimed that mortality is greater in Blacks than in Caucasians, but on careful analysis it appears that this is due to the stage of the disease at the time treatment is undertaken.

Detection of Carrier: In some families with multiple generations affected, quantitive esterase D levels may be informative. A DNA probe discovered in 1987 will be useful in detecting carriers by demonstrating deletion of 13q14. In all isolated cases, both parents must undergo dilated ophthalmoscopy with a binocular indirect ophthalmoscope and 360 degree scleral depression in a search for spontaneously involuted tumors.

Special Considerations: This is a highly malignant hereditary tumor, for which early diagnosis is vital. Leukokoria in infancy must be regarded as the most dangerous sign in all ophthalmology and should lead to thorough investigation for retinoblastoma. Once the tumor has extended outside the eye into the orbit, the chances of cure are slight, and few patients with metastatic retinoblastoma have survived. The differential diagnosis can be quite complex, and the most commonly confused conditions are larval granulomatosis (ocular toxocariasis), **Retina, Coats disease**, angiomatosis retinae, and granulomatous uveitis. Persistent hyperplastic vitreous, retrolental fibroplasia, congenital retinal folds, medullated nerve fibers, and colobomas can usually be identified readily when the children are examined under anesthesia.

The second most common presenting sign is strabismus and all children with this condition should have careful indirect ophthalmoscopic examination of the retina.

Support Groups: Atlanta; American Cancer Society

References:
Ellsworth RM: The practical management of retino-blastoma. Trans Am Ophthalmol Soc 1969; 67:462.
Reese AB: Tumors of the Eye, 3rd Ed. New York: Harper and Row, 1976.
Zimmerman LE: Retinoblastoma and retinocytoma. In: Spencer WH, ed.: Ophthalmic pathology: an atlas and textbook. Philadelphia: W.B. Saunders. 1985:1292–1351. * †
Cavenee WK, et al.: Prediction of familial predisposition to retinoblastoma. New Engl J Med 1986; 314:1201–1207.
Draper GY, et al.: Second primary neoplasms in patients with retinoblastoma. Br J Cancer 1986; 53:661–671. *
Friend SH, et al.: A human DNA segment with properties of the gene that predispose to retinoblastoma and osteosarcoma. Nature 1986; 323:643–646. *
Fung Y-KT, et al.: Structural evidence for the authenticity of the human retinoblastoma gene. Science 1987; 236:1657–1661.
Wiggs J, et al.: Prediction of the risk of hereditary retinoblastoma, using DNA polymorphisms within the retinoblastoma gene. New Engl J Med 1988; 318:151–157.
Yandell DW, et al.: Oncogenic point mutations in the human retinoblastoma gene: their application to genetic counseling. New Engl J Med 1989; 321:1689–1695.

Robert M. Ellsworth

Retinoic acid syndrome
See FETAL RETINOID SYNDROME
Retinoic fetal effects, experimental in animals
See FETAL RETINOID SYNDROME

RETINOPATHY OF PREMATURITY   0872

Includes:
  Fibroplasia retrolental
  Retrolental fibroplasia (RLF)

Excludes: Retrolental membranes, other causes of

Major Diagnostic Criteria: Bilateral retinal pathology that occurs in premature, low-birth-weight children who have usually received supplemental oxygen therapy immediately after birth. Typically, the earliest stages of the disease appear within the first month of life.
Standard classification for retinopathy of prematurity
Active stages:
Stage 1: Dilatation and tortuosity of retinal vessels.
Stage 2: Stage 1 plus neovascularization and some peripheral retinal clouding.
Stage 3: Stage 2 plus retinal detachment in the periphery of the fundus. Frequently, a retinal fold develops, extending from the disk to the retinal periphery. Of these folds, approximately 90% occur on the temporal side of the globe. Vitreous hemorrhage often occurs during this stage.
Stage 4: Hemispheric or circumferential detachment of the retina.
Stage 5: Complete retinal detachment with contracture and organization into a retrolental membrane. Massive vitreous hemorrhage may occur during retinal organization.
Late cicatricial grades:
Grade I: A small mass of opaque, gray tissue is present in the retinal periphery with an accompanying localized retinal detachment. In addition, there may be floating gray vitreous opacities with or without a pigment disturbance in the peripheral retina. Myopia is common, but vision may be normal or near normal.
Grade II: A mass of opaque, gray tissue, larger than in grade I cicatricial disease, is present in the retinal periphery with an accompanying localized retinal detachment. The disk may show

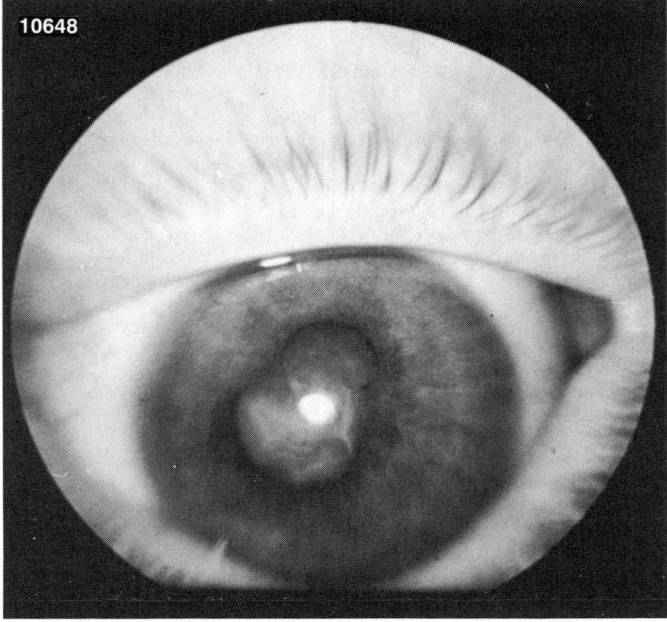

0872-10648:   Retrolental fibroplasia.

moderate distortion, with "dragging" of the major retinal vessels toward the periphery such that they become straighter than usual; this almost always occurs in the temporal direction. In addition, the macula may be displaced with obvious heterotopia. In these cases, the visual acuity ranges from 20/40 to 20/200.

Grade III: A large mass of opaque, gray tissue is present in the retina with a fold extending from this mass to the nervehead. When a retinal fold is present, the visual acuity is usually in the 20/200 to hand motion range. As the fold forms, there is often some hemorrhage along its edges; this hemorrhage is associated with a proliferation of the retinal pigment epithelium.

Grade IV: Extensive circumferential retinal pathology with a retrolental membrane occupying a portion of the retrolental space. The vision in these eyes is usually limited to hand motion or light perception.

Grade V: A total retrolental membrane covering the entire posterior surface of the lens. The entire retina is incorporated into the membrane. These patients have no light perception. Recently, a new, international classification system for retinopathy of prematurity has been proposed by a group of 23 ophthalmologists from 11 countries. This system defines retinopathy of prematurity according to three parameters: location, extent, and stage of the disease.

A. Location is defined by specific zones of retinal involvement, using the optic disk as the reference point for the center of each zone:

Zone 1: Posterior pole or inner zone. The limits of zone I are defined as two times the distance from the optic nervehead to the center of the macula in all directions (an arc of 60 degrees).

Zone II: This zone extends from the edge of zone I peripherally to a point tangential to the nasal ora serrata, extending in a circle to an area near the temporal equator.

Zone III: This zone includes the residual retinal crescent anterior to zone II.

B. Extent is defined as the specific clock hour position of retinal involvement.

C. Staging of the disease reflects the degree of associated vascular abnormalities:

Stage I, demarcation line: A relatively flat, white demarcation line separates avascular anterior retina from normal posterior retina. Abnormal branching vessels lead up to the edge of the demarcation line.

Stage II, ridge: The demarcation line extends up, as a ridge, out of the plane of the retina; it has height, width, and volume. The ridge may appear to be pink, with vascular tufts apparent posteriorly on the adjacent retina. In addition, vessels from the posterior retina may enter the ridge.

Stage III, ridge with extraretinal fibrovascular proliferation: Extraretinal fibrovascular proliferation tissue is present in addition to all of the stage II findings. This extraretinal tissue may be present continuous with, or adjacent to, the posterior aspect of the ridge, or it may develop in the vitreous, perpendicular to the plane of the retina.

Stage IV, retinal detachment: Stage III with accompanying secondary exudative with or without traction detachment of the retina.

Plus disease is a special subset of the four stages and is used in conjunction when progressive vascular incompetence is present, as evidenced by increasing dilation and tortuosity of the peripheral retinal vessels, engorgement of the iris vasculature, pupillary rigidity, and vitreous haze. When the posterior retinal veins enlarge and the arterioles become tortuous, a "+" is added to the appropriate stage (e.g., stage II+).

Clinical Findings: ROP occurs in premature, but generally otherwise normal, infants. These infants are usually born between 26 and 31 weeks gestation, with birth weights ranging from 800 to 1500g. In addition, most of them have received supplemental oxygen. The disease rarely occurs in full-term children of normal birth weight who have not received oxygen therapy. With some exceptions, the disease is bilateral and usually symmetric. There is an active phase early in life, which becomes clinically evident at 3–5 weeks after birth. The earliest sign is constriction of the retinal arterioles, which is followed by venous dilation, increased tortu-

osity, and neovascularization. Subsequently, retinal and vitreous hemorrhages may occur. These hemorrhages typically develop peripherally, particularly in the temporal half of the retina. An exudative phase can occur in which white patches of edema may develop followed by detachment of the peripheral retina. The process may end spontaneously at any stage.

Useful vision may be retained in those patients in whom pathologic changes are limited to peripheral cicatrization. In about 25% of the patients, a progressive cicatricial phase develops from the second to the fifth month of life and is characterized by organization and contracture of the entire retina. The end result is formation of retinal folds or the formation of a dense, gray-white membrane lying behind the lens completely obscuring all view of the fundus. As the retina undergoes progressive contraction, the ciliary processes are drawn into the mass and may be visible around the circumference of the lens without indentation of the globe. Since the retrolental membrane is frequently vascularized, it is possible that progressive traction on this membrane accounts for the hemorrhage that occasionally occurs. The iris is also involved in the process of neovascularization; large radial iris vessels and posterior synechiae are common. Eyes with advanced disease may develop glaucoma transiently; however, the contracture ultimately results in phthisis bulbi. After age six years, the condition of the eyes is usually stationary, although retinal detachments can occur until about age 10 years in patients who have grade III or IV cicatricial retinopathy of prematurity.

Complications: Secondary glaucoma may develop during the phase of vasoproliferation or intraocular hemorrhage. Heterochromia may occur as the result of anterior segment hemorrhage. Eccentric fixation may develop as a result of macular ectopia.

Associated Findings: High myopia, mental retardation (estimated to be present to some degree in as many as 40% of all cases).

Etiology: In premature infants, the retinal vasculature is not fully developed at birth and is abnormally sensitive to the vasoconstrictive effect of ambient oxygen.

Pathogenesis: Peripheral retinal hypoxia results from constriction of retinal arterioles. Abnormal surface retinal vessels develop as secondary vasoproliferation occurs in response to this hypoxia. These vessels tend to hemorrhage into the retina and vitreous. When the hemorrhage organizes, secondary traction, detachment of the retina, and ultimate contracture leading to phthisis bulbi can occur. In addition to vasoproliferation, the hypoxia may produce areas of complete vaso-obliteration with considerable capillary endothelial damage.

Sex Ratio: M1:F1

Occurrence: Undetermined but presumed rare.

Risk of Recurrence for Patient's Sib: Presumably not increased.

Risk of Recurrence for Patient's Child: Presumably not increased.

Age of Detectability: Birth to six weeks of age.

Gene Mapping and Linkage: Unknown.

Prevention: The ambient oxygen level in the incubator should be kept as low as possible concomitant with the well-being of the infant; in general, at a level of 40% or below. Catheterization of the umbilical artery is useful to monitor the blood pO$_2$ levels. Indirect ophthalmoscopy is not an effective way to monitor oxygen levels, because persistent vitreous haze in premature infants may make visualization difficult and there is very poor correlation between the arterial caliber as viewed with the ophthalmoscope and arterial oxygen tension values. Fluorescein angiography may detect early pathologic changes, but it is not practical in the monitoring of premature infants. Radiation and steroid therapies have been used but without definite effect.

Treatment: Light coagulation employed early in the active stages may arrest progression. Cryotherapy may also be useful in obliterating peripheral neovascular tufts in eyes that are technically difficult to treat by photocoagulation. The National Institutes of Health has sponsored an on-going multicenter trial of cryotherapy for retinopathy of prematurity; preliminary results have not been reported to date. Retinal detachment treated by scleral buckling has met with some limited success; however, follow-up has not been long or extensive. Vitamin E supplementation has not been shown to affect the incidence of ROP, but may decrease its severity.

Prognosis: Normal for life span. In stages 1 and 2, the active phase may regress spontaneously without serious retinal pathology. The healed grades I and II eyes may have normal maculae and essentially normal vision. In grades III and IV eyes, variable progressive loss of vision may occur as a result of retinal detachments in children aged five to 10 years. In grade V eyes, total loss of vision is typical.

Detection of Carrier: Unknown.

Special Considerations: In premature infants with an essentially normal cardiovascular system, there is fairly good data indicating that retinal changes will not occur if the ambient oxygen concentration is maintained at a level of 40% or less. The incidence of retinopathy of prematurity is definitely related to prematurity and birth weight.

Retinopathy of prematurity is more frequent and more severe in smaller infants. The rate at which a newborn is weaned from supplemental oxygen therapy does not seem to be related to the occurrence of retinopathy of prematurity. The development of the retina's vascular supply is unique. At the fourth month of gestation, vessels from the embryonic hyaloid system supply the retina. The normal retina does not fully vascularize until shortly after birth in the full-term, normal-birth-weight infant. Perhaps 1% of all cases of retinopathy of prematurity have occurred in infants receiving no significant oxygen therapy. This appears to be related to immaturity of the retinal vessels and peripheral anoxia in the absence of the vasoconstrictive effect of supplemental oxygen. In utero, the arterial oxygen saturation is only 50% or so. It has been suggested that the relative increase in oxygen saturation following birth may stimulate the sensitive premature retinal vessels to cause vasoproliferation and all of the pathologic changes associated with retinopathy of prematurity. Theoretically, a number of factors that can alter oxygen availability to the retina may also contribute to the development of ROP. Some of these factors include packed red blood cell transfusions, sepsis (increased oxygen release by macrophages), low pH, and very low temperatures. Current interest in retinopathy of prematurity centers around infants with the respiratory distress syndrome in whom there is pulmonary pathology and frequently right-to-left shunts. In these infants, the level of ambient oxygen does not reflect arterial oxygen concentration and it is only by monitoring arterial pO_2 that we may appreciate the oxygen levels in the retina. Safe limits of oxygen therapy have not been defined but, at the moment, it would seem that retinal pO_2 should be maintained at 100 mm Hg or less to avoid retinal pathology.

There is clinical evidence to show that systemic vitamin E therapy may be helpful in preventing the formation of neovascularization extending into the vitreous (stage 2 of active disease). It is thought that vitamin E may prevent free-radical damage to spindle cells (the cells that ultimately align, canalize, and differentiate to form nascent retinal blood vessels). The initiation of vitamin E therapy does not eliminate the occurrence of mild-to-moderate grades of ROP, but it may reduce its severity. However, vitamin E allegedly has multiple potential toxic effects, possibly due to its alteration of normal enzymatic levels.

References:
National Society for the Prevention of Blindness (Subcommittee, AB Reese, Chairman): Classification of retrolental fibroplasia. Am J Ophthalmol 1953; 36:1333.
Ashton N, et al.: Effect of oxygen on developing retinal vessels with particular reference to problem of retrolental fibroplasia. Br J Ophthalmol 1964; 38:387.
Patz A: New role of the ophthalmologist in prevention of retrolental fibroplasia. Arch Ophthalmol 1967; 78:565.
Brockhurst RJ, Chishti ML: Cicatricial retrolental fibroplasia: its occurrence without oxygen administration and in full term infants. Albrecht Von Graefes Arch Klin Ophthalmol 1975; 195:113.
Kalina RE, et al.: Retrolental fibroplasia: experience over two decades in one institution. Ophthalmologica 1982; 89:91.
Hittner HM, et al.: Suppression of severe retinopathy of prematurity with vitamin E supplementation. Ophthalmologica 1984; 91:1512–1523.
The Committee for the Classification of Retinopathy of Prematurity: An international classification of retinopathy of prematurity. Arch Ophthalmol 1984; 102:1130–1134.
Topilow HW, et al.: The treatment of advanced retinopathy of prematurity by cryotherapy and scleral buckling surgery. Ophthalmologica 1985; 92:379–387.
Bremer DL, et al.: The efficacy of vitamin E in retinopathy of prematurity. J Pediatr Ophthalmol Strab 1986; 23:132–136.

EL007   **Robert M. Ellsworth**
WE038   **Robert A. Weiss**
WU002   **Gloria Wu**

RETINOPATHY-HYPOTRICHOSIS SYNDROME   2627

Includes:
> Hypotrichosis-retinopathy
> Retinal dystrophy, posterior pole-congenital total
>   hypotrichosis
> Tapetoretinal degeneration-alopecia

Excludes: Ectodermal dysplasia-ectrodactyly-macular dystrophy (2793)

Major Diagnostic Criteria: Presence of retinal degeneration and hypotrichosis in the absence of ectrodactyly or syndactyly.

Clinical Findings: The hypotrichosis is noted during infancy in most cases and may be progressive. In two patients, hypotrichosis appeared in childhood. During childhood or early adolescence, patients manifest progressive decreased vision. The typical retinal changes are atrophy of the retinal epithelium in the posterior pole with pigment deposition in the peripapillar area and macular involvement. There may exist diffuse rarefaction of the retina and increased pigment mobilization in the periphery. Visual field examination may reveal large scotomas. The ERG shows photopic

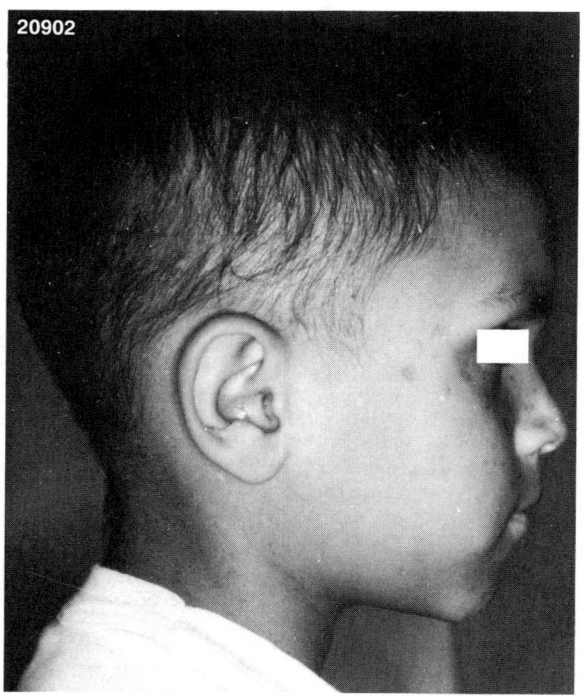

2627-20902:   Note the pattern and degree of hypotrichosis in this 6-year-old girl with retinopathy-hypotrichosis (RH) syndrome.

involvement; generally preserved for white and orange stimuli but extinct for red and blue stimuli. On testing for color vision, patients will generally show dyschromatopsia.

Complications: The retinal dystrophy is progressive and may lead to blindness.

Associated Findings: In one Brazilian family with six affected individuals, there was associated acrocyanosis in all cases.

Etiology: Presumably autosomal recessive inheritance.

Pathogenesis: Unknown.

POS No.: 3442, 4428

Sex Ratio: Presumably M1:F1. However, 15 of the 20 patients reported have been female.

Occurrence: Twenty patients, from eight families, have been observed. Four families (13 patients) are from Brazil, two from Germany, one from Hungary, and one from Sweden.

Risk of Recurrence for Patient's Sib:
See Part I, *Mendelian Inheritance*.

Risk of Recurrence for Patient's Child:
See Part I, *Mendelian Inheritance*.

Age of Detectability: During childhood.

Gene Mapping and Linkage: Unknown.

Prevention: None known. Genetic counseling indicated.

Treatment: Low-vision aids, cosmetic treatment (wig) for hypotrichosis.

Prognosis: Normal life span.

Detection of Carrier: Unknown.

References:
Wagner H: Makulaaffection vergesellchaftet mit Haarabnormität von Lanugotypus, beide vielleicht angeboren bei zwei Geschwistern. Graefes Arch Clin Exp Ophthalmol 1935; 134:71.
Björk A, Jahnberg P: Retinal dystrophy combined with alopecia. Acta Ophthalmol 1975; 53:781.
Kroll P: Beidseitige kongenitale Pigmentblattdystrophie des hinteren Augenpols bei gleichzeitiger Hypotrichosis congenita totalis. Klin Mbl Augenheilkd 1981; 178:118.
Mais FAQ, et al.: Distrofia do epitélio pigmentar retiniano do polo posterior associada com hipotricose congênita difusa. Arq Bras Oftalmol 1984; 47:137.
Pena SDJ, Ribeiro-Goncalves E: Sindrome autossomica recessiva de retinopatia e hipotricose. Ciencia e Cult 1987; 39:741.

PE017   **Sergio D.J. Pena**

Retinopathy-mental retardation
See RETINOPATHY-MICROCEPHALY-MENTAL RETARDATION

**RETINOPATHY-MICROCEPHALY-MENTAL
RETARDATION**   **2846**

Includes:
 Mental retardation-retinopathy-microcephaly
 Microcephaly-mental retardation-retinopathy
 Mirhosseini-Holmes-Walton syndrome
 Retinal pigmentary degeneration-microcephaly-mental
  retardation
 Retinopathy-mental retardation

Excludes:
 Bardet-Biedl syndrome (2363)
 Cockayne syndrome (0189)
 Cohen syndrome (2023)
 Laurence-Moon syndrome (0578)
 Pigmentary retinopathy in other conditions
 Usher syndrome (0983)

Major Diagnostic Criteria: Severe mental retardation, **Microcephaly**, and retinal pigmentary degeneration.

Clinical Findings: Neonatal hypotonia, failure to thrive during infancy, and slow psychomotor development are evident. Impairment of normal growth is probably part of the syndrome.

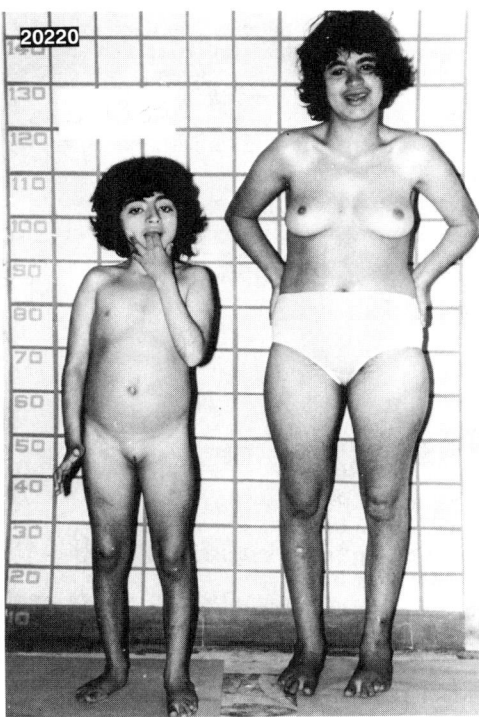

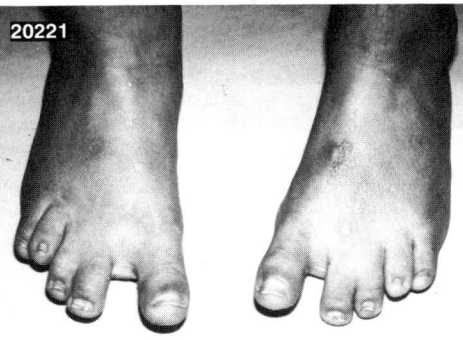

2846-20220: Facies with prominent supraorbital ridges, ptosis, short upper lip and short midface as well as the body habitus, short stature and microcephaly. **20221:** Syndactyly of the second and third toes, overlapping fourth toe, and wide gap between the hallux and the second toe.

The physical signs include dolichomicrocephalic skull, small forehead with prominence of the supraorbital ridges, short midface with some mandibular prognathism, bilateral ptosis, highly arched palate, hypoplastic philtrum, malformed teeth (hypoplastic or fused incisors, incisive-like canines), long and slender hands and feet, and scoliosis.

In one sibship, two sisters present bilateral cubitus valgus, genua recurvata, pes valgus, dorsipositioning of the 4th toe, wide gap between the hallux and the 2nd toe, while in the other sibship two brothers had cataracts. One male patient was found to have hypogonadism, probably due to testicular disfunction.

The ophthalmologic evaluation shows normal corneas, atrophy of the optic disc with peripheral pigmentary alteration of the fundi and severe myopic astigmatism. One male patient had both lenses totally cataractous while in the other the lenses had anterior and posterior axial irregular white subcapsular opacities.

The neurologic examination shows muscular strength diminished, muscular tone normal, hyperextensibility of the finger joints, deep tendon reflexes hyperactive, Babinsky sign positive, ataxic-paretic walk, severe retardation of speech and severe mental retardation in the two female patients. The male patients do not have hypertonia or hyperreflexia.

Glucose tolerance test is normal and cytogenetic study shows normal chromosomes (G-banding) in all patients.

Complications: Unknown.

Associated Findings: None known.

Etiology: Probably autosomal recessive inheritance, with possible variable expressivity. It has been suggested this and **Cohen syndrome** may be the same condition.

Pathogenesis: Unknown.

MIM No.: 26805

POS No.: 3540

Sex Ratio: M2:F2 (observed).

Occurrence: Two brothers in one family and two sisters in another family have been documented. The families were from Brazil and the United States.

Risk of Recurrence for Patient's Sib:
See Part I, *Mendelian Inheritance.*

Risk of Recurrence for Patient's Child:
See Part I, *Mendelian Inheritance.*

Age of Detectability: During childhood.

Gene Mapping and Linkage: Unknown.

Prevention: None known. Genetic counseling indicated.

Treatment: Unknown.

Prognosis: Life span is probably not affected.

Detection of Carrier: Unknown.

References:
Mirhosseini SA, et al.: Syndrome of pigmentary retinal degeneration, cataract, microcephaly, and severe mental retardation. J Med Genet 1972; 9:193–196.
Mendez HMM, et al.: The syndrome of retinal pigmentary degeneration, microcephaly, and severe mental retardation (Mirhosseini-Holmes-Walton syndrome): report of two patients. Am J Med Genet 1985; 22:223–228.

ME039   **Heirie Mendez**

RETINOSCHISIS   0871

Includes:
> Juvenile retinoschisis, X-linked
> Retinal cyst, congenital
> Retina, giant cyst of
> Retinoschisis of fovea
> Senile retinoschisis, autosomal recessive
> Typical retinoschisis, autosomal dominant
> Vitreoretinal dystrophy
> Vitreous, congenital vascular veils in

Excludes: Retinal detachment

Major Diagnostic Criteria: Typical retinal findings which fit one of three patterns and are usually easily seen.

Clinical Findings: The clinical signs and symptoms usually fit into one of three common pictures:
Typical retinoschisis commonly occurs in hyperopic young males; it is frequently bilateral and is often strikingly symmetric. The lesion begins most commonly in the inferior temporal quadrant or, somewhat less commonly, in the superior temporal quadrant, and it appears ophthalmoscopically as a thin, translucent, veil-like membrane extending up as a dome into the vitreous. The translucent membrane contains the retinal vessels and often has small, white dots, which represent glial strands extending across the cystic area. The vitreous is usually fluid, and posterior vitreous detachment is common. The process is often static for many years, although it may be slowly progressive.
Senile retinoschisis is related to typical retinoschisis. Senile reti-

noschisis is commonly noted in older patients on routine examination, and it is rarely symptomatic. It is bilateral in approximately 90% of cases, and may develop as a coalescence of peripheral cysts of Blessig. In the early stage, the cystic space is spanned by thin, gray fibers that gradually break, allowing the inner and outer leaves to separate and forming an elevated cyst. In senile retinoschisis, the split retina may extend 360 degrees around the retinal periphery, but it does not commonly progress posteriorly and may remain static for many years.

Juvenile retinoschisis, the third clinical variant of retinoschisis, frequently causes serious problems. The area involved by the schisis is very extensive, often including the macula. In some cases the entire retina becomes involved, with subsequent total detachment, preretinal organization, and a poor surgical prognosis. In earlier stages, the areas of schisis often exhibit large holes in the anterior leaf between vessels, and, if breaks develop in both the anterior and posterior leaves of the schisis, a true retinal detachment may occur. These eyes, with a combination of retinoschisis and retinal detachment, are particularly difficult to manage surgically. Patients with juvenile retinoschisis all have foveal retinoschisis, which adds to the visual defect and makes a surgical prognosis for useful vision more questionable. Both macular degeneration and splitting of the retina through the macula may contribute to the visual defect in these patients. The visual field shows a complete scotoma, with a sharp edge in the area of the schisis. On electrophysiologic testing, the electroretinogram (ERG) b wave is markedly depressed, but the a wave is characteristically normal except in severe cases.

Complications: Retinal detachment may complicate retinoschisis if holes are present in both the anterior and posterior leaf. Hemorrhage into the vitreous may occur as a result of traction on the retinal vessels, but may be mild and self-limited.

Associated Findings: Cystic macular degeneration, hyperopia, astigmatism, strabismus, nystagmus, optic atrophy, posterior cortical cataract, slight posterior capsular opacification, and liquification of the vitreous; rubeosis iridis and neovascular glaucoma have been reported in a case of X-linked juvenile retinoschisis as a complication of retinal detachment.

Etiology: Typical retinoschisis, usually by autosomal dominant inheritance. Senile retinoschisis, usually by autosomal recessive inheritance. Juvenile retinoschisis by X-linked recessive inheritance in almost all cases, although autosomal recessive, sporadic, and suspected autosomal dominant pedigrees have been reported.

Pathogenesis: Hereditary lamellar splitting in the layers of the retina usually occurs in the plane of the outer plexiform layer in typical and senile retinoschisis and in the nerve fiber layer in juvenile retinoschisis. The juvenile form of the disease may be related to congenital vascular veils in the vitreous, and may be due to a condensation of the vitreous, which was in contact with the inner layers of the optic cup. In addition, it is possible that there is some persistence of the secondary branches of the vasa propria hyaloidae.

In typical retinoschisis, *giant retinal cysts* are evident clinically. These cysts are probably caused by the secretion of hyaluronic acid-sensitive mucopolysaccharides by some of the cells in the inner portion of the retinal cyst. Once retinoschisis has begun because of this secretory mechanism, it may easily spread to peripheral areas of cystoid degeneration and progress posteriorly through normal retina.

Senile retinoschisis, especially the very mild, nonprogressive type, may simply represent a coalescence of peripheral microcysts without the secretory mechanism that appears to cause progression.

MIM No.: 18027, *26808, *31270

Sex Ratio: M1:F1 in both common and senile types. M1:F>0 for juvenile retinoschisis (female cases, although exceedingly rare, have been reported).

Occurrence: Incidence and prevalence of juvenile and typical retinoschisis is undetermined. While incidence of senile retinoschisis is undetermined, its prevalence is 7,000:100,000 (7%) of the population older than age 40 years.

Risk of Recurrence for Patient's Sib:
See Part I, *Mendelian Inheritance.*

Risk of Recurrence for Patient's Child:
See Part I, *Mendelian Inheritance.*

Age of Detectability: Juvenile retinoschisis may be detected at birth. The more common type of retinal cyst is usually seen in young men. Senile retinoschisis is seen in the fifth, sixth, and seventh decades of life.

Gene Mapping and Linkage: RS (retinoschisis) has been mapped to Xp22.2-p22.1.

Prevention: None known. Genetic counseling indicated.

Treatment: Light coagulation, cryotherapy (with possible drainage of subretinal fluid), vitrectomy for vitreous hemorrhage, and traction are indicated in some cases of juvenile retinoschisis and other selected cases. Since the fluid in the areas of schisis is extremely viscous, it is very difficult to drain by conventional detachment and drainage procedures. In many instances, especially in older adults, there is no or limited progression of the disease and treatment is rarely necessary. While approximately 8.9% of patients with senile retinoschisis develop localized, asymptomatic schisis detachments, the expected incidence of symptomatic progressive retinal detachment in the entire population with senile retinoschisis is only 0.05% (1:2,000). In general, there are three indications for treatment, as follows: 1) Most children with retinoschisis will require treatment; this form of the disease invariably progresses and possibly can be arrested, in some cases, before the macula is threatened. 2) Any patient who has demonstrable holes in both the inner and outer leaves of the schisis needs treatment; it is in these patients that complicated detachments can occur. 3) Patients who have retinal detachment in the fellow eye need treatment.

Two treatment modalities are effective. Light coagulation has been shown to cause collapse of these cysts. There are two rational approaches using light coagulation. The area of the "giant cyst" can be delimited with coagulations, which may function as a barrier to prevent peripheral and posterior spread; however, this barrier cannot be relied on to contain the schisis permanently. If, in addition to a delimiting row of coagulations, the entire area of the schisis is treated, the fluid will often resorb over a period of weeks or months. Apparently the heat has an effect that causes the schisis cavity fluid to resorb. The second approach is cryotherapy; again, the entire area of schisis is treated. At the present state of knowledge, it would seem that either light coagulation or cryotherapy is equally effective.

Prognosis: Normal for life span; guarded for vision in the X-linked form.

Detection of Carrier: Possibly by RFLP linkage.

References:
Mann I, MacRae A: Congenital vascular veils in the vitreous. Br J Ophthalmol 1938; 22:1–10.
Geiser EP, Falls HF: Hereditary retinoschisis. Am J Ophthalmol 1961; 51:1193.
Cibis PA: Retinoschisis: retinal cysts. Trans Am Ophthalmol Soc 1965; 63:417.
Yanoff M, et al.: Histopathology of juvenile retinoschisis. Arch Ophthalmol 1968; 79:49.
Conway BP, Welch RB: X-chromosome linked juvenile retinoschisis with hemorrhagic retinal cyst. Am J Ophthalmol 1977; 83:853.
Hung JY, Hilton GF: Neovascular glaucoma in a patient with X-linked juvenile retinoschisis. Ann Ophthalmol 1980; 12:1054–1055.
Yassur Y, et al.: Autosomal dominant inheritance of retinoschisis. Am J Ophthalmol 1982; 94:338.
Schulman J, et al.: Indications for vitrectomy in congenital retinoschisis. Br J Ophthalmol 1985; 69:482–486.
Byer NE: Long-term natural history study of senile retinoschisis with implications for management. Ophthalmologica 1986; 93:1127–1137.
Dahl N, et al.: DNA linkage analysis of X chromosome linked retinoschisis. (Abstract) Cytogenet Cell Genet 1987; HGM9.

EL007   **Robert M. Ellsworth**
WE038   **Robert A. Weiss**
WU002   **Gloria Wu**

Retinoschisis of fovea
See *RETINOSCHISIS*
Retinoschisis-early hemeralopia
See *EYE, GOLDMANN-FAVRE DISEASE*
Retraction syndrome
See *EYE, DUANE RETRACTION SYNDROME*
Retrocochlear hearing loss.
See *DEAFNESS*
Retrolental fibroplasia (RLF)
See *RETINOPATHY OF PREMATURITY*
Retromolar
See *TEETH, SUPERNUMERARY*
Retrosternal diaphragmatic hernia
See *DIAPHRAGMATIC HERNIA*

RETT SYNDROME   2226

Includes:
    Ataxia-dementia-autism
    Autism-dementia-ataxia-loss of purposeful hand use

Excludes:
    Autism, infantile (2128)
    Cerebellar ataxia
    Cerebral palsy (2931)

Major Diagnostic Criteria: 1) Normal prenatal, neonatal and early childhood (6–18 months) development and behavior; 2) after initial normal period, deceleration of psychomotor development and then, over a period of up to 18 months, deterioration of mental capacity (dementia with autistic features) and motor abilities, especially purposeful hand use; 3) acquisition of uncoordinated movement (ataxia) of the trunk and limbs, usually with some degree of spasticity and pyramidal tract signs; 4) development of major motor and minor motor seizures, usually associated with characteristic, though not specific EEG abnormalities; 5) subsequent period of more or less stable mental status, but slow and variable progression of the spasticity and seizures; 6) acquired microcephaly; and 7) to date only females have been described with this disorder.

Clinical Findings: 1) Normal birth weight, length and head circumference; 2) normal neonatal and early childhood development (6–18 months); 3) the subsequent progressive development of dementia with autistic elements, loss of purposeful hand movements, microcephaly, and later, seizures, generalized spasticity, ataxia, and episodic tachypnea and hyperventilation; 4) the loss of purposeful hand use is accompanied by stereotyped hand movements, usually characterized by flapping and wringing "hand-washing" motions; 5) the episodic hyperventilation, likewise, is highly stereotyped, with tachypnea, expiratory grunting and orofacial grimacing; 6) after the initial decline, a more or less static impoverishment of mental abilities (dementia); 7) more obvious and slow, but highly variable progression of the spasticity, ataxia and seizures; 8) EEG patterns are usually abnormal beyond three years of age. The waking background activity is slow, monotonous and without spatial differentiation, progressing at later ages to decreased voltage and general flattening with occasional bursts of high-amplitude slow waves, focal spikes or bilateral spike-wave complexes. The sleep pattern, on the other hand, shows frequent paroxysmal generalized slow spike-wave complexes; 9) cerebral CT scans may be normal or show nonspecific cortical atrophy; 10) although several of the original cases showed mild to modest hyperammonemia, this has not been a consistent finding.

In general, laboratory data, including karotypes, serum and urine amino acid and organic acid levels, serum and urine levels of copper and ceruloplasmin and other indicators of various types of inborn errors of metabolism, white blood cell and skin fibroblast lysozomal enzyme activities and ultrastructural appearances, have been normal or infrequently and nonspecifically abnormal; CSF catecholamine metabolite (i.e., homovanillic acid, 5-hydroxyindole acetic acid and 3-methoxy-4-hydroxyphenylethylene glycol) levels have been shown to be depressed (Zoghbi et al 1985).

Complications: Usually slow, variable progression of the neurological deficits, especially those related to the ataxia, corticospinal tract dysfunction and seizures; at times leading to severe quadriparesis and being wheelchair bound.

Associated Findings: None known.

Etiology: Uncertain, but limitation of known cases to females, including one pair of half-sisters (related through their mother), raises the possibility of an X-linked mutation (that is lethal in hemizygous males) or an abnormality related to X-chromosome inactivation (vis-a-vis the Lyon Principle). Identical twins are concordant, non-identical twins are discordant.

Pathogenesis: Undetermined, with no apparent clues except for the apparent preferential involvement of cerebral gray matter and the diminished levels of CSF catecholamines.

MIM No.: 31275

POS No.: 3796

Sex Ratio: M0:F1

Occurrence: Several hundred cases have been reported. Estimated at 1:15,000 in Sweden. Many cases have also been reported from France and Portugal.

Risk of Recurrence for Patient's Sib:
See Part I, *Mendelian Inheritance.*

Risk of Recurrence for Patient's Child:
See Part I, *Mendelian Inheritance.*

Age of Detectability: At six to 48 months of age.

Gene Mapping and Linkage: Unknown.

Prevention: None known. Genetic counseling indicated.

Treatment: Nonspecific supportive and nursing care, physical therapy, and anticonvulsants.

Prognosis: The prognosis is poor in terms of neurologic and mental function. Longevity is surely compromised, but accurate estimates are unavailable.

Detection of Carrier: Unknown.

Support Groups: MD; Fort Washington; International Rett Syndrome Association (IRSA)

References:
Rett A: Ueber ein eigenartiges hirnatrophisches Syndrom bei Hyperammoniamie in Kindersalter. Wien Med Wochenschr 1966; 116:723–738.
Hagberg B, et al.: A progressive syndrome of autism, dementia, ataxia and loss of purposeful hand use in girls: Rett's syndrome: report of 35 cases. Am J Neurol 1983; 14:471–479.
Kerr A, Stephenson JBP: Rett's syndrome in the west of Scotland. Brit Med Journal 1985; 291:579–582.
Zoghbi HY, et al.: Reduction of biogenic amine levels in the Rett syndrome. N Engl J Med 1985; 313:921–924.
Opitz JM, et al.: The Rett syndrome. Am J Med Genet 1986; 24(suppl 1):1–404.
Tariverdian G, et al.: A monozygotic twin pair with Rett syndrome. Hum Genet 1987; 75:88–90.
Journel H, et al.: Rett phenotype with X/autosome translocation: possible mapping to the short arm of chromosome X. Am J Med Genet 1990; 35:142–147.
Zoghbi HY, et al.: A *de novo* X;3 translocation in Rett syndrome. Am J Med Genet 1990; 35:148–151.

RI000   **Vincent M. Riccardi**

'Reye syndrome-like' manifestations
See VISCERA, FATTY METAMORPHOSIS
Reye-like syndrome, recurrent, due to MCAD
See ACYL-CoA DEHYDROGENASE DEFICIENCY, MEDIUM CHAIN TYPE

Rh hump
See TEETH, ENAMEL AND DENTIN DEFECTS FROM ERYTHROBLASTOSIS FETALIS
Rh incompatibility
See ERYTHROBLASTOSIS FETALIS
Rh null syndrome
See ANEMIA, HEMOLYTIC, RED CELL MEMBRANE DEFECTS
Rhabdomyosarcoma
See CANCER, SOFT TISSUE SARCOMA
Rheumatoid agglutinators (Raggs)
See ANTIBODIES TO HUMAN ALLOTYPES
Rheumatoid arthritis
See ARTHRITIS, RHEUMATOID
Rhinitis, ragweed pollen-induced
See RAGWEED POLLEN SENSITIVITY
Rhinolalia
See PALATOPHARYNGEAL INCOMPETENCE
Rhizomelic chondrodysplasia punctata
See CHONDRODYSPLASIA PUNCTATA, RHIZOMELIC TYPE
Rhizomelic dysplasia, familial
See OMODYSPLASIA

RHIZOMELIC SYNDROME, URBACH TYPE   **2816**

Includes:
    Skeletal dysplasia, Urbach rhizomelia of humeri
    Urbach skeletal dysplasia with rhizomelia of humeri

Excludes:
    Achondroplasia (0010)
    Brachydactyly (0114)
    Chondrodysplasia punctata, rhizomelic type (0154)
    Epiphyseal dysplasia, multiple (0358)
    Omodysplasia (3280)

Major Diagnostic Criteria: Rhizomelia of humeri, **Microcephaly**, saddle nose and congenital heart disease.

Clinical Findings: *Craniofacial:* **Microcephaly**; large anterior fontanelle; fine, sparse scalp hair; macroglossia; saddle nose; high-arched palate; micrognathia; short neck.

Skeletal: Short stature plus flat, thoracic vertebrae and abnormally shaped epiphyses of long bones; rhizomelia of humeri plus flared epiphyses; kyphosis; dislocated hips plus flat acetabulae; flexion contracture; digitalization of thumb plus bifid distal phalanx; clinodactyly plus hypoplasia of terminal phalanges of hands

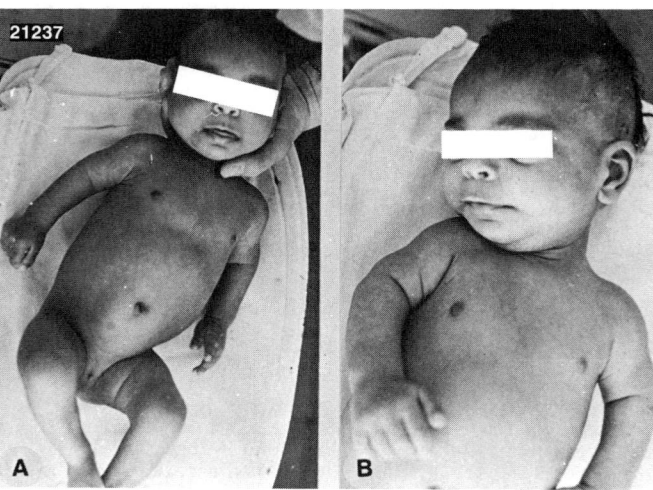

2816A-21237: Proband at four months shows microcephaly, macroglossia, short proximal upper extremities, flexion contracture of the knees, micrognathia, saddle nose and digitalization of the right thumb with a broad nail.

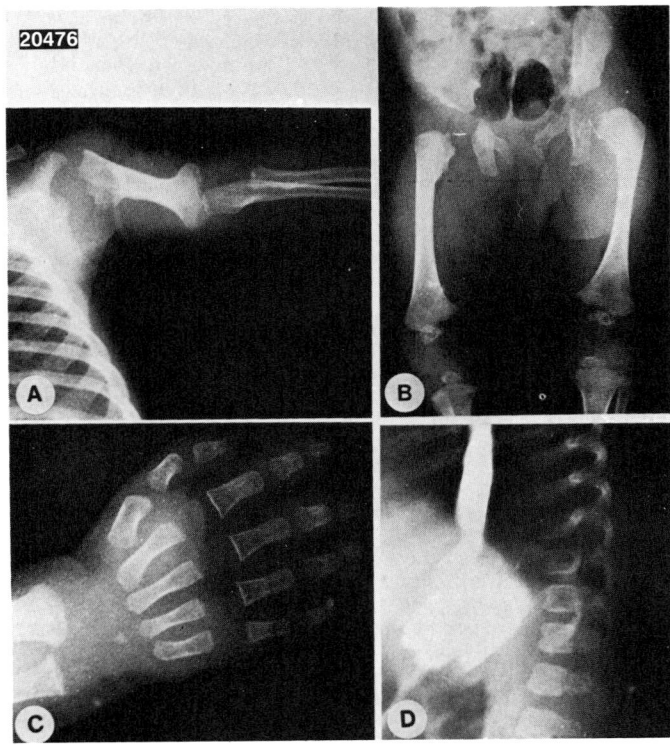

2816B-20476: Rhizomelic syndrome: A. Rhizomelia of humerus with flared epiphysis. B. Dislocated hips with flat acetabulae. C. Digitalization of the thumb with bifid distal phalanx. D. Flat thoracic vertebrae.

and feet; prominent calcaneous; additional irregular centers of epiphyses about the knees.

Other: Pulmonic stenosis, seborrheic dermatitis, and mental retardation.

Complications: Unknown.

Associated Findings: Short stature, mental retardation, and congenital heart disease.

Etiology: Possibly autosomal recessive inheritance. The parents of the first reported cases were consanguineous, but the precise relationship is not known.

Pathogenesis: Unknown.

MIM No.: 26825

POS No.: 3064

Sex Ratio: Presumably M1:F1.

Occurrence: Three siblings from one Arab family have been documented.

Risk of Recurrence for Patient's Sib:
See Part I, *Mendelian Inheritance.*

Risk of Recurrence for Patient's Child:
See Part I, *Mendelian Inheritance.*

Age of Detectability: *In utero* by ultrasound at five months gestation.

Gene Mapping and Linkage: Unknown.

Prevention: None known. Genetic counseling indicated.

Treatment: Symptomatic.

Prognosis: Unknown.

Detection of Carrier: Unknown.

Special Considerations: P. Maroteaux has proposed the term **Omodysplasia** based upon the Greek term for humerus, as a name for a disorder of variable expressivity in which hypoplasia of the distal humerus and subluxation of the radial head are major features. Omodysplasia is phenotypically distinct from the syndrome described above.

References:
Urbach D, et al.: A new skeletal dysplasia syndrome with rhizomelia of the humeri and other malformations. Clin Genet 1986; 29:83–87.

G0026   **Richard M. Goodman**

RHS syndrome
    See SMITH-LEMLI-OPITZ SYNDROME
Rib gap defects-micrognathia
    See CEREBRO-COSTO-MANDIBULAR SYNDROME
Ribbing disease
    See DIAPHYSEAL DYSPLASIA
Rice ear wax
    See EAR, CERUMEN VARIATIONS
Richner-Hanhart Syndrome
    See TYROSINEMIA II, OREGON TYPE
Rickets, familial vitamin D-resistant
    See HYPOPHOSPHATEMIA, X-LINKED
Rickets, hereditary hypocalcemic type IIa
    See RESISTANCE TO 1,25 DIHYDROXY VITAMIN D

**RICKETS, HEREDITARY HYPOPHOSPHATEMIC WITH
HYPERCALCIURIA (HHRH)**   **3020**

Includes:
    HHRH
    Hypercalciuria, idiopathic (some forms)
    Hypercalciuric rickets
    Hypophosphatemic rickets with hypercalciuria
Excludes:
    Hypercalciuria, familial idiopathic (2302)
    Hypophosphatemia, non X-linked (2040)
    Hypophosphatemia, X-linked (0517)
    Oncogenic hypophosphatemic osteomalacia

Major Diagnostic Criteria: Rickets/osteomalacia and elevated serum alkaline phosphatase; low serum phosphorus for age, elevated urine excretion and renal clearance of phosphate, and low TmP/GFR; elevated urine calcium excretion (0.30 g/g creatinine) and intestinal absorption of calcium; elevated plasma 1,25-$(OH)_2D$ for season and age; serum iPTH normal to low normal.

Clinical Findings: Onset of the disease is during early childhood in the homozygous phenotype. Signs and symptoms of rickets (in growing persons) and osteomalacia. Hypercalciuria, urinary tract calculi, and nephrolithiasis ("idiopathic hypercalciuria") can be the principal disease in heterozygotes.

Complications: Those of rickets/osteomalacia (pseudofractures, deformities, short stature, muscle weakness) and chronic hypercalciuria (urinary calculi and nephrolithiasis).

Associated Findings: None known.

Etiology: "Incomplete" autosomal recessive inheritance for bone disease. Autosomal dominant inheritance for hypercalciuria.

Pathogenesis: All manifestations can be explained by a selective impairment of phosphate reabsorption in the proximal nephron (convoluted segment) causing low serum phosphorus, elevated phosphate clearance, and low TmP/GFR. An adaptive response with increased renal synthesis of 1,25-$(OH)_2D$ causes the high serum hormone value. Increased hormone causes enhanced calcium absorption (intestine) and excretion (kidney), without hyperparathyroidism. Phosphorous deficiency causes defective bone mineralization and growth.

MIM No.: *24153

Sex Ratio: Presumably M1:F1; M2:F1 observed.

Occurrence: Nine members of one Bedouin pedigree have been documented. Other cases have been described in France, Japan, and a Bedouin tribe.

Risk of Recurrence for Patient's Sib:
See Part I, *Mendelian Inheritance.*

Risk of Recurrence for Patient's Child:
See Part I, *Mendelian Inheritance.*

Age of Detectability: Reported cases detected in early childhood. Could be detected as early as infancy.

Gene Mapping and Linkage: Unknown.

Prevention: None known. Genetic counseling indicated.

Treatment: Phosphate supplement in diet (1–2.5 g/day, in childhood, as neutral phosphate salts in four to five divided doses).

Prognosis: Excellent for normal mineralization of hard tissues and growth (with early therapy and good compliance). Life long treatment (age-adjusted dosage) is indicated.

Detection of Carrier: Carriers (presumed heterozygotes) have elevated urine calcium excretion (the "idiopathic hypercalciuria" phenotype), slightly depressed fasting serum phosphorus, slightly elevated plasma 1,25-$(OH)_2$D levels (>95 pg/ml), and low normal TmP/GFR (>1.15 SD units below normal mean).

Special Considerations: This condition has importance beyond its frequency. The homozygous phenotype has been observed in only nine members of one Bedouin tribe containing 21 presumed (or obligate) heterozygotes (Tieder et al., 1985, 1987) and perhaps also in one Japanese person (Nishiyama et al., 1986) and European cases (Tieder & Stark, 1979; Chen et al, 1989). The phenotype is important because 1) it demonstrates the predicted adaptive response to phosphate depletion (increased renal synthesis of 1,25-$(OH)_2$D); and 2) it identifies a gene product, probably at another cellular location in the proximal nephron different from those controlled by X-linked loci and another autosomal locus which also determine phosphate homeostasis (see **Hypophosphatemia, X-linked** and **Hypercalciuria, familial idiopathic**).

References:
Tieder M, Stark H: Forme familiale d'hypercalciurie idiopathique avec nanism, atteinte osseuse et renale chez l'enfant. Helv Paediat Acta 1979; 34:359–367.
Tieder M, et al.: Hereditary hypophosphatemic rickets with hypercalciuria. New Engl J Med 1985; 312:611–617.
Nishiyama S, et al.: A single case of hypophosphatemic rickets with hypercalciuria. J Pediatr Gastroenterol Nutr 1986; 5:826–829.
Tieder M, et al.: "Idiopathic" hypercalciuria and hereditary hypophosphatemic rickets. New Engl J Med 1987; 316:611–617.
Chen C, et al.: Hypercalciuric hypophosphatemic rickets, mineral balance, bone histomorphology, and therapeutic implications of hypercalciuria. Pediatrics 1989; 84:276–280.

SC050   **Charles R. Scriver**

Rickets, hereditary hypophosphatemic with hypercalciuria (some)
See HYPERCALCIURIA, FAMILIAL IDIOPATHIC

RICKETS, VITAMIN D-DEPENDENT, TYPE I   0873

Includes:
> Autosomal recessive vitamin D-dependency (ARVDD)
> Hypocalcemic, hypophosphatemic rickets with aminoaciduria
> Pseudovitamin D-deficiency rickets (PDR), hereditary
> Renal 25-hydroxyvitamin D1-hydroxylase deficiency
> Vitamin D-dependent rickets, hereditary
> Vitamin D-dependent rickets, type I
> Vitamin D-dependent rickets, type III, aminoaciduria

Excludes:
> **Cystinosis** (0238)
> **Hypophosphatemia, X-linked** (0517)
> Hypophosphatemic rickets associated with glucosuria
> Hypophosphatemic rickets associated with renal tubular acidosis
> **Rickets, hereditary hypophosphatemic with hypercalciuria (HHRH)** (3020)
> Rickets, vitamin D-deficient

Major Diagnostic Criteria: Radiologic rickets with hypocalcemia, aminoaciduria, and elevated alkaline phosphatase. The vitamin D requirement is usually 20,000 to 100,000 IU daily, considerably greater than that needed to prevent vitamin D-deficiency rickets. Exclusion of other disorders, including intestinal malabsorption, renal insufficiency, and renal tubular abnormalities. Concentrations in blood of 25-hydroxyvitamin D (25-[OH]D) are normal or elevated, and concentrations of 1,25-dihydroxyvitamin D (1,25-[OH]D) are low.

Clinical Findings: Clinical manifestations are similar to those of vitamin D-deficiency rickets. Symptoms usually appear before age one year and may occur as early as the first months of life. They include hypotonia, weakness, and growth failure. Motor retardation may be apparent or real. Enamel defects are seen in teeth that calcify postnatally. Pathologic fractures may occur. Later, bony deformities develop. Convulsions or tetany may be the presenting clinical feature. Rickets with a reliable history of adequate intake of vitamin D may be a clue to the diagnosis.

Prominent physical findings are shortness of stature, hypotonia, and the characteristic features of rickets, including thickening of the wrists and ankles, frontal bowing of lower limbs and positive Trousseau and Chvostek signs. X-ray findings are those of classic rickets. They may vary in severity, and they are indistinguishable from those of vitamin D-deficiency rickets.

The serum concentration of calcium is low, and serum phosphate level is low or normal. The levels of alkaline phosphatase and parathyroid hormone are elevated. Generalized aminoaciduria is characteristic.

Urinary cyclic AMP is elevated. GI absorption of calcium is depressed. Antirachitic activity as measured by bioassay is normal. Serum concentrations of 1,25-dihydroxyvitamin D_3 are low, while those of 25-(OH)D are normal or elevated.

Complications: Rachitic deformities, growth failure.

Associated Findings: Hypotonia, muscle weakness, tetany, convulsions. Enamel hypoplasia of teeth that form postnatally.

Etiology: Autosomal recessive inheritance.

Pathogenesis: A genetic defect in renal 25-hydroxycholecalciferol 1-hydroxylase, the enzyme responsible for the conversion of 25-hydroxyvitamin D to 1,25-dihydroxyvitamin D. This results in an attenuated response to normal amounts of vitamin D and the development of classic rickets and hypocalcemia.

MIM No.: *26470

POS No.: 3263

Sex Ratio: M1:F1

Occurrence: Over a half-dozen kindreds reported.

Risk of Recurrence for Patient's Sib:
See Part I, *Mendelian Inheritance.*

Risk of Recurrence for Patient's Child:
See Part I, *Mendelian Inheritance.*

Age of Detectability: Usually before age two years, and as early as the third or fourth month of life.

Gene Mapping and Linkage: VDD1 (vitamin D dependency 1) has been provisionally mapped to 12q14.

Prevention: None known. Genetic counseling indicated.

Treatment: Pharmacologic doses of vitamin D are required, and small physiologic quantities of 1,25-(OH)D or calcitriol are effective. Doses are 0.25 to 2.0 μg/day. Calcium therapy for hypocalcemic tetany or convulsions. Orthopedic correction of deformities.

Prognosis: Treatment results in complete healing of rickets, with normalization of plasma calcium and phosphate concentrations, remission of muscle hypotonia and weakness, and normalization of growth. Continuous treatment is required throughout childhood and probably for life.

Detection of Carrier: Unknown.

References:
Fraser D, Salter RB: The diagnosis and management of the various types of rickets. Pediatr Clin North Am 1958; 5:417–441.
Prader A, et al.: Eine besondere Form der primaeren Vitamin-D-

resistenten Rachitis mit Hypocalcaemie und autosomal-dominantem Erbgang: die Hereditaere Pseudo-mangelrachitis. Helv Paediatr Acta 1961; 16:452–468.

Fraser D, et al.: Pathogenesis of hereditary vitamin-D-dependent rickets: an inborn error of vitamin D metabolism involving defective conversion of 25-hydroxyvitamin D to 1-alpha, 25-dihydroxyvitamin D. New Engl J Med 1973; 289:817–822.

Balsan S, et al.: 1,25-Dihydroxyvitamin D, and 1,α-hydroxyvitamin D$_3$ in children: biologic and therapeutic effects in nutritional rickets and different types of vitamin D resistance. Pediatr Res 1975; 9:586–593.

Delvin EE, et al.: Vitamin D dependency: replacement therapy with calcitriol. J Pediatr 1981; 99:26–34.

Liberman UA, et al.: Resistance to 1,25-dihydroxyvitamin D: association with heterogeneous defects in cultured skin fibroblasts. J Clin Invest 1983; 71:192–200.

Nyhan WL: Diagnostic recognition of genetic disease. Philadelphia: Lea & Febiger, 1987:253–271. *

NY000   **William L. Nyhan**

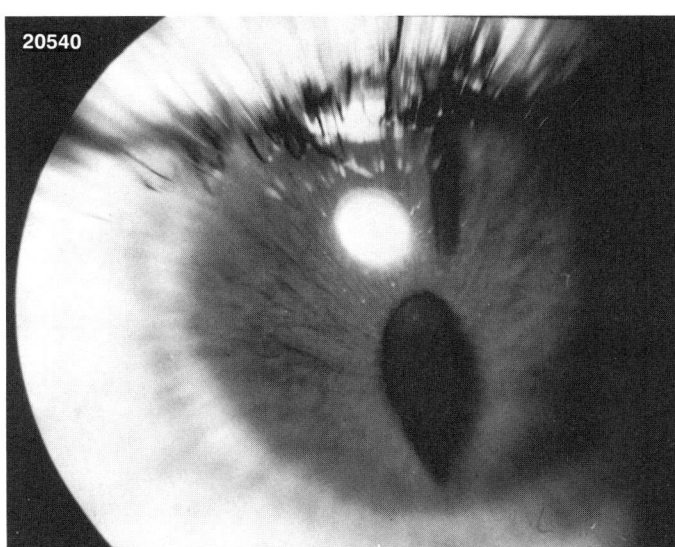

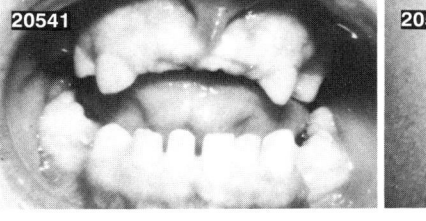 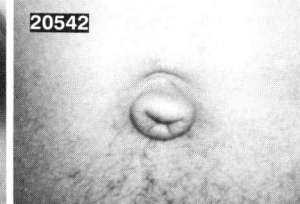

2139-20540: Rieger syndrome; note goniodysgenesis with irregular pupil. 20541: Hypodontia with absence of the incisors. 20542: Note failure of involution of the periumbilical skin.

RIEGER SYNDROME   2139

Includes:
 Goniodysgenesis-hypodontia
 Hypodontia-mesoectodermal dysgenesis of iris and cornea
 Iridogoniodysgenesis with somatic anomalies

Excludes:
 Axenfeld syndrome
 Eye, anterior segment dysgenesis (0439)

Major Diagnostic Criteria: Goniodysgenesis and hypodontia.

Clinical Findings: Affected individuals have mesodermal dysgenesis of the iris and cornea, congenital absence of the incisors and occasionally the premolars, and maxillary hypoplasia which is manifest as a flat midface.

Complications: Glaucoma, ectopic pupils.

Associated Findings: Failure of involution of the periumbilical skin.

Etiology: Autosomal dominant inheritance.

Pathogenesis: Undetermined, although a primary defect in the mesoderm could explain all features.

MIM No.: *18050

POS No.: 3380

Sex Ratio: M1:F1

Occurrence: Undetermined; extensive literature.

Risk of Recurrence for Patient's Sib:
 See Part I, *Mendelian Inheritance.*

Risk of Recurrence for Patient's Child:
 See Part I, *Mendelian Inheritance.*

Age of Detectability: Neonatal period if structural eye defects are visible, otherwise in early childhood because of visual difficulties or dental defects.

Gene Mapping and Linkage: Unknown.

Prevention: None known. Genetic counseling indicated.

Treatment: Early diagnosis offers the possibility to ameliorate the effects of glaucoma. Prostheses for incomplete dentition.

Prognosis: Good for life span and intelligence, but deteriorating vision may lead to total blindness.

Detection of Carrier: Unknown.

Special Considerations: Since many syndromes have been reported under the heading of Rieger syndrome, there is some confusion over the physical stigmata that are associated with it. In one series, for example, a number of patients with failure of involution of the periumbilical skin were thought to have herniae and were subjected to surgery unnecessarily.

References:

Rieger H: Beiträge zur Kenntniss seltener Mosbildungen der Iris. Graefe Arch Ophthalmol 1935; 133:602–635.

Alkemade PPH: Dysgenesis mesodermalis of the iris and cornea. Assen (Netherlands): Van Gorcum, 1969.

Fitch N, Kaback M: The Axenfeld syndrome and the Rieger syndrome. J Med Genet 1978; 15:30–34.

Jorgenson RJ, et al.: The Rieger syndrome. Am J Med Genet 1978; 2:307–318. * †

Chisholm IA, Chudley AE: Autosomal dominant iridogoniodysgenesis with associated somatic anomalies: four generation family with Rieger's syndrome. Br J Ophthal 1983; 67:529–534. †

J0027   **Ronald J. Jorgenson**

Right ventricular obstruction by aberrant muscular bands
  See VENTRICLE, DOUBLE CHAMBERED RIGHT
Right ventricular subinfundibular obstruction
  See VENTRICLE, DOUBLE CHAMBERED RIGHT
Rigid spine syndrome
  See HAUPTMANN-THANHAUSER SYNDROME
Riley-Day syndrome
  See DYSAUTONOMIA I, RILEY-DAY TYPE
Riley-Smith syndrome
  *See OVERGROWTH, MACROCEPHALY-HEMANGIOMA,
    RILEY-SMITH TYPE*
Ring 6
  See CHROMOSOME 6, RING 6
Ring 9
  See CHROMOSOME 9, RING 9
Ring 14
  See CHROMOSOME 14, RING 14
Ring 15
  See CHROMOSOME 15, RING 15
Ring 18
  See CHROMOSOME 18, RING 18
Ring 21
  See CHROMOSOME 21, RING 21
Ring 22
  See CHROMOSOME 22, RING 22
Ring-like corneal dystrophy
  See CORNEAL DYSTROPHY, REIS-BUCKLERS TYPE

ROBERTS SYNDROME   0875

Includes:

  Appelt-Gerken-Lenz syndrome
  Bone, absence deformities of long-cleft lip/palate
  Centromere abnormalities-chromatid apposition-Roberts
    spectrum
  Centromere spreading
  Centromere separation, premature
  Chromosome, abnormal centromere and chromatid
    apposition
  Limbs, deformities of long bones-cleft lip/palate
  Pseudothalidomide-SC syndrome
  Pseudothalidomide syndrome
  Roberts syndrome spectrum
  SC phocomelia syndrome
  Tetraphocomelia-ocular defects-cleft lip/palate-penile
    anomalies

Excludes:

  Caudal regression syndrome (3211)
  Femoral hypoplasia-unusual facies syndrome (2027)
  Fetal thalidomide syndrome (0386)
  Heart-hand syndrome (0455)

Major Diagnostic Criteria: Cytogenetic evidence of abnormal centromere and chromatid apposition (ACCA) or "puffing apart" in heterochromatic and centromeric regions of multiple chromosomes, usually most evident in acrocentric chromosomes and the long arms of chromosome Y. Interface nuclear morphology in fibroblasts is often disturbed and shows abnormal nuclear contours (blebbing) and micronuclei. The clinical signs of patients with ACCA are variable. Historically, the term, Roberts syndrome, is applied to patients with severe mid-facial clefting, hypoplastic nasal alae, facial hemangioma, ocular defects (mainly vascularization of the cornea) and absence/shortness-type limb malformations. A more severe spectrum of congenital malformations is found among stillborns, while in milder cases, facial clefts and limb defects are absent. Growth failure is severe in prenatal and postnatal life.

Clinical Findings: Among affected stillborns, abnormal brain segmentation, interocular encephaloceles, severe ocular malformations, maxillary agenesis, agenesis of nostrils, severe renal dysplasia, polycystic kidneys, and spina bifida have been found. Severely affected neonates characteristically have hypoplastic alae nasi, severe mid-facial clefts, and severe tetraphocomelia constituting the *Roberts syndrome* phenotype. In children who survive infancy, facial hemangioma, vascularized cornea, or microoph-

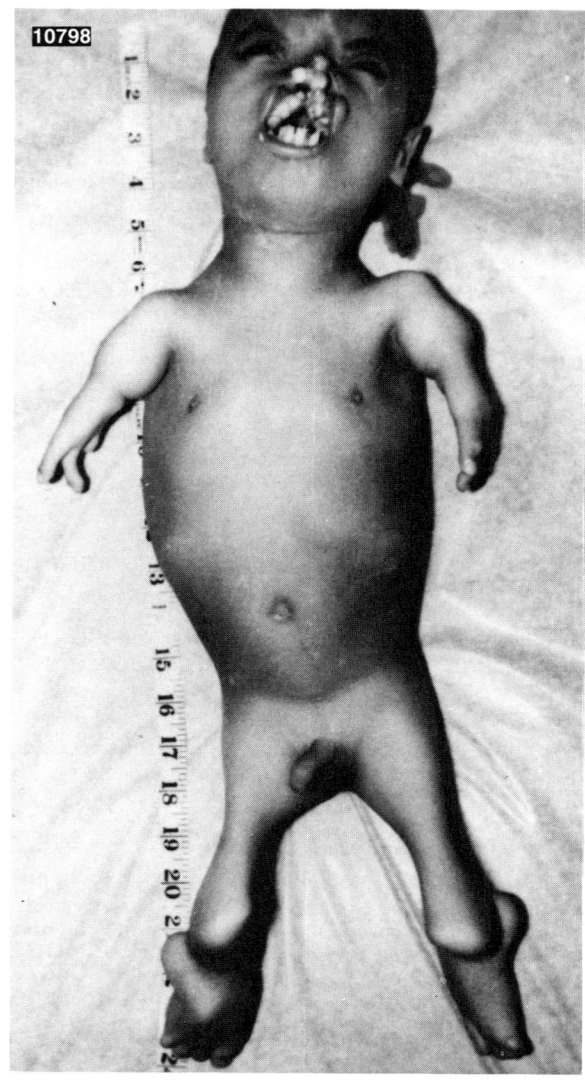

0875-10798: Note cleft lip and palate with protrusion of premaxilla and limb defects with shortened and deformed limbs.

thalmia, hypoplastic nasal alae (facial clefts are uncommon), micrognathia, mild mental retardation, severe failure to thrive, and milder degrees of tetraphocomelia were described as the *SC Phocomelia* or *Pseudothalidomide syndrome* or phenotype. The mildest clinical spectrum consists of stigmatic facies, vascularized cornea (Peters anomaly; see **Eye, anterior segment dysgenesis**), and mild mental retardation. Growth failure, mental retardation, ocular defects, and prominent penile or clitoral shaft are seen in severely and mildly affected patients.

Birth weight and length can be strikingly subnormal, and subsequent growth drastically lagging. Recorded birth weights of near term infants are illustrative (0.9, 1.04, 1.3, 1.4, 1.6 and 1.8 kg), as are small weights of survivors (at ages seven and 16 years the weight was 7.6 and 5.8 kg, respectively). The limb reduction defects invariably involve all four extremities, tend to be symmetric, and more severe in the upper limbs. The number of fingers is often reduced, radial aplasia or dysplasia is common, and lack of the first metacarpal, thumb, or first phalanx is frequent.

Frontal and interocular encephaloceles, maxillary agenesis, Peters anomaly, severe facial mid-line clefts, agenesis or hypoplastic nostrils, and hypoplastic alae nasi probably reflect the same pathogenesis. One mentally retarded patient with ACCA had no signs of Peters anomaly.

Among survivors, one female had her menarche at 11 years, later married and became pregnant but miscarried in the first trimester. Another female (IQ 70) experienced a full-term pregnancy at the age of 24, delivered a healthy girl, and later developed a malignant melanoma at the age of 32. She was also noted to have hypoplastic iris and scleralization of the peripheral cornea, dysmorphic facies, hypoplasia of the nasal tip, and nasal alae, no facial clefts, and multiple skeletal malformations affecting all limbs; her similarly affected sister died at 43, following a massive stroke.

Complications: Prenatal or perinatal death; respiratory and feeding difficulties related to cleft lip and palate; physical limitations due to limb defects; visual difficulties due to ocular malformations resulting from abnormal cleavage of the anterior chamber (Peter Anomaly); mental subnormality.

Associated Findings: High mortality among severely affected; mental retardation; failure-to-thrive; and decreased vision. One 23-month-old developed sarcoma botryoides, and a 32-year-old developed malignant melanoma.

Etiology: Autosomal recessive inheritance. Clinical heterogeneity is significant.

Pathogenesis: Unknown.

MIM No.: *26830

POS No.: 3378

Sex Ratio: M1:F1

Occurrence: At least 28 patients from 16 sibships demonstrating ACCA have been reported. Noted in many ethnic groups.

Risk of Recurrence for Patient's Sib:
See Part I, *Mendelian Inheritance.*

Risk of Recurrence for Patient's Child:
See Part I, *Mendelian Inheritance.*

Age of Detectability: Usually at birth, but possible prenatally by elevated maternal serum alpha-fetoprotein or by ultrasound confirming severe fetal failure to thrive, facial clefting, **Microcephaly**, and/or shortened extremeties. Incidental detection of ACCA in amniocytes has also led to the detection of a patient with mild manifestations.

Gene Mapping and Linkage: Unknown.

Prevention: None known. Genetic counseling indicated.

Treatment: Surgical repair of facial and limb defects and corneal grafts; special education.

Prognosis: Increased perinatal mortality among those severely affected. Those with milder congenital malformations may not be at risk for a shortened life span.

Detection of Carrier: Unknown.

Special Considerations: The frequency of ACCA is highest in the heterochromatic procentric region of chromosomes 16, 13–15, 21–22, and long arm of the Y and is strikingly rare in chromosome 11. Such a consistent pattern suggests a constitutive defect common to various chromosomal regions. Utilization of CREST antikinetochore antibodies demonstrated normal antigenicity but unusually large stained kinetochore regions. This suggests the presence of a decondensed or structurally altered kinetochore; a feature noticeable in metaphase but also in interphase cells. Cocultivation of patient and normal fibroblasts did not correct ACCA. Fusion hybrids (patient fibroblasts with Chinese hamster cell lines) apparently supplied the missing gene product needed to correct ACCA.

References:
Freeman MVR, et al.: The Roberts syndrome. Clin Genet 1974; 5:1–16.
Hermann J, Opitz JM: The SC phocomelia and the Roberts syndrome, vol. V: nosologic aspects. Eur J Pediatr 1977; 125:117–134.
Wertelecki W, et al.: Abnormal centromere-chromatid aposition (ACCA) and Peters anomaly. Ophthal Pediatr Genet 1985; 6:247–255. †
Krassikoff NE, et al.: Chromatid repulsion associated with Roberts/SC

phocomelia syndrome is reduced in malignant cells and not expressed in interspecies somatic-cell hybrids. Am J Hum Genet 1986; 39:618–630.
Parry DM, et al.: SC phocomelia syndrome, premature centramere separation and congenital cranial nerve paralysis in two sisters, one with malignant melanoma. Am J Med Genet 1986; 24:653–672.
Fryns JP, et al.: The Robert tetraphocomelia syndrome: identical limb defects in two siblings. Ann Genet 1987; 30:243–245.
Romke C, et al.: Roberts syndrome and SC phocamelia: a single genetic entity. Clin Genet 1987; 31:170–177. †
Jabs EW, et al.: Centromere separation and aneuploidy in human mitotic mutants: Roberts syndrome. In: Resnick M, Vig B, eds: Mechanisms of chromosome distribution and aneuploidy. New York: Alan R. Liss, 1989;111–118.
Robins DB, et al.: Prenatal detection of Roberts-SC phocomelia syndrome. Am J Med Genet 1989; 32:390–394.

WE029   **W. Wertelecki**

Roberts syndrome spectrum
See ROBERTS SYNDROME
Robertsonian translocation
See CHROMOSOME 13, TRISOMY 13
Robin anomaly (some)
See ARTHRO-OPHTHALMOPATHY, HEREDITARY, PROGRESSIVE, STICKLER TYPE
Robin anomaly, isolated
See CLEFT PALATE-MICROGNATHIA-GLOSSOPTOSIS
Robin sequence
See CLEFT PALATE-MICROGNATHIA-GLOSSOPTOSIS
Robin sequence with hyperphalangy
See DIGITO-PALATAL SYNDROME, STEVENSON TYPE
Robin sequence-aniridia-growth delay (RAG)
See RAG SYNDROME

ROBINOW SYNDROME   0876

Includes:
    Acral dysostosis-facial and genital abnormalities
    Costovertebral segmentation defect-mesomelia
    COVESDEM syndrome
    Dwarfism, mesomelic Robinow type
    Fetal face syndrome
    Mesomelic dysplasia, type Robinow
    Robinow-Silverman-Smith syndrome

Excludes:
    Aarskog syndrome (0001)
    Mesomelic skeletal dysplasias (other)
    Micropenis, in other conditions

Major Diagnostic Criteria: Most patients show at least three of the following four anomalies: the "fetal face," genital hypoplasia, forearm brachymelia, and moderate dwarfing.

Clinical Findings: *Fetal face:* So termed because it resembles the face of the fetus at eight weeks. The neurocranium is disproportionately large, while the viscerocranium is hypoplastic. Characteristic features are a bulging forehead; moderate hypertelorism; wide palpebral fissures; a short, upturned nose; and a broad, inverted V-shaped mouth. The facial characteristics become less striking at puberty.
Genital hypoplasia: In the male, the penis is often invisible in infancy and childhood unless the surrounding skin is retracted. Testicles are usually of normal size, although frequently undescended. During puberty the glans penis attains normal size, but the shaft remains unduly short. Nevertheless, sexual functioning is possible and procreation has been repeatedly documented. Androgen receptors and 5-α reductase of genital skin fibroblasts have been normal.
In the female, the clitoris and labia minora are hypoplastic. Sexual maturation and reproduction are normal. The pelvis is large enough to permit spontaneous vaginal delivery.
Forearm brachymelia: Usually obvious, sometimes demonstrable only by measurement, rarely absent. Mesomelic shortness of the lower extremities is less marked or absent.

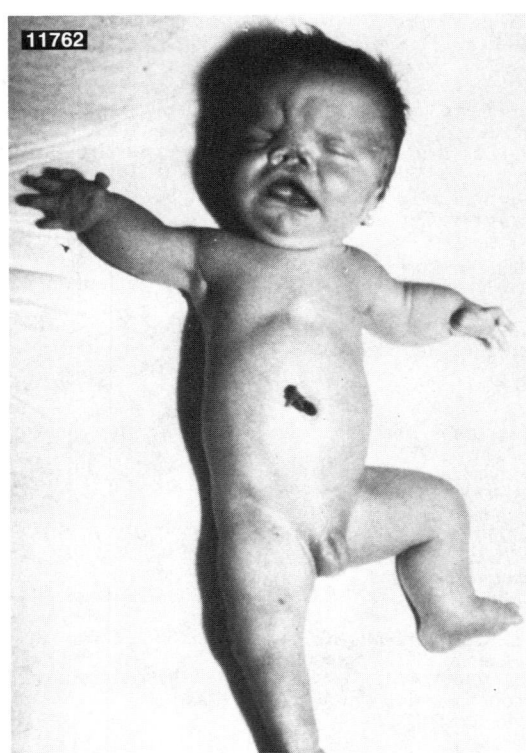

0876A-11762: Infant with characteristic triangular facies with broad forehead and forearm brachmelia.

Moderate dwarfing: Stature past infancy has ranged from the mean to -8 SD, and has averaged -3.1 SD.

Intelligence: Normal in most cases, mildly reduced in some, and severely impaired in a few.

Common but less frequent findings: Inguinal hernias, vertebral

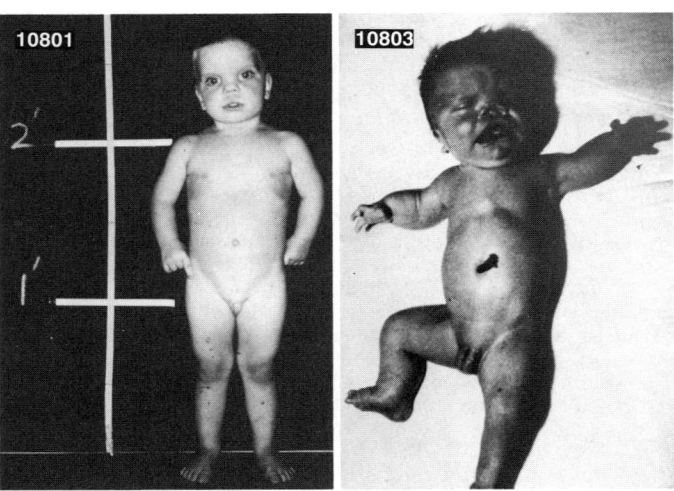

0876B-10801: Prominent forehead, ocular hypertelorism, short upturned nose, triangular mouth and brachymelia. **10803:** Affected infant shows similar facial features, very short forearms, severe penile hypoplasia.

segmentation defects, radial head dislocation, acromelic brachymelia (short metacarpals and phalanges), bifid or duplicated thumbs or big toes, ankyloglossia, crowding and malalignment of the anterior teeth, gingival hyperplasia, and delayed eruption of permanent teeth.

Complications: Scoliosis secondary to vertebral anomalies.

Associated Findings: Congenital heart disease (10% or less), cleft lip and palate, dislocated hips, hepatosplenomegaly, hyperostosis.

Etiology: Autosomal dominant or recessive inheritance. The two forms are usually distinct clinically and on X-ray. Most sporadic cases can be assigned to one of the two forms, although additional heterogeneity cannot be ruled out.

Patients with the recessive form (once called *Costovertebral segmentation defect with mesomellia,* or *COVESDEM*) tend to be more severely dwarfed, have more extensive vertebral anomalies, and more severe brachymelia. The recessive form is often associated with radio-ulnar dislocation and severe hypoplasia of the proximal radius and distal ulna.

Pathogenesis: The association of anomalies suggests a disturbance of embryogenesis around the 8th week.

MIM No.: *18070

POS No.: 3379

Sex Ratio: Probably M1:F1, although males are more likely to be recognized and reported because of the striking penile hypoplasia.

Occurrence: About 1:500,000, i.e., about six new cases per year in the United States. Prevalence slightly lower, since 5–10% of patients have died in infancy or early childhood. Some 41 published and 35 unpublished cases have been reviewed.

Risk of Recurrence for Patient's Sib:
See Part I, *Mendelian Inheritance.*

Risk of Recurrence for Patient's Child:
See Part I, *Mendelian Inheritance.*

Age of Detectability: At birth.

Gene Mapping and Linkage: Unknown.

Prevention: None known. Genetic counseling indicated.

Treatment: Orthopedic care for vertebral anomalies. Surgery for undescended testicles and inguinal hernias, orthodontia for dental malalignment, facial reconstruction in selected cases, psychologic support. Testosterone therapy for micropenis has not proven helpful.

Prognosis: Facial dysmorphism becomes less striking with age. Sexual functioning and reproduction appear good for both sexes, although male reproduction in the recessive form has not yet been documented.

Detection of Carrier: Unknown.

References:
Robinow M, et al.: A newly recognized dwarfing syndrome. Am J Dis Child 1969; 117:645–651.
Wadlington WB, et al.: Mesomelic dwarfism with hemivertebrae and small genitalia (the Robinow syndrome). Am J Dis Child 1973; 126:202–205.
Giedion A, et al.: The radiologic diagnosis of the fetal face (Robinow) syndrome (mesomelic dwarfism and small genitalia): report of 3 cases. Helv Paediatr Acta 1975; 30:409–423.
Lee PA, et al.: Robinow's syndrome: partial primary hypogonadism in pubertal boys, with persistence of micropenis. Am J Dis Child 1982; 136:327–330.
Shprintzen RJ, et al.: Male-to-male transmission of Robinow's syndrome: its occurrence in association with cleft lip and cleft palate. Am J Dis Child 1982; 136:594–597.
Bain MD, et al.: Robinow syndrome without mesomelic "brachymelia": report of 5 cases. J Med Genet 1986; 23:350–354.
Robinow M, Markert RJ: The fetal face (Robinow) syndrome: delineation of the dominant and recessive phenotypes. Proc Greenwood Genet Ctr 1988; 7:144 only.

R0004   **Meinhard Robinow**

Robinow-Silverman-Smith syndrome
  See ROBINOW SYNDROME
Robinow-Sorauf syndrome
  See CRANIOSYNOSTOSIS-FOOT DEFECTS, JACKSON-WEISS TYPE
Robinson ectodermal dysplasia-deafness
  *See ONYCHODYSTROPHY-CONIFORM TEETH-SENSORINEURAL
    HEARING LOSS*
Rod body myopathy
  See MYOPATHY, NEMALINE
Rod monochromatism
  See COLOR BLINDNESS, TOTAL
Rod-cone dystrophy
  See RETINITIS PIGMENTOSA
Rogers syndrome
  See HEART-HAND SYNDROME IV
Rokitansky sequence
  See MULLERIAN APLASIA
Rokitansky-Kuster-Hauser syndrome
  See MULLERIAN APLASIA
Rolandic epilepsy
  *See EPILEPSY, BENIGN CHILDHOOD WITH CENTROTEMPORAL
    EEG FOCUS (BEC)*
Rolland-Desbuquois syndrome
  See DWARFISM, DYSSEGMENTAL, ROLLAND-DESBUQUOIS TYPE
Romano-Ward syndrome
  *See ARRHYTHMIA, WITH LONG QT INTERVAL WITHOUT
    DEAFNESS*
Romberg syndrome
  See HEMIFACIAL ATROPHY, PROGRESSIVE
Rootless teeth
  See TEETH, DENTIN DYSPLASIA, RADICULAR
Roots, acquired concrescence of
  See TEETH, ROOT CONCRESCENCE
Rosenberg-Chutorian syndrome
  See DEAFNESS-POLYNEUROPATHY-OPTIC ATROPHY
Rosenfeld-Kloepfer syndrome
  See PACHYDERMOPERIOSTOSIS
Rosewater syndrome
  See ANDROGEN INSENSITIVITY SYNDROME, INCOMPLETE
Rosselli-Gulienetti syndrome
  See CLEFT LIP/PALATE-ECTODERMAL DYSPLASIA-SYNDACTYLY

ROTHMUND-THOMSON SYNDROME   2037

Includes:
  Cataract-poikiloderma atrophicans
  Poikiloderma atrophicans-cataract
  Telangiectasia-pigmentation-cataract syndrome
  Telangiectatic erythema, congenital

Excludes:
  Bloom syndrome (0112)
  Cockayne syndrome (0189)
  Dermal hypoplasia, focal (0281)
  Osteodysplastica gerodermia, Bamatter type (2099)
  Werner syndrome (0998)

Major Diagnostic Criteria: Skin atrophy, pigmentation, and telangiectasia appearing from third to sixth month of life; bilateral cataracts appearing from the fourth to the seventh year; hypogonadism with short stature and bony defects.

Clinical Findings: Bilateral cataracts developing at about age 4–7 years. The skin is normal at birth but develops cutis telangiectasia and atrophy about the third to sixth month of life, especially in the extensor surfaces of the hands, forearms, legs, thighs, and buttocks, with exposed surfaces being more severely affected. Once the initial inflammatory stage disappears, the affected areas present a combination of pigmentation, depigmentation, atrophy, and telangiectasia. Alopecia has been reported in 35% of the patients. Warty dyskeratosis with malignant transformation has been reported, and 25% of the patients have hypogonadism and nail dystrophy. Over 50% have short stature. A few patients do not have abnormal thumbs. Oral manifestations include microdontia, tooth crown and root malformations, and delayed and ectopic eruption.

Complications: Severe vision loss or blindness occurs within a few weeks as a result of the bilateral complete and semisolid eye cataracts. The small tooth roots cause the teeth to exfoliate

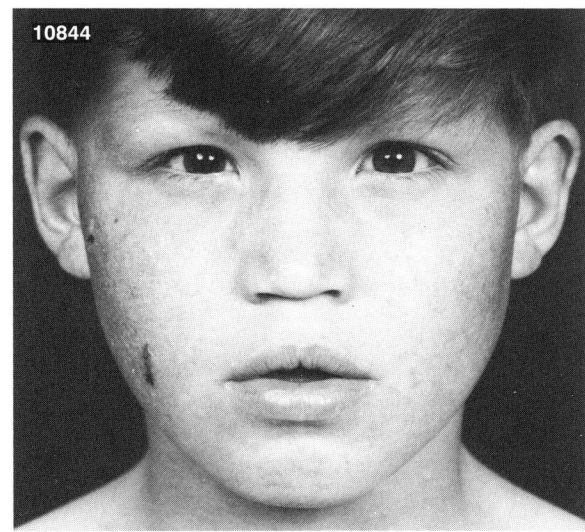

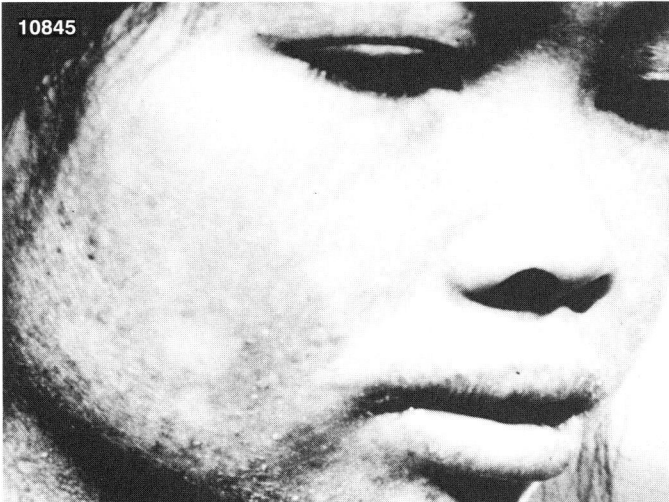

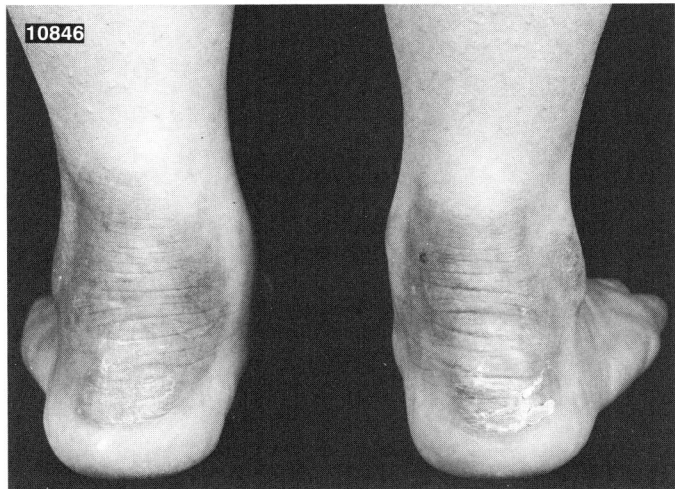

2037A-10844–46: Skin atrophy and hyperpigmentation.

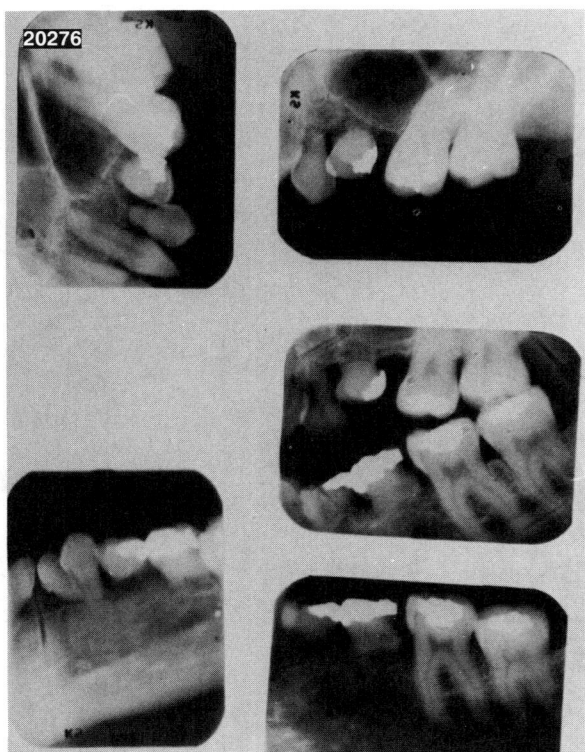

2037B-20276: Note short roots and bone loss.

prematurely. Blistered skin is frequently associated with sensitivity to sunlight.

Associated Findings: None known.

Etiology: Autosomal recessive inheritance, although over 70% of the patients have been female. The report of a mother and son with similar findings, however, raises the question of genetic heterogeneity.

Pathogenesis: Unknown.

MIM No.: *26840

POS No.: 3383

Sex Ratio: M3:F7

Occurrence: At least 65 patients have been documented, all Caucasians.

Risk of Recurrence for Patient's Sib:
See Part I, *Mendelian Inheritance.*

Risk of Recurrence for Patient's Child:
See Part I, *Mendelian Inheritance.*

Age of Detectability: Skin lesions develop by the third to sixth month of life, with confirmation as the child develops; eye problems by age 4–7 years.

Gene Mapping and Linkage: Unknown.

Prevention: None known. Genetic counseling indicated.

Treatment: Eye surgery, dental treatment.

Prognosis: Life span is within normal limits, unless squamous cell carcinoma is not identified. Reproduction seems to be impaired because of the scanty menstrual cycle in most affected females and juvenile genital organs in males. Nutrition may become important if these patients become edentulous. Early blindness should be anticipated.

Detection of Carrier: Unknown.

References:
Thomson MS: Poikiloderma congenitale. Br J Dermatol 1936; 48:221–234.
Bottomley WK, Box JM: Dental anomalies in the Rothmund-Thomson syndrome. Oral Surg 1976; 41:321–326.
Hall C, et al.: Rothmund-Thomson syndrome with severe dwarfism. Am J Dis Child 1980; 134:165–169. *
Dechenne C, et al.: A Rothmund-Thomson case with hypertension. Clin Genet 1983; 24:266–272.
Starr DG, et al.: Non-dermatological complications and genetic aspects of the Rothmund-Thomson syndrome. Clin Genet 1985; 27:102–104.

ES000   **Victor Escobar**

Rotor type hyperbilirubinemia
See HYPERBILIRUBINEMIA, CONJUGATED, ROTOR TYPE
Roussy-Levy syndrome
See NEUROPATHY, HEREDITARY MOTOR AND SENSORY, TYPE I
Rozycki syndrome
See DEAFNESS-VITILIGO-MUSCLE WASTING
Rubella malformation syndrome
See FETAL RUBELLA SYNDROME
Rubinstein syndrome
See RUBINSTEIN-TAYBI BROAD THUMB-HALLUX SYNDROME

RUBINSTEIN-TAYBI BROAD THUMB-HALLUX SYNDROME   0119

Includes:
>Brachydactyly-peculiar facies-mental retardation syndrome
>Broad thumb hallux syndrome
>Digitofacial-mental retardation syndrome
>Hallux-broad thumb syndrome
>Michail-Matsoukas-Theodorou-Rubinstein-Taybi syndrome
>Rubinstein syndrome
>Rubinstein-Taylor syndrome

Excludes:
>**Acrocephalosyndactyly type I** (0014)
>**Brachydactyly** (0114)

Major Diagnostic Criteria: No pathognomonic criterion has been found; however, the finding of broad terminal phalanges of the thumbs and hallucles, with or without angulation deformity; characteristic facial appearance with beaked or straight nose, broad nasal bridge, downward slant of palpebral fissures, peculiar "grimacing" smile and mild retrognathia; stature, head circumference, and bone age below the 50th percentile; mental, motor, language, and social retardation and incomplete or delayed descent of testes constitute the clinical syndrome.

Clinical Findings: *Developmental Defects*: Mental, motor, social and language retardation (100%); moderate to severe mental retardation (80%); growth defects: stature below 50th percentile (94%); stature at or below 3rd percentile (77%); bone age below 50th percentile (76%); head circumference below 50th percentile (93%); head circumference at or below 10th percentile (85%).
Cranio-Facial Defects: Highly arched palate (93%); Downward slanting of palpebral fissures (93%); beaked or straight nose (90%); apparent hypertelorism (85%); mild retrognathia (76%); abnormalities of external ear (74%); peculiar "grimacing" smile (72%); nasal septum extending below alae (72%); broad nasal bridge (71%); large anterior fontanel or delayed closure (64%); thick or highly arched eyebrows (56%); epicanthal folds (54%); prominent forehead (51%); parietal foramina (38%).
Digital Defects: Broad terminal phalanges of thumbs and/or hallucles (100%); broad terminal phalanges of other fingers (71%); abnormal thumb angulation with proximal (38%); phalanx anomalies; abnormal hallux angulation with anomalies of (20%); proximal phalanx or first metatarsal; duplicated distal phalanx of hallux (14%); duplicated proximal phalanx of hallux (10%).
Other Skeletal Defects: Stiff, awkward, unsteady gait (76%); pelvic vertebral anomalies (67%); large foramen magnum (65%); sternal or rib anomalies (56%); overlapping toes (54%); clinodactyly of 5th finger (54%).
Other Defects: Incomplete or delayed descent of testes (79%);

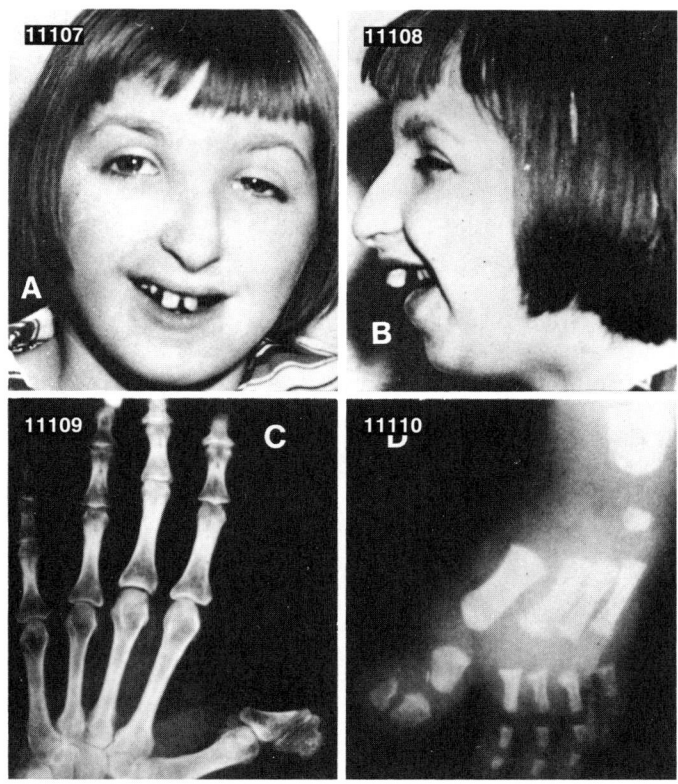

0119-11107: Facies at age 14 years shows downward slanting palpebral fissures, arched eyebrows, ptosis and prominent nose. **11108:** Lateral view of face shows beaked nose with nasal septum extending below alae and micrognathia. **11109:** Triangular and spatulate deformities of proximal and terminal phalanges. **11110:** Broad great toe with duplication of terminal phalanx.

strabismus (72%); EEG abnormalities (67%); hirsutism (64%); refractive error (63%); azygous or other abnormal lung lobation (53%); deep plantar crease in 1st interdigital area (53%); urinary tract disease and/or anomalies (50%); nevus flammeus of forehead, nape of neck or back (46%); simian crease (44%); long eyelashes (44%); congenital heart disease (36%); nasolacrimal duct obstruction (36%); heart murmur (33%); corpus callosum hypoplasia (28%) ptosis (18%); supernumerary nipples (13%).

Complications: Neonatal distress and/or recurrent respiratory tract infections (78%), feeding and swallowing difficulties in infancy (73%), gastroesophageal reflux, weak unusual cry in infancy; urinary tract infections, nephrolithiasis, hydronephrosis/hydroureter with or without reflux; stiff, awkward, unsteady gait; brisk tendon reflexes in lower limbs; inability to oppose thumb; EEG abnormalities, seizures, meningitis; relative obesity for height particularly involving the lower trunk; irregular crowded teeth, malocclusion; recurrent paronychiae; leukemia, brain tumor (ectopic pinealoma), and intraspinal neurilemoma. Stirt (1982) reported a risk of cardiac arrhythmia with the use of succinylcholine.

Associated Findings: Umbilical hernia, inguinal hernia; eczema, keloids; diabetes or abnormal glucose tolerance test; mild webbing of fingers and/or toes; contracture or dislocation of elbow; short metacarpal, sixth toe on fibular side of foot, hallux valgus, absence or subluxation of patella, coxa valga, genu valgum, valgus foot, pes planus, clubfoot; first degree hypospadias, angulated penis; wide-spaced nipples; short neck; subcortical atrophy, hydrocephalus, cavum septum pellucidum, myelomeningocele; premature

fusion of sternum; coloboma of iris, lens, and/or retina; exophthalmos or enophthalmos, cataract, congenital glaucoma, megalocornea; deviated nasal septum; macroglossia, forked or bifid tongue, bifid uvula, thin upper lip, long philtrum, lack of maxillary prominence with relative prognathism, enamel hypoplasia, talon cusps; stridor, low pitched-husky voice; persistent metopic suture, metopic synostosis, Luckenschädel, hyperostosis frontalis interna, flat occiput, brachycephaly. This list is not intended to be all-inclusive and the significance of many of the findings listed is uncertain.

Dermatoglyphic findings have included increased frequency of arches and decreased frequency of ulnar loops on fingertips, radial loops shifted to fingers other than second, additional triradius on apex of thumb or hallux, rare double pattern on thumbs, somewhat reduced total finger ridge count, large complex pattern in thenar/first interdigital area, hypothenar ulnar loops, distal axial triradius, increased atd angle pattern in second and/or third interdigital area of palm, missing c triradius, distorted and unusually long distal loop or a double loop in hallucal area with laterally displaced f triradius with or without e' triradius.

Etiology: Undetermined. The condition has been reported in several sets of twins, and some familial patterns have been noted. Although multifactorial inheritance has been proposed, Victor McKusick has found this "difficult to accept".

Pathogenesis: Unknown.

MIM No.: 26860

POS No.: 3384

CDC No.: 759.840

Sex Ratio: M1:F1

Occurrence: Simpson and Brissender (1973) estimated the population risk of 3:100,000 in the province of Ontario, Canada. Has been reported in 1:300–500 institutionalized persons with mental retardation over the age of five.

Reported among Caucasians, Orientals (Japanese) and Blacks. 250 cases from 22 countries have been documented.

Risk of Recurrence for Patient's Sib: Undetermined. A 1% risk figure has been suggested by Simpson (1973).

Risk of Recurrence for Patient's Child: Undetermined. No affected individual is know to have reproduced.

Age of Detectability: The syndrome can be detected in the newborn period by characteristic thumb, hallux and facial abnormalities, confirmed by X-ray findings of hands and feet.

Gene Mapping and Linkage: Unknown.

Prevention: None known. Genetic counseling indicated.

Treatment: Interdisciplinary evaluation and management should be considered to deal with the medical, social, psychological, and educational problems. Early management of respiratory and feeding problems. Appropriate medical and surgical care of associated defects, particularly those that require remediation. Antibiotics for infections and anticonvulsants for seizures. Individualized educational plan. Speech and language therapy. Surgery on hallux, particularly with duplication and/or angulation of phalanx may be required to get shoes that will fit properly. Functional results of surgery on angulated thumb deformity have not been published. Avoid obesity in late childhood and adolescence. Management of progressive malocclusion or other dental problems.

Prognosis: Of the 224 cases studied, age range was from one day to 62 years and 21 patients are known to have died. The causes of death and age at the time of death included respiratory distress syndrome (2 days, 8 days), cardiac failure (26 days, 4 months, 5–1/2 months, 2–1/2 years), respiratory infections (14 days, 42 days, 5 months, 18 months, 22 months, 26 months), meningitis (2 weeks), enteritis (2–1/2 years, 6 years), trauma and respiratory infection (9 years), brain tumor (ectopic pinealoma, 14 years), leukemia (25 months, 17 years), aspiration with seizures (33 years), respiratory distress after ventriculo-peritoneal (V-P) shunt (4 months).

Detection of Carrier: Unknown.

Support Groups: KA; Smith Center; Rubinstein-Taybi Parent Contact Group

The Center for Birth Defects Information Services wishes to thank Jack H. Rubinstein for his contributions to a previous version of this article.

References:
Rubinstein JH, Taybi H: Broad thumbs and toes and facial abnormalities: a possible mental retardation syndrome. Am J Dis Child 1963; 105:588–608.

Rubinstein J: The broad thumbs syndrome: progress report 1968. In: Bergsma D, ed: Proceedings conference on the clinical delineation of birth defects, Part II. Malformation syndromes. BD:OAS V(2), 1969:25–41.

Rubinstein JH: Broad thumb-hallux syndrome. In: Swoboda W, Stur O, eds: Proceedings of the international congress of pediatrics, Vienna, Austria, August 29– Sept. 4, 1971, Vienna, Verlag der Wiener Medizinischen Akademie, 1971:471–476.

Simpson NE, Brissender JE: The Rubinstein-Taybi syndrome: familial and dermatoglyphic data. Am J Hum Genet 1973; 25:225–229.

Kajii T, et al.: Monozygotic twins discordant for Rubinstein-Taybi syndrome. J Med Genet 1981; 18:312–314.

Stirt JA: Succinylcholine in Rubinstein-Taybi syndrome (Letter). Anesthesiology 1982; 57:429 (only).

Baraitser M, Preece MA: The Rubinstein-Taybi syndrome: Occurrence in two sets of identical twins. Clin Genet 1983; 23:318–320.

Berry AC: Rubinstein-Taybi syndrome. J Med Genet 1987; 24:562–566.

GR011   **Frank Greenberg**

Rubinstein-Taylor syndrome
See RUBINSTEIN-TAYBI BROAD THUMB-HALLUX SYNDROME
Rud syndrome
See SEIZURES-ICHTHYOSIS-MENTAL RETARDATION
Rudiger syndrome
See ECTRODACTYLY-ECTODERMAL DYSPLASIA-CLEFTING SYNDROME
Rudimentary uterine horn
See MULLERIAN FUSION, INCOMPLETE
Rufous albinism
See ALBINISM, OCULOCUTANEOUS, RUFOUS TYPE
Ruiter-Pompen-Wyers syndrome
See FABRY DISEASE
Rukavina type hereditary amyloidosis
See AMYLOIDOSIS, INDIANA TYPE
Russell-Silver syndrome
See SILVER SYNDROME
Russell-Silver syndrome, X-linked
See SILVER SYNDROME, X-LINKED
Rutherfurd syndrome
See GINGIVAL FIBROMATOSIS-CORNEAL DYSTROPHY
Rutledge lethal multiple congenital anomaly syndrome
See SMITH-LEMLI-OPITZ SYNDROME, TYPE II
Ruvalcaba syndrome
See OSTEODYSTROPHY-MENTAL RETARDATION, RUVALCABA TYPE
Ruvalcaba-Myhre-Smith syndrome
See OVERGROWTH, RUVALCABA-MYHRE-SMITH TYPE

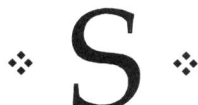

Sabinas brittle hair syndrome
See TRICHOTHIODYSTROPHY
Saccharopine dehydrogenase deficiency
See HYPERLYSINEMIA
Saccharopinuria
See HYPERLYSINEMIA
Sack type Ehlers-Danlos syndrome
See EHLERS-DANLOS SYNDROME
Sacral agenesis
See SACROCOCCYGEAL DYSGENESIS SYNDROME
Sacral agenesis, congenital
See CAUDAL REGRESSION SYNDROME
Sacral defects, anterior
See TERATOMA, PRESACRAL-SACRAL DYSGENESIS
Sacral dysgenesis-presacral teratoma
See TERATOMA, PRESACRAL-SACRAL DYSGENESIS
Sacral meningocele-conotruncal heart defects-head/neck anomalies
See MENINGOCELE-CONOTRUNCAL HEART DEFECT, KOUSSEFF TYPE
Sacral regression
See CAUDAL REGRESSION SYNDROME

SACROCOCCYGEAL DYSGENESIS SYNDROME   2380

Includes: Sacral agenesis

Excludes:
   Caudal regression syndrome (3211)
   Meningomyelocele (0693)
   Sirenomelia sequence (3191)
   Situs inversus viscerum (0888)
   Teratoma, presacral-sacral dysgenesis (2370)
   Vater association (0987)

Major Diagnostic Criteria: Sacrococcygeal dysgenesis (agenesis/dysplasia) associated with malformations of the lumbosacral vertebrae, ribs, and terminal spinal cord.

Clinical Findings: Most patients with the sacrococcygeal dysgenesis syndrome (SDS) are recognized at birth by the marked tapering of the lower trunk, particularly in the pelvic region, in association with severe hypoplastic lower limb defects. Sacrococcygeal dysgenesis (agenesis and/or dysplasia) is found on X-ray. While 12% of patients have dysmorphic cervicothoracic vertebrae, 51% have their most rostral abnormality in the lumbar spine, with a high ratio (10.5:1) of vertebral agenesis. SDS patients also have high incidences of CNS anomalies and of CNS-related complications such as urinary and anal incontinence (47%) and lower limb paraplegia (20%) which contrast sharply with the complete absence of anatomic malformations in these organ systems. The total associated anomalies in SDS are relatively low (3.3 per patient), as compared to **Sirenomelia sequence** (9.3 per patient), and **Vater association** (6.2 per patient).

Identification of SDS is further aided by concomitant demographic features: maternal diabetes reported in 26% of the patients; situs inversus in 4.6%; and patient survival in 97%. Twinning has a normal incidence of 1.3% in SDS patients.

Complications: Neurogenic bladder and sequelae; scoliosis.

Associated Findings: None known.

Etiology: Unknown. Autosomal dominant inheritance has been suggested in some cases.

Pathogenesis: Unknown.

MIM No.: 18294

CDC No.: 756.170

Sex Ratio: M1:F1

Occurrence: SDS occurred in 34% of 445 patients identified as having sacrococcygeal dysgenesis.

Risk of Recurrence for Patient's Sib: Unknown. Presumed low.

Risk of Recurrence for Patient's Child: Unknown. Two families with autosomal dominant transmission have been reported.

Age of Detectability: The severe lumbosacrococcygeal and complete sacrococcygeal forms are usually evident at birth, whereas patients with lesions below S3 are frequently not identified until later in life.

Gene Mapping and Linkage: Unknown.

Prevention: None known. Genetic counseling indicated.

Treatment: As indicated by defects, including orthopedic management of spine, pelvis, and lower limb defects, and surveillance for urinary tract complications.

Prognosis: Prognosis for life and intellect is dependent on the severity of the associated CNS anomalies. Urinary tract complications are usually either preventable or manageable if diagnosed and treated early in life.

Detection of Carrier: Unknown.

Special Considerations: In the past, sacrococcygeal dysgenesis syndrome (SDS) has been reported as *sacral agenesis*; however, the term SDS is preferable because not all patients have an absent sacrum, and because of the multi-system involvement.

References:
Duhamel B: From the mermaid to anal imperformation: the syndrome of caudal regression. Arch Dis Child 1961; 36:152–155.
Passarge E, Lenz W: Syndrome of caudal regression in infants of diabetic mothers: observations of further cases. Pediatrics 1966; 37:672–675.
Smith DW, et al.: Monozygotic twinning and the Duhamel anomalad (imperforate anus to sirenomelia): a nonrandom association between two aberrations in morphogenesis. BD:OAS XII(5). New York: March of Dimes Birth Defects Foundation, 1976:53–63.
Schinzel AAGL, et al.: Monozygotic twinning and structural defects. J Pediatr 1979; 95:921–930.
Duncan PA, et al.: Distinct caudal regression syndrome identified by associated malformation pattern and demographic features. (Abstract) Proc Greenwood Genet Center 1986; 5:142–143.

DU003   **Peter A. Duncan**
SH009   **Lawrence R. Shapiro**

Sacrococcygeal teratoma (benign or malignant)
See TERATOMA, SACROCOCCYGEAL TERATOMA

Saddle nose-deafness-myopia-cataract
See DEAFNESS-MYOPIA-CATARACT-SADDLE NOSE, MARSHALL TYPE

Saethre-Chotzen syndrome
See ACROCEPHALOSYNDACTYLY TYPE III

Sakati syndrome
See ACROCEPHALOPOLYSYNDACTYLY

Sakati-Nyhan syndrome
See ACROCEPHALOPOLYSYNDACTYLY

Saldino-Noonan short rib-polydactyly
See SHORT RIB-POLYDACTYLY SYNDROME, TYPE I

SALIVARY GLAND LYMPHANGIOMA — 2721

Includes: Lymphangioma of salivary gland

Excludes: Salivary gland, hemangioma (2726)

Major Diagnostic Criteria: Based on histologic appearance: lymphangioma simplex has capillary-sized channels; cavernous lymphangioma has dilated lymphatic channels; and cystic hygroma has channels of various sizes.

Clinical Findings: Asymptomatic, fluctuant mass located in any of the salivary glands.

Complications: May cause upper aerodigestive tract obstruction requiring a tracheotomy. Infection may occur. May result in severe cosmetic deformity.

Associated Findings: It is speculated that local infection may precipitate rapid growth.

Etiology: Unknown.

Pathogenesis: Glandular parenchyma is not replaced but rather it co-exists as islands of normal tissue surrounded by enlarged lymphatic spaces. Occasionally, there is spontaneous regression.

Sex Ratio: M1:F>1.

Occurrence: Undetermined but presumed rare.

Risk of Recurrence for Patient's Sib: Unknown.

Risk of Recurrence for Patient's Child: Unknown.

Age of Detectability: Commonly seen shortly after birth. More than one-half are present by age one year; 80–90% are present by age two years.

Gene Mapping and Linkage: Unknown.

Prevention: None known. Genetic counseling indicated.

Treatment: Since spontaneous regression is unlikely, surgical excision is the only acceptable mode. Prompt removal is necessary when the potential for airway compromise exists. May require tracheotomy.

Prognosis: Good for life span and intelligence. Function is dependent on the presence or absence of complications. Recurrence is uncommon when completely removed.

Detection of Carrier: Unknown.

References:
Batsakis JG, Regezi JA: Selected controversial lesions of salivary tissues. Otolaryngol Clin North Am 1977; 10:309–328.
Work WP: Cysts and congenital lesions of the parotid glands. Otolaryngol Clin North Am 1977; 10:339–344.
Work WP: Non-neoplastic disorders of the parotid gland. J Otolaryngol 1981; 10:35–40.
Sucupira MS, et al.: Salivary gland imaging and radionuclide dacryocystography in agenesis of salivary glands. Arch Otolaryngol 1983; 109:197–198.

MY003
OR005

Charles M. Myer III
Peter Orobello

Salivary gland virus infection
See FETAL CYTOMEGALOVIRUS SYNDROME

SALIVARY GLAND, AGENESIS — 2722

Includes:
Agenesis of the salivary gland
Mouth, dryness from salivary gland dysfunction
Xerostomia

Excludes: Salivary gland, acquired disorders of

Major Diagnostic Criteria: Xerostomia (dryness of the mouth) of unknown origin in a child.

Clinical Findings: Xerostomia. The diagnosis is confirmed by sodium pertechnetate imaging.

Complications: If undetected, sequelae resulting from xerostomia (i.e., poor oral hygiene, dental caries, dysphagia).

Associated Findings: The condition is seen in **Sjogren syndrome**.

Etiology: Unknown.

Pathogenesis: Unknown.

CDC No.: 750.230

Sex Ratio: Undetermined but presumably M1:F1.

Occurrence: Undetermined but presumably rare.

Risk of Recurrence for Patient's Sib: Unknown.

Risk of Recurrence for Patient's Child: Unknown.

Age of Detectability: During childhood.

Gene Mapping and Linkage: Unknown.

Prevention: None known.

Treatment: Early proper oral hygiene; artificial saliva, nutritional supplements, rigorous dental care and frequent dental examinations, and ophthalmologic screening.

Prognosis: Good for life span, intelligence and function.

Detection of Carrier: Unknown.

References:
Batsakis JG, Regezi JA: Selected controversial lesions of salivary tissues. Otolaryngol Clin North Am 1977; 10:309–328.
Work WP: Cysts and congenital lesions of the parotid glands. Otolaryngol Clin North Am 1977; 10:339–344.
Work WP: Non-neoplastic disorders of the parotid gland. J Otolaryngol 1981; 10:35–40.
Sucupira MS, et al.: Salivary gland imaging and radionuclide dacryocystography in agenesis of salivary glands. Arch Otolaryngol 1983; 109:197–198.

MY003
OR005
JA013

Charles M. Myer III
Peter Orobello
R. Kirk Jackson

Salivary gland, branchial cleft cysts
See BRANCHIAL CLEFT CYSTS

SALIVARY GLAND, DERMOID CYST — 2724

Includes: Dermoid cyst of the salivary gland

Excludes:
Branchial cleft cysts (2723)
Dermoid cyst, other
Immunologic diseases
Inflammatory disease, acute and chronic
Neoplastic diseases
Salivary gland, congenital cysts
Salivary gland, ductal cyst (2725)
Salivary gland, hemangioma (2726)
Salivary gland lymphangioma (2721)
Salivary gland, vascular tumors
Traumatic lesions

Major Diagnostic Criteria: An isolated mass deep within or near the surface of the parotid gland.

Clinical Findings: Isolated mass within the parotid gland which may cause mild ductal compression and secondary parotitis.

Complications: Infection, mass effect.

Associated Findings: None known.

Etiology: Anomalous development resulting in inclusion of all three germinal layers (ectoderm, mesoderm, and endoderm) in a cystic structure.

Pathogenesis: Keratinization of squamous epithelium, with associated skin appendages.

Sex Ratio: Undetermined but presumably M1:F1.

Occurrence: Undetermined but presumably rare.

Risk of Recurrence for Patient's Sib: Unknown.

Risk of Recurrence for Patient's Child: Unknown.

Age of Detectability: Usually during infancy.

Gene Mapping and Linkage: Unknown.

Prevention: None known. Genetic counseling indicated.

Treatment: Subtotal parotidectomy with facial nerve preservation.

Prognosis: Good for life span, intelligence, and function. Recurrence is likely unless entirely removed surgically.

Detection of Carrier: Unknown.

References:
Batsakis JG, Regezi JA: Selected controversial lesions of salivary tissues. Otolaryngol Clin North Am 1977; 10:309–328.
Schuller DE, McCabe BF: Salivary gland neoplasms in children. Otolaryngol Clin North Am 1977; 10:399–412.
Work WP: Cysts and congenital lesions of the parotid glands. Otolaryngol Clin North Am 1977; 10:339–344.
Work WP: Non-neoplastic disorders of the parotid gland. J Otolaryngol 1981; 10:35–40.

MY003
OR005

Charles M. Myer III
Peter Orobello

SALIVARY GLAND, DUCTAL CYST   2725

Includes: Ductal cyst of the salivary gland

Excludes: Salivary gland, others cysts of the

Major Diagnostic Criteria: Unilateral enlargement of the parotid gland during infancy.

Clinical Findings: Unilateral parotid enlargement. Sialography may be helpful in identifying the true nature of these lesions.

Complications: Repeated infections.

Associated Findings: None known.

Etiology: Unknown.

Pathogenesis: Most likely the result of a congenital retention cyst.

Sex Ratio: Undetermined but presumably M1:F1.

Occurrence: Undetermined but presumably rare.

Risk of Recurrence for Patient's Sib: Unknown.

Risk of Recurrence for Patient's Child: Unknown.

Age of Detectability: During infancy.

Gene Mapping and Linkage: Unknown.

Prevention: None known. Genetic counseling indicated.

Treatment: None necessary unless there are recurrent infections. Parotidectomy with preservation of the facial nerve is curative and should be performed only if necessary.

Prognosis: Good for life span, intelligence, and function. Risk of recurrence is low with complete surgical excision (parotidectomy).

Detection of Carrier: Unknown.

References:
Batsakis JG, Regezi JA: Selected controversial lesions of salivary tissues. Otolaryngol Clin North Am 1977; 10:309–328.
Work WP: Cysts and congenital lesions of the parotid glands. Otolaryngol Clin North Am 1977; 10:339–344.

Work WP: Non-neoplastic disorders of the parotid gland. J Otolaryngol 1981; 10:35–40.

MY003
OR005

Charles M. Myer III
Peter Orobello

SALIVARY GLAND, HEMANGIOMA   2726

Includes: Hemangioma, salivary gland

Excludes: Salivary gland lymphangioma (2721)

Major Diagnostic Criteria: Asymptomatic tumor of a salivary gland, gradually increasing in size.

Clinical Findings: Asymptomatic tumor of a salivary gland, gradually increasing in size, fluctuant to palpation and resulting in facial asymmetry. The tumor is usually confined to the intracapsular portion of the gland, with overlying skin only rarely involved. Enlarges with dependent positioning.

Complications: Excessivly rapid growth may result in functional impairment, infection, hemorrhage and/or ulceration.

Associated Findings: Other cutaneous hemangiomas may be present.

Etiology: Unknown.

Pathogenesis: Histologically, a continuum of maturation from capillary or cavernous forms to mixed and hypertrophic forms. The lobular architecture is maintained, but the parenchyma is replaced by endothelial proliferation with vascular differentiation. Acini and ductal structures are unaffected.

Sex Ratio: Seen predominantly in females.

Occurrence: Found in about 25% of a series of pediatric salivary gland tumors reviewed by Schuller and McCabe (1977).

Risk of Recurrence for Patient's Sib: Unknown.

Risk of Recurrence for Patient's Child: Unknown.

Age of Detectability: Usually discovered shortly after birth.

Gene Mapping and Linkage: Unknown.

Prevention: None known. Genetic counseling indicated.

Treatment: Controversial. Most surgeons prefer not to excise these lesions, since the majority will undergo spontaneous resolution. Excision is indicated with excessively rapid growth or presence of complications.

When appropriate, therapy involves subtotal parotidectomy with facial nerve preservation or total submandibular gland excision. Other methods of therapy include systemic steroids, pressure, and low-dose radiotherapy (not recommended due to possible malignant transformation).

Prognosis: Unknown.

Detection of Carrier: Unknown.

References:
Batsakis JG, Regezi JA: Selected controversial lesions of salivary tissues.
Schuller DE, McCabe BF: Salivary gland neoplasms in children. Otolaryngol Clin North Am 1977; 10:399–412.
Work WP: Cysts and congenital lesions of the parotid glands. Otolaryngol Clin North Am 1977; 10:339–344.
Work WP: Non-neoplastic disorders of the parotid gland. J Otolaryngol 1981; 10:35–40.

MY003
OR003

Charles M. Myer III
Peter Orobello

SALIVARY GLAND, MIXED TUMOR   0878

Includes:
 Adenoma, hereditary pleomorphic salivary
 Tumor, mixed, of salivary gland

Excludes:
 Branchogenic cyst
 Salivary gland tumors (other)

Major Diagnostic Criteria: Presence of mixed tumor of salivary gland in more than one member of a family.

Clinical Findings: A firm, well-circumscribed mass in the parotid gland without facial nerve involvement is found in the patient in the third decade of life. Excisional biopsy (minimal procedure is submandibular gland excision or lateral parotid lobectomy) reveals pathologic findings of a typical mixed benign tumor. In a series of 401 mixed tumors, Cameron (1959) found three families with tumors affecting more than one member. In one family, brother, sister and father were affected; in another, mother and daughter; and in the third, father and son. In this last family, the diagnosis of the father's tumor was made on clinical grounds, as he refused biopsy or excision. All the offspring were between 21 and 25 years of age.

Complications: Tumors rarely show malignant degeneration and rarely metastasize. Involvement of facial nerve with resultant paralysis is rare.

Associated Findings: None known.

Etiology: Undetermined. Possibly autosomal dominant inheritance.

Pathogenesis: Unknown.

Sex Ratio: Presumably M1:F1.

Occurrence: Undetermined but presumed rare.

Risk of Recurrence for Patient's Sib:
 See Part I, *Mendelian Inheritance.*

Risk of Recurrence for Patient's Child:
 See Part I, *Mendelian Inheritance.*

Age of Detectability: All patients were over 20 years of age at diagnosis.

Gene Mapping and Linkage: Unknown.

Prevention: None known. Genetic counseling indicated.

Treatment: Surgical excision by lateral lobe parotidectomy, total parotidectomy, or submandibular gland excision.

Prognosis: Generally good for normal life span, intelligence, and function if proper surgical treatment is employed. Metastases are rare, and untreated mixed tumors usually enlarge slowly.

Detection of Carrier: Unknown.

References:
Cameron JM: Familial incidence of 'mixed salivary tumors.' Scott Med J 1959; 4:455.

AU005   **Thomas Aufdemorte**

Salivary glands and lacrimal puncta, absence of
 See ALACRIMA-APTYALISM

SALLA DISEASE   2041

Includes:
 N-acetylneuraminic acid storage disease, infantile (one form)
 Sialic acid storage disease, infantile (one form)
 Sialuria, Finnish type

Excludes:
 Mucolipidosis I (0671)
 Sialic acid storage disease, infantile type (2222)

Major Diagnostic Criteria: Both the adult and infantile forms of Salla disease are characterized by alterations in the amount of free (unbound) sialic acid in various tissues and body fluids. Specifically, the urinary concentration of free sialic acid exceeds normal concentrations by 10 to 20 times. Excretion of sialic acid in heterozygotes is normal. Total sialic acid excretion is in the upper range of normal or slightly elevated. Urinary glycosaminoglycan excretion is normal. Cultured skin fibroblasts from affected patients are also characterized by increased levels of free sialic acid. Morphologic evidence of abnormal lysosomal storage occurs in several cell types, including skin biopsy specimens and cultured fibroblasts from patients with the infantile form of the disorder. Activities of the enzymes deficient in other types of lysosomal storage diseases, including sialidase, are normal.

Clinical Findings: There appears to be at least two distinct forms of this disease. In the milder form, the so-called Salla disease, affected individuals, born after an uncomplicated pregnancy, appear healthy for the first 6–18 months of life. Signs of progressive CNS deterioration usually appear during the first year. Motor and speech development are delayed; words are often dysarthric, and sentences, if any, are limited to a few words. The stage of moderate-to-severe mental retardation is reached between the ages of five and 10 years, with further deterioration occurring during the second decade. Most individuals have slightly coarse facies. Movements are clumsy, because most patients have ataxia and some muscular hypotonia. The liver and spleen, in general, are not enlarged; the eyes are normal. X-ray findings are limited to a thickened calvarium, while the long bones and vertebrae have a normal structure. The EEG is diffusely abnormal.

In contrast, infantile free sialic acid storage disease is characterized by a more rapid onset of clinical features. Patients with this form of the disease present at or soon after birth with coarse facies, hepatosplenomegaly, clear corneas, hypopigmentation, and diarrhea. The clinical course is one of rapid deterioration, with death in early childhood.

In both forms of the disease vacuolated lymphocytes are seen in the peripheral blood, vacuoles in dermal fibroblasts and histiocytes, as well as in epithelial cells of the blood capillaries, Schwann cells, and the secretory and myoepithelial cells of the sweat glands. Cultured fibroblasts from the infantile form also contain abnormal lysosomes. The activities of several lysosomal enzymes in cultured fibroblasts and in plasma are within normal limites. Urinary excretion of free sialic acid is significantly increased, whereas the total urinary sialic acid excretion is normal.

Complications: Unknown.

Associated Findings: None known.

Etiology: Autosomal recessive inheritance.

Pathogenesis: The enlarged storage lysosomes of different cell types (found in skin biopsy material) and the progressive course of the disease clearly indicate that Salla disease should be considered a lysosomal storage disease. Recent evidence strongly suggests that the defect in both Salla and infantile free sialic acid storage disease patients is due to an impairment of normal transport of free sialic acid out of cellular lysosomes as a result of an abnormality of the lysosomal membrane. Moreover, the demonstration of defective sialic acid egress indicates that this disease can be included in a small group of disorders characterized by the defective transport of small molecules across lysosomal membranes. The mechanism responsible for the increased excretion of free sialic acid in these patients remains unclear.

Activities of all lysosomal enzymes studied to date are normal in cultured fibroblasts of the Salla patients.

MIM No.: *26874

Sex Ratio: M1:F1

Occurrence: The milder form of Salla disease has been found almost exclusively in Finland, where close to 40 cases have been reported. In contrast, patients with the infantile form do not appear to have predilection for any particular ethnic group. Evidence to date, however, does suggest that the milder adult form is more common than the infantile form.

Risk of Recurrence for Patient's Sib:
 See Part I, *Mendelian Inheritance.*

Risk of Recurrence for Patient's Child:
See Part I, *Mendelian Inheritance*.

Age of Detectability: The age of usual clinical diagnosis is dependent, in large part, on the clinical form of the disorder. In the milder form of Salla disease, delayed development is usually suspected after 6–18 months of age. In contrast, the clinical manifestations of the infantile form are apparent at or very soon after birth. The biochemical abnormalities in all forms of the disease appear to be present throughout life. Prenatal diagnosis has been reported for both forms of the disorder.

Gene Mapping and Linkage: Unknown.

Prevention: None known. Genetic counseling indicated.

Treatment: Supportive.

Prognosis: Severe mental retardation before age 10 years seems to be the rule for the milder form of the disease. Additionally, the life span for the mild form of this disorder is probably close to normal, since the oldest living patient is now age 70 years. In contrast, the infantile form of the disorder is characterized by severe mental retardation and death at an early age.

Detection of Carrier: Unknown.

References:

Aula P, et al.: "Salla disease": a new lysosomal storage disorder. Arch Neurol 1979; 36:88–94.
Renlund M, et al.: Increased urinary excretion of free N-acetyl-neuraminic acid in thirteen patients with Salla disease. Eur J Biochem 1979; 101:245–250.
Hildreth J IV, et al.: N-acetylneuraminic acid accumulation in a buoyant lysosomal fraction of cultured fibroblasts from patients with infantile generalized N-acetylneuraminic acid storage disease. Biochem Biophys Res Commun 1986; 139:838–844.
Jonas AJ: Studies of lysosomal sialic acid metabolism. retention of sialic acid by Salla diseases lysosomes. Biochem Biophys Res Commun 1986; 137:175–181.
Mancini GMS, et al.: Free N-acetylneuraminic acid (NANA) storage disorders: evidence for defective NANA transport across the lysosomal membrane. Hum Genet 1986; 73:214–217.
Paschke E, et al.: Infantile sialic acid storage disease: the fate of biosynthetically labeled N-acetyl-(^{3}H)-neuraminic acid in cultured human fibroblasts. Pediatr Res 1986; 20:773–777.
Renlund M, et al.: Defective sialic acid egress from isolated fibroblast lysosomes of patients with Salla disease. Science 1986; 232:59–762.
Renlund M, Aula P: Prenatal detection of Salla disease based upon increased free sialic acid in amniocytes. Am J Med Genet 1987; 28:377–384.

TH021
RE016

George H. Thomas
Martin Renlund

Salmon patch
See NEVUS FLAMMEUS
Salonen-Herva-Norio syndrome
See HYDROLETHALUS SYNDROME
Sandhoff disease
See G(M2)-GANGLIOSIDOSIS WITH HEXOSAMINIDASE A AND B DEFICIENCY
Sandifer syndrome
See TORTICOLLIS
Sanfilippo syndrome
See MUCOPOLYSACCHARIDOSIS III
Santos syndrome
See HIRSCHSPRUNG DISEASE-POLYDACTYLY-DEAFNESS

SARCOIDOSIS 2966

Includes:
Besnier-Boek-Schaumann disease
Bilateral hilar involvement
EN-arthropathy-BHL syndrome
Mannen-Balcom syndrome

Excludes:
Cancer, Hodgkin disease, familial (2352)
Lupus erythematosus, systemic (2515)
Tuberculous lymphadenitis

Major Diagnostic Criteria: Bilateral hilar lymphadenopathy and pulmonary infiltration demonstrated in chest X-ray, elevated serum angiotensin converting enzyme, positive Kveim test, and noncaseating granulomas on biopsy.

Clinical Findings: Sarcoidosis is a systemic disease characterized by granulomatous inflammation of almost any organ or tissue, but with a marked predilection for lungs. The onset of the disease is usually between the second and third decades of life. Patients may present with malaise, fever, and dyspnea of insidious onset. In 10–15% of the patients, the onset is acute with erythema nodosum or acute polyarthritis developing in days or weeks, or sudden onset of an infiltrating granulomatous skin rash. Acute-onset sarcoidosis is usually a benign syndrome with a high incidence of spontaneous resolution. Subacute sarcoidosis is often asymptomatic and is initially recognized through health screening or routine chest X-rays. Patients generally have few extrathoracic lesions, and these recover spontaneously. Patients with chronic sarcoidosis patients have both intrathroracic and extrathoracic involvement.

Extrathoracic sarcoidosis: may present with symptoms referable to the skin, eyes, peripheral nerves, muscle, liver, or heart. The findings may include skin rash (erythema nodosum and plaque-like), peripheral neuropathy, myopathy, parotid gland enlargement, hepatosplenomegaly, lymphadenopathy, chronic arthritis, and lytic lesions of the bone.

Laboratory abnormalities: leukopenia, eosinophilia, and elevated sedimentation rate, hypergammaglobulinemia, hypercalcemia or hypercalciuria, elevated angiotensin-converting enzyme, and positive Kveim test (skin test). Biopsy material shows noncaseating granulomatous inflammation of tissues. Cutaneous changes may be seen in about 40%. Other studies to demonstrate pulmonary involvement include transbronchial lung biopsy and radioactive gallium scan.

X-ray findings: bilateral hilar adenopathy, paratracheal adenopathy, and parenchymal reticulonodular infiltrates.

Complications: Pulmonary fibrosis, chorioretinitis, congestive heart failure, pericardial effusion, cranial nerve palsies, and nephrolithiasis.

Associated Findings: Uveitis, iridocyclitis, peripheral neuropathies, liver and spleen enlargement, myocarditis, myopathies.

Etiology: Probably a combination of genetic and environmental factors. It is unclear whether one or several infectious agents are responsible or whether inhalation, ingestion, or dermal contact is the route of exposure. Agents that have been considered are viruses, typical and atypical mycobacteria, fungi, and fine pollen.

Pathogenesis: Sarcoidosis is a disorder of widespread, noncaseating granulomas that form in response to an unidentified stimulus. Pulmonary involvement is seen in 90% of the patients. The granulomas are composed of mostly epithelioid cells, but also of giant cells. Activated T lymphocytes and macrophages contribute to granuloma formation. These granulomas are rich in angiotensin-converting enzyme.

MIM No.: 18100

Sex Ratio: M1:F1.1

Occurrence: Sarcoidosis occurs worldwide and affects all ethnic groups. The incidence of sarcoidosis is 11:100,000 in United States, 3–4.5:100,000 in the United Kingdom, and 7:100,000 in Denmark. In the United States, the prevalence of sarcoidosis is much higher in Blacks than in whites.

Risk of Recurrence for Patient's Sib: Probably not increased.

Risk of Recurrence for Patient's Child: Probably not increased.

Age of Detectability: Generally between the second and third decades of life.

Gene Mapping and Linkage: Unknown.

Prevention: None known. Genetic counseling indicated.

Treatment: The preferred therapy for sarcoidosis is corticosteroids. The usual practice is to give 40 mg of prednisone daily for a 2-week period, then gradually tapering to 15 mg for a minimum of 6–8 months. Steroids are indicated in most extrathoracic sarcoidosis. Stage 0 and 1 intrathoracic sarcoidoses do not need treatment.

Prognosis: Corticosteroids produce a dramatic therapeutic effect in sarcoidosis. Lifetime, low-dose maintenance therapy may be required in some patients. Persistent prolonged untreated disease is less likely to be reversible.

Detection of Carrier: Unknown.

Special Considerations: Few familial aggregates have been found. However, no pattern of inheritance has been confirmed. HLA-DR-5 is highly associated with sarcoidosis.

References:
Sharma OP, et al.: Familial sarcoidosis: a possible genetic influence. Ann NY Acad Sci 1976; 278:386–400.
Bascom R, Johns CJ: The natural history and management of sarcoidosis. Adv Intern Med 1986; 31:213–241.
James DG: Sarcoidosis: past, present, and future concepts. Clin Dermatol 1986; 4:1–9.
Staton GW Jr., et al.: Comparison of clinical parameters, bronchoalveolar lavage, gallium-67 lung uptake, and serum angiotensin converting enzyme in assessing the activity of sarcoidosis. Sarcoidosis (Italy) 1986; 3:8–10.
Luke RA, et al.: Neurosarcoidosis: the long term clinical course. Neurology 1987; 37:461–463.
Nowack D, Goebel KM: Genetic aspects of sarcoidosis. Arch Intern Med 1987; 147:481–483.

KI016   **Smita Kittar**

Sarcoma family syndrome of Li and Fraumeni (some cases)
See CANCER, BREAST, FAMILIAL
Sarcosine dehydrogenase complex, deficiency of
See SARCOSINEMIA

SARCOSINEMIA   0503

Includes:
Hypersarcosinemia
Sarcosine dehydrogenase complex, deficiency of

Excludes:
Acidemia, ethylmalonic-adipic (2377)
Acidemia, glutaric acidemia II, neonatal onset (2289)

Major Diagnostic Criteria: Increased concentration of sarcosine in blood and urine without elevated concentrations of organic acids. Sarcosine levels in patient plasma range from 0.5 to 6.8 mg/dl; sarcosine excretion ranges from 0.13 to 0.84 mg/mg creatinine. Sarcosine is not usually detectable in the body fluids of normal individuals.

Clinical Findings: No consistent clinical syndrome has been associated with sarcosinemia. Most patients were initially investigated because of failure to thrive, poor feeding, delayed development, or mental retardation. This has led to a biased increase in patients with these conditions among reported sarcosinemia patients. When an unbiased method, neonatal urine screening, was used, Levy et al. (1984) found four unrelated patients; all had IQs in the normal range. However, one was emotionally disturbed, and one was dyslexic. No dysmorphic or other clinical abnormalities were found. A total of 19 patients from 16 different families have been reported. Of these, eight had normal intelligence, but three of these eight had significant psychiatric problems.

Complications: Unknown.

Associated Findings: None known.

Etiology: Probably autosomal recessive inheritance of an enzyme defect. There is evidence of genetic heterogeneity.

Pathogenesis: Sarcosine is not oxidized to glycine. Gerritsen (1972) found a deficiency of the enzyme sarcosine dehydrogenase in the liver of one patient. However, Scott (1974) found a value equal to that of controls in a liver biopsy from his patient. Sarcosine oxidation occurs primarily in the liver and kidney. The dehydrogenase is not present in either fibroblasts or circulating leukocytes.

MIM No.: *26890

Sex Ratio: Presumably M1:F1.

Occurrence: An incidence of 1:350,000 live births was calculated from Massachusetts data.

Risk of Recurrence for Patient's Sib:
See Part I, *Mendelian Inheritance.*

Risk of Recurrence for Patient's Child:
See Part I, *Mendelian Inheritance.*

Age of Detectability: Before age three months by urinalysis.

Gene Mapping and Linkage: Unknown.

Prevention: None known. Genetic counseling indicated.

Treatment: Supportive. Short-term therapy with folic acid was not effective in one patient of Glorieux et al. (1971); however, in the patient of Blom and Fernandes (1979), a decrease in urinary sarcosine excretion was seen after 8 weeks of treatment with high doses of folic acid. Sarcosinemia has been reported to occur in a patient with dietary folic acid deficiency.

Prognosis: Normal life span.

Detection of Carrier: Not always possible. Oral tolerance tests with sarcosine and dimethylglycine have been done. In some families the excretion of sarcosine from some probable carriers was increased after a sarcosine load. A difference in the ratio of urinary sarcosine to glycine after a sarcosine load has been suggested as another distinguishing criterion.

Special Considerations: Sarcosinemia is distinct from **Acidemia, glutaric acidemia II, neonatal onset** in which the activity of a large number of acyl-CoA dehydrogenases are deficient because of the defective activity of the associated electron transporting flavoprotein or its dehyrogenase. In this latter disease, sarcosine and a variety of other organic acids are elevated. In sarcosinemia there is normal excretion of organic acids.

References:
Gerritsen T, Waisman HA: Hypersarcosinemia: an inborn error of metabolism. New Engl J Med 1966; 275:66–69. *
Glorieux FH, et al.: Transport and metabolism of sarcosine in hypersarcosinemia and normal phenotypes. J Clin Invest 1971; 50:2313. *
Gerritsen T: Sarcosine dehydrogenase deficiency, the enzyme defect in hypersarcosinemia. Helv Paediatr Acta 1972; 27:33.
Scott CR: Sarcosinemia. In Nyhan WL, ed: Heritable disorders of amino acid metabolism. New York: John Wiley & Sons, 1974:324.
Blom W, Fernandes J: Folic acid dependent hypersarcosinemia. Clin Chem Acta 1979; 91:117.
Levy HL, et al.: Massachusetts metabolic disorders screening program: III. Sarcosinemia. Pediatrics 1984; 74:509. *
Sewell AC, et al.: Sarcosinaemia in a retarded amaurotic child. Europ J Pediat 1986; 144:508–510.

SM020   **Margaret L. Smith**

Sarcotubular myopathy
See MYOPATHY, SARCOTUBULAR
Sauk syndrome
See TAURODONTISM-SHORT ROOTED TEETH-MICROCEPHALIC DWARFISM
Say-Barber-Miller syndrome
See MICROCEPHALY-RETARDATION-SKELETAL AND IMMUNE DEFECTS

SAY-MEYER SYNDROME 3267

Includes:
   Trigonocephaly-short stature
   Trigonocephaly-short stature-developmental delay

Excludes:
   C syndrome (0121)
   Acrocephalosyndactyly type III (0229)

Major Diagnostic Criteria: The combination of trigonocephaly and growth failure and lack of limb defects should suggest the diagnosis.

Clinical Findings: All three affected boys in the one reported family had trigonocephaly, with a prominent vertical ridge on the forehead; **Microcephaly**, short stature; and developmental delay. Additional features include low birthweight (2), prominent eyes (1), hypotelorism (2), epicanthal folds (1), wide nasal bridge (1), beaked nose (1), highly arched palate (1), low-set ears (1), clinodactyly (1), **Hernia, inguinal** (1), and seizures (1). In one child, skull X-rays demonstrated craniosynostosis involving the sagittal, metopic, and left lambdoid sutures; in another the lambdoid and metopic were involved.

Complications: Unknown.

Associated Findings: None known.

Etiology: X-linked recessive inheritance is most likely.

Pathogenesis: Unknown.

MIM No.: 31432

Sex Ratio: M3:F0 (observed).

Occurrence: One family from Oklahoma has been documented.

Risk of Recurrence for Patient's Sib:
   See Part I, *Mendelian Inheritance.*

Risk of Recurrence for Patient's Child:
   See Part I, *Mendelian Inheritance.*

Age of Detectability: At birth by the presence of trigonocephaly.

Gene Mapping and Linkage: Unknown.

Prevention: None known. Genetic counseling indicated.

Treatment: Unknown.

Prognosis: All three boys had some degree of developmental delay, with the oldest (a 30-year-old) reported as being moderately mentally retarded. His height was 162 cm.

Detection of Carrier: Unknown.

References:
Say B, Meyer J: Familial syndrome of trigonocephaly associated with short stature and developmental delay. Am J Dis Child 1981; 135:711–712.

T0007   **Helga V. Toriello**

SBLA syndrome (some cases)
   See CANCER, BREAST, FAMILIAL
SC phocomelia syndrome
   See ROBERTS SYNDROME
Scalp cylindroma, types I and II
   See SCALP, CYLINDROMAS
Scalp defect-ectrodactyly
   See LIMB AND SCALP DEFECTS, ADAMS-OLIVER TYPE
Scalp defects from fetal exposure
   See FETAL EFFECTS FROM METHIMAZOLE AND CARBIMAZOLE

SCALP DEFECTS-POSTAXIAL POLYDACTYLY 2922

Includes: Polydactyly, postaxial type A-scalp defects
Excludes:
   Chromosome 13, trisomy 13 (0168)
   Limb and scalp defects, Adams-Oliver type (0459)
   Skin, localized absence of (0608)

Major Diagnostic Criteria: Postaxial polydactyly type A combined with a midline skin defect, localized on the vertex or the occipital region, frequently associated with defects of the calvarium or even the meninges. The size of the scalp defect may vary from a 2–3-mm diameter skin defect to a very extensive defect of the whole calvarium.

Clinical Findings: A midline scalp defect may occur as an isolated anomaly (see **Skin, localized absence of**) or may be associated with acral reduction anomalies of the limbs (see **Limb and scalp defects, Adams-Oliver type**). At least two reports have dealt with the association of congenital scalp defects and postaxial polydactyly type A.

Complications: Unknown.

Associated Findings: Scalp defects can be associated with various malformations of the central nervous system. These have been especially well documented after the advent of axial computed tomography, i.e., asymmetric ventricular enlargement and porencephalic cysts localized under the vertex defect.

Etiology: Presumably autosomal dominant inheritance with considerable variability in expression and penetrance.

Pathogenesis: Unknown.

MIM No.: 18125

POS No.: 4018

Sex Ratio: M1:F1

Occurrence: One kindred and one sporadic case have been reported in the literature.

Risk of Recurrence for Patient's Sib:
   See Part I, *Mendelian Inheritance.*

Risk of Recurrence for Patient's Child:
   See Part I, *Mendelian Inheritance.*

Age of Detectability: At birth.

Gene Mapping and Linkage: Unknown.

Prevention: None known. Genetic counseling indicated.

Treatment: Symptomatic.

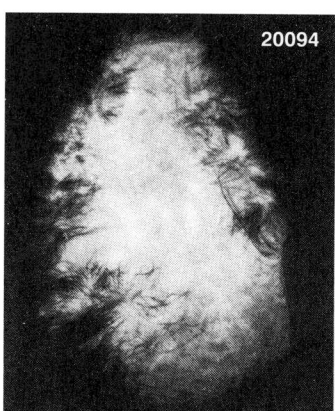 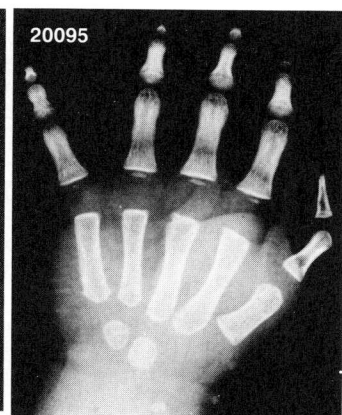

2922-20094: Large scalp defect covered by thin atrophic skin. 20095: Typical acral reduction defects of the hands.

Prognosis: In the first years of life, spontaneous bleeding and granulation of the skin defect occur, and, after the first years of life, the defect is covered by thin, atrophic skin. Calcification and mineralization of the bone defect progressively occur, and after some years the size of the bone defect may become relatively smaller than at birth.

Detection of Carrier: Unknown.

References:

Fryns JP, Van den Berghe H: Congenital scalp defects associated with postaxial polydactyly. Hum Genet 1979; 49:217–219.
Buttiens M, et al.: Scalp defect associated with postaxial polydactyly: confirmation of a distinct entity with autosomal dominant inheritance. Hum Genet 1985; 71:86–88.

FR030   **Jean-Pierre Fryns**

SCALP, CYLINDROMAS   0235

Includes:

Basal cell epithelioma, multiple benign nodular
    intraepidermal
Cylindromas of the scalp
Cylindromatosis
Endothelioma capitis of Kaposi
Hydradenoma
Hydradenoma, nonpapillary hyalinizing
Neuroepithelioma adenoids
Scalp cylindroma, types I and II
Spiegler-Brooke tumors
Syphonoma
Tomato tumor
Turban tumors of scalp

Excludes:

Epitheliomas, hereditary multiple cystic (2392)
Fibromatosis, juvenile hyaline (0411)

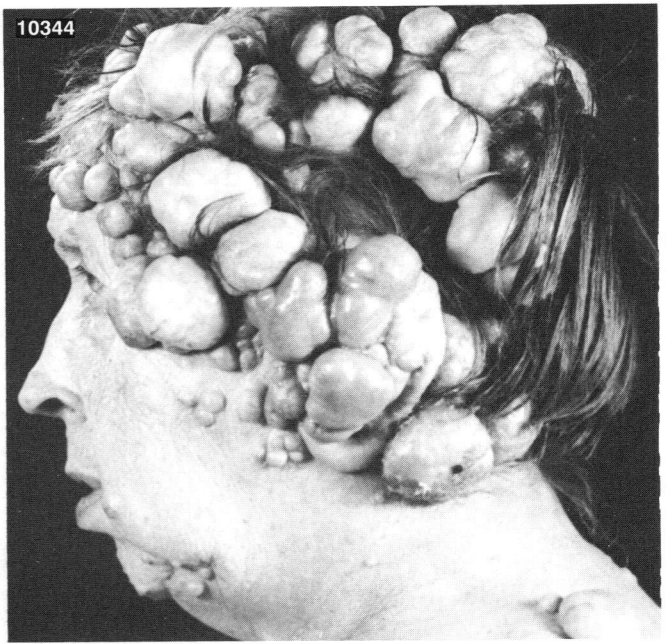

0235-10344: Cylindromatosis.

C0070

Major Diagnostic Criteria: A cylindroma is an epidermal appendage tumor in which differentiation toward apocrine or eccrine structure occurs. It occurs in two forms:

Type 1: Multiple sessile or pedunculated dome-shaped, smooth nodules on the scalp with occasional extension to the face, neck, and trunk. These lesions appear in early adulthood and increase in size and number. The size of these dominantly inherited tumors ranges from a few millimeters to several centimeters. They may become extensive on the scalp and give rise to the epithet "turban tumor."

Type 2: A solitary tumor of the scalp either sessile or pedunculated. Solitary cylindromas are not inherited.

Histologically, cylindromas, regardless of type, are composed of irregularly shaped islands of epithelial cells separated by a hyaline sheath or cylinder, hence the name, and a narrow band of collagen. These islands are composed of two types of cells, peripheral cells with small dark nuclei, representing undifferentiated cells, and central cells with large, pale nuclei, representing differentiation toward ductal cells.

Clinical Findings: These solitary or multiple smooth firm globular tumors of variable size are distinctive in appearance.

Complications: Bleeding and infection secondary to trauma can occur with both types of cylindromas. Malignant degeneration with metastatic spread to lymph nodes, viscera, and local extention have been noted with both types. It is to avoid these sequelae, as well as for esthetic consideration, that surgical excision is recommended.

Associated Findings: Type 1 cylindromas are commonly associated with multiple trichoepitheliomas.

Etiology: *Type 1:* Multiple cylindromas follow a pattern of autosomal dominant inheritance, but the possibility of X-linkage in a small number of families is not completely excluded.

Type 2: Solitary cylindromas have no hereditary pattern.

Pathogenesis: While histochemical and enzyme histochemical studies have not been convincing, electron microscopy studies and the association with trichoepitheliomas favor an apocrine, rather than an eccrine, differentiation.

MIM No.: 12385, 31310

Sex Ratio: Type 1, M<1:F1; type 2, M1:F1

Occurrence: More than 200 reported cases.

Risk of Recurrence for Patient's Sib:
See Part I, *Mendelian Inheritance.*

Risk of Recurrence for Patient's Child:
See Part I, *Mendelian Inheritance.*

Age of Detectability: Second or third decade of life.

Gene Mapping and Linkage: Unknown.

Prevention: None known. Genetic counseling indicated.

Treatment: Excision.

Prognosis: Prognosis is good for both type 1 and type 2 cylindromas, although case reports of malignant degeneration with subsequent metastatic spread argue for careful serial histologic examination of excised tumors. Regular follow-up is desirable.

Detection of Carrier: Unknown.

References:

Lever WF: Pathogenesis of benign skin tumors of cutaneous appendages and of basal cell epitheliomas. Arch Dermatol Syph 1948; 57:679–724.
Crain RC, et al.: Dermal eccrine cylindroma. Am J Clin Pathol 1961; 35:504–515.
Lyon JB, et al.: Malignant degeneration of turban tumor of the scalp. Trans St. John's Hosp Dermatol 1961; 46:74–77.
Hashimoto K, et al.: Histogenesis of skin appendage tumors. Arch Dermatol 1969; 100:356–369.
Harper PS: Turban tumor (cylindromatosis). BD:OAS; VII(8):338–341. White Plains: March of Dimes-Birth Defects Foundation, 1971. †

Brian Cook

Scalp, skull, and limbs; absence defect of Adams-Oliver
See LIMB AND SCALP DEFECTS, ADAMS-OLIVER TYPE
Scaphocephaly
See CRANIOSYNOSTOSIS
Scapula elevata
See SPRENGEL DEFORMITY
Scapuloilioperoneal atrophy-cardiopathy
See HAUPTMANN-THANHAUSER SYNDROME
Scarring epidermolysis bullosa
See EPIDERMOLYSIS BULLOSUM, TYPE III
Scheibe cochleosaccular degeneration of inner ear
See EAR, INNER DYSPLASIAS
Scheie syndrome
See MUCOPOLYSACCHARIDOSIS I-S
Scheuermann disease (vertebrae)
See JOINTS, OSTEOCHONDRITIS DISSECANS
Schimke X-linked mental retardation syndrome
See X-LINKED MENTAL RETARDATION-CHOREOATHETOSIS
Schimmelpenning-Feuerstein-Mims syndrome
See PROTEUS SYNDROME
Schindler disease
See ALPHA-N-ACETYLGALACTOSAMINIDASE DEFICIENCY
Schinzel syndrome
See ULNAR-MAMMARY SYNDROME
Schinzel type acrocallosal syndrome
See ACROCALLOSAL SYNDROME, SCHINZEL TYPE

SCHINZEL-GIEDION SYNDROME 2123

Includes:
Face, midface retraction-X-ray and renal anomalies-hypertrichosis
Hypertrichosis-midface retraction-X-ray and renal anomalies
Midface retraction-X-ray and renal anomalies-hypertrichosis
Renal and X-ray anomalies-midface retraction-hypertrichosis

Excludes:
Johanson-Blizzard syndrome (2026)
Mucopolysaccharidosis
Urofacial syndrome (2527)

Major Diagnostic Criteria: Midface retraction, hypertrichosis, skeletal anomalies, hydronephrosis, and failure to thrive.

Clinical Findings: In four reported cases, three involved post-term pregnancy, and polyhydramnios complicated one pregnancy. All affected children have had generalized hypertrichosis; widely patent cranial sutures and fontanelles; hypertelorism; midface retraction; low-set ears; short, broad neck with abundant skin; short forearms and legs; and in examined individuals, skeletal defects on X-ray, including steep short base of the skull, wide occipital synchondrosis, multiple wormian bones, hypoplastic first, and broad other ribs, hypoplastic distal phalanges, and hypoplastic/aplastic pubic bones. Additional features reported in affected individuals include facial hemangioma; high, prominent forehead; choanal stenosis; macroglossia; **Atrial septal defects**; hypoplastic nipples; post-axial polydactyly; narrow, hyperconvex nails; hypoplastic dermal ridges; talipes; and delayed tooth eruption. Genital anomalies are also common, and include short penis with cryptorchidism in males and deep interlabial sulcus in females.

One child died at one day of age; all the surviving children had growth retardation, seizures, and/or abnormal EEG, severe mental retardation, and recurrent apneic spells.

Complications: Unknown.

Associated Findings: None known.

Etiology: Autosomal recessive inheritance.

Pathogenesis: Unknown.

MIM No.: *26915

POS No.: 3025

Sex Ratio: Presumably M1:F1

Occurrence: About a dozen cases have been observed.

Risk of Recurrence for Patient's Sib:
See Part I, *Mendelian Inheritance.*

Risk of Recurrence for Patient's Child:
See Part I, *Mendelian Inheritance.*

Age of Detectability: At birth, by physical exam.

Gene Mapping and Linkage: Unknown.

Prevention: None known. Genetic counseling indicated.

Treatment: Supportive.

Prognosis: Affected individuals are severely retarded; death occurred at age one day, 16.5 months, and 19 months of age in three of four cases reported in the literature. The fourth case was permanently hospitalized at age 10 months.

Detection of Carrier: Unknown.

References:
Schinzel A, Giedion A: A syndrome of severe midface retraction, multiple skull anomalies, clubfeet, and cardiac and renal malformations in sibs. Am J Med Genet 1978; 1:361–375. * †
Donnai D, Harris R: A further case of a new syndrome including midface retraction, hypertrichosis, and skeletal anomalies. J Med Genet 1979; 16:483–486.
Kelley RI, et al.: Congenital hydronephrosis, skeletal dysplasia, and severe developmental retardation: the Schinzel-Giedion syndrome. J Pediatr 1982; 100:943–946.
Schinzel A: A syndrome of midface retraction, multiple radiological anomalies, renal malformations and hypertrichosis. (Letter) Hum Genet 1982; 62:382 only.

T0007 **Helga V. Toriello**

SCHISIS ASSOCIATION 2249

Includes:
Midline defects
Neural tube defects (some)

Excludes:
Amniotic bands syndrome (0874)
Chromosomal syndromes with similar phenotypes
Meningocele (0642)

Major Diagnostic Criteria: A combination of two or more schisis-type defects, i.e., neural tube defects including **Anencephaly**, **Encephalocele**, and spina bifida aperta-cystica (see **Meningomyelocele**); oral clefts including **Cleft lip** with or without **Cleft palate** and posterior cleft palate; **Omphalocele**, exomphalos, gastroschisis, or diaghragmatic defects without other major primary defects.

Clinical Findings: Birth weight is low, about 2,000 gm, and mean gestational age is short; about 36 weeks. The distribution of component schisis-type defects is: neural tube defects 42%, oral cleft 27%, omphalocele 19%, and diaphragmatic defects 12%.

Complications: About 40% of cases were found in stillborns. Component schisis-type defects provoke a number of secondary consequences and cause an extreme high mortality.

Associated Findings: Nearly all component defects have associated anomalies.

Etiology: Unknown. Specific polygenic systems may create a liability for different schisis-type defects, and some genes of these systems may participate in governing the closure speed of different developing tissues in general.

Pathogenesis: Schisis-type defects are so called *midline defects*, and this developmental field may have poorly buffered morphogenetic properties.

POS No.: 4137

Sex Ratio: M1:F3; varies with component defects.

Occurrence: 10:100,000 total births in Hungary. Owing to high perinatal mortality, prevalences are extremely low following the neonatal period.

Risk of Recurrence for Patient's Sib: 3.7%, however, there is a higher fetal death rate in sibs.

Risk of Recurrence for Patient's Child: No report exists of a patient having reproduced.

Age of Detectability: At birth, prenatal diagnosis including ultrasound examination and amniotic AFP and acetylcholinesterase determination is possible for some components.

Gene Mapping and Linkage: Unknown.

Prevention: None known. Genetic counseling indicated. Periconceptional multivitamin supplementation may have some benefit.

Treatment: No effective measure known in cases involving anencephaly. Surgical intervention in appropriate cases.

Prognosis: Usually lethal within the first days of life.

Detection of Carrier: Unknown.

Special Considerations: Breech presentation and caesarean section in the delivery of index patients are more common. Fetal deaths, miscarriages, and stillbirths have a higher rate in the previous and subsequent pregnancies of index patient's mothers.

References:
Czeizel A: Schisis-association. Am J Med Genet 1981; 10:25–34.
Opitz JM: The developmental field concept in clinical genetics. J Pediatr 1982; 101:805–809.

CZ001   **Andrew Czeizel**

Schizencephaly with head enlargement
  See HYDRANENCEPHALY
Schizophrenic disorders
  See MOOD AND THOUGHT DISORDERS
Schlichting syndrome
  See CORNEAL DYSTROPHY, POLYMORPHOUS POSTERIOR
Schmid metaphyseal dysostosis
  See METAPHYSEAL CHONDRODYSPLASIA, TYPE SCHMID
Schmid-Fraccaro syndrome
  See CAT EYE SYNDROME
Schmitt syndrome
  *See RADIAL HYPOPLASIA-TRIPHALANGEAL THUMBS-
  HYPOSPADIAS-DIASTEMA*
Schneckenbecken dysplasia
  See SKELETAL DYSPLASIA, SCHNECKENBECKEN TYPE
Schnyder crystalline corneal dystrophy
  See CORNEAL DYSTROPHY, SCHNYDER CRYSTALLINE
Schusterbrust
  See PECTUS EXCAVATUM
Schwartz-Jampel syndrome
  *See CHONDRODYSTROPHIC MYOTONIA, SCHWARTZ-JAMPEL
  TYPE*
Schwartz-Lelek syndrome (one form)
  *See CRANIOMETAPHYSEAL DYSPLASIA
  also DIAPHYSEAL DYSPLASIA*

SCIMITAR SYNDROME   0879

Includes:
  Lung, hypoplastic-systemic arterial supply-venous drainage
  Pulmonary venous return, partial anomalous

Excludes: Pulmonary venous connection, total anomalous (0842)

Major Diagnostic Criteria: A scimitar shadow on chest X-ray in the right hemithorax. Cardiac catheterization must demonstrate the anomalous right pulmonary vein draining caudally into the inferior vena cava. The right lower lobe, in some cases, has received its arterial supply from an anomalous vessel arising from the aorta below the diaphragm.

Clinical Findings: Various malformations of the pulmonary venous system have been reported. In the pediatric age group, the scimitar syndrome has been diagnosed most frequently in children being evaluated for recurrent respiratory infections or the presence of the heart in the right chest. In its most complete form, this syndrome consists of: anomalous pulmonary venous connection and drainage of part or the entire lung into the inferior vena cava, hypoplasia of the right lung, hypoplasia of the right pulmonary artery, dextrorotation or dextroposition of the heart; and anomalous subdiaphragmatic systemic arterial supply to the lower

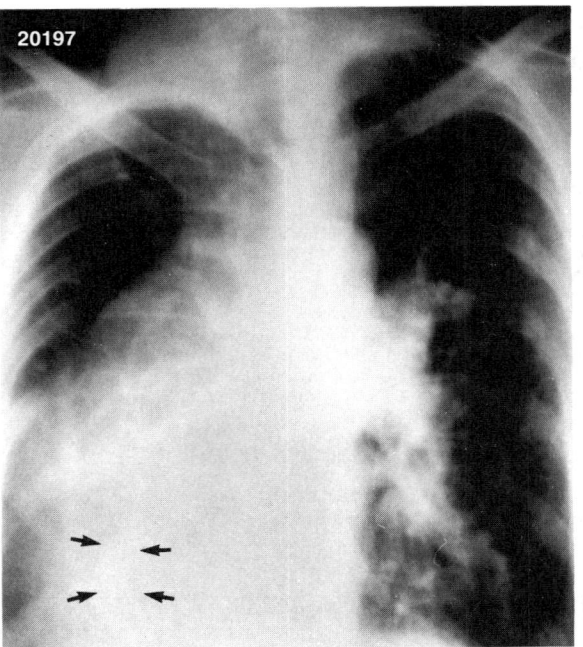

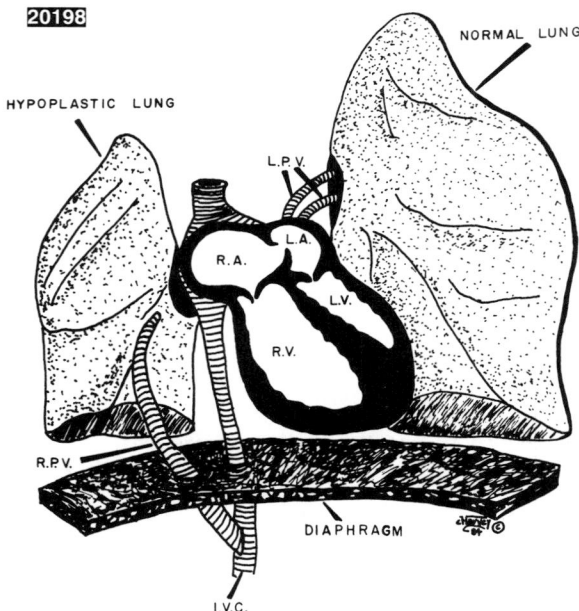

0879-20197: Chest X-ray shows cardiac shadow in the right chest (dextro-position) as well as a paracardiac shadow which is "scimitar-shaped" and widens as it approaches the right cardiophrenic angle. **20198:** Diagram shows the constellation of anomalies which produce the scimitar syndrome; note that the right hypoplastic lung and pulmonary vein drain into the inferior vena cava.

---

lobe of the right lung from the aorta or its main branches. The symptoms of this syndrome are related to the degree of hypoplasia of the right lung or associated cardiac anomalies. The presence of the anomalous pulmonary vein of the right lung draining into the inferior vena cava by itself does not usually give rise to symptoms. The diagnosis can be made on plain frontal chest X-ray: in the right hemithorax, a paracardiac shadow which is vertical, gently curved, and increased in width as it approaches the right cardiophrenic angle is seen. The shape of this shadow is similar to the shape of a scimitar. Also, the heart is usually in a dextroposition, and hypoplasia of the right lung in varying degrees may be seen. Bronchogram will demonstrate a variety of anomalies.

Complications: Recurrent pneumonia.

Associated Findings: Cardiac malformations are common. **Ventricular septal defect, Ductus arteriosus, patent, Heart, tetralogy of Fallot, Aorta, coarctation**, and absent right pulmonary artery have all been reported.

Etiology: Presumably multifactorial inheritance.

Pathogenesis: Unlike other pulmonary vein anomalies, the scimitar syndrome is accompanied by abnormalities of the right lung of varying degrees of severity. It should probably be considered an abnormal development of the right lung bud, representing a more primitive type of malformation than the usual anomalies of the pulmonary venous system.

MIM No.: 10670

Sex Ratio: M1:F1 in adults, preponderance of females in pediatric age group.

Occurrence: Over 100 cases have been documented.

Risk of Recurrence for Patient's Sib: Unknown.

Risk of Recurrence for Patient's Child: Unknown.

Age of Detectability: In infancy, by X-ray.

Gene Mapping and Linkage: Unknown.

Prevention: None known. Genetic counseling indicated.

Treatment: Antibiotics for recurrent pneumonia. Surgical resection of involved tissue or correction of cardiac anomalies.

Prognosis: Dependent on associated cardiac anomalies.

Detection of Carrier: Unknown.

Special Considerations: The scimitar syndrome is only one of a variety of pulmonary vein anomalies that are diverse in nature and frequently associated with other cardiac malformations. The clinical manifestations are varied but are frequently due to pulmonary venous and arterial hypertension. These anomalies have been classified on an anatomic basis into groups: stenotic lesions, accessory veins, and anomalous connection, either partial or total, in a variety of combinations.

References:

Neill CA, et al.: The familial occurrence of hypoplastic right lung with systemic arterial blood supply and venous draining: "Scimitar" syndrome. Bull Johns Hopkins Hosp 1960; 107:1–20.

Jue KL, et al.: Anomalies of great vessels associated with lung hypoplasia: the scimitar syndrome. Am J Dis Child 1966; 111:35–44.

Kiely B, et al.: Syndrome of anomalous venous drainage of the right lung into the inferiorvena cava: a review of 67 reported cases and three new cases in children. Am J Cardiol 1967; 20:102–116.

Nakib A, et al.: Anomalies of the pulmonary veins. Am J Cardiol 1967; 20:77–90.

Oakley D, et al.: Scimitar vein syndrome: report of nine new cases. Am Heart J 1984; 107–596–598.

K0018   **Boris G. Kousseff**

Sclera (blue)-hydrocephalus-nephrosis-thin skin-growth defect
See NEPHROSIS-HYDROCEPHALUS-THIN SKIN-BLUE SCLERA-GROWTH DEFECT
Scleroatrophic and keratotic dermatosis of limbs
See SCLEROTYLOSIS
Sclerocornea
See CORNEA PLANA

SCLERODERMA, FAMILIAL PROGRESSIVE   2154

Includes:
    Bleomycin induced scleroderma
    CREST syndrome
    L-5-hydroxytryptophan induced scleroderma
    Pentazocine induced scleroderma
    Progressive systemic sclerosis (PSS)
    Sclerosis, familial progressive systemic
    Trichloroethylene induced scleroderma
    Vinyl chloride induced scleroderma

Excludes:
    Graft vs host disease
    PSS following cosmetic surgery
    Scleroderma, non-familial
    Shulman syndrome

Major Diagnostic Criteria: The American Rheumatism Association (ARA) Scleroderma Criteria Cooperative Study Group suggested the following criteria: 1) proximal scleroderma is the single major criterion (91% sensitivity, 99% specificity); 2) sclerodactyly, pitting scars of fingertips or loss of substance of the finger pad, and bibasilar pulmonary fibrosis contribute as minor criteria; and 3) one major, or two or more minor criteria should be present to diagnose scleroderma.

Skin biopsy is essential to confirm the diagnosis. The characteristic microscopic features of scleroderma are: thickening or atrophy of dermis, thickening of cutis due to accumulation of layers of collagen in the dermis, obliteration of sweat glands and hair follicles, lymphocytic infiltration around sweat glands and roots of hair, hyalinization of walls of subcutaneous arterioles and perivascular infiltration by lymphocytes.

Recent studies on generalized scleroderma suggest the presence of two subsets:

1.) A diffuse cutaneous variety in which there is trunkal and acral skin involvement and early and significant interstital pulmonary fibrosis, renal failure, and diffuse involvement of the GI tract and of the myocardium. The presence of Anti-scl 70 antibody correlates highly with this clinical picture.

2.) A limited cutaneous variety charcterized by severe **Raynaud disease**, acral or no skin involvement, calcinosis, and telangiectasia. This subset is highly correlated with the presence of anti-centromere antibody.

Clinical Findings: Hardening of the skin of the hands, palms and chest; leathery feeling of the skin; generalized stiffness; inability to open mouth; polyarthralgia or polyarthritis, or both; blueness of hands and feet (see **Raynaud disease**); difficulty in swallowing; retrosternal chest pain and heartburn; constipation; crampy, abdominal pain.

Laboratory abnormalities that have been described include: elevated sedimentaion rate (ESR), anemia, hypergammaglobulinemia and the presence of antinuclear antibody (ANA) and rheumatoid factor (RF) in the serum.

Capillary nailfold microscopy is a simple procedure which shows characteristic abnormalities in the nailbed capillaries. These include enlargement of capillary loops, loss of capillaries (drop out), disruption of the orderly appearance of the normal capillary bed, and distortion and budding of the capillaries.

Pulmonary function studies show reduced vital capacity and defective diffusion (by carbon monoxide testing). Esophageal manometry shows decreased motility of the lower esophagus and defective functioning of lower esophageal sphincter.

Chest X-ray may show interstitial reticular pattern with prominence of pulmonary arterial segment and dilated heart. Gastrointestinal (GI) series with barium may show distended loops of bowel with air-fluid levels and dilated atonic colon. X-rays of the hands may show thinning of the pulp of the distal phalanges and partial absorption of bony tufts of the terminal phalanges and subcutaneous calcification.

Complications: **Raynaud disease**, with loss of fingertips and vasculitic ulcers of the tips of fingers; nodules over extensor aspects of elbows and knees which ulcerate; flexion deformity of fingers; respiratory failure with interstitial lung disease; right heart failure;

pulmonary hypertension; renal hypertension; renal failure; gastrointestinal obstruction.

Associated Findings: None known.

Etiology: Among the various chemicals that are known to induce a clinical picture of scleroderma are vinyl chloride, pentazocine, bleomycin, trichloroethylene and L-5-hydroxytryptophan. Occupational association with mining has been described. Also, recently, a scleroderma-like syndrome has been described from Spain following ingestion of adulterated cooking (rapeseed) oil. Some authors have also cited cases which suggest a genetic susceptibility to this condition.

Clinical, serological and pathological features of progressive systemic sclerosis (PSS) and **Lupus erythematosis, systemic** (SLE) have been described in different members of the same families. A mother with scleroderma, whose daughter had SLE, and a mother with SLE -- whose daughter had scleroderma, have both been described. There has also been a description of identical twins; one with PSS, and one with probable SLE. In another study of eight families containing one member with PSS and another with SLE, concordance for serological features was noted in familial pairs. Seven of the eight pairs in this study did not live in the same household at the onset of their diseases.

Pathogenesis: The etiology of scleroderma remains unknown. Abnormalities of collagen synthesis, collagen metabolism, humoral and cellular immune system, and vasoregulations have all been implicated. Clearly, the fibrosis of the skin and internal organs is due to the overproduction of collagen. There seems to be alterations in the metabolism and turn-over of collagen, and also probably synthesis of abnormal glycoproteins. Increase in quantitative immunoglobulins in the serum, the presence of rheumatoid factor and ANA, peripheral lymphopenia affecting T-cells, presence of T-cells in the tissue infiltrates, and the presence of sensitized lymphocytes in the circulation of patients with progressive systemic sclerosis suggest an immune basis for the pathogenesis of this disease. Also, a serum component capable of producing endothelial injury has been demonstrated in patients with progressive systemic sclerosis.

MIM No.: 18175

Sex Ratio: F3:M1

Occurrence: 5:10,000,000 per year

Risk of Recurrence for Patient's Sib: Unknown.

Risk of Recurrence for Patient's Child: Unknown.

Age of Detectability: Unknown.

Gene Mapping and Linkage: Unknown. Because the disease is more common in females, some authors have felt that this may be due to a mutant gene or genes on the X chromosome. However, in one report on familial scleroderma, all affected individuals were males, suggesting other inheritance factors.

Older studies have suggested a significant increase in frequency of HLA-A1, B-8, DR3, and DR5. However, more recent studies on large numbers of patients with progressive systemic sclerosis have failed to confirm these associations.

Scleroderma-like illness associated with vinyl chloride exposure is more common in individuals with HLA-DR5 (relative risk 3.5). The risk of progressive systemic sclerosis-like disease for males with DR5 antigen exposed to vinyl chloride is >90%.

Prevention: None known. Genetic counseling indicated.

Treatment: Nearly all patients need supportive therapy to control their **Raynaud disease**, arthritis, esophageal reflux and contractures. Right heart failure and renal disease may require intensive management. Renal failure may require aggressive antihypertensive treatment and renal dialysis. Specific therapy for progressive systemic sclerosis at present is d-Penicillamine.

Prognosis: The natural course is variable. Severe flexion contractures, particularly of the fingers, may be a major problem. Severe **Raynaud disease** may also lead to loss of fingertips or entire fingers and toes. Those with renal disease have the worst prognosis. Patients without visceral involvement may live a reasonably normal life. Prognosis is worse for those with involvement of lungs, kidney or heart at the time of diagnosis.

Detection of Carrier: Unknown.

Special Considerations: An inherited disease of Leghorn chicken, called, 'The University of California at Davis Line 200', has been described. The disease develops early in life with swelling and necrosis of the combs, digits, and the skin of these birds. Later on they develop fibrosis of the esophagus, heart, lungs and the small intestines -- just as in the human disease. These birds also develop antinuclear antibodies, rheumatoid factor, and antibodies to Type II collagen. Under the microscope, the skin shows intense mononuclear cell infiltration, dense deposition of collagen and obliteration of small arteries.

Increased frequency of chromosome breaks has been recognized in many rheumatic diseases. This has been particularly prominent in scleroderma. Chromosome abnormalities have been noted at rates of three times the control values in normals, and also in 95% of the patients examined. Cell cultures of both blood and skin have been shown to demonstrate these abnormalities. In a study of 21 relatives of patients with scleroderma, who also had Raynaud's phenomenon, all showed increased chromosome breaks. Subsequently, six of them developed scleroderma. Sister chromatid exchanges have also been described in scleroderma.

Chromosomal instability has been observed to be significantly increased in such occupations as goldminers with progressive systemic sclerosis. There is also increased chromosomal instability and breakage in patients with progressive systemic sclerosis with no known occupational exposure and in children of patients with progressive systemic sclerosis. These findings, together with the observation that certain chemicals can induce scleroderma-like syndrome, lend support to the concept of predisposition to progressive systemic sclerosis in the presence of certain environmental stimuli. Alternatively, certain chemicals can induce chromosome breaks which may or may not be related to the evolution of clinical disease.

Another interesting feature of this disease is the presence of anticentromere antibody (ACA) which has been noted in one variant of scleroderma called CREST syndrome. By special techniques, this antibody has been shown to be directed against the kinetochore discs of the chromosomes. It is occasionally seen in progressive systemic sclerosis also. In one study of 28 patients with scleroderma, fourteen had anticentromere antibody and fourteen did not have this antibody. Major chromosomal anomalies were noted in those with ACA more commonly that in those without ACA.

Support Groups: CA; Watsonville; United Scleroderma Foundation (USF)

References:

Greger RE: Familial progressive systemic scleroderma. Arch Dermatol 1975; 111:81–85.

Maricq HR: Widefield capillary microscopy: technique and rating scale for abnormalities seen in scleroderma and related disorders. Arthritis Rheum 1981; 24:1159–1165.

Sheldon WB, et al.: Three siblings with scleroderma (systemic sclerosis) and two with Raynaud's phenomenon from a single kindred. Arthritis Rheum 1981; 24:668–676.

LeRoy E, et al.: Scleroderm (systemic sclerosis): classification, subsets and pathogenisis. (Editorial) J Rheumatol 1988; 15:202–205.

McGregor AR: Familial clustering of scleroderma spectrum disease. Am J Med 1988; 84:1023–1032.

Steen VD, et al.: Clinical correlations and prognosis based on serum autoantibodies in patients with systemic sclerosis. Arthritis Rheum 1988; 31:196–203.

AT002   **Balu H. Athreya**
VA005   **Don C. Van Dyke**

SCLEROSTEOSIS 0880

Includes:
> Cortical hyperostosis-syndactyly
> Sklerosteose

Excludes:
> **Osteopetrosis, benign dominant** (0779)
> **Osteopetrosis, malignant recessive** (0780)
> **Endosteal hyperostosis** (0497)

Major Diagnostic Criteria: Gigantism, syndactyly, and X-ray demonstration of sclerosis and hyperostosis of the skull and axial skeleton.

Clinical Findings: Mandibular prognathism and frontal prominence become evident by the age of five years. These deformities progress, and in adulthood the face is severely distorted, with dental malocclusion, proptosis, and relative mid-facial hypoplasia. Affected children are tall for their age, and adults with the condition may have gigantism. The majority have partial or total

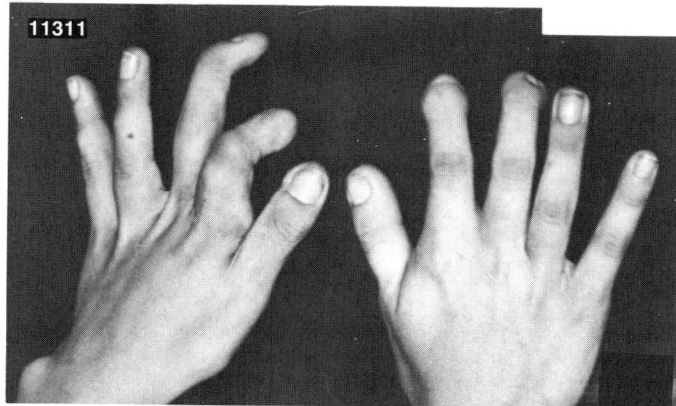

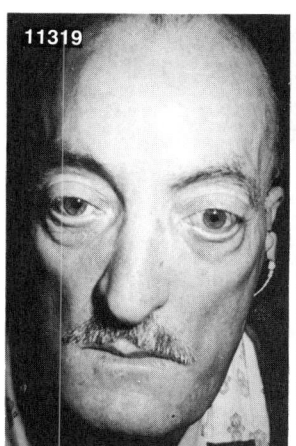 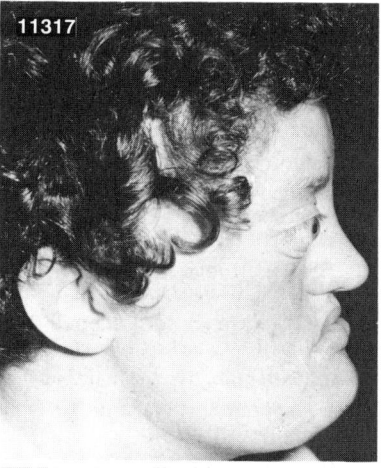

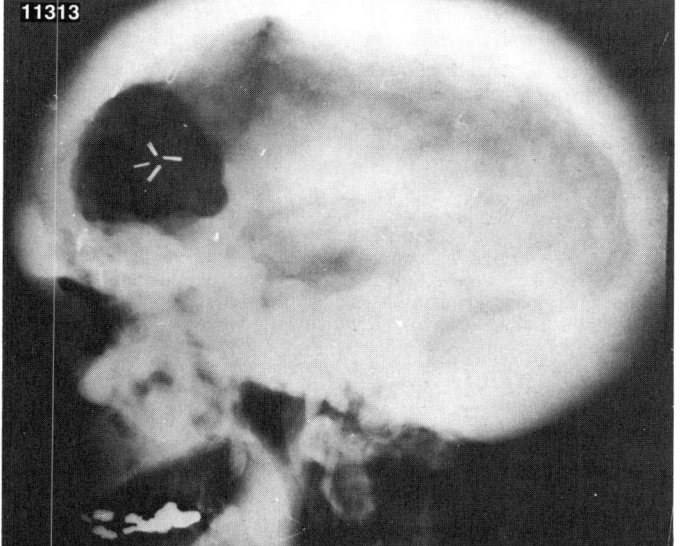

0880A-11319: Asymmetric enlargement of the mandible, facial palsy, proptosis and deafness. 11317: Profile of face shows broad mandible. 11313: Massive cranial hyperostosis and thickening of calvaria and skull base. Surgical clips are from a craniotomy.

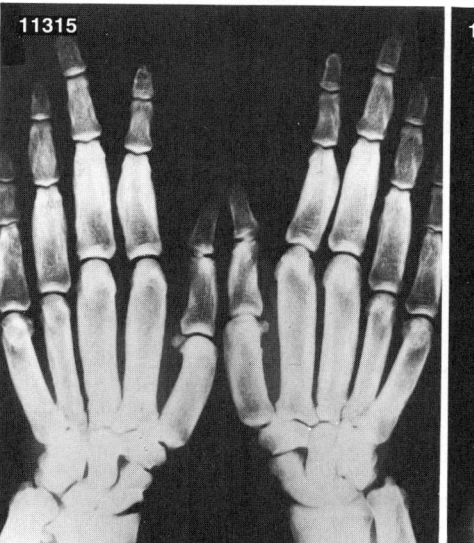 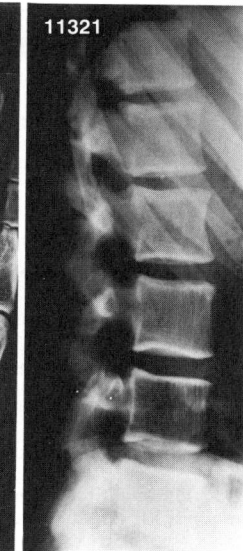

0880B-11311: Syndactyly and radial deviation of 2nd and 3rd fingers and dysplastic nails. 11315: Sclerosis and lack of diaphyseal constriction. 11321: Spinal sclerosis and straightening.

syndactyly, usually of the second and third fingers, with deviation of the terminal phalanges and hypoplasia of the nails on the corresponding digits. The bones are resistant to trauma and fractures are infrequent. On X-ray, the calvaria is widened and uniformly sclerotic. The base becomes very dense, and the cranial nerve foramina may be obliterated. The sinuses remain patent, and the sella turcica may be expanded. The mandible is dense and massive, with asymmetrical distortion and dental malocclusion. The vertebral end plates and pedicles are sclerotic, but the outlines of the bodies are not disturbed. The clavicles and ribs are widened and dense; the scapulae and pelvis are sclerotic but not expanded. The tubular bones are massive, with cortical hyperostosis and moderate alteration of their external contours.

Complications: Transient palsy of the seventh nerve occurs during infancy, and bilateral facial paralysis is usually permanent by adulthood. Progressive bony encroachment upon the middle ear cavities and auditory nerve canals often causes deafness in mid-childhood. Compression of the optic nerves is a late complication. Overgrowth of the calvarium leads to progressive diminution of the capacity of the cranial cavity, with elevation of intracranial pressure. Severe headache due to this mechanism often develops in early adulthood, and several patients have died suddenly from impaction of the medulla oblongata in the foramen magnum.

Associated Findings: None known.

Etiology: Autosomal recessive inheritance.

Pathogenesis: Unknown.

MIM No.: *26950

POS No.: 3386

Sex Ratio: M1:F1

Occurrence: About 60 cases have been documented, the majority in the Afrikaner population of South Africa. Sporadic cases, or siblings, have been recorded in the United States (including those from an inbred triracial group from southern Maryland known as the "We-Sorts"), Switzerland, Japan, and Brazil.

Risk of Recurrence for Patient's Sib:
See Part I, *Mendelian Inheritance.*

Risk of Recurrence for Patient's Child:
See Part I, *Mendelian Inheritance.*

Age of Detectability: At birth. Syndactyly or facial palsy in an "at risk" newborn are important diagnostic indicators. X-ray changes are evident by the age of five years.

Gene Mapping and Linkage: Unknown.

Prevention: None known. Genetic counseling indicated.

Treatment: Prophylactic craniectomy in early adulthood is necessary in most affected persons. Decompression of 7th and 8th cranial nerves gives inconsistent results. An external hearing aid may be beneficial. Syndactyly requires cosmetic repair. Orthodontic measures are indicated for dental malalignment.

Prognosis: Intelligence and general health are unimpaired. The majority of affected persons develop unilateral or bilateral facial palsy and deafness. Intracranial pressure rises in adulthood, and sudden death from impaction of the medulla oblongata in the foramen magnum is frequent unless circumvented by craniectomy.

Detection of Carrier: Heterozygotes have calvarial widening, with loss of distinction between the tables of the skull. The changes are variable in degree and not definitive.

Special Considerations: In a mildly affected person with sclerosteosis, the phenotype is very similar to that of severely affected individuals with van Buchem disease (see **Endosteal hyperostosis**). As the Afrikaners are derived from Dutch stock, it is possible that there is some fundamental genetic relationship between these two autosomal recessive disorders.

References:
Truswell AS: Osteopetrosis with syndactyly: a morphological variant of Albers-Schonberg's disease. J Bone Joint Surg 1958; 40B:208–218.
Beighton P, The radiology of sclerosteosis. Br J Radiol 1976; 49:934–939. †
Beighton P, et al.: The clinical features of sclerosteosis: a review of the manifestations in twenty-five affected individuals. Ann Intern Med 1976; 84:393–397. †
Beighton P, et al.: Sclerosteosis: an autosomal recessive disorder. Clin Genet 1977; 11:1–7.
Beighton P, Hamersma H: Sclerosteosis in South Africa. S Afr Med J 1979; 55:783–788. * †
Epstein S, et al.: Endocrine function in sclerosteosis. S Afr Med J 1979; 55:1105–1110.
Beighton P, et al.: The syndromic status of sclerosteosis and van Buchem's disease. Clin Genet 1984; 25:175–181. * †

BE008   **Peter Beighton**

SCLEROTYLOSIS   3076

Includes:
Scleroatrophic and keratotic dermatosis of limbs
TYS

Excludes: Keratosis palmaris et plantaris of Unna-Thost (3264)

Major Diagnostic Criteria: Atrophic fibrosis of the skin of the limbs, nail abnormalities, and keratodermia of the palms and soles in a symmetric distribution.

Clinical Findings: The hands are small, erythematous, and covered by thin cracked skin, giving a scleroatrophic appearance. Flattening of the thenar and hypothenar eminences with hyperkeratosis of the palms is present. The fingers are usually streamlined and in a slight flexural position, limiting extension. The nail changes are of the hypoplastic type, presenting with fissures and partial hippocratism. Hypohidrosis may be present. The same changes are exhibited on the feet, occurring symmetrically: acromicria, and keratodermia of the soles, particularly in the pressure points; diffuse erythrodermia; hypohidrosis; and nail abnormalities. The patients are in good health otherwise.

Complications: Development of a squamous cell carcinoma within a lesion has been reported by most investigators.

Associated Findings: None known.

Etiology: Autosomal dominant inheritance.

Pathogenesis: Unknown.

MIM No.: *18160

Sex Ratio: Presumably M1:F1.

Occurrence: Several kindreds have been reported (Huriez et al, 1969; Lambert et al, 1978; and Fischer, 1978) with over 50 affected individuals.

Risk of Recurrence for Patient's Sib:
See Part I, *Mendelian Inheritance.*

Risk of Recurrence for Patient's Child:
See Part I, *Mendelian Inheritance.*

Age of Detectability: Usually at birth.

Gene Mapping and Linkage: TYS (sclerotylosis) has been provisionally mapped to 4q.

Prevention: None known. Genetic counseling indicated.

Treatment: Emollient creams can be used to reduce the excessive dryness of the skin.

Prognosis: Guarded because of the degeneration of the skin lesions into squamous cell carcinoma usually observed after age 40 years.

Detection of Carrier: Unknown.

References:
Huriez CL, et al.: Genodermatose sclero-atrophiante et keratodermique des extremites. Ann Dermatol Syphilig 1969; 96:135–146.
Lambert D, et al.: La genodermatose sclero-atrophiante et keratodermique des extremites. Ann dermatol Venereol. 1977; 104:654–657.
Fischer S: La genodermatose scleroatrophiante et keratodermique des extremites (au sujet de trois nouveaux cas familiaux). Ann Dermatol Venereol 1978; 105:1079–1082.
Lambert D, et al.: Genodermatose sclero-atrophiante et Keratodermique des extremites. J Genet Hum 1978; 26:25–31.

MI038   **Giuseppe Micali**

Sebaceous nevus syndrome
  See NEVUS, EPIDERMAL NEVUS SYNDROME
Seborrheic alopecia
  See HAIR, BALDNESS, COMMON

SECKEL SYNDROME   0881

Includes:

Bird-headed dwarf (obsolete/pejorative)
Bird-headed dwarf, Montreal type
Bird-headed dwarfism, Virchow type
Dwarfism, Seckel type
Microcephalic primordial dwarfism
Nanocephalic dwarf

Excludes:

Alopecia-skeletal anomalies-short stature-mental retardation
  (2782)
Dwarfism, osteodysplastic primordial, Majewski-Ranke type
  (2582)
Dwarfism, osteodysplastic primordial, Majewski-Winter type
  (2581)
Microcephaly (0659)

Major Diagnostic Criteria: The diagnosis depends upon characteristic craniofacies: small head, large eyes, mental retardation, low birth weight, dwarfism, beaked nose, and other malformations.

Clinical Findings: Low birth weight for length of gestation, severe microcephaly, mental retardation, marked postnatal growth retardation, delayed bone age, large eyes, large beaklike nose, narrow face, dysplastic ears, and receding lower jaw. The brain shows a much simplified gross cerebral structure (pongidoid microcephaly), with relatively intact cerebellum.

Complications: Premature closure of cranial sutures.

Associated Findings: Hypoplastic thumb, dislocation of femoral heads or radial heads, clubfoot, scoliosis, strabismus, and gastrointestinal malformations. Chromosome breakage has been demonstrated in two patients, one of whom had pancytopenia.

Etiology: Autosomal recessive inheritance.

Pathogenesis: Some patients have had mitomycin C-produced chromosome breakage (Butler et al, 1987), and may account for a subgroup of Seckel cases.

MIM No.: *21060, 21070

POS No.: 3387

CDC No.: 759.820

Sex Ratio: M1:F1

Occurrence: Estimated at no more than 1:10,000 live births.

Risk of Recurrence for Patient's Sib:
  See Part I, *Mendelian Inheritance.*

Risk of Recurrence for Patient's Child:
  See Part I, *Mendelian Inheritance.*

Age of Detectability: At birth, or prenatally by serial ultrasound.

Gene Mapping and Linkage: Unknown.

Prevention: None known. Genetic counseling indicated.

Treatment: Unknown.

Prognosis: For life: good. For intelligence: mental retardation is a prominent feature of the syndrome. For function: function may be impaired by various anomalies such as dislocated femoral heads, clubfoot, and scoliosis.

Detection of Carrier: Unknown.

Special Considerations: Fitch et al (1970) described a similar but separate condition with normal birth weight and signs of premature senility which has been designated *bird-headed dwarfism, Montreal type.* Virchow (1896) also described a form of bird-headed dwarfism with low birthweight, but without mental retardation and associated malformations.

References:

Virchow R: Vostelling der birmesischen zwerge mit einem Salzburger Riesen. Z Ethnologie 1896 28:524–528.
McKusick VA, et al.: Seckel's bird-headed dwarfism. New Engl J Med 1967; 277:279–286.
Fitch N, et al.: A form of bird-headed dwarfism with features of premature senility. Am J Dis Child 1970; 120:260–264.
Fenolio KR, et al.: Prenatal diagnosis of Seckel syndrome. Am J Hum Genet 1982; 34:88A.
Majewski F, Goecke T: Studies of microcephalic primordial dwarfism: approaches to a delineation of Seckel syndrome. Am J Med Genet 1982; 12:7–21. *
Thompson E, Pembrey M: Seckel syndrome: an overdiagnosed syndrome. J Med Genet 1985; 22:192–201.
Butler MG, et al.: Do some patients with Seckel syndrome have hematological problems and/or chromosome breakage? Am J Med Genet 1987; 27:645–649.
Majoor-Krakauer DF, et al.: Microcephaly, micrognathia, bird-headed dwarfism: prenatal diagnosis of a Seckel-like syndrome. Am J Med Genet 1987; 27:183–188.

GR011   **Frank Greenberg**
                                                  Victor A. McKusick

Secondary diphallia
  See DIPHALLIA
Seemanova syndrome
  See CHROMOSOME INSTABILITY, NIJMEGEN TYPE
Segmental tracheal agenesis
  See TRACHEA, AGENESIS
Seip syndrome
  See LIPODYSTROPHY SYNDROME, BERARDINELLI TYPE
Seitelberg variant, Pelizaeus-Merzbacher syndrome
  See PELIZAEUS-MERZBACHER SYNDROME
Seitelberger disease
  See NEUROAXONAL DYSTROPHY, INFANTILE
Seizues, impulsive petit mal
  See SEIZURES, MYOCLONIC, JUVENILE JANZ TYPE
Seizures, benign familial neonatal-infantile
  See CONVULSIONS, BENIGN FAMILIAL NEONATAL

SEIZURES, CENTRALOPATHIC   0135

Includes:

Absence seizures
Centralopathic epilepsy
Epilepsy, centralopathic
Epilepsy, centrencephalic
Petit mal seizures
Petit mal automatism
Petit mal lapse ("absence")

Excludes:

Akinetic or atonic "drop" seizures
Automatisms and psychopathic behavior
Epilepsy due to focal cortical lesion
Grand mal epilepsy
Myoclonic petit mal
Petit mal grand mal epilepsy
Seizures (other)
Spastic ataxia, Charlevoix-Saguenay type (2566)

Major Diagnostic Criteria: The typical, bilaterally synchronous EEG, showing a three per-second spike-and-wave abnormality, is used to identify petit mal epilepsy in the context of concomitant alteration of consciousness.

Clinical Findings: There is considerable controversy as to the use of the term "centralopathic epilepsy," particularly since the introduction of the International Classification of the Epilepsies. Petit mal (absence) epilepsy is defined as a seizure disorder characterized by brief lapses in consciousness associated with a typical EEG and the absence of neurologic signs.

  The seizure may be so mild that it escapes notice; the child may be observed as inattentive or as daydreaming excessively. Seizures are usually abrupt in onset and may occur frequently for short periods of time. Recurrent seizures can cause loss of concentration and thus deterioration in school performance. The seizures typically begin between the ages of 5 and 10 years and are more common in females. There may be a slight pause, blinking of the eyes, a brief stare, and then resumption of activity. More severe seizures may cause lapses of speech and fluttering of the eyelids. Loss of sphincter control, change in color, and gross motor movements do not occur. At the conclusion of the attack, the patient continues the activity that immediately preceded the seizure. An aura does not occur. The diagnosis is made by the history and the typical EEG finding. Hyperventilation for a period of 3 or 4 minutes is often successful in eliciting a clinical seizure and producing typical EEG changes.

Complications: Grand mal seizures are relatively common in patients with petit mal epilepsy. Prolonged grand mal seizures may be associated with airway obstruction and anoxia.

Associated Findings: Frequent petit mal seizures can cause deterioration in memory and thus a decline in school performance. Rarely, patients with petit mal epilepsy develop status epilepticus and muteness, which may be misinterpreted as hysteria.

Etiology: Autosomal dominant inheritance in some families, although some investigators suggest the interaction of several genetic factors rather than a specific autosomal dominant mode of inheritance.

Pathogenesis: Until recently, it was generally accepted that petit mal epilepsy resulted from an abnormality in the subcortical structures, because electrical stimulation of midline areas in the experimental animal and man would often produce the typical EEG abnormality and clinical seizure. More recent studies suggest that petit mal epilepsy results from a cortical disturbance or abnormality, which produces bilateral foci, particularly from the frontal lobes. The delayed age of onset of the seizures may be related to maturation of the brain, including myelination of the corpus callosum and related structures, and the interaction of various neurotransmitters, all of which may be under genetic control.

MIM No.: *11710

Sex Ratio: M1:F1

Occurrence: 1:200.

Risk of Recurrence for Patient's Sib:
See Part I, *Mendelian Inheritance.* According to Metrakos and Metrakos (1961, 1966), there is a 50% chance that a patient's sib or offspring will inherit the gene for the spike and wave EEG trait and a 35% chance that the EEG will show a typical three per-second finding sometime during his or her lifetime. There is a 12% chance that the sib or offspring will have a convulsion at some time during his or her lifetime but only an 8% chance that a sib or child of a patient will actually develop petit mal epilepsy.

Risk of Recurrence for Patient's Child:
See Part I, *Mendelian Inheritance.* Petit mal epilepsy is probably the result of an autosomal dominant gene, which has low penetrance at birth but gains almost complete penetrance between ages 4 and 16 years and then rather rapidly declines. Twin studies have shown that when one monozygotic twin develops seizures, the chance of the other twin being affected is 80–90%. Dizygotic twins show only a 10% concordance.

Age of Detectability: Most readily detected between 4 and 16 years.

Gene Mapping and Linkage: Unknown.

Prevention: None known. Genetic counseling indicated.

Treatment: The use of specific drugs such as ethosuximide, clonazepam, or sodium valproate controls most seizures.
Special education may be necessary for the child with frequent and recurrent seizures that are not responsive to medication.

Prognosis: Most patients are seizure-free by age 15 to 20 years and may not require lifelong anticonvulsants.

Detection of Carrier: By EEG. Between ages 5 and 15 years approximately 40% of sibs have an abnormal EEG, but they may remain seizure-free clinically. The EEG finding is unusual beyond age 40 years.

Support Groups:
MD; Landover; Epilepsy Foundation of America

References:
Lennox WG: Heredity of epilepsy as told by relatives and twins. JAMA 1951; 146:529.
Penfield W, Jasper H: Epilepsy and the functional anatomy of the human brain. Boston: Little, Brown, 1954.
Metrakos K, Metrakos JD: Genetics of convulsive disorders: II. Genetic and electroencephalographic studies in centrencephalic epilepsy. Neurology 1961; 11:474–483.
Metrakos JD, Metrakos K: Childhood epilepsy of subcortical ("centrencephalic") origin. Clin Pediatr 1966; 5:536.
Gastaut H: Clinical and electroencephalographical classification of epileptic seizures. Epilepsia 1970; 11:102.
Doose H, et al.: Genetic factors in spike-wave absences. Epilepsia 1973; 14:57.
Newmark ME, Penry JK: Genetics of epilepsy: a review. New York: Raven, 1980.
Commission on Classification and Terminology of the International League Against Epilepsy. Proposal for classification of epilepsies and epileptic syndromes. Epilepsia 1981; 22:489–501.

HA053   **Robert H.A. Haslam**

Seizures, dominant benign neonatal
See CONVULSIONS, BENIGN FAMILIAL NEONATAL

SEIZURES, FEBRILE   2568

Includes: Febrile convulsions, simple and complex (complicated)

Excludes:
Convulsions, benign familial neonatal (3216)
Convulsions induced by gross abnormality of the brain
Convulsions induced by infections of the central nervous system

Major Diagnostic Criteria: Convulsions occurring in the presence of rectal temperature of over 38°C.

Clinical Findings: Simple febrile seizures are characterized by generalized and tonic-clonic seizures, usually of brief duration, (1–5 minutes in length). Less frequently, children have focal seizures or postictal Todds paralysis. In 2–3% of cases, the duration of the febrile seizure may last up to 30 minutes, which may indicate preexisting brain pathology. Occurrence of multiple febrile seizures is possible.

Complications: No children have died as a direct consequence of febrile seizures per se or their long term neurologic sequelae. However, individuals with febrile seizures of longer duration may be at increased risk to developing status epilepticus. The risk for development of future epilepsy is increased with repeated febrile seizures.

Associated Findings: Since infections of the respiratory tract and otitis media, accompanied by high fever, are common in young children (age 5 years or less), over 50% of febrile seizure patients are often seen with these conditions. Associated conditions include roseola, other infectious diseases, and in a small percentage (usually less than 5%) with intracranial infections. Approximately one-third of patients 3–6 years of age demonstrate three-per-second spike-and-wave-paroxysms, although this may not be evident at the time of the convulsion. These paroxysms occur more often in patients with a family history of convulsions.

Etiology: Family studies suggest that febrile seizures are a hereditary trait, with the mode of inheritance consistent with multifactorial transmission. However, recent evidence has indicated that transmission in families in which the proband has three or more febrile seizures is consistent with autosomal dominant inheritance. Transmission in families in which the proband has one or two febrile seizures is consistent with a multifactorial model, with a heritability liability of about 70%.

Pathogenesis: Unknown. Febrile-like seizures may be produced in laboratory animals by means of high temperature (hyperthermic seizures); however, the temperature increases in the animal models may be inordinately high with respect to those seen in the human patients. In addition, there have been reports of alterations in endorphin metabolism.

MIM No.: 12121, 21720

Sex Ratio: Presumably M1:F1. However, observed figures are M1.2:F1 for the United States and M1.6:F1 for Japan.

Occurrence: Convulsions associated with febrile illness are one of the most common acute neurologic disturbances seen in childhood. The population rate varies with the ethnic group and geographic location. There are high population rates in Japan (6.7%) and uniformly lower rates in Denmark (2.1%) and the United States (2.3%).

Risk of Recurrence for Patient's Sib: Overall, 8.0% of sibs will have convulsions with fever. The risk of febrile seizures for sibs is not significantly influenced by the sex of the proband. The greater the number of febrile convulsions in probands, the greater the risk for febrile convulsions in sibs. Complex features (focal seizures, Todds paralysis) in the proband are associated with increased risk for febrile seizures in sibs.

Risk of Recurrence for Patient's Child: Nearly 8.4% of children of probands are expected to have a febrile convulsion. Children of female probands, especially sons, have a higher risk than children of male probands. The greater the number of febrile convulsions in probands, the greater the risk for febrile convulsions in the children.

Age of Detectability: Usually clinically evident between birth and five years of age.

Gene Mapping and Linkage: Unknown.

Prevention: Patients with recurrent febrile seizures may be given long-term prophylactic anticonvulsants for one year from the last seizure, two years from the first seizure, or until five years of age.

Treatment: There is considerable debate in the literature concerning the utility of treatment for febrile seizures. The use of a loading dose of phenobarbital, at the time of prolonged febrile seizure, has been recommended for control of further febrile seizures, accompanied by clinical evaluation for the presence of structural brain abnormalities. Long-term treatment with phenobarbital does not appear to prevent epilepsy effectively following a febrile seizure. With the complication rate associated with drug usage as great as (or greater than) the risk of epilepsy, the cost/benefit of drug usage needs careful evaluation.

Prognosis: Good. However, nearly one-third of all patients with a first febrile seizure will have repeated febrile convulsions.

Detection of Carrier: Clinical evaluation and a careful family history.

Special Considerations: Patients with febrile seizures have a three-to-six fold increase in risk of epilepsy as compared with the general population. However, the majority of children with febrile seizures do not develop epilepsy. While twin studies of febrile seizures are inconclusive, there appears to be an increase in concordance of febrile seizures in monozygotic twins (31%) versus dizygotic twins (14%), consistent with a genetic as well as an environmental pathogenic mechanism.

Support Groups: MD; Landover; Epilepsy Foundation of America

References:
Schiottz-Christensen E: Genetic factors in febrile convulsions. Acta Neurol Scandinav 1972; 48:538–546.
van den Berg B: Studies on convulsive disorders in young children: incidence of convulsions among siblings. Develop Med Child Neurol 1974; 16:457–464.
Annegers JF, et al: The risk of epilepsy following febrile convulsions. Neurology 1979; 29:297–303. *
Hauser WA, et al: The risk of seizure disorders among relatives of children with febrile convulsions. Neurology 1985; 35:1268–1273. *
Annegers JF, et al: Prognostic factors for unprovoked seizures after febrile seizures. New Engl J Med 1987; 316:493–498.
Rich SS, et al: Complex segregation analysis of febrile convulsions. Am J Hum Genet 1987; 41:249–257.

RI016   **Stephen S. Rich**
HA073   **W. Allen Hauser**

SEIZURES, IN FEMALES, JUBERG-HELLMAN TYPE   2479

Includes: Juberg-Hellman syndrome

Excludes:
   Aicardi syndrome (2320)
   Convulsive disorder-mental retardation, benign familial neonatal
   Convulsive disorder with prenatal or early onset, familial
   Mental retardation-epilepsy-endocrine disorders

Major Diagnostic Criteria: 1) Convulsive disorder with age of onset from six to 18 months; 2) tonic-clonic seizures; 3) mental retardation ranging from profound to mild; and 4) electroencephalograms showing focal, diffuse, or paroxysmal abnormalities, or some combination thereof without unique or consistent patterns.

Clinical Findings: Female sex. Convulsive disorder without apparent mental retardation (12/29); convulsive disorder with mental retardation (8/29); asymmetry of the anterior horns (1/29); dilation of lateral ventricles (1/29); **Microcephaly** (1/29); focal electroencephalographic (EEG) abnormality (1/17); diffuse EEG abnormalities (2/17); focal and diffuse EEG abnormalities (2/17); focal and paroxysmal EEG abnormalities (3/17); diffuse and paroxysmal EEG abnormalities (2/17); and focal, diffuse, and paroxysmal EEG abnormalities (2/17).

Complications: Postictal paresis, facial asymmetry, and disturbance of gait.

Associated Findings: Strabismus, malformation of the hand with **Syndactyly** and digital deficiency.

Etiology: Possibly X-linked dominant inheritance with sex-limited expression.

Pathogenesis: Unknown.

MIM No.: 12125

Sex Ratio: M0:F1

Occurrence: One kinship originating with 15 affected sisters has been reported.

Risk of Recurrence for Patient's Sib:
   See Part I, *Mendelian Inheritance.*

Risk of Recurrence for Patient's Child:
   See Part I, *Mendelian Inheritance.*

Age of Detectability: Probably not before six months of age.

Gene Mapping and Linkage: Unknown.

Prevention: None known. Genetic counseling indicated.

Treatment: Anticonvulsant medications such as phenobarbital, diphenylhydantoin sodium, mephobarbital, and primidone. Early childhood educational intervention and special education.

Prognosis: Convulsive-free periods may last for years. Mental retardation will vary from mild to profound. Probably normal life span.

Detection of Carrier: Unknown.

Special Considerations: In the fourth generation, there is an unusually high proportion of affected females (15/18) among the offspring of transmitting males. In addition, 6/7 males with daughters past infancy transmitted the gene. An X-linked dominant gene with limitation of clinical manifestations to females is more likely than autosomal dominant inheritance in this family. The odds ratio is 562:1 favoring X-linked dominant inheritance over autosomal dominant, assuming high but not complete penetrance of either gene.

The author would like to express his appreciation to Herbert A. Lubs for his help in the follow-up of the family affected with this condition.

References:
Juberg RC, Hellman CD: A new familial form of convulsive disorder and mental retardation limited to females. J Pediatr 1971; 79:726–732. *

JU000   **Richard C. Juberg**

SEIZURES, MYOCLONIC, JUVENILE JANZ TYPE   2567

Includes:
    Epilepsy, juvenile myoclonic, Janz type
    Janz syndrome
    Juvenile myoclonic epilepsy (JME), Janz type
    Myoclonic epilepsy, benign
    Seizues, impulsive petit mal

Excludes: Seizures (other)

Major Diagnostic Criteria: Isolated bilateral, myoclonic jerks without loss of consciousness, most often of the upper extremities, sometimes also involving lower extremities, that occur usually in the mornings shortly after awakening or after sleep deprivation. Major seizures, generally tonic-clonic, are usually the initial complaint. About 30% of cases also show absence seizures.

Clinical Findings: Age of onset is seldom before 10 years. The most common pattern is for myoclonic jerks to start around age 14–15 years. However, patients usually do not recognize jerking as abnormal. Most often, the first tonic-clonic seizure will cause the patient to seek medical help. Patients may comment that they are "clumsy" or "spastic." Often only when asked if they "drop things" in the morning or suddenly "throw things across the room" will the fact that the patient has been having myoclonic jerks emerge. Myoclonic jerks will often start before the first tonic-clonic seizure, but the first occurrences of the two types of seizures may be close together in time. Absence, when it occurs, is almost always of the adolescent type, with a few absence attacks per day.

In almost all cases, the interictal EEG shows bursts of a 4–6-Hz multispike-and-wave pattern, sometimes lasting several seconds. On closed circuit television monitoring, these multispike-and-wave bursts can sometimes be seen to coincide with jerking.

Family history is sometimes positive for generalized epilepsy, either tonic-clonic seizures or absence, and occasionally for juvenile myoclonic epilepsy (JME) itself, but the family history is often negative. Research shows that a high percentage of family members have positive findings on EEG testing. Often, these findings show the same 4–6-Hz multispike-and-wave pattern seen interictally in patients, although jerking is not seen in the clinically unaffected family members. Other EEG abnormalities seen in family members are paroxysmal bursts of 3–5-Hz high-amplitude slowing. Perhaps 17% of sibs over age 20 years show EEG abnormalities, while only 1–5% of the general public show such abnormalities.

JME should be distinguished from the degenerative myoclonic epilepsies, which have a higher recurrence risk and poorer prognosis.

Complications: Usual complications of epilepsy. Uncontrolled seizures can be life-threatening and lead to accidents. Jerking can lead to accidents and falls. Complications that result from medications are frequent.

Associated Findings: None known.

Etiology: Possibly autosomal recessive inheritance with 60% penetrance. A two locus model of inheritance has also been suggested.

Pathogenesis: Unknown.

MIM No.: 25477

Sex Ratio: Presumably M1:F1.

Occurrence: Juvenile myoclonic epilepsy is thought to comprise 5–10% of all epilepsies, or a population prevalence of 5–10:10,000. This is probably an underestimate, since people manifesting the myoclonic jerks with no other seizures will seldom seek medical help. The condition affects all ethnic groups.

Risk of Recurrence for Patient's Sib: Empiric risk for any form of epilepsy in a sib is about 5–7%. If the sib has an EEG abnormality

and is older than age 20 years, risk is apparently not increased. The risk for sibs younger than age 20 years with an EEG abnormality is unknown.

Risk of Recurrence for Patient's Child: Unknown.

Age of Detectability: Clinical signs start at 10–20 years of age, most frequently around ages 13–15 years. Age when EEG abnormalities start is unknown.

Gene Mapping and Linkage: EJM (epilepsy, juvenile myoclonic) has been tentatively mapped to 6p.

Prevention: None known. Genetic counseling indicated.

Treatment: Valproic acid appears to be 95% effective in controlling both tonic-clonic and myoclonic seizures. Frequently, the EEG signs also disappear with valproic acid treatment. Adverse reactions to valproic acid monotherapy often dictate use of other drugs such as primidone or carbamazepine, but seizures with these medications will sometimes occur.

Prognosis: The condition is not progressive, though apparently life-long.

Detection of Carrier: Unknown.

Special Considerations: Heterogeneity may exist. Reports conflict about the proportions of patients with photosensitivity. Also, some patients have absence seizures while some do not. However, family members with epilepsy (but not JME) have been found to have tonic-clonic seizures without absence in some families, while in other families absence seizures occur without motor involvement. This may point to a similar underlying cause for both types of seizures in families with JME.

JME is frequently misdiagnosed, resulting in the prescription of inappropriate medication. As a result, while medications other than valproic acid will reduce the frequency of seizures, patients often achieve only fair or poor seizure control. In an effort to control seizures, levels of antiepileptic drugs may be increased to the point at which the patient feels constantly drowsy and, since onset is in the teenage years, the patient's education and social adjustment may suffer.

Support Groups:
    New York; National Myoclonus Foundation
    MD; Landover; Epilepsy Foundation of America

References:
Janz D: Inpulsiv-Petit mal. Dtsch Nervenheilkd 1957; 176:346–86.
Tsuboi T, Christian W: On the genetics of the primary generalized epilepsy with sporadic myoclonias of impulsive petit mal type: a clinical and electroencephalographic study of 399 probands. Humangenetik 1973; 19:155–182.
Delgado-Escueta A, Enrile-Bascal F: Juvenile myoclonic epilepsy of Janz. Neurology 1984; 34:285–294. *
Durner M, et al.: HLA and epilepsie mit impulsive petit mal. In: Speckman EJ, ed: Epilepsie 1987. Rheinbeck: Einhorn Presse, 1988.
Greenberg DA, et al.: Segregation analysis of juvenile myoclonic epilepsy. Genetic Epidemiology 1988; 5:81–94.
Greenberg DA, et al.: Juvenile myoclonic epilepsy (JME) may be linked to the BF and HLA loci on human chromosome 6. Am J Med Genet 1988; 31:185–192. *

GR012   **David A. Greenberg**

SEIZURES, PROGRESSIVE MYOCLONIC, LAFORA TYPE   2601

Includes:
    Epilepsy, myoclonus, Lafora type
    Lafora body disease
    Lafora disease
    Polyglucosan body disease, adult
    Myoclonus epilepsy with Lafora bodies progressive

Excludes:
    Action myoclonus-renal failure syndrome
    Dentatorubropallidoluysian degeneration, hereditary (3283)
    Dyssynergia cerebellaris myoclonica
    Gaucher disease (0406)

Kearns-Sayre disease (2070)
Mucolipidosis I (0671)
Neuronal ceroid-lipofuscinoses (NCL) (0713)
Seizures, myoclonic, juvenile Janz type (2567)
Seizures, progressive myoclonic, Unverricht-Lundborg type (2602)

Major Diagnostic Criteria: Progressive tonic-clonic seizures starting early in the second decade; myoclonus of variable severity; focal seizures, especially occipital attacks; and relentless cognitive decline. The diagnosis is confirmed by the finding of characteristic Lafora bodies, which may be found in eccrine sweat gland duct cells obtained by skin biopsy and stained for polysaccharides. The storage material is largely composed of complex carbohydrates, which are seen histologically as the typical inclusion bodies.

Clinical Findings: The children are initially normal. The first symptoms develop between 11–18 years of age, with a mean age of onset at 14 years. Myoclonic seizures may be virtually continuous or not very striking. Focal occipital seizures occur in about one-half the cases. There is a fairly rapid progressive cognitive decline in all patients. In rare cases, behavioural changes or school failure may be the first symptom, and seizures may be relatively infrequent.

Dysarthria and cerebellar signs appear as the disease progresses. Increased deep tendon reflexes may be found. Both hypotonia and rigidity of the limbs have been described, but spasticity is not seen. Fundoscopic examination is normal.

Death occurs 2–10 years after onset (mean six years), and the mean age at death is twenty years. Four patients are known in whom symptoms began in early adult life with a milder protracted course. These exceptional cases may represent a genetic type separate from the classical form.

The diagnosis may be suspected from the clinical picture. The electroencephalogram shows generalized spike and wave discharges activated by photic stimulation, and progressive slowing of background rhythms. Focal and multifocal posterior epileptiform discharges may also be seen. A modest amount of cerebral atrophy may be shown by neuroradiological studies.

Definitive diagnosis depends on the detection of the characteristic periodic acid Schiff-positive inclusion bodies which are present in various tissues including brain, liver, skeletal and cardiac muscle, and skin. Skin biopsy is the simplest and least invasive diagnostic procedure. Inclusion bodies are reliably found in eccrine sweat gland duct cells. The inclusion bodies consist largely of glucose polymers or polyglucosans with a small variable component of phophate and sulphate groups, and a minor amount of associated protein.

Complications: Fairly rapidly progressive pseudodementia, more striking as compared with the other progressive myoclonus epilepsies, is characteristic. The effect of antiepileptic drug toxicity in patients with **Seizures, myoclonic, juvenile Janz type** should be considered in the differential diagnosis.

Associated Findings: None known.

Etiology: Autosomal recessive inheritance. This has been confirmed by multiple cases in sibships, increased parental consanguinity, and absence of affected relatives in the direct line.

Pathogenesis: Unknown.

MIM No.: *25478

Sex Ratio: M1:F1

Occurrence: One of the more common forms of progressive myoclonus epilepsy; over 100 cases have been reported in the world literature. Most common in population groups where there is a high rate of consanguinity, such as in the Island of Réunion, North Africa and Québec, but it is also found in almost every population.

Risk of Recurrence for Patient's Sib:
See Part I, *Mendelian Inheritance.*

Risk of Recurrence for Patient's Child:
See Part I, *Mendelian Inheritance.* Affected individuals are not expected to survive to reproduce.

Age of Detectability: Preclinical dianosis can be carried out by skin biopsy in siblings of affected patients. Attempts at isolating a specific oligosaccharide in the urine of patients have failed.

Gene Mapping and Linkage: Unknown.

Prevention: None known. Genetic counseling indicated.

Treatment: Symptomatic treatment of seizures with emphasis on antimyoclonic drugs such as valproic acid and clonazepam, as well as general supportive care.

Prognosis: The disease progresses rapidly to severe dementia, quadriplegia, cachexia, and a vegetative state with death at a mean age of 20 years. Survival beyond the age of 25 years is extremely rare.

Detection of Carrier: Unknown.

Special Considerations: Storage of similar microscopic bodies restricted to processes of neurons and astrocytes has been found in some middle-aged patients with progressive lower and upper motor neuron deficits, marked sensory loss in the legs, neurogenic bladder, and dementia. The stored material may or may not be identical to that seen in Lafora body disease. This disorder is referred to as *adult polyglucosan body disease.*

Support Groups:
New York; National Myoclonus Foundation
MD; Landover; Epilepsy Foundation of America

References:
Lafora GR, Glueck B: Beitrag zur Histopathologie der myoklonischen Epilepsie. Z Gesamte Neurol Psychiatr 1911; 6:1–14.
Carpenter S, et al: Lafora's disease: peroxisomal storage in skeletal muscle. Neurology 1974; 24:531–538. †
Van Heycop ten Ham MW: Lafora disease: a form of progressive myoclonus epilepsy. In: Vinken PJ, Bruyn GW, eds: Handbook of Clinical Neurology, vol 15. Amsterdam: North Holland Publishing, 1974:382–422. *
Robitaille Y, et al: A distinct form of adult polyglucosan body disease with massive involvement of central and peripheral neuronal processes and astrocytes: a report of four cases and a review of the occurrence of polyglucosan bodies in other conditions such as Lafora's disease and normal ageing. Brain 1980; 103:315–336.
Carpenter S, Karpati G: Sweat gland duct cells in Lafora disease: diagnosis by skin biopsy. Neurology 1981; 31:1564–1568. * †
Roger J, et al: Le diagnostic Précoce de la maladie de Lafora: importance des manifestations paroxystiques visuelles et intérêt de la biopsie cutanée. Rev Neurol (Paris) 1983; 139:115–124.
Berkovic SF, Andermann F: The progressive myoclonus epilepsies. In: Pedley TA, Meldrum BS, eds: Recent Advances in Epilepsy. Edinburgh: Churchill Livingstone 1986:157–187. *
Berkovic SF, et al: Progressive myoclonus epilepsies: specific causes and diagnosis. New Eng J Med 1986; 315:296–305. *
Busard HLSM, et al.: Axilla skin biopsy: a reliable test for the diagnosis of Lafora's disease. Ann Neurol 1987; 21:599–601.

AN016   **Eva Andermann**
AN018   **Frederick Andermann**

SEIZURES, PROGRESSIVE MYOCLONIC, UNVERRICHT-LUNDBORG TYPE   2602

Includes:
Baltic myoclonus epilepsy
Dyssynergia cerebellaris myoclonica (some cases)
Myoclonus epilepsy, Unverricht-Lundborg type
Progressive myoclonus epilepsy without Lafora bodies
Ramsay-Hunt syndrome (some cases)
Unverricht-Lundborg disease

Excludes:
Action myoclonus-renal failure syndrome
Dentatorubropallidoluysian degeneration, hereditary (3283)
Ekbom syndrome
Gaucher disease (0406)
Kearns-Sayre disease (2070)
May-White syndrome
Mucolipidosis I (0671)

Neuronal ceroid-lipofuscinoses (NCL) (0713)
Seizures, myoclonic, juvenile Janz type (2567)
Seizures, progressive myoclonic, Lafora type (2601)

Major Diagnostic Criteria: Onset between 6–15 years of age; abundant, at times continuous, action and stimulus-sensitive myoclonus; generalized seizures; progressive ataxia with only mild dementia.

Clinical Findings: The disorder usually begins at about age 10 years, following a normal infancy and early childhood. The first symptoms are myoclonic jerks or generalized clonic-tonic-clonic seizures, with one following the other within several months or years. Absences and drop attacks occur infrequently. The myoclonic jerks are activated by movement (action myoclonus), and are also sensitive to stimuli such as light, noise and touch. The myoclonus becomes progressively severe, to the point where it interferes with the patients' ability to walk or feed themselves. Major seizures are clonic-tonic-clonic, often occur in the morning, and are not frequent.

Clinical features suggesting occipital onset of the seizures may occasionally be present. Unlike the myoclonus, the generalized seizures are relatively easily controlled by antiepileptic medication.

Dementia develops slowly, with the rate of the decline estimated at approximately one I.Q. point a year. A fixed neurological deficit develops gradually. This includes dysarthria, ataxia, and intention tremor, and is eventually seen in all cases. The disease progresses at a variable rate. In the past, death occurred at a mean age of 24 years; this was probably due to complications of epileptic seizures, unrecognized anticonvulsant toxicity, or respiratory infections due to recumbency and aspiration. Survival to adulthood is usual, some patients reaching the sixth decade. The longer survival is attributed to improved antiepileptic and antimyoclonic symptomatic treatment, in particular the replacement of phenytoin by valproate and clonazepam.

EEG investigations have shown generalized background disturbance and generalized epileptic activity with irregular photosensitive spike and wave or polyspike and wave patterns, and at times occipital focal epileptic discharges. Cortical somatosensory evoked potentials have shown slowing in short-latency median nerve components, suggesting mild involvement of the peripheral and spinal sensory connections, and more severe involvement of the thalamocortical pathways. The slowing increases with progression of the disease. Visual evoked potential latencies are also significantly delayed, but amplitudes are normal. Brainstem auditory evoked potentials show slight but significant prolongation in central conduction time. These findings suggest a multimodel disturbance in sensory projections to cortical areas; however, this may in part be attributed to the effect of anticonvulsant medication. Some cerebellar atrophy is demonstrated by CT scanning of the brain.

The diagnosis is clinical, with key features being the onset, the severity and continous nature of the myoclonus, and the absence of severe or early dementia. No definite biochemical abnormality has been demonstrated, although increased excretion of indican and decreased concentration of plasma tryptophan has been reported. Pathological studies reveal degenerative changes in the brain involving the Purkinje cells, mesial thalamic structures, and inferior olives. There are a few autopsy studies, and the characteristic anatomic picture is still debated.

Singe the diagnosis is clinical, and there is no definite biochemical or pathological marker for this disease, distinction from other types of progressive myoclonus epilepsy may be difficult. In particular, the patients may be diagnosed to suffer from Ramsey Hunt syndrome (dyssynergia cerebellaris myoclonica), in view of the combination of progressive myoclonus epilepsy and spinocerebellar symptoms. However, the Ramsay Hunt syndrome is no longer a useful diagnostic category, since it lacks etiologic specificity.

Complications: Related to antiepileptic medication, limitation imposed by the myoclonus, and complications of generalized seizures.

Associated Findings: Increased arterial blood pressure has been reported in 14% of patients in Finland.

Etiology: Autosomal recessive inheritance. In a series of 93 Finnish patients, Koskiniemi et al (1986) found three affected siblings in three families, two in twenty, and one in forty-four. No parents, offspring, half-siblings, or other family members in the direct line were affected. The parents were consanguineous in 15/68 families, or 22%. Many of the parents of different sibships were related to one another or originated from the same small communities, suggesting a possible founder effect.

Pathogenesis: Unknown.

MIM No.: *25480

Sex Ratio: M1:F1

Occurrence: The condition is common in Scandinavia, particularly in Finland, where the incidence has been estimated to exceed 1:20,000. Early cases were reported from Estonia and Sweden. The Finnish patients originate from small rural communities predominantly in the southeast part of Finland and in the adjacent province of East Karelia, which was annexed to Russia following the Second World War.

Eldridge et al (1983) have recently studied 27 patients in 15 families of various ethnic origins in the United States, only two of which had Scandinavian ancestors. There were two Black American families in Eldridge's study. Patients from other countries, including southern Europe, have also been reported.

Risk of Recurrence for Patient's Sib:
See Part I, *Mendelian Inheritance*. In the Finnish Study, the proportion of affected siblings over age 15 was calculated to be 0.260 by the *a priori* method, assuming complete truncate ascertainment.

Risk of Recurrence for Patient's Child:
See Part I, *Mendelian Inheritance*. Patients only exceptionally have children. Of 15 children of affected parents reported by Lundborg (1912) and by the Finnish group, three died in infancy, and one was mildly retarded. The remainder were healthy. Unfavourable outcomes do not appear to be related to degree of parental illness.

Age of Detectability: Children are normal at birth, and their early development is also normal.

Gene Mapping and Linkage: Unknown.

Prevention: None known. Genetic counseling indicated.

Treatment: A poor response to some antiepileptic drugs, mainly phenytoin, has been stressed by Eldridge et al (1983). Optimal treatment at the moment is valproic acid, alone or with clonazepam. Other specific antimyoclonic drugs such as piracetam and 5-hydroxytryptophan have been tried.

Prognosis: Average age at death has been 24 years. With improved antiepileptic and supportive treatment, the survival is now much longer, sometimes into the sixth decade.

Detection of Carrier: Unknown. In Finland, the heterozygote frequency is estimated as 1:70.

Special Considerations: Unverricht-Lundborg disease (Baltic myoclonus), first described by Unverricht in 1891, was the first type of progressive myoclonus epilepsy to be reported. Lundborg recognized the autosomal recessive nature of the disease, and it was the first human disease to be subjected to formal genetic analysis by Weinberg in 1912. However, its existence as a specific entity has only recently been re-confirmed. Reports of the last 90 years contain conflicting and confusing descriptions of clinical and pathological findings in cases regarded as similar to those initially described by Unverricht and Lundborg. Recent studies of patients from the Finnish aggregate by Koskiniemi and coworkers have clarified the features of the disease, and have distinguished it from other causes of progressive myoclonus epilepsy, mainly **Seizures, progressive myoclonic, Lafora type**.

Support Groups:
New York; National Myoclonus Foundation
MD; Landover; Epilepsy Foundation of America

References:
Unverricht H: Die myoclonie. Leipzig: Franz Deuticke, 1891:1–128.
Lundborg H: Der Erbgang der progressiven Myoklonus-Epilepsie. Z fr̈ die Ges Neur und Psychatrie 1912; 7:353–358.
Koskiniemi M, et al: Progressive myoclonus epilepsy: a clinical and histopathological study. Acta Neurol Scandinav 1974; 50:307–332. *
Norio R, Koskiniemi M: Progressive myoclonus epilepsy: genetic and nosological aspects with special reference to 107 Finnish patients. Clin Genet 1979; 15:382–398. *
Eldridge R, et al: Baltic myoclonus epilepsy: hereditary disorder of childhood made worse by phenytoin. Lancet 1983; 11:838–842. †
Berkovic SF, Andermann F: The progressive myoclonus epilepsies. In: Pedley TA, Meldrum BS, eds: Recent advances in epilepsy, vol 3. Edinbourgh: Churchill Livingstone, 1986:157–187. *
Berkovic SF, et al: Progressive myoclonus epilepsies: specific causes and diagnosis. New Eng J Med 1986; 315:296–305. *
Koskiniemi ML: Baltic myoclonus. In: Fahn S, et al, eds: Myoclonus: advances in neurology, vol 43. New York: Raven Press, 1986:57–64. *

AN016
AN018   **Eva Andermann**
                        Frederick Andermann

SEIZURES, VITAMIN B(6) DEPENDENCY   0991

Includes:
Pyridoxine dependency
Vitamin B(6) dependency with convulsions

Excludes: Vitamin B(6) deficiency states

Major Diagnostic Criteria: There is no specific biochemical or enzymatic phenotype to characterize this convulsive trait. Diagnosis must rest on control of seizures with 10–50 mg pyridoxine HCl intramuscularly, intravenously, or by mouth; positive family history; and no objective evidence for vitamin B_6 deficiency.

Clinical Findings: This familial convulsive disorder, also called "pyridoxine dependency," is known in at least 14 pedigrees. Symptoms appear in the perinatal period. Although convulsions in utero may occur, most patients develop grand mal seizures during the first week of life; occasionally onset is delayed for several weeks after birth. Hyperirritability, hyperacusis, and feeding difficulties accompany the seizures. The usual anticonvulsant drugs are ineffective. Pyridoxine (or other forms of vitamin B_6), given by any route, is the only agent that will control seizures. Electroencephalography can be used to monitor the effect of pyridoxine therapy; the response appears within minutes after administration of the vitamin. The majority of known patients are now severely retarded or have died for want of proper treatment; early treatment with pyridoxine is compatible with normal growth and development. The most important negative features of the syndrome are the absence of any cause or evidence for vitamin B_6 deficiency, or other causes for a convulsive disorder.

Complications: Retarded development or death.

Associated Findings: None known.

Etiology: Autosomal recessive inheritance of a mutation putatively affecting the enzymatic synthesis of a neuroregulatory (inhibitor) compound.

Pathogenesis: Endogenous metabolism of vitamin B_6 and synthesis of the coenzymatically active form, pyridoxal-5-phosphate, from dietary precursors (e.g., pyridoxine) are normal. The immediate clinical response to B_6 administration indicates adequate cellular uptake of the vitamin, as well as an intact B_6-dependent function awaiting activation. The exaggerated nutritional requirement for the vitamin to sustain normal activity of a particular cellular protein enzyme constitutes the pharmacologic dependency for vitamin B_6. It is hypothesized that the mutation may alter the normal relation of glutamic acid decarboxylase (the apoenzyme) with pyridoxal-5-phosphate (the coenzyme); the product of this enzyme's activity is gamma-aminobutyric acid, a presynaptic neuroinhibitor.

MIM No.: *26610

Sex Ratio: M1:F1

Occurrence: Undetermined, but probably more frequent than the limited number of cases in the literature would suggest.

Risk of Recurrence for Patient's Sib:
See Part I, *Mendelian Inheritance.*

Risk of Recurrence for Patient's Child:
See Part I, *Mendelian Inheritance.*

Age of Detectability: In the perinatal period.

Gene Mapping and Linkage: GAD (glutamate decarboxylase) has been provisionally mapped to 2.
There are different forms of the enzyme (multiple loci). Deficient brain GAD activity in vitamin B(6) dependency has not been proven.

Prevention: None known. Genetic counseling indicated.

Treatment: Coenzyme supplementation: vitamin B_6 as pyridoxine HCl, pharmacologic dosage (2–50 mg/day); dose must be titrated for individual patient. Dependency is permanent. Febrile conditions and infections may temporarily increase vitamin B_6 requirement.

Prognosis: Probably good, if treated early. This may require treating the mother with pyridoxine during pregnancy to prevent manifestation of the trait *in utero* in recurrent affected sibs. Late diagnosis and treatment has an 80% risk of retarded development or death.

Detection of Carrier: Unknown.

Special Considerations: The hereditary nutritional state, broadly termed "vitamin B_6 dependency," is a heterogeneous trait involving several distinctive and inherited abnormalities of different apoenzymes. In each case, it is possible that the normal relationship of the apoenzyme with its coenzyme is altered. Precedence for this concept is found in the mutations that affect the pyridoxal-5-phosphate binding site on the B_6-requiring enzyme, tryptophan synthetase, in *Neurospora crassa*. Since the original proposal by Scriver that "vitamin B_6 dependency with convulsions" is a phenotype reflecting the effect of mutation on a single enzyme (perhaps glutamate decarboxylase), rather than a primary abnormality of vitamin B_6 metabolism affecting many apoenzymes, other traits have been proposed as additional forms of "vitamin B_6 dependency." Thus, hereditary cystathioninuria, xanthurenicaciduria, and some forms of familial pyridoxine-responsive anemia can each be interpreted as inherited abnormalities of a specific enzyme. Discovery of many other forms of vitamin B_6 dependency can be anticipated in view of the many B_6-requiring enzyme reactions in amino acid, carbohydrate, and fatty acid metabolism; hyper-β-alaninemia, and some forms of homocystinuria may be further examples. The basis for pyridoxine responsiveness in each trait requires investigation. The glutamic acid decarboxylase in mammalian kidney (it was previously thought to be in brain only) has properties different from the brain enzyme.

References:
Bejsovec M, et al.: Familial intrauterine convulsions in pyridoxine dependency. Arch Dis Child 1967; 42:201–207.
Scriver CR, Whelan DT: Glutamic acid decarboxylase (GAD) in mammalian tissue outside the central nervous system, and its possible relevance to hereditary vitamin B_6 dependency with seizures. Ann NY Acad Sci 1969; 166:83–96.
Mudd SH: Pyridoxine-responsive genetic disease. Fed Proc 1971; 30:970–976.
Yoshida T, et al.: Vitamin B6 dependency of glutamic acid decarboxylase in the kidney from a patient with vitamin B6 dependent convulsion. Tohoku J Exp Med 1971; 104:195–198.
Bankier A, et al.: Pyridoxine-dependent seizures: a wider clinical spectrum. Arch Dis Child 1983; 58:415–418.
Goutieres F, Aircardi J: Atypical presentations of pyridoxine-dependent seizures: a treatable cause of intractable epilepsy in infants. Ann Neurol 1985; 17:117–120.

SC050   **Charles R. Scriver**

Seizures-adenoma sebaceum-mental retardation
See TUBEROUS SCLEROSIS
Seizures-hypotonic cerebral palsy-megalocornea-mental retardation
See MEGALOCORNEA-MENTAL RETARDATION SYNDROME

SEIZURES-ICHTHYOSIS-MENTAL RETARDATION   0741

Includes:
Ichthyosis-epilepsy-oligophrenia
Ichthyosis-neurologic disorder-hypogonadism
Oligophrenia-epilepsy-ichthyosis syndrome
Rud syndrome

Excludes:
Sjogren-Larsson syndrome (2030)
Xeroderma-mental retardation (1004)

Major Diagnostic Criteria: Seizures, ichthyosis, and mental retardation; the presence of all three apparently being essential. However, the syndrome may be suspected when there is onset of ichthyosis (usually within the first months of life) coupled with somatic and mental retardation. The onset of epilepsy may be delayed beyond the first 10 years of life, but in some instances, it has appeared as early as the first year of life.

Clinical Findings: There may be no observable findings at birth. Ichthyosis usually appears during the first two years of life. Ultimate IQ ranges from 30 to 80. Height is variable, with increased frequencies of either short or tall stature.

Complications: Severe cases of ichthyosis may show heat prostration in hot weather due to reduced sweating. The only other complications are those secondary to epilepsy and mental retardation.

Associated Findings: Retarded somatic development and hypogonadism (probably in most cases); sexual infantilism (about one-half of reported cases). The following conditions have each been reported once: macrocytic anemia, polyneuritis, partial gigantism of long bones, arachnodactyly, retinitis pigmentosa, hyperglycemia, hypothyroidism, macular atrophy, and alopecia totalis. Talipes equinovarus has been reported in some affected individuals.

Etiology: Possibly X-linked recessive inheritance.

Pathogenesis: The only gross structural defect is the ichthyotic skin. The only reported case that came to autopsy showed CNS changes of a nonspecific nature, typical of those associated with profound mental defect. Functional disorders are mental retardation and epilepsy (or EEG evidence of an epileptic diathesis in most cases in which EEGs were made).

MIM No.: 31277

POS No.: 3850

Sex Ratio: M2:F1

Occurrence: About 30 cases reported in the literature.

Risk of Recurrence for Patient's Sib:
See Part I, *Mendelian Inheritance.*

Risk of Recurrence for Patient's Child:
See Part I, *Mendelian Inheritance.*

Age of Detectability: Usually in childhood when all three clinical features are present.

Gene Mapping and Linkage: Unknown.

Prevention: None known. Genetic counseling indicated.

Treatment: Infrequent bathing and cleansing. Use of ointments for the ichthyosis; general treatment measures for epilepsy and mental retardation.

Prognosis: Life expectancy is probably shortened. No progressive mental impairment has been noted, but mental retardation appears to vary from severe to mild.

Detection of Carrier: Unknown.

Special Considerations: The concept of the Rud syndrome involves the perpetuation of what probably began as a translator's error. All complications over the misconceptions about Rud's original case descriptions can be resolved if we call the present syndrome the *Oligophrenia, epilepsy and ichthyosis syndrome,* and do not claim that it is necessarily the same as that described by Rud. See Maldonaldo et al (1975) for a discussion of this neuroichthyoses.

Support Groups: MD; Landover; Epilepsy Foundation of America

References:
Butterworth T, Strean LP: The ichthyosiform genodermatoses. Postgrad Med. 1965; 37:175–184.
Wells RS, Kerr CB: Genetic classification of ichthyosis. Arch Dermatol 1965; 92:1–6.
Nissley PS, Thomas GH: The Rud syndrome. BD:OAS VII(8). Baltimore: Williams & Wilkins Co. for The National Foundation-March of Dimes, 1971:246–248.
Maldonaldo RR, et al.: Neuroichthyosis with hypogonadism (Rud's syndrome). Int J Dermatol 1975; 14:347–349.
Munke M, et al.: Genetic heterogeneity of the ichthyosis, hypogonadism, mental retardation, and epilepsy syndrome: clinical and biochemical investigations on two patients with Rud syndrome and review of the literature. Eur J Pediat 1983; 141:8–13.
Wisniewski K, et al.: X-linked inheritance of the Rud syndrome. (Abstract) Am J Hum Genet 1985; 37:A83.

MY001   **Terry L Myers**

Seizures-mental retardation-alopecia
See ALOPECIA-SEIZURES-MENTAL RETARDATION, SHOKEIR TYPE
Seizures-skin lesions-mental retardation
See HYPOMELANOSIS OF ITO
Self-healing squamous cell epithelioma, multiple familial
See EPITHELIOMA, MULTIPLE SELF-HEALING SQUAMOUS
Sella turcica defect-pituitary dwarfism
See DWARFISM, PITUITARY WITH ABNORMAL SELLA TURCICA
SEMDJL
See SPONDYLOEPIMETAPHYSEAL DYSPLASIA-JOINT LAXITY
Seminiferous tubule dysgenesis
See KLINEFELTER SYNDROME
Seminoma
See TERATOMAS
Senile dementia of the Alzheimer type
See ALZHEIMER DISEASE, FAMILIAL
Senile dementia, familial
See ALZHEIMER DISEASE, FAMILIAL
Senile nanism
See PROGERIA
Senile retinoschisis, autosomal recessive
See RETINOSCHISIS
Senior-Loken syndrome
See RENAL DYSPLASIA-RETINAL APLASIA, LOKEN-SENIOR TYPE
Sensenbrenner-Dorst-Owens syndrome
See CRANIO-ECTODERMAL DYSPLASIA
Sensorimotor neuronopathy-agenesis of the corpus callosum
See CORPUS CALLOSUM AGENESIS-SENSORIMOTOR NEUROPATHY, FAMILIAL
Sensorineural deafness-chondrodystrophy
See CHONDRODYSTROPHY-SENSORINEURAL DEAFNESS, NANCE-INSLEY TYPE
Sensorineural hearing loss
See DEAFNESS
Senter syndrome
See ICHTHYOSIFORM ERYTHROKERATODERMA, ATYPICAL WITH DEAFNESS
Septal hypertrophy with obstruction, asymmetric
See HEART, SUBAORTIC STENOSIS, MUSCULAR

SEPTO-OPTIC DYSPLASIA   2018

Includes:
De Morsier syndrome
Optic-septo dysplasia

Excludes:
Optic nerve hypoplasia (0758)
Thyrotropin deficiency, isolated (0949)

Major Diagnostic Criteria: Two of the three characteristic features of absent septum pellucidum, optic nerve hypoplasia, or hypothalamic hypopituitarism.

Clinical Findings: The most common initial symptom is visual impairment with nystagmus as a neonate. The optic disk hypoplasia, bilateral or unilateral, may be difficult to define in infants due to variation in apparent optic disk size. Typically the optic disk is one-third to one-half the normal size, with a cuff-like or double-rim appearance; an outer margin shown by choroidal pigment, an inner hypoplastic margin with relatively large retinal vessels, and pale nerve tissue (Brook et al, 1972). Although blindness is common, visual loss may be mild. Bitemporal hemianopia, if present, is an important clue to defective fibers crossing the optic chiasm. Other findings include coloboma, strabismus, and microphthalmia. Diagnostic studies show normal electroretinogram (ERG) and abnormal visually evoked cortical responses (VER).

Endocrine abnormalities usually become apparent in early childhood, with a drop in growth rate and short stature; however an underlying endocrine deficiency may be responsible for the hypoglycemia with or without seizures, unexplained prolonged hyperbilirubinemia or failure to thrive common in the neonatal period. There is great variability in the multiplicity and severity of endocrine abnormalities. The most common is growth hormone deficiency (93%), followed by ACTH deficiency (57%), hypothyroidism (53%), and diabetes insipidus (Izenberg et al, 1984). Gonadotropin deficiency and sexual precocity have also been described. These hormonal problems are based on hypothalamic dysfunction.

The septum pellucidum is absent in roughly one-half of patients with optic nerve hypoplasia and hypopituitarism (Izenberg et al, 1984). Other CNS abnormalities noted on CT scan or air studies include atrophy of the optic nerve, dilation of the suprasellar and chiasmatic cisterns, enlargement of the pituitary stalk, empty sella, various grades of cortical atrophy, and absent or deficient corpus callosum.

The level of psychomotor development varies greatly from severe mental retardation, to learning disability, to normal mentation.

There is no characteristic craniofacies; however, a few patients had minor malformations; hypertelorism, flat nasal bridge, high-arched palate, and microphthalmus. Septo-optic dysplasia has been described in association with median cleft face syndrome, craniotelencephalic dysplasia, and digital anomalies.

Complications: Hypoglycemic seizures due to ACTH or growth hormone deficiency may lead to or aggravate mental retardation.

Associated Findings: None known.

Etiology: Usually sporadic. Most commonly the firstborn of young mothers.

Pathogenesis: Appears to be a developmental field defect affecting midline structures, mainly the optic nerves and chasma, posterior pituitary, anterior hypothalamus, and septum pellucidum. Insult occurs probably at 6 weeks gestation when differentiation of ganglion cells of the eye take place. Septo-optic dysplasia has been assumed to represent the mild end of the spectrum of holoprosencephaly.

MIM No.: 18223

POS No.: 3398

Sex Ratio: M1:F1

Occurrence: Undetermined but presumed rare.

Risk of Recurrence for Patient's Sib: Unknown. Probably not increased.

Risk of Recurrence for Patient's Child: Unknown.

Age of Detectability: As early as infancy and as late as the teen years.

Gene Mapping and Linkage: Unknown.

Prevention: None known. Genetic counseling indicated.

Treatment: All cases with optic nerve hypoplasia need follow-up for pituitary endocrine deficiency. There is a lag period of around 3.5 years from the diagnosis of Septo-optic dysplasia to the diagnosis of hypopituitarism. Prevention of recurrent hypoglycemic episodes or seizures should improve overall prognosis. Hormonal replacement therapy may prove beneficial.

Prognosis: Depends on other associated CNS pathology, and on the severity and multiplicity of the endocrine deficiency.

Detection of Carrier: Unknown.

References:

Brook CGD, et al.: Septo-optic dysplasia. Brit Med J 1972; 3:811–813.
Patel H, et al.: Optic nerve hypoplasia with hypopituitarism: septo-optic dysplasia with hypopituitarism. Am J Dis Child 1975; 129:175–180.
Arslanian SA, et al.: Hormonal, metabolic and neuroradiologic abnormalities associated with septo-optic dysplasia. Acta Endocrinol 1984; 107:282–288.
Izenberg I, et al.: The endocrine spectrum of septo-optic dysplasia. Clin Pediatr 1984; 23:632–636.
Blethen SL, Weldon VV: Hypopituitarism and septo-optic "dysplasia" in first cousins. Am J Med Genet 1985; 21:123–129.

J0010   **Virginia P. Johnson**

Sequeiros-Sack syndrome
  See ALOPECIA-SKIN ATROPHY-ANONYCHIA-TONGUE DEFECT
Serax^, fetal effects
  See FETAL BENZODIAZEPINE EFFECTS
Serine 84 amyloidosis
  See AMYLOIDOSIS, INDIANA TYPE
Sertoli-cell-only syndrome
  See GERM CELL APLASIA

SERUM ALLOTYPES, HUMAN   0476

Includes:
  A2m antigens
  Gamma globulin (Gm) antigens
  IgA constant heavy chain locus
  IgG heavy chain loci
  Immunoglobulin Am2
  Immunoglobulin Gm-1
  Immunoglobulin Gm-2
  Immunoglobulin Gm-3
  Immunoglobulin InV (Km)
  Inv (Km) antigens
  Kappa light chain of immunoglobulin

Excludes:
  Immunodeficiency, common variable type (0521)
  Immunodeficiency, IgG subclass deficiencies (2947)

Major Diagnostic Criteria: No clinical findings are associated with the presence of these antigens.

Clinical Findings: No clinical symptoms are attributable to the presence or absence of Gm or Inv allotypes, but the Am allotypes may be associated with transfusion reactions.

The Gm antigens are found on the heavy chains of IgG and the A2m antigens are found on the heavy chains of IgA2. The Inv(Km) antigens are found on the kappa light chains of the immunoglobulin molecules. Because IgG readily crosses the placenta, an individual's Gm and Inv types cannot ordinarily be determined before 6 months of age. IgA on the other hand does not cross the placenta, hence typing may be done in infants.

Complications: Unknown.

Associated Findings: None known.

Etiology: Normal antigen inheritance as autosomal codominant alleles. The antigens are inherited in different complexes (haplotypes) in each of the several races of man. Accordingly, they are extensively used for human population studies. They may also, in the hands of experts and with caution, be used for paternity testing and for identification of individuals.

Pathogenesis: Anti-IgA antibodies may occur as the result of transfusion or of the injection of Ig; possibly also as the result of immunization across the placenta, through a placental rupture.

MIM No.: *24050, 14683, *14690, *14691, *14700, *14701, *14702, *14707, *14710, *14711, *14712, *14713, *14716, *14717, *14718, *14720

Sex Ratio: M1:F1

Occurrence: These normal antigens are present in all races but with different frequencies. Worldwide distribution.

Risk of Recurrence for Patient's Sib: As for codominant alleles.

Risk of Recurrence for Patient's Child: As for codominant alleles.

Age of Detectability: After six months of age.

Gene Mapping and Linkage: IGHA1 (immunoglobulin alpha 1) has been mapped to 14q32.33.

IGHA2 (immunoglobulin alpha 2 (A2M marker)) has been mapped to 14q32.33.

IGHJ (immunoglobulin heavy polypeptide, joining region) has been mapped to 14q32.3.

IGHM (immunoglobulin mu) has been mapped to 14q32.33.

IGHV (immunoglobulin heavy polypeptide, variable region (many genes)) has been mapped to 14q32.33.

IGHG1 (immunoglobulin gamma 1 (Gm marker)) has been mapped to 14q32.33.

IGHG2 (immunoglobulin gamma 2 (Gm marker)) has been mapped to 14q32.33.

IGHG3 (immunoglobulin gamma 3 (Gm marker)) has been mapped to 14q32.33.

IGHG4 (immunoglobulin gamma 4 (Gm marker)) has been mapped to 14q32.33.

IGHEP1 (immunoglobulin epsilon pseudogene 1) has been mapped to 14q32.33.

IGHD (immunoglobulin delta) has been mapped to 14q32.33.

IGHE (immunoglobulin epsilon) has been mapped to 14q32.33.

IGKC (immunoglobulin kappa constant region) has been mapped to 2p12.

Prevention: Not necessary.

Treatment: Not necessary.

Prognosis: Normal life span.

Detection of Carrier: By means of an agglutination inhibition test.

References:
Giblett ER: Genetic markers in the human blood. Oxford: Blackwell Scientific Pub Ltd, 1969.
Steinberg AG: Globulin polymorphisms in man. Annu Rev Genet 1969; 3:25–52.
Grubb R: The genetic markers of human immunoglobulins. New York: Springer-Verlag, 1970.
Steinberg AG, Cook CE: The distribution of human immunoglobin allotypes. Oxford Univ Press, 1981. *
Steinberg AG: Immunoglobulin allotypes. In Atassi MZ, et al, eds: Molecular immunology. New York: Marcel Dekker, 1984:231–253. *

ST013   **Arthur G. Steinberg**

Serum carnosinase deficiency, disorders of
See CARNOSINEMIA
Serum ceruloplasmin, low
See HYPOCERULOPLASMINEMIA
Serum normal agglutinants (SNaggs)
See ANTIBODIES TO HUMAN ALLOTYPES
Serum prothrombin conversion accelerator deficiency
See FACTOR VII DEFICIENCY
Setleis syndrome
See ECTODERMAL DYSPLASIA, CONGENITAL FACIAL, SETLEIS TYPE
Seventeen-beta-hydroxysteroid dehydrogenase deficiency
See STEROID 17-KETOSTEROID REDUCTASE DEFICIENCY
Sever disease (os calcis)
See JOINTS, OSTEOCHONDRITIS DISSECANS
Severe combined immunodeficiency (SCID) with leukopenia
See IMMUNODEFICIENCY, SEVERE COMBINED
Severe combined immunodeficiency with ADA
See IMMUNODEFICIENCY, ADENOSINE DEAMINASE DEFICIENCY
Severe combined immunodeficiency, Nezelof type
See IMMUNODEFICIENCY, NEZELOF TYPE
Severe combined immunodeficiency, variant type
See IMMUNODEFICIENCY, NEZELOF TYPE
Severe combined immunodeficiency, X-linked (SCIDX)
See IMMUNODEFICIENCY, X-LINKED SEVERE COMBINED
Severe combined immunodeficiency-lack of HLA on lymphocytes
See IMMUNODEFICIENCY, SEVERE COMBINED
Sex reversal-polydactyly-renal hypoplasia-unilobular lung
See SMITH-LEMLI-OPITZ SYNDROME, TYPE II
Sex-linked neurodegenerative disease associated with monilethrix
See MENKES SYNDROME

Sexual ateleotic dwarfism
See GROWTH HORMONE DEFICIENCY, ISOLATED
Sexual development variations-asymmetry-short stature
See SILVER SYNDROME
Sexual headache, benign
See MIGRAINE
Sexual maturity (delayed)-short stature-mental retardation
See SHORT STATURE-MENTAL RETARDATION-DELAYED SEXUAL MATURITY
Sezary syndrome
See LEUKEMIA/LYMPHOMA, T-CELL
Shah-Waardenburg syndrome
See ALBINISM, WAARDENBURG TYPE-HIRSCHSPRUNG AGANGLIONOSIS
Shawl scrotum
See AARSKOG SYNDROME
Shell teeth
See TEETH, DENTINOGENESIS IMPERFECTA
Shokeir syndrome
See ALOPECIA-SEIZURES-MENTAL RETARDATION, SHOKEIR TYPE
Short chain acyl-CoA dehydrogenase deficiency (SCAD)
See ACYL-CoA DEHYDROGENASE DEFICIENCY, SHORT CHAIN TYPE
Short cord
See UMBILICAL CORD, SHORT
Short esophagus, most instances
See HERNIA, HIATAL
Short rib-polydactyly syndrome, Majewski type
See SHORT RIB-POLYDACTYLY SYNDROME, TYPE II
Short rib-polydactyly syndrome, Naumoff type
See SHORT RIB-POLYDACTYLY SYNDROME, VERMA-NAUMOFF TYPE
Short rib-polydactyly syndrome, Saldino-Noonan type
See SHORT RIB-POLYDACTYLY SYNDROME, TYPE I

SHORT RIB-POLYDACTYLY SYNDROME, TYPE I   0884

Includes:
Polydactyly-neonatal chondrodystrophy, type I
Saldino-Noonan short rib-polydactyly
Short rib-polydactyly syndrome, Saldino-Noonan type

Excludes:
Asphyxiating thoracic dysplasia (0091)
Chondroectodermal dysplasia (0156)
Osteochondrodysplasias, other lethal perinatal
Short rib-polydactyly syndrome, type II (0883)
Short rib-polydactyly syndrome, Verma-Naumoff type (2270)

Major Diagnostic Criteria: Lethal congenital dwarfism with marked limb reduction, narrow constricted thorax, short horizontal ribs, post-axial polysyndactyly, multiple systemic abnormalities, hydrops, and characteristic X-ray findings.

Clinical Findings: Severe hydrops at birth; marked limb reduction; narrow constricted thorax; pulmonary hypoplasia; protuberant abdomen; postaxial polysyndactyly with short "flipper"-like limbs; nail dysplasia; flat face and occiput resembling "Potter" facies (see **Renal agenesis, bilateral**) associated with oligohydramnios; low-set, flattened, deformed ears; severe cardiovascular abnormalities; gastrointestinal anomalies; gallbladder and cystic duct agenesis; pancreatic cysts and fibrosis; renal agenesis or cystic dysplasia; cloacal atresia (anal, urethral and vaginal); sexual ambiguity (complete suppression of secondary sexual differentiation may result in preponderance of phenotypic females).

X-ray abnormalities include short horizontal ribs; severely shortened tubular bones; marked metaphyseal dysplasia; ragged, pointed ends of tubular bones; longitudinal periosteal spurs projecting from the lateral aspects of the metaphyseal margins; ill-defined corticomedullary differentiation (a distinguishing feature from **Short rib-polydactyly syndrome** types II and III); small, rounded scapulae, small iliac bones with flattened acetabular roofs; vertebral abnormalities; incomplete and irregular ossification of the metacarpal and metatarsal bones and phalanges. Scapular, vertebral and pelvic abnormalities distinguish this condition from **Short rib-polydactyly syndrome** types II and III. Chondro-osseous changes include markedly irregular primary trabeculae. Histopathology is similar to that seen in **Short rib-polydactyly syndrome, Verma-Naumoff type**.

Complications: Respiratory insufficiency due to small thoracic cage and decreased pulmonary volume.

Associated Findings: None known.

Etiology: Autosomal recessive inheritance. Variable, heterogeneous expression and overlapping features with those of **Short rib-polydactyly syndrome** types II and III. Possible explanations for variability and overlapping features include point mutation at different loci, differing allelic mutations at the same locus, or variable expressivity of the same gene mutation.

Pathogenesis: Unknown.

MIM No.: *26353

POS No.: 3390

Sex Ratio: An excess of phenotypic females has been observed. Some males have had ambiguous genitalia.

Occurrence: About 40 cases have been documented.

Risk of Recurrence for Patient's Sib:
See Part I, *Mendelian Inheritance*.

Risk of Recurrence for Patient's Child:
See Part I, *Mendelian Inheritance*. Affected individuals are not expected to survive to reproduce.

Age of Detectability: At birth, by clinical examination. Prenatal diagnosis is possible by serial ultrasound during second trimester.

Gene Mapping and Linkage: Unknown.

Prevention: None known. Genetic counseling indicated.

Treatment: Unknown.

Prognosis: Patients are stillborn or die within hours after birth from respiratory insufficiency and other multiple abnormalities.

Detection of Carrier: Unknown.

References:
Saldino RM, Noonan CD: Severe thoracic dystrophy with striking micromelia, abnormal osseous development, including the spine and multiple visceral anomalies. Am J Roentgenol 1972; 114:257–263.
Spranger J, et al.: Short rib-polydactyly (SRP) syndromes, types Majewski and Saldino-Noonan. Z Kinderheilk 1974; 116:73–94.
Cherstvoy ED, et al.: Difficulties in classification of the short rib-polydactyly syndrome. Eur J Pediatr 1980; 133:57–61.
Sillence DO: Non-Majewski short rib-polydactyly syndrome. Am J Med Genet 1980; 7:223–229. *
International nomenclature of constitutional diseases of bone, Revision - May 1983. Ann Radiol 1984; 27:275–280.
Bernstein R, et al.: Short rib-polydactyly syndrome: a single or heterogeneous entity? a re-evaluation prompted by four new cases. J Med Genet 1985; 22:46–53.
Yang SS, et al.: Three conditions in neonatal asphyxiating thoracic dysplasia (Jeune) and the short rib-polydactyly syndrome spectrum: a clinicopathologic study. Am J Med Genet 1987; Suppl 3:191–207.
Frzen M, et al.: Comparative histopathology of the growth cartilage in short-rib polydactyly syndromes type I and type II and in chondroectodermal dysplasia. Ann Genet 1988; 31:144–150.

BE043   **Renée Bernstein**

SHORT RIB-POLYDACTYLY SYNDROME, TYPE II   0883

Includes:
Majewski short rib-polydactyly syndrome
Mohr-Majewski syndrome
Polydactyly-neonatal chondrodystrophy, type II
Short rib-polydactyly syndrome, Majewski type
Skeletal dysplasia, short rib-polydactyly syndrome type II

Excludes:
Asphyxiating thoracic dysplasia (0091)
Chondroectodermal dysplasia (0156)
Meckel syndrome (0634)
Oro-facio-digital syndrome, Mohr type (0771)

Osteochondrodysplasias, other lethal perinatal
Short rib-polydactyly syndrome, type I (0884)
Short rib-polydactyly syndrome, Verma-Naumoff type (2270)
Smith-Lemli-Opitz syndrome, type II (2635)

Major Diagnostic Criteria: Lethal congenital dwarfism with marked limb reduction, narrow constricted thorax, short horizontal ribs, preaxial and postaxial polysyndactyly, systemic abnormalities, hydrops, and characteristic X-ray findings.

Clinical Findings: Hydrops at birth; marked limb reduction; narrow constricted thorax; pulmonary hypoplasia; protuberant abdomen; polysyndactyly, preaxial and postaxial; nail dysplasia; craniofacial abnormalities with cleft upper lip or palate; short flat nose; low-set, deformed ears; rudimentary epiglottis; cardiovascular defects; renal dysplasia, polycystic kidneys; gastrointestinal tract anomalies; sexual ambiguity.

X-ray abnormalities include short horizontal ribs; severely shortened tubular bones with disproportionately short ovoid tibiae (the latter distinguising this condition from **Short rib-polydactyly syndrome** types I and III); moderate metaphyseal dysplasia; clearly demarcated corticomedullary differentiation (distinguishing this condition from **Short rib-polydactyly syndrome, type I**); minimal spurs, normal vertebrae and pelvic bones (also distinguishing this condition from **Short rib-polydactyly syndrome** types I and III). Chondro-osseous changes in proliferative columns and irregularity in columnization is less severe than in types I and II.

Complications: Respiratory insufficiency due to small thoracic cage and decreased pulmonary volume.

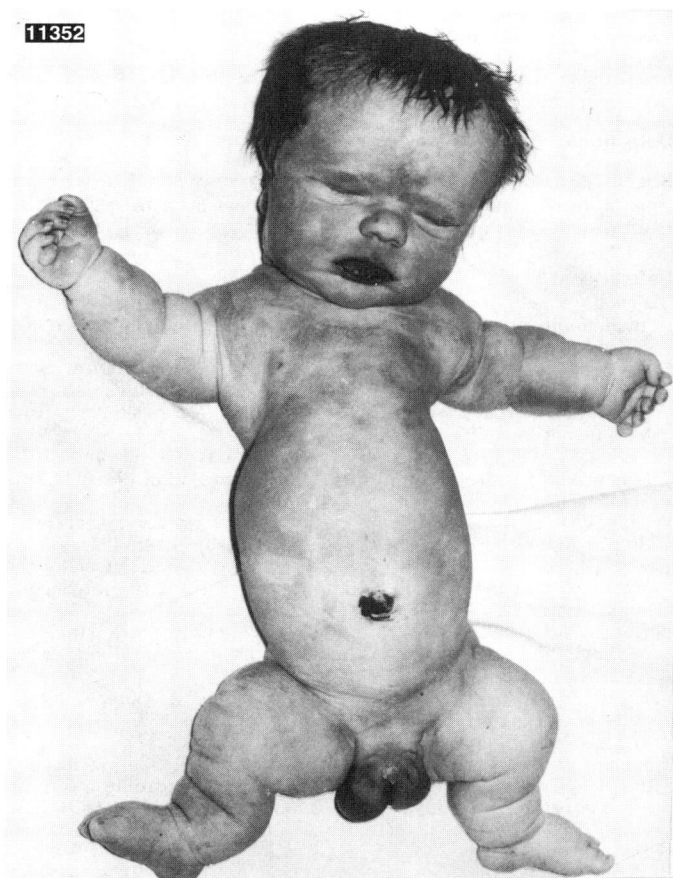

0883A-11352: Note shortened limbs, postaxial polydactyly, large head, narrow thorax and hypoplastic penis.

Associated Findings: None known.

Etiology: Autosomal recessive inheritance. Variable, heterogeneous expression and overlapping features with those of **Short rib-polydactyly syndrome** types I and III. The possible explanations for variability and overlapping features include point mutation at different loci, differing allelic mutations at the same locus, or variable expressivity of the same gene mutation. Silengo et al (1987) has suggested that this condition could be a severe expression of **Oro-facio-digital syndrome, Mohr type**.

Pathogenesis: Unknown.

MIM No.: *26352

POS No.: 3389

Sex Ratio: Presumably M1:F1. Some affected males have had ambiguous genitalia.

Occurrence: More than 40 cases have been documented in the literature.

Risk of Recurrence for Patient's Sib:
See Part I, *Mendelian Inheritance*.

Risk of Recurrence for Patient's Child:
See Part I, *Mendelian Inheritance*. Affected individuals are not expected to survive to reproduce.

Age of Detectability: At birth, by clinical examination. Prenatal diagnosis is possible by serial ultrasound during second trimester.

Gene Mapping and Linkage: Unknown.

Prevention: None known. Genetic counseling indicated.

Treatment: Unknown.

Prognosis: Patients are stillborn or die within hours after birth from respiratory insufficiency and other multiple abnormalities.

Detection of Carrier: Unknown.

Special Considerations: A transition type between the Mohr and the Majewski syndromes, called *Mohr Majewski syndrome*, has also been reported (Silengo et al, 1987).

References:
Majewski F, et al.: Polysyndaktylie, verküerzte gliedmassen und genitalfehlbildungen: kennzeichen cines sellstaendigen syndrome? Z Kinderheilk 1971; 111:118–138.
Spranger J, et al.: Short rib-polysyndaktyly (SRP) syndromes, types Majewski and Saldino-Noonan. Z Kinderheilk 1974; 116:73–94.
Chen H, et al.: Short rib-polydactyly syndrome, Majewski type. Am J Med Genet 1980; 7:215–222.
Cooper CP, Hall CM: Lethal short rib-polydactyly syndrome of the Majewski type: a report of three cases. Pediatr Radiol 1982; 144:513–517. *
Walley VM, et al.: Brief clinical report: short rib-polydactyly syndrome, Majewski type. Am J Med Genet 1983; 14:445–452.
Toftager-Larsen K, Benzie RJ: Fetoscopy in prenatal diagnosis of the Majewski and the Saldino-Noonan types of short rib-polydactyly syndromes. Clin Genet 1984; 26:56–60.
Bernstein R, et al.: Short rib-polydactyly syndrome: a single or heterogeneous entity? A re-evaluation prompted by four new cases. J Med Genet 1985; 22:46–53.
Silengo MC, et al.: Oro-facial-digital syndrome II: transition type between the Mohr and the Majewski syndromes. Clin Genet 1987; 31:331–336.
Yang SS, et al.: Three conditions in neonatal asphyxiating thoracic dysplasia (Jeune) and the short rib-polydactyly syndrome spectrum: a clinicopathologic study. Am J Med Genet 1987; Suppl 3:191–207.

BE043   **Renée Bernstein**

Short rib-polydactyly syndrome, type III
See SHORT RIB-POLYDACTYLY SYNDROME, VERMA-NAUMOFF TYPE

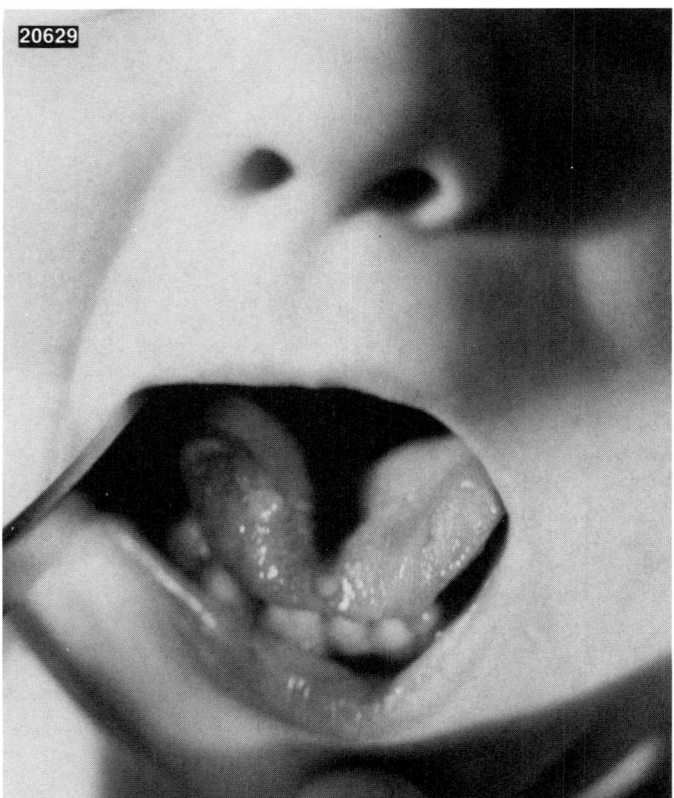

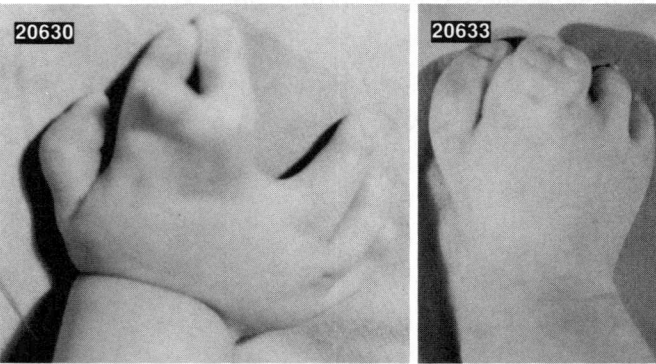

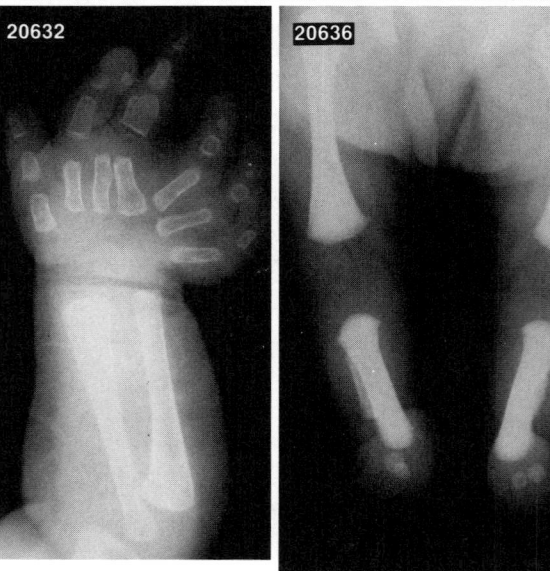

0883B-20629: Mohr-Majewski syndrome; note lobate tongue and teeth abnormalities. **20630:** Hand shows pre- and post-axial polydactyly. **20633:** Polysyndactyly of the foot. **20632:** X-ray of the right hand and forearm shows short and stubby radius and ulna, pre- and post-axial polydactyly, alterations in the number and shape of the phalanges, and retarded skeletal age. **20636:** Short and stubby tibia and fibula.

SHORT RIB-POLYDACTYLY SYNDROME, VERMA-NAUMOFF TYPE 2270

Includes:
Naumoff type short-rib polydactyly syndrome
Polydactyly-neonatal chondrodystrophy, type III
Short rib-polydactyly syndrome, Naumoff type
Short rib-polydactyly syndrome, type III
Skeletal dysplasia-short rib-polydactyly, type III
Verma-Naumoff short rib-polydactyly

Excludes:
Asphyxiating thoracic dysplasia (0091)
Chondroectodermal dysplasia (0156)
Osteochondrodysplasias, other lethal perinatal

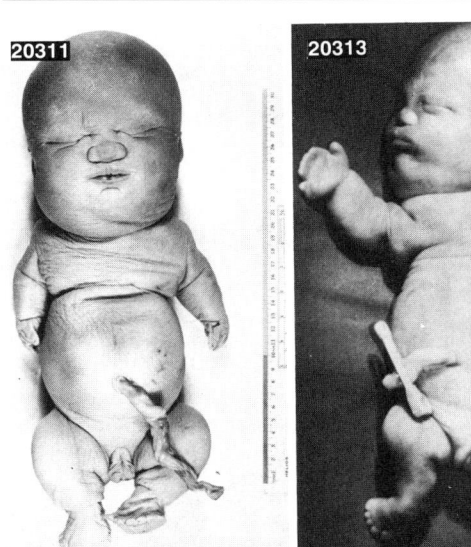

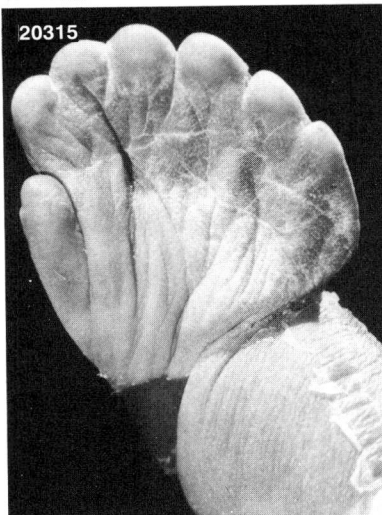

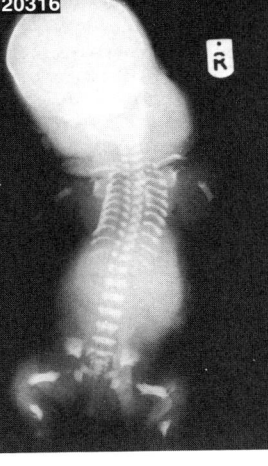

2270-20311: Stillborn infant with short-rib polydactyly syndrome type III; note short limbs, narrow thorax, hydropic and flattened facies with frontal bossing and depressed nasal bridge. **20313:** Appearance of a 28-week fetus who is the sib of the infant shown in 20311. **20315:** Pre- and postaxial polydactyly. **20316:** Short horizontal ribs, short tubular bones, widened metaphyses, longitudinal metaphyseal spurs, flat acetabulae and vertebral defects.

Short rib-polydactyly syndrome, type I (0884)
Short rib-polydactyly syndrome, type II (0883)

Major Diagnostic Criteria: Lethal dwarfism with marked limb reduction, narrow constricted thorax, short horizontal ribs, post-axial polysyndactyly, visceral abnormalities (particularly urogenital), hydrops, and characteristic X-ray findings.

Clinical Findings: Hydrops at birth; marked limb reduction; narrow constricted thorax; pulmonary hypoplasia; protuberant abdomen; **Polysyndactyly**, usually postaxial; mild nail dysplasia; flat occiput; frontal bossing; depressed nasal bridge ("saddle" nose); "Potter"-like facies, if there is associated oligohydramnios; low-set, flattened, deformed ears; occasional natal teeth and pseudoclefts of gums and lips; variable cardiovascular abnormalities; pancreatic fibrosis; renal dysplasia more common than renal agenesis; cloacal atresia (anal, urethral, and vaginal); and sexual ambiguity. The complete suppression of secondary sexual differentiation may result in preponderance of phenotypic females.

X-ray abnormalities include short, horizontal ribs; severely shortened, tubular bones; metaphyseal dysplasia; widened metaphases; longitudinal metaphyseal spurs; clearly demarcated corticomedullary differentiation (distinguishing feature from **Short rib-polydactyly syndrome, type I**); horizontal, trident lower iliac margins; flat acetabulae; vertebral abnormalities (pelvic and vertebral abnormalities differentiate **Short rib-polydactyly syndrome** (SRPS) types I and III from type II); shortened cranial base (unique to type III). Chondro-osseous changes include shortened or absent zone of proliferative chondrocytes with loss of columnization, and disorganized trabecular formation.

Complications: Respiratory insufficiency due to small thoracic cage and decreased pulmonary volume.

Associated Findings: None known.

Etiology: Autosomal recessive inheritance. Variable, heterogeneous expression and overlapping features with those of **Short rib-polydactyly syndrome** type I and type II. The possible explanations for variability and overlapping features include point mutations at different loci, differing allelic mutations at the same locus, or variable expressivity of the same gene mutation.

Pathogenesis: The generalized abnormalities of all organ systems suggest a defect in the regulation of cellular differentiation during early embryogenesis. Cytoplasmic periodic acid-Schiff (PAS) positive, diastase-resistant, inclusion bodies were observed in the chondrocytes of one patient with SRPS type III. These may represent products of abnormal synthesis or impaired secretion into the cartilagenous matrix. Other patients have not shown inclusion bodies.

MIM No.: 26351

POS No.: 3201

Sex Ratio: Based on phenotypic sex: M15:F9 (five males had ambiguous genitalia, and two phenotypic females are known to have a 46,XY karyotype and testes).

Occurrence: Over 60 cases have been documented.

Risk of Recurrence for Patient's Sib:
See Part I, *Mendelian Inheritance.*

Risk of Recurrence for Patient's Child:
See Part I, *Mendelian Inheritance.*

Age of Detectability: At birth. Prenatal diagnosis is possible by serial ultrasound during the second trimester.

Gene Mapping and Linkage: Unknown.

Prevention: None known. Genetic counseling indicated.

Treatment: Unknown.

Prognosis: Patients are stillborn or die within hours after birth from respiratory insufficiency and other multiple abnormalities.

Detection of Carrier: Unknown.

Special Considerations: The marked variability in the pattern of anomalies and, to a lesser extent, in X-ray findings, and the considerable overlap of supposedly characteristic features distinguishing the types of **Short rib-polydactyly syndrome** suggests that SRPS is a single syndrome, the different types representing a spectrum of the same pathogenetic mechanisms, which are most severely expressed in SRPS, type I, intermediate in type III, and least severe in type II.

References:
Verma IC, et al.: An autosomal recessive form of lethal chondrodystrophy with severe thoracic narrowing, rhizo-acromelic type of micromelia, polydactyly and genital anomalies. BD:OAS II(6). New York: March of Dimes Birth Defects Foundation, 1975:167–174.
Naumoff P, et al.: Short rib-polydactyly syndrome type 3. Radiology 1977; 122:443–447.
Sillence DO: Non-Majewski short rib-polydactyly syndrome. Am J Med Genet 1980; 7:2223–2229. *
Belloni C, Beluffi G: Short rib-polydactyly syndrome, type Verma-Naumoff. Fortschr Röntgenstr 1981; 134:431–435.
Bernstein R, et al.: Short rib-polydactyly syndrome: a single or heterogeneous entity? A re-evaluation prompted by four new cases. J Med Genet 1985; 22:46–53. †
Sillence D, et al.: Perinatally lethal short rib-polydactyly syndromes: variability in known syndromes. Pediatr Radiol 1987; 17:474–480. *
Yang SS, et al.: Three conditions in neonatal asphyxiating thoracic dysplasia (Jeune) and the short rib-polydactyly syndrome spectrum: a clinicopathologic study. Am J Med Genet 1987; Suppl 3:191–207.
Frzen M, et al.: Comparative histopathology of the growth cartilage in short-rib polydactyly syndromes type I and III and in chondroectodermal dysplasia. Ann Genet 1988; 31:144–150.

BE043   **Renée Bernstein**

Short stature in the African pygmy
See GROWTH DEFICIENCY, AFRICAN PYGMY TYPE
Short stature, X-linked, with skin pigmentation
See SILVER SYNDROME, X-LINKED
Short stature-alopecia-skeletal anomalies-mental retardation
See ALOPECIA-SKELETAL ANOMALIES-SHORT STATURE-MENTAL RETARDATION

SHORT STATURE-CEREBRAL ATROPHY-KERATOSIS FOLLICULARIS, X-LINKED   2340

Includes:
Cerebral atrophy-keratosis follicularis-short stature, X-linked
Keratosis follicularis-dwarfism-cerebral atrophy

Excludes:
Darier disease (2865)
Dyskeratosis congenita (2024)
Skin, keratosis follicularis spinulosa decalvans (2867)

Major Diagnostic Criteria: Congenital, proportionate, and progressive dwarfism; cerebral atrophy with **Microcephaly**, psychomotor retardation, and convulsions; and keratosis follicularis with alopecia.

Clinical Findings: Characteristic features are low birth weight (approximate average 2,415 g), early fetal-like face at birth, delayed somatic and psychomotor development, microcephaly, seizures, delayed dentition, micrognathia, generalized keratosis follicularis with alopecia. X-rays show osteoporosis and delayed bone age; EEG and pneumoencephalogram (PEG) are abnormal.

Complications: Microcephaly, psychomotor retardation, and convulsions are probably secondary to cerebral atrophy, whereas alopecia results from the keratosis follicularis.

Associated Findings: None known.

Etiology: Presumably X-linked recessive inheritance.

Pathogenesis: Unknown.

MIM No.: 30883

POS No.: 3934

Sex Ratio: M1:F0

Occurrence: Six members of one family have been documented.

Risk of Recurrence for Patient's Sib:
See Part I, *Mendelian Inheritance.*

Risk of Recurrence for Patient's Child:
See Part I, *Mendelian Inheritance.*

Age of Detectability: At birth.

Gene Mapping and Linkage: Unknown.

Prevention: None known. Genetic counseling indicated.

Treatment: Supportive and symptomatic, including anticonvulsant medication and special education.

Prognosis: Life expectancy is unknown but probably decreased. Of six reported patients, four were less than six years of age, and two died before two years of age from infections.

Detection of Carrier: Unknown.

References:
Cantú JM, et al.: A new X-linked recessive disorder with dwarfism, cerebral atrophy, and generalized keratosis follicularis. J Pediatr 1974; 84:564–567. * †

RI015   **Fernando Rivas**
CA011   **José María Cantú**

Short stature-ear abnormalities-elbow/hip dislocation
See AURICULO-OSTEODYSPLASIA
Short stature-facial and skeletal defects-mental retardation
See KABUKI MAKE-UP SYNDROME
Short stature-facial/skeletal anomalies-retardation-macrodontia
See KBG SYNDROME
Short stature-head/face anomalies-kyphoscoliosis-retardation
See COFFIN-LOWRY SYNDROME
Short stature-hypolipidemia-leukonychia
See HOOFT DISEASE

SHORT STATURE-MENTAL RETARDATION-DELAYED SEXUAL MATURITY   2338

Includes:
Mental retardation-sexual maturity (delayed)-short stature
Sexual maturity (delayed)-short stature-mental retardation

Excludes: Short stature-mental deficiency (in other conditions)

Major Diagnostic Criteria: Severe mental retardation, slow growth and maturation, and delayed sexual development with normal laboratory and endocrinologic findings.

Clinical Findings: The patients have proportionate dwarfism (height, weight, and cephalic circumference below the third percentile), infantile external genitalia, and severe mental deficiency (IQ: 11–21) with a calm behavior, permanent smile, and inability to communicate by any other means. Since the bone age is also severely delayed (about 5–6 years), the osseous development is somewhat compatible with the somatometric parameters.

The endocrinologic evaluation is normal, including response to specific stimulation. Chromosomal studies demonstrate that this mental retardation syndrome is not associated with **X-linked mental retardation, Fragile X syndrome.**

Complications: Unknown.

Associated Findings: None known.

Etiology: Recessive inheritance, either autosomal or X-linked.

Pathogenesis: Unknown.

Sex Ratio: M2:F0 (observed).

Occurrence: Two cases have been described in the literature.

Risk of Recurrence for Patient's Sib:
See Part I, *Mendelian Inheritance.*

Risk of Recurrence for Patient's Child:
See Part I, *Mendelian Inheritance.*

Age of Detectability: Since the delayed sexual maturation is a major finding, the patients must be older than 15 years of age.

Gene Mapping and Linkage: Unknown.

Prevention: None known. Genetic counseling indicated.

Treatment: Unknown.

Prognosis: Poor for independence because of the mental retardation.

Detection of Carrier: Unknown.

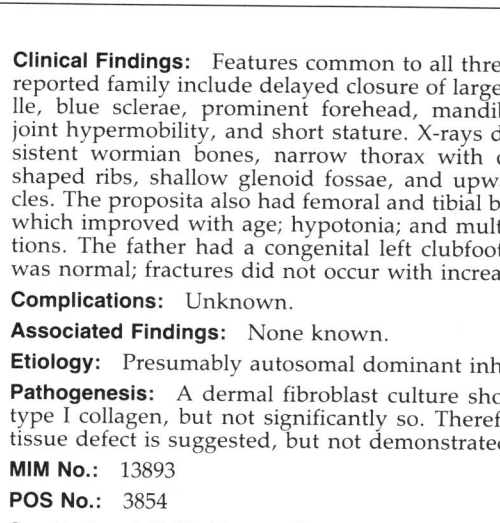

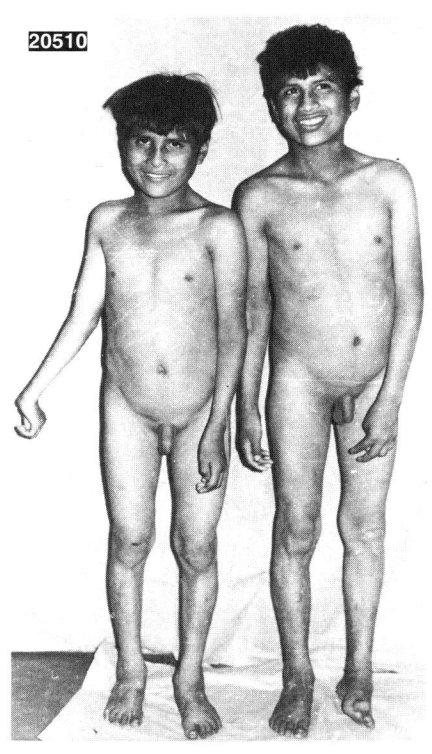

2338-20510: Note proportionate short stature in both brothers and the infantile external genitalia.

Clinical Findings: Features common to all three members of the reported family include delayed closure of large anterior fontanelle, blue sclerae, prominent forehead, mandibular hypoplasia, joint hypermobility, and short stature. X-rays demonstrated persistent wormian bones, narrow thorax with or without oddly shaped ribs, shallow glenoid fossae, and upward-bowing clavicles. The proposita also had femoral and tibial bowing in infancy, which improved with age; hypotonia; and multiple joint dislocations. The father had a congenital left clubfoot. Dentition in all was normal; fractures did not occur with increased frequency.

Complications: Unknown.

Associated Findings: None known.

Etiology: Presumably autosomal dominant inheritance.

Pathogenesis: A dermal fibroblast culture showed slightly less type I collagen, but not significantly so. Therefore, a connective tissue defect is suggested, but not demonstrated.

MIM No.: 13893

POS No.: 3854

Sex Ratio: M2:F1 (observed).

Occurrence: One family with three affected individuals has been reported.

Risk of Recurrence for Patient's Sib:
See Part I, *Mendelian Inheritance.*

Risk of Recurrence for Patient's Child:
See Part I, *Mendelian Inheritance.*

Age of Detectability: At birth by physical examination.

Gene Mapping and Linkage: Unknown.

Prevention: None known. Genetic counseling indicated.

Treatment: Supportive.

Prognosis: Intelligence, reproductive capability, and life span are normal.

Detection of Carrier: Unknown.

Special Considerations: Beighton (1981) reported a similar condition with blue sclerae, multiple wormian bones, and lack of fractures; however, the presence of dentinogenesis imperfecta and deafness and the lack of joint hypermobility help to distinguish the two conditions.

References:
Beighton P: Familial dentinogenesis imperfecta, blue sclera, and wormian bones without fractures: another type of osteogenesis imperfecta? J Med Genet 1981; 18:124–128.
MacLean JR, et al.: The Grant syndrome: persistent wormian bones, blue sclerae, mandibular hypoplasia, shallow glenoid fossae and campomelia - an autosomal dominant trait. Clin Genet 1986; 29:523–529.

T0007   **Helga V. Toriello**

References:
Cantú JM, et al.: Severe mental deficiency, proportionate dwarfism, and delayed sexual maturation: a distinct inherited syndrome. Hum Genet 1980; 56:231–234. *

C0064   **José Sánchez-Corona**
CA011   **José María Cantú**

Short stature-mental retardation-obesity-hypogonadism
See X-LINKED MENTAL RETARDATION-SHORT STATURE-OBESITY-HYPOGONADISM
Short stature-pterygia-dysmophic facies-mental retardation
See PTERYGIA-DYSMORPHIC FACIES-SHORT STATURE-MENTAL RETARDATION
Short stature-Rieger anomaly-lipodystrophy-diabetes
See LIPODYSTROPHY-RIEGER ANOMALY-SHORT STATURE-DIABETES
Short stature-sexual infantilism
See TURNER SYNDROME

SHORT STATURE-WORMIAN BONES-JOINT DISLOCATIONS   3014

Includes:
    Campomelia-wormian bones-blue sclerae-mandibular hypoplasia
    Grant syndrome
    Joint dislocations-wormian bones-short stature
    Osteogenesis imperfecta, possible variant
    Wormian bones-blue sclerae-mandibular hypoplasia-campomelia

Excludes: Osteogenesis imperfecta (0777)

Major Diagnostic Criteria: The combination of persistent wormian bones, blue sclerae, mandibular hypoplasia, and campomelia should suggest the diagnosis.

SHORT SYNDROME   2098

Includes:
    Growth retardation-Rieger anomaly
    Reiger anomaly-growth retardation

Excludes:
    Eye, anterior segment dysgenesis (0439)
    Lipodystrophy-Rieger anomaly-short stature-diabetes (2834)
    Lipodystrophy, sporadic
    Silver syndrome (0887)

Major Diagnostic Criteria: Most or all of the following findings are needed to make or suspect the diagnosis: low birth weight with subsequent short stature, liopatrophy of the face and upper limbs, delayed dental eruption, Rieger anomaly, and delayed speech development.

SHORT syndrome is a mnemonic for S = short stature, H = hyperextensibility or hernia (inguinal), O = ocular depression, R = Rieger anomaly, and T = teething (delayed).

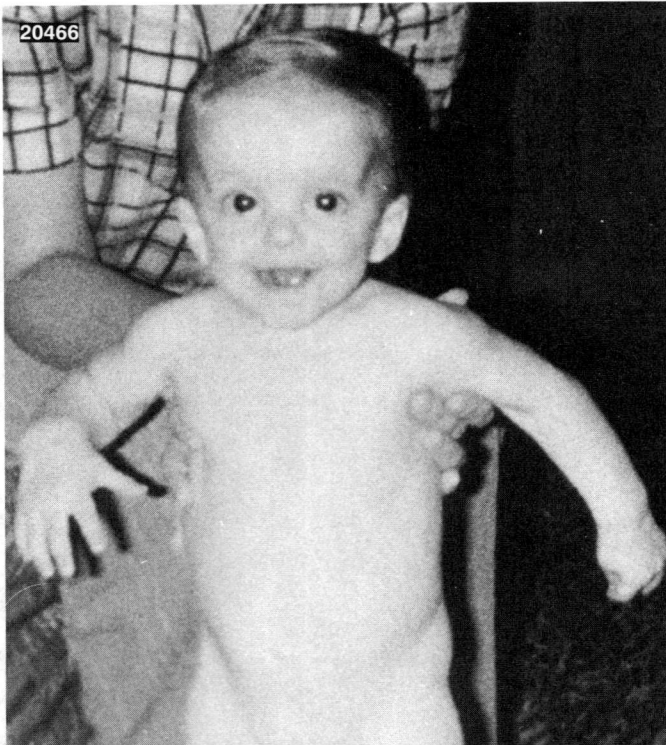

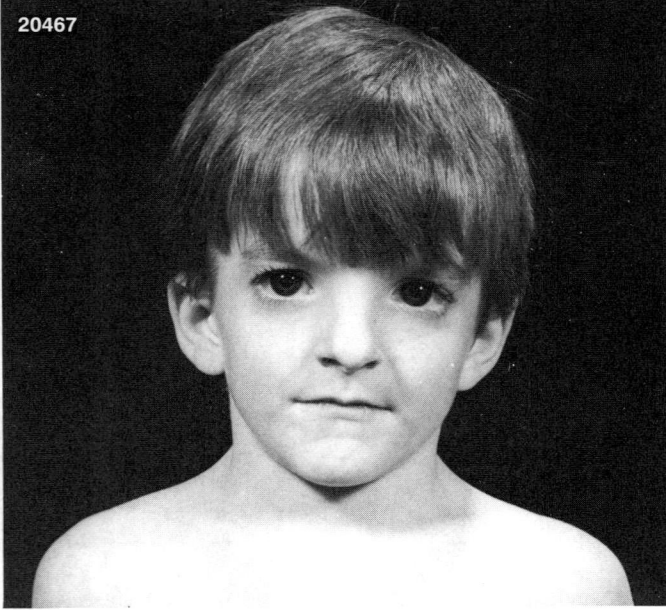

2098-20466–67: Reiger anomaly-growth retardation (SHORT syndrome); note triangular facies and hypoplastic nasal alae.

Clinical Findings: In the four reported cases, intrauterine growth retardation (3); slow weight gain (3); "triangular" face (4); telecanthus (2); deep-set eyes (4); Rieger anomaly (3); wide nasal bridge (4); hypoplastic alar cartilages (4); micrognathia (4); protuberant pinnae (4); clinodactyly (3); delayed dental eruption (4); lipoatrophy (4); joint hyperextensibility (4); short stature (4); functional cardiac murmur (2); inguinal hernia (2); delayed speech development (4); normal IQ (3); and delayed bone age on X-ray (4).

Complications: Frequent infections during infancy have been common.

Associated Findings: Sensorineural deafness was present in one patient.

Etiology: Probably autosomal recessive inheritance.

Pathogenesis: Unknown. Metabolic studies, growth hormone, somatomedin-C, thyroid studies, and banded chromosome studies have all been normal.

MIM No.: 26988

POS No.: 3496

Sex Ratio: M3:F1 (observed)

Occurrence: Four cases have been reported.

Risk of Recurrence for Patient's Sib:
See Part I, *Mendelian Inheritance.*

Risk of Recurrence for Patient's Child:
See Part I, *Mendelian Inheritance.*

Age of Detectability: At birth, by physical examination.

Gene Mapping and Linkage: Unknown.

Prevention: None known. Genetic counseling indicated.

Treatment: Screening for hearing ability, treatment of infections, and ocular examination are all indicated.

Prognosis: Mentation is normal, life span is unlikely to be impaired.

Detection of Carrier: Unknown.

References:
Gorlin RJ: A selected miscellany. BD:OAS XI(2). New York: March of Dimes Birth Defects Foundation, 1975:46–48.
Sensenbrenner JA, et al.: A low birthweight syndrome? Reiger syndrome. BD:OAS XI(2). New York: March of Dimes Birth Defects Foundation, 1975:423–426.
Toriello HV, et al.: Report of a case and further delineation of the SHORT Syndrome. Am J Med Genet 1985; 22:311–314.

T0007   **Helga V. Toriello**

Short-limbed campomelic syndrome, normocephalic type
See *KYPHOMELIC DYSPLASIA*
Short-rib syndrome, Beemer type
See *DWARFISM, SHORT-RIB, BEEMER TYPE*
Short-segment coarctation
See *AORTA, COARCTATION, INFANTILE TYPE*

SHOVAL-SOFFER SYNDROME   **3258**

Includes:
Male hypogonadism-mental retardation-skeletal anomalies
Skeletal anomalies-male hypogonadism-mental retardation
Testicular deficiency, familial

Excludes:
Bardet-Biedl syndrome (2363)
Crandall syndrome (3257)
Deafness-pili torti, Bjornstad type (2015)
Laurence-Moon syndrome (0578)

Major Diagnostic Criteria: The combination of mental retardation, cervical spine and rib anomalies, and hypogonadism.

Clinical Findings: In the two reported affected males, mental retardation and moderate short stature were present. Hypogonadism was present, in that both males had decreased facial and chest hair, breast development, female fat distribution, and small penis and testes. Histologic examination of the testes revealed two types of seminiferous tubules: those affected by true germinal aplasia, and those which were fibrotic. X-ray studies demonstrated rib anomalies, including cervical ribs and/or fusion; and cervical vertebral anomalies, including atlanto-occipital fusion, reversed lordotic curve, and hypertrophic spondylitis.

Complications: Unknown.

Associated Findings: One patient had a thyroid nodule which was either a cyst or adenoma.

Etiology: Possibly X-linked recessive inheritance.

Pathogenesis: Unknown.

MIM No.: 30750

Sex Ratio: M1:F0

Occurrence: One family with two affected male sibs has been reported.

Risk of Recurrence for Patient's Sib:
See Part I, *Mendelian Inheritance.*

Risk of Recurrence for Patient's Child:
See Part I, *Mendelian Inheritance.*

Age of Detectability: Unknown. The reported patients were 36 and 47 years at the time of report.

Gene Mapping and Linkage: Unknown.

Prevention: None known. Genetic counseling indicated.

Treatment: Unknown.

Prognosis: Prognosis for life span is apparently normal; mental retardation is moderate in severity.

Detection of Carrier: Unknown. Some of the female relatives exhibited mild mental retardation.

References:
Sohval AR, Soffer LJ: Congenital familial testicular deficiency. Am J Med 1953; 14:328–248.

T0007   **Helga V. Toriello**

Shprintzen syndrome
See VELO-CARDIO-FACIAL SYNDROME
Shprintzen-Goldberg syndrome
See PHARYNX/LARYNX HYPOPLASIA-OMPHALOCELE,
SHPRINTZEN-GOLDBERG TYPE
also CRANIOSYNOSTOSIS-ARACHNODACTYLY-HERNIA
'Shunt' hyperbilirubinemia
See HYPERBILIRUBINEMIA, CONJUGATED
Shurtleff syndrome
See MARSHALL-SMITH SYNDROME

SHWACHMAN SYNDROME   0885

Includes:
Bone marrow dysfunction-pancreatic insufficiency-short
    stature
Lipomatosis of pancreas, congenital
Metaphyseal dysplasia-pancreatic hypoplasia-marrow
    dysfunction
Pancreatic hypoplasia-marrow dysfunction-metaphyseal
    dysplasia
Shwachman-Bodian syndrome
Shwachman-Diamond-Oski-Khaw syndrome

Excludes:
Cystic fibrosis (0237)
Johanson-Blizzard syndrome (2026)
Pancreatic insufficiency, secondary

Major Diagnostic Criteria: Short stature, developmental delay, exocrine pancreatic insufficiency, short ribs with metaphyseal dysplasia, and isolated or combined decreases in red cell, white cell, or platelet counts.

Clinical Findings: Patients typically present with either short ribs and bone dysplasia in the newborn period, or developmental delay, short stature, malabsorption, recurrent infections, or hematologic abnormalities in childhood. Pancreatic insufficiency confirmed by quantitative assay of duodenal fluid appears to be the most consistent finding, but is not always accompanied by symptoms. Older patients frequently have normal stool patterns. Short stature, unaffected by nutritional status, is found in most cases, and mild-to-moderate developmental delay is also often evident.

Bone marrow dysfunction is probably always present, but is not always manifested by abnormal peripheral blood counts. Defective granulopoiesis has been demonstrated in vitro in patients who were not neutropenic at the time of the study. Anemia, neutropenia, and thrombocytopenia occur singly or in combination, and can be persistent, cyclic, or intermittent in nature.

Bone dysplasia is common, and may improve with time. The X-ray features are fairly specific, and the lesions found in bone biopsy material appear to differ from other metaphyseal dysplasias.

Saliva production is decreased, but this does not appear to lead to significant clinical symptoms.

Complications: Malabsorption of fat and protein, diarrhea, failure to thrive, hypoproteinemia, recurrent bacterial infections, coxa vara deformity, and cirrhosis of the liver. Hearing loss may occur secondary to recurrent otitis media. Leukemia occurs with increased frequency in older patients.

Associated Findings: **Colon, aganglionosis,** endocardial fibroelastosis, **Syndactyly,** supernumerary metatarsals, imperforate anus with rectourethral fistula, galactosuria, clitoral hypertrophy, increased circulating fetal hemoglobin, and defective leukocyte mobility.

Etiology: Autosomal recessive inheritance. Spontaneous chromosome breakage has been reported in one patient.

Pathogenesis: The decreases in bone matrix and pancreatic enzymes, coupled with the presence of inclusions in chondrocytes and pancreatic acinar cells, suggest a defect in polypeptide secretion. This appears to be supported by a decreased production of saliva and salivary amylase, and numerous amorphous particles in the tear layer on slit-lamp examination.

It has been suggested that abnormal polymorphonuclear chemotaxis reflects defective cytoskeletal integrity.

MIM No.: *26040

POS No.: 3453

Sex Ratio: M1:F1

Occurrence: The second most common cause of pancreatic insufficiency in childhood. Over 100 cases have been reported.

Risk of Recurrence for Patient's Sib:
See Part I, *Mendelian Inheritance.*

Risk of Recurrence for Patient's Child:
See Part I, *Mendelian Inheritance.*

Age of Detectability: During the newborn or infancy periods.

Gene Mapping and Linkage: Unknown.

Prevention: None known. Genetic counseling indicated.

Treatment: Orally administered pancreatic enzyme replacement improves digestion and absorption of peptides and fats. Early attention to febrile illnesses, including bacterial cultures, is necessary to prevent overwhelming infection. No therapy has been successful in reversing neutropenia, thrombocytopenia, or anemia, but specific replacement of blood components is useful for symptomatic patients. Appropriate orthopedic attention to the metaphyseal dysplasia, especially that involving the hip, may prevent deformity.

Prognosis: The long-term prognosis is uncertain. Some patients appear to do very well; others have major difficulties, and death in childhood from overwhelming infection or leukemia is common. The severity of symptoms from the other manifestations of the disorder varies greatly.

Detection of Carrier: Unknown.

References:
Bodian M, et al.: Congenital hypoplasia of the exocrine pancreas. Acta Paediatr 1964; 53:282–293.
Shwachman H, et al.: The syndrome of pancreatic insufficiency and bone marrow dysfunction. J Pediatr 1964; 65:645–663.
McLennan TW, Steinback HL: Shwachman's syndrome: the broad spectrum of bony abnormalities. Radiology 1974; 112:167–173.
Aggett PJ, et al.: Shwachman's syndrome: a review of 21 cases. Arch Dis Child 1980; 55:331–347. †

Hill RE, et al.: Steatorrhea and pancreatic insufficiency in Shwachman syndrome. Gastroenterology 1982; 83:22–27.

Rothbaum RJ, et al.: Unusual surface distribution of concanavalin A reflects a cytoskeletal defect in neutrophils in Shwachman's syndrome. Lancet 1982; II:800–801.

Tada H, et al.: A case of Shwachman syndrome with increased spontaneous chromosome breakage. Hum Genet 1987; 77:289–291.

DI001 **John H. Di Liberti**
WH007 **Peter F. Whitington**

Shwachman-Bodian syndrome
See SHWACHMAN SYNDROME
Shwachman-Diamond-Oski-Khaw syndrome
See SHWACHMAN SYNDROME
Shy-Magee disease
See MYOPATHY, CENTRAL CORE DISEASE TYPE
Sialangiectasis
See PAROTITIS, PUNCTATE
Sialectasis
See PAROTITIS, PUNCTATE
Sialic acid storage disease, infantile (one form)
See SALLA DISEASE

SIALIC ACID STORAGE DISEASE, INFANTILE TYPE — 2222

Includes:
> N-acetylneuraminic acid storage disease
> Sialuria, French type
> Sialuria, severe infantile

Excludes:
> **Galactosialidosis** (3110)
> **Mucolipidosis I** (0671)
> **Mucolipidosis II** (0672)
> **Mucolipidosis III** (0673)
> **Salla disease** (2041)

Major Diagnostic Criteria: Typical clinical findings with early onset accumulation of free sialic acid in tissues, and hypersecretion of free sialic acid in urine.

Clinical Findings: Clinical findings are present at birth or soon thereafter and include coarse facies, epicanthus, anteverted nostrils, clear corneas, hypopigmented hair, hepatosplenomegaly, diarrhea, anemia, inactivity, slow growth, and profound developmental impairment.

Abnormalities on X-ray include punctate calcifications of epiphyses and minimal changes of dysostosis multiplex.

Laboratory findings include anemia, clear vacuoles in lymphocytes and other tissues, urinary hypersecretion of free sialic acid, accumulation of free sialic acid in tissues, and nonspecific increase in activities of some lysosomal enzymes.

Complications: Unknown.

Associated Findings: None known.

Etiology: Autosomal recessive inheritance.

Pathogenesis: Unknown. Storage of sialic acid in this condition does not appear to be related to a deficiency of a lysosomal hydrolase. A transport defect has been suggested.

MIM No.: 26992

Sex Ratio: Presumably M1:F1.

Occurrence: Less than a dozen cases have been documented.

Risk of Recurrence for Patient's Sib:
See Part I, *Mendelian Inheritance.* A family history has been noted in only a few instances; in one the mother of a girl with the syndrome had extreme short stature at birth and extending into adult life, along with precocious sexual development, café-au-lait spots, and mild syndactyly. In another, three affected sibs were reported.

Risk of Recurrence for Patient's Child:
See Part I, *Mendelian Inheritance.* No affected individuals have survived to reproduce.

Age of Detectability: At birth. Prenatal diagnosis may be possible by quantification of free sialic acid in amniotic fluid and amniocytes.

Gene Mapping and Linkage: Unknown.

Prevention: None known. Genetic counseling indicated.

Treatment: Curative therapy is not available. Supportive therapy has been ineffective. Care for associated symptoms as indicated.

Prognosis: Progressive emaciation and loss of environmental contact result in early death.

Detection of Carrier: Unknown.

Special Considerations: *Sialuria, French type* (Stevenson et al, 1982), observed in a single case, is sialuria of infantile onset and severe manifestations. Free sialic acid is elevated in urine, serum, and cellular cytosol. This condition is distinct from **Sialic acid storage disease, infantile type** and from **Salla disease**.

References:
Hancock LW, et al.: Generalized N-acetylneuraminic acid storage disease: quantification and identification of the monosaccharide accumulating in brain and other tissues. Neurochem Res 1982; 38:803–809.

Stevenson RE, et al.: Sialuria: clinical and laboratory features of a severe infantile form. Proc Greenwood Genet Center 1982; 1:73–78.

Tondeur M, et al.: Infantile form of sialic acid storage disorder: clinical, ultrastructural and biochemical studies in two siblings. Eur J Pediatr 1982; 139:142–147.

Stevenson RE, et al.: Sialic acid storage with sialuria: clinical and biochemical features in the severe infantile type. Pediatrics 1983; 72:441–449.

Baumkotter J, et al.: N-acetylneuraminic acid storage disease. Hum Genet 1985; 71:155–159.

Mancini GMS, et al.: Free N-acetylneuraminic acid (NANA) storage disorders. Hum Genet 1986; 73:214–217.

SC053 **Richard J. Schroer**
ST021 **Roger E. Stevenson**

Sialidase deficiency
See MUCOLIPIDOSIS I
Sialidosis
See MUCOLIPIDOSIS I
Sialidosis type II, juvenile-onset form
See GALACTOSIALIDOSIS
Sialuria, Finnish type
See SALLA DISEASE
Sialuria, French type
See SIALIC ACID STORAGE DISEASE, INFANTILE TYPE
Sialuria, severe infantile
See SIALIC ACID STORAGE DISEASE, INFANTILE TYPE
Siamese twins
See TWINS, CONJOINED
Sicca syndrome
See SJOGREN SYNDROME
Sickle cell anemia
See ANEMIA, SICKLE CELL
Sideroblastic anemia, autosomal recessive
See ANEMIA, SIDEROBLASTIC
Sideroblastic anemia, congenital hereditary
See ANEMIA, CONGENITAL SIDEROBLASTIC, NOT B(6) RESPONSIVE
Sideroblastic anemia, hereditary X-linked
See ANEMIA, CONGENITAL SIDEROBLASTIC, NOT B(6) RESPONSIVE
Sideroblastic anemia, X-linked
See ANEMIA, SIDEROBLASTIC
Sideroblastic anemia, X-linked-ataxia
See ANEMIA, SIDEROBLASTIC
Sideroblastic anemia-exocrine pancreatic dysfunction
See ANEMIA, SIDEROBLASTIC
Sideroblastic anemia-glucose-6-phosphate dehydrogenase deficiency
See ANEMIA, SIDEROBLASTIC
Sideroblastic anemia-Xg(a) blood group antigen
See ANEMIA, SIDEROBLASTIC
Sideroblastic hypochromic aplastic anemia, congenital
See ANEMIA, CONGENITAL SIDEROBLASTIC, NOT B(6) RESPONSIVE
Siderophilin deficiency
See ATRANSFERRINEMIA

Siemens disease
See MAL DE MELEDA
Siemerling-Creutzfeldt disease
See ADRENOLEUKODYSTROPHY, X-LINKED
Silent microcephaly
See MICROCEPHALY, ISOLATED AUTOSOMAL DOMINANT TYPE

SILVER SYNDROME   0887

Includes:
   Asymmetry, congenital-short stature-sexual development variations
   Dwarfism, Silver-Russell type
   Russell-Silver syndrome
   Sexual development variations-asymmetry-short stature
   Silver-Russell syndrome

Excludes:
   Cerebral defects, diffuse static
   Fibrous dysplasia, polyostotic (0391)
   Hemihypertrophy (0458)
   Neurofibromatosis (0712)
   Silver syndrome, X-linked (2829)
   Turner syndrome (0977)

Major Diagnostic Criteria: Significant skeletal asymmetry, short stature, small size for gestational age, and variations in the clinical and laboratory pattern of sexual development. A combination of three or more of these findings probably should be present for a clinical diagnosis to be made. The presence of several of the minor manifestations (short incurved fifth fingers, triangular facies, turned-down corners of the mouth, café-au-lait spots and syndactyly) tend to make the diagnosis more certain.

Clinical Findings: Short stature, significant skeletal asymmetry, variations in the pattern of sexual development, and small size despite being born at term. Other findings include café-au-lait areas of the skin, unusually short and incurved fifth fingers, triangular shape of the face, turned-down corners of the mouth, and syndactyly of the toes. Variable combinations of findings have been reported, and no single finding was noted in all patients.

At birth affected infants are unusually small for gestational age. In those cases in which the pattern of subsequent growth could be evaluated, it usually paralleled the normal growth curve but remained below the third percentile level. The children who were observed into puberty continued to be short. The pattern of puberty and adolescent growth is essentially normal but may occur at a marginally earlier time than normal. Mature height has been described as being comparable to the height reduction at the time the diagnosis was made in earlier childhood. However, some patients have experienced catch-up growth prior to adolescence.

The asymmetry, when present, can be quite variable in extent and degree. In some, one entire side of the body was significantly larger than the other; in others, the extent of the asymmetry was limited and involved only the skull, spine, or all or part of a limb. The asymmetry is probably present at birth, but may not be appreciated for variable periods of time.

Variations in the pattern of sexual development include elevated levels of serum and urinary gonadotropins in prepubertal children of both sexes. Sexual development may be precocious or may occur disproportionately early in relation to other physiologic evidences of maturity. Precocious sexual development is much more likely to occur in affected girls than in boys.

The café-au-lait spots are usually sharply circumscribed, smooth, light brown, and vary in size from less than 1 cm to over 30 cm in diameter. The spots are usually not raised, but in one instance, the entire pigmented area was wrinkled and slightly elevated. The borders of most café-au-lait areas are smooth, but some have jagged edges. Affected children may sweat excessively.

The heads of children with the Silver syndrome may be disproportionately large for the small facial mass ("pseudohydrocephaly"), tapering to a narrow jaw and producing the characteristic triangular-shaped face. The lips are often thin, with the corners of the mouth turned down ("shark mouth"). Delay in the closure of the anterior fontanelle has been noted.

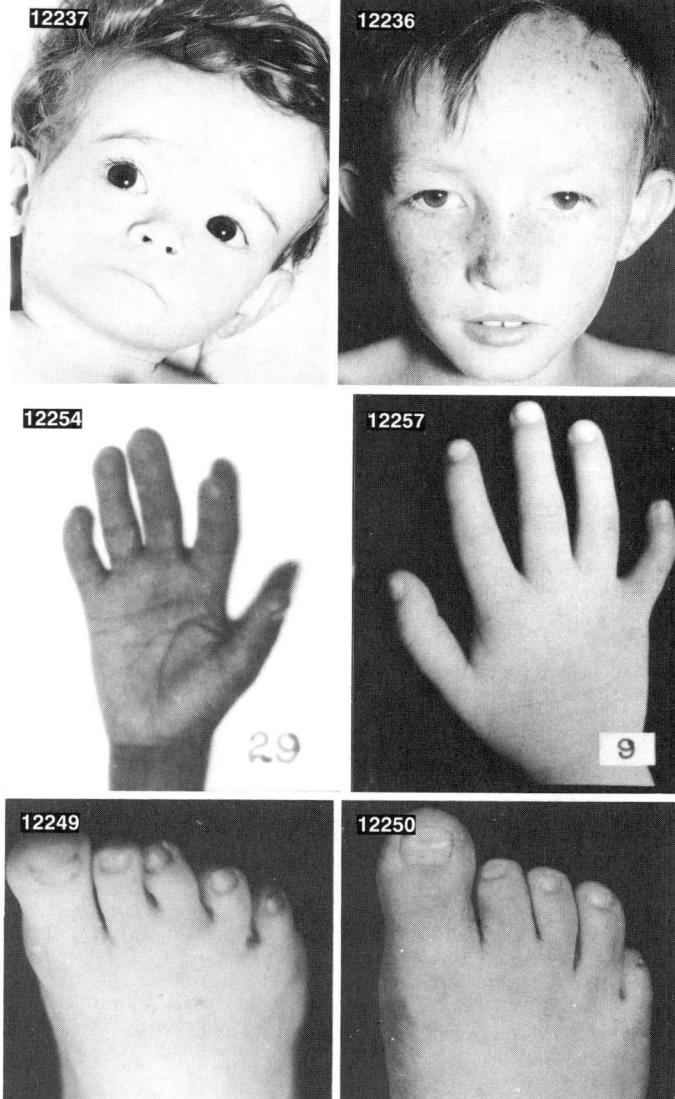

0887-12237–36: Typical facies with broad forehead tapering down to a narrow chin with triangular facies. **12254–57:** Clinodactyly of the fifth finger. **11249–50:** Disproportionate toes and syndactyly of toes 2–3.

Abnormalities of the limbs include incurving of the fifth fingers and variable, usually slight, syndactyly between the second and third toes. Other variations in the size and configuration of the toes are not uncommon. In most cases subcutaneous tissue is sparse. Abnormal genitalia, especially cryptorchidism, are not uncommon. Most affected children have normal intelligence. Bone age is retarded but generally to a lesser degree than height age.

In children who do not exhibit significant skeletal asymmetry or variations in the pattern of sexual development, the combination of small size at birth, shortness of stature, café-au-lait areas of the skin, and unusually short and incurved fifth fingers, is relatively common and may represent a partial form of the syndrome.

Serum gonadotropins and the excretion of urinary gonadotropins may be increased for age. In the first decade, the level of urinary gonadotropins may be increased to that found in normal women during the reproductive period of life. Hypoglycemia has been noted on several occasions. One patient with this syndrome has been described with elevated blood levels of β-hydroxybutyrate and acetoacetate, and massive excretion of these compounds and of C_6-C_{12} dicarboxylic acids.

Epiphyseal maturation has been retarded in approximately one-half of the cases. There may be a difference in osseous maturation on the two sides of the body.

In at least two instances, elevated serum levels of growth hormone have been found. In several other cases the serum levels of growth hormone have been decreased, but most children with the syndrome have normal growth hormone values.

Defects of the skeleton, including poorly formed thoracic vertebrae which differed from those seen in the ordinary type of hemivertebra, surface irregularities of the lumbar vertebrae, which resemble those seen in juvenile kyphosis, irregularity and indentation of the metaphyses of the phalanges and hypoplasia, and absence of various phalanges, the sacrum, and the coccyx have all been described.

Complications: Although a significant association between **Hemihypertrophy** in children who are not short, and tumors of the kidneys (see **Cancer, Wilms tumor**) and adrenals (see **Cancer, neuroblastoma**) and **adrenal hyperplasia** has been noted, none of the reported cases of the Silver syndrome has been associated with malignancy of the kidneys and adrenals. Asymmetry of the spine and lower limbs may produce disturbances of gait. Precocious puberty may be psychologically disturbing to the child and parents.

Associated Findings: Urinary tract abnormalities and cardiac defects have been described in a few cases.

Etiology: Possibly autosomal recessive inheritance, or dominant inheritance with incomplete penetrance. An X-linked form has also been reported (see **Silver syndrome, X-linked**).

Pathogenesis: The finding of elevated levels of growth hormone in a few cases suggests that the short stature may result in part from a relative unresponsiveness to this hormone. Although growth hormone assays have been normal in most patients studied, several instances of idiopathic growth hormone deficiency, one case of Silver syndrome with growth hormone deficiency in a patient with a craniopharyngioma, and a few cases of elevated levels of growth hormone have been reported. The pathogenesis of both the asymmetry and the other clinical findings is undetermined. Some patients have had diploid-triploid mosaicism during some point in their development.

MIM No.: 27005

POS No.: 3385

CDC No.: 759.820

Sex Ratio: M1:F1

Occurrence: Close to 200 cases have been documented. All races and ethnic groups appear susceptible.

Risk of Recurrence for Patient's Sib:
See Part I, *Mendelian Inheritance*. A family history has been noted in only a few instances; in one the mother of a girl with the syndrome had extreme short stature at birth and extending into adult life, along with precocious sexual development, café-au-lait areas, and mild syndactyly. In another, three affected sibs were reported.

Risk of Recurrence for Patient's Child: Unknown.

Age of Detectability: Ordinarily at birth, but may not be recognized for several months.

Gene Mapping and Linkage: Unknown.

Prevention: None known. Genetic counseling indicated.

Treatment: Treatment is symptomatic. Corrective shoes, braces, and physical therapy may be necessary, but functional impairment may be minimal despite significant asymmetry. Patients, especially female patients and their parents, should be prepared for the precocious sexual development that may occur. Periodic examination should be carried out to determine the possible presence of a tumor of the kidney or adrenal.

Prognosis: Apparently normal for life span. Functional impairment will depend on the degree of asymmetry. In most instances no functional disturbance occurs. Approximately one-third of patients have been reported as showing some degree of mental retardation.

Detection of Carrier: Unknown.

Special Considerations: Parents of affected individuals and health professionals interested in Silver Syndrome are encouraged to contact the newly-formed ACRSS support Group listed below by writing Lois Vaughan, 5781 Vine Street, Oak Forest, IL, 60452.

Support Groups: NJ; Madison (22 Hoyt Street 07940); Association for Children with Russell-Silver Syndrome (ACRSS)

References:
Silver HK, et al.: Syndrome of congenital hemihypertrophy, shortness of stature, and elevated urinary gonadotropins. Pediatrics 1953; 368–375. †
Russell A: A syndrome of "intra-uterine dwarfism" recognizable at birth with cranio-facial synostosis, disproportionately short arms, and other anomalies. Proc R Soc Med 1954; 47:1040–1044. †
Silver HK: Asymmetry, short stature, and variations in sexual development: a syndrome of congenital malformations. Am J Dis Child 1964; 107:495–515. *
Tanner JM, et al.: The natural history of the Silver-Russell syndrome: a longitudinal study of thirty-nine cases. Pediatr Res 1975; 9:611–623.
Graham JM Jr., et al.: Diploid-triploid mixoploidy: clinical and cytogenetic aspects. Pediatrics 1981; 68:23–28. †
Gardner L: The lesions of polyploidy: relation to congenital asymmetry and the Russell-Silver syndrome. Am J Dis Child 1982; 136:292–293. †
Nishi Y, et al.: Silver-Russell syndrome and growth hormone deficiency. Acta Pediatr Scand 1982; 71:1035–1036.
Cassidy SB, et al.: Russell-Silver syndrome and hypopituitarism. Am J Dis Child 1986; 140:155–159. †
Davies PSW, et al.: Adolescent growth and pubertal progression in the Silver-Russell syndrome. Arch Dis Child 1988; 63:130–135. †
Willems PJ, et al.: Activation of fatty acid oxidation in the Silver-Russell syndrome and the Brachmann - de Lange syndrome. Am J Med Genet 1988; 30:865–873. †
Duncan PA, et al.: Three-generation dominant transmission of the Silver-Russell syndrome. Am J Med Genet 1990; 35:245–250.

SI012   **Henry K. Silver**

SILVER SYNDROME, X-LINKED   **2829**

Includes:
  Russell-Silver syndrome, X-linked
  Short stature, X-linked, with skin pigmentation
  Skin pigmentation-short stature, X-linked

Excludes:
  Silver syndrome (0887)
  Neurofibromatosis (0712)

Major Diagnostic Criteria: Short stature and brown pigmentation of the skin. Males have the clinical appearance of **Silver syndrome**.

Clinical Findings: Based on one family with two affected brothers, their mother, and two of her sisters: both males had intrauterine growth retardation, with birth weights of 1,890 and 1,960 g, respectively, at term. The head appeared large and the face triangular. Growth was slow, with both height and weight staying some 2 to 2.5 SD below the mean into middle childhood. One boy had frequent minor infections in infancy and then developed asthma with repeated short admissions to the hospital. Intellectual development was normal.

Abnormal pigmentation of the skin appeared in the second year with a few small spots, some of which were brown and some achromic. Thereafter, over a couple of years, diffuse light-brown pigmentation developed over the lower trunk, arms, and thighs, containing a few achromic and some dark-brown spots. Diffuse depigmentation was seen in the groin. There was no blistering or lichenification, but the achromic areas were easily sunburned.

Nothing abnormal was found in the history of the three affected females, but none achieved an adult height of more than 160 cm whereas their four unaffected sisters were 168 cm tall. All three women had 30 to 50 café-au-lait spots on the trunk and arms with a few achromic spots. All looked similar to each other, with a somewhat large mouth and prominent upper jaw.

Complications: Unknown.

Associated Findings: The severe asthma seen in one boy may have been coincidental.

Etiology: Presumably X-linked inheritance.

Pathogenesis: Unknown.

MIM No.: 31278

CDC No.: 759.820

Sex Ratio: M1:F1

Occurrence: One family from The Netherlands, living in Canada, has been reported.

Risk of Recurrence for Patient's Sib:
See Part I, *Mendelian Inheritance.*

Risk of Recurrence for Patient's Child:
See Part I, *Mendelian Inheritance.*

Age of Detectability: After the characteristic pigmentation appears in the second year of life.

Gene Mapping and Linkage: Unknown.

Prevention: None known. Genetic counseling indicated.

Treatment: Unknown.

Prognosis: Normal life span. Adult height of affected males is likely to be short.

Detection of Carrier: Possibly by relatively short stature and café-au-lait spots.

Special Considerations: The delineation of this variant of **Silver syndrome** supports the suggestion of others that the syndrome is heterogeneous. Usually the condition is a sporadic event in a family, and many such cases may well not be genetic. Familial cases have been reported and interpreted as indicating autosomal dominant inheritance with incomplete penetrance. Some of these families have shown a pattern of inheritance that is also consistent with X-linked inheritance.

References:
Partington MW: X-linked short stature with skin pigmentation: evidence for heterogeneity of the Russell-Silver syndrome. Clin Genet 1986; 29:151–156. * †

PA026   **M.W. Partington**

Silver-Russell syndrome
See SILVER SYNDROME
Silverman-Handmaker dwarfism
See DWARFISM, DYSSEGMENTAL, SILVERMAN-HANDMAKER TYPE
Simian crease, incomplete
See SKIN CREASE, SINGLE PALMAR
Simpson dysmorphia syndrome
See SIMPSON-GOLABI-BEHMEL SYNDROME

SIMPSON-GOLABI-BEHMEL SYNDROME   2826

Includes:
Bulldog syndrome
Dysplasia-gigantism syndrome, X-linked
Golabi-Rosen syndrome
Overgrowth, Golabi-Rosen type
Overgrowth-mental retardation syndrome, X-linked
Simpson dysmorphia syndrome
X-linked mental retardation-overgrowth syndrome
Excludes:
Beckwith-Wiedemann syndrome (0104)
Cebebral gigantism (0137)
Marshall-Smith syndrome (2193)
Overgrowth, Ruvalcaba-Myhre-Smith type (2120)
Proteus syndrome (2382)
Weaver syndrome (2036)

Major Diagnostic Criteria: The combination of overgrowth, unusual facial appearance, digital anomalies, and minor skeletal anomalies.

Clinical Findings: Six families have been reported. Anomalies present in most affected individuals include pre- and post-natal overgrowth; hypotonia; **Microcephaly**; **Eye, hypertelorism**; short, broad nose; large mouth with thick lips; submucous cleft or high-arched palate; midline groove or notch of the lower lip, tongue and/or **Hernia, inguinal**; cryptorchidism; broad halluces and thumbs; hypoplastic or absent index fingernails; high palmar pattern intensity; and normal to mildly delayed intellectual and motor development. Occasional abnormalities include hypodontia; pre-auricular dimples or tags; cadiac defects; supernumerary nipples; gastrointestinal abnormalities, including intestinal malrotation or constipation; renal anomalies, including "large", lobulated or cystic kidneys, duplicated renal pelvis, or mild hydronephrosis; postaxial polydactyly; small calf muscles; skin hyperpigmentation; and hyperinsulinemia attributable to an increased number of islets of Langerhans.

A family reported by Opitz et al (1988) included three affected males; the propositus of that family did not have overgrowth and was severely mentally retarded. Behmel et al (1988) suggest that the phenotype in the affected individuals of this family represents the "severe end of the spectrum".

Complications: Unknown.

Associated Findings: Present in one or two patients each were **Cleft lip**, **Omphalocele**, ocular coloboma, seizures, and limited extension of elbows and knees.

Etiology: Presumably X-linked recessive inheritance.

Pathogenesis: Unknown.

MIM No.: 30605, 31287

POS No.: 3325

Sex Ratio: M1:F0

Occurrence: Six families and one sporadic case have been described.

Risk of Recurrence for Patient's Sib:
See Part I, *Mendelian Inheritance.*

Risk of Recurrence for Patient's Child:
See Part I, *Mendelian Inheritance.*

Age of Detectability: At birth, by physical exam and presence of overgrowth.

Gene Mapping and Linkage: SDYS (Simpson dysmorphia syndrome) has been provisionally mapped to X.

Prevention: None known. Genetic counseling indicated.

Treatment: Supportive. Surgery may also be indicated.

Prognosis: Postnatal mortality is relatively high. In survivors, motor development is essentially normal, although clumsiness is present in childhood. Intellectual development is usually normal or mildly delayed.

Detection of Carrier: Carrier females may have some of the pheotypic features, including mild expression of the facial features, **Syndactyly**, hypoplastic index fingernails, and tall stature.

References:
Simpson JL, et al.: A previously unrecognized X-linked syndrome of dysmorphia. BD:OAS; XI(2). New York: March of Dimes Birth Defects Foundation, 1973:18–24.
Golabi M, Rosen L: A new X-linked mental retardation overgrowth syndrome. Am J Med Genet 1984; 17:345–358.
Opitz JM: The Golabi-Rosen syndrome. Am J Med Genet 1984; 17:359–366.
Tsukahara M, et al.: A Weaver-like syndrome in a Japanese boy. Clin Genet 1984; 25:73–78.
Behmel A, et al.: A new X-linked dysplasia gigantism syndrome: follow-up in the first family and a second Austrian family. Am J Med Genet 1988; 30:275–285.
Neri G, et al.: Simpson-Golabi-Behmel syndrome: an X-linked encephalo-tropho-schisis syndrome. Am J Med Genet 1988; 30:287–299.

Opitz JM, et al.: Simpson-Golabi-Behmel syndrome: follow-up of the Michigan family. Am J Med Genet 1988; 30:301–308.

T0007   **Helga V. Toriello**

Sindig-Larsen-Johansson disease (patella)
See JOINTS, OSTEOCHONDRITIS DISSECANS
Single transverse fold
See SKIN CREASE, SINGLE PALMAR

SINGLETON-MERTEN SYNDROME   2087

Includes:
> Aorta, idiopathic calcification
> Dental and bone defects
> Merten-Singleton syndrome
> Muscle weakness
> Skeletal defects with aortic calcification and muscle weakness

Excludes:
> **Ectodermal dysplasia** (see all)
> **Hypophosphatasia** (0516)
> **Mucopolysaccharidosis**
> **Oculo-dento-osseous dysplasia** (0737)
> **Progeria** (0825)
> **Thalassemia** (0939)
> **Xanthomatosis, cerebrotendinous** (2395)

Major Diagnostic Criteria: A combination of the following features should be present for a clinical diagnosis of the Singleton-Merten syndrome to be strongly suspected; all were found in the few cases reported: poor physical development, generalized muscular weakness, severe dental dysplasia in deciduous and permanent teeth. X-ray findings showed linear calcification of the proximal aorta and aortic valve; generalized osteoporosis; widened medullary spaces in the metacarpals, metatarsals, and phalanges.

Clinical Findings: Pregnancy, delivery, and early postnatal development are normal. The first signs and symptoms appear in infancy (4–24 months). The initial complaint is generalized muscular weakness (100%), which may follow an acute febrile illness (50%). Somatic growth and motor development are delayed (75%), while mental development is normal (100%). Severe dental dysplasia: carious deciduous teeth with premature loss; dysplasia and delayed development of permanent teeth (100%). Generalized osteoporosis is associated with thin cortices, expanded medullary cavities, and poorly defined trabeculae of the short tubular bones of the hands and feet (100%). Progressive calcification of the proximal aorta was apparent on X-ray by 4 to 12 years of age (100%), and calcific aortic valvular stenosis developed in mid to late childhood (100%). Mitral valve calcification was also frequently present (75%). Systolic murmurs were present early in life; however, valvular calcifications were not seen until later. The cardiac abnormalities led to left heart failure, which was the immediate cause of death in all patients.

In addition to the above problems, there may be psoriaform skin eruption in late childhood (50%) and erosion of the terminal phalanges without destructive psoriatic arthritis; soft tissue calcification (50%); calcification of the bursa, proximal radius, and ulna (1/4); and subungual calcification (1/4); hypertension (25%); heart block (25%).

There are no abnormalities in serum calcium, phosphorus, and alkaline phosphatase. Electromyograms are normal. Muscle biopsy shows nonspecific atrophy of the muscle fibers. No metabolic or hematologic disorders have been documented (100%). Death due to left heart failure occurred at 4–18 years of age.

Complications: Eye problems (50%): glaucoma and photosensitivity, are presumably related to viral or psoriatic keratitis. Orthopedic deformities (including shallow acetabular fossa, subluxation of femoral head, coxa valga, equinovarus foot deformity) are presumed secondary to generalized muscle weakness. Acro-osteolysis may be a complication of psoriaform eruption.

Associated Findings: None known.

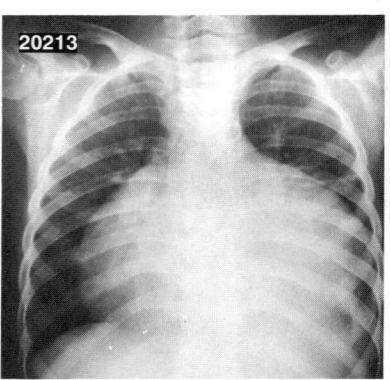 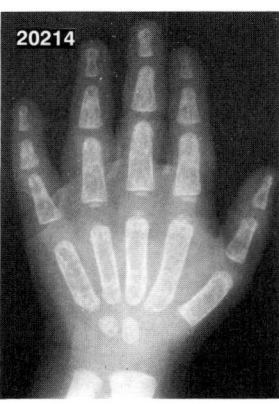

2087-20213: The heart is enlarged; there is tubular calcification of the ascending aorta and aortic arch. **20214:** The metacarpals and phalanges are osteoporotic with thinned cortices, accentuated trabeculae, and expansion of the medullary cavities.

Etiology: Unknown. Possibly autosomal dominant inheritance.

Pathogenesis: The basic pathogenesis of skeletal and cardiovascular changes is unknown. Autopsy findings show extensive calcification of the intima and media of the proximal aorta. There is myocardial degeneration and necrosis without evidence of inflammatory cells.

MIM No.: 18225

POS No.: 4024

Sex Ratio: M1:F3

Occurrence: Four cases have been published. Other patients with calcification of the ascending aorta and aortic valve due to idiopathic or infectious aortitis are reported in adults without the skeletal, dental, or muscular stigmata of Singleton-Merten syndrome.

Risk of Recurrence for Patient's Sib: All cases have been sporadic.

Risk of Recurrence for Patient's Child: No affected individuals have survived to reproduce.

Age of Detectability: Usually in infancy (less than age two years) the condition may be suspected clinically by generalized muscle weakness and poor development and abnormal dentition. Systolic murmurs develop early, but cardiovascular calcifications are not seen until four years of age or later. Skeletal changes are present in early infancy.

Gene Mapping and Linkage: Unknown.

Prevention: None known. Genetic counseling indicated.

Treatment: None known; symptomatic treatment of cardiac disease, but there is no experience with valve replacement. Supportive treatment for muscular weakness and complications, including orthopedic deformities.

Prognosis: Death from cardiac failure 4–16 years after onset.

Detection of Carrier: Unknown.

References:
Singleton EB, Merten DF: An unusual syndrome of widened medullary cavities of the metacarpals and phalanges, aortic calcification and abnormal dentition. Pediatr Radiol 1973; 1:2–7. *
McLoughlin MJ, et al.: Idiopathic calcification of the ascending aorta and aortic valve in two young women. Br Heart J 1974; 36:96–100.
Gay B Jr, Kuhn JP: A syndrome of widened medullary cavities of bone, aortic calcification, abnormal dentition, and muscular weakness (the Singleton-Merten syndrome). Radiology 1976; 118:389–395.
Rangaswami N, et al.: Idiopathic linear calcification of the ascending aorta in an adolescent. Am J Dis Child 1979; 133:860–861.

Rosenthal T, et al.: Aortic calcification in young women: a case report. Angiology 1979; 30:53–55.

Theman TE, et al.: Morphological findings in idiopathic calcification of the ascending aorta and aortic valve affecting a young woman. Histopathology 1979; 3:181–190.

ME031   **David F. Merten**

Sinoatrial block, congenital complete
See ARRHYTHMIA, HEART BLOCK, CONGENITAL COMPLETE

SINUS, ABSENT PARANASAL   0797

Includes:

Agenesis of paranasal sinuses, unilateral
Paranasal sinuses, absent
Sinuses, absence of frontal
Sinuses, absence of frontal-microcornea-glaucoma

Excludes: Paranasal sinuses, hypoplastic

Major Diagnostic Criteria: Absence of paranasal sinuses on X-ray, if the patient is past the age at which the sinuses are present on X-rays. (The average age at which the paranasal sinuses become easily identifiable on X-rays is maxillary, one year; frontal, 6–8 years; ethmoid, one year; sphenoid, four years.)

In adults with absence on X-ray of only one sinus, the possibility of neoplastic and inflammatory disease must be eliminated before a diagnosis of agenesis can be assumed. This may necessitate surgical exploration.

Clinical Findings: Transillumination of involved frontal or maxillary sinuses is not possible. However, this is of little help in small children because the sinuses are not large enough normally to transilluminate well. Palpation of the face over the paranasal sinuses will be normal. Examination of the nose may reveal abnormalities of the turbinates on the ipsilateral side of the unilateral agenesis. Waters view, lateral view, Caldwell view, and basal view X-rays will show absence of some or all paranasal sinuses.

Complications: Unknown.

Associated Findings: In one family; microcornea, glaucoma, and absent frontal sinuses.

Etiology: Unknown.

Pathogenesis: Unknown.

Sex Ratio: Presumably M1:F1.

Occurrence: Undetermined but presumed rare.

Risk of Recurrence for Patient's Sib: Unknown.

Risk of Recurrence for Patient's Child: Unknown.

Age of Detectability: At 1–8 years, when paranasal sinuses appear on X-ray.

Gene Mapping and Linkage: Unknown.

Prevention: None known. Genetic counseling indicated.

Treatment: None for absent paranasal sinuses, but in patients with absent frontal sinuses, microcornea, and open-angle glaucoma, insidious blindness may develop unless the glaucoma is treated.

Prognosis: Normal for life span and intelligence.

Detection of Carrier: Unknown.

Special Considerations: There is one reported case of panagenesis of paranasal sinuses and one known case of unilateral absent paranasal sinuses. The case of unilateral agenesis was associated with an ipsilateral hypertrophied middle turbinate resulting in obstruction of the nasal airway on that side. There was also an absence of the inferior turbinate on the same side. A single family presented with *absent frontal sinuses, microcornea, and glaucoma*. In this particular family, no male-to-male transmission was present in the three generations affected; therefore, the type of dominant transmission is unknown.

References:

Gob, AS, Acquarelli, MJ: Unilateral absent paranasal sinuses with hypertrophied middle turbinate. West J Med 1966; 7:239–241.

Mocellin, L.: Panagenesis of the paranasal sinuses: report of a case. Arch Otolaryngol 1968; 88:311–314.

Holmes, LB, Walton, DS: Hereditary microcornea, glaucoma and absent frontal sinuses: a family study. J Pediatr 1969; 74:968–972.

GE000   **Robert N. Gebhart**

Sinuses, absence of frontal
See SINUS, ABSENT PARANASAL
Sinuses, absence of frontal-microcornea-glaucoma
See SINUS, ABSENT PARANASAL
Sinusitis-dextrocardia-bronchiectasis syndrome
See DEXTROCARDIA-BRONCHIECTASIS-SINUSITIS SYNDROME
Sipple syndrome
See ENDOCRINE NEOPLASIA, MULTIPLE TYPE II

SIRENOMELIA SEQUENCE   3191

Includes:

Symmelia
Sympodia
Uromelia

Excludes:

Caudal regression syndrome (3211)
Vater association (0987)

Major Diagnostic Criteria: Sirenomelia is an anomalous development of the caudal region of the body, with varying degrees of "fusion" of the lower extremities with or without long bones being present.

Clinical Findings: Complete or nearly complete fusion of the lower limbs is the most striking feature of sirenomelia. However, other congenital anomalies usually exist. Hemivertebrae have been observed involving cervical, thoracic and lumbar vertebrae. Spina bifida and meningomyelocele have also been noted. Abnormalities of the pelvis can include fused iliac bones with a poorly formed acetabula. Characteristically a single umbilical artery with hypoplasia of the aorta below the origin of the umbilical artery is present. The external genitalia in males can vary from rudimentary perineal skin tags to almost normal penis and scrotum. Rudimentary ovaries, and anomalous uterus and vagina are occasionally seen in females. Reported urinary tract anomalies include either unilateral or bilateral renal agenesis, renal artery agenesis, renal dysplasia, rudimentary ureters and agenesis of the bladder. Imperforate anus and blind ending rectum are invariably present.

Based on osseous findings, sirenomelia has been classified into seven types: *Type I*, all bones of thigh and lower leg present and unfused; *Type II*, fused fibulae; *Type III*, fibulae absent; *Type IV*, partially fused femora and fused fibulae; *Type V*, partially fused femora; *Type VI*, fused femora and fused tibiae; and *Type VII*, fused femora and absent tibiae. Another classification based on the leg and foot defects include three types: *Symelus* (sympus dipus-two feet), legs almost perfectly united and terminating in a double foot with soles on the anterior surfaces; *Uromelus* (sympus monopus-one foot), incompletely united legs ending in an incomplete single foot with the sole on the anterior surface, and *Sirenomelus* (Sympus apus-no foot), incomplete union of the legs with absence of a distinct foot.

Complications: Unknown.

Associated Findings: Lung hypoplasia is present in a high number of affected cases and is probably due to the associated oligohydramnios. Tracheoesophageal fistula can also be seen. Cardiovascular malformations occur in approximately 25% of the cases and range from **Ventricular septal defect** to acardius amorphus.

Etiology: Unknown. To date all cases have been sporadic. The incidence of the condition in monozygotic twins is increased (100 to 150-fold over that in dizygotic twins or singletons). This suggests that the cause of sirenomelia in twins may be associated with the twinning process itself. The concordance rate in monozygotic twins is low.

Pathogenesis: Unknown. Major theories are: *The fusion theory*, the oldest attempt to explain this anomaly, suggests that the lower extremities develop in lateral contact to each other and subsequently become fused. *The classical theory* proposes a deficiency of the caudal axial area in the embryo, allowing the approximation of the side plates from where the limbs develop. The close positioning of the lower limbs permits their fusion with a direct proportional relation between the distance of the lumb buds and the severity of the condition. *The single umbilical artery theory* states that the resulting vascular insufficiency does not allow the normal process of lower limb development. *The vascular steal theory* proposes that sirenomelic malformations result from diversion of the blood flow from caudal structures of the embryo to the placenta. Distal tissues to the steal have demised vascular supply and are arrested or are totally absent at some stage of fetal development. *Extrinsic pressure* is the fifth theory and suggests that any mechanical pressure on the caudal portion of the embryo will impede normal rotation of the limb buds as it has been observed in chick embryos exposed to such influences. Finally, the *neural tube distention theory* has been suggested. Presumably an overdistention of the neural tube in the caudal region expands the roof plate of the tube, displacing and laterally rotating the mesoderm, which allows the fusion of the limb buds.

POS No.: 3399

Sex Ratio: M2.7:F1

Occurrence: From 1.5–4.2:100,000 births. In a series of 331 monozygotic twins, 27 had sirenomelia, with concordance in only two pair.

Risk of Recurrence for Patient's Sib: Unknown.

Risk of Recurrence for Patient's Child: Affected individuals are not expected to survive to reproduce.

Age of Detectability: Second trimester ultrasound findings suggesting this condition include renal agenesis, oligohydramnios, difficulty visualizing the lower extremities or separate legs, and intrauterine growth retardation.

Gene Mapping and Linkage: Unknown.

Prevention: None known. Genetic counseling indicated.

Treatment: Supportive.

Prognosis: Poor. The majority of affected individuals are either stillborn or die shortly after birth.

Detection of Carrier: Unknown.

Special Considerations: A number of investigators have suggested that sirenomelia is a part of the **Caudal regression syndrome**. However, the uniqueness of the clinical findings in sirenomelia justify separation into a separate condition, although there may be a single specific etiological mechanism producing this condition and caudal regression syndrome. At the present time the two most likely mechanisms would be deficiency of caudal mesoderm and vascular disruption. The problem with the vascular etiology theory is that the vascular abnormalities observed in sirenomelia could be secondary to decreased blood flow needs in the caudal region and lower extremities of the embryo, rather than the defects being produced by vascular insufficiency. Aberrant development of the caudal developmental field includes **Vater association**, **Urorectal septum malformation sequence**, exstrophy of the bladder, exstrophy of the cloaca, **Mullerian aplasia**, sirenomelia, **Caudal regression syndrome**, and cloacal dysgenesis.

References:

Stevenson RE, et al.: Vascular steal: the pathogenetic mechanism producing sirenomelia and associated defects of the viscera and soft tissues. Pediatrics 1986; 78:451–457.

Stocker JT, Heifetz SA: Sirenomelia: a morphological study of 33 cases and review of the literature. Perpect Pediatr Pathol 1987; 10:7–50. * †

ES004
WE005
WI063

Luis F. Escobar
David D. Weaver
Jeffrey Winn

Site-specific colorectal cancer, Lynch syndrome I
See CANCER, COLORECTAL
Situs inversus intestinalis (complete, partial)
See SITUS INVERSUS VISCERUM

SITUS INVERSUS VISCERUM 0888

Includes: Situs inversus intestinalis (complete, partial)

Excludes:
Dextrocardia
Dextrocardia-bronchiectasis-sinusitis syndrome (0285)

Major Diagnostic Criteria: X-ray evaluation of the gastric bubble in the right upper abdomen. Air insufflation of the stomach after passing a nasogastric tube will assist in this diagnostic evaluation. The presence of dextrocardia on the chest X-ray film may be helpful in establishing this diagnosis. In incomplete situs inversus the liver will be palpable in the left upper quadrant of the abdomen on physical examination, whereas in partial situs inversus the liver will be in the normal position. Contrast barium X-ray studies will demonstrate the sigmoid colon to be in the right lower quadrant in cases of complete situs inversus.

Clinical Findings: In total situs inversus there is complete transposition of the viscera with the stomach on the left side. Isolated situs inversus of the stomach is extremely rare. Approximately 70% of the patients with situs inversus will have other congenital anomalies of the gastrointestinal tract. Forty percent of affected patients have other major congenital malformations of the heart. Other malformations in this syndrome include clubfeet, choanal atresia, cleft palate, absent humerus, meningomyelocele, and cutaneous hemangioma. Birth weight is only slightly lower than average.

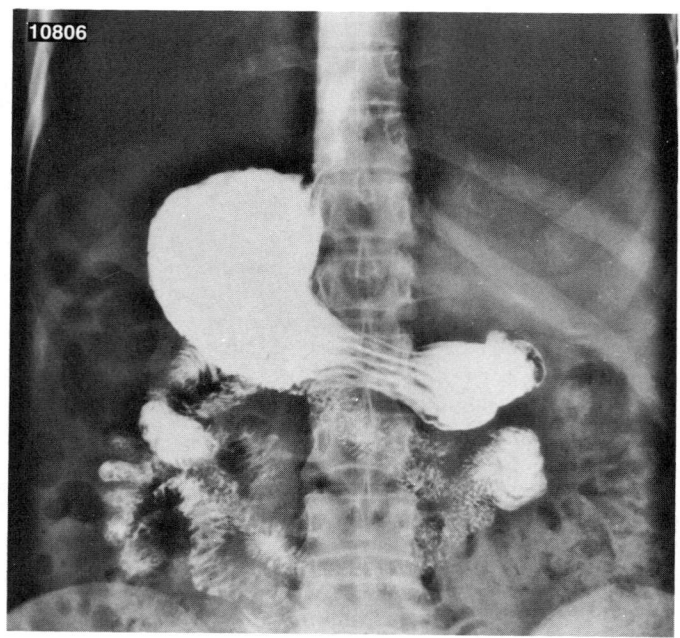

0888-10806: Upper GI series showing mirror image positioning of liver, stomach, and intestines in visceral situs inversus.

Complications: Complications are determined by the other congenital malformations that accompany situs inversus. Serious complications have resulted from failure to recognize the presence of situs inversus while attempting surgical correction of other visceral malformations.

Associated Findings: Congenital heart disease, including **Heart, tetralogy of Fallot**, **Heart, transposition of great vessels**, **Pulmonary valve, stenosis**, septal defects, and others occur twice as frequently when dextrocardia is present. Approximately 50% of the intra-abdominal anomalies require operative correction within the first few months of life. The most common malformations are rotation abnormalities with or without volvulus, **Biliary atresia**, splenic agenesis, duodenal atresia or stenosis, annular pancreas, imperforate anus, anterior portal vein, jejunal atresia and stenosis, gastric duplications, **Colon, aganglionosis**, and left vena cava.

Etiology: Possibly autosomal recessive or dominant inheritance. Sporadic cases are frequent.

Pathogenesis: Mirror-image transposition of the internal organs may affect thoracic and abdominal viscera together or independently. Because of sequential or dependent organogenesis, a rotational abnormality will affect all subsequent phases of development and associated dependent organs. For example, rotation of the stomach to the right results in transposition of the intestine. The left vitelline and umbilical veins are larger than their mates and have been regarded as determining the early positions of the heart and liver. More recent studies suggest that the rotation of the viscera may depend upon controlling factors in the gut which are operative before the liver bud appears.

MIM No.: 27010

CDC No.: 759.3

Sex Ratio: M6:F4

Occurrence: Estimated 1:6,000–8,000 for complete; the partial type is less frequent.

Risk of Recurrence for Patient's Sib:
See Part I, *Mendelian Inheritance.* Occurrence has been as high as 50% in some families.

Risk of Recurrence for Patient's Child:
See Part I, *Mendelian Inheritance.* Occurrence has been as high as 50% of the offspring.

Age of Detectability: Usually within the first few weeks of life, based on the severity of associated malformations.

Gene Mapping and Linkage: Unknown.

Prevention: None known. Genetic counseling indicated.

Treatment: Early recognition and prompt, accurate management of the associated congenital malformations are necessary. The majority of the malformations are very serious, and prompt diagnosis and surgical management are indicated for either intra-abdominal or cardiac lesions. Recognition of situs inversus is imperative for surgical management.

Prognosis: Depends on the associated congenital malformations.

Detection of Carrier: Unknown.

References:
Chib P, et al.: Unusual occurrence of dextrocardia with situs inversus in succeeding generations of a family. J Med Genet 1977; 14:30–32.
Zlotogora J, Elina E: Asplenia and polysplenia syndromes with abnormalities of lateralization in the sibships. J Med Genet 1981; 18:301–302.
Mishalne H, Mahnouski V: Congenital asplenia and anomalies of the gastrointestinal tract. Surgery 1982; January:38–41.
Arnold GL, Bixler D: Probable autosomal recessive inheritance of polysplenia, situs inversus and cardiac defects in an Amish family. Am J Med Genet 1983; 16:35–42.
Niikawa N, et al.: Familial clustering of situs inversus totalis and asplenia and polysplenia syndrome. Am J Med Genet 1983; 16:43–47.
Rott HO: Genetics of Kartagener's syndrome. Eur J Respir Dis 1983; 127:1–4.
Zlotogora J, et al.: Familial situs inversus and congenital heart defects. Am J Med Genet 1987; 26:181–184.

BE049   **Arthur S. Besser**

Six-pyruvoyl tetrahydropterin synthase deficiency
See BIOPTERIN SYNTHESIS DEFICIENCY

SJOGREN SYNDROME   2101

Includes:
Mikulicz syndrome
Sicca syndrome

Excludes:
Parotitis, punctate (0799)
Salivary gland, agenesis (2722)

Major Diagnostic Criteria: Xerostomia and xerophthalmia with (secondary Sjögren syndrome) or without (primary Sjögren syndrome) **Arthritis, rheumatoid** or other autoimmune disease. Also, either unilateral or bilateral salivary gland swelling, usually involving the parotid (80% of primary, 30–40% of secondary). Arthritis is the most frequent initial symptom in secondary Sjögren syndrome. The pathologic hallmark of the disorder is marked lymphocytic infiltration of the salivary glands.

Clinical Findings: Primary Sjögren syndrome involves the exocrine glands only, while secondary Sjögren syndrome is associated with a definable autoimmune disease, most commonly **Arthritis, rheumatoid**.

The major clinical manifestations of the disorder affect the eye and the salivary glands. Other systemic findings may also be seen. Ophthalmologic findings are secondary to atrophy of the secretory epithelium of both the major and minor lacrimal glands leading to desiccation of the cornea and conjunctiva (keratoconjunctivitis sicca). The cornea may undergo severe damage. Common symptoms include discomfort and dryness of the eyes, burning, a scratchy or sandy sensation, redness, photophobia, changes in visual acuity, and failure to produce tears.

Salivary gland abnormalities include firm, tender enlargement of one or more parotid or submandibular glands. Salivary glands become atrophic, and saliva becomes deficient in quantity, leading to xerostomia. The lips and oral mucous membranes may also become atrophic. Other common symptoms include difficulty speaking, swallowing, and eating, and loss of taste and smell.

Systemic clinical findings include dry skin, achlorhydria, interstitial pneumonitis, hepatosplenomegaly, **Raynaud disease**, genital dryness, hyposthenuria, myositis, pancreatitis, anemia, lymphadenopathy, dry sparse hair, alopecia, impairment of esophageal motility, and abnormalities of renal tubular function.

Laboratory findings include the presence of polyclonal hypergammaglobulinemia, numerous autoimmune antibodies (both organ-specific and non-organ-specific) and circulating IgG immune complexes, which may include a positive rheumatoid factor (70%) and a positive LE preparation (15–20%). Impaired cell-mediated immunity can be seen. Increased sedimentation rate (67%), anemia (33%), and leukopenia or eosinophilia (25%) can also occur.

Diagnosis of the ophthalmologic components of the disorder is possible by the rose bengal ocular staining technique, which can detect keratoconjunctivitis sicca, and the Schirmer test. The latter test uses filter paper strips placed under the eyelids to measure the quantity of tears secreted, and is the most widely used ocular test for diagnosis.

Sialography or nuclear scanning with technetium 99m can be used to assess salivary gland function.

Confirmation of the diagnosis may be obtained by salivary gland biopsy, which reveals massive lymphoid infiltration, with atrophy of the acinar tissue, and ductal alterations characterized by the formation of epimyoepithelial islands. Labial glands are a convenient source to biopsy. The lymphocytic infiltration is quantifiable and correlates well with the severity of the disease and the clinical manifestations.

Complications: Mucosal ulcerations and an increased incidence of dental caries can occur as a result of xerostomia. Xerophthalmia can lead to corneal ulcerations and perforation. An increased incidence of otitis media, bronchitis, pneumonia, pancreatitis, and atrophic gastritis can also be seen. There is also an increased incidence (44 times the expected rate) of lymphoma, usually of the histiocytic or mixed histiocytic-lymphocytic type. Lymphoma is more commonly seen in patients with a history of parotid enlargement, splenomegaly, lymphadenopathy, and/or parotid irradiation.

Associated Findings: Biliary cirrhosis, other liver abnormalities, autoimmune liver disease, laryngeal involvement, membranous glomerulonephritis, nephrocalcinosis, renal insufficiency, uremia, osteomalacia, secondary amyloidosis, and diffuse peripheral neuropathy.

Etiology: Familial occurrence has been infrequently observed. Increased HLA-B8 and HLA-DW3 has been observed in primary Sjögren syndrome.

Pathogenesis: Lymphocyte-mediated destruction of the exocrine glands. Laboratory findings suggest that one of the underlying defects is B-cell hyperreactivity with or without abnormalities of immunoregulation.

MIM No.: 27015

Sex Ratio: M1:F9

Occurrence: 1:200

Risk of Recurrence for Patient's Sib: Unknown.

Risk of Recurrence for Patient's Child: Unknown.

Age of Detectability: Average age of onset is 50 years, but childhood cases have been reported.

Gene Mapping and Linkage: Unknown.

Prevention: None known. Genetic counseling indicated.

Treatment: Symptomatic. Artificial saliva, artificial tears, antibiotic therapy of infections, good dental hygiene, and analgesics for the pain and tenderness associated with sudden enlargement of the salivary glands.

Prognosis: Varies with severity of the disease and complications.

Detection of Carrier: Unknown.

References:
Lichtenfeld JL, et al.: Familial Sjogren's syndrome with associated primary salivary gland lymphoma. Am J Med 1976; 60:286–292.
Shearn MA: Sjogren's syndrome. Med Clin North Am 1977; 61:271–282.
Kassan SS: Increased risk of lymphoma in sicca syndrome. Ann Intern Med 1978; 89:888–892.
Moutsopoulos HM, et al.: Genetic differences between primary and secondary sicca syndrome. New Engl J Med 1979; 301:761–763. *
Moutsopoulos HM, et al.: Sjogren's syndrome (sicca syndrome): current issues. Ann Intern Med 1980; 92:212–226.
Rice DH: Advances in diagnosis and management of salivary gland diseases. West J Med 1984; 140:238–249.
Reveille JD, et al.: Primary Sjogren's syndrome and other autoimmune diseases in families: prevalence and immunogenetic studies in six kindreds. Ann Intern Med 1984; 101:748–756.

IR000   **Mira Irons**

SJOGREN-LARSSON SYNDROME   2030

Includes:
Fatty alcohol:NAD+ oxidoreductase (FAO), deficiency of
Ichthyosis-oligophrenia-spasticity
Oligophrenia-ichthyosis-spasticity
Spasticity-ichthyosis-oligophrenia

Excludes:
Chondrodysplasia punctata
Ichthyosis, linearis circumflexa (2858)
Phytanic acid storage disease (0810)
Seizures-ichthyosis-mental retardation (0741)

Major Diagnostic Criteria: The triad of congenital ichthyosiform dermatitis, mental deficiency, and spastic paresis of the extremities.

Clinical Findings: In infancy, redness of the skin is first apparent; later, a typical fish-scale appearance (congenital ichthyosiform erythroderma) becomes visible. The areas most affected are the neck, lower abdomen, axillae, and flexures of the elbows.

Almost all patients reported in the literature have been described as retarded, although there are three cases in which the patients have been said to have IQs between 70 and 79 (borderline mental retardation).

Neurologically, the spasticity is usually of the symmetric diplegic type. About 75% of the patients are confined to wheelchairs. Muscle tone is increased in the limbs and in the muscles of the mouth and bulbar region so that speech and feeding may be a problem.

As early as age two years, a degenerative defect in the retinal pigment epithelium can be detected in about 50% of the affected children. These chorioretinal lesions are of varying size in and about the macula.

Complications: Activities of daily living are difficult due to both spasticity and to the limited mental capacities of the patients.

Associated Findings: Seizures, speech disorders, muscular degeneration.

Etiology: Autosomal recessive inheritance.

Pathogenesis: Cultured skin fibroblasts show impaired hexadecanol oxidation due to fatty alcohol:NAD+ oxidoreductase (FAO) deficiency.

MIM No.: *27020

POS No.: 3400

CDC No.: 757.120

Sex Ratio: M1:F1

Occurrence: Reported from many countries. Sjögren and Larsson (1957) established the syndrome by an exhaustive survey of inhabitants of northern Sweden, which yielded 28 cases in 14 sibships. Incidence in Sweden has been estimated as 6:1,000,000. In Vasterbotten County, Sweden, the prevalence is 8.3:100,000; the gene frequency is 0.01.

Risk of Recurrence for Patient's Sib:
See Part I, *Mendelian Inheritance.*

Risk of Recurrence for Patient's Child:
See Part I, *Mendelian Inheritance.*

Age of Detectability: The rash can appear in the neonatal period; signs become apparent in the first year of life. Prenatal diagnosis is possible.

Gene Mapping and Linkage: Unknown.

Prevention: None known. Genetic counseling indicated.

Treatment: Symptomatic treatment of skin lesions; infant physical and educational intervention for central nervous system manifestations.

Prognosis: Prognosis depends on the severity of the CNS symptoms. In a wheelchair-bound, severely retarded individual, the prognosis is more guarded than in a less severely affected patient.

Detection of Carrier: By FAO deficiency in skin fibroblasts or leukocytes.

Special Considerations: The dramatic nature of the skin lesions has led to confusion among the many different syndromes presenting with ichthyosis. Sjögren-Larsson is a distinct syndrome, different from the multiple other syndromes with fish-scale appearance of the skin.

References:
Sjögren T, Larsson T: Oligophrenia in combination with congenital ichthyosis and spastic disorders: a clinical and genetic study. Acta Psychiatr Neurol Scand (suppl 113) 1957; 32:1–112.
McLennan JE, et al.: Neuropathological correlates in Sjögren-Larsson syndrome. Brain 1974; 97:693.
Jagell S, et al.: Specific changes in the fundus typical for the Sjögren-

Larsson syndrome: an ophthalmological study of 35 patients. Acta Ophthalmol 1980; 58:321–330.

Jagell S, et al.: Sjögren-Larsson syndrome in Sweden: a clinical, genetic and epidemiological study. Clin Genet 1981; 19:233–256.

Jagell S, Linden S: Ichthyosis in the Sjögren-Larsson syndrome. Clin Genet 1982; 21:243–252.

Kousseff BG, et al.: Prenatal diagnosis of Sjogren-Larsson syndrome. J Pediatr 1982; 101:998–1001.

Rizzo WB, et al.: Sjogren-Larsson syndrome: deficient fatty alcohol: NAD+ oxidoreductase (FAO) activity in mixed leukocytes. (Abstract) Am J Hum Genet 1987; 41:A16 only.

C0018 **Mary Coleman**

Skeletal and facial defects-short stature-mental retardation
See KABUKI MAKE-UP SYNDROME
Skeletal and laryngeal anomalies-motor and sensory neuropathy
See NEUROPATHY, CONGENITAL MOTOR & SENSORY-SKELETAL-LARYNGEAL DEFECTS
Skeletal anomalies-joint dislocations-unusual facies
See LARSEN SYNDROME
Skeletal anomalies-male hypogonadism-mental retardation
See SHOVAL-SOFFER SYNDROME
Skeletal anomalies-short stature-mental retardation-alopecia
See ALOPECIA-SKELETAL ANOMALIES-SHORT STATURE-MENTAL RETARDATION

SKELETAL BOWING-CORTICAL THICKENING-BONE FRAGILITY-ICTHYOSIS 2937

Includes:
Bone fragility-skeletal bowing-cortical thickening-ichthyosis
Cortical thickening-skeletal bowing-bone fragility-ichthyosis
Ichthyosis-skeletal bowing-cortical thickening-bone fragility
Osteosclerosis-ichthyosis-fractures

Excludes:
Diaphyseal dysplasia (0290)
Skeletal dysplasia, Weismann-Netter-Stuhl type (2542)

Major Diagnostic Criteria: Endosteal cortical thickening of the long tubular bones and icthyosis.

Clinical Findings: A bone disorder characterized by cortical thickening of the diaphyses of long tubular bones and bowing of the weight-bearing bones. All have had ichthyosis, and three also had an unusual proclivity to fractures. The clinical symptoms were waddling gait, muscle weakness, and leg pains.

Complications: Fractures and deformity of long bones.

Associated Findings: None known.

Etiology: Presumably autosomal dominant inheritance. No male-to-male transmission has been observed, and no affected male has had children; hence, X-linked inheritance cannot be excluded.

Pathogenesis: Unknown.

MIM No.: 16674

CDC No.: 756.480

Sex Ratio: M1:F1

Occurrence: Six cases in two generations of a family from northern Norway have been documented.

Risk of Recurrence for Patient's Sib:
See Part I, *Mendelian Inheritance.*

Risk of Recurrence for Patient's Child:
See Part I, *Mendelian Inheritance.*

Age of Detectability: During early childhood.

Gene Mapping and Linkage: Unknown.

Prevention: None known. Genetic counseling indicated.

Treatment: Orthopedic correction of deformities.

Prognosis: Good, with only moderate handicap.

Detection of Carrier: Unknown.

References:
Koller M-E, et al.: A familial syndrome of diaphyseal cortical thickening of the long bones, bowed legs, tendency to fracture and ichthyosis. Pediatr Radiol 1979; 8:179–182.

AA002 **Dagfinn Aarskog**

Skeletal defects with aortic calcification and muscle weakness
See SINGLETON-MERTEN SYNDROME
Skeletal defects-dysmorphic facies-aural atresia
See AURAL ATRESIA-DYSMORPHIC FACIES-SKELETAL DEFECTS
Skeletal defects-dysmorphic facies-torsion dystonia
See BLEPHARO-NASO-FACIAL SYNDROME
Skeletal disorder-deafness
See METAPHYSEAL DYSOSTOSIS-DEAFNESS
Skeletal dysplasia
See DWARFISM

SKELETAL DYSPLASIA, 3-M TYPE 2569

Includes: Three-M slender-boned nanism

Excludes:
Bloom syndrome (0112)
Dwarfism (other primordial)
Silver syndrome (0887)

Major Diagnostic Criteria: Low birth weight, short stature, craniofacial dysmorphia, and minor musculoskeletal malformations.

Clinical Findings: Low birth weight is a constant feature in postnatal growth deficiency leading to proportionate dwarfism. The head may appear large, but measures at the 50th percentile. The craniofacies is said to be hatchet-shaped with dolichocephaly, triangular face, hypoplastic maxilla, and prominent mouth and chin. The neck is short with prominent trapizii. Sternal abnormalities, winged scapulae, and diastasis recti are common.

On X-ray, the long bones appear slender with diaphyseal constriction and exaggerated modeling. The vertebral bodies may appear long, but reduced in anteroposterior and transverse diameters. The ribs are slender, and the pelvis and iliac wings are small. Bone maturation is delayed.

Complications: Unknown.

Associated Findings: Spina bifida, short fifth fingers, and hypospadias have been reported.

Etiology: Autosomal recessive inheritance.

Pathogenesis: Unknown.

MIM No.: *27375

POS No.: 3613

CDC No.: 756.480

Sex Ratio: M1:F1

Occurrence: Less than two dozen cases have been reported.

Risk of Recurrence for Patient's Sib:
See Part I, *Mendelian Inheritance.*

Risk of Recurrence for Patient's Child:
See Part I, *Mendelian Inheritance.*

Age of Detectability: At birth.

Gene Mapping and Linkage: Unknown.

Prevention: None known. Genetic counseling indicated.

Treatment: Unknown.

Prognosis: Good for general health and life span.

Detection of Carrier: Subtle facial dysmorphia and slender long bones may be seen in some carriers.

References:
Miller JD, et al.: The 3-M syndrome: a heritable low birthweight dwarfism. BD:OAS XI(5). New York: March of Dimes Birth Defects Foundation, 1975:39–47. * †

Cantu JM, et al.: 3-M slender boned nanism. Am J Dis Child 1981; 135:95–98.

Winter RM, et al.: The 3-M syndrome. J Med Genet 1984; 21:124–128. †

Hennekam RCM, et al.: Further delineation of the 3-M syndrome with a review of the literature. Am J Med Genet 1987; 28:195–209.

J0027   **Ronald J. Jorgenson**

Skeletal dysplasia, acromicric
See ACROMICRIC DYSPLASIA

SKELETAL DYSPLASIA, BOOMERANG DYSPLASIA   2522

Includes: Boomerang skeletal dysplasia

Excludes: Dwarfism, other lethal neonatal

Major Diagnostic Criteria: Lethal neonatal dwarfism with diagnostic X-ray and characteristic clinical features.

Clinical Findings: This form of neonatal dwarfism is associated with hydramnios, prematurity, and death *in utero* or shortly thereafter. The trunk is shortened with a small chest. All the extremities are shortened and the lower ones are bowed anteriorly. There is equinovarus deformity of the feet. The head is large, with peculiar facial appearances, and a small mandible. The palpebral fissures are horizontal, and there are epicanthal folds. The nose has a broad nasal root, and severe hypoplasia of the septi nasi and lateral cartilages. The nares are small and oval, with a slanted long axis. The philtrum is prominent. X-ray findings include a boomerang-like, triangular, or oval shape of the long bones. The radii and fibulae are missing. Ossification of the cervical and thoracic spine is retarded. In the pelvis, the iliac wings are well developed, but the iliac bodies are hypoplastic and the pubic bones are absent. Moderate to severe hypoplastic/dysplastic changes are present in the feet.

Complications: Intrauterine or neonatal death.

Associated Findings: None known.

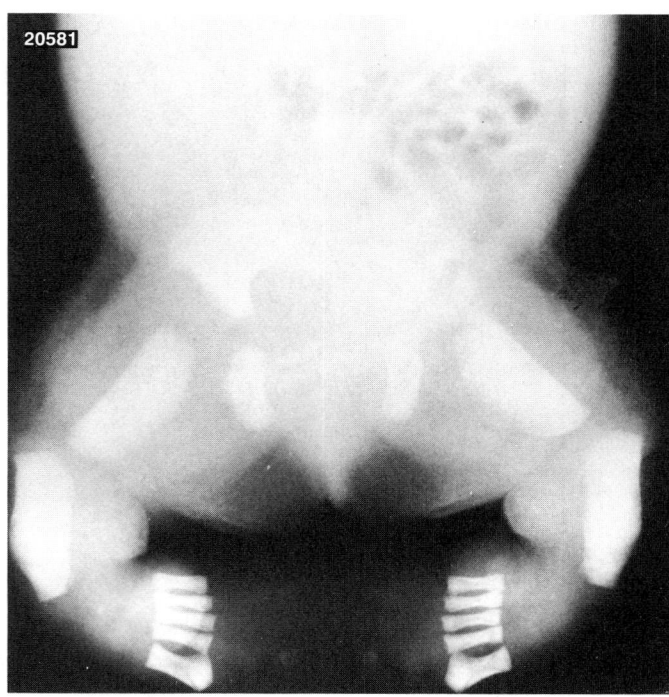

2522B-20581: Boomerang dysplasia; note boomerang-shaped long bones; the pelvis shape is characteristic and one leg bone is missing.

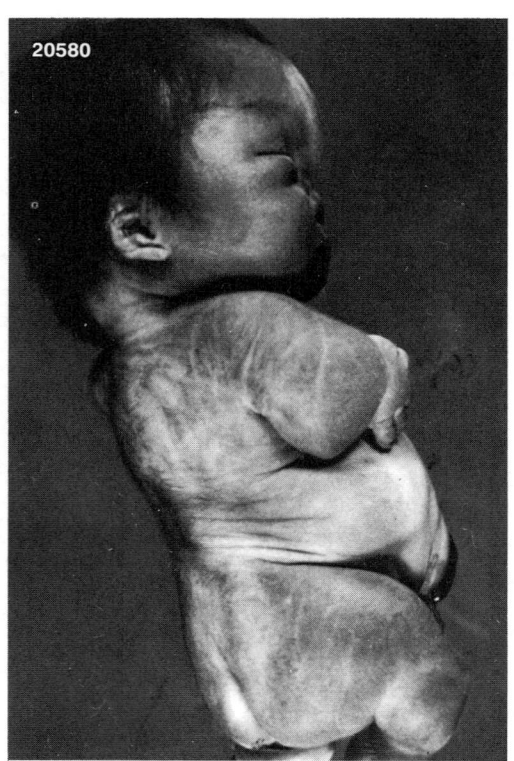

2522A-20580: Boomerang dysplasia; note extreme shortening of the limbs and protrusion of the triangular bones of the extremities.

Etiology: Unknown. Possibly autosomal recessive inheritance.

Pathogenesis: Growth plates are not evenly distributed, and giant cells may be found in the serial sections.

POS No.: 3813

Sex Ratio: M3:F0 (observed).

Occurrence: Three cases have been reported in the literature, and at least as many additional cases have been observed.

Risk of Recurrence for Patient's Sib:
See Part I, *Mendelian Inheritance.*

Risk of Recurrence for Patient's Child: Affected individuals are not expected to survive to reproduce.

Age of Detectability: At birth. Prenatal diagnosis by ultrasound in the second trimester is possible.

Gene Mapping and Linkage: Unknown.

Prevention: None known. Genetic counseling indicated.

Treatment: Unknown.

Prognosis: Fatal in neonatal period.

Detection of Carrier: Unknown.

References:
Kozlowski K, et al.: New forms of neonatal death dwarfism: report of 3 cases. Pediatr Radiol 1981; 10:155–160.
Tenconi R, et al.: Boomerang dysplasia: a new form of neonatal death dwarfism. Fortsch Röntgenstr 1983; 138:378–380.
Kozlowski K, et al.: Boomerang Dysplasia. Brit J Radiol 1985; 58:369–371.

K0021   **K.S. Kozlowski**

SKELETAL DYSPLASIA, DE LA CHAPELLE TYPE 2631

Includes:

    de la Chapelle skeletal dysplasia
    Neonatal osseous dysplasia I

Excludes:

    Achondrogenesis
    Achondroplasia (0010)
    Atelosteogenesis (2521)
    Mesomelic dysplasia, Langer type (0646)
    Skeletal dysplasia, boomerang dysplasia (2522)
    Thanatophoric dysplasia (0940)

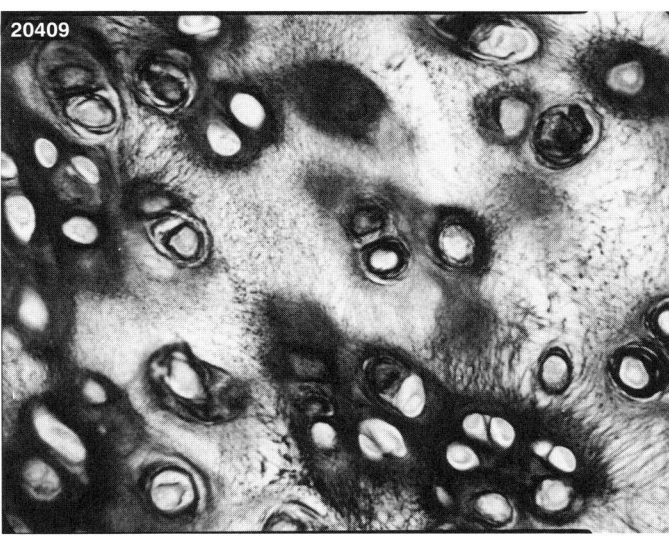

2631B-20409: High-power view of the concentric "lacunar halos" surrounding chondrocytes in the resting zone of skeletal cartilage (methenamine silver nitrate-alcian blue; ×544).

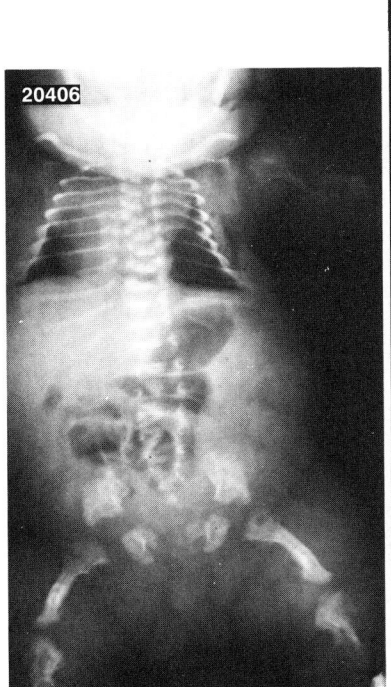

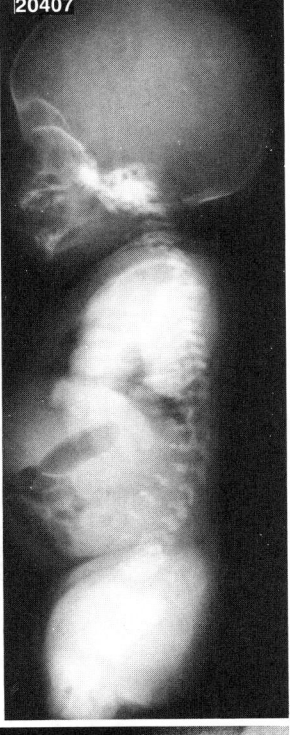

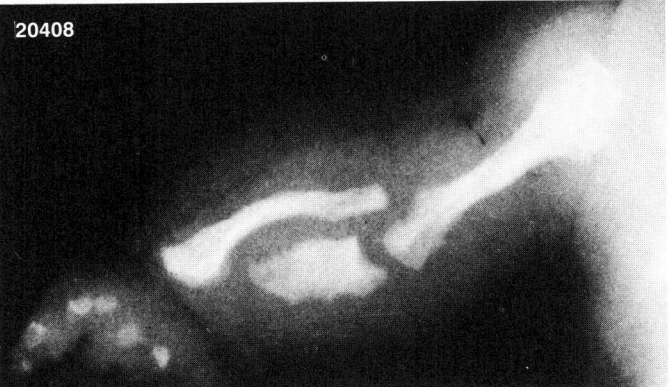

2631A-20406: Note short limbs, platyspondyly, and hypoplastic pelvis. 20407: Vertebral bodies have small ossification centers with irregular contours and anterior tongue-like projections in the lateral view. 20408: The ulna is represented by an irregular and almost triangular remnant.

Major Diagnostic Criteria: X-ray features of this lethal neonatal skeletal dysplasia are distinctive and comprise the major diagnostic criteria. The skull, scapulae, and clavicles are not markedly abnormal. However, there is severe spinal deformity with platyspondyly. Vertebral bodies have small ossification centers with irregular contours and anterior tongue-like projections in lateral view. There is a wide cleft between each vertebral body and its respective posterior arch. The acetabulum is flat and horizontal. Bones of the limbs are moderately shortened. Ulnae and fibulae are represented as a very distinctive, almost triangular osseous remnant. The proximal humeral metaphysis is relatively broad. Bones of the hands and digits are small and poorly ossified. "Lacunar halos" have been identified as a distinctive histopathologic feature and have also been seen in some forms of **Achondrogenesis** but not in several other skeletal dysplasias.

Clinical Findings: Affected newborn infants present with immediate apnea. The presence of a dwarfing condition is readily apparent (crown-heel length, 35–40 cm). The head is normocephalic except for **Cleft palate**. The chest is small, and there is moderately severe micromelia with small hands, equinovarus deformity, and widely spaced first and second toes. Scoliosis is sometimes evident from external examination. At autopsy the larynx is seen to be malformed and stenotic, and cartilage from respiratory structures is abnormal. Tracheal and bronchial rings are soft, permitting easy collapse of the major airways. Identification of distinctive "lacunar halos" in skeletal cartilage is aided with methenamine silver nitrate-alcian blue stain.

Complications: Death has occurred at birth in all cases and is attributed to a triad of respiratory tract malformations: laryngeal stenosis, tracheobronchomalacia, and pulmonary hypoplasia.

Associated Findings: Double ossification centers in the phalanges were observed in the original case, but were not present in affected sibs or in an unrelated case. Other abnormalities have been observed, but none of these has been a consistent finding: duplicated renal artery, hydronephrosis, ectopic thymus, multiple endocrine neoplasia, and bifid ureter.

Etiology: Autosomal recessive inheritance.

Pathogenesis: Presumably a defect in the synthesis of a normal component of cartilage, although no biochemical or molecular genetic studies have been reported.

MIM No.: *25605

POS No.: 3847
CDC No.: 756.480
Sex Ratio: M1:F1
Occurrence: Four cases from two families have been reported.
Risk of Recurrence for Patient's Sib:
See Part I, *Mendelian Inheritance.*
Risk of Recurrence for Patient's Child:
See Part I, *Mendelian Inheritance.*
Age of Detectability: At birth, or may be detected prenatally by ultrasonography.
Gene Mapping and Linkage: Unknown.
Prevention: None known. Genetic counseling indicated.
Treatment: Attempts at tracheal intubation have failed, apparently due to collapse of floppy tracheal airways, thus obviating attempts at newborn resuscitation.
Prognosis: Lethal at birth.
Detection of Carrier: Unknown.
Special Considerations: There should be no confusion with the term *de la Chapelle syndrome*, which refers to phenotypic males with an apparent 46,XX karyotype resulting from translocation or other mutations of genes determining sex phenotype.

References:
de la Chapelle A, et al.: Une rare dysplasia osseuse letale de transmission recessive autosomique. Arch Fr Pediatr 1972; 29:759–770.
Whitley CB, et al.: de la Chapelle dysplasia. Am J Med Genet 1986; 25:29–39.

WH008 **Chester B. Whitley**

Skeletal dysplasia, fibrochondrogenesis
See FIBROCHONDROGENESIS

SKELETAL DYSPLASIA, FUHRMANN TYPE 2696

Includes:
Femoral bowing-fibula aplasia/hypoplasia-poly-, syn-, oligodactyly
Fibula aplasia/hypoplasia-femoral bowing-poly-, syn-, oligodactyly
Fuhrmann skeletal dysplasia

Excludes:
Bones, congenital bowing of the long
Campomelic dysplasia (0122)
Chondroectodermal dysplasia (0156)
Femoral hypoplasia-unusual facies syndrome (2027)
Fibula, congenital absence of (2229)
Grebe syndrome (0445)

Major Diagnostic Criteria: Aplasia or hypoplasia of the fibulae associated with acromelic duplication or reduction defects and femoral bowing or shortening.

Clinical Findings: Fuhrmann et al (1980) described a severe skeletal dysplasia in four full sibs. Variability of expression and asymmetry of the severity of the defects were seen among the affected children. The lower extremities and the pelvis were severly dysplastic, with the upper extremity involvment including postaxial polysyndactyly, cutaneous **Syndactyly**, **Camptodactyly**, and clinodactyly. The fingernails were variably involved, but the toenails in all the sibs were reduced to scar-like bands of tissue or were absent. The axial skeleton, craniofacies, viscera, and central nervous system were spared. The fourth sib was diagnosed prenatally with ultrasound and aborted at 17–19 weeks gestation. This infant had atypical lobation of the lungs noted at autopsy.

X-ray features included hypoplasia of the pelvic bones, often associated with congenital dislocation of the hips in the more severely affected sibs to slight flaring of the ilia in the mildest case. The femora were bowed or shortened in all cases (asymmetrically in the mildest case). The fibulae were absent during early childhood, but in the one surviving sib rudimentary ossification was noted at age nine years. The feet demonstrated reduction deformities involving the metatarsals and phalanges and coalescence of the tarsals. The hands demonstrated postaxial hexadactyly, phalangeal hypoplasia, metacarpal coalescence, and interphalangeal ankyloses. The humeri, radii, ulnae, and vertebrae were normal in all sibs.

Complications: All sibs had short stature caused by the lower limb deformities. Two of the sibs died of infection in early childhood, but this was thought to be unrelated to their skeletal dysplasia.

Associated Findings: None known.

Etiology: Presumably autosomal recessive inheritance. The parents were members of a small ethnic minority group from neighboring villages, but consanguinity was not established.

Pathogenesis: Chondro-osseous tissue was examined in the abortus. Localized perichondral ossification described as atypical was seen in several sites, but no specific abnormalities of endochondral ossification were found. Reactive ossification with an unusual trabecular pattern was seen at the diaphyseal angulation. Fuhrmann et al (1980) speculated that the pattern of defects was consistent with a developmental field defect.

MIM No.: 22893
POS No.: 3519
CDC No.: 756.480
Sex Ratio: M3:F1 (observed).
Occurrence: Four sibs of a Turkish-Arabian family working in Germany have been documented.
Risk of Recurrence for Patient's Sib:
See Part I, *Mendelian Inheritance.*
Risk of Recurrence for Patient's Child:
See Part I, *Mendelian Inheritance.*
Age of Detectability: Prenatally.
Gene Mapping and Linkage: Unknown.
Prevention: None known. Genetic counseling indicated.
Treatment: Orthopedic surgery.
Prognosis: Unknown.
Detection of Carrier: Unknown.

References:
Fuhrmann W, et al.: Poly-, syn-, and oligodactyly, aplasia or hypoplasia of fibula, hypoplasia of pelvis and bowing of femora in three sibs-a new autosomal recessive syndrome. Eur J Pediatr 1980; 133:123–129.
Fuhrmann W, et al.: A new autosomal recessive skeletal dysplasia syndrome: prenatal diagnosis and histopathology. In: Papadatos CJ, Bartsocas CS, eds: Skeletal dysplasias. New York: Alan R. Liss, 1982:519–524.

H0025 **O.J. Hood**
H0033 **William A. Horton**

Skeletal dysplasia, Grebe type
See GREBE SYNDROME
Skeletal dysplasia, humerospinal dysostosis
See DYSOSTOSIS, HUMEROSPINAL
Skeletal dysplasia, Kniest-like
See KNIEST-LIKE DYSPLASIA
Skeletal dysplasia, kyphomelic dysplasia
See KYPHOMELIC DYSPLASIA
Skeletal dysplasia, neonatally lethal short-limbed, Glasgow type
See THANATOPHORIC DYSPLASIA, GLASGOW TYPE

SKELETAL DYSPLASIA, SCHNECKENBECKEN TYPE   2632

Includes:
Chondrodysplasia, lethal neonatal with snail-like pelvis
Schneckenbecken dysplasia
Snail-like pelvis dysplasia

Excludes:
Achondrogenesis, Parenti-Fraccaro type (0009)
Achondrogenesis, Houston-Harris type (2870)
Achondrogenesis, Langer-Saldino type (0008)
Kniest-like dysplasia (2799)
Thanatophoric dysplasia (0940)
Thanatophoric dysplasia, Glasgow type (2821)

Major Diagnostic Criteria: Lethal neonatal dwarfism with characteristic clinical, X-ray, and histopathologic features.

Clinical Findings: This disorder is a form of lethal neonatal dwarfism associated with second trimester polyhydramnios and prematurity. Most published cases were stillborn. On clinical grounds alone, these cases cannot be distinguished from the other known lethal, short-limb dysplasias. The skull is relatively large, with flat face, short trunk, and very short limbs. As shown on X-ray, the skull is normally ossified. The vertebral bodies are hypoplastic and flat. Punctate ossification of a round nature is seen in the lateral projection. There is marked spinal stenosis. The ribs are short and splayed. The iliac wings are "snail-like" (*schneckenbecken* in German) in configuration, with a very unusual medial projection of bone forming the head of the "snail." The ischium is not ossified. The long bones are very short; most had a dumbbell-like appearance without significant metaphyseal abnormalities. There is often ossification of talus and calcaneous.

Complications: Intrauterine or neonatal death.

Associated Findings: None known.

2632-20071: X-ray of an affected fetus showing flattened vertebral bodies, snail-like ilia and dumbbell-shaped long bones. Note the precocious ossification in the ankle.

Etiology: Autosomal recessive inheritance.

Pathogenesis: Pathologic examination of cartilage has demonstrated resting chondrocytes with round central nucleus and absence of a lacunar space. The matrix often appeared normal. Ultrastructurally, most chondrocytes have their cell membranes immediately adjacent to the interterritorial matrix leaving no lacunar space. The rough endoplasmic reticulum is not dilated.

MIM No.: *26925

POS No.: 3852

CDC No.: 756.480

Sex Ratio: M1:F1

Occurrence: Nine cases have been documented.

Risk of Recurrence for Patient's Sib:
See Part I, *Mendelian Inheritance.*

Risk of Recurrence for Patient's Child:
See Part I, *Mendelian Inheritance.*

Age of Detectability: At birth, or prenatally by ultrasound.

Gene Mapping and Linkage: Unknown.

Prevention: None known. Genetic counseling indicated.

Treatment: Unknown.

Prognosis: Fatal during the neonatal period.

Detection of Carrier: Unknown.

References:
Rimoin DL: The chondrodystrophies. Adv Hum Genet 1975; 5:1.
Borochowitz Z, et al.: A distinct lethal neonatal chondrodysplasia with snail-like pelvis: Schneckenbecken dysplasia. Am J Med Genet 1986; 25:47–59.
Knowles S, et al.: A new category of lethal short limbed dwarfism. Am J Med Genet 1986; 25:41–46.

B0025   **Zvi Borochowitz**

Skeletal dysplasia, short rib dwarfism, Beemer type
See DWARFISM, SHORT-RIB, BEEMER TYPE
Skeletal dysplasia, short rib-polydactyly syndrome type II
See SHORT RIB-POLYDACTYLY SYNDROME, TYPE II
Skeletal dysplasia, Urbach-rhizomelia of humeri
See RHIZOMELIC SYNDROME, URBACH TYPE

SKELETAL DYSPLASIA, WEISMANN-NETTER-STUHL TYPE   2542

Includes:
Bowing of legs, anterior, with dwarfism
Legs, bowing of anterior-dwarfism
Toxopachyosteose diaphysaire tibio-peroniere
Weismann-Netter-Stuhl syndrome

Excludes:
Campomelic dysplasia (0122)
Diaphyseal dysplasia (0290)
Femoral hypoplasia-unusual facies syndrome (2027)
Rickets (all forms)
Syphilitic sabre shins

Major Diagnostic Criteria: The diagnosis rests on the X-ray findings: 1) Anterior bowing of tibiae and fibulae, often (35%) associated with lateral bowing of femora, usually bilateral and symmetric, occasionally unilateral. The apex of the tibial curve is at the junction of the middle and lower one-third, and the fibular bowing is slightly lower. The cortex of both bones is thickened throughout, especially on the concave side. The marrow cavity is widened. There is no anterior periosteal overgrowth as in syphilis. There are no signs of present or past rickets. 2) Proportionate short stature (adult stature 120–156 cm). 3) Delayed onset of walking (18 months to five years). 4) Absence of pain, discomfort, or disability. 5) Normal laboratory findings.

Clinical Findings: The tibial bowing is readily recognized on inspection and palpation. Most patients state that it has been present as long as they can remember. In a few patients the

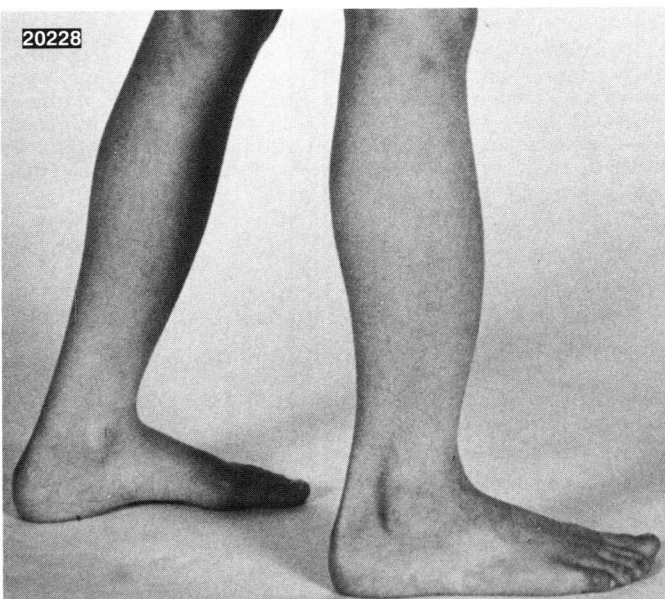

2542A-20228: Note the anterior bowing of the tibia.

bowing has been documented at birth, suggesting that onset may be prenatal. No explanation for the delayed onset of walking has been offered. The angulation does not seem to progress with age. Most cases have been discovered incidentally in patients admitted to hospitals for other reasons. Serum calcium, phosphorus, and alkaline phosphatase levels have been normal. Life span is not impaired; the oldest patient was 93 years old at the time of diagnosis. No patient had any discomfort or disability attributable to the bowing. Gait is normal.

Occasional X-ray findings are mild bowing of the radius and sometimes the ulna, square iliac wings, and a horizontal sacrum.

Complications: Unknown.

2542B-21450: X-ray showing lateral bowing of the femora.
21451: X-ray showing anterior bowing of the femora.

Associated Findings: Mental retardation, generally mild, has been reported in 20% of the cases.

Etiology: Autosomal or X-linked dominant inheritance. Male-to-male transmission has not been documented. Penetrance is unknown.

Pathogenesis: Unknown.

MIM No.: 11235

POS No.: 3461

CDC No.: 756.480

Sex Ratio: Presumably M1:F1; observed, M1:F:0.7

Occurrence: Forty-one cases have been reported in the literature.

Risk of Recurrence for Patient's Sib:
See Part I, *Mendelian Inheritance.*

Risk of Recurrence for Patient's Child:
See Part I, *Mendelian Inheritance.*

Age of Detectability: Usually at birth.

Gene Mapping and Linkage: Unknown.

Prevention: None known. Genetic counseling indicated.

Treatment: Unknown.

Prognosis: Normal life span. No functional impairment except for the delayed onset of walking.

Detection of Carrier: Unknown.

References:
Weismann-Netter R, Stuhl L: D'une ostéopathie congénitale éventuellement familiale. Presse Med 1954; 62:1618–1621. * †
Keats TE, Alavi SM: Toxopachyostéose diaphysaire tibio-péronière (Weismann-Netter syndrome). Am J Roentgenology 1970; 109:568–574.
Amendola MA, et al.: Weismann-Netter-Stuhl syndrome: toxopachyostéose diaphysaire tibio-péronière. Am J Roentgenology 1980; 135:1211–1215. †

R0004   **Meinhard Robinow**

Skeletal dysplasia-Robin anomaly-polydactyly
See *CLEFT PALATE-DYSMORPHIC FACIES-DIGITAL DEFECTS, MARTSOLF TYPE*
Skeletal dysplasia-short rib-polydactyly, type III
See *SHORT RIB-POLYDACTYLY SYNDROME, VERMA-NAUMOFF TYPE*
Skeletal dysplasia-sparse hair-dental anomalies
See *CRANIO-ECTODERMAL DYSPLASIA*
Skeletal malformations-heart disease-conductive hearing loss
See *MITRAL REGURGITATION-DEAFNESS-SKELETAL DEFECTS*
Skeletal malocclusion, class III
See *MANDIBULAR PROGNATHISM*
Skeletal maturation (fast)-dysmorphic facies-failure to thrive
See *MARSHALL-SMITH SYNDROME*
Skeletal-dermo-facio-cardio syndrome
See *DERMO-FACIO-CARDIO-SKELETAL SYNDROME*
Skeletal-neuro-facio syndrome
See *FACIO-NEURO-SKELETAL SYNDROME*
Skeleto-branchio-genital syndromes
See *BRANCHIO-SKELETO-GENITAL SYNDROME*
Skewfoot
See *FOOT, METATARSUS VARUS*
Skin (thin)-hydrocephalus-nephrosis-blue sclera-growth defect
See *NEPHROSIS-HYDROCEPHALUS-THIN SKIN-BLUE SCLERA-GROWTH DEFECT*
Skin atrophy, linear
See *ALOPECIA-SKIN ATROPHY-ANONYCHIA-TONGUE DEFECT*
Skin changes-typical facies-heart defect
See *CARDIO-FACIAL-CUTANEOUS SYNDROME*

SKIN CREASE, SINGLE PALMAR 2607

Includes:
> Crease, single palmar
> Four-finger line
> Palm, single line
> Palmar crease, single transverse
> Simian crease, incomplete
> Single transverse fold
> Sydney line
> Transverse crease, single

Excludes:
> Proximal crease variations
> Thenar crease variations

Major Diagnostic Criteria: Fusion of the proximal and distal horizontal creases of the palm.

Clinical Findings: Flexion of the fingers during the second month of gestation normally results in the formation of two horizontal creases, distal and proximal. Fusion of the two lines into a single palmar transverse crease is seen in 2–3% of the adult population. Two lines that approach and are joined by a third line or bridge are called an incomplete single palmar crease. The proximal horizontal palmar crease may traverse the entire palm in a final variant known as a Sydney line. All three findings are related and may be combinatorially found in a single individual.

Complications: Single palmar creases do not affect function of the hand.

Associated Findings: A single palmar crease is commonly associated with **Chromosome 21, trisomy 21** and has been reported to be increased in frequency among premature infants, stillborns, babies dying in the neonatal period, and infants with multiple congenital anomalies, **Fetal rubella syndrome, Chromosome 18, trisomy 18, Smith-Lemli-Opitz syndrome, Rubinstein-Taybi broad thumb-hallux syndrome,** and other conditions.

Etiology: Heterogeneous. A higher frequency is seen in patients with chromosomal anomalies, congenital anomalies, stillbirth, neonatal death and prematurity. Siblings and other first degree relatives have a higher frequency of single palmar creases than expected by chance alone. At least one family has been reported in which the single palmar crease and its variants appears follow autosomal dominant inheritance with decreased penetrance.

Pathogenesis: The single palmar crease is presumed to result from abnormal flexion of the fingers and hand during the first and second months of gestation. Normal infants with single palmar creases have not demonstrated abnormal hand movements or skeletal anomalies.

Sex Ratio: M1:F<1. Among otherwise normal children, there appears to be a higher frequency of the single palmar crease in males. In one pedigree in which the single palmar crease appears to segregate as an autosomal dominant trait, penetrance is 10% in females and 100% in males, suggesting that in this family the single palmar crease is a sex-influenced trait.

Occurrence: The incidence of the single palmar crease in neonates in the American population varies between 3–9%. Only 2–3% of older children and adults are so affected. The decline in prevalence results from the attrition of children with serious congenital abnormalities, and possibly from changes in palmar creases that occur with use of the hand. The prevalence of the single palmar crease varies with ethnic group, ranging as high as 13% in some isolated Chinese subpopulations.

Risk of Recurrence for Patient's Sib: Accurate risks of recurrence in otherwise normal patients are still not determined. Based on a limited number of studies, risk ranges between 14 and 28%, with some variation by sex.

Risk of Recurrence for Patient's Child: 14–28% in a normal offspring.

Age of Detectability: Evident by the second month of gestation.

Gene Mapping and Linkage: Unknown.

Prevention: None known. Genetic counseling indicated.

Treatment: Unnecessary, since a single palmar crease will not alone impair the function of the hand of an affected individual.

Prognosis: Because the incidence of the single palmar crease is increased in neonates with complex malformation syndromes, the presence of a single palmar crease should raise the physician's suspicion of abnormality. In the absence of other findings, in the presence of a positive family history of single palmar crease, or when the presence of the single palmar crease is first noted in a normal child of school age, the single palmar crease should be considered to be a normal variant. With the passage of time, the single palmar crease may become an incomplete single palmar crease or separate to form two normal creases.

Detection of Carrier: Clinical examination.

References:
Davies PA, Smallpiece V: The single transverse palmar crease in infants and children. Dev Med Child Neurol 1963; 5:491–496.
Johnson CF, Optiz E: The single palmar crease and its clinical significance in a child development clinic: observations and correlations. Clin Pediatr 1971; 10:392–403.
Dar H, et al.: Palmar crease variants and their clinical significance: a study of newborns at risk. Pediatr Res 1977; 11:103–108.

SC058   **Harry W. Schroeder, Jr.**

SKIN CREASES, ABSENT DISTAL INTERPHALANGEAL 2488

Includes: Interphalangeal skin creases, absent distal

Excludes:
> Interphalangeal crease, single, with deformity of middle phalanx
> **Poland syndrome** (0813)
> **Symphalangism** (1001)

Major Diagnostic Criteria: Absence of interphalangeal distal creases without any associated malformations.

Clinical Findings: Complete absence of the distal interphalangeal creases of fingers 2, 3, and 4 on the volar and dorsal sides of both hands. There are no nail abnormalities. No bone abnormalities or fusions are found on X-ray examination. Limitation of flexion of the distal interphalangeal joints may be present.

Complications: Difficulties with finger extension have been reported in two cases.

Associated Findings: Mental retardation was present in one case, but may have been fortuitous.

Etiology: Autosomal dominant inheritance with complete penetrance and variable expressivity.

Pathogenesis: One patient presented with absent distal skin creases, **Camptodactyly,** and clinodactyly. This subject was the mother of a child born with preaxial polydactyly type 1 and the **Poland syndrome.** Whether these anomalies represent a mild expression of the Poland syndrome remains to be determined.

Sex Ratio: Presumably M1:F1

Occurrence: Two kindreds have been reported.

Risk of Recurrence for Patient's Sib:
See Part I, *Mendelian Inheritance.*

Risk of Recurrence for Patient's Child:
See Part I, *Mendelian Inheritance.*

Age of Detectability: Patients have been recognized at ages six and 13 years of age.

Gene Mapping and Linkage: Unknown.

Prevention: None known. Genetic counseling indicated.

Treatment: Unknown.

Prognosis: Good except for two patients in whom decreased flexion of the fingers seemed to be progressive; the patients complained of not being able to play a musical instrument.

Detection of Carrier: Unknown.

Special Considerations: The condition described has some resemblance to a family described with distal symphalangism (Inman et al, 1924; Steinberg and Reynolds, 1948) in which all the patients, except for one (aged three years) presented with bone fusion and absent interphalangeal skin creases.

References:
Inman OL et al.: Four generations of symphalangism. J Hered 1924; 15:329–334.
Daniel GH: A case of hereditary anarthrosis of the index finger, with associated abnormalities in the proportion of the fingers. Ann Eugen 1936; 7:281–297.
Steinberg AG, Reynolds EL: Further data on symphalangism. J Hered 1948; 39:23–27.
Fried K, Mundel G: Absence of distal interphalangeal creases of fingers with flexion limitation. J Med Genet 1976; 13:127–130.
Lambert D et al.: Absence of distal interphalangeal fold causing difficulty in extending fingers. J Med Gen 1977; 14:466–467.
Halal F: Minor manifestations in preaxial polydactyly type 1 and Poland complex. Am J Med Genet 1981; 8:221–228.

MJ038   **Giuseppe Micali**

Skin creases, multiple benign circumferential of the limbs
See MICHELIN TIRE BABY SYNDROME

SKIN CREASES, RETICULATE PIGMENTED FLEXURES, DOWLING-DEGOS TYPE   2393

Includes:
  Dark dot disease
  Dowling-Degos disease (DDD)
  Genodermatose en cocarde of Degos
  Haber syndrome (some)
  Kitamura acropigmentatio reticularis
  Reticular pigmented anomaly of flexures

Excludes:
  Follicular hamartoma, familial multiple
  Skin, acanthosis nigricans (0005)
  Skin, erythrokeratolysis hiemalis (2862)

Major Diagnostic Criteria: Characteristic, progressive, pigmented maculae in the flexural areas.

Clinical Findings: Reticulate pigmented anomaly of the flexures initially affects the axilla and the groin; later in life, other areas, including the intergluteal and inframammary folds, neck, trunk, arms, and wrists, may be involved. The pigmented lesions consist of punctate macules dappled peripherally (2–5 mm); confluence of lesions toward the vault of the axillae and the center of the genitocrural fold is frequent. A shiny and wrinkled appearance of the affected areas sometimes may give an impression of atrophy. Additional signs include the presence of small, pitted, acneform scars around the mouth and scattered dark comedo-like hyperkeratotic follicular lesions on the neck and axillary margins (the so-called *dark dot follicles*). The pigmentation is progressive and asymptomatic; once established, it is thought to be permanent.

Complications: In some patients, sun exposure may lead to an exacerbation of the hyperpigmentation. Friction and pressure may also induce pigmentation.

Associated Findings: Moderate mental retardation (three cases) and epidermal or trichilemmal cysts (four cases) have been reported. Multiple large seborrheic warts were present in one case.

Etiology: Possibly autosomal dominant inheritance with possibly variable penetrance and expressivity.

Pathogenesis: Unknown. It is undetermined whether the epidermal proliferation is related to an excess production of melanosomes or a passive retention of melanin.

MIM No.: 17985

Sex Ratio: M1:F1

Occurrence: Undetermined but presumed rare.

Risk of Recurrence for Patient's Sib:
  See Part I, *Mendelian Inheritance.*

Risk of Recurrence for Patient's Child:
  See Part I, *Mendelian Inheritance.*

Age of Detectability: Possibly during childhood, but the majority of cases are detected during the third to fourth decade of life.

Gene Mapping and Linkage: Unknown.

Prevention: None known. Genetic counseling indicated.

Treatment: Unknown.

Prognosis: A benign genodermatosis, but there are cosmetic problems caused by a diffuse hyperpigmentation in some patients.

Detection of Carrier: Unknown.

Special Considerations: Since it has been noted that Dowling-Degos disease, *Haber syndrome*, and *Kitamura acropigmentatio reticularis* show a very similar histopathologic pattern (epidermal digitate budding, extensive proliferation of the epidermal walls), it has been proposed to include all of these under a spectrum of diseases with different clinical features, but sharing a unique histologic picture.

References:
Dowling GB, Freudenthal W: Acanthosis nigricans. Br J Dermatol 1938; 50:467–471.
Degos R, Ossipowski B: Dermatose pigmentaire reticulee des plis. Ann Dermatol Syphilol 1954; 81:147–151.
Howell JB, Freeman RG: Reticular pigmented anomaly of the flexures. Arch Dermatol 1978; 114:400–403.
Jones EW, Grice K: Reticulatd pigmented anomaly of the flexures: Dowling-Degos disease, a new genodermatosis. Arch Dermatol 1978; 114:1150–1157.
Grosshans E, et al.: Ultrastructure of early pigmentary changes in Dowling-Degos disease. J Cutan Pathol 1980; 7:77–87.
Brown WG: Reticulated pigmented anomaly of the flexures: case reports and genetic investigation. Arch Dermatol 1982; 118:490–493.
Kikuchi I, et al.: The broad spectrum of Dowling-Degos disease, including Haber's syndrome: a hereditary abnormal reactivity to stimulation, increasing with age? J Dermatol (Tokyo) 1983; 10:361–375.
Rebora A, Crovato F: The spectrum of Dowling-Degos disease. Br J Dermatol 1984; 110:627–630.
Rebora A, Crovato F: Pigmentatio reticularis faciei et colli. Arch Dermatol 1985; 121:968 only.
Crovato F, Rebora A: Reticulate pigmented anomaly of the flexures associating reticulate acropigmentation. J Am Acad Dermatol 1986; 14:359–361.
Reymond JL, et al.: Dowling-Degos disease (reticulate pigmentation of the flexures) [in French] Ann Dermatol Venereo 1986; 113:249–251

MI038   **Giuseppe Micali**

Skin lesions, papular
  See SKIN, ELASTOSIS PERFORANS SERPIGINOSA
Skin lesions-seizures-mental retardation
  See HYPOMELANOSIS OF ITO

SKIN PEELING SYNDROME   2864

Includes:
  Deciduous skin, idiopathic
  Keratolysis exfoliativa congenita
  Skin peeling, familial continual

Excludes:
  Ichthyosiform hyperkeratosis, bullous congenital (2852)
  Ichthyosis, linearis circumflexa (2858)
  Pemphigus foliaceus
  Skin, erythrokeratolysis hiemalis (2862)
  Staphylococcal scalded skin syndrome

Major Diagnostic Criteria: Periodic or continuous shedding of whole sheets of stratum corneum. Histopathology demonstrates a split within the lower stratum corneum.

Clinical Findings: Ichthyosis is reported in most patients from birth, but the onset may be delayed until late childhood in some cases. All cases exhibit the ability to manually peel large sheets of intact stratum corneum. Palms and soles may be hyperkeratotic but do not peel. Other clinical features, such as the presence or absence of erythroderma, pruritis, easily plucked anagen hairs, or seasonal exacerbation, are variable. Histopathology in patients with erythroderma demonstrates a psoriasiform dermatitis with hyperkeratosis and parakeratosis, while in nonerythrodermic patients the epidermis is unremarkable except for hyperkeratosis. The split occurs within the lower stratum corneum.

Complications: Unknown.

Associated Findings: Short stature. Generalized aminoaciduria with decreased plasma tryptophan levels.

Etiology: Autosomal recessive inheritance is evidenced by reports of consanguinity, more than one affected sib, and absence of vertical transmission. Variability of onset and other clinical features may reflect underlying genetic heterogeneity.

Pathogenesis: Unknown. A generalized aminoaciduria with low plasma tryptophan levels has been reported in some patients. Electron microscopy of the skin in one study demonstrated an intracellular cleavage within the stratum corneum with dense intercellular globular deposits, believed to represent lipid-like material.

MIM No.: *27030

CDC No.: 757.900

Sex Ratio: M1:F1

Occurrence: About 20 cases have been reported in the literature, including cases from India, Kuwait, and the United States.

Risk of Recurrence for Patient's Sib:
See Part I, *Mendelian Inheritance.*

Risk of Recurrence for Patient's Child:
See Part I, *Mendelian Inheritance.*

Age of Detectability: Usually during infancy, but may be delayed until the end of the second decade.

Gene Mapping and Linkage: Unknown.

Prevention: None known. Genetic counseling indicated.

Treatment: Unknown.

Prognosis: Lifelong once established.

Detection of Carrier: Unknown.

Special Considerations: The acquired disorders of pemphigus foliaceus and staphylococcal scalded skin syndrome show cleavage at the stratum granulosum-stratum corneum interface.

References:
Kurban AK, Azar HA: Familial continual skin peeling. Br J Dermatol 1969; 81:191–195. * †
Levy SB, Goldsmith LA: The peeling skin syndrome. J Am Acad Dermatol 1982; 7:606–613. * †
Abdel-Hafez K, et al.: Familial continual skin peeling. Dermatologica 1983; 166:22–31.
Silverman AK, et al.: Continual skin peeling syndrome: an electron microscopic study. Arch Dermatol 1986; 122:71–75. †

WI013   **Mary L. Williams**

Skin peeling, familial continual
See SKIN PEELING SYNDROME
Skin pigmentation-short stature, X-linked
See SILVER SYNDROME, X-LINKED

SKIN TUMORS, MULTIPLE GLOMUS 0416

Includes: Glomus tumors, multiple

Excludes:
Solitary glomangioma
Solitary glomus tumor

Major Diagnostic Criteria: Positive diagnosis by biopsy. The characteristic histopathologic features are endothelial-lined dilated vascular spaces which are surrounded by one or more layers of the oval glomus tumor (smooth muscle) cells.

Clinical Findings: Multiple flesh-colored to blue nodules in the skin, 0.3 to 3.0 cm in diameter. They may occasionally involve deeper structures such as bone. The lesions are usually regional but may be generalized. The lesions are soft, movable, and sometimes tender. No changes are ordinarily seen in the overlying epidermis.

Complications: Unknown.

Associated Findings: A case has been reported with deformities of the affected limb consisting of hypoplasia with precocious closure of the epiphyses and bradymetacarpia. Another case had some atrophy of the affected limb and (by arteriography) many abnormal ballooning blood vessels at the end of arteries and arteriovenous anastomoses corresponding to tumors.

Etiology: Autosomal dominant inheritance has been seen in several families.

Pathogenesis: Possibly a benign hyperplasia of the normal cutaneous arteriovenous anastomosis.

MIM No.: *13800

CDC No.: 757.900

Sex Ratio: M1+:F1

Occurrence: About 50 cases in the medical literature.

Risk of Recurrence for Patient's Sib:
See Part I, *Mendelian Inheritance.*

Risk of Recurrence for Patient's Child:
See Part I, *Mendelian Inheritance.*

Age of Detectability: The average age of development of the regional type is 29 years and that of the generalized type 40 years. One-third of all cases appear before age 20. Some cases have been apparent at birth.

Gene Mapping and Linkage: Unknown.

Prevention: None known. Genetic counseling indicated.

Treatment: Surgical excision of the lesion.

Prognosis: Normal for life span and intelligence. Functional disability may result from pain or rarely, deformity of the limb. The lesions have no malignant potential.

Detection of Carrier: Unknown.

References:
Sluiter JT, Postma C: Multiple glomus tumors of the skin. Acta Dermatol Venereol (Stockh) 1959 39:98.
Gorlin RJ, et al.: Multiple glomus tumor of the pseudocavernous hemangioma type. Arch Derm 1960; 82:776–778.
Gordon B, Hyman AB: Multiple nontender glomus tumors: report of a case with 33 lesions. Arch Dermatol 1961; 83:640.
Goodman TF Jr, Abele DC: Multiple glomus tumors: a clinical and electron microscopic study. Arch Dermatol 1971; 103:11.
Beasley SW, et al.: Hereditary multiple glomus tumours. Arch Dis Child 1986; 61:801–802.

WA046   **Silas Wallk**

SKIN, ACANTHOSIS NIGRICANS   0005

Includes:

    Acanthosis nigricans
    Drug-induced insulin resistance
    Insulin resistance, autosomal dominant type
    Insulin resistance, drug induced type
    Malignant acanthosis nigricans (AN)

Excludes:

    Acanthosis nigricans, Hirschowitz type
    Dermatosis papulosa nigra
    Generalized cutaneous papillomatosis
    Leprechaunism (0587)

Major Diagnostic Criteria: A skin eruption characterized by velvety hyperkeratotic macules, which can be accompanied by various degrees of pigmentation, affecting the entire skin but preferentially the axilla, neck, genitalia, and oral cavity. Acanthosis nigricans (AN) can be accompanied by an internal malignancy, especially an adenocarcinoma of the stomach, or can be associated with insulin resistance, Crouzon Seip, and Beare syndromes; drug

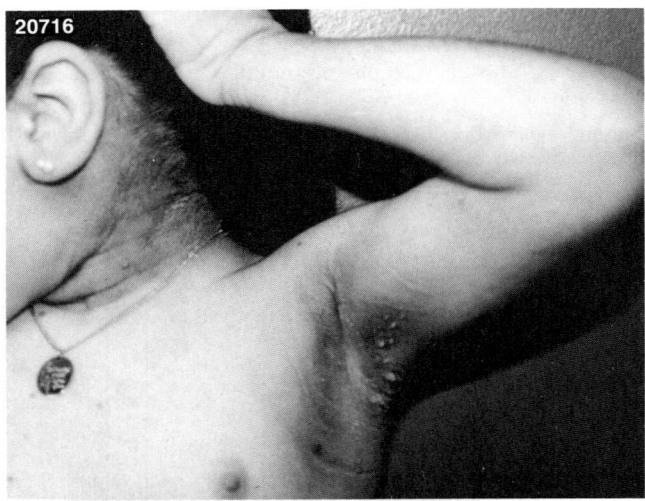

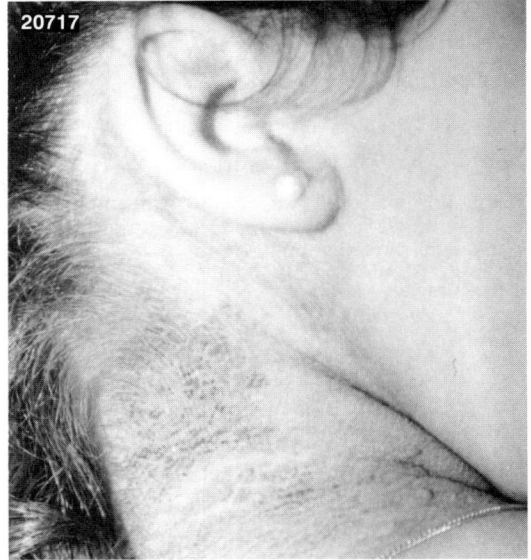

0005-20716–17: Acanthosis nigricans; note dark, hyperpigmented, raised lesion in the axilla and the neck.

eruptions and miscellaneous diseases; or it could be inherited as an autosomal dominant.

Clinical Findings: The classical presentation consists of dark-brown, velvety, hyperkeratotic macules; there may be slight discoloration or the entire skin may be affected. The body regions affected by AN, in descending order of frequency, are as follows: axillae, neck, genitalia, groin and inner thighs, umbilicus, perianal area, other flexural surfaces, and areolas. Pigmentation of either the axillae or the neck, or both, usually occurs before other areas are involved. Normal skin margins are accentuated.

Multiple, rapidly growing seborrheic keratoses (sign of Leser-Trélat) and florid cutaneous papillomatosis are part of the clinical findings.

About 40% of those cases associated with internal malignancy have oral manifestations, especially of the tongue and lips. The tongue may have hypertrophy and elongation of papillae, deep fissures, and papillomatous growths. Oral lesions are non-pigmented. Lip, buccal mucosa, and palate may be similarly affected. Occasional cases affecting the gingiva may resemble idiopathic fibromatosis. Marked perioral papillomatosis is a frequent finding. Only 15% of cases not associated with internal malignancy have oral manifestations.

In the neoplastic association type, about 75% of the associated tumors are abdominal adenocarcinomas, of which 60% arise in the stomach. Adenocarcinomas of the uterus, pancreas, intestine, and, to a lesser extent, bladder, lung, and breast, can also be associated with AN. These carcinomas have a high degree of malignancy. In about 20% of cases, AN precedes the malignancy by up to 16 years. It parallels the cancer in proportion to the degree of spread; it may regress with radiation therapy or with surgical removal of the tumor, and it may reflourish with recurrence of the adenocarcinoma. Generalized skin hyperpigmentation and pruritus occur in about 40% of cases of the neoplastic association type, and palmar and plantar hyperkeratosis is seen in about 25% of these cases. The vaginal, conjunctival, esophageal, and pharyngeal mucosas can be the site of papillary and verrucous lesions.

The insulin-resistant types have been divided in two groups. Type A (HAIR-AN syndrome) is mostly observed in adolescent or young females, and is characterized by hyperandrogenism, insulin resistance, and AN. Virilization, polycystic ovaries, and accelerated growth are also present. Leprechaunism also falls into this type. Type B is observed in older females with autoimmune disorders. Other endocrinopathies and obesity are also associated with AN, as well as some cases of Bloom, Crouzon, Seip and Beare syndromes. Injection of some drugs, such as nicotinic acid, also may induce AN.

Complications: In the neoplastic association type, metastasis and complications due to radiation therapy are expected.

In the insulin-resistant types, complications are derived from the basic defect.

Associated Findings: Deep skin margins on the neck can be seen in some patients.

The gingiva, especially the interdental papillae, may become so enlarged as to almost cover the teeth, resembling idiopathic fibromatosis.

Etiology: Autosomal dominant or recessive inheritance. It has been suggested that this condition is produced by a peptide or group of peptides. In some patients it is due to genetic defects in insulin receptor pathways.

Pathogenesis: It is assumed that the responsible peptides may be produced by the adenocarcinomas and might be present in the endocrinopathies. Growth hormone, adrenocorticotropin and luteinizing hormones have also been thought responsible for the skin changes of AN.

MIM No.: *10060, *18730, 20017, *24309, *26970

CDC No.: 757.900

Sex Ratio: M1:F1 in neoplastic association type; M1:F5 in insulin-resistant types.

Occurrence: Some 1,500 cases have been reported to date.

Risk of Recurrence for Patient's Sib:
See Part I, *Mendelian Inheritance.*

Risk of Recurrence for Patient's Child:
See Part I, *Mendelian Inheritance.*

Age of Detectability: More then 80% of affected persons with the neoplastic association type are over 40 years old at the time of onset. Patients with the insulin-resistant types are generally diagnosed during childhood or early adolescence.

Gene Mapping and Linkage: Unknown.

Prevention: None known. Genetic counseling indicated.

Treatment: Neoplastic association type requires oncologic treatment; AN may regress with radiation therapy or with surgical excision of the malignancy involved. Insulin-resistant types will regress with the adequate hormonal treatment.

Prognosis: For the neoplastic association type, the mortality rate is 100% and the average survival period after discovery is less than 2 years. For the nonneoplastic association types, the patients have a normal life span.

Detection of Carrier: By clinical examination.

Special Considerations: Acanthosis nigricans appears not only as a sign of Type A and Type B insulin resistance, but as a sign of the insulin resistance seen in **Leprechaunism**.

References:

Rigel DS, Jacobs MI: Malignant acanthosis nigricans: a review. J Dermatol Surg Oncol 1980; 6:923–927.

Andreev VC, et al.: Generalized acanthosis nigricans. Dermatologica 1981; 163:19–24.

Barbieri RL, Ryan KJ: Hyperandrogenism, insulin resistance, and acanthosis nigricans syndrome: a common endocrinopathy with distinct pathophysiologic features. Am J Obstet Gynecol 1983; 147:90–101.

Flier JS: Metabolic importance of acanthosis nigricans. Arch Dermatol 1985; 121:193–194.

Flier JS, et al.: Acanthosis nigricans in obese women with hyperandrogenism: characterization of an insulin-resistant state distinct from the type A and B syndromes. Diabetes 1985; 34:101–107.

SE007   **Heddie O. Sedano**

Skin, acrokeratosis verruciformis
See ACROKERATOSIS VERRUCIFORMIS

SKIN, ATOPY, FAMILIAL   3150

Includes:
    Allergic diathesis
    Allergic rhinitis
    Asthma, inherited
    Atopic dermatitis
    Atopic diathesis with asthma and hayfever
    Atopic hypersensitivity
    Eczema, atopic
    Hayfever, atopic
    Prurigo Besnier

Excludes:
    Croup and Acute epiglotitis
    Cystic fibrosis (0237)
    Hypersensitivity pneumonitis
    Infections of the bronchopulmonary system, all
    Laryngotracheobronchitis
    Lichen simplex chronicus

Major Diagnostic Criteria: *Atopic dermatitis:* Usually demonstrates some of the following basic features: pruritis; typical morphology and distribution; flexural lichenification or linearity in adults; facial and extensor involvement in infants and children; chronic or chronically relapsing eczematous dermatitis; personal or family history of atopy (asthma, allergic rhinitis, or atopic dermatitis). Other features include xerosis, immediate skin test reactivity, elevated serum IgE, early age of onset, tendency toward cutaneous infections, tendency towards nonspecific hand or foot derma-

titis, nipple eczema, cheilitis, recurrent conjunctivitis, Dennie-Morgan infraorbital fold, keratoconus, anterior and or posterior subcapsular cataracts, orbital darkening, facial pallor/facial erythema, pityriasis alba, anterior neck folds, itch when sweating, intolerance to wool and lipid solvents, perifollicular accentuation, food intolerance, a course influenced by environmental/emotional factors, and white dermographism.

Asthma: 1) presence of significant, obstructive ventilatory abnormality in tests of ventilatory mechanics, 2) presence in some patients of associated cough, chest tightness, wheezing, or dyspnea.

Clinical Findings: *Atopic dermatitis:* usually onset is in infancy, occurring frequently at about three months of age. The lesions involve the face at first, but spreading to trunk and extremities does occur. It is always an eczematous inflammation. This may resolve or evolve into the classic pattern of chronic lichenification in antecubital area and popliteal fossa. By the end of the second year of life, many patients have healed, but others continue into the childhood phase, which includes, in addition to face and flexural involvement, involvement of the hands, feet, and sometimes the buttocks and backs of the thighs. The condition is chronic but may alternate between symptom-free intervals and relapses.

Asthma: The attacks of infants are generally associated with respiratory infections. Between infections, the infant is generally free of chest symptoms, although some infants may have persistent wheezing.

Complications: *Of bronchial asthma:* infections, such as otitis media, sinusitis, bronchitis, pneumonitis, atelectasis, pneumomediastinum and pneumothorax, growth complications, psychologic problems, bronchopulmonary aspergillosis, respiratory failure.

Of atopic dermatitis: decreased cell-mediated immunity and malfunctioning chemotaxis are associated with increased occurrence of staphylococcal, viral (including warts, herpes simplex, and molluscum contagiosum), and dermatophytic infections of the skin. Chronically affected areas of the skin may show hyperpigmentation and even depigmentation, related to excessive rubbing and inflammation. Ocular complications include mild conjunctivitis to bilateral cataracts. Cataracts may affect 5–10% of severely affected individuals.

Associated Findings: **Urticaria, dermo-distortive type**, **Migraine headaches**, drug sensitivity, **Ichthyosis vulgaris**, keratosis pilaris, vitiligo, and **Hair, alopecia areata**.

Etiology: Probably autosomal dominant inheritance, with clinical expression dependent on interaction with other factors. Previously, most authors had generally accepted "multifactorial environmental influences on a genetic predisposition". There is also evidence for autosomal recessive inheritance, and for the contribution of several HLA-linked interactive genes.

Pathogenesis: For *asthma*, bronchial hyperreactivity. For *atopic eczema*, the role of IgE has been considered in depth, including total serum IgE levels and the propensity to produce IgE in response to common, usually inhaled allergens. Yet patients with agammaglobulinemia do manifest atopic disease. The primary cause of the disease remains unknown. The immunological problems may be secondary to a more pervasive disorder of metabolism.

MIM No.: 20920

Sex Ratio: *Eczema*, M2:F1 in several studies. Until puberty, *asthma* is approximately twice as common in boys as in girls. The more severe the asthma, the greater preponderance of male over female children. As age increases, there is a reversal of this trend, with female cases predominating in older age groups.

Occurrence: *Asthma:* prevalence ranges from a low of 0.06% in Finland, to 1.4% in Sweden, to 8.9% in United States, to 11.4% in Australia.

Atopic dermatitis: prevalence is 3.1% among children up to five years of age in England. 19:1,000 among children in United States.

The frequency of eczema in patients with asthma or allergic rhinitis is poorly documented.

The frequency of allergic respiratory symptoms in patients with atopic eczema is approximately 1:3.

Risk of Recurrence for Patient's Sib: Multiple factors will determine an individual's risk. One study reported an average risk of 32% if only one other sibling is affected, and the parents are not affected (Kjellman, 1977).

Risk of Recurrence for Patient's Child: For atopy, risk figures vary from 15% to 72%, based upon the types of atopy and if one or both parents are affected (Kjellman, 1977).

Age of Detectability: *Atopic eczema*: during infancy or early childhood; rarely before six weeks of age.

Gene Mapping and Linkage: APY (atopy (allergic asthma and rhinitis)) has been provisionally mapped to 11q12-q13.
There is a possible HLA linkage.

Prevention: None known. Genetic counseling indicated.

Treatment: *For atopic dermatitis*: topical corticosteroids, tar preparation. Avoidance of extremes in environmental temperature and humidity; avoidance of wool and synthetic fibers on the skin.
For asthma: bronchodilators.

Prognosis: Although most deaths from *asthma* occur in adults, a significant number do occur in children. Asthma may spontaneously disappear with increasing age after a number of years, and the percentage of patients who continue to have severe disease is relatively low.
Atopic dermatitis: figures for persistence of disease vary from 70% in severe cases to 10% overall.
Allergic rhinitis: usually persists for many years, and is less likely to remit than asthma.

Detection of Carrier: Unknown.

References:
Kjellman II: Atopic disease in seven-year-old children: incidence in relation to family history. Acta Paediatr Scand 1977; 66:465–470.
Hanifin JM: Atopic Dermatitis. J Allergy Clin Immunol 1984; 73:211–226.
Saarinen Ulla M: Prophylaxis for atopic disease: role of infant disease. Clin Rev Allergy 1984; 2:151–167.
Borecki IB, et al.: Demonstration of a common major gene with pleiotropic effects on immunoglobulin E levels and allergy. Genet Epidemiol 1985; 2:327–328.
Siegel C: Asthma in infants and children. J Allergy Clin Immunol 1985; 76:1–15.
Rajka G: Natural history and clinical manifestations of atopic dermatitis. Clin Rev Allergy 1986; 4:3–26.
Blumenthal MN, Amos DB: Genetic and Immunologic Basis of atopic responses. Chest 1987; 91:176S–184S.
Cookson WL, Hopkin JM: Dominant and inheritance of atopic immunoglobulin-E responsiveness. Lancet 1988; I:86–88.

FI031   **Cheryl Nagel Fialkoff**

Skin, atrophy-anonychia-alopecia-tongue defect
See ALOPECIA-SKIN ATROPHY-ANONYCHIA-TONGUE DEFECT

SKIN, CUTANEOUS MELANOSIS, DIFFUSE   2309

Includes:
Cutaneous melanosis (diffuse)
Hyperpigmentation, familial progressive
Melanoderma, familial generalized

Excludes:
Neurocutaneous melanosis (2014)
Skin, hyperpigmentation, familial (2362)

Major Diagnostic Criteria: Diffuse macular pigmentary darkening which intensifies and becomes more widespread over time. Affected individuals are otherwise healthy.

Clinical Findings: Children are born with spotted reticulated, striated, and whorled hyperpigmentation including the oral mucosa but sparing palms, soles, conjunctiva (which later become pigmented as the child ages). There is at birth hyperpigmentation of the forehead, lateral face, back, extensor surface of extremities,

and scrotum. Pigmentary darkening and new dark macules develop later (Chernosky et al, 1971). Melanosomes are increased in size and number compared to normal.

Complications: Unknown.

Associated Findings: None known.

Etiology: Possibly X-linked or autosomal dominant inheritance.

Pathogenesis: Unknown.

CDC No.:   757.900

Sex Ratio: Presumably M1:F1

Occurrence: Described in at least one kindred.

Risk of Recurrence for Patient's Sib:
See Part I, *Mendelian Inheritance*.

Risk of Recurrence for Patient's Child:
See Part I, *Mendelian Inheritance*.

Age of Detectability: As early as childhood.

Gene Mapping and Linkage: Unknown.

Prevention: None known. Genetic counseling indicated.

Treatment: None required.

Prognosis: Normal lifespan is expected.

Detection of Carrier: Unknown.

Special Considerations: A variant is one reported case in a Mexican child born white who then became progressively dark to resemble a black panther with intense Black melanosis of all skin, hair and mucosa (see **Skin, hyperpigmentation, familial**). Melanocyte numbers were normal. Electron microscope showed increased numbers of melanosomes in keratinocytes.

References:
Chernosky HE, et al.: Familial Progressive Hyperpigmentation. Arch Derm 1971; 103:581.
Ruiz-Maldonaldo R, et al.: Universal Acquired Melanosis: the Carbon Baby. Arch Derm 1978;114:775.

M0040   **David B. Mosher**

SKIN, CUTANEOUS MELANOSIS: MONGOLIAN SPOT   3206

Includes:
Child spot
Congenital dermal melanocytosis (CDM)
Mongolian spot
Cutaneous melanosis: mongolian spot

Excludes:
Nevus of Ota (0716)
Nevus of Ito

Major Diagnostic Criteria: Mongolian spot is a congenital circumscribed melanocytosis which is very common in Orientals and much less so in Caucasians. The sacrum is the classic site of involvement but extra-sacral locations occur.

Clinical Findings: There are several types of mongolian spots. The classic or common mongolian spot (MS) occurs over the back and lumbosacral regions; the extra-sacral or aberrant spot which is less frequent occurs elsewhere. There is a well circumscribed variant with sharp discrete margins. A persistent type also occurs ("persistent mongolian spot"). Up to 90% of Asiatics and Amerindians, but less than 10% of Caucasians, are affected. The persistent MS occurs in 3–4%. The classic MS is a blue-green uniformly colored with indistinct, feathered margins and involves the buttock and lumbosacral region bilaterally and not the anus. Lesions may be centimeters in diameter and may cover the entire low back and buttocks. Sharp margins are seen in large lesions. Extra-sacral MS are found on the face or extremities or elsewhere.
A **Cleft lip** - MS type is also described (but not in Caucasians). A special type includes atypical blue nevus type 2, which is an overlap of MS and nevus spots. Overlap with **Nevus flammeus** also occurs.
Studies have shown the dermal melanosis to be present micro-

scopically in the three month fetus and macroscopically at seven months. Pigment density appears greatest at one year and diminishes slowly thereafter; the size of the macule however, reaches maximal dimensions at age two years. Microscopic presence of melanocytes is routine (melanocytes may be DOPA negative). Regression is usually more characteristic of smaller lesions.

Complications: Unknown.

Associated Findings: None known.

Etiology: Unknown.

Pathogenesis: Persistence may be related to the presence of a fibrous sheath which is gradually lost and dislodged in a regressing lesion.

Sex Ratio: M1:F1

Occurrence: Reported in as high as 90% of Asians, but only 10% of Caucasians. Other population groups range between these figures.

Risk of Recurrence for Patient's Sib: Presumably not increased.

Risk of Recurrence for Patient's Child: Presumably not increased.

Age of Detectability: At birth.

Gene Mapping and Linkage: Unknown.

Prevention: None known. Genetic counseling indicated.

Treatment: Cosmetic coverup with Covermark^ (Lydia O'Leary) or Dermablend^ (Flori Roberts). Treatment by laser therapy may be useful in cases of persistent MS.

Prognosis: Some 96–97% fade nearly or completely by age ten years.

Detection of Carrier: Unknown.

Special Considerations: A different type of dermal melanocytosis has been described by Lever in a case of what appeared to be a mongolian spot of the nose at age eight. Extensive dermal melanocytosis was found on biopsy. At age 13, metastatic melanoma was discovered in liver and lymph nodes. Autopsy showed diffuse dermal, visceral and cranial melanosis but only melanophages were present in visceral and cranial tissues.

References:
Morooka K: On the Mongolian spot in the Japanese. Acta Anat Jpn 1931; 3:1371.
Hidano A: Persistent Mongolian spot in the adult. Arch Dermatol 1971; 103:680.
Levene A: Disseminated dermal melanocytosis terminating in melanoma: a human condition resembling equine melanotic disease. Br J Derm 1979; 101:197.
Fitzpatrick TB, et al., eds: Dermal melanocytosis (Mongolian spot) in biology and disease of dermal pigmentation. Tokyo: Tokyo Press, 1981:83–94.

M0040   **David B. Mosher**

Skin, Darier disease
See DARIER DISEASE

SKIN, ELASTOSIS PERFORANS SERPIGINOSA   0339

Includes:
   Elastoma intrapapillarea perforans verruciforme
   Elastosis perforans serpiginosa
   Keratosis follicularis serpiginosa
   Miescher elastoma
   Skin lesions, papular

Excludes:
   Skin, Kyrle disease (0561)
   Skin, porokeratosis (0819)

Major Diagnostic Criteria: Keratotic papules characterized histologically by extrusion of dermal elastic tissue through the epidermis.

Clinical Findings: Skin colored, slightly erythematous keratotic papules arranged in arcs, circles, or without particular configuration. These lesions spread peripherally and may become hypopigmented and centrally atrophic. Most frequently observed on the neck and upper extremities.

Complications: Development of keloidal scar following surgical manipulation or electrodesiccation of the skin lesions.

Associated Findings: In 26% of the reported cases, elastosis perforans serpiginosa has occurred in association with various heritable disorders such as **Chromosome 21, trisomy 21, Ehlers-Danlos syndrome, Pseudoxanthoma elasticum, Rothmund-Thomson syndrome, Marfan syndrome,** and **Osteogenesis imperfecta.** In several instances, elastosis perforans serpiginosa occurred in patients with **Hepatolenticular degeneration** and **Cystinuria** during treatment with penicillamine.

Etiology: Possibly autosomal dominant inheritance.

Pathogenesis: Localized increase of dermal elastic fibers with secondary epidermal and follicular epithelial hyperplasia and transepithelial elimination of the elastic fibers through multiple perforating channels.

MIM No.: 13010

CDC No.: 757.900

Sex Ratio: M4:F1

Occurrence: Over 120 cases reported.

Risk of Recurrence for Patient's Sib:
   See Part I, *Mendelian Inheritance.*

Risk of Recurrence for Patient's Child:
   See Part I, *Mendelian Inheritance.*

Age of Detectability: Ninety percent of the patients with elastosis perforans serpiginosa are younger than 30 years of age.

Gene Mapping and Linkage: Unknown.

Prevention: None known. Genetic counseling indicated.

Treatment: Cyrotherapy and tape stripping can be useful therapies. Corticosteroids, local or intralesional, have had little effect. Surgery or electroderscation can result in keloid formation.

Prognosis: Normal life expectancy.

Detection of Carrier: Unknown.

References:
Mehregan AH: Elastosis perforans serpiginosa: a review of the literature and report of 11 cases. Arch Dermatol 1968; 97:381.
Mehregan AH: Perforating dermatoses: a clinicopathologic review. Int J Dermatol 1977; 16:19.
Bardach H, et al.: "Lumpy-bumpy" elastic fibers in the skin and lungs of a patient with a penicillamine-induced elastosis perforans serpiginosa. J Cutan Pathol 1979; 6:243.
Sfar Z, et al.: Deux cas d'elastomes verruciformes apres administration prolongee de D-penicillamine. Ann Dermatol Venereol 1982; 109: 813–814.
Ayala F, Donofrio P: Elastosis perforans serpiginosa: report of a family. Dermatologica 1983; 166:32–37.
Patterson JW: The perforating disorders. J Am Acad Derm 1984; 10:561–581.

S0009   **Lawrence M. Solomon**

**SKIN, ERYTHROKERATODERMIA, PROGRESSIVA
SYMMETRICA   2863**

Includes:
   Erythematokeratotic phacomatosis
   Erythrokeratodermia figurata, congenital familial, in
      plaques

Excludes:
   Giroux-Barbeau syndrome (2866)
   Skin, erythrokeratodermia, variable (0361)
   Skin, erythrokeratolysis hiemalis (2862)
   Skin, pityriasis rubra pilaris (0811)
   Skin, psoriasis vulgaris (0833)

Major Diagnostic Criteria: Onset in infancy and early childhood of symmetric hyperkeratotic erythematous plaques on head, buttocks, and extremities. **Skin, psoriasis vulgaris** and **Skin, pityriasis rubra pilaris** must be excluded by response to therapy and histopathology.

Clinical Findings: Well-demarcated erythematous, hyperkeratotic plaques that are absolutely symmetrically distributed on the head, buttocks, and extremities, but sparing the trunk. The lesions are not present at birth; they begin in infancy, stabilize after 1–2 years, and often partially regress at puberty. The palms and soles may be involved, and the lesions may be pruritic. Histologically, a psoriasiform dermatitis is present, but the disorder differs from psoriasis both in its fixed, absolute symmetry and in its truncal sparing. Moreover, Auspitz sign is absent and Munro microabscesses are not found histologically. Finally, the disorder, unlike psoriasis, is resistant to most topical therapies.

Complications: Unknown.

Associated Findings: None known.

Etiology: Autosomal dominant inheritance with incomplete penetrance and variable expressivity. Several sporadic cases have been reported from consanguineous kindreds, suggesting that a recessive form may also occur.

Pathogenesis: Unknown. The epidermis is hyperproliferative. Electron microscopic studies show lipid vacuoles within the stratum corneum and perinuclear swollen mitochondria in stratum granulosum. These findings may not be specific for this disorder, but may reflect the hyperproliferative state.

CDC No.: 757.190

Sex Ratio: M1:F1

Occurrence: Approximately 25 cases have been reported, including ten from Mexico.

Risk of Recurrence for Patient's Sib:
See Part I, *Mendelian Inheritance.*

Risk of Recurrence for Patient's Child:
See Part I, *Mendelian Inheritance.*

Age of Detectability: By early childhood.

Gene Mapping and Linkage: Unknown.

Prevention: None known. Genetic counseling indicated.

Treatment: Responds partially, if at all, to conventional topical therapies. Improvement with oral synthetic retinoids (e.g., etretinate) is reported. However, the risk/benefit ratio of these agents must be carefully considered on an individual basis, particularly their teratogenicity and long-term effects on bones, and treatment should be reserved for disabling cases (see **Fetal retinoid syndrome**).

Prognosis: Partial or complete regression may occur at puberty.

Detection of Carrier: Careful skin examination coupled with history will help to detect minimally affected family members.

References:
Ruiz-Maldonado R, et al.: Erythrokeratodermia progressiva symmetrica: report of 10 cases. Dermatologica 1982; 164:133–141. * †
Nazzaro V, Blanchet-Bardon C: Progressive symmetric erythrokeratoderma: histological and ultrastructural study of patient before and after treatment with etretinate. Arch Dermatol 1986; 122:434–440. †

WI013   **Mary L. Williams**

SKIN, ERYTHROKERATODERMIA, VARIABLE   0361

Includes:
    Erythrokeratoderma figurata, congenital familial, in plaques
    Erythrokeratoderma variabilis Mendes da Costa
    Ichthyosis-erythema annulare centrifugum
    Keratosis rubra figurata
    Mendes da Costa syndrome

Excludes:
    Erythema, familial annual
    Erythema perstans
    Ichthyosiform erythrokeratoderma, atypical with deafness (2861)
    Skin, erythrokeratodermia, progressiva symmetrica (2863)

Major Diagnostic Criteria: This disorder of cornification is characterized by sharply demarcated, geographic erythemas of shifting configuration and fixed, keratotic plaques bearing no relationship to the variable erythemas in conjunction with characteristic histopathology of laminated hyperkeratosis, acanthosis, and papillomatosis.

Clinical Findings: The dermatosis is composed of two parts: first, discrete, irregular configurate patches of erythema that are extremely variable in size, position, duration, and number. These are subject to environmental influences, such as cold, heat, and wind, or to emotional upsets and are relatively transient in nature. Second, there are fixed hyperkeratotic plaques that are sharply demarcated and persistent. These yellow-brown hyperkeratotic plaques have irregular outlines and usually arise on normal skin. In most instances only focal hyperkeratotic plaques are present, but occasionally the hyperkeratosis may be generalized, including the palms and soles. Hair, nails, and mucous membranes are

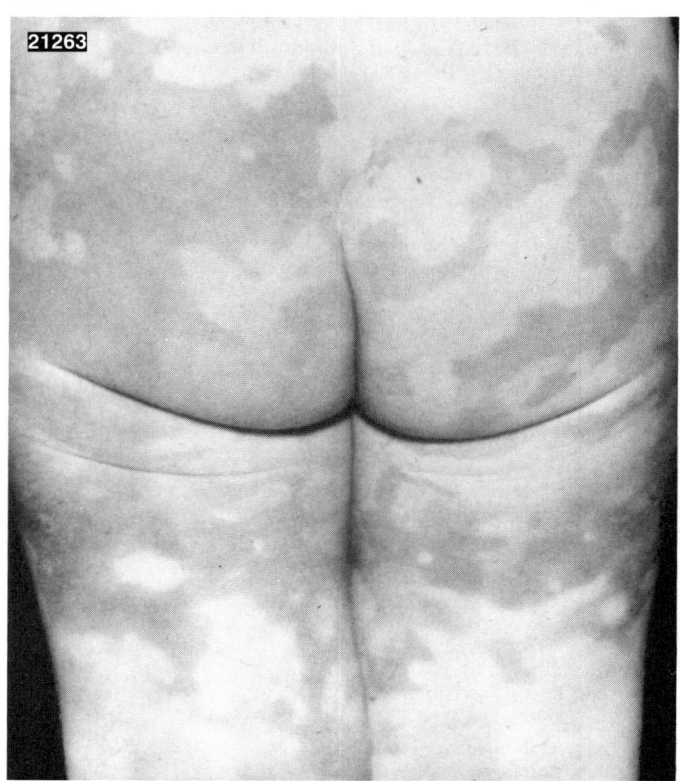

0361-21263: Erythrokeratodermia; note the irregular erythematous patches which occur with hyperkeratotic plaques which are not necessarily related to the erythema.

normal. The histopathology of the hyperkeratotic plaques demonstrates marked orthohyperkeratosis and focal parakeratosis with a prominent granular cell layer and severe papillomatosis with suprapapillary thinning. This "church-spire" configuration is characteristic but not diagnostic.

Complications: Approximately one-third of the case reports do not mention the presence of erythema. In those cases in which it has been noted, it tends to localize to the face, buttocks, and extensor aspect of the limbs. The hyperkeratotic lesions have a similar distribution, and while they usually develop on normal skin, they may occasionally arise from persistent erythrodermic areas. Their tendency is to persist indefinitely, although rarely they may involute spontaneously. The palms and soles show a variable keratoderma. The Koebner phenomenon (isomorphic response, induction of new lesions at sites of skin trauma) has been elicited in some of these cases. The underlying cause is unknown.

Associated Findings: There are isolated reports of perceptive deafness, developmental and growth retardation, and motor dysfunction.

Etiology: Usually autosomal dominant inheritance of variable expressivity. The majority of pedigrees are consistent with an autosomal dominant transmission, but other modes of inheritance cannot be excluded in some families. Thorough examination of the parents, sibs, and descendants of an affected individual is important because of the variable expressivity. Some reports describe a generalized hyperkeratosis in conjunction with variable erythrodermas; an autosomal dominant inheritance pattern was documented in one instance.

Pathogenesis: Autoradiographic studies reveal a normal epidermal proliferation rate, indicating that this is a "retention type" of hyperkeratosis. Ultrastructural examination reveals decreased numbers of lamellar bodies in the upper stratum spinosum and granular layer and increased numbers of unmyelinated nerves in the papillary dermis. Enzyme histochemical and immunohistochemical investigations have shown a decreased number of epidermal Langerhans cells, a cell of monocyte lineage responsible for antigen recognition and processing.

MIM No.: *13320

CDC No.: 757.190

Sex Ratio: M1:F1

Occurrence: Some 150 cases of variable erythrokeratodermia have been reported, the majority being from Europe.

Risk of Recurrence for Patient's Sib:
See Part I, *Mendelian Inheritance.*

Risk of Recurrence for Patient's Child:
See Part I, *Mendelian Inheritance.*

Age of Detectability: At birth in approximately 30% of cases. The majority of the remainder note the onset during the first year of life, but it may be delayed until after the third year of life.

Gene Mapping and Linkage: EKV (erythrokeratodermia variabilis) has been provisionally mapped to 1.

Prevention: None known. Genetic counseling indicated.

Treatment: Topical corticosteroids may be helpful for the erythematous lesions. Palliation of the hyperkeratotic plaques can be achieved with topical retinoic acid, salicylic acid gel, or 5% lactic acid in hydrophilic ointment. Oral synthetic retinoids, particularly etretinate are helpful. Their long-term administration, however, is necessary to control this disorder of cornification, and use of these agents must be carefully considered against their many toxicities.

Prognosis: The general tendency is for the process to increase in severity until puberty and then remain stationary or show gradual signs of improvement. The general health remains unaffected.

Detection of Carrier: Careful examination of family members.

References:
Brown J, Kierland RR: Erythrokeratodermia variabilis: report of 3 cases and review of the literature. Arch Dermatol 1966; 93:194–201. * †
Schellander FG, Fritsch PO: Variable erythrokeratodermia: an unusual case. Arch Dermatol 1969; 100:744–748. †
Cram DL: Erythrokeratoderma variabilis and variable circinate erythrokeratodermis. Arch Dermatol 1970; 101:68–73. * †
Vandersteen PR, Muller SA: Erythrokeratoderma variabilis: an enzyme histochemical and ultrastructural study. Arch Dermatol 1971; 103:362–370.
Gewirtzman GB, et al.: Erythrokeratodermia variabilis. Arch Dermatol 1978; 114:259–261.
Hacham-Zadeh S, Even-Paz Z: Erythrokeratodermia variabilis in a Jewish Kurdish family. Clin Genet 1978; 13:404.
Bond MJ, et al.: Erythrokeratodermia variabilis in a patient followed through the first year of life. Cutis 1982; 30:633. †
Rappaport IP, et al.: Erythrokeratodermia variabilis treated with isotretinoin: a clinical, histological and ultrastructural study. Arch Dermatol 1986; 122:441–445.

WI013
VA010
Mary L. Williams
Paul R. Vandersteen

SKIN, ERYTHROKERATOLYSIS HIEMALIS   2862

Includes:
> Genodermatose en cocarde of Degos
> Erythrokeratolysis hiemalis
> Keratolytic winter erythema
> Oudtshoorn skin

Excludes:
> Erythema, familial annular
> **Lyme disease** (3212)
> **Skin creases, reticulate pigmented flexures, Dowling-Degos type** (2393)
> **Skin, erythrokeratodermia, variable** (0361)
> **Skin peeling syndrome** (2864)

Major Diagnostic Criteria: The combination of cyclic attacks of symmetric erythematous plaques that peel from the center outward in conjunction with characteristic histopathology of spinous cell necrosis.

Clinical Findings: This disorder is characterized by cyclic attacks of symmetrically distributed, erythematous plaques that peel full-thickness stratum corneum from the center outward. The onset may begin in infancy or may be delayed until adolescence. The disorder tends to improve by middle age. The disorder is often worse in winter and may be precipitated by fever or surgical operations. Characteristically, the palms and soles are involved, but the disorder of cornification may spill over to dorsal surfaces or occur elsewhere on the body. Histologically, an unusual pattern of necrosis of the spinous cell layers with overlying parakeratosis is present above a zone of basaloid proliferation. As a normal epidermis reforms, the damaged malphigian and corneal layers are lifted outward.

Complications: Attacks may be precipitated by fever or surgical operations.

Associated Findings: None known.

Etiology: Autosomal dominant inheritance with high penetrance.

Pathogenesis: Focal necrobiosis of spinous cell layers results in absence of stratum granulosum and parakeratosis. The basal cells underlying these necrobiotic foci proliferate to form six to eight cell layers, and differentiation to spinous cells appears to be blocked.

CDC No.: 757.190

Sex Ratio: Presumably M1:F1.

Occurrence: This disorder has been described primarily in descendants of nineteenth century farmers in the Oudtshoorn district of the Cape of South Africa.

Risk of Recurrence for Patient's Sib:
See Part I, *Mendelian Inheritance.*

Risk of Recurrence for Patient's Child:
See Part I, *Mendelian Inheritance.*

Age of Detectability: Usually clinically evident by adolescence, but may have its onset in infancy.

Gene Mapping and Linkage: Unknown.

Prevention: None known. Genetic counseling indicated. Avoidance of precipitating factors.

Treatment: Unknown.

Prognosis: Improves with age. Usually resolved or of trivial severity after middle age.

Detection of Carrier: History and clinical examination should allow detection of affected adults.

References:
Findlay GH, Morrison JGH: Erythrokeratolysis hiemalis-keratolytic winter erythema or "Oudtshoorn skin": a new epidermal genodermatosis with its histological features. Br J Dermatol 1978; 98:491–495.

WI013   **Mary L. Williams**

Skin, generalized folded with an underlying lipomatous nevus
See MICHELIN TIRE BABY SYNDROME

SKIN, HYPERKERATOSIS, FOCAL PALMOPLANTAR AND GINGIVAL   2096

Includes:
Gingival hyperkeratosis-hyperkeratosis palmoplantaris
Keratosis, focal palmoplantar and gingival
Palmoplantar hyperkeratosis-gingival hyperkeratosis

Excludes:
Hyperkeratosis palmoplantaris-periodontoclasia (0494)
Hyperkeratosis (other)

Major Diagnostic Criteria: The combination of hyperkeratosis palmoplantaris and attached gingival hyperkeratosis in a kindred.

Clinical Findings: *Skin:* Hyperkeratosis appears around puberty and progresses with age. There is focal-to-widespread hyperkeratosis of the soles of the foot, generally more prominent over the weightbearing areas (the heels, toe pads, and metatarsal heads). These may be painful and can affect ambulation. Hyperkeratosis also occurs on the palms and appears related to trauma. Hyperhidrosis is found in the hyperkeratotic areas. Subungual and circumungual keratin deposits can be found in the toenails at about 4–5 years of age, followed by fingernail changes at ages 8–9 years. Follicular keratoses of the sebaceous areas of the face are common.

Oral: Sharply marginated hyperkeratosis involves the labial and lingual attached gingiva. The hard palate, beneath denture-bearing areas, and the lateral bodies or dorsum of the tongue may also be affected. Oral hyperkeratotic areas appear in early childhood and progress in severity with age.

Microscopic examination shows paranuclear bodies in the spinous and granular cell layers of the keratinocytes of the gingival epithelium. Ultrastructure changes show these to be condensed tonofilaments.

Complications: Painful hyperkeratosis of the soles may interfere with ambulation.

Associated Findings: Many disorders may be associated with hyperkeratosis palmoplantaris. Generalized oral hyperkeratosis, especially of the buccal mucosa, is often reported.

Etiology: Autosomal dominant inheritance.

Pathogenesis: Unknown.

MIM No.: *14873

CDC No.: 757.900

Sex Ratio: M1:F1

Occurrence: Seven kindreds have been documented.

Risk of Recurrence for Patient's Sib:
See Part I, *Mendelian Inheritance.*

Risk of Recurrence for Patient's Child:
See Part I, *Mendelian Inheritance.*

Age of Detectability: During childhood, usually by age five years.

Gene Mapping and Linkage: Unknown.

Prevention: None known. Genetic counseling indicated.

Treatment: Unknown.

Prognosis: Good for life span and intelligence; ambulation may be inhibited.

Detection of Carrier: By clinical examination.

References:
Raphael AL, et al.: Hyperkeratosis of gingival and plantar surfaces. Periodontics 1968; 6:118–120.
Fred HL, et al.: Keratosis palmaris et plantaris. Arch Intern Med 1974; 113:866–871.
Gorlin RJ: Focal palmoplantar and marginal gingival hyperkeratosis in a syndrome. BD:OAS XII(5). New York: March of Dimes Birth Defects Foundation, 1976:239–242.
Roth W, et al.: Hereditary painful callosities. Arch Dermatol 1978; 114:591–592.
Laskaris G, et al.: Focal palmoplantar and oral mucosa hyperkeratosis syndrome: a report concerning five members of a family. Oral Surg 1980; 50:250–253.
Young WG, et al.: Focal palmoplantar and gingival hyperkeratosis syndrome: report of a family, with cytologic, ultrastructural and histochemical findings. Oral Surg 1982; 53:473–482.

G0038   **Robert J. Gorlin**

Skin, hyperkeratotic papules or plaques
See SKIN, POROKERATOSIS

SKIN, HYPERPIGMENTATION, FAMILIAL   2362

Includes:
"Carbon baby"
Hyperpigmentation, familial progressive
Melanosis, universal
Skin, universal melanosis

Excludes:
Acromelanosis progressiva
Dermal melanocytosis
Hyperpigmentation of eyelids
Hyperpigmentation of Fuldauer and Kuijpers
Intestinal polyposis, juvenile type (2259)
Melasma, idiopathic
Neurocutaneous melanosis (2014)
Polyposis-alopecia-pigmentation-nail defects (3040)
Reticulate pigmented anomaly of the flexures
Skin, cutaneous melanosis

Major Diagnostic Criteria: *Autosomal dominant:* scattered, hyperpigmented macular spots, streaks, and whorls that gradually enlarge in size and are associated with the development of *de novo* areas of hyperpigmentation. *Autosomal recessive:* normally pigmented skin that develops diffuse hyperpigmentation. Normal vision.

Clinical Findings: Two types of familial hyperpigmentation have been described.
Autosomal dominant: Multiple macular hyperpigmented spots, streaks, and whorls involving the face, trunk, genitalia, and extensor surfaces of the extremities are present at birth and increase in size with time. New areas of hyperpigmentation develop. The increase in hyperpigmentation is rapid in childhood, but then slows in adolescence and is very slow in adults. The oral-buccal mucosa and conjunctiva are involved, as are the palms and soles, and more than 80% of the body is eventually hyperpigmented, with the remaining skin normally pigmented. Areas of hyperpigmented and normally pigmented skin may give a marbled appearance. The retina is not involved, and vision is normal. No other abnormalities are present. Histologic examina-

tion of the skin shows an increase in melanin pigment, particularly in the basal cell layer, by light microscopy and normal melanocytes, with larger, more numerous melanosomes, by electron microscopy.

Autosomal recessive: The skin is normally pigmented at birth. A gradual increase in skin pigment starts at ages 4–12 months and progresses to age five years, after which the hyperpigmentation partially recedes. The hyperpigmentation starts with the scalp, the external genitalia and groin, or the abdomen and spreads to involve the face, trunk, and extremities with minimal involvement of the palms and soles. Mucosal pigment is present. The hair is normal or variably pigmented. As the pigment recedes, the child is left with zones of skin, involving large parts of the body, that vary from normal pigmentation to yellow-to-dark pigmentation. Multiple small, white macules develop in the groin and on the trunk, with areas of coalescence. No other abnormalities are present. Histologic examination of the skin shows an increase in number and size of melanocytes in the basal layer and the dermis by light microscopy. The irregularly shaped cells are filled with pigmented melanosomes and can be found in clumps.

Complications: Unknown.

Associated Findings: None known.

Etiology: Autosomal dominant and autosomal recessive inheritance have both been reported.

Pathogenesis: Unknown.

MIM No.: 14525, *15580

CDC No.: 757.900

Sex Ratio: Presumably M1:F1.

Occurrence: More than a dozen families have been reported.

Risk of Recurrence for Patient's Sib:
See Part I, *Mendelian Inheritance.*

Risk of Recurrence for Patient's Child:
See Part I, *Mendelian Inheritance.*

Age of Detectability: The first year of life.

Gene Mapping and Linkage: Unknown.

Prevention: None known. Genetic counseling indicated.

Treatment: Unknown.

Prognosis: Undetermined. Probably normal life span.

Detection of Carrier: Unknown.

Special Considerations: These two conditions appear to be the result of separate genes affecting melanocyte physiology. A condition called *carbon baby* has been described by Ruiz-Maldonado et al (1978) and may be similar to autosomal recessive familial hyperpigmentation as described above. In the carbon baby, diffuse hyperpigmentation began at age six months and continued until all of the skin and mucous membranes were black, at which time the white undergarments turned gray after being worn. The pigmentation had not receded by age four years. Electron microscopy showed normal melanocyte number with an increase in normal-sized melanosomes. This Mexican boy had two normally pigmented brothers.

References:

Wende GW, Bauckus HH: A hitherto undescribed generalized pigmentation of the skin appearing in infancy in brother and sister. J Cutan Genitourinary Dis 1919; 37:685–701.
Carleton A, Biggs R: Diffuse mesodermal pigmentation with congenital cranial abnormality. Br J Derm 1948; 60:10.
Pegum JS: Diffuse pigmentation in brothers. Proc R Soc Med 1955; 48:179–180.
Chernosky ME, et al.: Familial progressive hyperpigmentation. Arch Dermatol 1971; 103:581–591.
Ruiz-Maldonado R, et al.: Universal acquired melanosis. Arch Dermatol 1978; 114:775–778.
Bashito HM, et al.: General dermal melanocytosis. Arch Derm 1981; 117:791.

Richard A. King

SKIN, KERATOSIS FOLLICULARIS SPINULOSA DECALVANS   2867

Includes:
Ichthyosis follicularis
Keratosis follicularis spinulosa decalvans cum ophiasi

Excludes:
Darier disease (2865)
Ichthyosiform erythrokeratoderma, atypical with deafness (2861)

Major Diagnostic Criteria: Progressive follicular hyperkeratosis on face and scalp resulting in progressive cicatricial alopecia.

Clinical Findings: Noninflammatory follicular hyperkeratosis begins in infancy on the face and progress during childhood to involve the trunk and extremities. In later childhood and adolescence scarring alopecia develops on the eyebrows and scalp. Many patients also develop hyperkeratosis of the palms and soles in adolescence. Photophobia is common and may be due to punctate corneal defects. Atopic diathesis also occurs.

Complications: Permanent hair loss due to scarring alopecia develops in most patients.

Associated Findings: Photophobia, corneal defects, and atopic diathesis.

Etiology: Autosomal dominant inheritance, possibly with more severe manifestations in males. Families with an X-linked pattern of inheritance have also been reported. Sporadic cases have been reported.

Pathogenesis: Unknown.

MIM No.: *30880

CDC No.: 757.900

Sex Ratio: M1:F<1. A predominance of males has been reported in the literature.

Occurrence: Undetermined. Established literature.

Risk of Recurrence for Patient's Sib:
See Part I, *Mendelian Inheritance.*

Risk of Recurrence for Patient's Child:
See Part I, *Mendelian Inheritance.*

Age of Detectability: In sporadic cases, diagnosis may not be apparent until adolescence when full progression of the disease is evident. In families at risk, facial follicular hyperkeratoses are usually evident in infancy.

Gene Mapping and Linkage: Unknown.

Prevention: None known. Genetic counseling indicated.

Treatment: Topical agents to loosen keratoses (e.g., 5–10% lactic acid) usually are ineffective. Due to their long-term toxicity, use of oral synthetic retinoids should be considered experimental at present.

Prognosis: Progressive scarring alopecia; otherwise, normal life span and intelligence.

Detection of Carrier: By clinical examination.

Special Considerations: In patients with photophobia, **Ichthyosiform erythrokeratoderma, atypical with deafness** should be excluded. An X-linked recessive disorder with more extensive follicular hyperkeratoses, absence of scarring alopecia, absent or atrophic sebaceous glands, and hyperkeratotic plaques of extensor extremities has been delineated by Eramo et al. (1985). Moreover, localized forms of follicular hyperkeratoses with scarring but without photophobia have also been reported.

References:

Kuokkanen K: Keratosis follicularis spinulosa decalvans in a family from Northern Finland. Acta Dermatovener (Stockholm) 1941; 51: 156–160.
Rand R, Baden HP: Keratosis follicularis spinulosa decalvans: report of two cases and literature review. Arch Dermatol 1983; 119:22–26.
Eramo LR, et al.: Ichthyosis follicularis with alopecia and photophobia. Arch Dermatol 1985; 121:1167–1174.

Mary L. Williams

SKIN, KYRLE DISEASE 0561

Includes:

Hyperkeratosis follicularis et parafollicularis in cutem penetrans

Kyrle disease

Excludes:

Hyperkeratosis lenticularis perstans

Perforating folliculitis

Major Diagnostic Criteria: Follicular and parafollicular hyperkeratotic papules. Kyrle sign; a central keratotic plug which, when removed, leaves a corresponding crater.

Clinical Findings: *Distribution:* Widespread, symmetrical, especially arms and legs. Sparing of palms, soles, and mucous membranes.

Morphology: Papules 1–8 mm diameter, follicular or parafollicular, with central hyperkeratotic plug up to 1.5 cm diameter protruding from a crateriform depression. Lesions may be linear or they coalesce into plaques or verrucous streaks. Verrucous streaks usually occur on flexural surfaces.

Natural History: Lesions occur in crops that last several weeks and heal with with minimal or no scarring. The condition is asymptomatic.

Pathology: Epithelial invagination filled by a plug of hyperkeratosis and parakeratosis and containing basophilic cellular debris. Adjacent to plug, epidermis may be acanthotic or atrophic. Granulomatous dermal reaction with infiltrate of neutrophils and lymphocytes and foreign body giant cells. A mild perivascular infiltrate may be seen.

Complications: Unknown.

Associated Findings: *Ocular:* Posterior subcapsular cataracts. Yellow-brown anterior corneal opacities.

Systemic: Diabetes mellitus, chronic renal failure, cardiac failure, pachyonychia congenita. These conditions usually occur in association with nongenetic Kyrle disease.

Etiology: Possibly autosomal dominant inheritance, but most often nongenetic. (No male-male transmission reported.)

Pathogenesis: Unknown.

MIM No.: 14950

CDC No.: 757.900

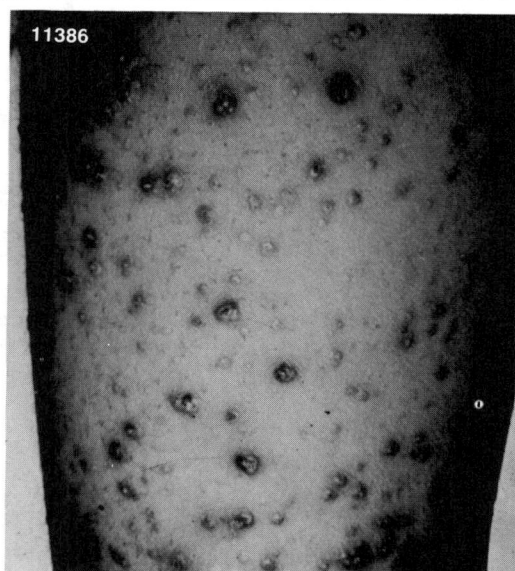

0561-11386: Kyrle disease.

Sex Ratio: M1:F1

Occurrence: Undetermined but presumably rare.

Risk of Recurrence for Patient's Sib:

See Part I, *Mendelian Inheritance.*

Risk of Recurrence for Patient's Child:

See Part I, *Mendelian Inheritance.*

Age of Detectability: Onset in third to seventh decade of life.

Gene Mapping and Linkage: Unknown.

Prevention: None known. Genetic counseling indicated.

Treatment: Vitamin A 100,000 units daily; topical keratolytic ointments.

Prognosis: Usually good. Associated systemic disease may alter life expectancy.

Detection of Carrier: Unknown.

References:

Constantine VS, Carter VH: Kyrles disease I. clinical findings in five cases and a review of the literature. Arch Dermatol 1968; 97:624–632.

Constantine VS, Carter VH. Kyrles disease I. histologic findings in five cases and review of the literature. Arch Dermatol 1968; 97:633–639.

Tessler HH, et al.: Ocular findings in a kindred with Kyrle disease. Arch Ophthal 1973; 90:278–280.

Der Kaloustian UM, Kurban AK: Genetic diseases of the skin. Berlin: Springer Verlag, 1979.

Patterson JW: The perforating disorders. J Am Acad Derm 1984; 10:561–581.

Rook A, et al.: Textbook of dermatology, 4th ed. Oxford: Blackwell Scientific Publications, 1986.

WI055

Ingrid M. Winship

SKIN, LEIOMYOMAS, MULTIPLE 0890

Includes:

Leiomyomata, hereditary multiple, of skin

Leiomyomata, multiple cutaneous

Excludes: Skin nodules, other

Major Diagnostic Criteria: Cutaneous leiomyomata are known to occur as solitary or multifocal skin tumors arising from the pilar arrector muscles of the skin.

Clinical Findings: Cutaneous leiomyomata are known to occur as solitary or multifocal skin tumors arising from the pilar arrector muscles of the skin. They are usually less than 15 mm in diameter and appear as a collection of pink to reddish-brown firm intradermal nodules. These benign tumors grow slowly over a period of several years, mostly beginning in late infancy, with new lesions forming as others stabilize. They may occur on any cutaneous surface but most commonly on thighs, lips, and buttocks.

Complications: Unknown.

Associated Findings: Uterine leiomyomata, occurring before the age of 20 years, were documented in a number of female patients.

Etiology: Autosomal dominant inheritance with incomplete penetrance.

Pathogenesis: Recently, a severely mentally retarded adult female with chromosome 9p trisomy/18pter monosomy was reported. In addition to a **Chromosome 9, trisomy 9p** phenotype, this patient presented with multiple cutaneous leiomyomata, raising the question whether the occurrence of the chromosomal anomaly and the multiple skin tumors indicates another example of a specific chromosomal deletion (18pter) in a dominantly inherited multiple human tumor.

Histologic examination identifies the skin lesions as benign tumors of smooth muscle fibers, originating in the pilomotor muscle.

MIM No.: *15080

CDC No.: 757.900

Sex Ratio: M1:F1

Occurrence: Undetermined but presumed rare.

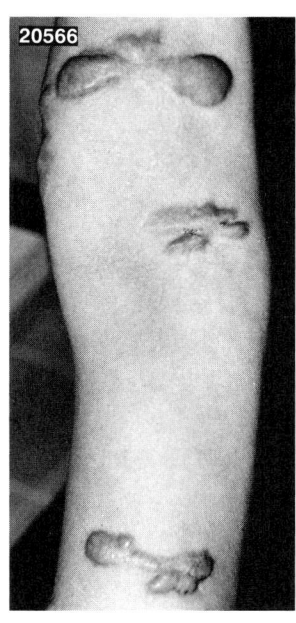
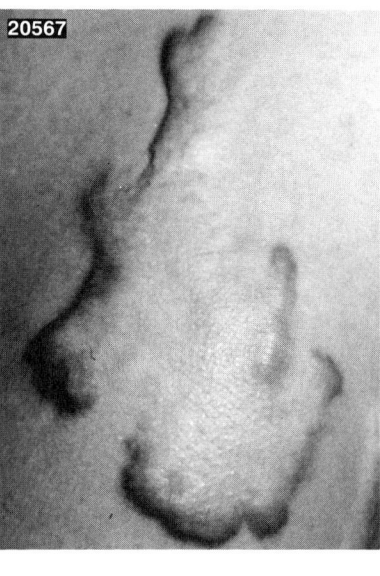

0890-20566–67: Note nodular and linear type of multiple cutaneous leiomyomata.

Risk of Recurrence for Patient's Sib:
See Part I, *Mendelian Inheritance.*

Risk of Recurrence for Patient's Child:
See Part I, *Mendelian Inheritance.*

Age of Detectability: About one-half are detectable before 20 years of years.

Gene Mapping and Linkage: Unknown.

Prevention: None known. Genetic counseling indicated.

Treatment: Surgical excision if symptomatic.

Prognosis: Normal for life span and health.

Detection of Carrier: Unknown.

References:
Berendes U, et al.: Segmentary and disseminated lesions in multiple hereditary cutaneous leiomyoma. Hum Genet 1971; 13:81–82.
Engelke H, Christopher E: Leiomyomatosis cutis et uteri. Acta Derm Venereol Stockh 1979; 59(Suppl 85):52–54.
Fryns JP, et al.: 9p Trisomy/18 distal monosomy and multiple cutaneous leiomyomata. Hum Genet 1985; 70:284–286.

FR030   **Jean-Pierre Fryns**

SKIN, LIPOID PROTEINOSIS   0599

Includes:
    Hyalinosis cutis et mucosae
    Lipoglycoproteinosis
    Lipoproteinosis
    Urbach-Wiethe disease

Excludes: Porphyria, protoporphyria (0362)

Major Diagnostic Criteria: Typical skin and mucosal lesions due to an increased deposition of a hyaline material in the dermis. This deposition may also involve other organs. Hoarseness may be noted early in the course of the condition.

Clinical Findings: Skin lesions usually appear during childhood as vesiculopustular lesions on the face and distal extremities. These lesions usually heal with residual depressed acneiform scars. With time, the deposition of hyaline material increases and gradually the susceptible skin and mucosa become irregularly filled with yellowish, pale hyaline deposits in plaques, and papules, nodules on the face and neck. Areas of increased friction (hands, elbows, and knees) are most affected and may be covered with hyperpigmented, hyperkeratotic patches. A characteristic finding is the presence of papules on the eyelid margins, producing "itchy eyes" and a distortion of the eyelashes. However, cutaneous changes may occur on any part of the skin. Patchy alopecia of the scalp or beard is a relatively common finding. The mucous membranes that are most involved include the mouth, larynx, and pharynx. The soft palate may appear thickened and the tongue is often firm and difficult to protrude. Laryngeal examination usually shows a thickened epiglottis, swollen arytenoids, and aryepiglottic folds. Increased stiffness of the vocal cords resulting in hoarseness is a pathognomic sign, often being the first clinical manifestation. Narrowing of the pharynx may occur. An obstruction of the Stensen duct by the infiltrate may cause recurrent parotitis and faulty dentition. Lesions can also be found in the gastrointestinal tract but are usually asymptomatic. Wart-like lesions of unknown origin may be present in the trachea and main bronchi. The neurologic findings are characterized by hippocampal calcifications on either side of the sella turcica or as bilateral calcifications lateral or just above the dorsum sellae. Intracranial calcifications have been found in 52% of the cases. Epilepsy may occur, but seems to be a less common finding than intracranial calcifications as a neurologic sign. The ocular manifestations include moniliform blepharitis (two-thirds of the cases) and, rarely, corneal opacities, glaucoma, and drusen.

Complications: Narrowing of the larynx and pharynx may require tracheostomy to ensure adequate ventilation.

Associated Findings: Diabetes mellitus, conductive deafness, mental retardation. Severe loss of memory with intact intellect has been reported without involvement of both hippocampi. Pseudomembranous conjunctivitis was present in one case.

Etiology: Autosomal recessive inheritance.

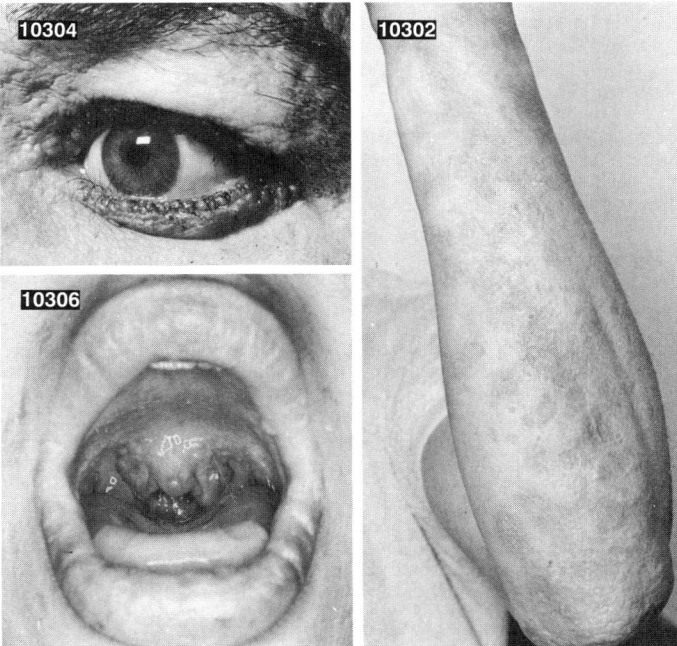

0599-10304: Characteristic row of nodules along left lower eyelid. 10306: Thickening of lip and nodular lesions on pharynx. 10302: Large atrophic scars on the forearm.

Pathogenesis: Biochemical and electron microscopic (EM) studies have shown that the hyaline deposit arises from basal laminae produced by endothelial cells, pericytes, Schwann cells, perineural cells, myofibroblasts, smooth muscle cells, and epithelial cells. The reason for the multilamination of the basal laminae is still obscure. EM studies show that the hyaline substance is composed of a very fine network of procollagen filaments interlinked with amorphous granular material. Recently it was confirmed that the affected dermis contains excessive amounts of matrix glycoproteins and decreased quantities of collagen fibers. Some authors suggest that multilamination may represent either a particular lysosomal storage disease due to single or multiple enzyme defects resulting in defective degradation or a disorder in which cellular activity (fibroblasts and epithelial and endothelial cells) is altered such that fibrous collagens are underproduced and basement membrane collagens overproduced.

MIM No.: *24710

CDC No.: 757.900

Sex Ratio: M1:F1

Occurrence: Over 280 cases have been described, and most of the patients appear to be of European descent. Cases have been reported most often in South Africa. It is there that the responsible gene is thought to have been introduced by a German settler and his sister.

Risk of Recurrence for Patient's Sib:
See Part I, *Mendelian Inheritance.*

Risk of Recurrence for Patient's Child:
See Part I, *Mendelian Inheritance.*

Age of Detectability: During the first few years of life. Hoarseness is often present at birth.

Gene Mapping and Linkage: Unknown.

Prevention: None known. Genetic counseling indicated.

Treatment: Carbon dioxide laser treatment of thickened vocal cords has proved to be effective for hoarseness. Anticonvulsants should be prescribed for affected individuals who develop epilepsy. Tracheostomy is necessary in some cases due to laryngeal obstruction.

Prognosis: The disease usually runs a chronic and benign course, generally with no shortening of life span.

Detection of Carrier: Unknown.

References:
Fabrizi G, et al.: Urbach-Wiethe disease: light and electron microscopic study. J Cutan Pathol 1980; 7:8–20.
Bauer EA, et al.: Lipoid proteinosis: in vivo and in vitro evidence for a lysosomal storage disease. J Invest Dermatol 1981; 76:119–125.
Ishibashi A: Hyalinosis cutis et mucosae: defective digestion and storage of basal lamina glycoprotein synthesized by smooth muscle cells. Dermatologica 1982; 165:7–15.
Haneke E, et al.: Hyalinosis cutis et mucosae in siblings. Hum Genet 1984; 68:342–345.
Harper JI, et al.: Lipoid proteinosis: an inherited disorder of collagen metabolism? Br J Dermatol 1985; 113:145–151.
Yakout YM, et al.: Radiological findings in lipoid proteinosis. J Laryngol Otol 1985; 99:259–265.
Barthelemy H, et al.: Lipoid proteinosis with pseudomembranous conjunctivitis. J Am Acad Dermatol 1986; 14:367–371.
Moy LS, et al.: Lipoid proteinosis: ultrastructural and biochemical studies. J Am Acad Dermatol 1987; 16:1193–1201.
Pierard GE, et al.: A clinicopathologic study of six cases of lipoid proteinosis. Am J Dermopathol 1988; 10:300–305.

Giuseppe Micali

SKIN, LOCALIZED ABSENCE OF   0608

Includes:
    Aplasia cutis congenita (ACC)
    Carmi syndrome
    Gastrointestinal atresia-aplasia cutis congenital
    Localized absence of skin
    Skull and scalp, congenital defect

Excludes:
    Dermal hypoplasia, focal (0281)
    Epidermolysis bullosum, type III (2562)
    Parietal foramina, symmetric

Major Diagnostic Criteria: Localized absence of skin of scalp, trunk and limbs.

Clinical Findings: Localized absence of skin at birth. Most commonly seen on scalp, usually at the apex on or near the midline. Presents as ulcer with absence of both skin and hair. Serous membrane may cover subcutaneous tissue. Crusting is followed by healing in a few weeks leaving a fine depressed hairless scar. A similar condition may involve the trunk and limbs, particularly the lower legs.

Complications: Underlying skull, meninges and brain may be included in defect.

Associated Findings: Unilateral ear anomalies, facial paresis and dermal sinuses may occur. Rarely associated with gastrointestinal atresias or other malformations.

    Localized absence of skin occasionally seen in **Chromosome 13, trisomy 13, Chromosome 18, trisomy 18, Chromosome 4, monosomy 4p, Dermal hypoplasia, focal,** recessive dystrophic **Epidermolysis bullosa,** symmetric parietal foramina, **Johanson-Blizzard syndrome** and **Limb and scalp defects, Adams-Oliver type**.

Etiology: Autosomal dominant inheritance of a predominantly "scalp defect". Autosomal recessive inheritance of some instances of scalp/skull defects, and trunk and limb sites. Most represent isolated cases.

Pathogenesis: Localized developmental abnormality of skin. Amniotic adhesions no longer accepted as cause.

MIM No.: *10760, 20770, *20773.

CDC No.: 757.395

Sex Ratio: M1:F1

Occurrence: Approximately 250 cases reported.

Risk of Recurrence for Patient's Sib:
See Part I, *Mendelian Inheritance.*

Risk of Recurrence for Patient's Child:
See Part I, *Mendelian Inheritance.*

Age of Detectability: At birth by examination of skin.

Gene Mapping and Linkage: Unknown.

Prevention: None known. Genetic counseling indicated.

Treatment: If defect covers large area, skin grafting may be required.

Prognosis: Excellent except in rare patients with associated complications.

Detection of Carrier: Unknown.

References:
Deekin JH, Caplan RM: Aplasia cutis congenita. Arch Dermatol 1970; 102:386–389.
McMurray BR, et al.: Hereditary aplasia cutis congenita and associated defects: three instances in one family and a survey of reported cases. Clin Pediatr 1977; 16:610–614.
Dubosson J-D, Schneider P: Manifestation familiale d'une aplasie cutanee circonscrite du vertex (ACCV), associele dans un cas a une malformation candiaque. J Genet Hum 1978; 26:351–365.
Anderson CE, et al.: Autosomal dominantly inherited cutis aplasia congenita, ear malformations, right-sided facial paresis, and dermal sinuses. BD:OAS XV(5b) New York: March of Dimes Birth Defects Foundation, 1979:265–270.

Carmi R, et al.: Aplasia cutis congenita in two sibs discordant for pyloric atresia. Am J Med Genet 1982; 11:319–328.
Sybert VP: Aplasia cutis congenita: a report of 12 new families and review of the literature. Pediatr Dermatol 1985; 3:1–14.
Frieden IJ: Aplasia cutis congenita: a clinical review and proposal for classification. J Am Acad Dermat 1986; 14:646–660.

LA007   **Roger L. Ladda**

Skin, Naegeli syndrome
See ECTODERMAL DYSPLASIA, NAEGELI TYPE

SKIN, PAINFUL PLANTAR CALLOSITIES   2895

Includes:
    Brauer keratoderma palmoplantar
    Buschke-Fischer keratoderma palmoplantar
    Callosities, painful plantar
    Plantar callosities, autosomal dominant painful

Excludes: Skin (other defects)

Major Diagnostic Criteria: Noncongenital plantar callosities.

Clinical Findings: Plantar callosities that arise with upright ambulation and persist (these are always present over the pressure points of the soles). Warm and oily feet. Bullae at the edge of the callosities are formed when the patients walk too much, contain a malodorous liquid, and tend to quickly burst. In one large Brazilian kindred (Rachid et al, 1987), no instance of palmar callosities was mentioned even in individuals engaged in heavy manual labor. Osteoarticular X-ray aspects were normal.

Complications: Discomfort and pain during walking.

Associated Findings: None known.

Etiology: Autosomal dominant inheritance.

Pathogenesis: Unknown.

MIM No.: *11414

CDC No.: 757.900

Sex Ratio: Presumably M1:F1.

Occurrence: One Caucasian family was verified to have 31 affected persons (13 men and 18 women) in six generations. About 50 cases of possible variants have been reported in the literature.

Risk of Recurrence for Patient's Sib:
    See Part I, *Mendelian Inheritance.*

Risk of Recurrence for Patient's Child:
    See Part I, *Mendelian Inheritance.*

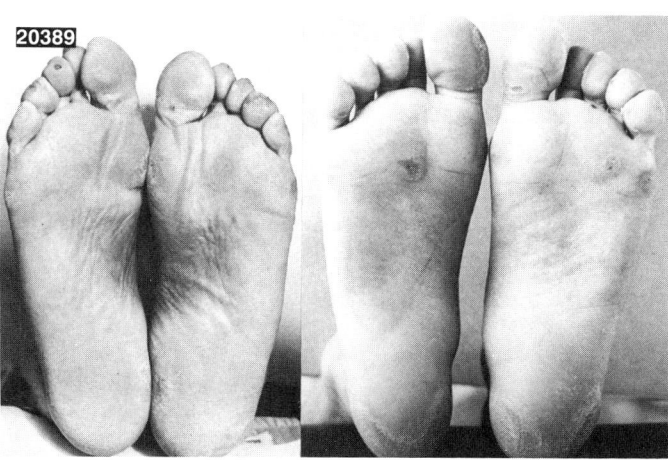

2895-20389: Feet of two patients with plantar callosities.

Age of Detectability: During childhood, after upright ambulation, by physical examination.

Gene Mapping and Linkage: Unknown.

Prevention: None known. Genetic counseling indicated.

Treatment: Hot water and brine alleviate the pain; aromatic tretinoin taken orally may also relieve this genodermatosis.

Prognosis: Normal life span. The callosities and bullae never bleed and tend to regress during winter.

Detection of Carrier: Unknown.

Special Considerations: Some authors consider *Brauer keratoderma palmoplantar, Buschke-Fischer keratoderma palmoplantar,* and other conditions which may or may not involve palmar callosites to be variants of the above described condition. The present author restricts this diagnosis to a condition with *only* plantar callosities.

References:
Roth W, et al.: Hereditary painful callosities. Arch Derm 1978; 114: 591–592.
Dupré A, et al.: Treatment of hereditary painful callosities with tretinoin. Arch Dermatol 1979; 115:638–639.
Baden HP, et al.: Hereditary callosities with blisters: report of a family and review. J Am Acad Derm 1984; 11:409–415.
Rachid A, et al.: Autosomal dominant painful plantar callosities. Am J Med Genet 1987; 26:185–187. * †

FR033   **Newton Freire-Maia**

SKIN, PALMO-PLANTAR ERYTHEMA   0792

Includes:
    Erythema palmare hereditarium
    Erythema palmo-plantar
    Lane disease
    Palmo-plantar erythema
    Red palms

Excludes: N/A

Major Diagnostic Criteria: Constant erythema of palmar surfaces of fingers.

Clinical Findings: Constant symmetrical bright mottled erythema over the thenar and hypothenar eminence, palmar surface at the base of the fingers, and the palmar surfaces of the fingers. May involve the soles. Asymptomatic red zone sharply demarcated at wrist crease and side of hands.

Complications: Unknown.

Associated Findings: Keratosis palmaris et plantaris diffusa in certain affected families. May be associated with liver disease, rheumatoid arthritis, chronic immunologic diseases, aging, pregnancy.

Etiology: While McKusick reports observing the trait in successive generations, etiology is still unclear. Possibly of multifactorial etiology.

Pathogenesis: Unknown.

MIM No.: *13300

CDC No.: 757.900

Sex Ratio: Presumably M1:F1.

Occurrence: Undetermined but presumed rare.

Risk of Recurrence for Patient's Sib: Unknown.

Risk of Recurrence for Patient's Child: Unknown.

Age of Detectability: Unknown.

Gene Mapping and Linkage: Unknown.

Prevention: None known. Genetic counseling indicated.

Treatment: None required.

Prognosis: Benign asymtomatic condition.

Detection of Carrier: Unknown.

Special Considerations: The condition was first described in two patients in 1929. The lesion is indistinguishable from, if not precisely the same phenomenon as, palmar erythema of liver disease, normal pregnancy, rheumatoid arthritis, and perhaps many other diseases. Even such nonspecific states as aging may show red palms. The evidence that it is hereditary is very thin indeed; the heritable etiology of palmar erythema seems to be unfortunately perpetuated from book to book and in published papers since its first casual appearance in 1929.

References:

Lane JE: Erytheme palmare hereditarium. Arch Dermatol Syph (Chic) 1929;20:445–448.

Olivier J: Erytheme jpalmo-plantaire hereditarire: maladie de Lane. Arch Belg Derm Syph 1956;12:202–207.

Bland JH, et al.: Palmar erythema and spider angiomata in rheumatoid arthritis. Ann Intern Med 1958;48:1026–1032.

LA007   **Roger L. Ladda**

SKIN, PARANA HARD SKIN SYNDROME   3051

Includes: Parana hard skin syndrome

Excludes: Stiff skin syndrome (2629)

Major Diagnostic Criteria: Progressive rigidity of skin, commencing in the second to third month of life, with subsequent growth retardation.

Clinical Findings: At two to three months of age, the skin and subcutaneous tissue progressively harden, forming an immovable cast. All but the eyelid, neck and ear skin is involved. As the skin hardens, growth decelerates with eventual joint, chest, and abdominal wall immobility. Additional findings include hirsutism, hyperpigmentation of the skin, and enlargement of the parotid glands.

Complications: Lichenification of skin in flexure areas and pulmonary insufficiency are the most common complications.

Associated Findings: None known.

Etiology: The occurrence of this condition in siblings and in an offspring of a consanguineous mating suggests autosomal recessive inheritance.

Pathogenesis: Unknown. Histologic studies of the skin have been uninformative.

MIM No.: 26053

POS No.: 4006

Sex Ratio: M1:F1

Occurrence: Reported in eight persons from seven families in the Parana region of Brazil.

Risk of Recurrence for Patient's Sib:
See Part I, *Mendelian Inheritance.*

Risk of Recurrence for Patient's Child:
See Part I, *Mendelian Inheritance.*

Age of Detectability: Evident by three months of age.

Gene Mapping and Linkage: Unknown.

Prevention: None known. Genetic counseling indicated.

Treatment: Symptomatic; known treatmens are probably ineffective in preventing the progressive skin hardening.

Prognosis: The skin hardening is progressive, death as a result of pulmonary insufficiency appears to be inevitable. Intellect appears unimpaired.

Detection of Carrier: Possibly by clinical examination.

References:

Cat I, et al: Parana hard-skin syndrome: study of seven families. Lancet 1974; I:215–216.

T0007   **Helga V. Toriello**

Skin, pemphigus, benign familial
See PEMPHIGUS, BENIGN FAMILIAL

SKIN, PITYRIASIS RUBRA PILARIS   0811

Includes:
Lichen acuminatus
Lichen ruber acuminatus
Pityriasis pilaris
Pityriasis rubra pilaris

Excludes:
Exfoliative dermatitis-pityriasis rubra pilaris
Ichthyosis
Keratosis pilaris
Phrynoderma
Skin, erythrokeratodermia, progressiva symmetrica (2863)
Skin, psoriasis vulgaris (0833)

Major Diagnostic Criteria: Pathognomonic black horny follicular plugs on the backs of the fingers; hyperkeratosis of palms and soles. The yellowish or grayish-red to orange or salmon-yellow color of the plaques, with islands of normal skin, and the dry scaliness of the face and scalp, are diagnostic.

Clinical Findings: Persistent, dry, horny, acuminate, follicular papules on the dorsal surfaces of the first and second phalanges. These are symmetrically distributed, pinhead in size, brownish-red to rosy-yellow in color, and enclose a dry lusterless atrophic hair in their keratotic centers. The horny central plugs are often capped by a black point. Multiplication and coalescence of papules form plaques, which are symmetrically distributed. The plaques are sharply marginated, with small islands of normal skin within the affected areas. The skin looks like goose flesh and feels like a nutmeg grater.

Nails are dull, rough, brittle, and frequently transversely striated. They are lusterless, and gray or yellow in color. Palms and soles exhibit firm thick reddish-yellow hyperkeratosis, which scales freely, and often become fissured. The face is red, thickened, inelastic, and often there is ectropion of the lower lids.

Complications: Unknown.

Associated Findings: Liver disease, neuromuscular dysfunction, rheumatism, psoriasis, and hormonal dysfunction.

Etiology: Autosomal dominant inheritance with incomplete penetrance. Most cases are sporadic. The hereditatry form tends to be less severe and more limited in extent, and does not show lesions at birth.

Pathogenesis: Unknown.

MIM No.: *17320

CDC No.: 757.900

Sex Ratio: M1:F1

Occurrence: Familial cases reported in a few families.

Risk of Recurrence for Patient's Sib:
See Part I, *Mendelian Inheritance.*

Risk of Recurrence for Patient's Child:
See Part I, *Mendelian Inheritance.*

Age of Detectability: From infancy to 70 years of age, without any significant age predilection.

Gene Mapping and Linkage: Unknown.

Prevention: None known. Genetic counseling indicated.

Treatment: Difficult to evaluate because of natural exacerbations and remissions. Vitamin A by mouth ranging from 50,000 to 200,000 units per day. Metrotrexate has been used. Vitamin A alcohol in Lubriderm^ topically has been used successfully.

Prognosis: In 75 patients; 8% resolved completely; 60% improved, 24% remitted and exacerbated, 7% did not change, and 1% became worse.

Detection of Carrier: Unknown.

References:

Lamar LM, Gaethe G: Pityriasis rubra pilaris. Arch Dermatol 1964; 89:515–522.

Davidson CL Jr., et al.: Pityriasis rubra pilaris: a follow-up study of 57 patients. Arch Dermatol 1969; 100:175–178.

Gross DA, et al.: Pityriasis rubra pilaris: report of a case and analysis of the literature. Arch Dermatol 1969; 99:710–716.

Beamer JE, et al.: Pityriasis rubra pilaris. Cutis 1972; 10:419–421.

MY001   **Terry L. Myers**

SKIN, POROKERATOSIS   0819

Includes:
  Disseminated superficial actinic porokeratosis (DSAP)
  Hyperkeratosis eccentrica
  Keratoatrophoderma, chronic progressive
  Linear porokeratosis
  Porokeratosis, linear
  Porokeratosis, plantaris
  Porokeratosis of Mibelli
  Skin, hyperkeratotic papules or plaques

Excludes:
  Keratoderma of palms and soles
  Nevus, epidermal nevus syndrome (0593)

Major Diagnostic Criteria: Hyperkeratotic papules or plaques most frequently noted on dorsum of hands and feet. Histologic examination demonstrates cornoid lamella. Biopsy is required to confirm the diagnosis.

Clinical Findings: The primary lesion is a small hyperkeratotic papule, which gradually enlarges to form a plaque with a raised wall-like border and a depressed center (crater-like). Some lesions remain small, while others may attain a large size. Any part of the integument, even the mucosa, may be involved. The areas most affected are the hands and feet, especially the dorsal surfaces, and the face and neck.

Since the early classic description of porokeratosis by Mibelli, several clinical variants of the disease have been reported. Most investigators now accept the classification of Chernosky (1967), which includes three subdivisions:

1. *Porokeratosis of Mibelli*, which includes the keratotic verrucous form. These centrifugally spreading patches are surrounded by narrow horny ridges with central atrophy, which produce crater-like lesions.

2. *Disseminated superficial actinic porokeratosis (DSAP)* lesions develop in the third to fourth decade, and occur almost only in the sun-exposed areas of the skin.

3. *Porokeratosis palmaris et plantaris disseminata* occurs first in the second or third decade, on the palmar and plantar surfaces; a rare finding in the other two types of porokeratosis. The lesions spread to other body parts and are not limited to sun-exposed areas. The annular or gyrate plaques have elevated borders.

Complications: Malignant degeneration (epidermoid carcinoma) has been reported.

Associated Findings: None known.

Etiology: Autosomal dominant inheritance, possibly with reduced penetrance in females.

Pathogenesis: Undetermined. No relationship to sweat duct, contrary to what is implied by the present name of the disease. Several investigators believe that porokeratosis arises from abnormal clones of keratinocytes, and that the tendency to develop these clones is inherited.

MIM No.: *17580, 17585, *17590

CDC No.: 757.900

Sex Ratio: M2:F1 (observed).

Occurrence: Undetermined but presumed rare. Many cases are mild and may escape notice. Wide ethnic distribution.

Risk of Recurrence for Patient's Sib:
  See Part I, *Mendelian Inheritance*.

Risk of Recurrence for Patient's Child:
  See Part I, *Mendelian Inheritance*.

Age of Detectability: Any age.

Gene Mapping and Linkage: Unknown.

Prevention: None known. Genetic counseling indicated.

Treatment: Excision if feasible. Favorable response to topical 5-fluorouracil has been obtained in some cases of disseminated superficial actinic porokeratosis. Cryosurgery has been found useful for plantar lesions.

Prognosis: Normal for life span and intelligence. Involvement of the face may present cosmetic problems. Although characteristically progressive, lesions may spontaneously involute.

Detection of Carrier: Unknown.

Special Considerations: The name porokeratosis is derived either from the Greek prefix poro (callus) or because Mibelli, the Italian dermatologist who first described the condition, thought that it derived from the sweat glands (pores). A study of cultured fibroblasts from affected areas shows a variety of chromosomal aberrations without any consistent specific abnormality.

References:

Chernosky ME, Freeman RG: Disseminated superficial actinic porokeratosis (DSAP). Arch Dermatol 1967; 96:611–624. * †

Mikhail GR, Wertheimer FW: Clinical variants of porokeratosis (Mibelli). Arch Dermatol 1968; 98:124–131. * †

Guss SB, et al.: Porokeratosis plantaris et disseminata. A third type of porokeratosis. Arch Dermatol 1971; 104:366–373. †

Pirozzi JJ, Rosenthal A: Disseminated superficial actinic porokeratosis: analysis of an affected family. Br J Dermatol 1976; 95:429–432.

Limmer BL: Cryosurgery of porokeratosis plantaris discreta. Arch Dermatol 1979; 115:582–583.

McDonald SG, Peterka ES: Porokeratosis (Mibelli): treatment with topical 5-fluorouracil. J Am Acad Dermatol 1983; 8:107–110.

0819-10307–08: Porokeratosis with classic plaque form and dike-like keratotic borders.

MI005   **George R. Mikhail**

SKIN, PSORIASIS VULGARIS   0833

Includes:
Psoriasis
Pustular psoriasis

Excludes:
Ankylosing spondylitis (2516)
Fetal syphilis syndrome (0385)
Parapsoriasis
Pityriasis rosea
Seborrheic dermatitis
Skin, erythrokeratodermia, progressiva symmetrica (2863)
Skin, pityriasis rubra pilaris (0811)

Major Diagnostic Criteria: Lesions of typical morphology and distribution: erythematous scaling plaques, most frequently on elbows, knees, and scalp. When clinical presentation is atypical, histologic confirmation may be necessary.

Clinical Findings: *Skin:* erythematous plaques on the skin with silver scale; pinpoint bleeding typically on removal of the scale cases. Distribution is usually generalized with a predisposition for the elbows, knees, scalp, and genitalia. Lesions may be symmetric. Palms and soles may be hyperkeratotic. Koebner phenomenon (isomorphic response) well known. Other morphologies of lesions in psoriasis are erythroderma and pustulosis. Pustular psoriasis may be a medical emergency.
Nails: finger- and toenails frequently involved in the form of pitting, dystrophy, and onycholysis.
Joints: arthritis, usually asymmetric and more often monoarticular than polyarticular. Five patterns of arthropathy are recognized.
Onset: childhood to adulthood.
Course/Progression: chronic fluctuating course with remissions and exacerbations.
Expressivity: very variable within family members and in each patient in subsequent episodes.
Histology: parakeratosis with or without hyperkeratosis; hypogranulosis; uniform elongation of rete ridges or dermal papillae; Munro microabscesses.

Complications: Generalized pustular psoriasis may be a medical emergency. This exfoliative erythroderma may be associated with high-output cardiac failure, hypoalbuminemia, and hypothermia.

Associated Findings: High uric acid level. β-Hemolytic streptococcus may be associated with guttate psoriasis.

Etiology: Multifactorial. Autosomal dominant inheritance with variable penetrance has been reported.

Pathogenesis: Lesions are characterized by increased epidermal mitotic rate and decreased cell turnover time, parakeratosis, epidermal hyperplasia, minimal inflammation, and prominent subepidermal capillaries.
Emotional stress plays a large role in the precipitation of psoriasis in susceptible individuals.
Certain drugs are known to aggravate psoriasis, notably indomethacin, β-adrenergic blocking agents, lithium, and antimalarial drugs.

MIM No.: *17790

CDC No.: 757.900

Sex Ratio: M1:F1

Occurrence: 3:100 in the United States. Common in Caucasians and infrequent in Blacks.

Risk of Recurrence for Patient's Sib: 7.5% if neither parent is affected; 16% if one parent is affected; 50% if both parents are affected.

Risk of Recurrence for Patient's Child: 16% if one parent affected; 50% if both parents affected.

Age of Detectability: Onset usually in young adulthood, with a range from early childhood to old age.

Gene Mapping and Linkage: Certain HLA loci have been linked with psoriasis. HLA-B13, HLA-B17 (worldwide); HLA-BW16, HLA-B37 (restricted to certain population groups); HLA-BW16, HLA-B17, HLA-DW11 (correlate with extensive psoriasis); HLA DW11 (susceptibility to psoriasis is questionable).

Prevention: Avoidance of precipitants; e.g., trauma to the skin, emotional stress, and triggering drugs.

Treatment: *Topical:* Antimitotic agents include tar derivatives, anthralin derivatives, and corticosteroids. Keratolytic agents include salicylic acid; urea; ultraviolet light A, spectrum 320–400; ultraviolet light B.
Photochemotherapy: PUVA-8 methoxypsoralens; 8-MOP + UVA (320–400).
Systemic: methotrexate; vitamin A derivatives, retinoids (severe teratogenic effects have been reported with the use of retinoids in early pregnancy. See **Fetal retinoid syndrome**), Corticosteroids probably introduce greater risks than benefits in almost all patients.

Prognosis: Life span is normal. IQ not affected. The natural history of psoriasis is one of remissions and exacerbations. With complete clearing of lesions, longstanding remissions may be achieved.

Detection of Carrier: Unknown.

References:
Abele DC, et al.: Heredity and psoriasis: study of a large family. Arch Derm 1963; 88:38–47.
Watson W, et al.: The genetics of psoriasis. Arch Dermatol 1972; 105:197–207.
Saiag P, et al.: Psoriatic fibroblasts induce hyperproliferation of normal keratinocytes in a skin equivalent model in vitro. Science 1985; 230:669–672.
Dermis DJ: Clinical dermatology, 13th revision. Philadelphia: Harper & Row, 1986.
Rook A, et al.: Textbook of dermatology, ed 4. Oxford: Blackwell, 1986.

WI055   **Ingrid M. Winship**

Skin, stiff skin syndrome
See STIFF SKIN SYNDROME
Skin, tight
See RESTRICTIVE DERMATOPATHY
Skin, universal melanosis
See SKIN, HYPERPIGMENTATION, FAMILIAL

SKIN, VITILIGO   0993

Includes:
Achromia, primary
Halo nevi
Leukoderma acquisitum centrifugum of Sutton
Leukoderma, primary
Nevus anemicus
Vitiligo

Excludes:
Achromia secondary to causes of melanocyte destruction
Albinism
Deafness-vitiligo-muscle wasting (0275)
Depigmentation occurring as a sign of nongenetic disorders
Nevus, congenital (2165)

Major Diagnostic Criteria: Progressive, primary melanin depigmentation of skin.

Clinical Findings: A small area of normally hyperpigmented skin loses pigmentation. It rapidly enlarges peripherally with sharp margins, reaching a stable size that then may remain static, slowly enlarge and coalesce with other depigmented areas, or repigment.
The condition should be distinguished from *nevus anemicus*, which consists of a patch of pale skin of normal texture, usually on the trunk, described in four generations of a family by Cardose et al (1975).

Complications: Sunburn of depigmented skin. Cosmetic defect.

Associated Findings: Halo nevus (Chisa, 1965), which may or may not be a part of this condition.

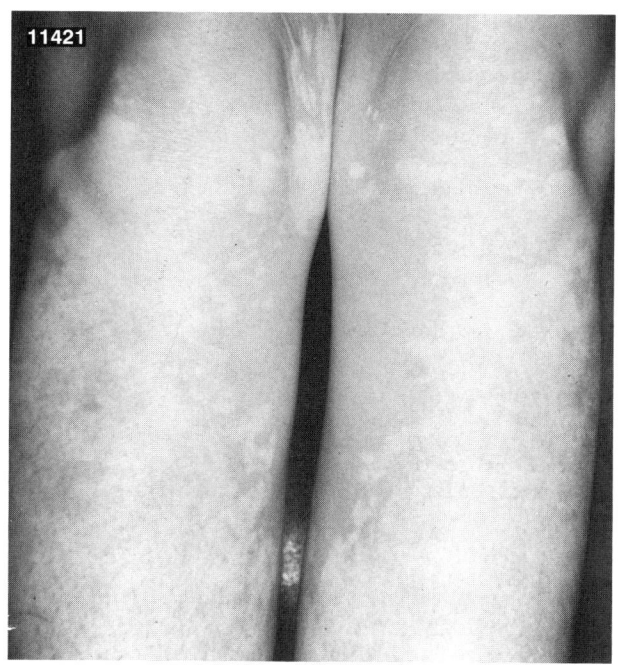

0993-11421: Vitiligo.

Etiology: Presumably polygenic.

Pathogenesis: Melanocytes are absent from the depigmented areas. The mechanism of their loss has not been established.

MIM No.: 19320, 23430, 16305

CDC No.: 757.900

Sex Ratio: Presumably M1:F1

Occurrence: 1:200 has been reported in two studies.

Risk of Recurrence for Patient's Sib: Variable, depending on the number of cases in close relatives and on the amount of inbreeding. Only 2.7% of first degree relatives are found to be affected when all families are considered together. This figure may represent the maximal risk when the patient has no affected relatives. In some reported families, the frequency of affected first degree relatives is nearly 50%. This figure may represent the maximal risk in families with numerous affected relatives and parental consanguinity. The average risk based on polygenic theory should be 6.8%, which may be the approximate risk when the patient has an affected relative or when the patient's parents are consanguineous.

Risk of Recurrence for Patient's Child: Variable, depending on the number of cases in close relatives and on the amount of inbreeding. Only 2.7% of first degree relatives are found to be affected when all families are considered together. This figure may represent the maximal risk when the patient has no affected relatives. In some reported families, the frequency of affected first degree relatives is nearly 50%. This figure may represent the maximal risk in families with numerous affected relatives and parental consanguinity. The average risk based on polygenic theory should be 6.8%, which may be the approximate risk when the patient has an affected relative or when the patient's parents are consanguineous.

Age of Detectability: Any time of life, but about one-half have onset before 20 years of age.

Gene Mapping and Linkage: Unknown.

Prevention: None known. Genetic counseling indicated.

Treatment: Sun screens should be used on the depigmented areas when outdoors. Cosmetic camouflage may be used to cover small depigmented areas. Psoralen derivatives followed by long-wave ultraviolet light treatment causes gradual repigmentation, which spreads outward from hair follicles. The improvement may be only temporary. When the vitiligo is extensive, the remaining pigmented skin may be depigmented with hydroquinone monobenzyl ether. Potential hazards of these medications must be included in advice about therapy.

Prognosis: Most cases are lifelong, but a few have spontaneous repigmentation. Shunning and humiliation may contribute to psychoneurosis in some untreated cases. The depigmented areas may be prone to sunlight-associated skin cancers.

Detection of Carrier: Unknown.

References:

Chisa N: Multiple halo nevi in siblings. Arch Derm 1965; 92:404–405.
Cardoso H, et al.: Familial naevus anemicus. (Abstract) Am J Hum Genet 1975; 27:24A only.
Hafez M, et al.: The genetics of vitiligo. Acta Dermatol Venereol (Stockh) 1983; 63:249–251.
Witkop CJ: Abnormalities of pigmentation. In: Emery AEH, Rimoin DL, eds: Principles and practice of medical genetics. New York: Churchill Livingstone, 1983:635 only.
Das SK, et al.: Studies on vitiligo. II. Familial aggregation and genetics. Genet Epidemiol 1985; 2:255–262.

TH017
UR001

T.F. Thurmon
S.A. Ursin

SMITH-FINEMAN-MYERS SYNDROME   **2845**

Includes:

Mental retardation, Smith-Fineman-Myers type
X-linked mental retardation, Smith-Fineman-Myers type

Excludes: **X-linked mental retardation** (others)

Major Diagnostic Criteria: Mental retardation with minor physical anomalies; growth and developmental retardation as well as distinctive facial and skeletal signs.

Clinical Findings: The three known male patients were short in stature (less than the 3–10th percentile), severely mentally retarded (a recorded IQ of 21 for a non-familial case), and are lightly

2845-20083: Note the similar facial features in these two unrelated boys.

pigmented with multiple freckles. Facial appearance is most significant for prominence of the maxilla and central incisors with contrasting micrognathia. Other craniofacial findings include dolichocephaly and elongation of the face, upslanting and/or short palpebral fissures, ptosis, strabismus, hyperopia, optic nerve hypoplasia (one case), decreased nasolabial folds, flat philtral pillars, patulous lower lip, and bifid uvula (one case). The facial appearance is reminiscent of patients with **Dubowitz syndrome** or **Marden-Walker syndrome**, but features are more distinctive in these syndromes.

Skeletal features include a thin habitus, minor chest abnormalities such as **Pectus excavatum**, short sternum and rib flaring, bridged palmar creases, femoral anteversion, foot deformities such as hallux valgus, toe **Camptodactyly** and overriding, longitudinal sole creases, metatarsus varus and pes planus, and back changes such as scoliosis and lordosis.

Skeletal X-rays may show delayed bone age, absence of the mastoid process, prominence of the frontal sinuses, overtubulation of the long bones, and scoliosis. Pneumoencephalography of affected brothers showed moderate cortical atrophy but brain biopsies were normal. A brain CAT Scan on an isolated case was essentially normal (thickened calvaria and **Microcephaly**). Metabolic screens and karyotypes were normal.

Complications: Psychomotor retardation is severe but non-progressive. There is early delay in attainment of milestones, and later, behavior difficulties and self-stimulation with little capacity for social interaction. Hypotonia and hyperreflexia evolve into hypertonia and spasticity. Mixed seizures developed as early as age 11 months, and were present in all three patients.

Associated Findings: Feeding difficulties and infections complicate infancy. The affected brothers were small for gestational age. There was increased fetal and neonatal loss in the family of the isolated case.

Etiology: Probably X-linked inheritance (70%) or possibly autosomal recessive inheritance (30%). The family history of an isolated case is suggestive of X-linked inheritance because a sister had a "learning disability" and a maternal aunt had mental retardation attributed to "birth trauma".

Pathogenesis: Unknown.

MIM No.: 30958

POS No.: 3257

Sex Ratio: M3.F0 (observed).

Occurrence: Three cases have been reported; all male from the United States west, including one pair of affected brothers.

Risk of Recurrence for Patient's Sib:
See Part I, *Mendelian Inheritance.*

Risk of Recurrence for Patient's Child:
See Part I, *Mendelian Inheritance.*

Age of Detectability: The diagnosis in an isolated case would be extremely difficult until clinical features have evolved. When growth and psychomotor retardation with hypotonia have be-

come apparent, recognition of facial and skeletal features, probably by school-age, would allow diagnosis.

Gene Mapping and Linkage: Unknown.

Prevention: None known. Genetic counseling indicated.

Treatment: Anticonvulsants may be required for control of seizures.

Prognosis: The three males are institutionalized and are capable of only minimal self-care. Seizures have been controlled with medication. The skeletal features are relatively asymptomatic, although scoliosis is progressive in one patient and may eventually cause pulmonary compromise. Otherwise there is no apparent limitation of life span.

Detection of Carrier: Unknown.

References:
Smith RD, Fineman RM, Myers GG: Short stature, psychomotor retardation, and unusual facial appearance in two brothers. Am J Med Genet 1980; 7:5–9. * †
Stephenson L, Johnson JP: Smith-Fineman-Myers Syndrome: report of a third case. Am J Med Genet 1985; 22:301–304. * †

J0012

John P. Johnson

SMITH-LEMLI-OPITZ SYNDROME   0891

Includes:
RHS syndrome
SLOS (Smith-Lemli-Opitz syndrome)

Excludes:
Meckel syndrome (0634)
Smith-Lemli-Opitz syndrome, type II (2635)

Major Diagnostic Criteria: Up to one-half of the infants with Smith-Lemli-Opitz Syndrome (SLOS) manifest prenatal onset of growth retardation (for weight and/or length). Characteristic craniofacial features include microcephaly, narrow high forehead with prominent metopic suture (a high, square "Daniel Webster" forehead), broad nasal bridge, short nose with anteverted nostrils, bilateral epicanthal folds, ptosis, broad maxillary alveolar ridges, cleft of the posterior palate, micrognathia, and abnormally shaped and/or positioned pinnae. Approximately 70% of 46,XY males with SLOS have abnormalities of the external genitalia which include varying degrees of hypospadias, cryptorchidism, and/or frank ambiguous genitalia. Abnormalities of external genitalia in 46,XX females with SLOS have not been reported. The most characteristic limb abnormalities are postaxial polydactyly (seen in 20–30% of cases) and cutaneous syndactyly of toes 2–3 (seen in 75–95% of cases). Relatively nonspecific major malformations occur in a number of other organ systems, including urinary tract defects in approximately 50% (renal hypoplasia, ureteral or urethral constriction, hydronephrosis, cystic kidney disease); congenital heart disease in approximately 20% (endocardial cushion defects, **Heart, tetralogy of Fallot**, **Ventricular septal defect**); and **Pyloric stenosis** in 15–25% of cases. Detailed neuropathologic information is limited, but characteristic findings include ventriculomegaly plus hypoplasia of the cerebral hemispheres, the cerebellum, and/or the brainstem.

Clinical Findings: Postnatal growth retardation and failure to thrive occur in over 90% of individuals with SLOS. Severe feeding problems with regurgitation and poor sucking also occur in over 90% of affected individuals. Hypotonia is frequent in the newborn period, although hypertonia may develop later. Moderate-to-severe mental retardation is to be expected, although one patient with near normal intelligence has been reported. There is currently insufficient information to comment about secondary sexual development or reproductive capacity.

Complications: Gastroesophageal reflux and aspiration resulting in bronchopneumonia.

Associated Findings: **Colon, aganglionosis** has been reported in several cases.

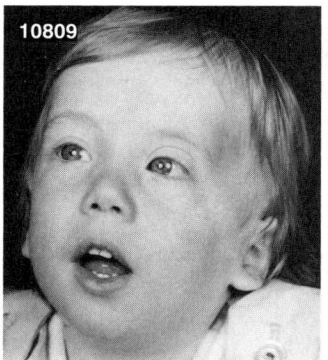
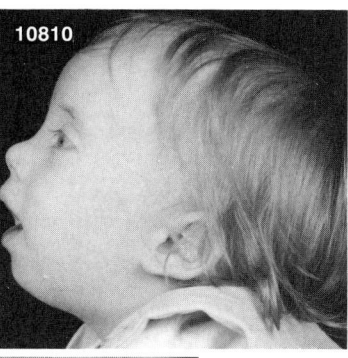
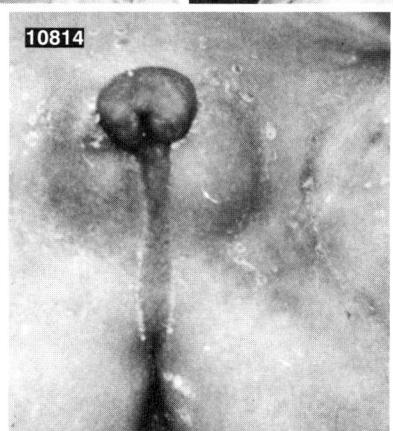

0891-10809–10: 18-month-old male with ptosis and small jaw. 10814: Hypospadias and hypoplastic scrotum.

Etiology: Autosomal recessive inheritance.

Pathogenesis: Unknown.

MIM No.: *27040

POS No.: 3391

CDC No.: 759.820

Sex Ratio: Presumably M1:F1. Diagnosed more frequently in males, which probably reflects the greater ease of recognition in the presence of genital abnormalities.

Occurrence: Estimated at about 1:40,000.

Risk of Recurrence for Patient's Sib:
See Part I, *Mendelian Inheritance.*

Risk of Recurrence for Patient's Child:
See Part I, *Mendelian Inheritance.* Most affected individuals do not reproduce.

Age of Detectability: In the newborn period. A specific prenatal diagnostic test is not currently available, although ultrasonographic detection of genital anomalies is possible.

Gene Mapping and Linkage: Unknown.

Prevention: None known. Genetic counseling indicated.

Treatment: Unknown.

Prognosis: Approximately one-fourth of all affected individuals die within the first two years of life. Most survivors demonstrate moderate to severe mental retardation.

Detection of Carrier: Unknown.

Special Considerations: The synonym *RSH syndrome* was derived from the surnames of three families originally observed by John Opitz.

References:
Smith DW, et al.: A newly recognized syndrome of multiple congenital anomalies. J Pediatr 1964; 64:210–217.
Opitz JM, et al.: The RSH Syndrome. BD:OAS II(2). New York: March of Dimes Birth Defects Foundation, 1969:43–52.
Johnson VP: Smith-Lemli-Opitz syndrome: review and report of two affected siblings. Z Kinderheilk 1975; 119:221–234. *
Lowry RB, Yong SL: Borderline normal intelligence in the Smith-Lemli-Opitz (RSH) syndrome. Am J Med Genet 1980; 5:137–143.
Patterson K, et al.: Hirschsprung disease in a 46,XY phenotypic infant girl with Smith-Lemli-Opitz syndrome. J Pediatr 1983; 103:425–427.
Curry CJR, et al.: Smith-Lemli-Opitz syndrome type II multiple congenital anomalies with male pseudohermaphriditism and frequent early lethality. Am J Med Genet 1987; 26:45–57.
Joseph DB, et al.: Genitourinary abnormalities associated with Smith-Lemli-Opitz syndrome. J Urol 1987; 137:719–721.
Opitz JM, et al.: Smith-Lemli-Opitz (RSH) syndrome bibliography. Am J Med Genet 1987; 28:745–750.

P0021   **Barbara Pober**

SMITH-LEMLI-OPITZ SYNDROME, TYPE II   **2635**

Includes:
 Lung, unilobular-polydactyly-sex reversal-renal hypoplasia
 Polydactyly-sex reversal-renal hypoplasia-unilobular lung
 Renal hypoplasia-unilobular lung-polydactyly-sex reversal
 Rutledge lethal multiple congenital anomaly syndrome
 Sex reversal-polydactyly-renal hypoplasia-unilobular lung

Excludes:
 Aneuploidies (some)
 Chondroectodermal dysplasia (0156)
 Hydrolethalus syndrome (2279)
 Hypothalamic hamartoblastoma syndrome, congenital (2285)
 Meckel syndrome (0634)
 Oculo-encephalo-hepato-renal syndrome (3242)
 Short rib-polydactyly syndrome
 Smith-Lemli-Opitz syndrome (0891)

Major Diagnostic Criteria: Three of the following major malformations: **Cleft palate**, **Polydactyly**, congenital heart disease, cataracts, small tongue, or severe genital ambiguity or pseudohermaphroditism in XY males. A clinical course characterized by frequent early lethality, severe feeding problems, metabolic derangement, and, occasionally, the oligohydramnios sequence. Less frequently seen are **Colon, aganglionosis**, large adrenals, pancreatic islet hypertrophy, unilobated lungs.

Clinical Findings: Unlike the **Smith-Lemli-Opitz syndrome** as originally described, Smith-Lemli-Opitz type II is characterized by major structural abnormalities, male pseudohermaphroditism and early death. Pregnancies frequently have been marked by growth retardation and decreased fetal movement, and oligohydramnios has been noted in several instances. Breech presentation occurred in about 50%, and birth asphyxia was extremely common. Three of 43 reported cases died as a consequence of pulmonary hypoplasia secondary to renal agenesis or cystic dysplasia. Congenital heart disease was seen in over 75%, cataracts (50%), postaxial polydactyly (85%), **Cleft palate** (70%), and male pseudohermaphroditism (70%), and genital ambiguity (30%). The incidence of islet cell hyperplasia was approximately 40%, and unilobated lungs were noted in 57% of autopsied cases. Mild **Microcephaly** has been seen in many Smith-Lemli-Opitz type II patients. **Hydrocephaly** and the absence of the corpus callosum have been noted in several patients. Most infants with this presentation have died prior to three months of age. The exact cause of death is frequently not clear, but in those surviving beyond the first few days, poor suck and feeding, projectile vomiting, abdominal distention, profound developmental delay, occasional liver disease, and recurrent respiratory infections are common.

Complications: Recurrent respiratory infections, pyloric stenosis, and hepatic dysfunction.

Associated Findings: Toe **Syndactyly**, redundant neck skin, short limbs, facial hemangiomata, and joint contractures.

2635-21508: Note facial profile with microcephaly and micrognathia. 21509: Polydactyly. 21510: Synda of second and third toes; note also polydactyly.

Etiology: Autosomal recessive inheritance.

Pathogenesis: The occasional findings of renal cysts, large adrenals and hepatic dysfunction are suggestive of a possible **Peroxisomal** defect. However, initial investigations of long-chain fatty acid levels and plasmalogen synthesis have revealed no abnormalities. The frequency of low estriol levels in late pregnancy, and aberrant sexual differentiation and large adrenals at autopsy, point to a possible defect in fetal adrenal metabolism.

MIM No.: *26867

POS No.: 3645

CDC No.: 759.820

Sex Ratio: Presumably M1:F1. The presence of genital ambiguity in affected males has strongly biased the ascertainment of males with this syndrome.

Occurrence: Close to 50 that appear to fulfill criteria for the diagnosis have been reported in the literature.

Risk of Recurrence for Patient's Sib:
See Part I, *Mendelian Inheritance.*

Risk of Recurrence for Patient's Child:
See Part I, *Mendelian Inheritance.* Affected individuals are not expected to survive to reproduce.

Age of Detectability: At birth, or prenatally by the 24th week of pregnancy. Ultrasound can be used to assess fetal movement, determine fetal sex, and to assess renal and cardiac function. Amniocentesis for fetal sexing may be appropriate. Measurements of estriols may also be useful but there is no data on these levels in at-risk pregnancies in the second trimester.

Gene Mapping and Linkage: Unknown.

Prevention: None known. Genetic counseling indicated.

Treatment: Surgery for complications such as **Pyloric stenosis** and **Colon, aganglionosis**.

Prognosis: Most affected infants have died in the first week of life. The longest survivor died at age 19 months. Severe growth failure and mental retardation have been characteristic in those surviving beyond the first weeks of life.

Detection of Carrier: Unknown.

References:
Rutledge JC, et al.: A "new" lethal multiple congenital anomaly syndrome. Am J Med Genet 1984; 19:255–264. * †
Donnai D, et al.: The lethal multiple congenital anomaly syndrome of polydactyly, sex reversal, renal hypoplasia, and unilobar lungs. J Med Genet 1986; 23:64–71.
Belmont JW, et al.: Two cases of severe lethal Smith-Lemli-Opitz syndrome. (Letter) Am J Med Genet 1987; 26:65–67.
Curry CJR, et al.: Smith-Lemli-Opitz syndrome-type II: multiple congenital anomalies with male pseudohermaphroditism and frequent early lethality. Am J Med Genet 1987; 26:45–57. *

CU009
RU017

Cynthia J.R. Curry
Joe C. Rutledge

Smith-Magenis syndrome
See CHROMOSOME 17, INTERSTITIAL DELETION 17p
Smith-McCort dwarfism
See DYGGVE-MELCHIOR-CLAUSEN SYNDROME
Smith-Strang disease
See METHIONINE MALABSORPTION
Smoking, cigarette, fetal effects
See FETAL EFFECTS OF MATERNAL CIGARETTE SMOKING
Snail-like pelvis dysplasia
See SKELETAL DYSPLASIA, SCHNECKENBECKEN TYPE
Sneezing from light exposure
See ACHOO SYNDROME
Snow-capped teeth
See TEETH, SNOW-CAPPED
Solitary polyp syndrome
See CANCER, COLORECTAL
Somatomedin C deficiency
See GROWTH DEFICIENCY, AFRICAN PYGMY TYPE
Sorsby syndrome
See MACULAR COLOBOMA-BRACHYDACTYLY
Sotos syndrome
See CEBEBRAL GIGANTISM
South African porphyria
See PORPHYRIA, VARIEGATE

SPASTIC ATAXIA, CHARLEVOIX-SAGUENAY TYPE   **2566**

Includes:
Autosomal recessive spastic ataxia of Charlevoix-Saguenay (ARSACS)
Charlevoix-Saguenay spastic ataxia

Excludes:
Ataxia, Friedreich type (2714)
Ataxia-telangiectasia (0094)
Ataxia (others)
Marinesco-Sjogren syndrome (2031)
Optic atrophy, infantile heredofamilial (0755)
Paraplegia, familial spastic (0295)
Sjogren-Larsson syndrome (2030)
Troyer syndrome

Major Diagnostic Criteria: Onset between 1–2 years of age; spasticity; dysarthria; distal muscle wasting; truncal ataxia; foot deformities; absence of sensory evoked potentials in the lower limbs; nystagmus; retinal striation reminiscent of early **Optic atrophy, Leber type**; and the frequent presence of **Mitral valve prolapse**.

Clinical Findings: Although most patients have normal early milestones, none ever walk normally. The parents note unsteadiness and frequent falls when affected children begin to walk. Dysarthria with slurring of speech is always present. Horizontal nystagmus is always present, often with predominance on one side. There is occasionally a more irregular vertical nystagmus. There is also a gross defect of conjugate pursuit ocular movements. These are dysmetric, saccadic, and restricted to the horizontal plane.

Muscle tone is markedly increased in the lower limbs, with polykinetic knee jerks and occasionally clonus at this level. Chaddock and Babinski signs are easily elicited in all cases. Posterior column signs in the lower limbs are found in all patients, with decreased or absent vibration sense in the toes and to a lesser extent at the ankles.

Position sense in the toes is mildly impaired. Cutaneous sensation is normal in all patients. Distal leg atrophy is present in most patients, and this sometimes extends to the anterior compartment of the leg. Pes cavus is frequently seen. Wasting of the small muscles is seen in almost half of the patients. Incontinence of urine or feces is a frequent important feature.

Mean I.Q.'s are in the low normal range, with significant impairment of non-verbal vs. verbal tasks. Visual acuity and fundoscopy are normal, except for striking and markedly increased visibility of the retinal nerve fibers, resembling early stages of **Optic atrophy, Leber type**.

The progression of the disease is relatively slow. The ataxia can be stable for long periods, and then seems to worsen over a period of a few years. Vibration sense gradually diminishes. There are progressive deformities of the feet and hands. The nonverbal performance scales are also negatively correlated with age.

The diagnosis can be suspected from the geographic origin, the early onset of ataxia, the slow progression, and normal or increased deep tendon reflexes in the lower extremities. The main clinical features differentiating these patients from those with classical **Ataxia, Friedreich type** (FA) are constant nystagmus; spasticity with increased deep tendon reflexes; the absence of scoliosis; the presence of retinal striations; incontinence of bladder and/or bowels; absence of hypertrophic cardiomyopathy; and high frequency of **Mitral valve prolapse**.

Motor nerve conduction is slowed in ARSACS, whereas it is normal in FA. Sensory nerve conduction is absent or markedly impaired in both conditions. The EMG shows more signs of denervation in ARSACS, despite the fact that the evolution is slower. The CT scan in ARSACS demonstrates signs of cerebellar atrophy almost limited to the superior parts of the vermis and anterior lobes, whereas in FA, the X-ray signs are variable and less obvious.

Sural nerve biopsy in two patients revealed a severe loss of large myelinated axons contrasting with a normal myelinated fiber density, suggesting a developmental abnormality of peripheral nerve. No diagnostic biochemical abnormalities are known.

Complications: Deformities of the feet and hands, including clawing of the toes; pes cavus; equinovarus deformities of the feet, alone or with supination (club feet); marked atrophy of the muscles, leading to claw hands; and internal rotation and scissoring of the lower limbs due to spasticity. Some patients require surgery for Achilles tendon elongation.

Associated Findings: None known.

Etiology: Autosomal recessive inheritance. This is confirmed by multiple cases in sibships, absence of affected parents or offspring, increased parental consanguinity, and the finding of a common ancestral couple in a number of sibships.

Pathogenesis: Unknown.

MIM No.: *27055

Sex Ratio: M3:F2 (observed, based on 42 patients).

Occurrence: Not described outside of the Charlevoix-Saguenay region of Québec, which represents a genetic isolate. The prevalence in this region is unknown. Over 200 cases have been observed.

Risk of Recurrence for Patient's Sib:
See Part I, *Mendelian Inheritance*.

Risk of Recurrence for Patient's Child:
See Part I, *Mendelian Inheritance*.

Age of Detectability: The disease can be suspected soon after the child starts to walk, particularly if there is a positive family history and/or the child originates from the Charlevoix-Saguenay region of Québec.

Gene Mapping and Linkage: Unknown.

Prevention: None known. Genetic counseling indicated.

Treatment: Symptomatic. Lengthening of Achilles tendons and surgical correction of the foot and hand deformities may indicated.

Prognosis: The disease is slowly progressive, and survival to the fifth and sixth decade of life is not uncommon. A number of patients have reproduced.

Detection of Carrier: Unknown.

Special Considerations: It is important to distinguish this very specific and clinically homogeneous form of spastic ataxia from the many similar syndromes that have been previously described, such as Troyer syndrome (Cross and McKusick, 1967).

Support Groups:
New York; National Myoclonus Foundation
MD; Landover; Epilepsy Foundation of America

References:
Cross HE, McKusick VA: The Troyer syndrome: a recessive form of spastic paraplegia with distal muscle wasting. Arch Neurol 1967; 16:473–485.
Bouchard JP, et al: Autosomal recessive spastic ataxia of Charlevoix-Saguenay. Can J Neuro Sci 1978; 5:61–69. *
Bouchard JP, et al: Electromyography and nerve conduction studies in Friedreich's ataxia and autosomal recessive spastic ataxia of Charlevoix-Saguenay. Can J Neurol Sci 1979; 6:185–189.
Bouchard JP, et al: Electroencephalographic findings in Friedreich's ataxia and autosomal recessive spastic ataxia of Charlevoix-Saguenay (ARSACS). Can J Neurol Sci 1979; 6:191–194.
Dionne J, et al: Oculomotor and vestibular findings in autosomal recessive spastic ataxia of Charlevoix-Saguenay. Can J Neurol Sci 1979; 6:177–184.
Langelier R, et al: Computed tomography of posterior fossa in hereditary ataxias. Can J Neurol Sci 1979; 6:195–198.
Peyronnard JM, et al: The neuropathy of Charlevoix-Saguenay ataxia: an electrophysiological and pathological study. Can J Neurol Sci 1979; 6:199–203.
Barbeau A: A tentative classification of recessively inherited ataxias. Can J Neurol Sci 1982; 9:95–98.

AN016   **Eva Andermann**

Spastic diplegia, from extrinsically caused iodine disorder
See CRETINISM, ENDEMIC, AND RELATED DISORDERS
Spastic infantile paralysis (cerebral)
See CEREBRAL PALSY
Spastic paraplegia, hereditary
See PARAPLEGIA, FAMILIAL SPASTIC
Spastic paraplegia, pure hereditary
See PARAPLEGIA, FAMILIAL SPASTIC
Spastic paraplegia, X-linked, complicated
See PARAPLEGIA, FAMILIAL SPASTIC
Spastic paraplegia-palmoplantar hyperkeratosis-retardation
See HYPERKERATOSIS PALMOPLANTARIS-SPASTIC PARAPLEGIA-RETARDATION
Spastic pseudosclerosis
See CREUTZFELDT-JAKOB DISEASE
Spasticity-ichthyosis-oligophrenia
See SJOGREN-LARSSON SYNDROME
Speech fluency disorder
See STUTTERING
Speech, hypernasal
See PALATOPHARYNGEAL INCOMPETENCE
Sperocytosis, hereditary
See SPHEROCYTOSIS

SPHEROCYTOSIS   **0892**

Includes:
Anemia, spherocytic, congenital
Minkowski-Chauffard syndrome
Sperocytosis, hereditary

Excludes:
Anemia, hemolytic, red cell membrane defects (2646)
Anemias, congenital nonspherocytic
Elliptocytosis (2665)

Major Diagnostic Criteria: Chronic hemolytic anemia of variable severity, with the presence of a variable number of spherocytic and microspherocytic erythrocytes on blood smear. Mean corpuscular hemoglobin concentration (MCHC) often elevated (>34 g/dl). Elevated autohemolysis of erythrocytes upon incubation for 48 hours at 37 degree C, with partial correction in the presence of glucose. Increased sensitivity to lysis of erythrocytes in hypotonic media (osmotic fragility), which is accentuated by incubation for 24 hours at 37 degree C. Absence of erythrocyte autoantibodies.

Clinical Findings: The anemia is of variable severity, ranging from normal hemoglobin levels with modestly elevated reticulocytes in some individuals to severe anemia with overt jaundice and markedly elevated reticulocyte counts in others. Severity of anemia is often variable among affected family members. Hemolytic jaundice is common in neonates with hereditary spherocytosis, but the etiology is often not recognized at this age. Anemia is generally more severe in the first year of life, occasionally requiring transfusions, but few patients over age one year require chronic transfusions. Splenomegaly is extremely common (75–100%). A family history of spherocytosis, splenectomies, or cholelithiasis is often elicited. Severely affected individuals may have "hemolytic facies" due to expansion of the medullary spaces in the cranial bones.

Complications: The most common potentially life-threatening complications in the individual with an intact spleen are acute exacerbations of anemia. These include aplastic crises characterized by rapidly worsening anemia and reticulocytopenia. The bone marrow shows a marked decrease in erythroid precursors, with a few giant proerythroblasts present. A human parvovirus has been found to cause the majority of aplastic crises and selectively inhibit erythroid cell production in marrow culture. Simultaneous depression of granulocytes and platelets has been reported. Prompt red cell transfusion is generally required. Normal erythrocyte production resumes spontaneously in 7–10 days. Hyperhemolytic crises manifested by worsening anemia, increased jaundice, dark urine, reticulocytosis, and possibly increasing spleen size may be associated with other illnesses such as viral infections. Overt hypersplenism with leukopenia and thrombocytopenia may occur. As many as 50% of patients may develop cholelithiasis or cholecystitis, particularly in the teen and adult years. Other complications of hemolytic anemia such as leg ulcers may occur. Hemochromatosis has been reported, but may represent independent inheritance of an unrelated illness. Following splenectomy, there is an approximately 3% risk for overwhelming postsplenectomy septicemia, which carries a high fatality rate of about 50%. The causative organism is generally pneumococcus. The risk for septicemia exists for an indefinite period following splenectomy.

Associated Findings: None known.

Etiology: Usually autosomal dominant inheritance, although in about 20% of cases the parents are apparently not affected. In some cases this is due to variable penetrance, since there are some families with hematologically normal parents and more than one affected child. Autosomal recessive inheritance of severe spherocytosis due to partial spectrin deficiency has been reported.

Pathogenesis: Hereditary spherocytosis is classified as an inherited erythrocyte membrane protein defect. A variety of biochemical and physiologic abnormalities have been reported in the erythrocytes of these individuals. The most consistent of these is a passive increase in transmembrane sodium leak, which is compensated by increase in ATP-dependent sodium extrusion. Hence, metabolic activity (glucose consumption) is increased, intracellular pH is lower than normal, and 2,3-diphosphoglycerate levels are often depressed. However, the severity of the cation leak does not correlate with the severity of the hemolysis in vivo. The hemolytic process is clearly related to splenic function, since splenectomy usually cures the anemia despite the persistence of the morphologic red cell defect. The spleen is felt to "condition" the red cells so that repetitive passage of a cell through the spleen leads to progressive loss of membrane lipid, with concomitant decrease in surface:volume ratio. The mechanism of this conditioning is unknown. With progressive spherocytic transformation, the cell becomes less deformable, ultimately trapped in the narrow (3 μm) splenic cords. Increased cell fragmentation under conditions of high shear stress has been seen in some forms of hereditary spherocytosis. Several different membrane protein

defects have now been found, consistent with the heterogeneity in clinical severity and inheritance modes. Partial spectrin deficiency with spectrin levels as low as 26–29% of normal has been found in recessively inherited spherocytosis. Interestingly, some degree of spectrin loss may occur in all spherocytosis and correlates with the severity of the hemolysis. Defective binding of spectrin to protein 4.1 in some kindreds with spherocytosis appears to be caused by a defect in the alpha-spectrin V or beta-spectrin IV domain. An abnormal spectrin with increased binding avidity to the cell membrane has also been reported.

MIM No.: *18290, *27097

CDC No.: 282.000

Sex Ratio: M1:F1

Occurrence: The most common form of inherited hemolytic anemia in persons of Northern European descent, with a prevalence of 1:5,000. Does occur in other populations.

Risk of Recurrence for Patient's Sib:
See Part I, *Mendelian Inheritance.*

Risk of Recurrence for Patient's Child:
See Part I, *Mendelian Inheritance.*

Age of Detectability: At birth or during early childhood in many cases, although individuals with milder anemia often are discovered as older children or even adults. Prenatal diagnosis has not been reported.

Gene Mapping and Linkage: SPH1 (spherocytosis 1 (clinical type II)) has been mapped to 8p21.1-p11.22.
    ANK (ankyrin) has been provisionally mapped to 8p21-p11.

Prevention: None known. Genetic counseling indicated.

Treatment: Splenectomy is definitive treatment. Following splenectomy, red cell survival becomes nearly normal, eliminating the anemia and hemolysis in most individuals. Even severely anemic individuals improve clinically, although the anemia may only be partially relieved. Splenectomy reduces the risks for aplastic and hyperhemolytic crises and gallbladder disease. Because of the risk for postsplenectomy sepsis, careful consideration of splenectomy must be made based on the severity of the anemia. Chronically anemic individuals, particularly those with jaundice, hyperhemolytic events, hypersplenism, poor growth and exercise intolerance, gallbladder disease and so forth, will derive the greatest benefit. Splenectomy is generally deferred until the patient is five years or older due to the unacceptably high incidence of sepsis following splenectomy in infants. Administration of pneumococcal vaccine, preferably prior to splenectomy, as well as prophylactic penicillin administration following splenectomy, may reduce the risk for later sepsis. In the individual with an intact spleen, an aplastic or hyperhemolytic crisis may necessitate red cell transfusion. Folic acid therapy is useful in the recovery phase of aplastic crisis, when transient folate deficiency may occur. Symptomatic gallbladder disease may require cholecystectomy.

Prognosis: Following splenectomy, spherocytosis is generally compatible with a normal life-style, although about 2% of these individuals will succumb to overwhelming bacterial infection.

Detection of Carrier: In dominantly inherited spherocytosis, most heterozygotes are clinically affected. Occasionally, a parent may have a detectable increase in passive red cell sodium flux without evidence of spherocytes, possibly representing incomplete penetrance. In the recessive form of spherocytosis, reduced red cell spectrin occurs in heterozygotes, but such testing is currently available only on an experimental basis.

Special Considerations: The presence of spherocytes on a blood smear indicates a population of cells with reduced surface:volume ratio and may result from a variety of congenital or acquired illnesses. Such cells may exhibit increased osmotic fragility, regardless of their origin. Therefore, until definitive tests for intrinsic red cell membrane abnormalities become clinically available, the diagnosis of hereditary spherocytosis can only be made when due consideration is given to other causes of spherocyte formation. For example, hereditary spherocytosis in the neonate may be difficult to distinguish from erythroblastosis fetalis due to a maternal-fetal ABO incompatibility. A further difficulty in establishing the diagnosis of hereditary spherocytosis in the newborn is that neonatal red cells ordinarily exhibit *decreased* osmotic fragility compared to erythrocytes from older individuals. A diagnosis of spherocytosis in a neonate should always be confirmed by retesting at age six months or older.

References:

Wiley JS: Co-ordinated increase of sodium leak and sodium pump in hereditary spherocytosis. Br J Haematol 1972; 22:529–542.

Agre P, et al.: Deficient red cell spectrin in severe, recessively inherited spherocytosis. New Engl J Med 1982; 306:1155–1161.

Goodman SR, et al.: Identification of the molecular defect in the erythrocyte membrane skeleton of some kindreds with hereditary spherocytosis. Blood 1982; 60:772–784.

Burke BE, Shotton DM: Erythrocyte membrane skeleton abnormalities in hereditary spherocytosis. Br J Haematol 1983; 54:173–187.

Agre P, et al.: Partial deficiency of erythrocyte spectrin in hereditary spherocytosis. Nature 1985; 314:380–383.

Becker PS, Lux SE: Hereditary spherocytosis and related disorders. Clin Hematol 1985; 14:15–43.

Chilicote RR, et al.: Association of red cell spherocytosis with deletion of the short arm of chromosome 8. Blood 1987; 69:156–159.

LA041   **Richard J. Labotka**

Spherocytosis, hereditary
See ANEMIA, HEMOLYTIC, RED CELL MEMBRANE DEFECTS

SPHEROPHAKIA-BRACHYMORPHIA SYNDROME   0893

Includes:
  Mesodermal dysmorphodystrophy, brachymorphic type, congenital
  Weill-Marchesani syndrome

Excludes: Short stature, constitutional-dislocated lens and pupil

Major Diagnostic Criteria: Congenital spherophakia, with or without dislocated lenses, and short stature.

Clinical Findings: Characterized by microspherophakia and progressive dislocation of the lens in patients of pyknic habitus. The height is usually below the third percentile. The patients show brachycephaly, pug nose, depressed nasal bridge, and short pudgy hands and feet. There may be articular stiffness and limitation of extension. Affected persons have marked myopia.

Complications: Acute pupillary block glaucoma.

Associated Findings: Subvalvular fibromuscular aortic stenosis was reported in one 11-year-old girl.

Etiology: Presumably autosomal recessive inheritance with partial expression in the heterozygote, although dominant inheritance has been suggested in some pedigrees.

Pathogenesis: Undetermined. Acute glaucoma may arise through several mechanisms. The anterior displacement of the lens may block the pupil and hinder the aqueous flow. In this case dilation of the pupil may relieve the symptoms. Glaucoma may also arise as a complication of a dislocated lens through irritation of the ciliary body. Complete luxation into the anterior chamber is occasionally seen, and may lead to corneal decompensation.

MIM No.: *27760

POS No.: 3043

CDC No.: 743.310

Sex Ratio: M1:F1

Occurrence: 1:100,000, with world-wide distribution.

Risk of Recurrence for Patient's Sib:
  See Part I, *Mendelian Inheritance.*

Risk of Recurrence for Patient's Child:
  See Part I, *Mendelian Inheritance.*

Age of Detectability: At birth, if suspected.

Gene Mapping and Linkage: Unknown.

Prevention: None known. Genetic counseling indicated.

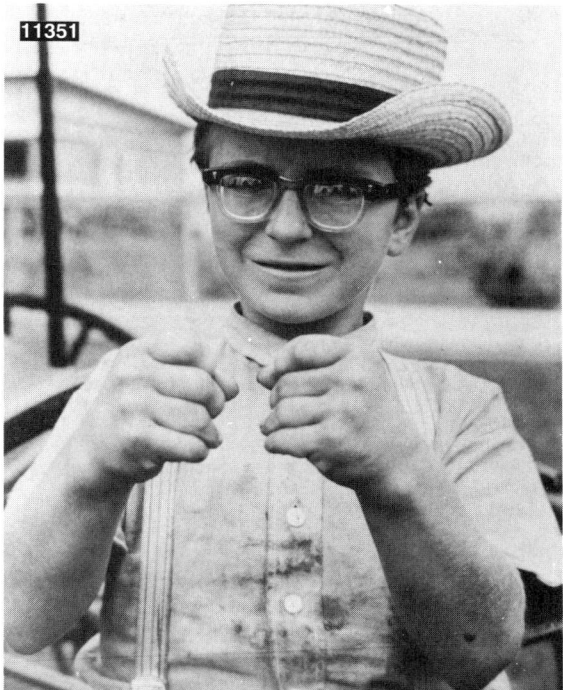

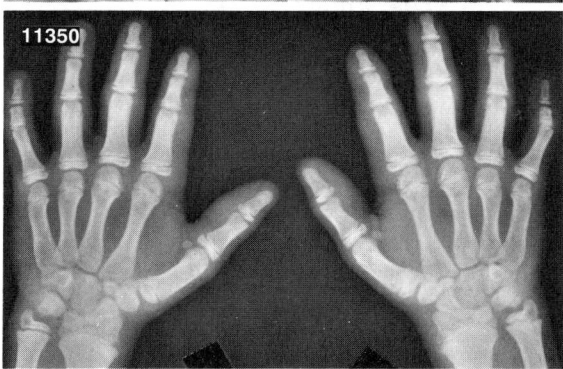

0893-11351: Pug nose, short hands with knobby joints, and restriction in flexion. 11350: All bones are short, especially middle phalanges of 5th fingers.

Treatment: Control of intraocular pressure; prophylactic iridotomy or lens extraction if glaucoma present.

Prognosis: Good for life span and intelligence, reduced visual function.

Detection of Carrier: By clinical examination, looking for a distinctly short pyknic habitus without the ocular findings in first degree relatives.

References:

Kloepfer HW, Rosenthal JW: Possible genetic carriers in the spherophakia - brachymorphia syndrome. Am J Hum Genet 1955; 7:398–425.

Rennert OM: The Marchesani syndrome: a brief review. Am J Dis Child 1969; 117:703–705.

Jensen AD, et al.: Ocular complications in the Weill-Marchesani syndrome. Am J Ophthal 1974; 77:261–269.

Ferrier S, et al.: Le syndrome de Marchesani (spherophakie-brachymorphie). Helv Paediatr Acta 1980; 35:185–198.

Young ID, et al.: Weill-Marchesani syndrome in a mother and son. Clin Genet 1986; 30:475–480.

MA054   Irene H. Maumenee

Sphingomyelin lipidosis
See NIEMANN-PICK DISEASE
Sphingomyelinase deficiency
See NIEMANN-PICK DISEASE
Spiegler-Brooke tumors
See EPITHELIOMAS, HEREDITARY MULTIPLE CYSTIC
also SCALP, CYLINDROMAS
Spielmeyer-Sjogren disease (juvenile NCL)
See NEURONAL CEROID-LIPOFUSCINOSES (NCL)
Spielmeyer-Vogt disease (juvenile NCL or JNCL)
See NEURONAL CEROID-LIPOFUSCINOSES (NCL)
Spina bifida cystica with paralysis
See MENINGOMYELOCELE
Spina bifida cystica without neurologic deficit
See MENINGOCELE
Spina bifida-anencephaly
See BRAIN, ARNOLD-CHIARI MALFORMATION
Spinal achnoid cysts-distichiasis-lymphedeme, hereditary
See DISTICHIASIS-LYMPHEDEMA SYNDROME
Spinal and bulbar muscular atrophy
See SPINAL MUSCULAR ATROPHY
Spinal ataxia, heredofamilial
See ATAXIA, FRIEDREICH TYPE
Spinal cord cavitation
See SYRINGOMYELIA

SPINAL CORD, NEURENTERIC CYST   0894

Includes:
Cyst of the spinal cord associated with posterior mediastinal cyst
Neurenteric cyst of spinal cord

Excludes: Diastematomyelia (0292)

Major Diagnostic Criteria: Progressive neurologic deficit consisting of weakness and sensory loss from pressure on the spinal cord of a cyst demonstrated by sonography or myelography.

Clinical Findings: Depending upon the level of the persisting embryonic defect, a progressive neurologic loss occurs, as well as a paralysis of the legs, bladder, and bowel. Sensory loss is present in the newborn or during the first few years of life. If there is an associated posterior mediastinal cyst, cardiothoracic symptoms are present. There is generally no skin lesion over the area of the affected spinal cord. Butterfly vertebrae are also seen.

Complications: Failure to sweat below the level of the lesion; temperature control is difficult.

Associated Findings: Bowel duplications, mediastinal or cervical cysts; diastematomyelia.

Etiology: Unknown.

Pathogenesis: There is a persistent connection between the alimentary tract and the midline neural structures with this mesodermal defect. One hypothesis is that primitive notocordal plate tissue carries entoderm into the vertebral canal, and enterogenous cysts occur within the spinal canal in the lower cervical or upper thoracic level. The association of enterogenous cysts with vertebral anomalies suggests errors in embryonic development. A midline ectoendodermal adhesion obstructing the axial mesoderm and persisting as a neurenteric connection through the vertebral defect in the second week of life is postulated. During the third week the axial mesoderm would have to either split or detour in order to pass the ectoendodermal adhesion. This might result in defects in the vertebral bodies, with the adhesion remaining as a postnatal cyst and a diastematomyelia or band between the alimentary canal and spinal cord.

CDC No.: 742.580

Sex Ratio: Presumably M1:F1.

Occurrence: Undetermined but presumed rare.

Risk of Recurrence for Patient's Sib: Unknown.

Risk of Recurrence for Patient's Child: Unknown.

Age of Detectability: Unknown.

Gene Mapping and Linkage: Unknown.

Prevention: None known.

Treatment: Surgical excision or drainage of the spinal cyst is possible. If a cyst is present in the mediastinum or neck, it may be removed during a secondary operation. Prevention of kidney disease secondary to bladder paralysis.

Prognosis: Depends on the degree of paralysis and the rapidity of onset.

Detection of Carrier: Unknown.

References:
Bale PM: A congenital intraspinal gastroenterogenous cyst and diastematomyelia. J Neurol Neurosurg Psychiatry 1973; 36:1011.

SH007   **Kenneth Shapiro**

Spinal dysraphism syndrome
See LIPOMENINGOCELE

SPINAL MUSCULAR ATROPHY   0895

Includes:
Bulbospinal muscular atrophy, X-linked
Finkel late-adult spinal muscular atrophy
Kennedy disease
Kugelberg-Welander disease
Muscular atrophy, adult spinal
Muscular atrophy, juvenile spinal
Muscular atrophy, spinal, intermediate type
Spinal and bulbar muscular atrophy
Spinal muscular atrophy, benign-hypertrophy of calves
Spinal muscular atrophy, childhood isolated
Spinal muscular atrophy, distal type
Spinal muscular atrophy, facioscapulohumeral type
Spinal muscular atrophy, infantile acute form
Spinal muscular atrophy, infantile chronic form
Spinal muscular atrophy, proximal, adult type
Spinal muscular atrophy, type I
Spinal muscular atrophy, type II
Spinal muscular atrophy, type III
Spinal muscular atrophy, type IV
Werdnig-Hoffmann disease

Excludes:
Amyotrophic lateral sclerosis (2067)
Charcot-Marie-Tooth disease
G(M2)-gangliosidosis with hexosaminidase A and B deficiency (0433)
G(M2)-gangliosidosis with hexosaminidase A deficiency (0434)
Guillain-Barre syndrome
Hypotonia, benign congenital
Muscular atrophy, spinal and bulbar, X-linked Kennedy type (2493)
Muscular dystrophy (see all)

Major Diagnostic Criteria: Hypotonia, weakness, and decreased or absent deep tendon reflexes with characteristic electromyogram (EMG) and muscle biopsy findings.

Clinical Findings: A number of forms of spinal muscular atrophy (SMA) have been described, with the infantile type I (*Werdnig-Hoffmann*) and juvenile type III (*Kugelberg-Welander*) being perhaps the best recognized.

In the infantile form (*type I*), symptoms may begin in utero with decreased fetal movement, at birth, or in the first months of life. Hypotonia, weakness, decreased spontaneous activity, and decreased or absent deep tendon reflexes are some of the first signs. There is no sensory loss. Intercostal muscles are nearly always involved, while the diaphragm is spared, resulting in "paradoxic" respirations. Common findings include muscle atrophy; fasciculations, particularly of the tongue; and a characteristic "frog" position with abducted hips and flexed knees. There is a failure to attain age-appropriate motor milestones. The course is rapidly progressive, with death occurring within 1 to 2 years of diagnosis, usually due to pulmonary infection or respiratory insufficiency.

In the juvenile form (*type III*), onset is usually after the second year and may occur as late as adolescence or adulthood. The course may be slowly progressive, but is often static, and there may be slight improvement with age. The proximal muscles are affected first, and may initially mimic Duchenne muscular dystrophy. A fine tremor of outstretched arms is often present. Life span may be normal. Intellectual development is normal.

An intermediate form (*chronic childhood spinal muscular atrophy, type II*), probably genetically distinct from the juvenile form, presents in infancy usually between six to 24 months, and has a prolonged course extending over several years.

Both slowly progressive and rapidly progressive adult onset forms have been recognized.

Other, probably distinct, forms known as distal SMAs involve only distal muscles and have a slow clinical progression.

Laboratory findings include normal cerebrospinal-fluid. Muscle enzymes are usually normal but may be mildly elevated in the juvenile form. Electromyogram (EMG) shows a denervation pattern with large amplitude, polyphasic potentials of long duration, reduced interference pattern on voluntary movement, and fibrillation potentials at rest. Nerve conduction times are normal or minimally prolonged. Muscle biopsy shows groups of angular atrophied fibers interspersed with large bundles of exclusively type I (usually) or type II fibers. "Type grouping" can be demonstrated with appropriate histochemical stains. Atrophy of anterior horn cells of the spinal cord and peripheral nerve degeneration are seen.

Electron microscopic findings include disorganized fibrils, filaments, and sarcomeres, as well as mitochondrial changes, nuclear clumping, and areas of regeneration.

In several families, hexosaminidase deficiency (see **G(M2)-gangliosidosis**) has been associated with clinical and laboratory findings of SMA.

Complications: Recurrent lower respiratory infection, scoliosis, osteoporosis, and other orthopedic deformities.

Associated Findings: Urinary incontinence, cardiomyopathy, cardiac arrhythmia, arthrogryposis. One family was reported in which weakness was confined mainly to the face and pectoral girdle musculature (Fenichel et al, 1967). Hausmanowa-Petrusewicz (1984) reported an absence of tonsillar tissue.

Etiology: Autosomal recessive inheritance (most cases of types I, II, and III) is most common, but some cases of types II and III, many cases of adult onset type IV, and some of the distal varieties are by autosomal dominant inheritance. For an X-linked form, see **Muscular atrophy, spinal and bulbar, X-linked Kennedy type.**

Pathogenesis: Degeneration of anterior horn cells of the spinal cord and brain stem, with subsequent distinctive changes in the associated muscles.

MIM No.: 15859, *15860, 18296, 18297, *18298, *25330, *25340, *25355, 27112, 27115

CDC No.: 335.000

Sex Ratio: Presumably M1:F1. Males are more frequently reported, although males with the juvenile form may be less severely involved. This accounts, in part, for the belief that some cases may be X-linked.

Occurrence: Incidence 4:100,000 live births in northeast England (infantile form). Prevalence 12:1,000,000 in northeast England (juvenile form). The Kugelberg-Welander form has been frequently reported in an inbred Scottish population and on Reunion Island.

Risk of Recurrence for Patient's Sib:
See Part I, *Mendelian Inheritance.*

Risk of Recurrence for Patient's Child:
See Part I, *Mendelian Inheritance.*

Age of Detectability: Before two years of age in the infantile form; two years to adulthood in the juvenile form. An adult form with onset in the fifth or sixth decade has been reported (Jansen et al, 1986).

Gene Mapping and Linkage: SBMA (spinal and bulbar muscular atrophy (Kennedy disease)) has been mapped to Xq13-q22.

Prevention: None known. Genetic counseling indicated.

Treatment: Physical therapy, respiratory care, scrupulous treatment of respiratory infections, and orthopedic care.

Prognosis: In the infantile and adult forms: death within one to two years of onset. In the juvenile form: prolonged survival and sometimes normal life span.

Detection of Carrier: Unknown.

Special Considerations: The nosology of the spinal muscular atrophies has provoked considerable discussion. Several genetic and clinical entities are readily recognized, but there are several other forms. Pearn (1978) distinguished at least ten separate SMA syndromes and postulates 15 or more mutant genes. Until basic defects are identified, distinctions remain imprecise. Although age of onset, clinical course, pattern of muscle involvement, and mode of inheritance are useful distinguishing characteristics for prognosis and counseling purposes, they must be interpreted carefully, since overlapping may occur among the various forms. Families are known in which different members are affected by clinically distinct forms of SMA. Bouwsma et al (1986), Zerres et al (1987), and others have supported Becker's allelic model as an explanation for some unusual pedigrees.

Support Groups:
New York; Muscular Dystrophy Association (MDA)
IL; Highland Park (P.O. Box 1465); Families of Spinal Muscular Atrophy

References:
Fenichel GM, et al.: Neurogenic atrophy simulating facioscapulohumeral dystrophy. Arch Neurol 1967; 17:257–260.
Emery AEH: The nosology of the spinal muscular atrophies. J Med Genet 1971; 8:481–494.
Pearn JH: Incidence, prevalence and gene frequency studies of childhood spinal muscular atrophy. J Med Genet 1978; 15:409–433.
Johnson WG: Hexosaminidase deficiency: a cause of recessively inherited motor neuron diseases. Adv Neurol 1982; 36:159–164.
Hausmanowa-Petrusewicz I, et al.: Chronic proximal spinal muscular atrophy of childhood and adolescence: sex influence. J Med Genet 1984; 21:447–450.
Hausmanowa-Petrusewicz I, et al.: Chronic proximal spinal muscular atrophy of childhood and adolescence: problems of classification and genetic counseling. J Med Genet 1985; 22:350–353.
Bouwsma G, et al.: Unusual pedigree pattern in seven families with spinal muscular atrophy. Clin Genet 1986; 30:145–149.
Jansen PHP, et al.: A rapidly progressive autosomal dominant scapulohumeral form of spinal muscular atrophy. Ann Neurol 1986; 20:538–540.
Zerres K, et al.: Becker's allelic model to explain unusual pedigrees with spinal muscular atrophy. (Letter) Clin Genet 1987; 31:276–277.

BA039   **Louis E. Bartoshesky**

Spinal muscular atrophy, benign-hypertrophy of calves
See SPINAL MUSCULAR ATROPHY
Spinal muscular atrophy, childhood isolated
See SPINAL MUSCULAR ATROPHY
Spinal muscular atrophy, distal type
See SPINAL MUSCULAR ATROPHY
Spinal muscular atrophy, facioscapulohumeral type
See SPINAL MUSCULAR ATROPHY
Spinal muscular atrophy, infantile acute form
See SPINAL MUSCULAR ATROPHY
Spinal muscular atrophy, infantile chronic form
See SPINAL MUSCULAR ATROPHY
Spinal muscular atrophy, proximal, adult type
See SPINAL MUSCULAR ATROPHY
Spinal muscular atrophy, type I
See SPINAL MUSCULAR ATROPHY
Spinal muscular atrophy, type II
See SPINAL MUSCULAR ATROPHY

Spinal muscular atrophy, type III
  See SPINAL MUSCULAR ATROPHY
Spinal muscular atrophy, type IV
  See SPINAL MUSCULAR ATROPHY
Spinal muscular atrophy-hypertrophy of the calves
  *See MUSCULAR ATROPHY, SPINAL AND BULBAR, X-LINKED
  KENNEDY TYPE*
Spine, rigid spine syndrome
  See HAUPTMANN-THANHAUSER SYNDROME

SPINE, SCOLIOSIS, IDIOPATHIC   3003

Includes:
  Discogenic scoliosis
  Scoliosis, genetic

Excludes:
  Scoliosis, paralytic
  Scoliosis associated with other disorders

Major Diagnostic Criteria: Spinal curvature with associated rotation that is *structural.* Curvature may or may not be progressive in both growing and skeletally mature individuals. The abnormality is confirmed by X-ray of the spine taken in the erect position.

Clinical Findings: Trunk asymmetry with curvature of the spine in the thoracic, thoracolumbar, or lumbar regions, the right thoracic pattern being the most common. The most frequent type of idiopathic scoliosis is classified as *adolescent* with onset at more than ten years of age. Two other types of scoliosis are seen; *infantile* is seen from birth to age three years and is typically a left thoracic curve. The curvatures may be resolving or progressive. *Juvenile idiopathic scoliosis* is diagnosed from ages three to ten years.

Typically, in the adolescent idiopathic group, the patients are taller and heavier than their peers without scoliosis. The natural history and risk of progression are intimately involved with skeletal maturity or its lack, and the adolescent growth spurt. It has been shown that increase in the rate of progression of curves does occur during the adolescent growth spurt, although the reasons for this are not clear. Conversely, an adolescent who is at or near skeletal maturity and who has a relatively small curve is at very little risk for progression of the curve.

Complications: With some curvatures, significant cosmetic deformity occurs, including trunk shift, waist asymmetry, pelvic obliquity, rib hump, uneven shoulders, and asymmetric neck line. Large curvatures in the thoracic spine are associated with restrictive lung disease. Pain and neurologic deficits can be found in older individuals, particularly with larger curves. Continued progression of curving can occur in skeletally mature individuals with larger curves (i.e., greater than 45 degrees).

Associated Findings: Some degree of ligamentous laxity, **Mitral valve prolapse.**

Etiology: The cause of idiopathic scoliosis is unclear, but vestibular system dysfunction, posterior spinal cord column malfunction, and abnormalities in vibratory sense can be implicated. Other findings not clearly determined to be causes are abnormal collagen, hormonal abnormalities, and muscle abnormalities.

Pathogenesis: Initial curving and deformity occurs through the soft tissues. With further progression, rotation and other secondary deformities (e.g., rib hump) develop. With further increase in size, secondary changes in vertebrae (e.g., wedging) can occur.

MIM No.: 18180

CDC No.: 754.200

Sex Ratio: M1:F4–7. From school screening data, small curves (less than 20 degrees) are seen equally among boys and girls. Larger curves (greater than 20 degrees) occur more frequently in girls.

Occurrence: The prevalence of scoliosis has been studied using chest and school screening data. Chest X-rays are accurate for thoracic curves but do not show the lumbar spine and thus underestimate the incidence (1.9% for curves greater than 10 degrees). School screening data reveal an incidence 1.1 to 3.2%.

Risk of Recurrence for Patient's Sib: Probably greater than general population. Although there is some controversy about this, a positive family history occurred with twice the frequency in children with progressive curves compared with that in children with stable curves.

Risk of Recurrence for Patient's Child: Unknown. Probably greater than that of the general population.

Age of Detectability: *Infantile,* birth to three years; *juvenile,* 3–10 years; *adolescent,* greater than ten years.

Gene Mapping and Linkage: Unknown.

Prevention: None known. Genetic counseling indicated.

Treatment: Observation is recommended for small curves (i.e., less than 25 degrees) in growing children. For progressive curves of 25 to 40–45 degrees, nonoperative treatment (e.g., a brace) is advised to prevent curve progression. For curves greater than 45 degrees and for those that progress despite bracing, surgery is recommended to correct the curve and to prevent further progression. Various approaches (e.g., anterior vs. posterior) and types of instrumentation (e.g., Harrington, C-D, Zielke) are available.

Prognosis: The importance of detection is to prevent severe curve progression. The predictive factors for progression in growing children are curve size, the Risser sign, and the skeletal age at diagnosis. Other important factors are menstrual history and curve pattern. Curve progression in adults relates primarily with size and pattern of curve.

Detection of Carrier: By clinical examination.

Support Groups:
  CA; Orange; Scoliosis Research Society
  MA; Belmont; National Scoliosis Foundation
  NY; Manhasset; The Scoliosis Association

References:
Bobechko WP, et al.: Electrospinal instrumentation for scoliosis: current status. Orthop Clin North Am 1979; 10:927–941.
Carr WA, et al.: Treatment of idiopathic scoliosis in the Milwaukee brace. J Bone Joint Surg 1980; 62A:599–612.
Weinstein SL, et al.: Idiopathic scoliosis. J Bone Joint Surg 1981; 63A:702–712.
Axelgaard J, et al.: Correction of spinal curvatures by transcutaneous electrical muscle stimulation. Spine 1983; 8:463–481.
Bunnell WP: The natural history of idiopathic scoliosis. 19th Ann Meet SRS, Orlando, FL: 1984.
Lonstein JE, Carlson JM: The prediction of curve progression in untreated idiopathic scoliosis during growth. J Bone Joint Surg 1984; 66A:1061–1071.
Smith MK, et al.: Idiopathic scoliosis and mitral valve prolapse. J Fam Pract 1984; 19:2, 229.
Bradford DS, Hensinger RM: The pediatric spine. New York: Thieme, 1985.
Bradford DS, et al.: Moe's textbook of scoliosis and other spinal deformities, ed 2. Philadelphia: W.B. Saunders, 1987.
Connor JM, et al.: Genetic aspects of early childhood scoliosis. Am J Med Genet 1987; 27:419–424.

LU015   **John P. Lubicky**

SPINE, SPONDYLOLISTHESIS AND SPONDYLOLYSIS   3004

Includes:
  Dysplastic spondylolisthesis and spondylolysis
  Isthmic spondylolisthesis and spondylolysis
  Spondylolisthesis, spine
  Spondylolysis, spine

Excludes:
  Spondylolisthesis; degenerative, traumatic, and pathologic
  Spondylolysis; degenerative, traumatic, and pathologic

Major Diagnostic Criteria: *Spondylolysis* is a defect in the pars interarticularus, resulting in a discontinuity of the body and pedicle with the remainder of the neural arch. This is confirmed by oblique X-rays of the vertebrae, tomography, or computed tomography (CT) with reconstruction. *Spondylolisthesis* is the slipping forward of one vertebrae onto another. This is confirmed by lateral erect X-rays. Isthmic spondylolisthesis is the forward shift of the cranial vertebrae on the inferior one in association with either a lytic defect of the pars or an elongation of an intact pars interarticularus. *Dysplastic spondylolisthesis* is the forward shift of the upper vertebrae on a lower vertebrae in association with a congenital deficiency of the facet articulation that allows the slippage to occur. These conditions are confirmed by plain X-ray and by tomography or CT scans. The degree of spondylolisthesis is graded according to the percentage of slip.

Grade I is a slippage of 0–25%, *grade II* is a slippage of 25–50%, *grade III* is a slippage of 50–75%, and *grade IV* is a slippage greater than 75%. Spondyloptosis is the complete displacement of the upper vertebrae anterior to the vertebrae below. The percentage of slip is the ratio of the millimeters of displacement of the olisthetic vertebrae over the width of the C5 vertebrae as measured in the standing lateral X-ray. The slip angle is determined by a line drawn parallel to the inferior end-plate of the olisthetic vertebrae and a line drawn perpendicular to the posterior cortex of the vertebrae below.

Clinical Findings: Symptoms are generally uncommon during childhood and adolescence. If present, symptoms fall into two categories. The first is mild low back pain or aching in the low back and buttocks related to activities and is generally decreased with rest. The second form of presentation is low back pain with an associated significant radicular component into the posterior thigh and occasionally into the calves. The second form of presentation is generally not associated with the grade I slips. In the higher grades of slippage, an observable and palpable step-off can be felt at the level of spondylolisthesis. Occasionally in the symptomatic patient pressure over the involved arch may reproduce the patient's symptoms. The patient with a high degree of slip has a more characteristic clinical presentation. The sacrum becomes more vertical secondary to pelvic rotation, creating heart-shaped buttocks on examination. The lumbar spine goes into a secondary hyperlordotic position. The hip joints are forced into hyperextension, and the knees remain flexed. Varying degrees of spasm of the hamstrings are generally present. These deformities are thought to be due to the hyperkyphotic deformity of the olisthetic vertebrae.

Neurologic deficits may be present. These generally involve the L5 root, but may involve all of the sacral roots in severe cases. Scoliosis may be associated with spondylolisthesis. This is not a structural curve in the early stages, but may develop some structural characteristics in time. Spina bifida oculta is seen in over 90% of children with spondylolitic spondylolisthesis and in over 70% of adolescents.

Complications: Hyperlordosis of the lumbar spine with associated hamstring tightness can be seen in high-degree slips. The exact cause of hamstring tightness is not known. The abnormal gait pattern associated with these findings is described as stiff leg short-strided. A radiculopathy may be seen, including motor weakness in the rare patient. In the rare dysplastic spondylolisthesis, a low cauda equina syndrome may be seen. This generally is not found in the spondylolitic spondylolistheses.

Associated Findings: Generally there are no associated findings other than the X-ray findings of spina bifida oculta and scoliosis.

Etiology: Family studies suggest that spondylolitic spondylolisthesis is an inherited trait. The exact mode of transmission has not been defined. Most investigators believe the inheritance pattern to be either autosomal dominant with reduced penetrance, multifactorial, or genetic heterogeneity with multiple Mendelian traits.

Pathogenesis: Development of the spondylolitic defect probably takes place in an area of dysplasia in the cartilagenous model of the arch. Assumption of the upright position is probably associated with the development of the actual defect. Spondylolysis has not been identified in the person who does not leave the recumbent position. There is excess stress to the area of the pars, which may be associated with a stress fracture of the pars.

MIM No.: 18420

CDC No.: 756.130

Sex Ratio: M2:F1

Occurrence: Six percent of the Caucasian population have X-ray evidence of spondylolysis as an adult: 8% in males and 4% in females. The frequency in various ethnic groups has been reported to be less than 3% in Blacks and greater than 50% in Eskimos. The high frequency in the Eskimo population may be due to the posture assumed while performing many of their tasks.

Risk of Recurrence for Patient's Sib:
See Part I, *Mendelian Inheritance.*

Risk of Recurrence for Patient's Child:
See Part I, *Mendelian Inheritance.*

Age of Detectability: The youngest reported patient was four months old. Most patients are first seen in early childhood at ages 5–6. Many cases are not clinically evident throughout life.

Gene Mapping and Linkage: Unknown.

Prevention: None known. Genetic counseling indicated.

Treatment: Most patients are asymptomatic and require no treatment. Patients with grade I and II slips are allowed full activities. Patients with grade III and IV slips should be followed with serial X-rays, and, if progression of the slip is documented, fusion should be performed. Patients with symptoms are generally treated with rest followed by appropriate stretching and strengthening exercises for the trunk and lower extremities. A brace may be useful at times in controlling symptoms. Patients who present with significant hamstring tightness and pain and who do not respond to the above regimen usually respond to fusion. The question of reduction of severe degrees of slips, i.e., grades III and IV, is controversial. Those patients with a high slip angle should attempt to reduce at least the slip angle by postural means at the time of fusion.

Prognosis: Good in most patients. Pain and deformity can usually be helped by surgical intervention, if needed.

Detection of Carrier: Unknown.

References:

Taillard W: Le spondylolisthesis chez l'enfant et l'adolescent (Etude de 50 cas). Acta Orthop Scand 1954; 24:115–144.
Wiltse LL: The etiology of spondylolisthesis. J Bone Joint Surg 1962; 44A:539–560.
Neugebauer FL: The classic: a new contribution to the history and etiology of spondyl-olisthesis. Clin Orthop 1976; 117:4–22.
Wynn-Davies R, Scott JHS: Inheritance and spondylolisthesis: a radiographic family survey. J Bone Joint Surg 1979; 61B(3):301–305.
Fredrickson D, et al.: The natural history of spondylolysis and spondylolisthesis. J Bone Joint Surg 1984; 66A:669–707.

FR041   **Bruce E. Fredrickson**
LU015   **John P. Lubicky**

Spinocerebella ataxia with dysmorphism
See *ATAXIA-DYSMORPHIC FACIES-TRICHODYSPLASIA*
Spinocerebellar ataxia with dementia and amyloid plaques
See *GERSTMANN-STRAUSSLER SYNDROME*
Spinocerebellar ataxia-sideroblastic anemia
See *ANEMIA, SIDEROBLASTIC*

SPINOCEREBELLAR DEGENERATION-CORNEAL DYSTROPHY   2619

Includes:
Corneal-cerebellar syndrome
Corneal dystrophy-spinocerebellar degeneration

Excludes:
Amyloidosis, Finnish type (2145)
Ataxia, Friedreich type (2714)
Corneal dystrophy, endothelial (0208)
Fabry disease (0373)
Mucopolysaccharidosis

Major Diagnostic Criteria: Moderate mental retardation, bilateral corneal opacification starting in the second year of life and leading to severe visual impairment, and slowly progressive cerebellar abnormalities with variable dorsal column and upper motor neuron involvement.

Clinical Findings: Corneal opacification is noted during the second year of life and is slowly progressive. During the third decade, recurrent eye pain may start, along with photophobia, foreign body sensation, and lacrimation. Visual acuity is reduced to counting fingers at one meter and to noticing hand motion.

Neurologically, the following may be present: unsteady tandem gait, head tremor, ataxia on finger-to-nose and heel-to-shin tests, exaggeration of myotatic tendon reflexes in the upper and lower limb, hyperreflexia, slight increase in the muscle tone, with fairly good muscle power. Sensory findings are normal. Eye movements are normal, without nystagmus. Plantar reflexes may be extensor or flexor. IQ is 50–60.

The EEG may reveal localized or diffuse slow waves or prominent, high-voltage waves. Nerve conduction studies may show delayed motor conduction in the peroneal nerve and delayed distal latency. Electromyography and audiometry are normal. There may be a slight increase in alpha-1, alpha-2 serum protein fractions and an increase in IgG, IgA, and IgM.

Histologic examination shows findings of corneal dystrophy, including corneal edema, thickening of Descemet membrane, and degenerative pannus. High-resolution light and electron microscopy of muscle shows variation in muscle fiber size and subsarcolemmal mitochondrial aggregates intermixed with lysosomes and lipid droplets, myelin figures, and increased thickness of the basement membrane of capillaries. A moderate degree of glycogen, giant mitochondria with dense, crystalline, filamentous inclusions may be seen. The sural nerve shows an increase in connective tissue between fibers and reduction in the number of myelinated nerve fibers.

Complications: Unknown.

Associated Findings: Cervical lordosis, lumbar rotoscoliosis, or severe osteoarthritis of the hip joint may be found.

Etiology: Autosomal recessive inheritance. The two sisters reported with this condition had consanguineous parents.

Pathogenesis: Unknown.

MIM No.: 27131

POS No.: 3534

Sex Ratio: Presumably M1:F1.

Occurrence: Two sisters were reported from Lebanon.

Risk of Recurrence for Patient's Sib:
See Part I, *Mendelian Inheritance.*

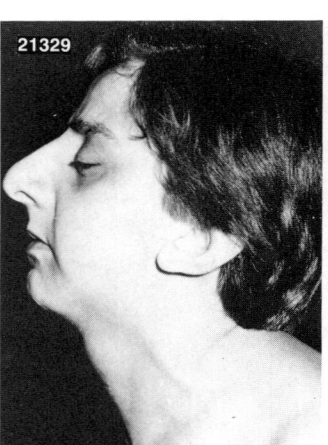 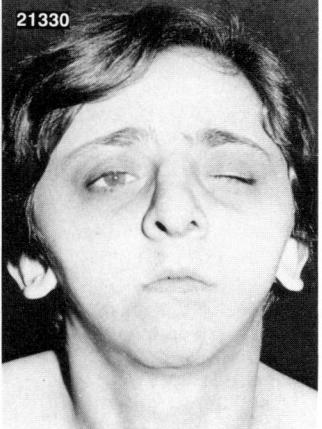

2619-21329–30: Facial view shows corneal dystrophy and ptosis.

Risk of Recurrence for Patient's Child:
See Part I, *Mendelian Inheritance.*

Age of Detectability: The corneal opacities begin during the second year of life, and the neurologic findings appear toward the end of the first decade of life.

Gene Mapping and Linkage: Unknown.

Prevention: None known. Genetic counseling indicated.

Treatment: Corneal grafting can be performed. However, vision cannot be improved more than 20/100 because of amblyopia.

Prognosis: Normal life span. However, both the decreased vision and the neurologic problems are disabling and limit the independence of the patient.

Detection of Carrier: Unknown.

References:
Der Kaloustian VM, et al.: Familial spinocerebellar degeneration with corneal dystrophy. Am J Med Genet 1985; 20:325–339.

DE030   **Vazken M. Der Kaloustian**

Spinopontine atrophy
   See MACHADO-JOSEPH DISEASE
Spirochete, fetal effects of maternal Lyme disease
   See FETAL EFFECTS FROM LYME DISEASE

SPLEEN, CONGENITAL ISOLATED HYPOSPLENIA   2600

Includes:
   Hyposplenia, congenital isolated
   Splenic agenesis, isolated congenital

Excludes: Asplenia syndrome (0092)

Major Diagnostic Criteria: The presence of Howell-Jolly bodies in an infant with repeated infections or on routine examination should make the physician suspicious of congenital splenic hypoplasia or agenesis. Other findings in the blood smear are polycythemia, Heinz bodies, siderocytes, target cells, and normablasts. A chest X-ray in an older infant or child may demonstrate an absence of the splenic shadow. Absence or hyposplenia can be confirmed with radioisotope imaging of the spleen.

Clinical Findings: With the absence of other congenital anomalies, splenic hypoplasia or agenesis will present with repeated episodes of sepsis, usually of the upper respiratory tract or lungs.

Complications: Persistent or recurrent, difficult-to-treat infections may cause death.

Associated Findings: **Mucopolysaccharidosis** has been reported in one series of patients with congenital hyposplenia.

Etiology: Possibly autosomal recessive inheritance, although autosomal dominant inheritance has also been suggested. Consanguinity was present in the sibship reported by Kevy et al (1968)

Pathogenesis: Compression or a stretching force on the developing splenic artery at about the fourth week of gestation may prevent the spleen from developing. At birth the spleen is noted to weigh 1g or less.

MIM No.: *27140

CDC No.: 759.010

Sex Ratio: M1:F1

Occurrence: Undetermined but presumed rare. Familial patterns have been reported in one sibship and two generations of another family.

Risk of Recurrence for Patient's Sib:
See Part I, *Mendelian Inheritance.*

Risk of Recurrence for Patient's Child: Unknown.

Age of Detectability: Usually within the first few weeks to the first few months of life.

Gene Mapping and Linkage: Unknown.

Prevention: None known. Genetic counseling indicated.

Treatment: Early recognition and prompt diagnosis and treatment of sepsis will save the patient's life. Prophylactic antibiotics and vaccination for *Pneumococcus* and *Haemophilus* infections after age two years should be implemented.

Prognosis: Depends on early recognition and treatment of sepsis. In a series of patients with the asplenic syndrome, there is an improved survival with asplenia or hyposplenia.

Detection of Carrier: Unknown.

References:
Kevy SV, et al.: Hereditary splenic hypoplasia. Pediatrics 1968; 42:752–758.
Gray SW, Skandalakis JE: Embryology for surgeons. Philadelphia: W.B. Saunders, 1972.
Dehner LP: Pediatric surgical pathology. St. Louis: C.V. Mosby, 1975.
Biggar WD, Remirez RA: Congenital asplenia: immunologic assessment and a clinical review of eight surviving patients. Pediatrics 1981; 67:548–551.
Monie IW: The asplenia syndrome: an explanation for absence of the spleen. Teratology 1982; 25:215–219.
Gates AJ, Black SH: Isolated congenital hyposplenia (ICH) in two generations of a non-consanguineous family. (Abstract) Am J Hum Genet 1986; 39:A61 only.

BE049   **Arthur S. Besser**

SPLEEN, CYSTS   0240

Includes:
Cysts, true, benign
Epidermoid cysts
Epithelial cysts
Mesothelial cysts-squamous metaplasia

Excludes:
Cystic lymphangioma
Degenerative (post-traumatic) cysts
Dermoid tumor with cystic degeneration
Parasitic cyst
Polycystic hemangioma
Serous cyst
Splenic capsular fusion with pancreatic pseudocyst

Major Diagnostic Criteria: Cyst (usually unilocular) of spleen with lining consisting of a single cell layer of flattened cells, most likely mesothelium.

Clinical Findings: Cysts are minimal or absent in early life despite the assumption that splenic cysts have congenital origin. Splenic cysts have not been identified in series of autopsies of stillbirths, infants and children. They produce symptoms only when they cause splenic enlargement as a result of fluid accumulation within the cyst lumen. The most common presenting symptom is dull left upper quadrant pain. Next most common is a mass in the left upper quadrant. Other presentations include rupture (up to 25% in some series), dyspnea and early satiety due to gastric compression. Overt abdominal protuberance has been described.
The X-ray triad of a normal intraveneous pyelogram, inferior displacement of the splenic flexure of the colon and medial displacement of the left gastric border is diagnostic of splenic enlargement. Imaging techniques reveal the cystic nature of the lesion. Ultrasound, computerized tomography and radionucleide liver-spleen scan (^{99m}Tc-sulfocolloid or ^{198}Au) are each capable of determining the nature and size of splenic cysts. The histologic type is confirmed at surgical splenectomy.
The cyst is often large - ranging from 6 to more than 30 cm in diameter. It has a thin squamous epithelial-like lining and contains sero-sanguinous to toothpaste-like fluid ranging in color from light yellow to dark brown. The wall is occasionally calcified. Cysts most often involve the upper pole of the spleen.

Complications: Rupture of the cyst with intraperitonal hemorrhage is the most common and life-threatening complication. Splenic cyst rarely has been associated with hypersplenism.

Associated Findings: None known.

Etiology: Unknown.

Pathogenesis: The most likely mechanism is inclusion of primative coelomic mesothelium into the splenic primordium during early organogenesis. Against this hypothesis is the fact that the splenic primordium arises as a specialized condensation of mesenchyme within the leaves of the dorsal mesogastrium and therefore is not open to inclusions from a mesothelial surface. An alternative hypothesis is invagination of capsular surface mesothelium during later development. Against this, it is interesting to note that cysts have not been reported in accessory spleens despite their incidence of up to 35% in adult autopsies. In either case, the mesothelial remnant undergoes squamous metaplasia to form the characteristic epithelial lining. The lining secretes fluid into the cystic lumen producing the expanded cyst which is clinically evident.

CDC No.: 759.080

Sex Ratio: M1:F1.5–10

Occurrence: Fewer than 200 splenic cysts reported.

Risk of Recurrence for Patient's Sib: Not increased.

Risk of Recurrence for Patient's Child: Not increased.

Age of Detectability: Six months to seventy years (usually in second to fourth decade) by clinical examination.

Gene Mapping and Linkage: Unknown.

Prevention: None known. Genetic counseling indicated.

Treatment: Surgical cystectomy is needed. Because of the risk of hemorrhage from the spleen, total splenectomy has been successfully performed for treatment of cysts. Subtotal splenectomy is recommended because of the risk of post-splenectomy sepsis or reduced immune competence.

Prognosis: Excellent unless rupture and hemorrhage occur or surgical therapy is complicated by hemorrhage.

Detection of Carrier: Unknown.

References:
Bostick WL, Lucia SP: Nonparasitic, noncancerous cystic tumors of the spleen. AMA Arch Pathol 1949; 47:215–222.
Fowler RH: Collective review: non-parasitic cystic tumors of the spleen. Int Abstr Surg (Surg Gynec Obstet) 1953; 96:209–227.
Browne MK: Epidermoid cysts of the spleen. Brit J Surg 1963; 50:838–841.
Hoffman E: Non-parasitic splenic cysts. Am J Surg 1968; 93:765–770.
Blank E, Cambell JR: Epidermoid cysts of the spleen. Pediatrics 1973; 51:75–84.
Ough YD, et al.: Mesothelial cysts of the spleen with squamous metaplasia. Am J Clin Pathol 1981; 75:666–669.
Dachman AH, et al.: Nonparasitic spleen cysts: a report of 52 cases with radiologic-pathologic correlation. Am J Roentgen 1986; 147: 537–542.
Khan AH, et al.: Partial splenectomy for benign cystic lesions of the spleen. J Pediatr Surg 1986; 21:749–752.

SH054   **Douglas R. Shanklin**
WH007   **Peter F. Whitington**
                                               John R. Esterly

Splenic agenesis
See ASPLENIA SYNDROME
Splenic agenesis, isolated congenital
See SPLEEN, CONGENITAL ISOLATED HYPOSPLENIA

SPLENOGONADAL FUSION-LIMB DEFECT 3053

Includes:

> Limb deficiency-splenogonadal fusion
> Micrognathia-limb deficiency-splenogonadal fusion
> Splenogonadal fusion, isolated

Excludes:

Hypoglossia-hypodactylia (0451)

Major Diagnostic Criteria: The combination of terminal transverse limb defects and splenogonadal fusion.

Clinical Findings: Lower limb involvement, ranging from unilateral missing lower leg to total absence of both legs. Upper limbs were also involved (13/17), with severity ranging from missing fingers on one hand to total lack of both arms. Orofacial anomalies also occur, with micrognathia (7/17) the most common finding. Anal atresia or stenosis occurred in three cases.

Complications: Bowel obstruction, **Hernia, inguinal**, and cryptorchidism.

Associated Findings: Reported in one affected individual each were plagiocephaly, misshapen and posteriorly rotated ears, anodontia, V-shaped palate, congenital heart defect, unilateral diaphragmatic agenesis, **Diaphragmatic hernia**, polymicrogyria, and bifid vertebrae C6-T3.

Etiology: Unknown. No familial cases have been reported; no affected individuals have reproduced. Autosomal dominant inheritance has therefore not been ruled out.

Pathogenesis: Unknown. Several theories have been proposed to explain the co-occurrence of splenogonadal fusion and limb defects; none entirely satisfactory.

MIM No.: 18330

POS No.: 4025

Sex Ratio: M15:F2 observed.

Occurrence: Seventeen cases have been reported in the literature.

Risk of Recurrence for Patient's Sib:
See Part I, *Mendelian Inheritance.*

Risk of Recurrence for Patient's Child:
See Part I, *Mendelian Inheritance.*

Age of Detectability: At birth, although prenatal diagnosis is theoretically possible.

Gene Mapping and Linkage: Unknown.

Prevention: None known. Genetic counseling indicated.

Treatment: Supportive.

Prognosis: Although 8/14 individuals died within the first year of life or were stillborn, two other individuals were aged 10 and 15 years at the time of last report. The ten-year-old was mildly mentally retarded; the 15-year-old was of apparently normal intellect.

Detection of Carrier: Unknown.

Special Considerations: It has been suggested by Pauli and Greenlaw (1982) that splenogonadal fusion-limb defect and **Hypoglossia-hypodactylia** may have a similar, if not identical, pathogenesis and therefore represent different expressions of the same basic defect. It is also suggested that splenogonadal fusion without limb defects is pathogenetically related to splenogonadal fusion with limb defects, and simply represent differences in the timing of the occurrence of the initial insult.

References:

Putschar WGJ, Manion WC: Splenic-gonadal fusion. Am J Path 1956; 32:15–35.

Hives JR, Eggum PR: Splenic-gonadal fusion causing bowel obstruction. Arch Surg 1961; 83:887–889.

Pauli RM, Greenlaw A: Limb deficiency and splenogonadal fusion. Am J Med Genet 1982; 13:81–90. †

Gouw ASH, et al.: The spectrum of spleno-gonadal fusion. Eur J Pediatr 1985; 144:316–323.

T0007

Helga V. Toriello

SPONDYLOCOSTAL DYSOSTOSIS-VISCERAL DEFECTS-DANDY WALKER CYST 2924

Includes:

> Dandy-Walker cyst-spondylocostal dysostosis-visceral defects
> Micromelia (lethal)-spondylocostal dysostosis-skeletal anomalies
> Visceral defects-Dandy-Walker cysts-spondylocostal dysostosis

Excludes: Achondrogenesis

Major Diagnostic Criteria: Severe micromelia, **Cleft palate**, rocker-bottom feet, generalized **Brachydactyly**, **Hydrocephaly** with **Corpus callosum agenesis** and Dandy-Walker cyst, pulmonary hypoplasia, intestinal malrotation, right heart hypoplasia, dysplastic small kidneys, stenosis of the ureterovesicular junction, and uterovaginal duplication.

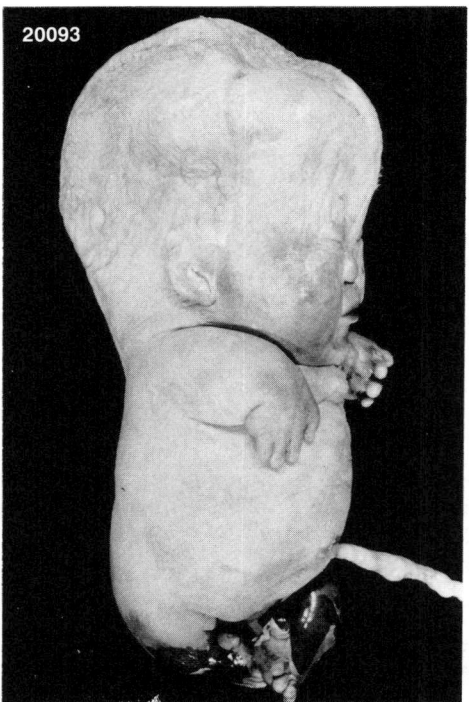

2924-20093: Micromelic dwarfism with marked hydrocephaly, short trunk and narrow chest.

Clinical Findings: Based on two cases; severe micromelia, **Cleft palate**, rocker-bottom feet, generalized **Brachydactyly**, **Hydrocephaly** with **Corpus callosum agenesis** and Dandy-Walker cyst, pulmonary hypoplasia, intestinal malrotation, right heart hypoplasia, dysplastic small kidneys, stenosis of the ureterovesicalar junction, and uterovaginal duplication.

Complications: Unknown.

Associated Findings: In addition to the short-limbed dwarfism and the spondylocostal dysostosis, identical external and internal malformations were present in both stillborns. Polyhydramnios was evident in the third trimester of pregnancy.

Etiology: Two isolated patients have been reported. As for other types of lethal short-limbed dwarfism, autosomal recessive inheritance is possible.

Pathogenesis: Histologic examination of the growth plates revealed that the reserve cartilage was hypercellular, often with clumping of the resting chrondrocytes into lacunae containing three to four cells. The cartilage matrix and the individual chondrocytes appeared normal. The endochondral ossification was disturbed, with markedly narrowed zones of proliferation and hypertrophy.

POS No.: 3659

Sex Ratio: M1:F1 (based on the two known patients).

Occurrence: Undetermined but presumably rare. Two patients have been reported.

Risk of Recurrence for Patient's Sib:
See Part I, *Mendelian Inheritance.*

Risk of Recurrence for Patient's Child:
See Part I, *Mendelian Inheritance.* Affected individuals are not expected to survive to reproduce.

Age of Detectability: Prenatal ultrasound diagnosis is, in principle, feasible in the second trimester of pregnancy by the presence of short-limbed dwarfism, central nervous system malformations, and polyhydramnios.

Gene Mapping and Linkage: Unknown.

Prevention: None known. Genetic counseling indicated.

Treatment: Supportive.

Prognosis: Lethal syndrome due to the short-limbed dwarfism, short trunk, narrow chest, and severity of the central nervous system malformations.

Detection of Carrier: Unknown.

References:
Shih LY, et al.: Dwarfism associated with prenatal ventriculomegaly. Prenatal Diagn 1983; 3:69–73.
Moerman PH, et al.: A new lethal chondrodysplasia with spondylocostal dysostosis, multiple internal anomalies and Dandy-Walker cyst. Clin Genet 1985; 27:160–164.

FR030
Jean-Pierre Fryns

Spondylocostal dysplasia
See SPONDYLOTHORACIC DYSPLASIA

SPONDYLOCOSTAL DYSPLASIA   0896

Includes:
Costovertebral segmentation anomalies
Hemivertebrae, autosomal dominant multiple
Jarcho-Levin syndrome
Polydysspondyly

Excludes:
Facial cleft, lateral (0374)
Incontinentia pigmenti (0526)
Klippel-Feil anomaly (2032)
Larsen syndrome (0570)
Nevoid basal cell carcinoma syndrome (0101)
Oculo-auriculo-vertebral anomaly (0735)
Spondylothoracic dysplasia (0900)

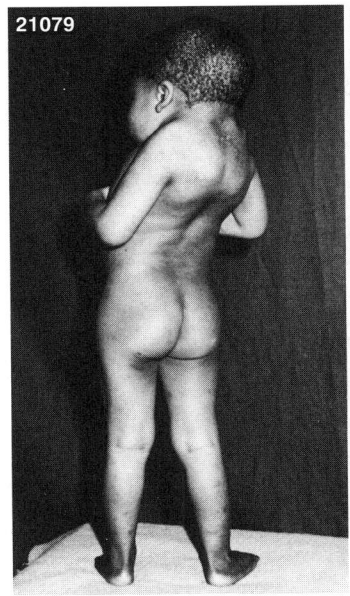 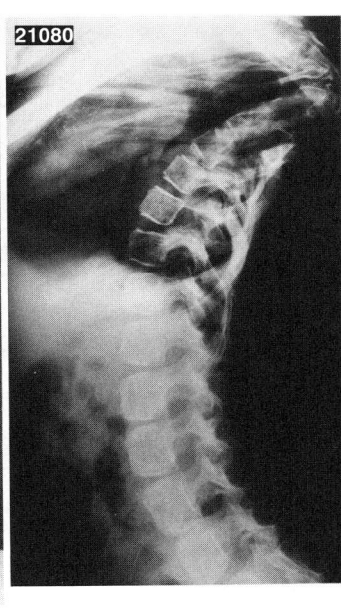

0896-21079: An affected girl aged 5 years. Her neck is short and she has a lumbar lordosis and mild dorsal kyphoscoliosis. 21080: Lateral X-ray of the spine showing unusually tall vertebral bodies in the upper lumbar and lower thoracic regions.

Major Diagnostic Criteria: A shortened trunk associated with segmentation anomalies of the vertebrae and ribs, with a normal skull and limbs.

Clinical Findings: Short-trunked dwarfism associated with multiple anomalies of the vertebrae and ribs. The skull and limbs are normal. The upper/lower segment ratio is decreased for age, and the arm span is greater than the height. The neck is thick and short, and rotary movements are limited. Patients are usually asymptomatic in childhood, but increasing limitation of motion of the spine with back pain can occur in adults. X-rays show gross disorganization of vertebral segmentation, with a reduced number of vertebrae, fused or "block" vertebrae, hemivertebrae and sagitally cleft or "butterfly" vertebrae. The ribs and their vertebral pedicles are reduced in number, and many of those present are hypoplastic or fused. The bones of the skull and limbs are normal.
A relatively mild form of recessively inherited spondylocostal dysplasia has also been reported which is difficult to distinguish clinically from dominant spondylocostal dysplasia.

Complications: Increasing limitation of spinal movement, which may be associated with back pain and referred pain secondary to nerve root compression.

Associated Findings: None known.

Etiology: Usually autosomal dominant inheritance, although a milder recessive form has also been reported. In one report of a similar condition in a mother and daughter, both carried a 14–15 chromosome translocation.

Pathogenesis: Unknown.

MIM No.: *12260

POS No.: 3390, 3410, 3393

Sex Ratio: M1:F1

Occurrence: About a dozen families have been reported.

Risk of Recurrence for Patient's Sib:
See Part I, *Mendelian Inheritance.*

Risk of Recurrence for Patient's Child:
See Part I, *Mendelian Inheritance.*

Age of Detectability: At birth, by clinical and X-ray examination.

Gene Mapping and Linkage: Unknown.

Prevention: None known. Genetic counseling indicated.

Treatment: The effects of bracing or spinal fusion to prevent scoliosis and nerve root compression have not been systematically evaluated.

Prognosis: Normal life span.

Detection of Carrier: By clinical examination of first degree relatives.

References:
Van de Sar A: Hereditary multiple hemivertebrae. Docum Med Geogr Trop 1952; 4:23–28.
Rimoin DL, et al.: Spondylocostal dysplasia: a dominantly inherited form of short-trunked dwarfism. Am J Med 1968; 45:948–953.*†
Ayme S, Preus M: Spondylocostal/spondylothoracic dysostosis: the clinical basis for prognosticating and genetic counseling. Am J Med Genet 1986; 24:599–606.
Lorenz P, Rupprecht E: Spondylocostal dysostosis: dominant type. Am J Med Genet 1990; 35:219–221.†

B0025

Zvi Borochowitz
David L. Rimoin

Spondylodysplasia with pure brachyolmia
See BRACHYOLMIA, HOBAEK TYPE
Spondylodysplasia, dominant type
See BRACHYOLMELIA, DOMINANT TYPE
Spondylodysplasia, Maroteaux type
See BRACHYOLMELIA, MAROTEAUX TYPE
Spondyloenchondrodysplasia
See SPONDYLOMETAPHYSEAL DYSPLASIA WITH ENCHONDROMATOUS CHANGES

SPONDYLOEPIMETAPHYSEAL DYSPLASIA   2313

Includes:
Spondyloepimetaphyseal dysplasia, Irapa type (SEMDIT)
Spondyloepimetaphyseal dysplasia, Minnesota type
Spondylometepiphyseal dysplasia (SMED)
Spondylometaepiphyseal dysplasia

Excludes:
Metaphyseal chondrodysplasia (all)
Spondyloepimetaphyseal dysplasia, Strudwick type (3059)
Spondyloepiphyseal dysplasia congenita (0897)
Spondyloepimetaphyseal dysplasia-joint laxity (2244)
Spondyloepiphyseal dysplasia, late (0898)

Major Diagnostic Criteria: Disproportionate short stature with X-ray changes involving the spine, epiphyses, and metaphyses.

Clinical Findings: The term *spondyloepimetaphyseal dysplasia* (SEMD) is used broadly to include any skeletal dysplasia involving the spine, epiphyses, and metaphyses. Several clinical syndromes meeting this criterion have been reported. This article will focus on two specific conditions:
The *Irapa type* of SEMD was first described by Arias et al. in 1976. Three Mexican sibs with the same entity were described by Hernandez et al (1980). Like **Spondyloepimetaphyseal dysplasia, Strudwick type**, these children have severe short-trunk dwarfism with platyspondyly, **Pectus carinatum**, increased lumbar lordosis, genu valga, and pes planus. Features distinguishing Irapa type include short metacarpals and metatarsals with a relatively spared second metatarsal.
SEMD, *Minnesota type*, has been identified in 26 individuals from 19 families. This disorder was not clinically recognized until ages 1–2 years, although X-ray changes were present at birth. The extremities and trunk became noticeably short between ages 1–2 years. The neck is short and the chest is barrel shaped. Hip and knee flexion contractures, genu valga, and pes planus develop in early childhood. Kyphoscoliosis is progressive and requires surgery in the more severe cases. Odontoid hypoplasia to aplasia has been noted in all individuals, and some require cervical spine fusion. Whether life span is altered is not known, but respiratory insufficiency does occur.

X-ray findings of the Minnesota-type SEMD include marked platyspondyly with mild-to-moderate kyphoscoliosis, odontoid hypoplasia to aplasia, wide and short proximal femora, irregular ossification centers at the knee, marked metaphyseal widening and irregularity, and flat epiphyses.
SEMD, Minnesota type, has been previously misclassified as a variant of **Pseudoachondroplastic dysplasia** or, occasionally, as **Mucopolysaccharidosis IV**. Unlike the other SEMDs, clinical recognition usually occurs between ages one and two years, but X-ray changes are present in the newborn.

Complications: Severe scoliosis and cord compression are consequences of the vertebral malformations. Myopia was found in one patient, but ophthalmologic evaluations were not done routinely. The vitreoretinal degeneration and retinal detachments of SED congenita do not appear to be a feature of these disorders. Inguinal and umbilical hernias have occurred, and they probably reflect the underlying connective tissue disorder.

Associated Findings: Midface hemangioma, bilateral congenital hydronephrosis.

Etiology: Families with unaffected parents and multiple affected sibs have been reported with SEMDIT, suggesting autosomal recessive inheritance.
SEMD, Minnesota type, by autosomal dominant inheritance. Four families with parent-to-child transmission have been documented. Sporadic cases have also been reported.

Pathogenesis: Biochemical alterations in type II collagen have been reported in three cases of unclassified SEMD.

MIM No.: *27165

Sex Ratio: M1:F1 (Minnesota type). Arias et al. (1976) observed a predominance of affected males in their Irapa population.

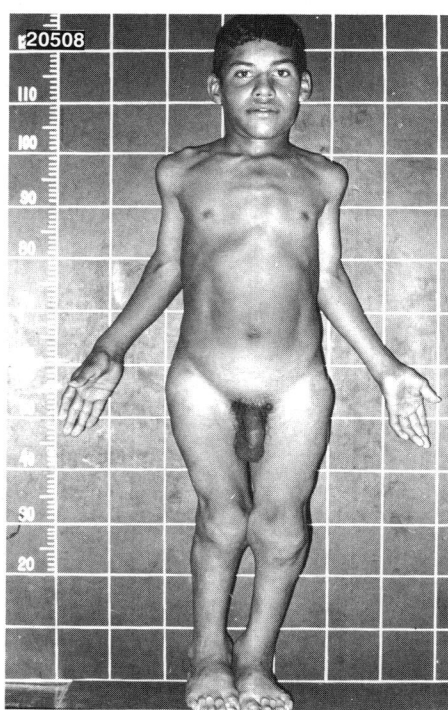

2313-20508: Spondyloepimetaphyseal dysplasia; note disproportionate short stature, rhizomelic shortening of the limbs and a semiflexed posture.

Occurrence: At least 19 reported cases of SEMDIT; and 26 cases SEMD, Minnesota type. Unclassified SEMD has also been reported.

Risk of Recurrence for Patient's Sib:
See Part I, *Mendelian Inheritance.*

Risk of Recurrence for Patient's Child:
See Part I, *Mendelian Inheritance.*

Age of Detectability: SEMDIT is clinically detectable at birth; SEMD, Minnesota type, is detectable during the first 1–2 years of life.

Gene Mapping and Linkage: Unknown.

Prevention: None known. Genetic counseling indicated.

Treatment: Symptomatic management of orthopedic complications. Special attention must be paid to the potential of cervical vertebral abnormalities and secondary cord compression.

Prognosis: The natural history has not been well delineated. The most serious complications are cord compression and respiratory insufficiency. Only one of the cases of Anderson et al. (1982) was mentally retarded; this was a child with congenital hydronephrosis who underwent multiple surgeries very early in infancy. On the whole, intelligence is normal.

Detection of Carrier: Unknown.

Special Considerations: Genetic heterogeneity undoubtedly exists in this group of patients. This is evidenced by the existence of not only of clinically distinct types of SEMD, but also of multiple persons with short stature and X-ray changes involving the spine, epiphyses, and metaphyses who do not fit into any currently accepted classification. Families have been observed that conform to both autosomal dominant and autosomal recessive modes of inheritance. Thus, genetic counseling in this condition must cover the possibilities of either dominant or recessive inheritance. In addition, the potential of metaphyseal involvement later in life should be considered in any infant in whom the diagnosis is made.

References:

Murdoch JL, Walker BA: A "new" form of spondylometaphyseal dysplasia. BD:OAS V(4). New York: March of Dimes Birth Defects Foundation, 1969:368–370.

Arias S, et al.: Irapa osteochondrodysplastic dwarfism: an ethnic marker gene for a subgroup or polymorphic differentiation in one locus. Exerpta Med Int Congress Ser 1976; 397:173 only.

Hernandez A, et al.: Autosomal recessive spondylo-epi-metaphyseal dysplasia (Irapa type) in a Mexican family: delineation of the syndrome. Am J Med Genet 1980; 5:179–188.

Arias S: Osteochondrodysplasia Irapa type: an ethnic marker gene in two subcontinents. Am J Med Genet 1981; 8:251–253.

Spranger JW, Maroteaux P: Genetic heterogeneity of spondyloepiphyseal dysplasia congenita? Am J Med Genet 1982; 13:241–242.

Murray L, et al.: Abnormal type II collagen in the spondyloepi- and spondyloepimetaphyseal dysplasias. Clin Res 1985; 33:118a.

FR005

Clair A. Francomano

Spondyloepimetaphyseal dysplasia, Irapa type (SEMDIT)
See SPONDYLOEPIMETAPHYSEAL DYSPLASIA
Spondyloepimetaphyseal dysplasia, Minnesota type
See SPONDYLOEPIMETAPHYSEAL DYSPLASIA

SPONDYLOEPIMETAPHYSEAL DYSPLASIA, STRUDWICK TYPE   3059

Includes:
> Dappled metaphysis syndrome
> SMED Strudwick
> Spondylometaphyseal dysplasia, Brazilian type
> Spondylometaepiphyseal dysplasia, Strudwick type
> Spondylometaepiphyseal dysplasia congenita
> Strudwick syndrome

Excludes:
> **Spondyloepimetaphyseal dysplasia** (2313)
> **Spondyloepimetaphyseal dysplasia-joint laxity** (2244)

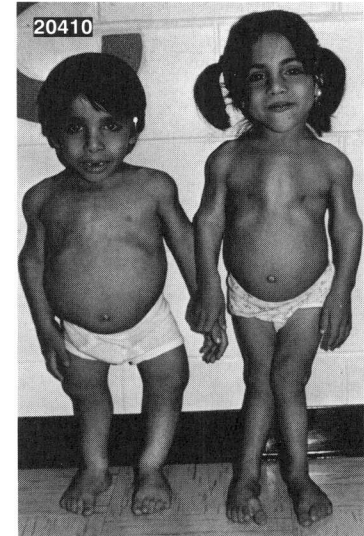
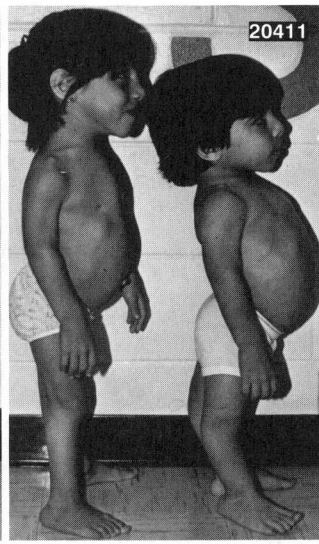
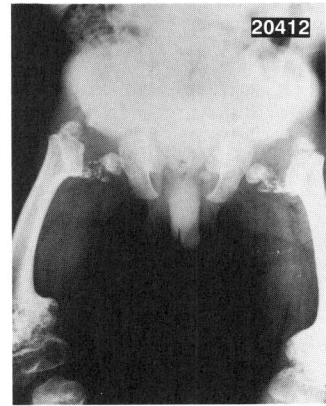
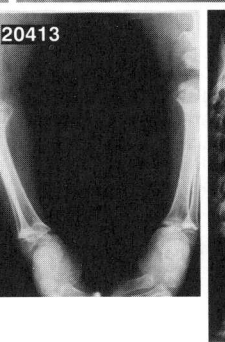
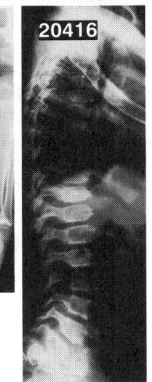

3059-20410: Spondylometepiphyseal dysplasia, Strudwick type; note short trunk-short limb type of short stature with normal facies and genua valga. **20411:** Lateral view shows lordosis and pectus carinatum. **20412:** Hypoplastic pelvis, coxa vara with wide, irregular metaphyses and shortened femurs in the brother. **20413:** Tibiae vara, metepiphyseal changes. **20416:** Hypoplastic flattened vertebrae with anterior beaking, and accentuated lordosis.

Spondyloepiphyseal dysplasia congenita (0897)
Spondylometaphyseal chondrodysplasia, Kozlowski type (0899)

Major Diagnostic Criteria: Short trunk-short limb dwarfism with delayed epiphyseal maturation present at birth. The face appears normal. Exacerbated lordosis, scoliosis, genua valga, **Pectus carinatum**, and pes planus appear later.

Clinical Findings: The most common major and characteristic features are the disproportionate short stature at birth and normal-appearing skull and facies. A **Cleft palate** may be present. Clubfeet, hernias, dislocated hips, and hydronephrosis are additional nonspecific anomalies. With age, lordosis, scoliosis, pectus carinatum with rib flaring and Harrison groove, knock knees, and pes planus appear. With exertion, arthralgias are common.

X-ray findings include epiphyseal delay at birth and club-shaped femora; ribs with splayed, bulbous anterior ends; hypoplastic olecranon and odontoid and fragmented appearance of the epiphyses during infancy and early childhood. Metaphyseal "dappling" of alternating osteosclerosis and radiolucencies appears usually after age three years. It starts on the proximal femur and subsequently involves the proximal humeri, distal radii, ulnae, and both ends of tibiae and fibulae. The dappling is greater in the ulna than in the radius and in the fibula compared with the tibia; this is in contrast to other metaphyseal dysplasias. Platyspondyly is almost always present after age one year. Pear-shaped vertebrae are seen as a result of posterior hypoplasia of vertebral bodies. Scoliosis is usually a late sign, after age ten years.

In a few patients with the condition, chondro-osseous studies have shown abnormal iliac crest growth plate. Clustering of chondrocytes in the proliferative and hypertrophic zones with short osseous trabeculae arising at irregular intervals were noted. Inclusion bodies were observed in many chondrocytes. Costochondral junction study in a patient showed hypocellularity of the growth plate with very few hypertrophic or proliferative cells.

Electron microscope studies of cartilage have shown chondrocytes with dilated rough endoplasmic reticulum, filled with granular material. The matrix appeared normal.

Complications: Genua valga may be so severe that it limits ambulation and requires surgery. Amortization of the hip is another complication. The hypoplastic odontoid could lead to C1-C2 dislocation and cord compression. The **Cleft palate** leads to recurrent ear infections and possible conductive hearing loss.

Associated Findings: Myopia, hydronephrosis, **Mitral valve prolapse**, and hemangioma have been reported on occasion.

Etiology: Probably autosomal recessive inheritance.

Pathogenesis: The abnormalities of the growth plate with hypocellularity are probably responsible for the stunted growth. The inclusion bodies in the chondrocytes suggest metabolic rearrangement most likely involving the collagen (Murray & Rimoin, 1985), but the exact pathogenetic mechanism remains unknown.

MIM No.: 27167

POS No.: 3561

Sex Ratio: M1:F1

Occurrence: Fewer than 30 cases have been reported.

Risk of Recurrence for Patient's Sib:
See Part I, *Mendelian Inheritance.*

Risk of Recurrence for Patient's Child:
See Part I, *Mendelian Inheritance.*

Age of Detectability: At birth or during infancy. Prenatal diagnosis should be possible.

Gene Mapping and Linkage: Unknown.

Prevention: None known. Genetic counseling indicated.

Treatment: Palliative corrective surgery for the orthopedic deformities.

Prognosis: As in the other severe skeletal dysplasias, life span may be shortened; accurate data, however, are not available.

Detection of Carrier: Unknown.

Special Considerations: The eponym Strudwick is derived from the prototype patient seen at Johns Hopkins Hospital.

References:
Murdoch JL, Walker BA: A "new" form of spondylometaphyseal dysplasia. BD:OAS V(4). New York: March of Dimes Birth Defects Foundation, 1969:368–370.
Diamond L: Spondylometaphyseal dysplasia (Brazilian type). BD:OAS X(12). New York: March of Dimes Birth Defects Foundation, 1974: 412–415.
Anderson CE, et al.: Spondylometaepiphyseal dysplasia, Strudwick type. Am J Med Genet 1982; 13:243–256.
Spranger JW, Maroteaux P: Genetic heterogeneity of spondyloepiphyseal dysplasia congenita? Am J Med Genet 1982; 13:241–242.
Kousseff BG, Nichols P: Autosomal recessive spondylometepiphyseal dysplasia, type Strudwick. Am J Med Genet 1984; 17:547–550.
Murray LW, Rimoin DL: Type II collagen abnormalities in the spondyloepi- and spondyloepimetaphyseal dysplasias. (Abstract) Am J Hum Genet 1985; 37:A13.

Boris G. Kousseff

SPONDYLOEPIMETAPHYSEAL DYSPLASIA-JOINT LAXITY   2244

Includes:
Joint laxity-spondyloepimetaphyseal dysplasia
SEMDJL

Excludes:
Skeletal dysplasias and joint laxity syndromes, other
Spondyloepimetaphyseal dysplasia (2313)
Spondyloepimetaphyseal dysplasia, Strudwick type (3059)

Major Diagnostic Criteria: X-ray evidence of generalized spondyloepimetaphyseal dysplasia, hypermobility, and characteristic facies.

Clinical Findings: Dwarfism; articular hypermobility; spinal malalignment; thoracic asymmetry; elbow deformity (bilateral dislocation of the radial heads); foot deformity (bilateral talipes equinovarus). *Facies*: oval face, long upper lip, protuberant eyes, variable blue sclera. *Hands*: spatulate terminal phalanges, especially of the thumbs, gross joint laxity permitting abnormal positioning. *Skin*: soft, doughy texture with some hyperelasticity.

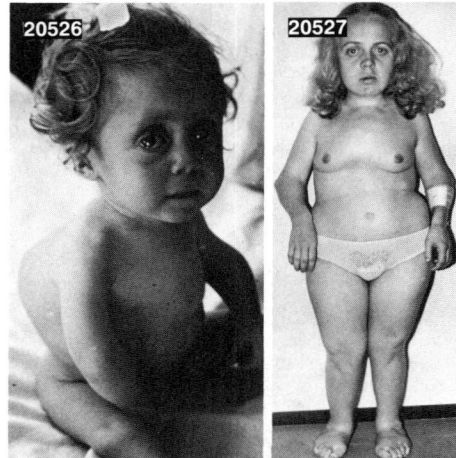

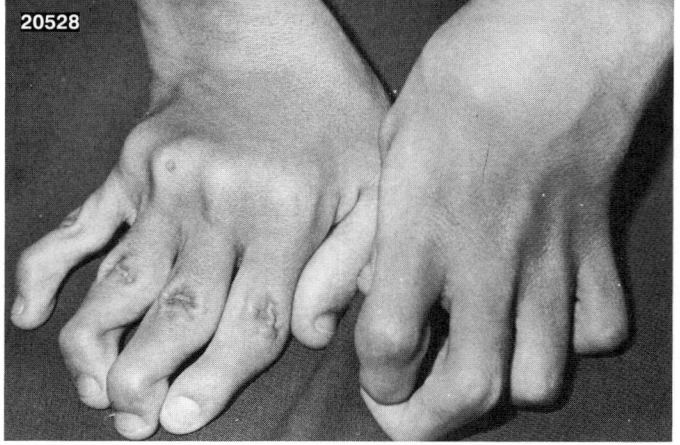

2244-20526: Spondyloepimetaphyseal dysplasia-joint laxity; note this 2-year-old girl with characteristic facies, elbow deformity due to dislocation of the radial heads and kyphosis.   **20527:** Short stature, dislocation of the radial heads, genu valgum, pes planus and the characteristic facies with prominent eyes and a long upper lip.   **20528:** Unusual hand positioning as a result of gross joint laxity. The terminal phalanges are spatulate.

Complications: Spinal cord compression, cardio-respiratory failure.

Associated Findings: Cleft palate; (31%); high palate (12%); cardiac defect (**Ventricular septal defect, Atrial septal defects**, MI) (28%); genu valgus (weight bearing) (80%); **Hip, congenital dislocated** (27%), **Myopia, congenital.**

Etiology: Autosomal recessive inheritance.

Pathogenesis: Possibly a structural defect in collagen.

MIM No.: *27164

POS No.: 4257

Sex Ratio: M1:F1

Occurrence: Twenty known cases, all in the Afrikaner population of South Africa. 1:40,000 live births. The condition is potentially lethal. Several of the affected families have German antecedents and it is possible that the gene reached the Afrikaner population (Dutch ancestry) from Germanic sources.

Risk of Recurrence for Patient's Sib:
See Part I, *Mendelian Inheritance.*

Risk of Recurrence for Patient's Child:
See Part I, *Mendelian Inheritance.*

Age of Detectability: At birth, or possibly by ultrasound in second trimester.

Gene Mapping and Linkage: Unknown.

Prevention: None known. Genetic counseling indicated. Antenatal recognition of limb or spine malalignment may be possible in early pregnancy by ultrasonic monitoring.

Treatment: Surgical stabilization of progressive spinal malalignment is indicated in the majority of patients. This operation is difficult, and long-term results are indifferent. Orthopedic measures may be required for congenital dislocation of hips, talipes equinovarus and genu valgum following weight bearing.

Prognosis: Only two of the 20 known patients have survived to early adulthood. Eight have died during childhood and the 10 survivors all have significant handicap.

Detection of Carrier: Unknown.

References:
Beighton P, Kozlowski K: Spondylo-epimetaphyseal dysplasia with joint laxity and severe, progressive kyphoscoliosis. Skel Radiol 1980; 5:205–212.
Beighton P, et al.: Spondylo-epimetaphyseal dysplasia with joint laxity and severe, progressive kyphoscoliosis. S Afr Med J 1983; 64:772–775.
Beighton P, et al.: The manifestations and natural history of spondylo-epimetaphyseal dysplasia with joint laxity. Clin Genet 1984; 26:308–317.
Kozlowski K, Beighton P: Radiographic features of spondylo-epimetaphyseal dysplasia with joint laxity and severe, progressive kyphoscoliosis: review of 19 cases. Fortschr Röntgenstr 1984; 141:337–341.
Beighton P, et al.: International nosology of heritable disorders of connective tissue, Berlin, 1986. Am J Med Genet 1988; 29:581–594.

BE008   **Peter Beighton**

SPONDYLOEPIPHYSEAL DYSPLASIA CONGENITA   0897

Includes: Dwarfism, short-trunk with retarded ossification

Excludes:
  Mucopolysaccharidosis IV (0678)
  Spondyloepiphyseal dysplasia, late (0898)
  Spondyloepiphyseal dysplasia (others)

Major Diagnostic Criteria: Short-trunk type of dwarfism; retarded ossification of the vertebral bodies and proximal femur; coxa vara; and normally shaped hand bones.

Clinical Findings: Flat face, myopia or retinal detachment (approximately 50% of cases); muscular hypotonia in infancy; occasionally cleft palate or clubfoot; short-trunk type of dwarfism,

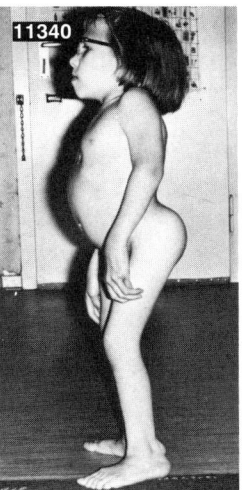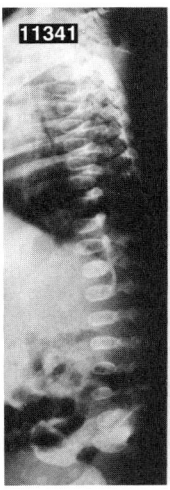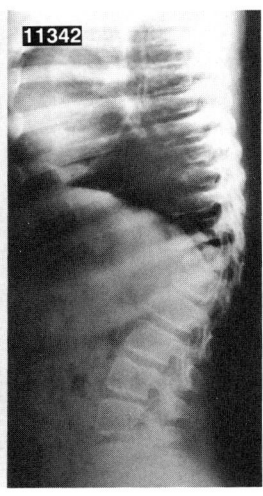

0897-11340: Short trunk dwarfism, lumbar lordosis which is accentuated. Facies are flat and glasses are worn to correct myopia. 11341: At age 2 months: flat vertebral bodies, dorsal wedging of thoracic and upper lumbar bodies. 11342: At age 13 years: platyspondyly in dorsal spine and kyphosis.

---

barrel-chest, genu valga or vara; waddling gait; and normal-sized hands and feet.

X-rays show retarded ossification of the spine and proximal femora with flattened, anteriorly pointed vertebral bodies; lack of ossification of the pubic and ischial bones in young infants; grossly retarded or absent ossification of the femoral head and neck in older patients; severe varus deformity of the femoral neck; varying degrees of epiphyseal and metaphyseal irregularities of the long tubular bones; and retarded ossification of the hand bones which are normally shaped.

A number of patients with clinical and X-ray features of spondyloepiphyseal dysplasia have been described who died at or shortly after birth. Histologically, these patients seem to differ from those with bona fide spondyloepiphyseal dysplasia congenita, exhibiting features reminiscent of hypochondrogenesis. At least one patient with these histologic features is known to have survived to the age of 12 years and at that age had more severe bone changes than other patients with spondyloepiphyseal dysplasia congenita. In particular, there was considerable involvement of the metaphyses at the knees and wrists, and the hand bones were not entirely normal. The condition is probably heterogenous.

Complications: Retinal detachment may lead to blindness. Premature and severe arthritic changes occur in the hips. Hypoplasia of the odontoid process of C2 and lax ligaments predispose to atlantoaxial instability and spinal cord compression. Kyphoscoliosis, hyperextensible finger joints, and joint dislocation.

Associated Findings: Recurrent otitis has been observed. Moderate sensorineural hearing loss (30–60 db), especially marked in high tones. Associated ocular findings include myopia, strabismus, cataracts, buphthalmos, and secondary glaucoma.

Etiology: Autosomal dominant inheritance with considerable variability in phenotypic expression. Sporadic cases are common.

Pathogenesis: Histologic studies show a hypocellular matrix and a lack of column formation, with an irregular array of broad, short spicules of calcified cartilage and bone. Electron microscopic examination of cartilage reveals widely distended cisterns of rough endoplasmic reticulum in the chondrocytes.

Murray and Rimoin (1985) found abnormal mobility of type II collagen cyanogen bromide peptides which may be a consequence of excessive posttranslation modification which in turn results from impediments in the formation of the collagen helix.

Lee et al (1989) identified a structural defect in collagen, type II (COL2A1) among the members of a large family with spondyloepiphyseal dysplasias.

MIM No.: *18390

POS No.: 3394

CDC No.: 756.460

Sex Ratio: M1:F1

Occurrence: Estimated at about 1:100,000.

Risk of Recurrence for Patient's Sib:
See Part I, *Mendelian Inheritance.*

Risk of Recurrence for Patient's Child:
See Part I, *Mendelian Inheritance.*

Age of Detectability: At birth.

Gene Mapping and Linkage: COL2A1 (collagen, type II, alpha 1) has been mapped to 12q14.3.

Prevention: None known. Genetic counseling indicated.

Treatment: Early correction of clubfoot deformity, closure of cleft palate; prevention of retinal detachment by regular ophthalmologic examinations and coagulation of early retinal tears. Careful neurologic examinations to detect early signs of cervical cord compression. Symptomatic orthopedic care.

Prognosis: The patients reach adulthood and may reproduce. The adult height varies between 84 and 128 cm. Mental development is normal. Patients who die at or shortly after birth probably have a different disorder.

Detection of Carrier: The phenotype is usually well expressed and easily detectable by clinical and X-ray studies.

References:
Macpherson RI: Spondyloepiphyseal dysplasia congenita. Pediatr Radiol 1980; 9:217–224.
Spranger J, Langer LO: Spondyloepiphyseal dysplasia congenita. Radiology 1980; 94:313–322.
Wynne-Davies R, Hall C: Two clinical variants of spondylo-epiphyseal congenita. J Bone Joint Surg 1982; 64B:435–441.
Harrod MJE, et al.: Genetic heterogeneity in spondyloepiphyseal dysplasia congenita. Am J Med Genet 1984; 18:311–320.
Murray TG, et al.: Spondyloepiphyseal dysplasia congenita: light and electron microscope studies of the eye. Arch Ophthal 1985; 103:407–411.
Murray TG, Rimoin DL: Type II collagen abnormalities in the spondyloepi- and spondyloepimetaphyseal dysplasias. (Abstract) Am J Hum Genet 1985; 37:A13.
Lee B, et al.: Identification of the molecular defect in a family with spondyloepiphyseal dysplasia. Science 1989; 244:978–980.

MY001   **Terry L. Myers**
SP007   **Jürgen W. Spranger**

Spondyloepiphyseal dysplasia tarda, Toledo type
See SPONDYLOEPIPHYSEAL DYSPLASIA, LATE

SPONDYLOEPIPHYSEAL DYSPLASIA, LATE   0898

Includes:
Chondroitin sulfate sulfotransferase deficiency
Chondro-osteodystrophy
Dwarfism, dysplasia spondyloepiphysaria tarda
Dysplasia spondyloepiphysaria tarda
PAPA-Chondroitin sulfate sulfotransferase deficiency
Spondyloepiphyseal dysplasia, X-linked form
Spondyloepiphyseal dysplasia tarda, Toledo type

Excludes:
Mucopolysaccharidosis IV (0678)
Spondyloepiphyseal dysplasia congenita (0897)
Spondyloepiphyseal dysplasia-mental retardation (3127)

Major Diagnostic Criteria: Short trunk dwarfism, with characteristic spinal and hip involvement, of late childhood or early adolescence onset. Skeletal X-rays confirm the diagnosis.

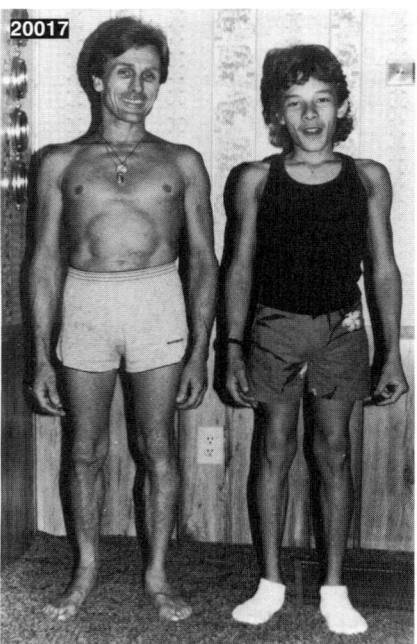

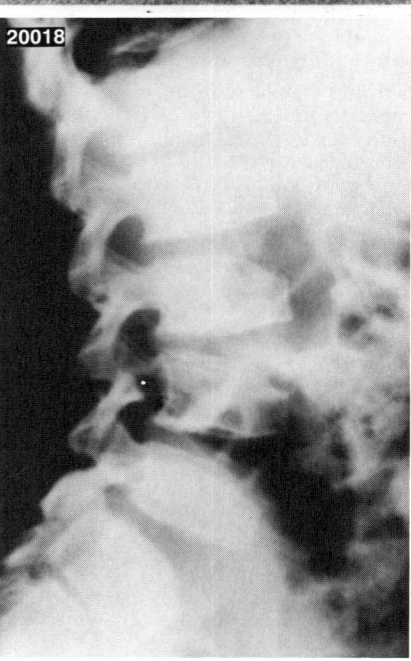

0898A-20017: Uncle and nephew with short-spine type of disproportionate short stature; limb lengths are relatively normal. **20018:** Characteristic humped-up platyspondylotic vertebral bodies on this lateral view of the lumbar spine.

Clinical Findings: In the typical case, disproportionate short stature secondary to vertebral loss of height. Adult height ranges from 130–155 cm. Premature osteoarthrosis, primarily of the spine and hips, frequently leads to restricted mobility. Less frequently, shoulders, knees and ankles are involved. Laboratory studies are usually normal. Skeletal X-rays rays show flattening of the vertebral bodies with a hump-shaped build-up of ivory-like bone in the central and posterior portions of the superior and inferior plates. There is a complete lack of visible bone in the areas of the ring

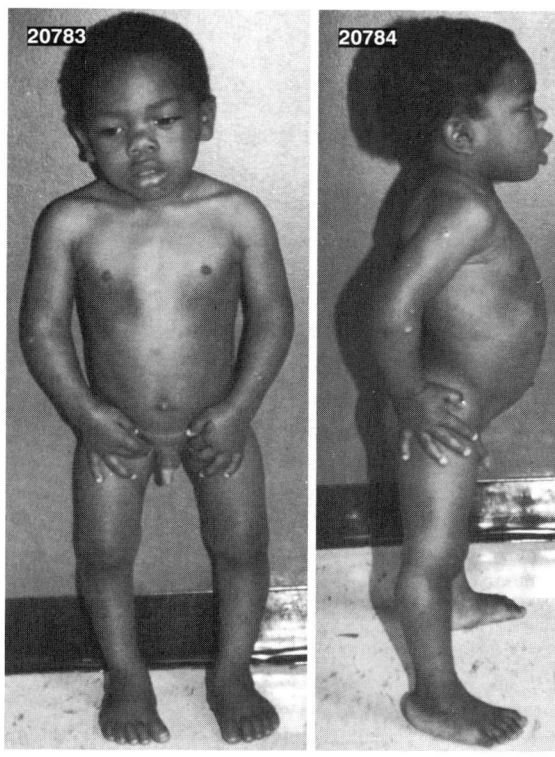

0898B-20783–84: Spondyloepiphyseal dysplasia; note short trunk, bowed legs, mild lordosis.

apophyses (projection from vertebrae). The disk spaces appear narrow, and at first glance may appear calcified, but the calcification is actually part of the vertebral body itself. Premature disk generation does occur. The platyspondyly extends throughout the thoracic and cervical spine to the C 2 level with less marked involvement of the end plates. The thoracic cage appears increased in both transverse and anteroposterior diameters. The bony pelvis is small. The acetabuli are deep and the femoral necks short. Mild dysplastic changes are seen in all large joints, especially the hips. Premature osteoarthosis of the hips, with extensive cyst formation, may develop in the third or fourth decade. The bones of the hands appear normal.

In addition to the more common X-linked form of this condition, a few families have been described with an autosomal dominant form. other cases have been reported with an autosomal recessive form which has been termed *chondro-osteodystrophy*. A *Toledo type* variant of the recessive form, with corneal opacity and anomalies of urinary mucopolysaccharides, is sometimes called *(PAPA)-Chondroitin sulfate sulfotransferase deficiency* (Toledo, 1978).

Complications: Premature osteoarthosis of the hips almost always occurs in adulthood, and may lead to disabling pain and restricted mobility. Pain in the back and shoulders is also reported.

Associated Findings: One patient has been reported with poikiloderma and lymphoma. Deutan color blindness segregated with this condition in the three affected males of one family. A large kindred with numerous affected individuals included two males with protan color blindness.

Etiology: Usually X-linked recessive inheritance with variable expressivity and almost complete penetrance. Autosomal dominant and recessive inheritance has also been reported.

Pathogenesis: Unknown.

MIM No.: *31340, *27160, *27163, *18410

POS No.: 3395

CDC No.: 756.460

Sex Ratio: M1:F0 in the X-linked form. Presumably M1:F1 in the dominant and recessive forms.

Occurrence: Undetermined. Reported in several kindreds and ethnic groups.

Risk of Recurrence for Patient's Sib:
See Part I, *Mendelian Inheritance.*

Risk of Recurrence for Patient's Child:
See Part I, *Mendelian Inheritance.*

Age of Detectability: Late childhood or early adolescence, by short trunk dwarfism and typical skeletal X-rays.

Gene Mapping and Linkage: SEDL (spondyloepiphyseal dysplasia, late) has been provisionally mapped to Xp22.

Prevention: None known. Genetic counseling indicated.

Treatment: Palliative; physical therapy for the joint stiffness and pain. Total hip replacement is considered for severely disabled patients.

Prognosis: Normal life span and intelligence. Premature osteoarthrosis may lead to disabling pain and restricted mobility in mid or late adulthood.

Detection of Carrier: Clinical examination of first degree relatives.

References:
Maroteaux P, et al.: La dysplasie spondylo-epiphysaire tardive. Presse Med 1957; 65:1205–1208.
Langer LO: Spondyloepiphyseal dysplasia tarda. Radiology 1964; 82:833–839.
Bannerman RM, et al.: X-linked spondyloepiphyseal dysplasia tarda: clinical and linkage data. J Med Genet 1971; 8:291–301.
Spranger J, Langer LO: Spondyloepiphyseal dysplasia. BD:OAS X(9). Miami: Symposia Specialists for The National Foundation March of Dimes, 1974:19.
Toledo SPA, et al.: Recessively inherited, late onset, spondylar dysplasia and peripheral corneal opacity with anomalies in urinary mucopolysaccharides. Am J Med Genet 1978; 2:385–395.
Kousseff BG, et al.: Spondyloepiphyseal dysplasia tarda and deutan color blindness in a family. (Abstract) 7th Internat Congress of Hum Genet, Berlin, 1986:258.

K0018   **Boris G. Kousseff**

Spondyloepiphyseal dysplasia, pseudoachondroplastic type
See PSEUDOACHONDROPLASTIC DYSPLASIA
Spondyloepiphyseal dysplasia, X-linked form
See SPONDYLOEPIPHYSEAL DYSPLASIA, LATE

SPONDYLOEPIPHYSEAL DYSPLASIA-MENTAL RETARDATION   **3127**

Includes: Mental retardation-spondyloepiphyseal dysplasia

Excludes: Spondyloepiphyseal dysplasia, late (0898)

Major Diagnostic Criteria: The combination of **Spondyloepiphyseal dysplasia, late** with mental retardation, particularly in a female, helps to distinguish this condition from others.

Clinical Findings: Normal birth weights and lengths with normal or near-normal early development in one patient and delayed milestones in the remaining two known patients. Physical examinations done when these affected females were adults demonstrated short stature (<3rd percentile), joint limitation, and mild-to-moderate mental retardation. X-ray studies revealed absent dens epistrophei (2/3), platyspondyly (3/3), anterior protrusion in the lumbar region (3/3), flared iliac bones with short sacrosciatic notch (3/3), coxa valga (3/3), and abnormal epiphyses of the femur and humerus (3/3).

Complications: Degenerative joint changes.

Associated Findings: None known.

Etiology: Probably autosomal recessive inheritance.

Pathogenesis: Unknown.

MIM No.: 27162

POS No.: 4280

Sex Ratio: M0:F3 (observed).

Occurrence: Reported in three sisters in an inbred Bedouin family.

Risk of Recurrence for Patient's Sib:
See Part I, *Mendelian Inheritance.*

Risk of Recurrence for Patient's Child:
See Part I, *Mendelian Inheritance.*

Age of Detectability: Probably during late childhood.

Gene Mapping and Linkage: Unknown.

Prevention: None known. Genetic counseling indicated.

Treatment: Orthopedic intervention may be indicated.

Prognosis: Mental retardation is present. Life span is unknown, although unlikely to be significantly affected.

Detection of Carrier: Unknown.

References:
Kohn G, et al.: Spondyloepiphyseal dysplasia tarda: a new autosomal recessive variant with mental retardation. J Med Genet 1987; 24:366–377.

T0007   **Helga V. Toriello**

Spondyloepiphyseal-spondyloperipheral dysplasia
See SPONDYLOPERIPHERAL DYSPLASIA
Spondylohumerofemoral hypoplasia, giant cell
See ATELOSTEOGENESIS
Spondylolisthesis, spine
See SPINE, SPONDYLOLISTHESIS AND SPONDYLOLYSIS
Spondylolysis, spine
See SPINE, SPONDYLOLISTHESIS AND SPONDYLOLYSIS
Spondylometaepiphyseal dysplasia
See SPONDYLOEPIMETAPHYSEAL DYSPLASIA
Spondylometaepiphyseal dysplasia congenita
See SPONDYLOEPIMETAPHYSEAL DYSPLASIA, STRUDWICK TYPE
Spondylometaepiphyseal dysplasia, Strudwick type
See SPONDYLOEPIMETAPHYSEAL DYSPLASIA, STRUDWICK TYPE

SPONDYLOMETAPHYSEAL CHONDRODYSPLASIA, KOZLOWSKI TYPE   0899

Includes:
Chondrodysplasia, spondylometaphseal, Kozlowski type
Dwarfism, Kozlowski type
Kozlowski chondrodysplasia, spondylometaphyseal

Excludes:
Metatropic dysplasia (0656)
Mucopolysaccharidosis IV (0678)
Spondyloepimetaphyseal dysplasia
Spondylometaphyseal chondrodysplasias, other types

Major Diagnostic Criteria: Short stature and X-ray signs of platyspondyly and metaphyseal osteochondrodysplasia.

Clinical Findings: Progressive, moderate short stature with predominant shortening of the trunk, waddling gait, kyphosis, and normal head. Adult height is about 140 cm. X-rays show generalized platyspondyly with unique shape of the vertebral bodies, metaphyseal osteochondrodysplasia, and retarded carpal and tarsal bone age.

Complications: Kyphosis; scoliosis; early, severe osteoarthritic changes.

Associated Findings: None known.

Etiology: Autosomal dominant and autosomal recessive inheritance has been reported.

Pathogenesis: Undetermined. Fibrous appearance of cartilage matrix.

MIM No.: 18425, *27166

POS No.: 3396

Sex Ratio: M1:F1

Occurrence: Over a dozen possible cases have been reported, but diagnostic classifications are still tentative.

Risk of Recurrence for Patient's Sib:
See Part I, *Mendelian Inheritance.*

Risk of Recurrence for Patient's Child:
See Part I, *Mendelian Inheritance.*

Age of Detectability: Preschool, by X-ray features.

Gene Mapping and Linkage: Unknown.

Prevention: None known. Genetic counseling indicated.

Treatment: Physiotherapy, orthopedic treatment.

Prognosis: Normal life span.

Detection of Carrier: Unknown.

Special Considerations: A number of patients with spine and metaphyseal dysplastic changes have been described who differ from the standard profile of this condition in X-ray appearance and distribution of the lesions. Although an attempt has been made to divide these cases into certain subtypes, their classification is still in question.

References:
Kozlowski K, et al.: La dysostose spondylo-metaphysaire. Presse Med 1967; 75:2769–2774.
Kozlowski K: Spondylo-metaphyseal dysplasia. Prog Pediatr Radiol 1973; 4:229–308.
Kozlowski K: Metaphyseal and spondylo-metaphyseal dysplasias. Clin Orthop 1976; 114:83–93.
Kozlowski K, et al.: Spondylo-metaphyseal dysplasias (Report of a case of common type and three pairs of siblings of "new varieties"). Austr Radiol 1976; 20:154–164.
Schorr S, et al.: Spondyloenchondrodysplasia. Radiology 1976; 118:133–139.
Kozlowski K, et al.: Spondylo-metaphyseal dysplasia (report of a case of common type and three cases of "new varieties"). Röfo 1979; 130:222–230.
Kozlowski K, et al.: Spondylo-metaphyseal dysplasia (Report of 7 cases and essay of classification). In: Papadatos CJ, Bartsocas CS, eds: Skeletal dysplasias. New York: Alan R. Liss, 1982:89–101.
Ouadfel-Meziane A, et al.: Sponndylometaphyseal dysplasia: report of three familial cases. Ann Genet 1987; 30:216–220.

K0021   **K.S. Kozlowski**

SPONDYLOMETAPHYSEAL DYSPLASIA WITH ENCHONDROMATOUS CHANGES   2595

Includes: Spondyloenchondrodysplasia

Excludes:
Enchondromatosis (0345)
Enchondromatosis and hemangiomas (0346)
Enchondromatosis with irregular vertebral lesions
Metachondromatosis (0650)
Mucopolysaccharidosis IV (0678)
Spondyloepimetaphyseal dysplasia, Strudwick type (3059)
Spondylometaphyseal chondrodysplasia, Kozlowski type (0899)
Spondylometaphyseal dysplasia (other)

Major Diagnostic Criteria: Disproportionate short stature with short trunk and limbs. Typical radiolucencies in the metaphyses, which extend into the shafts of the long bones. Spinal changes mainly confined to the posterior part of the vertebral bodies with severe platyspondyly. With time, irregular end-plates become apparent. Calcification of the basal ganglia, spasticity, and mental retardation may be variably present.

Clinical Findings: Birth length may be normal. Low birth weight was observed in the patients reported by Schorr et al (1976). Short stature probably becomes apparent only in the second year, but X-ray changes are already present at age six months. The growth rate is slow, with normal pubertal spurt. Patients may reach 150 cm, but most patients will probably be shorter. Kyphosis with increased lumbar lordosis is frequent and affects final height. The wrists, elbows, and knees appear widened, and joint and limb pains may be present. There may be difficulties in psychosocial adaptation. Mental retardation and spasticity are variably present.

The typical X-ray changes include radiolucent "masses" resembling enchondromas, which extend from the irregular metaphyses into the shafts of the long bones. The distal ulna and proximal fibula seem more severely affected than the corresponding radius and tibia. The elbow is almost spared, and the hips are moderately involved. In the spine similar radiolucencies are confined mainly to the posterior part of the vertebral bodies around the growth plate, as evidenced by computerized tomographic (CT) studies. Severe platyspondyly is present, but the vertebral bodies are not widened and present a cut-off anterior border. The iliac crests and sacrum are also involved. Three out of five patients who had brain CT scans showed calcification of the basal ganglia, not apparent on a plain skull X-ray.

At age six months, rachitic-like metaphyseal changes were already present. At age 31 months, typical radiolucencies were seen, and with time sclerotic streaks tend to appear and extend into the shafts of the long bones.

In the spine, irregularities of the end-plates tend to appear, and in the second decade a typical appearance of "vertebra within a vertebra" may develop.

Complications: Kyphosis, increased lumbar lordosis, and genu valgus.

Associated Findings: Three patients had mental retardation. Four patients had neurological manifestations ranging from spasticity of the lower limbs to quadriparesis.

Etiology: Autosomal recessive inheritance.

Pathogenesis: It has been suggested that the changes are cartilagenous in nature, but there is no histopathological evidence to support this view. A needle iliac crest biopsy did not enter a cartilagenous island. By light microscope, the chondrocytes showed non-specific changes only. Electron microscope studies showed inclusions within the rough endoplasmatic reticulum similar to those seen in **Kniest dysplasia**.

MIM No.: *27155

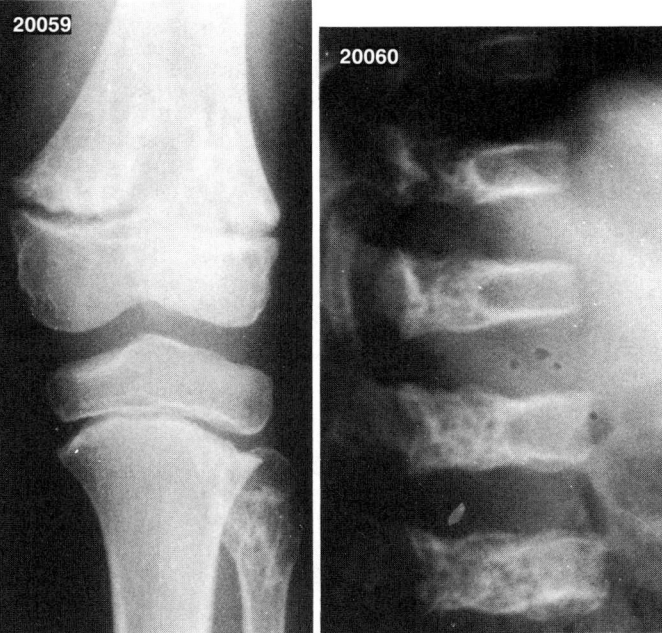

2595-20059: Metaphyseal changes are seen in this knee X-ray. 20060: Flattened and narrowed vertebral bodies.

POS No.: 4026

Sex Ratio: Presumably M1:F1.

Occurrence: Two sibs were reported by Schorr et al (1976), two patients by Sauvegrain et al (1982). The total number of reported patients is under twenty. Frydman et al studied six patients including two pairs of sibs. Two of the reported families are Iraqi Jews (four patients), and three are Palestinian Arabs (four patients). Menger et al (1989) reported on four patients and reviewed other reports.

Risk of Recurrence for Patient's Sib:
See Part I, *Mendelian Inheritance*.

Risk of Recurrence for Patient's Child:
See Part I, *Mendelian Inheritance*.

Age of Detectability: Clinically evident in the second year of life. X-ray changes were already present at age six months and probably earlier.

Gene Mapping and Linkage: Unknown.

Prevention: None known. Genetic counseling indicated.

Treatment: Physical therapy to prevent spine deformities. Analgesics for joint and limb pains. Psychologic support as indicated. Limb lengthening procedures may be appropriate.

Prognosis: Probably normal life span. Physical handicaps are related to the short stature and to the severity of kyphosis. Sauvegrain et al (1982), Menger et al (1989) and Frydman et al each observed one patient with mental retardation. Neurological manifestations ranging from spasticity to quadriparesis were seen in four patients.

Detection of Carrier: Unknown.

Special Considerations: The mother of two affected sibs and her sister and nephew had a stature below the third percentile without evidence of skeletal involvement (Frydman et al, 1986). This observation may indicate that the abnormal gene may have some effect in the heterozygote.

Other types of spondylometaphyseal dysplasia with enchondromatous-like changes also exist (i.e. see Sauvegrain et al, 1982).

References:
Schorr S, et al.: Spondyloenchondrodysplasia. Radiology 1976; 118: 133–139.
Sauvegrain J, et al.: Chondromes multiples avec atteinte rachidienne. Spondylo-enchondroplasie et autres formes. J Radiol 1982; 61:495–501.
Frydman M, et al.: Spondylometaphyseal dysplasia with "enchondromatous-like" changes: a distinctive type. 7th International Congress of Human Genetics, Berlin, September 22–26, 1986:257.
Menger H, et al.: Spondyloenchondrodysplasia. J Med Genet 1989; 26:93–99.

FR034 **Moshe Frydman**

Spondylometaphyseal dysplasia, Brazilian type
See SPONDYLOEPIMETAPHYSEAL DYSPLASIA, STRUDWICK TYPE
Spondylometepiphyseal dysplasia (SMED)
See SPONDYLOEPIMETAPHYSEAL DYSPLASIA

SPONDYLOPERIPHERAL DYSPLASIA 3054

Includes:
Spondyloepiphyseal-spondyloperipheral dysplasia
Spondyloperipheral dysplasia with short ulna

Excludes:
Acromesomelic dysplasia
Brachydactyly (0114)
Exostoses-anetodermia-brachydactyly type E (2764)
Pseudohypoparathyroidism
Pseudo-pseudohypoparathyroidism

Major Diagnostic Criteria: The combination of brachydactyly E, shortened long bones, and vertebral defects should suggest the diagnosis.

Clinical Findings: The hand and foot abnormalities, when present, are consistent with brachydactyly E, with short, broad metacarpals and metatarsals, short distal phalanges, and short fifth finger middle phalanges. Most affected individuals have short stature at or below the 10th percentile, with normal facial features. Spine and long bone anomalies are variable, ranging from no vertebral or long bone involvement to short or absent distal ulnae, humeri, tibiae, and femora. Coxarthrosis and epiphyseal dysplasia of the humerus have also been described. The spine anomalies are described as biconcavity with or without platyspondyly.

Complications: Joint and back pain and limitation of supination of various joints are relatively common complications; subchronic synovitis may also occur.

Associated Findings: None known.

Etiology: Autosomal dominant inheritance seems more likely than autosomal recessive, in that Sybert et al (1979) reported affected individuals in five generations.

Pathogenesis: Unknown.

MIM No.: 27170

POS No.: 4027

Sex Ratio: M1:F1

Occurrence: Three families have been reported, two in the United States and one in Czechoslovakia. A single case from South Africa has also been reported.

Risk of Recurrence for Patient's Sib:
See Part I, *Mendelian Inheritance.*

Risk of Recurrence for Patient's Child:
See Part I, *Mendelian Inheritance.*

Age of Detectability: During childhood.

Gene Mapping and Linkage: Unknown.

Prevention: None known. Genetic counseling indicated.

Treatment: Supportive, with orthopedic treatment possibly indicated.

Prognosis: Life span and intellect are apparently normal.

Detection of Carrier: Unknown.

References:

Kelly TE, et al.: An unusual familial spondyloepiphyseal dysplasia: "spondyloperipheral dysplasia." I: BD:OAS XIII(3B). New York: March of Dimes Birth Defects Foundation, 1977:149–165.

Sybert VP, et al.: Variable expression in a dominantly inherited skeletal dysplasia with similarities to brachydactyly E and spondyloepiphyseal-spondyloperipheral dysplasia. Clin Genet 1979; 15; 160–166. * †

Vanek J: Spondyloperipheral dysplasia. J Med Genet 1983; 20:117–121. †

Goldblatt J, Behari D: Unique skeletal dysplasia with absence of the distal ulnae. Am J Med Genet 1987; 28:625–630.

T0007   Helga V. Toriello

Spondyloperipheral dysplasia with short ulna
See SPONDYLOPERIPHERAL DYSPLASIA

SPONDYLOTHORACIC DYSPLASIA   0900

Includes:
Costovertebral dysplasia
Hemivertebrae, autosomal recessive multiple
Jarcho-Levin syndrome
Occipito-facial-cervico-thoracic-abdomino-digital dysplasia
Spondylocostal dysplasia
Vertebral anomalies

Excludes:
Robinow syndrome (0876)
Spondylocostal dysplasia (0896)

Major Diagnostic Criteria: Severe vertebral dysplasia and fusion giving markedly short trunk and "crab-like" appearance on X-ray.

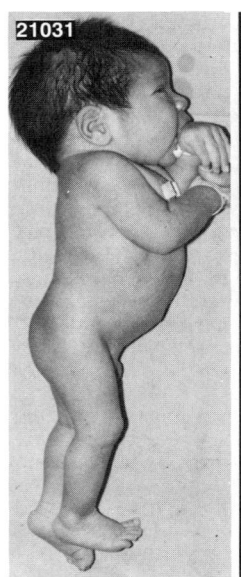
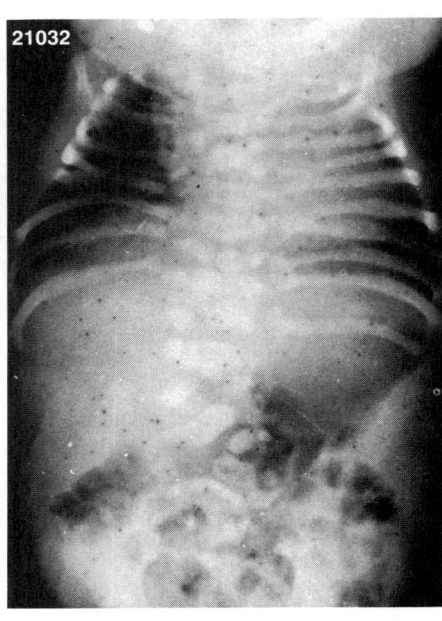

0900-21031: Spondylothoracic dysplasia; note short trunk and protuberant abdomen. **21032:** Chest X-ray shows crab-like chest deformity from vertebral and rib anomalies.

Clinical Findings: Congenital short trunk with protuberant abdomen and relatively long limbs, which may be of normal length. The trunk is short because of anomalous vertebral development (hemivertebrae, partially absent vertebral bodies, fused vertebrae) and incomplete segmentation of the ribs. The thorax has a bizarre "crab-like" appearance on X-ray, with ribs splaying out from fused vertebrae. The neck is short, also because of anomalous vertebrae, with a low posterior hairline and limited movement. The occiput is prominent. The facies are round, somewhat puffy, with the chin resting on the chest. Long fingers and toes, even hammer toes, have been reported. Many patients have hernias. Nonskeletal anomalies reported include bilobed bladder, hydronephrosis, cerebral polygyria, anal atresia, submucous cleft palate, single umbilical artery, bilateral hydroceles, and inguinal hernia.

Complications: Affected children often die in infancy as a result of pulmonary insufficiency and pneumonia.

Associated Findings: None known.

Etiology: Autosomal recessive inheritance. Consanguinity, and affected sibs of both sexes, have been reported.

Pathogenesis: These particular spinal and rib anomalies probably have their origin in early embryonic development during vertebral segmentation; about the fourth to six week. Secondary anomalies in trunk and thorax shape occur.

MIM No.: *27730

POS No.: 3410

Sex Ratio: M16:F11 (observed).

Occurrence: 27 infants have been reported in 17 families. Most patients have been Puerto Rican.

Risk of Recurrence for Patient's Sib:
See Part I, *Mendelian Inheritance.*

Risk of Recurrence for Patient's Child:
See Part I, *Mendelian Inheritance.* Affected individuals are not expected to survive to reproduce.

Age of Detectability: At birth. Prenatal diagnosis by ultrasound should be possible.

Gene Mapping and Linkage: Unknown.

Prevention: None known. Genetic counseling indicated.

Treatment: Respiratory support.

Prognosis: Most reported cases have died in infancy.

Detection of Carrier: Clinical examination of first degree relatives.

Special Considerations: Less severe vertebral segmentation anomalies have been reported in similar but different conditions with autosomal dominant and recessive inheritance.

References:

Perez-Comas A, et al.: Occipito-facial-cervico-thoracic-abdomino-digital dysplasia. Jarcho-Levin syndrome of vertebral anomalies: a report of six cases and a review of the literature. J Pediatr 1974; 85:388–391.

Poor MA, et al.: Nonskeletal malformations in one of three siblings with Jarcho-Levin syndrome of vertebral anomalies. J Pediatr 1983; 103:270–272.

Cassidy SB, et al.: Natural history of Jarcho-Levin syndrome. (Abstract) Proc Greenwood Genet Center 3:92–94.

Young ID, Moore JR: Spondylocostal dysostosis. J Med Genet 1984; 21:68–69.

HA014   **Judith G. Hall**

Sponge kidney
See KIDNEY, MEDULLARY SPONGE KIDNEY
Spongioblastoma multiforme
See CANCER, GLIOMA, FAMILIAL
Spongy glioneuronal dystrophy
See ALPERS DISEASE
Spoon nails
See NAILS, KOILONYCHIA
Sporadic Burkitt lymphoma
See LYMPHOMA, BURKITT TYPE
'Spotted bones'
See OSTEOPOIKILOSIS
Spotted corneal dystrophy
See CORNEAL DYSTROPHY, MACULAR TYPE
Sprengel anomaly-hydrocephalus-costovertebral dysplasia
See HYDROCEPHALUS-COSTOVERTEBRAL DYSPLASIA-SPRENGEL ANOMALY

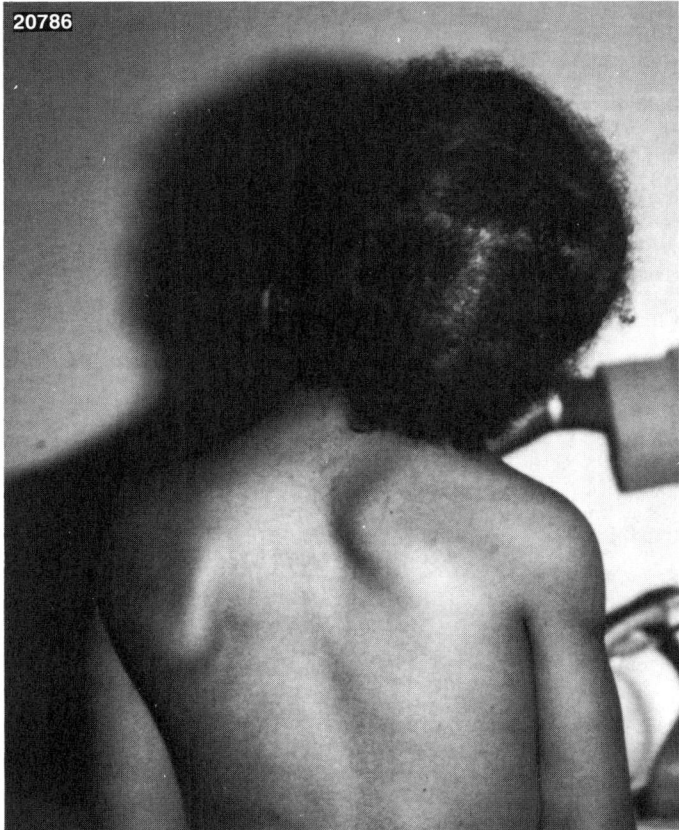

0901-20786: Sprengel deformity; note high, triangular scapula.

SPRENGEL DEFORMITY   0901

Includes:
High scapula
Scapula elevata

Excludes: Klippel-Feil anomaly (2032)

Major Diagnostic Criteria: Clinical or X-ray evidence of elevated scapula.

Clinical Findings: The scapula is located higher than its usual T2 - T7 position and is usually hypoplastic, having the "fetal shape" of an equilateral triangle. It lies closer to the midline, producing a lump in the web of the neck, and is rotated such that the glenoid fossa faces downward, restricting abduction of the affected arm. Involvement may be bilateral. A communication of bone, cartilage, or fibrous tissue between the scapula and adjacent vertebrae is found in 25–50% of patients. Over one-half the cases (67%) have associated skeletal anomalies or shoulder muscle hypoplasia.

Among those families showing autosomal dominant transmission, some demonstrate the scapula deformity alone in all affected members, while in other families the entire spectrum of associated anomalies may be found, with wide variation among affected members.

Complications: Limitation of motion (elevation) of ipsilateral arm, related to degree of scapular deformity.

Associated Findings: Scoliosis, hemivertebrae, fused vertebrae, spina bifida occulta, cervical ribs, missing ribs, fused ribs, chest deformities, situs inversus, clavicular anomalies, cleft palate, and hypoplasia of the muscles of the shoulder girdle.

Etiology: Most cases occur sporadically, but autosomal dominant inheritance has been reported.

Pathogenesis: The defect presumably results from failure of the mesenchymal anlage of the scapula to descend from its cervical position to the normal thoracic position during the second month of gestation.

MIM No.: *18440

CDC No.: 755.556

Sex Ratio: Presumably M1:F1. M1:F2 observed in sporadic cases.

Occurrence: About 20 families have been reported.

Risk of Recurrence for Patient's Sib:
See Part I, *Mendelian Inheritance.* Low risk for sporadic cases.

Risk of Recurrence for Patient's Child:
See Part I, *Mendelian Inheritance.*

Age of Detectability: At birth, or during childhood.

Gene Mapping and Linkage: Unknown.

Prevention: None known. Genetic counseling indicated.

Treatment: Surgery may not be needed in mild cases; however, in those severely affected, both function and cosmetic appearance can be improved by reconstructive surgery. This usually involves removal of the omovertebral communication and excision of the superomedial part of the scapula.

Conservative treatment, including exercise, passive stretching and voluntary elevation of the unaffected scapula, has been used but appears to be of little value.

Prognosis: Life span and intelligence are normal. Functional disability is related to degree of scapula deformity and associated anomalies.

Detection of Carrier: Unknown.

References:
Otter GD: Bilateral Sprengel's syndrome with situs inversus totalis. Acta Orthopaedica Scand 1970; 41:402–410.
Wilson MG, et al.: Dominant inheritance of Sprengel's deformity. J Pediatr 1971; 79:818–821.
Cavendish ME: Congenital elevation of the scapula. J Bone Joint Surg [Br] 1972; 54B:395–408.
Chung SM, Nissenbaum MM: Congenital and developmental defects of the shoulder. Orthop Clin North Am 1975; 6:381–392.
Hodgson SV, Chiu DC: Dominant transmission of Sprengel's shoulder and cleft palate. J Med Genet 1981; 18:263–265.

H0033   **William A. Horton**
H0025   **O.J. Hood**

Sprue
    See GLUTEN-SENSITIVE ENTEROPATHY
Spun-glass hair and crystalline cataract
    See HAIR, UNCOMBABLE-CRYSTALLINE CATARACT
Stable Factor deficiency
    See FACTOR VII DEFICIENCY
Stale fish syndrome
    See TRIMETHYLAMINURIA
Stammering
    See STUTTERING
Stanescu osteosclerosis
    See CRANIOFACIAL DYSOSTOSIS-DIAPHYSEAL HYPERPLASIA
Stapes ankylosis and perilymphatic gusher-deafness
    See DEAFNESS WITH PERILYMPHATIC GUSHER
Stapes fixation-deafness
    See DEAFNESS WITH PERILYMPHATIC GUSHER
Stapes fixation-oligodontia-cleft palate
    See CLEFT PALATE-STAPES FIXATION-OLIGODONTIA
Stargardt disease
    See RETINA, FUNDUS FLAVIMACULATUS
Startle disease
    See HYPEREKPLEXIA
Startle syndromes
    See JUMPING FRENCHMAN OF MAINE
Stationary nightblindness with high myopia congenital
    See NIGHTBLINDNESS, CONGENITAL STATIONARY, X-LINKED RECESSIVE
Stationary nightblindness with normal fundus congenital
    See NIGHTBLINDNESS, CONGENITAL STATIONARY, AUTOSOMAL RECESSIVE
Stature, short
    See DWARFISM
Status Bonnevie-Ullrich
    See NOONAN SYNDROME
Steatocystoma-pachyonychia congenita
    See PACHYONYCHIA CONGENITA-STEATOCYSTOMA MULTIPLEX
Steely hair disease
    See MENKES SYNDROME
Steinert disease
    See MYOTONIC DYSTROPHY
Stenosis at the conus elasticus
    See LARYNX, ATRESIA
Stenosis of anterior nares
    See NOSE, ANTERIOR ATRESIA
Stenosis of aqueduct of Sylvius
    See HYDROCEPHALY
Stenosis of ostium infundibulum
    See VENTRICLE, OBSTRUCTION WITHIN RIGHT VENTRICLE OR ITS OUTFLOW TRACT
Stenosis, combined subglottic
    See SUBGLOTTIC STENOSIS
Stenosis, hard subglottic
    See SUBGLOTTIC STENOSIS
Stenosis, soft subglottic
    See SUBGLOTTIC STENOSIS
Stenosis, subglottic
    See SUBGLOTTIC STENOSIS
Stephens syndrome (ophthalmoplegia-ataxia-peripheral neuropathy)
    See KEARNS-SAYRE DISEASE

STERNAL MALFORMATION-VASCULAR DYSPLASIA ASSOCIATION   3055

Includes:
    Hemangiomata-cleft sternum
    Leiber sternal clefts and telangiectasia/hemangiomas
    Vascular dysplasia-sternal malformation association

Excludes:
    Cleft sternum without associated anomalies
    Heart, cordis ectopia (0335)
    Pentalogy of Cantrell (3121)

Major Diagnostic Criteria: The combination of cleft sternum and hemangiomata.

Clinical Findings: The sternal defect ranged in severity from cleft of the upper one-third to cleft of the entire sternum. Hemangiomas usually affect the face, neck, and chin. Most were present at birth, although in one case the hemangioma did not become noticeable until age three months. In most cases, the vascular lesions are limited to the skin; however, one child also had a respiratory tract hemangioma, and a second had an intra-abdominal hemangioma.

Complications: Infection is the most common complication. If internal hemangiomas are present, site-dependent complications such as respiratory compromise and gastrointestinal bleeding can also occur.

Associated Findings: Micrognathia was present in two individuals; absent pericardium and unilateral **Cleft lip** were found in one individual each.

Etiology: Only one pair of affected sibs has been described; all other cases have been sporadic. Multifactorial inheritance or heterogeneity has not been ruled out.

Pathogenesis: A midline defect affecting mesodermal structure and proliferation of angioblastic tissue has been postulated. The components of this anomaly are thought to arise between 8–10 weeks of gestation.

POS No.: 3504

Sex Ratio: Presumably M1:F1.

Occurrence: About 15 cases have been reported.

Risk of Recurrence for Patient's Sib: Among 15 patients, two were sibs. Risk may therefore be small, but not neglible.

Risk of Recurrence for Patient's Child: Unknown.

Age of Detectability: At birth.

Gene Mapping and Linkage: Unknown.

Prevention: None known. Genetic counseling indicated.

Treatment: Surgical correction of the sternal defect may be indicated; corticosteroids may stop the progression of the hemangiomas; treatment of complications, such as infection, is also indicated.

Prognosis: Barring any complications, prognosis for normal growth, intellectual development, and life span is good.

Detection of Carrier: Unknown.

References:
Hague KN: Isolated asternia: an independent entity. Clin Genet 1984; 25:362–365.
Hersh JH, et al.: Sternal malformation/vascular dysplasia association. Am J Med Genet 1985; 21:177–186.
Opitz JM: Editorial comment on the papers by Hersh et al. and Kaplan et al. on sternal cleft. Am J Med Genet 1985; 21:201–202.

T0007   **Helga V. Toriello**

Sternocleidomastoid torticollis
    See TORTICOLLIS
Sternogladiolar prominence
    See PECTUS CARINATUM
Sternomastoid torticollis
    See TORTICOLLIS

STEROID 3 BETA-HYDROXYSTEROID DEHYDROGENASE DEFICIENCY 0909

Includes: Adrenal hyperplasia II

Excludes: Adrenal steroidogenesis, other enzyme deficiencies in

Major Diagnostic Criteria: Ambiguous genitalia in both males and females, vomiting, dehydration, and low serum sodium and chloride constitute the major manifestations. Elevated 17-ketosteroid (17-KS) excretion, predominately dehydroepiandrosterone (DHEA) or its derivatives, preponderance of δ5 urinary steroid compounds, mild virilization in females or under-masculinization in males, and suppression of abnormal steroids with exogenous glucocorticoids.

Clinical Findings: This is a rare form of congenital adrenal hyperplasia (CAH) in which the enzyme defect occurs early in adrenal steroidogenesis and affects the mineralocorticoid, glucocorticoid, and sex steroid pathways. Thus, in severe enzyme deficiency, salt loss, hyponatremia, hyperkalemia, vomiting, and dehydration are characteristic. In patients with partial defects, mineralocorticoid deficiency may not become apparent without stress, but hyponatremia becomes manifest during salt deprivation, particularly during withdrawal of supplemental glucocorticoids. Gradation in the severity of salt loss occurs even in affected sibs emphasizing the clinical heterogeneity in this syndrome,

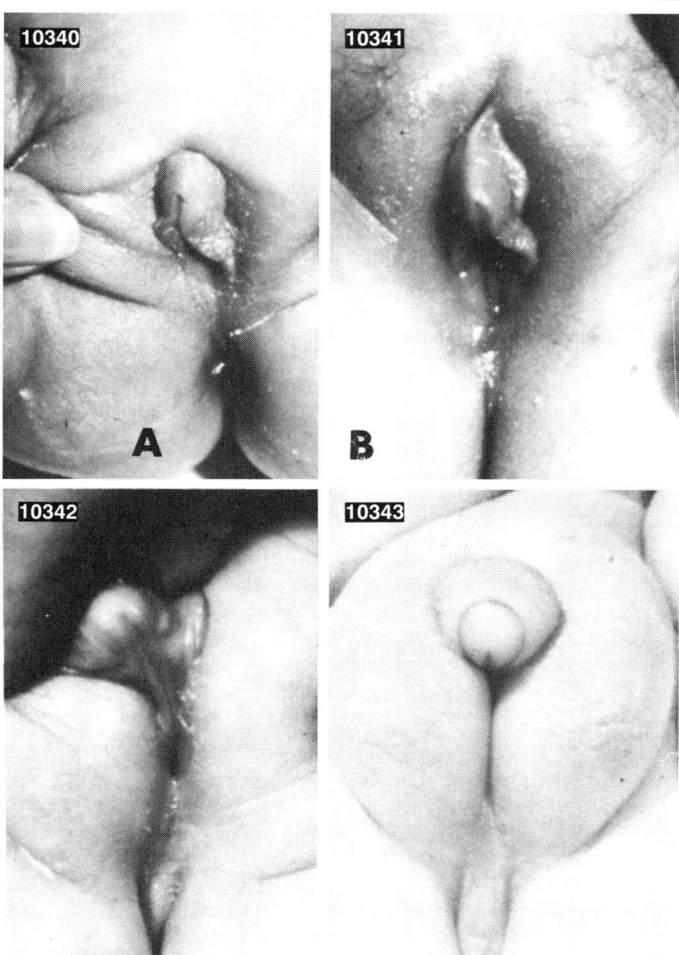

0909-10340–41: Mild clitoral hypertrophy and pubic hair development in a female. 10342–43: Bifid scrotum, severe hypospadias, and small phallus in a male.

which has been diagnosed in a 40-year-old woman. The external genitalia show variable degrees of abnormality in both males and females. Males have hypospadias, often perineal or second degree in type, and a bifid scrotum, with or without cryptorchidism. Females have labial fusion; clitoral hypertrophy, which is often mild; and mild but progressive hirsutism. This inadequate masculinization in males and mild virilization in females results from the accumulation and defective conversion of DHEA, a weak androgen, to androstenedione and, subsequently, to testosterone.

Laboratory tests reveal a high urinary excretion of 17-ketosteroids in which DHEA or its metabolites predominate. 17-hydroxycorticosteroids and aldosterone excretion are typically low but may be normal in patients with partial defects, where plasma cortisol and cortisol production rates have been shown to be within the normal range. Pregnenolone and its derivatives (δ5-pregnenetriol, 16α-hydroxy pregnenolone, 17α hydroxy pregnenolone) rather than pregnanolone derivatives (pregnanetriol), predominate in urine, reflecting the lack of enzyme isomerase activity required to shift the double bond from the C5-C6 position in the B-ring, to the C4-C5 position in the A ring of the steroid nucleus. The enzyme defect also occurs in the fetal testes (and ovary) and persists into later life, so that the response to exogenous (and presumably endogenous) gonadotropin is subnormal. However, in individuals with partial defects, there is evidence for increasing 3β-HSD activity with age, the enzyme activity being extra-adrenal, and probably hepatic in origin. Consequently, with increasing age, a large amount of pregnanetriol may appear in the urine, but this does not represent the coexistence of a double enzyme defect in 3β-HSD and 21-hydroxy activity. It should be noted that in severe enzyme deficiency, six of the seven initially reported patients died despite adequate glucocorticoid and salt replacement. The adrenal glands are hypertrophied, and histologically they appear laden with lipid.

Complications: Salt loss, dehydration, hypoglycemia, and death may occur. Involvement of the gonads may preclude spontaneous puberty or fertility.

Associated Findings: None known.

Etiology: Autosomal recessive inheritance.

Pathogenesis: The enzyme defect appears to affect the adrenals, as well as the gonads. There is a difference in the timing of maximal enzyme activity in the testis and ovary. Thus 3β-HSD activity in the testes is maximal at about the third intrauterine month, whereas in the ovaries and adrenal glands it becomes maximal at about the fourth month. Consequently, the abnormalities in male external genitalia are more severe.

An animal model of 3β-HSD deficiency has been produced in rats by the administration of a C-19 substrate analog to the mother. Partial prevention of hypospadias in affected male rats has been achieved by testosterone administration in utero; the anatomic defect in affected female offspring was prevented by *in utero* administration of corticosterone.

MIM No.: *20181

CDC No.: 255.200

Sex Ratio: M1:F1

Occurrence: About a dozen cases have been documented.

Risk of Recurrence for Patient's Sib:
See Part I, *Mendelian Inheritance.*

Risk of Recurrence for Patient's Child:
See Part I, *Mendelian Inheritance.*

Age of Detectability: May be detected from birth to adult life; most frequently in the first years of life, by virtue of salt loss, with ambiguity of external genitalia. Antenatal diagnosis has not been demonstrated.

Gene Mapping and Linkage: HSDB3 (hydroxy-delta 5-steroid dehydrogenase, 3 beta- and steroid delta-isomerase) has been provisionally mapped to 1p13-p11.

Prevention: None known. Genetic counseling indicated.

Treatment: Treatment with glucocorticoid and mineralocorticoids should be instituted early, particularly in view of the reported high mortality in severely affected patients. Because the defect affects the gonads, replacement with sex steroids at puberty will be required. Surgical correction of hypospadias or clitoromegaly may be required.

Prognosis: Normal life span in patients with partial defects; death has been reported in severely affected infants despite adequate replacement therapy. Reproductive function will be impaired.

Detection of Carrier: Unknown.

Special Considerations: MN; Wrenshall (c/o Diana Johnson, 10 Co Hwy 4); Congenital Adrenal Hyperplasia Group

References:

Goldman AS: Experimental congenital adrenocortical hyperplasia: persistent postnatal deficiency in activity of 3β-hydroxysteroid dehydrogenase produced in utero. J Clin Endocrinol 1967; 27:1041.

Zachmann M, et al.: Unusual type of congenital adrenal hyperplasia probably due to deficiency of 3β-hydroxysteroid dehydrogenase. case report of a surviving girl with steroid studies. J Clin Endocrinol 1970; 30:719.

Bongiovanni AM, et al.: Urinary excretion of pregnanetriol and δ5-pregnenetriol in two forms of congenital adrenal hyperplasia. J Clin Invest 1971; 50:2751.

Kenny FM, et al.: Partial 3β-hydroxysteroid dehydrogenase (3βHSD) deficiency in a family with congenital adrenal hyperplasia: evidence for increasing 3β-HSD activity with age. Pediatrics 1971; 48:756.

Zachmann M, et al.: 3 β-hydroxysteroid dehydrogenase deficiency: follow-up study in a girl with pubertal bone age. Hormone Res 1979; 11:292–302.

Rosenfeld RL, et al.: Pubertal presentation of congenital δ5–3β-hydroxysteroid dehydrogenase deficiency. J Clin Endocrinol Metab 1980; 51:345.

Miller WL, Levine LS: Molecular and clinical advance in congenital adrenal hyperplasia. J Pediat 1987; 111:1–17.

White PC, et al.: Congenital adrenal hyperplasia. New Engl J Med 1987; 316:1519 (first part) and 1580 (second part).

New MI, et al.: The adrenal hyperplasias. In: Scriver CR, et al, eds: The metabolic basis of inherited disease, 6th ed. New York: McGraw-Hill, 1989:1881–1918.

SP004   **Mark A. Sperling**

STEROID 5 ALPHA-REDUCTASE DEFICIENCY   3062

Includes:

Genital ambiguity, pseudovaginal perineoscrotal hypospadias
Male pseudohermaphroditism due to 5 alpha-reductase deficiency
Pseudohermaphroditism, familial incomplete male, type 2
Pseudovaginal perineoscrotal hypospadias

Excludes:

Genital ambiguity in XY males, external (other)
Receptor-dependent androgen-responsive defects
Testis differentiation defects
Testosterone production defects

Major Diagnostic Criteria: Perineal hypospadias with separate urethral and vaginal openings within a urogenital sinus. The testes are usually cryptorchid. At puberty, there is impressive genital and somatic virilization, without gynecomastia. Plasma testosterone is normal or elevated, but its level in relation to 5α-dihydrotestosterone is high. Plasma luteinizing hormone is high; follicle stimulating hormone may be high. Urinary 5α-reduced metabolites of testosterone and of various other C-19 and C-21 steroids are low. Decreased or defective 5α-reductase activity in fresh tissue slices or cultured genital skin fibroblasts.

Clinical Findings: The infant is born with external genitalia that are predominantly feminine in character, but is otherwise well. Plasma testosterone level is normal or elevated basally and augments normally in response to a course of human chorionic gonadotropin. In either case the plasma testosterone: 5α-dihy-

drotestosterone ratio is higher than normal. The epididymes, vasa deferentia, and seminal vesicles (all Wolffian duct derivatives) are present, but the prostate is impalpable or hypoplastic. Müllerian duct derivatives are absent. At puberty, the voice deepens, skeletal muscle development is normal, the phallus grows, the scrotum becomes rugose and pigmented, pubic hair growth is impressive, and the testes often descend. Spermatogenesis may be near normal in testes that have not been cryptorchid. The subjects have erections and ejaculates. They do not have temporal hairline recession, facial and body hair are less than normal, and acne is rare. Despite a female sex-of-rearing, subjects have a remarkable tendency to adopt a male sexual identity and orientation at puberty.

Complications: None, except those in the psychosexual sphere, and particularly if inadequate reinforcement of the female sex-of-rearing allows affected subjects to adopt a male identity at puberty.

Associated Findings: None known.

Etiology: Autosomal recessive inheritance.

Pathogenesis: 5α-reductase is the enzyme responsible for converting testosterone to 5α-dihydrotestosterone (DHT). Deficient activity of the enzyme in androgen target tissues yields a phenotype that distinguishes testosterone-dependent from DHT-dependent events in male sexual development. Since Wolffian differentiation is normal, it is testosterone-dependent. Indeed, 5α-reductase enzyme activity does not appear in Wolffian-derived structures until they have passed their critical period in differentiation. Contrarily, masculinization of the neutral external genital primordia and prostate morphogenesis are DHT dependent. Hence their development is blocked. Not surprisingly, 5α-reductase enzyme activity appears in these structures before their critical period of differentiation. The fact that growth and maturation of the external genitalia occur at puberty suggests that these structures acquire a degree of responsiveness to testosterone that they lack in utero. The elevated plasma level of luteinizing hormone suggests that DHT is important for negative feedback of LH release. The absence of clinical features in female homozygotes means that testosterone is sufficient for normal female sexual development.

MIM No.: *26460

Sex Ratio: M1:F1 biochemically, but M1:F0 clinically.

Occurrence: Uncommon, but precise data are unavailable.

Risk of Recurrence for Patient's Sib:
See Part I, *Mendelian Inheritance.*

Risk of Recurrence for Patient's Child:
See Part I, *Mendelian Inheritance.*

Age of Detectability: At birth in XY homozygotes.

Gene Mapping and Linkage: Unknown.

Prevention: None known. Genetic counseling indicated. In theory, DHT replacement could prevent the dysmorphogenesis, but there is no way, currently, to detect affected male fetuses early enough to use this form of prophylaxis.

Treatment: Diagnosis in early infancy and an early decision on sex-of-rearing are basic to good treatment. If a male sex-of-rearing is chosen, topical application of DHT cream to the external genitalia will facilitate staged surgical reconstruction in the male direction. At puberty, intramuscular testosterone in doses sufficient to raise the plasma DHT level into the normal range have been beneficial. An excessively high level of DHT must be avoided as it reduces the plasma testosterone level secondarily and thereby causes loss of libido and impotence.

Prognosis: Normal life span.

Detection of Carrier: Asymptomatic male and female carriers are often detectable by their intermediately abnormal levels of urinary 5α-reduced metabolites of testosterone and other C-19 or C-21 steroids.

Special Considerations: Measurement and characterization of 5α-reductase activity in cultured genital skin fibroblasts may be useful for ruling out the diagnosis. However, the normal level of

5α-reductase activity in these cells is very variable. In some laboratories, the lower level of normal is at the limit of sensitivity of the assay. Hence, in these laboratories such cells cannot be used to rule in the diagnosis. Normal cultured nongenital skin fibroblasts are even more likely to have very low levels of 5α-reductase activity. They should not be used for ruling in the diagnosis.

The remarkable tendency for affected subjects, reared as females, to adopt a male sexual identity at puberty indicates that exposure of the brain to testosterone prenatally, in early postnatal life, and at puberty is sufficient to overcome a female sex-of-rearing, unless the latter is strongly reinforced.

References:
Peterson RE, et al.: Male pseudohermaphroditism due to steroid 5α-reductase deficiency. Am J Med 1977; 62:170–191.
Pinsky L, et al.: 5α-reductase activity of genital and non-genital skin fibroblasts from patients with 5α-reductase deficiency, androgen insensitivity, or unknown forms of male pseudohermaphroditism. Am J Med Genet 1978; 1:407–416.
Imperato-McGinley J, et al.: Androgens and the evolution of male-gender identity among male pseudohermaphrodites with 5α-reductase deficiency. New Engl J Med 1979; 300:1233–1237.
Imperato-McGinley J, et al.: Steroid 5α-reductase deficiency in a 65 year old male pseudohermaphrodite: the natural history, ultrastructure of the testes and evidence for inherited enzyme heterogeneity. J Clin Endocrinol Metab 1980; 50:15–22.
Price P, et al.: High dose androgen therapy in male pseudohermaphroditism due to 5α-reductase deficiency and disorders of the androgen receptor. J Clin Invest 1984; 74:1496–1508.
Imperato-McGinley J, et al.: Decreased urinary C19 and C21 steroid 5α-metabolites in parents of male pseudohermaphrodites with 5α-reductase deficiency: detection of carriers. J Clin Endocrinol Metab 1985; 60:553–558.
Imperato-McGinley J, et al.: The diagnosis of 5α-reductase deficiency in infancy. J Clin Endocrinol Metab 1986; 63:1313–1318.

PI005 **Leonard Pinsky**

STEROID 11 BETA-HYDROXYLASE DEFICIENCY　　0902

Includes:
Adrenal hyperplasia IV
Adrenogenital syndrome with hypertension
Hypertensive form of adrenal hyperplasia
P450C11B1, deficiency of

Excludes: Enzyme deficiencies in adrenal steroid biosynthesis, other

Major Diagnostic Criteria: Progressive virilization, excessive 17-KS and 17-OHCS excretion, and markedly elevated concentration of compound-S in plasma or urine which is suppressed during glucocorticoid replacement.

Clinical Findings: Progressive virilization and all the sequelae of excessive androgen formation, including ambiguity of the external genitalia in genetic and gonadal females, as described for 21-hydroxylase deficiency. However, salt loss, hyponatremia, and hyperkalemia do not occur. Hypertension may occur but is not universally present, suggesting a spectrum in the severity of enzyme deficiency. The enzyme involved catalyzes the conversion of 11-deoxycortisol (compound-S) to cortisol (compound-F) in the glucocorticoid pathway, and deoxycorticosterone (DOC) to corticosterone (compound-B) in the mineralocorticoid pathway. Consequently, the plasma concentrations of compound-S and DOC are elevated, as are the respective urinary excretion products, whereas plasma and urinary cortisol and aldosterone may be diminished. Urinary excretion of 17-ketosteroids is elevated, reflecting excessive adrenal androgen production, which is unaffected by the enzyme block and stimulated by excessive ACTH that results from inadequate cortisol secretion. Urinary 17-hydroxycorticosteroids (17-OHCS) are also elevated since compound-S and its urinary metabolite, tetrahydro-S, both contain the 17, 21 dihydroxy, 20 keto grouping, which reacts in the standard 17-OHCS measurements. Pregnanetriol excretion in urine may be modestly elevated.

Salt restriction is not associated with a rise in aldosterone, even after suppression of DOC by administered cortisol, suggesting that the same enzyme is involved in both glucocorticoid and mineralocorticoid pathways. Plasma renin levels are low. Mild cases may present in adult life and simulate the Stein-Leventhal syndrome.

Complications: Ambiguity of the external genitalia may result in false gender assignment in genetic females; lack of electrolyte disturbances may delay the diagnosis in males. Progressive virilization, premature epiphyseal closure, and final short stature, as well as preclusion of normal puberty and fertility may result from the untreated condition. Hypertension is a direct result of excessive production of DOC, a potent mineralocorticoid.

Associated Findings: Gynecomastia has been described in an affected male infant.

Etiology: Autosomal recessive inheritance.

Pathogenesis: The enzyme block prevents the normal synthesis of cortisol, resulting in excessive ACTH stimulation and adrenal hyperplasia. The androgenic pathway is unaffected by the block; consequently, production of dehydroepiandrosterone, androstenedione, and testosterone is increased, producing virilization, rapid growth, and accelerated bone maturation. DOC also is secreted in large quantities, resulting in salt and water retention, volume expansion, and hypertension, with low renin secretion. Both the enzymatic block and the suppressed renin contribute to low aldosterone secretion.

A block in 11-hydroxylation may occur in some adrenocortical carcinomas, thus totally simulating the clinical features and plasma and urinary steroid patterns observed with the congenital enzyme deficiency. However, under these circumstances glucocorticoid replacement will not suppress the oversecretion of the specific steroids. The possibility of carcinoma must always be considered in "late onset" cases. Metapyrone (SU4885) is a drug that also blocks 11-hydroxylation; use is made of this agent in studying the intactness of the hypothalamic-pituitary-adrenal axis.

MIM No.: *20201

CDC No.: 255.200

Sex Ratio: M1:F1

Occurrence: Undetermined but presumed rare. About 40 cases reported in Jews of Moroccan and Iranian extraction.

Risk of Recurrence for Patient's Sib:
See Part I, *Mendelian Inheritance.*

Risk of Recurrence for Patient's Child:
See Part I, *Mendelian Inheritance.*

Age of Detectability: From birth to adult life. Intrauterine diagnosis has been demonstrated, based on maternal urine or amniotic fluid hormone measurements.

Gene Mapping and Linkage: CYP11B1 (cytochrome P450, subfamily XIB, polypeptide 1 (steroid 11-beta-hydroxylase)) has been mapped to 8q21-q22.
CYP11B2 (cytochrome P450, subfamily XIB, polypeptide 2 (steroid 11-beta-hydroxylase)) has been provisionally mapped to 8q21-q22.

Prevention: None known. Genetic counseling indicated.

Treatment: Replacement therapy with cortisol arrests virilization and restores blood pressure to normal. Intrauterine diagnosis is theoretically feasible, as is intrauterine therapy with cortisol to minimize virilization. Primary and definitive surgical repair may be required for ambiguous genitalia in genetic females.

Prognosis: Normal for life span, reproduction, and intelligence when diagnosed early and appropriate treatment is instituted.

Detection of Carrier: Theoretically, via levels of compound-S achieved after ACTH stimulation, but in practice this has not proven useful. Unlike the 21-hydroxylase defect, there is no association with the HLA system that would permit identification of the heterozygote, or antenatal diagnosis or detection of an unrecognized homozygote (see **Steroid 21-hydroxylase deficiency**).

Special Considerations: MN; Wrenshall (c/o Diana Johnson, 10 Co Hwy 4); Congenital Adrenal Hyperplasia Group

References:
McLaren NK, et al.: Gynecomastia with congenital virilizing adrenal hyperplasia (11-β-hydroxylase deficiency). J Pediat 1975; 86:597.
Cathelineau G, et al.: Adrenocortical 11β-hydroxylation defect in adult women with post menarchial onset of symptoms. J Clin Endocrinol Metab 1980; 51:287.
Pang S, et al.: Hormonal studies in obligate heterozygotes and siblings of patients with 11β-hydroxylase deficiency congenital adrenal hyperplasia. J Clin Endocrinol Metab 1980; 50:586.
Rosler A, et al.: Clinical variability of congenital adrenal hyperplasia due to 11-beta-hydroxylase deficiency. Hormone Res 1982; 16:133–141.
Zachmann M, et al.: Clinical and biochemical variability of congenital adrenal hyperplasia due to 11β-hydroxylase deficiency: a study of 25 patients. J Clin Endocrinol Metab 1983; 56:222.
Hochberg Z, et al.: Growth and pubertal development in patients with congenital adrenal hyperplasia due to 11-beta-hydroxylase deficiency. Am J Dis Child 1985; 139:771–776.
Miller WL, Levine LS: Molecular and clinical advance in congenital adrenal hyperplasia. J Pediat 1987; 111:1–17.
White PC, et al.: Congenital adrenal hyperplasia. New Engl J Med 1987; 316:1519 (first part) and 1580 (second part).
New MI, et al.: The adrenal hyperplasias. In: Scriver CR, et al, eds: The metabolic basis of inherited disease, 6th ed. New York: McGraw-Hill, 1989:1881–1918.

SP004   **Mark A. Sperling**

STEROID 17 ALPHA-HYDROXYLASE DEFICIENCY   0903

Includes:
Adrenal hyperplasia V
Hypertensive congenital adrenal hyperplasia

Excludes:
Adrenal hyperplasia, other forms
Hyperaldosteronism, familial glucocorticoid suppressible (0484)

Major Diagnostic Criteria: Diminished 17-hydroxylated steroids and sex steroids, hypertension, and lack of secondary sexual characteristics in phenotypic females or males with ambiguous genitalia. Secretion of DOC (deoxycorticosterone) is elevated but can be suppressed with administration of glucocorticoids. The cortisol response to ACTH and the sex steroid hormone responses to chorionic gonadotropin are diminished or absent.

Clinical Findings: Hypertension and the absence of secondary sexual characteristics. The enzyme defect prevents the formation of cortisol or any of its 17-hydroxylated precursors, as well as the formation of sex steroids, the latter defect apparently shared by the gonad. Mineralocorticoid formation is not affected.

In females, there is no ambiguity of the external genitalia at birth, but secondary sexual characteristics (breasts, and pubic and axillary hair) fail to develop and primary amenorrhea may be the presenting complaint. Acute abdominal pain secondary to infarction of cystic enlarged ovaries has been reported in sibs. As might be expected from a defect interfering with adrenal and testicular androgen formation and thus male sexual differentiation, genotypic males have congenitally ambiguous genitalia. The penis is small or rudimentary, hypospadias is present, and the labia majora fail to fuse, creating a shallow vagina. Cryptorchidism may be present.

Laboratory tests reveal hypokalemic alkalosis, low cortisol concentrations in plasma or 17-OHCS excretion in urine, and low-to-absent 17-ketosteroids (17-KS), estrogens, and testosterone. Plasma ACTH levels are elevated, and there is no response or a subnormal response in serum cortisol, or urinary 17-OHCS, or 17-KS following administration of ACTH. Similarly there is little or no gonadal response to administration of chorionic gonadotropin. Endogenous serum gonadotropin concentrations are high in older

individuals. In contrast, circulating corticosterone (compound-B) and deoxycorticosterone (DOC) levels are elevated. Plasma renin is low, as is aldosterone, suggesting salt and water retention and volume expansion by DOC, with resultant suppression of the renin/angiotensin/aldosterone pathway. This is confirmed by finding normal renin and aldosterone concentrations after suppressive doses of glucocorticoids. Partial defects with normokalemia have been described, but hypertension, diminished or absent sexual hair, and amenorrhea have been characteristic in all females, who consequently present in the mid-to-late teen years. In genetic males with the complete defect, the external genitalia will be entirely female, and diagnosis can be delayed until puberty, unless hypertension and hypokalemia are recognized. Males with the partial defect will be recognized earlier by virtue of ambiguity of the external genitalia.

A defect in 17-hydroxylation has been found in an infant with a corticosterone-secreting adrenal tumor nonsuppressible by glucocorticoids. Glucocorticoid-responsive hyperaldosteronism should and can be differentiated because 17-hydroxy corticosteroids and 17-ketosteroids are intermittently elevated.

Complications: Hypertension and hypokalemia result from excessive DOC secretion. Phenotypically normal female external genitalia in genetic males may result in false gender assignment. Impaired sexual development and fertility occur in both sexes.

Associated Findings: None known.

Etiology: Autosomal recessive or possibly X-linked recessive inheritance.

Pathogenesis: A defect in 17-hydroxylation affecting adrenal and gonadal steroidogenesis.

MIM No.: *20211

CDC No.: 255.200

Sex Ratio: M1:F1

Occurrence: At least 40 cases have been reported in the literature.

Risk of Recurrence for Patient's Sib:
See Part I, *Mendelian Inheritance.*

Risk of Recurrence for Patient's Child:
See Part I, *Mendelian Inheritance.* Fertility impaired.

Age of Detectability: From birth to adult life; most frequently in the second decade as a result of lack of pubertal development. Antenatal diagnosis has not yet been demonstrated.

Gene Mapping and Linkage: CYP17 (cytochrome P450, subfamily XVII (steroid 17-alpha-hydroxylase)) has been provisionally mapped to 10.

Prevention: None known. Genetic counseling indicated.

Treatment: Therapy with replacement doses of glucocorticoids returns blood pressure and serum potassium level to normal; it corrects inhibition of the renin/angiotensin/aldosterone pathway. Estrogen therapy in females and testosterone treatment in males brings about normal secondary sexual development. Corrective surgery may be necessary in males with ambiguity of the external genitalia.

Prognosis: Normal for life span and intelligence, but fertility may be impaired. Malignant hypertension may develop if the condition is not treated.

Detection of Carrier: Hypertension and mild elevation of aldosterone partially supppressible by glucocorticoids were reported in the mother of an affected patient in whom the 17-hydroxylase defect seemed limited to the adrenal.

References:
Weinstein RL, et al.: Deficient 17-hydroxylation in a corticosterone producing adrenal tumor from an infant with hemihypertrophy and visceromegaly. J Clin Endocrinol 1970; 30:457.
DeLange WE, et al.: Primary amenorrhea with hypertension due to 17-hydroxylase deficiency. Acta Med Scand 1973; 193:565.
Waldhäusl W, et al.: Combined 17α-and 18-hydroxylase deficiency associated with complete male pseudohermaphroditism and hypoaldosteronism. J Clin Endocrinol Metab 1978; 46:236.

Yazaki K, et al.: Hypokalemic myopathy associated with 17-alpha-hydroxylase deficiency: a case report. Neurology 1982; 32:94–97.
Morimoto I, et al.: An autopsy case of 17α-hydroxylase deficiency with malignant hypertension. J Clin Endocrinol Metab 1983; 56:915.
Miller WL, Levine LS: Molecular and clinical advance in congenital adrenal hyperplasia. J Pediat 1987; 111:1–17.
White PC, et al.: Congenital adrenal hyperplasia. New Engl J Med 1987; 316:1519 (first part) and 1580 (second part).
New MI, et al.: The adrenal hyperplasias. In: Scriver CR, et al, eds: The metabolic basis of inherited disease, 6th ed. New York: Mc-Graw-Hill, 1989:1881–1918.

SP004   **Mark A. Sperling**

STEROID 17,20-DESMOLASE DEFICIENCY   0904

Includes: Pseudohermaphroditism, male, steroid 17,20-desmolase deficiency

Excludes:
Enzymatic defects in testosterone biosynthesis, other
Steroid 3 beta-hydroxysteroid dehydrogenase deficiency (0909)
Steroid 17 alpha-hydroxylase deficiency (0903)

Major Diagnostic Criteria: The condition is to be considered in an infant with ambiguous genitalia, low to absent 17-ketosteroids and with no response to HCG or ACTH stimulation. Other steroids are normal and adrenals and gonads are present. The karyotype is 46,XY. The testicular tissue is unable to convert precursors at the 17,20-desmolase step.

Clinical Findings: The hallmark of this syndrome is ambiguous genitalia in genetic males. Although long suspected, the condition has only recently been described. The propositi were male cousins with ambiguous genitalia and XY karyotype. A maternal uncle had been reared as a female; his karyotype was XY, testicles had been surgically removed, and a rudimentary uterus was present as well as one fallopian tube. Excretion of all androgens, including dehydroepiandrosterone and testosterone, was minimal or undetectable, even after administration of human chorionic gonadotropin (HCG) at a dose of G5,000 U/m² for 5 days. In contrast, secretion of glucocorticoids and mineralocorticoids was essentially normal. In vitro, testicular tissue from an affected patient readily converted 17-ketosteroids to testosterone, excluding 17-ketoreductase deficiency, but testosterone could not be formed from other precursors such as pregnenolone, progesterone, or their 17-hydroxylated equivalents. Thus, the defect appears to be at the 17,20-desmolase step. Infertility is to be expected in these individuals. Affected females have normal internal and external genitalia and failure of pubertal development, with infertility due to inability to form estrogen. With a complete defect, genetic males may have female external genitalia.

Complications: Infertility.

Associated Findings: None known.

Etiology: Autosomal recessive inheritance. Until recently, lack of reports of affected females made it difficult to rule out X-linked inheritance.

Pathogenesis: The clinical features are explicable on the basis of 17,20-desmolase deficiency affecting the adrenal and gonad.

MIM No.: *30915

CDC No.: 255.200

Sex Ratio: Presumably M1:F1, although most cases reported to date have been male.

Occurrence: Undetermined but presumably rare.

Risk of Recurrence for Patient's Sib:
See Part I, *Mendelian Inheritance.*

Risk of Recurrence for Patient's Child:
See Part I, *Mendelian Inheritance.* Fertility is severely impaired.

Age of Detectability: Birth to adult life. Males are likely to present in the perinatal period because of ambiguous genitalia; females

will present because of failure to develop secondary sexual changes.

Gene Mapping and Linkage: TDD (testicular 17,20-desmolase deficiency) has been mapped to X.

Other researchers believe that the same polypeptide subserves this condition and **Steroid 17 alpha-hydroxylase deficiency,** and CYP17 (cytochrome P450, steroid 17-alpha-hydroxylase) has been provisionally mapped to 10.

Prevention: None known. Genetic counseling indicated.

Treatment: In females, treatment with estrogen should permit sexual development but will not restore fertility. In males with severe ambiguity of genitalia, plastic reconstruction of female external genitalia, removal of testes, and rearing in the female role would seem to be indicated, since construction of adequate male genitalia and repair of hypospadias may be technically impossible. When ambiguity is less severe, plastic repair of external genitalia, and treatment with testosterone to bring about pubertal changes at the appropriate time are indicated.

Prognosis: Normal life span, but fertility is severely impaired.

Detection of Carrier: Unknown.

References:
Zachmann M, et al.: Testicular 17,20-desmolase deficiency causing male pseudohermaphroditism. Acta Endocrinol [Suppl] (Copen) 1971; 155:65–80.
Zachmann M, et al.: Steroid 17,20-desmolase deficiency: a new cause of male pseudohermaphroditism. Clin Endocrinol 1972; 1:369–385.
Goebelsmann U: Male pseudohermaphroditism consistent with 17, 20-desmolase deficiency. Gynecol Invest 1976; 7:138–156.
Zachmann M, et al.: Two types of male pseudohermaphroditism due to 17,20-desmolase deficiency. J Clin Endocrinol Metab 1982; 55:487.
Larrea F, et al.: Hypergonadotrophic hypogonadism in an XX female subject due to 17,20 steriod desmolase deficiency. Acta Endocrinol 1983; 103:400.
Miller WL, Levine LS: Molecular and clinical advance in congenital adrenal hyperplasia. J Pediat 1987; 111:1–17.
New MI, et al.: The adrenal hyperplasias. In: Scriver CR, et al, eds: The metabolic basis of inherited disease, 6th ed. New York: Mc-Graw-Hill, 1989:1881–1918.

SP004   **Mark A. Sperling**

STEROID 17-KETOSTEROID REDUCTASE DEFICIENCY   2299

Includes:
Male pseudohermaphroditism due to 17-KSR deficiency
Neutral 17-beta-hydroxysteroid oxidoreductase deficiency
Polycystic ovary disease due to 17-KSR deficiency
Pseudohermaphroditism, male-gynecomastia
Seventeen-beta-hydroxysteroid dehydrogenase deficiency

Excludes:
Androgen insensitivity syndrome, incomplete (0050)
Enzymatic defects in testosterone biosynthesis, other
Gonadal dysgenesis, XY type (0437)
Steroid 5 alpha-reductase deficiency (3062)

Major Diagnostic Criteria: Elevated androstenedione (δ⁴)A to testosterone ratio in plasma in a 46,XY male with female or ambiguous external genitalia. Similar laboratory criteria apply to a female with clinical features of polycystic ovary disease (PCOD).

Clinical Findings: Affected males usually appear to be phenotypic females at birth, although some degree of ambiguity may be present. Testes may or may not be present in the inguinal canal. At puberty, virilization takes place normally. Although the enzyme deficiency leads to deficient testosterone and hence dihydrotestosterone production, Wolffian structures are present, indicating that less testosterone is necessary for this developmental step than for masculinization of the external genitalia. Testicular biopsy material from adults shows absent or markedly decreased spermatogenesis and marked peritubular sclerosis. Serum gonadotropin levels are high. At puberty, males may develop gynecomastia. The diagnosis is uncommonly made prior to puberty unless a sib is affected. Some women with polycystic ovary disease (PCOD) have been found to have the enzyme deficiency in the ovary. Serum testosterone level in females may be proportionately higher because nongonadal peripheral 17-ketosteroid reductase (KSR) enzymatic activity is intact and by inference is a separate enzyme. The sclerocystic ovaries apparently result from deficient ovarian estradiol production (derived normally from testosterone) with a secondary LH increase and cystic changes. Definite diagnosis in either sex would require demonstration of absent or deficient 17-KSR activity in gonadal tissue.

Complications: Psychosocial problems may develop in males because of sexual ambiguity and confusion in gender assignment.

Associated Findings: Testicular carcinoma has been reported in a male with persistent cryptorchidism.

Etiology: Probably autosomal recessive inheritance, given that some families have been consanguineous. Most reports are of affected males, because of the genital ambiguity. Depending on the severity of the enzyme defect, affected females could go undetected.

Pathogenesis: The clinical features in both sexes are explicable on the basis of deficient gonadal (δ^4)A to testosterone conversion.

MIM No.: *26430

CDC No.: 255.200

Sex Ratio: Probably M1:F1, if careful sibship studies are made, although ascertainment through genital ambiguity yields far more affected males.

Occurrence: Undetermined but presumably rare. Large kinships were reported in an inbred Arab community in Israel. A Venezuelan sibship and about a dozen other widely distributed cases have been reported.

Risk of Recurrence for Patient's Sib:
See Part I, *Mendelian Inheritance.*

Risk of Recurrence for Patient's Child:
See Part I, *Mendelian Inheritance.* Males are infertile. Because of the rarity of the condition, the risk to fertile females is negligible.

Age of Detectability: From birth to adulthood, with most males being diagnosed at puberty. Many females are likely undiagnosed or otherwise categorized as having PCOD.

Gene Mapping and Linkage: Unknown.

Prevention: None known. Genetic counseling indicated.

Treatment: Males reared as females should have gonadectomy and reconstructive genital surgery is necessary. Estrogen therapy will be required for life. Females may require therapy for PCOD. Some males have switched gender roles at puberty with success, analogous to men with **Steroid 5 alpha-reductase deficiency.**

Prognosis: Normal life span with impaired fertility. Cryptorchid testes may become malignant.

Detection of Carrier: Unknown.

References:
Saez JM, et al.: Familial male pseudohermaphroditism with gynecomastia due to testicular 17-ketosteroid reductase defect. I. Study in vivo. J Clin Endocrinol 1971; 32:604–610.
Lanes R, et al.: Sibship with 17-ketosteroid reductase (17-KSR) deficiency and hypothyroidism: lack of linkage of histocompatibility leucocyte antigen and 17-KSR loci. J Clin Endocrinol Metab 1983; 57:190–196.
Balducci R, et al.: Familial male pseudohermaphroditism with gynecomastia due to 17-beta-hydroxysteroid dehydrogenase deficiency: a report of 3 cases. Clin Endocrinol 1985; 23:439–444.
Pang S, et al.: Hirsutism, polycystic ovarian disease, and ovarian 17-ketosteroid reductase deficiency. New Engl J Med 1987; 316:1295–1301.
Ecksteria B, et al.: The nature of the defect in familial male pseudohermaphroditism in males of Gaza. J Clin Endocrinol Metab 1989; 68:477–485.

R. Neil Schimke

STEROID 18-HYDROXYLASE DEFICIENCY 0905

Includes:
Adrenal 18-hydroxylase deficiency
Aldosterone deficiency I
Corticosterone methyl oxidase type I deficiency

Excludes:
Adrenal hypoaldosteronism of infancy, transient isolated (0023)
Adrenal hypoplasia, congenital (0024)
Angiotensin-unresponsive hypoaldosteronism
Steroid 18-hydroxysteroid dehydrogenase deficiency (0906)

Major Diagnostic Criteria: Infants with this condition have clinical features of hypoaldosteronism with vomiting, dehydration, hyponatremia, and hyperkalemia. There are no abnormalities in the production of glucocorticoids and sex steroids, but there is overproduction of corticosterone and little or no 18-OH corticosterone.

Clinical Findings: These patients characteristically present in infancy with features of mineralocorticoid deficiency: dehydration, vomiting, failure to thrive, hyponatremia, and hyperkalemia. The original report concerned three cousins from an inbred family: two girls and one boy, all with normal external genitalia. There was no abnormal hyperpigmentation. Investigation revealed normal urinary excretion of 17-hydroxycorticosteroids and 17-ketosteroids, with a normal response to stimulation by ACTH. Aldosterone excretion was undetectable, and there was no response to ACTH or salt deprivation. However, urinary excretion of corticosterone and its metabolites was markedly increased, whereas only small amounts of 11-deoxycorticosterone (DOC) were detected, even after ACTH stimulation, and 18-hydroxycorticosterone or its metabolites were absent. The defect therefore involves the 18-hydroxylation step from corticosterone to 18-OH corticosterone; the second to last step in aldosterone biosynthesis. The adrenal gland of one affected patient showed a poorly developed zona glomerulosa and a hypertrophied juxtaglomerular apparatus. Despite the severe reduction in aldosterone synthesis, patients on a normal salt intake can maintain marginal sodium balance with serum sodiums of 120–130 mEq/liter; salt deprivation is poorly tolerated. There is an excellent response to supplementation with salt and a mineralocorticoid. As with other defects involving aldosterone secretion, there is an amelioration of the salt-losing tendency with increasing age, so that electrolyte balance can be maintained by a high salt intake without addition of mineralocorticoid, although the basic biochemical defect persists. Milder forms of this entity also exist, since hypoaldosteronism and increased excretion of corticosterone consistent with an 18-hydroxylase defect has been reported in young adults. The possibility that transient hypoaldosteronism of infancy represents a maturational delay in 18-hydroxylation has been separately discussed (see **Adrenal hypoaldosteronism of infancy, transient isolated.**)

Complications: In newborns, death may result from failure to replace fluids, salt, and mineralocorticoid.

Associated Findings: None known.

Etiology: Autosomal recessively inheritance.

Pathogenesis: The final two steps in aldosterone biosynthesis involve the hydroxylation of carbon 18 of corticosterone followed by oxidation (dehydrogenation) of the same carbon to produce aldosterone. Since cortisol and sex steroid synthesis is unaffected, there is no elevation in ACTH or hyperpigmentation, and the external genitalia are normal. Although large quantities of corticosterone and some DOC are produced, they are weak mineralocorticoids relative to aldosterone. Hyponatremia, hyperkalemia, and volume depletion ensue, with an attempt to stimulate aldosterone via the renin-angiotensin system, thus accounting for renal juxtaglomerular hyperplasia. The reduced or absent 18-hydroxycorticosterone, with overproduction of corticosterone, confirms the locus of the defect. More recently, the traditional concepts concerning the final two steps of aldosterone biosynthesis from corticosterone have been revised. Although a two-step, mixed oxidation-reduction reaction is likely, the actual intermediate may not be 18-hydroxycorticosterone itself. Thus, the suggested terminology for the defects in the two biosynthetic steps for aldosterone are corticosterone methyloxidase defects types 1 and 2. When corticosterone only is elevated, (and not suppressible by exogenous glucocorticoid to distinguish it from 17-hydroxylase deficiency) the defect is type 1. When the defect is characterized by overproduction of both corticosterone and 18-hydroxycorticosterone, the defect is type 2.

MIM No.: *20340

CDC No.: 255.200

Sex Ratio: M1:F1

Occurrence: At least six cases reported; three from common ancestry.

Risk of Recurrence for Patient's Sib:
See Part I, *Mendelian Inheritance.*

Risk of Recurrence for Patient's Child:
See Part I, *Mendelian Inheritance.*

Age of Detectability: Usually in the newborn period or in the first year of life, but milder defects may be detected at any age.

Gene Mapping and Linkage: Unknown.

Prevention: None known. Genetic counseling indicated.

Treatment: Treatment with salt supplementation and a mineralocorticoid, such as DOC, is necessary in the first few years of life. Later, patients appear able to maintain normal electrolyte balance by adjusting their sodium intake without mineralocorticoid supplements.

Prognosis: Excellent for life span, intelligence, and reproduction if electrolyte disturbance is recognized and appropriately treated.

Detection of Carrier: Unknown.

Special Considerations: Hypoaldosteronism, with apparent selective inhibition of the 18-hydroxylation step has been reported after prolonged administration of heparin. In adults over 40 years of age with hypoaldosteronism and biochemical findings compatible with defective aldosterone synthesis, cardiovascular complications of hypokalemia have been a prominent presenting feature.

References:
Rösler A, et al.: The nature of the defect in a salt-wasting disorder in Jews of Iran. J Clin Endocrinol Metab 1977; 44:279.
Veldhuis JD: Inborn error in the terminal step of aldosterone biosynthesis: corticosterone methyl oxidase type II deficiency in a North American pedigree. New Engl J Med 1980; 303:117.
Rosler A: The natural history of salt-wasting disorders of adrenal and renal origin. J Clin Endocrinol Metab 1984; 59:689.
Miller WL, Levine LS: Molecular and clinical advance in congenital adrenal hyperplasia. J Pediat 1987; 111:1–17.
White PC, et al.: Congenital adrenal hyperplasia. New Engl J Med 1987; 316:1519 (first part) and 1580 (second part).
New MI, et al.: The adrenal hyperplasias. In: Scriver CR, et al, eds: The metabolic basis of inherited disease, 6th ed. New York: McGraw-Hill, 1989:1881–1918.

SP004   **Mark A. Sperling**

STEROID 18-HYDROXYSTEROID DEHYDROGENASE
DEFICIENCY   0906

Includes:
Adrenal 18-hydroxysteroid dehydrogenase deficiency
Aldosterone deficiency II
Corticosterone methyl oxidase type II deficiency

Excludes:
Adrenal hypoaldosteronism of infancy, transient isolated (0023)
Adrenal hypoplasia, congenital (0024)
Angiotensin-unresponsive hypoaldosteronism
Steroid 18-hydroxylase deficiency (0905)

Major Diagnostic Criteria: Varying degrees of severity of vomiting and dehydration accompanied by salt loss and hyperkalemia are the early manifestations of this syndrome. The genitalia are normal. The condition is due to hypoaldosteronism, with elevated

production of 18-hydroxycorticosterone and normal cortisol and sex steroid levels.

Clinical Findings: This defect is identical in its chemical findings to that caused by **Steroid 18-hydroxylase deficiency**. Growth failure, with hyponatremia and hyperkalemia that ameliorate with increasing age, and hypoaldosteronism, are its hallmarks. The genitalia are normal and the response to salt and mineralocorticoid supplementation is excellent.

Complications: The degree of salt loss and hyperkalemia will determine the extent of early complications.

Associated Findings: None known.

Etiology: Autosomal recessive inheritance.

Pathogenesis: Identical to that described for **Steroid 18-hydroxylase deficiency** except that the defect involves the final step in aldosterone biosynthesis. Biochemically, the defect involves the final oxidation (dehydrogenation) of 18-hydroxycorticosterone to aldosterone. Thus, the steroid patterns differ only in that production of 18-hydroxycorticosterone is increased, but that of aldosterone remains low, despite stimuli such as ACTH. As indicated for the 18-hydroxylase deficiency syndrome, the term methyloxidase defect type II has been suggested to describe this condition, which is characterized by overproduction of both corticosterone and 18-hydroxycorticosterone.

MIM No.: *20341

CDC No.: 255.200

Sex Ratio: M1:F1

Occurrence: Over 25 cases document. Most frequent in Iranian Jews.

Risk of Recurrence for Patient's Sib:
See Part I, *Mendelian Inheritance.*

Risk of Recurrence for Patient's Child:
See Part I, *Mendelian Inheritance.*

Age of Detectability: Usually in the newborn period or in the first year of life, but milder defects may be detected at any age.

Gene Mapping and Linkage: Unknown.

Prevention: None known. Genetic counseling indicated.

Treatment: Treatment with salt supplementation and a mineralocorticoid, such as DOC, is necessary in the first few years of life. Later, patients appear able to maintain normal electrolyte balance by adjusting their sodium intake without mineralocorticoid supplements.

Prognosis: Excellent, if treatment with mineralocorticoid and salt is instituted.

Detection of Carrier: Unknown.

References:
Rösler A, et al.: The nature of the defect in a salt-wasting disorder in Jews of Iran. J Clin Endocrinol Metab 1977; 44:279–291.
Veldhuis JD, et al.: Inborn error in the terminal step of aldosterone biosynthesis: corticosterone methyloxidase type II deficiency in a North American pedigree. New Engl J Med 1980; 303:117–121.
Rösler A: The natural history of salt-wasting disorders of adrenal and renal origin. J Clin Endocrinol Metab 1984; 59:689.
Miller WL, Levine LS: Molecular and clinical advance in congenital adrenal hyperplasia. J Pediat 1987; 111:1–17.
White PC, et al.: Congenital adrenal hyperplasia. New Engl J Med 1987; 316:1519 (first part) and 1580 (second part).
New MI, et al.: The adrenal hyperplasias. In: Scriver CR, et al, eds: The metabolic basis of inherited disease, 6th ed. New York: McGraw-Hill, 1989:1881–1918.

SP004   **Mark A. Sperling**

Steroid 18-oxidation, delayed biochemical maturation of
*See ADRENAL HYPOALDOSTERONISM OF INFANCY, TRANSIENT
ISOLATED*

STEROID 20–22 DESMOLASE DEFICIENCY   0907

Includes:
> Adrenal hyperplasia I
> Lipoid adrenal hyperplasia with male
>   pseudohermaphroditism
> P450 side-chain cleavage enzyme, deficiency of

Excludes: Adrenal hyperplasia, other forms

Major Diagnostic Criteria: Vomiting, hyperkalemia, dehydration, and shock in a neonate with low serum sodium and chloride are the earliest manifestations. Males may have ambiguous genitalia. There is virtual absence of all steroids in their urine or blood. Definitive diagnosis is not feasible without performing stimulation tests with ACTH and HCG; both should be abnormal, without a rise in pregnenolone. A presumptive diagnosis can be made if the adrenals show the characteristic histology.

Clinical Findings: This defect affects the critical initial reaction in the conversion of cholesterol to pregnenolone, a step involving cleavage of the cholesterol side chain from carbon 20 to carbon 22. The entire cleavage process, although termed a desmolase, may represent a series of enzyme reactions shared by the adrenal and gonad and mediated by a P450 enzyme catalyzing side-chain cleavage (P450 SCC). Because of the early site in the assembly of all steroids, salt and water loss, and glucocorticoid insufficiency are universal findings. The external genitalia are normal in females, but males may have ambiguity, supporting the contention that the gonad is affected and thus precludes masculinization during fetal life. Laboratory investigation reveals virtual absence of urinary steroids, including pregnenolone, and low secretion rates of cortisol and aldosterone. Extended survival is possible, but death is frequent, despite seemingly adequate replacement with glucocorticoids, mineralocorticoids, and salt. At necropsy, the adrenals are markedly enlarged, and the cells are distended with cholesterol. Consanguinity has been frequent in the parents of affected individuals.

Complications: Death is frequent, even with adequate therapy.

Associated Findings: None known.

Etiology: Autosomal recessive inheritance.

Pathogenesis: The clinical features are explicable from the site and severity of the enzyme block affecting the adrenal and gonad, and the deficiency of glucocorticoids, mineralocorticoids, and sex steroids. The specific process, known as cholesterol side-chain

cleavage, is catalyzed by a specific form of cytochrome P-450; P450 (CSS), which is localized to the inner mitochondrial membrane.

MIM No.: *20171

CDC No.: 255.200

Sex Ratio: M1:F1

Occurrence: About 35 cases, with about a dozen surviving, have been documented in the literature.

Risk of Recurrence for Patient's Sib:
> See Part I, *Mendelian Inheritance.*

Risk of Recurrence for Patient's Child:
> See Part I, *Mendelian Inheritance.* Surviving affected individuals will probably be infertile.

Age of Detectability: Usually in the newborn period as a result of salt loss or ambiguous genitalia. Antenatal diagnosis has not been demonstrated.

Gene Mapping and Linkage: CYP11A (cytochrome P450, subfamily XIA) has been mapped to 15.

Prevention: None known. Genetic counseling indicated.

Treatment: Early recognition and replacement therapy with glucocorticoid, mineralocorticoid, and salt are essential for survival. Replacement therapy with estrogen or testosterone will be required to achieve secondary sexual characteristics in those reaching the age of puberty. In genetic males with severe ambiguity of the external genitalia, closely resembling those of a female, plastic reconstruction to achieve male characteristics is, at best, difficult. Consideration should therefore be given to raising the individual as a female with appropriate surgical correction of the external genitalia.

Prognosis: Prognosis has been poor in severely affected individuals. Infertility is likely in those surviving to adult life.

Detection of Carrier: Unknown.

Special Considerations: Aminoglutethimide, a toxic drug used rarely to inhibit steroidogenesis in adrenal carcinoma, acts by inhibiting the desmolase system and experimentally can simulate lipoid adrenal hyperplasia.

Support Groups: MN; Wrenshall (c/o Diana Johnson, 10 Co Hwy 4); Congenital Adrenal Hyperplasia Group

References:
Camacho AM, et al.: Congenital adrenal hyperplasia due to a deficiency of one of the enzymes involved in biosynthesis of pregnenolone. J Clin Endocrinol 1968; 28:153–161.
Moragas A, Ballabriga A: Congenital lipoid hyperplasia of the fetal adrenal gland. Helv Paediatr Acta 1969; 24:226.
Kirkland RT: Congenital lipoid adrenal hyperplasia in an eight-year-old phenotypic female. J Clin Endocrinol Metab 1973; 36:488–496.
Miller WL, Levine LS: Molecular and clinical advance in congenital adrenal hyperplasia. J Pediat 1987; 111:1–17.
Nebert DW, et al.: The P450 gene superfamily: recommended nomenclature. DNA 1987; 6:1–11.
White PC, et al.: Congenital adrenal hyperplasia. New Engl J Med 1987; 316:1519 (first part) and 1580 (second part).
New MI, et al.: The adrenal hyperplasias. In: Scriver CR, et al, eds: The metabolic basis of inherited disease, 6th ed. New York: McGraw-Hill, 1989:1881–1918.

SP004   **Mark A. Sperling**

0907-21392: Simplified scheme of steroidogenesis in the adrenal gland.

STEROID 21-HYDROXYLASE DEFICIENCY   0908

Includes:
> Adrenal hyperplasia III
> Adrenal hyperplasia-1, congenital virilizing
> Female pseudohermaphroditism
> Macrogenitosomia praecox
> Male pseudo-precocious puberty

Excludes: Adrenal steroidogenesis, other enzyme deficiencies in

Major Diagnostic Criteria: Elevated 17-ketosteroids (17-KS) and pregnanetriol excretion or markedly elevated plasma 17α-hydroxyprogesterone (50–450 times normal) and ACTH levels in patients with progressive virilization from birth. Abnormal steroid secretion must be suppressed following glucocorticoid administration.

Affected female infants show a variable degree of masculinization; males appear normal, but the external genitalia may be hyperpigmented in both sexes. Vomiting and dehydration may occur in the salt-losing variety.

Clinical Findings: This is the most common variant of congenital adrenal hyperplasia (CAH) resulting from a defect in the enzyme that catalyzes the conversion of progesterone or 17α-hydroxy progesterone to deoxycorticosterone or 11-deoxycortisol, respectively; a step requiring hydroxylation of the carbon at the 21 position of the steroid nucleus. The androgen pathway is not blocked, so the fetus is exposed to excessive androgens from about the third month of intrauterine life. Consequently, newborn females show variable degrees of masculinization of the external genitalia, ranging from mild clitoral hypertrophy to complete labioscrotal fusion simulating a scrotum, male phallus with urethra opening at its tip, absence of palpable gonads within the "scrotal sac," and presence of a prostate. However, ovaries and a uterus are present and the chromosomal sex is female. Excessive skin pigmentation may be present around the genitalia or nipples, reflecting increased ACTH (MSH). In newborn males no abnormality is apparent, although some may have phallic enlargement. However, progressive virilization occurs in both sexes, resulting in rapid initial growth; accelerated bone age development, with premature fusion of epiphyses and final short stature, progressive clitoral or penile enlargement, early development of pubic and axillary hair, acne, hirsutism, voice changes, male habitus, and male gender identification. Males have been referred to as an infant "Hercules." Untreated females fail to undergo pubertal changes due to suppression of gonadotropins by androgen excess. In males, the same mechanism prevents testicular enlargement, allowing differentiation from true precocious puberty secondary to ectopic or inappropriate pituitary gonadotropin secretion. However, rarely, there may be adrenal rests within the testes, subject to ACTH stimulation, which may result in symmetric or nodular testicular enlargement and suggest precocious puberty or testicular neoplasia. In females with ambiguous genitalia the diagnosis is usually established in infancy or early childhood; occasional cases have been identified in the second decade and as late as the sixth decade of life. Complete external virilization of newborn females may delay diagnosis and lead to false gender assignment with consequent psychologic sequelae.

Patients with partial or mild defects in 21-hydroxylase deficiency have normal serum electrolytes and may have normal levels of cortisol and aldosterone production, the latter rising with a low salt diet. The serum cortisol response to ACTH may be minimal, indicating existing maximal stimulation by endogenous ACTH. Adrenal capacity is limited, however, since many of these patients develop salt loss during stress or during diagnostic sodium restriction, with hyponatremia, hyperkalemia, vomiting, severe dehydration, and vascular collapse.

Complete or severe 21-hydroxylase deficiency manifests itself early in the neonatal period with vomiting, renal salt loss, hyponatremia, hyperkalemia, and dehydration. A misdiagnosis of pyloric stenosis may be made in newborn males; death of an older sib in infancy, particulary during stress, may be recorded.

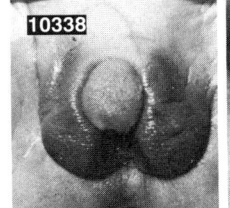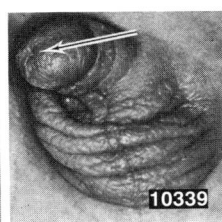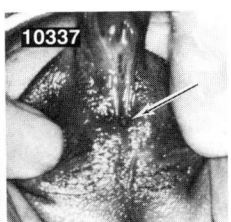

0908-10337–39: Complete and incomplete virilization of the external genitalia in genetic females.

There is no direct correlation between the degree of virilization or external genital ambiguity and completeness of the 21-hydroxylase defect. However, plasma and urinary cortisol and its metabolites are decreased, as is aldosterone; salt restriction is poorly tolerated and does not produce further increments in aldosterone secretion.

The clinical division of patients into "salt-losers" and "non-salt losers" is relatively arbitrary, and it is highly likely that the mild and severe forms represent a spectrum of a single enzyme deficiency, although debate on this issue continues. All affected subjects display abnormalities in sodium balance, ranging from borderline depletion, detectable by elevated levels of plasma renin activity in the simple virilizers, to overt salt-loss and hypovolemia in the clinical salt-losers. There is a high degree of correlation among the degree of salt-loss, plasma renin activity and ACTH levels, suggesting a relationship between the renin-angiotensin system and the pituitary-adrenal axis. These findings have important clinical implications because they suggest that both salt-losers and simple virilizers would benefit from treatment with mineralocorticoids for optimal hormonal control of the disease, including suppression of excessive androgen production with lower than conventionally recommended doses of glucocorticoids. Independent studies confirm these concepts. It is therefore strongly recommended that all patients with the 21-hydroxylase deficiency receive some mineralocorticoid supplement in addition to glucocorticoid therapy.

Irrespective of clinical type, all affected patients have elevated urinary excretion of 17-ketosteroids and pregnanetriol, the excretory product of 17α-hydroxyprogesterone. Plasma levels of these substances as well as testosterone, derived from peripheral conversion of androgen precursors, are elevated. Urinary 17-hydroxycorticosteroids or plasma cortisol may be low or normal, depending on the severity of the block.

Complications: Lack of cortisol and aldosterone may result in hypoglycemia, and severe electrolyte disturbances with dehydration and shock, particularly during stress. Ambiguity of genitalia may result in false gender assignment for genetic females. Progressive virilization, early epiphyseal closure with short stature, preclusion of normal pubertal changes, and infertility are direct sequelae of the untreated condition, or of poor patient compliance. Adenomatous changes within the adrenal or adrenal rest tissue in distant sites, such as testes, may also occur with inadequate treatment.

Associated Findings: Renal anomalies have been associated with this syndrome.

Etiology: Autosomal recessive inheritance.

Pathogenesis: The pathogenesis of all the features is explicable from the site and severity of the enzyme block, deficiency of cortisol or aldosterone, and oversecretion of androgens. In about 95% of cases, 21-hydroxylation is impaired in the zona fasciculata of the adrenal cortex so that 17-hydroxyprogesterone is not converted to 11-deoxycortisol. ACTH levels increase, resulting in excess cortisol precursors which are shunted into excessive production of androgens, resulting in virilization.

MIM No.: *20191

CDC No.: 255.200

Sex Ratio: M1:F1

Occurrence: Varies with geographic locale: 1:500 in certain Eskimos, 1:5,000 in Switzerland, 1:15,000 in the United States Caucasians.

Risk of Recurrence for Patient's Sib:
See Part I, *Mendelian Inheritance.*

Risk of Recurrence for Patient's Child:
See Part I, *Mendelian Inheritance.*

Age of Detectability: Molecular probes can now be used to establish the diagnosis in the fetus. Successful antenatal detection and neonatal screening have been reported. Amniotic fluid screening shows elevated 17-alpha-hydroxyprogesterone, delta-4-androstenedione, and pregnanetriol levels; maternal serum screening after 34 weeks shows increased concentration of 17-

alpha-hydroxyprogesterone; a genetic linkage with HLA-B antigens is determined on cultured amniotic fluid cells.

Gene Mapping and Linkage: CYP21 (cytochrome P450, subfamily XXI) has been mapped to 6p21.3.

Prevention: Diagnosis of an affected female early in gestation by molecular probes or HLA typing permits attempts at preventing virilization by high-dose glucocorticoid therapy to the mother.

Treatment: Replacement therapy with cortisol arrests the progressive virilization. A mineralocorticoid (DOC or 9α-fluorohydrocortisone), with additional salt intake, may be necessary in the salt-losing form; a mineralocorticoid should also be provided for non-salt-losers. Supplemental cortisol is necessary during acute stress. Antenatal diagnosis, with cortisol injections into the amniotic fluid or fetus, may minimize virilization.

Initial plastic surgical repair of ambiguous genitalia is achieved between the first to third years of life in order to permit appropriate gender identification and sex rearing. Definitive plastic repair can be achieved after puberty. Psychologic counseling may be required for parents and in late-diagnosed cases with ambiguous genitalia.

It is generally agreed that if diagnosis is missed for the first 3–4 years, a completely virilized female with penile urethra and apparent cryptorchidism should be perpetuated in male rearing and identification.

Prognosis: Normal for life span, reproduction, and intelligence, when diagnosed early and appropriately treated.

Detection of Carrier: Urinary pregnanetriol excretion after ACTH infusion has been reported to be elevated in the parents of affected children when compared with controls. This test has not been commonly employed. The close linkage between the gene for 21-hydroxylase deficiency and the HLA-B locus provides a method for detection of carriers or for prenatal diagnosis once an index case is established. cDNA probes can be used to detect carriers.

Support Group: MN; Wrenshall (c/o Diana Johnson, 10 Co Hwy 4); Congenital Adrenal Hyperplasia Group.

References:
Migeon CJ, et al.: The attenuated form of congenital adrenal hyperplasia as an allelic form of 21-hydroxylase deficiency. J Clin Endocrinol Metab 1980; 51:647–649.
Kohn B, et al.: Late-onset steroid-21-hydroxylase deficiency: a variant of classical congenital adrenal hyperplasia. J Clin Endocrinol Metab 1982; 55:817–827.
Hughes IA, et al.: Prenatal diagnosis of congenital adrenal hyperplasia. J Med Genet 1987; 24:344–347.
Miller WL, Levine LS: Molecular and clinical advance in congenital adrenal hyperplasia. J Pediat 1987; 111:1–17.
Mulaikal R, et al.: Fertility rates in female patients with congenital adrenal hyperplasia due to 21-hydroxylase deficiency. New Engl J Med 1987; 316:178–182.
White PC, et al.: Congenital adrenal hyperplasia. New Engl J Med 1987; 316:1519–1524 (first part) and 1580–1586 (second part).
Killeen AA, et al.: Diagnosis of classical steroid 21-hydroxylase deficiency using an HLA-B locus-specific DNA-probe. Am J Med Genet 1988; 29:703–712.
Miller WL: Gene conversions, deletions and polymorphisims in congenital adrenal hyperplasia. Am J Hum Genet 1988; 42:4–7.
New MI, et al.: The adrenal hyperplasias. In: Scriver CR, et al, eds: The metabolic basis of inherited disease, 6th ed. New York: McGraw-Hill, 1989:1881–1918.
Pang S, et al.: Prenatal treatment of congenital adrenal hyperplasia due to 21-hydroxylase deficiency. New Engl J Med 1990; 322:111–115.

SP004   **Mark A. Sperling**

Steroid sulfatase deficiency disease (SSDD)
See ICHTHYOSIS, X-LINKED WITH STEROID SULFATASE DEFICIENCY

STEROID, BINDING GLOBULIN ABNORMALITIES   0222

Includes:
>CBG-transcortin abnormalities
>Corticosteroid-binding globulin abnormalities
>Corticosteroid-binding globulin, decreased
>Corticosteroid-binding globulin, increased
>Transcortin deficiency

Excludes:
>Disease-induced changes in CBG
>Drug-induced changes in CBG

Major Diagnostic Criteria: No known signs or symptoms accompany this biochemical variant. Low or elevated total plasma cortisol with a normal amount of free cortisol are found in plasma and urine in the absence of disease or drugs affecting CBG. Measurement of free cortisol in urine, or determination of binding capacity of plasma for radioactively labeled cortisol akin to the T3 resin uptake test may be required.

Clinical Findings: Congenital abnormalities in cortisol-binding globulin (CBG) do not reflect a disease state and are not associated with any abnormality in adrenal function or symptomatology. They are detected as laboratory findings in individuals who have low or high concentrations of cortisol in plasma, but are otherwise normal. However, the laboratory findings may suggest hyper- or hypofunction of the adrenal and spur unnecessary investigations.

Complications: Unknown.

Associated Findings: None known.

Etiology: CBG deficiency is familial and transmitted by autosomal dominant or X-linked recessive inheritance. CBG excess is also familial but the mode of transmission is uncertain. The most common cause of CBG excess is pregnancy and estrogen-containing medication.

Pathogenesis: Cortisol-binding globulin (CBG-transcortin) is a plasma glycoprotein with high affinity for cortisol as well as progesterone, deoxycorticosterone, corticosterone and some synthetic glucocorticoids. About 75% of plasma cortisol is reversibly bound by CBG, 15% is bound to albumin, and about 10% remains free and biologically active, being constantly replenished from CBG. Decreased CBG is associated with a low total cortisol, and increased CBG with a high total cortisol; in both circumstances, free cortisol remains normal, urinary excretion of free cortisol is also normal, and cortisol production and the response to ACTH remain normal. In liver disease and nephrotic syndrome, CBG, and consequently total cortisol, are low; in pregnancy and with estrogen therapy CBG and total cortisol are high.

MIM No.: 12250

Sex Ratio: M1:F<1 in CBG deficiency; M1:F1 in CBG excess

Occurrence: About a dozen familial cases documented; 8 in three generations of one family.

Risk of Recurrence for Patient's Sib:
>See Part I, *Mendelian Inheritance.* For CBG excess, undetermined.

Risk of Recurrence for Patient's Child:
>See Part I, *Mendelian Inheritance.* For CBG excess, undetermined.

Age of Detectability: At birth.

Gene Mapping and Linkage: Unknown.

Prevention: None known. Genetic counseling indicated.

Treatment: Not required.

Prognosis: Excellent.

Detection of Carrier: Unknown.

References:
Doe RP, et al.: Familial decrease in corticosteroid-binding globulin. Metabolism 1965; 14:940.
Lohrenz FN, et al.: Adrenal function and serum protein concentrations in a kindred with decreased corticosteroid-binding globulin (CBG) concentration. J Clin Endocrinol Metab 1967; 27:966.
Lohrenz FN, et al.: Idiopathic or genetic elevation of corticosteroid-binding globulin? J Clin Endocrinol Metab 1968; 28:1073–1075.

Hadjian AJ, et al.: Cortisol binding to proteins in plasma in the human neonate and infant. Pediatr Res 1975; 9:40.

Derncor P, et al.: Unexplained high transcortin levels in patients with various hematological disorders and their relatives: a connection between these high transcortin levels and HLA antigen B 12. J Clin Endocrinol Metab 1980; 50:421.

Dunn JF, et al.: Transport of steroid hormones: binding of 21 endogenous steroids to both testosterone-binding globulin and corticosteroid-binding globulin in human plasma. J Clin Endocrinol Metab 1981; 53:58.

Pugeat MM: Transport of steroid hormones: interaction of 70 drugs with testosterone-binding globulin and corticosteroid-binding globulin in human plasma. J Clin Endocrinol Metab 1981; 53:69.

SP004   **Mark A. Sperling**

Stevenson syndrome
  See DIGITO-PALATAL SYNDROME, STEVENSON TYPE
Stickler syndrome
  See ARTHRO-OPHTHALMOPATHY, HEREDITARY, PROGRESSIVE, STICKLER TYPE
Stiff man syndrome (obsolete; pejorative)
  See HALLERVORDEN-SPATZ DISEASE

STIFF SKIN SYNDROME   2629

Includes:
  Fascial dystrophy
  Skin, stiff skin syndrome

Excludes:
  Arthrogryposis
  Dwarfism-stiff joints (2033)
  Hallervorden-Spatz disease (2526)
  Kuskokwin syndrome (0560)
  Lipomatosis, systemic
  Neck/face, lipomatosis (0601)
  Sclerema
  Scleroderma, familial progressive (2154)
  Skin, parana hard skin syndrome (3051)

Major Diagnostic Criteria: Thick, indurated skin over most of the body associated with firm muscles, joint stiffness, and contractures present from birth or early childhood.

Clinical Findings: Features are limited to the soft tissues and are usually present from birth. Skin has rock hard consistency without evidence of atrophy or vascular change. Central areas, buttocks, shoulders, and proximal limbs are more severely affected. Underlying muscles appear firm but have normal strength. Joint stiffness and contractures may occur. Viscera are not affected.

Complications: Limitation at joints, impaired ventilation secondary to chest wall involvement.

Associated Findings: None known.

Etiology: Autosomal dominant inheritance.

Pathogenesis: Basic metabolic defect. The inital report of increased dermal glycosaminoglycan deposition has not been confirmed. Abnormal production and extracellular organization of collagen in the fascia has been identified in one patient.

MIM No.: *18490

POS No.: 3469

Sex Ratio: M1:F1

Occurrence: About a dozen families have been reported.

Risk of Recurrence for Patient's Sib:
  See Part I, *Mendelian Inheritance.*

Risk of Recurrence for Patient's Child:
  See Part I, *Mendelian Inheritance.*

Age of Detectability: At birth or during the early years.

Gene Mapping and Linkage: Unknown.

Prevention: None known. Genetic counseling indicated.

Treatment: Unknown.

Prognosis: Undetermined. The degree of incapacitation appears minimal in the reported cases.

Detection of Carrier: Unknown.

References:
Esterly ND, McKusick VA: Stiff skin syndrome. Pediatrics 1971; 47:360–369.
Singer HS, et al.: The stiff skin syndrome: new genetic and biochemical investigations BD:OAS XIII(3B). New York: March of Dimes Birth Defects Foundation, 1977:254–255.
Jablonska S, et al.: Congenital fascial dystrophy: a noninflammatory disease of fascia: the stiff skin syndrome. Pediatr Derm 1984; 2:87–97.

ST021   **Roger E. Stevenson**

Stiff baby syndrome, hereditary
  See HYPEREKPLEXIA
Stiff man syndrome, congenital
  See HYPEREKPLEXIA
Stilbestrol-R, fetal effects
  See FETAL DIETHYLSTILBESTROL (DES) EFFECTS
Stilling-Turk-Duane syndrome
  See EYE, DUANE RETRACTION SYNDROME
Stimulus-evoked epilepsy
  See EPILEPSY, REFLEX
Stippled epiphyses
  See CHONDRODYSPLASIA PUNCTATA, X-LINKED DOMINANT TYPE
Stomach cancer
  See CANCER, GASTRIC FAMILIAL

STOMACH, DIVERTICULUM   0911

Includes: Gastric diverticulum, congenital

Excludes:
  Gastric cysts
  Stomach, duplication (0912)

Major Diagnostic Criteria: There are no consistent symptoms or signs, and diagnosis is made by X-ray findings using contrast material.

Clinical Findings: No characteristic clinical findings are present. Usually X-ray diagnosis shows an outpouching from juxtacardiac posterior gastric wall involving all layers of the gastric wall. occurs. This may occur near the pylorus in the presence of a high small bowel obstruction, probably as an acquired lesion.

Complications: Severe vomiting. In one instance, intussusception of the diverticulum resulted in gangrenous perforation and peritonitis.

Associated Findings: None known.

Etiology: Unknown.

Pathogenesis: May originate as a duplication, or result from pressure effects of pyloric or duodenal obstruction.

CDC No.: 750.740

Sex Ratio: Presumably M1:F1.

Occurrence: Undetermined. Usually asymptomatic and discovered by chance X-ray, at gastroscopy or operation, or incidentally at necropsy.

Risk of Recurrence for Patient's Sib: Unknown.

Risk of Recurrence for Patient's Child: Unknown.

Age of Detectability: At any age.

Gene Mapping and Linkage: Unknown.

Prevention: None known.

Treatment: Surgical excision rarely indicated.

Prognosis: Unknown.

Detection of Carrier: Unknown.

References:
Ogur GL, Kolarsick AJ: Gastric diverticula in infancy. J Pediatr 1951; 39:723.

Burke MB: Gastric diverticula in childhood: a report of two cases and a review of the literature. J Singapore Paediatr Soc 1965; 7:101–106.

SI004 **William K. Sieber**

STOMACH, DUPLICATION 0912

Includes:
> Cardioduodenal duct
> Gastric enterocystoma
> Stomach, reduplication of

Excludes:
> Dorsal enteric remnants
> Ectopic pancreas involving gastric wall
> **Esophagus, duplication** (0368)
> **Meckel diverticulum** (0633)
> Mediastinal gastric cysts
> **Stomach, diverticulum** (0911)

Major Diagnostic Criteria: Palpable abdominal mass with X-ray evidence of origin from the gastric wall. Usually gastric origin can be established only at operation. Sonography and technetium scan may identify gastric lining of cystic mass.

Clinical Findings: May present as an asymptomatic upper abdominal mass, a mass with vomiting or GI bleeding; may simulate pyloric stenosis (with symptoms beginning at birth and an easily palpable pyloric "tumor"); or may present as diffuse peritonitis due to rupture of the duplication. An abdominal mass is almost always palpable. X-ray studies with contrast material sometimes clarify the diagnosis but usually demonstrate only pressure effects along the greater curvature and obstruction. These findings, with depression of the splenic flexure, are suggestive of gastric duplication.

Complications: Pyloric obstruction, rupture of the duplication and resulting generalized peritonitis, sepsis, and autodigestion with erosion into surrounding viscera may cause gastrocolic fistula and other bizarre fistulizations.

Associated Findings: Carcinomatous degeneration of the duplication, usually solitary; occasionally there are other duplications of alimentary tract.

Etiology: Possibly error of recanalization.

Pathogenesis: Embryonic, possible persistence of solid stage, with failure of coalescence of the vacuoles that form lumen.

CDC No.: 750.750

Sex Ratio: M1:F8 (observed on one series).

Occurrence: About 65 cases have been reported in the literature.

Risk of Recurrence for Patient's Sib: Unknown.

Risk of Recurrence for Patient's Child: Unknown.

Age of Detectability: Often during the neonatal period, by physical examination, but small cysts may be detected only if they become symptomatic in later life.

Gene Mapping and Linkage: Unknown.

Prevention: None known. Genetic counseling indicated.

Treatment: Laparotomy and surgical excision of the duplication and the associated site of attachment to the normal gastric wall may require simple excision, or subtotal or even total gastrectomy. Internal drainage by anastomosis of the cyst to the true gastric lumen has relieved symptoms.

Prognosis: Excellent when surgically removed. Carcinoma has been reported in long-standing duplications.

Detection of Carrier: Unknown.

References:
Kremer RM, et al.: Duplication of the stomach. J Pediatr Surg 1970; 5:360–364.
Pruksapang C, et al.: Gastric duplications. J Pediatr Surg 1979; 14:83–85.
Spence RK, et al.: Coexistent gastric duplication and accessory pan-

creas: clinical manifestations, embryogenesis, and treatment. J Pediatr Surg 1986; 21:68–70.

SI004 **William K. Sieber**

STOMACH, HYPOPLASIA 0913

Includes: Microgastria

Excludes: Agastrica

Major Diagnostic Criteria: Stomach hypoplasia is diagnosed by upper GI examination and is always associated with failure of rotation of the stomach, without differentiation into fundus, body, and pyloric areas. The esophagus is usually dilated and takes over some storage function.

Clinical Findings: Vomiting, hematemesis, malnutrition, and secondary anemia are noted at birth, and these intensify.

Complications: Malnutrition.

Associated Findings: None known.

Etiology: Unknown.

Pathogenesis: Unknown.

CDC No.: 750.780

Sex Ratio: Presumably M1:F1.

Occurrence: Undetermined but presumed arre.

Risk of Recurrence for Patient's Sib: Unknown.

Risk of Recurrence for Patient's Child: Unknown.

Age of Detectability: Usually in neonatal period, by X-ray exam.

Gene Mapping and Linkage: Unknown.

Prevention: None known. Genetic counseling indicated.

Treatment: Continuous slow feeding. Surgical enlargement of stomach and correction of reflux may be helpful in selected patients.

Prognosis: General poor health has been the rule, with early death in most. Two cases followed for long periods slowly developed a functional stomach.

Detection of Carrier: Unknown.

References:
Blank E, et al.: Congenital microgastria: a case report with a 26 year follow-up. Pediatrics 1973; 51:1037.
Hochberger, et al.: Congenital microgastria: a follow-up observation over six years. Pediatr Radiol 1974; 2:207.
Anderson KD, Guzzetta PC: Treatment of congenital microgastria and dumping syndrome. J Pediatr Surg 1983; 18:747.
Mandell GA, et al.: A case of microgastria in association with splenicgonadal fusion. Pediatr Radiol 1983; 13:95–98.

SI004 **William K. Sieber**

STOMACH, PYLORIC ATRESIA 0910

Includes:
> Antral atresia
> Antral web
> Aplasia of pylorus, congenital
> Fibromuscular atresia of antrum
> Gastric atresia
> Gastric outlet obstruction, incomplete
> Prepyloric membrane
> Pyloric atresia
> Pyloric diaphragm, incomplete

Excludes:
> Duodenal atresia (supraampullary)
> **Duodenum, atresia or stenosis** (0300)
> **Pyloric stenosis** (0848)
> **Pyloroduodenal atresia, hereditary** (2617)

Major Diagnostic Criteria: Nonbilious vomiting with X-ray identification of the antrum as the site of obstruction. Often identified only at time of surgery.

Clinical Findings: Nonbilious vomiting in a new born infant having a scaphoid lower abdomen and a distended stomach. Maternal hydramnios is common. X-ray examination examination discloses only a large air-filled stomach with no second "bubble." Incomplete diaphragms can be identified only by upper GI series, or by gastroscopy. In such infants partial obstruction produces clinical findings identical with pyloric stenosis, but originating at birth.

Complications: Hypokalemic alkalosis, dehydration, starvation.

Associated Findings: Two non-inherited cases had **Chromosome 21, trisomy 21**. **Epidermolysis bullosum** associated with complete pyloric atresia was reported in four cases.

Etiology: Partial obstruction, as discussed in this article, is of undetermined etiology. Complete atresia by autosomal recessive inheritance (see **Pyloroduodenal atresia, hereditary**).

Pathogenesis: Error of recanalization of the gastric lumen.

CDC No.: 750.780

Sex Ratio: M11:F15 (observed).

Occurrence: 1:1,000,000 births; about 1% of reported gastrointestinal atresias.

Risk of Recurrence for Patient's Sib: Unknown.

Risk of Recurrence for Patient's Child: Unknown.

Age of Detectability: From birth to as late as adulthood.

Gene Mapping and Linkage: Unknown.

Prevention: None known. Genetic counseling indicated.

Treatment: Laparotomy, gastroduodenostomy, gastrojejunostomy, or excision of pyloric membrane have all been successful in relieving the obstruction. When associated with **Epidermolysis bullosum, type II**, no treatment is advised.

Prognosis: Good.

Detection of Carrier: Unknown.

References:
Bronsther B, et al.: Congenital pyloric atresia: a report of three cases and a review of the literature. Surg 1971; 69:130–136.
Woolley MM, et al.: Congenital partial gastric antral obstruction. Ann Surg 1974; 180:265–271.
Weitzel A, et al.: Two cases of pyloric atresia. Z Kinderchir 1984; 39:396–398.
Rosenbloom MS, Ratner M: Congenital pyloric atresia and epidermolysis bullosa letalis in premature siblings. J Pediat Surg 1987; 22:374–376.

SI004 **William K. Sieber**

Stomach, reduplication of
See STOMACH, DUPLICATION

STOMACH, TERATOMA   0914

Includes:
Dermoid cyst of stomach
Gastric teratoma
Tridermal gastric teratoma
Tridermic teratoma of stomach

Excludes: N/A

Major Diagnostic Criteria: Large upper abdominal mass with calcification by X-ray suggests the diagnosis. Confirmed only by gross and microscopic pathology.

Clinical Findings: Abdominal mass. GI bleeding is sometimes present (3 of 17 cases). X-ray studies characteristically show areas of calcification in large, bulky tumors that may cause gastric obstruction. Respiratory difficulty and intestinal obstruction may be present secondary to pressure from the large abdominal mass.

Complications: Gastric bleeding and/or obstruction, respiratory distress due to increased intra-abdominal pressure.

Associated Findings: None known.

Etiology: Unknown.

Pathogenesis: Unknown.

POS No.: 3399

CDC No.: 750.780

Sex Ratio: M1:F>0.

Occurrence: About 30 cases have been reported; all but one being male.

Risk of Recurrence for Patient's Sib: Undetermined but apparently small.

Risk of Recurrence for Patient's Child: Undetermined but apparently small.

Age of Detectability: Usually at birth or during infancy.

Gene Mapping and Linkage: Unknown.

Prevention: None known. Genetic counseling indicated.

Treatment: Surgical excision of the tumor by partial or total gastrectomy.

Prognosis: Fifteen of 16 patients recovered following surgical resection of the tumor.

Detection of Carrier: Unknown.

References:
DeAngelis VR: Gastric teratoma in a newborn infant: total gastrectomy with survival. Surgery 1969; 66:794–795.
Ohgami H, et al.: Gastric teratoma in infancy and childhood: report of three cases and review of literature. Jpn J Surg 1973; 3:218–220.
Haley T, et al.: Gastric teratoma with gastrointestinal bleeding. J Pediatr Surg 1976; 21:949–950.
Purvis JM, et al.: Gastric teratoma: first reported case in a female. J Pediatr Surg 1979; 14:86–88.

SI004 **William K. Sieber**

Stomach-duodenum-small intestine-rectum, duplication of
See INTESTINAL DUPLICATION
Stomatitis areata migrans
See TONGUE, GEOGRAPHIC
Stomatocytosis, hereditary
See ANEMIA, HEMOLYTIC, RED CELL MEMBRANE DEFECTS

STORAGE DISEASE, NEUTRAL LIPID TYPE   2859

Includes:
Chanarin-Dorfman syndrome
Chanarin syndrome
Cornification, disorder of, neutral lipid storage type (DOC 12)
Ichthyotic neutral lipid storage disease
Ichthyosiform erythroderma with leukocyte vacuolization
Neutral lipid storage disease with ichthyosis
Triglyceride storage disease-impaired fatty acid oxidation

Excludes:
Cholesteryl ester storage disease (0151)
Ichthyosis, congenital erythrodermic (2855)
Myopathy-metabolic, carnitine deficiency, primary and secondary (0124)
Myopathy-metabolic, carnitine palmityl transferase deficiency (0125)
Phytanic acid storage disease (0810)
Wolman disease (1003)

Major Diagnostic Criteria: Affected patients exhibit a generalized ichthyosiform erythroderma in conjunction with lipid vacuoles in circulating granulocytes and monocytes. Lipid storage is widespread in tissues and can also be demonstrated in skin, muscle, or liver biopsy material or within cultured fibroblasts.

Clinical Findings: Generalized ichthyosis, myopathy, and vacuolated leukocytes. Clinically, the disorder of cornification most closely resembles **Ichthyosis, congenital erythrodermic** of mild-to-moderate severity. Some patients have also exhibited atopic-like dermatitis.

Prominent lipid vacuoles are seen in virtually every circulating granulocyte and monocyte, and the diagnosis can be established readily by direct examination of a peripheral blood smear. Lipid vacuoles are also present within numerous cell types, including those of the skin, where vacuoles are found within dermal cells and within the basal and granular cell layers of the epidermis. Lipid vacuoles are also present within cells of the gastrointestinal epithelia, skeletal muscle, and liver. Despite widespread evidence of tissue lipid storage, serum lipid levels are usually normal and systemic manifestations may be subtle. Myopathy may be discovered only upon detailed testing, but serum muscle enzyme levels are elevated. All patients who have undergone liver biopsy have exhibited severe fatty change, but this may not be reflected in liver function studies. Both neurosensory deafness and cataracts are present in some patients. Mild developmental delay and growth retardation may also be features of this syndrome.

Complications: Liver dysfunction, weakness, and intolerance to fasting.

Associated Findings: Atopic-like dermatitis occurs in some patients.

Etiology: Autosomal recessive inheritance.

Pathogenesis: Since electron microscopy demonstrates non-membrane-enclosed lipid droplets, the disorder is unlikely to be a lysosomal storage disease. The stored lipid is triglyceride. Studies on cultured cells *in vitro* suggest a novel defect in fatty acid metabolism distinct from other known abnormalities of triglyceride metabolism, including Wolman disease (acid lipase deficiency) and carnitine deficiency. Some investigators have suggested an impairment of long-chain fatty acid oxidation, but this has been disputed by others.

Electron microscopic studies of epidermis have shown a unique abnormality of lamellar body structure in which the normal lamellae are disrupted by electron-lucent, globular inclusions. These distortions may be responsible for the abnormality in cohesion in this disorder.

MIM No.: *27563

POS No.: 4111

Sex Ratio: Presumably M1:F1; observed, M8:F6.

Occurrence: Fourteen patients with this syndrome have been reported; the majority of these were of Middle Eastern or Mediterranean descent.

Risk of Recurrence for Patient's Sib:
See Part I, *Mendelian Inheritance.*

Risk of Recurrence for Patient's Child:
See Part I, *Mendelian Inheritance.*

Age of Detectability: Usually evident at birth. Prenatal diagnosis has not been attempted but may be possible if amniocytes also store lipid or by fetal blood sampling if fetal leukocytes store lipid.

Gene Mapping and Linkage: Unknown.

Prevention: None known. Genetic counseling indicated.

Treatment: No specific therapy is recognized.

Prognosis: Probably normal for life span. Visual and hearing deficits or myopathy may be disabling. Intelligence may be normal or impaired.

Detection of Carrier: Carriers exhibit similar lipid vacuoles within some of their eosinophils.

Special Considerations: A peripheral blood smear from all patients with generalized ichthyosis should be examined because systemic symptoms may not be pronouced in these patients.

References:
Dorfman ML, et al.: Ichthyosiform dermatosis with system lipidosis. Arch Dermatol 1974; 110:261–266.
Chanarin I, et al.: Neutral lipid storage disease: a new disorder of lipid metabolism. Br Med J 1975; 1:553–555. *
Elias PM, Williams ML: Neutral lipid storage disease with ichthyosis: defective lamellar body contents and intercellular dispersion. Arch Dermatol 1985; 121:1000–1008. †
Williams ML, et al.: Ichthyosis and neutral lipid storage disease. Am J Med Genet 1985; 20:711–726. * †
Williams ML, et al.: Neutral lipid storage disease with ichthyosis: lipid content and metabolism in fibroblasts. J Inherit Metab Dis 1988; 11:131–143.

WI013   **Mary L. Williams**

'Stork bite' mark
See *NEVUS FLAMMEUS*
Strabismus, Duane type
See *EYE, DUANE RETRACTION SYNDROME*
Straight-chain C6-C10-omega-dicarboxylic aciduria
See *ACYL-CoA DEHYDROGENASE DEFICIENCY, MEDIUM CHAIN TYPE*
Strangulated hernia
See *HERNIA, INGUINAL*
Straussler disease
See *GERSTMANN-STRAUSSLER SYNDROME*
Strawberry nevus
See *HEMANGIOMAS OF THE HEAD AND NECK*
Streblodactyly
See *CAMPTODACTYLY*
Streblomicrodactyly
See *CAMPTODACTYLY*
Streeter bands
See *AMNIOTIC BANDS SYNDROME*
Streptomycin, fetal effects
See *FETAL AMINOGLYCOSIDE OTOTOXICITY*
Streptomycin-sensitivity deafness
See *DEAFNESS, STREPTOMYCIN-SENSITIVITY*
Striatonigral degeneration, autosomal dominant
See *MACHADO-JOSEPH DISEASE*
Stridor, congenital
See *LARYNGOMALACIA*
Stroke-like episodes
See *MYOPATHY, MITOCHONDRIAL-ENCEPHALOPATHY-LACTIC ACIDOSIS-STROKE*
Stromal dystrophy of the cornea, congenital hereditary
See *CORNEAL DYSTROPHY, STROMAL, CONGENITAL HEREDITARY*
Strudwick syndrome
See *SPONDYLOEPIMETAPHYSEAL DYSPLASIA, STRUDWICK TYPE*
Strumpell familial spastic paraplegia
See *PARAPLEGIA, FAMILIAL SPASTIC*
Strumpell-Lorrain syndrome
See *PARAPLEGIA, FAMILIAL SPASTIC*
Stuart-Prower Factor deficiency
See *FACTOR X DEFICIENCY*
'Stub thumb'
See *BRACHYDACTYLY*

STURGE-WEBER SYNDROME   0915

Includes:
>   Encephalofacial angiomatosis
>   Encephalotrigeminal angiomatosis
>   Fourth phacomatosis
>   Meningeal capillary angiomatosis

Excludes:
>   **Neurofibromatosis** (0712)
>   **Tuberous sclerosis** (0975)
>   **Von Hippel-Lindau syndrome** (0995)

Major Diagnostic Criteria: Port-wine angioma of the face following the distribution of the trigeminal nerve and accompanied by seizures and intracranial calcifications.

Clinical Findings: Capillary angioma over the first or all of the three divisions of the fifth cranial nerve is always present at birth. There may be glaucoma on the side of the angioma due to the outflow occlusion of the angle. Generalized seizures begin at 1–2 years of age. Intracranial calcifications do not appear until after 2 years of age, although CT scans may demonstrate calcification earlier. The skull is smaller on the side of the abnormality; 15% of affected individuals have bilateral angiomas and bilateral neurologic involvement.

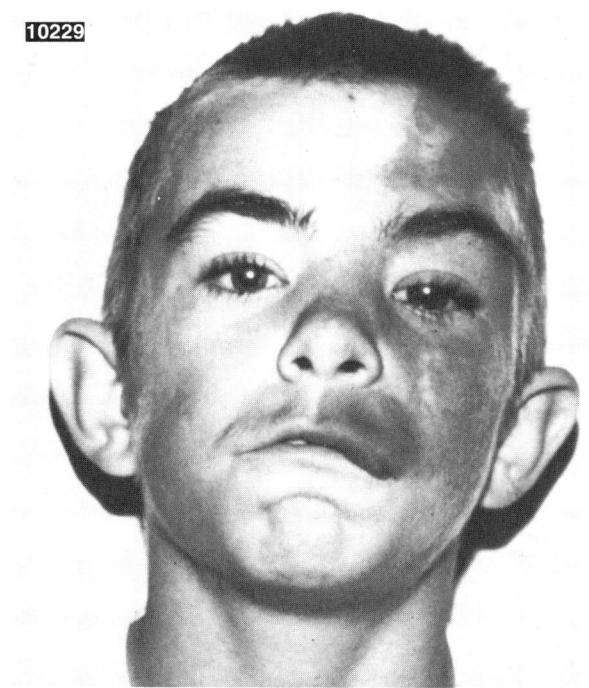

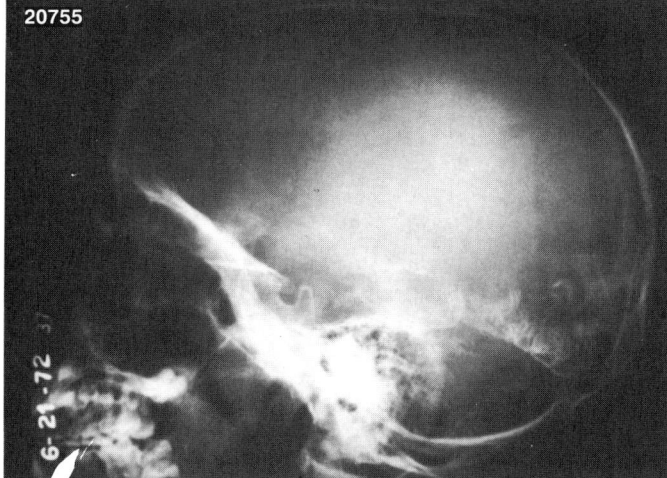

0915-10229: Typical unilateral distribution of port wine stain.
20755: Skull X-ray shows double contour or "railroad track" pattern of intercranial calcifications.

Complications: Seizures, mental retardation.

Associated Findings: Sometimes associated with **Angio-osteohypertrophy syndrome. Nevus of Ota** has been reported.

Etiology: Unknown.

Pathogenesis: The intracranial calcifications are not in blood vessel walls, but in the second and third layers of cortex, presumably due to tissue anoxia. The calcifications consist of characteristic serpiginous double tracks. An alternate explanation for calcification is transudation of protein through abnormal vessels and calcium binding. Degeneration of neurons and gliosis follows. The homolateral eye may be enlarged because of congenital glaucoma (buphthalmos). The iris of such an eye may remain blue, although the normal eye is brown, due to angiomatosis of the choroid. Hemiplegia is present, in many cases opposite the

side of the nevus. Hemianopsia is frequently found in patients who can be tested.

MIM No.: 18530
POS No.: 3397
CDC No.: 759.610
Sex Ratio: Presumably M1:F1.
Occurrence: Undetermined but presumed rare.
Risk of Recurrence for Patient's Sib: Unknown.
Risk of Recurrence for Patient's Child: Unknown.
Age of Detectability: Facial lesions determine the diagnosis at birth. In patients diagnosed on the basis of seizures, one-half were diagnosed before one year of age.
Gene Mapping and Linkage: Unknown.
Prevention: None known. Genetic counseling indicated.
Treatment: In uncontrolled seizure states, cortical resection or hemispherectomy is indicated. Results of this therapy are reasonably good.
Prognosis: Normally progressive. If seizures become frequent, mental retardation occurs. Normal development may occur in slowly progressive patients or in those without major CNS involvement.
Detection of Carrier: Unknown.

References:

Weber FP: Notes on association of extensive haemangiomatous naevus of skin with cerebral (meningeal) haemangioma, especially cases of facial vascular naevus with contralateral hemiplegia. Proc R Soc Med 1929; 22:25.
Furukawa T, et al.: Sturge-Weber and Klippel-Trenaunay syndrome with nevus of Ota and Ito. Arch Derm 1970; 102:640–645.
Boltshauser E, et al.: Sturge-Weber syndrome with bilateral intracranial calcification. J Neurol Neurosurg Psychiatry 1976; 39:429.
Hoffman HJ, et al.: Hemispherectomy for Sturge-Weber syndrome. Child Brain 1979; 5:223.

SH007   **Kenneth Shapiro**

STUTTERING   **3060**

Includes:
    Dysfluency
    Speech fluency disorder
    Stammering

Excludes: Cluttering

Major Diagnostic Criteria: The diagnosis of stuttering is based on a purely behavioral analysis. In fact, the disorder is essentially defined by its symptoms, or, in other words, the symptoms and the disease are synonymous. Stuttering is generally defined as the interruption of the normal flow of speech by repetitions or prolongations of whole words or parts of words or by prolonged silences (or "blocks"), which may be accompanied by a struggle response, ticks, and grimaces.

Clinical Findings: Stuttering has been noted to begin most often in early childhood (at ages 4–5 years) and at that point tends to be characterized by easy repetitions of parts of words or whole words. Struggle behavior (visible and audible blockings of speech with accompanying grimacing) and increased severity of stuttering begins to occur later in childhood and continues to worsen through adolescence unless treated successfully. Males are far more likely to stutter than are females, and a strong familial pattern has been reported. To date, no specific structural phenotype has been documented.

A number of studies have shown physiologic responses associated with stuttering, such as increased anxiety levels and altered EEG patterns (e.g., increased beta wave production versus alpha waves), but many investigators believe that much of the physiologic response is secondary to the altered speech pattern, and the stress it causes the stutterer. To date, no physiologic phenotype has been demonstrated conclusively. Many other structural, physiologic, medical, and behavioral disorders have been hypothesized, but none have been scientifically confirmed.

Stuttering may be inconsistent. For example, many stutterers will be more dysfluent in certain environments or situations. Most stutterers are fluent when singing.

Complications: Stutterers may withdraw from situations demanding strong communication skills. They may also develop strong anxiety responses in situations that center around communicative ability, such as telephone conversation, meeting strangers, and other social interactions. Struggle responses appear later in the stutterer and are generally thought to be operantly learned behaviors.

Associated Findings: Though dysfluent speech may occur in individuals with a variety of neurogenic disorders such as **Neurofibromatosis**, stuttering generally occurs as an isolated findings in individuals who are reportedly otherwise normal.

Etiology: A number of hypotheses have been forwarded regarding the etiology of stuttering, including autosomal dominant inheritance, purely environmental factors, X-linked recessive inheritance, and sex-modified transmission of an autosomal dominant trait. At present, multifactorial inheritance seems to provide the best model for the majority of stutterers, though etiologic heterogeneity cannot be ruled out. In fact, it has not been established that all stuttering is in fact the same disorder, thus raising questions about the validity of considering it a "disease" versus merely a "symptom" of an underlying biologic dysfunction.

Pathogenesis: Unknown.

MIM No.: 18445

Sex Ratio: Reports range from M2:F1 to M10:F1. The most likely figure is approximately M4:F1.

Occurrence: Childhood dysfluency has been reported in up to 5% of males and 2% of females, although the incidence of fully expressed stuttering in the general population is undetermined. The condition is relatively common and known to occur in all cultures. An estimated prevelance of 0.7 has been reported. Stuttering is said to be unusually frequent in the Japanese, low in Polynesians, and almost completely absent in American Indians.

Risk of Recurrence for Patient's Sib: If neither parent is affected, males, 18%; females, 2%. If father is affected, males, 26%; females, 12%. If mother is affected, males, 33%; females, <1%.

Risk of Recurrence for Patient's Child: For males, 22%; females, 9%

Age of Detectability: After onset of speech, but not usually until past three years of age.

Gene Mapping and Linkage: Unknown.

Prevention: None known. Genetic counseling indicated.

Treatment: Speech therapy.

Prognosis: Life span is normal. Speech therapy is often, though not always, effective.

Detection of Carrier: Unknown.

Special Considerations: Stuttering may not be a single disorder, but rather a symptom of many possible biologically based problems of speech or voice coordination. However, its organic basis cannot be refuted, and extrinsic or environmental factors may be contributory, but not pathogenetic.

References:
Young A: Onset, prevalence, ar⌐ recovery from stuttering. J Speech Hear Disord 1975; 40:49–58.
Kidd KK: A genetic perspective on stuttering. J Fluence Disord 1977; 2:259–269.
Kidd KK, et al.: Vertical transmission of susceptibility to stuttering with sex-modified expression. Proc Natl Acad Sci USA 1978; 78:606–610.
Kidd KK, et al.: The possible causes of the sex ratio in stuttering and its implications. J Fluency Disord 1978; 3:13–23.
Chakravartti R, et al.: Hereditary factors in stammering. J Genet Hum 1979; 27:319–328.
Kidd KK, et al.: Familial stuttering patterns are not related to one measure of severity. J Speech Hear Res 1980; 23:539–545.
Cox NJ, Kidd KK: Can recovery from stuttering be considered a genetically milder subtype of stuttering? Behav Genet 1983; 13:129–139.
Cox NJ, et al.: Segregation analyses of stuttering. Genet Epidemiol 1984; 1:245–253.
Cox NJ, et al.: Some environmental factors and hypotheses for stuttering in families with several stutterers. J Speech Hear Res 1984; 27:543–548.

SH040
SA045

Robert J. Shprintzen
Vicki L. Sadewitz

Subacute myelo-optico neuropathy (SMON)
See NEUROPATHY, MYELO-OPTICO, SUBACUTE TYPE
Subacute necrotizing encephalomyelopathy (SNE)
See ENCEPHALOPATHY, NECROTIZING
Subacute spongiform encephalopathy
See CREUTZFELDT-JAKOB DISEASE
also GERSTMANN-STRAUSSLER SYNDROME
Subaortic stenosis, discrete
See HEART, SUBAORTIC STENOSIS, FIBROUS
Subaortic stenosis, fibrous
See HEART, SUBAORTIC STENOSIS, FIBROUS
Subaortic stenosis, idiopathic hypertrophic
See HEART, SUBAORTIC STENOSIS, MUSCULAR
Subaortic stenosis, muscular
See HEART, SUBAORTIC STENOSIS, MUSCULAR
Subclavian artery supply disruption sequence (SASDS)
See POLAND SYNDROME
Subclavian artery, anomalous origin of contralateral
See ARTERY, ANOMALOUS ORIGIN OF CONTRALATERAL SUBCLAVIAN
Subclavian artery, isolation from aorta
See AORTA, ISOLATION OF SUBCLAVIAN ARTERY FROM AORTA
Subcostosternal hernia
See DIAPHRAGMATIC HERNIA
Subendocardial fibroelastosis, right ventricular
See VENTRICLE, ENDOCARDIAL FIBROELASTOSIS OF RIGHT VENTRICLE
Suberylglycinuria
See ACYL-CoA DEHYDROGENASE DEFICIENCY, MEDIUM CHAIN TYPE

SUBGLOTTIC HEMANGIOMA 0918

Includes: Hemangioma, subglottic

Excludes:
Respiratory distress from other causes
Subglottic stenosis (0919)

Major Diagnostic Criteria: The clinical history and typical endoscopic appearance are considered sufficiently diagnostic for therapy, pending biopsy confirmation.

Clinical Findings: Because these hemangiomas are located subglottically affected infants typically have a history of dyspnea and inspiratory stridor which may become biphasic, yet the cry and voice remain clear. The fluctuating character of the respiratory distress, varying from day to day or even hour to hour, particularly with crying or exertion, is considered strongly diagnostic. The absence of marked temperature elevation, leukocytosis, and pharyngeal inflammation distinguish this disease from tracheobronchitis. Cutaneous hemangioma, particularly of the head and neck, should prompt immediate suspicion of a similar lesion in the subglottis in any child with respiratory distress; however about one-half of all patients will have no external hemangioma.

Soft tissue X-rays of the neck are generally nonspecific, although larger lesions may be seen on airway films. Typically, there is an asymmetric narrowing in the subglottis. Barium swallow may show posterior displacement of the esophagus from the air column in the subglottic area. Laryngoscopy and bronchoscopy allow visualization of the hemangioma, which usually appears as a sessile mass between the true vocal cord and the lower limit of the cricoid cartilage located in the posterolateral portion of the subglottis. The color varies from pink to blue; depending on the lesion's vascularity and relative depth beneath the mucosa. Such hemangiomas are readily compressible, differentiating them from other tumors of the larynx. Biopsy is generally condemned as dangerous and unnecessary because hemorrhage may be very difficult to control.

Complications: Acute respiratory failure or "sudden death" in about one-half of cases.

Associated Findings: Failure to gain weight; a characteristic of chronic respiratory obstruction.

Etiology: Unknown.

Pathogenesis: Usually a cavernous hemangioma with mature endothelium on only one side of the subglottic area, but may circumscribe the entire lumen.

Sex Ratio: M1:F2 (observed).

Occurrence: Between 1913 and 1986, 356 cases of infantile subglottic hemangioma were reported in the English literature.

The actual incidence has been difficult to establish because autopsy gross examination of infants succumbing to acute respiratory failure from this disease reveals no abnormality of the trachea or larynx. This finding is explained by the submucosal locations of these tumors, and when emptied of blood the lumen contour is restored with normal-appearing mucosa. With the recent increased awareness of this lesion, some centers advocate routine sections of the larynx and trachea in all cases of "sudden death" of unknown etiology in infants.

Risk of Recurrence for Patient's Sib: Unknown.

Risk of Recurrence for Patient's Child: Unknown.

Age of Detectability: Usually asymptomatic at birth. However, over 90% will develop symptoms before age three months.

Gene Mapping and Linkage: Unknown.

Prevention: None known. Genetic counseling indicated.

Treatment: Systemic steroids have produced dramatic regression of tumors in two to four weeks; and recurrence has been controlled by a second course of steroids. Excision of the tumor by laryngofissure is reserved for those tumors requiring tracheostomy that have not regressed after serveral years. Laser excision may be appropriate before attempting an open procedure. Smaller lesions may be treated with the carbon dioxide laser.

Tracheostomy is necessary with moderate-to-severe respiratory distress. Low-dose irradiation or injection of sclerosing agents are probably ineffective and may be dangerous to the developing larynx.

Prognosis: The lesions usually cease growth by age nine months, followed by gradual regression. A normal life span is expected if the patient survives infancy.

Detection of Carrier: Unknown.

Special Considerations: The association with cutaneous hemangioma and hemangioma of other organs is well documented. This includes hemangioma of the parotid gland, mediastinum, abdominal viscera, central nervous system, and retina. With multiple hemangiomas, there may be sufficient shunting of blood from the arterial to the venous system to cause right heart failure. Thrombocytopenia may result from the trapping of platelets within a large hemangioma.

References:
Calcaterra VC: An evaluation of the treatment of subglottic hemangioma. Laryngoscope 1968; 78:195.
Cohen SR: Unusual lesions of the larynx, trachea and bronchial tree. Ann Otol Rhinol Laryngol 1969; 78:476.
Cracovaner AJ: Anomalies of the larynx. In: Maloney WH, ed: Otolaryngology. Hagerstown: Harper and Row, 1969:42.
Choa OI, et al.: Subglottic hemangioma in children. J Laryngol Otol 1986; 100:447–454.
Shikhani AH, et al.: Infantile subglottic hemangiomas: an update. Ann Otol Rhinol Laryngol 1986; 95:336–347.

Thomas Aufdemorte

SUBGLOTTIC STENOSIS 0919

Includes:
Stenosis, combined subglottic
Stenosis, hard subglottic
Stenosis, soft subglottic
Stenosis, subglottic

Excludes: Acquired subglottic stenosis

Major Diagnostic Criteria: Stridor and cyanosis due to a developmental defect of the conus elasticus or the cricoid cartilage, which produces stenosis (when the infant's transverse subglottic diameter is less than 4 mm). The diagnosis is made by endoscopic examination.

Clinical Findings: Symptoms are variable according to the degree of stenosis, the presence of other anomalies, and superimposed infection. Symptoms may begin at birth with stridor and cyanosis. Other infants will be asymptomatic until superimposed low-grade infections cause recurrent bouts of respiratory difficulty, commonly misdiagnosed as croup. Lateral X-ray of the neck may show a decrease in anteroposterior (AP) diameter of the subglottic airway. Direct laryngoscopy and bronchoscopy are the most important studies for establishing the diagnosis. In the infant's larynx the subglottic region is cone-shaped and the smallest part of the larynx. The cricoid cartilage is somewhat funnel-shaped, with an AP diameter greater than that of the trachea. Later development produces the ring-shaped cricoid.

Soft stenosis: Narrowing of the normally cone-shaped conus elasticus produces a diffuse stenosis. This "hypertrophy" is composed of increased amounts of connective tissue and large dilated mucous glands, with a normal epithelial covering.

Hard stenosis: Caused by the cricoid cartilage, the lumen is compressed in inward "overgrowth" of its cartilaginous walls.

Combined stenosis: A subglottic stenosis can be caused by both soft (conus elasticus) and hard (cricoid cartilage) components.

Complications: Airway obstruction, exercise intolerance.

Associated Findings: None known.

Etiology: Unknown.

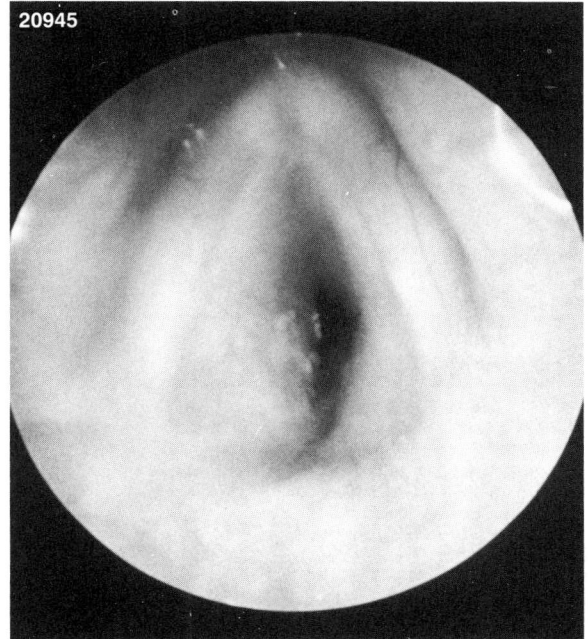

0919-20945: Subglottic stenosis.

Pathogenesis: Possible hypotheses include failure of the lateral infraglottic branchial fused masses to recanalize (soft stenosis) or recanalization after chondrification centers for the cricoid cartilage appear. An alternate theory suggests developmental arrest and formation of the stenosis from mesodermal elements.

Sex Ratio: M1:F1

Occurrence: Undetermined but presumed rare.

Risk of Recurrence for Patient's Sib: Unknown.

Risk of Recurrence for Patient's Child: Unknown.

Age of Detectability: Usually at or shortly after birth, but may not be detected until infant develops a respiratory infection or "croup". May become apparent following intubation if the child cannot be extubated or develops an obstruction.

Gene Mapping and Linkage: Unknown.

Prevention: None known. Genetic counseling indicated.

Treatment: In very mild stenosis no treatment is needed, other than aggressive therapy of upper respiratory infections. Functionally significant stenosis will require a tracheotomy until laryngeal growth produces an adequate airway. In Holinger's series of 53 infants with subglottic stenosis (1967), 39 required tracheotomy because of progressive respiratory difficulty.

Prognosis: Good if mild or if recognized and promptly treated. It is presently thought that most or all of these stenoses will "cure" themselves with growth. If the condition is severe and untreated, the patient may die of acute upper airway obstruction. A marginal airway may become inadequate during a respiratory infection. If tracheotomy is required, there is significant morbidity and mortality in infants and young children.

Detection of Carrier: Unknown.

References:
Holinger PH, et al.: Congenital anomalies of the larynx. Ann Otol Rhinol Laryngol 1954; 63:581–606.
Cavanagh F: Congenital laryngeal web. Proc R Soc Med 1965; 58:272–277.
Holinger PH, Brown WT: Congenital webs, cysts, laryngoceles, and other anomalies of the larynx. Ann Otol Rhinol Laryngol 1967; 76:744–752.
Cotton RT, Myer III, CM: Contemporary surgical management of laryngeal stenosis in children. Am J Otolaryngol 1984; 5:360–368.

MY003   **Charles M. Myer III**

Subglottic web
  See LARYNX, WEB
Subluxation of lens
  See LENS, ECTOPIC
Subluxed nasal septum, congenital
  See NOSE, DISLOCATED NASAL SEPTUM
Submerged teeth
  See TEETH, ANKYLOSED
SUC syndrome
  See UMBILICAL CORD, SHORT UMBILICAL CORD SYNDROME
Succedaneous teeth, agenesis of
  See TEETH, PEGGED OR ABSENT MAXILLARY LATERAL INCISOR
Succinic semialdehyde dehydrogenase deficiency
  See ACIDEMIA, GAMMA-HYDROXYBUTYRIC
Succinylcholine apnea
  See CHOLINESTERASE, ATYPICAL
Sucrase insufficiency
  See SUCRASE-ISOMALTASE DEFICIENCY
Sucrase intolerance, congenital
  See SUCRASE-ISOMALTASE DEFICIENCY
Sucrase-alpha dextrinase insufficiency
  See SUCRASE-ISOMALTASE DEFICIENCY

SUCRASE-ISOMALTASE DEFICIENCY   0920

Includes:
  Anisomaltasia
  Asucrosia
  Disaccharide intolerance I
  Isomaltase insufficiency
  Isomaltase-sucrase deficiency
  Sucrase-alpha dextrinase insufficiency
  Sucrase insufficiency
  Sucrase intolerance, congenital
  Sucrose-isomaltose malabsorption, congenital

Excludes:
  Lactase deficiency, congenital (0566)
  Lactase deficiency, primary (0567)
  Secondary sucrase-isomaltase deficiency

Major Diagnostic Criteria: Fermentative diarrhea from the earliest time of sucrose, dextrin, or starch ingestion, which disappears when these foods are eliminated and which does not occur with feedings of monosaccharides or lactose. Deliberate feeding of measured doses of sucrose, isomaltose, or palatinose yields flat serum glucose curve, abdominal discomfort, and explosive stool of pH below 5.0. The disaccharide can usually be identified in blood, urine, and stool after feeding for a tolerance test. If one is certain that the condition is congenital, these criteria may suffice if the patient's condition precludes peroral biopsy. However, demonstration of normal intestinal histology and decreased or absent sucrase and isomaltase activity is essential in most instances.

Clinical Findings: Symptoms of fermentative diarrhea and failure to thrive begin with initial ingestion of sucrose or dextrins. This would be virtually at birth in infants on modified milk formulas, or with weaning and introduction of sucrose or fruits containing sucrose. Severity of symptoms varies among individuals, but they are usually more severe in infants and young children. In most patients sucrosuria is present on ingestion of this disaccharide. Symptoms clear as soon as the offending disaccharide is removed from the diet. Patients with intolerance to sucrose are virtually universally described as simultaneously intolerant to isomaltose, the 1–6α-linked diglucose, which is found at the branching points of polysaccharide molecules (dextrins, starches).

The stool is fluid and frothy from contained gas, as it is passed. The pH of fresh stool is always below 5.0 if sucrose or dextrins have been ingested, and it may contain reducing sugars (glucose or fructose). These monosaccharides and sucrose or isomaltose may be identified in the stool by chromatography. Ingestion of a standard dose of sucrose (1.5–2.0 g/kg or 45–60 m/m^2) always results in a flat 3-hour "tolerance curve" for serum glucose, or with increased breath hydrogen excretion. The test dose almost universally produces clinical discomfort and explosive diarrhea during the observation period.

The Zurich group initially demonstrated that all patients with sucrose intolerance were also intolerant to isomaltose. It is this defect that causes the inability to tolerate dextrins and starches in young infants. Since adequate supplies of isomaltose are not available to demonstrate the flat absorption curve in routine loading tests, palatinose (1–6α-linked glucose and fructose), a bacterial product, is substituted. This disaccharide is split by the same α-glycosidase as is isomaltose. In addition to sucrosemia and sucrosuria, patients with this deficiency of sucrase-isomaltase demonstrate isomaltose in blood and urine after dextrin and starch feedings, and also palatinose in these fluids after its ingestion for tolerance testing.

The importance of the isomaltase deficiency is variously regarded by different authors. In our own experience, patients must remain on a sucrose-free diet for life to avoid symptoms. However, starches appear to be tolerated in reasonably normal amounts, once patients are beyond the early months of life. This is probably because isomaltose makes up only approximately 10% of the average starch molecule.

Peroral biopsy specimen of the upper small intestinal mucosa is histologically normal, but it contains decreased sucrase and isomaltase activities when these are compared with the activities of maltases 1 and 2 (not maltase 3, 4, and 5) and of lactase, or when assayed in relation to unit weight, or to protein content of the tissue.

Complications: Dehydration, electrolyte, and acid-base disturbance in almost all cases. Failure to thrive or death in all cases, if correct diagnosis is not made and treatment is not instituted early enough.

Associated Findings: Renal calculi.

Etiology: Autosomal recessive inheritance of sucrase and isomaltase deficiency. The combined deficiencies of two enzymes (sucrase-isomaltase) is unusual in genetic defects. It has been suggested that a common regulator gene, or inhibitor, is shared by both enzyme molecules. More probably, they are not separate but represent two activity centers of the same molecule. Gray (1975) suggests that the defect be viewed, for this reason, as sucrase-α dextrinase deficiency, since free isomaltose is not present in the intestinal lumen.

Pathogenesis: Ingested sucrose or isomaltose, which results from amylolytic action on polysaccharides, are not hydrolyzed to the component monosaccharides in the upper small intestine, as in normal individuals, and pass undigested to the colon. In this organ these disaccharides are hydrolyzed and fermented. The resultant mixture contains two and three carbon volatile acids, glucose, fructose (if sucrose has been ingested), and often the undigested disaccharide(s). The increase in osmolarity of the colonic contents induces a net flux of water to the lumen. A combination of the irritant effect of the excessive fermentation, increased colonic gas, and distension of the bowel walls by the increase in fluid, results in explosive passage of the loose stool.

MIM No.: *22290

Sex Ratio: Presumably M1:F1.

Occurrence: As high as 1:100 in Greenland Eskimos, and probably increased in Alaskan Eskimos. 2:1,000 in North Americans. Intestinal sucrase deficiency is a cause of diarrhea in adults.

Risk of Recurrence for Patient's Sib:
See Part I, *Mendelian Inheritance.*

Risk of Recurrence for Patient's Child:
See Part I, *Mendelian Inheritance.*

Age of Detectability: In early infancy, by loading with sucrose and isomaltose or palatinose and assay of enzymes in intestinal mucosal biopsy specimen.

Gene Mapping and Linkage: SI (sucrase-isomaltase) has been provisionally mapped to 3q25-q26.

Prevention: None known. Genetic counseling indicated.

Treatment: Avoidance of sucrose in diet. Dextrins and starches should also be avoided in very young infants. Toddlers and older children tolerate these quite well, but sucrose is either never tolerated, or, in some instances, may begin to be taken without concomitant symptoms in the second decade of life.

Fluid and electrolyte support may be necessitated during the diarrheal activity in undiagnosed infants.

Prognosis: Normal life span, if patient is diagnosed and treated. In many patients, the symptoms disappear with aging. In a few instances, if not recognized in infancy, patients may die of severe inanition and electrolyte disturbances.

Detection of Carrier: Although some parents have been demonstrated to have decreased sucrase-isomaltase activities in peroral biopsy specimens, the tolerance of such individuals for loading with the appropriate disaccharides is usually better than that of children. This confusing finding cannot yet be interpreted to mean either that they represent heterozygote carriers or that they are affected but have undergone the improvement in clinical symptomatology, which is characteristic with growing out of childhood.

References:
Prader A, Auricchio S: Defects of intestinal disaccharide absorption. Ann Rev Med 1965; 16:345–385.

Davidson M: Disaccharide intolerance. Pediatr Clin North Am 1967; 14:93–107.

Antonowicz I, et al.: Congenital sucrase-isomaltase deficiency. Pediatrics 1972; 49:847–853.

Gray GM: Carbohydrate digestion and absorption. New Engl J Med 1975; 292:1225–1230.

Gray GM, et al.: Sucrase-isomaltase deficiency. New Engl J Med 1976; 294:750–753.

Harms H-K, et al.: Enzyme-substitution therapy with yeast saccharomyces cerevisiae in congenital sucrase-isomaltase deficiency. New Engl J Med 1987; 316:1306–1309.

Lloyd ML, Olsen WA: A study of the molecular pathology of sucrase-isomaltase deficiency. New Engl J Med 1987; 316:438–442.

DA017   **Murray Davidson**

Sucrose-isomaltose malabsorption, congenital
See SUCRASE-ISOMALTASE DEFICIENCY
Sudden infant death syndrome (SIDS), one theory of
See MYOPATHY, MALIGNANT HYPERTHERMIA
Sugarman syndrome
See ORO-FACIO-DIGITAL SYNDROME, SUGARMAN TYPE
Sugio-Kajii syndrome
See TRICHO-RHINO-PHALANGEAL SYNDROME, TYPE III
Sulcus mentalis
See FACE, CHIN FISSURE

SULFATASE DEFICIENCY, MULTIPLE   2860

Includes:
Mucosulfatidosis
Sulfatidosis, juvenile, Austin type

Excludes:
Metachromatic leukodystrophies (0651)
Mucopolysaccharidosis

Major Diagnostic Criteria: Early onset developmental delay; hepatomegaly; ichthyosis developing after 2–3 years of age; dysostosis multiplex; and deficiency of two or more sulfatases demonstrated in biologic fluids and/or cultured skin fibroblasts.

Clinical Findings: Most patients come to medical attention during the first two years of life for evaluation of delayed development and/or mild to moderate organomegaly. In a few carefully studied cases, slow development was documented from infancy. Severe acrocyanosis may occur intermittantly. On physical exam there may be mildly coarsened facial features. Mild corneal clouding is sometimes detected by slit lamp exam but is not severe enough to be detected with the hand ophthalmoscope. Some patients have exhibited vertical nystagmus. There is usually moderate hepatomegaly or hepatosplenomegaly, camptodactyly, and limited extension of the elbows and hips. The deep tendon reflexes are absent or reduced. The characteristic ichthyotic skin rash which usually is not present until 2–3 years of life, waxes and wanes and is particularly prominent over the trunk.

The peripheral leukocytes often have abnormal granulation. X-rays reveal dysostosis multiplex. There is mild to moderate mucopolysacchariduria and sulfatiduria. Urinary arylsulfatase A is deficient. Nerve conduction velocities are slow.

Complications: Seizures have occurred in several reported cases.

Associated Findings: Some patients have had broad thumbs and great toes.

Etiology: Autosomal recessive inheritance.

Pathogenesis: The primary defect responsible for this deficiency of at least seven sulfatases including six lysosomal and one microsomal enzyme is not known. Complementation studies in somatic cell hybrids indicate that the structural genes for these sulfatases are intact. A defect in a shared regulatory or stabilizing factor or a defect in a common co-factor or post-translational modification could account for the biochemical phenotype of multiple enzymatic deficiencies. The observations that cultured skin fibroblasts from multiple sulfatase deficiency patients express near normal levels of sulfatase activity under certain culture conditions and that several of the sulfatases in these cells have markedly reduced half-lives supports the notion of a defect in a shared stabilizing factor.

The sulfatases which have been shown to be deficient in this disorder and the disease associated with specific deficiency of each are shown below:

SULFATASE	ASSOCIATED SYNDROME
Iduronate sulfatase	*Mucopolysaccharidosis II*
Heparan N-sulfatase	*Mucopolysaccharidosis III* (Sanfilippo A)
N-acetylglucosamine 6-sulfatase	*Mucopolysaccharidosis III* (Sanfilippo D)
Galactose 6-sulfatase	*Mucopolysaccharidosis IV*
N-acetylgalactosamine 4-sulfatase (arylsulfatase B)	*Mucopolysaccharidosis VI*
Arylsulfatase A	*Metachromatic leukodystrophies*
Steroid sulfatase (arylsulfatase C)	*Ichthyosis, X-linked with steroid sulfatase deficiency*

Certain aspects of the clinical phenotype can be attributed mainly to deficiency of one particular sulfatase by comparison with the phenotypes of the inherited isolated sulfatase deficiencies. For example, the ichythosis resembles that of isolated steroid sulfatase deficiency, the peripheral nerve involvement resembles that of arylsulfatase A deficiency and the dysostosis multiplex resembles that observed in deficiencies of iduronate sulfatase, heparan N-sulfatase, N-acetylglucosamine 6-sulfatase and N-acetylgalactosamine 4-sulfatase.

MIM No.: *27220

Sex Ratio: M1:F1

Occurrence: Fewer than 25 cases have been reported. Some reports of **Mucopolysaccharidosis II** in females may actually represent this disorder.

Risk of Recurrence for Patient's Sib:
See Part I, *Mendelian Inheritance*.

Risk of Recurrence for Patient's Child:
See Part I, *Mendelian Inheritance*. No affected individuals are known to have reproduced.

Age of Detectability: Clinically evident within the first few months of life. Biochemical abnormalities are present *in utero*.

Gene Mapping and Linkage: Unknown.

Prevention: None known. Genetic counseling indicated.

Treatment: Unknown.

Prognosis: Life span of reported cases ranged from a few months to 12 years.

Detection of Carrier: Some but not all heterozygotes have had reduced levels of one or more sulfatases, but this is so variable as to be unreliable.

References:

Austin JH: Studies of metachromatic leukodystrophy. Arch Neurol 1973; 28:258–264.

Fluharty AL, et al.: Arylsulfatase A modulation with pH in multiple sulfatase deficiency disorder fibroblasts. Am J Hum Genet 1979; 31:574–580.

Burk RD, et al.: Early manifestations of multiple sulfatase deficiency. J Pediatr 1984; 104:574–578.

Fedde K, Horwitz AL: Complementation of multiple sulfatase deficiency in somatic cell hybrids. Am J Hum Genet 1984; 36:623–633.

Steckel F, et al.: Synthesis and stability of arylsulfatase A in fibroblasts from multiple sulfatase deficiency. Eur J Biochem 1985; 151:141–145.

Steckel F, et al.: Multiple sulfatase deficiency: degradation of arylsulfatase A and B after endocytosis in fibroblasts. Eur J Biochem 1985; 151:147–152.

Horwitz AL, et al.: Rapid degradation of steroid sulfatase in multiple sulfatase deficiency. Biochem Biophys Res Comm 1986; 135:389–396.

VA000   **David Valle**

Sulfatide lipidosis
See METACHROMATIC LEUKODYSTROPHIES
Sulfatidosis, juvenile, Austin type
See SULFATASE DEFICIENCY, MULTIPLE
Sulfatidosis, juvenile, Austin type (Some forms)
See MUCOPOLYSACCHARIDOSIS II
Sulfatidosis, juvenile, Austin type (some forms)
See METACHROMATIC LEUKODYSTROPHIES
Sulfite oxidase/xanthine dehydrogenase/aldehyde oxidase deficiency
See MOLYBDENUM CO-FACTOR DEFICIENCY
Sulfo-iduronate sulfatase deficiency
See MUCOPOLYSACCHARIDOSIS II
Sulfocysteinuria
See ACIDURIA, SULFITE OXIDASE DEFICIENCY
Sulfonamides, fetal effects of
See OPTIC NERVE HYPOPLASIA
Summerskill disease
See CHOLESTASIS, INTRAHEPATIC, RECURRENT BEGIGN
Summerskill-Tygstrup disease
See CHOLESTASIS, INTRAHEPATIC, RECURRENT BEGIGN
Summitt syndrome
See ACROCEPHALOPOLYSYNDACTYLY
Superior vena cava syndrome
See CANCER, THYMOMA
Supernumerary puncta and canaliculi
See EYELID, PUNCTA AND CANALICULI, SUPERNUMERARY
Supraaortic stenosis
See AORTIC STENOSIS, SUPRAVALVAR
Supraglottic web
See LARYNX, WEB
Supramitral ring
See MITRAL VALVE STENOSIS
Suprapineal recess
See BRAIN, MIDLINE CAVES
Supraumbilical (paraumbilical) hernia
See HERNIA, UMBILICAL
Supravalvar aortic stenosis
See WILLIAMS SYNDROME
also AORTIC STENOSIS, SUPRAVALVAR
Supravalvular pulmonary stenosis
See PULMONARY ARTERY, COARCTATION
Supraventricular tachycardia paroxysmal
See ARRHYTHMIA, SUPRAVENTRICULAR TACHYCARDIAS, CONGENITAL
Supraventricular tachycardias, congenital
See ARRHYTHMIA, SUPRAVENTRICULAR TACHYCARDIAS, CONGENITAL
Surdocardiac syndrome
See CARDIO-AUDITORY SYNDROME
Sutural cataract
See CATARACT, AUTOSOMAL DOMINANT CONGENITAL
Suxamethonium sensitivity
See CHOLINESTERASE, ATYPICAL

SWEATING, GUSTATORY   0448

Includes:
Auriculotemporal syndrome
Frey syndrome
Gustatory sweating
Hyperhidrosis, gustatory

Excludes:
Parotid duct fistula
Postencephalitic gustatory sweating
Posttraumatic and postoperative gustatory sweating
Syringomyelia (0924)

Major Diagnostic Criteria: A lifelong history of facial and neck sweating, with or without flushing, during or after eating, in a person who has no medically or surgically induced neurologic deficits. A strong positive family history is usually present.

Clinical Findings: At the time of or just after eating or drinking, perspiration of the face and neck is noted. The face and neck areas may show associated flushing. No increase of sweating or flushing is noted in other areas of the body. The symptoms appear with any food or beverage, but there are no symptoms or findings to suggest specific food allergy. There is no history of trauma or surgery in the area, nor of encephalitis or neurologic deficits. Generally the symptoms have been lifelong or date from infancy; often a family history can be obtained.

Complications: Social embarrassment or in extreme cases withdrawal from social contacts might occur.

Associated Findings: None known.

Etiology: Probably autosomal dominant inheritance.

Pathogenesis: Unknown.

MIM No.: 14410

Sex Ratio: M>1:F1 (observed).

Occurrence: Undetermined. The known cases have been in American Blacks as reported by Mailander (1967); and 3 generations of Zuni Indians with the syndrome have been studied by Jacobs. However, there is no reason to believe that other ethnic groups might not also be affected.

Risk of Recurrence for Patient's Sib:
See Part I, *Mendelian Inheritance.*

Risk of Recurrence for Patient's Child:
See Part I, *Mendelian Inheritance.*

Age of Detectability: In infancy.

Gene Mapping and Linkage: Unknown.

Prevention: None known. Genetic counseling indicated.

Treatment: Intratympanic section of Jacobsen nerve (ninth cranial nerve) might be successful in interrupting the efferent innervation to the parotid gland. This is postulated on the theory that aberrant autonomic innervation occurs. It is thought that the sweat glands and blood vessels of the skin are innervated by parasympathetic rather than sympathetic fibers. A topical preparation, such as 3% scopolamine cream, may be useful in instances where the sweating is not profuse. In mild cases simple assurance to the patient that he does not have a serious or life-threatening disorder may be sufficient. Intracranial section of the 9th cranial nerve is not justified for this benign disease. X-ray therapy of the skin would require near-cancerocidal doses to destroy the sweat glands and also is not indicated. In some instances, elevation of a skin flap overlying the parotid gland is useful.

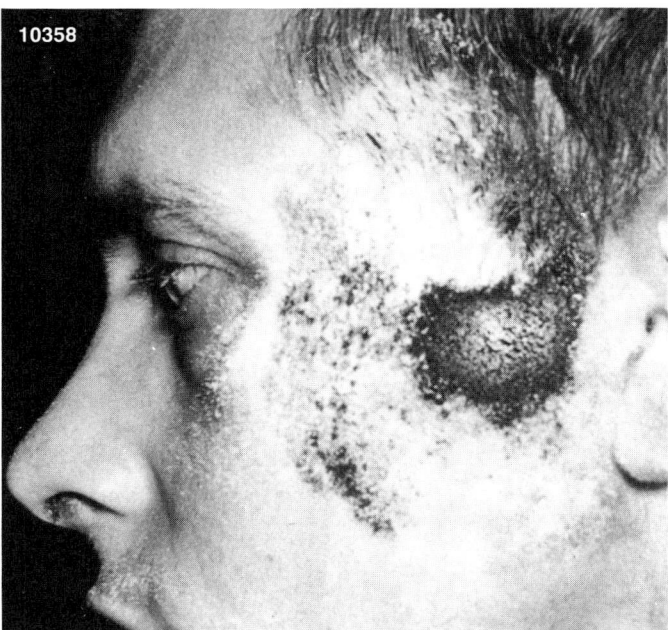

0448-10358: Gustatory sweating.

Prognosis: Good for normal life span. Total function of the patient is limited only if he tends to withdraw from society.

Detection of Carrier: Unknown.

Special Considerations: As pointed out by Mailander, the incidence of this disorder may be higher than reported since affected individuals may tend to deny the symptoms or withdraw from society. Also, in both ethnic groups in which this condition has been described there is a tendency to ignore such physical complaints or at least not to bring them to medical attention. Often this is an incidental finding when the patient is receiving medical care for an unrelated problem. An erroneous diagnosis of parotid fistula or neuropsychiatric disease is often made and proper therapy not instituted.

The author wishes to thank Kent F. Jacobs for his help in preparing this article.

References:
Mailander JC: Hereditary gustatory sweating. J Am Med Assoc 1967; 201:203–204.

BE028   **LaVonne Bergstrom**

Sweaty feet syndrome
See ACIDEMIA, ISOVALERIC
Swedish genetic porphyria
See PORPHYRIA, ACUTE INTERMITTENT
Swedish type distal myopathy
See MUSCULAR DYSTROPHY, DISTAL
Swedish-type hereditary amyloidosis
See AMYLOIDOSIS, TRANSTHYRETIN METHIONINE-30 TYPE
Swiss type hereditary amyloidosis
See AMYLOIDOSIS, INDIANA TYPE
Swiss-cheese cartilage syndrome
See KNIEST DYSPLASIA
Swyer syndrome
See GONADAL DYSGENESIS, XY TYPE
Sydney line
See SKIN CREASE, SINGLE PALMAR
Sylvian seizures
See EPILEPSY, BENIGN CHILDHOOD WITH CENTROTEMPORAL EEG FOCUS (BEC)
Symbrachydactyly-ipsilateral aplasia of head of pectoralis muscle
See POLAND SYNDROME
Symmelia
See SIRENOMELIA SEQUENCE
Symphalangism
See SYNOSTOSIS

SYMPHALANGISM   **1001**

Includes:
Cushing symphalangism
Deafness (conduction)-multiple synostoses
Deafness-symphalangism, Herrmann type
Facio-audio-osymphalangism
Herrmann symphalangism-brachydactyly syndrome
Synostoses, multiple-brachydactyly
Synostoses (multiple)-conduction deafness
Symphalangism, C.S. Lewis type
Symphalangism-brachydactyly
Symphalangism, distal
Symphalangism, proximal
Thumbs, stiff
WL symphalangism-brachydactyly syndrome

Excludes:
Brachydactyly (0114)
Diastrophic dysplasia (0293)
Poland syndrome (0813)
Skin creases, absent distal interphalangeal (2488)
Synostosis (1522)

Major Diagnostic Criteria: *Symphalangism* refers to general ankylosis of the joints of fingers or toes. Several forms exist, and many of these are or appear to be inherited. In addition, the condition

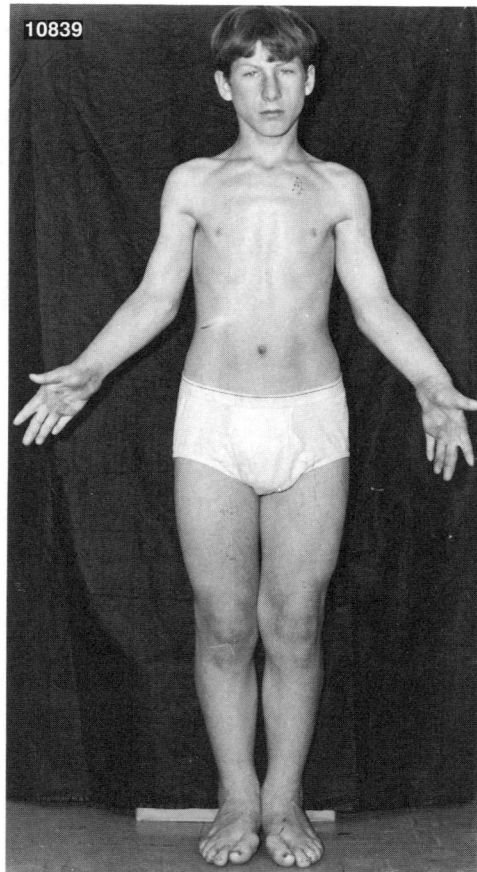

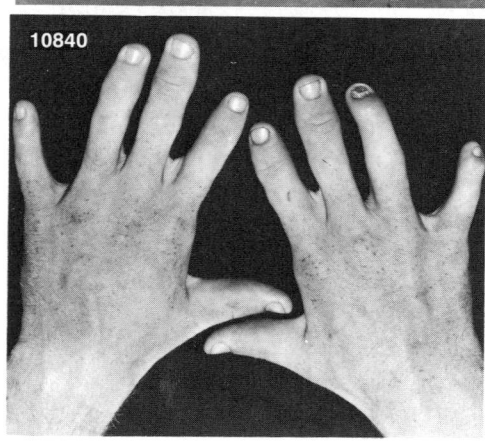

1001A-10839: Characteristic facies with long nose and thin upper lip. 10840: Proximal symphalangism and brachydactyly.

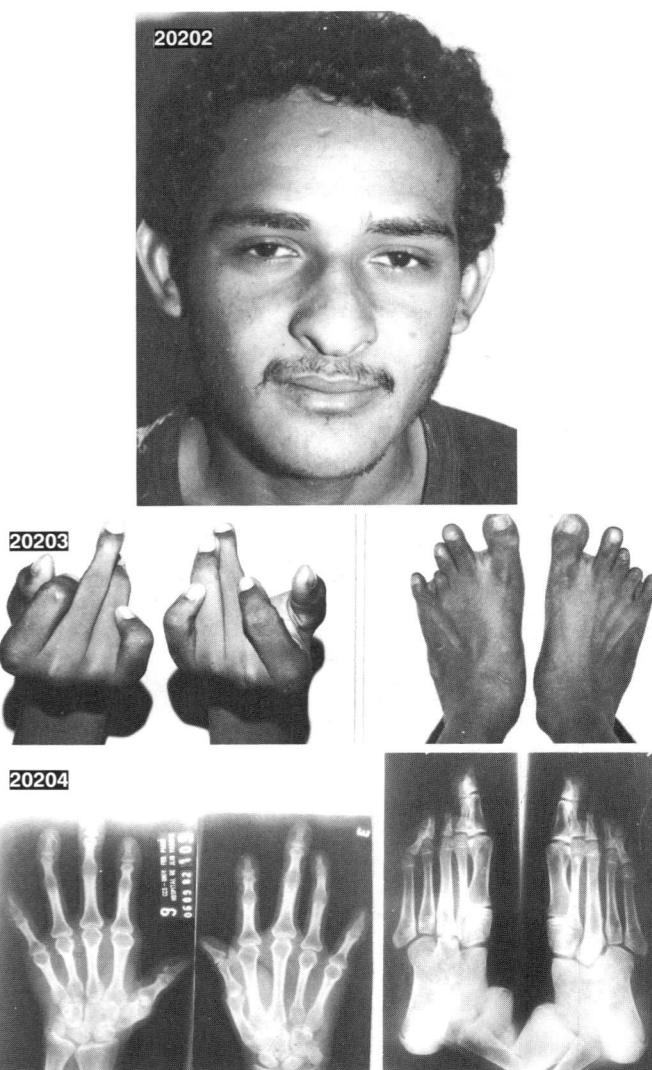

1001B-20202: Typical facies with hypoplastic nasal alae and short upper lip. 20203: Note symphalangism, clinodactyly, absence of part of the toes, and a wide gap between the first and second toes. 20204: X-rays of the hands and feet show symphalangism, carpal and tarsal synostosis, partial synostosis of the first and second metacarpals, tarsometatarsal synostosis, and agenesis of the phalanges.

can be observed in combination with other findings including brachydactyly, deafness, and other hand and foot anomalies.

The *Symphalangism-brachydactyly syndrome* (also known as *Deafness-symphalangism, Herrmann type, Synostoses, multiple-brachydactyly*, and the *WL symphalangism-brachydactyly syndrome*, is a specific disorder consisting of 1) Symphalangism, proximal, 100%; 2) Brachydactyly, especially involving the thumb and great toe, 100%; 3) Prominent cylindrical nose with hypoplastic alae nasi, 100%; 4) Carpal and tarsal coalitions, 100%; 5) Hypoplastic/absent middle phalanges, 100%; 6) Cubitus valgus or limited range of motion at the elbow, 86%; 7) Conductive deafness, 72+%.

Clinical Findings: C.S. Lewis suffered from a specific form of symphalangism to which he attributed his decision to became an author (Lewis, 1955, p. 12). This "still thumbs" variant has also been observed in association with brachydactyly and mental retardation.

Both *distal* (Matthews et al, 1987) and *proximal* (Cremers et al, 1985) symphalangism have been described. Learman et al (1981) reported an Arabic kindred with proximal symphalangism and syndactyly, clinodactyly, hypoplasia of the thenar and hypothenar eminences, and unique dermatoglyphics.

Cushing symphalangism, which involves absence of the proximal interphalangeal joints, has been traced back, perhaps erroneously, to the Earl of Shrewsbury in the 15th century. Conductive hearing loss has also been reported in this condition (Cremers, et al, 1985).

Multiple synostoses is a feature of the *WL symphalangism-brachydactyly syndrome*, so designated by Herrmann (1974) from the names of the two husbands of the mother of the children described in his account. The syndrome itself was first reported by W.G. Fuhrmann in a 1966 issue of *Humangenetik*.

This pleiotropic syndrome is characterized by proximal symphalangism, brachydactyly, absence of distal portions of digits, dermatoglyphic abnormalities, shortness of first metacarpals/metatarsals, synostosis of carpal/tarsal bones, dislocation of the head of the radius, conductive hearing deficit, and a particular facial appearance. The face is long and narrow, with a prominent, long, hemicylindrical nose and a thin upper lip. The hearing deficit is apparently due to ankylosis of the stapes. Patients are of normal height but may have abnormal body proportions due to short arms. The syndrome shows considerable intrafamily variability. In early infancy, symphalangism may be apparent clinically (stiffness, absence of flexion and extension creases at the joint) but not on X-ray.

Complications: Limited joint mobility in fingers, wrists, elbows and feet; gait abnormalities.

Associated Findings: Strabismus, radial head dislocation, radiohumeral synostosis, and mild cutaneous syndactyly.

Etiology: Autosomal dominant inheritance.

Pathogenesis: Unknown.

MIM No.: 18565, *18570, 18575, *18580, *18640, *18650

POS No.: 3402

Sex Ratio: M1:F1

Occurrence: About 20 cases of WL symphalangism-brachydactyly syndrome have been reported from about six families, including one from Japan. A large Brazilian kindred with 28 cases of WL or a closely related condition was reported by da-Silva et al (1984). There is an extensive literature on other variants of symphalangism, but no consensus on their occurrence.

Risk of Recurrence for Patient's Sib:
See Part I, *Mendelian Inheritance.*

Risk of Recurrence for Patient's Child:
See Part I, *Mendelian Inheritance.*

Age of Detectability: Usually at birth.

Gene Mapping and Linkage: Unknown.

Prevention: None known. Genetic counseling indicated.

Treatment: The abnormalities of the arms, hands, and feet do not usually require surgical procedures. Patients with symphalangism should have a hearing evaluation (which may need to be repeated) to rule out a hearing deficit and a comprehensive skeletal survey to rule out further skeletal abnormalities. Hearing aids, stapedectomy, and insertion of a prosthesis may improve hearing.

Prognosis: Symphalangism, carpal synostoses and hearing loss are slowly progressive.

Detection of Carrier: Possibly by clinical examination of first degree relatives.

References:
Lewis CS: Surprised by joy. New York: Harcourt, Brace and World, 1955.
Maroteaux P, et al.: La maladie des synotoses multiples. Nouv Presse Med 1972; 1:3041–3047.†
Herrmann J: Symphalangism and brachydactyly syndrome: report of the *WL symphalangism-brachydactyly syndrome*: review of literature and classification. BD:OAS X(5). Miami: Symposia Specialists for The National Foundation-March of Dimes, 1974:23–53. †
Learman Y, et al.: Symphalangism with multiple anomalies of the hands and feet. Am J Med Genet 1981; 10:245–255.
Higashi K, Inoue S: Conductive deafness, symphalangism, and facial abnormalities: the WL syndrome in a Japanese family. Am J Med Genet 1983; 16:105–109. †
da-Silva EO, et al.: Multiple synostosis syndrome: study of a large Brazilian kindred. Am J Med Genet 1984; 18:237–247.
Cremers C, et al.: Proximal symphalangia and stapes ankylosis. Arch Otolaryng 1985; 111:765–767.
Hurvitz SA, et al.: The facio-audio-symphalangism syndrome: report of a case and review of the literature. Clin Genet 1985; 28:61–68.
Matthews S, et al.: Distal symphalangism with involvement of the thumbs and great toes. Clin Genet 1987; 32:375–378.

LU001
R0007
HE023
DA025

Mark Lubinsky
Luther K. Robinson
Jürgen Herrmann
Elias O. da-Silva

Symphalangism, C.S. Lewis type
See SYMPHALANGISM
Symphalangism, distal
See SYMPHALANGISM
Symphalangism, proximal
See SYMPHALANGISM
Symphalangism-brachydactyly
See SYMPHALANGISM
Sympodia
See SIRENOMELIA SEQUENCE
Syncephalus
See TWINS, CONJOINED
Syncope and QT prolongation without deafness
See ARRHYTHMIA, WITH LONG QT INTERVAL WITHOUT DEAFNESS

SYNDACTYLY 0923

Includes:
Metacarpal 4–5 fusion
Syndactyly type I (zygodactyly)
Syndactyly type II (synpolydactyly)
Syndactyly type III (ring and little finger syndactyly)
Syndactyly type IV (Haas type and Cenani-Lenz type)
Syndactyly type V (with metacarpal and metatarsal fusion)

Excludes:
Acrocephalosyndactyly type I (0014)
Amniotic bands syndrome (0874)
Poland syndrome (0813)
Syndactyly with multifactorial inheritance

Major Diagnostic Criteria: Syndactyly indicates webbing between digits. Genetic types may be identified by determining if the abnormalities fit into a known characteristic patterns, and identifying similarly affected relatives.

Clinical Findings: In *syndactyly, type I* (zygodactyly), there is usually webbing between the 3rd and 4th fingers, either complete

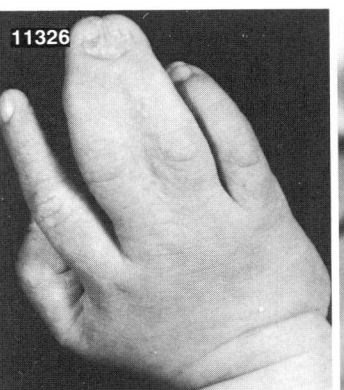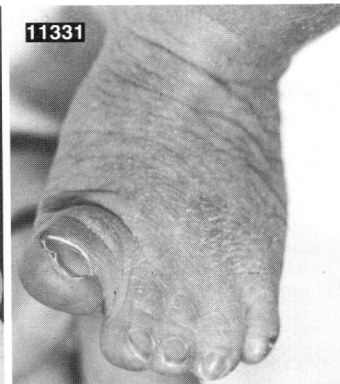

0923-11326: Syndactyly with bony fusion between fingers 3 and 4. **11331:** Complete syndactyly between toes 2, 3 and 4, and partial syndactyly between hallux and 2nd toe.

reaching to the nails, or partial, and occasionally associated with fusion of the distal phalanges of these fingers. Other fingers are sometimes also involved, but the 3rd and 4th fingers are the most commonly affected. In the feet, there is usually webbing between the 2nd and 3rd toes, either complete or partial.

In *syndactyly, type II* (synpolydactyly), there is usually syndactyly of the 3rd and 4th fingers associated with polydactyly of all components or of part of the 4th finger in the web. In the feet, there is polydactyly of the 5th toe.

In *syndactyly, type III* (ring and little finger syndactyly), syndactyly between the ring and the little fingers is usually complete and bilateral. The 5th finger is short, with absent or rudimentary middle phalanx. Feet are usually not affected in this type. This type of syndactyly is the hand malformation in oculodentoosseous dysplasia.

In *syndactyly, type IV* (Haas type) there is complete cutaneous fusion of the fingers, giving the hands a cup-like appearance. In Cenani-Lenz type the complete syndactyly is associated with bizarre disorganization of metacarpals and phalanges; the radius and ulna are either fused, short, or rudimentary. Feet are similarly affected.

In *syndactyly, type V*, there is an associated metacarpal and metatarsal fusion. The metacarpals and metatarsals most commonly fused are the 3rd and 4th or the 4th and 5th. Soft tissue syndactyly usually affects the 3rd and 4th fingers and the 2nd and 3rd toes. Syndactyly is usually more extensive and complete.

Complications: Unknown.

Associated Findings: None known.

Etiology: Autosomal dominant inheritance of most types. Fusion of metacarpals 4–5 is inherited as an X-linked recessive trait in some families. Cenani-Lenz syndactyly by autosomal recessive inheritance.

Pathogenesis: Unknown.

MIM No.: *18590, *18600, *18610, 18620, *18630, *21278, *30963

CDC No.: 755.1

Sex Ratio: M1:F1

Occurrence: Syndactyly type I (zygodactyly) is the most common, with an incidence of 1:3,000 live births in North Americans.

Risk of Recurrence for Patient's Sib:
See Part I, *Mendelian Inheritance.*

Risk of Recurrence for Patient's Child:
See Part I, *Mendelian Inheritance.*

Age of Detectability: At birth.

Gene Mapping and Linkage: MF4 (metacarpal 4–5 fusion) has been mapped to X.

Prevention: None known. Genetic counseling indicated.

Treatment: Surgical intervention.

Prognosis: Normal life span.

Detection of Carrier: Unknown.

References:
Haas SL: Bilateral complete syndactylism of all fingers. Am J Surg 1940; 50:363–366.
Johnston O, Kirby VV: Syndactyly of the ring and little finger. Am J Hum Genet 1955; 7:80–82.
Cross HE, et al.: Type II syndactyly. Am J Hum Genet 1968; 20:368–380.
Holmes LB, et al.: Metacarpal 4–5 fusion with X-linked recessive inheritance. Am J Hum Genet 1972; 24:562–568.
Temtamy SA, McKusick VA: The genetics of hand malformations. BD:OAS IV(3). New York: march of Dimes Birth Defects Foundation, 1978.
Castila EE, et al.: Syndactyly: frequency of specific types. Am J Med Genet 1980; 5:357–364.
Pfeiffer RA, Meisel-Stosiek M: Present nosology of the Cenani-Lenz type of syndactyly. Clin Genet 1982; 21:74–79.
Robinow M, et al.: Syndactyly type V. Am J Med Genet 1982; 11:475–482.
Merlob P, Grunebaum M: Type II syndactyly or synpolydactyly. J Med Genet 1986; 23:237–241.

TE004   **Samia A. Temtamy**

Syndactyly type I (zygodactyly)
See SYNDACTYLY
Syndactyly type II (synpolydactyly)
See SYNDACTYLY
Syndactyly type III (ring and little finger syndactyly)
See SYNDACTYLY
Syndactyly type IV (Haas type and Cenani-Lenz type)
See SYNDACTYLY
Syndactyly type V (with metacarpal and metatarsal fusion)
See SYNDACTYLY

SYNDACTYLY, CENANI TYPE   2976

Includes:
  Cenani-Lenz syndactyly
  Cenani syndactylism
Excludes:
  Acrocephalosyndactyly
  Poland syndrome (0813)
  Syndactyly (other)
  Syndactyly associated with congenital constriction rings
  Syndactyly with multifactorial inheritance

Major Diagnostic Criteria: Complete syndactyly of the digits, giving a mitten-like appearance to the hands. Fusion of all the carpal bones and disorganization of the metacarpals and phalanges.

Clinical Findings: The fingers are enclosed in the webbing and are deformed. The digits in some appear pea-shaped. Radioulnar synostosis is common, and the radius and ulna may be short or rudimentary. The feet may be similarly affected.

Complications: Unknown.

Associated Findings: None known.

Etiology: Autosomal recessive inheritance.

Pathogenesis: Unknown.

MIM No.: *21278

POS No.: 3887

Sex Ratio: M1:F1

Occurrence: About a dozen cases have been documented.

Risk of Recurrence for Patient's Sib:
See Part I, *Mendelian Inheritance.*

Risk of Recurrence for Patient's Child:
See Part I, *Mendelian Inheritance.*

Age of Detectability: At birth. Prenatal ultrasonography may detect this condition.

Gene Mapping and Linkage: Unknown.

Prevention: None known. Genetic counseling indicated.

Treatment: Surgical intervention.

Prognosis: Normal life span.

Detection of Carrier: Unknown.

References:
Cenani A, Lenz W: Total Syndaktylie und totale radioulnare Synostose bei zwei Bruedern. Ein Beitrag zur Genetik der Syndaktylien. Z Kinderheilkd 1967; 101:181–190.
Drohm D, et al.: Totale syndaktylie mit mesomeler Armverkerzung, radioulnaeren und metacarpalen Synostosen und Disorganisation der Phalangen ("Cenani-Syndaktylie"). Klin Paediatr 1976; 188:359–365.
Temtamy SA, McKusick VA: The genetics of hand malformations. New York: Alan R. Liss, 1978:320–322.
Dodinval P: Oligodactyly and multiple synostoses of the extremities: two case in sibs. Hum Genet 1979; 48:183–189.

Pfeiffer RA, Meisel-Stosiek M: Present nosology of the Cenani-Lenz type of syndactyly. Clin Genet 1982; 21:74–79.

HE006 **Jacqueline T. Hecht**

Syndactyly-anophthalmos
See ANOPHTHALMIA-LIMB ANOMALIES
Syndactyly-cleft lip/palate-ectodermal dysplasia
See CLEFT LIP/PALATE-ECTODERMAL DYSPLASIA-SYNDACTYLY
Syndactyly-cleft lip/palate-oligodontia-hair defects
See CLEFT LIP/PALATE-OLIGODONTIA-SYNDACTYLY-HAIR DEFECTS
Syndactyly-cleft lip/palate-pili torti
See PILI TORTI-CLEFT LIP/PALATE-SYNDACTYLY
Syndactyly-cryptophthalmos
See FRASER SYNDROME

SYNDACTYLY-MICROCEPHALY-MENTAL RETARDATION, FILIPPI TYPE 2820

Includes:
   Filippi syndrome
   Microcephaly-syndactyly-mental retardation, Filippi type
Excludes:
   Aarskog syndrome (0001)
   Blepharo-naso-facial syndrome (2088)
   Cranio-digital syndrome-mental retardation, Scott type (2831)
   KBG syndrome (0554)
   Syndactyly, type I (zigodactyly) syndromes, other
   Tricho-rhino-phalangeal syndrome, type II (0967)
   Waardenburg syndromes (0997)

Major Diagnostic Criteria: Unusual facial appearance, **Microceph-aly**, retarded somatic and mental development, inability to speak, and **Syndactyly** type I of fingers and toes.

Clinical Findings: Growth retardation and low birth weight. Height, weight, and head size are generally below the third percentile. Broad and prominent nasal root and diminished alar flare give an unusual facial appearance. Striking **Syndactyly** of fingers 3 and 4, clinodactyly of finger 5, and **Syndactyly** of toes 2,3, and 4 are present; however, one girl showed an absence of finger syndactyly and presence of bilateral simian creases.

   Mental retardation is severe to mild: with IQ between 30 and 60. Prepubertal genitalia with bilateral cryptorchidism and incomplete descent of testes are present in males. Inarticulate sounds or some utterance of sounds are recorded with no hearing deficit. Skeletal X-rays show moderately retarded bone age (two years below normal) in one male; brachymesophalangy of the fifth fingers; and syndactyly, limited to the soft tissues. Chromosomes have been normal (G and Q bands).

Complications: Defective speech and language development.

Associated Findings: None known.

Etiology: Possibly autosomal recessive inheritance with some variability in expression.

Pathogenesis: Unknown.

MIM No.: 27244

POS No.: 3725

Sex Ratio: Presumably M1:F1; M2:F1 observed.

Occurrence: Three of eight sibs (two boys and one girl) of healthy, unrelated parents from Italy have been documented.

Risk of Recurrence for Patient's Sib:
   See Part I, *Mendelian Inheritance.*

Risk of Recurrence for Patient's Child:
   See Part I, *Mendelian Inheritance.*

Age of Detectability: In early infancy.

Gene Mapping and Linkage: Unknown.

Prevention: None known. Genetic counseling indicated.

Treatment: Training in language through auditory or manual learning techniques, and oral speech training.

Prognosis: Normal life span. Mental retardation is severe to mild.

Detection of Carrier: Unknown.

References:
Filippi G: Unusual facial appearance, microcephaly, growth and mental retardation, and syndactyly: a new syndrome? Am J Med Genet 1985; 22:821–824.

FI030 **Giorgio Filippi**

SYNDACTYLY-POLYDACTYLY-EAR LOBE SYNDROME 3042

Includes:
   Ear lobe-syndactyly-polydactyly syndrome
   Goldberg-Pashayan syndrome
   Polydactyly-syndactyly-ear lobe syndrome
Excludes:
   Polydactyly (isolated)
   Polysyndactyly-dysmorphic craniofacies, Greig type (2925)
   Zygodactyly

Major Diagnostic Criteria: The combination of **Polydactyly** of hands and sometimes feet, **Syndactyly** of the toes, and minor earlobe anomalies should suggest the diagnosis.

Clinical Findings: Ten affected individuals from a single family have been described. Earlobe anomalies consisted of a deep, horizontal groove (7/10) or a nodule (2/10). Five individuals had bilateral postaxial polydactyly of the hands, with the extra digit ranging from a soft tissue nubbin to a well-formed finger. Foot anomalies included hallux syndactyly (6/10), syndactyly of toes 2–3 (5/10), preaxial polydactyly (7/10), MTP delta phalanx (4/10), and accessory metatarsal (4/10), occurring alone or in combination. However, only four individuals had all three anomalies (earlobe, foot, and hand); the other six had only one or two of the above-listed findings.

Complications: Unknown.

Associated Findings: None known.

Etiology: Autosomal dominant inheritance. This condition was originally reported in three generations of one kindred, with male-to-male transmission occurring twice.

Pathogenesis: Unknown.

MIM No.: *18635

POS No.: 3901

Sex Ratio: M1:F1

Occurrence: One United States family with ten affected members has been reported.

Risk of Recurrence for Patient's Sib:
   See Part I, *Mendelian Inheritance.*

Risk of Recurrence for Patient's Child:
   See Part I, *Mendelian Inheritance.*

Age of Detectability: At birth by the presence of hand and foot anomalies.

Gene Mapping and Linkage: Unknown.

Prevention: None known. Genetic counseling indicated.

Treatment: Surgical removal of extra digits or release of syndactyly, if indicated.

Prognosis: Life span and intellect are not affected.

Detection of Carrier: Unknown.

References:
Goldberg MJ, Pashayan HM: Hallux syndactyly, ulnar polydactyly, abnormal ear lobes: a new syndrome. BD:OAS XII(5). New York: March of Dimes Birth Defects Foundation, 1976:255–266.

T0007 **Helga V. Toriello**

Syngnathism, congenital
  See CLEFT PALATE-PERSISTENCE OF BUCCOPHARYNGEAL
    MEMBRANE
Synkinetic ptosis
  See JAW-WINKING SYNDROME
Synopthalmia
  See CYCLOPIA
Synostoses (multiple)-conduction deafness
  See SYMPHALANGISM
Synostoses, multiple-brachydactyly
  See SYMPHALANGISM

SYNOSTOSIS   1522

Includes: Symphalangism

Synostosis denotes the presence of bony fusions that cause limitation of joint movement, eg. extension, flexion, supination and pronation. The long bones of the upper extremities are most often affected but carpals, tarsals, and phalanges can also be involved. Synostosis specifically denotes either fusion of sutures, as in the calvarium or fusion of two long bones as in **Radial-ulnar synostosis**. *Symphalangism* describes fusion of the phalanges and coalition refers to fusion of the carpal or tarsal bones. Bony fusions may be difficult to detect in the newborn or in early childhood but decreased range of movement and reduction of the joint space on X-ray are suggestive of synostosis.

Bony fusions can occur from trauma or arise secondarily from abnormal bone growth such as that occuring in **Exostoses, multiple cartilaginous**. In this condition, the bony outgrowths can cause bridging and synostosis which leads to bony deformation and decreased range of joint movement. Bony fusions may be isolated abnormalities or part of single gene and chromosomal syndromes. For example, **Radial-ulnar synostosis** is an autosomal dominant condition, but radioulnar synostosis also commonly occurs in the 48,XXXY, 49,XXXXY and **Acrofacial dysostosis, Nager type**. Multiple joints can be involved such as that seen in **Synostosis, multiple synostosis syndrome** where symphalangism, carpal and tarsal coalitions and occasionally radiohumeral synostosis occur. Symphalangism is also present in dwarfing conditions such as **Diastrophic dysplasia** and **Kniest dysplasia**.

The pathogenesis of bony fusions is unknown. Atrophy and fibrosis of the supernator and pronator muscles and thickened interosseous membranes have been found in the radioulnar synostosis suggesting longterm joint immobility. Isolated unilateral synostosis generally is not genetic, but bilateral involvement usually has a genetic etiology. Indeed **Radial-ulnar synostosis** is an autosomal dominant condition; and autosomal recessive and dominant patterns of inheritance have been reported for conditions associated with radiohumeral synostosis. When synostosis occurs as part of a condition, recurrence of the bony abnormality is related to the frequency that it occurs in the condition and the recurrence of the condition.

Treatment of bony fusions is limited. Surgery is generally not recommended except where there is a possibility of obtaining a more functional fixed position of an extremity. Physical therapy early in life is not recommended for dwarfing conditions as it may cause the fusions to worsen.

HE006   **Jacqueline T. Hecht**

Synostosis, humero-radial
  See HUMERO-RADIAL SYNOSTOSIS
Synostosis, radial cubital
  See RADIAL-ULNAR SYNOSTOSIS
Synotia-agnathia-microstomia
  See AGNATHIA-MICROSTOMIA-SYNOTIA

SYNOVITIS, FAMILIAL HYPERTROPHIC   2155

Includes:
  Arthritis, "E" family
  Arthropathy-camptodactyly syndrome
  Camptodactyly-arthropathy syndrome
  Jacobs syndrome
  Pericarditis-arthropathy-camptodactyly (CAP) syndrome

Excludes:
  Arthritis, rheumatoid (2517)
  Thumbs, trigger

Major Diagnostic Criteria: 1) Onset soon after birth of trigger thumbs followed by flexion contractures of other proximal interphalangeal joints; 2) development of painless effusions at large joints (especially knees, wrists and ankles) during early childhood; 3) no fever, rash, iritis, visceromegaly, nodules, leucocytosis, systemic illness; 4) normal growth and development; 5) no radiographic destructive changes; femoral necks unusually broad and with varus deformity (present in three other families; not commented on in other reported cases; 6) distinctive microscopic pathology with large hypertrophic avascular synovial villi with giant cells but no underlying inflammation. Some villi are lined by or replaced by fibrin-like material; 7) similar findings in affected tendon sheaths extend into the underlying tendons causing tight adhesions of tendon sheaths to tendons. These are difficult to lyse. A large amount of fibrous tissue is seen in underlying normal tendons.

Clinical Findings: Trigger thumbs are the first manifestation noted during the first few months of life, followed soon thereafter by flexion contractures in the proximal interphalangeal joints of other fingers. A diagnosis of tenosynovitis is made and tendon sheath releases are often performed. Joint effusions are then noted at the knee and typical pathologic findings have been demonstrated in biopsy material taken from the knee as early as age 20 months. Synovial "pouches" become apparent at the wrists and effusions are apparent in the ankle joints. While the children have no pain at first, during the second decade pain and morning stiffness become more apparent and progressive limitations are noted at the hips with exaggerated lumbar lordosis.

In early childhood the erythrocyte sedimentation rate (ESR) is normal, but in one affected family the ESR was elevated during later childhood. Elevation of the ESR has not been noted in other families.

There is a paucity of X-ray findings in childhood, but in three families there was a striking varus deformity of the femoral necks.

Complications: During the third decade of life one affected individual developed extraordinary chondrocalcinosis with progressively increasing amounts of calcium being demonstrable on X-ray in joint spaces. This patient had increasingly frequent attacks of pseudogout. One of her sibs was said to have a similar problem, although this could not be demonstrated on X-ray.

Associated Findings: Acute pericarditis, and in some cases constrictive pericarditis, has been seen as a feature of this syndrome in three recent reports; one patient had a brief attack of pericarditis thought to be tuberculous.

Etiology: Although the number of affected individuals in each reported family (6/11;3/5;3/3;2/2) suggested autosomal dominant inheritance with absence of the disease in any parent being explained by incomplete penetrance, affected individuals in the oldest family now have seven unaffected children. This observation, plus the absence of disease in the parents, and the fact that at least initially the disease was only recognized when multi-family cases presented, now makes recessive inheritance much more likely. Of the 14 reported cases only three were male, but all families had a predominance of female children.

Pathogenesis: Possibly a chemical defect affecting synovial lining cells. There are no reports of attempts to grow the cells in tissue culture.

MIM No.: *20825

Sex Ratio: M1:F5 original reports; M4:F7 patients with pericarditis.

Occurrence: About two dozen cases have been reported.

Risk of Recurrence for Patient's Sib:
See Part I, *Mendelian Inheritance.*

Risk of Recurrence for Patient's Child:
See Part I, *Mendelian Inheritance.*

Age of Detectability: May be suspected at two months of age; diagnosis possible in the second year in a first case in a family, but by two months of age in subsequent cases.

Gene Mapping and Linkage: Unknown.

Prevention: None known. Genetic counseling indicated.

Treatment: Diagnosis enables avoidance of hazardous medications prescribed for juvenile rheumatoid arthritis, including corticosteroids which have been administered to many affected children. Appropriate surgery (finger tendon releases) can be performed and inappropriate surgery (open synovial biopsies) can be avoided. In later life if chondrocalcinosis appears with symptoms of pseudogout treatment can be tailored to maneuvers appropriate for crystal arthropathy rather than rheumatoid arthritis, gout or infection.

Prognosis: Normal function is the rule throughout childhood but tendon sheath releases are required for satisfactory use and appearance of fingers. More severely affected individuals develop rather severe limitation of motion of the hips which is progressive during the second and third decades and disability may be expected to increase thereafter.

Detection of Carrier: The mother of the index family always had an elevated erythrocyte sedimentation rate and developed increasing but undefined arthritic complaints during the fifth decade of life.

Special Considerations: It remains to be determined whether this disorder is to be included as one of the forms of familial pyrophosphate arthropathy; however, none of the described forms begin in early childhood or have the markers of the disease observable in all of these children. It is possible that the crystal arthritis seen in the one older individual, and perhaps developing in others, is a non-specific secondary effect of the defect rather than a clue to etiology and pathogenesis of the disorder.

A similar disorder, *Familial arthritis and camptodactyly* (Malleson et al.: Arthritis Rheum 1981; 24:1199–1204) is distinguished by biopsy evidence of inflammation in the synovium, a finding strikingly absent in all reported cases of familial hypertrophic synovitis.

References:
Athreya BH, Schumacher HR: Pathologic features of a familial arthropathy associated with congenital flexion contractures of fingers. Arthritis Rheum 1978; 21:429–437.
Malleson P, et al.: Familial arthritis and camptodactyly. Arthritis Rheum 1981; 24:1199–1204.
Jacobs JC: Pediatric rheumatology for the practitioner. New York: Springer-Verlag, 1982:151–154.
Martinez-Lavin M, et al.: A familial syndrome of pericarditis arthritis and camptodactyly. New Engl J Med 1983; 309:224–225.
Ochi T, et al.: The pathology of the involved tendons in patients with familial arthropathy and congenital camptodactyly. Arthritis Rheum 1983; 26:896–900.
Bulutlar G, et al.: A familial syndrome of pericarditis, arthritis, camptodactyly, and coxa vera. Arthritis Rheum 1986; 29:436–438.
Laxer RM, et al.: The camptodactyly-arthropathy-pericarditis syndrome: case report and literature review. Arthritis Rheum 1986; 29:439–444.

JA012   **Jerry C. Jacobs**

Synovitis-granulomatous-uveitis-cranial neoropathies, familial
See GRANULOMATOSIS-POLYSYNOVITIS, FAMILIAL SYSTEMIC
Syphilis, prenatal
See FETAL SYPHILIS SYNDROME
Syphonoma
See SCALP, CYLINDROMAS

SYRINGOMYELIA   0924

Includes:
Gliosis
Spinal cord cavitation

Excludes:
Intramedullary spinal cord tumor
Myopathy
Neuropathy

Major Diagnostic Criteria: Progressive muscular atrophy of the upper extremities associated with anesthesia and trophic changes.

Clinical Findings: Syringomyelia most commonly involves the cervical enlargement of the spinal cord. The pathologic process of cavitation most frequently originates in the region of the anterior white commissure. The symptoms and signs result from expanding cavitation and subsequent gliosis.

Rapidly progressive scoliosis is relatively common. Atrophy and weakness of the intrinsic hand muscles may be the first finding, but progressive wasting of arm, trunk, and neck musculature follows. The upper limbs are flaccid and areflexic. The corticospinal tracts are often compromised, so that spasticity, weakness, hyperreflexia, and extensor plantar responses are noted in the lower limbs.

Sensory symptoms, particularly loss of pain and temperature sensation, are the result of destruction of the lateral spinothalamic tracts. Analgesia is usually more apparent than tactile anesthesia. Trophic changes include Charcot joints, abnormalities of perspiration, and skin ulceration. The most frequent age of presentation is during the third and fourth decades.

Cervical spine X-rays may show widening of the interpediculate distance, particularly in the sagittal diameter. Bony erosion is rare. The CSF protein may be elevated. Myelography frequently shows an abnormally enlarged spinal cord. CT may demonstrate the lesion, but MRI is the procedure of choice to demonstrate the location and extent of cystic lesion.

Complications: Poser (1956) examined 245 cases of syringomyelia and found a 16% incidence of associated intramedullary tumors. Mild trauma to the cord has been reported to cause bleeding within the cavity followed by marked deterioration in function. Syringobulbia may occur due to upward extension of the process from the cervical spinal cord into the medulla producing lower cranial nerve abnormalities and bulbar signs causing aspiration, pneumonia, and death.

Associated Findings: Spina bifida, **Klippel-Feil anomaly**, cervical ribs, **Brain, Arnold-Chiari malformation, Hydrocephaly**, webbed fingers, abnormal hair distribution, basilar impression and invagination, and hypospadias.

Etiology: Both autosomal dominant and autosomal recessive inheritance have been suggested, with little evidence. Most cases are non-familial.

Pathogenesis: Syringomyelia may be the result of an abnormality of embryogenesis. The abnormality may be the result of an arrest in the development of the spinal cord before complete differentiation of gray and white matter occurs. An alternate theory suggests that during development of the cord there is a failure of the normal migration of spongioblasts from the central canal region. These cells later develop the capability of proliferating and causing cavitation. Netsky (1953) suggested that syringomyelia is the result of developmental anomalies of the intramedullary blood supply, which leads to infarction, gliosis, and cavity formation.

MIM No.: 18670, 27248

CDC No.: 336.000

Sex Ratio: M1:F1

Occurrence: Hundreds of cases have been reported.

Risk of Recurrence for Patient's Sib: Unknown.

Risk of Recurrence for Patient's Child: Unknown.

Age of Detectability: Usually between the ages of 20 and 40 years, primarily by physical examination, CT, and myelography.

The condition may be detected in infancy, particularly when a spinal MRI is obtained in connection with evaluation for an associated spina bifida, occult dysraphism, and craniovertebral anomalies.

Gene Mapping and Linkage: Unknown.

Prevention: None known. Genetic counseling indicated.

Treatment: Laminectomy and appropriate drainage of the rapidly enlarging cavity is indicated in the presence of progressive neurologic signs. Trophic skin changes require treatment.

Prognosis: Slowly progressive. Bulbar paralysis may lead to chronic aspiration and death. Has been fatal in over one-half of all cases.

Detection of Carrier: Unknown.

References:

Jackson M: Familial lumbosacral syringomyelia and the significance of developmental errors of the spinal cord and column. Med J Aust 1949; 1:433.

Netsky M: Syringomyelia: a clinical pathologic study. Arch Neurol Psychiatry 1953; 70:741.

Poser CM: Relationship between syringomyelia and neoplasm. Springfield: Charles C Thomas, 1956.

Bentley SJ, et al.: Familial syringomyelia. J Neurol Neurosurg 1975; 38:346–349.

Dichiro G, et al.: Computerized axial tomography in syringomyelia. New Engl J Med 1975; 292:13.

Gimenez-Roldan S, et al.: Familial communicating syringomyelia. J Neuro Sci 1978; 36:135–146.

HA053   **Robert H.A. Haslam**

Systemic carnitine deficiency due to MCAD
  See ACYL-CoA DEHYDROGENASE DEFICIENCY, MEDIUM CHAIN TYPE

Systemic elastorrhexis
  See PSEUDOXANTHOMA ELASTICUM

Systemic G(M2)-gangliosidosis
  See G(M2)-GANGLIOSIDOSIS WITH HEXOSAMINIDASE A AND B DEFICIENCY

Systemic lupus erythematosis (SLE)
  See LUPUS ERYTHEMATOSUS, SYSTEMIC

❖ T ❖

T-cell antigen receptor, alpha subunit (TCRA)
  See *LEUKEMIA/LYMPHOMA, T-CELL*
T-cell chronic lymphocytic leukemia
  See *LEUKEMIA/LYMPHOMA, T-CELL*
T-cell leukemia/lymphoma, adult
  See *LEUKEMIA/LYMPHOMA, T-CELL*
T-cell prolymphocytic leukemia
  See *LEUKEMIA/LYMPHOMA, T-CELL*
T-lymphocyte deficiency
  See *IMMUNODEFICIENCY, NEZELOF TYPE*
Tabatznik syndrome
  See *HEART-HAND SYNDROME II*
Tabes of Friedreich
  See *ATAXIA, FRIEDREICH TYPE*
Tachycardia, junctional
  See *ARRHYTHMIA, SUPRAVENTRICULAR TACHYCARDIAS, CONGENITAL*
Takahara syndrome
  See *ACATALASEMIA*
Talipes calcaneovalgus
  See *FOOT, CONGENITAL CLUBFOOT*
Talipes equinovarus, congenital idiopathic
  See *FOOT, TALIPES EQUINOVARUS (TEV)*
Tangier disease
  See *ANALPHALIPOPROTEINEMIA*
Tapazole^, fetal effects
  See *FETAL EFFECTS FROM METHIMAZOLE AND CARBIMAZOLE*
Tapetochoroidal dystrophy, progressive
  See *CHOROIDEREMIA*
Tapetoretinal degeneration-alopecia
  See *RETINOPATHY-HYPOTRICHOSIS SYNDROME*
TAR syndrome
  See *THROMBOCYTOPENIA-ABSENT RADIUS*
Tarsomegaly
  See *DYSPLASIA EPIPHYSEALIS HEMIMELICA*
Tarui disease
  See *GLYCOGENOSIS, TYPE VII*
Taste blindness
  See *TASTING DEFECT, PHENYLTHIOCARBAMIDE*
Taste threshold to bitter compounds containing the N-C-S group
  See *TASTING DEFECT, PHENYLTHIOCARBAMIDE*

TASTING DEFECT, PHENYLTHIOCARBAMIDE   0809

Includes:
  Phenylthiocarbamide tasting
  Phenylthiourea insensitivity
  PTC taster defect
  Taste blindness
  Taste threshold to bitter compounds containing the N-C-S group

Excludes: Taste threshold to other substances, hereditary differences.

Major Diagnostic Criteria: Inability to taste dilute phenylthiocarbamide (PTC). There is a bimodal population curve for detecting increasing concentrations of PTC. Tasters can detect bitterness at 50 parts per million (ppm), whereas nontasters can detect only concentrations of about 400 ppm.

Clinical Findings: The threshold for the bitter taste of substances containing the N-C=S group, such as phenylthiocarbamide, propylthiouracil, and naturally occurring goitrogens, such as goitrin, is bimodal in many populations. The only other substance which elicits this bimodal threshold is anetholtrithione.

Goitrin or other thioureas occur in cabbage, kale and rutabaga in quantities too dilute to evoke a bitter taste. When eaten in excess, they may cause goiters by inhibiting both iodide organification and iodotyrosine coupling in thyroglobulin. This is especially true for small animals and human infants fed milk from cows eating large quantities of these or similar foods. The goitrogenic effect is independent of the taster status of the individual.

Complications: Unknown.

Associated Findings: Tasters having the HLA-B8 antigen have a six-fold greater incidence of Graves' disease, whereas nontasters are more likely to be hypothyroid, with nodular goiter. Most athyrotic cretins are nontasters.

Depression is more common among tasters according to a subjective test of depression severity (Beck's Depression Inventory). There is an increased incidence of nontasters associated with **Diabetes mellitus**.

Congenital cataracts, aphakic retinal detachment, and both convergent and divergent squint are associated with a higher incidence of nontasters. There is also an increased incidence of nontasters in people with primary simple **Glaucoma**, and of tasters in people with closed angle glaucoma; individuals with congenital glaucoma are more likely to be tasters.

Some studies indicate an increased incidence of nontasters among alcoholics, but the effect of alcohol on taste sensitivity in general is unknown.

Etiology: Homozygosity of a recessive gene, t. Individuals who are heterozygous (Tt) and homozygous for T are tasters.

Pathogenesis: Unknown.

MIM No.: *17120

Sex Ratio: M1:F1

Occurrence: About 30% among individuals of western European descent; lower or almost non-existent in some African, Chinese, American Indian, Brasilian Indian and Eskimo populations. The highest gene frequency of t (0.76) was reported among the Kayastha Indian community, but their smoking and eating habits may predispose them to general taste insensitivity.

Risk of Recurrence for Patient's Sib: 25% if neither parent is a nontaster; 50% if one parent is a nontaster; 100% if both parents are nontasters.

Risk of Recurrence for Patient's Child: 100% if spouse is a nontaster; 50% if spouse is heterozygous; 0% if spouse is TT.

Age of Detectability: In infancy. There is a slight diminution of taste sensitivity with advancing age.

Gene Mapping and Linkage: PTC (phenylthiocarbamide tasting) is ULG1.

Linked to Kell with a lod score of 10.78 for a theta = 0.045.

Prevention: None known. Genetic counseling indicated.

Treatment: Appropriate treatment for associated conditions is required.

Prognosis: Excellent.

Detection of Carrier: Taster parent or taster child of an affected individual. There is no reliable distinction between TT and Tt individuals, although heterozygotes have somewhat diminished thresholds.

Special Considerations: Some associations have been single studies of limited population groups. Although statistical significance has been demonstrated, panethnicity has not. The odor of PTC solutions may contribute to taste perception.

References:
Harris H, Kalmus H: The measurement of taste sensitivity to phenylthiourea (PTC). Ann Eugen 1949; 15:24–31.
Conneally PM, et al.: Linkage relations of the loci for Kell and phenylthiocarbamide (PTC) taste sensitivity. Hum Hered 1976; 26:267–271.
Farid NR, et al.: HLA and phenylthiocarbamide (PTC) tasting in autoimmune thyroid disease. Tissue Antigens 1977; 10:414–416.
David R, Jenkins T: Genetic markers in glaucoma. Brit J Ophthalm 1980; 64:227–231.
Padma T, Murty JS: Association of genetic markers with some eye diseases. Acta Anthropogenetica 1983; 7:1–12.
Swinson RP: Genetic markers and alcoholism. Recent developments in Alcoholism 1983; 1:9–24.
Whittemore PB: Phenylthiocarbamide (PTC) tasting and reported depression. J Clin Psychol 1986; 42:260–263.

VI006   **Jaclyn M. Vidgoff**
KA006   **Hans Kalmus**

Taurodontism
See TEETH, TAURODONTISM

TAURODONTISM-SHORT ROOTED TEETH-MICROCEPHALIC DWARFISM   3232

Includes:
Dwarfism, microcephalic-taurodontism-short rooted teeth
Sauk syndrome
Teeth, short rooted-taurodontism-microcephalic dwarfism

Excludes:
Angelman syndrome (2086)
Beckwith-Wiedemann syndrome (0104)
Bloom syndrome (0112)
Chromosome XXY, XXYY, and XXXXY syndromes with taurodontism
Cockayne syndrome
De Lange syndrome (0242)
Meckel syndrome (0634)
Neu-laxova syndrome (2092)
Oculo-cerebro-facial syndrome, Kaufman type (2179)
Rubinstein-Taybi broad thumb-hallux syndrome (0119)
Seckel syndrome (0881)
Teeth, taurodontism (0926)
Tricho-dento-osseous syndrome (0965)
Tricho-rhino-phalangeal syndrome

Major Diagnostic Criteria: Taurodontism and short rooted teeth in conjunction with microcephalic dwarfism.

Clinical Findings: Low-birth-weight (1,040–2,068), small placental, microcephalic dwarfism. The facies are small and delicate. The nose is thin but not prominently beaked. The eyes are proportional in size to the face, and the ear lobes are distinct. The mandible is usually small with a class II occlusion and maxillary overbite, and the chin is not small or retruded. There is no cleft palate.

This syndrome is characterized by the dentition. There is true microdontia. The teeth are small in proportion to the small face. The incisors do not meet at contact points. The enamel is of

normal thickness relative to the booth size. The teeth have been reported to be mobile and can shed spontaneously.

On X-ray, the molars are taurodont and may contain pulpal calcifications. The roots of the anterior teeth are short and may be foreshortened by external resorption. Periapical radiolucent areas develop on anterior teeth with apical resorption without a history of trauma.

Complications: The most obvious complications are the premature loss of teeth, progressive malposition of teeth, and the development of diastemas between teeth. Affected individuals are retarded but usually shy and passive.

Associated Findings: Class II malocclusion and pulpal calcifications.

Etiology: Possibly autosomal recessive inheritance. In all instances, parents and parental relatives have been unaffected. Karyotypes have been 46,XY in male patients. G-banded karyotypes, chromosomal breakage, and sister chromatid exchanges have been normal.

Pathogenesis: Unknown.

Sex Ratio: M3:F1

Occurrence: The condition has been documented in four cases; American Caucasians, French-Canadians, and Japanese.

Risk of Recurrence for Patient's Sib:
See Part I, *Mendelian Inheritance.* Observed figure is 40%.

Risk of Recurrence for Patient's Child: Unknown. Affected individuals have not been known to reproduce.

Age of Detectability: After the age of seven for the permanent dentition, by radiographic examination.

Gene Mapping and Linkage: Unknown.

Prevention: None known. Genetic counseling indicated.

Treatment: Routine oral hygiene.

Prognosis: Unknown.

Detection of Carrier: Unknown.

References:
Sauk JJ, et al.: Taurodontism, diminished root formation and microcephalic dwarfism. Oral Surg 1973; 36:231–235.
Gardner DG, Girgis B: Taurodontism, short roots, and external resorption, associated with short stature and a small head. Oral Surg 1977; 44:271–273.
Tsuchiya H, et al.: Analysis of the dentition and orofacial skeleton in Seckel's bird-headed dwarfism. J Max-Fac Surg 1981; 9:170–175.

SA029   **John J. Sauk**
WI043   **Carl J. Witkop, Jr.**

Taussig-Bing syndrome
See VENTRICLE, DOUBLE-OUTLET RIGHT WITH ANTERIOR SEPTAL DEFECT
Tay syndrome
See TRICHOTHIODYSTROPHY
Tay-Sachs disease
See G(M2)-GANGLIOSIDOSIS WITH HEXOSAMINIDASE A DEFICIENCY
Tay-Sachs with visceral involvement
See G(M1)-GANGLIOSIDOSIS, TYPE 1
TC2 deficiency
See TRANSCOBALAMIN II DEFICIENCY
Tear duct, blocked
See NASOLACRIMAL DUCT OBSTRUCTION
Teeth (anomalies)-skeletal dysplasia-sparse hair
See CRANIO-ECTODERMAL DYSPLASIA
Teeth (conical)-polydactyly-nail dysplasia-short limbs
See ACROFACIAL SYNDROME, CURRY-HALL TYPE
Teeth (coniform)-onychodystrophy-deafness
See ONYCHODYSTROPHY-CONIFORM TEETH-SENSORINEURAL HEARING LOSS
Teeth (pseudoanodontia)-growth retardation-alopecia
See GROWTH RETARDATION-ALOPECIA-PSEUDOANODONTIA-OPTIC ATROPHY
Teeth retention
See TEETH, IMPACTED

TEETH, AMELOGENESIS IMPERFECTA 0046

Includes:

Amelogenesis imperfecta, hypocalcification type
Amelogenesis imperfecta, hypomaturation type
Amelogenesis imperfecta, hypoplastic type
Amelogenesis imperfecta, pigmented hypomaturation type
Enamel hypoplasia, hereditary
Enamel, hypoplastic-hypocalcified with taurodontism
Enamel, hypoplastic-hypomaturation
Enamel, hypoplastic-hypomaturation-taurodontism
Microdontia, generalized

Excludes:

Enamel defects associated with extrinsic causes
Enamel defects associated with generalized diseases
Enamel defects associated with syndromes
Isolated taurodontism-trichodentoosseous, isolated
Teeth, enamel hypoplasia (0342)
Teeth, snow-capped (2136)

Major Diagnostic Criteria: All or most teeth have defective enamel and other possible causes have been eliminated.

Clinical Findings: Clinical, X-ray and histologic features vary according to type of amelogenesis. Both primary and permanent dentitions are affected unless otherwise noted. Anterior open bite is common in the severe hypoplastic and hypocalcified types. Several types have been deliniated:

Type I, Hypoplastic The enamel does not develop to normal thickness. On X-ray, the enamel contrasts normally from dentin.

Type IA, The hypoplastic, pitted autosomal dominant type has enamel with random pits from pinpoint to pinhead size, located primarily on labial or buccal surfaces in permanent teeth, often arranged in rows and columns. Some teeth may appear normal in both dentitions.

Type IB, The hypoplastic, local autosomal dominant type may affect only primary teeth or teeth in both dentitions. Pits and grooves of hypoplastic enamel occur in a horizontal fashion across the middle third of the tooth. All or only some teeth show this defect. Most frequently affected are the incisors, premolars, or primary molars.

Type IC, The hypoplastic, local autosomal recessive type is more severe than the dominant type. Nearly all teeth are affected in both dentitions. Type IC has been described by Chosack et al (1979).

Type ID, The hypoplastic, smooth autosomal dominant type, in which the enamel is generally thin so the crowns frequently do not meet at contact points. The enamel is hard, glossy, smooth, and varies from white to yellow-brown in color, except at contact points, where it may be hypocalcified and stained. X-rays show a thin layer of enamel outlining the crown. Unerupted teeth that undergo intraalveolar resorption are frequent. Small calcified bodies may be seen adjacent to unerupted teeth. Anterior open bite occurs in about 50%.

Type IE, The hypoplastic, smooth X-linked dominant type affects males who have enamel that is thin, brown to yellow-brown, smooth, and shiny. Carrier females have alternating vertical bands of normal and abnormal enamel (Lyon effect). X-rays of male teeth show a thin layer of enamel outlining the crowns. Unerupted teeth with resorption of crowns are less frequently seen here than in types ID, IF, IG, and IIA. Anterior open bite occurs in most males and in about one-half of affected females. X-rays of female teeth show vertical banding of the enamel.

Type IF, The hypoplastic, rough autosomal dominant type is associated with a thin, brown, very hard enamel, which has a granular vitreous surface. Contact between adjacent teeth is lacking. On X-ray, the teeth are outlined by a thin layer of enamel. There is high contrast between the enamel and dentin. Unerupted teeth with resorption of crowns may occur. Anterior open bite occurs in about 50% of cases.

Type IG, The enamel agenesis autosomal recessive type has a rough, granular tooth surface and is light yellow-brown in color. Adjacent teeth lack contact. There is no X-ray evidence of enamel, and many teeth are unerupted and partially resorbed in the alveolus. On microscopic examination the only evidence of enamel is the laminated agate-like vitreous calcification on the dentin surface. Anterior open bite occurs frequently, 9:11. It is not known if this type is different from enamel agenesis and nephrocalcinosis.

Type II, Hypomaturation The enamel is of normal thickness but has a mottled appearance, is slightly softer than normal enamel, and chips from the crown. On X-ray, the enamel has approximately the same radiodensity as dentin.

Type IIA, The hypomaturation, pigmented autosomal recessive type has enamel that is clear to cloudy, mottled, agar-brown in color, and of normal thickness. The enamel fractures from the dentin and is softer than normal, admitting a probe point under pressure. X-rays show lack of contrast between enamel and dentin. Unerupted teeth with resorption of the crowns are uncommon. Anterior open bite occurs infrequently.

Type IIB, The hypomaturation, X-linked recessive type. In affected males, the enamel of the primary teeth is ground glass white, whereas the enamel of the permanent teeth is mottled yellow. The enamel is soft and will admit the point of a probe under pressure. The condition Lyonizes in females, where the primary teeth have random alternating vertical bands of abnormal ground glass white enamel with bands of translucent normal enamel. The permanent teeth have random alternating vertical bands of either opaque white or opaque yellow enamel with bands of translucent normal enamel. Transillumination aids the diagnosis in females. In males, the X-ray contrast between enamel and dentin is reduced in comparison with normal enamel; in females, no defects are observed.

Type IIC and IID See **Teeth, snow-capped.**

Type III, Hypocalcified The enamel initially develops normal thickness, is orange-yellow at eruption, and consists of poorly calcified matrix, which is rapidly lost, leaving dentin cores. On X-ray, the enamel is less radiopaque than dentin.

Type IIIA, The hypocalcified, autosomal dominant type is characterized by unerupted and newly erupted teeth covered by a light yellow-brown to orange-colored enamel of normal thickness. After eruption, the enamel becomes brown to black from food stains. It is friable, soft, and rapidly lost by attrition. By 10–12 years of age, only dentin cores remain. The cervical enamel may be better calcified. It is associated with anterior open bite frequently (22:26). The teeth are sensitive to temperature changes. On X-ray, the enamel is less radiopaque than the dentin. The crowns have a moth-eaten appearance with a radiodense line of calcified enamel at the cervical edge. Teeth accumulate heavy deposits of calculus.

Type IV, Hypoplastic-hypocalcified with taurodontism The enamel is less than normal in thickness and mottled. Molar teeth have a taurodontic shape. On X-ray, the enamel has approximately the same radiodensity as dentin.

Type IVA, The hypoplastic-hypomaturation type associated with taurodontic molar teeth is distinct from the **Tricho-dento-osseous**

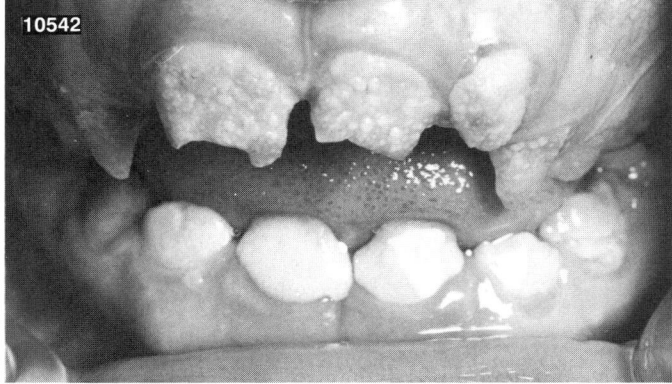

0046-10542: Amelogenesis imperfecta, hypocalcified type.

syndrome, lacking the nail, hair, and bone changes of the latter. The enamel is mottled, has a yellow-brown color, and is pitted and thin. Large pulp chambers may occur in single rooted teeth. On X-ray, the enamel is thin and rough and has about the same radiodensity as dentin.

Complications: Among 50 patients: psychologic distress may occur or be aggravated by unsightly teeth 40/50; early tooth loss 46/50; prone to periodontal disease 25/50; sensitivity to hot and cold 24/50; pulpal exposure from attrition 8/50.

Associated Findings: Anterior open bite was found in 22/26 with the hypocalcified autosomal dominant type; in 22/22 men and in 18/30 women with the hypoplastic, smooth X-linked dominant type; and in 15/29 with the hypoplastic rough autosomal dominant type.

Etiology: Inherited as autosomal dominant, autosomal recessive, or X-linked depending upon type. It is not known whether the autosomal traits and the X-linked traits represent genes at different loci or if they represent alleles.

Pathogenesis: Structural defects in enamel formation. The primary protein defect is unknown. In the hypoplastic forms there is a failure of ameloblasts to lay down an enamel matrix of full thickness. It is my opinion that in the thin enamel type the defect is primarily in the ameloblast, while in the pitted forms there may be a vascular defect of the enamel organ. In the hypocalcified types full thickness of the enamel matrix is produced but fails to calcify normally. Scanning electron microscopy shows a defect in the so-called enamel sheath in hypomaturation types. Degeneration of the end-stage enamel organ is associated with resorption of unerupted tooth crowns.

MIM No.: *10450, *10453, 13090, *20470, *30110, *30120

Sex Ratio: Autosomal dominant and recessive types M1:F1; X-linked dominant type M1:F2; X-linked recessive type M1:F0 (if females who have a mild defect detectable by special examination are included, M1:F2).

Occurrence: 1:16,000 in North American Caucasians.

Risk of Recurrence for Patient's Sib:
See Part I, *Mendelian Inheritance.*

Risk of Recurrence for Patient's Child:
See Part I, *Mendelian Inheritance.*

Age of Detectability: At the time of eruption of teeth; 1–2 years by visual examination.

Gene Mapping and Linkage: AIH2 (amelogenesis imperfecta 2, hypocalcification (autosomal dominant)) has been tentatively mapped to unassigned.
AIH1 (amelogenesis imperfecta 1, hypomaturation or hypoplastic (?=AMG & AMGS)) has been mapped to Xp22.
AMG (amelogenin (?=AMGS & AIH)) has been mapped to Xp22.31-p22.1.
Types IE and IIB are X-chromosomal.

Prevention: None known. Genetic counseling indicated.

Treatment: Excellent results in all types with full crown restorations and composite resins for less severe types. Orthodontic procedure for open bite. Desensitizing toothpaste may be used.

Prognosis: Early loss of teeth by attrition, pulp exposure, and periodontal disease if untreated. With restoration, normal life span of teeth can be maintained.

Detection of Carrier: In the recessive type this is not possible. In the X-linked recessive type, alternating vertical stripes of normal translucent enamel and opaque yellow-white abnormal enamel occur, which can best be seen on transillumination.

Special Considerations: Dental restoration at an early age is recommended to avoid psychosocial trauma. Nearly all patients (80 of the 100 patients seen to date) have shown marked psychosocial affects from their unsightly teeth. With treatment there has been a marked improvement in their personality and social relations with others; however, a few individuals who had used their defect to elicit attention from family members had negative reactions after restoration.

References:
Witkop CJ Jr, Rao SR: Inherited defects in tooth structure. BD:OAS 1971:VII(7):153–184. †
Winter GB, Brook AH: Enamel hypoplasia and anomalies of the enamel. Dent Clin North Am 1975; 19:3–24. †
Witkop CJ Jr, Sauk JJ Jr: Defects of enamel. In: Stewart RE, Prescott GH, eds: Oral facial genetics. St. Louis: CV Mosby Co., 1976:151–226. * †
Chosack A, et al.: Amelogenesis imperfecta among Israeli Jews and the description of a new type of local hypoplastic autosomal recessive amelogenesis imperfecta. Oral Surg 1979; 47:148–156. †
Congleton J, Burkes EJ: Amelogenesis imperfecta with taurodontism. Oral Surg 1979; 48:540–544. †
Escobar VH, et al.: A clinical, genetic, and ultrastructural study of snow-capped teeth: amelogenesis imperfecta, hypomaturation type. Oral Surg 1981; 52:607–614. †

WI043   **Carl J. Witkop, Jr.**

TEETH, ANKYLODONTIA, MULTIPLE HERITABLE TYPE   **2243**

Includes:
　Ankylodontia, multiple heritable type
　Dental eruption, arrested
　Eruption failure of the permanent dentition
　Hypercementosis

Excludes: N/A

Major Diagnostic Criteria: Malocclusion characterized by partial eruption of the permanent dentition; percussion dullness of the teeth; X-ray hypercementosis, and absence of periodontal ligament space.

Clinical Findings: Malocclusion characterized by partial eruption of the permanent dentition; percussion dullness of the teeth; X-ray hypercementosis, and absence of periodontal ligament space.

Complications: Unknown.

Associated Findings: None known.

Etiology: Autosomal dominant inheritance with high penetrance.

Pathogenesis: Unknown.

Sex Ratio: M1:F1

Occurrence: Six cases from two families have been reported.

Risk of Recurrence for Patient's Sib:
See Part I, *Mendelian Inheritance.*

Risk of Recurrence for Patient's Child:
See Part I, *Mendelian Inheritance.*

Age of Detectability: After six years of age.

Gene Mapping and Linkage: Unknown.

Prevention: None known. Genetic counseling indicated.

Treatment: Unknown. Orthodontic therapy ineffective.

Prognosis: Masticatory function compromised; difficult dental extractions.

Detection of Carrier: Clinical examination confirmed by X-ray.

References:
Humerfelt A, Reitan K: Effects of hypercementosis on the movability of teeth during orthodontic treatment. Angle Orthod 1966; 36:179–189.
Shokeir MHK: Complete failure of eruption of all permanent teeth: an autosomal dominant disorder. Clin Genet 1974; 5:322–326.
Israel H: Early hypercementosis and arrested dental eruption: heritable multiple ankylodontia. J Craniofac Genet Dev Biol 1984; 4:243–246.

IS002   **Harry Israel**

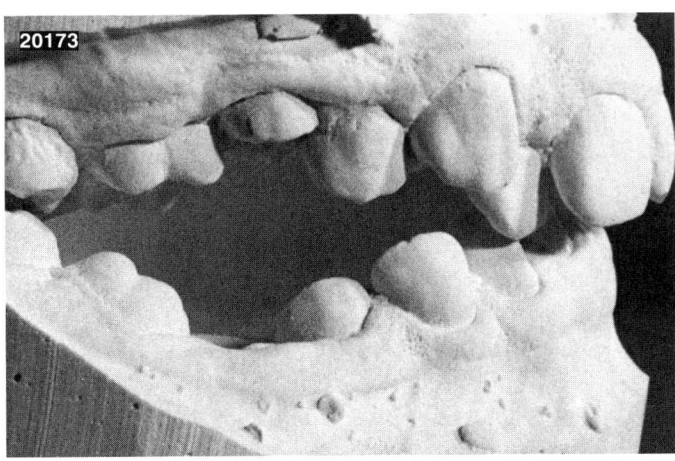

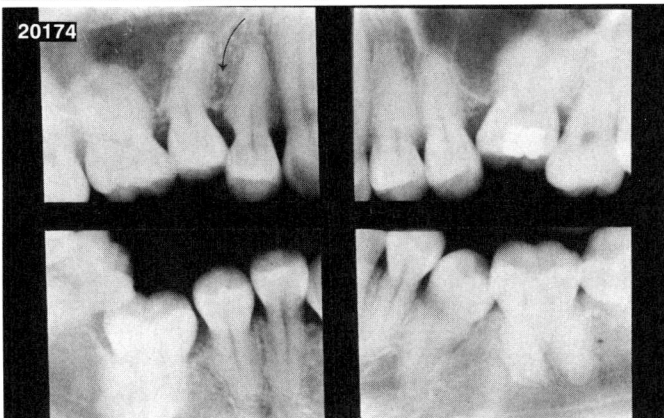

2243-20173: The extreme degree of arrested dental development has created severe malocclusion. 20174: Hypercementosis and reduction of the periodontal ligament spaces are evident throughout. The arrow defines an especially obvious site.

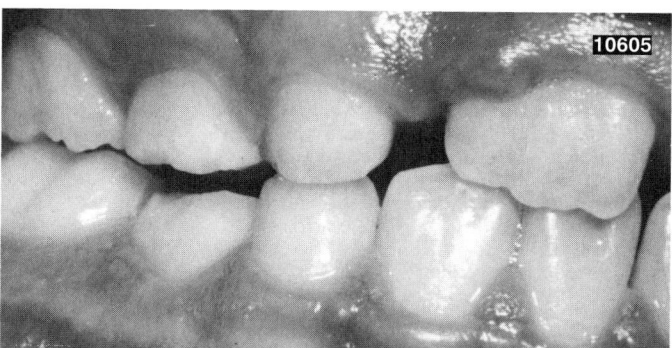

0927-10605: Ankylosed mandibular first primary molar.

TEETH, ANKYLOSED   0927

Includes:
> Ankylosed teeth
> Submerged teeth

Excludes:
> **Teeth, dens invaginatus** (0276)
> **Teeth, dilacerated** (0929)
> **Teeth, fused** (0930)
> **Teeth, geminated** (0931)
> **Teeth, impacted** (0932)
> **Teeth, molar reinclusion** (2137)
> **Teeth, root concrescence** (0928)

Major Diagnostic Criteria: The occlusal surface of the affected tooth is situated below the plane of occlusion, and the tooth lacks mobility to manual rocking.

Clinical Findings: A fusion of tooth cementum and bone, occurring anywhere along path of eruption, either before or after emergence of tooth into the mouth. The condition may affect any tooth, but the mandibular first primary molar is most frequently involved. Ankylosis becomes clinically apparent by 1) occlusal plane of tooth beneath the plane of occlusion of adjacent teeth, 2) clinical crown height less than that of adjacent teeth, and 3) immobility to manual rocking. A solid sound on percussion and X-ray evidence of partial obliteration of periodontal ligament are nonessential criteria for diagnosis. The interproximal alveolar bone height is below that of adjacent unaffected teeth.

Complications: Difficulty extracting the affected tooth, noneruption of succedaneous tooth, supereruption of opposing tooth/ teeth, tipping of adjacent teeth, loss of arch length, and possible development of malocclusion or local periodontal pathology.

Associated Findings: Subsequent to dental caries, there may be pulpal exposure, periapical infection, granuloma, cyst formation, and loss of teeth, followed by possible drifting and development of malocclusion. On occasion, ankylosis of primary teeth may be associated with congenitally missing succedaneous teeth. Lack of alveolar bone height may predispose to local periodontal pathology. Enamel opacity, hypoplasia, and malformed teeth in association with ankylosed molars have been reported in the permanent dentition.

Etiology: Undetermined, but a genetic or congenital gap in periodontal ligament is cited as an intrinsic causative factor. Chemical or thermal irritation, disturbed local metabolism, infection, local mechanical trauma, and reimplantation of evulsed tooth are cited as extrinsic causative factors.

Pathogenesis: The affected tooth has an area of cemental root resorption repaired by osteoid-like tissue which is continuous with alveolar bone. Periodontal ligament may become increasingly obliterated in affected area.

Sex Ratio: M1:F1

Occurrence: Reported in a United States study to affect 6.9% of primary molar teeth; very rare in secondary teeth unless they are traumatized. The prevalence in other world population groups is reported to range from 14.2% to 35.2%.

Risk of Recurrence for Patient's Sib: Significantly increased over population incidence.

Risk of Recurrence for Patient's Child: Unknown.

Age of Detectability: When adjacent teeth have reached occlusal plane, by clinical or X-ray examination.

Gene Mapping and Linkage: Unknown.

Prevention: Avoidance of extrinsic causative factors.

Treatment: Extraction of affected tooth, artificial restoration of proximal and occlusal contacts, or leaving tooth undisturbed. In some instances extraction may be delayed and the tooth utilized as a space maintainer until the succedaneous tooth is ready to erupt. Presence of succedaneous tooth should be established prior to extracting the affected tooth. Extraction of an ankylosed tooth usually requires vertical sectioning of the tooth and surgical removal of each section. Affected mandibular first primary molars are likely to exfoliate normally, and early extraction is not indicated. Affected maxillary and mandibular second primary molars tend to become severely affected, with marked absence of alveolar bone growth, and they do not exfoliate normally. Such teeth should be extracted.

Prognosis: *Treated:* Excellent. If there is no succedaneous tooth, a partially restored ankylosed tooth can serve well indefinitely. Periodic replacement of the restoration may be required as changes occur in surrounding alveolar bone. Alveolar bone height will always be lower than that of adjacent unaffected teeth.

Untreated: Tooth will not erupt to the plane of occlusion and surrounding alveolar bone height will not develop. Mandibular first primary molars are likely to exfoliate normally. Maxillary and mandibular second primary molars tend to become severely affected and tend not to exfoliate normally. In addition, there may be complications as listed above. The condition does not appear to affect longevity of patient.

Detection of Carrier: Unknown.

References:

Via WF: Submerged deciduous molars: familial tendencies. J Am Dent Assoc 1964; 69:127–129.

Biederman WB: The problem of the ankylosed tooth. Dent Clin North Am 1968; 24:409–424.

Brearley LJ, McKibben DH Jr: Ankylosis of primary molar teeth. I. Prevalence and characteristics. II: a longitudinal study. J Dent Child 1973; 40:54–63.

Darling AI, Levers BGH: Submerged human deciduous molars and ankylosis. Arch Oral Biol 1973; 18:1021–1040.

Messer LB, Cline JT: Ankylosed primary molars: results and treatment recommendations from an eight-year longitudinal study. Pediatr Dent 1980; 2:37–47.

Koyoumdjisky-Kaye E, Steigman S: Ethnic variability in the prevalence of submerged primary molars. J Dent Res 1982; 61:1401–1404.

MC021

D. H. McKibben, Jr.
Louise Brearley Messer

TEETH, ANODONTIA, PARTIAL OR COMPLETE 2134

Includes:
Hypodontia
Oligodontia, isolated
Teeth, congenitally missing

Excludes:
Anodontia associated with syndromes, diseases, or extrinsic causes
Ectodermal dysplasia (all)
Hypodontia in/from syndromes, diseases, or extrinsic causes
Oligodontia, not isolated
Schizodontism
Teeth, ankylosed (0927)
Teeth, impacted (0932)
Teeth, microdontia (0660)
Teeth, pegged or absent maxillary lateral incisor (0934)
Teeth, root concrescence (0928)

Major Diagnostic Criteria: Congenital absence of one or more teeth in the primary or the permanent dentition in the absence of associated systemic malformations.

Clinical Findings: Congenital agenesis of one or more teeth may occur in both the deciduous and permanent dentitions, although it appears more often in the permanent teeth. The most commonly affected teeth are the third molars: one, two, or all of them may be absent. The maxillary lateral incisors and second mandibular bicuspids are also frequently missing. The mandibular lateral incisors and first molars are rarely affected.

When deciduous teeth are involved, the succedaneous permanent teeth will usually be missing as well. Various degrees and combinations as to right or left side may occur within individuals and within kindreds. Because of the missing teeth, occlusion is usually defective in these children. An oral soft tissue examination generally shows no abnormalities. X-ray examination must be carried out to confirm the agenesis and a detailed dental history obtained in order to rule out extractions and trauma.

A positive family history for one or more missing teeth in combination with the lack of an environmental insult to explain causation are usual. In many kindreds, congenital absence of teeth and microdontia occur simultaneously either in the same individual, or in different individuals i.e., one person will have microdontia and another has agenesis. This finding suggested that microdontia and hypodontia/anodontia were expressions of the same genetic character and may constitute phenotypic variations of a continuous spectrum of tooth size diminution.

Complications: The most obvious complications are malocclusion, drifting of teeth, diastemas between present teeth. In severe cases, the patients are almost edentulous and their facial appearance becomes an important factor. Nutritional deficiencies might occur in these children, since they are unable to chew.

The most commonly mentioned finding in children with severe hypodontia is their psychologic status. The lack of teeth gives them an undesirable facial profile. Several reports show these children to be shy, secluded, and isolated from their peers. Fortunately, the number of severely affected children is low. Most affected individuals only have one or two missing teeth.

Associated Findings: Possibly microdontia.

Etiology: Family studies suggest that hypodontia/anodontia is a hereditary trait, although the mode of transmission is unclear. Many investigators consider hypodontia to be the result of a single gene, often transmitted as an autosomal dominant with incomplete penetrance and variable expressivity, or as an X-linked dominant phenotype. Others consider it to be a multifactorial trait. The best data suggested that hypodontia was an autosomal dominant phenotype. These data have been reanalyzed twice, using different methods. The autosomal dominant hypothesis was confirmed in one, while in the other, a multifactorial model provided a better fit to the data.

Pathogenesis: Absence of tooth development is the major reason hypodontia occurs, but why teeth fail to develop is unclear. However, destruction of the dental lamina, space limitations, and competition for minimum nutritional requirements causing regressions and agenesis, functional abnormalities of the dental epithelium, and failure of induction of the underlying mesenchyme have all been implicated in the production of hypodontia.

MIM No.: *10660, *20678, 31350

Sex Ratio: Presumably M1:F1. (M1:F1.3 observed).

Occurrence: Varies among different populations. The prevalence of hypodontia of the secondary dentition of Caucasians ranged from 2.3 to 9.6%; Hawaiians, 1.7%; American Blacks, 2.0%; Japanese, 1.1%; and Chinese, 0.15%. The frequency of the individual teeth involved also varies: the third molars are the most commonly affected teeth, followed by maxillary lateral incisors, then lower mandibular bicuspids.

The incidence of anodontia is 0.5% of Swedish children. Hypodontia is found in the primary dentition of 5% of Japanese children; and in between 0.1 and 0.7% of Caucasians.

Risk of Recurrence for Patient's Sib:
See Part I, *Mendelian Inheritance.* Empiric risk is 0.82.

Risk of Recurrence for Patient's Child:
See Part I, *Mendelian Inheritance.*

Age of Detectability: After eight years of age for the permanent dentition, by X-ray examination.

Gene Mapping and Linkage: Unknown.

Prevention: None known. Genetic counseling indicated.

Treatment: Prosthetic replacement and orthodontic treatment.

Prognosis: Normal life span. Patients adapt quite well to the use of prosthetic devices.

Detection of Carrier: Examination of relatives for evidence of the trait.

Special Considerations: The term, "hypodontia" should be used to describe the absence of one or more teeth. The term "oligodontia" is commonly used in the literature and is intended in many cases to be used interchangeably with hypodontia. However, the term oligodontia should be reserved for those instances when hypodontia is part of a multi-system condition or syndrome. Furthermore, the term oligodontia may be used preferably to describe the absence of numerous teeth (compared with relatively fewer teeth implied by the use of the term hypodontia). Anodontia, the complete absence of teeth, is the most extreme example of oligodontia.

Although hypodontia seems to be a hereditary trait which more likely follows an autosomal dominant inheritance pattern, its phenotypic expression in members of the same family is variable.

The ratios of affected to normal individuals are also variable and suggest that, although this is a genetic trait, environmental effects and gene-gene interaction also play a significant role in its production and expression.

References:

Dahlberg AA: Inherited congenital absence of six incisors, deciduous and permanent. J Dent Res 1937; 16:59–62.

Juarez CK, Spence A: The genetics of hypodontia. J Dent Res 1974; 53:781–783.

Graber LW: Congenital absence of teeth: a review with emphasis on inheritance patterns. J Am Dent Assoc 1978; 96:266–275.

Burzynski N, Escobar V: Classification and genetics of numeric anomalies of the dentition. BD:OAS XIX(1). New York: March of Dimes Birth Defects Foundation, 1983:95–106.

Witkop CJ, Jr.: Agenesis of succedaneous teeth: an expression of the homozygous state of the gene for the pegged or missing maxillary lateral incisor trait. Am J Med Genet 1987; 26:431–436.

ES000   **Victor Escobar**

Teeth, anterior permanent, flame-shaped pulp chambers
 See TEETH, DENTIN DYSPLASIA, CORONAL
Teeth, carnivore-like
 See TEETH, LOBODONTIA
Teeth, congenital
 See TEETH, NATAL OR NEONATAL
Teeth, congenitally missing
 See TEETH, ANODONTIA, PARTIAL OR COMPLETE
Teeth, conical, multiple
 See TEETH, LOBODONTIA
Teeth, conical-clefting-ectropion
 See CLEFTING-ECTROPION-CONICAL TEETH
Teeth, connate
 See TEETH, FUSED

TEETH, DEFECTS FROM TETRACYCLINE   0341

Includes:

Brown teeth
Enamel and dentin defects from tetracycline
Grey teeth
Tetracycline discoloration of enamel and dentin
Yellow teeth

Excludes:

Teeth, amelogenesis imperfecta (0046)
Teeth, dentinogenesis imperfecta (0279)
Teeth, enamel and dentin defects from erythroblastosis fetalis (0340)

Major Diagnostic Criteria: Yellow, brown or grey discoloration of teeth, distributed in horizontal bands and exhibiting yellow fluorescence under ultraviolet light.

Clinical Findings: Yellow, brown or grey discoloration of enamel and dentin of teeth. Seen most frequently in primary dentition. In severe cases, some enamel of primary molars and cuspids and secondary incisors and molars may be hypoplastic or missing. Incidence is variable, depending upon use of tetracyclines in community in early years of child's life and length of period of administration. Exposure to sunlight may change yellow color to brownish grey. In ultraviolet light affected areas fluoresce pale to bright yellow, although fluorescence may be lost in teeth whose color has changed to brownish grey.

Complications: Attrition of the hypoplastic tooth structure.

Associated Findings: Staining of bones.

Etiology: Tetracycline administered during the period of tooth calcification. Primary dentition is affected when drug is given during the last 2 months of intrauterine life to 9 months of age. The anterior teeth of the secondary dentition may be affected if administration occurs between birth and 5 years. The degree of involvement depends on total dose. Where this exceeds 100 mg/kg (30–35 mg/kg/day) in first few months of life, discoloration and hypoplasia of enamel of primary dentition can be expected in 90% or more cases. Where drug is given to premature infants shortly after birth, hypoplasia of enamel is more likely to occur.

Involvement of secondary dentition is less common and unlikely with a normal single course of administration but may affect severely the anterior teeth if drug is given over a period of months during the first 5 years of life.

Tetracycline hydrochloride, demethylchlortetracycline and chlortetracycline produce a yellower discoloration than oxytetracycline which causes a paler creamy color. Incidence with long acting new tetracyclines not known.

Pathogenesis: Tetracycline is deposited in developing dentin and enamel.

Sex Ratio: M1:F1

Occurrence: Variable. Depends upon the use of tetracyclines in the community. Prevalence varies with year and age of children. When last studied in the United States, in children 4–12 years of age, 1:24 (urban) and 1:71 (rural) in 1964 and 1:7 (urban) in 1966. Use of tetracycline in pregnant women has since been discontinued.

When total dose exceeds 100 mg/kg in the first 12 months, discoloration and hypoplasia of primary dentition occurs in at least 90% of cases. Dose required to produce changes in secondary dentition not known.

Risk of Recurrence for Patient's Sib: Related directly to tetracycline exposure.

Risk of Recurrence for Patient's Child: Related directly to tetracycline exposure.

Age of Detectability: After eruption of teeth.

Gene Mapping and Linkage: N/A

Prevention: Do not give tetracycline in any form during last 2 months of pregnancy or during first 5 years of life.

Treatment: In general, no treatment. Esthetic crowns may be considered for older children with severe discoloration or hypoplasia of anterior secondary teeth.

Prognosis: No effect on general health. Teeth may change color and become either darker or lighter with exposure to sunlight. Psychosocial problems may develop in person with severely stained and hypoplastic teeth.

Detection of Carrier: Unknown.

References:

Wallman IS, Hilton HB: Teeth pigmented by tetracycline. Lancet 1962; I:827.

Witkop CJ Jr, Wolf RO: Hypoplasia and intrinsic staining of enamel following tetracycline therapy. JAMA 1963; 185:100.

WA015   **I.S. Wallman**

TEETH, DENS INVAGINATUS   0276

Includes:

Dens invaginatus
Dens telescopes
Dilated composite odontome
Gestant odontome
Radix in radice

Excludes:

Dens evaginatus
Teeth, lobodontia (0607)

Major Diagnostic Criteria: An anomalous invagination of tooth structure, involving the crown or root, in which the outer surface of enamel or cementum is continuous with the inner layer. Diagnosis confirmed by X-ray.

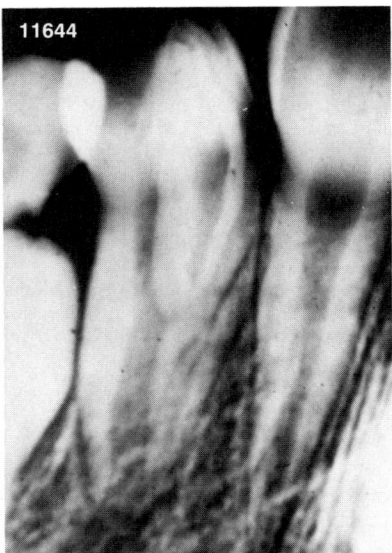

0276-11644: X-ray shows "tooth within a tooth" appearance.

Clinical Findings: This is a relatively common dental anomaly that is often bilateral. The maxillary permanent dentition is usually affected: most commonly the lateral incisors and less frequently the central incisors, premolars, and molars. It is occasionally found in mandibular permanent teeth, usually premolars. It has been reported in supernumerary teeth and is exceedingly rare in the deciduous dentition. Most cases of dens invaginatus involve the crown. Clinically the crown may be normal or conical, peg-, or barrel-shaped, with a pit or groove on the lingual/occlusal surface. X-ray examination is necessary for accurate diagnosis and management and is especially beneficial prior to tooth eruption.

The invagination may have a direct communication with the pulp chamber or it may have a thin wall of dental hard tissue. This area is susceptible to the accumulation of debris and bacterial invasion with subsequent pulpal necrosis. Pulpal necrosis may occur in the newly erupted tooth.

Classification of dens invaginatus is as follows:
Type 1: confined to tooth crown, an accentuated lingual pit may be considered a minor form.
Type 2: involves crown and root.
Type 3: involves crown and root and has a periapical or periodontal foramen.

On X-ray examination there are small, inverted, pear-shaped areas of enamel within the pulp cavity, which may extend to the apex in the more severe forms. This often suggests the appearance of a tooth within a tooth. The more severe forms are likely to be associated with dilation of the tooth.

Complications: Pulpal necrosis may occur before root formation is complete. A periapical abscess, cyst, or granuloma may occur.

Associated Findings: Has been reported in association with **Teeth, microdontia** and **Teeth, taurodontism** with **Teeth, dentinogenesis imperfecta**, and with ameloblastoma.

Etiology: Possibly autosomal dominant inheritance.

Pathogenesis: One or more invaginations of the enamel organ or Hertwig's epithelial root sheath into the dental papilla of the developing tooth. It is theorized that these invaginations may result from focal growth retardation or proliferation or from increased external pressure.

MIM No.: 12530

Sex Ratio: M1:F1

Occurrence: 0.04–10% is reported incidence (3% of 3,000 Swedish children and 1.7% of Saudi Arabians). Prevalence is 0.25–5.2%.

Risk of Recurrence for Patient's Sib:
See Part I, *Mendelian Inheritance*. Observed frequency, 32%.

Risk of Recurrence for Patient's Child:
See Part I, *Mendelian Inheritance*. Observed frequency, 43%.

Age of Detectability: Prior to eruption by X-ray examination.

Gene Mapping and Linkage: Unknown.

Prevention: None known. Genetic counseling indicated.

Treatment: Eruption of a tooth exhibiting dens invaginatus may be anticipated if detected by X-ray. Upon eruption, or after removal of the soft tissue just prior to eruption, the invagination on the labial/occlusal surface may be prophylactically sealed or a dental restoration placed.

Teeth with pulpal necrosis may require apexification if root formation is incomplete, conventional root canal therapy with or without apicoectomy and retrograde restoration, or, in the extreme case, extraction.

Prognosis: Prophylactic dental restoration will prevent pulpal necrosis in most cases. Once pulpal involvement occurs the tooth may be retained in the majority of cases by using a variety of endodontic procedures. In addition to the pulpal considerations, anomalous crown shapes may compromise periodontal health and require restorative procedures. Extraction is necessary in only the rare case today.

Detection of Carrier: Unknown.

References:
Oehlers FAC: Dens invaginatus (dilated composite odontome). I. variations of the invagination process and associated crown forms. Oral Surg 1957; 10:1204–1218.
Grahnen H: Dens invaginatus I. A clinical, roentgenological and genetic study of permanent upper lateral incisors. Odontol Rev 1959; 10:115–137.
Ferguson FS: Successful apexification technique in an immature tooth with dens in dente. Oral Surg 1980; 49:356–359.
De Smit A, Demaut L: Nonsurgical endodontic treatment of invaginated teeth. J Endodont 1982; 8:506–511.
Ruprecht A, et al.: The incidence of dental invagination. J Pedodont 1986; 10:265–272.

ZU002   **Susan L. Zunt**

TEETH, DENTIN DYSPLASIA, CORONAL   **0277**

Includes:
  Coronal dentin dysplasia
  Dentin dysplasia, coronal
  Dentin dysplasia, type II
  Pulp stones
  Teeth, anterior permanent, flame-shaped pulp chambers
  Teeth, pulpal dysplasia
  Teeth, thistle-shaped pulp chambers

Excludes:
  Branchio-skeleto-genital syndrome (0118)
  Calcinosis
  Dentino-osseous dysplasia (0280)
  Ehlers-Danlos syndrome (0338)
  Fibrous dysplasia of dentin
  Osteogenesis imperfecta (0777)
  Teeth, dentin dysplasia, radicular (0278)
  Teeth, dentinogenesis imperfecta (0279)
  Teeth, odontodysplasia (0739)

Major Diagnostic Criteria: Opalescent, brownish-blue primary teeth and normal-appearing permanent teeth. On X-ray, primary teeth have obliterated pulp chambers; anterior permanent teeth have flame- or thistle-shaped pulp chambers; molars have bow-tie-shaped pulp chambers.

Must be differentiated from **Teeth, dentinogenesis imperfecta** in which teeth of both dentitions are opalescent.

Clinical Findings: Primary teeth are brownish-blue with a translucent opalescent sheen and are identical in appearance with teeth seen in **Teeth, dentinogenesis imperfecta (0279)**. Permanent teeth are

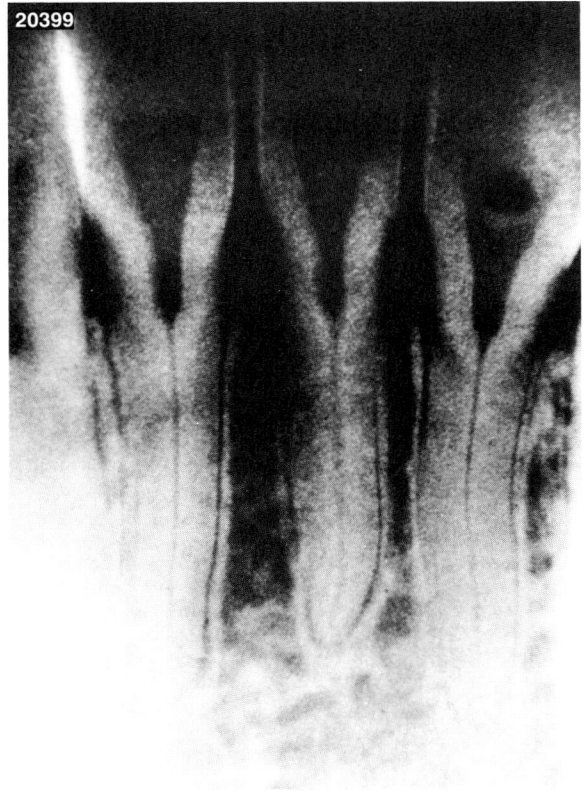

0277A-20399:   Thistle-tube pulps in dentin dysplasia.

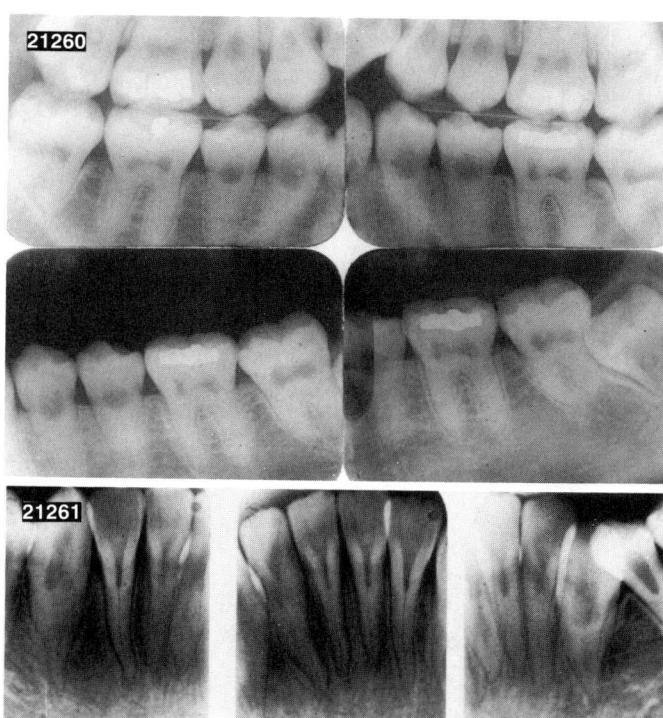

0277C-21260–61:   Dentin dysplasia, coronal; permanent molars have bow-tie–shaped chambers and premolars and incisors have large flame-shaped chambers with flat apical floors. Teeth are of normal color.

normal in color, size, and shape. By X-ray, the primary teeth have obliterated pulp chambers and reduced root canals. Anterior permanent teeth have flame-shaped pulp chambers, often with a radicular extension with or without pulp stones. Molar teeth have bow-tie-shaped pulp chambers. Root formation in permanent teeth is usually normal. Primary teeth abrade rapidly.

Complications: Crowns of primary teeth rapidly lost by attrition.

Associated Findings: None known.

Etiology: Autosomal dominant inheritance.

Pathogenesis: Undetermined. The dentin of primary teeth is amorphous, resembling a gray granular gelatin with vestiges of tubule formation. The permanent teeth coronally have normal tubular dentin. The radicular dentin has a transition zone in which tubular, atubular, and fibrous dentin is admixed. Osteo- and

tubular denticles may occur in the pulp chamber, which is flame-shaped. With age, the pulp chamber becomes partially obliterated in permanent teeth.

MIM No.:   *12542

Sex Ratio: M1:F1

Occurrence: Rare. Approximately 80 kindreds have been reported or are known.

Risk of Recurrence for Patient's Sib:
See Part I, *Mendelian Inheritance*.

Risk of Recurrence for Patient's Child:
See Part I, *Mendelian Inheritance*.

Age of Detectability: At age nine to 18 months, upon eruption of primary teeth by visual and X-ray examination.

Gene Mapping and Linkage: Unknown.

Prevention: None known. Genetic counseling indicated.

Treatment: Crowning of primary teeth. Resin bonded restorations.

Prognosis: Premature loss of teeth may be slightly increased.

Detection of Carrier: Unknown.

Special Considerations: Pulpal dysplasia is a different condition. It has been seen in two families, and the individuals who have this condition have an associated growth and developmental retardation which is not associated with **Teeth, dentin dysplasia, coronal.**

References:
Shields EP, et al.: A proposed classification for heritable human dentine defects with a description of a new entity. Arch Oral Biol 1973; 18:543–553.
Giansanti JS, Allen JD: Dentin dysplasia, type II, or dentin dysplasia, coronal type. Oral Surg 1974; 38:911–917.

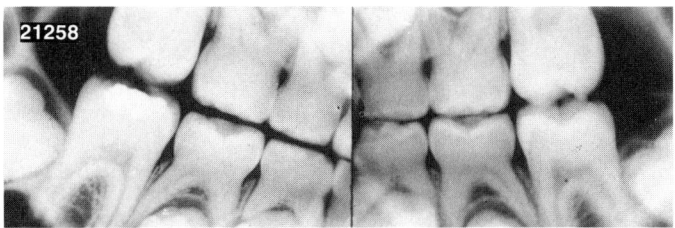

0277B-21258:   Dentin dysplasia, coronal; primary teeth have obliterated pulp chambers shown in the primary molars. Primary teeth are an opalescent brown color and resemble those seen in dentinogenesis imperfecta both clinically and radiographically.

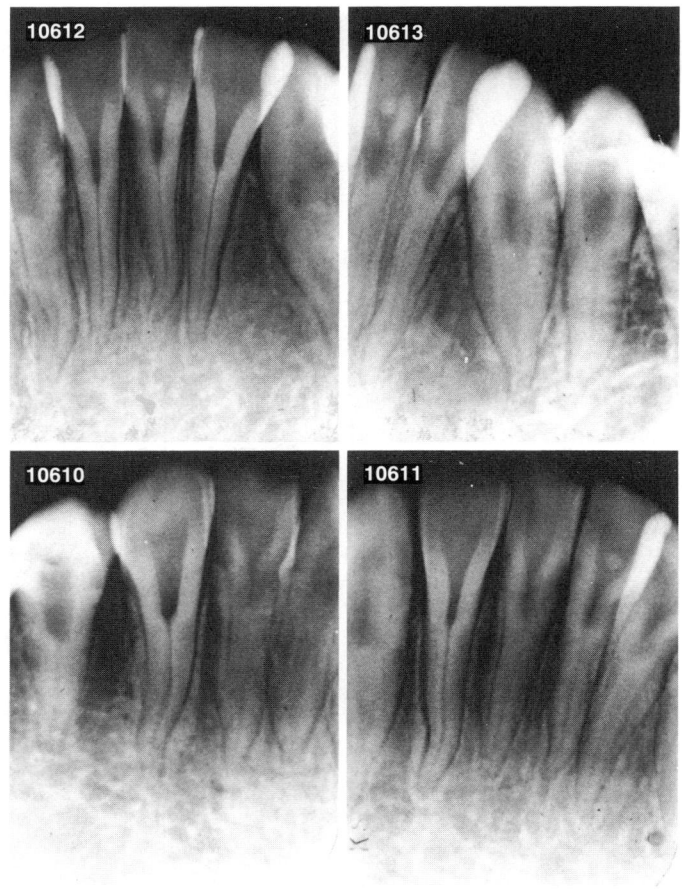

0277D-10610–13:   Thistle-shaped pulp chambers.

Witkop CJ Jr: Hereditary defects of dentin. Dent Clin North Am 1975; 19:25–45.
Melnick M, et al.: Dentin dysplasia, type II: a rare autosomal dominant disorder. Oral Surg 1977; 44:592–599. * †

WI043   **Carl J. Witkop, Jr.**

TEETH, DENTIN DYSPLASIA, RADICULAR   0278

Includes:
  Dentin dysplasia, radicular
  Dentin dysplasia, type I
  Nonopalescent opalescent dentine
  Radicular dentin dysplasia
  Rootless teeth

Excludes:
  Branchio-skeleto-genital syndrome (0118)
  Calcinosis
  Dentino-osseous dysplasia (0280)
  Ehlers-Danlos syndrome (0338)
  Fibrous dysplasia of dentin
  Osteogenesis imperfecta (0777)
  Teeth, dentin dysplasia, coronal (0277)
  Teeth, dentinogenesis imperfecta (0279)
  Teeth, odontodysplasia (0739)

Major Diagnostic Criteria: Generally, teeth are normal in color, but on X-ray examinations they lack pulp chambers or have

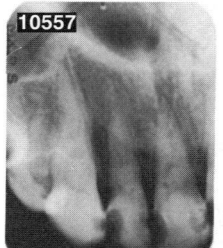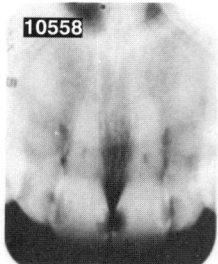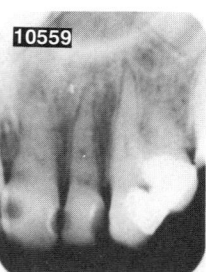

0278A-10557–59:   Radicular dentin dysplasia.

half-moon-shaped pulp chambers and short or abnormally shaped roots.

Clinical Findings: Both dentitions are affected. Teeth are usually normal in color and contour of crowns but may have a bluish-brown hue. Teeth are frequently malaligned in arch with a history of drifting. X-ray changes include absent or half-moon-shaped pulp chambers in 100%, short or abnormally shaped roots in 80%, radiolucent areas around roots in 20%. Coronal dentin and enamel are histologically normal. Radicular and pulp areas filled with foci of dentin formed in the dental papilla surrounded by dentin formed from the normal root development. The histologic picture resembles a stream flowing around boulders. Vascular channels cap the foci of dentin formed in the papilla. Periapical lesions are radicular cysts. Teeth may exfoliate spontaneously or with minor trauma.

Complications: Spontaneous exfoliation of teeth, premature loss of teeth, and destruction of jaws by cyst expansion.

Associated Findings: None known.

Etiology: Autosomal dominant inheritance. Five of 30 propositi have had normal parents, which may indicate either genetic heterogeneity, variable expressivity, or high mutation rate.

Pathogenesis: A defect in the epithelial root sheath, in which epithelial cells invade the dental papilla and induce mesenchymal cells at many foci to undergo transformation to odontoblasts. These odontoblasts lay down multiple areas of dentin, which fuse and become surrounded by a layer of more normal radicular

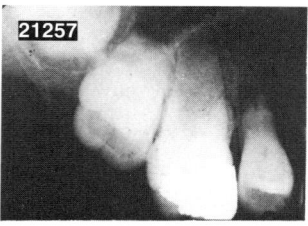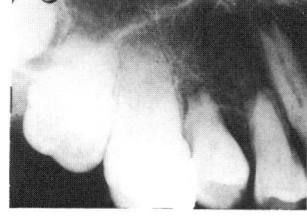
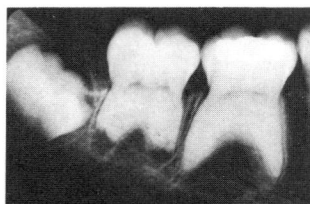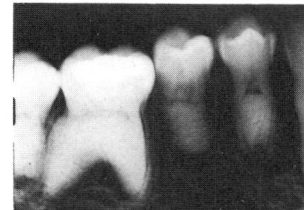

0278B-21257: Radicular dentin dysplasia; pulp chambers are obliterated except for a crescent-shaped area below the coronal dentin. Roots are short and some are surrounded by a radiolucent area in the bone.

dentin, resulting in complete or nearly complete obliteration of pulp chambers, root canals, and short abnormal roots. Epithelial rests undergo cystic degeneration, forming periapical cysts.

MIM No.: *12540

Sex Ratio: M1:F1

Occurrence: 1:50,000 among North American Caucasians.

Risk of Recurrence for Patient's Sib:
See Part I, *Mendelian Inheritance.*

Risk of Recurrence for Patient's Child:
See Part I, *Mendelian Inheritance.*

Age of Detectability: By X-ray examination at time of eruption of teeth, age 9 to 18 months.

Gene Mapping and Linkage: Unknown.

Prevention: None known. Genetic counseling indicated.

Treatment: Prosthetic replacement of teeth, extraction, and surgical treatment of cysts.

Prognosis: No apparent effect on life span. Usually complete loss of teeth by third to fourth decades.

Detection of Carrier: Unknown.

Special Considerations: Clinically and histologically identical teeth also occur in dentino-osseous dysplasia and in the branchio-skeleto-genital syndrome. This type of dentin dysplasia also occurs in the tricho-onycho-dental syndrome, which has hair, nail, and enamel defects. A similar but less severe dentin defect also occurs in some types of Ehlers-Danlos syndrome, enamel and interradicular dentin dysplasia, tumoral calcinosis with hyperphosphatemia, and in dermatomyositis.

References:
Bruszt P: Sur deux cas de dysplasie dentinaire. Bull Group Int Rech Sci Stomatol Odontol 1969; 12:107–119.
Witkop CJ Jr, Rao S: Inherited defects in tooth structure. In BD:OAS; VII(7). Baltimore: William & Wilkins, 1971, 153–184. *
Sauk JJ Jr, et al.: An electron optic analysis and explanation for the etiology of dentinal dysplasia. Oral Surg 1972; 33:763–771. *
Shields ED, et al.: Heritable defects in dentine; description, differentiation and classification. Arch Oral Biol 1973; 18:543–553.
Witkop CJ Jr: Hereditary defects of dentin. Dent Clin North Am 1975; 19:25–45. †
Melnick M, et al.: Dentin dysplasia type I: a scanning electron microscope analysis of the primary dentition. Oral Surg 1980; 50:335–339.

WI043   **Carl J. Witkop, Jr.**

TEETH, DENTINOGENESIS IMPERFECTA   0279

Includes:
Dentinogenesis imperfecta, Brandywine type
Dentinogenesis imperfecta, Mayflower type
Dentinogenesis imperfecta, Shields type II, III
Opalescent dentin
Shell teeth
Teeth, hereditary brown

Excludes:
Branchio-skeleto-genital syndrome (0118)
Calcinosis
Dentino-osseous dysplasia (0280)
Ehlers-Danlos syndrome (0338)
Fibrous dysplasia of dentin
Osteogenesis imperfecta (0777)
Teeth, dentin dysplasia, coronal (0277)
Teeth, dentin dysplasia, radicular (0278)
Teeth, odontodysplasia (0739)

Major Diagnostic Criteria: Lack of any pulp chambers on X-ray examination in opalescent teeth of both dentitions.

Clinical Findings: Two types of dentinogenesis may exist: a milder form frequently tracing ancestry to descendants of the Mayflower (DI type II) and a more severe form, the Brandywine

type (DI, type III). The phenotypes frequently overlap, and DI type III may only be a stage in development of DI, type II.

All teeth in both dentitions are affected. Teeth are bluish-brown to brown in color with opalescent sheen. Crowns are bulbous-shaped. Enamel hypoplasia occurs in about 20%. The enamel fractures and easily abrades so the teeth wear rapidly, and, in adults, only roots may remain. Lack of history of repeated fractures and absence of other signs of osteogenesis imperfecta.

Pulp chambers and root canals are absent on X-ray examination. A few patients may show normal or large chambers or canals in primary teeth as a variation in expressivity. Short, thin roots.

Histologically, there are scanty, atypical tubules of varying width and length and globular dentin. Lack of scalloping occurs in most cases at the dentinoenamel junction. Cell remnants are embedded in dentin.

Complications: There is secondary hypoplasia of the alveolar process, probably from loss of occlusal tooth surface, resulting in large gingivae and alveolar ridges. Premature loss of teeth results from attrition, pulp exposure, and fractures of crown. Occasional periapical cyst formation occurs, but less frequently than that seen in dentin dysplasia.

Associated Findings: None known.

Etiology: Autosomal dominant inheritance with low mutation rate and with variable expression.

Pathogenesis: A defect in odontoblasts, which form a defective periodic acid Schiff (PAS)-positive matrix. Odontoblasts differentiate and lay down 1–2 mm of fairly normal-appearing tubules adjacent to the dentinoenamel junction. This layer of odontoblasts degenerates, and, new layer differentiates from mesenchyme and lays down 1–2 mm of atypical dentin. This process continues until tooth is completely filled. The dentin matrix does not calcify properly, lacking phosphophoryn, a calcium-binding protein. Abnormal peripulpal dentin contains reticulin and type III collagen, normally not present except in the mantle layer.

MIM No.: *12549, 12550

Sex Ratio: M55:F45. Several large studies of over 600 affected persons and their normal sibs have shown a consistent and statistically significant deviation of the expected 1:1 ratio.

Occurrence: Prevalence 1:8,000 in the general North American population. Occurs in isolates in higher prevalence. Highest known, Brandywine isolate of Maryland, 1:15. Reported nearly exclusively in people of Caucasian ancestry, especially tracing ancestry to France. Unreported in pure Black, Asiatic, or Australoid populations.

Risk of Recurrence for Patient's Sib:
See Part I, *Mendelian Inheritance.*

Risk of Recurrence for Patient's Child:
See Part I, *Mendelian Inheritance.*

Age of Detectability: Upon eruption of teeth at age 9–18 months, by visual and X-ray examination.

Gene Mapping and Linkage: DGI1 (dentinogenesis imperfecta 1) has been mapped to 4q12-q23.

Prevention: None known. Genetic counseling indicated.

Treatment: Crowning usually fails unless teeth are well formed. Children aged 4–15 years: Do not extract teeth. Place full denture prosthesis over teeth to maintain alveolar ridge. Adults: Full-mouth extraction and prosthetic replacements. Caution! Teeth are soft and crush under forceps pressure. Extract by elevation. Recommend treatment at early age, as the unsightly teeth affect psychosocial development. Alveolectomy may be needed in older children and adults prior to prosthetic replacement.

Prognosis: No effect on life span. Early loss of teeth. Risk of alveolar infection. Untreated cases can be associated with social difficulties.

Detection of Carrier: Unknown.

Special Considerations: Genetic heterogeneity may exist in this category. Shields et al (1973) feel that the Brandywine triracial isolate type with an occasional child showing large pulp chambers in primary teeth is a different disease than that found in most families. Studies to date have not shown definitive collagen, glycosaminoglycan, or phosphophoryn differences in the Brandy-wine type and what these authors term dentinogenesis imperfecta, type II (hereditary opalescent dentin), or in a similar tooth defect in **Osteogenesis imperfecta** (DI type I).

An occasional variation in the expressivity of this gene is encountered in kindreds of the classic disease. These variants usually affect primary teeth, which demonstrate normal-sized or very large pulp chambers (*shell teeth*). Sections reveal a reduced or absent layer of odontoblasts on the pulpal surface in these instances. Several reports of isolated cases have designated such cases as a separate entity; however, permanent teeth of relatives usually show the classic disease picture. Must be differentiated from dentin dysplasia, which usually has a remnant of pulp chamber visible on X-ray examination.

Two large studies indicate that there is a significantly increased reproductive fitness of 30–35% of affected individuals over their unaffected sibs and the population from which they were derived. Among a triracial isolate, all of the excess was attributable to excess male reproduction and among North American Caucasians to excess female reproduction, possibly indicating psychosocial factors involved with unsightly teeth.

References:

Witkop CJ Jr, et al.: Medical and dental findings in the Brandywine isolate. Ala J Med Sci 1966; 3:382–403.
Witkop CJ Jr: Manifestations of genetic disease in the human pulp. Oral Surg 1971; 32:278–316. * †
Shields ED, et al.: A proposed classification for heritable human dentine defects with a description of a new entity. Arch Oral Biol 1973; 18:543–553.
Sauk JJ, et al.: Immunohistochemical localization of type III collagen in the dentin of patients with osteogenesis imperfecta and hereditary opalescent dentin. J Oral Pathol 1980; 9:210–220.
Takagi Y, Veis A: Matrix protein difference between human normal and dentinogenesis imperfecta dentin. In: Veis A, ed: The chemistry and biology of mineralized connective tissue, vol 22. New York: Elsevier North Holland, 1981:233–243.
Ball SP, et al.: Linkage between dentinogenesis imperfecta and Gc. Ann Hum Genet 1982; 46:35–40.
Levin LS, et al.: Dentinogenesis imperfecta in the Brandywine isolate. Oral Surg Oral Med Oral Path 1983; 56:267–274.

WI043

Carl J. Witkop, Jr.

TEETH, DIASTEMA, MEDIAN INCISAL   0291

Includes:
> Diastema, dental medial
> Median incisal diastema
> Midline diastema

Excludes: Teeth, microdontia (0660)

Major Diagnostic Criteria: A space of 1 mm or greater between normal sized maxillary central incisors. The labial frenum may be observed to extend into the incisive papilla so that tugging on the labial frenum results in blanching of the interdental papilla.

Clinical Findings: A true diastema is caused by a persistent tectolabial frenum following the eruption of the permanent teeth. It does not spontaneously recede. True diastema occurs in approximately 10% of individuals without an abnormally positioned labial frenum. Conversely, a marginally situated labial frenum without diastema can be observed. Physiologic spacing of mixed dentition at an early age is not true median diastema. Mandibular central incisors may show diastema too.

Complications: Undetermined. Orthodontic closure of the interincisal diastema is not mechanically difficult, but the stability of the closure has been problematic.

Associated Findings: Median diastema is a frequent finding in individuals with mental retardation.

Etiology: Hereditary factors are suggested; possibly autosomal dominant inheritance. Forty-three percent of all subjects with diastema had similarly affected parents and sibs. Twin studies

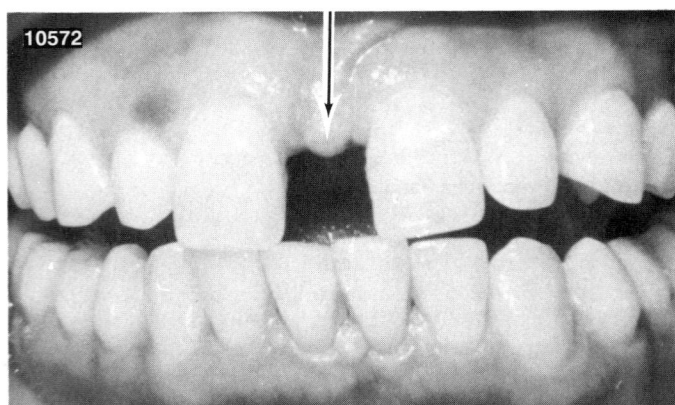

0291-10572: Diastema.

show a high concordance rate among monozygotic and a low rate among dizygotic twins. Single gene inheritance is most likely. Anterior teeth spacing or separation may also be caused by a larger arch size, abnormal tongue posture, discrepancy in tooth size, missing lateral incisors, or the presence of supernumeraries.

Pathogenesis: The tectolabial frenum consists of two parts: a connective tissue septum in the maxillary suture, which separates the upper dental ridge in median sagittal plane, and the frenular plate, which corresponds to the somewhat later-appearing labial frenum. The deciduous incisor buds are separated during the rise of the septum, which, under normal conditions, regresses or involutes. In most cases, involution of the septum occurs at the same time as resorption of the frenular plate. Any discrepancy in timing will result in a diastema.

MIM No.: 12590

Sex Ratio: Higher prevalence in females at age 6 years, but the opposite is seen at age 14 years (possibly because girls mature earlier than boys).

Occurrence: True diastema occurs in approximately ten percent of individuals without an abnormally positioned labial frenum. Ninety-seven percent of 6-year-old children exhibit a maxillary midline diastema followed by a sharp decrease in occurrence (45% of 9-year-olds, 9% of 16-year-olds) due to eruption of permanent maxillary anterior teeth. Diastemas greater than 0.5 mm were found in 22.33% of the adult subjects (aged 18 to 60 years).

Risk of Recurrence for Patient's Sib:
> See Part I, *Mendelian Inheritance.*

Risk of Recurrence for Patient's Child:
> See Part I, *Mendelian Inheritance.*

Age of Detectability: After the complete eruption of the dentition has occurred (for deciduous teeth, around three years ± 6 months; for permanent teeth, about 21 years ± 6 months, including third molars).

Gene Mapping and Linkage: Unknown.

Prevention: None known. Genetic counseling indicated.

Treatment: As a general rule, if a diastema persists after the maxillary canines erupt, then a frenectomy with or without space closure is considered. It is best to perform a frenectomy after orthodontic space closure since the scar tissue that forms after the surgical procedure is more resilient than the original frenum. If the diastema exceeds 4 to 5 mm prior to canine eruption, the probability is high that bodily tooth movement will be necessary to accomplish closure and root paralleling.

Prognosis: Excellent.

Detection of Carrier: Unknown.

References:
Banker CA, et al.: Alternative methods for the management of persistent maxillary central diastema. Gen Dent 1982; 30:136–139.
Teo CS: Maxillary median diastema: aetiology and incidence. Singapore Dent J 1983; 8:59–63.
McVay TJ, Latta GH, Jr: Incidence of the maxillary midline diastema in adults. J Prosthet Dent 1984; 52:809–811.

PA047   **Raj-Rajendra A. Patel**

TEETH, DILACERATED   0929

Includes: Dilacerated teeth

Excludes:
   Teeth, ankylosed (0927)
   Teeth, fused (0930)
   Teeth, geminated (0931)
   Teeth, impacted (0932)
   Teeth, root concrescence (0928)
   Teeth, supernumerary (0936)
   Twinning of teeth

Major Diagnostic Criteria: Clinical or X-ray evidence of displacement of tooth crown due to abnormal curvature in development.

Clinical Findings: Displacement of the tooth crown in relation to root, characterized by clinically obvious malalignment of varying severity. Hard and soft tissues of the crown or root may show defective formation. The crown may show hypoplasia or hypocalcification. Appearance on X-ray depends upon severity of the condition and the spatial relationship of oral tissues, X-ray film, and beam. The most frequently affected teeth in descending order

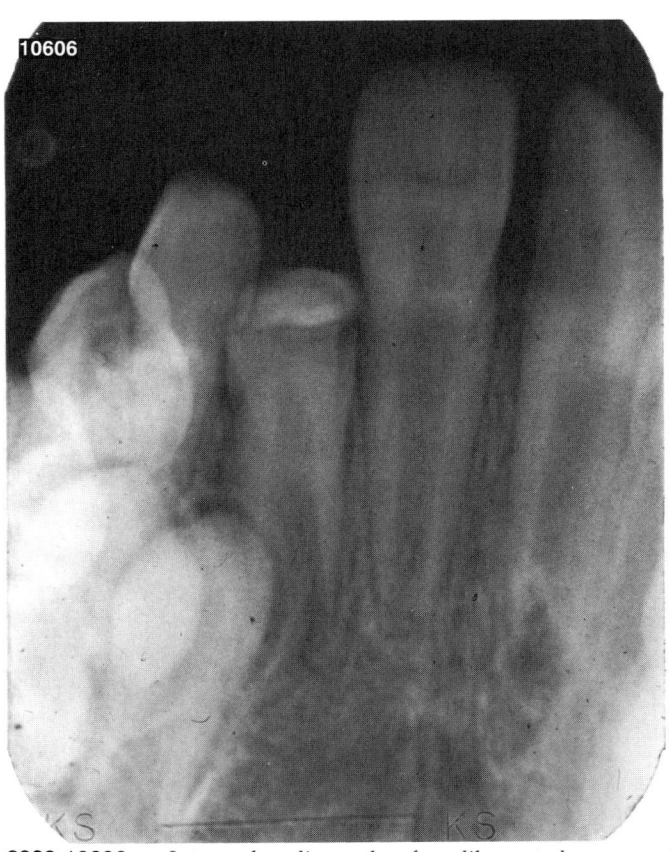

0929-10606: Intraoral radiograph of a dilacerated crown of maxillary permanent lateral incisor.

of involvement are: 1) mandibular third molars, 2) maxillary bicuspids, 3) mandibular secondary incisors, and 4) maxillary secondary incisors. Primary teeth are very rarely affected.

Complications: Psychosocial problems may arise due to unesthetic anterior affected tooth/teeth; dental caries may occur in hypoplastic defects, if present; continued root formation may be arrested; affected tooth or associated teeth may not erupt; and infection, dentigerous cyst formation, and ameloblastomatous change may develop in relation to an unerupted dilacerated tooth/teeth.

Associated Findings: Subsequent to dental caries, there may be pulpal exposure, periapical infection, granuloma, cyst formation, and loss of teeth followed by possible drifting and development of malocclusion.

Etiology: Trauma to developing tooth, prior to completion of root formation, results in coronal displacement. Displacement of crown or the developing root(s) may occur 1) during traumatic intrusion or extrusion of primary teeth; 2) during removal of primary teeth; 3) in cases of tooth size-arch size discrepancy resulting in tooth crowding; and 4) subsequent to pressure from adjacent pathologic processes (e.g. cyst).

Pathogenesis: At the point of crown-root deflection, enamel or dentin may exhibit abnormal matrix formation or calcification. Crown enamel and dentin may show hypoplasia or hypocalcification. Root apex may exhibit arrested cellular differentiation.

Sex Ratio: M1:F1

Occurrence: Undetermined but presumed rare.

Risk of Recurrence for Patient's Sib: Unknown.

Risk of Recurrence for Patient's Child: Unknown.

Age of Detectability: Variable, depending upon time of individual tooth formation. Condition is detectable on X-ray during early crown or root formation.

Gene Mapping and Linkage: Unknown.

Prevention: Avoidance of trauma to unerupted or erupting teeth; careful surgical removal of primary teeth, and early diagnosis and treatment of pathologic processes adjacent to dental structures.

Treatment: Orthodontic correction of tooth size-arch size deficiencies to avoid dental crowding. Other therapy may include removal of involved tooth and fabrication of prosthetic replacement, if indicated. Where possible, appropriate restoration of tooth structure to provide function, or, if asymptomatic and acceptable to the patient, leave undisturbed. Endodontic therapy, if indicated, is difficult to perform satisfactorily. Root fracture may occur during extraction of involved tooth.

Prognosis: Prognosis of condition depends upon severity of crown-root malalignment, extent of tooth eruption, and condition of clinical crown. With increasing severity of any of these factors, the prognosis of involved tooth worsens. Unless pathology such as infection, dentigerous cyst formation, and ameloblastomatous change develop in relation to an unerupted, dilacerated tooth, the condition does not interfere with longevity.

Detection of Carrier: Unknown.

References:
Large ND: Anomalies of the teeth and regressive alterations of the teeth. In: Tiecke RW, ed: Oral pathology. 1st ed. New York: McGraw-Hill, 1965:233.
Shafer WG, et al.: A textbook of oral pathology, 3rd ed. Philadelphia: W.B. Saunders, 1974:37.
Stewart RE, et al.: Pediatric dentistry, 1st ed. St. Louis: Mosby, 1982:99–100.

WA011   **Paul O. Walker**
SC054   **Mary E. Schwind**

Teeth, double
   See TEETH, FUSED
Teeth, double shoveling
   See TEETH, INCISORS, SHOVEL-SHAPED

TEETH, ENAMEL AND DENTIN DEFECTS FROM ERYTHROBLASTOSIS FETALIS 0340

Includes:
Blueberry muffin rash
Enamel shelf teeth
Erythroblastosis fetalis and staining of enamel and dentin
Hemolytic disease of newborn
Rh hump

Excludes:
Teeth, amelogenesis imperfecta (0046)
Teeth, defects from tetracycline (0341)
Teeth, odontodysplasia (0739)

Major Diagnostic Criteria: Primary teeth with green, brown, or blue hue and history of parental blood group incompatibilities.

Clinical Findings: Intrinsic staining of enamel and dentin of the deciduous teeth occurs with or without enamel hypoplasia. The stain ranges from green, brown, black, or yellow to blue or a mixture of any of these. Orange stain has also been demonstrated. The green stain does not affect the crowns of the deciduous teeth uniformly. The centrals are completely discolored, but the lateral incisors, cuspid, and molars may be only partially stained. Enamel hypoplasia results in defects involving the incisal edges of the anterior teeth and the middle of the crown of the cuspids, where a typical ring-like defect, called *Rh hump*, appears. Icterus gravis, hydrops fetalis, and anemia of the newborn with erythroblastosis represent different grades of clinical severity of the same syndrome of hemolytic anemia affecting the fetus. Chalky enamel surface seen in fluorosis, yellow tetracycline stain observed in permanent teeth, red fluorescence seen in porphyria, and green stain common in other forms of neonatal jaundice must be all considered in the differential diagnosis.

Complications: Possible psychosocial complex may arise due to unesthetic appearance of primary teeth. Dental caries may occur in hypoplastic defects, if present.

Associated Findings: Dermal erythropoiesis (2 to 8 mm in size, bluish, red, or magenta macules, and infiltrated papules, known as *blueberry muffin rash*). If they begin in early childhood, other hereditary hemolytic diseases such as **Anemia, sickle cell** and **Thalassemia** may result in pigmentation of the permanent teeth.

Etiology: Hemolysed erythrocytes liberate hemosiderin pigment, which may become deposited in developing dentin matrices. Ameloblasts apparently are damaged by bilirubin deposited in the dental organ, producing enamel hypoplasia in some cases.

Pathogenesis: Hemolytic anemia develops in the infants when an Rh-positive fetus is nurtured in the womb of an Rh-negative mother who has developed anti-Rh antibodies previously. When the antibodies pass the placental membrane and enter the fetal circulation, they agglutinate fetal erythrocytes, bind complement, and cause hemolysis. The same immunologic lesion may evolve as a consequence of ABO isoantigen incompatibility, in which the fetus is A, B, or AB and the mother lacks A or B isoantigens.

CDC No.: 282.000

Sex Ratio: M1:F1

Occurrence: Erythroblastosis fetalis actually occurs in about 10% of pregnancies, but the observed rate is only 0.5%. The low incidence may be explained by the inability of the mother to form antibodies in the presence of an Rh-positive fetus, failure of transplacental transfer of the antigen, or a low level of antibodies in the peripheral blood. Only 22% of patients with ABO incompatibility present enamel hypoplasia. The Rh hump occurs in 1:2,000 children.

Risk of Recurrence for Patient's Sib: If Rh immune globulin is administered to the mother, sensitization is 1% or less; if not administered, risk increases with successive pregnancies.

Risk of Recurrence for Patient's Child: Rh incompatibility occurs in 1:200 pregnancies.

Age of Detectability: At eruption of primary teeth (First deciduous tooth, central incisor, erupts at around 6 to 7 months).

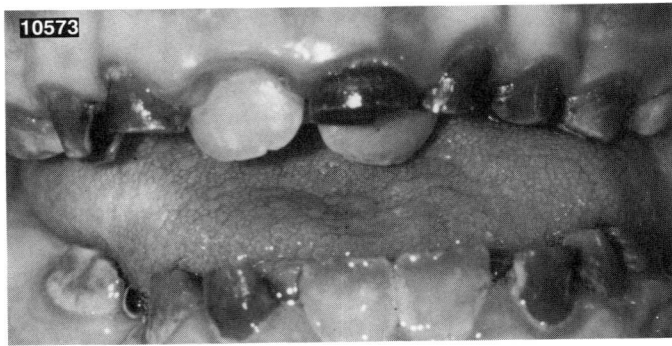

0340-10573: Bilirubin staining of teeth.

Gene Mapping and Linkage: Rhesus blood group locus on chromosome 1 (1p32–1pter). ABO blood group locus on chromosome 9 (9pter-9q33).

Prevention: Administer Rh immune globulin (RhIG) to unsensitized Rh-negative women after abortion, amniocentesis, ectopic pregnancy, or delivery of an Rh-positive infant.

Treatment: Since it affects only the deciduous teeth, the defect presents only a temporary cosmetic problem; esthetics and function may be restored by complete coverage with crowns.

Prognosis: Excellent once the oral condition has been treated. Untreated, unesthetic primary teeth may predispose toward childhood psychopathology. Dental caries may occur in hypoplastic defects, if present. Perinatal mortality rate in alloimmunization twin pregnancies is about 9.2%.

Detection of Carrier: Parental blood grouping and Rh determination will identify the potential in children to develop this condition.

References:
Shafer WG, et al.: A textbook of oral pathology, ed 4. Philadelphia: W.B. Saunders, 1983.
Frigoletto FD, et al.: Ultrasonographic fetal surveillance in the management of the isoimmunized pregnancy. N Engl J Med 1986; 315:430–432.

PA047   **Raj-Rajendra A. Patel**

TEETH, ENAMEL HYPOPLASIA 0342

Includes:
Enamel aplasia, chronologic
Hutchinson incisors
Intrauterine and neonatal enamel hypoplasia
Mulberry molars
Peg-shaped lateral incisor
Turner tooth

Excludes:
Heritable disorders of enamel and dentin
Hypoplastic defects of enamel from exanthematous disease
Porphyria, erythropoietic (0821)
Teeth, amelogenesis imperfecta (0046)
Teeth, defects from tetracycline (0341)
Teeth, enamel and dentin defects from erythroblastosis fetalis (0340)

Major Diagnostic Criteria: A quantitative defect of enamel visually and morphologically identified as involving the surface of the enamel (an external defect) and associated with a reduced thickness of enamel.

Clinical Findings: The defective enamel may occur as (1) shallow or deep pits, or rows of pits arranged horizontally in a linear fashion across the tooth surface or generally distributed over the whole or part of the enamel surface; (2) small or large, wide or narrow grooves; (3) partial or complete absence of enamel over small or considerable areas of dentin.

Complications: Dental caries is more likely to occur in hypoplastic enamel.

Associated Findings: A qualitative defect of enamel identified visually as an abnormality in the translucency (opacity) of enamel, characterized by a white or discolored (cream, brown, yellow) area, due to hypoplastic enamel.

Etiology: Several systemic factors are associated with enamel hypoplasia, as follows:

Birth trauma: Breech presentation, multiple pregnancy, caesarian section, prolonged labor.

Infections; maternal, postnatal: Syphilis, rubella, measles, chicken pox, scarlet fever, pneumonia, and gastrointestinal infections such as *Salmonella* gastroenteritis.

Maternal metabolic diseases: Hypoxia, toxemia of pregnancy, diabetes.

Perinatal metabolic diseases: Hyperbilirubinemia, neonatal asphyxia, hypocalcemia, prematurity complications, hypopituitarism.

Postnatal metabolic diseases: Hypothyroidism, hypoparathyroidism, congenital cardiac diseases, gastrointestinal malabsorption, nephrotic syndrome, chronic renal failure, biliary atresia.

Nutritional disorders, maternal, perinatal, and postnatal: Vitamin D deficiency, celiac disease.

Chemicals, maternal, perinatal, and postnatal: Tetracycline, thalidomide, lead intoxication, excessive fluoride.

Pathogenesis: Uncertain, but the mechanism appears to involve multifactorial events. Offending agent possibly damages the ameloblasts directly. The lesion appears to be a defect of matrix growth and maturation, probably involving a partial and momentary failure of the operating cycle of an ameloblast. Faulty formation of enamel matrix due to degenerative changes in the ameloblastic layer results in enamel hypoplasia.

Sex Ratio: Presumably M1:F1

Occurrence: The incidence of at least one tooth with defective enamel in normal children is approximately 63%. However, enamel hypoplasia of primary teeth is found in 21% of children born with low birth weight (<1,500 g). The prevalence of all acquired enamel defects according to Pindborg (1982) is about 14% in primary teeth and between 3% and 15% in permanent teeth.

Risk of Recurrence for Patient's Sib: Low, provided no environmental insults are present.

Risk of Recurrence for Patient's Child: Low, provided no environmental insults are present.

Age of Detectability: Defects can be seen in areas corresponding to both prenatal and postnatal tooth formation. Diagnosis is made by visual, clinical, and X-ray examination for primary teeth at ages 2–5 years, and for permanent teeth at ages 6–7 years.

Gene Mapping and Linkage: N/A

Prevention: Maintain proper nutritional status during pregnancy; prevent maternal infections, metabolic diseases, toxemia of pregnancy, and febrile childhood diseases.

Treatment: Regular topical applications of fluoride on defective enamel increase resistance to dental decay. Shallow pits and grooves can be filled with sealants; deeper defects, with composite restorative material. Full crown coverage is desirable for severe cases.

Prognosis: Depends on severity of enamel defect. Some defects weaken the enamel structurally, and others create difficult restorative or cosmetic problems. In the most severe cases teeth are extracted.

Detection of Carrier: Unknown.

Special Considerations: Chronic fetal distress, as manifested by a significantly subnormal birth weight, is almost always associated with severe damage to the enamel organ. Postnatal enamel is more susceptible to disturbances in mineralization than is prenatal enamel.

References:

Ainamo J, Cutress TW: An epidemiological index of developmental defects of dental enamel (DDE Index). Int Dent J 1982; 32:159–167.

Pindborg JJ: Aetiology of developmental enamel defects not related to fluorosis. Int Dent J 1982; 32:123–134. *

Noren JG: Enamel structure in deciduous teeth from low-birth-weight infants. Acta Odontol Scand 1983; 41:355–362.

Daculsi G, et al.: High-resolution study by transmission electron microscopy of a microhypoplasia of the human enamel surface. Arch Oral Biol 1984; 29:210–203.

Sarnat H, Moss SJ: Diagnosis of enamel defects. NY State Dent J. 1985; 51:103–104. *

Seow WK: Oral complications of premature birth. Aust Dent J, 1986; 31:23–29.

PA047   **Raj-Rajendra A. Patel**

Teeth, enlarged
See TEETH, MACRODONTIA

TEETH, EPULIS, CONGENITAL   0360

Includes:

Epulis, congenital
Gingival granular cell tumor, congenital
Granular cell epulis, congenital
Granular cell fibroblastoma, congenital
Granular cell myoblastoma, congenital
Granular cell tumor (WHO terminology)

Excludes:

Granular cell myoblastoma
Granular cell neurofibroma

Major Diagnostic Criteria: Soft tissue mass of the anterior maxilla or mandible that is present at birth. Ninety percent occur in females. Diagnosis requires histologic confirmation.

Clinical Findings: Uncommon, benign soft tissue nodule present in newborns, including the premature infant. Usually a solitary lesion, occasionally multiple (10%). Usually in the incisor or canine region of the maxilla or mandible (ratio: 2 maxilla : 1 mandible). Usually a broad-based soft tissue nodule, but may be pedunculated. Usually covered with intact, normal-appearing mucosa, but may be ulcerated. Size: 1–2 cm diameter average, range 0.3–7.5 cm. Some tumors will regress in size if untreated, but this is not always the case.

Histology: Sheets of uniform granular cells with a delicate plexiform capillary network and stromal fibroblasts. Lack of both a prominent neural component and psuedoepitheliomatous hyperplasia of the overlying squamous epithelium differentiates this from granular cell tumors (granular cell myoblastoma). Occasional nests of odontogenic epithelium may be observed. Cytoplasmic PAS-positive, diastase-resistant granules are present. Immunohistochemical studies have been negative for S-100 protein, carcinoembryonic antigen, and estrogen receptors.

X-ray findings: Occasional speckled calcifications.

Complications: May interfere with nursing and breathing. Rarely affects the developing dentition. Polyhydramnios resulting from obstructed fetal swallowing.

Associated Findings: None known.

Etiology: Unknown.

Pathogenesis: Controversy persists as to whether this lesion is a hamartoma or a neoplasm and as to the histogenesis. Fuhr and Krogh (1972) reviewed the major theories of origin, which included neurogenic, myogenic, fibroblastic, histiocytic, and odontogenic. Several investigators have suggested that the congenital epulis of the newborn represents a degenerative process of mesenchymal tissue that may be hormonally moderated, i.e., by estrogen. Ultrastructural and immunohistochemical studies are suggestive of a mesenchymal origin for this tumor.

The congenital epulis of the newborn is thought by most investigators to be a separate and distinct clinicohistopathologic entity and not a type of granular cell tumor (granular cell myoblastoma). Granular cell tumors exhibit strong ultrastructural and immunohistochemical evidence of neurogenic origin.

Sex Ratio: M1:F9

Occurrence: About 200 cases in the world literature.

Risk of Recurrence for Patient's Sib: No familial tendency reported.

Risk of Recurrence for Patient's Child: Unknown.

Age of Detectability: Present at birth. Has been seen in premature infants, and intrauterine ultrasonographic detection at 35 weeks has been reported.

Gene Mapping and Linkage: Unknown.

Prevention: None known. Genetic counseling indicated.

Treatment: Conservative surgical excision, avoiding the developing dentition, is the treatment of choice. Tumors removed later in the neonatal period have been reported to be smaller, with histologic evidence suggestive of involution. Spontaneous regression and regression of incompletely excised tumors are not uncommon.

Prognosis: Excellent for health and life span. Recurrence has not been reported of this benign tumor. Rarely, the developing deciduous dentition may be affected. There are occasional reports of continued difficulty in breathing following surgical excision. There is no evidence of malignant transformation, a malignant counterpart, or metastasis.

Detection of Carrier: Unknown.

References:

Custer RP, Fust JA: Congenital epulis. Am J Clin Pathol 1952; 22:1044–1053.

Fuhr AH, Krogh PH: Congenital epulis of the newborn. J Oral Surg 1972; 30:30–35.

Lack EE, et al.: Gingival granular cell tumors of the newborn. Am J Surg Pathol 1981; 5:37–46.

Lack EF, et al.: Gingival granular cell tumor of the newborn ("congenital epulis"): ultrastructural observations relating to histogenesis. Hum Pathol 1982; 13:686–689.

Lifshitz MS, et al.: Congenital granular cell epulis. Cancer 1984; 153:1845–1848.

Rainy JB, Smith IJ: Congenital epulis of the newborn. J Pediatr Surg 1984; 19:305–306.

ZU002

Susan L. Zunt

Teeth, fetal
  See TEETH, NATAL OR NEONATAL

TEETH, FUSED 0930

Includes:
  Incisor, single upper central
  Maxillary incisor, single central
  Teeth, connate
  Teeth, double

Excludes:
  Teeth, dens invaginatus (0276)
  Teeth, ankylosed (0927)
  Teeth, root concrescence (0928)
  Teeth, geminated (0931)

Major Diagnostic Criteria: A developmental anomaly consisting of the union of two or more normally separate teeth by confluent dentin or, rarely, enamel. X-ray evidence is required to confirm the diagnosis.

Clinical Findings: More common in primary than permanent dentition. Usually involves two normally separate teeth, or a tooth plus a supernumerary. The usual primary location is at the anterior mandible, while the location in permanent teeth is usually the anterior maxilla or mandible. May be unilateral or bilateral. Fusion of primary teeth is often followed by hypodontia in the permanent successors. Clinical examination reveals a wide tooth often with a longitudinal groove. X-ray films are necessary

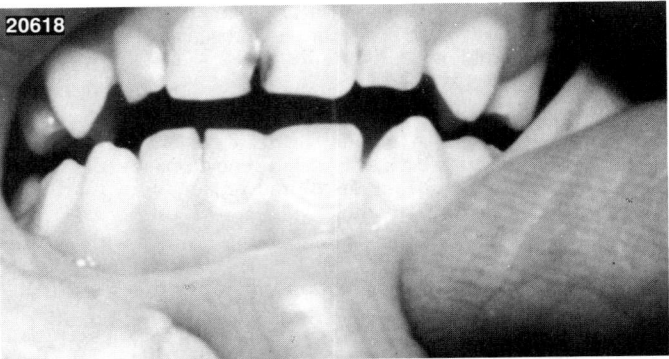

0930-20618: Teeth, fused; note fusion of the central and lateral incisors.

to establish the diagnosis and dental management. The root canals may be separate or fused.

Complications: Esthetics may be compromised when anterior teeth are involved. This may result in psychological problems. Dental caries may develop in the longitudinal groove. Fused primary teeth may influence the permanent dentition by retarding eruption, dental arch space discrepancy and malocclusion. The abnormal shape of fused teeth may predispose to periodontal disease.

Associated Findings: Increased incidence in **Fetal thalidomide syndrome**. Winter et al (1988) reported single upper central incisor as a feature of a possible "new" ectodermal dysplasia. Found in humans with abnormal brain development, and the mouse with hypervitaminosis A, trypan blue injection, and riboflavin deficiency.

Etiology: Possibly autosomal recessive or autosomal dominant inheritance with incomplete penetrance. May result from external pressure or forces causing contact between developing tooth buds.

Pathogenesis: Union of two separate developing tooth buds. The degree of fusion, incomplete to complete, is dependent on the stage at which the contact occurs.

MIM No.: 14725, 27300

Sex Ratio: M1:F1

Occurrence: Approximately 1:100 incidence; prevalence is approximately 0.6% of the Caucasian population; higher in the Japanese (2.5%) and American Indian. Primary dentition: 0.5–2.5%. Permanent dentition: 1%.

Risk of Recurrence for Patient's Sib: Unknown. Higher than general population.

Risk of Recurrence for Patient's Child: Unknown. Higher than general population.

Age of Detectability: Before eruption, by X-ray.

Gene Mapping and Linkage: Unknown.

Prevention: None known. Genetic counseling indicated.

Treatment: Children with fusion of primary teeth require dental evaluation for esthetics, caries prevention and treatment, and dental arch space management. Attempts to maintain the primary fused tooth may be important if the permanent successor is missing. The treatment of fused teeth in the permanent dentition may involve several dental therapeutic modalities, including orthodontics, endodontics, and prosthodontics. Some fused teeth may be separated. In some cases it may be necessary to extract the fused teeth and recommend prosthetic replacement.

Prognosis: Depends on the degree of confluence of dentin and pulp, and the morphology and X-ray features.

Detection of Carrier: Unknown.

References:
Brook AH, Winter GB: Double teeth: a retrospective study of "geminated" and "fused" teeth in children. Br Dent J 1970; 129:123–130.
McKibben DR, Brearley LJ: Radiographic determination of the prevalence of selected dental anomalies of children. J Dent Child 1971; 38:390–398.
Jarvinen S, et al.: Epidemiologic study of joined primary teeth in Finnish children. Community Dent Oral Epidemiol 1980; 8:201–202.
Delany GM, Goldblatt LI: Fused teeth: a multidisciplinary approach to treatment. J Am Dent Assoc 1981; 103:732–734.
Bazan MT: Fusion of maxillary incisors across the midline: clinical report. Pediatr Dent 1983; 5:220–221.
Gregg TA: Surgical division and pulpotomy of a double incisor tooth. Br Dent J 1985; 159:254–256.
Winter RM, et al.: Sparse hair, short stature, hypoplastic thumbs, single upper central incisor and abnormal skin pigmentation: a possible "new" form of ectodermal dysplasia. Am J Med Genet 1988; 29:209–216.

ZU002   **Susan L. Zunt**

TEETH, GEMINATED   **0931**

Includes: Geminated teeth

Excludes:
    Teeth, ankylosed (0927)
    Teeth, dens invaginatus (0276)
    Teeth, dilacerated (0929)
    Teeth, fused (0930)
    Teeth, impacted (0932)
    Teeth, root concrescence (0928)

Major Diagnostic Criteria: An enlarged bifid or cloven crown on a single root. Number of teeth normally in the arch is neither increased nor decreased.

Clinical Findings: Single tooth structure with two completely or incompletely separated crowns that have a single root and a single or partially divided pulp chamber. Clinical crown may exhibit hypoplasia or hypocalcification of enamel or dentin. There is a normal number of teeth in the affected area. The condition is usually limited to mandibular (primary or secondary) incisors.

Complications: Delayed eruption of affected or succedaneous tooth. Unesthetic anterior teeth may predispose toward psychopathology. Dental caries may occur in hypoplastic defects, if present. Abnormal coronal morphology may predispose toward malocclusion or periodontal pathology.

Associated Findings: Subsequent to dental caries, there may be pulpal exposure, periapical infection, granuloma, cyst formation, and loss of teeth, with possible drifting and resultant malocclusion.

Etiology: Undetermined. Some cases appear familial.

Pathogenesis: Invagination of dental lamina of tooth germ, resulting in double crown, ranging in morphology from an accessory cusp to bifid appearance.

Sex Ratio: Presumably M1:F1

Occurrence: Undetermined but presumed rare.

Risk of Recurrence for Patient's Sib: Unknown.

Risk of Recurrence for Patient's Child: Unknown.

Age of Detectability: Variable, depending upon age of calcification of the affected tooth. Detected preeruptively on X-ray or posteruptively on clinical examination.

Gene Mapping and Linkage: Unknown.

Prevention: None known. Genetic counseling indicated.

Treatment: Extract affected tooth (presence of succedaneous tooth should be ascertained prior to removing affected primary tooth). Endodontic therapy may be difficult, if root canal is partially divided. It is not always possible to differentiate between gemination and a case in which there has been fusion between a normal tooth and a supernumerary tooth); appropriate restoration of tooth crown, if possible; removal of minimally affected part of crown; or leave tooth undisturbed.

Prognosis: Depends on the extent and location of coronal separation, the extent of occlusal disharmony, and the periodontal condition of the affected tooth. A minimally involved tooth with good occlusion and a healthy periodontium has an excellent prognosis. Affected teeth with malocclusion or periodontal pathology have poor prognosis. The condition does not appear to affect life span.

Detection of Carrier: Unknown.

References:
Large ND: Anomalies of the teeth and regressive alterations of the teeth. In: Tiecke RW, ed: Oral pathology, ed 1. New York: McGraw-Hill, 1965:235 only.
Shafer WG, et al.: A textbook of oral pathology, ed 3. Philadelphia: W.B. Saunders, 1974:35–36.
Stewart RE, et al.: Pediatric dentistry, ed 1. St. Louis: Mosby, 1982:100 only.

WA011   **Paul O. Walker**
SC054   **Mary E. Schwind**

Teeth, ghost
    See TEETH, ODONTODYSPLASIA
Teeth, hereditary brown
    See TEETH, DENTINOGENESIS IMPERFECTA
Teeth, hypoplastic enamel
    See AMELO-CEREBRO-HYPOHIDROTIC SYNDROME
Teeth, immature
    See TEETH, NATAL OR NEONATAL

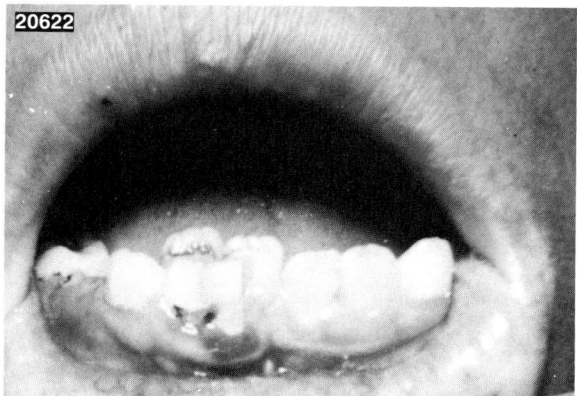

0931-20622: Teeth, geminated primary lateral incisors.

TEETH, IMPACTED   **0932**

Includes:
    Impacted teeth
    Teeth retention
    Dentes incluses

Excludes:
    Teeth, ankylosed (0927)
    Teeth, dens invaginatus (0276)
    Teeth, dilacerated (0929)
    Teeth, fused (0930)
    Teeth, geminated (0931)
    Teeth, root concrescence (0928)

Major Diagnostic Criteria: A tooth that is completely or partially unerupted and is positioned against another tooth, bone, or soft tissue so that its further eruption is unlikely. Unerupted teeth include embedded and impacted teeth, which are not seen clinically but are quite apparent on X-ray.

Clinical Findings: Any tooth may become impacted; most commonly involved are the third molars, followed by cuspids. The pericoronal space becomes an ideal trap for bacteria, food residue, and cell debris. The dentist often finds pericoronitis associated with a partially erupted mandibular third molar. In the upper jaw, impacted teeth have been found in the vicinity of the maxillary sinus and, occasionally, in the nose. Lower wisdom teeth may be located in the ascending ramus, at the base of the mandible, in the condylar neck, and in the coronoid process.

Complications: An impacted tooth may cause infection, resorption of the adjacent roots, idiopathic pain, trismus, and, due to lack of function in arch, may produce loss of arch length and malocclusion.

Associated Findings: Supernumerary teeth occur in 0.3%-3.8% of the population.

Etiology: A logical explanation for impacted teeth is the gradual evolutionary reduction in the size of the human mandible and maxilla. The modern diet does not require a decided effort in mastication, and thus growth stimulus of the jaws is lost. Impactions occur because of malpositioning of the tooth bud or obstruction in the path of eruption. Local causative factors include lack of space due to underdeveloped jaws, malocclusion of adjacent teeth, prolonged retention with or without premature loss of primary teeth, and local pathosis such as supernumerary teeth, cysts, and odontogenic tumor. Rare syndromic conditions may also show impactions, such as **Cleidocranial dysplasia, Intestinal polyposis, type III, Craniosynostosis, Progeria, Achondroplasia,** and **Teeth, amelogenesis imperfecta.** The etiology of tooth impaction is related to an arch-length deficiency, except for maxillary cuspid palatal impaction.

Pathogenesis: Undetermined. It is possible that malposition of the tooth follicle can lead to the premature exhaustion of the eruptive forces, and to a malposition of the erupted tooth.

MIM No.: 30828

Sex Ratio: Impacted canines occur more frequently among females than among males (M1:F2.5).

Occurrence: Impacted teeth are an increasingly common problem. Andreasen et al. (1986) summarized incidence figures mentioned in various studies: The overall incidence of all impactions reported in 1961 is 16.7%. In a recent study done in 1985, 96.5% of the patients showed X-ray evidence of one or more unerupted or impacted teeth; 98% of these were third molar impactions, 0.9–2% were cuspids, and 0.27% were first premolars. These surveys were performed in the United States.

Risk of Recurrence for Patient's Sib: Not increased except in unusual familial cases.

Risk of Recurrence for Patient's Child: Not increased except as part of an associated syndrome.

Age of Detectability: Following calcification of tooth crown, by X-ray.

Gene Mapping and Linkage: Unknown.

Prevention: Extraction of supernumerary teeth in the pathway of eruption facilitates spontaneous eruption. Mechanical space maintainers should be used after premature loss of teeth.

Treatment: Surgical removal of impacted teeth. More than 55% of extractions are done between the ages of 16 and 25 years, when indicated.

Prognosis: There is no association between impacted teeth and systemic disease.

Detection of Carrier: Possibly by clinical examination in familial cases.

References:
Mercuri LG, O'Neill R: Multiple impaced and supernumerary teeth in sisters. Oral Surg 1980; 50:293 only.
Goldberg MH, et al.: Complications after mandibular third molar surgery: a statistical analysis of 500 consecutive procedures in private practice. J Am Dent Assoc 1985; 111:227–229.
Tetsch P, Wagner W: Operative extraction of wisdom teeth. Littleton, CO: PSG, 1985.
Andreasen JO, et al.: Oral health care: more than caries and periodontal disease. A survey of epidemiological studies on oral disease. Int Dent J 1986; 36:207–214.
Nitzan DW, et al.: The effect of aging on tooth morphology: a study on impacted teeth. Oral Surg 1986; 61:54–60.

PA047   **Raj-Rajendra A. Patel**

TEETH, INCISORS, SHOVEL-SHAPED   2135

Includes:
Incisors, barrel-shape
Teeth, double shoveling
Teeth, semi-shovel

Excludes:
Teeth, crown malformations (other)
Teeth, pegged or absent maxillary lateral incisor (0934)

Major Diagnostic Criteria: Incisor teeth with prominent elevation or hypertrophy of the marginal ridges, enclosing the lingual fossa.

Clinical Findings: Elevation or hypertrophy of the marginal ridges enclosing the lingual fossa is the characteristic feature of shovel-shaped incisors. The enamel is not hypertrophied on the marginal ridges; dentin is also involved in their formation. Bilateral symmetry is usually seen and, when central upper incisors are affected, the lateral incisors are commonly affected. As a result of the high marginal ridges sometimes being extremely elevated, a so-called barrel-shaped incisor can be seen. There is a prominent, common variant called double shovel-shape, in which the labial marginal ridges are also strongly elevated. These teeth tend to look wide and large for the patient's mouth. Sometimes the mandibular incisors and canines can also be affected, but the lingual fossa is never as prominent as it is in the maxillary incisors.

Complications: Unknown.

Associated Findings: Because of the enlargement of the marginal ridges, the lingual fossa becomes accentuated and a deep pit can be seen there. As a result, caries is a common complication which often is not detected until too late, after pulpal exposure has occurred.

Etiology: Undetermined. Several models for explaining genetic control of shoveling have been proposed: 1) Autosomal dominant inheritance with variable expressivity, 2) two autosomal alleles without dominance, and 3) polygenic inheritance.

The extent to which genetic factors determine the degree of shovel shapes has been studied by considering different familial correlations. The parent-offspring correlations, when compared to the full-sib correlation, suggest that there is no dominance deviation in the variation of shoveling. They also suggest that about 68% of the variation seen in shoveling can be explained by the additive effect of genes.

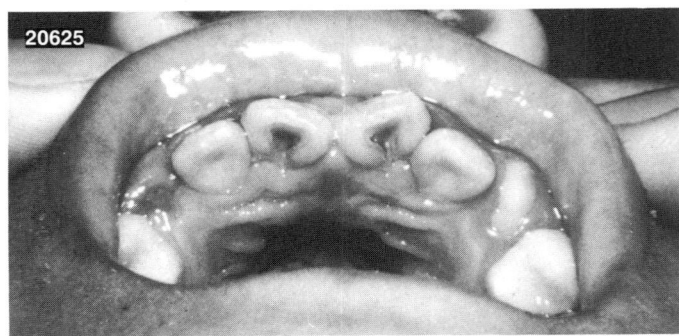

2135-20625: Teeth, incisors, shovel-shaped; note also mesiopalatal rotation.

Pathogenesis: Primate incisors display a cingulum formed by a mesial, a cervical and a distal marginal tuberculum. In a shovel-shaped tooth, the marginal ridges are well developed and the median ridge is reduced.

MIM No.: 14740

Sex Ratio: M1:F1

Occurrence: Depends on the population being studied. For Caucasians, an average incidence over several populations is 37.9%; for Japanese, 95.5%; and for the American Indian, 99.0%.

Risk of Recurrence for Patient's Sib:
See Part I, *Mendelian Inheritance.*

Risk of Recurrence for Patient's Child:
See Part I, *Mendelian Inheritance.*

Age of Detectability: As soon as the incisors erupt in the mouth; about six to seven years of age.

Gene Mapping and Linkage: Unknown.

Prevention: None known. Genetic counseling indicated.

Treatment: Pulpal complications due to caries should be prevented by doing prophylactic restorations of the lingual fossa when indicated.

Prognosis: Normal life span.

Detection of Carrier: By oral examination.

References:
Lee GTR, Goose DH: The inheritance of dental traits in a Chinese population in the United Kingdom. J Med Genet 1972; 9:336–339.
Kirveskari P: Morphological traits in the permanent dentition of the living skolt lapps. Proceedings of the Finnish Dental Society 1974; (Suppl II)70.
Portin P, Alvesalo L: The inheritance of shovel shape incisors in maxillary incisors. Am J Phys Anthrop 1974; 41:59–62.
Blanco R, Chakraborti R: Genetics of shovel-shaped maxillary central incisors. Am J Phys Anthrop 1976; 44:233–236.
Escobar V, et al.: Genetic structure of the Queckchi Indians. Hum Hered 1979; 29:134–142.

ES000   **Victor Escobar**

TEETH, LOBODONTIA   0607

Includes:
Lobodontia
Teeth, carnivore-like
Teeth, conical, multiple
"Wolf teeth"

Excludes:
Hypodontia
Teeth, dens invaginatus (0276)
Teeth, enamel hypoplasia (0342)
Teeth, microdontia (0660)

Major Diagnostic Criteria: Multiple dental anomalies of the teeth resulting in a dentition resembling that of a carnivore.

Clinical Findings: Multiple anomalies of the teeth resulting in a dentition resembling that of a carnivore. All observed cases have had multitubercular molar crowns, generalized reduction of crown size, accentuation of mesiobuccal cusps of molars and buccal cusps of premolars, accentuation of cingulum of premolars and incisors, suppression in height of other molar and premolar cusps and large diastemata in upper and lower canine regions. Some, but not all cases, have in addition, multiple dens in dente or deep palatal invaginations, single conical molar roots, agenesis of teeth, ectopic eruption of teeth, and shovel-shaped incisors.

Complications: Pulpal inflammation, degeneration and periapical involvement in teeth with dens in dente.

Associated Findings: None known.

Etiology: Autosomal dominant inheritance.

Pathogenesis: Undetermined. The morphologic alterations peculiar to this entry are genetically determined, and clinical com-

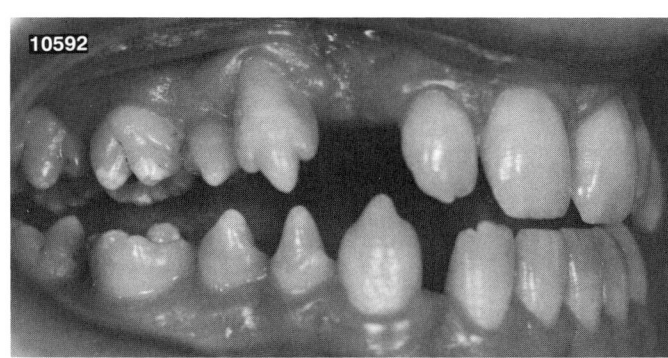

0607-10592: Note cone-shaped mandibular premolars and fang-like maxillary canine.

plications such as pulpal degeneration in teeth with dens in dente probably occur after eruption into the oral cavity.

MIM No.: *18700

Sex Ratio: Presumably M1:F1 (observed M7:F5).

Occurrence: Estimated to be less than 1:1,000,000. Three kindreds have been documented.

Risk of Recurrence for Patient's Sib:
See Part I, *Mendelian Inheritance.*

Risk of Recurrence for Patient's Child:
See Part I, *Mendelian Inheritance.*

Age of Detectability: At two years by clinical and X-ray examination of deciduous teeth.

Gene Mapping and Linkage: Unknown.

Prevention: None known. Genetic counseling indicated.

Treatment: Root canal therapy for teeth with dens in dente; use of occlusal sealants following eruption. Occlusal table should be restored, and cusps preserved.

Prognosis: Apparently normal life span.

Detection of Carrier: Unknown.

References:
Robbins IM, Keene HJ: Multiple morphologic dental anomalies: report of a case. Oral Surg 1964; 17:683–690.
Mayhall JT: Analysis of dental form regression syndrome. IADR program and abstract #373, 1967.
Shuff RY: A patient with multiple conical teeth. Dent Practit 1972; 22:414–417.
Brook AN, Winder M: Lobodontia: a rare inherited dental anomaly. Br Dent J 1979; 147:213–215.
Dahlberg AA: Rationale of identification based on biological factors of the dentition. Am J Forensic Med Pathol 1984; 5(4).

DA002   **Albert A. Dahlberg**
KE003   **Harris J. Keene**

Teeth, localized arrested development
See TEETH, ODONTODYSPLASIA

TEETH, MACRODONTIA   0617

Includes:
Megadontia
Teeth, enlarged

Excludes:
Conjoined teeth
Hemihypertrophy (0458)
Teeth, fused (0930)

Major Diagnostic Criteria: Teeth are significantly larger than normal. Mesiodistal and buccolingual measurements exceed range of normal variation.

Clinical Findings: Teeth that are larger than normal can be classified as follows: (1) True-generalized or generalized proportional macrodontia is a condition in which all teeth are larger than normal. It has been associated with pituitary gigantism and hemihypertrophy. (2) Relative-generalized or generalized disproportional macrodontia is the result of the presence of normal or slightly larger than normal teeth in small jaws. This disparity in size gives the illusion of macrodontia. (3) Localized macrodontia is a condition in which one or a few large teeth exist in relation to an otherwise normal dentition and body size. It usually involves the mandibular third molar. True macrodontia of a single tooth should not be confused with conjoined teeth or fusion of teeth, in which early in odontogenesis, the union of two or more teeth results in a single large tooth. In hemihypertrophy of the face, a variant of this localized macrodontia may occasionally be seen in which the teeth of the involved side are considerably larger than those of the unaffected side.

Complications: Crowding and irregular alignment of the dentition (malocclusion) result when relative-generalized macrodontia occurs. Large teeth may get impacted and may later show dentigerous cyst formation.

Associated Findings: Macrodontia occurs in syndromes in which there may be numerous other features such as mental retardation, hypogonadism, midface hypoplasia, and limb deformities, among others. For example: **KBG syndrome**, **Klinefelter syndrome**, and **Sturge-Weber syndrome**.

Etiology: The size of teeth is only one variable in a complex system of craniofacial development, the components of which generally show a continuous size variation. Twin studies have established a genetic component in tooth size variability. Family studies have demonstrated consistently that important environmental effects are superimposed upon genetic effects to determine tooth size. From animal experimentation, these environmental influences were shown to be largely maternal, such as cytoplasmic inheritance, prenatal uterine environment (influenced by maternal diet), and postnatal maternal effects. No genetic basis for tooth size asymmetry has been detected, and tooth pairs (e.g., maxillary canines, mandibular first premolars) may be assumed to be under identical genetic control with respect to size. Asymmetry is thus considered to be the result of a phenotypic environmental disturbance during tooth development.

Pathogenesis: Secretion of an abnormally high level of growth hormone may result in increased size of all body tissues, including teeth and jaws. This is apparently what happens in true-generalized macrodontia associated with pituitary gigantism.

Sex Ratio: M1:F1

Occurrence: Undetermined.

Risk of Recurrence for Patient's Sib: Probably very low.

Risk of Recurrence for Patient's Child: Probably very low.

Age of Detectability: At the time of eruption of deciduous and permanent teeth.

Gene Mapping and Linkage: Unknown.

Prevention: None known. Genetic counseling indicated.

Treatment: No treatment is necessary or indicated except in cases where there is malocclusion, or when impacted teeth are present. Then, extraction and orthodontic treatment is recommended.

Prognosis: Excellent.

Detection of Carrier: Unknown.

References:
Harzer W: A hypothetical model of genetic control of tooth-crown growth in man. Arch Oral Biol 1987; 32:159–162.

PA047   **Raj-Rajendra A. Patel**

TEETH, MESIOPALATAL TORSION OF CENTRAL INCISORS

Includes:
> Counterwing teeth
> Incisors, mesiopalatal torsion of central
> Incisors, rotation of upper central
> Mesiolabial rotation of upper central incisors
> Mesiopalatal rotation of upper central incisors
> Wing teeth

Excludes:
> Bite, open
> **Teeth, supernumerary** (0936)
> Teeth, crowding

Major Diagnostic Criteria: The upper central incisors must be in a correct alignment within the dental arch, with the distal part of the crown rotated labially, bringing the mesial part to a palatal position in the absence of crowding.

Clinical Findings: Mesiopalatal rotation of upper central incisors presents as a rotation of the upper central incisors within their bony sockets. The distal part of the crown is rotated labially, bringing the mesial part to a lingual position. The reverse position or mesiolabial rotation also occurs. This latter position gives the impression of a pointed prominence to the upper incisor region. The teeth shapes are normal, and they are correctly positioned in the maxillary dental arch.

Complications: Malocclusion.

Associated Findings: Although this condition usually occurs as an isolated finding, its presence suggests malocclusion and esthetic disharmony.

Etiology: Risk of recurrence figures have been derived from a study of 166 families. A segregation analysis suggests an autosomal dominant trait, with variable expression and a penetrance of 84%.

Pathogenesis: Fetal material suggests that the rotation of the incisors as seen clinically in erupted teeth is a continuation of a rotation seen during early embryonic development. One can then hypothesize that the mechanism for rotation of the incisors from the position seen in fetal life to the adult position is defective and does not allow for this movement. Linkage studies have placed this trait in close association with blood group P and chromosome 6. This linkage association lends support to the existence of this trait as a separate genetic entity.

MIM No.: 14735

Sex Ratio: M1:F1

Occurrence: Incidence and prevalence depend on the population studied. In the average American Indian, 23–44%; among

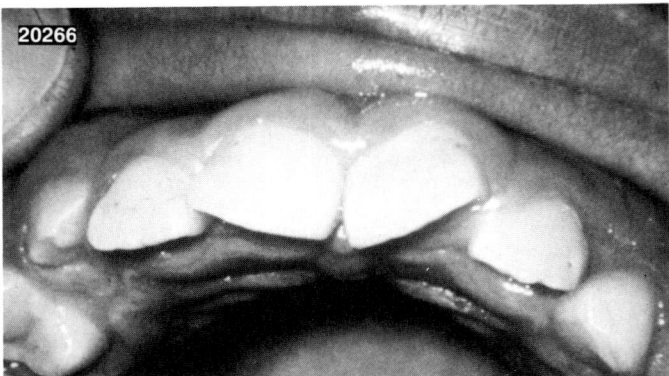

2133-20266: Note winged teeth resulting from the mesiopalatal torsion of the central incisors.

Caucasions, 6%; Chinese 5.2%; Japanese, 5.6%, and Hawaiians, 22%.

Risk of Recurrence for Patient's Sib: Empiric risk: 58% if one parent is affected; 40% if both parents are normal.

Risk of Recurrence for Patient's Child: Empiric risk :40%.

Age of Detectability: After the teeth erupt in the mouth.

Gene Mapping and Linkage: Linkage studies have placed this trait in close association with blood group P on chromosome 6.

Prevention: None known. Genetic counseling indicated.

Treatment: Interceptive orthodontics. In older children and adult patients, orthodontic treatment can be performed if the degree of rotation is severe enough to require treatment. However, one should bear in mind that tooth rotations around their axes are one of the most difficult orthodontic problems, since teeth tend to revert to their original position once the orthodontic appliances have been removed.

Prognosis: An association with several other traits characteristic of Indian populations has been reported, especially **Teeth, incisors, shovel-shaped**. Because of the deep lingual fossae, these teeth are more susceptible to caries and pulpal involvement. Otherwise, longevity of the tooth is not affected.

Detection of Carrier: By oral examination.

References:

Escobar V, et al.: The inheritance of bilateral rotation of maxillary central incisors. Am J Phys Anthrop 1976; 45:109–116.
Escobar V: A genetic study of upper central incisor rotation (wing teeth) in the Pima Indians. PhD thesis, Department of Medical Genetics. Indianapolis: Indiana University School of Medicine, 1979.

ES000   **Victor Escobar**

TEETH, MICRODONTIA   0660

Includes:

> Microdontia
> Teeth, small

Excludes:

> **Chondroectodermal dysplasia** (0156)
> **Chromosome 21, trisomy 21** (0171)
> Ectodermal dysplasia, anhidrotic
> **Eye, anterior segment dysgenesis** (0439)
> **Fetal radiation syndrome** (0383)
> **Incontinentia pigmenti** (0526)
> **Teeth, amelogenesis imperfecta** (0046)
> **Teeth, pegged or absent maxillary lateral incisor** (0934)

Major Diagnostic Criteria: The involved tooth or teeth must be small enough to be outside the usual limits of variation.

Clinical Findings: The involved tooth or teeth are small in size, well beyond usual limits of variation. Microdontia is manifested in 2 forms: true generalized microdontia which is extremely rare, occurring in some cases of pituitary dwarfism and, secondly, microdontia involving a single tooth or groups of teeth. The latter commonly affects the lateral incisors and maxillary molars and, along with the reduction in size, these teeth often exhibit a change in shape.

Complications: Cosmetic problem may have psychologic effects.

Associated Findings: Microdontia of the whole dentition may occur in syndromes, for example, **Chromosome 21, trisomy 21**, congenital heart disease, and pituitary dwarfism.

Microdontia may occur as a partial manifestation in a number of conditions including: **Cleft lip**, **Turner syndrome**, focal dermal hypoplasia, lipoid proteinosis, some forms of **Mucopolysaccharidosis**, **Oculo-auriculo-vertebral anomaly**, progeria, **Craniofacial dysostosis**, **Ehlers-Danlos syndrome**, **Sturge-Weber syndrome**, **Teeth, odontodysplasia**, **Osteogenesis imperfecta**, **Teeth, dentinogenesis imperfecta**, oculomandibulodyscephaly, and monilethrix. Small cone-shaped teeth may occur in many syndromes in which teeth are missing, especially those generally classed as **Ectodermal dysplasia**.

The most common form of microdontia (1.2 to 3.2% of general population) are peg maxillary lateral incisors. This is a discrete genetic trait which is manifest as either peg or missing maxillary lateral incisors. This tooth is also found in microform in **Acrocephalopolysyndactyly** (type III). Loss of the central mamelon of developing incisors in patients with congenital syphilis results in small screwdriver-shaped teeth. Absent or small mandibular incisors are nearly a constant feature of the **Hypoglossia-hypodactylia**. Microdontia of a specific tooth, the maxillary second primary molar, occurs in **Williams syndrome**.

Etiology: A hypothesis proposed by Harzer (1987) states 1) autosomal and X-linked genes determine the basic structures of tooth germ, whereas additional genes may promote size compensations during early odontogenesis; and 2) the tooth germ and the surrounding bone structures are genetically interdependent with regard to size determination so that there is a growth hierarchy. In one study, an association between hypodontia and microdontia was established. These findings may be explained as a multifactorial model having a continuous scale, related to tooth number and size, with thresholds. Reduced or hypoplastic maxillary laterals are a variable expression of the gene for congenitally missing lateral incisors. The genetic contribution to variation of mesiodistal diameter is greater both for individual teeth and tooth groups than it is to buccolingual diameter. However, there is a general decrease in heritability from anterior to posterior in the upper jaw and no clear trend in the lower jaw.

Pathogenesis: Unknown. Some disturbance impending on the full development of the tooth germ or germs involved either by disturbing enamel organ development or secondarily by faulty formation of dentin or enamel.

Sex Ratio: M1:F1.6

Occurrence: Prevalence of microdontia for males is 1.9%, for females is 3.1%, and for both sexes is 2.5%. True generalized microdontia is rare. Individual microdontia is more common, reaching 4% for third molars.

Risk of Recurrence for Patient's Sib: Incidence among first degree relatives of all probands is 29.1%.

Risk of Recurrence for Patient's Child: Unknown.

Age of Detectability: At eruption of teeth by dental examination.

Gene Mapping and Linkage: Unknown.

Prevention: None known. Genetic counseling indicated.

Treatment: Requires a collective effort in preventive dentistry, restorative dentistry, oral surgery, orthodontics, and prosthodontics.

Prognosis: Excellent for isolated microdontia.

Detection of Carrier: Unknown.

References:

Steinberg AG, et al.: Hereditary generalized microdontia. J Dent Res 1961; 40:58.
Shafer WG, et al.: A textbook of oral pathology, 2nd ed. Philadelphia, W.B. Saunders, Co., 1963:34.
Woof CM: Missing maxillary lateral incisors: a genetic study. Am J Hum Genet 1971; 23:289.
Freire-Maia N, Pinheiro M: Ectodermal dysplasias: a clinical and genetic study. New York: Alan R Liss, 1984.
Harzer W: A hypothetical model of genetic control of tooth-crown growth in man. Arch Oral Biol 1987; 32:159–162.

WI043   **Carl J. Witkop, Jr.**
PA047   **Raj-Rajendra A. Patel**

TEETH, MOLAR REINCLUSION   2137

Includes:
Ankylosis of teeth
Dental ankylosis
Molars, reincluded
Reinclusion of permanent molars, familial

Excludes:
Teeth, dilacerated (0929)
Teeth, impacted (0932)

Major Diagnostic Criteria: Molar teeth which, during or after a period of active eruption, stop their relative occlusal movement and remain below the occlusal plane.

Clinical Findings: Teeth are considered to be reincluded if, after a short period of active eruption and occlusal function, they fail to maintain their occlusal position in relation to other teeth. This leads to the false impression that they are depressed (being reincluded) into the jawbone while, in fact, they are remaining stationary while their neighbors continue to move occlusally. The only affected teeth so far appear to be both upper and lower molars, which present clinically as a posterior open bite. Although ankylosis (fusion of cementum to alveolar bone) has been blamed for the occurrence of "submerged teeth," this is not a finding in patients with familial reinclusion of permanent molars. Linkage studies, using blood and serum groups as markers, have provisionally assigned the "molar reinclusion" gene to the same linkage group as the gene locus of blood group P.

Complications: Unknown.

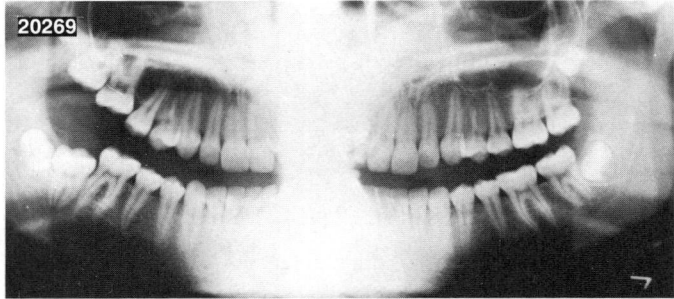

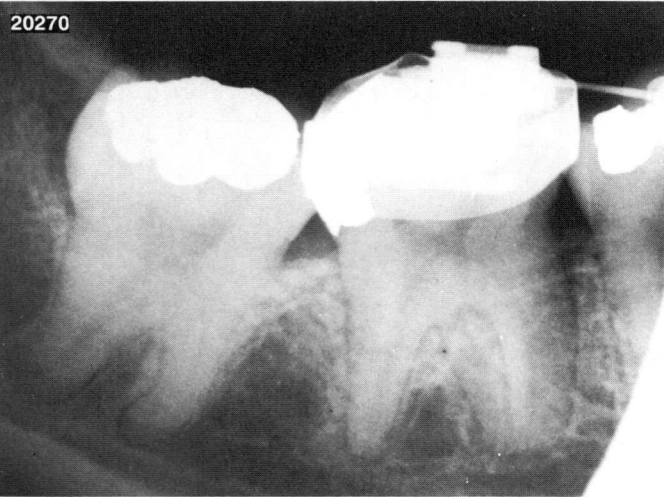

2137-20269: Submerged upper and lower molars. **20270:** Note the presence of the peridontal ligament in this close-up of the same teeth as shown in **20269.**

Associated Findings: Supereruption of opposing teeth with tipping of adjacent teeth and development of malocclusion. Reported patients have been identified because of an open posterior bite on the affected site.

When the infraocclusion is severe, soft tissue covers these teeth again. Since they did break through the epithelium initially, an epithelial-lined tract occurs which communicates the tooth with the oral cavity. This raises the possibility of local periodontal pathology.

Etiology: Twelve families regarded as examples of a genetic entity different from tooth ankylosis suggest autosomal dominant inheritance.

Pathogenesis: The primary biochemical defect which prevents these teeth from reaching their normal position in the dental arch is unknown. However, tooth ankylosis as a result of environmental or congenital injury to the periodontal membrane has been suggested as the etiologic factor. Yet, histologic and scanning electron microscopy studies have failed to reveal any indications of ankylosis. Proffitt and Vig (1981) suggest that a primary defect in the periodontal ligament or its vascular supply may be involved.

MIM No.: *15795

Sex Ratio: M1:F1

Occurrence: Nine families are from the Netherlands, two from the United States, and one from India have been documented. However, scattered in the literature on ankylosed teeth, one can find references of familial cases which may represent this condition.

Risk of Recurrence for Patient's Sib:
See Part I, *Mendelian Inheritance.*

Risk of Recurrence for Patient's Child:
See Part I, *Mendelian Inheritance.*

Age of Detectability: In the late teens, when adjacent teeth have reached their final occlusal plane.

Gene Mapping and Linkage: Unknown.

Prevention: None known. Genetic counseling indicated.

Treatment: Orthodontic treatment may be successful in correcting this condition, since tooth ankylosis is not present. However, Proffitt and Vig (1981) suggest that orthodontic treatment of such teeth can produce ankylosis. Surgical removal of bone and soft tissue covering the teeth have proved successful when inducing eruption of these molars. At least one case is known in which teeth did not erupt in spite of orthodontic treatment, and had to be surgically removed.

Prognosis: Treated, the prognosis is good. Orthodontic treatment may bring these teeth into normal occlusion. Once this has happened, surrounding alveolar bone will develop. Since there appear to be no other associated findings, life span is not affected.

Detection of Carrier: Unknown.

Special Considerations: Orthodontic treatment should always be attempted. If ineffective because of the possibility of undetectable ankylosis, surgical luxation of the tooth might be attempted. This has been suggested to permit resumption of eruption by breaking the bony bridge.

References:
Biederman W: Etiology and treatment of tooth ankylosis. Am J Ortho 1962; 48:670–684.
Bosker H, Nijenhuis LW: Possible linkage between a gene causing reinclusion of molar I and blood group P. Cytogenet Cell Genet 1975; 14:255–256.
Bosker H, et al.: Familial reinclusion of permanent molars. Clin Genet 1978; 13:314–320.
Kapoor AK, et al.: Bilateral posterior open bite. Oral Surg 1981; 52:21–22.
Poffitt WR, Vig KL: Primary failure of eruption: a possible cause of posterior open bite. Am J Ortho 1981; 80:173–190.

ES000   **Victor Escobar**

TEETH, NATAL OR NEONATAL   **0933**

Includes:

Precocious dentition
Teeth, congenital
Teeth, fetal
Teeth, immature
Teeth, present at birth

Excludes: Inclusion cysts of the oral mucosa in the newborn (3236)

Major Diagnostic Criteria: One or two teeth are present at birth or in first month of life.

Clinical Findings: Natal teeth are present at birth (75%). Neonatal teeth appear in the first 30 days of life (25%). Usually, one or two natal/neonatal teeth are seen in the anterior mandibular incisor area (85%).

A dental X-ray may be helpful in determining the maturity of the natal/neonatal tooth and whether it represents early eruption of a deciduous (90%) or a supernumerary (10%) tooth. The parent can hold the infant and positioned dental X-ray film during the exposure.

Natal teeth are slightly more common in females than males. The natal tooth's structure may resemble primary teeth, but it is more often a small, chalky white to yellow, conical structure with enamel defects. These teeth are often hypomineralized, cartilaginous in texture, and wear or fracture easily. Most natal/neonatal teeth are in the anterior mandibular incisor area (85%). Seventy percent of natal/neonatal teeth are firm in the alveolus, while 30% are mobile. These mobile teeth may be immature anomalous dental structures with little or no root development that may exfoliate in 10–15 days if untreated. Some of the initially mobile teeth will become firm if left in situ. A localized swelling of the alveolar mucosa is observed overlying neonatal teeth.

Failure of root formation with disruption of Hertwig epithelial root sheath, a large vascular dental pulp, irregular dentin, and cementum hypoplasia or agenesis have also been reported.

Complications: With teeth present, these complications include sublingual and/or lingual frenula ulceration resulting in feeding difficulties and irritability, as well as laceration or irritation of nursing mother's nipples. There is a potential for aspiration or swallowing (the latter has little clinical significance) of mobile natal/neonatal teeth, but neither has been reported.

With extraction, neonatal hypoprothrombinemia or bleeding defects should be excluded. Excessive hemorrhage has been reported following extraction, including one infant who had received vitamin K at birth. Lost space in the dental arch may be significant. Rarely, extraction may damage the underlying developing permanent tooth.

Associated Findings: Facial clefts, **Cyclopia, Pachyonychia congenita-steatocystoma multiplex, Oculo-mandibulo-facial syndrome,** and **Chondroectodermal dysplasia.**

A few unique syndromes have been identified with natal teeth as a feature (Harris et al, 1976; McDonald and Reed, 1982).

Etiology: Undetermined. Familial tendency identified in 15–24% of reported cases.

Pathogenesis: Superficial location of a developing tooth is the most accepted theory.

MIM No.: 18705

CDC No.: 520.600

Sex Ratio: M1:F>1

Occurrence: 1:2,000–6,000 live births

Risk of Recurrence for Patient's Sib: Overall risk in the absence of established inheritance pattern is 15%.

Risk of Recurrence for Patient's Child: Overall risk in the absence of established inheritance pattern is 15%.

Age of Detectability: Natal teeth: at birth; neonatal teeth: within 30 days of birth.

Gene Mapping and Linkage: Unknown.

Prevention: None known. Genetic counseling indicated.

Treatment: If the natal/neonatal teeth are causing the infant discomfort, refusal to eat, ulceration or they exhibit incomplete immature development with excessive mobility, extracton can be accomplished with topical or local anesthesia. Supernumerary teeth should be extracted in most cases. Natal/neonatal teeth that are components of the deciduous dentition should be maintained for as long as possible.

Dental evaluation by a pedodontist is strongly recommended.

Prognosis: Immature, mobile, supernumerary natal or neonatal teeth often require extraction. If these teeth are part of the normal complement of deciduous teeth, an attempt should be made to maintain them. Often the mobility will decrease as root development proceeds.

The presence of natal/neonatal teeth may herald significant dental arch space management problems. Dental consultation with a pediatric dentist is recommended.

In general, the patient has a good medical prognosis if natal/neonatal teeth are an isolated finding. Modification of the prognosis results with the presence of the less frequently associated conditions.

Detection of Carrier: Unknown.

Special Considerations: The nursing mother may be at risk for injury, although this may resolve with continued breast feeding, i.e., the child becomes conditioned not to bite.

Among the Chinese, the presence of natal teeth is considered very bad luck and the parents may require reassurance.

King Louis XIV and other significant historical figures were born with teeth (Bodenhoff and Gorlin, 1963).

References:

Bodenoff J, Gorlin RJ: Natal and neonatal teeth: folklore and fact. Pediatrics 1963; 32:1087–1098.

Harris DJ, et al.: Natal teeth, patent ductus arteriosus and intestinal pseudo-obstruction: a lethal syndrome in the newborn. Clin Genet 1976; 9:479–482.

Anneroth G, et al.: Clinical, histologic and microradiographic study of natal, neonatal and preerupted teeth. Scand J Dent Res 1978; 86:58–66.

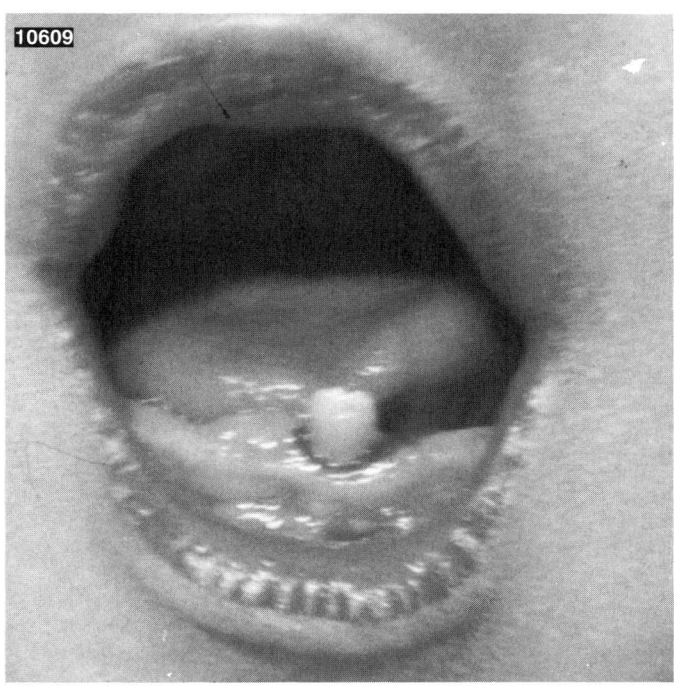

0933-10609:   Natal tooth.

McDonald RM, Reed WB: Natal teeth and steatocystoma multiplex complicated by hidradenitis suppurative. Arch Dermatol 1982; 112: 1132–1134.

Ronk SL: Multiple immature teeth in a newborn. J Pedod 1982; 6:254–260.

McDonald RE, Avery DR: Dentistry for the child and adolescent, 4th ed. St. Louis: C.V. Mosby, 1983:114–116.

Leung AKC: Natal teeth. Am J Dis Child 1986; 140:249–251.

ZU002   **Susan L. Zunt**

TEETH, ODONTOBLASTIC DYSPLASIA, FOCAL   2109

Includes:
     Dentin dysplasia type III
     Odontoblastic dysplasia, focal

Excludes:
     Dentino-osseous dysplasia (0280)
     Osteogenesis imperfecta (0777)
     Teeth, dentin dysplasia, coronal (0277)
     Teeth, dentin dysplasia, radicular (0278)
     Teeth, dentinogenesis imperfecta (0279)
     Teeth, odontodysplasia (0739)

Major Diagnostic Criteria: Extensive pulp stone formation in all permanent teeth which are otherwise clinically and on X-ray within normal limits.

Clinical Findings: Extensive pulp stones are present in the pulp chambers and/or canals of all permanent teeth. The root canals in many anterior teeth are distorted in proximity to these pulpal masses. Pulp stone formation in posterior teeth is so extensive that only a very thin radiolucent line distinguishes the pulpal wall boundaries. All permanent teeth are normal in size, shape, color, enamel hardness, vitality (electrical) and radiographic dentin-enamel contrast. Light and scanning electron microscopy reveal the pulp stones to be true denticles composed of a chaotic array of dysplastic dentinal tubules attached to the floor of the pulp chamber. Similar but separate excrescences of dysplastic dentin are identified on the dentinal walls of the pulp canals. Histologically, the bulk of the enamel, dentin and cementum are within normal limits.

Complications: Unknown.

Associated Findings: None known.

Etiology: Unknown.

Pathogenesis: Appears to be a primary dentin defect in which the dysplastic pulpal masses originate from circumscribed groups of odontoblasts at the pulpal wall which produce chaotic dentin.

Sex Ratio: Presumably M1:F1.

Occurrence: Only one case has been reported.

Risk of Recurrence for Patient's Sib: Unknown.

Risk of Recurrence for Patient's Child: Unknown.

Age of Detectability: In young adulthood.

Gene Mapping and Linkage: Unknown.

Prevention: None known. Genetic counseling indicated.

Treatment: None necessary.

Prognosis: Unknown.

Detection of Carrier: Unknown.

Special Considerations: Focal odontoblastic dysplasia shares with **Teeth, dentin dysplasia, coronal** extensive pulp stone formation in all teeth present. However, differences between the reported cases exist relative to the apparent site of origin of the pulp stones, dentition involved, shape of pulp chamber and crowns, and associated stature and mental defects. It may be that these two conditions will be found to be variations of the same process.

References:
Eastman JR, et al.: Focal odontoblastic dysplasia: dentin dysplasia type III? Oral Surg 1977; 44:909–914.

G0009   **Lawrence I. Goldblatt**

TEETH, ODONTODYSPLASIA   0739

Includes:
     Odontodysplasia
     Odontogenesis imperfecta
     Odontogenic dysplasia
     Regional odontodysplasia
     Teeth, ghost
     Teeth, localized arrested development
     Unilateral dental malformation

Excludes:
     Teeth, amelogenesis imperfecta (0046)
     Teeth, dentin dysplasia, coronal (0277)
     Teeth, dentin dysplasia, radicular (0278)
     Teeth, dentinogenesis imperfecta (0279)
     Teeth, shell

Major Diagnostic Criteria: Segments of primary or permanent dentition exhibit hypoplasia and hypocalcification of enamel and dentin. Affected teeth show reduced radiodensity (described as

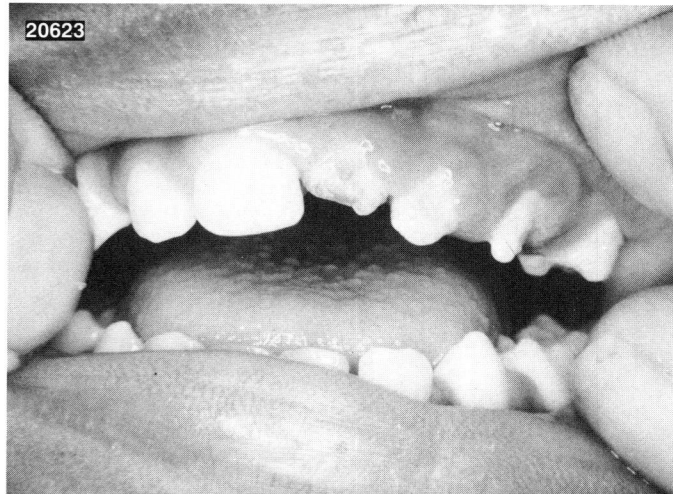

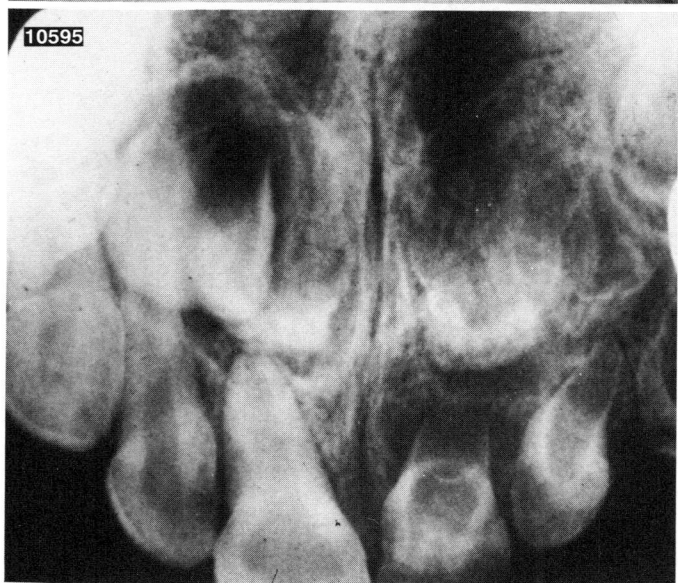

0739-20623–10595: Teeth, odontodysplasia.

"ghostly") and abnormally large pulp chambers with calcific inclusions.

Clinical Findings: Dysgenesis of enamel, dentin, and pulp, with hypoplasia and hypocalcification of enamel and dentin. Primary or secondary teeth may be affected independently, with only a portion of the teeth being involved. It is unlikely that the succedaneous tooth will be formed normally if the primary tooth is involved. Condition appears to occur more frequently in the maxillary arch; it affects the primary teeth equally, but the incisors and cuspids of the permanent teeth are more commonly involved. Affected teeth may remain unerupted, with associated enlarged follicles. Affected teeth are characterized by defective formation of both enamel and dentin, and are 1) smaller than normal, 2) of abnormal morphology, and 3) delayed or partially erupted. Histologically, there may be calcifications within the pulp or follicle. Corpuscular structures comprising concentric layers of collagenous connective tissue may occur in the follicle.

X-rays show reduced radiodensity and abnormally large pulpal chambers with calcific inclusions and short or hypoplastic roots. Root formation may be near-normal or much delayed.

Complications: Delayed eruption of primary or secondary teeth. Unesthetic anterior teeth may predispose to psychosocial concerns. Dental caries may occur in hypoplastic defects. Brittleness of teeth may predispose to coronal fractures.

Associated Findings: Subsequent to dental caries, there may be pulpal exposure, periapical infection, granuloma, cyst formation, and loss of teeth with possible drifting and resultant malocclusion.

Etiology: Undetermined. Both prenatal and early postnatal influences appear to be important. Intrinsic causative factors suggested are localized viral infection, abnormal vascular supply, localized tissue ischemia, and somatic mutation. Trauma or ionizing radiation do not appear to be tenable causes.

Pathogenesis: Initial event unknown; affected teeth show thin, hypoplastic, and hypocalcified enamel exhibiting irregular, aprismatic, matrix formation, with embedded cellular debris. Dentin shows tubular irregularity, with amorphous clefts of debris. The pulp may exhibit inflammation and calcific inclusions. The dental follicle may show corpuscular structures comprising concentric layers of collagenous connective tissue and calcifications. There may be delayed root formation, with large pulp chambers and root canals.

Sex Ratio: Estimated M1:F2

Occurrence: About 65 reported cases.

Risk of Recurrence for Patient's Sib: Probably not increased.

Risk of Recurrence for Patient's Child: Probably not increased.

Age of Detectability: Detected pre-eruptively by X-ray, or post-eruptively by clinical examination.

Gene Mapping and Linkage: Unknown.

Prevention: None known.

Treatment: Removal of affected primary teeth. Removal of affected, pulpally-involved secondary teeth and fabrication of artificial replacements for function and esthetics. An affected secondary tooth bud may be removed, attached to soft tissue of affected primary tooth, during extraction. Teeth may fracture readily. Affected teeth may be associated with a firm, painless, soft tissue swelling of the labial and lingual gingiva.

Prognosis: Treated: excellent for primary dentition, but succedaneous teeth may be involved. Untreated: associated complications may occur. Oral condition does not appear to interfere with patient's longevity.

Detection of Carrier: Unknown.

References:
Lustmann J, et al.: Odontodysplasia report of two cases and review of the literature. Oral Surg 1975; 39:781–793.
Herold RCB, et al.: Abnormal tooth tissue in human odontodysplasia. Oral Surg 1976; 42:357–365.
Bixler D: Heritable disorders affecting dentin. In: Stewart RE, Prescott GH, eds: Oral and facial genetics. St. Louis: C.V. Mosby, 1976:242–244.

Walton L, et al.: Odontodysplasia: report of three cases with vascular nevi overlying the adjacent stem of the face. Oral Surg 1978; 46:676–684.

WA011
SC054

**Paul O. Walker
Mary E. Schwind**

TEETH, PEGGED OR ABSENT MAXILLARY LATERAL INCISOR   0934

Includes:
Lateral incisors, absence of
Maxillary lateral incisor, hypodontia of
Maxillary lateral incisor, pegged or missing
Succedaneous teeth, agenesis of

Excludes:
Chromosome 21, trisomy 21 (0171)
Hypodontia-cleft lip
Teeth, anodontia, partial or complete (2134)
Teeth, microdontia (0660)
Teeth, pegged or absent associated with other syndromes

Major Diagnostic Criteria: Small maxillary lateral incisors.

Clinical Findings: The maxillary lateral incisor teeth may be small, peg-shaped, or congenitally missing. Various degrees and combinations as to right or left side may occur within individuals and within kindreds. Teeth in both dentitions may be affected, but the secondary teeth are most commonly affected.

Complications: Diastema of maxillary central incisors, or diastema between the canines and central incisors. Drifting of teeth.

Associated Findings: Congenital absence of premolar teeth (10–20%), and a higher incidence of pegged or congenitally missing third molar.

Etiology: Usually autosomal dominant inheritance.

While the trait shows an autosomal dominant inheritance pattern, the expression shows a threshold effect for missing teeth, i.e. below a certain size the pegged tooth gene seems to be expressed as a missing tooth and does not show smaller and smaller pegged teeth. At the other end of the continuum of tooth size, kindred studies show persons with normal-sized lateral incisors who apparently can pass the gene to offspring. The ratio between pegged and missing teeth varies by population: Swedes 1:1, United States Caucasians 1:1, Orientals 1:0.09. In United States Caucasians, a 2:1 preference for the left side is reported. Several families have been observed in which both parents had pegged permanent maxillary lateral incisors, and the children had severe oligodontia involving primarily agenesis of succedaneous permanent teeth. These kindreds are compatible with the hypothesis of the homozygous expression of the gene.

Pathogenesis: Absence or reduction in the size of tooth germ.

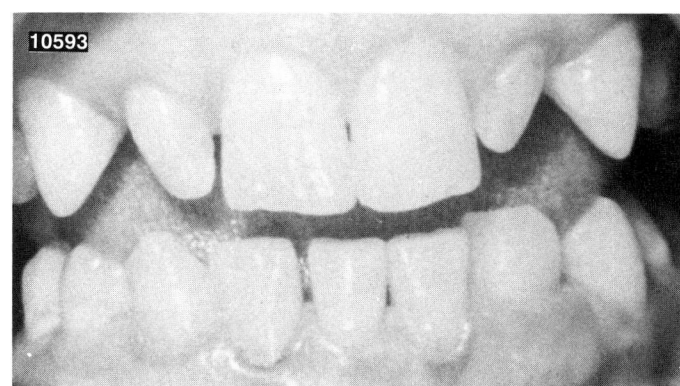

0934-10593: Peg-shaped maxillary lateral incisors.

MIM No.: *15040

Sex Ratio: Presumably M1:F1 (M1:F1.4 observed).

Occurrence: 1–3:100 in Caucasions and 6–7:100 in Orientals.

Risk of Recurrence for Patient's Sib:
See Part I, *Mendelian Inheritance.*

Risk of Recurrence for Patient's Child:
See Part I, *Mendelian Inheritance.*

Age of Detectability: Six to eight years of age, for permanent dentition.

Gene Mapping and Linkage: Unknown.

Prevention: None known. Genetic counseling indicated.

Treatment: Prosthetic replacement and orthodontic treatment.

Prognosis: Normal life span.

Detection of Carrier: Unknown.

References:

Witkop CJ Jr.: Studies of intrinsic disease in isolates with observations on penetrance and expressivity of certain anatomical traits. In: Pruzansky S, ed: Congenital anomalies of the face and associated structures. Springfield: Charles C Thomas, 1961:291–368.

Meskin LH, Gorlin RJ: Agenesis and peg-shaped permanent maxillary lateral incisors. J Dent Res 1963; 42:1476–1479.

Grahnen H: Hypodontia in the permanent dentition. Odont Rev 1965; 7(suppl 3):419–421.

Sutter J: L'Atteinte des incisives latérales supérieures. étude d'une mutation à l'échelle démographique. Paris: Presse Univ Fr, 1966.

Woolf CM: Missing maxillary lateral incisors: a genetic study. Am J Hum Genet 1971; 23:289–296.

Witkop CJ Jr: Agenesis of succedaneous teeth: an expression of the homozygous state of the gene for the pegged or missing maxillary lateral incisor trait. Am J Med Genet 1987; 26:431–436. †

WI043   **Carl J. Witkop, Jr.**

TEETH, PERIODONTITIS, JUVENILE   0806

Includes:

Bone atrophy, diffuse
Cementopathia, deep
Precocious periodontitis
Periodontitis, generalized juvenile
Periodontitis, localized juvenile
Periodontosis (misnomer)

Excludes:

Acatalasemia (0006)
Agranulocytosis

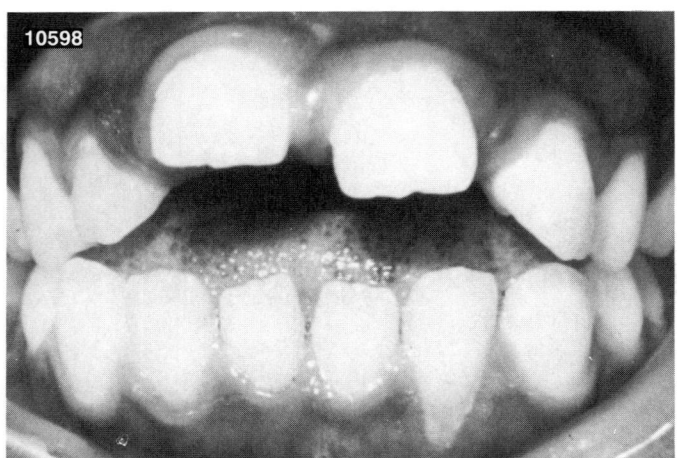

0806A-10598: Malpositioned teeth in periodontosis.

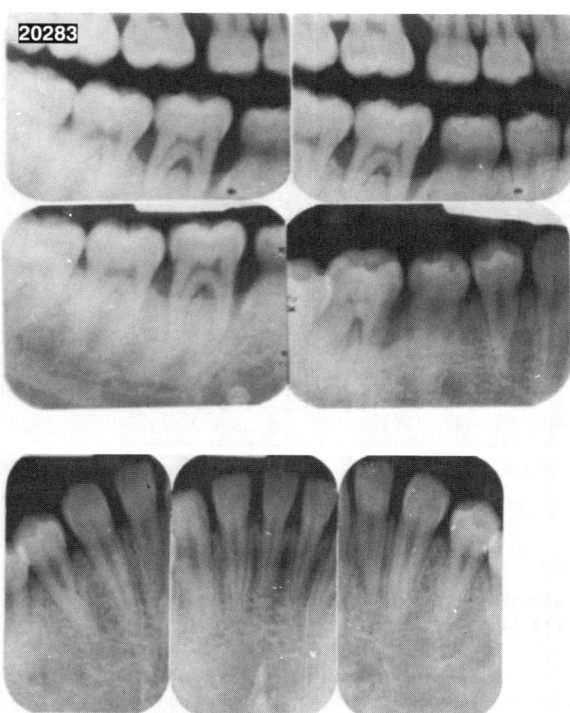

0806B-20283: Note periodontal bone destruction in central incisors and first molars of both arches in a 20-year-old white female.

Chediak-Higashi syndrome (0143)
Chromosome 21, trisomy 21 (0171)
Compromised blood supply
Diabetes mellitus, insulin dependent type (0549)
Histiocytosis
Hypergammaglobulinemia IgE
Hyperkeratosis palmoplantaris-periodontoclasia (0494)
Hypophosphatasia (0516)
Hypovitaminosis D
Lazy leukocyte syndrome
Leukemia
Neutropenia, cyclic (0714)

Major Diagnostic Criteria: Rapid idiopathic loss of connective tissue attachment and alveolar bone at more than one tooth in the permanent and sometimes the deciduous dentition in children. Destruction of the alveolar bone is initiated in the incisor and first molar areas, but may extend into the adjacent alveolus later in the disease, causing migration and loss of teeth. There are insufficient local irritants in the mouth to account for the degree of alveolar bone destruction, and no other associated anomalies are present.

Conditions that need to be present to confirm the diagnosis of juvenile periodontitis include 1) good general health as determined by a physical examination, including a chest X-ray, CBC and WBC, urinalysis, sedimentation rate, hemoglobin, and hematocrit; 2) bone loss of 2 mm or more around more than one tooth, detectable on X-ray; 3) local irritants absent or not commensurate with amount of bone loss. 4) age of less than 30 years.

Clinical Findings: Juvenile periodontitis is a rapidly progressive periodontal disease seen in adolescents who are otherwise in good health. The age of detection is usually around 11–13 years, but it has been shown that the defect is also present in the primary dentition.

In the early stages of the disease, only the first molars and incisors are affected (localized periodontitis), but as the disease progresses the periodontal tissues of other teeth become involved until the whole dentition is affected (generalized or postjuvenile periodontitis). Two types of generalized juvenile periodontitis have been suggested to exist: a chronic disseminated and slowly progressive disease and an acute disseminated and rapidly progressive condition.

In the initial stages, the disease is a painless condition that is followed by tooth migration and mobility in the apparent absence of inflammation. The gingival tissues appear to be normal in size, color, and texture, but upon gentle probing severe loss of attachment and bleeding is evident. Despite the deep periodontal pockets present at one or more proximal surfaces of affected teeth, gingival tissues usually remain positioned nearly normal in relation to the cementoenamel junction. The amount of periodontal destruction observed cannot be accounted for by the minimal amounts of supragingival and subgingival calculus deposits found. Often, a heavy sulcular fluid is present, giving the appearance of an exudate. Caries have been reported to be minimal in these patients. Periapical X-rays show a bilateral pattern of bone loss involving mainly the incisors and first molars. Destruction of the interdental septa is vertical, angular, or arc-like rather than horizontal. On the first molars, alveolar resorption is seen frequently on the mesial aspect of the root.

Complications: Rapid progression and premature loss of teeth in a relatively young individual with severe alveolar bone destruction. The incidence of recurrence after treatment is high if a frequent and strict maintenance schedule is not followed.

Associated Findings: Alveolar ridge destruction may cause difficulties wearing lower dentures due to poor retention. For treatment to be successful, there is a strong need for optimal oral hygiene by the patient.

Etiology: The etiology of juvenile periodontitis is unclear. Bacterial, genetic, and immunologic theories have been proposed to explain this condition.

Using anaerobic culturing techniques, two main bacteria associated with juvenile periodontitis have consistently been identified: 1) *Actinobacillus actinomycetemcomitans (Aa)* and 2) several species of *Capnocytophaga*. *Capnocytophaga* is capable of reducing neutrophil chemotaxis as well as phagocytosis. *Aa* can alter neutrophil phagocytotic function and cell morphology. Most young patients subjected to an infection develop antibodies to associated bacteria, but may demonstrate an arrested localized form of juvenile periodontitis into adulthood. Those who do not develop sufficient antibody levels will progress into the generalized form. Recently, Genco (1986) has shown that in about 70% of patients with localized juvenile periodontitis the polymorphonuclear neutrophil leukocytes (PMNs) have a decreased number of surface receptor sites for circulating antibodies. This defect seems to be familial, effectively reduces chemotaxis, and is often present prior to the onset of periodontitis. The question still remains, nevertheless, as to whether the PMN defect is caused by the bacteria or by a genetic factor that allows the bacteria more easily to infect susceptible individuals. The answer may depend on the fact that after periodontal treatment, the PMN activity of juvenile periodontitis patients returns to normal levels, suggesting the possibility that no genetic predisposition is required to contract the disease.

Evidence to support the heritable nature of juvenile periodontitis relies on the important role that individual patient susceptibility seems to play in the production of the disease, on particular associations of juvenile periodontitis with certain blood groups, on specific human leukocyte antigen (HLA) associations which if present suggest a role for genes at the major histocompatibility locus (MHC), and on the recent provisional assignment to a locus on the long arm of chromosome 4. Both autosomal dominant and autosomal recessive, as well as X-linked dominant, patterns of inheritance have been proposed to explain the transmission of juvenile periodontitis. The consensus, however, is that bacterial cross colonization plays a major role in the familial distribution of juvenile periodontitis, making a genetic pattern (if any) more difficult to identify.

Pathogenesis: The histopathologic changes observed have been correlated by different authors with the clinical sequence of events. First, degeneration of the principal fibers of the periodontal membrane occurs. The membrane widens, and bone is resorbed. Capillary proliferation is observed, and loose connective tissue develops. The epithelial attachment does not proliferate, and no inflammatory response is observed. As the disease progresses, proliferation of epithelial attachment and mild cellular infiltrate by plasma cells occur. Finally, the epithelial attachment separates from the roots, and deep pockets develop.

The cementum is thin and may present areas of resorption. The alveolar bone is irregular, and evidence of idiopathic osteoblastic activity and osteoclastic resorption is present. The spongiosa may be replaced by fibrous tissue.

Studies of PMN motility show abnormally low levels of PMN chemotaxis-directed migration. Microbiologic analysis shows predominant populations of *A. actinomycetemcomitans*, *Bacteroides ochraceus*, and gram-positive cocci and rods. The results of serum antibody titers (IgG, IgM, and IgA) in patients with juvenile periodontitis show increased antibody activity (IgG) to *A. actinomycetemcomitans* but low antibody levels to *B. gingivalis*, while the opposite is true for adult-onset periodontitis. Juvenile periodontitis patients also had impaired lymphocyte blastogenic responses to selected gram-negative organisms. They also have neutrophilic granulocytes in the circulating blood, with an impaired capacity to react to chemotactic stimuli. This neutrophil dysfunction may be caused by a cell-associated defect of long duration. These findings, together with available culture data, imply that localized juvenile periodontitis and juvenile periodontitis are microbiologically distinct diseases.

Circulating antibodies to antigens of pathogenic strains of *A. actinomycetemcomitans* have been found in a large percentage of localized juvenile periodontitis patients and in a small percentage of generalized juvenile periodontitis patients. Those patients who develop high levels of antibodies will demonstrate an arrested localized form of juvenile periodontitis into adulthood, whereas those who do not will progress into a more severe generalizd form of the acute disseminated form. This suggests that there may be a genetically controlled host resistance or susceptibility to the disease.

MIM No.: *17065, 26095

Sex Ratio: Reported to be in the range M1:F1 to M1:F41, but most studies consider that the true ratio is around M1:F3.

Occurrence: Varies with geographic areas and with populations, being higher for populations of African and Middle Eastern descent. The relative frequency in the United States is 0.02% for whites, 0.8% for Blacks, and 0.2% for Asians.

Risk of Recurrence for Patient's Sib: Empiric risk based on observed ratio is 0.17%.

Risk of Recurrence for Patient's Child: Unknown.

Age of Detectability: Usually about ages 11–13 years, when severe idiopathic bone loss can be detected in X-rays of incisors and first molars of otherwise healthy children.

Gene Mapping and Linkage: JPD (juvenile periodontitis) has been provisionally mapped to 4.

Prevention: None known. Genetic counseling indicated.

Treatment: About two-thirds of the patients with localized disease respond favorably to conventional periodontal treatment, involving 1) administration of tetracycline 250 mg qid for 2 weeks prior to surgery, 2) excision of the deepened pockets, 3) root curettage with removal of granulation tissue after flap elevation, and 4) plaque control. After surgery, the patients are instructed to rinse with chlorhexidine mouth wash for 2 minutes, twice a day, for the first 2 weeks after surgery. Professional tooth cleaning is carried out by a dental hygienist or dentist once every 3 months.

Treatment of localized juvenile periodontitis results in resolution of gingival inflammation, substantial gain in attachment, and refilling of bone in the angular defects. These patients are prone to recurrence, especially during the first 2 years after treatment. Treatment for the generalized form of juvenile periodontitis is less effective but is recommended, since some arresting of the disease process does occur.

Prognosis: The disease usually progresses with early loss of teeth. Treatment is necessary to arrest the disease process.

Detection of Carrier: Prior to ages 11–13 years, when the initial signs usually occur, it is not possible to detect individuals at risk for juvenile periodontitis. The discovery that neutrophil chemotaxis deficiency often precedes localized juvenile periodontitis may help to identify those children under age 12 years who are not yet affected.

Special Considerations: As the descriptive criteria for juvenile periodontitis have become more specific, diagnostic technology has been developed to confirm the diagnosis with blood studies, immunologic studies, and bacterial analyses. Despite these advances, confusion remains among clinicians on the use of the terms *periodontosis* and *juvenile periodontitis*. The term *periodontosis* was coined in 1942 by Orban and Weinmann to designate a condition seen in young individuals who had very little calculus for the amount of alveolar bone destruction seen and seemed to be essentially noninflammatory. Contemporary observers, however, had difficulty differentiating this type of periodontal disease from other forms in which additional findings were being observed. As a result, in 1963, the term *juvenile periodontitis* was created to identify other forms of periodontal disease in which an environmental component was observed. Despite this separation, much confusion and skepticism about the existence of a disease entity called *periodontosis* remained, and at the 1966 World Workshop in periodontics the American Academy of Periodontology issued the statement that "There is insufficient evidence to identify periodontosis as a specific disease entity. . . ." By consensus, the Academy agreed to place the word *periodontosis* in parentheses after the term juvenile periodontitis. Although every so often the terms are still used interchangeably, the name *juvenile periodontitis* is more accurate than *periodontosis* because current evidence suggests an associated bacterial etiology and because insufficient information exists to show a definitive genetic pattern of inheritance.

References:
Fourel J: Periodontosis: a periodontal syndrome. J Periodontol 1972; 43:240–255.
Melnick M, et al.: Periodontosis: a phenotypic and genetic analysis. Oral Surg 1976; 42:32–41.
Cullinan MO, et al.: The distribution of HLA-A and B antigens in patients and their families with periodontosis. J Periodont Res 1980; 15:177–184.
Lindhe J, Slots J: Juvenile periodontitis (periodontosis). In: Lindhe J, ed: Textbook of clinical periodontology. Philadelphia: W.B. Saunders, 1983:188–201.
Saxen L, Nevalinna HR: Autosomal recessive inheritance of juvenile periodontitis: test of a hypothesis. Clin Genet 1984; 25:332–335.
Long JC, et al.: Segregation analysis of early onset periodontitis. Am J Hum Genet 1985; 37:A200.
Page RC, et al.: Clinical and laboratory studies of a family with high prevalence of juvenile periodontitis. J Periodontol 1985; 56:602–610.
Roulton D, et al.: Linkage analysis of dentinogenesis imperfecta and juvenile periodontitis: creating a 5 point map of 4q. Am J Hum Genet 1985; 37:A206.
Genco R: New genetic evidence for juvenile periodontitis. Dentistry Today 1986; 4:1.
Beaty TH, et al.: Genetic analysis of juvenile periodontitis in families ascertained through an affected proband. Am J Hum Genet 1987; 40:443–452.

ES000
M0044

Victor Escobar
Regan L. Moore

Teeth, poor eruption-corneal dystrophy-gingival fibromatosis
See GINGIVAL FIBROMATOSIS-CORNEAL DYSTROPHY
Teeth, present at birth
See TEETH, NATAL OR NEONATAL
Teeth, pulpal dysplasia
See TEETH, DENTIN DYSPLASIA, CORONAL

TEETH, ROOT CONCRESCENCE   0928

Includes:
  Cementum, environmental defects in
  Concrescence of roots of teeth
  Roots, acquired concrescence of
  True concrescence

Excludes:
  Teeth, ankylosed (0927)
  Teeth, dilacerated (0929)
  Teeth, fused (0930)
  Teeth, geminated (0931)
  Teeth, impacted (0932)

Major Diagnostic Criteria: The roots of two or more teeth are united by cementum after the formation of the crowns. Only if this condition has occurred during tooth development is it called *true concrescence*. A union of two teeth by cementum after the completion of root formation is termed *acquired concrescence*. In both cases, there is no interdentinal combination and the crowns are not affected. Diagnosis can frequently be established by X-ray examination.

Clinical Findings: The most common location for true concrescence is between the second and third molars in the maxilla. Concrescence may occur in both impacted and erupted teeth. Concrescence is almost impossible to detect clinically, since the crowns of affected teeth appear clinically normal.

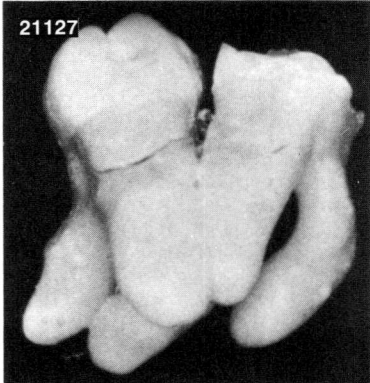

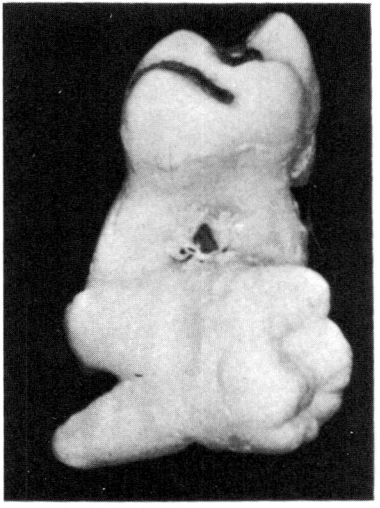

0928-21127: Concrescence of the molars.

Complications: 1) Delayed eruption of teeth as a consequence of root resorption or ankylosis of the root surface to the underlying bone. 2) Delayed eruption of succedaneous teeth. 3) Involved teeth often have periodontal involvement.

Associated Findings: None known.

Etiology: Undetermined. One hypothesis poses either a lack of space or dislocation of tooth germs as probable causes. No genetic inheritance has been established. True concrescence between maxillary second and third molars occurs in an arch where lack of space is most common. Etiology of acquired concrescence includes hypercementosis associated with either chronic infections or other systemic diseases such as Paget disease of bone.

Pathogenesis: Two elements must be fulfilled. First is the close approximation of the roots of adjacent teeth. This may result from simple crowding or from the constant changing of positions during the eruptive process. Second is the deposition of additional cementum. Union of the cementum of teeth is usually in the apical two-thirds of the root and is of an acellular type. Concrescence may occur before or after teeth have erupted. Microscopically, affected teeth are found to have separate pulp canals and roots.

Sex Ratio: M1:F1.

Occurrence: Undetermined. The prevalence of supernumerary teeth in Caucasian populations ranges between 0.15 and 1%. Ninety percent or more occur in the maxilla.

Risk of Recurrence for Patient's Sib: Unknown.

Risk of Recurrence for Patient's Child: Unknown.

Age of Detectability: Since crowns are not affected, concrescence of roots is not usually detected clinically. Concrescence may be observed on X-ray when the tooth involved or the region is X-rayed for other diagnostic purposes.

Gene Mapping and Linkage: Unknown.

Prevention: None known. Genetic counseling indicated.

Treatment: Concrescence alone does not require treatment, because the affected teeth are normal except for the union of cemental tissue. If these teeth are either in malocclusion or impacted, extraction is indicated.

Prognosis: If the teeth are fully erupted into good occlusion with healthy periodontium, prognosis is excellent. The condition is clinically not significant unless one of the attached teeth is to be extracted.

Detection of Carrier: Unknown.

References:
Eversole LR: Clinical outline of oral pathology: diagnosis and treatment, ed 2. Philadelphia: Lea & Febiger, 1984. †
Mader CL: Concrescence of teeth: a potential treatment hazard. Gen Dent 1984; 32:52–55.
Braham RL, Morris ME: Textbook of pediatric dentistry, ed 2. Baltimore: Williams & Wilkins, 1985. *

PA047   **Raj-Rajendra A. Patel**

Teeth, semi-shovel
See TEETH, INCISORS, SHOVEL-SHAPED
Teeth, short rooted-taurodontism-microcephalic dwarfism
See TAURODONTISM-SHORT ROOTED TEETH-MICROCEPHALIC DWARFISM
Teeth, small
See TEETH, MICRODONTIA

TEETH, SNOW-CAPPED   **2136**

Includes:
   Amelogenesis imperfecta, hypomaturation type
   Snow-capped teeth
Excludes:
   Teeth, amelogenesis imperfecta (0046)
   Fluorosis

Major Diagnostic Criteria: Areas of white-opaque enamel on incisal third of all teeth associated with areas of brown pigmentation.

Clinical Findings: On clinical examination, affected teeth have a smooth surface, which is hard and resists penetration by a sharp instrument. The enamel appears normal and does not chip away from the dentin. The defect in the enamel seems to be limited to the incisal and occlusal third of the teeth, with areas of defective enamel either opaque white or brownish in color. The pattern of severity varies from individual to individual, but in every affected individual all permanent teeth are clinically affected. The junction between clinically normal and abnormal enamel is well defined. The condition seems to be present at eruption, and both the primary and secondary dentitions are affected. Some patients present with tooth sensitivity to heat, cold, touch, and sweet. No unusual X-rays findings occur.

Complications: As in other amelogenesis imperfectas, the unsightly teeth may produce psychological changes in the child's personality.

Associated Findings: Difficulties in chewing, since some of the patients have tooth sensitivity to touch and/or sweets.

Etiology: X-linked recessive inheritance.

Pathogenesis: Low magnification SEM examination shows porosities of variable size distributed randomly over the abnormal enamel surface. Interestingly enough, if the tooth is etched with HCL and the prismless layer of the enamel is removed, the underlying enamel appears to have a normal structure. This confirms previous suggestions that the genetic defect is limited to the prismless layer of the enamel.

MIM No.: *30110

Sex Ratio: M1:F0. A few females are mildly affected.

Occurrence: Prevalence of 1:2,000 for the general population has been suggested without definitive data.

Risk of Recurrence for Patient's Sib:
   See Part I, *Mendelian Inheritance.*

Risk of Recurrence for Patient's Child:
   See Part I, *Mendelian Inheritance.*

Age of Detectability: Visual examination after eruption of teeth.

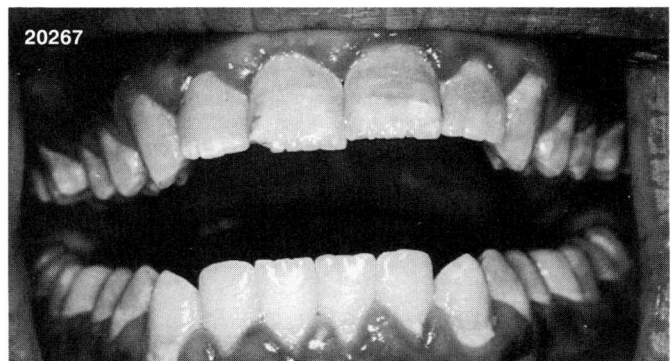

2136-20267: Note the "snow-capped" appearance of the teeth on the incisal third of all teeth. This is characteristically seen in amelogenesis imperfecta hypomaturation type III.

Gene Mapping and Linkage: AIH1 (amelogenesis imperfecta 1, hypomaturation or hypoplastic (?=AMG & AMGS)) has been mapped to Xp22.

Prevention: None known. Genetic counseling indicated.

Treatment: Unknown.

Prognosis: Excellent. No effect on life span.

Detection of Carrier: Unknown.

Special Considerations: No data regarding the biochemical defect in snow-capped teeth have been published, nor have sufficient numbers of families been reported to permit complete characterization of gene expression. However, both intra- and interfamilial variation is present in this trait. The differential diagnosis should always include fluorosis. However, while fluorosis is usually bright and shiny, snow-capped teeth enamel is dull and white.

References:

Witkop CJ Jr, Sauk JJ Jr: Defects of enamel. In: Stewart RE, Prescott GH, eds: Oral facial genetics. St. Louis: C.V. Mosby, 1976.
Escobar V, et al.: A clinical, genetic, and ultrastructural study of snow-capped teeth: amelogenesis imperfecta, hypomaturation type. Oral Surg 1981; 52:609–614.

ES000   **Victor Escobar**

TEETH, SUPERNUMERARY   0936

Includes:
- Distomolar
- Hyperodontia
- Mesiodens
- Paramolar
- Peridens
- Polydontia
- Retromolar
- Teeth, supplementary

Excludes:
- **Cleidocranial dysplasia** (0185)
- **Intestinal polyposis, type III** (0536)
- Odontomas

Major Diagnostic Criteria: Teeth in addition to those of the normal series (20 deciduous and 32 permanent teeth). Supernumerary teeth (ST) are usually abnormal in size and shape and may or may not erupt (remain impacted). They usually have no deciduous precursor and no replacing tooth. Morphologic features include diminutive, blunted, conical, and multicusped teeth.

Clinical Findings: ST may develop in any tooth-bearing area, but occur most frequently in the anterior and molar regions of the maxilla and the premolar region of the mandible either unilaterally or bilaterally. ST are usually single, but multiple ST have been reported and are unusual in the deciduous dentition. The number of supernumerary primary teeth is underestimated, so it is likely that many teeth exfoliate without being recognized as ST. Most common of all ST is a *mesiodens* between maxillary central incisors. The majority have conical crowns and short roots. A *paramolar* arises alongside the maxillary molars and is usually buccally placed, whereas a *distomolar* (or a *retromolar*) develops distal to a third molar. A *peridens* is one that has erupted outside the dental arches, e.g., into the nose, which termed a *nasal tooth*. Other locations include palate, orbit, coronoid process, and maxillary antrum. The ratio of frequency of all ST in the maxilla versus in the mandible is 8:1, and that of unerupted to erupted is 5:1.

Complications: Malocclusion, ectopic or delayed eruption, and impaction and resorption of adjacent teeth due to the presence of ST have been observed. The possibility of ameloblastoma formation in the walls of the follicle exists. It is speculated that cysts such as the median alveolar, median mandibular, lateral periodontal, and even globulomaxillary cysts are variants of a supernumerary primordial cyst.

Associated Findings: ST may be associated with facial cleft. They are also seen in stromes such as **Cleidocranial dysplasia, Oro-facio-digital syndrome, Cherubism, Klippel-Feil anomaly, Cataract-brachydactyly-oto-dental defects, Fabry disease, Chondroectodermal dysplasia, Incontinentia pigmenti,** and **Tricho-rhino-phalangeal syndrome.** The incidence of concurrent hyperodontia and hypodontia ranges from 8–41:10,000.

Etiology: It has been suggested that ST develop from a third tooth bud arising from the dental lamina near the permanent tooth bud, or possibly from splitting of the permanent bud itself. This latter view is somewhat unlikely, since the associated permanent teeth are usually normal in all respects. In some cases there appears to be a hereditary tendency for the development of ST. Mesiodens has been reported as transmitted by autosomal dominant inheritance with lack of penetrance. It has been suggested that hyperodontia is controlled by a number of different loci, and a polygenic scheme should be considered.

Pathogenesis: It is contended that supernumerary buds originate either from an occasional accessory proliferation of the dental lamina or from whorls of epithelial cells that persist from the breaking up of epithelial cords. These epithelial clusters also have the potential to produce tooth-like tumors (odontomas) and cyst linings, as determined by the stage of differentiation of enamel organ.

MIM No.: 18710

Sex Ratio: M2:F1. In one pedigree (Finn, 1967) all 14 females were affected while the three males were not.

Occurrence: Prevalence of ST among males is 2.4%, among females is 1.7%, and for both sexes is 2.1%. Incidence among first degree relatives of all probands is 19.7%. Overall frequency of ST ranges from 0.3–3.8%. Hyperodontia is seen in approximately 0.5% of children. Occurrence of supernumerary premolars is 1:10,000 individuals. Multiple ST occur in 14% of all cases that have ST.

Risk of Recurrence for Patient's Sib:
See Part I, *Mendelian Inheritance.* Probably not increased, except in association with a syndrome, or in the rare familial instance. Careful examination of relatives is indicated.

Risk of Recurrence for Patient's Child:
See Part I, *Mendelian Inheritance.* In sporadic, isolated ST, there is no increased risk.

Age of Detectability: Often diagnosed for the first time at ages 6–8 years by routine, full-mouth X-rays.

Gene Mapping and Linkage: Unknown.

Prevention: None known. Genetic counseling indicated.

Treatment: Extraction is the recommended course of treatment for ST. However, a success rate of 95% with autologous transplantation of ST has been reported.

Prognosis: Excellent. In certain cases there is no immediate indication for surgical removal. However, the patient should receive a regular clinical and X-ray examination.

Detection of Carrier: Possibly by clinical examination.

References:

Finn SB: Clinical pedodontics. Philadelphia: W.B. Saunders, 1967.
Grover PS, Lorton L: The incidence of supernumerary teeth. Gen Dent 1984; 32:224–227.

PA047   **Raj-Rajendra A. Patel**

Teeth, supplementary
See TEETH, SUPERNUMERARY

TEETH, TAURODONTISM   0926

Includes:
"Bull teeth"
Hypertaurodontism
Hypotaurodontism
Mesotaurodontism
Taurodontism

Excludes:
Hyperphosphatasia-mental retardation, Mabry type
Hypophosphatemia, X-linked (0517)
Teeth, amelogenesis imperfecta (0046)
Teeth, odontodysplasia (0739)
Teeth, taurodontism (0926)
Tricho-dento-osseous syndrome (0965)

Major Diagnostic Criteria: Multirooted teeth with vertically enlarged pulp chambers and apical displacement of the furcation of the roots.

Clinical Findings: The large pulp chambers of taurodontic teeth ("bull teeth") are most striking in the molars. The crowns of teeth appear normal. The condition is detected on X-ray. The furcations of the roots of molar and premolar teeth are displaced apically. The body and root of the teeth have a block rectangular shape. This is a relatively frequent trait particularly among Eskimos, American Indians, Bantus, and extinct hominids (Neanderthal). Classified on extent of the apical displacement of the furcation of roots as hypotaurodontism, mesotaurodontism, and hypertaurodontism.

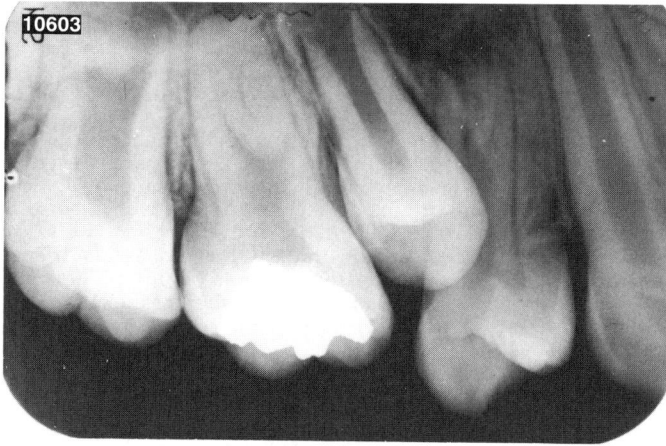

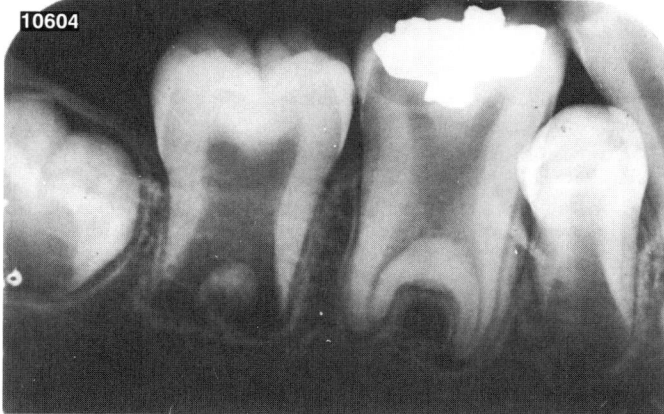

0926-10603–04:   Taurodontism.

Complications: When occurring with associated syndromes, pulp exposures with abcess formation and tooth loss are frequent.

Associated Findings: Taurodont teeth occur in X chromosome aneuploidy (90%); other chromosome abnormalities, e.g. **Chromosome 21, trisomy 21** (55%); other autosomal translocations and trisomy; **Oto-dental dysplasia**; **Tricho-dento-osseous syndrome**, **Amelo-onycho-hypohidrotic syndrome**, and **Oro-facio-digital syndrome, Mohr type**. Moller et al (see Gorlin et al, 1975) reported taurodontia in combination with absent teeth and sparse hair, as well as other findings often seen in hypohidrotic forms of **Ectodermal dysplasia**.

Teeth with large pulp chambers occur in **Hypophosphatemia, X-linked**, vitamin-D-refractory rickets (including renal types such as **Renal tubular syndrome, Fanconi type**), in the shell teeth variant of **Teeth, dentinogenesis imperfecta**; and in **Teeth, odontodysplasia**, and internal resorption. The anthropologic explanation for the high frequency of this trait in certain populations past and present is that it has a selective value; where teeth are used as tools (skin tanning), the taurodont tooth is less liable to pulp exposure from attrition than the cynodont tooth.

Etiology: Probably multifactorial inheritance, if not associated with syndrome of other known inheritance. Of the 22 completely examined kindreds, 19 show no affected parents, and none of the parents are known to be consanguineous. Twelve of the 21 have other affected sibs. Genetic heterogeneity is likely, and evidence for either dominant or recessive transmission is suggested in some kindreds when the condition is a part of an associated syndrome.

Pathogenesis: The primary alteration is unknown. The Hertwig epithelial root sheath fails to invaginate at the proper point below the crown to form roots in multirooted teeth, resulting in teeth with large pulp chambers such that the distance from the bifurcation or trifurcation of roots to the cementoenamel junction is greater than the occlusal-cervical distance. When associated with chromosomal anomalies, taurodontism probably reflects a defect in genetic homeostasis due to altered cell division and induction timing.

MIM No.:   27270, 27298

Sex Ratio: M1:F1

Occurrence: At least hypotaurodontism occurs in about 2:100 in the Caucasian population of the United States. Occurs in all races. Occurs in higher frequencies among Eskimos (20%) and Aleuts; in African Boskopoid, and Australoid (30%). Frequently noted in fossil hominid remains, particularly Neanderthal (20–60%). Found in 90% of X-chromosomal aneuploid patients, and in 55% of **Chromosome 21, trisomy 21** patients.

Risk of Recurrence for Patient's Sib: Based on 24 North American Caucasian propositi and corrected for ascertainment: 22%.

Risk of Recurrence for Patient's Child: Unknown.

Age of Detectability: From three to 12 years of age, by X-ray examination.

Gene Mapping and Linkage: Unknown.

Prevention: None known. Genetic counseling indicated.

Treatment: Taurodontic teeth frequently have pulp horns approaching the dentino-enamel junction. Pulp may be exposed when abrasion of the enamel exposes pulp horn at the dentin level. Teeth may require onlay capping to prevent pulp exposure, abcess formation, and tooth loss.

Prognosis: Normal life span.

Detection of Carrier: Unknown.

References:
Witkop CJ Jr: Manifestations of genetic diseases in the human pulp. Oral Surg 1971; 32:278–316. * †
Gorlin RJ, et al.: A selected miscellany. BD:OAS XI(2). New York: March of Dimes Birth Defects Foundation, 1975:39–50.
Jaspers MT, Witkop CJ Jr: Taurodontism, an isolated trait associated with syndromes and X-chromosomal aneuploidy. Am J Hum Genet 1980; 32:396–413. * †
Jaspers MT: Taurodontism in the Down syndrome. Oral Surg 1981; 51:632–636.

Jorgenson RJ: The conditions manifesting taurodontism. Am J Med Genet 1982; 11:435–442.

Witkop CJ, et al.: Taurodontism: an anomaly of teeth reflecting disruptive developmental homeostasis. Am J Med Genet 1988; 4:85–97.

WI043   Carl J. Witkop, Jr.

Teeth, thistle-shaped pulp chambers
    See TEETH, DENTIN DYSPLASIA, CORONAL
Tegison^, fetal effects of
    See FETAL RETINOID SYNDROME
Tegretal^, fetal exposure
    See FETAL CARBAMAZEPINE EXPOSURE
Tel-Hashomer camptodactyly syndrome
    See CAMPTODACTYLY SYNDROME, TEL HASHOMER TYPE
Telangiectasia macularis eruptiva perstans
    See URTICARIA PIGMENTOSA (UP)
Telangiectasia, congenital retinal
    See RETINA, COATS DISEASE

TELANGIECTASIA, OSLER HEMORRHAGIC   2021

Includes:
    Hemorrhagic telangiectasia, hereditary
    Osler disease
    Osler-Weber-Rendu disease
    Rendu-Osler disease
    Rendu-Osler-Weber disease
Excludes:
    Ataxia-telangiectasia (0094)
    Calcinosis-Raynaud-scleroderma-telangiectasia (CRST)
    Fabry disease (0373)
    Nevus, blue rubber bleb nevus syndrome (0113)
    Telangiectasia, hereditary benign

Major Diagnostic Criteria: The classic triad consists of cutaneous or mucosal telangiectasias; recurrent nasal or gastrointestinal hemorrhage with normal coagulation factors; and a positive family history. About 20% of patients have a negative family history.

Clinical Findings: The majority of patients have telangiectasias of the skin and mucous membranes. The telangiectasias appear as red to purple 2 mm to 2 cm papules or nodules that blanch with pressure. Additionally, there may be spider-like forms consisting of a central dot with radiating venules. The most common locations for the telangiectasias are the face, oral and nasopharyngeal membranes, tips of the digits, subungual and periungual

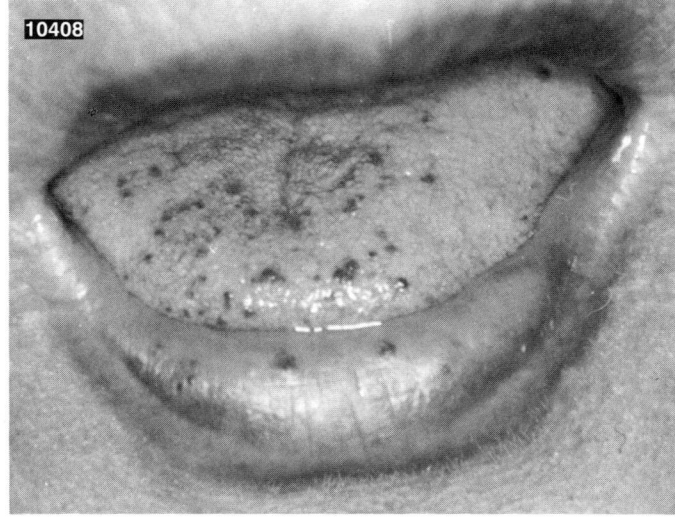

2021-10408: Telangiectasia on the tongue.

areas, palms, and soles. The frequency of patients demonstrating telangiectasias increases with age, to 90% by sixty years of age. The most common complaint, however, is epistaxis, which occurs in 78% of affected patients. Roughly one third of this group have had nasal hemorrhage severe enough to require tranfusion. The second most common complaint (44%) is gastrointestinal hemorrhage secondary to intestinal telangiectasias.

The usual onset is in the fifth decade of life, although bleeding has been reported in infancy. Liver abnormalities (30%) have been reported, including hepatic telangiectasias, passive hepatic congestion, arteriovenous fistulas, connective tissue formation with fibrosis, and atypical cirrhosis. Vascular malformations of the brain and spinal cord are relatively common (27%). Presenting symptoms may be headache, recurrent syncope, diplopia, vertigo, visual or auditory disturbances, dysarthria, or paresthesias. Approximately 20% of affected patients have hemoptysis secondary to pulmonary arteriovenous malformations. These may be demonstrable on standard chest X-rays. Vascular malformations of the retina, thyroid, heart, spleen, pancreas, kidneys, prostate, cervix, bladder, urethra, diaphragm, vertebrae, aorta, and other major arteries have been reported.

Complications: Anemia requiring tranfusions; high-output cardiac failure secondary to anemia or systemic arteriovenous shunt; cyanosis secondary to large pulmonary arteriovenous malformations; polycythemia; transient ischemic attacks; stroke; seizures; brain abscess (almost all associated with pulmonary arteriovenous malformations); and portal-systemic encephalopathy.

There have been several reports of a lethal homozygous form of this condition in which affected infants rapidly develop generalized telangiectasia and die within the first few months of life.

Associated Findings: Duodenal ulcer, **Von Willebrand disease**, cleidocranial dysostosis, and hepatocellular carcinoma.

Etiology: Autosomal dominant inheritance.

Pathogenesis: Hereditary hemorrhagic telangiectasia is a generalized vascular dysplasia. The telangiectasias are small collections of thin-walled blood vessels without muscular or elastic layers. Because of the lack of supporting connective tissue, these vessels are easily subject to traumatic or spontaneous rupture. On electron microscopy, the affected vessels have been shown to be dilated venules. Erythrocytes extravasate through gaps in the vascular endothelial cell junctions. These gaps are caused by defective overlapping of the endothelial cytoplasmic villi. Microthrombi are present within these gaps and are presumed to be necessary for closure of the endothelial junction. Additional abnormalities have been demonstrated in the perivascular tissues: abnormally large fibrils, increased amounts of amorphous material, and marked edema. It is not known whether the endothelial junction gap is due primarily to an intrinsic abnormality in the endothelial cell or whether it is secondary to defects in the periendothelial support structure.

MIM No.: *18730

POS No.: 3760

Sex Ratio: M1:F1

Occurrence: 1-2:100,000. Has been reported in all races, but is most common in Caucasians.

Risk of Recurrence for Patient's Sib:
    See Part I, *Mendelian Inheritance.*

Risk of Recurrence for Patient's Child:
    See Part I, *Mendelian Inheritance.*

Age of Detectability: The median age at diagnosis is 44 years. Fifty percent of patients develop epistaxis in first decade of life.

Gene Mapping and Linkage: Unknown.

Prevention: None known. Genetic counseling indicated.

Treatment: Mainly supportive and not curative. Trauma to the oral mucosa should be avoided, and a very soft toothbrush should be used. Local treatment in the form of compression, cauterization, vasoconstriction, or lubrication is the most common means of controlling bleeding. Tranfusion and iron supplementation are prescribed for severe hemorrhage. Systemic estrogen has been given with limited success as treatment for recurrent epistaxis. On electron microscopy, estrogen has been shown to re-establish continuity of the endothelium of affected vessels. For severe epistaxis, septal dermoplasty is advocated. This protects vessels from trauma by the application of a split-thickness skin graft over superficial nasal vessels. In symptomatic patients (with cyanosis, polycythemia, brain abscess, hemothorax, or severe hemoptysis), pulmonary arteriovenous fistulas have been treated with surgical excision or balloon embolization. Gastrointestinal hemorrhage rarely responds to electrocautery. Surgical removal of intestinal telangiectatic areas is not recommended, except in cases of life-threatening bleeding. Cerebral arteriovenous malformations have been treated with surgery, embolization, and proton beam irradiation.

Prognosis: Except in severe cases, patients with this disorder generally lead normal lives. Rarely, patients may have frequent and severe bleeding episodes.

Detection of Carrier: Unknown.

Special Considerations: *Calcinosis-Raynaud-scleroderma-telangiectasia (CRST)*, a probable collagen vascular disease, is a phenocopy of this condition, and may also be familial (Frayha et al, 1977).

Support Groups:
CA; Palo Alto; Hereditary Hemorrhagic Telangiectasia Foundation (HHTF)
MA; Amherst (c/o Dr. Bruce Jacobson, Biochemistry Dept., Univ. of Mass.); Hereditary Hemorrhagic Telangiectasia Registry

References:
Hodgson CH, et al.: Hereditary hemorrhagic telangiectasia and pulmonary arteriovenous fistula. New Engl J Med 1959; 261:625–636.
Hashimoto K, et al.: Hereditary hemorrhagic telangiectasia. An electron microscopy study. Oral Surg 1972; 34:751–762.
Frayha RA, et al.: Familial CRST syndrome with sicca complex. J Rheumatol 1977; 4:53–58.
Martini A: The liver in hereditary hemorrhagic telangiectasia: an inborn error of vascular structure with multiple manisfestations. Gut 1978; 19:531–537.
Roman G, et al.: Neurological manifestations of hereditary hemorrhagic telangiectasia (Rendu-Osler-Weber disease): report of two cases and review of the literature. Ann Neurol 1978; 4:130–144.
Bartolucci EG, et al.: Oral manifestations of hereditary hemorrhagic telangiectasia. J Periodontol 1982; 53:163–167.
Reilly PJ, et al.: Clinical manifestations of hereditary hemorrhagic telangiectasia. Am J Gastroenterol 1984; 79:363–367.
Cooke DAP: Renal arteriovenous malformation demonstrated angiographically in hereditary haemorrhagic telangiectasia (Rendu-Osler-Weber disease). J Roy Soc Med 1986; 79:744–746.
Plauchu H, et al.: Age-related clinical profile of hereditary hemorrhagic telangiectasia in an epidemiologically recruited population. Am J Med Genet 1989; 32:291–297.

BI001   **Diana W. Bianchi**

Telangiectasia-pigmentation-cataract syndrome
See ROTHMUND-THOMSON SYNDROME
Telangiectatic erythema, congenital
See ROTHMUND-THOMSON SYNDROME
Telangiectatic osteosarcoma
See OSTEOSARCOMA
Telecanthus
See BLEPHAROPTOSIS-BLEPHAROPHIMOSIS-EPICANTHUS INVERSUS-TELECANTHUS
Telecanthus with associated abnormalities
See HYPERTELORISM-HYPOSPADIAS SYNDROME

TELECANTHUS, HEREDITARY   2425

Includes:
Eyes, interpupillary distance
Face, interpupillary distance
Juberg-Hirsch syndrome

Excludes:
Hypertelorism-hypospadias syndrome (0505)
Hypertelorism-microtia-facial cleft-conductive deafness (0506)

Major Diagnostic Criteria: 1) Telecanthus (separation of the medial canthi more than 2 SD from mean for age, sex, and ethnic group); 2) dacryostenosis; 3) dacryagogatresia; 4) cleft lip and palate; 5) occult cleft lip; 6) asymmetric nares, 7) hypodontia.

Clinical Findings: Telecanthus (8/9); dacryostenosis or dacryagogatresia (3/9); occult cleft lip (2/9); cleft lip and palate (1/9); epicanthi (2/9); iridic coloboma (1/9); anisocoria (1/9); strabismus (2/9); asymmetric, external nares (4/9); hypoplastic columella nasi (3/9); rectangular uvula (1/9); bifid uvula (1/9); anomalous teeth (2/9); congenital absence of mandibular teeth (2/9); congenital absence of maxillary teeth (3/9). Sphenoidal bone abnormality, such as heaviness or asymmetry, may be seen, as well as the central hiatus of the maxillary and palatal bones seen with the palatal defect.

Complications: A speech defect may be associated with palatal deficiency. Severe dental crowding with anterior and posterior crossbite may result from a palatal defect. Malocclusion may accompany congenital absence of teeth.

Associated Findings: Penile chordee was present in one male. Clinodactyly of the 3rd, 4th, and 5th digits was present in one male.

Etiology: Autosomal dominant inheritance with incomplete penetrance and variable expressivity.

Pathogenesis: Unknown.

MIM No.: 18735

Sex Ratio: M3:F6 (observed in one kindred).

Occurrence: One kindred reported.

Risk of Recurrence for Patient's Sib:
See Part I, *Mendelian Inheritance.*

Risk of Recurrence for Patient's Child:
See Part I, *Mendelian Inheritance.*

Age of Detectability: At birth.

Gene Mapping and Linkage: Unknown.

Prevention: None known. Genetic counseling indicated.

Treatment: Plastic and reconstructive surgery, orthodontics, ophthalmologic surgery, speech therapy.

Prognosis: Normal life span.

Detection of Carrier: By physical examination.

References:
Pryor H.B.: Objective measurement of interpupillary distance. Pediatrics 1969; 44:973–977.
Juberg RC, Hirsch R: Expressivity of heritable telecanthus in five generations of a kindred. Am J Hum Genet 1971; 23:547–554. * †
Juberg RC, et al.: Normal values for intercanthal distance of 5 to 11-year-old American blacks. Pediatrics 1975; 55:431–436.

JU000   **Richard C. Juberg**

Telecanthus-hypospadias syndrome
See HYPERTELORISM-HYPOSPADIAS SYNDROME
Temazepam, fetal effects
See FETAL BENZODIAZEPINE EFFECTS
Temporal bone cholesteatoma
See EAR, CHOLESTEATOMA OF TEMPORAL BONE
Temporal "forceps marks" scarring and unusual facies
See ECTODERMAL DYSPLASIA, CONGENITAL FACIAL, SETLEIS TYPE
Temporal lobe, agenesis
See BRAIN, ARACHNOID CYSTS

Tenosynovitis, progressive-contractures-systemic involvement
  See ARTHRITIS-ARTERITIS SYNDROME
Terata Anacatadidymus
  See TWINS, CONJOINED
Terata Anadidymus
  See TWINS, CONJOINED
Terata Catadidymus
  See TWINS, CONJOINED
Teratoid cyst of the orbit, congenital
  See EYE, ORBITAL TERATOMA, CONGENITAL
Teratoid tumor of head or neck
  See NECK/HEAD, DERMOID CYST OR TERATOMA
Teratologic syndrome of visceral heterotaxy
  See ASPLENIA SYNDROME
Teratoma
  See ORAL DERMOIDS

TERATOMA, PRESACRAL-SACRAL DYSGENESIS   2370

Includes:
  Hemisacrum, familial type II
  Meningocele, anterior sacral
  Sacral defects, anterior
  Sacral dysgenesis-presacral teratoma
Excludes:
  Sacral defect with anterior sacral meningocele, X-linked
  Teratoma, sacrococcygeal teratoma (0877)

Major Diagnostic Criteria: Presacral teratoma plus sacral defect, or a positive family history and a sacral defect.

Clinical Findings: This variable dominant disorder may differ from family to family. Classically, it includes presacral teratoma, sacral dysgenesis, sacral dimple, and anal stenosis as primary anomalies. Anterior meningocele and tethered cord may also be seen in some cases, and teratoma may be absent. Many affected individuals are asymptomatic.

Complications: Constipation, retrorectal abcess, meningitis, and functional urinary tract anomalies ranging from reflux to neurogenic bladder. Malignant degeneration can occur but is relatively infrequent, with a rate estimated at 5%.

Associated Findings: None known.

Etiology: Autosomal dominant inheritance with variable expression.

Pathogenesis: It is tempting to ascribe the clinical findings associated with the teratoma to a physical effect of the mass during development. However, the teratoma is not always present even when these other findings are. For example, one family investigated had two members with teratomas and sacral findings, one with an anterior meningocele, and another with severe anal stenosis and sacral anomaly; the latter two without any evidence of teratoma. This would therefore seem to suggest a dominant variable developmental field defect, probably acting at the stage of determination, rather than morphogenesis.

MIM No.: *17645

POS No.: 4155

Sex Ratio: M1:F1

Occurrence: About ten families have been reported.

Risk of Recurrence for Patient's Sib:
  See Part I, *Mendelian Inheritance.*

Risk of Recurrence for Patient's Child:
  See Part I, *Mendelian Inheritance.*

Age of Detectability: Prenatal detection has been accomplished using ultrasound.

Gene Mapping and Linkage: Unknown.

Prevention: None known. Genetic counseling indicated.

Treatment: Physical anomalies should be treated surgically as needed. Although the teratomas are generally benign, the still present risk for malignancy is enough to warrant their removal. The possibility of a tethered cord, meningitis, or neurological deficits should be cause for rapid intervention, but family members may be reluctant to have surgery for asymptomatic findings. Surgical treatment of urinary tract problems may be necessary. Appropriate chemotherapy and other treatment for malignancy is indicated.

Prognosis: If complications do not arise, prognosis is excellent. Most complications are manageable or avoidable.

Detection of Carrier: X-ray of the sacral area and ultrasound of the pelvis.

Special Considerations: The frequency of teratomas in different families seems to vary. These may very well represent different alleles, and it is possible that the teratoma may not occur at all, or only very rarely, in some kindreds.

Support Groups: Atlanta; American Cancer Society

References:
Ashcraft KW, et al.: Familial presacral teratomas. BD:OAS XI(5). New York: March of Dimes Birth Defects Foundation, 1975:143–146.
Bolande RP: Childhood tumors and their relationship to birth defects. In: Mulvihill JJ, et al, ed: Genetics of human cancer. New York: Raven Press, 1977:43–75.
Durkin-Stamm MV, et al.: An unusual dysplasia-malformation-cancer syndrome in two patients. Am J Med Genet 1978; 1:279–289.
Yates VD, et al.: Anterior sacral defects: an autosomal dominantly inherited condition. J Pediatr 1983; 102:239–242.
Welch JP, Aterman K: The syndrome of caudal dysplasia: a review, including etiologic considerations and evidence of heterogeneity. Pediat Pathol 1984; 2:313–327.

LU001   **Mark Lubinsky**

TERATOMA, SACROCOCCYGEAL TERATOMA   0877

Includes:
  Currarime triad
  Sacrococcygeal teratoma (benign or malignant)
Excludes:
  Sacromeningocele
  Teratoma, presacral-sacral dysgenesis (2370)

Major Diagnostic Criteria: Most frequently seen as a tumor projecting at the sacrococcygeal area. Lobulated tumor mass in presacral space. Histopathologic confirmation is required.

All teratomas include cellular elements derived from embryonic ectoderm, endoderm, and mesoderm. The most common tissues observed in the mature (benign) form of teratoma are those of the respiratory, gastro-intestinal, and nervous systems, and are clearly recognizable as to cell type and organ system. Fully developed limbs, segments of normal intestine, and well-formed teeth have been found in benign tumors. The incidence of calcification with benign tumors is 35%. Incomplete maturation of various components is observed in immature teratomas, while neoplastic tissue, usually adenocarcinomas (53%), is identified in patients with malignant teratomas.

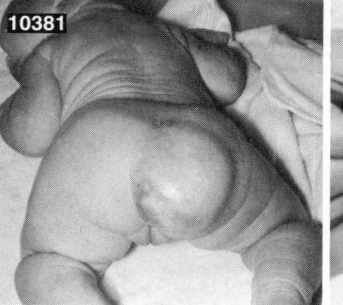 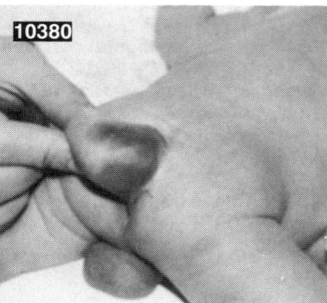

0877-10381–80:   Sacrococcygeal teratoma.

Clinical Findings: Sacrococcygeal teratomas are classified by their location. The most common type (47%) is predominantly external (sacrococcygeal), with only a minimal presacral component; type 2 (34%) tumors present externally but with a significant intrapelvic extension; type 3 (9%) are apparent externally, but the predominant mass is pelvic and extends into the abdomen; the type 4 (10%) tumor is entirely presacral with no external presentation. The visible tumor presents as a lobulated mass, bulging into the perineum, distorting and displacing the anus and external genitalia to a more anterior position. The tumors are composed of both solid and cystic areas, and are enclosed within a fibrous capsule. The extent of presacral extension can be ascertained by rectal digital examination and plain X-rays demonstrating anterior displacement of the rectal gas column. The majority (76%) of sacrococcygeal teratomas present within the first two months of life, at which time the incidence of pelvic obstructive symptoms, including bowel and bladder dysfunction, is 7%, and the risk of malignancy is 10.1%. Symptoms are present in 80% of infants when the teratoma is discovered after two months of age, and the incidence of malignancy in this group is 91.7%.

Complications: Ulceration and infection; ulceration and hemorrhage may occur in association with hemangiomatous component; malignancy (related to age of first detection: newborn and first two months of life 10.1%; after first two months 91.7%).

Associated Findings: None known.

Etiology: Unknown.

Pathogenesis: A sacrococcygeal teratoma begins as a zone of totipotent cells derived from the distal primitive streak and remnants of Hensen node. These undergo disorganized growth in contiguity with the developing coccygeal area.

Benign tumors, while arising from the sacrococcygeal region, have both an intrapelvic and external perineal component. Approximately 6% will grow outward and be pedunculated in appearance. The malignant tumors are primarily intrapelvic in location.

MIM No.: *17645

CDC No.: 238.040

Sex Ratio: M1:F3

Occurrence: 1:40,000 live births. One ten-year national study identified 105 cases.

Risk of Recurrence for Patient's Sib: Unknown.

Risk of Recurrence for Patient's Child: Unknown.

Age of Detectability: At birth or under two months of age in 76%; older than two months, 24%. Prenatally, there is increased amniotic fluid alpha-fetoprotein; ultrasound shows soft-tissue mass attached to lower pole of fetus and hydramnios; amniography shows soft-tissue mass with smooth encapsulated outline.

Gene Mapping and Linkage: Unknown.

Prevention: None known. Genetic counseling indicated.

Treatment: Treatment is operative removal of the tumor with reconstruction of the perineal region. Since these tumors are intimately associated with the perichondrium of the coccyx, coccygectomy is mandatory to avoid local recurrence of the tumors. The entire mass can be excised through a perineal incision in most patients; a combined abdominosacral procedure is necessary to remove all the intrapelvic component of large dumbbell-shaped tumors.

Reexcision of recurrent tumors, plus radiotherapy and chemotherapy, if recurrence is malignant.

Prognosis: Overall operative mortality is 4%. *Benign teratoma* cure following complete excision of tumor with coccygectomy has been 100%. Recurrence rate without coccygectomy is 31.3%. *Malignant teratoma*: 60% die within 10 months of operation; only 11% survive without apparent residual disease.

Detection of Carrier: Unknown.

Special Considerations: A syndrome of presacral teratoma with anorectal stenosis and recognizable sacral defect, sometimes called *Currarime triad*, has been described in 17 individuals from six kindreds (Yates et al, 1983).

Support Groups: Atlanta; American Cancer Society

References:
Donnellan WA, Swenson O: Benign and malignant sacrococcygeal teratomas. Surgery 1968; 64:834–846.
Dillard BM, et al.: Sacrococcygeal teratoma in children. J Pediatr Surg 1970; 5:53–59.
Altman RP, et al.: Sacrococcygeal teratoma: American Academy of Pediatrics surgical section survey for 1973. J Pediatr Surg 1974; 9:389–398.
Noseworthy J, et al.: Sacrococcygeal germ cell tumors in childhood: an updated experience with 118 patients. J Pediatr Surg 1981; 16:358–364.
Yates VD, et al.: Anterior sacral defects: an autosomal dominantly inherited condition. J Pediat 1983; 102:239–242.

T0009 **Robert J. Touloukian**

TERATOMAS 2919

Includes:
Dermoid cyst
Epignathus
Pineal teratomas
Seminoma
Testical tumors

Excludes:
Fetus in fetu
Hamartomas
Mixed tumors

Major Diagnostic Criteria: Teratomas are tumors formed from totipotent cells with ectodermal, mesodermal, and endodermal derivatives. The dermoid, or hair-filled cyst, of the ovary is a teratoma variant with well-differentiated skin appendages.

Clinical Findings: Derivatives of skin, teeth, respiratory mucosa, alimentary mucosa, various endocrine glands, and the central nervous system are common constituents of teratomas. They differ from hamartomas, which represent proliferation of tissue appropriate to the region of origin, and choristomas with tissue not normally found in the region of origin by virtue of their tissue heterogeneity. Teratomas occur most often in a para-axial, gonadal, or midline location from the brain to sacral area. Based on a survey of 142 cases in infants and children, the primary sites for teratomas included the sacrococcyx (84 cases), ovaries (15), testicles (15), mediastinum (14), retroperitoneum (7), cervix (3), gastrointestinal tract (1), palate (epignathus; 1), vagina (1), and uterine cervix (1). Teratomas are classified histologically as benign (mature adult tissue only), immature (embryonic tissue present but not malignant tissue), and malignant (frankly malignant tissue present in addition to mature or embryonic tissue). By these criteria, malignancy occurred in 40 of the 142 cases cited above (28%) and was highly correlated with elevated serum alpha-fetoprotein. Some authors cite a high incidence of malignant degeneration in benign teratomas as justification for aggressive therapy.

Sacrococcygeal teratomas present most commonly in infancy. About one-half are benign. There is a poor prognosis for malignant tumors, especially in older patients. Ovarian and testicular teratomas are usually detected in the first two years of life. Ovarian teratomas are more likely to be malignant in children, while the reverse is true of testicular teratomas. Most mediastinal teratomas occur in adults, while retroperitoneal teratomas are restricted almost exclusively to early childhood. Gastric, orbital, pulmonary, cardiac, and hepatic teratomas have been reported as rarities.

Complications: Nonresectable malignant teratomas are usually fatal despite radiation or chemotherapy. Fetal epignathous tumors may cause polyhydramnios. Ovarian teratomas may present with abdominal pain and vomiting after torsion.

Associated Findings: Fetal teratomas may cause or be associated with congenital malformations, such as **Hydrocephaly** with intracranial tumors, urogenital anomalies, or **Meningomyelocele** with sacrococcygeal tumors. In addition to adjacent malformations that might occur secondary to tumor compression, a general increased incidence (nine percent of patients) of noncontiguous congenital malformations has been reported.

Etiology: While most teratomas are sporadic, several families with an autosomal dominant predisposition to ovarian dermoid cysts have been reported. These families, plus the existence of mouse mutations that cause a high incidence of either ovarian or testicular teratomas, suggest genetic factors as part of the etiology of teratomas. Hereditary teratomas may be underreported because of their benign phenotype or spontaneous regression.

The bilaterality, early onset, and familial occurrence of ovarian teratomas suggest that chromosome deletions or genetic mutations will eventually be demonstrated for these and other teratomas.

Pathogenesis: While the presence of vertebral organization may be used to distinguish the fetus in fetu from teratomas, a relationship of both to twinning has been hypothesized. Ovarian teratomas may be viewed as an example of parthenogenesis through self-fertilization; one report postulates failure of extrusion of the second polar body at meiosis. Consistent chromosomal rearrangements or oncogene mutations have not yet been defined in teratomas.

MIM No.: 27312, 27330.

CDC No.: 238.000

Sex Ratio: M1:F2–3 for sacrococcygeal teratomas; M1:F1 for nongonadal tumors.

Occurrence: Teratomas constitute approximately three percent of childhood tumors.

Risk of Recurrence for Patient's Sib: Undetermined but presumably rare.

Risk of Recurrence for Patient's Child: Undetermined but presumably rare.

Age of Detectability: Teratomas are the most common neoplasms in newborns and may be detected prenatally by ultrasonography or maternal serum alpha-fetoprotein measurement.

Gene Mapping and Linkage: Unknown.

Prevention: None known. Genetic counseling indicated.

Treatment: Extirpation of accessible, benign lesions is recommended to prevent malignant degeneration. Malignant lesions are removed surgically followed by radiotherapy with or without regimens of chemotherapy, including vincristine, adriamycin, actinomycin D, cyclophosphamide, and bleomycin.

Prognosis: Prognosis ranges from survival averaging sixteen months for malignant sacrococcygeal teratoma, to excellent for benign or contained lesions.

Detection of Carrier: Unknown.

Support Groups: Atlanta; American Cancer Society

References:
Warkany J: Congenital malformations. Chicago: Yearbook Medical, 1971:1239–1246.
Hecht F, et al.: Ovarian teratomas and genetics of germ-cell formation. Lancet 1976; II:1311.
Chervenak FA, et al.: Diagnosis and management of fetal teratomas. Obstet Gynecol 1985; 66:666–671.
Siman A, et al.: Familial occurrence of mature ovarian teratomas. Obstet Gynecol 1985; 66:278–279.
Billmire DF, Grosfeld JL: Teratomas in childhood: analysis of 142 cases. J Pediatr Surg 1986; 21:548–551.
von der Maase H, et al.: Carcinoma in situ of contralateral testis in patients with testicular germ cell cancer: study of 27 cases in 500 patients. Brit Med J 1986; 293:1398–1401.

WI024   **Golder N. Wilson**

Teratomas of the orbit
See NECK/HEAD, DERMOID CYST OR TERATOMA

THALASSEMIA   0939

Includes:
    Cooley anemia
    Hemoglobin Lepore syndromes
    Mediterranean anemia
    Microcythemia

Excludes:
    Anemia, congenital sideroblastic, not B(6) responsive (2659)
    Anemia, sideroblastic (1518)
    Hematologic disease from iron or other nutritional deficiency
    Seizures, vitamin B(6) dependency (0991)

Major Diagnostic Criteria: Pallor, microcytic anemia, and jaundice, which vary with the type of thalassemia. Most clinically significant forms of β thalassemia are accompanied by "compensatory" changes, expressed as an increase in the percentage of hemoglobins A_2 and/or F. Forms of α thalassemia associated with moderate-to-severe clinical disease often are accompanied by the presence of abnormal hemoglobins composed entirely of non-α chains. These include hemoglobin H (β_4) and hemoglobin Barts (γ_4).

Clinical Findings: All clinically significant forms of thalassemia are accompanied by anemia and erythrocyte microcytosis. Enlargement of the liver and/or spleen may also be present. Anemia may vary from very mild to a degree of severity sufficient to require periodic transfusions in order to sustain life. Clinical features of major forms of thalassemia by type include:

β *Severe* (β^0) *heterozygous*: Possible splenomegaly and mild icterus.

β *Severe* (β^0) *homozygous*: Pallor, jaundice, bone deformities with

Table 0939-1 Clinical and Hematologic Features of the Major Forms of Thalassemia

Type	Hemoglobin findings	Hematologic changes	Clinical features
Heterozygous			
β Severe (β^0)(high A_2)	A_2, 3.5%–7.5% F, 1%–6%	Erythrocyte microcytosis and hypochromia, mild-to-moderate anemia	Possible splenomegaly and mild icterus
β Mild (β^+)(high A_2)	A_2, 3.5%–7.5%	Erythrocyte microcytosis and hypochromia, mild or absent anemia	Usually none
β Silent carrier	A_2 and F normal (F-containing cells sometimes detectable by slide elution test)	Hematologically normal	None
$\beta\delta$ (high F)	A_2, normal or low F, 5%–20%	Erythrocyte microcytosis and hypochromia, mild or absent anemia	Usually none
$\gamma\delta\beta$	Normal	Newborn: microcytosis, hemolytic anemia with normoblastemia Adult: same as heterozygous β^0	Newborn: hemolytic disease with splenomegaly Adult: same as heterozygous β^0
α Severe (α_1)(-,-)	Adult: normal Newborn: Barts, 5%–10%	Erythrocyte microcytosis and hypochromia, mild anemia	Usually none
α Mild (α_2)(-,α) (α Silent carrier)	Adult: normal Newborn: Barts, 1%–2%	Usually normal	Usually none
α_1/α_2 compound Heterozygous (Hb H disease)(-,-/-,α)	H (β_4), 5%–25% Barts (γ_4), 1%–3%	Erythrocyte hypochromia, poikilocytosis, anisocytosis; inclusion bodies demonstrable by supravital staining; moderate anemia	Pallor, jaundice, hepatosplenomegaly
Homozygous			
β Severe (β^0)	F, 30%–95%	Markedly abnormal red cell morphology with microcytosis and hypochromia, nucleated red cells, severe anemia	Pallor, jaundice, bone deformities with abnormal facies, hepatosplenomegaly, usually transfusion-dependent
β Mild (β^+)	F, 40%–80%	Poikilocytosis, anisocytosis, target cells; moderate anemia	Pallor, hepatosplenomegaly, jaundice; transfusions not usually required
$\beta\delta$ (high F)	F, 100%	Poikilocytosis, anisocytosis, hypochromia, microcytosis; mild-to-moderate anemia	Mild jaundice, hepatosplenomegaly usually present
α Severe (α_1)(-,-/-,-)	Barts, 80%–90% A and F, absent	Red cell hypochromia, anisocytosis, poikilocytosis; severe anemia	Hydrops fetalis with severe edema, hepatosplenomegaly, congestive heart failure; usually still-birth or death within first 24 hr.
α Mild (α_2)(-,α/-,α)	(same findings as heterozygous α_1)(see above)		

abnormal facies, hepatosplenomegaly, usually transfusion-dependent.

β Mild (β^+) homozygous: Pallor, hepatosplenomegaly, jaundice; transfusions not usually required.

$\beta\delta$ heterozygous: Usually clinically normal.

$\beta\delta$ homozygous: Pallor, hepatosplenomegaly.

α^0 (-,-) heterozygous: Usually normal.

α^+ (-,α) heterozygous: Usually normal.

Hemoglobin H disease (-,-/-,α): Pallor, jaundice, hepatosplenomegaly.

α^0 homozygous (-,-/-,-): Hydrops fetalis with severe edema, hepatosplenomegaly, congestive heart failure, usually stillbirth or death within 24 hours after birth.

Hematologic changes of major forms of thalassemia by type include:

β Severe (β^0) heterozygous: Erythrocyte microcytosis and hypochromia, mild-to-moderate anemia; increased levels of hemoglobin A_2 and hemoglobin F.

β Severe (β^0) homozygous: Markedly abnormal red cell morphology with marked hypochromia, nucleated red cells, severe anemia; hemoglobin F 80–95%.

β Mild (β^+) homozygous: Poikilocytosis, anisocytosis, target cells, moderate anemia; hemoglobin F 40–80%.

$\beta\delta$ heterozygous: Erythrocyte microcytosis and hypochromia, mild or absent anemia; hemoglobin A_2 normal or low with hemoglobin F 5–20%.

$\beta\delta$ homozygous: Poikilocytosis, anisocytosis, hypochromia, microcytosis, moderate anemia; hemoglobin F 100%.

α^0 (-,-) heterozygous: Usually normal.

α^+ (-,α) heterozygous: Usually normal.

Hemoglobin H disease (-,-/-,α): Erythrocyte hypochromia, poikilocytosis, anisocytosis, inclusion bodies demonstrable by supravital staining, moderate anemia; hemoglobin H (β_4) 5–25%.

α^0 homozygous (-,-/-,-): Red cell hypochromia, anisocytosis, poikilocytosis, severe anemia; hemoglobin Barts 80–90%.

Complications: *Anemia:* "Ineffective erythropoiesis" is characteristic of severe forms of thalassemia. The bone marrow erythroid elements are greatly increased, and utilization of iron and other erythropoietic nutrients is accelerated significantly, but inadequate numbers of mature erythrocytes are released into the peripheral blood. This series of events is thought to result from intramedullary destruction of erythroid precursors. In addition to the disordered erythropoiesis in these conditions, a major hemolytic component is also present, attributed to enhanced reticuloendothelial trapping of erythrocytes as a result of inclusion body formation. The red cell inclusions represent precipitated globin material, resulting from the unbalanced synthesis of complementary (α and non-α) globin chains of hemoglobin.

Enlargement of liver and spleen: These changes result from several associated features of thalassemia. These include extramedullary hematopoiesis, congestive changes related to anemia and myocardial dysfunction, and proliferation of reticuloendothelial elements due to hemosiderin deposition.

Cortical thinning of bone with associated fractures and deformities: These changes appear to be related to the massive expansion of erythroid bone marrow.

Iron overload: As a result of chronic anemia, patients with thalassemia absorb considerably increased quantities of iron. For this reason, and particularly because of the large quantities of iron that are derived from blood transfusions, these patients often develop severe complications, including liver dysfunction with cirrhosis; pancreatic iron loading, which in some cases is associated with overt diabetes; and myocardial dysfunction, which, not infrequently, leads to the development of intractable arrhythmias and death.

Associated Findings: None known.

Etiology: Autosomal recessive inheritance. All of the thalassemia disorders represent biosynthetic defects, which result in a deficiency of synthesis of one or more of the globin chains of hemoglobin. More than 75 distinct molecular abnormalities give rise to thalassemia. These include partial or total deletion of the globin genes; mutations involving the promoter regions of the genes; mutations involving splice junction regions at exon-intron boundaries; mutations causing abnormal splicing of the mRNA precursors; "nonsense" mutations, which cause premature termination of globin chain synthesis; and mutations involving translation initiation and termination codons. A number of structurally abnormal hemoglobins are also expressed with the thalassemia phenotype. These include hemoglobin E, the Lepore hemoglobins, and a group of hyper-unstable variants.

Pathogenesis: The genetic abnormalities that underlie these conditions result in a biosynthetic deficiency of the affected globin chain(s), with an accompanying decrease in the concentration of hemoglobin in the erythroid cells due to the globin deficiency. As an additional consequence, a relative excess of the noninvolved globin chain is produced within the hemoglobin-synthesizing cells. Because uncombined globin chains are unstable in solution, this globin material undergoes intracellular precipitation, leading to inclusion body formation. This, in turn, leads to greatly accelerated cellular destruction, with a major hemolytic process that may aggravate the primary degree of anemia.

MIM No.: 27350

Sex Ratio: M1:F1

Occurrence: The thalassemias occur predominantly in tropical and subtropical areas of Europe, Africa, and Asia. In regions of high gene frequency, an occurrence of greater than 1:100 births has been documented. All forms of thalassemias are uncommon in Northern European and in Western Hemispheric native populations. The prevalence is highly variable, depending on the population group.

Risk of Recurrence for Patient's Sib:
See Part I, *Mendelian Inheritance.*

Risk of Recurrence for Patient's Child:
See Part I, *Mendelian Inheritance.*

Age of Detectability: All forms of α thalassemia are fully expressed and detectable at birth. Antenatal detection in the second trimester fetus can be accomplished by fetal blood sampling or by restriction endonuclease mapping studies using fetal cells derived from amniotic fluid. This can be accomplished as early as 8–10 weeks by chorionic villus biopsy.

The β thalassemias are normally not clinically expressed until 3–6 months of age. Detection at birth and prenatal detection in the first or second trimester fetus are accomplished by globin synthesis studies, by DNA analysis, or in appropriate families by linkage studies with a DNA polymorphism.

Gene Mapping and Linkage: The α-globin locus has been mapped to 16p13.3, and the β-globin locus to 11p15.5. Several mutant hemoglobin α-chain genes have been shown to exist in close linkage with α-thalassemia gene deletions. These include Hb G Philadelphia (68 Lys), Hb Q (65 His), Hb Hasharon (47 His), Hb Nigeria (81 Cys), Hb J Tongariki (115 Asp), and Hb J Capetown (92 Gln). A β-chain mutant, Hb Vicksburg (75 deleted), appears to be linked to a β-thalassemia gene.

Prevention: None known. Genetic counseling indicated.

Treatment: In patients with severe β thalassemia, periodic transfusions may be required to sustain life. Use of transfusions containing "neocytes" or young red blood cells with a longer life span may allow reduction of the numbers of transfusions required. By application of "hypertransfusion" regimens, whereby transfusions are administered to a sufficient degree and at frequent intervals so as to maintain a near-normal hemoglobin concentration in the blood, many of the secondary complications, particularly cardiac dysfunction and skeletal changes can be largely prevented. This form of therapy, however, serves to increase the degree of iron storage. Treatment that minimizes iron storage is becoming important in the treatment of thalassemias requiring transfusions. Desferrioxamine is given by long-term infusion via a mechanical pump. Bone marrow transplantation, when successful, is curative.

Prognosis: The application of intensive transfusion therapy in patients with severe β thalassemia has greatly improved the quality of life for these patients, but the increased iron burden that this form of therapy produces has come to represent the major cause of death of these patients, as a result of cardiac or hepatic failure. Median survival for the transfusion-dependent thalassemia patient has been approximately 20 years, but the introduction of improved methods of chelation therapy holds promise that increased survival will be achieved.

Detection of Carrier: Most forms of heterozygous α and β thalassemia are accompanied by microcytosis, mild anemia, and morphologic abnormalities of the erythrocytes. "Silent-carrier" forms of these disorders have also been identified, and these individuals may have no apparent hematologic abnormality. Heterozygous β thalassemia can be confirmed by the findings of elevated levels of hemoglobins A$_2$ or F. The heterozygous forms of α thalassemia, on the other hand, typically have no abnormality of hemoglobin composition. These usually require an investigation of family members and studies of globin chain synthesis or restriction endonuclease mapping studies for confirmation of the diagnosis. Some of the forms of hereditary persistence of fetal hemoglobin may be difficult to distinguish from heterozygous β-thalassemia syndromes.

Special Considerations: The hemoglobin Lepore syndromes are caused by hemoglobin types containing abnormal non-α chains that are hybrid molecules which contain parts of the fused δ-globin and β-globin chains. These mutant hemoglobins produce the clinical and hematologic features of a thalassemia syndrome. When present in combination with a gene for β thalassemia, these syndromes may present as severe, transfusion-dependent thalassemia. The Lepore hemoglobins are identified by electrophoresis and exhibit a mobility, at alkaline pH, similar to that of sickle hemoglobin. Hemoglobin Constant Spring, an extended α chain variant, produces the phenotype of α thalassemia, and has been observed in a large percentage of individuals with Hb H disease. Its electrophoretic mobility at alkaline pH is slower than that of Hb A$_2$.

Support Groups:
New York; Cooley's Anemia Blood and Research Foundation for Children
New York; Cooley's Anemia Foundation, Inc.
NY; Douglaston; AHEPA Cooley's Anemia Foundation

References:
Propper RD, et al.: Continuous subcutaneous administration of desferrioxamine in patients with iron overload. New Engl J Med 1977; 297:418–423.
Propper RD, et al.: New approaches to the transfusion management of thalassemia. Blood 1980; 55:55–60.
Weatherall DJ, Clegg JB: The thalassemia syndromes, 3rd ed. Oxford: Blackwell Scientific Publications, 1981.
Modell B, Berdoukas V: The clinical approach to thalassemia. London: Grune & Stratton, 1984.
Honig GR, Adams JG III: Human hemoglobin genetics. Vienna: Springer-Verlag, 1986.
Lucarelli G, et al.: Marrow transplantation in patients with advanced thalassemia. New Engl J Med 1987; 316:1050–1055.
Weatherall DF, et al.: The hemoglobinopathies. In: Scriver CR, et al, eds: The metabolic basis of inherited disease. New York: McGraw-Hill, 1989:2281–2340.

H0024   **George R. Honig**

Thalidomide external ear malformation
See EAR, MICROTIA-ATRESIA
Thalidomide, fetal effects
See FETAL THALIDOMIDE SYNDROME
Thanatophoric dwarfism
See THANATOPHORIC DYSPLASIA

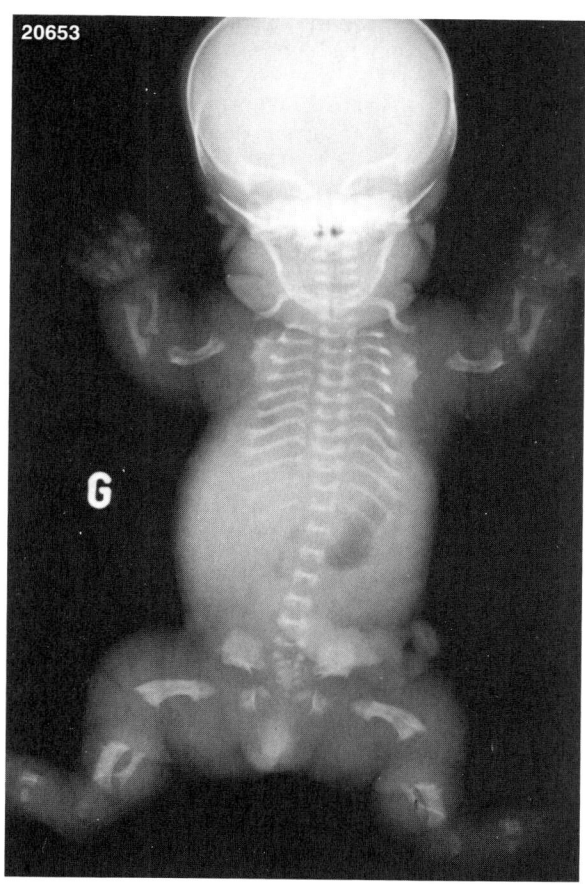

0940-20653: Thanatophoric dysplasia in a newborn; note short long bones and ribs, flattening of the vertebral bodies, and horizontal acetabular roofs.

THANATOPHORIC DYSPLASIA   0940

Includes:
Dwarfism, thanatophoric
Thanatophoric dwarfism

Excludes:
Asphyxiating thoracic dysplasia (0091)
Craniosynostosis, Kleeblattschadel type (0555)
Dwarfism, short-limb, other forms in the newborn
Skeletal dysplasia, Schneckenbecken type (2632)
Thanatophoric dysplasia, Glasgow type (2821)

Major Diagnostic Criteria: Severe neonatal short-limb dwarfism with characteristic X-ray features, including vertebral and pelvic abnormalities, and a narrow thorax with short cupped ribs and irregular metaphyses.

Clinical Findings: Birth length ranges from 36 to 46 cm. Limbs are very short and extend away from an essentially normal-sized trunk with thighs abducted and externally rotated. The fingers are very short and conically shaped. The head is relatively large, with a prominent forehead and depressed nasal bridge. The thorax is small, and respiratory distress occurs. Hypotonia and numerous skin folds are present; the primitive reflexes are absent. Death within the first few days is usual, although survival for over six months has been reported.

X-ray findings include vertebral bodies that have a small vertical diameter, with the narrowest area in the middle of the body in both anteroposterior (AP) and lateral projections. The intervertebral spaces are large. The posterior vertebral elements are well ossified. The interpediculate distance is narrowed in the mid or lower lumbar spine. The ilia have a short vertical dimension. The transverse diameter is greater than the vertical. The inferior margin of the ilia is horizontal and the sacrosciatic notches small. The pubic and ischial bones are broad and short. The thorax is narrow in both AP and transverse diameters, with short ribs, the ends of which are cupped. The long bones are very short; relatively broad, and bowed with irregular, spur-like flaring of the metaphyses. Hand and foot bones are very short and broad. There are no abnormal laboratory findings. The presence of a cloverleaf skull probably reflects variability, rather than heterogeneity.

Complications: Most reported affected infants die of respiratory complications. On autopsy, some have showed an impression on the spinal cord made by the small foramen magnum.

Associated Findings: **Hydrocephaly** has been reported.

Etiology: Probably polygenic inheritance, with a high rate of new dominant mutations. Gross changes of thanatophoric dwarfism appear similar but more marked than those of heterozygous achondroplasia. Presumed cases of homozygous achondroplasia have gross deformity intermediate between those of thanatophoric dwarfism and heterozygous achondroplasia. No infant with changes of thanatophoric dwarfism has been born to a couple with one achondroplastic mate. Although several kindreds have been reported where two or more siblings are affected by "thanatophoric dysplasia," analysis of X-rays and chondroosseous histopathology has demonstrated that they do not have this entity, except for two affected sibs with the additional feature of cloverleaf skull. All other documented cases of thanatophoric dysplasia have been sporadic.

Pathogenesis: Characteristic generalized disruption of growth plate with persistant mesenchymal-like tissue.

MIM No.: *18760

POS No.: 3411

CDC No.: 756.447

Sex Ratio: Presumably M1:F1.

Occurrence: 1:42,000. Most affected individuals die in infancy.

Risk of Recurrence for Patient's Sib:
See Part I, *Mendelian Inheritance.* The empiric risk has been computed at 2%.

Risk of Recurrence for Patient's Child:
See Part I, *Mendelian Inheritance.* Affected individuals are not expected to survive to reproduce.

Age of Detectability: At birth, by X-ray. Prenatally, by ultrasonography showing shortened limbs, small chest, relatively large head with thickened scalp, protuberant abdomen, hydramnios.

Gene Mapping and Linkage: Unknown.

Prevention: None known. Genetic counseling indicated.

Treatment: Unknown.

Prognosis: Fatal in first year of life, usually in first week.

Detection of Carrier: Unknown.

References:

Maroteaux P, et al.: Le nanisme thanatophore. Presse Med 1967; 75:2519–2524.
Langer LO Jr, et al.: Thanatophoric dwarfism: a condition confused with achondroplasia in the neonate, with brief comments on achondrogenesis and homozygous achondroplasia. Radiology 1969; 92: 285–294.
Rimoin DL: The chondrodystrophies. Adv Hum Genet 1975; 5:1–118.
Maroteaux P, et al.: The lethal chondrodysplasias. Clin Orthop 1976; 114:31–45.
Nissenbaum M, et al.: Thanatophoric dwarfism: two case reports and survey of the literature. Can Pediatr 1977; 16:690–697.
Elejalde BR, de Elejalde MM: Thanatophoric dysplasia: fetal manifestations and prenatal diagnosis. Am J Med Genet 1985; 22:669–683.
Martinez-Frias ML, et al.: Thanatophoric dysplasia: an autosomal dominant condition. Am J Med Genet 1988; 31:815–820.

B0025
LA016

Zvi Borochowitz
Leonard O. Langer, Jr.
David L. Rimoin

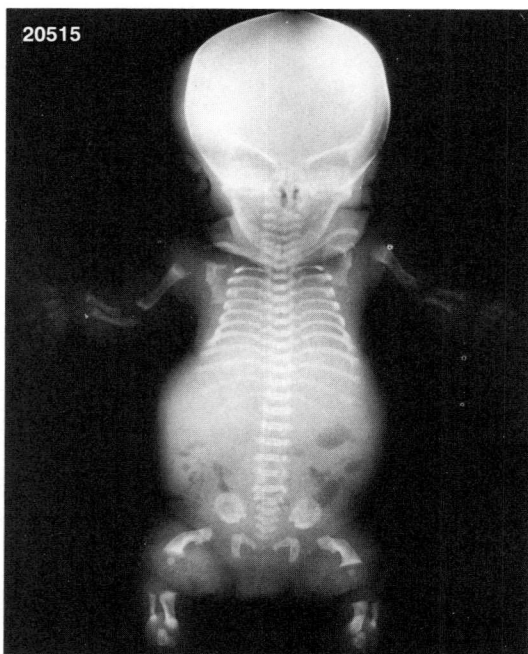

THANATOPHORIC DYSPLASIA, GLASGOW TYPE   2821

Includes: Skeletal dysplasia, neonatally lethal short-limbed, Glasgow type

Excludes:
    Skeletal dysplasia (other)
    Thanatophoric dysplasia (0940)

Major Diagnostic Criteria: Severe neonatal short-limb dwarfism with characteristic X-ray features.

Clinical Findings: Birth length about 36 cm, with severe micromelia. The head is relatively normal, but facies are flattened. Neonatal death occurs from respiratory insufficiency. Cataracts and unexplained hepatosplenomegaly were present in one child.

X-ray findings include shortness of all long bones, with curved femora, moderate rib shortness, a short skull base, hypoplastic mandible, hypoplasia of the ilia, pubic, and ischial bones, and mild platyspondyly.

Complications: Neonatal death due to respiratory insufficiency.

Associated Findings: Polyhydramnios may occur.

Etiology: Possibly autosomal recessive inheritance.

Pathogenesis: Marked disturbance of enchondral ossification with reduced numbers of proliferating and hypertrophic chondrocytes, irregular thickness and reduction in number of advancing cartilaginous columns in the metaphysis, and a fine zone of mesenchymal tissue blocking off the epiphyseal plate from the marrow cavity.

MIM No.: 27368

Sex Ratio: Presumably M1:F1.

Occurrence: Two females sibs from the West of Scotland have been documented.

Risk of Recurrence for Patient's Sib:
See Part I, *Mendelian Inheritance.*

Risk of Recurrence for Patient's Child:
See Part I, *Mendelian Inheritance.* Affected individuals are not expected to survive to reproduce.

Age of Detectability: During the second trimester by ultrasonic measurement of long bone lengths.

Gene Mapping and Linkage: Unknown.

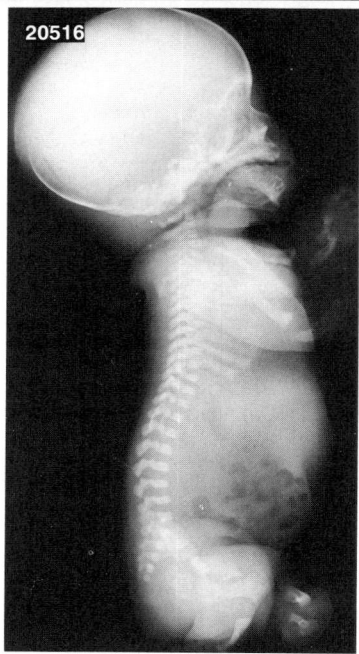

2821-20515–16: Thanatophoric dysplasia, Glasgow type: note short limbs with curved femora, and small pelvic bones. Lateral view demonstrates platyspondyly and micrognathia.

Prevention: None known. Genetic counseling indicated.

Treatment: Unknown.

Prognosis: Fatal during the newborn period.

Detection of Carrier: Unknown.

Special Considerations: Differentiation from **Thanatophoric dysplasia** is vital in view of the high recurrence risk for this condition. Short curved "telephone-receiver" femora are seen in both conditions, but other X-ray features, notably the spinal changes, serve to distinguish between the two conditions.

References:
Connor JM, et al.: Lethal neonatal chondrodysplasias in the West of Scotland 1970–1983 with a description of a thanatophoric, dysplasialike, autosomal recessive disorder, Glasgow variant. Am J Med Genet 1985; 22:243–253. * †

C0066   **J. Michael Connor**

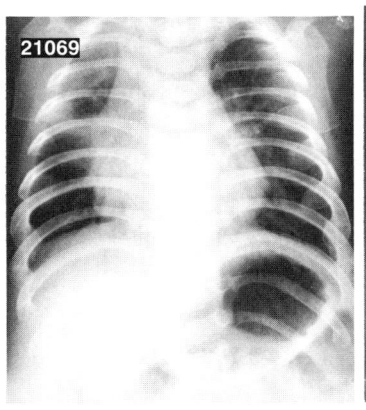 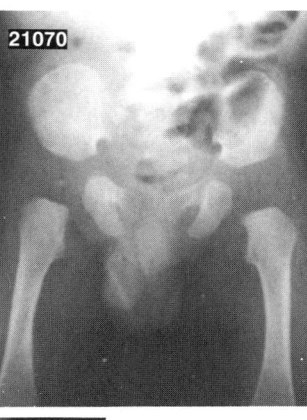

Thenar hypoplasia
  See POLYDACTYLY
Thiamine-responsive MSUD
  See MAPLE SYRUP URINE DISEASE
Thick lips-oral mucosa
  See ACROMEGALOID FACIAL APPEARANCE SYNDROME
Thiemann disease (phalangeal epiphyses)
  See JOINTS, OSTEOCHONDRITIS DISSECANS
Third and fourth pharyngeal pouch syndrome
  See IMMUNODEFICIENCY, THYMIC AGENESIS
Thode mental retardation
  See X-LINKED MENTAL RETARDATION-Xq DUPLICATION
Thompson-Baraitser syndrome
  See OCULO-ENCEPHALO-HEPATO-RENAL SYNDROME
Thomsen congenital myotonia
  See MYOTONIA CONGENITA
Thoracic aorta, coarctation of lower
  See AORTA, COARCTATION
Thoracic dysplasia, asphyxiating
  See ASPHYXIATING THORACIC DYSPLASIA

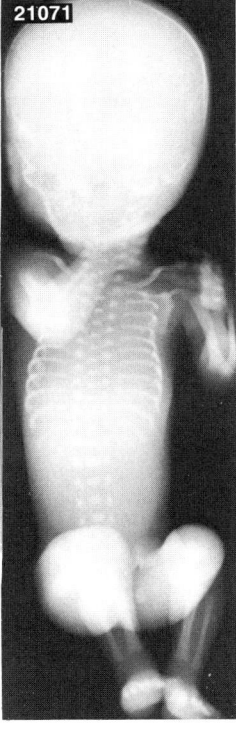

THORACIC DYSPLASIA-HYDROCEPHALUS   3129

Includes: Hydrocephaly-thoracic dysplasia

Excludes: Asphyxiating thoracic dysplasia (0091)

Major Diagnostic Criteria: **Hydrocephaly** with a narrow thorax and short ribs.

Clinical Findings: The condition has been described in two sibs, one liveborn and one diagnosed prenatally. Present in both were **Hydrocephaly**, narrow thorax with short ribs, and short limbs, with the shortness being primarily rhizomelic. Mental retardation was present in the living child, and is also likely a component of this condition.

Complications: Death from respiratory insufficiency.

Associated Findings: None known.

Etiology: Possibly autosomal recessive inheritance.

Pathogenesis: Unknown.

MIM No.: 27373

POS No.: 4191

Sex Ratio: Presumably M1:F1.

Occurrence: Two sibs from a family of Pakistani ethnic origin has been documented.

Risk of Recurrence for Patient's Sib:
  See Part I, *Mendelian Inheritance.*

Risk of Recurrence for Patient's Child:
  See Part I, *Mendelian Inheritance.*

Age of Detectability: At birth. Prenatal diagnosis using ultrasound is possible.

Gene Mapping and Linkage: Unknown.

Prevention: None known. Genetic counseling indicated.

Treatment: Shunting of **Hydrocephaly**.

Prognosis: Poor. The liveborn child died at age 18 months.

Detection of Carrier: Unknown.

References:
Winter RM, et al.: A previously undescribed syndrome of thoracic dysplasia and communicating hydrocephalus in two sibs, one diagnosed prenatally by ultrasound. J Med Genet 1987; 24:204–206.

T0007   **Helga V. Toriello**

3129-21069: Chest X-ray at 4 months shows short, horizontal ribs and narrow thorax. **21070:** Iliac bones are small and there is mild metaphyseal flaring of the femora. **21071:** Postmortem X-ray of an affected 19-week-old fetus shows short, horizontal, angulated ribs.

Thoracic tracheoesophageal fistula, congenital isolated H-type
  See TRACHEOESOPHAGEAL FISTULA
Thoracic tracheoesophageal fistula-esophageal atresia
  See TRACHEOESOPHAGEAL FISTULA
Thoracic-pelvic-phalangeal dystrophy
  See ASPHYXIATING THORACIC DYSPLASIA
Thoracoabdominal ectopia cordis
  See PENTALOGY OF CANTRELL
Thoracolaryngopelvic dysplasia
  See THORACOPELVIC DYSOSTOSIS
Thoracopagus
  See TWINS, CONJOINED

THORACOPELVIC DYSOSTOSIS 2775

Includes:
> Barnes syndrome
> Thoracolaryngopelvic dysplasia

Excludes: Asphyxiating thoracic dysplasia (0091)

Major Diagnostic Criteria: Characteristic X-ray features are short ribs; small, round ileum with a small and shallow sciatic notch; and poor development of the acetabulum. Significant respiratory distress in the neonatal period improves with age. A constricted pelvis is noted in adults.

Clinical Findings: Infants usually present with a small chest and respiratory distress of variable severity, which is rarely fatal. Respiratory support may be needed in the neonatal period, but milder cases improve with age and achieve near-normal respiratory function, a much better outcome than would be anticipated from the neonatal state. The chest remains narrow, and lung volumes may be reduced.

Laryngeal hypoplasia of variable severity is may also be noted. Although this was not mentioned by Bankier and Danks (1983), the small larynx in the child came to light by difficult intubation for an anesthetic at a later date. A small larynx has been a feature in the other reports, and Burn et al (1986) rightly pointed out that this condition may be the same as that of *thoracolaryngopelvic dysplasia*, originally reported by Barnes et al (1969).

The two adult women who were reported had a constricted pelvis, necessitating delivery of infants by cesarean section. Stature has been in the normal range. Other reported skeletal changes include slight difference in lower limb length, high clavicles, narrow thoracic cage, and mild thoracic scoliosis. The facies and other organs appear normal, and intelligence is in the normal range.

Complications: Unknown.

Associated Findings: None known.

Etiology: Possibly autosomal dominant inheritance.

Pathogenesis: Unknown.

MIM No.: 18777

POS No.: 3606

Sex Ratio: Presumably M1:F1.

Occurrence: Three families have been reported.

Risk of Recurrence for Patient's Sib:
See Part I, *Mendelian Inheritance.*

Risk of Recurrence for Patient's Child:
See Part I, *Mendelian Inheritance.*

Age of Detectability: During the newborn period.

Gene Mapping and Linkage: Unknown.

Prevention: None known. Genetic counseling indicated.

Treatment: Respiratory support, including artificial ventilation, may be necessary during the neonatal period. Mild cases improve and need no further respiratory treatment. Operative intervention has been reported in more severe cases, splitting the sternum and inserting bone grafts. This, together with more lengthy ventilatory support, achieved improvement, but death from respiratory failure and cor pulmonale have occurred in childhood. Tracheostomy has been used for severe laryngeal hypoplasia. Women are advised of the need of delivery by cesarean section because of constricted pelvis.

Prognosis: Good for those who survive the respiratory distress during the neonatal period without operative intervention.

Detection of Carrier: Clinical and X-ray examination.

References:
Barnes ND, et al.: Thoracic dystrophy. Arch Dis Child 1969; 44:11–17.
Bankier A, Danks DM: Thoracic-pelvic dysostosis: a "new" autosomal dominant form. J Med Genet 1983; 20:276–279.
Burn J, et al.: Autosomal dominant thoracolaryngopelvic dysplasia: Barnes syndrome. J Med Genet 1986; 23:345–349.

BA062   **Agnes Bankier**

Thorax cuneiforme
See PECTUS CARINATUM
Thost-Unna disease
See KERATOSIS PALMARIS ET PLANTARIS OF UNNA-THOST
Three methylcrotonyl-CoA carboxylase deficiency, isolated
See ACIDURIA, BETA-METHYL-CROTONYL-GLYCINURIA
Three-jointed thumb
See THUMB, TRIPHALANGEAL
Three-M slender-boned nanism
See SKELETAL DYSPLASIA, 3 M TYPE
Three-methylcrotonylglycinuria
See ACIDURIA, BETA-METHYL-CROTONYL-GLYCINURIA
Thrombasthenia
See THROMBASTHENIA, GLANZMANN-NAEGELI TYPE

THROMBASTHENIA, GLANZMANN-NAEGELI TYPE 2683

Includes:
> Diacyclothrombopathia IIb-IIIa
> Glanzmann thrombasthenia
> Glycoprotein complex IIb-IIIa, deficiency of
> Platelet fibinogen receptor deficiency
> Platelet glycoprotein IIb-IIIa deficiency
> Thrombasthenia
> Thrombocytopathic purpura

Excludes:
> **Albinism, oculocutaneous, Hermansky-Pudlak type** (0033)
> Bernard-Soulier giant platelet syndrome
> Gray platelet syndrome
> Platelet release abnormality
> **Von Willebrand disease** (0996)

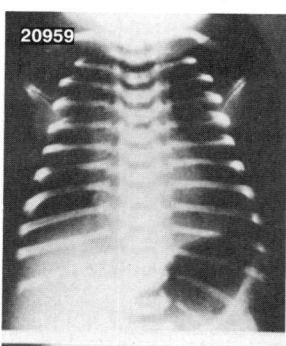
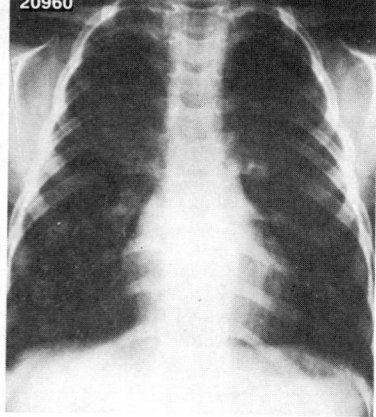
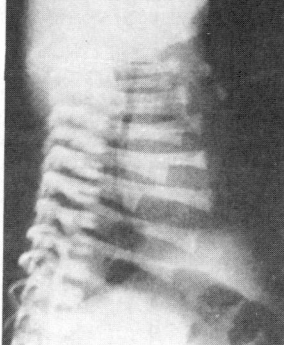
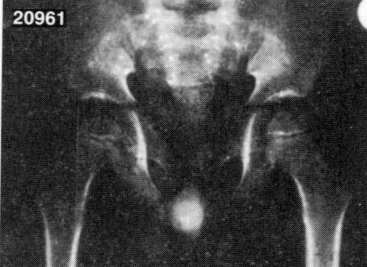

2775-20959: Thoracopelvic dysostosis; note short ribs in an affected infant. **20960**: "Bell-shaped" thorax in an older child. **20961**: Narrow pelvic inlet in the adult; note short, round ileum, and shallow sciatic notch.

Major Diagnostic Criteria: A hemorrhagic disorder characterized by low or normal platelet number; prolonged bleeding time; abnormal platelet aggregation responses to ADP, epinephrine, and collagen; abnormal clot retraction; and deficient platelet fibrinogen.

Clinical Findings: A lifelong bleeding diathesis. The hemorrhagic disorder varies in severity among families from a relatively mild disease manifesting with prolonged bleeding only at surgery or severe injury to a more aggressive hemorrhagic disorder characterized by purpurae and mucosal bleeding not associated with obvious trauma.

Complications: Those arising from the hemorrhagic manifestations of the disease. Bleeds can be exsanguinating when affecting an oral, nasal, or gastrointestinal mucosal site. Internal hemorrhages may involve vital structures or musculoskeletal limb structures.

Associated Findings: None known.

Etiology: Usually autosomal recessive inheritance, with infrequent "dominant pedigrees" possibly reflecting a heterozygous expression.

Pathogenesis: A platelet membrane defect identified with this disorder involving the platelet membrane glycoprotein complex IIb/IIIa (GP IIb/IIIa). Two subgroups have been documented. This classification is based on the low levels of GP IIIa with virtual absence of GP IIb and bound fibrinogen in subgroup type I and the reduced levels of GP IIb/IIIa in subgroup II. This subgroup is associated with limited amounts of fibrinogen binding. Variations have also been described on the basis of the extent of fibrinogen bound within the alpha granules.

MIM No.: *27380, 18780

Sex Ratio: M1:F1

Occurrence: The prevalence of this disease is higher in populations in which consanguinity is more likely. Established literature; considered second most frequent bleeding disorder in Jordan.

Risk of Recurrence for Patient's Sib:
See Part I, *Mendelian Inheritance.*

Risk of Recurrence for Patient's Child:
See Part I, *Mendelian Inheritance.*

Age of Detectability: At birth.

Gene Mapping and Linkage: GP2B (glycoprotein IIb (IIb/IIIa complex, platelet, CD41B)) has been mapped to 17q21.32.

Prevention: None known. Genetic counseling indicated.

Treatment: Platelet transfusion.

Prognosis: Depends on the severity of the hemorrhagic diathesis. In its severest form, prognosis is guarded.

Detection of Carrier: Quantitation of GP IIb/IIIa is not a routinely available procedure, but has the potential to detect the heterozygous state.

References:
Stormorken H, et al.: Diagnosis of heterozygotes in Glanzmann's thrombasthenia. Thromb Haemost 1982; 48:217–221.
George JN, et al.: Molecular defects in interactions of platelet with the vessel wall. New Engl J Med 1984; 311:1084–1098.
Giltay JC, et al.: Normal synthesis and expression of endothelial IIb/IIIa in Glanzmann's thrombasthenia. Blood 1987; 69:809–812.
Nurden AT, et al.: A variant of Glanzmann's thrombasthenia with abnormal glycoprotein IIb-IIIa complexes in the platelet membrane. J Clin Invest 1987; 79:962–969.
Nurden AT: Platelet membrane glycoproteins and their clinical aspects. In: Verstraete M, et al., eds: Thrombosis and haemostasis. Leuven: University Press, 1987:93–125.

G0055   **Edward Gomperts**

Thrombocytopathic purpura
See THROMBASTHENIA, GLANZMANN-NAEGELI TYPE

THROMBOCYTOPENIA-ABSENT RADIUS 0941

Includes:
> Amegakaryocytic thrombocytopenia-bilateral absence of the radii
> Megakaryocytopenia-radius aplasia
> Radius absent-thrombocytopenia
> TAR syndrome
> Tetraphocomelia-thrombocytopenia syndrome
> Thrombocytopenia-bilateral absence of the radii

Excludes:
> **Chromosome 18, trisomy 18** (0160)
> **Fetal thalidomide syndrome** (0386)
> **Heart-hand syndrome** (0455)
> **Pancytopenia syndrome, Fanconi type** (2029)

Major Diagnostic Criteria: Thrombocytopenia < 100,000 platelets/cubic mm. Bilateral absence of radius.

Clinical Findings: *Hematologic:* The affected newborn often has purpura, nosebleeds, bloody stools, and hematemesis. Thrombocytopenia probably 100% at some time. More than 90% have

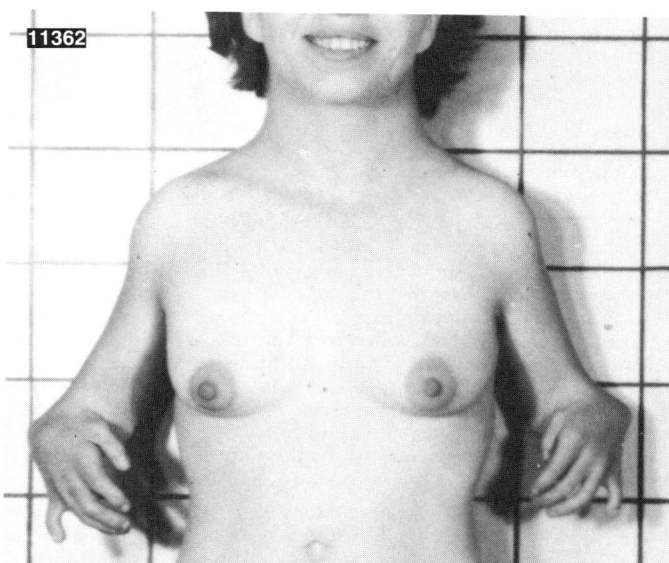

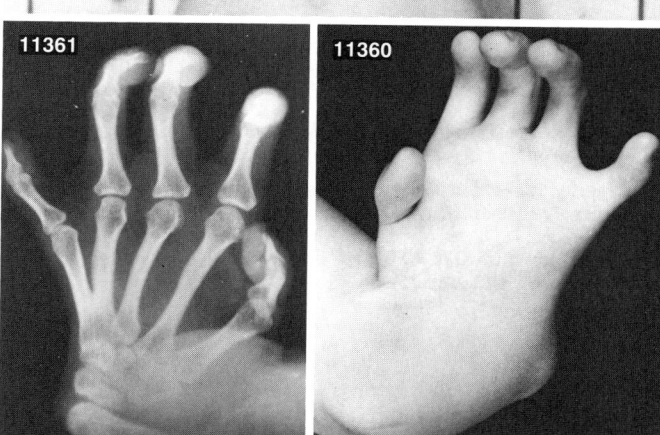

0941-11362: Symmetric, short upper limbs with radial deviation of hands and hypoplastic shoulder girdle. **11361:** Absent radius and middle phalanx of 5th finger. **11360:** Short forearm, radial deviation of hand, syndactyly, flexion contractures and abduction of 5th finger.

symptoms in the first four months of life. Megakaryocytes are small, basophilic, vacuolated, and nongranulated when thrombocytopenia is present. Thrombocytopenia is episodic, probably sometimes precipitated by stress, infections, and surgery. Platelet counts, often 15,000–30,000 in infancy, improve to almost normal range by adulthood. Platelet aggregation and survival are reduced.

Leukemoid reactions are recorded in 60–70% of patients during the first year of life. White blood counts may exceed 35,000, with a shift to left; and thrombocytopenia is worse during such reactions. The patient often has hepatosplenomegaly during leukemoid reaction.

Eosinophilia is recorded in bone marrow and peripheral smears in more than one-half of the patients.

Anemia, particularly during the first year of life, may have a hemolytic component or be related to blood loss. The frequency of anemia is undetermined.

Skeletal: The radius is always absent bilaterally. Hands are probably abnormal in all cases, with limited extension, radial deviation, hypoplastic carpals and phalanges, but thumbs always present. If the thumbs are absent, some other diagnosis must be considered. The muscles that normally attach to the radius attach instead to the wrist and pull it radially, leading to radial subluxation of the wrist. The ulnas are probably somewhat shorter and malformed in all cases; and absent bilaterally in 20%, unilaterally in 8%. The humerus is abnormal in at least one-half of the cases; absent in 5%, resulting in phocomelia. Other anomalies include dislocated hips, tibial torsion, subluxation of knees, stiff knee, dislocated patella, overriding fifth toe, rib and spine anomalies, hypoplasia of mandible and maxilla, and, rarely, severe reduction of leg long bones (giving tetraphocomelia). Short stature for family is frequent.

Cardiac anomalies are present in 30%; the most common being **Heart, tetralogy of Fallot** and **Atrial septal defects**.

Other anomalies are rare; mental retardation with intracranial bleeds, and glaucoma.

Complications: Significant symptomatic bleeding because of thrombocytopenia; death in 35–40%, almost all associated with bleeding, particularly intracranial, and almost all before one year of age; delayed motor development because of hand deformities, eventually good function, nerve compression, and arthritis at older age because of hand malformation; subluxation of wrist and knees may need splinting. Congestive failure secondary to heart defects and anemia; abnormal dermatoglyphics present in all cases, increased frequency of simian lines, decreased flexion creases.

Associated Findings: Mental retardation seen in 7% probably secondary to intracranial bleeding; cow milk allergy may be related and precipitates episodes of thrombocytopenia, eosinophilia, leukemoid reactions, and hemolysis; diarrheal illness common during the first year of life. *Tetraphocomelia*, simulating **Fetal thalidomide syndrome**, was reported in one infant (Anyane-Yeboa et al, 1985).

Etiology: Autosomal recessive inheritance. No increased consanguinity has been reported.

Pathogenesis: Undetermined. Gene action must occur early in gestation, between fourth and eighth weeks, to affect radial formation, blood-forming elements, and chambers of the heart. The condition may be fatal intrauterinely in some affected male embryos, since the M:F ratio is less than expected.

MIM No.: *27400

POS No.: 3412

CDC No.: 759.840

Sex Ratio: M5:F7 observed, possibly due to the condition being fatal intrauterinely in some affected males.

Occurrence: Over 100 cases are known, with no specific geographic or ethnic group distribution.

Risk of Recurrence for Patient's Sib:
See Part I, *Mendelian Inheritance*. Intra and interfamilial variability present with regard to extent of skeletal, hematologic, and cardiac involvement.

Risk of Recurrence for Patient's Child:
See Part I, *Mendelian Inheritance*. Patients are fertile and no patient-to-child transmission has yet been observed.

Age of Detectability: At birth, or prenatally from the 16 weeks by ultrasound.

Gene Mapping and Linkage: Unknown.

Prevention: None known. Genetic counseling indicated.

Treatment: Avoid infections, stress and surgery during first year, because these may precipitate severe thrombocytopenia. Supportive hematologic; i.e., platelet transfusions from a single donor if possible, whole blood transfusions; corrective orthopedic, braces for forearms early, surgery if indicated; elimination of cow's milk during infancy if indicated; cardiac care as indicated.

Prognosis: Appears to be good if the child survives the first year. May need strenuous supportive therapy for thrombocytopenia during the first year. Women have heavy menses. Probably normal life span, if patient survives childhood.

Detection of Carrier: Unknown.

Special Considerations: The possibility that this condition represents a genetic compound (e.g. one Fanconi anemia gene and one as-yet-undefined gene that could be lethal in homozygous states) would explain the lack of consanguinity in a rare recessive disorder. There is an interesting report from Turkey (Altay et al, 1975) of a possibly affected man fathering a son with classic Fanconi anemia.

Support Groups: NJ; Linwood; Thrombocytopenia Absent Radius Syndrome (TARSA)

References:
Hall JG, et al.: Thrombocytopenia with absent radius (TAR). Medicine 1969; 48:411–439.
Altay C, et al.: Fanconi's anemia in offspring of patient with congenital radial and carpal hypoplasia. New Engl J Med 1975; 293:151.
Ray R, et al.: Brief clinical report: lower limb anomalies in the thrombocytopenia absent-radius (TAR) syndrome. Am J Med Genet 1980; 7:523–528.
Stephens TD: Muscle abnormalities associated with radial aplasia. Teratology 1983; 27:1–6.
Anyane-Yeboa K, et al.: Tetraphocomelia in the syndrome of thrombocytopenia with absent radii. Am J Med Genet 1985; 20:571–576.
Hall JG: Thrombocytopenia and absent radius (TAR) syndrome. J Med Genet 1987; 24:79–83.

HA014   **Judith G. Hall**

Thrombocytopenia-bilateral absence of the radii
   See *THROMBOCYTOPENIA-ABSENT RADIUS*
Thrombocytopenia-Dohle bodies in neutrophils
   See *LEUKOCYTE, MAY-HEGGLIN ANOMALY*
Thrombocytopenia-hemangioma syndrome
   See *HEMANGIOMA-THROMBOCYTOPENIA SYNDROME*

THROMBOCYTOPENIC PURPURA AND LIPID HISTIOCYTOSIS   0942

Includes:
   Idiopathic thrombocytopenic purpura
   Lipid histiocytosis of spleen
   Lipidosis-thrombocytopenia-angiomata of the spleen
   Thrombocytopenic purpura, autoimmune

Excludes:
   Follicular lipoidosis
   Gaucher disease (0406)
   Lipid histiocytosis associated with diabetes
   Lipid histiocytosis associated with hyperlipemic states
   Lipid histiocytosis associated with malignancy
   Lipid histiocytosis associated with thalassemia
   Sea-blue histiocyte syndrome
   Sphingolipidoses other

Major Diagnostic Criteria: Thrombocytopenia and histologic demonstration of splenic histiocytosis.

Clinical Findings: The general findings are those usual for chronic, so-called *idiopathic thrombocytopenic purpura (ITP)* (Karpatkin 1985); easy bruising, cutaneous petechiae and ecchymoses, epistaxis, and other mucous membrane hemorrhages. The platelet count is low, and antiplatelet antibodies can be demonstrated in the serum of 70% or more of ITP patients. The serum lipids are normal. Bone marrow shows increased megakaryocytes; lipid histiocytes in the marrow are rare. The spleen is usually not enlarged clinically.

The process of lipid histiocytosis occurring in patients with ITP can be recognized only upon examination of the extirpated spleen, rarely on bone marrow examination. In various studies it has been reported to be present in 2–30% of splenectomized cases. Although the incidence of this phenomenon has increased sharply since the introduction of corticosteroid therapy for ITP, the true nature of this relationship is not known. On direct analysis, the splenic lipids are found to be generally increased, perhaps somewhat more prominently in the phospholipid fraction. Increased destruction of formed blood elements is thought to be pertinent, with platelet breakdown the most likely source of the sequestered lipid material.

Complications: Hemorrhage.

Associated Findings: Postsplenectomy infection.

Etiology: Unknown. The possible role of corticosteroids is undetermined.

Pathogenesis: Lipid-containing vacuolated histiocytes are found in the splenic pulp. By electron microscopy, these can be seen to contain osmiophilic lamellated inclusions in the cytoplasm.

MIM No.: 18803

Sex Ratio: M1:F1

Occurrence: Undetermined but presumed rare. Observed mainly in Caucasians.

Risk of Recurrence for Patient's Sib: Unknown.

Risk of Recurrence for Patient's Child: Unknown.

Age of Detectability: From three years of age to adulthood, based on experience to date from the examination of splenic specimens.

Gene Mapping and Linkage: Unknown.

Prevention: None known. Genetic counseling indicated.

Treatment: Management of purpura or hemorrhage.

Prognosis: Dependent on control of hemorrhage.

Detection of Carrier: Unknown.

The author wishes to thank the late Lottie Strauss for her contributions to an earlier version of this article.

References:

Saltzstein SL: Phospholipid accumulation in histiocytes of splenic pulp associated with thrombocytopenic purpura. Blood 1961; 18:73–88.

Hill JM, et al.: Secondary lipidosis of spleen associated with thrombocytopenia and other blood dyscrasias treated with steroids. Am J Clin Pathol 1963; 39:607–615.

Quinton S, et al.: Histiocytosis of spleen, lymph node, and bone marrow, associated with thrombocytopenia, splenomegaly and splenic angiomata. Am J Clin Pathol 1967; 47:484–489.

Tavassole M, McMillan R: Structure of the spleen in idiopathic thrombocytopenic purpura. Am J Clin Pathology 1975; 64:180–191.

Cohn J, Tygstrup I: Foamy histiocytosis of the spleen in patients with chronic thrombocytopenia. Scand J Hematol 1976; 16:33–37.

Luk SC, et al.: Platelet phagocytosis in the spleen of patients with idiopathic thrombocytopenic purpura (ITP). Histopathology 1980; 4:127–136.

Karpatkin S: Autoimmune thrombocytopenic purpura. Sem Hemat 1985; 22:260–288.

Diebold J, Audoin J: Association of splenoma, peliosis, and lipid histiocytosis in spleen or accessory spleen removed in two patients with chronic idiopathic thrombocytopenic purpura after long term treatment with steroids. Path Res Practice 1988; 183:446–452.

Stephen J. Qualman

Thrombocytopenic purpura, autoimmune
  See THROMBOCYTOPENIC PURPURA AND LIPID HISTIOCYTOSIS
Thrombophilia due to deficiency of AT III, hereditary
  See ANTITHROMBIN III DEFICIENCY
Thrombophilia, inherited
  See PROTEIN C DEFICIENCY
Thromboses, and protein S deficiency
  See PROTEIN S DEFICIENCY
Thrombotic disease, congenital
  See PROTEIN C DEFICIENCY
Thrombotic microangiopathy, familial
  See HEMOLYTIC-UREMIC SYNDROME
Thrombotic thrombocytopenic purpura, familial
  See HEMOLYTIC-UREMIC SYNDROME
Thumb defects
  See RADIAL DEFECTS
Thumb extensors, aplastic or hypoplastic
  See THUMB, CLASPED
Thumb polydactyly
  See POLYDACTYLY

THUMB, ADDUCTED THUMB SYNDROME   **2075**

Includes:
  Adducted thumb syndrome
  Thumbs, congenital clasped

Excludes:
  Arthrogryposis, distal types (2280)
  Cranio-carpo-tarsal dysplasia, whistling face type (0223)
  Thumb, clasped (0175)
  X-linked mental retardation-clasped thumb (2291)

Major Diagnostic Criteria: The combination of craniostenosis, microcephaly, cleft palate, swallowing difficulty, and adducted thumbs should suggest the diagnosis.

Clinical Findings: Breech delivery (2/9); feeding difficulties in the neonatal period (9/9); respiratory difficulties in the neonatal period (6/9); hypotonia (4/9); hirsutism (5/9); craniosynostosis or craniostenosis (6/9); microcephaly (8/9); prominent occiput (5/9); ophthalmoplegia (5/9); downslanting palpebral fissures (3/9); cleft soft palate/bifid uvula/high-arched palate (8/95); micrognathia (3/9); low-set, poorly formed ears (8/9); laryngomalacia (2/9); pectus excavatum (3/9); adducted thumbs (9/9); **Foot, talipes equinovarus (TEV)** or calcaneovalgus (8/9); torticollis (2/9); other joint contractures (4/9); radial arch hypothenar pattern (3/9); muscle fibrillations (4/9); seizures (6/9); and mental retardation (5/9).

X-ray findings have included hypoplastic metacarpals and clubbed ribs. Autopsies have revealed dysmyelination of the central nervous system.

Complications: Pneumonia was a frequent complication.

Associated Findings: Each of the following was present in only one patient: epicanthal folds, distichiasis, entropion, short first metacarpal, **Ventricular septal defect**, and **Hernia, inguinal**.

Etiology: Probably autosomal recessive inheritance.

Pathogenesis: Most of the findings, including the facial features, are secondary to the CNS defects. Christian et al (1971) suggested that the basic defect could be abnormal lipid synthesis or an abnormal structural protein necessary to myelin synthesis. However, the basic defect is unknown.

MIM No.: *20155

POS No.: 3591

CDC No.: 755.500

Sex Ratio: Presumably M1:F1.

Occurrence: Nine cases have been reported; three from an Amish kindred.

Risk of Recurrence for Patient's Sib:
  See Part I, *Mendelian Inheritance*.

Risk of Recurrence for Patient's Child:
  See Part I, *Mendelian Inheritance*.

Age of Detectability: At birth by physical examination and lack of thumb extension during Moro reflex.

Gene Mapping and Linkage: Unknown.

Prevention: None known. Genetic counseling indicated.

Treatment: Supportive care.

Prognosis: Poor. Six patients died during the first year of life. One living child was two years at the time of the report and had an IQ of 90; a second living child was four years and was severely retarded (not yet able to stand or crawl).

Detection of Carrier: Unknown.

References:
Christian JC, et al.: The adducted thumbs syndrome. Clin Genet 1971; 2:95–103.
Fitch N, Levy EP: Adducted thumb syndromes. Clin Genet 1975; 8:190–198. *
Majoor-Krakaver O, Weicker H: Das "adducted-thumb-syndrome", poster session 17. Tagung der Gesellschaft fur anthropologie und Humangenetik Gottingen 1981; 23:269.
Kunze J, et al.: Adducted thumb syndrome: report of a new case and a diagnostic approach. Eur J Pediatr 1983; 141:122–126. *

T0007   **Helga V. Toriello**

THUMB, CLASPED   0175

Includes:
>   Adducted thumbs
>   Extensor pollicis brevis or longus
>   Extensor pollicis longus, congenital absence of
>   Pollex varus
>   Thumb-clutched hand
>   Thumb extensors, aplastic or hypoplastic
>   Thumb, flexion adduction deformity of
>   Ulnar deviation of fingers syndrome

Excludes:
>   **Arthrogryposes** (0088)
>   "Cortical" thumbs
>   **Cranio-carpo-tarsal dysplasia, whistling face type** (0223)
>   **Radial defects** (0853)
>   **Thumb, adducted thumb syndrome** (2075)
>   **X-linked mental retardation-clasped thumb** (2291)

Major Diagnostic Criteria: An isolated inability to extend the thumb, secondary to hypoplasia or aplasia of the extensor muscles and tendons.

Clinical Findings: An isolated aplasia or hypoplasia, usually bilateral, of the extensor muscles and tendons of the thumb, resulting in persistently flexed or adducted first metacarpals bilaterally; proximal phalanx of the thumb is flexed forward and partially subluxed. Most common defect involves the extensor pollicis brevis, with an accompanying impairment of extension at the metacarpophalangeal joint. Defects of the extensor pollicis longus have also been described.

Since persistent adduction of the thumb may result from any imbalance in extension and flexion forces, due to structural or neurologic defects, it may be observed in conjunction with generalized joint abnormalities or as part of other distinct syndromes.

Complications: Without treatment, atrophy of the intrinsic thumb muscles and soft tissue contractures occur, resulting in limited function.

Associated Findings: Ulnar deviation or flexion deformities of other fingers, excessively long 4th and 5th digits, congenital dislocation of hip, scoliosis, torticollis, foot deformities.

Etiology: Possibly X-linked inheritance.

Pathogenesis: Unknown.

MIM No.: 31410

CDC No.: 755.500

Sex Ratio: M27:F15 (observed)

Occurrence: At least 42 cases have been reported in the literature.

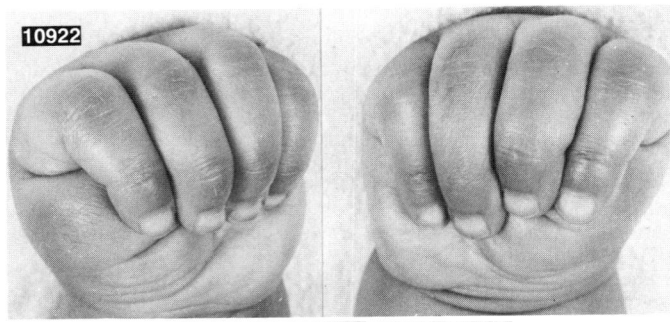

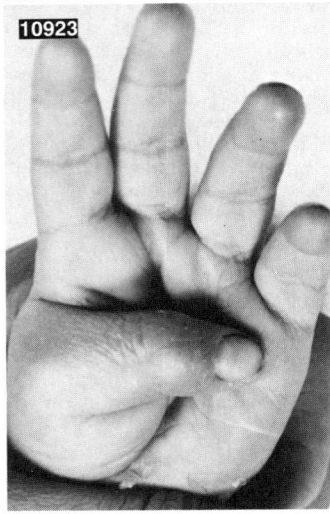

0175-10922: Clasped thumb deformity at age 1 year. **10923:** Clasped thumb in an older child.

Risk of Recurrence for Patient's Sib:
See Part I, *Mendelian Inheritance.*

Risk of Recurrence for Patient's Child:
See Part I, *Mendelian Inheritance.*

Age of Detectability: At birth or during infancy.

Gene Mapping and Linkage: Unknown.

Prevention: None known. Genetic counseling indicated.

Treatment: Early splinting of the thumb in extension and adduction may give good results. Unresponsive or untreated cases may need surgery for release of soft tissues or tendon transplants or transfers.

Prognosis: Mild-to-moderate impairment in function, improved with early treatment.

Detection of Carrier: Unknown.

Special Considerations: Adducted thumbs may occur with other phalangeal extensor defects and with clubfeet, with an apparent dominant inheritance, or in generalized arthrogryposis. Hypoplasia of the radial ray or neurologic impairment may result in an adducted thumb, as seen in X-linked hydrocephalus. It has also been noted in **Thumb, adducted thumb syndrome** with cleft palate, microencephaly, and dysmyelination; and in **X-linked mental retardation-clasped thumb** with aphasia and shuffling gait; and in **Cranio-carpo-tarsal dysplasia, whistling face type**. In familial trigger thumb, the defect is bilateral and the flexion is at the interphalangeal joint, not at the metacarpophalangeal joint.

References:
Weckesser EC, et al.: Congenital clasped thumb (congenital flexion-adduction deformity of the thumb). A syndrome, not a specific entity. J Bone Joint Surg 1968; 50A:1417–1428.
Fitch N, Levy EP. Adducted thumb syndromes. Clin Genet 1975; 8:190–198.
Anderson TE, Breed AL: Congenital clasped thumb and the Moro reflex (letter). J Pediat 1981; 99:664–665.
Wood VE: Congenital thumb deformities. Clin Orthop 1985; 195:7–25.

AT002   **Balu H. Athreya**
VA005   **Don C. Van Dyke**

Thumb, congenital clasped-mental retardation
See X-LINKED MENTAL RETARDATION-CLASPED THUMB
Thumb, flexion adduction deformity of
See THUMB, CLASPED
Thumb, long-brachydactyly syndrome
See BRACHYDACTYLY-LONG THUMB SYNDROME

THUMB, TRIPHALANGEAL   2276

Includes:
  Delta phalanx
  Hyperphalangeal thumb
  Three-jointed thumb
  Triphalangeal thumb, nonopposable

Excludes:
  Phalangeal duplication of the thumb
  Pseudotriphalangism

Major Diagnostic Criteria: Triphalangeal thumb (TPT) is a type of hyperphalangy in which a middle extra phalanx is interposed between the two normal phalanges of the thumb.

Clinical Findings: In general, TPT appears elongated, with three phalanges and an additional interphalangeal joint. Ulnar deviation at the terminal phalanx is common. Typically, an extra set of skin creases overlies the additional interphalangeal joint. A narrow first web space may be detrimental to the functional ability of the thumbs, as they lose dexterity. An enlarged first web space is uncommon. Horizontal patterns of dermal ridges are present in the thenar region. TPT may be unilateral or bilateral (in the majority of cases). In general, unilateral TPT is sporadic and bilateral is familial.

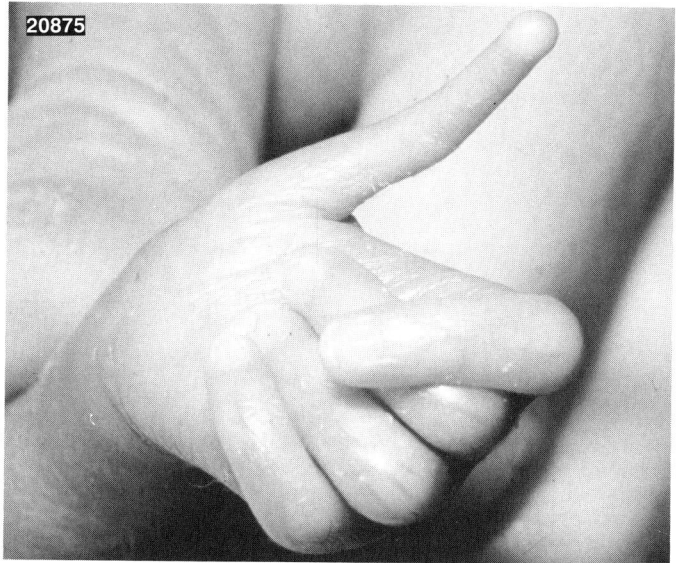

2276-20875: Thumb, triphalangeal; note finger-like thumb.

There are two types of TPT. *True TPT*: a four-fingered hand with TPT; and a *Finger-like TPT*: a five-fingered hand. True TPT usually has a normal position, with a normal thenar muscle; it is an opposable thumb having an almost normal rotation. A finger-like TPT lies at the same plane as the other digits, has a hypoplastic or absent thenar muscle, and functionally is a nonopposable thumb, with restriction of movement at the distal interphalangeal joint.

On X-ray, a TPT appears elongated, with an additional middle phalanx and interphalangeal joint. The extra phalanx may have three shapes: a small, triangular phalanx called *delta phalanx*; a rectangular shape; or a normal, regular phalanx. The shape of the abnormal phalanx is a definite factor in the direction of the deviation of the distal phalanx. The "delta phalanx" routinely causes deviation. Usually the distal phalanx has an ulnar deviation. Radial deviation *varus thumb* is very rare.

Patients with a small ossicle (delta phalanx) as a middle phalanx usually have opposable thumbs, but when the middle phalanx is rectangular or regular, opposition is generally very difficult. A true opposable TPT has a first metacarpal slightly shorter than usual, and its epiphyseal plate is at the proximal end, similar to the phalanges (as in the normal thumb). The finger-like nonopposable TPT has a long first metacarpal, and its epiphyseal plate is at the distal end.

Complications: Without treatment, the supernumerary component tends to displace the normal components and to increase the deviation of the terminal phalanx, resulting in limited function. The hand becomes less efficient, both in heavy manual work and in more delicate activities.

Associated Findings: **Polydactyly** of the thumb or other digits, **Syndactyly**, radial hypoplasia, and split hand. Polydactyly of the big toe or the fifth toe, split foot, dislocation of the patella, and tibial hypoplasia have also been reported. Extraskeletal associated anomalies include congenital heart disease, iris coloboma, hypoplasia of the lacrimal puncta, deafness, cleft lip and/or palate, imperforate anus, anemia, thrombocytopenia, **Hypomelanosis of Ito**, and mental retardation.

Etiology: May be sporadic, familial, or part of a complex malformation syndrome. The sporadic occurrence of TPT is relatively uncommon.

The wedge-shaped delta phalanx is more frequently sporadic and also more frequently unilateral. Two-thirds have a positive family history, typically of autosomal dominant inheritance with marked penetrance and variable expressivity. The inheritance of TPT in a syndrome depends on the specific syndrome in which it appears.

Pathogenesis: Unknown.

MIM No.: 19060

CDC No.: 755.500

Sex Ratio: M1:F1

Occurrence: The general incidence of all types of TPT has been estimated at 1:25,000.

Risk of Recurrence for Patient's Sib:
See Part I, *Mendelian Inheritance.*

Risk of Recurrence for Patient's Child:
See Part I, *Mendelian Inheritance.*

Age of Detectability: At birth.

Gene Mapping and Linkage: Unknown.

Prevention: None known. Genetic counseling indicated.

Treatment: The treatment of a true opposable TPT is mainly connected with the angular deformity. With minimal angulation, minimal or slight impaired function, and without associated anomalies, there is no need for treatment. However, most cases of true TPT require extirpation of the extra phalanx.

The nonopposable, finger-like TPT is a difficult functional problem, which must be corrected by surgery. Pollicization with large dorsal flaps, or metacarpal osteotomy or metacarpal removal, has been performed. TPT associated with other local anomalies (especially polydactyly) is a major surgical problem. The treatment must be early (by the age of two years); frequently a better result is obtained by removing the TPT, even if function appears better than in the biphalangeal thumb.

Prognosis: Isolated (nonsyndromatic) true TPT has a good functional prognosis. The nonopposable, finger-like TPT function can be improved by surgery, but functional results are not always satisfactory. Life span is normal in both types.

Detection of Carrier: Unknown.

Special Considerations: TPT has been described in the literature as part of numerous syndromes, but many of these descriptions are incomplete, and the type of thumb anomaly is not precisely defined. In the reports with a good description, the TPT was of a nonopposable finger-like type and not a true opposable TPT.

References:

Swanson AB, Brown KS: Hereditary triphalangeal thumb. J Hered 1962; 53:259–265.

Miura T: Triphalangeal thumb. Plastic Reconstr Surg 1976; 58:587–594. †

Theander G, Carstam N: Triphalangism and pseudotriphalangism of the thumb in children. Acta Radiol 1979; 20:223–232. *

Wood VE: Treatment of the triphalangeal thumb. Clin Orthop Rel Res 1979; 120:188–200. *

Lamb DW, et al.: Five-fingered hand associated with partial or complete tibial absence and pre-axial polydactyly. J Bone Joint Surg 1983; 65B:60–63.

Qazi Q, Kassner EG: Triphalangeal thumb. J Med Genet 1988; 25:505–520.

ME034
RE025

Paul Merlob
Salomon H. Reisner

Thumb, triphalangeal-acrofacial dysostosis-cleft lip/palate
See ACROFACIAL DYSOSTOSIS-CLEFT LIP/PALATE-TRIPHALANGEAL THUMB

THUMB, TRIPHALANGEAL-BRACHYECTRODACTYLY   2884

Includes:
Brachyectrodactyly-triphalangeal thumb
Ectrodactyly-brachydactyly-triphalangeal thumb
Triphalangeal thumb-brachyectrodactyly syndrome

Excludes:
Anus-hand-ear syndrome (0072)
Deafness-onycho-osteo-dystrophy-retardation-seizures (DOORS) (0262)
Ectrodactyly (0336)
Fetal thalidomide syndrome (0386)
Heart-hand syndrome (0455)
Vater association (0987)

Major Diagnostic Criteria: **Thumb, triphalangeal**, with or without **Polydactyly** and index fingernail dysplasia associated with **Ectrodactyly** or **Brachydactyly** and/or **Syndactyly** of the toes.

Clinical Findings: The typical hand malformations are triphalangy of the thumbs and index fingernail dysplasia. The foot anomalies range from true split foot to variable hypoplasia of toe 3 with or without syndactyly. A wide variability in clinical expression has been observed in the familial cases. One affected individual had normal hands and minimal brachydactyly of toe 3. The nail dysplasia of the index finger has proved to be the only feature of the syndrome in two affected relatives of a typical patient. Careful examination of all the family members of a given case is therefore essential.

Complications: Orthopedic problems may be anticipated in patients with severe foot involvement.

Associated Findings: None known.

Etiology: Autosomal dominant inheritance with variability of clinical expression. The mutation rate is unknown; two of 23 cases are sporadic and possibly result from a fresh gene mutation.

Pathogenesis: The combination of absence deformities, such as ectrodactyly, with duplication anomalies, such as triphalangeal thumb and polydactyly, has been induced in experimental animals by teratogen exposure. In mice, interchangeability between polydactyly and oligodactyly has been observed in genetically induced malformations as well. In humans, **Fetal thalidomide syndrome** represents the best example of limb malformations in which reductional and duplication anomalies occur, depending on the time of exposure to the teratogen.

In this syndrome, the hand malformation is almost always of the duplication type, whereas in the feet only absence anomalies are seen. This suggests that the gene mutation affects the limb

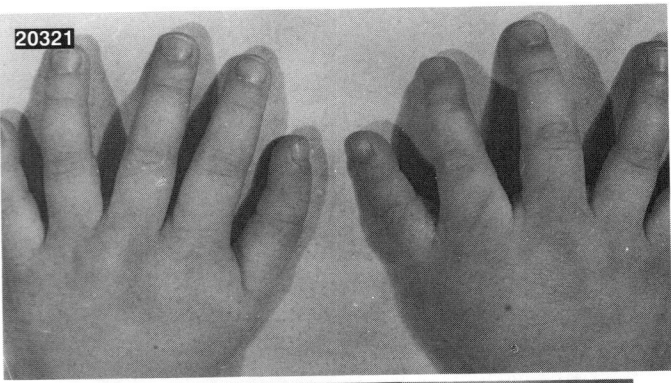

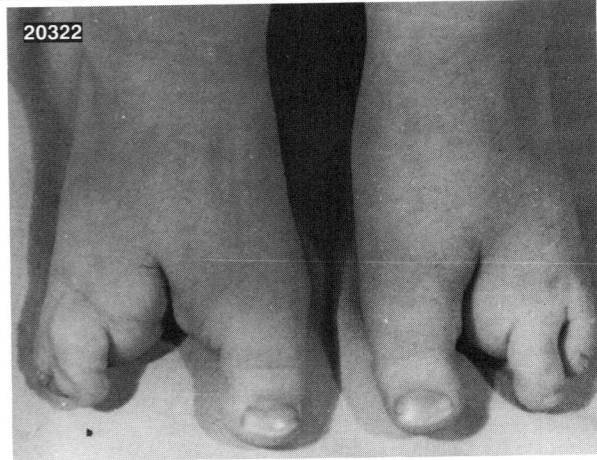

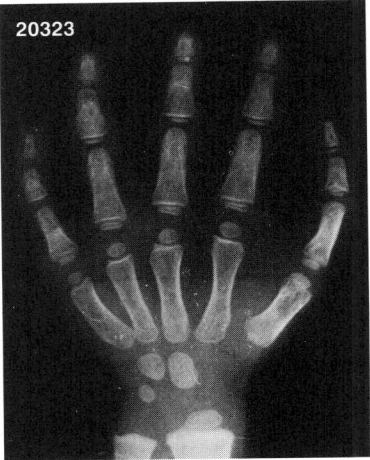

2884-20321: Note finger-like thumb; the preaxial polydactyly of the right hand has been surgically corrected. **20322:** Ectrosyndactyly of the feet. **20323:** Hand X-ray shows triphalangeal thumb.

development at a definite stage, although the actual mechanism is still unknown.

MIM No.: 19068

POS No.: 3962

Sex Ratio: M8:F15 (observed).

Occurrence: Twenty-three cases have been reported in the literature.

Risk of Recurrence for Patient's Sib:
See Part I, *Mendelian Inheritance.*

Risk of Recurrence for Patient's Child:
See Part I, *Mendelian Inheritance.*

Age of Detectability: At birth. Cases with reduced clinical expression may be detected only by familial studies.

Gene Mapping and Linkage: Unknown.

Prevention: None known. Genetic counseling indicated.

Treatment: Orthopedic management of foot deformities; plastic surgery may be indicated.

Prognosis: Normal life span.

Detection of Carrier: By clinical examination.

References:

Carnevale A, et al.: A new syndrome of thriphalangeal thumbs and brachy-ectrodactyly. Clin Genet 1980; 18:244–252. * †
Majewski F, et al.: Triphalangeal thumb ectrodactyly in a sporadic case. Clin Genet 1981; 20:310–314.
Cirillo Silengo M, et al.: Triphalangeal thumb and brachyectrodactyly syndrome: confirmation of autosomal dominant inheritance. Clin Genet 1987; 31:13–18.

SI033
FR040

Margherita C. Silengo
Piergiorgio Franceschini

THUMB, TRIPHALANGEAL-DUPLICATED GREAT TOES   2277

Includes:
> Hyperphalangism of thumbs-duplication of thumbs and big toes
> Polydactyly of thumbs/hallux-extra phalanges in the thumbs
> Polydactyly, preaxial II
> Triphalangeal thumbs-duplication of great toes
> Triphalangeal thumb, opposable

Excludes:
> **Thumb, triphalangeal** (2276)
> **Thumb, triphalangeal-brachyectrodactyly** (2884)
> **Tibial hypoplasia/aplasia-ectrodactyly** (2388)

Major Diagnostic Criteria: A triphalangeal thumb with duplication of big toes in a familial nonsyndromic association.

Clinical Findings: The abnormality appears only in the thumbs and great toes. The thumbs have all the characteristics of a true triphalangeal thumb. They appear long, with three phalanges, an additional interphalangeal joint, and an extra set of skin creases. Ulnar deviation of the terminal phalanx is common. The position of the thumb, the thenar region, and the first webspace are normal. The thumbs are opposable, although there is restriction in movement at the distal interphalangeal joint. The other fingers are normal. The great toes are duplicated, with cutaneous **Syndactyly**. The other four toes are normal.

On X-ray, the thumbs appear elongated, with an additional middle phalanx and interphalangeal joint. The middle extra phalanx of the thumbs at birth may be composed of two small ossification centers. The first metacarpal is shorter than usual, with the epiphyseal plate at its proximal end. Hexadactyly with five metatarsals is noted on X-rays of the feet. The first metatarsal is more distally placed than usual, is very large, and has a broad distal end. The great toes are duplicated and composed of two separate phalangeal bones. Cutaneous syndactyly is visible between the duplicated parts of the great toes. The rest of the skeletal survey shows no abnormalities.

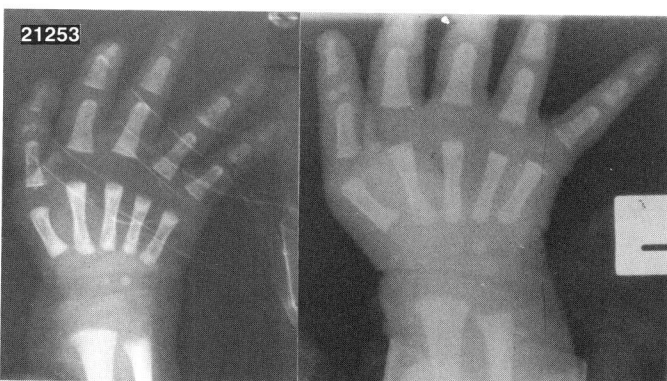

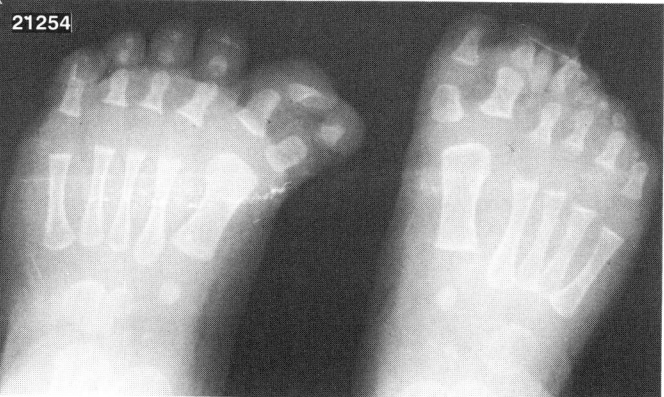

2277-21253: Bilateral triphalangeal thumbs. **21254:** Bilateral duplication of the great toes.

This is the typical presentation of this thumb-hallux association. However, there is great variability in expression between the patients and within the same patient. Some patients have a finger-like thumb in place of a true triphalangeal thumb; others have both types, a true triphalangeal thumb on one hand and a finger-like thumb in the other one.

Complications: Without treatment, the hand may become less efficient, both in heavy manual work and in more delicate activities.

Associated Findings: None known.

Etiology: Autosomal dominant inheritance with marked penetrance and great variability in expression.

Pathogenesis: Unknown.

MIM No.: *17450

POS No.: 4201

CDC No.: 755.500

Sex Ratio: Presumably M1:F1 (M3:F4 observed).

Occurrence: About five kinships have been documented.

Risk of Recurrence for Patient's Sib:
See Part I, *Mendelian Inheritance.*

Risk of Recurrence for Patient's Child:
See Part I, *Mendelian Inheritance.*

Age of Detectability: At birth.

Gene Mapping and Linkage: Unknown.

Prevention: None known. Genetic counseling indicated.

Treatment: A true triphalangeal thumb needs extirpation of the extra phalanx, while a finger-like thumb will be corrected by pollicization. Duplication of the great toes should be treated before the child begins walking. Amputation of the most medial toe, together with removal of the wide metatarsal head, is indicated.

Prognosis: Normal life span. Without early and adequate treatment, functional impairment with worsening restriction of movement.

Detection of Carrier: Unknown.

References:
Manoiloff EO: A rare case of hereditary hexadactylism. Am J Phys Anthropol 1931; 15:503–508.
Hefner RA: Hereditary polydactyly associated with extra phalanges in the thumb. J Hered 1940; 31:25–27.
Komai T, et al.: A Japanese kindred of hyperphalangism of thumbs and duplication of thumbs and big toe. Folia Hered Pathol 1953; 2:307–312.
Temtamy S, McKusick VA: The genetics of hand malformations. New York: Alan R. Liss, 1978.
Merlob P, et al.: Familial opposable triphalangeal thumbs associated with duplication of the big toes. J Med Genet 1985; 22:78–80. * †

ME034
GR038
RE025

Paul Merlob
Michael Grunebaum
Salomon H. Reisner

THYROGLOSSAL DUCT REMNANT   0945

Includes:
    Duct, thyroglossal remnant
    Lingual thyroid
    Thyroglossal duct, cyst or sinus
Excludes:
    Branchial cleft cysts (2723)
    Nasopharyngeal cysts (0706)
    Neck/head, dermoid cyst or teratoma (0283)
    Lipoma
    Suppurative lesions

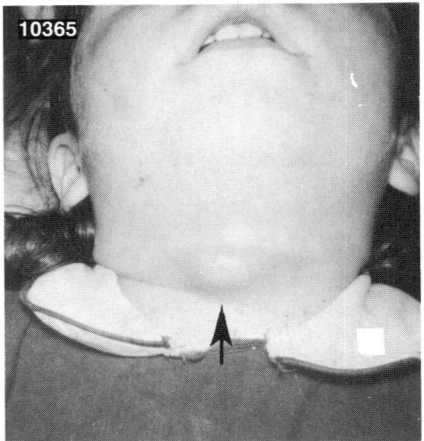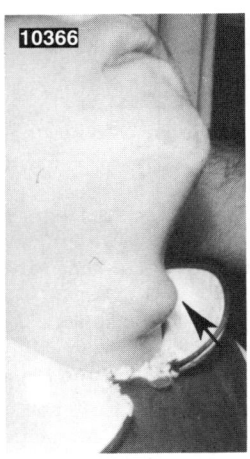

0945A-10365: Thyroglossal duct remnant.   10366: Lateral view.

Major Diagnostic Criteria: Lingual mass, or midline neck cyst or mass, moving with deglutition or tongue protrusion, with or without associated infection.

Clinical Findings: Midline or slightly lateral solid or cystic mass or sinus in the anterior neck, located anywhere from the tongue base to the suprasternal region. A thyroglossal cyst may be present laterally in the neck or into the larynx. A tract from the cyst to the foramen cecum may remain patent, allowing cyst fluid to drain into the mouth. When this occurs the cyst may become smaller. However, in most cases, the duct is closed and persists as a fibrous cord that may be palpated from the neck mass to the center of the hyoid bone. A sinus opening onto the anterior neck may occasionally discharge a few drops of fluid. When the patient swallows or protrudes the tongue, the cyst may appear to move upward in the neck.

The thyroglossal duct, cyst, and tract are remnants of the

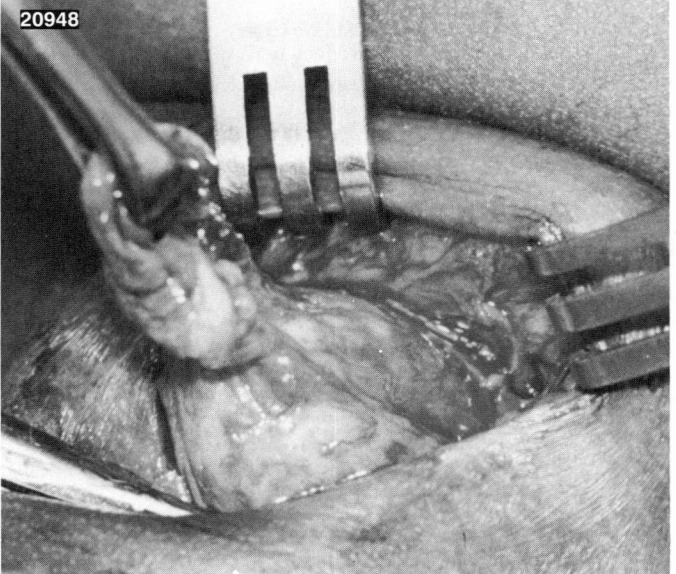

0945B-20948: Thyroglossal duct cyst.

embryologic descent of the developing thyroid gland from the pharynx to the neck. In some instances several tiny ducts may be found. Rarely descent does not occur and a mass at the foramen cecum may not be a thyroglossal duct cyst, but a lingual thyroid.

An I^{125} thyroid scan should be done in the case of lingual mass. If the lingual thyroid is the only thyroid tissue in the body; the radioactive isotope uptake will be in the area of the base of the tongue. Most patients with a lingual thyroid are euthyroid, although in a series of cretins 63.6% had ectopic thyroid. The majority of patients are asymptomatic. 65–70% have no other thyroid tissue. Diagnosis may be made by fine needle aspiration for cytology.

Grossly the lingual thyroid is hemispheric, about 2 cm in diameter, pink, and covered by squamous epithelium through which vascular markings are visible. The most common histology is fetal or microvillar adenomatous pattern, closely followed by normal thyroid microscopic appearance. The thyroglossal cyst and duct may be lined with squamous, ciliated respiratory, pseudostratified columnar, columnar, cuboidal, or transitional epithelium. More than one type of epithelium may be present. Subepithelial aggregations of lymphocytes may be seen. The epithelial lining may be replaced by fibrous tissue. Thyroid follicles may be seen in 2–36% of specimens. The contents may be mucoid, grumous, or pasty.

Complications: Infection (50%); recurrence (15–20%); osteomyelitis of hyoid bone; airway obstruction.

Associated Findings: Papillary adenocarcinoma (less than 100 reported cases).

Etiology: Unknown.

Pathogenesis: Failure of the thyroglossal anlage to descend to the normal location of the thyroid gland. Persistence of a cystic dilation of embryonic thyroglossal duct.

CDC No.: 759.220

Sex Ratio: M1:F4–5

Occurrence: 31 cases in 86,000 consecutive admissions to Mayo Clinic. In a series of routine autopsies, 10% had ectopic thyroid tissue.

Risk of Recurrence for Patient's Sib: Unknown.

Risk of Recurrence for Patient's Child: Unknown.

Age of Detectability: Usually in early childhood, by physical examination.

Gene Mapping and Linkage: Unknown.

Prevention: None known. Genetic counseling indicated.

Treatment: En bloc surgical excision of cyst and a core of tissue in continuity with the middle one-third of hyoid bone and to the foramen cecum (Sistrunk, 1920). Treatment of infection with antibiotics. Primary excision is recommended rather than incision and drainage. Medical treatment consists of I^{131} ablation of the lingual thyroid followed by hormonal suppression. However, excision of the lingual thyroid and implantation of slices into the sternocleidomastoid muscle has been successful. Surgical treatment may be reserved for cases where hemorrhage, cystic degeneration, suspected malignancy, or failure of medical therapy has occurred.

Endotracheal intubation or tracheotomy may be needed if the airway is obstructed. For carcinoma of the thyroglossal remnant; total thyroidectomy, bilateral neck explorations, followed by I^{131} and hormonal suppression.

Prognosis: Good if adequately excised.

Detection of Carrier: Unknown.

References:
Sistrunk WE: The surgical treatment of cysts of the thyroglossal tract. Ann Surg 1920; 71:121–122. *
Swan H, et al.: Autotransplantation of the lingual thyroid. Arch Surg 1958; 76:458–464.
Sadé J, Rosen G: Thyroglossal cysts and tracts: a histological and histochemical study. Ann Otol Rhinol Laryngol 1968; 77:139–145.
Ward PH, Strahan RW, et al.: The many faces of thyroglossal duct. Trans Am Acad Ophth & Otol 1970; 74:310–318 *.
Weider DJ, Parker W: Lingual thyroid: review, case reports and therapeutic guidelines, Ann Otol Rhinol Laryngol 1977; 86:841–848.
Hawkins DB, et al.: Cysts of the thyroglossal duct. Laryngoscope 1982; 92:1254–1258.

BE028   **LaVonne Bergstrom**

Thyroglossal duct, cyst or sinus
  See *THYROGLOSSAL DUCT REMNANT*
Thyroid 1, transforming sequence
  See *CANCER, THYROID, FAMILIAL PAPILLARY CARCINOMA OF*
Thyroid hormone organification defect IIB
  See *DEAFNESS-GOITER*
Thyroid hormone, familial resistance to
  See *THYROID, HORMONE RESISTANCE*
Thyroid hormone, generalized tissue resistance to
  See *THYROID, HORMONE RESISTANCE*
Thyroid hormone, insensitivity to
  See *THYROID, HORMONE RESISTANCE*
Thyroid hormone, partial resistance to
  See *THYROID, HORMONE RESISTANCE*
Thyroid hormone, pituitary resistance to
  See *THYROID, HORMONE RESISTANCE*
Thyroid hormone, refractoriness to
  See *THYROID, HORMONE RESISTANCE*
Thyroid hormone, target hormone resistance to
  See *THYROID, HORMONE RESISTANCE*
Thyroid hormonogenesis, genetic defect in
  See *DEAFNESS-GOITER*
Thyroid hormonogenesis, genetic defect in, I
  See *THYROID, IODIDE TRANSPORT DEFECT*
Thyroid hormonogenesis, genetic defect in, IIA
  See *THYROID, PEROXIDASE DEFECT*
Thyroid hormonogenesis, genetic defect in, IV
  See *THYROID, IODOTYROSINE DEIODINASE DEFICIENCY*
Thyroid hormonogenesis, genetic defect in, V
  See *THYROID, THYROGLOBULIN DEFECTS*
Thyroid organification defects (some types)
  See *THYROID, PEROXIDASE DEFECT*
Thyroid peroxidase deficiency
  See *THYROID, PEROXIDASE DEFECT*

THYROID, DYSGENESIS   0946

Includes:
  Agoitrous cretinism
  Agoitrous hypothyroidism
  Athyreotic hypothyroidism
  Athyrosis
  Cretinism, agoitrous
  Cretinism, athyreotic
  Cretinism, sporadic nongoitrous
  Cryptothyroidism

Excludes:
  Cretinism, endemic (3167)
  Thyroid dyshormonogenesis, all forms
  Thyroid, iodotyrosine deiodinase deficiency (0543)
  Thyroid, peroxidase defect (0947)
  Thyrotropin deficiency, isolated (0949)
  Thyrotropin unresponsiveness (0948)

Major Diagnostic Criteria: Cord blood or filter paper spot T4 concentration < 7 μg/dl and TSH concentration > 60 μU/ml. After one week of age, serum T4 is below the range for age and TSH > 10 μU/ml. Serum T3 concentrations are variable. Thyroidal radioiodine uptake and scan may be confirmatory.

Clinical Findings: Infants with thyroid dysgenesis may have ectopic or hypoplastic thyroid tissue or total thyroid agenesis. Thus, there is a spectrum of severity of thyroid hormone deficiency. Some thyroid tissue is present in as many as 70–80% of cases. Infants with inadequate thyroid tissue are born with low (hypothyroid) circulating levels of thyroxine (T4) and high TSH concentrations. Significant but low levels of T4 usually are present in infants with residual functioning thyroid tissue, and serum TSH levels are increased. Thyroid scanning techniques are not sensitive enough to detect small volumes of residual tissue in some infants, but significant circulating concentrations of triiodothyronine (T3) during the neonatal period in the face of low serum T4 concentrations suggest the presence of residual functioning thyroid tissue. Significant levels of circulating thyroglobulin also indicate the presence of thyroid tissue.

Although signs and symptoms of hypothyroidism may occur in the newborn period, the clinical diagnosis is difficult and is made early (before 8–12 weeks) in only 30% of affected infants. Suggestive early signs and symptoms include a large posterior fontanel, prolonged "physiologic" hyperbilirubinemia, mild myxedema of the face and neck, respiratory distress in a full-term infant, hypothermia (< 35.5° C rectal), bradycardia (rate < 100), constipation, lethargy, poor feeding, noisy breathing, and persistent nasal stuffiness. The more classic signs and symptoms of macroglossia, abdominal distention, umbilical hernia, hypotonia, dry hair and skin, puffy facies, and hoarse cry appear later in infancy and indicate prolonged hypothyroidism. In children, delayed growth, delayed skeletal maturation, and delayed dental development are the most sensitive indicators of thyroid hormone deficiency. Hypofunction of a variety of organ systems may be detected by careful study but offer only nonspecific, secondary evidence for thyroid hormone deficiency. Congenital hypothyroidism leads to intellectual deficit and clinical brain dysfunction if thyroid replacement therapy is not begun before 45 days of age; 95% of infants begun on treatment before this time develop normal intellect, whereas only 10% or less develop normally if treatment is delayed beyond one year.

Complications: Mental retardation, growth retardation, delayed bone and dental maturation.

Associated Findings: Nearly all athyreotic cretins are PTC non-tasters.

Etiology: Usually sporadic. A few familial cases have been described, associated with maternal autoimmune thyroid disease. Also a few cases have occurred after administration of therapeutic doses of radioiodine for treatment of thyrotoxicosis. In these cases, the pregnancy was of 10–20 weeks duration at the time of therapy, and pregnancy was not suspected.

Pathogenesis: Failure of normal embryologic development of the thyroid gland primordium. Hypoplasia may be associated with ectopy or residual thyroid gland tissue, which may be located at the base of the tongue, between the base of the tongue and the hyoid bone, or between the hyoid bone and the normal position below the thyroid cartilage. Ectopic location of residual thyroid tissue occurs in 60–80% of cases. Residual tissue is hyperplastic with a high cell/colloid ratio and little visible colloid. The reduced volume of thyroid tissue results in deficiency of T4 secretion and compensatory increase in secretion of TSH from the pituitary gland. T3 secretion may be increased from the intensely stimulated residual tissue, and the normal or near-normal serum T3 levels offer some protection against severe thyroid hormone deficiency.

MIM No.: *21870

POS No.: 3521

CDC No.: 759.210

Sex Ratio: M1:F4

Occurrence: 1:5,526 in whites; 1:32,377 in blacks.

Risk of Recurrence for Patient's Sib: Very small. There is some evidence to suggest that the risk may be increased if the mother has a high titer of antithyroid, and particularly TSH receptor, antibody.

Risk of Recurrence for Patient's Child: Very small.

Age of Detectability: At birth, by cord blood or filter paper spot screening for T4 and TSH concentrations.

Gene Mapping and Linkage: Unknown.

Prevention: Avoidance of radioiodine treatment of thyrotoxicosis in pregnancy. Counseling for women with high thyroid antibody titer.

Treatment: Treatment with thyroid hormone to prevent complications.

Prognosis: Normal life span with early diagnosis and treatment; mental deficiency and growth retardation without therapy. The prognosis for mental development becomes poorer as treatment is delayed.

Detection of Carrier: Unknown.

References:
Dussault JH, et al.: Thyroid function in neonatal hypothyroidism. J Pediatr 1976; 89:541.
Klein AH, et al.: Neonatal thyroid function in congenital hypothyroidism. J Pediatr 1976; 89:545.
Brown AL, et al.: Racial differences in the incidence of congenital hypothyroidism. J Pediatr 1981; 99:934–936.
New England Congenital Hypothyroidism Collaborative. Neonatal hypothyroid screening: status of patients at 6 years. J Pediatr 1985; 107:915–919.
Rovet J, et al.: Intellectual outcome in children with fetal hypothyroidism. J Pediatr 1987; 110:700–704.
Muir A, et al.: Thyroid scanning, ultrasound and serum thyroglobulin in determining the origin of congenital hypothyroidism. Am J Dis Child 1988; 142:214–216.
New England Congenital Hypothyroidism Collaborative: Elementary school performance of children with congenital hypothyroidism. J Pediatr 1990; 116:27–32.

FI017   **Delbert A. Fisher**

Thyroid, familial papillary carcinoma
See CANCER, THYROID, FAMILIAL PAPILLARY CARCINOMA OF

THYROID, HORMONE RESISTANCE   **0257**

Includes:
Refetoff syndrome
Thyroid hormone, familial resistance to
Thyroid hormone, generalized tissue resistance to
Thyroid hormone, insensitivity to
Thyroid hormone, partial resistance to
Thyroid hormone, pituitary resistance to
Thyroid hormone, refractoriness to
Thyroid hormone, target hormone resistance to
Thyrotropin secretion, inappropriate

Excludes:
Cretinism, endemic (3167)
Deafness-goiter (0249)
Epiphyseal dysplasia, multiple (0358)
Euthyroid hyperthyroxinemia
Familial dysalbuminemic hyperthyroxinemia (FDH)
Graves disease, neonatal
Inborn errors of thyroid hormone synthesis
Thyrotropin-secreting pituitary adenoma
Thyrotropin unresponsiveness (0948)
Thyroxine-binding globulin defects (0950)

Major Diagnostic Criteria: Goiter and thyroid overactivity associated with high levels of free (protein-unbound) circulating thyroid hormone, non-suppressed thyrotropin (thyroid stimulating hormone, TSH), absence of thyrotoxicosis and diminished response to exogenous thyroid hormone.

Clinical Findings: The first description of this defect was in three siblings of consanguineous parents, who presented with deaf-mutism, delayed bone maturation, goiter, high levels of protein-bound iodine and the absence of stigmata of thyrotoxicosis. Subsequent case reports have shown a heterogeneity of features in terms of growth, bone maturation, hearing and mental development, as well as in the severity of the defect. Most patients have small goiters but none have ophthalmopathy or dermopathy typical of Graves' disease. The hallmark is elevated levels of circulating thyroid hormone (thyroxine and triiodothyronine), in the presence of eumetabolism, with normal concentration of thyroxine-binding globulin and non-suppressed thyrotropin. Both thyroxine and triiodothyronine are the L-isomers. Free thyroxine in blood is elevated. The 24-hour thyroidal radioiodide uptake is high and is non suppressible with replacement doses of thyroid hormone. The extrathyroidal thyroxine and triiodothyronine pools and their rates of degradation are elevated. Penetration of thyroxine into tissues and its conversion to triiodothyronine are normal. Circulating thyrotropin levels are normal or just above the normal range and increase in response to the administration of thyrotropin-releasing hormone. Thyroid-stimulating immunoglobulins are absent as are thyroglobulin and thyroid microsomal antibodies. Administration of replacement doses of thyroid hormone fail to supress the response of thyrotropin to thyrotropin-releasing hormone. Glucocorticoids and dopaminergic drugs, given in usual doses, produce their suppressive effect on thyrotropin. Some patients have demonstrable abnormalities of their nuclear receptor for thyroid hormone.

Complications: Probably deafness, bony dysgenesis and sequelae of hypothyroidism in patients given treatment aimed to reduce the circulating thyroid hormone level.

Associated Findings: Sensorineural hearing loss has been described in several cases and may be a complication of hypothyroidism during early life. Other abnormalities, probably not related to thyroid hormone activity have been observed less frequently. These are: winged scapulae, vertebral abnormalities, pigeon breat, prurigo Besnier, congenital ichthyosis and bull's eye type macular atrophy.

Etiology: Possibly represents the manifestation of a number of defects beginning at the interaction of thyroid hormone with its receptor and encompassing all subsequent steps leading to the expression of thyroid hormone action. The defect may be familial (30 families) or sporadic (7 cases). Both autosomal recessive and autosomal dominant modes of inheritance have been suggested. Consanguinity is known to have occurred in 4 families. Some cases may represent *de novo* mutations.

Pathogenesis: The condition appears to be a congenital metabolic defect of resistance to the action of thyroid hormone which affects tissues to a variable degree and that has been partially compensated by the production of excess hormone. Since thyroid hormone is probably essential for normal embryonic development and post-natal growth and maturation, complete thyroid hormone unresponsiveness by all tissues would presumably be incompatible with life. In some cases there may be demonstrable abnormalities at the level of the nuclear thyroid hormone receptor. The latter probably represents one of a spectrum of biochemical abnormalities responsible for the observed resistance to the hormone. Bioassys in cultured skin fibroblasts from affected subjects have not been always diagnostic. However, recent work has shown that in fibroblasts from 6 out of 7 patients with resistance to thyroid hormone, triiodothyronine suppressed fibronectin synthesis clearly less than in fibroblasts from normal subjects. The test may prove to be useful in the tissue diagnosis of the defect.

MIM No.: *18857, *27430

POS No.: 3910

Sex Ratio: M1:F1

Occurrence: Undetermined; 120 cases have been reported affecting individuals with a wide spectrum of ethnic backgrounds.

Risk of Recurrence for Patient's Sib:
See Part I, *Mendelian Inheritance.*

Risk of Recurrence for Patient's Child:
See Part I, *Mendelian Inheritance.*

Age of Detectability: Infancy, although often not detected until adulthood. The diagnosis can be made at any age on the basis of a small goiter with elevated serum thyroid hormone levels in the presence of euthyroidism and non-suppressed thyrotropin.

Gene Mapping and Linkage: Unknown.

Prevention: None known. Genetic counseling indicated.

Treatment: Avoid all treatment designed to correct the hyperthyroidism and thus normalize the thyroid hormone levels in serum. Treatment with supraphysiologic doses of thyroid hormone is reserved for patients with hypometabolism and growth retardation and for patients who have received therapy causing irrevers-

ible reduction of the hormonal reserve of the thyroid gland. Special training for deaf-mutism.

Prognosis: Variable but life span is probably normal. Thyroid hormone deprivation during early age may result in diminished mental and physical development.

Detection of Carrier: Unknown.

Special Considerations: The distinguishing features of this syndrome includes thyrotropin-mediated elevation of circulating levels of free thyroid hormone in the presence of clinical euthyroidism. Isolated tissue responses suggestive of hypothyroidism may be present, especially during early life. Administration of replacement doses of thyroid hormone fails to suppress thyrotropin, and supraphysiologic doses fail to induce signs of thyrotoxicity or produce the normal metabolic responses to thyroid hormone excess. Uptake of thyroid hormone and conversion of thyroxine to triiodothyronine are normal. A variant of the syndrome with resistance to thyroid hormone selective to the pituitary gland has been described. In the latter condition, patients have thyrotropin induced thyrotoxicosis with hypermetabolism. A condition with little clinical significance but which can be confused with thyrotoxicosis is familial dysalbuminemic hyperthyroxinemia (FDH). FDH has several subtypes and is frequent in Hispanics of Puerto Rican origin (Ruiz et al, 1982).

References:

Refetoff S, et al.: Familial syndrome combining deaf-mutism, stippled epiphyses, goiter and abnormally high PBI: Possible target organ refractoriness to thyroid hormone. J Clin Endocrinol Metab 1967; 27:279–294.

Refetoff S, et al.: Studies of a sibship with apparent hereditary resistance to the intracellular action of thyroid hormone. Metabolism 1972; 21:723–756.

Bernal J, et al.: Abnormalities of triiodothyronine binding to lymphocyte and fibroblast nuclei from patients with peripheral resistance to thyroid hormone action. J Clin Endocrinol Metab 1978; 47:1266–1272.

Brooks MH, et al.: Familial thyroid hormone resistance. Am J Med 1981; 71:414–421.

Weintraub BD, et al.: Inappropirate secretion of thyroid stimulating hormone. Ann Intern Med 1981; 95:339–351.

Refetoff S: Syndromes of thyroid hormone resistance. Am J Physiol 1982; 243:E88–E98.

Eil C, et al.: Nuclear binding of [125]-triiodothyronine in dispersed cultured skin fibroblasts from patients with resistance to thyroid hormone. J Clin Endocrinol Metab 1982; 55:502–510.

Ruiz M, et al.: Familial dysalbuminemic hyperthyroxinemia: a syndrome that can be confused with thyrotoxicosis. New Engl J Med 1982; 306:635–639.

Ceccarelli P, et al.: Resistance to thyroid hormone diagnosed by the reduced response of fibroblasts to the triiodothyronine-induced suppression of fibronectin synthesis. J Clin Endocrinol Metab 1987; 65:242–246.

RE007   **Samuel Refetoff**
EI002   **Charles Eil**

THYROID, IODIDE TRANSPORT DEFECT   0542

Includes:
> Goiter, familial (some forms)
> Hypothyroidism, congenital (some forms)
> Iodide accumulation, transport or trapping defect
> Iodide transport defect, partial
> Thyroid hormonogenesis, genetic defect in, I

Excludes:
> **Goiter, goitrogen induced** (0435)
> **Thyroid, dysgenesis** (0946)
> **Thyroid, iodotyrosine deiodinase deficiency** (0543)
> **Thyrotropin unresponsiveness** (0948)
> Other types of thyroid dyshormonogenesis

Major Diagnostic Criteria: Congenital hypothyroidism, or compensated hypothyroidism; an absent or very reduced RAI uptake in the presence of normal or increased serum TSH levels, and low salivary to plasma iodide ratio. Known goitrogens must be absent from the diet.

Clinical Findings: Patients are generally hypothyroid, usually presenting during infancy with developmental, growth, and skeletal retardation. Other signs of congenital hypothyroidism, such as lethargy, constipation, macroglossia, dry skin, umbilical hernia, and cretinoid facies may be present. Goiter may be evident at birth, but usually appears in early childhood. Laboratory findings include a low T4 with a low radioactive iodine (RAI) uptake with no increase after exogenous TSH administration. The defect may be complete or partial, indicating genetic heterogeneity.

Complications: Congenital hypothyroidism, with mental and physical retardation.

Associated Findings: Occasionally mechanical airway obstruction secondary to a large goiter.

Etiology: Autosomal recessive inheritance. Heterogeneity in the iodide transport defect exists. Three patients with a defect in thyroidal iodide transport but with some residual concentrating ability of their salivary glands and gastric mucosa have been described. Clinically, they are congenitally hypothyroid, and the defect in these cases also appears to be transmitted as an autosomal recessive trait. Whether they represent a different mutation at the same gene locus involved in the complete defect, or a separate basic defect of iodide transport, is unknown.

Pathogenesis: The transport defect may be due either to an altered postulated membrane iodide receptor or carrier, or an altered energy supply to this active transport system.

MIM No.: *27440

Sex Ratio: M1:F1

Occurrence: Presumably rare. However, since the defect can be treated with a high iodide intake, it may not be apparent in areas of high dietary iodide intake.

Risk of Recurrence for Patient's Sib:
See Part I, *Mendelian Inheritance.*

Risk of Recurrence for Patient's Child:
See Part I, *Mendelian Inheritance.*

Age of Detectability: Clinical symptoms of congenital hypothyroidism are usually apparent during the first one-half year of life. Occasionally goiter is present at birth. Serum T4 or TSH screening may be diagnostic at birth.

Gene Mapping and Linkage: Unknown.

Prevention: None known. Genetic counseling indicated.

Treatment: Early replacement therapy with thyroxine to prevent hypothyroidism. Iodide therapy also has been successfully utilized. Surgical removal of goiter if airway obstruction is present. Educational programs for the problem of mental retardation.

Prognosis: Prevention of mental retardation is dependent on early treatment in infancy.

Detection of Carrier: Unknown.

References:
Medeivos-Neto, G.A. et al.: Partial defect of iodide trapping mechanism in two siblings with congenital goiter and hypothyroidism. J Clin Endocrinol Metab 1972; 35:370–377.
Stanbury, J.B. and Chapman, E.M.: Congenital hypothyroidism with goiter. Absence of an iodide-concentrating mechanism. Lancet 1960 I:1162–1165.
Stanbury, J.B.: Familial goiter. In: Wyngaarden JB, Fredrickson DS, eds: The metabolic basis of inherited disease, 4th ed. New York: McGraw-Hill, 1978:206–239.
Couch RM, et al.: Congenital hypothyroidism caused by defective iodide transport. J Pediatr 1985; 106:950–953.
Wolff J: Congenital goiter with defective iodide transport. Endocrin Rev 1983; 4:240–254.
Couch RM, et al.: Congenital hypothyroidism caused by defective iodide transport. J Pediatr 1985; 106:950–953.

       R. Neil Schimke

THYROID, IODOTYROSINE DEIODINASE DEFICIENCY   0543

Includes:
 Deiodinase deficiency
 Goiter, familial (some forms)
 Hypothyroidism, congenital (some forms)
 Iodotyrosine dehalogenase deficiency
 Iodotyrosine deiodinase deficiency, partial
 Iodotyrosine deiodinase deficiency, peripheral
 Thyroid hormonogenesis, genetic defect in, IV
 Thyroidal deiodination deficiency

Excludes:
 Goiter, goitrogen induced (0435)
 Thyroid, dysgenesis (0946)
 Thyroid, iodide transport defect (0542)
 Other types of thyroid dyshormonogenesis

Major Diagnostic Criteria: Congenital hypothyroidsim, or compensated hypothyroidism with a rapid and high thyroid uptake and turnover of RAI; no deiodination of injected, labeled MIT (monoiodotyrosine) or DIT (diiodotyrosine); and probably MIT and DIT and their derivatives in abnormally high concentration in plasma and urine.

Clinical Findings: Patients with the complete form of iodotyrosine deiodinase deficiency, presumably homozygous for the trait, have the typical clinical appearance of congenital hypothyroidism. There is a variable age of onset in the development of goiter, that may be present at birth, but usually develops during childhood. Clinical laboratory findings are a low serum T4 with a rapid and high uptake and turnover of radioactive iodine. MIT and DIT and their derivatives are probably present in abnormally high concentrations in the plasma and urine. Exogenous intravenous administration of MIT or DIT results in their excretion unchanged in the urine, indicating deficient peripheral deiodination of these compounds as well.

Some presumedly heterozygous relatives of these patients, especially females, have goiters but are euthyroid. They display a partial impairment in peripheral deiodination when given exogenous DIT intravenously.

Complications: Congenital hypothyroidism, with resultant mental and growth retardation.

Associated Findings: Occasionally airway obstruction due to an enlarged goiter.

Etiology: Autosomal recessive inheritance. Homozygous state manifesting congenital hypothyroidism; heterozygotes, especially females, may manifest euthyroid goiter.

Pathogenesis: The iodotyrosine deiodinase enzyme is not involved in the direct synthesis of T_4 or T_3, but functions as a salvage mechanism for iodide recovery from thyroglobulin-bound MIT and DIT not utilized in synthesis. A defect in this enzyme results in continued loss of iodinated precursors and depletion of available iodine stores, with resultant hypothyroidism. Consistent with this is the observation that replacement therapy with a large excess of iodide can reestablish a euthyroid state.

MIM No.: *27480

Sex Ratio: M1:F1

Occurrence: Undetermined. Since iodide therapy can ameliorate the disorder, it may not be clinically apparent in areas with a high dietary iodide intake.

Risk of Recurrence for Patient's Sib:
See Part I, *Mendelian Inheritance.*

Risk of Recurrence for Patient's Child:
See Part I, *Mendelian Inheritance.*

Age of Detectability: Symptoms of congenital hypothyroidism usually are apparent during the first half-year of life, usually with goiter. Serum T4 screening should detect this at birth.

Gene Mapping and Linkage: Unknown.

Prevention: None known. Genetic counseling indicated.

Treatment: Early replacement therapy with thyroxine to prevent congenital hypothyroidism. Iodide treatment has been successful, although large doses are often necessary. Surgical removal of a goiter may be necessary, due to pressure symptoms. Educational programs for the problem of mental retardation.

Prognosis: Good, with early treatment of hypothyroidism. Poor mental development, if treated late.

Detection of Carrier: Intravenous radioiodine-labeled diiodotyrosine (DIT) test may distinguish the heterozygous state.

Special Considerations: Heterogeneity of iodotyrosine deiodinase defects has become apparent. Patients have been described with a partial deiodination deficiency, a deficient thyroidal deiodination with normal peripheral deiodination, and a peripheral defect with a normal thyroidal iodotyrosine deiodinase activity. Clinically, these patients usually have been euthyroid with goiter. The genetic etiology of each of these types is unclear. They may represent other mutations at the same locus, or at a different locus, perhaps affecting different tissue isoenzymes or enzyme subunits.

References:
Stanbury, JB, et al.: Familial goiter and related disorders. In: Stanbury JB, et al. eds: The Metabolic Basis of Inherited Disease, 5th Ed. New York: McGraw-Hill, 1983:231–269.

SC016   **R. Neil Schimke**

THYROID, PEROXIDASE DEFECT   0947

Includes:
> Goiter, familial
> Hypothyroidism, congenital
> Iodide peroxidase deficiency
> Thyroid organification defects (some types)
> Thyroid peroxidase deficiency
> Thyroid hormonogenesis, genetic defect in, IIA

Excludes:
> **Deafness-goiter** (0249)
> Hashimoto thyroiditis
> Thyroglobulin synthesis, abnormal
> **Thyroid, dysgenesis** (0946)
> Thyroid dyshormonogenesis, other
> Thyroid nonperoxidase deficient organification defects, other

Major Diagnostic Criteria: Hypothyroidism or compensated hypothyroidism, with a rapid discharge of radioiodine after administration of thiocyanate or perchlorate. In addition, *in vitro* demonstration of defective peroxidase activity.

Clinical Findings: Clinical heterogeneity is apparent in patients with thyroid peroxidase deficiency. One group, congenitally hypothyroid, presents in early infancy or childhood with mental, growth, and skeletal retardation, and a typical cretinoid appearance. The appearance of goiter is variable, but it usually appears during early childhood. Clinical laboratory findings include a low serum thyroxine, and patients demonstrate a rapid discharge of radioactive iodine, of variable amounts, from the thyroid after oral administration of thiocyanate or perchlorate. This indicates an abnormally large pool of inorganic iodide in the thyroid; this iodide is not organically bound to thyroglobulin, whereas in the normal individual virtually no iodide is dischargeable. Other conditions, such as Hashimoto thyroiditis, or a hyperactive thyroid remnant, may result in a partial perchlorate discharge and must be differentiated by other tests.

Another group of patients have presented with goiter but are clinically and chemically euthyroid. They demonstrate a partial radioactive iodine discharge with perchlorate or thiocyanate administration. These patients usually can be distinguished clinically from the **Deafness-goiter** syndrome by the presence of normal hearing.

Complications: Mental and physical retardation due to congenital hypothyroidism.

Associated Findings: Occasionally, airway obstruction secondary to a large goiter.

Etiology: Usually autosomal recessive inheritance. The genetics of a partial defect, with euthyroid goiter, is unclear; though dominant inheritance has been postulated in some families.

Pathogenesis: Thyroid peroxidase, in the presence of the necessary substrates, functions to oxidize inorganic iodide and transfer it to organically bound iodine. Several defects in peroxidase enzymatic activity have been defined. In the first, there is a quantitatively decreased activity that cannot be restored by the addition of hematin, the prosthetic group of the enzyme. This defect has been found among the group of patients with congenital hypothyroidism who also demonstrate complete *in vivo* perchlorate discharge.

A second defect is the peroxidase apoenzyme prosthetic group defect. No in vitro peroxidase activity is present; however, upon the addition of hematin, its prosthetic group, enzymatic activity is partially restored. Thus this defect appears to affect the binding site and thereby the affinity of the apoenzyme for its prosthetic group. These patients demonstrate only partial impairment of organification in vivo. These patients have shown a spectrum of severity; some compensated and euthyroid, and some hypothyroid.

Defects in iodide organification may result from a defect in the peroxidase enzyme. In addition, a defective thyroglobulin molecule, a defective hydrogen peroxide generating system, or abnormal cytoarchitecture may also result in impaired organification. Such defects may be responsible for the organification failure in non-peroxidase-deficient conditions, such as **Deafness-goiter**. In addition, many of the original patients described with organification defects may prove to have a peroxidase enzyme defect or a separate organification defect.

The thyroid microsomal antigen involved in autoimmune thyroid disease is, at least in part, thyroid peroxidase (TPO) (Seto et al, 1987).

MIM No.: *27450

Sex Ratio: M1:F1 in the congenital hypothyroid group. Among those patients with euthyroid goiter, there is a predominance of females.

Occurrence: Unknown.

Risk of Recurrence for Patient's Sib:
> See Part I, *Mendelian Inheritance.*

Risk of Recurrence for Patient's Child:
> See Part I, *Mendelian Inheritance.*

Age of Detectability: Clinically, symptoms of hypothyroidism are usually apparent during early infancy. Goiter may be present in infancy, but usually is not apparent until childhood. Serum thyroxine or TSH screening may detect hypothyroidism at birth.

Gene Mapping and Linkage: TPO (thyroid peroxidase) has been mapped to 2pter-p12.

Prevention: None known. Genetic counseling indicated.

Treatment: Early treatment with thyroid replacement if hypothyroid, and to reduce size of the goiter. Educational programs for problems of mental retardation.

Prognosis: Good in euthyroid goiter. Poor for mental development in congenital hypothyroidism, unless treated in early infancy.

Detection of Carrier: Unknown.

References:
Seto P, et al.: Isolation of a complementary DNA clone for thyroid microsomal antigen. J Clin Invest 1987; 80:1205–1208.
Dumont JE, et al.: Thyroid disorders. In: Scriver CR, et al, eds: The metabolic basis of inherited disease, 6th ed. New York: McGraw-Hill, 1989:1843–1880. *
New England Congenital Hypothyroidism Collaborative: Elementary school performance of children with congenital hypothyroidism. J Pediatr 1990; 116:27–32.

SC016   **R. Neil Schimke**

THYROID, THYROGLOBULIN DEFECTS 3061

Includes:
Goiter, congenital
Goitrous hypothyroidism
Hypothyroidism, congenital
Thyroglobulin, absent
Thyroglobulin synthesis, defect in
Thyroid hormonogenesis, genetic defect in, V

Excludes:
Deafness-goiter (0249)
Thyroid, dysgenesis (0946)
Thyroid dyshormonogenesis (other)
Thyroid organification defects

Major Diagnostic Criteria: Congenital primary hypothyroidism or compensated primary hypothyroidism with a normal thyroid scan; increased radioiodine uptake; absent or abnormal thyroglobulin by thyroid biopsy.

Clinical Findings: Infants are usually detected by thyroid screening with a low-normal or low thyroxine (T4) level and elevated serum TSH. A thyroid scan with ^{123}I or technetium reveals a normal or enlarged thyroid gland. A serum thyroglobulin measurement by radioimmunoassay may show a low or absent level. A perchlorate discharge test usually will be negative but can be positive in patients with a thyroglobulin defect. Infants are usually treated with T4 until ages 2–3 years or later, when a definitive workup to define the defect can be conducted off T4 replacement with no risk to brain development. If untreated, these infants develop growth retardation, a cretinoid appearance, delayed skeletal growth and maturation, and mental retardation.

Definitive characterization of the defect requires thyroid radioiodine uptake studies to document increased uptake and turnover of radioiodine, testing for labeled monoiodotyrosine (MIT) and diiodotyrosine (DIT) in urine to exclude a thyroid iodotyrosine deiodinase defect, a perchlorate discharge test to exclude a peroxidase system defect, and thyroid biopsy. Histologic examination reveals hyperplasia with decreased or absent colloid and decreased or absent thyroglobulin by immunohistochemistry studies. Labeled aminoacid incorporation studies of thyroid tissue *in vitro* show little or no thyroglobulin. Measurements of thyroglobulin mRNA will help to resolve the level of the defect. A labeled cDNA probe can be used to test for the presence of the thyroglobulin gene.

Complications: Mental and physical retardation due to congenital hypothyroidism.

Associated Findings: If untreated, large goiter.

Etiology: Defects associated with both autosomal dominant and autosomal recessive inheritance have been identified.

Pathogenesis: The thyroid gland synthesizes thyroglobulin (TG) as substrate for iodothyronine (T4 and T3) biosynthesis. Thyroglobulin, which provides the tyrosyl residues for iodotyrosine synthesis, is an iodinated glycoprotein with a molecular weight approximating 660,000 daltons and a sedimentation coefficient of 19.4 (19S). It is composed of two 12S subunits each of which is comprised of two to four peptide chains. The predominant protein in thyroid colloid is 19S TG, and the thyroid gland normally contains 50–100 mg TG for every 1g of gland. MIT, DIT, T3 and T4 are present within TG as iodoaminoacyl residues that can be cleaved by proteolytic enzymes. The tyrosyl residues, which are the iodine acceptors of TG, comprise about three percent of the weight of the protein, and about two-thirds of these are spatially oriented to be susceptible to iodination. Synthesis of T4 and T3 does not occur in the absence of thyroglobulin synthesis, and, if the thyroglobulin molecule is abnormal in structure, MIT and DIT might not be spatially oriented for coupling.

Thyroglobulin synthesis could be deficient due to a gene deletion, a gene defect leading to defective transcription, a post-transcription translation defect, or production of an abnormal thyroglobulin. Patients have been reported with reduced or absent thyroglobulin, low molecular weight thyroglobulin, a thyroglobulin-like protein that was incompletely glycosylated, a thyroglobulin that was resistant to iodination, and an abnormal intracellular transport of thyroglobulin into the colloid space. These patients often secrete other iodinated proteins into blood (such as iodoalbumin) and excrete iodinated aminoacids (iodohistidine) in urine.

MIM No.: *18845, 27490

Sex Ratio: M1:F1

Occurrence: Undetermined but presumed rare.

Risk of Recurrence for Patient's Sib:
See Part I, *Mendelian Inheritance.*

Risk of Recurrence for Patient's Child:
See Part I, *Mendelian Inheritance.*

Age of Detectability: At birth, by elevated TSH level.

Gene Mapping and Linkage: TG (thyroglobulin) has been mapped to 8q24.

Prevention: None known. Genetic counseling indicated.

Treatment: Early treatment with thyroid replacement, if hypothyroid, to reduce size of the goiter. Educational programs for problems of mental retardation.

Prognosis: Good if treated in early infancy.

Detection of Carrier: Unknown.

References:
Desai KB, et al.: Familial goiter with absence of thyroglobulin and synthesis of thyroid hormones from thyroidal albumin. J Endocrinol 1974; 60:389–397.
Monaco F, et al.: Isolation and characterization soluble and particulate thyroid iodoproteins in human congenital goiter. Horm Res 1974; 5:141–155.
Lissitzky S, et al.: Defective thyroglobulin export as a cause of congenital goiter. Clin Endocrinol 1975; 4:363–392.
Dinsart C, et al.: Thyroglobulin complimentary DNA as a means to investigate congenital goiters with impaired thyroglobulin synthesis. Ann Endocrinol 1979; 39:133 only.
Silva JE, et al.: Low molecular weight thyroglobulin leading to a goiter in a 12 year old girl. J Clin Endocrinol Metab 1984; 58:526–534.
Dumont JE, et al.: Thyroid disorders. In: Scriver CR, et al, eds: The metabolic basis of inherited disease, 6th ed. New York: McGraw-Hill, 1989:1843–1880. *

FI017 **Delbert A. Fisher**

Thyroid-stimulating hormone, resistance to
See THYROTROPIN UNRESPONSIVENESS
Thyroidal deiodination deficiency
See THYROID, IODOTYROSINE DEIODINASE DEFICIENCY

THYROTOXICOSIS 3230

Includes:
Graves disease
Hyperthyroidism

Excludes:
Euthyroid hyperthyroxinemia
HCG-related hyperthyroidism
Hyperthyroidism as part of Hashimoto disease
Iatrogenic hyperthyroidism
Jod-Basedow disease
Pituitary resistance to thyroxine, selective
Toxic adenoma
Toxic multinodular goiter (some)
TSH-producing tumor with hyperthyroidism

Major Diagnostic Criteria: Elevated serum levels of T4 and T3, and elevated radioiodine uptake in the thyroid, along with depressed serum TSH level. Thyroid enlargement is generally but not invariably present, particularly in the elderly. Symptoms vary.

Clinical Findings: The classic clinical picture consists of hyperactivity, nervousness, and tremor in a patient with a smooth, symmetrically enlarged thyroid gland. The patient is often hyperreflexic, irritable, and has lost weight despite a voracious appetite.

Heat intolerance and increased sweating may be evident as well. Graves ophthalmopathy, onycholysis and pretibial myxedema may be present, or may occur in the absence of clinical thyrotoxicosis. The typical laboratory findings are elevated serum levels of T4 and T3, and elevated radioiodine uptake in the thyroid, along with depressed serum TSH level. Severe, untreated Graves disease may eventuate in thyroid storm with extreme muscle weakness, hyperpyrexia, and cardiovascular collapse. The ophthalmopathy usually accompanies the hyperthyroid state, but there is no correlation regarding relative severity. Moreover, the ocular changes may preceed overt thyrotoxicosis, or even occur many years after the thyroid has been successfully treated.

Complications: Untreated disease may result in extreme cachexia secondard to the hypermetabolic state and gastrointestinal hypermotility. High output heart failure may occur. Menstrual irregularities may be present. In young children, growth may be impaired. Enlargement of extraocular muscles, when ophthalmopathy is present, results in restrictive strabismus, and crowding of structures in the orbit may lead to compressive optic neuropathy.

Associated Findings: Other autoimmune endocrine diseases may preceed, occur with, or succeed Graves disease, the most common being **Diabetes mellitus** and idiopathic autoimmune Addison disease. Associated conditions also include myasthenia gravis, pernicious anemia and, periodic paralysis (the latter being reported most commonly in Japanese patients).

Etiology: Multifactorial inheritance pattern.

Pathogenesis: Graves disease is the prototype of an autoimmune disease. The thyrotoxicosis is secondary to circulating thyroid stimulating immunoglobulins (TSI) that arise presumably because of some defect in immune surveillance. There is an association with HLA antigens, particularly B8 and D3 in North America and Europe. In Japan, the association is with B35/D12. As with other autoimmune diseases, the consensus is that multilocus genetic factors interact with some environmental component, probably viral, to produce the disease. Graves disease may be etiologically heterogenous. The ophthalmopathy is likely related to crossreactivity of the TSI with some component of the extra ocular muscles, possibly the acetylcholine receptor.

MIM No.: 27500

Sex Ratio: M1:F5

Occurrence: 30–50:100,000 in females, 6–8:100,000 in males. The lifetime risk is about 5% for females and 1% for males.

Risk of Recurrence for Patient's Sib: Average risk about 5%. If a female relative is HLA identical with an affected individual, this risk is probably about 15%. The risk for male sibs is correspondingly lower.

Risk of Recurrence for Patient's Child: Unknown. Probably about the same as sibling risk overall, although impressive pedigrees consistent with sex-influenced autosomal dominant patterns have been reported. These may be due to reporting bias in conjunction with a common disease. Neonatal Graves disease is due to transplacental passage of TSI (pseudodominant inheritance).

Age of Detectability: At any point over the lifetime.

Gene Mapping and Linkage: Unknown.

Prevention: None known. Genetic counseling indicated.

Treatment: Oral thionamides, radioactive iodine, and thyroidectomy are all appropriate treatment modalities. Steroids may be useful in early ophthalmopathy. Radiation therapy or decompression of the orbit surgically may be necessary if compressive neuropathy occurs.

Prognosis: Excellent for thyroid disease. Not predictible insofar as ocular complications are concerned.

Detection of Carrier: Unknown.

References:
Adams DD, et al.: On the nature of the genes influencing the prevalence of Graves' disease. Life Sci 1983; 31:3–13.
Brennan MD, Gorman C: Thyroid dysfunction and ophthalmopathy.
In: Gorman CA, et al, eds: The eye and orbit in thyroid disease. New York: Raven Press, 1984:49–58.
Solomon DH: Treatment of Graves' hyperthyroidism. In: Ingbar SH, Braverman LE, eds: Wermer's the thyroid, 5th ed. Philadelphia: J.B. Lippencott, 1986:987–1014.
Utiger RD: Treatment of Graves' ophthalmopathy. New Engl J Med 1989; 321:1403–1405.

SC016   **R. Neil Schimke**

THYROTROPIN DEFICIENCY, ISOLATED   0949

Includes:
  Hypothalamic hypothyroidism
  Isolated TSH deficiency
  Pituitary cretinism
  Thyrotropin, biologically inactive

Excludes:
  Cretinism, endemic (3167)
  Cretinism, sporadic nonendemic
  Dwarfism, panhypopituitary (0303)
  Immunodeficiency, thymic agenesis (0943)
  Parathormone resistance (0830)
  Thyroid, dysgenesis (0946)

Major Diagnostic Criteria: Documentation of low circulating thyroid-stimulating hormone (TSH) and thyroxine concentrations. An isolated TSH deficiency is often a component of pseudohypoparathyroidism (see **Parathormone resistance**), and proper genetic counseling requires exclusion of this latter disorder.

Clinical Findings: The severity of (TSH) deficiency and secondary hypothyroidism varies; but in most cases the symptoms are mild, and the diagnosis is not made until adulthood. The symptoms are usually vague and not suggestive of thyroid disease, i.e. dizziness, weakness, constipation, angina pectoris, and so on. Severely affected individuals may rarely manifesting mental retardation, hypometabolism, dry puffy skin, husky voice, and delayed dental and skeletal maturation have been described. The diagnosis is established by confirming both low serum TSH and thyroxine levels.

Complications: Dependent upon severity of secondary hypothyroidism. Untreated severe disease will lead to profound mental and physical retardation.

Associated Findings: None known.

Etiology: Almost all cases have been sporadic, but there have been at least two pairs of female sibs reported from a consanguineous mating, which suggests autosomal recessive inheritance.

Pathogenesis: Various defects in the hypothalamic-pituitary axis have been postulated, and both hypothalamic and pituitary primary defects probably exist.

MIM No.: 27510

Sex Ratio: M1:F1

Occurrence: More than a dozen cases have been reported; many of them Japanese.

Risk of Recurrence for Patient's Sib:
  See Part I, *Mendelian Inheritance.*

Risk of Recurrence for Patient's Child:
  See Part I, *Mendelian Inheritance.*

Age of Detectability: Although usually not suspected until adulthood, the condition may be diagnosed at birth.

Gene Mapping and Linkage: Unknown.

Prevention: None known. Genetic counseling indicated.

Treatment: Replacement therapy with thyroxine.

Prognosis: Depends on severity of secondary hypothyroidism.

Detection of Carrier: Unknown.

References:
Odell WD: Isolated deficiencies of anterior pituitary hormones, symptoms and diagnosis. J Am Med Assoc 1966; 197:1006–1016.

Miyai D, et al.: Familial isolated thyrotropin deficiency with cretinism. New Engl J Med 1971; 285:1043–1048.
Rimoin DL, Schimke RN: Genetic disorders of the endocrine glands. St. Louis: C.V. Mosby, 1971:11–65.
Kohno H, et al.: Pituitary cretinism in two sisters. Arch Dis Child 1980; 55:725–727.

H0033
H0025

William A. Horton
O.J. Hood

Thyrotropin secretion, inappropriate
See THYROID, HORMONE RESISTANCE

THYROTROPIN UNRESPONSIVENESS 0948

Includes:

Hypothyroidism, congenital
Thyroid-stimulating hormone, resistance to
TSH resistance

Excludes:

Thyroid, dysgenesis (0946)
Thyroid dyshormonogenesis, other
Thyrotropin deficiency, isolated (0949)

Major Diagnostic Criteria: Congenital hypothyroidism with an elevated serum thyroid-stimulating hormone (TSH), a normal-sized thyroid, normal radiodine (RAI) uptake, and lack of response to exogenous thyrotropin administration.

Clinical Findings: Mental and growth retardation and other typical stigmata of congenital hypothyroidism. The thyroid gland is of normal size. Clinical laboratory findings include low serum thyroxine, markedly elevated serum TSH, and normal baseline RAI uptake. Administration of exogenous TSH does not increase serum thyroxine, RAI uptake, or glandular size. *In vitro* study of thyroid slices reveal no stimulation with the addition of TSH.

Complications: Congenital hypothyroidism, with accompanying mental and growth retardation.

Associated Findings: None known.

Etiology: Possibly autosomal recessive inheritance.

Pathogenesis: Thyrotropin has multiple effects on the thyroid, including stimulating cell division and thyroglobulin synthesis. An altered thyrotropin receptor site, or a defect in a subsequent step, such as a second messenger system, may be responsible for this disorder.

MIM No.: 27520

Sex Ratio: Presumably M1:F1.

Occurrence: About a dozen cases have been reported.

Risk of Recurrence for Patient's Sib:
See Part I, *Mendelian Inheritance.*

Risk of Recurrence for Patient's Child:
See Part I, *Mendelian Inheritance.*

Age of Detectability: Clinically, symptoms of congenital hypothyroidism are usually apparent during the first one-half year of life. Newborn serum thyroxine or TSH screening may suggest the disorder at birth. Complete delineation requires *in vitro* study.

Gene Mapping and Linkage: TSHR (thyroid stimulating hormone receptor) has been provisionally mapped to 22q11-q13.

Prevention: None known. Genetic counseling indicated.

Treatment: Early thyroxine replacement. Educational programs for problems of mental retardation.

Prognosis: Poor for mental and physical development if not treated early; however, this may be improved with early detection and therapy.

Detection of Carrier: Unknown.

References:
Dumont JE, et al.: Thyroid disorders. In: Scriver CR, et al, eds: The metabolic basis of inherited disease, 6th ed. New York: McGraw-Hill, 1989:1843–1880.

SC016

R. Neil Schimke

Thyrotropin, biologically inactive
See THYROTROPIN DEFICIENCY, ISOLATED
Thyroxine-binding capacity of serum, increase or decrease
See THYROXINE-BINDING GLOBULIN DEFECTS
Thyroxine-binding globulin (TBG) of serum
See THYROXINE-BINDING GLOBULIN DEFECTS

THYROXINE-BINDING GLOBULIN DEFECTS 0950

Includes:

Thyroxine-binding capacity of serum, increase or decrease
Thyroxine-binding globulin (TBG) of serum

Excludes:

Thyroxine-binding capacity of serum, acquired variation
Thyroxine-binding capacity of serum, chemically indiced variation

Major Diagnostic Criteria: Persistent high or low levels of thyroxine-binding globulin (TBG) or serum thyroxine in the absence of drug administration, and demonstration of a familial pattern.

Clinical Findings: No clinical disease or associated congenital abnormality has been observed in patients with familial excess or deficiency of TBG. The abnormalities produce either an increase or decrease in serum thyroid hormone concentrations and alter the pool sizes and half-time of disappearance of radioiodine-labeled thyroid hormones in the extrathyroidal pools. The rates of peripheral utilization of thyroid hormones, however, are normal. Normal circulating concentrations of TBG range from about 2–5 mg/dl; values of 2–9 mg/dl are seen in the newborn. Normal serum thyroxine (T4 concentrations range from 4.5 to 12.5 µg/dl; values in the newborn are 7–17 µg/dl. Patients with absent TBG have T4 levels in the hypothyroid range without evidence of hypothyroidism. Patients with low levels of TBG have low or low-normal TBG levels with low or low-normal serum T4 concentrations. TBG levels in adult patients with increased TBG range from 5 to 10 mg/dl, and T4 values from 13 to 25 µg/dl. Serum TSH values are normal.

At least six variants have been described: including TBG-A found in 40% of Australian aborigines; TBG-S found in Blacks, Eskimos, Melanesians, Polynesians, and Indonesians, but not in Caucasians; and the TBG-Gary; TBG-Quebec; TBG-Montreal; and the heat-stable TBG-Chicago (Murata et al, 1986; Takamatsu and Refetoff, 1986).

Complications: Unknown.

Associated Findings: Retarded mental and motor development has been reported.

Etiology: Presumably X-linked dominant or codominant inheritance of a biochemical defect, although autosomal dominant inheritance has been reported. The defect probably represent mutations at a single X-linked locus.

Pathogenesis: TBG, like glucose-6-phosphate dehydrogenase (see **Glucose-6-phosphate dehydrogenase deficiency**), is subject to both genetically determined increases and decreases in its concentration. The genetic defect presumably results in abnormal binding of T4 with or without alteration in the rate of hepatic TBG synthesis. Thorson et al (1966) presented evidence for two thyroid-binding globulins, thus creating the potential for heterogeneity in both high and low TBG.

MIM No.: *31420, *18860

Sex Ratio: While a sex-linked condition, intermediate TBG levels are seen in females.

Occurrence: At least 1:5,000 births (1:2,800 males). TBG excess is the rarer condition, with only a dozen or so kinships reported.

Risk of Recurrence for Patient's Sib:
See Part I, *Mendelian Inheritance.*

Risk of Recurrence for Patient's Child:
See Part I, *Mendelian Inheritance.*

Age of Detectability: For absent TBG: at birth by measuring serum thyroxine or TBG-binding capacity. For decreased or increased TBG: at one month by measuring serum thyroxine or TBG-binding capacity.

Gene Mapping and Linkage: TBG (thyroxin binding globulin) has been mapped to Xq21-q22.

Prevention: None known. Genetic counseling indicated.

Treatment: Early recognition is important in order to prevent unnecessary treatment for hypothyroidism.

Prognosis: Normal life span.

Detection of Carrier: By reduced levels of TBG or serum thyroxine.

References:

Thorson SC, et al.: Evidence for the existence of two thyroxine-binding globulin moieties. J Clin Endocr 1966; 26:181–188.
Rivas ML, et al.: Genetic variants of thyroxine-binding globulin (TBG). BD:OAS VII(6). New York: March of Dimes Birth Defects Foundation, 1971:34–41.
Hodgson SF, Wahner HW: Hereditary increased thyroxin binding globulin capacity. Proc Mayo Clinic 1972; 47:720–724.
Refetoff S, et al.: Study of four new kindreds with inherited thyroxine-binding globulin abnormalities. J Clin Invest 1972; 51:848–867.
Bigazzi M, et al.: Inherited X-chromosome linked thyroxin binding gloubin deficiency in a homozygous female. J Endocr Invest 1980; 4:349–352.
Grimald S, et al.: Polymorphism of human thyroxin-binding globulin. J Clin Endocr Metab 1983; 57:1186–1192.
Murata Y, et al.: Inherited abnormality of thyroxin-binding globulin with no demonstrable thyroxin-binding activity and high serum levels of denatured thyroxin-binding globulin. New Engl J Med 1986; 314:694–699.
Takamatsu J, Refetoff S: Inherited heat-stable variant thyroxin-binding globulin (TBG-Chicago). J Clin Endocr Metab 1986; 63:1140–1144.
Jenkins MB, Steffes MW: Congenital thyroxin binding globulin deficiency: incidence and inheritance. Hum Genet 1987; 77:80–84.

FI017   **Delbert A. Fisher**

Tibia, absence of, with polydactyly
  See MESOMELIC DYSPLASIA, WERNER TYPE
Tibia, bilateral aplasia of with polydactyly and absent thumbs
  See MESOMELIC DYSPLASIA, WERNER TYPE
Tibia, hypoplasia of, with polydactyly
  See MESOMELIC DYSPLASIA, WERNER TYPE
Tibial aplasia
  See TIBIAL APLASIA/HYPOPLASIA

TIBIAL APLASIA/HYPOPLASIA   2387

Includes:
  Tibial aplasia
  Tibial hemimelia
  Tibial hypoplasia

Excludes:
  Mesomelic dysplasia, Werner type (0649)
  Mesomelic dysplasia (other)
  Tibial hemimelia-fibular and ulnar dimelia
  Tibial hemimelia-fibular dimelia-mirror feet (diplopodia)
  Tibial hypoplasia/aplasia-ectrodactyly (2388)

Major Diagnostic Criteria: Abnormalities limited to unilateral or bilateral tibial hypoplasia/aplasia with or without hypoplasia/aplasia of preaxial bones of the foot.

Clinical Findings: Isolated tibial hemimelia is characterized in X-rays by unilateral or bilateral tibial hypoplasia or aplasia with or without preaxial hypoplasia or aplasia of bones of the feet. Affected individuals do not have other skeletal or nonskeletal abnormalities. Delayed and difficult ambulation and short stature are the primary clinical problems.

Complications: Clubfoot, fibular dislocation, fibular curving, and fibular hypertrophy or hyperplasia.

Associated Findings: None known.

Etiology: Both autosomal dominant and autosomal recessive inheritance, as well as sporadic cases, have been identified.

Pathogenesis: Unknown.

MIM No.: 27522

CDC No.: 755.365

Sex Ratio: M1:F1

Occurrence: Undetermined but presumed rare.

Risk of Recurrence for Patient's Sib:
See Part I, *Mendelian Inheritance.*

Risk of Recurrence for Patient's Child:
See Part I, *Mendelian Inheritance.*

Age of Detectability: At birth. Prenatal diagnosis may be possible by ultrasound.

Gene Mapping and Linkage: Unknown.

Prevention: None known. Genetic counseling indicated.

Treatment: Orthopedic devices, surgery, and rehabilitation.

Prognosis: Good, with adjustment to physical disability.

Detection of Carrier: Unknown.

Special Considerations: Tibial hypoplasia and tibial aplasia (agenesis) are separated clinically by X-ray findings, but a radiolucent cartilaginous tibial anlage may later ossify or may be detected at surgery. The presence or absence of any tibia may influence the choice of orthopedic surgery and devices and determine the ultimate form and function of the affected limb.

Tibial hemimelia may be the only manifestation of **Tibial hypoplasia/aplasia-ectrodactyly**, or may represent a separate entity.

Most cases of isolated tibial hemimelia are sporadic, but there are families with both vertical and horizontal transmission. Unaffected parents have had multiple children with isolated tibial hemimelia that has subsequently segregated as an autosomal dominant suggesting germinal mosaicism. There is no method of identifying the isolated case as autosomal dominant, autosomal recessive, or sporadic.

References:

Clark MW: Autosomal dominant inheritance of tibial meromelia: report of a kindred. J Bone Joint Surg 1975; 57A:262–264. †
Jones D, et al.: Congenital aplasia and dysplasia of the tibia with intact fibula: classification and management. J Bone Joint Surg 1978; 60B:31–39. †
Schroer RJ, Meyer LC: Autosomal dominant tibial hypoplasia-aplasia. Proc Greenwood Genet Center 1983; 2:27–31. * †
McKay M, et al.: Isolated tibial hemimelia in sibs: an autosomal-recessive disorder? Am J Med Genet 1984; 17:603–607. * †
Richieri-Costa A: Tibial hemimelia-cleft lip/palate in a Brazilian child born to consanguineous parents. Am J Med Genet 1987; 28:325–329. †

SC053   **Richard J. Schroer**

Tibial aplasia/hypoplasia-ectrodactyly
  See TIBIAL HYPOPLASIA/APLASIA-ECTRODACTYLY
Tibial hemimelia
  See TIBIAL APLASIA/HYPOPLASIA
Tibial hemimelia-split hand/split foot
  See TIBIAL HYPOPLASIA/APLASIA-ECTRODACTYLY
Tibial hypoplasia
  See TIBIAL APLASIA/HYPOPLASIA

TIBIAL HYPOPLASIA/APLASIA-ECTRODACTYLY   2388

Includes:
    Ectrodactyly-tibial hemimelia
    Gollop-Wolfgang syndrome
    Hypoplasia/aplasia of tibia and/or ulna with split-hand/split
      foot
    Tibial aplasia/hypoplasia-ectrodactyly
    Tibial hemimelia-split hand/split foot

Excludes:
    Ectrodactyly (0336)
    Ectrodactyly-ectodermal dysplasia-clefting syndrome (0337)
    Limb and scalp defects, Adams-Oliver type (0459)
    Tibial aplasia/hypoplasia (2387)

Major Diagnostic Criteria: Split hand/split foot and tibial or ulnar hypoplasia/aplasia.

Clinical Findings: Split hand/split foot and long bone hypoplasia/aplasia are associated in the same individual or members of the same family. The split hand may be severe or isolated 3–4 syndactyly. Tibial and ulnar are the most common long bone deficiencies. The tibial (preaxial) deficiency may be isolated hypoplasia of the hallux. More severe limb deficiencies, peromelia and transverse hemimelia, have been reported.

Complications: Dislocations and contractures of knees and elbows; club foot.

Associated Findings: Polydactyly, distal hypoplasia, duplication or bifurcation of femur, and hypoplasia of patella.

Etiology: Autosomal dominant and autosomal recessive inheritance have been reported.

Pathogenesis: Unknown.

MIM No.: *18360

POS No.: 3974

CDC No.: 755.250, 755.365, 755.350

Sex Ratio: M1:F1

Occurrence: Undetermined but presumed rare.

Risk of Recurrence for Patient's Sib:
    See Part I, *Mendelian Inheritance.*

Risk of Recurrence for Patient's Child:
    See Part I, *Mendelian Inheritance.*

Age of Detectability: At birth.

Gene Mapping and Linkage: Unknown.

Prevention: None known. Genetic counseling indicated.

Treatment: Orthopedic devices, surgery, and rehabilitation.

Prognosis: Good, with adjustment to physical disability.

Detection of Carrier: Unknown.

Special Considerations: The majority of familial cases of split-hand/split-foot and tibial and/or ulnar deficiency are consistent with autosomal dominant inheritance. Nonpenetrance and variable expressivity including isolated syndactyly or isolated hypoplastic great toes have been reported. Tibial deficiency and ulnar deficiencies have been reported both separately and together in different families. Autosomal recessive inheritance, suggested by affected children of normal parents, is questionable because of the marked variability of expression, including nonpenetrance of the autosomal dominant variety. Split-hand/split-foot with long bone aplasia may be a severe manifestation of isolated split-hand/split-foot, or may represent one or more etiologically separate entities.

References:
Temtamy S, McKusick V: The genetics of hand malformations. New York: Alan R. Liss Inc, 1978:53–71. †
Bujdoso G, Lenz W: Monodactylous splithand-splitfoot: a malformation occurring in three distinct genetic types. Eur J Pediatr 1980; 133:207–215. †
Majewski F, et al.: Aplasia of tibia with split-hand/split-foot deformity:

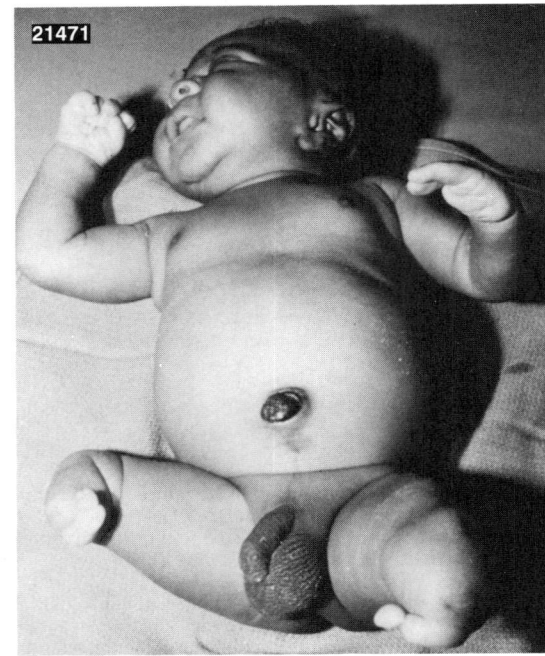

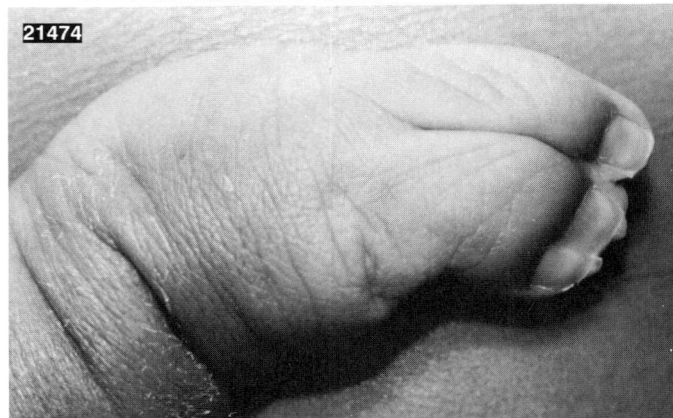

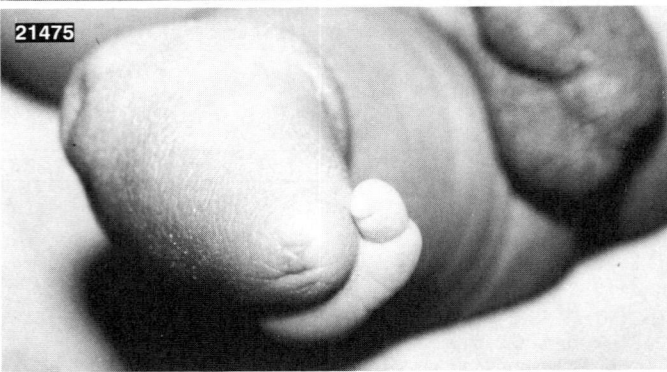

2388A-21471: Normal head and trunk measurements with normal external genitalia. There are severe limb reduction defects with a hypoplastic left forearm. **21474:** There are three digits on the left hand with syndactyly. **21475:** Note the skin dimples, malformed digits and hypoplastic distal segment of the right leg.

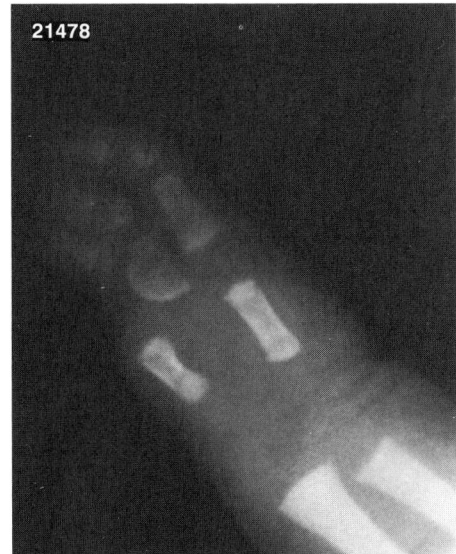

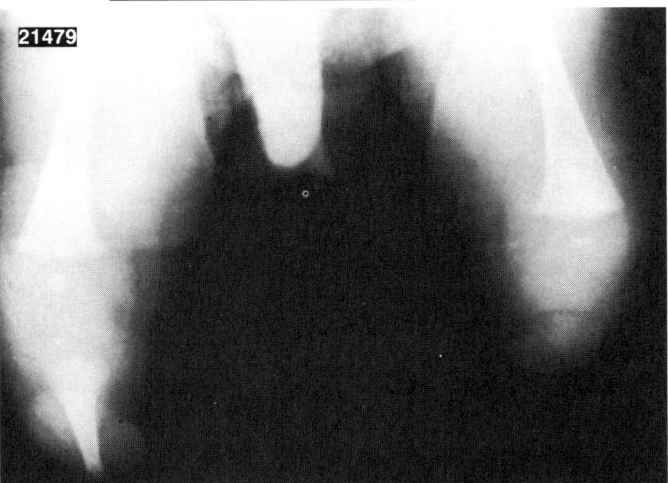

2388B-21478: X-ray shows deformity of the left hand with fusion of the proximal phalanges into a block and three digit syndactyly. **21479:** X-ray shows hypoplastic right tibia and aplasia of the left tibia and fibula. The left femoral epiphysis is similarly hypoplastic compared to the right.

report of six families with 35 cases and considerations about variability and penetrance. Hum Genet 1985; 70:136–147. * †

Schroer RJ: Split-hand/split-foot. Proc Greenwood Genet Center 1986; 5:65–75. †

Richieri-Costa A, et al.: Tibial hemimelia: report on 37 new cases, clinical and genetic considerations. Am J Med Genet 1987; 27:867–884. * †

SC053   **Richard J. Schroer**

Tick-borne meningopolyneuritis.
   See FETAL EFFECTS FROM LYME DISEASE
Tics, multiple motor and vocal
   See TOURETTE SYNDROME
Tight skin contracture syndrome
   See RESTRICTIVE DERMATOPATHY
TKCR syndrome
   See CERVICO-DERMO-GU SYNDROME, GOEMINNE TYPE
Tobramycin, fetal effects
   See FETAL AMINOGLYCOSIDE OTOTOXICITY

Tobrex∧, fetal effects
   See FETAL AMINOGLYCOSIDE OTOTOXICITY
Toe, recurring fibroma
   See DIGITAL FIBROMA, RECURRING IN INFANTS & CHILDREN
Toes, polysyndactyly-Hirschsprung disease-cardiac defect
   See HIRSCHSPRUNG DISEASE-CARDIAC DEFECT
Tomaculous neuropathy
   See NEUROPATHY, HEREDITARY WITH PRESSURE PALSIES
Tomato tumor
   See SCALP, CYLINDROMAS
Tongue curling
   See TONGUE, FOLDING OR ROLLING
Tongue gigantism
   See MACROGLOSSIA

TONGUE, ANKYLOGLOSSIA   0061

Includes:
   Ankyloglossia
   Tongue-tie
   Tongue, pseudocleft

Excludes:
   Hypoglossia-hypodactylia (0451)
   Palatoglossal adhesion

Major Diagnostic Criteria: Tongue movement is restricted so that with the mouth opened to its fullest extent, effort to raise the tongue tip fails to bring it above the level of a line between the commissures of the mouth. Upon forward protrusive effort the tip of the tongue demonstrates a central groove.

Clinical Findings: A variation of the lingual frenum resulting in an elevated and short band-like structure adherent at a higher than normal position of attachment on the alveolar ridge behind the central incisors causing a restriction of elevation and protrusion of tongue.

Complications: Some varieties may produce spacing of mandibular central incisors, periodontal disease, and some limitations in cleansing excursions of the tongue. There is no interference with infant nursing or later masticatory functions. If any disorder in speech is produced by ankyloglossia, it is extremely minor.

Associated Findings: None known.

Etiology: Possibly autosomal dominant inheritance.

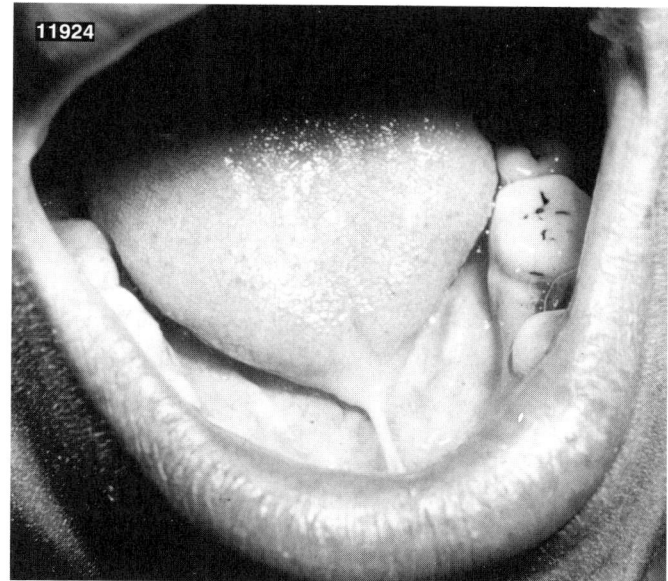

0061-11924: Ankyloglossia.

Pathogenesis: A developmental variation in the lingual frenum of the tongue such that the fibrous band of the midline raphe of the tongue, which anteriorly forms the lingual frenum, attaches anteriorly to tongue tip and high onto the alveolar process.

MIM No.: 10628

CDC No.: 750.000

Sex Ratio: M1:F1

Occurrence: Estimated at 1:330. Familial cases reported in the Dutch and German literature.

Risk of Recurrence for Patient's Sib: Unknown.

Risk of Recurrence for Patient's Child: Unknown.

Age of Detectability: At birth.

Gene Mapping and Linkage: Unknown.

Prevention: None known. Genetic counseling indicated.

Treatment: A decision for surgical release should be based upon associated dental disorders or dental prosthetic needs. The speech benefits of a release procedure should not be overestimated since they are probably insignificant. However, affected musical wind instrument players may benefit from surgical release.

Prognosis: Excellent.

Detection of Carrier: Unknown.

References:

McEnery ET, Gaines FP: Tongue-tie in infants and children. J Pediatr 1941; 18:252.

Stucke K: Zur frage der verkürzung der zungenbänochens. Aertgl Wschr 1946; 1:259.

Keizer D: Dominant erfeljik ankyloglosson. Ned Tijdschr Geneeskd 1952; 96:2203–2205.

Wilson RA, et al.: Ankyloglossia superior: palatoglossal adhesion in the newborn infant. Pediatrics 1963; 31:1051.

Witkop CJ Jr, Barros L: Oral and genetic studies of Chileans, 1960. I. Oral anomalies Am J Phys Anthropol 1963; 21:15.

Block JR: The role of the speech clinician in determining indications for frenulotomy in cases of ankyloglossia. NY State Dent J 1968; 34:479.

Young EC, et al.: Examining for tongue-tie. Clin Pediatr 1979; 18:298.

Nevin NC, et al.: Ankyloglossum superious syndrome. J Oral Surg 1980; 50:254.

HA067   **James R. Hayward**

Tongue, bifid
See TONGUE, CLEFT

TONGUE, CLEFT   0952

Includes:
Tongue, bifid
Tongue, trifid

Excludes:
Hypoglossia-hypodactylia (0451)
Oro-facio-digital syndrome I (0770)
Tongue, ankyloglossia (0061)
Tongue, pseudocleft

Major Diagnostic Criteria: Tongue divided into two or more lobes.

Clinical Findings: True cleft of the tongue divides the tongue into two or more lobes, in contrast to pseudocleft tongue in which the body appears to be divided into two lobes due to the pull of a short frenum. Cleft tongue may be part of a continuum of cleft mandible. However, both occur as isolated conditions.

Complications: The cleft does not usually interfere with speech unless associated with cleft lip and/or palate.

Associated Findings: Cleft lip, cleft palate, cleft mandible, heart defects, polydactyly, cryptorchidism, strabismus, absent hyoid, facial asymmetry, polypoid growth attached to tongue apex, and cervical webbing.

Etiology: All reported cases appear to have been sporadic.

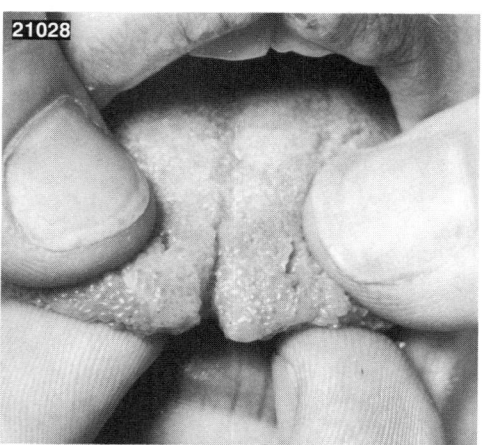

0952-21028: Cleft tongue.

Pathogenesis: Failure of fusion during embryogenesis of lateral tongue processes from a defect involving the first branchial arch.

CDC No.: 750.140

Sex Ratio: M5:F7 (observed).

Occurrence: Less than two dozen cases reported.

Risk of Recurrence for Patient's Sib: Presumably low, since condition is usually sporadic.

Risk of Recurrence for Patient's Child: Presumably low, since condition is usually sporadic.

Age of Detectability: At birth.

Gene Mapping and Linkage: Unknown.

Prevention: None known. Genetic counseling indicated.

Treatment: Surgical repair.

Prognosis: Isolated cleft tongue does not seem to interfere with longevity. Prognosis appears to be dependent upon associated defects.

Detection of Carrier: Unknown.

References:

Hubinger HL: Bifid tongue: report of case. J Oral Surg 1952; 10:64–66. †

Gorlin R, et al.: Syndromes of the head and neck, ed 2. New York: McGraw-Hill, 1976:178–179.

WE013   **Bernd Weinberg**

TONGUE, FISSURED   0953

Includes:
Fissured tongue
Lingua fissurata types I, II, and III

Excludes:
Tongue, cleft (0952)
Tongue, geographic (0954)
Tongue, plicated (0956)

Major Diagnostic Criteria: Multiple fissures on the tongue, other than the normal variation of a single shallow, central fissure at the insertion of the median raphe.

Clinical Findings: Many persons have one or two superficial midline fissures which are normal variations of the mucosal insertion of the median raphe of the tongue. Fissured tongue can be of several types arising from a variety of causes:

Type I: A deep central furrow, which probably represents a part of a continuum of normal midline raphe on one hand, and cleft tongue at the other.

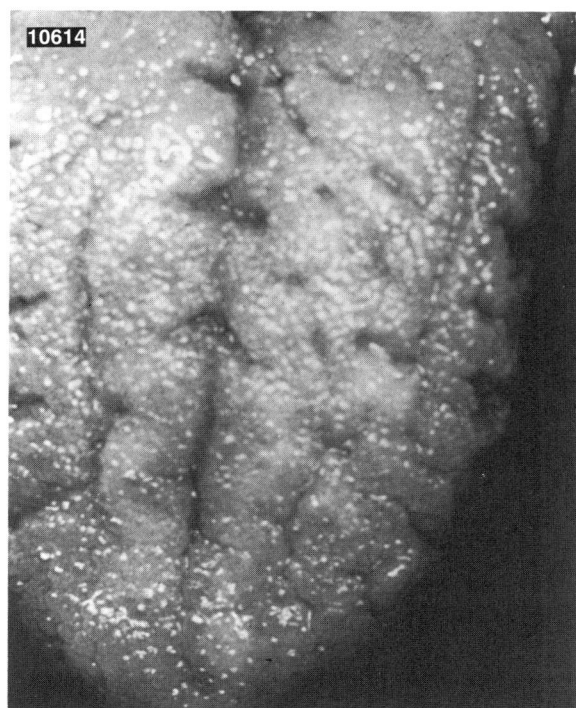

10614

0953-10614: Fissured tongue.

Type II: Multiple narrow fissures running parallel or obliquely at right angles to the midline raphe.

Type III: Deep, broad fissures parallel to the midline raphe in which the lingual papillae are absent and the base has a dense band of connective tissue scar. May be distinguished from **Tongue, plicated** by age and size distribution.

Complications: Unknown.

Associated Findings: Type III fissures are associated with cleft palate. May be governed by the same gene as **Tongue, geographic** and **Tongue, plicated**.

Etiology: Possibly autosomal dominant inheritance. It has been suggested that familial cases may be caused by the same gene responsible for **Tongue, geographic** and **Tongue, plicated**. Some cases may be caused by intrauterine infections.

Pathogenesis: *Type I*: Fissures represent incomplete fusion of the lateral halves of the tongue or binding of the mucosa to the central raphe of the tongue.

Type II: Unknown, but are probably acquired. When congenital they may be secondary to intrauterine infections, such as syphilis, and when they develop postnatally they are probably associated with a wide variety of infections and malnutrition.

Type III: Found in some patients with cleft palate including submucous clefts and is thought to be due to a misplacement of tongue-palatal shelf relationship during palatal development. Normally, initial palatal development takes place such that the palatal shelves grow downward between the lateral borders of the tongue and the cheek, and then snap into a horizontal relationship with each other. These fissures appear to result from the inferior borders (which become the midline margins after snapping into horizontal relationship) of the palatal shelves developing on the surface of the tongue instead of lateral to the tongue borders.

MIM No.: 13740

CDC No.: 750.180

Sex Ratio: M1:F1 in all three types.

Occurrence: Prevalence of Types I and II combined is about 1:20 over all age groups. Type III, about 1:10 to 1:8 cases with cleft palate.

Risk of Recurrence for Patient's Sib: Unknown.

Risk of Recurrence for Patient's Child: Unknown.

Age of Detectability: Type III: at birth. Type I and some Type II: from infancy to adulthood, by clinical examination.

Gene Mapping and Linkage: Unknown.

Prevention: None known. Genetic counseling indicated.

Treatment: Unknown.

Prognosis: Excellent for life and function.

Detection of Carrier: Unknown.

References:

Biegert J: Anthropologisch-erbbiologische unterschung der menschlichen zunge. Z Morph Anthrop 1954; 46:371–399. *

Witkop CJ Jr, Barros L: Oral and genetic studies of Chileans, 1960. I. oral anomalies. Am J Phys Anthropol 1963; 21:15–24.

Gorlin RJ: Developmental anomalies of face and oral structures. In: Gorlin RJ, Goldman HM, eds: Thoma's oral pathology, vol. I. 6th ed. St. Louis: C.V. Mosby, 1970:30–95.

WI043   **Carl J. Witkop, Jr.**

TONGUE, FOLDING OR ROLLING   **0951**

Includes:
    Cloverleaf tongue
    Tongue curling

Excludes: Tongue, ankyloglossia (0061)

Major Diagnostic Criteria: Ability to fold back the tongue or to roll the tongue so as to form a tube.

Clinical Findings: Ability to fold the tongue tip back upon itself or to roll or curl the sides of the tongue inward to form a tube. Both movements are performed by the intrinsic muscles of the tongue with no mechanical assistance. The two abilities are independent of each another.

Cloverleaf tongue, a possible variant, consists of the ability to fold the tongue in a particular cloverleaf configuration (Whitney, 1950).

Complications: Unknown.

Associated Findings: None known.

Etiology: Undetermined. Some researchers have suggested autosomal dominant inheritance, but other studies have refuted this conclusion.

Pathogenesis: Dependent upon genetic characteristics enabling unusual movement of the intrinsic muscles of the tongue.

MIM No.: 18930, 12910

CDC No.: 750.180

Sex Ratio: Presumably M1:F1. The ability to roll the tongue has been found in 63% of males and 66.84% of females. In males, this skill appears to be associated with the ability to move the ears.

Occurrence: In a sample of black individuals it was found that 70.79% of males could roll or curl their tongues but not fold it back upon itself, that 2.10% of the males could fold but not roll their tongues, and that 10.27% could both fold and roll their tongues. In the same sample it was found that 65.25% of females could roll but not fold, that 2.44% could fold but not roll, and that 17.26% could both fold and roll their tongues.

In a sample of various groups to determine the ability to roll the tongue, the following percentages were obtained: American whites 65.62, Chinese 62.2, Dutch 65.98, Jewish, 53.33.

Risk of Recurrence for Patient's Sib: Unknown.

Risk of Recurrence for Patient's Child: Unknown.

Age of Detectability: Early childhood.

Gene Mapping and Linkage: Unknown.

Prevention: N/A

Treatment: None required.

Prognosis: Normal for life span and intelligence with no known functional disability. No investigations have been made into a possible relationship between this ability and speech function.

Detection of Carrier: Unknown.

References:

Urbanowski A, Wilson J: Tongue curling. J Hered 1947; 38:365–366.

Hsu TC: Tongue upfolding; a newly reported heritable character in man. J Hered 1948; 39:187–188.

Liu T, Hsu T: Tongue-folding and tongue-rolling in a sample of the Chinese population. J Hered 1949; 40:19–21.

Whitney DD: Clover-leaf tongues. J Hered 1950; 41:176 only.

Lee JW: Tongue-folding and tongue-rolling in an American Negro population sample. J Hered 1955; 46:289–291.

Hernandez M: La movilidad del pabellon auditivo. Trab Anthropol 1980; 18:199–203.

MY003

Charles M. Myer III

TONGUE, GEOGRAPHIC 0954

Includes:

> Annulus migrans
> Glossitis, benign migratory
> Lingua plicata
> Stomatitis areata migrans
> Tongue, wandering rash of

Excludes:

> **Ankylosing spondylitis** (2516)
> Erythema multiforme
> **Glossitis, median rhomboid** (0417)
> Glossitis, resulting from nutritional deficiencies
> Lichen planus
> Lingual lesions of aphthae
> Pemphigus
> Syphilis
> **Tongue, fissured** (0953)
> **Tongue, plicated** (0956)
> Tuberculosis

0954-21029: Geographic tongue.

Major Diagnostic Criteria: The diagnosis is readily made from the striking appearance of discrete, smooth, red patches on the silver-gray, rough, dorsal surface of the tongue. "Migration" or evanescence of the patches over a period of days is diagnostic in otherwise doubtful cases. Rarely, the pattern may seem static for days or weeks, but even here, biopsy is seldom necessary to rule out other lesions.

Clinical Findings: Characteristic lesions are discrete, reddened, smooth, irregularly shaped patches on the dorsal and lateral surfaces of the anterior two-thirds of the tongue. The borders are often slightly raised and white or pale yellow in color. The pattern often resembles the configuration of a map; hence, the term "geographic" tongue. The lesions usually "migrate" by healing on one border while advancing on another. They tend to undergo exacerbations and regressions, and may often be completely absent for varying periods of time. About one-fourth of affected persons have tenderness, burning; occasionally, these symptoms are severe.

Complications: Unknown.

Associated Findings: It has been suggested that this condition may be associated with some of the same genes responsible for **Tongue, fissured** and **Tongue, plicated**. A history of allergy was found in 40% of the cases. A few cases have been reported in which identical lesions have appeared on other areas of the oral mucosa (*stomatitis areata migrans*) and even on the skin (*annulus migrans*).

Etiology: Familial occurrence best explained by multifactorial inheritance. Nutritional deficiency and infection are unlikely factors. Emotional stress is a contributing factor. Allergy seems worthy of investigation, as total and allergen-related serum IgE levels are higher in affected individuals.

Pathogenesis: Lesions progress through three stages: acute inflammation; chronic inflammation and desquamation; and regeneration and recornification. All three may be present in different areas of a given lesion.

Microscopically, the early lesions or advancing borders of older lesions show acute inflammation of the superficial mucosa, with intercellular edema and neutrophilic infiltration of the epithelium. The central areas are noncornified, with flattened or atrophic papillae, and show chronic inflammation. Many lesions show a striking resemblance to pustular psoriasis. In general, other laboratory tests are of no known diagnostic value.

MIM No.: 13740

CDC No.: 750.180

Sex Ratio: M1:F1

Occurrence: The incidence is somewhat higher than the prevalence because lesions are evanescent in many affected individuals. Prevalence is 1:83 among whites and Blacks between five and 70 years of age in surveys of several thousand people, each involving school children or dental patients in the United States. Higher occurrences have been reported in Japan and Israel, but these represent incidence rather than prevalence, and were conducted in wartime when nutritional deficiencies and stress were likely to have caused tongue lesions easily confused with those of geographic tongue.

Risk of Recurrence for Patient's Sib: Empirical risk 11%; higher if one or more parents are affected.

Risk of Recurrence for Patient's Child: Empirical risk 14%.

Age of Detectability: Has been observed in infants.

Gene Mapping and Linkage: Unknown.

Prevention: None known. Genetic counseling indicated.

Treatment: Reassurance. Soothing mouth wash for symptoms.

Prognosis: No effect on life span.

Detection of Carrier: Unknown.

References:

Redman RS, et al.: Psychological component in the etiology of geographic tongue. J Dent Res 1966; 45:1403–1408.

Richardson ER: Incidence of geographic tongue and median rhomboid glossitis in 3,319 Negro college students. Oral Surg 1968; 26:623–625.
Redman RS, et al.: Hereditary component in the etiology of geographic tongue. Am J Hum Genet 1972; 24:124–133.
Hume WJ: Geographic stomatitis: a critical review. J Dent 1975; 3:25–43. *
Eidelman E, et al.: Scrotal tongue and geographic tongue: polygenic and associated traits. Oral Surg 1976; 42:591–596. *
Marks R, Czary D: Geographic tongue: sensitivity to the environment. Oral Surg 1984; 58:156–159.

RE003   **Robert S. Redman**

Tongue, isolated congenital enlarged
   See MACROGLOSSIA
Tongue, large and protruding
   See MACROGLOSSIA
Tongue, median cleft
   See CLEFTS, LOWER MEDIAN LIP, MANDIBLE AND TONGUE
Tongue, pigmented fungiform papillae of
   See TONGUE, PIGMENTED PAPILLAE

TONGUE, PIGMENTED PAPILLAE   0955

Includes:
   Tongue, prominent pigmented papillae of
   Tongue, pigmented fungiform papillae of

Excludes:
   Intestinal polyposis
   Pigmentation, mucocutaneous
   Pigmentation, physiologic
   Tongue pigmentation

Major Diagnostic Criteria: Long-term history of presence of pigmented fungiform papillae of tongue. It is important to differentiate this condition from **Intestinal polyposis, type II.**

Clinical Findings: Brown to brownish-red pigmentation localized to tips of fungiform papillae. Lesions located primarily on tip and lateral margins of tongue. Occasionally, brown macules, 1–2 mm in diameter, on soft palate; distribution extending to junction of hard and soft palate. Routine blood and urine laboratory studies, serum electrolytes, and X-ray films of the chest and skull are normal.

Complications: Unknown.

Associated Findings: None known.

Etiology: Autosomal recessive inheritance, with about 89% penetrance in adults.

Pathogenesis: Undetermined. The pigmentary defect is present at birth and persists through life. The pigmentation is limited to the fungiform papillae of the tongue, with the occasional exception of pigmented macules of the soft palate. There is no correlation between this condition and the state of nutrition of the mother or the patient.

MIM No.: *27525

CDC No.: 750.180

Sex Ratio: M1:F9 (observed).

Occurrence: 1:12 African Blacks; 1:50 African whites. No data is available for other populations.

Risk of Recurrence for Patient's Sib:
   See Part I, *Mendelian Inheritance.*

Risk of Recurrence for Patient's Child:
   See Part I, *Mendelian Inheritance.*

Age of Detectability: Usually within first three months of life, by clinical observation. Rarely seen in the newborn.

Gene Mapping and Linkage: Unknown.

Prevention: None known. Genetic counseling indicated.

Treatment: None required.

Prognosis: Normal for life span, intelligence, and function.

Detection of Carrier: Unknown.

References:
Kaplin EJ, W'srand MB: The clinical tongue. Lancet 1961; I:1094.
Koplon BS, Hurley HJ: Prominent pigmented papillae of the tongue. Arch Dermatol 1967; 95:394.
Rao DC, Lew R: Complex segregation analysis of tongue pigmentation. Hum Hered 1978; 28:317–320.

AU005   **Thomas Aufdemorte**

Tongue, Pleomorphic lipoma
   See NECK/FACE, LIPOMATOSIS

TONGUE, PLICATED   0956

Includes: Scrotal tongue

Excludes:
   Cheilitis granulomatosa, Melkersson-Rosenthal type (2083)
   Chromosome 21, trisomy 21 (0171)

Major Diagnostic Criteria: Lingual papillae are divided into multiple groups by definite shallow fissures.

Clinical Findings: The tongue has a wrinkled or cerebriform appearance. The papillae of the tongue are divided into multiple groups or islands by definite small shallow fissures, which may not be apparent without folding the tongue so the surface mucosa is stretched. The small fissures involve the dorsal mucosa, including the edges of the tongue. **Tongue, geographic** may be superimposed giving a patchy or map-like appearance, with areas showing relatively short, smooth-appearing mucosa surrounded by longer white papillae at the borders. The two conditions are associated in about 20% of cases. The condition is asymptomatic.

Complications: Unknown.

Associated Findings: Plicated tongue occurs in **Cheilitis granulomatosa, Melkersson-Rosenthal type**, and in about 30% of patients with **Chromosome 21, trisomy 21**. Hanhart (1934) reported a 47% frequency in psychotic patients. The autosomal dominant form is associated with migraine headaches in some families.

Etiology: While many kindreds show autosomal dominant inheritance, it is not known if all cases are inherited. In most

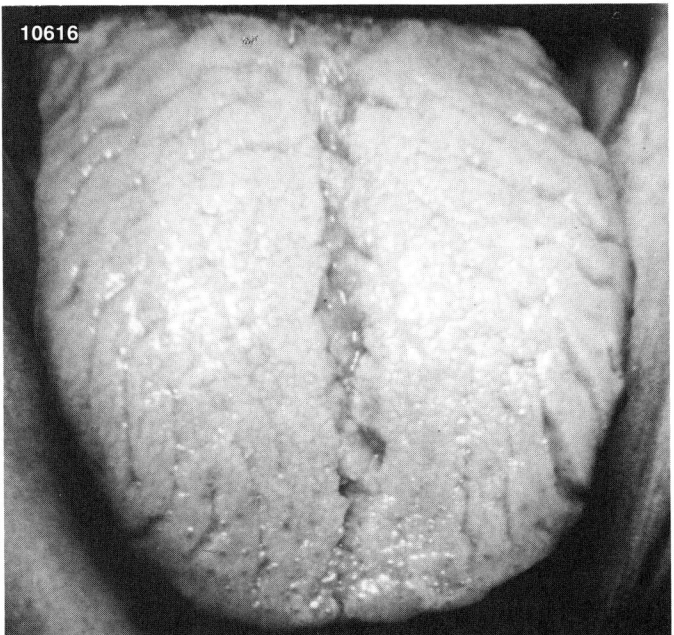

0956-10616: Plicated tongue.

instances, this is probably an age-related developmental polygenic anomaly. Since plicated tongue and **Tongue, Geographic** occur together with high frequency in first degree relatives, the mode of inheritance of each remains unclear and suggests etiologic heterogeneity and/or genes in common to both traits.

Pathogenesis: Undetermined. Condition is rare before age four years. Cerebriform pattern becomes more pronounced around puberty. One study showed a inconclusive association with blood group O. An association between plicated tongue and persons with low serum vitamin A levels has not been substantiated in later studies.

MIM No.: 13740

CDC No.: 750.180

Sex Ratio: M2.24:F1.68.

Occurrence: Prevalence 1:20 to 1:12 in all age groups combined. Shows increasing frequency with age, from about 1:100 in children to 1:8 in adults over 40. Rare before age four years.

Risk of Recurrence for Patient's Sib:
See Part I, *Mendelian Inheritance.*

Risk of Recurrence for Patient's Child:
See Part I, *Mendelian Inheritance.*

Age of Detectability: Frequency and severity of plicated tongue increases with age. Most cases are detectable by 12 years of age, by clinical examination.

Gene Mapping and Linkage: Unknown.

Prevention: None known. Genetic counseling indicated.

Treatment: None indicated. Vitamin A has been used with questionable success.

Prognosis: Excellent. Does not reduce longevity.

Detection of Carrier: Unknown.

References:
Hanhart E: Die faltenzunge (lingua plicata) als stigma nervöser minderwertigkeit. Verh Schweiz Naturforsch Ges 1934; 115:432–433.
Witkop CJ Jr, Barros L: Oral and genetic studies of Chileans 1960. I. Oral anomalies. Am J Phys Anthropol 1963; 21:15–24.
Gorlin RJ: Developmental anomalies of face and oral structures. In: Gorlin RJ, Goldman HM, eds: Thoma's oral pathology, 6th ed. vol. 1. St. Louis: C.V. Mosby, 1970:30–95. †
Eidelman E, et al.: Scrotal tongue and geographic tongue: polygenic and associated traits. Oral Surg 1976; 42:591–596. *

WI043   **Carl J. Witkop, Jr.**

Tongue, prominent pigmented papillae of
See TONGUE, PIGMENTED PAPILLAE
Tongue, trifid
See TONGUE, CLEFT
Tongue, wandering rash of
See TONGUE, GEOGRAPHIC
Tongue-tie
See TONGUE, ANKYLOGLOSSIA
Tooth and nail syndrome
See HYPODONTIA-NAIL DYSGENESIS
Tooth-hair-bone-nail dysplasia
See TRICHO-DENTO-OSSEOUS SYNDROME
Toothless man of Sind
See ECTODERMAL DYSPLASIA, CHRIST-SIEMENS-TOURAINE TYPE

TORSION DYSTONIA   **0957**

Includes: Dystonia musculorum deformans

Excludes:
Cerebral palsy (2931)
Dystonia, drug induced
Dystonic lipidosis
Hallervorden-Spatz disease (2526)
Hepatolenticular degeneration (0469)
Huntington disease (0478)
Hysteria
Niemann-Pick disease (0717)

Parkinsonism, early onset
X-linked mental retardation-basal ganglion disorder (2841)

Major Diagnostic Criteria: The diagnosis is clinical, and is suspected by the appearance of involuntary movement or posturing of one part of the body; often plantar flexion inversion movement of a foot combined with a pattern of progression. Family history may assist the diagnosis.

Clinical Findings: The disease has at least two hereditary types: autosomal recessive, and autosomal dominant. The autosomal recessive type has been described in Ashkenazi Jews with an earlier age of onset and a more rapid course. The dystonic posturing of the extremity is at first intermittent but gradually becomes constant. The symptoms spread to other extremities, eventually the neck and the trunk. The affected limbs assume a fixed, continuously maintained, abnormal attitude upon which athetotic fluctuations are superimposed later in the progression of the disease.

Autosomal dominant torsion dystonia has been reported mostly in non-Jewish families, particularly those from Sweden and French Canada. It has a more variable age of onset. It fluctuates in course and has more involvement of the axial musculature. In one-fourth of these patients, torticollis is the initial symptom.

The disease is a progressive movement disorder. Symptoms may be worse under stress. The movements may be triggered by the motion of any other part of the body or ultimately may appear spontaneously. Extrapyramidal movements cease during sleep.

Complications: Activities of daily living can be limited due to the involuntary movements and the dystonic posturing of the extremities. Eventually arthritis may develop in the affected limbs.

Associated Findings: The vast majority of patients have normal mental intelligence and are fully aware of their condition as they gradually become functionally handicapped in the motor area.

Etiology: Autosomal recessive or autosomal dominant inheritance.

Pathogenesis: Norepinephrine concentrations are markedly and consistently decreased in the lateral and posterior hypothalamus, mammillary body, subthalamic nucleus, and locus ceruleus. The cause of the neurochemical abnormality is undetermined.

MIM No.: *12810, *22450

Sex Ratio: M1:F1

Occurrence: In the autosomal recessive form, 1:20,000 live births are reported in Ashkenazi Jewish families.

Risk of Recurrence for Patient's Sib:
See Part I, *Mendelian Inheritance.*

Risk of Recurrence for Patient's Child:
See Part I, *Mendelian Inheritance.*

Age of Detectability: In the autosomal recessive type, onset is between four and 16 years of age. In the autosomal dominant type, there is a greater variation in the age of detectability.

Gene Mapping and Linkage: DYT1 (dystonia, torsion 1 (autosomal dominant)) has been provisionally mapped to 9q32-q34.
DYT2 (dystonia, torsion 2 (autosomal recessive)) is unassigned.

Prevention: None known. Genetic counseling indicated.

Treatment: A number of treatment modalities are available, but there is no consistently successful treatment. The most frequently used modalities include stereotactic surgery, L-dopa, bromocriptine, baclofen, lissuride, and diazepam.

Prognosis: Eventually the patients become bedridden and exhausted by constant muscular activity. The usual cause of death is intercurrent infection.

Detection of Carrier: Unknown.

Support Groups:
CA; Beverly Hills; Dystonia Medical Research Foundation
NY; Melville; Dystonia Foundation
CANADA: BC; Vancouver; Dystonia Medical Research Foundation

References:
Eldridge R: The torsion dystonias: literature review and genetic and clinical studies. Neurology 1970; 20:1–78.
Marsden CD, et al.: Natural history of idiopathic torsion dystonia. Adv Neurol 1976; 14:177–187.
Zilber N, et al.: Inheritance of ideopathic torsion dystonia among Jews. J Med Genet 1984; 21:13–20.
Hornykiewicz O, et al.: Brain neurotransmitters in dystonia musculorum deformans. New Engl J Med 1986; 315:347–353.

C0018   **Mary Coleman**

Torsion dystonia-skeletal and facial defects
See BLEPHARO-NASO-FACIAL SYNDROME

TORTICOLLIS   2940

Includes:
    Muscular torticollis
    Postural torticollis
    Sandifer syndrome
    Sternocleidomastoid torticollis
    Sternomastoid torticollis
    Wryneck

Excludes:
    Cervical hemivertebrae
    Cervico-dermo-gu syndrome, Goeminne type (2174)
    Klippel-Feil anomaly (2032)
    Oculo-auriculo-vertebral anomaly (0735)

Major Diagnostic Criteria: The affected sternocleidomastoid muscle is shortened so that the head is tipped forward and the chin is pointed away from the affected muscle. The muscle may feel hard or woody. A mass may be palpated in the body of the muscle in about 20% of cases.

Clinical Findings: Typically, the head is held in a neutral posture at birth, but tips into the wry position over the subsequent days or weeks. The active range of neck motion may vary with muscle shortening and will become intermittently more severe when the child is irritated, fatigued, or ill. Torticollis will generally remain persistent until ages 4–6 months and will then spontaneously, slowly improve. The pathology of the muscle mass discloses fibrous reaction without hemorrhage. The presence or size of the mass has no prognostic significance.

Complications: Torticollis often precedes the progressive development of a rhomboidal head shape with flattening of the face ispilateral to the shortened neck muscle and contralateral flattening of the occipitoparietal area (see **Plagiocephaly**).

Although there is some speculation that persistent torticollis affects overall gross motor development, no studies have clearly demonstrated this to be the case.

Associated Findings: Torticollis may be associated with other prenatal deformities, including scoliosis, metatarsus adductus, calcaneovalgus, and possibly dislocated hip. Hypotonia and other intrinsic neuromuscular disorders that predispose fetuses to constraint may be found.

Etiology: Congenital deformation without genetic predisposition is the usual situation. However, several multigeneration pedigrees have been reported, variably suggesting autosomal dominant, recessive, and polygenic inheritance.

Pathogenesis: There is general agreement that congenital torticollis is produced as a prenatal injury to the sternocleidomastoid muscle. The precise mechanism(s) of that injury are undetermined.

MIM No.: 18960

CDC No.: 756.860

Sex Ratio: M1:F1

Occurrence: Estimated at 6:10,000 live births, although some authors believe subtle damage to the sternomastoid is found in as many as 200:10,000 infants.

Risk of Recurrence for Patient's Sib:
See Part I, *Mendelian Inheritance*. Generally, deformities occur through an interaction of increased fetal size, decreased intrauterine space, and decreased fetal movement. Each pregnancy must be assessed for contributing factors.

Risk of Recurrence for Patient's Child:
See Part I, *Mendelian Inheritance*. Undetermined but presumed low unless familial.

Age of Detectability: Usually evident within the first 2–4 weeks of life.

Gene Mapping and Linkage: Unknown.

Prevention: None known. Genetic counseling indicated.

Treatment: Generally, torticollis resolves spontaneously by 6–12 months of life. When wryneck is persistent after 9–12 months of life, physical therapy will usually resolve the situation. In rare cases, a surgical release of the muscle after age three years may be necessary.

Prognosis: Normal neck movement can generally be expected.

Detection of Carrier: Careful clinical evaluation of the maternal pelvis and uterus may detect problems predisposing to constraining the fetus, and family histories may help to identify the rare families with multiply affected members.

Special Considerations: *Sandifer syndrome*, first described in 1969, is the rare association of GE reflux-torticollis to the left (Sutcliffe, 1969; Ramenofsky et al, 1978). Its cause is unknown, but since the wry neck resolves with the correction of reflux it is assumed to be neurologic.

References:
Sutcliffe J: Torsion spasms and abnormal postures in children with hiatus hernia: Sandifer's syndrome. Prog Pediatr Radiol 1969; 2:190–197.
Dunn PM: Congenital sternomastoid torticollis: an intrauterine postural deformity. Arch Dis Child 1974; 49:824–825.
Clark RN: Diagnosis and management of torticollis. Pediatr Ann 1976; 5:43–60.
Ramenofsky ML, et al.: Gastroesophageal reflux and torticollis. J Bone Joint Surg 1978; 60-A:1140–1141.
Clarren SK: Plagiocephaly and torticollis: etiology, natural history, and helmet treatment in 43 patients. J Pediatr 1981; 98:92–95.
Smith DW: Recognizable patterns of human deformities. Philadelphia: W.B. Saunders, 1981. * †
Dunne KB, Clarren SK: The origin of prenatal and postnatal deformities. Pediatr Clin North Am 1986; 33:1277–1297. †
Thompson F, et al.: Familial congenital muscular torticollis: case report and review of the literature. Clin Orthop Rel Res 1986; 202:193–196.

CL006   **Sterling K. Clarren**

TOURETTE SYNDROME 2305

Includes:
> Gilles de la Tourette syndrome
> Tics, multiple motor and vocal

Excludes:
> **Hallervorden-Spatz disease** (2526)
> **Hepatolenticular degeneration** (0469)
> **Huntington disease** (0478)
> Klazomania
> Tardive dyskinesia
> **Torsion dystonia** (0957)

Major Diagnostic Criteria: Tourette syndrome (TS) is clinically diagnosed on the basis of the presence of multiple motor tics (e.g., eye blinks, facial grimaces, head jerks, shoulder shrugs, arm movements, trunk movements) and multiple vocal tics (e.g. throat clearing, sniffing, hissing, coughing, sucking, yelping, ejaculation of inappropriate words or phrases including coprolalia). The onset is usually before age 21 years, and the symptoms must persist for at least one year.

Clinical Findings: Motor tics typically appear well before vocal tics. The motor tics usually show a rostral-caudal progression, so that tics involving the face and head usually precede those involving the trunk or extremeties. Symptoms vary in their complexity, frequency, and degree of social role dysfunction they produce. In most cases this is a lifelong chronic illness, with symptoms waxing and waning over time.

Complications: Coprolalia develops in approximately one-third of the patients. This and other severe symptoms can be socially disabling. Although not life threatening, this illness can markedly limit the individual's choices for a satisfying and productive life.

Associated Findings: Over one-half of the patients seen in a clinic will have attention problems that can interfere with school work. In addition, a large percentage (50–75%) will also develop obsessions and compulsions. In fact, in later life the obsessions and compulsions may be the most troublesome features of the illness.

Etiology: Autosomal dominant inheritance with incomplete penetrance, although a substantial number of patients (10–35%) do not have a positive family history and appear to be isolated cases.

Pathogenesis: Unknown.

MIM No.: *13758

Sex Ratio: Approximately M3:F1.

Occurrence: The incidence has been estimated to be between 1:2,000 and 1:3,000 for males, and between 1:5,000 and 1:10,000 for females, but most investigators believe that this syndrome tends to be underdiagnosed.

Risk of Recurrence for Patient's Sib:
See Part I, *Mendelian Inheritance.* Tourette syndrome, 10%; chronic multiple tics, 20%; obsessive compulsive disorders, 10%.

Risk of Recurrence for Patient's Child:
See Part I, *Mendelian Inheritance.*

Age of Detectability: The age of onset can range from two to 21 years, with mean onset at seven years of age.

Gene Mapping and Linkage: GTS (Gilles de la Tourette syndrome) is unassigned.

Prevention: None known. Genetic counseling indicated.

Treatment: Currently haloperidol is frequently used to control symptoms; a number of other medications, including pimozide, piperidine, clonazepam, and clonidine have also been tried with variable results.

Prognosis: Chronic lifelong illness in most cases.

Detection of Carrier: Unknown.

Special Considerations: This syndrome is particularly difficult to diagnose, since a wide variety of symptoms can usher in the syndrome.

Support Groups:
> NY; Bayside; Tourette Syndrome Association (TSA)
> AUSTRALIA: Victoria; Elsternick; Tourette Syndrome Association of Australia
> CANADA: Ontario; Willowdale; Tourette Syndrome Foundation of Canada
> DENMARK: Lyngby; Tourette Syndrome Association of Denmark
> ENGLAND: Essex; Ilford; Tourette Syndrome Association of Great Britain
> THE NETHERLANDS: Rhood; Tourette Syndrome Association of The Netherlands

References:
Comings DE, Comings BG: Tourette syndrome: clinical and psychological aspects of 250 cases. Am J Hum Genet 1985; 37:435–450.
Pauls DL, Leckman JF: The inheritance of Gilles de la Tourette's syndrome and associated behaviors: evidence for autosomal dominant transmission. New Engl J Med 1986; 315:993–997.
Shapiro AK, et al.: Gilles de la Tourette Syndrome, 2nd ed. New York: Raven Press, 1988.

PA048   **David Pauls**
C0018   **Mary Coleman**

Townes-Brocks syndrome
See ANUS-HAND-EAR SYNDROME
Toxopachyosteose diaphysaire tibio-peroniere
See SKELETAL DYSPLASIA, WEISMANN-NETTER-STUHL TYPE
Toxoplasmosis, infantile
See FETAL TOXOPLASMOSIS SYNDROME

TRACHEA, AGENESIS 2848

Includes:
> Segmental tracheal agenesis
> Tracheal aplasia
> Tracheal atresia

Excludes:
> **Tracheal agenesis-multiple anomaly association** (2849)
> Tracheal stenosis

Major Diagnostic Criteria: Congenital absence of all or part of the trachea.

Clinical Findings: Tracheal agenesis manifests at birth with severe respiratory distress and difficulty with resuscitation. Many cases are born at or near term after uncomplicated pregnancies. Occasionally polyhydramnios or intrauterine growth retardation may lead to fetal assessment and diagnosis of associated anomalies, though the tracheal agenesis is not usually suspected before birth. There may be complete or, less commonly, partial absence of the trachea. Several classifications of tracheal agenesis subtypes have been described. The classification of Floyd et al (1962) documents three main types: *type I*, in which part of the distal trachea is preserved and communicates with the esophagus; *type II*, in which the main stem bronchi are connected below the normal carina by an interbronchial segment communicating by a fistula to the esophagus; and *type III*, in which the main stem bronchi enter the esophagus separately. Rarer forms include those with complete pulmonary agenesis and segmental defects. Type II is the most common form, seen in approximately 60% of cases.

In the more than 50 cases of tracheal agenesis reported to date, the defect has usually been fatal within a few hours, though operations aimed at stabilizing the child and providing a permanent airway have been attempted. The longest survival reported is six weeks.

Complications: This condition has been uniformly fatal.

Associated Findings: Associated anomalies in the respiratory system include **Larynx, atresia** (15%) and **Lung, aberrant lobe** (20%). Over 80% of reported cases have had major anomalies in other systems, especially the cardiovascular (65%), genitourinary (45%), gastrointestinal (30%), and musculoskeletal (30%) systems. Central nervous system and craniofacial anomalies are rarely reported.

Etiology: Unknown.

Pathogenesis: Presumably involves faulty development of the tracheobronchial tree. The laryngotracheal groove develops as a ventral projection of the floor of the foregut caudal to the pharyngeal pouches. The lung buds develop as this outgrowth extends caudally. Along the lateral margins of the outgrowth, the tracheoesophageal grooves form, grow inward, and join in a caudocephalad direction to produce the tracheoesophageal septum. Failure of the cephalic portion of the laryngotracheal groove to form would result in total or partial absence of the trachea, though the bronchi and lungs would remain. Incomplete fusion of the tracheoesophageal folds would allow abnormal persistence of communication between the trachea or bronchi and the esophagus.

Sex Ratio: M1.5:F1 for all reported cases, but M3:F1 for isolated tracheal agenesis.

Occurrence: Over 50 cases have been reported in the world literature, and the defect has been seen in all ethnic groups. A population-based survey in Manitoba indicated an incidence of approximately 1:80,000 live births.

Risk of Recurrence for Patient's Sib: Presumably low. No recurrences have been documented, although detailed family studies have not been undertaken.

Risk of Recurrence for Patient's Child: Defect has been lethal in all cases.

Age of Detectability: At or soon after birth. May go unrecognized as tracheal agenesis if postmortem examination is not carried out.

Gene Mapping and Linkage: Unknown.

Prevention: None known. Genetic counseling indicated.

Treatment: Surgical intervention has been attempted in several patients. Initial therapy has involved utilization of the esophagus as a conduit to the bronchi or insertion of an endobronchial tube. Survival has varied from 23 hours to six weeks. Definitive repair will be complicated by lack of suitable homologous or prosthetic tracheal replacements and is unlikely to be successful until a graft is available that can provide suitable ciliated epithelium, withstand normal pressure changes, and allow for normal growth and development. In most cases survival is jeopardized by the presence of other serious birth defects, especially complex congenital heart anomalies.

Prognosis: With currently available therapy, this condition is lethal.

Detection of Carrier: Unknown.

References:

Floyd J, et al.: Agenesis of the trachea. Am Rev Respir Dis 1962; 86:557–560.
Hopkinson JM: Congenital absence of the trachea. J Pathol 1972; 107:63–66. †
Buchino JJ, et al.: Tracheal agenesis: a clinical approach. J Pediatr Surg 1982; 17:132–137.
Evans JA, et al.: Tracheal agenesis and associated malformations: a comparison with tracheoesophageal fistula and the VACTERL association. Am J Med Genet 1985; 21:21–34.*

EV001   **Jane A. Evans**

Tracheal agenesis association
See TRACHEAL AGENESIS-MULTIPLE ANOMALY ASSOCIATION

TRACHEAL AGENESIS-MULTIPLE ANOMALY ASSOCIATION   2849

Includes:
Tracheal agenesis association
Tracheal-renal-alimentary-cardiovascular-limb association

Excludes:
Trachea, agenesis (2848)
Vater association (0987)

Major Diagnostic Criteria: Presence of tracheal agenesis should alert the physician to the possibility of associated anomalies, especially in the cardiovascular, genitourinary, gastrointestinal, and musculoskeletal systems. Although not recognized as a specific syndrome, a child with tracheal agenesis and a major anomaly in one or more of these additional systems may be an example of a specific tracheal-renal-alimentary-cardiovascular-limb association.

Clinical Findings: Over 80% of reported cases of tracheal agenesis have additional major anomalies. The most common of these are **Lung, aberrant lobe** (26%), imperforate anus (see **Anorectal malformations**) (21%), **Ventricular septal defect** (33%), **Atrial septal defects** (21%), single umbilical artery (29%), and single kidney (21%). **Larynx, atresia**, duodenal atresia (see **Duodenum, atresia or stenosis**), pancreatic anomalies, cystic dysplastic kidney, aberrant internal genitalia, and radial ray defects are also relatively common (10–20%).

This association has obvious similarities to **Vater association**, but differs in the nature and frequency of anomalies. In particular, defects of the axial skeleton and external genital anomalies are relatively rare (<10%) in the tracheal agenesis association, and the heart defects tend to be more complex (e.g., **Heart, truncus arteriosus, Heart, transposition of great vessels**, hypoplastic left heart).

Patients with the tracheal-renal-alimentary-cardiovascular-limb association rarely have defects in other systems. However, tracheal agenesis has also been seen in one patient with sirenomelia (see **Sirenomelia sequence**), and infants with total absence of the pulmonary system have had other major anomalies, including neural tube defects, urethral atresia, and hemimelia.

Children with tracheal agenesis and other major anomalies are frequently premature (50% are less than 37 weeks gestation), and approximately 20% show intrauterine growth retardation. Polyhydramnios has been noted in some cases with associated duodenal atresia. In many, however, multiple anomalies are not suspected until birth, when the tracheal agenesis causes severe respiratory distress and difficulty with resuscitation. All cases have been fatal within a few hours or days, although surgical intervention has allowed survival to a maximum of six weeks.

Complications: Death at or shortly after birth.

Associated Findings: None known.

Etiology: Unknown.

Pathogenesis: Unknown. Several potential mechanisms could explain the pattern of anomalies observed in some of the patients. For example, some cases with aberrant lung lobation, congenital heart defects and spleen anomalies may represent defects of laterality similar to the asplenia/polysplenia spectrum. Review of patients with bilateral right or left sidedness has shown an increased incidence of defects, such as tracheoesophageal anomalies, gastric hypoplasia, agenesis of the gallbladder, annular pancreas, duodenal stenosis, imperforate anus, **Kidney, horseshoe**, and hydroureter, that are also seen in the tracheal agenesis association.

At least two cases of tracheal agenesis with associated anomalies have been seen in one of monozygous twins; the co-twins were normal. It is possible in these cases that the multiple anomalies have a basis in vascular interchange between twins.

A third mechanism may, as with **Vater association**, involve disorganization and faulty migration of cells from the primitive streak, though this hypothesis is purely speculative at this time. The tracheal agenesis association probably represents a polytopic field defect.

POS No.: 3405

Sex Ratio: Approximately M1.2:F1.

Occurrence: Over 40 cases of tracheal agenesis with other major defects have been reported. About 20 of these involve children with tracheal agenesis and two or more other anomalies seen in the more restricted tracheal-renal-alimentary-cardiovascular-limb association. Incidence is approximately 1:100,000.

Risk of Recurrence for Patient's Sib: Probably low, although detailed family studies have not been carried out. The published reports of tracheal agenesis patients document two cases of **Anencephaly** and one of **Ventricular septal defect** among 43 sibs, suggesting a possible susceptibility to midline defects in these families.

Risk of Recurrence for Patient's Child: No affected individuals have survived to reproduce.

Age of Detectability: At birth, when obvious external anomalies such as radial ray defects and imperforate anus may also be noted. The precise nature of the tracheal anomaly and other internal defects may only become apparent at postmortem examination.

Gene Mapping and Linkage: Unknown.

Prevention: None known. Genetic counseling indicated.

Treatment: Attempts have been made to treat the tracheal agenesis surgically, but survival beyond age six weeks has not been achieved. Long-term survival is unlikely until suitable tracheal replacements are available, and will in many cases be complicated by congenital heart defects and other associated anomalies.

Prognosis: All patients have died by age six weeks.

Detection of Carrier: Careful histories documenting relatives with other midline defects may help to indicate families at increased risk.

References:
Fonkalsrud EW, et al.: Surgical treatment of tracheal agenesis. J Thorac Cardiovasc Surg 1963; 45:520–525.
McNie DJM, Pryse-Davies J: Tracheal agenesis. Arch Dis Child 1970; 45:143–144.
Hopkinson JM: Congenital absence of the trachea. J Pathol 1972; 107:63–66. †
Evans JA, et al.: Tracheal agenesis and associated malformations: a comparison with tracheoesophageal fistula and the VACTERL association. Am J Med Genet 1985; 21:21–34. *

EV001   **Jane A. Evans**

Tracheal aplasia
See TRACHEA, AGENESIS
Tracheal atresia
See TRACHEA, AGENESIS
Tracheal lobe
See LUNG, ABERRANT LOBE
Tracheal-renal-alimentary-cardiovascular-limb association
See TRACHEAL AGENESIS-MULTIPLE ANOMALY ASSOCIATION
Tracheo-laryngo-esophageal cleft
See LARYNGO-TRACHEO-ESOPHAGEAL CLEFT

TRACHEOESOPHAGEAL FISTULA   0960

Includes:
Cervical tracheoesophageal fistula, congenital isolated H-type
Esophageal atresia-tracheoesophageal fistula
Thoracic tracheoesophageal fistula, congenital isolated H-type
Thoracic tracheoesophageal fistula-esophageal atresia

Excludes:
Bronchopulmonary foregut malformations-esophageal communication
Intralobar sequestration-esophageal communications
Tracheoesophageal fistula acquired due to caustic ingestion
Tracheoesophageal fistula acquired due to surgery
Tracheoesophageal fistula acquired due to trauma

Major Diagnostic Criteria: Repeated bouts of pneumonia and gastric dilation suggest a tracheoesophageal fistula. Contrast material swallowed with careful positioning under fluoroscopic control may demonstrate the fistula. Tamponading of the distal esophagus by balloon catheter may force the contrast material (barium or metriziamide) through the fistula. Esophagobronchoscopy with installation of methylene blue into the endotracheal tube under anesthesia is necessary if contrast studies do not demonstrate the fistula.

Clinical Findings: Repeated episodes of aspiration syndrome or pneumonia and choking or coughing when feeding are almost always present. Liquids cause greater difficulty than solids. The repeated episodes of bronchopneumonia beginning early in life are diffuse, patch-like infiltrates. Marked abdominal distention occurs following crying and coughing. The distention is due to air escaping through the fistula into the GI tract.

Complications: Aspiration and suffocation. Repeated episodes of pneumonitis and sepsis. Failure to thrive. Chronic pulmonary insufficiency and disability.

Associated Findings: None known.

Etiology: Van Staey et al (1984), after studying 33 pedigrees, concluded that "with the exception of [cases attributable to] chromosomal or of a known monogenic or teratogenic syndrome, the recurrence risk fit into a multifactorial scheme."

Pathogenesis: Failure of closure of laryngotracheal groove. Continued passage of saliva or food from the esophagus through the fistula into the bronchus causes chemical pneumonitis with subsequent sepsis, death, or chronic pulmonary insufficiency.

MIM No.: 18996

CDC No.: 750.3

Sex Ratio: M1:F1

Occurrence: 1:75,000 to 1:100,000 live births.

Risk of Recurrence for Patient's Sib: Unknown.

Risk of Recurrence for Patient's Child: Unknown.

Age of Detectability: Newborn through early infancy. The diagnosis is usually established by one year of age.

Gene Mapping and Linkage: Unknown.

Prevention: None known. Genetic counseling indicated.

Treatment: In patients with a cervical esophageal fistula, which occurs in about two-thirds of the cases, suture ligation and division of the fistula can be performed in the cervical region through a neck exploration under general anesthesia. A right thoracotomy is performed for thoracic fistulas with suture ligation and division of the fistula.

Prognosis: Excellent, if the diagnosis is made before chronic lung disease or disability occurs.

Detection of Carrier: Unknown.

References:
Ravitch M, et al.: Pediatric surgery, ed 3. Chicago: Yearbook Medical, 1979.
Van Staey M, et al.: Familial congenital esophageal atresia: personal case report and a review of the literature. Hum Genet 1984; 66:260–266.
Welch K, et al.: Pediatric surgery, ed 4. Chicago: Yearbook Medical, 1986.

BE049   **Arthur S. Besser**

Tracheoesophageal fistula with or without esophageal atresia
See ESOPHAGUS, ATRESIA AND TRACHEOESOPHAGEAL FISTULA

TRACHEOMALACIA   2505

Includes: Tracheomalacia, secondary

Excludes:
    Bronchomalacia (2995)
    Chondromalacia, congenital
    Larsen syndrome, lethal type (2800)
    Polychondritis

Major Diagnostic Criteria: Bronchoscopy is essential for definitive diagnosis. Bronchoscopic findings include weak cartilaginous support of the trachea with anterior-posterior expiratory collapse, anterior-posterior inspiratory collapse with exertion, and a widened posterior membranous wall. When it is associated with tracheoesophageal fistula, the tracheal cartilages have an indented half-circle shape, and the posterior membranous wall is widened.

Clinical Findings: Clinical features vary from mild to severe depending on the location, length, and degree of airway collapse. Features include inspiratory and/or expiratory stridor, wheezing, cough (sometimes barking), hyperextension of the neck, recurrent respiratory infections, difficulty clearing endobronchial secretions, sometimes reflex apnea, respiratory distress, croup, and cyanosis.

Patients with tracheoesophageal fistula have a 30% incidence of secondary tracheomalacia. In mild cases, symptoms begin about age 5–6 months. Moderate cases develop during the first 2–6 months. In severe cases, symptoms of stridor at rest, and occasionally cardiac arrest, develop during the first two months of life.

Primary tracheomalacia in premature infants is noted after extubation. In mature, normal infants, severe symptoms may develop in the first few weeks of life.

Complications: Reflex apnea, respiratory arrest, cardiac arrest, and recurrent pneumonia.

Associated Findings: Primary tracheomalacia is seen in premature infants, otherwise normal infants, and in association with **Chondrodysplasia**.

Secondary tracheomalacia is associated with **Tracheoesophageal fistula**, innominate artery "compression", vascular ring, and congenital cyst or tumor.

Etiology: Endoscopic evaluations suggest congenital disease for primary tracheomalacia. The cartilage to muscle ratio of 2:1 is grossly abnormal (the normal ratio is 4.5 to 1). See also **Tracheoesophageal fistula**.

Pathogenesis: Unknown. When associated with innominate artery compression, it is not known if the artery is in an abnormal location producing localized tracheomalacia, or if normally positioned artery compresses a soft trachea.

CDC No.: 748.320

Sex Ratio: Undetermined but presumably M1:F1.

Occurrence: Undetermined but presumed rare.

Risk of Recurrence for Patient's Sib: Unknown.

Risk of Recurrence for Patient's Child: Unknown.

Age of Detectability: During the first few weeks or months of life.

Gene Mapping and Linkage: Unknown.

Prevention: None known. Genetic counseling indicated.

Treatment: For severe innominate artery compression, suspension of artery from posterior sternum, or reimplantation.

Prognosis: Excellent for mild to moderate cases. Fair to good for severe cases.

Detection of Carrier: Unknown.

References:
Baxter JD, Dunbar JS: Tracheomalacia. Ann Otol Rhinol Laryngol 1963; 72:1013–1023.
Cogbill TH, et al.: Primary tracheomalacia. Ann Thorac Surg 1983; 35:538–541.

Benjamin B: Tracheomalacia in infants and children. Ann Otol Rhinol Laryngol 1984; 93:438–442.

HU015   **Richard Hubbell**
MY003   **Charles M. Myer III**

Tracheomalacia, secondary
   See TRACHEOMALACIA
Tragus, of ear, absent
   See EAR, ABSENT TRAGUS
Tranebjaerg mental retardation
   See X-LINKED MENTAL RETARDATION-PSORIASIS
Tranquilizer, fetal effects (some)
   See FETAL BENZODIAZEPINE EFFECTS

TRANSCOBALAMIN II DEFICIENCY   2624

Includes:
    Transcobalamin II, hereditary abnormal (TC2)
    Vitamin B(12) binding protein defects

Excludes:
    Anemia, pernicious congenital (2656)
    Vitamin B(12) malabsorption (0992)

Major Diagnostic Criteria: Failure to thrive; irritability; beefy red, smooth tongue; macrocytic anemia; occasionally pancytopenia. Immunologic alteration may predispose to infection. Serum B_{12} levels are typically normal, but have been reported to be low. Diagnosis is established by demonstrating absent transcobalamin II by immunologic means or by demonstrating nonfunctional transcobalamin II (TC II) in binding or delivery assays.

Clinical Findings: Children have presented with clinical signs from several weeks to several months of age. Part of the variability in the age of presentation has resulted from variable use of oral vitamin supplements. Either folate or vitamin B_{12} orally can delay manifestations of the disease.

Children present with symptoms and signs as a result of either anemia or infection. Pallor, weakness, and irritability are common. Diarrhea, pneumonia, and failure to thrive have been reported. Laboratory evaluation reveals megaloblastic anemia: red cells are macrocytic, and neutrophils are hypersegmented. Bone marrow aspiration typically shows severe megaloblastic changes in both the erythroid and myeloid series. Two patients have been reported with erythroid hypoplasia or aplasia. The marrow picture can be confused with leukemia or myelodysplastic syndrome (preleukemia).

Complications: Administration of folate may improve the anemia associated with TC II deficiency, but will exacerbate neurologic impairment. Two patients so treated developed severe neurologic impairment, one with associated mental retardation.

Associated Findings: Immunodeficiency has been reported in two patients. One exhibited agammaglobulinemia and inability to make antibody to specific antigenic challenge. The second presented with *Pneumocystis carinii* pneumonia and exhibited failure to produce antibody to specific antigenic stimuli. In both cases, therapeutic doses of cobalamin led to complete restoration of immune function.

Etiology: Autosomal recessive inheritance. More commonly, children inherit an allele from each parent, which results in production of no immunologically or functionally detectable TC II. One patient inherited one silent allele and one allele that coded for a protein that was immunologically reactive as TC II but that could not function in vitamin B_{12} transport.

Pathogenesis: Lack of functional TC II results in severe impairment in availability of vitamin B_{12} metabolites to cells.

MIM No.: *27535

Sex Ratio: M1:F1 (six girls and four boys have been described).

Occurrence: Ten cases have been documented in the literature.

Risk of Recurrence for Patient's Sib:
   See Part I, *Mendelian Inheritance*.

Risk of Recurrence for Patient's Child:
See Part I, *Mendelian Inheritance.*

Age of Detectability: Cord blood can be used to assay for TC II.

Gene Mapping and Linkage: TCN2 (transcobalamin II; macrocytic anemia) has been mapped to 22q.

Prevention: None known. Genetic counseling indicated.

Treatment: Pharmacologic doses of cyanocobalamin or hydroxycobalamin completely correct the defect. Cobalamin circulates in plasma either free or bound to albumin and reaches tissues in adequate levels. Lifetime treatment is required. Most patients have been treated with intramuscular cobalamins. A single patient has been maintained exclusively on oral hydroxycobalamin but there are theoretical concerns about this approach. Treated patients grow and develop normally.

Prognosis: With prompt diagnosis and treatment, life span is normal. Delayed diagnosis or inadvertant administration of folate may result in neurologic impairment or mental retardation.

Detection of Carrier: Heterozygotes will have 50% of the immunologic or functional TC II detectable in normal individuals.

References:
Hakami N, et al.: Neonatal megaloblastic anemia due to inherited transcobalamin II deficiency in two siblings. New Engl J Med 1971; 285:1163–1170. *
Hitzig WH: Hereditary transcobalamin-II deficiency: clinical findings in a new family. J Pediatr 1974; 85:622–628.
Seligman PA, et al.: Studies of a patient with megaloblastic anemia and an abnormal transcobalamin II. New Engl J Med 1980; 303:1209–1212.
Hall CA: Congenital disorders of vitamin B12 transport and their contributions to concepts. Yale J Biol Med 1981; 54:485–495.
Meyers PA, Carmel R: Hereditary transcobalamin II deficiency with subnormal serum cobalamin levels. Pediatrics 1984; 74:866–871.
Rosenblatt DS, et al.: Expression of transcobalamin II by amniocytes. Prenatal Diag 1987; 7:35–39.

ME040 **Paul Meyers**

TRANSPORT, RENAL, DEFECTS OF 1501

Includes: Renal transport defects

The human body is composed of organs and systems. They, in turn, contain cells that have subcellular compartments. Membranes delineate these different spaces. Chemical composition differs in each membrane-defined compartment. Control of the molecular traffic across membranes is one mechanism by which specific composition of particular compartments is achieved.

Disorders of transfer across plasma membranes are more common, but there are confirmed Mendelian disorders affecting transport across *intra*cellular membranes. **Cystinosis, Salla Disease,** and a form of Vitamin B12-dependent methylmalonic aciduria each have impaired lysosomal efflux; of cystine (the disulfide), sialic acid, and free cobalamin (cblF complementation group) respec-

tively. **Glycogenosis, Type Ib** is a disorder of glucose-6-phosphate transfer across endoplasmic reticulum.

Transmembrane transport of molecules is accomplished by several processes that achieve and maintain the distributions of freely soluble substances on opposite sides of membranes. Diffusion does not do this; gated channels, ion gradient or voltage-coupled carriers, and receptor-mediated endocytotic processes can. The ability of mediated processes to recognize specific ions, substrates, and ligands is a function of their macromolecular component(s). Their specificity is determined by the genes that encode the polypeptide component of the transporter or channel. It follows that mutations at loci coding for structural components of transport systems may modify the associated functions (inborn errors of transport).

As a general principle, mutations affecting brush-border membrane systems are not expressed in parenchymal cells. On the other hand, basolateral membrane transporters in epithelial cells and plasma membrane transporters of parenchymal cells serve homologous functions (fluxes between extracellular and intracellular fluids), and one might expect a mutation affecting a carrier in the basolateral membrane to be expressed also in parenchymal cells (and vice versa). The defect in efflux on the cationic amino acid carrier in lysinuric-protein intolerance is an example: the mutant phenotype is expressed in basolateral membranes of kidney and small intestine and the plasma membrane of skin fibroblasts.

A major stimulus for the recognition of "inborn errors of transport" was awareness first of renal glucosuria and then of various renal hyperaminoacidurias. Many renal transport disorders have counterparts in intestinal absorption. Refinements in the classification of renal transport systems lead to a topologic view of transport systems in the nephron. Systems in brush-border and basolateral membranes have different roles to play and different specificities for substrates. Systems in convoluted and straight segments of proximal nephron are likely to have different properties, even when they transport the same substrate or group of substrates (see Table 1501–1). The relative importance of the transport system in the maintenance of metabolic homeostasis determines the extent of the phenotypic effect of the mutation affecting it.

A partial classification of mendelian disorders of membrane transport is given in Tables 1501–1 and 1501–2. Most of the phenotypes listed are disorders of carriers and channels for low-molecular weight organic substrates and ions.

References:
Scriver CR, et al, eds: The metabolic basis of inherited disease, 6th ed. New York: McGraw-Hill, 1989:

SC050 **Charles R. Scriver**

Table 1501-1 Mendelian Disorders of Amino Acid Transport

| Name | Amino Acid Affected | Kidney Site (Putative)[a] | | Other organs | Inheritance |
		Segment[b]	Membrane[c]		
Classical **Cystinuria**	Cystine, Lysine Ornithine, Arginine	PS	BBM	Intestine (some pedigrees)	AR (incompletely reces- sive for some alleles)
Isolated **Cystinuria**	Cyst(e)ine	PC	BBM		AR
Hyperdibasic aminoaciduria-1	Lysine, Ornithine, Argi- nine	PC	BBM	Intestine	AD
Hyperdibasic aminoaciduria-2	Lysine, Ornithine, Argi- nine	PC/PS	BLM	Fibroblast Intestine Liver(?)	AR
Hyperlysinuria, isolated	Lysine	PS(?)	BBM(?)	Intestine	AR
Hartnup disorder	Neutrals (excluding imi- noacids & glycine)	PC	BBM	Intestine	AR
Familial **Iminoglycinuria**	Proline, Hydroxyproline, Glycine	PC(?)	BBM(?)	Intestine	AR (incompletely reces- sive for some alleles)
Isolated **Histidinuria**	Histidine	PS(?)	BBM(?)	Intestine (some pedigrees)	AR
Aciduria, dicarboxylic aminoacid- uria	Glutamic & aspartic acids	PC	BBM		AR
Methionine malabsorption	Methionine			Intestine	AR(?)
Tryptophan malabsorption	Tryptophan			Intestine	AR(?)
Cystinosis	Cystine (disulphide)			Lysosome (efflux)	AR
Fanconi Syndrome(s) Primary & Secondary forms[d]	Amino acids (all), other organic substrates and electrolytes	PC,PS(?) BBM, BLM?			AR (many loci)

[a]Site refers to proximal nephron segment (convoluted or straight) and membrane (brush-border or basolateral). In no case has there been confirmation by direct measurement of site affected.
[b]PC, proximal convoluted segment; PS, proximal straight segment.
[c]BBM, brush-border membrane; BLM, basolateral membrane.
[d]Fanconi syndromes (secondary Mendelian forms) include **Cystinosis, Fructose-1-phosphate aldolase deficiency, Galactosemia, Tyrosinemia, Hepatolenticular degeneration, Oculo-cerebro-renal syndrome,** and **Rickets, Vitamin D-dependent, type I.**

Table 1501-2 Other Mendelian Disorders of Membrane Transport

Name	Substrate Affected	Tissue Affected	Inheritance
Renal **glycosuria**	Glucose	Kidney (PC?[a])	AR (multiple alleles)
Glucose-galactose malabsorption	Glucose, galactose	Kidney (PS?) Intestine	AR
Salla disease	Sialic acid	Lysosome (efflux)	AR
Glycogenosis, Type I	Glucose-6-P	Endoplasmic reticulum (?)	AR
Renal hypouricemia	Uric acid	Kidney (Proximal & distal tubule sites)	AR (multiple loci?, alleles)
Hypophosphatemia, X-linked	Phosphate	i. Kidney, (bone?) ii. Kidney, inner ear, (bone?)	XL Dominant (2 loci)[b]
Hypophosphatemia, non X-linked	Phosphate	Kidney	AD (and AR) (alleles?)
Bartter Syndrome	Chloride (primary) Potassium (sec- ondary)	Kidney (Henle loop, thick ascending limb?)	AR
Hypomagnesemia, primary	Mg^{2+}	Kidney, intestine	AR & XLD forms
Renal tubular acidosis	H$^+$	Kidney (distal tubule)	AD
Renal bicarbonate reabsorptive defect	HCO$_3^-$	Kidney (Proximal tubule)	XLD AR (forms) (various loci? & alleles?)
Thyroid, iodide transport defect	I$^-$	Thyroid, salivary glands	AR
Diarrhea, congenital chloride	Cl$^-$	Intestine	AR
Diabetes insipidus, vasopressin resistant	H$_2$O	Kidney (collecting duct)	XLR
Hypercholesteremia	LDL-Cholesterol	Parenchymal cells (Plasma membrane receptor)	AD
Vitamin B(12) malabsorption	Vitamin B$_{12}$	Intestine	AR
Vitamin B(12) lysosomal transport defect	Free B$_{12}$	Lysosome (efflux)	AR
Folate malabsorption	Folic acid	Intestine, (other tissues?)	AR
Myopathy-metabolic, carnitine deficiency	Carnitine	Kidney (other tissues?)	AR

[a]PC, PS: See Table 1501-1
[b]Corresponding loci in mouse are *Hyp* and *Gy*.

Tranxene^, fetal effects
  See FETAL BENZODIAZEPINE EFFECTS
Trapezoidocephaly-synostosis syndrome
  See ANTLEY-BIXLER SYNDROME
Treacher Collins syndrome
  See MANDIBULOFACIAL DYSOSTOSIS
Treacher Collins-Franceschetti syndrome
  See MANDIBULOFACIAL DYSOSTOSIS
Treacher Collins mandibulofacial dysostosis, recessive type
  See MANDIBULOFACIAL DYSOSTOSIS, TREACHER-COLLINS TYPE, RECESSIVE
Tremor, benign essential
  See TREMOR, HEREDOFAMILIAL

TREMOR, HEREDOFAMILIAL 0964

Includes: Tremor, benign essential

Excludes:
  Hepatolenticular degeneration (0469)
  Huntington disease (0478)
  Multiple sclerosis, familial (2598)
  Parkinson disease
  Tremor-duodenal ulcer syndrome (0963)

Major Diagnostic Criteria: A symmetric familial tremor is present in an otherwise healthy individual in whom medical and neurologic causes of the tremor have been excluded.

Clinical Findings: The tremor is most commonly noted between the ages of 40 and 50 years. Although rarely documented at the age extremes, essential tremor may begin in the neonate and the elderly. The tremor begins in the hands and arms in a symmetric fashion. It then may involve the facial muscles and tongue. When the tremor involves the head and neck, it has been termed "senile" tremor. If severe, dysarthria may result. The trunk and legs are least commonly involved. The tremor is more pronounced during movement and maintenance of postures against gravity, diminishes at rest and disappears during sleep. Fatigue and emotion may enhance the tremor, and alcohol may relieve it. The tremor is of variable amplitude; the frequency is 3–12 per second. The tremor may be progressive or remain unchanged throughout life. Remissions are rare. There are no associated neurologic signs in the majority of patients.

Complications: Approximately 20% eventually develop rigidity of varying degrees.

Associated Findings: None known.

Etiology: Autosomal dominant inheritance with complete penetrance by the age of 70.

Pathogenesis: Many theories have been advanced: 1) autosomal dominant tremor is a monosymptomatic form of Parkinson disease. Larsson and Sjögren's large study (1960) did not support this view; 2) Minor (1936) suggested the tremor was a triad which included fecundity and longevity. 3) More recent experimental studies have suggested an abnormality of monoamines in the rubro-olivo-cerebello-rubral tracts. No consistent neuropathology has been described.

MIM No.: *19030

Sex Ratio: M1:F1

Occurrence: In Sweden, it has been estimated that the gene frequency is 1:10,000. In the parish of Xa-sjö, the gene frequency approaches 1:22.

Risk of Recurrence for Patient's Sib:
  See Part I, *Mendelian Inheritance.*

Risk of Recurrence for Patient's Child:
  See Part I, *Mendelian Inheritance.*

Age of Detectability: Tremor is usually evident by the fifth decade of life.

Gene Mapping and Linkage: Unknown.

Prevention: None known. Genetic counseling indicated.

Treatment: If tremor is severe, appropriate job placement may be helpful. Most patients with autosomal dominant tremor do not seek medical advice. Many patients report that the tremor is mitigated by ethanol. Propanolol, a β-adrenergic blocking agent, and primidone may be effective. The primidone effect is felt to be from a metabolite, phenylethylmalonamide.

Prognosis: Good for life span. Function affected by degree of tremor and rigidity.

Detection of Carrier: Unknown.

References:
Minor L: Heredo-familiare nervenkrankheiten ohne anatomischen befundi: das erbliche zittern. In: Bumke O, Foerster O, eds: handbuch der neurologie. Berlin: Springer, 1936; 16:974–1005.
Critchley M: Observations on essential heredofamilial tremor. Brain 1949; 72:113–139.
Larsson M, Sjögren H: Essential tremor: a clinical and genetic population study. Acta Psychiatry Scand 1960; 144 (Suppl 36):1–176.
Marshall J: Observations on essential tremor. J Neurol Neurosurg Psychiatry 1962; 25:112–125.
Vanasse M, et al.: Shuddering attacks in children: an early clinical manifestation of essential tremor. Neurology 1976; 26:1027–1030.
O'Brien MD, et al.: Benign familial tremor treated with primidone. Br Med J 1981; 282:178–180.

HA053   **Robert H.A. Haslam**
MC035   **Ross McLeod**

TREMOR-DUODENAL ULCER SYNDROME 0963

Includes:
  Duodenal ulcer-tremor syndrome
  Tremor-nystagmus-duodenal ulcer

Excludes:
  Narcolepsy (3287)
  Tremor of head-nystagmus
  Tremor, heredofamilial (0964)
  Tremor of limbs-nystagmus
  Tremor of other etiology

Major Diagnostic Criteria: Slowly progressive "essential" tremor, "congenital" nystagmus, and duodenal ulceration.

Clinical Findings: Nystagmus is present from birth or is noted in childhood (4–8 years). Rotary nystagmus occurs at rest, intensified by lateral gaze, and accompanied by refractive errors. Slowly progressive tremor starts in childhood, but more often after puberty, involving fingers, hands, shoulders, and head; it is increased with fatigue or emotional upset, but temporarily alleviated by alcohol. Signs of cerebellar dysfunction may be present, i.e., slight ataxia, unsteadiness, incoordination, and clumsiness. Symptoms and signs of duodenal ulceration usually appear later in life but may precede the neurologic syndrome. Unusual need for sleep, with a narcolepsy-like propensity for falling asleep, is noted in some patients.

Complications: Complaints and bleeding from duodenal ulceration. Physical handicap from increasing tremor and from cerebellar dysfunction. Social and mental deterioration because of alcoholism and physical disability have been reported.

Associated Findings: None known.

Etiology: Autosomal dominant inheritance with fairly uniform expressivity. In a few patients, partial manifestations were noted.

Pathogenesis: The presence of cerebellar signs in severely affected persons may point to a possible pathogenetic relationship to the genetic cerebellar atrophies. The combination of neurologic dysfunction, duodenal ulceration, and narcolepsy is explained by some disturbance of the autonomic nervous system.

MIM No.: *19031

POS No.: 4166

Sex Ratio: M2:F1 (observed in the family reported)

Occurrence: The syndrome was reported in a family of Swedish-Finnish descent.

Risk of Recurrence for Patient's Sib:
  See Part I, *Mendelian Inheritance.*

Risk of Recurrence for Patient's Child:
See Part I, *Mendelian Inheritance.*

Age of Detectability: In childhood or adolescence.

Gene Mapping and Linkage: Unknown.

Prevention: None known. Genetic counseling indicated.

Treatment: Dietary treatment and surgery for duodenal ulceration; prevention of alcoholism; physiotherapy.

Prognosis: Life expectancy usually is normal; the neurologic syndrome is slowly progressive. Some patients are incapacitated early in life by tremor and ataxia.

Detection of Carrier: Possibly by clinical examination of first degree relatives.

References:

Neuhäuser G, et al.: Essential tremor, nystagmus and duodenal ulceration. a "new" dominantly inherited condition. Clin Genet 1976; 9:81–91.

Rotter JL, Rimoin DL: The genetic syndromology of peptic ulcer. Am J Med Genet 1981; 10:315–321.

NE012   **Gerhard Neuhäuser**

Tremor-nystagmus-duodenal ulcer
See TREMOR-DUODENAL ULCER SYNDROME
Trevor disease
See DYSPLASIA EPIPHYSEALIS HEMIMELICA
Triazolam, fetal effects
See FETAL BENZODIAZEPINE EFFECTS
Trichloroethylene induced scleroderma
See SCLERODERMA, FAMILIAL PROGRESSIVE

TRICHO-DENTO-OSSEOUS SYNDROME   0965

Includes:
Bone-hair-nail-tooth dysplasia
Enamel hypoplasia-taurodontism-tight hair-cortical
    sclerosteosis
Hair-bone-nail-tooth dysplasia
Nail-hair-bone-tooth dysplasia
Tooth-hair-bone-nail dysplasia

Excludes:
Amelo-onycho-hypohidrotic syndrome (0045)
CHANDS (3039)
Tricho-dermodysplasia-dental defects (2903)
Tricho-odonto-onychial dysplasia (2889)

Major Diagnostic Criteria: Enamel dysplasia, taurodontism (see **Teeth, taurodontism**), excessively curly hair in infancy, and excessively radiodense bones.

Clinical Findings: The enamel of both primary and secondary teeth is thin, soft, and yellowish brown in color. The molars are taurodont in form. Tooth eruption may be delayed or some teeth may be congenitally missing. The teeth have large pulp chambers and often become abscessed within the first years of life.

The hair in infancy is curly but not woolly, and the lashes and eyebrows are long. In some cases the hair tends to straighten with age. The nails are thin and show splitting of the superficial layers; sometimes only a few toenails show the defect.

Multiple fractures due to sclerosis of cortical bone occurs in about 30% of cases. The base of the skull, mastoids, and zones of provisional calcification in the long bones are the areas most commonly involved.

Complications: Attrition of teeth, with exposure of pulps and abscess formation and premature loss of teeth.

Associated Findings: Mandibular prognathism and a shallow nasal bridge is found in some families.

Etiology: Autosomal dominant inheritance. Three variants have been documented.

Pathogenesis: A defect in ectodermal cells involving the morpho-differentiation of tooth, hair, and nail form and structure.

MIM No.: *19032

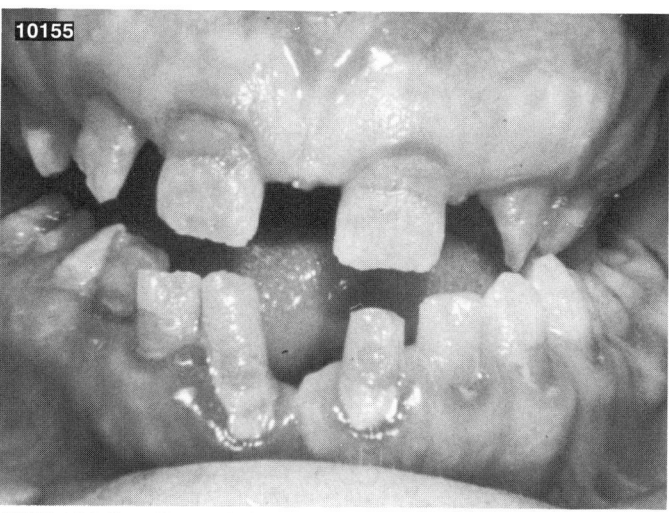

0965-10155:   Enamel dysplasia.

POS No.: 3414

Sex Ratio: M1:F1

Occurrence: About a dozen kindreds reported; some possibly of Irish extraction.

Risk of Recurrence for Patient's Sib:
See Part I, *Mendelian Inheritance.*

Risk of Recurrence for Patient's Child:
See Part I, *Mendelian Inheritance.*

Age of Detectability: At six months to one year of age, at tooth eruption.

Gene Mapping and Linkage: Unknown.

Prevention: None known. Genetic counseling indicated.

Treatment: Early restoration of teeth, and prosthetic replacement of lost or congenitally missing teeth.

Prognosis: Does not affect life span. Premature loss of teeth in untreated case.

Detection of Carrier: Mildly affected individuals may be found by clinical examination.

Special Considerations: The features that differentiate the three types of tricho-dento-osseous (TDO) syndrome are that the long bones are predominantly involved in TDO-I, the cranial bones are predominantly involved in TDO-III, while both are involved in TDO-II. Furthermore, the hair is woolly and easily detachable in TDO-II.

References:

Robinson GC, et al.: Hereditary enamel hypoplasia: its association with characteristic hair structure. Pediatrics 1966; 37:498–502.

Lichtenstein J, et al.: The tricho-dento-osseous (TDO) syndrome. Am J Hum Genet 1972; 24:569–582. * †

Jorgenson RJ, Warson RW: Dental anomalies in the trich-dento-osseous syndrome. Oral Surg 1973; 36:693–700. †

Quattromani F, et al.: Clinical heterogeneity in the tricho-dento-osseous syndrome. Hum Genet 1983; 64:116–121.

Shapiro SD, et al.: Tricho-dento-osseous syndrome: heterogeneity or clinical variability. Am J Med Genet 1983; 16:225–236. *

J0027   **Ronald J. Jorgenson**
                                         Hermine M. Pashayan

TRICHO-DERMODYSPLASIA-DENTAL DEFECTS 2903

Includes:
Dental defects-trichodermodysplasia
Ectodermal dysplasia, tricho-dermodysplasia-dental defects
Trichodermodysplasia-dental alterations

Excludes:
Dermo-odontodysplasia (2763)
Ectodermal dysplasia (anhidrotic types)
Ectodermal dysplasia, hidrotic (0334)
Odonto-onychodermal dysplasia (2618)

Major Diagnostic Criteria: Trichodysplasia, dental anomalies, and skin alterations.

Clinical Findings: Fine, dry, slow-growing, brittle, and lusterless hair; generalized hypotrichosis; delayed eruption of deciduous teeth; hypodontia of both dentitions; small and peg-shaped upper central incisors; recurrent epistaxis; palmoplantar keratosis; facial wens; café-au-lait spots on the back; and bilateral inward (tibial) deflection of the fourth toes.

Complications: Unknown.

Associated Findings: Dystrophic toenails; partial absence of the alveolar wall of the mandible (one patient); and retroverted uterus (one patient).

Etiology: Autosomal dominant or possibly X-linked dominant inheritance. A mother and her only two children (one girl and one boy) were described.

Pathogenesis: Defective formation of several derivatives of the embryonic ectoderm suggests that this condition must be classified as an ectodermal dysplasia.

POS No.: 4226

Sex Ratio: Presumably M1:F1; M1:F2 observed.

Occurrence: Three members of one Brazilian family have been documented.

Risk of Recurrence for Patient's Sib:
See Part I, *Mendelian Inheritance.*

Risk of Recurrence for Patient's Child:
See Part I, *Mendelian Inheritance.*

Age of Detectability: During childhood, by physical examination.

Gene Mapping and Linkage: Unknown.

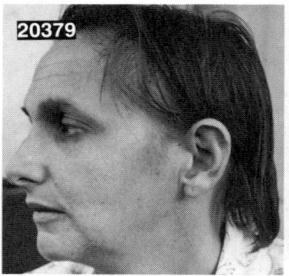
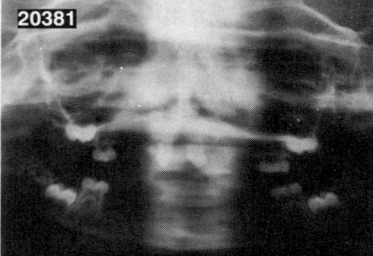
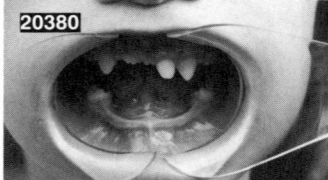
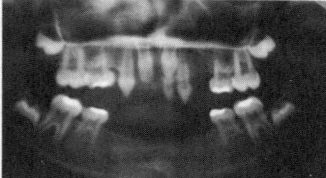

2903-20379: Affected woman at 36 years of age; note scalp hypotrichosis, sparse eyebrows (especially the distal 2/3), and facial wens. **20381:** Orthopantomogram of an affected boy at 4 years of age. **20380:** Oral findings in an affected girl at age 7 years.

Prevention: None known. Genetic counseling indicated.

Treatment: Prosthetic replacement and orthodontic treatment.

Prognosis: Life span is not affected.

Detection of Carrier: Unknown.

Special Considerations: The vertebral problems presented by the mother do not seem to be a part of the condition, since they are also present in her own mother but not in the other members of the kindred.

References:
Freire-Maia N: Ectodermal dysplasias. Hum Hered 1971; 21:309–312.
Freire-Maia N: Ectodermal dysplasias revisited. Acta Genet Med Gemellol 1977; 26:121–131.
Freire-Maia DV, et al.: Tricodermodisplasia com alterações dentárias. Ciênc Cult (suppl) 1985; 37:746.
Pinheiro M, et al.: Trichodermodysplasia with dental alterations: an apparently new genetic ectodermal dysplasia of the tricho-odonto-onychial subgroup. Clin Genet 1986; 29:332–336.

PI008 **Marta Pinheiro**

TRICHO-ODONTO-ONYCHIAL DYSPLASIA 2889

Includes: Ectodermal dysplasia, tricho-odonto-onychial type

Excludes:
Ectodermal dysplasia, Christ-Siemens-Touraine type (0333)
Ectodermal dysplasia, hidrotic (0334)
Odonto-onychodysplasia-alopecia (2890)
Tricho-dermodysplasia-dental defects (2903)

Major Diagnostic Criteria: Alopecia at the parietal region, generalized hypotrichosis, dental abnormalities, onychodystrophy, and skin alterations.

Clinical Findings: Dry, brittle, and sparse scalp hair at the temporal and occipital regions; alopecia at the parietal region; scanty eyebrows, eyelashes, and axillary and pubic hair; enamel hypoplasia leading to secondary anodontia; dystrophic finger- and toenails; yellowish or brownish toenails; extranumerary nipples; dermatoglyphics with palmar and digital ridge dissociation; palmoplantar keratosis; xeroderma on limbs; pigmented nevi; ephelides, actinic keratosis, papules, and crusts on scalp; skull deficiency (6 x 8 cm) in the frontoparietal region of one patient.

Complications: Psychologic problems due to partial alopecia; feeding problems due to dental loss.

Associated Findings: None known.

Etiology: Probably autosomal recessive inheritance.

Pathogenesis: Defective formation of several derivatives of the embryonic ectoderm suggests that this condition must be classified as an ectodermal dysplasia.

MIM No.: 27545

POS No.: 3603

Sex Ratio: Presumably M1:F1; M0:F4 observed.

Occurrence: Four sisters in one Brazilian sibship of 13 have been documented.

Risk of Recurrence for Patient's Sib:
See Part I, *Mendelian Inheritance.*

Risk of Recurrence for Patient's Child:
See Part I, *Mendelian Inheritance.*

Age of Detectability: At birth, by physical examination.

Gene Mapping and Linkage: Unknown.

Prevention: None known. Genetic counseling indicated.

Treatment: Early aggressive dental care to reduce spread of caries and avoid decay; wigs are cosmetically and psychologically helpful. Skull deficiency in one patient required plastic surgery, skin grafts, and flap rotation of skin.

Prognosis: Normal for life span.

Detection of Carrier: Unknown.

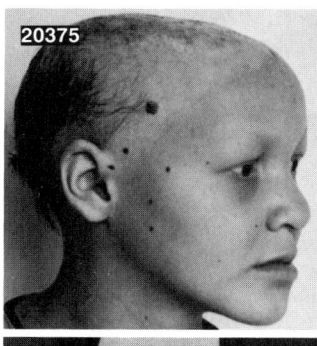
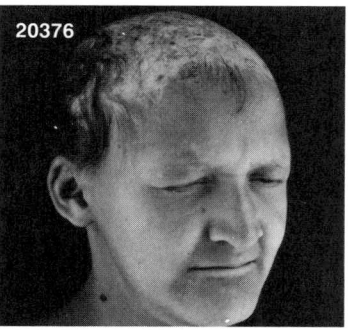
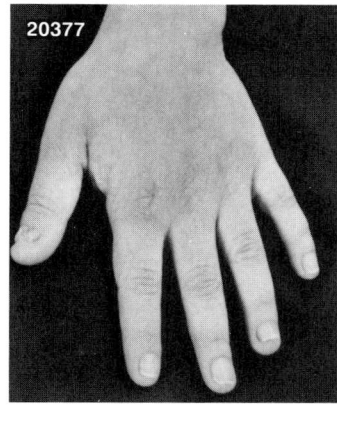
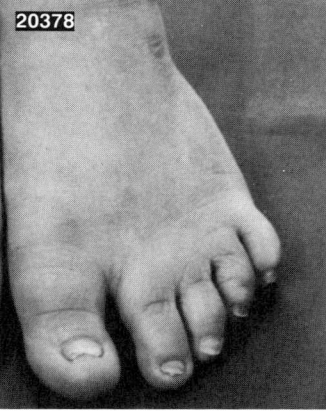

2889-20375: Affected 16-year-old female; note the extensive area of alopecia on the top of the head with only a peripheral fringe of hair in the temporal and occipital regions. She had a skull deficiency that measured 6 × 8 cm in the fronto-parietal region which was also traumatically altered. Note also the absence of eyebrows and lashes, mandibular prognathism, and a large number of pigmented nevi. **20376:** Affected 22-year-old woman; note central alopecia with hypotrichosis of the peripheral fringe, eyebrows, and lashes as well as ephelides, actinic keratosis, papules and crusts on the scalp. **20377:** Dystrophic nails. **20378:** Dystrophic toenails.

References:
Pinheiro M, et al.: Trichoodontoonychial dysplasia: a new meso-ectodermal dysplasia. Am J Med Genet 1983; 15:67–70.

PI008   **Marta Pinheiro**

Tricho-onycho-dysplasia-neutropenia
See ONYCHO-TRICHODYSPLASIA-NEUTROPENIA

TRICHO-ONYCHODYSPLASIA-XERODERMA 2892

Includes:
Ectodermal dysplasia, tricho-onychodysplasia-xeroderma type
Onycho-trichodysplasia-xeroderma
Xeroderma-tricho-onychodysplasia

Excludes:
Ectodermal dysplasia, hidrotic (0334)
Odonto-onychodysplasia-alopecia (2890)
Tricho-dermodysplasia-dental defects (2903)
Trichodysplasia-xeroderma (2894)

Major Diagnostic Criteria: Hair and nail alterations, and xeroderma.

Clinical Findings: Absent hair and nails at birth, but normal hair later; dystrophic fingernails and toenails; mild-to-severe generalized xeroderma with permanent and abundant scaling over the entire body; tendency to fissures in hands and feet.

Complications: Psychologic problems due to skin alterations.

Associated Findings: None known.

Etiology: Probably autosomal recessive inheritance. Parental consanguinity has been noted.

Pathogenesis: Defective formation of some derivatives of the embryonic ectoderm and absence of malformations show that this condition is a pure ectodermal dysplasia.

Sex Ratio: Presumably M1:F1.

Occurrence: One Caucasian Brazilian 23-year-old boy belonging to a sibship of five from nonconsanguineous parents has been reported. One of his sisters, who died at age three months, was reported to have been equally affected. He also has a first and second cousin, the daughter of first cousins, who was reported more severely affected.

Risk of Recurrence for Patient's Sib:
See Part I, *Mendelian Inheritance.*

Risk of Recurrence for Patient's Child:
See Part I, *Mendelian Inheritance.*

Age of Detectability: At birth, by physical examination.

Gene Mapping and Linkage: Unknown.

Prevention: None known. Genetic counseling indicated.

Treatment: Avoidance of exposure to the sun, ordinary xeroderma care.

Prognosis: Normal life span.

Detection of Carrier: The mother of two affected individuals presented discrete xeroderma.

References:
Freire-Maia N, et al.: Trichoonychodysplasia with xeroderma: an apparently hitherto undescribed pure ectodermal dysplasia. Rev Bras Genet 1985; 8:775–778.

PI008   **Marta Pinheiro**

Tricho-rhino-auriculo-phalangeal multiple exostoses dysplasia
See TRICHO-RHINO-PHALANGEAL SYNDROME, TYPE II
Tricho-rhino-phalangeal syndrome, dominant type I
See TRICHO-RHINO-PHALANGEAL SYNDROME, TYPE I
Tricho-rhino-phalangeal syndrome, recessive form
See TRICHO-RHINO-PHALANGEAL SYNDROME, TYPE I

TRICHO-RHINO-PHALANGEAL SYNDROME, TYPE I 0966

Includes:
Tricho-rhino-phalangeal syndrome, dominant type I
Tricho-rhino-phalangeal syndrome, recessive form

Excludes:
Dysostosis, other forms of radiographic peripheral
Tricho-rhino-phalangeal syndrome, type II (0967)
Tricho-rhino-phalangeal syndrome, type III (2847)

Major Diagnostic Criteria: Short stature, with deformities of the joints of the fingers and hands, characteristic X-ray changes, sparse scalp hair, pear-shaped nose, and long philtrum.

Clinical Findings: Short stature (variable: adult heights have ranged from 99 cm for females to 162 cm for males). Sparse, slowly growing scalp hair; eyebrows heavier medially than laterally; long philtrum; and a pear-shaped nose (of variable severity). There is usually a deformity at the proximal interphalangeal (IP) joints of hands.
X-ray findings: Cone-shaped epiphyses of phalanges, with ivory epiphyses (in 75%); premature fusion of involved epiphyses to the shaft. There is a scattered pattern of involvement, with middle

phalanges most commonly involved. The metacarpals may be short (frontal projection). No abnormal laboratory findings.

Complications: Thin hair, crooked fingers, and misshaped nose may be of cosmetic concern to affected individual, especially females. **Hip, osteonecrosis, capital femoral epiphysis** has been reported and several adults, with compatible residual deformity.

Associated Findings: Progressive arthritic changes of the dorsal spine, elbows, and fingers may occur in midlife.

Etiology: Usually autosomal dominant inheritance with great variability of expression, but autosomal recessive inheritance has also been reported. Recent reports have documented complex chromosomal rearrangements which have been linked to a deleted segment; 8q24.12 (Buhler et al, 1987).

Pathogenesis: Unknown.

MIM No.: *19035, 27550

POS No.: 3415

Sex Ratio: Presumably M1:F1.

Occurrence: Over a dozen kindreds have been reported, including several of Japanese extraction.

Risk of Recurrence for Patient's Sib:
See Part I, *Mendelian Inheritance*.

Risk of Recurrence for Patient's Child:
See Part I, *Mendelian Inheritance*.

Age of Detectability: In late childhood, by a combination of X-ray and clinical methods.

Gene Mapping and Linkage: A link to 8q24.12 has been suggested (Buhler et al, 1987).

Prevention: None known. Genetic counseling indicated.

Treatment: A wig, if thin hair is of concern to the affected individual. Treatment for **Hip, osteonecrosis, capital femoral epiphysis** if this occurs.

Prognosis: Normal life span.

Detection of Carrier: Possibly by clinical examination of first degree relatives.

References:
Giedion A: Cone-shaped epiphyses of the hands and their diagnostic value: the tricho-rhino-phalangeal syndrome. Ann Radiol (Paris) 1967; 10:322–329.
Giedion A, et al.: Autosomal dominant transmission of the tricho-rhino-phalangeal syndrome. Helv Paediat Acta 1973; 28:249–259.
Pashayan H, et al.: The tricho-rhino-phalangeal syndrome. Am J Dis Child 1974; 127:257–261.
McCloud DJ, Solomon LM: The tricho-rhino-phalangeal syndrome. Brit J Derm 1977; 96:403–407.
Peltola J, Kuokkanen K: Tricho-rhino-phalangeal syndrome in five succesive generations: report on a family in Finland. Acta Derm Venerol 1978; 58:65–68.
Sugiura Y: Tricho-rhino-phalangeal syndrome associated with Perthes-disease-like bone change and spondylolisthesis. Jpn J Hum Genet 1978; 23:23–30.
Ferrandez A, et al.: The trichorhinophalangeal syndrome: report of 4 familial cases belonging to 4 generations. Helv Paediat Acta 1980; 35:559–567.
Howell CJ, Wynne-Davies R: The tricho-rhino-phalangeal syndrome: a report of 14 cases in 7 kindreds. J Bone Joint Surg 1986; 68B:311–314.
Buhler EM, et al.: A final word on the tricho-rhino-phalangeal syndromes. Clin Genet 1987; 31:273–275.

B0025
LA016

Zvi Borochowitz
Leonard O. Langer, Jr.
David L. Rimoin

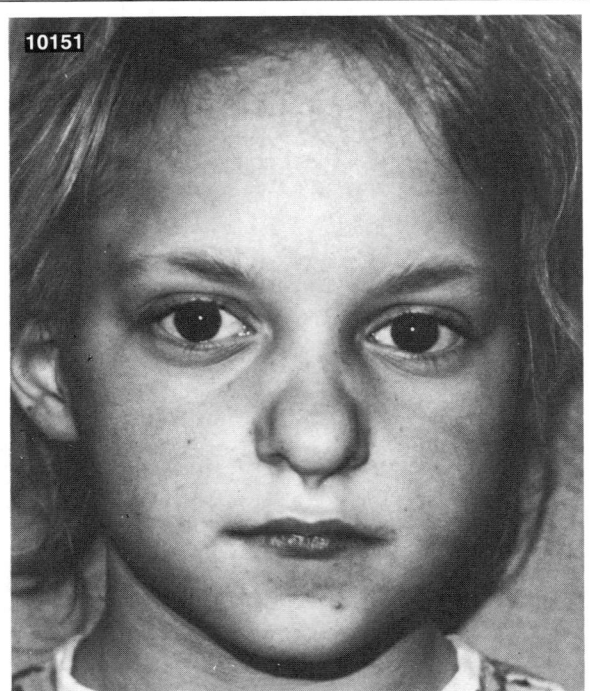

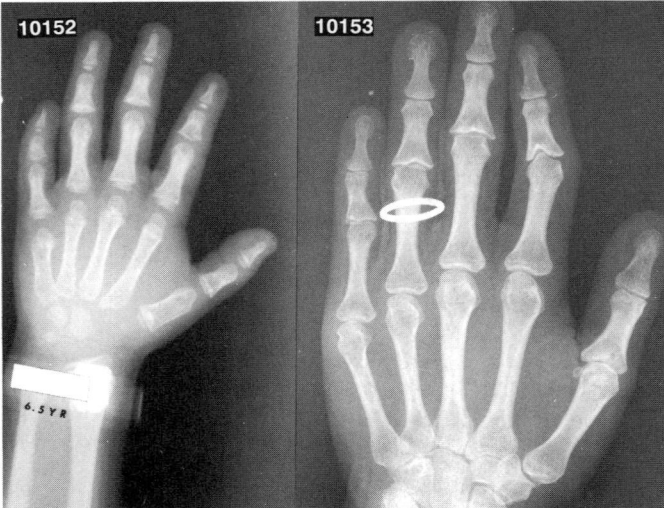

0966-10151: Typical facies with bulbous, pear-shaped nose with prominent philtrum. **10152:** Typical cone and ivory epiphyses in child's X-ray. **10153:** In adult, some residual deformity from old cones.

TRICHO-RHINO-PHALANGEAL SYNDROME, TYPE II   **0967**

Includes:
Acrodysplasia with exostoses
Giedion-Langer syndrome
Langer-Giedion syndrome
Tricho-rhino-auriculo-phalangeal multiple exostoses dysplasia

Excludes:
Exostoses, multiple cartilaginous (0685)
Metachondromatosis (0650)
Tricho-rhino-phalangeal syndrome, type I (0966)
Tricho-rhino-phalangeal syndrome, type III (2847)

Major Diagnostic Criteria: Bulbous nose, cone epiphyses, and multiple exostoses.

Clinical Findings: Craniofacial features include a broad nasal bridge; a bulbous, pear-shaped nose with tented, thickened alae;

prominent elongated philtrum; apparent mandibular micrognathia; thin upper lip; and large, laterally protruding ears. Scalp hair is thin, but eyebrows may be normal or even bushy laterally. There is mild microcephaly in 60%, mild-to-severe mental retardation in 70% of affected individuals, with disproportionate speech delay in at least one-half, and multiple cartilaginous exostoses with onset before the fifth year. The exostoses are present in the same distribution as in **Exostoses, multiple cartilaginous**, although some observers consider them to be quite different. They usually increase in number until skeletal maturation, and may lead to asymmetric limb growth. Spinal curvature may be seen. Ribs may be thin. Short stature of postnatal onset, cone-shaped epiphyses of the Giedion type 12 with clinobrachydactyly, and redundant or loose skin, which improves with age, are seen.

Other features seen in some patients include laxity or hypermobility of joints and hypotonia; changes in capital femoral epiphyses (see **Hip, osteonecrosis, capital femoral epiphysis**); exotropia, ptosis, ocular hypertelorism; winged scapulae; fractures; pigmented nevi increasing with age; recurrent respiratory infections; hearing deficit; colobomata of iris; partial syndactyly of 4th and 5th fingers; heart anomalies; and GU anomalies.

Complications: Compression of nerves or vessels, and limitation of movement or asymmetric growth of limbs, may occur secondary to exostoses.

Associated Findings: Respiratory infections and fractures.

Etiology: All cases have been sporadic except one father/daughter pair and one pair of like-sexed twins. No consanguinity or advanced parental age have been observed. Buhler et al (1987) concluded that the condition is due to a chromosomal deletion in the segment 8q24.11 to 8q24.13.

Pathogenesis: Facial and nose shape, epiphyseal changes, and exostoses are probably due to abnormal growth of endochondrial bone; however, a common mechanism to explain the hair abnormalities and mental retardation is undetermined.

MIM No.: 15023

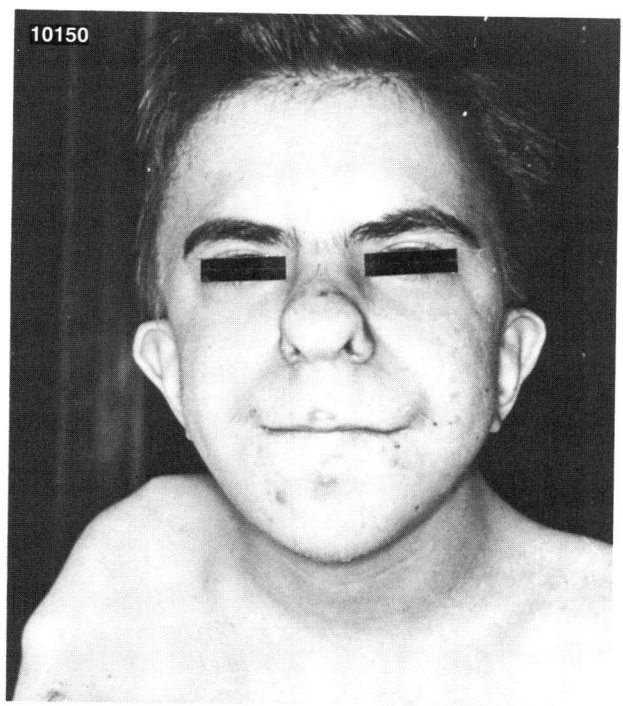

0967-10150: Characteristic nose, bushy eyebrows and long philtrum.

POS No.: 3416

Sex Ratio: M3:F1

Occurrence: About 50 cases have been reported in the literature.

Risk of Recurrence for Patient's Sib: Unknown.

Risk of Recurrence for Patient's Child: Apparently low.

Age of Detectability: At birth for facial characteristics; epiphyseal changes by three years of age, exostosis by five years of age.

Gene Mapping and Linkage: LGCR (Langer-Giedion syndrome chromosome region) has been mapped to 8q24.11-q24.13.

Prevention: None known. Genetic counseling indicated.

Treatment: Orthopedic excision of impinging exostoses; special school for developmental delay, with emphasis on speech development.

Prognosis: Depends on degree of mental retardation, if present.

Detection of Carrier: Unknown.

Special Considerations: It is important to distinguish this disorder from **Tricho-rhino-phalangeal syndrome, type I** and **Exostoses, multiple cartilaginous** because of the poorer prognosis, sporadic nature, frequent mental retardation, and other complications seen in this condition, as well as possible translocation carriers in the family if a chromosomal deletion is present.

References:
Murachi S, et al.: Familial tricho-rhino-phalangeal syndrome type II. Clin Genet 1981; 19:149–155.
Langer LO Jr, et al.: The tricho-rhino-phalangeal syndrome. Am J Med Genet 1984; 19:81–111.
Buhler EM, et al.: A final word on the tricho-rhino-phalangeal syndromes. Clin Genet 1987; 31:273–275.

HA014

Judith G. Hall

TRICHO-RHINO-PHALANGEAL SYNDROME, TYPE III   2847

Includes: Sugio-Kajii syndrome

Excludes:
  Acrodysostosis (0016)
  Osteodystrophy-mental retardation, Ruvalcaba type (2076)
  Peripheral dysostosis, other forms of
  Tricho-rhino-phalangeal syndrome, type I (0966)
  Tricho-rhino-phalangeal syndrome, type II (0967)

Major Diagnostic Criteria: Clinical features of **Tricho-rhino-phalangeal syndrome, type I** plus a severe form of generalized shortness of all phalanges, metacarpals and metatarsals.

Clinical Findings: Craniofacial dysmorphology (6/6) including somewhat light-colored sparse hairs, hypoplastic alae nasi, pear-shaped nose, a long, broad and prominent philtrum, protruding upper lip, malar hypoplasia, prominent maxilla, delayed eruption of teeth, and malocclusion is almost identical to that of **Tricho-rhino-phalangeal syndrome, type I**. Cone-shaped epiphyses of phalanges with premature fusion of the epiphysis and clinodactyly are common (3/4, an infant excluded). Characteristic findings which may differ from **Tricho-rhino-phalangeal syndrome, type I** include severe short stature (4/5), broad hip in post-adolescent female patients (3/3), osteochondritis of the spine (2/3), and severely short and stubby fingers with shortness of all metacarpals, metatarsals and phalanges (5/5), the end of which appears a mushroom shape on X-ray films. There is no mental retardation (6/6).

Complications: Limitation of joint movements, **Pectus carinatum**, and thoracic scoliosis are sometimes seen.

Associated Findings: None known.

Etiology: Autosomal dominant inheritance with variability in expression.

Pathogenesis: Unknown.

POS No.: 4413

Sex Ratio: M2:F4 (observed).

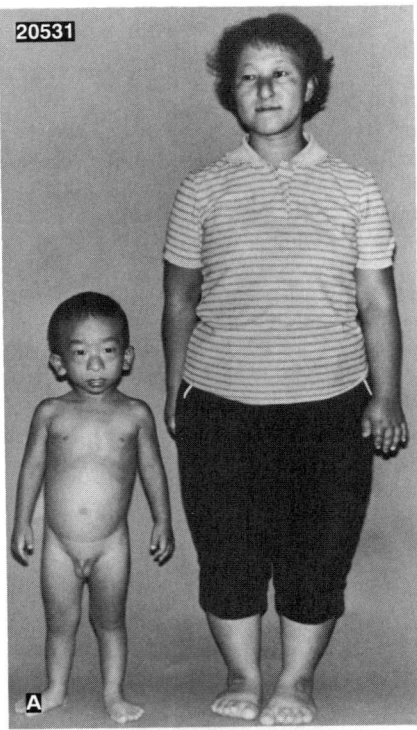

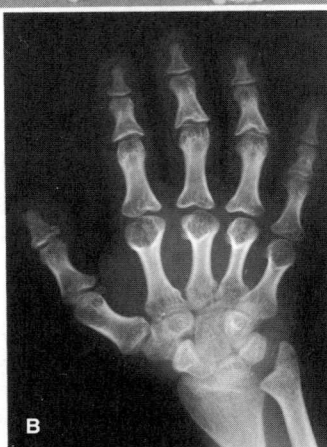

2847-20531: Tricho-rhino-phalangeal syndrome, type III; A. Note affected mother and son with characteristic facies, short stature and short stubby fingers. B. X-ray of the hand shows shortened phalanges and metacarpals.

Occurrence: Six affected Japanese have been documented; five from a family and one sporadic case.

Risk of Recurrence for Patient's Sib:
See Part I, *Mendelian Inheritance.*

Risk of Recurrence for Patient's Child:
See Part I, *Mendelian Inheritance.*

Age of Detectability: Possibly in early infancy.

Gene Mapping and Linkage: Unknown.

Prevention: None known. Genetic counseling indicated.

Treatment: As with **Tricho-rhino-phalangeal syndrome, type I.**

Prognosis: Normal life span.

Detection of Carrier: Unknown.

References:
Sugio Y, Kajii T: Ruvalcaba syndrome: autosomal dominant inheritance. Am J Med Genet 1984; 19:741–753. †
Niikawa N, Kamei T: The Sugio-Kajii syndrome: proposed tricho-rhino-phalangeal syndrome type III. Am J Med Genet 1986; 24:759–760. * †

NI010   **Norio Niikawa**

TRICHODENTAL DYSPLASIA WITH REFRACTIVE ERRORS   2813

Includes:
Ectodermal dysplasia, euhidrotic-refractive errors
Kopysc syndrome
Trichodental dysplasia-hyperopia

Excludes:
Ectodermal dysplasia
Hair, atrichia congenita (2346)
Hair, hypotrichosis (3151)
Tricho-dento-osseous syndrome (0965)
Tricho-dermodysplasia-dental defects (2903)

Major Diagnostic Criteria: The combination of abnormally shaped teeth, hypotrichosis, and hyperopia, with normal nails and sweating.

Clinical Findings: Sparse, brittle scalp hair; broad nose; cone-shaped teeth (both deciduous and permanent affected); and skin anomalies consisting of perifollicular papules affecting the trunk and limbs and reticular hyperpigmentation on the neck nape. In each case, hyperopia was diagnosed at age six years. One patient also had astigmatism and amblyopia. Microscopic examination of hair revealed pili annulati (alternating light and dark rings of pigmentation).

Complications: Unknown.

Associated Findings: None known.

Etiology: Probably autosomal recessive inheritance.

Pathogenesis: One of the ectodermal dysplasias, although the basic genetic defect is unknown.

MIM No.: 26202

Sex Ratio: Presumably M1:F1.

Occurrence: Reported in a brother and sister in one family from Poland.

Risk of Recurrence for Patient's Sib:
See Part I, *Mendelian Inheritance.*

Risk of Recurrence for Patient's Child:
See Part I, *Mendelian Inheritance.*

Age of Detectability: During the first year of life by the presence of thin scalp hair and cone-shaped teeth.

Gene Mapping and Linkage: Unknown.

Prevention: None known. Genetic counseling indicated.

Treatment: Correction of the ocular defect is indicated. Dental or orthodontic treatment may also be indicated.

Prognosis: Life span and intellect are apparently unaffected.

Detection of Carrier: Unknown.

References:
Kopysc Z, et al.: A new syndrome in the group of euhidrotic ectodermal dysplasia: pilodental dysplasia with refractive errors. Hum Genet 1985; 70:376–378.

T0007   **Helga V. Toriello**

Trichodental dysplasia-hyperopia
See TRICHODENTAL DYSPLASIA WITH REFRACTIVE ERRORS
Trichodermodysplasia-dental alterations
See TRICHO-DERMODYSPLASIA-DENTAL DEFECTS
Trichodysplasia hereditary
See HAIR, HYPOTRICHOSIS

Trichodysplasia-dysmorphic facies-ataxia
See ATAXIA-DYSMORPHIC FACIES-TRICHODYSPLASIA

TRICHODYSPLASIA-XERODERMA 2894

Includes: Xeroderma-trichodysplasia

Excludes: Hair, hypotrichosis (3151)

Major Diagnostic Criteria: Trichodysplasia with structural changes, and xeroderma.

Clinical Findings: Variable degree of scalp hypotrichosis (from almost alopecia to an apparently normal amount of hair with a small alopetic area); coarse, brittle, slow-growing, and excessively dry scalp hair; irregularly sparse eyebrows; short and scanty eyelashes; absent beard; sparse axillary and pubic hair; scalp hair shafts with pili torti, scaling, longitudinal grooves, longitudinal splitting, and peeling; variable degree of universal xeroderma.

Complications: Psychologic problems due to hair alterations.

Associated Findings: None known.

Etiology: Probably autosomal dominant inheritance with variable expression. The many instances of male-to-male transmission and the presence of normal daughters of affected men rule out X-linked dominant inheritance.

Pathogenesis: Probably a defect in ectodermal cells involving the morphodifferentiation of skin and hair structure.

MIM No.: 19036

POS No.: 4440

Sex Ratio: Presumably M1:F1; M36:F29 observed.

Occurrence: A Brazilian family of mixed Portuguese, Paraguayan, Bolivian and Amerindian origin was verified to have 65 affected members in five generations.

Risk of Recurrence for Patient's Sib:
See Part I, *Mendelian Inheritance.*

Risk of Recurrence for Patient's Child:
See Part I, *Mendelian Inheritance.*

Age of Detectability: At birth, by physical examination.

Gene Mapping and Linkage: Unknown.

Prevention: None known. Genetic counseling indicated.

Treatment: Use of wigs is cosmetically and psychologically helpful; skin emollients.

Prognosis: Normal life span.

Detection of Carrier: Unknown.

References:
Pinheiro M, Freire-Maia N: Trichodysplasia-xeroderma: an autosomal dominant condition. Clin Genet 1987; 31:62–67.

PI008 **Marta Pinheiro**

Trichoepithelioma
See PILOMATRIXOMA
Trichoepitheliomas, multiple
See EPITHELIOMAS, HEREDITARY MULTIPLE CYSTIC

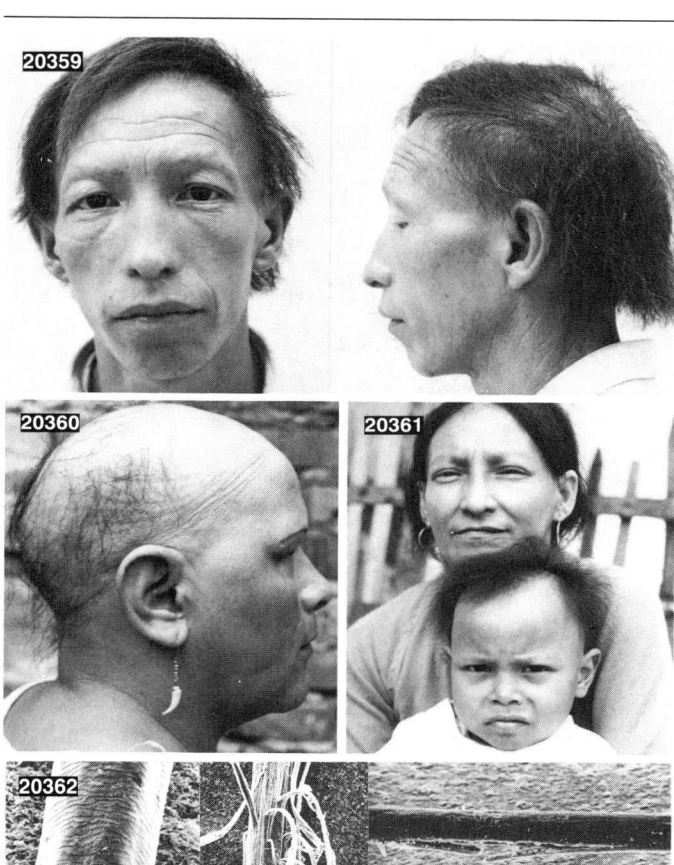

2894-20359–61: Note varying degrees of hypotrichosis involving the scalp, eyebrows and lashes. **20362:** Scanning electron micrograph showing defects of the hair shafts: longitudinal grooves, peeling, longitudinal splitting, dystrophic bulb, scaling and pili torti.

TRICHOMEGALY-RETARDATION-DWARFISM-RETINAL PIGMENTARY DEGENERATION 2294

Includes:
Eyelashes (long)-mental retardation
Oliver-McFarlane syndrome

Excludes:
Albinism, ocular (0032)
Albinism, oculocutaneous
Bardet-Biedl syndrome (2363)
Ectodermal dysplasia
Trichomegaly, congenital

Major Diagnostic Criteria: Long and sparse eyelash and eyebrow hair, pigmentary degeneration of the retina, growth retardation.

Clinical Findings: Intrauterine growth retardation is present, and postnatal growth is slow, with poor weight gain and eventual short stature. Bone maturation is delayed. Frontal and occipital bossing are present. Long eyelash (up to 40 mm) and eyebrow hair is present at birth or within the first year. The eyelashes can be curved and sparse. Diffuse retinal pigmentary degeneration is present by age two years, and visual acuity is reduced to 20/200 or more. Nystagmus may be present. The electroretinogram is absent, and the pigmentary degeneration lacks the characteristic bone corpuscles found in **Retinitis pigmentosa**.

Scalp hair is sparse (i.e., patchy or frontal alopecia) in the first decade of life, and total scalp alopecia has been noted in a 37-year-old patient. A scalp skin biopsy from one patient showed degenerating hair follicles with lymphocytic histiocytic infiltration, typical of alopecia areata. Slow dental eruption was present in one patient, resulting in small, discolored teeth at age 30 months, while dentition was normal in one four-year-old patient. Cryptorchidism and hypogonadism with lack of secondary sexual characteristics has been described in the two reported adult cases. Developmental delay and mental retardation have been present in three of six cases, normal intelligence in one of six, and no developmental information for one of six. Gait ataxia, generalized clumsiness, and titubation of the head, associated with cerebellar atrophy demonstrated by computed tomography of the head, were present in the 37-year-old patient. Neurologic problems other than those involving the visual system were not described in the remaining five reported cases.

Nonbanded chromosome analyses were normal in three cases. An abnormality, possibly representing partial 13q trisomy resulting from a familial translocation was reported in one case in 1972.

Complications: Progressive reduction in visual acuity resulting from retinal pigmentary degeneration.

Associated Findings: Hypothyroidism (2/6) and growth hormone deficiency (1/6) have been described. The sella was described as "empty" in the 37-year-old male with hypothyroidism and growth hormone deficiency.

Etiology: Unknown. The six reported cases have been sporadic with no affected sibs.

Pathogenesis: Unknown.

MIM No.: 27540

POS No.: 3442

CDC No.: 270.200

Sex Ratio: 5M:1F (observed).

Occurrence: A half-dozen cases have been documented.

Risk of Recurrence for Patient's Sib: Unknown.

Risk of Recurrence for Patient's Child: Unknown. Both reported adults had hypogonadism and absent testes and are presumed to be sterile.

Age of Detectability: At birth or within the first year of life.

Gene Mapping and Linkage: Unknown.

Prevention: None known. Genetic counseling indicated.

Treatment: Hormone therapy for endocrine deficiencies.

Prognosis: Unknown. Adult cases were reported at ages 19 and 37 years.

Detection of Carrier: Unknown.

References:
Oliver GL, McFarlane DC: Congenital trichomegaly. Arch Ophthalmol 1965; 74:169–171.
Cant JS: Ectodermal dysplasia. J Pediatr Ophthalmol 1967; 4:13–17.
Corby DG, et al.: Trichomegaly, pigmentary degeneration of the retina, and growth retardation. Am J Dis Child 1971; 121:344–345.
Delleman JW, Van Walbeek K: The syndrome of trichomegaly, tapetoretinal degeneration and growth disturbances. Ophthalmologica 1975; 171:313–315.
Patton MA, et al.: Congenital trichomegaly, pigmentary retinal degeneration, and short stature. Am J Ophthalmol 1986; 101:490–491.
Sampson JR, et al.: Oliver McFarlane syndrome: a 25 year follow-up. Am J Med Genet 1989; 34:199–201. †

Richard A. King

KI007

Trichopoliodystrophy
See MENKES SYNDROME
Trichorrhexis nodosa syndrome
See TRICHOTHIODYSTROPHY

TRICHOTHIODYSTROPHY 2559

Includes:
> Amish brittle hair syndrome
> Hair-brain syndrome
> Hair defect-photosensitivity-mental retardation
> Hair, sparse, short, thin and brittle
> Hair, "tiger tail"
> Ichthyosis-trichothiodystrophy
> Pollitt syndrome
> Sabinas brittle hair syndrome
> Tay syndrome
> Trichorrhexis nodosa syndrome
> Trichothiodystrophy-ichthyosis
> Trichothiodystrophy-neuro-cutaneous syndrome

Excludes:
> **Cockayne syndrome** (0189)
> **Ichthyosis, linearis circumflexa** (2858)
> **Marinesco-Sjogren syndrome** (2031)
> **Oculo-mandibulo-facial syndrome** (0738)

Major Diagnostic Criteria: A group of related conditions involving brittle hair with reduced sulfur content; and other possible

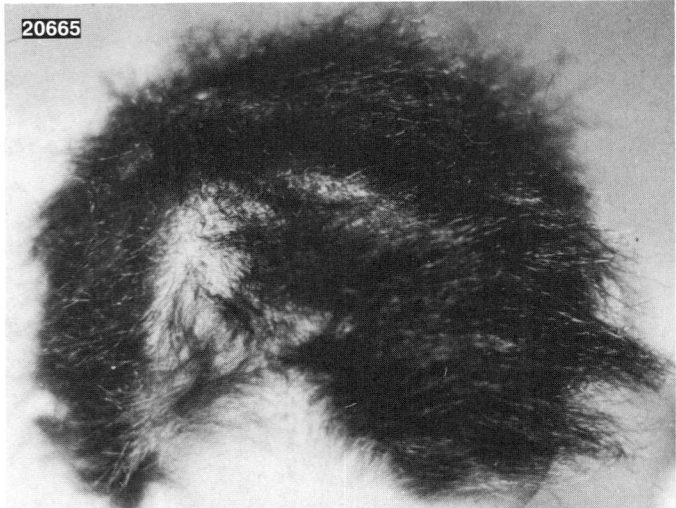

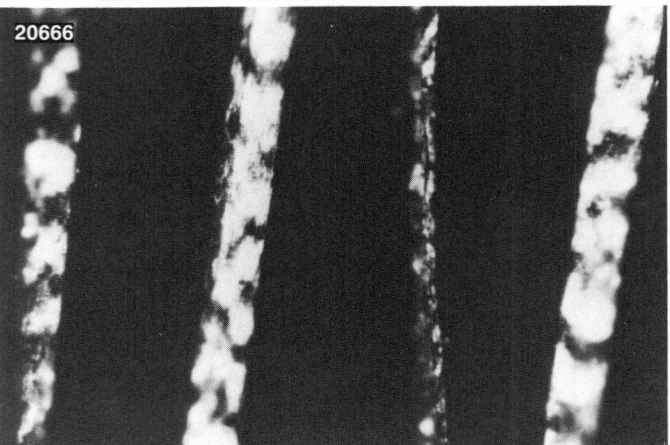

2559-20665: Sparse, stubbly and easily broken scalp hair. **20666:** "Zig-zag" pattern of dark and bright zones demonstrated by polarizing microscopy of the hair shaft.

associated features including mental retardation, short stature, decreased fertility, ichthyosis, photosensitivity, and peculiar face.

Clinical Findings: Delivery is frequently preterm. Birth weight is low for pregnancy age. Physical development is definitely slow. Short stature; **Microcephaly**; mild, nonprogressive mental impairment; poor motor coordination, and unsteady gait may be seen. Some patients show signs of neurologic abnormality (ataxia, intention tremor). Neurosensory hearing loss and cataract are rarely reported. Face is peculiar, with receding chin and small nose. Ichthyosis or ichthyosiform erythroderma are common.

The most dramatic and consistent findings are the hair abnormalities. The hair is sparse, short, thin, and brittle. Analysis with light, polarizing, and scanning electron microscopy shows pili torti, trichoschisis, trichorrhexis nodosa, and a peculiar pattern of alternating dark and bright bands, giving a "tiger tail" appearance. Nails are frequently dysplastic. Cystine and cysteic acid of hair and nails content is lower (50%) than normal. Postpubertal patients have delayed and reduced development of secondary sexual characters. Fertility is reduced.

In about one-half of the reported families, the patients present a marked sensitivity to sunlight and photophobia; freckle-like lesions in the sun-exposed areas usually occur. Cultured cells from these patients are hypersensitive to UVC light and are defective in the repair of UV-induced DNA damage. This defect is due to the presence of the same mutation responsible for **Xeroderma pigmentosum**, complementation group D as demonstrated by complementation analysis of UDS in hybrid cells.

Complications: Susceptibility to infections.

Associated Findings: None known.

Etiology: Usually autosomal recessive inheritance.

Pathogenesis: The reduced content of sulfur-rich matrix proteins may account for the hair shaft disruption; however, the pathogenetic mechanisms of this and other symptoms are unknown.

MIM No.: *21139, 23403, *23405, *24217, 27555

POS No.: 3456

Sex Ratio: M1:F1

Occurrence: At least sixty-nine patients, belonging to 38 families, have been reported. In ten of these families, the parents of affected individuals are apparently unrelated; consanguinity data are missing on five families. In the remaining 23 families consanguinity has been demonstrated and accounts for the high prevalence of the syndrome in specific regions (northern Indiana, Sabinas, Mexico, and northeastern Italy, where 25, 12, and four patients, respectively, can be traced to common ancestors).

Risk of Recurrence for Patient's Sib:
See Part I, *Mendelian Inheritance.*

Risk of Recurrence for Patient's Child:
See Part I, *Mendelian Inheritance.*

Age of Detectability: Early infancy; prenatal diagnosis of the DNA repair defect can be performed in pregnancies at-risk for trichothiodystrophy associated with **Xeroderma pigmentosum** D.

Gene Mapping and Linkage: Unknown.

Prevention: None known. Genetic counseling indicated. Prevention of actinic damage by avoiding sunlight in patients with photosensitivity.

Treatment: As indicated for infections or other symptomatic problems. Lubricants for hair. Avoid use of dyes, straighteners, permanents, and hot combs.

Prognosis: Varies with the specific symptoms. Reduced life span, intelligence, and sexual function have been reported.

Detection of Carrier: Unknown.

Special Considerations: The notable finding regarding trichothiodystrophy is the association with **Xeroderma pigmentosum**. Studies of DNA repair performed on patients displaying photosensitivity showed a reduced capacity to repair UV-induced DNA damage caused by XP, complementation group D, mutation. Unexpectedly in trichothiodystrophy patients, precancerous skin

lesions and tumors, which characterize the pathology of age-matched xeroderma pigmentosum, complementation group D, patients have never been observed. The association of xeroderma pigmentosum and trichothiodystrophy in more than one patient in a kindred and in different unrelated families could indicate a linkage between the loci involved in the two syndromes.

The various acronyms PIBIDS, IBIDS, and BIDS have been used to designate combinations of photosensitivity, ichthyosis, brittle hair, impaired intelligence, decreased fertility, and short stature.

References:

Tay CH: Ichthyosiform erythroderma, hair shaft abnormalities, and mental and growth retardation. Arch Dermatol 1971; 104:4–13.

Jackson CE, et al.: Brittle hair with short stature, intellectual impairment and decreased fertility: an autosomal recessive syndrome in an Amish kindred. Pediatrics 1974; 54:201–207.

Happle R, et al.: The Tay syndrome (congenital ichthyosis with trichothiodystrophy). Eur J Pediatr 1984; 141:149–152.

Price VH, et al.: Trichothiodystrophy: sulfur-deficient brittle hair as a marker for a neuroectodermal symptom complex. Arch Dermatol 1984; 116:1375–1384.

Stefanini M, et al.: Xeroderma pigmentosum (complementation group D mutation) is present in patients affected by trichothiodystrophy with photosensitivity. Hum Genet 1986; 74:107–112.

NU002   **Fiorella Nuzzo**
B0051   **Carla Borrone**

Trichothiodystrophy-ichthyosis
See TRICHOTHIODYSTROPHY
Trichothiodystrophy-neuro-cutaneous syndrome
See TRICHOTHIODYSTROPHY
Trichothiodystrophy-sun sensitivity
See XERODERMA PIGMENTOSUM
Trichterbrust
See PECTUS EXCAVATUM
Tricuspid incompetence
See TRICUSPID VALVE, INSUFFICIENCY
Tricuspid regurgitation
See TRICUSPID VALVE, INSUFFICIENCY

TRICUSPID VALVE, ATRESIA   **0968**

Includes:
 Atresia of tricuspid valve
 Atretic atrioventricular (AV) valve of the right atrium
 Heart, tricuspid valve atresia
 Ventricle, hypoplasia of right

Excludes:
 Pulmonary valve, atresia (0837)
 Tricuspid valve, stenosis (0970)
 Ventricular inversion when valve of the left atrium is atretic

Major Diagnostic Criteria: Although tricuspid atresia is a great mimicker of other forms of cyanotic heart disease, the following findings are virtually pathognomonic in a patient who exhibits cyanosis: reversed Q loop in the horizontal plane (deeper Q waves in lead V_5 than V_6), diminished vascularity by X-ray and left axis deviation and the two aforementioned signs, plus the added X-ray finding of juxtaposition of the atrial appendages.

A selective right atriogram is the procedure of choice to confirm the diagnosis. All cases reveal the typical sequence of opacification: right atrium, left atrium, left ventricle. In cases with normally related great vessels and transposition with noninversion, there is a clear zone, termed "right ventricular window," just below and medial to the lower margin of the right atrium. In patients with inversion, the right ventricular window is absent because the right ventricle is located superiorly and anteriorly. A selective left ventriculogram is recommended for precise location of the origin of the great arteries, the type of obstruction to pulmonary flow if present, the contractile state of the left ventricle, the position of the right ventricle, and the size of **Ventricular septal defect**.

Includes cases with ventricular inversion in which the atretic right atrioventricular (AV) valve is bicuspid or mitral-like and the functioning left AV valve is tricuspid. Thus, the term "tricuspid atresia'' is retained for all cases in which the AV valve of the right atrium is atretic, regardless of its anatomy.

Clinical Findings: Despite considerable variation in the anatomic and physiologic manifestations from case to case, certain features are common to all: atresia of the AV valve of the right atrium; patent atrial septum; an enlarged mitral orifice; a hypertrophied left ventricle which functions as a single ventricle; and a rudimentary and essentially nonfunctioning right ventricle. Tricuspid atresia is divided into two main categories according to the relationship of the aorta and the pulmonary trunk: those with normally related great vessels and those with transposition of the great vessels. Tricuspid atresia with transposition may be subdivided into two additional categories: those with and without inversion of the ventricles. Regardless from which morphologic ventricle the pulmonary trunk arises, obstruction to pulmonary flow occurs under the following circumstances: atresia of the pulmonary valve with the pulmonary arteries perfused through a patent ductus arteriosus or via bronchial arteries: stenosis of the pulmonary valve; a narrowed subpulmonary tract or a combination of the latter two. Among cases with normally related great vessels, obstruction to pulmonary flow may occur because of a small ventricular septal defect. Lastly, patients with transposition may exhibit the additional abnormality, double outlet right ventricle. The aorta is anterior and arises from a rudimentary right ventricle, while the pulmonary trunk arises partially or entirely from the right ventricle. Regardless, the left AV valve tissue is not in continuity with either semilunar valve. Juxtaposition of the atrial appendages-levoposition of the right atrial appendage occurs in a relatively high percentage of cases with transposition and noninversion. A right aortic arch is present in 7–8% of cases. Dextrocardia or dextroversion, with atria in situs solitus position, also occurs with increased frequency especially where there is shunt vascularity.

The hemodynamic alterations, and consequently the clinical manifestations, will vary according to the magnitude of pulmonary flow, the position of the great vessels and the type of ventricular arrangement, inversion or noninversion. Whatever the anatomic type, in all cases of tricuspid atresia there is a right-to-left shunt at the atrial level. The right atrium becomes enlarged and hypertrophied since it functions as the sole pumping chamber for blood from the venae cavae. It pushes all the systemic venous blood through either the foramen ovale or through an atrial septal defect. The right ventricle is usually so diminutive as to be functionally ineffective. Consequently, the left ventricle becomes the single propelling chamber for delivery of blood into both great arteries. As the left atrium is the common mixing chamber into which all the saturated (pulmonary venous) and desaturated (systemic venous) blood is poured, the peripheral arterial saturation depends on the relative amounts of each. Other factors that diminish peripheral arterial saturation are ventricular failure and obstruction to aortic flow.

The presence of cyanosis, the EKG and the thoracic X-ray are the vital clinical data. The auscultatory findings are of little help. Cyanosis is common to most patients. Those with decreased pulmonary flow may exhibit hypoxic spells as well. In patients with increased pulmonary flow, cyanosis may be clinically absent. Congestive heart failure often occurs during infancy, especially when pulmonary flow is increased. Older children exhibit the usual stigmata of the cyanotic child: clubbing, growth retardation and frequent bouts of bronchitis. EKG evidence of left axis deviation is present in at least 90% of the cases. The exceptions are usually patients with excess pulmonary flow in whom a normal axis may be present. Usual signs are left ventricular hypertrophy and diminished or absent signs of right ventricular activity. Pure right ventricular hypertrophy is never seen. Patients with normally related great vessels show Q waves in the left precordial leads, whereas those with transposition rarely show Q waves in the left precordial leads. The presence of deeper Q waves in the lead V_5 than V_6 in a cyanotic patient is virtually pathognomonic of tricuspid atresia with normally related great vessels. The thoracic roentgenogram is extremely variable, and may mimic virtually any form of cyanotic heart disease. The pulmonary flow may be excessive (uncommon), normal (rare), or diminished (common).

The classic and most common variety resembles **Heart, tetralogy of Fallot.** There are certain roentgen findings, when occurring in a cyanotic patient, that are suggestive of tricuspid atresia: juxtaposition of the atrial appendages, dextroversion or dextrocardia (in whom the atria are situs solitus), and right aortic arch which occurs in approximately 7–8% of cases.

The echocardiogram shows an absent tricuspid valve (although motion of the right atrial floor can be confused as valve), dilation of the left ventricular cavity, a small right ventricular cavity and a thickened right ventricular anterior wall. Caution must be exercised as this is a diagnosis of exclusion.

Cardiac catheterization will confirm the presence of a right-to-left shunt at the atrial level, degree of peripheral arterial desaturation, and often the presence or absence of obstruction to pulmonary flow, if the catheter is placed within the pulmonary trunk.

Complications: Death may occur from congestive heart failure and pneumonia, clubbing, severe hypoxic spells, growth retardation, or frequent bouts of bronchitis.

Associated Findings: None known.

Etiology: Presumably multifactorial inheritance.

Pathogenesis: The formation of the right AV valve probably occurs during the 4th intrauterine week. Although embryogenesis is not fully understood, normal rotation of the ventricular septum probably fails and the right AV orifice is sacrificed, so that the embryologic AV valve results in an enlarged mitral valve at the expense of an atretic tricuspid valve.

MIM No.: 27720

CDC No.: 746.100

Sex Ratio: Presumably M1:F1

Occurrence: Approximately 1:5,000 live births. Prevalence < 1 in 5,000 in the pediatric population.

Risk of Recurrence for Patient's Sib: Estimated at about 1%.

Risk of Recurrence for Patient's Child: Unknown. Reproductive fitness is greatly diminished.

Age of Detectability: From birth, by selective angiocardiography.

Gene Mapping and Linkage: Unknown.

Prevention: None known. Genetic counseling indicated.

Treatment: In patients with obstruction to pulmonary flow, procedures are aimed at increasing pulmonary blood flow, which can be accomplished by a side-to-side anastomosis of the ascending aorta to the right pulmonary artery (Waterson-Cooley shunt) or by the creation of a subclavian artery-pulmonary artery shunt (Blalock-Taussig operation). In older children, an anastomosis between the superior vena cava and the distal right pulmonary artery (Glenn procedure) is preferred by some. Those patients with excess flow to the pulmonary arteries may require a banding to decrease pulmonary flow and prevent hyperresistant changes occurring in the vasculature. Some of these, plus patients with only a moderate degree of obstruction to pulmonary flow, may be managed medically. A few such patients reach adult age. Symptomatic therapy for congestive heart failure and pneumonia may be necessary.

Prognosis: The prognosis closely depends upon the anatomic type and in particular, the magnitude of pulmonary blood flow. Most individuals, regardless of type, expire during infancy unless palliative surgery is performed. Those with some form of severe pulmonary stenosis expire due to severe hypoxia; those with excess pulmonary flow expire secondary to congestive heart failure, pneumonia, etc. Those individuals who survive infancy without palliation do so because they developed high pulmonary vascular resistance, or there is only a moderate degree of obstruction to pulmonary flow, regardless of origin of the pulmonary trunk.

Detection of Carrier: Unknown.

References:

Glenn WW, et al.: Circulatory bypass of the right side of the heart. VI. shunt between superior vena cava and distal right pulmonary artery: report of clinical application in 38 cases. Circulation 1965; 31:172.

Elliott LP, et al.: The roentgenology of tricuspid atresia. Semin Roentgenol 1968; 3:399.

Meyer RA, Kaplan S: Echocardiography in the diagnosis of hypoplasia of the left or right ventricles in the neonate. Circulation 1972; 46:55.

Rosenthal A, Dick M: Tricuspid atresia. In: Adams FH, Emmanoullides GC, eds: Heart disease in infants, children, and adolescents, 3rd ed. Baltimore: Williams & Wilkins Co., 1983:271–283. *

EL004   **Larry P. Elliott**
                                           Irwin F. Hawkins, Jr.

Tricuspid valve, downward displacement
See TRICUSPID VALVE, EBSTEIN ANOMALY

TRICUSPID VALVE, EBSTEIN ANOMALY   0332

Includes:
Ebstein anomaly of tricuspid valve
Eskatlith∧, fetal effects
Lithium, fetal effects
Lithobid∧, fetal effects
Lithone∧, fetal effects
Tricuspid valve, downward displacement

Excludes:
Ebstein anomaly in cases of ventricular inversion
Fetal lithium effects (2732)
Other forms of congenital tricuspid valve incompetence

Major Diagnostic Criteria: In the acyanotic individual, selective angiocardiography or cardiac catheterization with the intracavitary electrode catheter are necessary to establish a definitive diagnosis. The diagnosis of Ebstein anomaly becomes mandatory in the cyanotic individual who has bouts of tachycardia with decreased pulmonary vascular markings on chest X-rays, an ECG showing either large P waves, a prolonged PR interval and a precordial QRS pattern suggesting RBBB or having no definite criteria for either right or left ventricular hypertrophy, or the type B WPW pattern.

Clinical Findings: The pathology of Ebstein anomaly is extremely variable. The two characteristic features are redundancy of valve tissue and adherence of a variable portion of the septal and posterior cusps to the right ventricular wall. Redundancy involves all cusps, although the anterior cusp is always much less affected. The area of adherence may be small, in which case the true origin of the cusps at the atrioventricular annulus is close to the apparent origin; or it may extend all the way down to the ring formed by the parietal band, crista supraventricularis, septal and moderator bands and anterior papillary muscle. That portion of the ventricle between the annulus and the apparent origin of the valve is said to be "atrialized," as it more or less forms a common chamber with the right atrium. The myocardium of the atrialized portion of the right ventricle may be fairly well developed in mild forms of the anomaly. In severe forms it may be fibrous. Both the pathology and pathophysiology are variable. In rare cases of Ebstein anomaly, the valve mechanism may function almost normally. With increasing severity of the anomaly, there is valvar insufficiency and/or stenosis. In time, right atrial pressure is elevated, the right atrium becomes markedly enlarged and a right-to-left shunt is established through an anatomically patent foramen ovale or, rarely, an atrial septal defect.

The malformation may be so pronounced as to cause intrauterine or neonatal death. Symptoms and signs are commonly present during the first month of life, particularly cyanosis, murmurs, congestive heart failure and bouts of tachycardia. Symptoms in the older child and adult are dyspnea on exertion, profound weakness or fatigue, cyanosis, bouts of tachycardia and in the terminal stages, cardiac failure. Auscultation is variable. Often the widely split components of the first sound are followed by a systolic murmur, two widely split components of the second sound and frequently a prominent third or fourth sound, producing a "triple" or "quadruple" rhythm. A diastolic murmur may surround either S₃ or S₄, or both.

The EKG either shows a right bundle branch block pattern or the Wolff-Parkinson-White (type B) pattern often with right atrial enlargement and a prolonged PR interval. The vectorcardiogram classically shows P loop changes of right atrial enlargement and slowing of the terminal rightward, superior and anterior QRS forces consistent with RBBB. The radiologic features in infancy are variable ranging from slight to massive cardiac enlargement and often resemble severe pulmonic stenosis with an intact ventricular septum and a right-to-left shunt. In patients of all age groups, certain X-ray features are seen: there are varying degrees of right heart enlargement; the pulmonary artery segment is usually inapparent; no left atrial enlargement; the aortic knob is normal or small; pulmonary vascular markings are normal or decreased, and even with chronic congestive heart failure, pleural effusion is not seen.

The M-mode echocardiogram shows dilation of the right ventricular cavity and delayed tricuspid closure with respect to mitral diastolic closure. The tricuspid valve excursion is exaggerated and its echo representation is displaced leftward. Many patients have paradoxic septal motion. The 2-dimensional echocardiogram will demonstrate the "displaced" tricuspid valve.

Cardiac catheterization, to be diagnostic, must demonstrate that a portion of the right ventricle functions as the right atrium. When, with an intracavitary electrode catheter, right ventricular muscle potentials are recorded in the presence of a right atrial pressure, the diagnosis is established. The hemodynamic findings depend on whether there is tricuspid insufficiency, or stenosis, or both. In cyanotic individuals, the right-to-left shunt is localized to the atrial level. Angiocardiography is best performed in the right ventricle. This outlines clearly the enlarged right atrium, the atrialized right ventricle and the functional right ventricle. The true and apparent annulus divide the inferior margin of the cardiac border in the AP view into three distinct compartments.

Complications: Cerebral abscess, thromboembolic phenomena and organ pathology secondary to chronic congestive failure.

Associated Findings: These most commonly are a ventricular septal defect or pulmonary stenosis or atresia. Extracardiac anomalies are rare.

Etiology: Multifactorial inheritance. Lithium has been proposed as a specific environmental trigger (see **Fetal lithium effects**).

Pathogenesis: Ebstein anomaly is probably an abnormality of the process of undermining of the embryonic right ventricular myocardium which normally leads to the formation of the tricuspid valve apparatus. In Ebstein anomaly, it remains incomplete and never reaches the annulus. Thus, the normal development of chordae and papillary muscles does not take place, or remains abortive. The relatively normal development of the anterior cusp is probably related to its very early liberation.

MIM No.: 22470

CDC No.: 746.200

Sex Ratio: M1:F1

Occurrence: Approximately 1:200 births with congenital heart disease. Risk of congenital heart disease, most often Ebstein anomaly, is 10% for infants of mothers taking lithium in the first weeks of pregnancy. Prevalence 1:50,000 to 1:20,000 in the pediatric population.

Risk of Recurrence for Patient's Sib: Empiric risk 1.0%

Risk of Recurrence for Patient's Child: Unknown.

Age of Detectability: From birth, particularly with selective right ventricular angiocardiography or the intracavitary electrode catheter.

Gene Mapping and Linkage: Unknown.

Prevention: Genetic counseling is indicated. Mothers on lithium should review options with a knowledgeable counselor.

Treatment: Replacement of abnormal tricuspid valve with a prosthesis, appropriate drugs or electrical conversion for bouts of tachycardia. Symptomatic therapy for congestive heart failure. Antibiotic therapy for cerebral abscess.

Prognosis: Variable, depending on the degree of pathologic anatomy and resultant distortion of physiology. Ebstein anomaly may cause neonatal death or be compatible with a normal life span.

Detection of Carrier: Unknown.

References:
Donegan CC Jr, et al.: Familial Ebstein's anomaly of the tricuspid valve. Am Heart J 1968; 75:375–379.
Nora JJ, et al.: Lithium, Ebstein's anomaly, and other congenital heart defects. Lancet 1974; II:594–595. *
Park JM, et al.: Ebstein's anomaly of the tricuspid valve associated with prenatal exposure to lithium carbonate. Am J Dis Child 1980; 134:704–708.
Silverman NH, Snider AR: Two-dimensional echocardiography in congenital heart disease. Connecticut: Appleton-Century-Crofts, 1982.
Van Mierop LHS, et al.: Anomalies of the tricuspid valve resulting in stenosis or incompetence. In: Adams FH, et al., eds: Heart disease in infants, children, and adolescents, ed 3. Baltimore: Williams & Wilkins, l983. *
Pierard LA, et al.: Persistent atrial standstill in familial Ebstein's anomaly. Brit Heart J 1985; 53:594–597.

N0003   **James J. Nora**

TRICUSPID VALVE, INSUFFICIENCY   0969

Includes:
   Heart, tricuspid valve insufficiency
   Tricuspid incompetence
   Tricuspid regurgitation

Excludes:
   Heart, endocardial cushion defects (0347)
   Tricuspid insufficiency secondary to bacterial/fungal
      endocarditis
   Tricuspid insufficiency secondary to Ebstein anomaly
   Tricuspid insufficiency secondary to rheumatic heart
      disease
   Tricuspid insufficiency secondary to trauma
   Tricuspid valve insufficiency, transient neonatal

Major Diagnostic Criteria: Cyanosis, dyspnea, and cardiomegaly are present. Angiocardiography is the procedure of choice with cine- or biplane angiograms from the right ventricle demonstrating reflux into the right atrium. The normally inserted tricuspid valve distinguishes this lesion from **Tricuspid valve, Ebstein anomaly.** Other diagnoses within the differential include **Pulmonary valve, stenosis, Pulmonary valve, atresia** with tricuspid insufficiency with a normally sized right ventricle.

Clinical Findings: The pathologic anatomy in congenital tricuspid insufficiency varies. It may be due to a primary malformation (dysplasia) of the valve, shortened chordae tendineae, or defective papillary muscles with fibrosis. In some cases, the septal cusp remains adherent to the ventricular septum.

Isolated congenital tricuspid insufficiency is an extremely rare cardiac lesion. The most common presenting signs and symptoms include dyspnea, cyanosis, cardiomegaly and right-sided congestive heart failure. A pulsatile, enlarged liver and neck vein distention with prominent v waves have been observed.

A loud pansystolic murmur is invariably heard along the lower right or left sternal border with transmission to the back. The increase in intensity on inspiration is of tricuspid origin. An associated mid and late diastolic rumble represents relative tricuspid stenosis.

The X-ray findings are dependent on the severity of the lesion. In the symptomatic patient, the usual findings include massive cardiac enlargement with either normal or diminished vascularity of the lung fields. The right atrium is huge and in postmortem studies is 2–3 times the normal size. The right ventricular cavity is also increased in size.

The EKG commonly shows tall, peaked P waves, particularly in lead II, right axis deviation, and a q^R or $rs^{R'}$ pattern over the right precordium, indicating right atrial enlargement and right ventricular hypertrophy. Also seen in some cases is a right bundle branch block pattern.

The echocardiogram in the Ebstein abnormality is described elsewhere (see **Tricuspid valve, Ebstein anomaly**). In tricuspid insufficiency, it shows a dilated right ventricle, and septal motion may be paradoxic.

Selective right ventricular angiocardiography demonstrates reflux of contrast material into the right atrium during ventricular systole. A right-to-left atrial shunt through a patent foramen ovale is often an associated finding.

The right atrial mean pressure is invariably elevated; and the right atrial pressure pulse has a systolic plateau with a prominent V wave and a rapid y descent. In the symptomatic neonate, right ventricular pressure is often at systemic levels, and is associated with pulmonary hypertension.

Complications: Most infants improve with digitalis, diuretics, and oxygen as the pulmonary vascular resistance falls. Follow-up of many of these children has shown relatively normal hemodynamics with mild tricuspid insufficiency.

Associated Findings: None known.

Etiology: Unknown.

Pathogenesis: Undetermined, but probably due to the abnormal or incomplete elaboration of the septal cusp of the tricuspid valve. This may be adherent to the septum, or possess only very short chordae tendineae.

CDC No.: 746.105

Sex Ratio: Presumably M1:F1

Occurrence: About 20 cases reported in the world literature.

Risk of Recurrence for Patient's Sib: Unknown.

Risk of Recurrence for Patient's Child: Unknown.

Age of Detectability: From birth, by selective angiocardiography.

Gene Mapping and Linkage: Unknown.

Prevention: None known. Genetic counseling indicated.

Treatment: Those instances of functional tricuspid insufficiency revert to normal when the underlying abnormality is corrected. Oxygen, which dilates the pulmonary vascular bed and thus results in a lowering of pulmonary vascular resistance, has a role in management. Surgical intervention has rarely been attempted, and usually has a fatal outcome.

Symptomatic therapy may be a treatment for right-sided congestive heart failure including digitalization and diuretics, and oxygen.

Prognosis: Unknown.

Detection of Carrier: Unknown.

References:
Reisman M, et al.: Congenital tricuspid insufficiency: a cause of massive cardiomegaly and heart failure in the neonate. J Pediatrics 1965; 66:869–876.
Ahn AJ, Segal BL: Isolated tricuspid insufficiency: clinical features, diagnosis and management. Prog Cardiovasc Dis 1966; 9:166–193. *
Goldberg SJ, et al.: Pediatric and adolescent echocardiography. Chicago: Year Book Medical Publishers, 1975.

HE014   **William E. Hellenbrand**
BE029   **Michael A. Berman**
TA002   **Norman S. Talner**

TRICUSPID VALVE, STENOSIS   **0970**

Includes: Heart, narrowing of tricuspid orifice

Excludes:
Tricuspid stenosis from large atrial level shunts
Tricuspid stenosis secondary to rheumatic heart disease
Tricuspid stenosis secondary to right atrial myxomas
Tricuspid valve, atresia (0968)
Tricuspid valve, Ebstein anomaly (0332)

Major Diagnostic Criteria: The clinical, X-ray, and electrocardiographic manifestations of tricuspid stenosis with right ventricular hypoplasia are often identical to those of **Tricuspid valve, atresia**. Two dimensional echocardiography with Doppler analysis and/or cardiac catheterization with selective angiocardiography are needed to differentiate these two anomalies.

Clinical Findings: Isolated tricuspid stenosis is extremely rare, with few proven cases reported in the literature. With moderate-to-severe tricuspid stenosis, right atrial hypertension occurs, resulting in hypertrophy and dilatation of the chamber. Atrial dilatation promotes continued patency of the foramen ovale which allows for right atrial decompression but results in systemic venous blood gaining access to the systemic arterial circulation. The majority of children with congenital tricuspid stenosis have diminished pulmonary flow and may present in early infancy with cyanosis. Cyanotic spells associated with paroxysmal dyspnea may occur in these patients within the first six months of life. Enough blood may bypass the right ventricle through a large atrial communication such that there is insufficient flow across the tricuspid valve to produce a detectable murmur. When right atrial to right ventricular blood flow is of sufficient magnitude, atrial contraction may be reflected as a presystolic precordial impulse at the left sternal border, a jugular venous ''a'' wave, or a hepatic presystolic pulsation. A short mid-to-late diastolic rumble can only rarely be appreciated. Other murmurs will reflect associated lesions, particularly pulmonary stenosis, ventricular septal defect, or patent ductus arteriosus.

X-rays of the chest reveal decreased pulmonary vascularity and signs of an enlarged right atrium. The plain films cannot be distinguished from the **Heart, tetralogy of Fallot, Tricuspid valve, Ebstein anomaly**, and certain forms of **Tricuspid valve, atresia**.

The most constant findings on electrocardiography are peaked ''P'' waves, indicating right atrial enlargement. QRS axis and signs of left ventricular hypertrophy are variable, depending on the degree of right ventricular hypoplasia.

The two-dimensional echocardiogram shows a narrowed tricuspid valve orifice and a small, or even hypoplastic, right ventricular cavity. In severe forms, tricuspid valve motion may be absent and thus be indistinguishable from tricuspid atresia. In such circumstances Doppler analysis may be able to demonstrate flow through the valve, thus excluding tricuspid atresia.

Cardiac catheterization helps to confirm the diagnosis of tricuspid stenosis as well as to further evaluate associated defects. Passage of the catheter from the right atrium to the right ventricle on occasion may be difficult since the preferred pathway is into the left atrium. Simultaneous right atrial and right ventricular tracings should demonstrate a diastolic pressure difference, but such simultaneous records are rarely obtained. Generally, pullback tracings from the right ventricle to the right atrium are used for detection of the pressure difference.

Selective right atrial and right ventricular angiocardiography aid in the demonstration of the abnormality and associated defect(s). Frequently, the right atrial injection will show thickening of the valve and right-to-left atrial shunt.

Complications: Cyanosis, secondary to right-to-left shunt via a patent foramen ovale or associated **Atrial septal defects**. Systemic venous congestion manifested by peripheral edema and ascites. Infrequently, a superior vena caval type of syndrome may develop.

Associated Findings: None known.

Etiology: Unknown.

Pathogenesis: Probably due to partial fusion of the tricuspid valve primordia at an early age.

CDC No.: 746.100

Sex Ratio: Presumably M1:F1.

Occurrence: 3:1,000 cases of autopsied congenital heart disease.

Risk of Recurrence for Patient's Sib: Unknown. Strong familial tendency reported, but no accurate recurrence risk is known.

Risk of Recurrence for Patient's Child: Unknown.

Age of Detectability: From birth, with echocardiography and/or selective angiocardiography. Prenatal diagnosis may be possible through the use of fetal echocardiography and Doppler analysis.

Gene Mapping and Linkage: Unknown.

Prevention: None known. Genetic counseling indicated.

Treatment: Valvotomy or prosthetic valve replacement. Associated lesions must be considered individually. Infants with cyanosis and right ventricular hypoplasia or other lesions (e.g. pulmonary artery hypoplasia), which are not amenable to immediate surgical correction, may benefit from a systemic to pulmonary artery anastomosis. The use of an atrial-to-pulmonary artery conduit (Fontan procedure) or right atrial-right ventricular outflow conduit has been suggested for patients surviving infancy who are not candidates for valve reconstruction or replacement.

Prognosis: Influenced primarily by the severity of the stenosis, degree of right ventricular hypoplasia, and the nature of associated intracardiac abnormalities.

Detection of Carrier: Possibly by echocardiography and Doppler analysis.

References:
Calleja HB, et al.: Congenital tricuspid stenosis. Am J Card 1960; 6:821–829.
Medd WE, et al.: Isolated hypoplasia of the right ventricle and tricuspid valve in siblings. Br Heart J 1961; 23:25–30.
Dabachi F, et al.: Hypoplasia of the right ventricle and tricuspid valve in siblings. J Pediatr 1967; 71:869–874.
Dimich I, et al.: Congenital tricuspid stenosis-case treated by heterograft replacement of the tricuspid valve. Am J Cardiol 1973; 31:89–92.
Bharati S, et al.: Anatomic variations in underdeveloped right ventricle related to tricuspid atresia and stenosis. J Thoracic Cardiovasc Surg 1976; 72:383–400.
Van Mierop LHS, et al.: Ebstein's anomaly. In: Moss' heart disease in infants, children and adolescents, 4th ed. Baltimore: William and Wilkins, 1989.

RI012   **Richard E. Ringel**
HE014   **William E. Hellenbrand**
BR039   **Joel I. Brenner**
BE029   **Michael A. Berman**

TRIGONENCEPHALY, AUTOSOMAL DOMINANT TYPE   3030

Includes:
    Craniosynostosis of metopic sutures
    Metopic suture synostosis

Excludes:
    C syndrome (0121)
    Say-Meyer syndrome (3267)

Major Diagnostic Criteria: Trigonocephaly with normal mental development and positive family history should suggest the diagnosis.

Clinical Findings: In six affected individuals from the same family, trigonocephaly limited to metopic suture involvement was present. In the two examined individuals, an S-curved lower lid (2/2), Microcephaly (1/2), short inner canthal distance (1/2), and preauricular skin tag (1/2) were also present. Mental development in all affected individuals was normal.

Complications: Unknown.

Associated Findings: An omphalocele was present in one affected individual.

Etiology: Possibly autosomal dominant inheritance with variable expressivity and possible reduced penetrance.

Pathogenesis: Unknown.

MIM No.: 19044

CDC No.: 754.070

Sex Ratio: M5:F1 (observed).

Occurrence: One family from Israel has been reported.

Risk of Recurrence for Patient's Sib:
    See Part I, *Mendelian Inheritance.*

Risk of Recurrence for Patient's Child:
    See Part I, *Mendelian Inheritance.*

Age of Detectability: Possibly at birth or during infancy, by the abnormal skull shape.

Gene Mapping and Linkage: Unknown.

Prevention: None known. Genetic counseling indicated.

Treatment: Unknown.

Prognosis: Life span and intellectual development appear to be unimpaired.

Detection of Carrier: Unknown.

References:
Frydman M, et al.: Trigonocephaly: a new familial syndrome. Am J Med Genet 1984; 18:55–59.

T0007   **Helga V. Toriello**

Trigonocephaly "C" syndrome
    See C SYNDROME
Trigonocephaly-short stature
    See SAY-MEYER SYNDROME
Trigonocephaly-short stature-developmental delay
    See SAY-MEYER SYNDROME
Trihydroxycoprostanic acidemia
    See ACIDEMIA, TRIHYDROXYCOPROSTANIC
Trimethadione, fetal effects of
    See FETAL TRIMETHADIONE SYNDROME

TRIMETHYLAMINURIA   3241

Includes:
    Fish odor syndrome
    Stale fish syndrome

Excludes: N/A

Major Diagnostic Criteria: Excretion of trimethylamine in urine.

Clinical Findings: A prominent odor of rotting fish, particularly in areas of active sweating, such as the axillae and feet. This may become more severe after puberty. There are no physical manifestations, however severe psychosocial problems have been described, such as aggressive behavior, poor school performance, and depression.

Complications: Unknown.

Associated Findings: One patient has been described with **Noonan syndrome**, neutropenia, anemia, splenomegaly, and an intermittent fishy odor, and with elevated levels of trimethylamine in the urine.

Etiology: Autosomal recessive inheritance.

Pathogenesis: Trimethylamine is normally formed in man, in the gut, by the action of bacteria on ingested choline (from eggs, liver, legumes) and trimethylamine-oxide (from some species of salt water fish). It is then transported to the liver and oxidized to form trimethylamine oxide, which is then excreted in the urine. Patients with this disorder have diminished activity of hepatic trimethylamine-n-oxide synthetase, causing accumulation of trimethylamine, which is responsible for the fishy odor.

MIM No.: *27570

Sex Ratio: M1:F1

Occurrence: Eighteen cases have been reported in the literature. A random study of 169 people, however, detected two carriers, suggesting that the condition may be more common than initially thought.

Risk of Recurrence for Patient's Sib:
    See Part I, *Mendelian Inheritance.*

Risk of Recurrence for Patient's Child:
    See Part I, *Mendelian Inheritance.*

Age of Detectability: Can be variable, depending on ingestion of substrates. Two cases have been reported in which the odor was present from infancy, while the mother was breast feeding and had eaten eggs or fish.

Gene Mapping and Linkage: Unknown.

Prevention: None known. Genetic counseling indicated.

Treatment: Usually dietary restriction of fish and choline containing foods eliminates the odor. However, two patients have also required antibiotics to reduce intestinal bacterial degradation of choline and trimethylamine.

Prognosis: Excellent.

Detection of Carrier: Oral challenge with 600 mg. of trimethylamine can detect partial impairment of N-oxidation in carriers.

References:
Humbert JR, et al.: Trimethylaminuria: the fish-odour syndrome. Lancet 1970; II:770–771.
Higgins T, et al.: Trimethylamine-n-oxide synthesis: a human variant. Biochem Med 1972; 6:392–396.
Calvert GD: Trimethylaminuria and inherited Noonan Syndrome. Lancet 1973; I:320–321.
Lee CWG, et al.: Trimethylaminuria: fishy odors in children. New Eng J Med 1976; 295:937–938.
Danks DM, et al.: Trimethylaminuria: diet does not always control the fishy odor. New Eng J Med 1976; 295:962 only.
Todd WA: Psychosocial problems as the major complication of an adolescent with trimethylaminuria. J Pediatr 1979; 94:936–937.
Nyhan WL: Abnormalities in amino acid metabolism in clinical medicine. Stanford, CT: Appleton-Century-Crofts, 1984:360–362.
Shelley ED, Shelley WB: The fish-odour syndrome: trimethylaminuria. J Am Med Asso 1984; 251:253–255.

Al-Waiz, et al.: Trimethylaminuria (fish-odour syndrome): an inborn error of oxidative metabolism. Lancet 1987; II:634–635.
Al Waiz, et al.: Trimethylaminuria (fish-odour syndrome): a study of an affected family. Clin Sci 1988; 74:231–236.

MA095   **Deborah L. Marsden**

TRYPSINOGEN DEFICIENCY   0973

Includes:
Isolated trypsinogen deficiency
Trypsin-1

Excludes:
Cystic fibrosis (0237)
Intestinal enterokinase deficiency (0533)
Secondary pancreatic exocrine insufficiency
Shwachman syndrome (0885)

Major Diagnostic Criteria: Malabsorption and protein calorie malnutrition cause failure to thrive, edema, and anemia in infancy. Demonstration of trypsinogen deficiency is required. Basal and secretin-stimulated duodenal aspirates contain subnormal activities of peptidases but normal amylase and lipase. After incubation with enterokinase, there is no increase in trypsin activity. After incubation with bovine trypsin, there is normal activity of carboxypeptidase, chymotrypsin, and elastase but no augmentation of tryptic activity. The maneuvers indicate an absence of pancreatic trypsinogen.

Clinical Findings: Reported patients presented in infancy with failure to thrive, hypoproteinemia, edema, and anemia, i.e., the pattern of protein-calorie malnutrition. Generalized malabsorption was evident in each. There was no evidence for serum protein loss in urine or stool. Fecal nitrogen and fat excretion were increased. Pancreatic exocrine function was characteristically disturbed.
Confusion may occur in two circumstances: 1) the severely malnourished infant with generalized pancreatic exocrine dysfunction and subnormal activities of all exocrine enzymes; 2) trypsinogen activation may be accomplished by incubation with bovine trypsin (4° C for 16 hours) in some patients. This test is not reliable and should not be used to diagnose absence of trypsinogen. Enterokinase alone should be used in the incubation as a pro-enzyme activator.

Complications: Protein malabsorption, hypoproteinemia, edema, secondary pancreatic exocrine dysfunction, generalized malabsorption, failure to grow and gain weight, and anemia.

Associated Findings: None known.

Etiology: Autosomal recessive inheritance.

Pathogenesis: Normal trypsinogen is secreted by the pancreas and is converted within the intestinal lumen to trypsin. Trypsin, in turn, activates other propeptidases to their active enzymatic forms. Deficiency of trypsinogen results in subnormal activities of all peptidases. Lipase and amylase are secreted as active enzymes, and are not deficient in trypsinogen deficiency disease.

MIM No.: *27600

Sex Ratio: M2:F1

Occurrence: About a half-dozen cases have been documented.

Risk of Recurrence for Patient's Sib:
See Part I, *Mendelian Inheritance.*

Risk of Recurrence for Patient's Child:
See Part I, *Mendelian Inheritance.*

Age of Detectability: In infancy.

Gene Mapping and Linkage: TRY1 (trypsin 1) has been mapped to 7q32-qter.

Prevention: None known. Genetic counseling indicated.

Treatment: Provision of pancreatic enzymes by oral replacement; elemental diets are useful in providing nutrition in infancy.

Prognosis: Excellent.

Detection of Carrier: Unknown.

References:
Townes PL: Trypsinogen deficiency disease. J Pediatr 1965; 66:275–285.
Morris MD, Fisher DA: Trypsinogen deficiency disease. Am J Dis Child 1967; 114:203–208.
Townes PL, et al.: Further observations on trypsinogen deficiency disease: report of a second case. J Pediatr 1967; 71:220–224.
Emi M, et al.: Cloning, characterization and nucleotide sequences of two cDNAs coding human pancreating trypsinogens. Gene 1986; 41:305–310.

WH007   **Peter F. Whitington**

TRYPTOPHAN MALABSORPTION   0974

Includes:
> Blue diaper syndrome
> Hypercalcemia, familial with nephrocalcinosis and
> indicanuria

Excludes:
> **Hartnup disorder** (0453)
> Intestinal malabsorption syndromes
> **Phenylketonuria** (0808)

Major Diagnostic Criteria: Severe prolonged hypercalcemia can be provoked by L-tryptophan in affected probands. There is excess tryptophan in the feces of the patient. Tryptophan derivatives increased in the urine (e.g., indoleacetic acid, indolelactic acid, indolylacetyl glutamine, indole acetamide, and indican) are of intestinal origin. These derivatives are secondary to retention of tryptophan in the intestinal lumen.

Blue staining of diapers is caused by indigotin, presumably formed by enzymatic conversion of indolic compounds in urine. The source of the urinary enzyme(s) may be from damaged renal tissue. Fecal *Pseudomonas aeruginosa* contamination of urine on diaper may produce a phenocopy.

Plasma tryptophan concentration is normal; the rise following oral L-tryptophan load (100 mg/kg) is less than normal. Renal clearance of tryptophan is normal under endogenous conditions.

Clinical Findings: Hypercalcemia and nephrocalcinosis are associated with a defect in intestinal absorption of L-tryptophan. Two brothers had a similar clinical course involving failure to thrive, recurrent unexplained fever, infections, irritability, and constipation. Bluish discoloration of the diapers was observed continuously from early infancy. The first-born died after a mastoidectomy; the second was alive at 44 months. The vitamin D intake was 1,400 units daily in both patients (maximum RDA: 400 units), but no clinical signs of the infantile hypercalcemia syndrome were apparent.

Complications: Hypercalcemia, producing nephrocalcinosis. The defect in tryptophan absorption is, in some undetermined way, correlated with the occurrence of hypercalcemia.

Associated Findings: None known.

Etiology: Undetermined, but possibly autosomal recessive or X-linked recessive inheritance of a biochemical defect.

Pathogenesis: Proposed deficiency of substrate-specific intestinal membrane transport system for L-tryptophan.

MIM No.: 21100

Sex Ratio: In the only reported pedigree, there were two affected male siblings, one female sib with no symptoms (but "occasionally blue diapers"), and one normal male sib.

Occurrence: One family has been reported.

Risk of Recurrence for Patient's Sib:
> See Part I, *Mendelian Inheritance.*

Risk of Recurrence for Patient's Child:
> See Part I, *Mendelian Inheritance.*

Age of Detectability: In infancy.

Gene Mapping and Linkage: Unknown.

Prevention: None known. Genetic counseling indicated.

Treatment: Reduced protein intake; advisable to limit vitamin D intake to 400 units/day. Treatment for hypercalcemia; avoidance of dietary alkali and high milk intake is prudent.

Prognosis: Limited if hypercalcemia is complicated by nephrocalcinosis.

Detection of Carrier: Both parents in the only reported pedigree were free of abnormal biochemical manifestations or clinical symptoms.

Special Considerations: The indoluria may resemble that present in **Hartnup disorder**, but a specific hyperaminoaciduria distinguishes the latter trait. Indoluria also occurs in phenylketonuria, apparently because phenylalanine competes with tryptophan for intestinal absorption. In neither primary disease is there hypercalcemia. Tryptophan malabsorption and indoluria accompany many forms of intestinal malabsorption.

References:

Drummond KN, et al.: The blue diaper syndrome: familial hypercalcemia with nephrocalcinosis and indicanuria. A new familial disease, with definition of the metabolic abnormality. Am J Med 1964; 37:928–948.
Michael AF, et al.: Tryptophan metabolism in man. J Clin Invest 1964; 43:1730–1746.
Libit SA, et al.: Fecal Pseudomonas aeruginosa as a cause of the blue diaper syndrome. J Pediatr 1972; 81:546–560.

SC050   **Charles R. Scriver**

TSH resistance
> See THYROTROPIN UNRESPONSIVENESS
Tuberculosis, INH inactivation peripheral neuropathy
> See NEUROPATHY, HERITABLE ISONIAZIDE TYPE (INH)
Tuberose sclerosis
> See TUBEROUS SCLEROSIS

TUBEROUS SCLEROSIS   0975

Includes:
> Adenoma sebaceum-seizures-mental retardation
> Bourneville syndrome
> Epiloia
> Mental retardation-seizures-adenoma sebaceum
> Pringle disease
> Seizures-adenoma sebaceum-mental retardation
> Tuberose sclerosis

Excludes: Neurofibromatosis (0712)

Major Diagnostic Criteria: Adenoma sebaceum, seizures, and mental retardation constitute the classic symptom complex. There are many variations of the disease, even within the same family.

Clinical Findings: Tuberous sclerosis is a multisystem disease classically characterized by the triad of adenoma sebaceum, epilepsy, and mental retardation. Many variations have been documented. The disease may present in infancy with infantile spasms and tufts of white hair or faintly depigmented nevi, which are shaped in the form of an ash leaf and vary in size. These nevi are differentiated from vitiligo by the presence of melanocytes in the lesion, although the number of pigmented melanocytes is lower than in adjacent normomelanotic skin. Depigmented nevi are often difficult to appreciate, but ultraviolet light (a Wood lamp) may be helpful in their identification. In the preschool child the most common symptom is epilepsy. Although the seizures are primarily generalized tonic-clonic, focal motor, complex partial, and petit mal variants have been observed. Mental retardation of a moderate to severe degree occurs in about one-half of the cases.

Skin lesions are present in the majority of cases and include adenoma sebaceum, shagreen plaques, subungual fibromata, depigmented nevi, subcutaneous nodules, and café-au-lait spots in decreasing frequency. In the very young infant only the depigmented nevi or hair patch may be present. Retinal tumors consisting of mulberry lesions and plaques of glia (phakoma) have been noted in as many as 70%. Oral lesions include gingival fibromas and small enamel pits on the teeth, and the iris may have hypopigmented spots. Attention is brought to their disease by the complications of tuberous sclerosis or family members with tuberous sclerosis.

CT scan of the brain shows cerebral calcification, most frequently subependymally in the walls of the third and lateral ventricles, especially in the region of the basal ganglia. Subependymal nodules can be seen on MRI in the majority of patients. Skull X-rays demonstrate intracranial calcification in approximately 50%. The EEG is not characteristic. X-rays of the hands reveal cystic areas of rarefaction, particularly in the phalanges (30–60%). A chest X-ray may rarely demonstrate symmetric coarse markings, which appear as multiple cysts. Occasionally an intravenous pyelogram or abdominal CT will suggest a renal mass

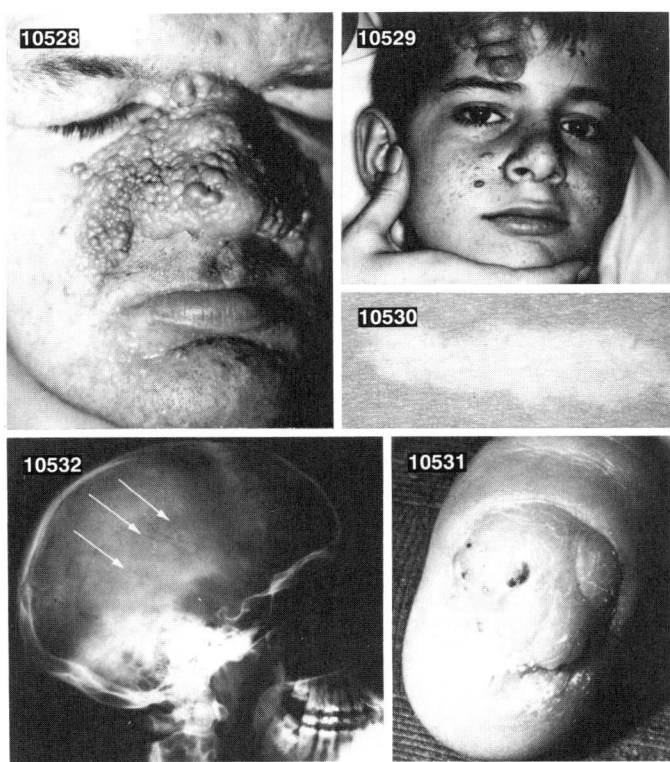

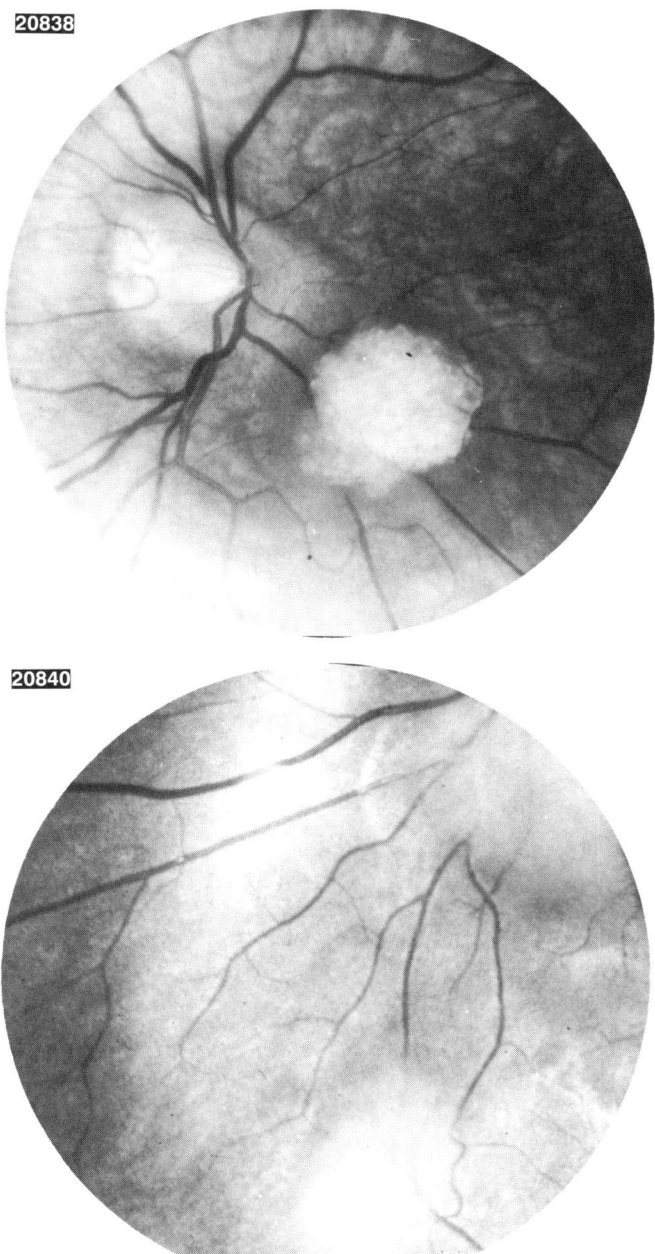

0975A-10528: Angiofibromas. 10529: Polypoid fibrous masses on forehead. 10530: Patch of vitiligo. 10531: Subungual fibroma. 10532: Skull X-ray showing intracranial calcifications.

(angiomyolipoma), or a renal ultrasound will detect polycystic kidneys. Facial adenoma sebaceum are actually angiofibromas, with consistent histologic features and on biopsy show a benign hamartomatous tumor composed of many cellular elements, including sebaceous glands, smooth muscle, blood vessels, and hair follicles.

Complications: Infrequently, the cerebral glial nodules undergo malignant transformation to a giant cell astrocytoma. More commonly the nodules may by their position or growth cause obstruction of the CSF pathway and an increase in intracranial pressure secondary to hydrocephalus. Optic atrophy may be the end result. Other eye complications include congenital blindness, cataract, and chorioretinitis. The rupture of a cyst within the lung parenchyma may produce a pneumothorax. More commonly, progressive dyspnea, hemoptysis, and pulmonary hypertension occur if the lung is involved. Tumors located within the kidney can cause obstruction, leading to pyelonephritis and uremia, and true polycystic kidneys can be rarely associated. Up to one-half may have rhabdomyomas of the heart which can be detected in the fetus at risk by echocardiogram.

Associated Findings: None known.

Etiology: Autosomal dominant inheritance, although it has been estimated that as many as 85% of the cases are the result of new mutations. Paternal age is not increased.

Pathogenesis: Unknown.

MIM No.: *19110

POS No.: 3417

CDC No.: 759.500

Sex Ratio: M1:F1

0975B-20838: Classical phakoma (mulberry). 20840: Flat, smooth phakoma.

Occurrence: 1:10,000 to 1:50,000 in all populations and ethnic groups studied.

Risk of Recurrence for Patient's Sib:
See Part I, *Mendelian Inheritance.*

Risk of Recurrence for Patient's Child:
See Part I, *Mendelian Inheritance.* The most severe cases do not reproduce because of death at an early age.

Age of Detectability: Shortly after birth, when the combination of infantile spasms and depigmented skin lesions is present. Calcifications and/or subependymal masses seen on CT scan may be confirmatory. At age two to five years, by physical examination and appropriate X-rays. Prenatal diagnosis has been reported (Journel et al, 1986).

Gene Mapping and Linkage: TSC1 (tuberous sclerosis 1) has been provisionally mapped to 9q.

Exclusion of linkage to 9p has been demonstrated for some families (Kandt et al, 1989).

Prevention: None known. Genetic counseling indicated.

Treatment: Anticonvulsants for the treatment of seizures. Dermatologic cosmetic procedures for facial angiofibromas. Occasional surgical removal of a strategically placed glial nodule of the brain. Treatment of the complications.

Prognosis: Asymptomatic patients with skin lesions and normal intelligence probably have a normal life span in the absence of renal failure or brain tumors. This is in contrast to severely retarded children with infantile spasms who probably have a progressive course with early death.

Detection of Carrier: Unknown.

Special Considerations: Careful investigation of first degree relatives of those affected should be undertaken prior to genetic counseling. This should include examination for pitted enamel hypoplasia (Lygidakis and Lindenbaum, 1987), of skin for cutaneous lesions, examination by an ophthalmologist for retinal phakomata, and CT scan of cranium and possibly kidneys. If these investigations are negative, the recurrence risk is low for subsequent sibs, in keeping with a new mutation. Two rare cases of affected sibs with unaffected parents have been reported.

Support Groups:
MA; Rockland; American Tuberous Sclerosis Association
IL; Winfield; National Tuberous Sclerosis Association
AUSTRALIA: NSW; Bulli; The Australian Tuberous Sclerosis Society
THE NETHERLANDS: Duiven; Stichting Tubereuze Sclerosis Nederland
SCOTLAND: Glasgow; Tuberous Sclerosis Association of Great Britain

References:
Monaghan HP, et al.: Tuberous sclerosis complex in children. Am J Dis Child 1981 135:912–917.
Baraitser M: The genetics of neurological disorders. New York: Oxford University Press, 1982.
Gutman I, et al.: Hypopigmented iris spot: an early sign of tuberous sclerosis. Am Acad Ophthalmol 1982; 89:1155–1159.
Cassidy SB, et al.: Family studies in tuberous sclerosis. J Am Med Assoc 1983; 249:1302–1304.
Sugita K, et al.: Tuberous sclerosis: report of two cases studied by computerized cranial tomography within one week after birth. Brain Dev 1985; 7:438–443.
Journel H, et al.: Prenatal diagnosis of familial tuberous sclerosis following detection of cardiac rhabdomyoma by ultrasound. Prenatal Diagnosis 1986; 6:283–289.
Fryer AE, et al.: Forehead plaque: a presenting skin sign in tuberous sclerosis. Arch Dis Child 1987; 62:292–304.
Grether P, et al.: Wilms' tumor in an infant with tuberous sclerosis. Ann Genet 1987; 30:183–185.
Hall JG, Byers PH: Genetics of tuberous sclerosis. (Letter) Lancet 1987; 28:751 only.
Lygidakis NA, Lindenbaum RH: Pitted enamel hypoplasia in tuberous sclerosis patients and first degree relatives. Clin Genet 1987; 32:216–221.
Roach ES, et al.: Magnetic resonance imaging in tuberous sclerosis. 1987; 44:301–303.
Gomez MR, ed: Tuberous sclerosis, 2nd ed. New York: Raven Press, 1988.
Kandt RS, et al.: Absence of linkage of tuberous sclerosis to the ABO blood group locus. Exp. Neurol 1989; 104:223–228.

HA053   **Robert H.A. Haslam**

Tubular ectasia
See KIDNEY, MEDULLARY SPONGE KIDNEY
Tubular male pseudohermaphroditism
See MULLERIAN DERIVATIVES IN MALES, PERSISTENT

Tubular nostril congenital
See NOSE, PROBOSCIS LATERALIS

TUBULAR STENOSIS   0976

Includes:
Dwarfism-congenital medullary stenosis
Dwarfism-cortical thickening of tubular bones
Hypocalcemia-dwarfism-cortical thickening of tubular bones
Kenny-Caffey syndrome
Kenny disease
Medullary stenosis, congenital
Tubular stenosis, Kenny type

Excludes:
Cleidocranial dysplasia (0185)
Osteopetrosis, benign dominant (0779)
Osteopetrosis, malignant recessive (0780)
Parathormone resistance (0830)
Pyknodysostosis (0846)
Silver syndrome (0887)

Major Diagnostic Criteria: Proportionate dwarfism; ophthalmologic abnormalities; epidsodic hypocalcemia; and characteristic X-ray findings, including cortical thickening and medullary stenosis of the long bones.

Clinical Findings: Small stature is often of prenatal origin. The anterior fontanel is usually quite large in early childhood, very late in closing, and associated with a widely split metopic suture. The forehead is prominent and appears especially so because the eyes are usually small. Hyperopia is characteristically present, and strabismus or pseudopapilledema may occur. Intelligence is usually normal.

Episodes of hypocalcemia and hyperphosphatemia often are present in infancy but may occur at any age. Such episodes may be precipitated by illness or surgery, and may cause tetany or seizures.

X-ray features are distinctive: narrow long bone diaphyses, with narrowing of the marrow cavities and thickening of the cortex. The metaphyses are overfunnelized, and there is absence of the diploic space in the skull. Skeletal maturation during childhood is delayed. Vertebrae, round bones, and facial bones are normal.

Complications: Episodes of hypocalcemic tetany or seizures may occur, especially in infancy or during periods of stress.

Associated Findings: Idiopathic hypoparathyroidism and other parathyroid anomalies. Abnormal hearing and dental anomalies have been reported.

Etiology: Autosomal dominant inheritance with variable expressivity.

Pathogenesis: Unknown.

MIM No.: *12700

POS No.: 3086

Sex Ratio: M1:F1

Occurrence: About 20 cases have been reported, all Caucasian.

Risk of Recurrence for Patient's Sib:
See Part I, *Mendelian Inheritance.*

Risk of Recurrence for Patient's Child:
See Part I, *Mendelian Inheritance.*

Age of Detectability: In infancy.

Gene Mapping and Linkage: Unknown.

Prevention: None known. Genetic counseling indicated.

Treatment: Vitamin D and calcium have been used succesfully to treat symptomatic hypocalcemia.

Prognosis: Apparently good for normal life span and intelligence, although one patient died unexpectantly at 19 years of age. Adult height has been 121–155 cm in affected females.

Detection of Carrier: Unknown.

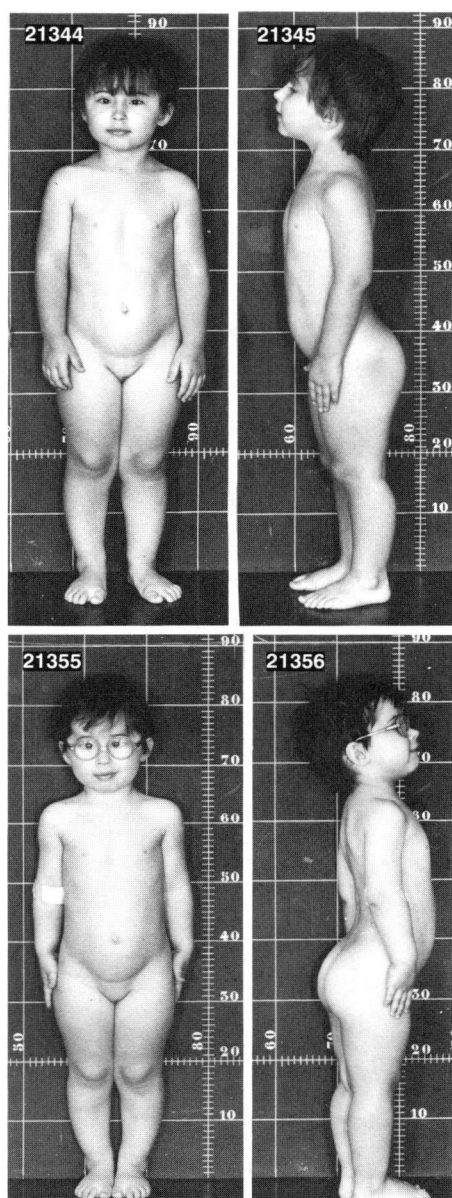

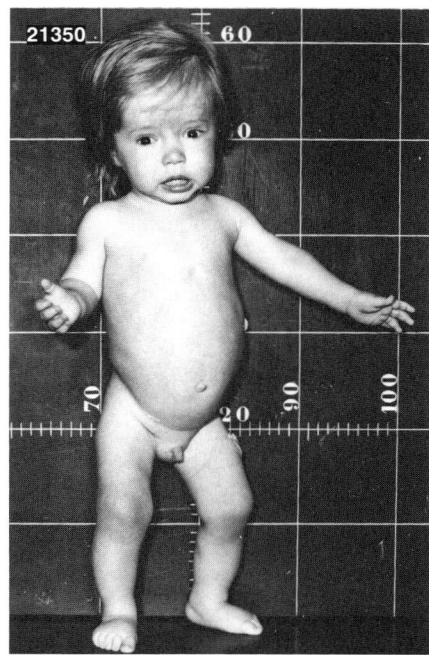

0976B-21350: Affected 1½-year-old male; note marked short stature, macrocephaly, and prominent forehead.

0976A-21344–56: Affected girls at 6½ (upper) and 6 years (lower) of age; note marked short stature, macrocephaly, mildly dysmorphic facies and microphthalmos.

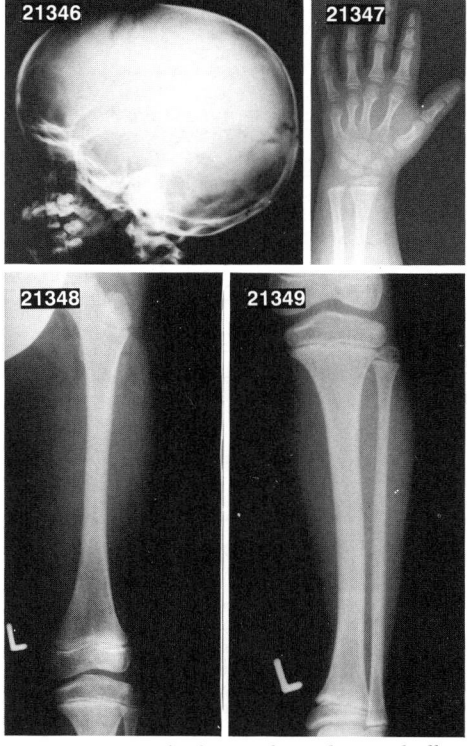

0976C-21346–49: X-ray findings show large skull with open anterior fontanel, absent diploic space and prominent forehead, medullary stenosis, mild brachymetacarpism, and cortical thickening of tubular bones.

References:
Kenny FM, Linarelli L: Dwarfism and cortical thickening of tubular bones. Am J Dis Child 1966; 111:201–207.
Caffey J: Congenital stenosis of medullary spaces in tubular bones and calvaria in two proportionate dwarfs - mother and son; coupled with transitory hypocalcemic tetany. Am J Roentgenol 1967; 100:1–11.
Boynton JR, et al.: Ocular findings in Kenny's syndrome. Arch Ophthalmol 1979; 97:896–900.
Lee WK, et al.: The Kenny-Caffey syndrome: growth retardation and hypocalcemia in a young boy. Am J Med Genet 1983; 14:773–782.
Larsen JL, et al.: Unusual cause of short stature. Am J Med 1985; 78:1025–1032.
Fanconi S, et al.: Kenny syndrome: evidence for idiopathic hypopara-

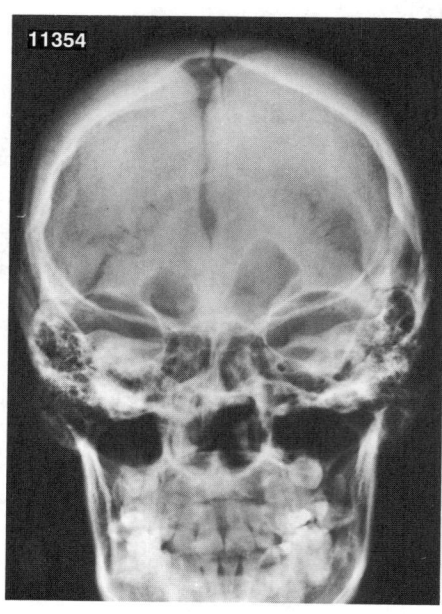
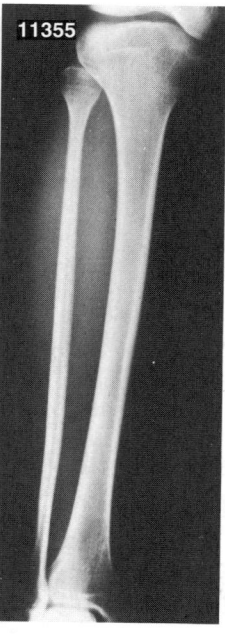

0976D-11354: Markedly thickened bony calvaria with wide open anterior fontanel and unfused metopic suture. **11355:** Stenosis of the diaphyseal portion of long bones, medullary canals severely constricted; in the fibula, almost obliterated.

thyroidism in two patients and for abnormal parathyroid hormone in one. J Pediatr 1986; 109:469–475.

FR017

J.M. Friedman

Tubular stenosis, Kenny type
See TUBULAR STENOSIS
Tubulointerstitial nephropathy, chronic idiopathic
See KIDNEY, NEPHRONOPHTHISIS-MEDULLARY CYSTIC DESEASE
Tuftsin deficiency
See IMMUNODEFICIENCY, TUFTSIN DEFICIENCY TYPE
Tumor, juxtavagal
See CAROTID BODY TUMOR
Tumor, mixed, of salivary gland
See SALIVARY GLAND, MIXED TUMOR
Tumors of the central nervous system, site-specific aggregation
See CANCER, NEUROEPITHELIAL AND MENINGEAL
Tune deafness
See DEAFNESS, TUNE
Turban tumors
See EPITHELIOMAS, HEREDITARY MULTIPLE CYSTIC
Turban tumors of scalp
See SCALP, CYLINDROMAS
Turbinate deformity
See NOSE, TURBINATE DEFORMITY

TURCOT SYNDROME   2739

Includes:
   Brain tumor-adenomatous polyposis syndrome
   Central nervous system tumors-polyposis of colon
   Colon (familial polyposis)-CNS tumors
   Glioma-polyposis
Excludes:
   Brain tumors-small numbers of colorectal adenomas in the
      young
   Cancer, glioma, familial (2839)
   Intestinal polyposis, type I (0535)
   Intestinal polyposis, type III (0536)

Major Diagnostic Criteria: Central nervous system tumor (medulloblastoma, glial cell tumor, or pituitary adenoma) in a patient affected with or at risk for adenomatous polyposis syndrome. These histopathologic types of brain tumors appear to be one of the several extraintestinal manifestations of **Intestinal polyposis, type I** which is characterized >100 colorectal adenomas, autosomal dominant inheritance, and a chromosomal marker on 5q21-q22.

Clinical Findings: The clinical findings are those of a brain tumor, with the neurologic manifestations dependent on the anatomic site. Clinical evidence of the brain tumor can either precede or follow onset of manifestations of adenomatous polyposis syndrome. Examination of parents, sibs, and offspring for evidence of adenomatous polyposis syndrome, including its extracolonic manifestations, may confirm the familial nature of the illness. However, affected members of the same family may demonstrate different patterns of extracolonic disease.

Complications: The clinical picture is usually dominated by the manifestations of the brain tumor. Colorectal carcinoma can result from polyposis if a preventive colectomy is not performed.

Associated Findings: Other extracolonic manifestations of adenomatous polyposis syndrome may be present, including epidermal inclusion cysts, **Retina, congenital hypertrophy of retinal pigment epithelium**, occult radio-opaque jaw lesions, and carcinomas of the thyroid and other extracolonic sites. Café-au-lait spots have been reported in several patients.

Etiology: **Intestinal polyposis, type I** is an autosomal dominantly inherited condition. Extracolonic manifestations, including brain tumors, are variable components of undetermined etiology.

Pathogenesis: Unknown.

MIM No.: *27630

Sex Ratio: M1:F1

Occurrence: Adenomatous polyposis syndrome (see **Intestinal polyposis, type I**) has an incidence of about 1:7,500 to 1:22,000 live births. Turcot syndrome occurs in less than 5% of pedigrees with adenomatous polyposis. Fewer than 100 cases have been documented.

Risk of Recurrence for Patient's Sib:
   See Part I, *Mendelian Inheritance.* For brain tumor, uncertain; rare sibs with Turcot syndrome have been reported.

Risk of Recurrence for Patient's Child:
   See Part I, *Mendelian Inheritance.* No cases of brain tumor in offspring of a patient with Turcot syndrome have been reported in the literature.

Age of Detectability: Adenomatous polyposis syndrome may be detectable *in utero* by use of the recently described chromosomal markers. Some clinical markers are apparent in childhood (elevated colonic mucosal ornithine decarboxylase activity, **Retina, congenital hypertrophy of retinal pigment epithelium**, presence of occult radio-opaque jaw lesions). The brain tumor may present clinically before or after the manifestations of adenomatous polyposis syndrome.

Gene Mapping and Linkage: APC (adenomatosis polyposis coli) has been mapped to 5q21-q22.

Prevention: None known. Genetic counseling indicated.

Treatment: Appropriate therapy for **Intestinal polyposis, type I** and brain tumor.

Prognosis: Outcome usually depends on results of the therapy of the brain tumor.

Detection of Carrier: N/A

Special Considerations: The literature contains reports of sibs with brain tumors and small numbers of colorectal adenomas occurring at a young age (Baughman syndrome). The relationship of this syndrome to Turcot syndrome must await the results of DNA studies.
   Although the eponym *Turcot syndrome* is used after the 1959 publication of J. Turcot et al., the first patient with this syndrome was reported in the literature in 1949 by H.W. Crail.

Support Groups: Atlanta; American Cancer Society

References:
Crail HW: Multiple primary malignancies arising in the rectum, brain, and thyroid. Naval Medical Bulletin 1949; 49:123–128.
Turcot J, et al.: Malignant tumors of the central nervous system associated with familial polyposis of the colon: report of two cases. Dis Colon Rectum 1959; 2:465–468.
Baughman FA Jr., et al.: The glioma-polyposis syndrome. New Engl J Med 1969; 281:1345–1346.
Bodmer WF, et al.: Localization of the gene for familial polyposis on chromosome 5. Nature 1987; 328:614–616.
Costa OL, et al.: Turcot syndrome: autosomal dominant or recessive transmission? Dis Colon Rectum 1987; 30:391–394.
Jarvis L, et al.: Turcot's syndrome: a review. Dis Colon Rectum 1988; 31:907–914.

HA078   **Stanley R. Hamilton**

Turner phenotype with normal karyotype
See NOONAN SYNDROME

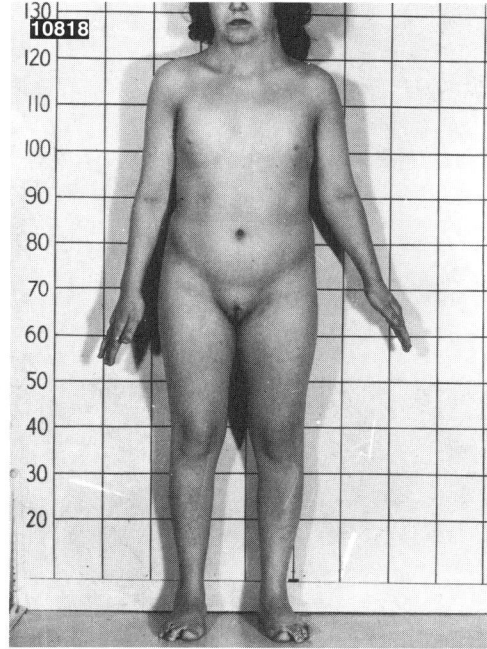

TURNER SYNDROME   0977

Includes:

    Chromosome X, monosomy X
    Chromosome 45,X syndrome
    Mosaic Turner syndrome
    Short stature-sexual infantilism
    Ullirch-Turner syndrome

Excludes:

    Chromosome 22, trisomy mosaicism (2478)
    Gonadal dysgenesis, XX type (0436)
    Gonadal dysgenesis, XY type (0437)
    Noonan syndrome (0720)

Major Diagnostic Criteria: A female should be tested for the diagnosis of Turner syndrome if during the newborn period she has edema of the hands and feet and excessive skin of the neck or if during childhood she has short stature, left-sided cardiac or aortic problems, particularly coarctation or dilation of the aorta. During the teenage period, the diagnosis should be suspected if there is delayed adolescence and primary amenorrhea, particularly if associated with short stature. In each of these situations, a karyotype should be obtained to establish or exclude Turner syndrome.

Since features found in the Turner syndrome are also seen in other conditions, a chromosomal analysis demonstrating partial or complete monosomy X or monosomy X mosaicism is mandatory to make the diagnosis. Cytogenetic analyses from several tissue sources may be necessary to detect a mosaic form of Turner syndrome. A buccal smear is not an adequate laboratory test to diagnose Turner syndrome and should never be used.

Clinical Findings: The frequency of the cardinal clinical features of Turner syndrome are small stature, often evident at birth (100%); ovarian dysgenesis with concomitant amenorrhea and sterility (>90%); lymphedema, with puffiness of the dorsum of the hands and feet, often noted at birth (40%); broad chest, sometimes with pectus excavatum, with widely spaced and often hypoplastic or inverted nipples (>80%); anomalous ears, most often prominent (80%); low posterior hairline with short-appearing neck (80%); narrow maxilla (palate) (80%); micrognathia (>70%); cubitus valgus (70%); narrow, hyperconvex, and deeply set nails (70%); renal anomalies (the most common being horseshoe kidney and double or cleft renal pelvis) (60%); redundant skin of the neck or webbed neck (50%); short metacarpals and metatarsals of the fourth digits (50%); pigmented nevi (50%); hearing impairment (50%); cardiac and aortic defects, including bicuspid aortic valves and coarctation, dilation, and rupture of the aorta (20–40%); and unexplained hypertension (27%).

Less common features of Turner syndrome include ptosis of the eyelids, hypertelorism, and vertebral and other skeletal anomalies. Dermatoglyphic features include an increase in hypothenar patterns, a distally placed palmar axial triradius, and large fin-

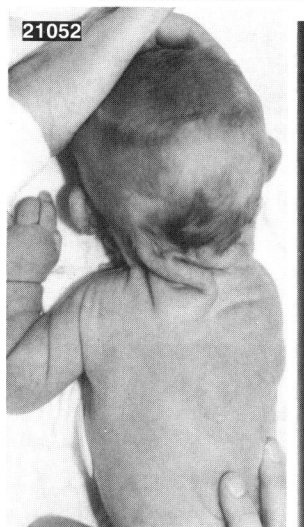
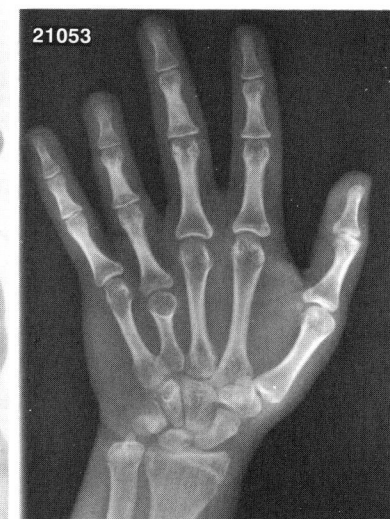

0977A-10818: Female with 45,X karyotype and webbed neck, shield-like chest, cubitus valgus and sexual infantilism.   21052: Newborn infant with 45,X karyotype and cystic hygroma.   21053: Hand X-ray of an adult with short 4th metacarpal and a resulting short 4th finger.

gertip patterns, most commonly whorls, with an increase in total ridge count. A transverse palmar crease (simian crease) is seen more often than in the general population. Secondary amenorrhea occurs infrequently and generally early.

Hypoplastic left heart syndrome occurs more frequently in Turner syndrome and may represent the extreme of the left-sided heart lesions seen in these patients. In addition, the incidence of congenital heart disease in Turner syndrome patients with webbing of the neck appears to be increased. For instance, Clark (1984) found that 30% of 106 patients with neck webbing had congenital heart disease, while only 9% of 87 patients without the webbing had a significant heart defect. One explanation for this is that

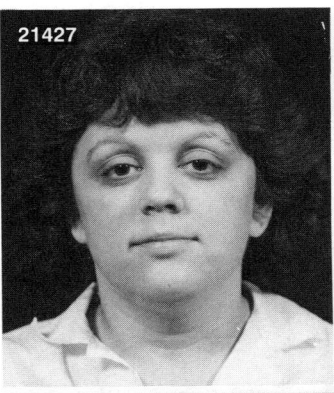
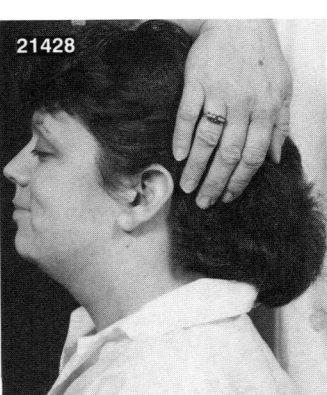
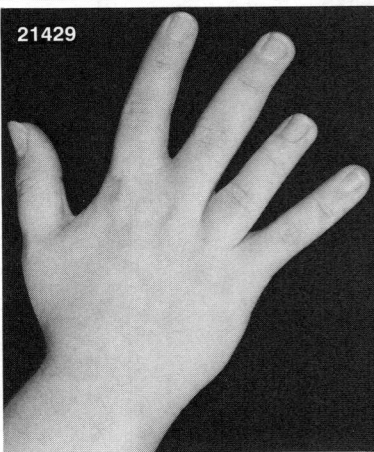
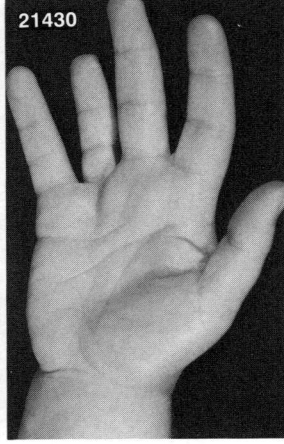

0977B-21427–28: AP and lateral views of a 24-year-old woman with 45,X/46,Xr(X)/46, X,i(Xq). This patient has a high arched palate, but does not have neck webbing. **21429:** Right hand shows short 4th finger due to a short 4th metacarpal. **21430:** Palm of the right hand shows a rearrangement of the creases of the base of the 4th finger.

lymphedema compresses the ascending aorta, altering the intracardiac blood flow.

Earlier studies suggested an increased incidence in mental retardation among females with Turner syndrome. It is now recognized that this is not the case, but affected individuals may have a deficiency in spatial ability that will affect their performance on standard IQ tests. Verbal skills are reportedly normal.

In general, no single one of the above clinical findings is found in every patient, and, likewise, no one patient exhibits every clinical feature listed.

Complications: Coarctation, hypertension, and aortic dilation may require treatment. Aortic dissection may develop as a result of the aortic dilation and may be lethal if not treated promptly. Females with 45,X or 45,X/46,XX karyotypes are generally not considered at increased risk for gonadal neoplasias. However, with 45,X/46,XY mosaicism, the Y-bearing cell line does predispose these patients to these neoplasias. Thus, any Turner syndrome patient with a Y chromosome cell line must have her gonads surgically removed.

Psychologic problems may result from sexual infantilism, short stature, primary amenorrhea, and sterility.

Associated Findings: Turner females may have an increase incidence of thyroiditis, diabetes mellitus, and collagen-vascular disease.

Etiology: The most frequent karyotype in Turner syndrome is 45,X, i.e. complete monosomy X. Mosaic individuals may be 45,X/46,XX, in which case the effects of the monosomic cell line may be mitigated by the normal cell line. In addition, structural abnormalities of the X chromosome may produce partial monosomy of either the p or q arms or both. When one of the short arms is deleted, the Turner phenotype is invariably present, while normal gonadal development and function is generally preserved. However, this function is lost if the deletion extends to the proximal region of Xp11. Monosomy for Xq produces gonadal dysgenesis when the breakpoint is at or proximal to Xq21, with about one-half of the patients showing signs of Turner syndrome. Pure gonadal dysgenesis has been observed when the breakpoint is at or distal to Xq22 (Passarge and Schmidt, 1983).

Karyotypes found in patients with Turner syndrome

Karyotype	Description	Percent of cases
45,X	Complete monosomy X	57 %
46,X,i(Xq) and mosaics with i(xq)	Isochromosome of the long arm of the X chromosome (monosomy Xp)	17 %
Mosaics 45,X/46XX; 45,X/47,XXX; etc	Mosaic monosomy	12 %
45,X/46XY	Mosaic monosomy X with Y-bearing cell line	4 %
Other (del(Xp), r(X), mosaics)	Xp monosomy, ring X	10 %

Pathogenesis: Monosomy X may occur as a result of nondisjunction during gametogenesis in either the mother or the father, or it may be the result of errors in mitosis after fertilization. An increased incidence of Turner syndrome births among older mothers has not been demonstrated. In fact, in testable cases, the paternal-derived sex chromosome is more often missing than the maternal X chromosome. This would suggest that a meiotic error in spermatogenesis or a loss of the paternal X or Y chromosome through mitotic error is the more usual cause.

It is unclear why either deletions of the short arm of an X chromosome or a missing X chromosome produces the Turner phenotype. It is clear that monosomy X is highly lethal prenatally, since cytogenetic investigations of spontaneous abortions indicate that more than 95% of Turner conceptuses do not reach term.

With regard to oogenesis and development of ovaries in Turner syndrome, evaluation of 45,X embryos and fetuses has shown that ovarian development is normal. Subsequently, the rate of degeneration of the primary oocytes appears to be increased over that in 46,XX females. Consequently, by puberty there are few, if any, oocytes remaining in the ovaries of Turner individuals. However, there is the occasional Turner female who develops secondary sexual characteristics and menses and may be fertile. In these women, the germ cell attrition rate is most likely less, and oocytes are present at puberty and beyond. These cases may represent the extreme end of the spectrum of germ cell degeneration, or they may be cases of Turner mosaicism. Turner mosaics frequently have normal puberty, are often fertile, but have earlier onset of menopause.

Patients with 45,X/46,XY mosaicism may have clitoral enlargement at birth and virilize to an extent at puberty. The pathogenesis of gonadal tumors in these individuals is not understood.

The lymphedema seen in Turner syndrome results from atresia, hypoplasia, and delayed development of the lymphatic system. The edema seen in fetuses is frequently profound and may be detected prenatally by ultrasound as hydrops fetalis or cystic hygroma.

POS No.: 3104

CDC No.: 758.610, 758.600

Sex Ratio: M0:F1

Occurrence: A minimum estimate of 1:5,000 live births.

Risk of Recurrence for Patient's Sib: Very low unless an identical twin.

Risk of Recurrence for Patient's Child: More than 99% of Turner syndrome patients are sterile. A study of pregnancies among women with 45,X and various mosaic karyotypes identified 54 pregnancies that resulted in 16 miscarriages, one termination, 12 abnormal children, three stillborns, and 22 normal live-born. The abnormalities included neural tube defects, **Chromosome 21, trisomy 21**, and Turner syndrome mosaicism. These observations may represent biases in ascertainment in that most of these children were first identified at birth as having congential or chromosomal abnormalities that resulted in the chromosomal analysis of their mothers. As might be expected, the reproductive record of Turner women who were identified first is better than those recognized retrospectively.

Age of Detectability: Prenatally through adulthood.

Gene Mapping and Linkage: See *Gene Map.*

Prevention: None known. Genetic counseling indicated.

Treatment: Cyclic estrogen replacement therapy is usually begun in the second decade of life in patients lacking sexual development. The therapy should be delayed for as long as possible to allow for maxium growth in height. However, much delay may not be possible for psychologic reasons if the girl is disturbed because she is not maturing at the same rate as her peers. Some authorities recommend the use of anabolic steroids for several years prior to the onset of estrogen therapy in an effort to increase the growth rate. More recent studies report the use of synthetic human growth hormone with encouraging preliminary results. In one study, administering human growth hormone in conjunction with anabolic steroids produced the greatest growth response.

Surgical intervention may be necessary for cardiovascular and renal anomalies, ptosis of the eyelids, and webbing of the neck. Surgical removal of any remaining gonadal tissue is indicated if a Y-bearing cell line is present. Vision and hearing defects may need to be corrected, and orthondontic treatment for dental malocclusion may be necessary. Supportive counseling or psychotherapy may be necessary because of short stature, lack of sexual development, and sterility. If learning disabilities occur, special education may be required.

Although the vast majority of women with Turner syndrome have been incapable of reproduction, they usually have normal uteruses. There are now cases reported in which embryos were transplanted in the uteruses of the Turner individuals who then carried the resulting pregnancies to term. Appropriate prepregnancy and intrapregnancy hormonal support was needed in each case.

Prognosis: Life span is presumably normal if there are no cardiovascular and renal anomalies, hypertension, and gonadal tumors, or if these conditions are treated.

Detection of Carrier: Unknown.

Special Considerations: The clinical features listed are based on cases with 45,X karyotypes. If a 46,XX cell line exists, these features may mitigate the effects of the monosomy X cell line. Thus, the frequency of sexual development, menses, and fertility is greater in the mosaic female, and other physical problems may be absent or less severe. Additionally, the mean ultimate height of mosaic patients is greater than that of nonmosaic Turner syndrome patients.

In nonmosaic patients with 46, X,i(Xq) karyotype, the phenotype is not significantly different from that seen in nonmosaic monosomy X. The severity of the phenotypic alterations in 46,X,r(X) and 46,X,del(Xp) patients may roughly correlate with the extent of deletion of the short arm of X. A deletion of the long arm of the X chromosome does produce gonadal dysgenesis, with resulting sexual infantilism, amenorrhea, and sterility. While the majority of patients with Xq deletions do not exhibit the typical phenotypic features of Turner syndrome, there are reported patients with short stature and the somatic features of Turner syndrome who have Xq deletions. Phenotypic variation appears to correlate with the break point on the long arm.

Support Groups:
CA; Sacramento; Turner's Syndrome Society of Sacramento
MD; Baltimore; Human Growth Foundation
NJ; Somerset; Turner's Syndrome Support Group
CANADA: Ontario; Downsview; Turner's Syndrome Society

References:
Turner HH: A syndrome of infantilism, congenital webbed neck, and cubitus valgus. Endocrinology 1938; 23:566. *
Palmer CG, Reichmann A: Chromosomal and clinical findings in 100 females with Turner syndrome. Hum Genet 1976; 35:35–49.
Simpson JL: Disorders of sexual differentiation. Chicago: Year Book Medical Publishers, 1977:259–302. *
Dewhurst J: Fertility in 47,XXX and 45,X patients. J Med Genet 1978; 15:132–135.
Passarge P, Schmidt A: Functional consequences of X-chromosome loss in the human female. In: Sandberg A, ed: Cytogenetics of the mammalian X chromosome, Part B: X chromosome anomalies and their clinical manifestations. New York: Alan R. Liss, 1983:301–320.
Bender B, et al.: Cognitive development of unselected girls with complete and partial X monosomy. Pediatrics 1984; 73:175–182.
Clark EB: Neck web and congenital heart defects: a pathogenic association in 45 X-O turner syndrome? Teratology 1984, 29:355–361.
Hassold T, et al.: Determination of the parental origin of sex-chromosome monosomy using restriction fragment length polymorphisms. Am J Hum Genet 1985; 37:965–972.
Lin AE, et al.: Aortic dilation, dissection, and rupture in patients with Turner syndrome. J Pediatr 1986; 109:820–826.
Rosenfeld RG, et al.: Methionyl human growth hormone and oxandrolone in Turner syndrome: preliminary results of a prospective randomized trial. J Pediatr 1986; 109:936–943. *
Knudtzon J, Aarskog D: 45,X/46,XY mosaicism: a clinical review and report of ten cases. Eur J Pediatr 1987; 146:266–271.
Massarano AA, et al.: Ovarian ultrasound appearances in Turner syndrome. J Pediatr 1989; 114:568–573.

DA029
WE005
**Margaret A. Davee
David D. Weaver**

Turner syndrome phenotype
See NECK, CYSTIC HYGROMA, FETAL TYPE
Turner syndrome, familial
See NOONAN SYNDROME
Turner tooth
See TEETH, ENAMEL HYPOPLASIA
Turner-Kieser syndrome
See NAIL-PATELLA SYNDROME
Turricephaly
See CRANIOSYNOSTOSIS
Twin-to-twin transfusion
See FETAL MONOZYGOUS MULTIPLE PREGNANCY DYSPLACENTATION EFFECTS

TWINS, CONJOINED   **0202**

Includes:
Conjoined twins
Craniopagus
Dicephalus
Diprosopus
Dipygus
Ischiopagus
Monozygotic twins, conjoined
Omphalopagus
Pygopagus
Rachipagus
Siamese twins
Syncephalus
Terata anacatadidymus
Terata anadidymus
Terata catadidymus
Thoracopagus

Excludes: Parasitic twinning

Major Diagnostic Criteria: Fusion of some portion of monovular or monozygotic twins.

Clinical Findings: Diagnosis evident by physical examination. The visceral conjunction between the co-twins requires X-ray,

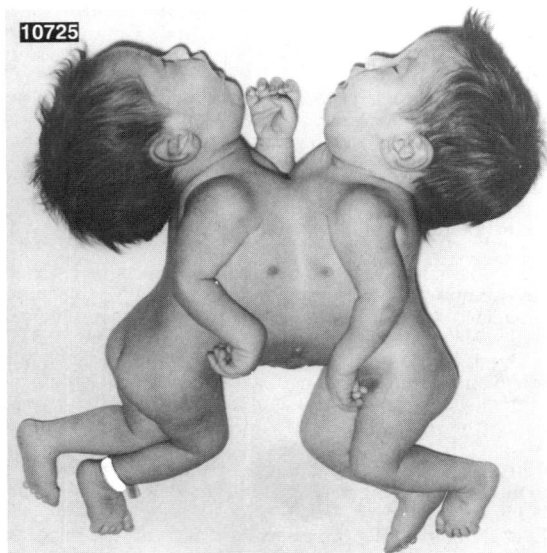

0202A-10725:   Lateral view of thoracopagus twins.

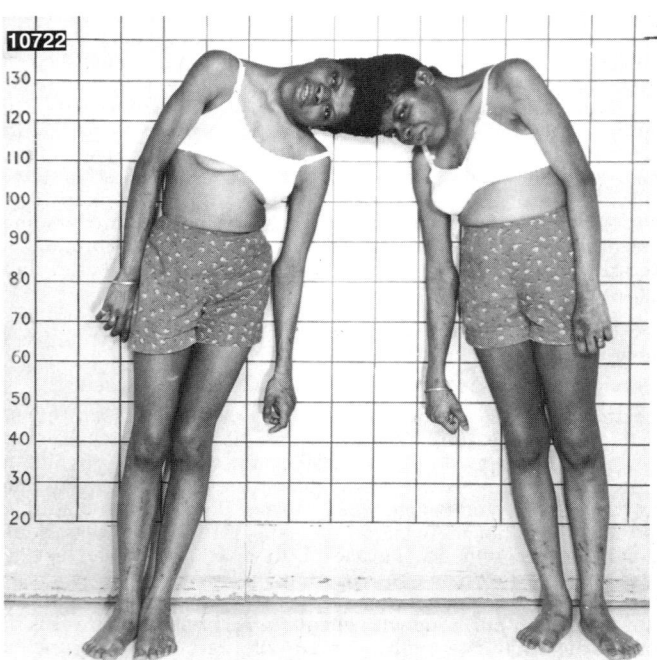

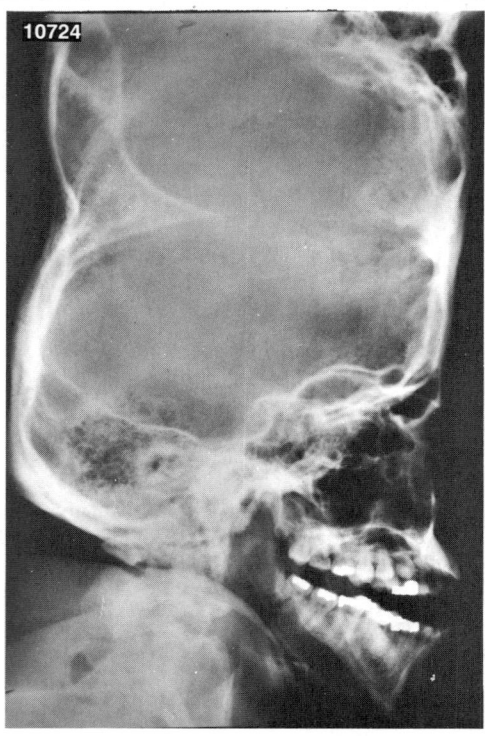

isotope and ultrasound techniques to outline anatomic and functional interdependence. Diagnosis can be made in utero by the use of X-ray or ultrasound techniques. Common types of fusion include:

Terata catadidymus - fusion caudally

Diprosopus - single trunk and limbs, varying duplication of face and head

Dicephalus - single trunk and limbs, duplication of head

Ischiopagus - Fusion at ischia, the axis of the 2 bodies being at 180° - 6% +

Pygopagus - fusion in sacral region - 19% +

Terata anadidymus - fusion in cephalic region

Dipygus - fusion limited to region proximal to pelvis

Syncephalus - Single head, separation below head

Craniopagus - fusion at the head - 2% +

Terata anacatadidymus - fusion in midportion of body

Thoracopagus - fusion in sternal region - 74% +

Omphalopagus - fusion in abdominal region

Rachipagus - fusion back to back in sagittal plane, fusion limited to upper trunk and cervical region

Rudolph et al (1967) reviewed 117 cases; the basic problem in thoracopagus is whether separate hearts allow surgery. In ischiopagus, pygopagus and craniopagus decisions need to be made concerning which twin will benefit from single shared organs.

Complications: All cases with conjoined hearts have died with or without the aid of surgery. Unexplained postoperative deaths have occurred, therefore, careful postoperative monitoring is required.

Associated Findings: Nearly all cases of dicephalus and diprosopus have associated neural tube defects.

Etiology: Conjoined twins are the product of a single ovum. They are monovular or monozygotic twins. Teratogenesis occurs by incomplete fission during the process of twinning. While monozygotic twinning is considered uninfluenced by genetic factors, Harvey et al (1977) has reported on ten families with multiple pairs of monozygotic twins. Derom et al (1987) has reported a significant increase in the frequency of zygotic splitting producing monozygotic twins and triplets after artificial induction of ovulation.

Pathogenesis: According to Zimmermann (1967), the morula becomes a blastocyst on day 6 of ovulation age. Within this vesicle, 0.2–0.3 mm in length, the inner cell mass develops at one

0202B-10722:   Conjoined craniophagus twins at 23 years of age. 10724:   Lateral view of skulls showing bony fusion and projecting bony shelf.

pole. The inner cell mass is totipotent for morphogenesis and organogenesis. For a short time, this cell mass has the potentialities of forming a single or dual embryologic primordium or germinal disk. The caudal end, appearing between 15 and 18 days of embryonic age, represents the primitive streak which is the primordium of all intraembryogenic mesoderm. Terata are the result either of disordered morphogenesis or organogenesis. By day 20 the process of either normal twinning or conjoined twinning will be initiated. The end of the 3rd week of development age marks the end of the period of incomplete fission. The anomalous twinning can occur at any point of incomplete division of the inner cell mass accounting for the variations in types of conjoined twins.

MIM No.: 27641

CDC No.: 759.4

Sex Ratio: M3:F7

Occurrence: 0.06:1000 live births in India and Africa; 0.004:1000 live births in Europe and the Americas. Prevalence rare.

Risk of Recurrence for Patient's Sib: Undetermined but presumably rare.

Risk of Recurrence for Patient's Child: Undetermined but presumably rare.

Age of Detectability: At birth or prenatally.

Gene Mapping and Linkage: Unknown.

Prevention: None known. Genetic counseling indicated.

Treatment: Extent of cardiac anomalies not detectable before 8 weeks of fetal development. The presence of twins with a single fetal EKG is the most serious condition.

Surgical separations have been successfully performed on all conjoined twins with exception of those thoracopagus with conjoined hearts. Although experience is scanty, it is probable that other anomalies of fission can be managed by existing rehabilitation procedures.

Prognosis: Although conjoined twins have lived as long as 63 years without separation, surgical separation is the management of choice. Psychologic studies of unoperated twins reveal serious limitations to the quality of life. The rehabilitation of any postoperative defects due to incomplete fission of shared organs and tissues is vital to the success of the surgical approach. The general experience has been that optimal surgical management requires a well-rehearsed surgical and pediatric team. In the absence of a single heart, the procedure should not be carried out under emergency conditions. At present, there are no survivors following division of a single heart, however, it is expected that this will become possible with continuing advances in cardiovascular surgery.

Detection of Carrier: Unknown.

Special Considerations: Steps in evaluation of operability: 1) Physical examination to differentiate thoracopagus and omphalopagus twins; operative separation of omphalopagus twins. 2) EKG with standard leads to determine ventricular independence; operative separation of those with separate QRS complexes (25%). 3) Angiography with physiologic study to determine great vessel and atrial communication; operative separation of conjoined atrium (10%) and 4) Ethical considerations; e.g. whether only one twin can survive with existing shared ventricular structure (68%).

Support Groups:
RI; Providence; The Twins Foundation
MD; Rockville; National Organization of Mothers of Twin Clubs

References:
Nichols BL, et al.: General clinical management of thoracopagus twins. In: Bergsma D, ed: Conjoined twins. BD:OAS 1967; III(1):28. White Plains: The National Foundation-March of Dimes.
Rudolph AJ, et al.: Obstetric management of conjoined twins. In Bergsma D, ed: Conjoined twins. BD:OAS 1967; III(1):38. White Plains: The National Foundation-March of Dimes.
Zimmermann AA: Embryologic and anatomic considerations of conjoined twins. In Bergsma D, ed: Conjoined twins. BD:OAS 1967; III(1):18. White Plains: The National Foundation-March of Dimes.
Harvey MAS, et al.: Familial monozygotic twinning. J Pediat 1977; 90:246–248.
Benirscke K, et al.: Conjoined twins: nosology and congenital malformations. BD:OAS 1978; XIV(6A):179. White Plains: The National Foundation-March of Dimes.
Edmonds LD, Layde PM: Conjoined twins in the United States, 1970–1977. Teratology 1982; 25:301.
Derom C, et al.: Increased monozygotic twinning rate after ovulation induction. Lancet 1987; I:1236–1238.
Cunniff C, et al.: Laterality defects in conjoined twins. Am J Med Genet 1988; 31:669–677.

NI003 **Buford L. Nichols**

TWINS, CONJOINED, TERATOGENICITY **2928**

Includes:
Clomaphene ovulation induction and conjoined twins
Griseofulvin exposure and conjoined twins
Valproic acid and conjoined twins

Excludes: Fetal effects (other)

Major Diagnostic Criteria: Possible teratogenic exposure causing conjoined twinning.

Clinical Findings: Several suspicious periconceptional drug exposures have been reported with conjoined twinning. Two cases of conjoined twins with periconceptional maternal griseofulvin exposure have been separately reported to the Food and Drug Administration. Griseofulvin is an orally administered agent for fungus infections, usually epidermal. Because of the rarity of conjoined twins (about 1:20,000 pregnancies), and the infrequency of maternal first trimester griseofulvin exposure (about 1:2,000), this coincidence is unlikely to have occurred by chance. Both of the outcomes with griseofulvin exposure were thoracopagus, which consitute about 18% of conjoined twins. Record studies of 86 other cases of conjoined twins did not find a griseofulvin exposure, but this is inadequate to rule out an association, because of the rarity of griseofulvin exposure.

Seven cases of conjoined twinning have been reported with clomaphene ovulation induction (two published). Only one set occurred in cohort studies totalling 5,519 clomaphene inductions. This indicates this is a rare occurrence with clomaphene induction. Clomaphene is a much more frequent pregnancy exposure than griseofulvin. Two of the clomaphene exposed cases were detected among 61 conjoined twins in two birth defect registries. Case control study of conjoined twins is necessary to determine if clomaphene exposure is more frequent than expected.

One set of conjoined twins with associated spina bifida has been reported to FDA with maternal exposure to an antiepileptic combination including valproic acid. Valproic acid is known to be associated with spina bifida, and spina bifida is known to be associated with conjoined twinning.

Complications: Unknown.

Associated Findings: None known.

Etiology: Where a drug teratogen is associated with conjoined twinning, the etiology could be either the agent or the indication for which the agent is given. Subfertility for which clomaphene is given could be the actual true association. In this case, an association may be found with subfertility management other than clomaphene. Epilepsy for which valproic acid is given, or fungus infections for which griseofulvin is given, have less causal plausibility.

Pathogenesis: Interference with completion of twinning fission of blastula from 15–20 days following ovulation. Griseofulvin is known to be an animal teratogen. It affects microtubules, which have a role in spindle formation. Other agents having such an effect include vincristine, podophyllotoxin, and colchicine.

Sex Ratio: Presumably M1:F1.

Occurrence: For these suspicious exposures, data is inadequate to establish that conjoined twinning is a result of exposure, but adequate to show that association is infrequent.

Risk of Recurrence for Patient's Sib: Unknown.

Risk of Recurrence for Patient's Child: Unknown.

Age of Detectability: Prenatal detection by ultrasound is possible.

Gene Mapping and Linkage: Unknown.

Prevention: Because griseofulvin treatment is seldom urgent, use should be avoided in early pregnancy. With accidental exposure, most outcomes are likely to be normal.

Treatment: Unknown.

Prognosis: Unknown.

Detection of Carrier: N/A

Special Considerations: The FDA Division of Drug Experience urges exposure inquiries and reports on any conjoined twins.

This article expresses the views of the author and is not an official statement of the Food and Drug Administration.

References:

Carlson DH, et al.: Cephalothoracopagus syncephalus: prenatal roentgenographic diagnosis. Pediat Radiol 1975; 3:50–52.
Edmunds LD, Layde PM: Conjoined twins in the U.S., 1970–1977. Teratology 1982; 25:301–308.
Brenbridge AN, Teja K: Sonographic findings in the prenatal diagnosis of cephalothoracopagus syncephalus. J Reprod Med 1987; 32:59–62.
Knudsen LB: No association between griseofulvin and conjoined twinning. Lancet 1987; II:1097.
Rosa FW, et al.: Griseofulvin teratology including two thoracopagus conjoined twins. Lancet 1987; I:171. *

R0018   **Franz W. Rosa**

Twins, parasitic conjoined without spinal columns
  See LIMBS, SUPERNUMERARY
Two-Chambered right ventricle
  See VENTRICLE, DOUBLE CHAMBERED RIGHT
Two-oxoglutaric aciduria
  See ACIDEMIA, 2-OXOGLUTARIC
Tylosis
  See KERATOSIS PALMARIS ET PLANTARIS OF UNNA-THOST
Tylosis with malignancy
  See HOWEL EVANS SYNDROME
Typical retinoschisis, autosomal dominant
  See RETINOSCHISIS
Typus degenerativus Amstelodamensis
  See DE LANGE SYNDROME
Typus Edinburgensis
  See EDINBURGH MALFORMATION SYNDROME
Tyrosinase negative oculocutaneous albinism
  See ALBINISM, OCULOCUTANEOUS, TYROSINASE NEGATIVE
Tyrosinase positive oculocutaneous albinism
  See ALBINISM, OCULOCUTANEOUS, TYROSINASE POSITIVE
Tyrosine 77 amyloidosos
  See AMYLOIDOSIS, ILLINOIS TYPE
Tyrosine aminotransferase deficiency
  See TYROSINEMIA II, OREGON TYPE
Tyrosine transaminase deficiency
  See TYROSINEMIA II, OREGON TYPE
Tyrosinemia and tyrosyluria, hereditary
  See TYROSINEMIA I

TYROSINEMIA I   **0978**

Includes:

> Four-hydroxyphenylpyruvic acid oxidase deficiency
> Fumarylacetoacetase deficiency
> Hepatorenal tyrosinemia
> Tyrosinemia and tyrosyluria, hereditary
> Tyrosinemia III
> Tyrosinosis, acute and chronic

Excludes:

> Tyrosinemia and tyrosyluria associated with disease states
> Tyrosinemia and tyrosyluria, transient of newborn
> **Tyrosinemia II, Oregon type** (2009)

Major Diagnostic Criteria: Clinical evidence of hepatic cellular damage and renal tubular defect, in association with hypertyrosinemia and a distinctive aminoaciduria. There is persistent elevation of the concentration of tyrosine in plasma above 3 mg/dl with normal or slightly elevated levels of plasma phenylalanine,

(phenylalanine/tyrosine ratio less than 1.0) and urinary hyperexcretion of tyrosyl compounds (p-hydroxyphenyllactic, p-hydroxyphenylpyruvic, and p-hydroxyphenylacetic acids) in the fasting state. Concentrations of alpha-fetoprotein in the blood are elevated. The currently accepted diagnostic feature is the excretion of large amounts of succinylacetone in the urine.

Differential diagnosis should include hereditary fructose intolerance, galactosemia, neonatal hepatitis, and congenital CMV infection.

Transient tyrosinemia of the newborn also presents with elevated concentrations of tyrosine in plasma, along with normal or slightly elevated phenylalanine and tyrosyluria. This condition appears to have no significant clinical sequelae. The elevation of tyrosine and tyrosyluria in this condition occur within the first 2 weeks of life and usually persists for one to two months, but it may persist for longer periods. The alteration of tyrosine metabolism seen in this condition is indicative of delayed maturation of liver enzyme systems and not a true inborn error of metabolism. It is more apt to occur in immature infants who ingest high-protein formula without vitamin C. Administration of high doses of vitamin C results in rapid return to normal of elevated plasma tyrosine levels. See **Tyrosinemia II, Oregon type**.

Clinical Findings: There are two variant patterns: acute and chronic.

The *acute form* is represented by most of the reported patients. Onset of symptoms occurs under one year of age. The presenting symptoms frequently are general manifestations such as temperature elevation, lethargy, and irritability; failure to thrive, however, has been the presenting complaint in nearly all cases. Hepatomegaly with or without abdominal distention, jaundice, or hepatic cirrhosis, has been found in more than 80% of patients. Vomiting, edema, ascites, and peculiar odor occur in at least one-half of the cases. Progressive hepatic failure may result in jaundice, anemia, ecchymosis, hemorrhage, melena, hematuria hypoproteinemia, diarrhea and, as noted in nearly one-third of patients, often in the terminal stage, demise is rapid.

The *chronic form* of hereditary tyrosinemia has been reported in a relatively small number of patients. Symptoms develop secondary to renal tubular dysfunction, and patients present with rickets and a less severe degree of hepatic cirrhosis. Most of these patients died under ten years of age; exceptions include a few recently reported patients between the ages of 12 and 20 years, several of whom have benefited from dietary treatment and hepatic transplantation.

Mental retardation and neurologic abnormalities are not constant findings.

Biochemical determinations in affected persons with acute or chronic hereditary tyrosinemia show elevated plasma levels of tyrosine above 3 mg/dl, with range of 3–12 mg/dl, (normal: < 1 mg/dl) and constant hyperexcretion of tyrosyl compounds (p-hydroxyphenyllactic acid, p-hydroxyphenylpyruvic acid, and p-hydroxyphenylacetic acid) in the fasting state. Increased levels of succinylacetone and succinylacetic acid in serum and urine, and increased urinary excretion of δ-aminolevulinic acid have been reported in the majority of recent cases.

Plasma levels of phenylalanine are usually not elevated.

Other significant urinary findings are a generalized aminoaciduria; hyperphosphaturia; proteinuria; and the presence of reducing substances, usually glucose.

Hypophosphatemia; reduced prothrombin-proconvertin index; hypoglycemia; elevated concentrations of alpha-fetoprotein; and elevated methionine in serum are frequent laboratory findings, particularly in terminal stages of hepatic failure.

X-rays demonstrate the characteristic bony changes of rickets.

Complications: Hepatic cirrhosis, resulting in hepatic failure and death in over 80% of cases; a complex renal tubular defect, producing a generalized aminoaciduria; hypophosphatemic rickets, more common in chronic form of hereditary tyrosinemia; and a coagulation defect, evidenced by ecchymosis, melena, hematuria, and prothrombin abnormality in about one-third of the cases.

Associated Findings: Hepatoma (hepatocarcinoma) has been reported in over 30% of patients with tyrosinemia I who survive beyond two years of age; evidence suggests this is due to factors other than cirrhosis. The median age of death is reported to be five years, with a range from four to 25 years.

A few individuals have been reported with intermittent attacks of severe pain in the abdomen and legs, hypertensive crisis, and increased urinary excretion of δ-aminolevulinic acid.

A single case of diabetes mellitus has been reported. There is theoretical speculation that hyperkalemia, hypophosphatemia, and hypermethioninemia may contribute to pancreatic dysfunction; pancreatic islet cell hyperplasia and hypoglycemia have been observed. Tyrosinemia I has been reported in a child with partial monosomy 4p-.

Etiology: Autosomal recessive inheritance. Specific data are not available to answer whether or not the observed impairment of enzyme activity of p-hydroxyphenylpyruvic acid oxidase, or of fumarylacetoacetase, represents the primary expression of the abnormal gene. Finding acute and chronic cases in a single family strengthens the hypothesis that there is one disease process, which has variable clinical manifestations.

The one individual with "tyrosinosis" reported by Medes appears to represent a different inborn error of metabolism, with the enzymatic block resulting in hyperexcretion of p-hydroxyphenylpyruvic acid, which is greater than the excretion of other tyrosyl compounds. This strongly suggests that the site of the block was in p-hydroxyphenylpyruvic acid oxidase, but the disorder is clearly different from that found in patients with "hereditary tyrosinemia." Medes' patient had myasthenia gravis but was essentially unaffected by the biochemical abnormality (tyrosinosis). A patient with mild retardation, seizures, abnormal EEG, and CT scan associated with defective activity of p-hydroxyphenylpyruvic acid oxidase and normal tyrosine aminotransferase and fumarylacetoacetase activities has been reported. This patient may represent the same disorder described by Medes, although the case has been cataloged as a new varient of hypertyrosinemia; *Tyrosinemia III* or *Four-hydroxyphenylpyruvic acid oxidase deficiency*.

Pathogenesis: Several enzyme defects have been established in hepatic, renal and other organ tissues in affected patients. A marked deficiency of the enzyme p-hydroxyphenylpyruvic acid oxidase in hepatic and renal tissues has been reported whenever enzyme assays have been determined. This enzyme defect results in tyrosinemia and tyrosyluria. Data suggest that the decreased enzyme activity of p-HPPA oxidase found in this disorder may be secondary to liver disease, rather than causitive.

A deficiency of the enzyme fumarylacetoacetic acid hydrolase (fumarylacetoacetase), catalyzing the last step in the degradation of tyrosine, has been documented. This enzyme activity is markedly deficient in hepatic and renal tissue of affected patients, as well as in lymphocytes, skin fibroblasts, and cultured amniotic fluid cells. The resultant accumulation of its metabolites, succinylacetoacetate, succinylacetone, and furmarylacetone, partially explain multiple other enzyme deficiencies observed in this disease. These data have led to the suggestion that fumarylacetoacetase deficiency may be the primary enzyme defect in the pathogenesis of this disorder.

Methionine adenosyltransferase, cystathionine synthase, and tyosine aminotransferase (TAT) are reportedly decreased in the liver of patients with this condition.

The molecular defect of this disorder remains unclear. Clinical and biochemical variability observed in these patients point to the possibility that it may be due to a defect in a regulatory gene common for p-hydroxyphenylpyruvic acid oxidase and fumarylacetoacetase.

MIM No.: *27670, *27671

Sex Ratio: M1:F1

Occurrence: Varies among different populations. An estimated 146:100,000 live births, and an estimated 1 carrier for every 14 persons has been determined in an isolated French Canadian population, as compared to an overall incidence of 8:100,000 in the French Canadian population of Quebec. Newborn screening in Norway and Sweden established a prevalence of 1:120,000 and

1:100,000 respectively. Approximately 100 cases, acute and chronic form, have been reported in the literature; most during the past 25 years.

Risk of Recurrence for Patient's Sib:
See Part I, *Mendelian Inheritance*.

Risk of Recurrence for Patient's Child:
See Part I, *Mendelian Inheritance*. Affected individuals are not expected to survive to reproduce.

Age of Detectability: *Acute form*: hyperexcretion of tyrosyl compounds in urine and elevated plasma tyrosine has been reported as early as 2–3 weeks of age in one patient with a known affected sib.

Chronic form: onset of symptoms reported as early as six months of age, but most cases detected between one and three years of age.

Recent studies demonstrate increased succinylacetone in urine and serum at birth, and prenatally in amniotic fluid; activity of fumarylacetoacetase measured in cultured amniotic fibroblast cells is decreased (<5% of controls) in affected fetuses, thus allowing prenatal diagnosis. The feasibilty of enzymatic diagnosis in chorionic villus has been suggested. The δ-aminolevulinate dehydratase-inhibition test, an indirect measure of succinylacetone, provides another method for prenatal diagnosis in at-risk families.

Gene Mapping and Linkage: FAH (fumarylacetoacetate) has been provisionally mapped to 15q23-q25.

Prevention: None known. Genetic counseling indicated.

Treatment: Low phenylalanine - low tyrosine diets have been tried, and some improvement in biochemical and clinical aspects of the disorder have been reported. Dietary treatment should begin early in life, and careful monitoring of plasma tyrosine, phenylalanine, and methionine is advised, with use of currently recommended formula, because of the high methionine concentrations. Cholestasis was reported in one patient, possibly associated with hypermethioninemia, suggesting the need to monitor serum bile acids as well.

Hepatic transplant, reported in several patients, offers the best opportunity for survival. Replacement of the liver corrects the hepatic enzyme deficiency, but kidney and other tissues remain potentially affected. Renal tubular dysfunction has reportedly continued after otherwise successful liver transplantation.

Supportive and symptomatic treatment for GI disturbances, electrolyte imbalance, hypoglycemia, anemia, bleeding, and rickets.

Prognosis: *Untreated acute form*: Most patients die before one year of age, and frequently within one month after the onset of symptoms.

Untreated chronic form: Few patients are reported to have survived beyond ten years of age.

Treated patients on restricted phenylalanine-tyrosine diets may have an increased life expectancy, but data on long-term follow-up are inadequate. There is improvement of general symptoms, including disappearance of acidosis and ascites. The renal tubular lesion and rickets improve, and a growth spurt may occur. Significant improvement of liver disease has been recorded, but results are highly variable and possibly depend on the extent of prior irreversible hepatic damage, acute vs. chronic form, or on yet undetermined pathologic factors. Even when restrictive diets are started early in life, outcomes suggest that diet alone is not effective in preventing serious and fatal progression of liver and renal disease.

Hepatic transplantation appears to correct the enzyme defect, but renal and other tissue deficiencies persist in renal lesions of variable severity.

Detection of Carrier: Levels of fumarylacetoacetase in red blood cells, lymphocytes, and fibroblasts of parents yield intermediate enzyme values, consistent with heterozygosity.

Special Considerations: Tyrosinemia, tyrosinosis, and tyrosyluria have been interchangeably used in the literature to describe conditions with increased tyrosine in blood and urine, but it has become increasingly clear that a number of different conditions are described under these names. Some are probably true inborn errors of metabolism, and some represent maturational delay.

Several variant forms of hereditary hypertyrosinemia have been reported; patients demonstrating tyrosinemia, tyrosyluria, reduced p-hydroxyphenylpyruvic acid oxidase, and normal fumarylacetoacetase activity without hepatorenal dysfunction, or oculodermal lesions but with varied neurological symptoms, and normal FAH enzyme levels. One patient has been reported to have intermittent CNS symptoms associated with deficient activity of hepatic four-hydroxyphenylpyruvate dioxygenase; and two children with severe metabolic acidosis excreted unique tyrosine metabolites, hawkinsin, and four-hydroxycyclo-hexylacetic acid in urine (see **Hawkinsinuria**).

References:

Halvorsen S, et al.: Tyrosinosis: a study of 6 cases. Arch Dis Child 1966; 41:238–249. †

Shear CS, et al.: Tyrosinosis and tyrosinemia. In: Nyhan WL, ed: Amino acid metabolism and genetic variation. New York: McGraw-Hill, 1967:97–114. †

Gartner JC, et al.: Orthotopic liver transplantation in children: two-year experience with 47 patients. Pediatrics 1984; 74:140–145.

Nyhan WL: The tyrosinemias. In: Nyhan WL, ed: Abnormalities in amino acid metabolism in clinical medicine. Norwalk, CT: Appleton-Century-Crofts, 1984:149–169. *

Berger R: Biochemical aspects of type I hereditary tyrosinemia. In Bickel H, Wachtel U, eds: Inherited diseases of amino acid metabolism: recent progress in the understanding, recognition and management. New York: Thieme, 1985:191–202.

Kvittingen EA, et al.: Prenatal diagnosis of hereditary tyrosinemia by determination of fumarylacetoacetase in cultured amniotic fluid cells. Pediatr Res 1985; 19:334–337.

Starzl TE, et al.: Changing concepts: liver replacement for hereditary tyrosinemia and hepatoma. J Pediatr 1985; 106:604–606.

Tuchman M, et al.: Contribution of extrahepatic tissues to biochemical abnormalities in hereditary tyrosinemia type I. J Pediatr 1987; 110:399–403.

Goldsmith LA, Laberge C: Tyrosinemia and related disorders. In: Scriver CR, et al, eds: The metabolic basis of inherited disease, 6th ed. New York: McGraw-Hill, 1989:547–562. *

SH017
NY000

Carol S. Shear
William L. Nyhan

TYROSINEMIA II, OREGON TYPE   2009

Includes:

Cytosolic tyrosine transaminase deficiency
Keratosis palmoplantaris-corneal dystrophy
Oculocutaneous tyrosinemia or tyrosinosis
"Oregon type" tyrosinosis
Richner-Hanhart Syndrome
Tyrosine aminotransferase deficiency
Tyrosine transaminase deficiency
Tyrosinemia with eye and skin lesions, familial
Tyrosinemia-plantar and palmar keratosis-ocular keratitis

Excludes:

Tyrosinemia I (0978)
Tyrosinemia and tyrosyluria, transient of the newborn
Tyrosinemia and tyrosyluria associated with disease states

Major Diagnostic Criteria: The diagnosis should be considered in patients with persistent elevation of the concentration of tyrosine in plasma (.1–.6mg/100dl) hyperexcretion of tyrosine, and tyrosyluria. The additional presence of the characteristic oculocutaneous lesions is diagnostic. Hepatic and renal functions are normal.

Clinical Findings: The predominant clinical features of the disease are ocular keratitis, hyperkeratosis and erosions of palms, soles, fingertips and toes. Mental retardation is commonly seen. The association of these clinical abnormalities with tyrosinemia, tyrosinuria, and tyrosyluria comprise this disorder. There is variable expressivity among patients described which suggests genetic heterogeneity.

Ocular symptoms such as photophobia, hyperlacrimation, red-

ness and pain are present as early as two weeks of age. Most affected patients develop keratitis early in the first year of life, although onset is variable. A few patients have not manifested symptoms until eight or nine years of age, and others have not had any evidence of eye disease. The ocular lesions are mostly limited to the corneal epithelium and have been described as dendritic keratitis. Nonspecific inflammatory changes of the cornea and conjunctiva have been described, as well as corneal nebulae, and superficial or deep corneal ulcers. Patients have been misdiagnosed as having herpes-simplex keratitis. Fluorescein staining is absent or minimal. Cultures have been negative for herpes-simplex virus, bacteria and fungi. Treatment with topical antibiotics, corticosteroids or lubricants has been ineffective. Chronic eye disease in the untreated patient may result in cataracts, corneal scarring and opacification, nystagmus, exotropia, and visual impairment.

Skin lesions usually appear weeks or months after the onset of eye symptoms and may be painful. Initially, pinpoint papular lesions appear on fingers, toes, palms and soles; later they increase in size (5–10mm) and become hyperkeratotic. Some lesions are punctate erosions which may become crusted, hyperkeratotic, erythematous or pustular. Most often, the lesions are found on the distal phalanges or thenar and hypothenar eminences. The distribution may be linear. The skin lesions may clear spontaneously or worsen independent of topical or systemic therapies or other environmental factors. Many reported patients have been described as moderately to severely retarded. Others have demonstrated educational delay and behavioral abnormalities, presumably secondary to visual impairment. Microcephaly has been noted in at least four patients. Two patients displayed growth retardation and seizures; one patient reported had multiple congenital anomalies.

In affected patients the elevated concentrations of tyrosine in plasma range from 16–62mg/dl. Increased urinary excretion of tyrosine exceeds 2.5mg/mg creatine and has been reported as high as 3.2mg. p-tyramine, n-acetyltyrosine, p-hydroxyphenyllactic acid, p-hydroxyphenylacetic acid, and p-hydroxyphenylpyruvic acid may be found in the urine.

Complications: The chronic, inflammatory ocular lesions may result in corneal clouding, cataracts or glaucoma, and may lead to visual impairment or blindness. Subungual hyperkeratosis can produce separation of the nails and painful plantar lesions may limit or interfere with walking. **Microcephaly**, growth retardation, hyperactivity, aberrant behavior, and self-mutilation also have been reported.

Associated Findings: None known.

Etiology: Autosomal recessive inheritance.

Pathogenesis: Deficiency of cytoplasmic hepatic tyrosine aminotransferase (L-tyrosine-2-oxyglutarate aminotransferase) has been reported. This enzyme catalyzes the conversion of tyrosine to p-hydroxyphenylpyruvic acid (p-HPPA). Hepatic tyrosine aminotransferase is found in the mitochondria and in the cytoplasm; only the cytoplasmic enzyme is deficient. Patients with tyrosinemia II generally have higher concentrations of tyrosine in plasma than do patients with **Tyrosinemia I**.

A causal relationship has been demonstrated between the hypertyrosinemia of the eye and skin in that a low tyrosine-low phenylalanine diet which lowers the level of tyrosine in plasma results in healing lesions. Conversely, an increase in blood tyrosine is followed by recurrence of the lesions. Experiments with an animal model have demonstrated parallel findings of epithelial corneal and dermal lesions. Rats fed excessive diets of tyrosine developed focal corneal lesions in which the presence of bifringent needle-shaped crystals, resembling tyrosine crystals, were demonstrated (electron and polarizing microscopy). The crystals may be responsible for cell disruption, and the release of lysosomal enzymes causing the acute inflammatory response seen in the corneal epithelium. Similar histologic changes have been observed in dermal lesions. Tyrosine crystals placed in the skin or peritoneal cavity do not produce an inflammatory response. However, it has been postulated that when tyrosine crystallizes within the cells, an inflammatory response is initiated. Increased synthesis of tonofibrils and keratohyalin, and large numbers of micro-tubules, have been observed. The reason for the predilection of lesions for ocular and volar epithelium in humans with tyrosinemia II and in rats with experimental tyrosinemia is unknown.

MIM No.: *27660

Sex Ratio: M1:F1

Occurrence: About 50 patients have been reported since this syndrome recognized in the early 1960s. Affected patients have been of Italian, Norwegian, Anglo-Saxon and American Black ethnic origin.

Risk of Recurrence for Patient's Sib:
See Part I, *Mendelian Inheritance.*

Risk of Recurrence for Patient's Child:
See Part I, *Mendelian Inheritance.*

Age of Detectability: Hypertyrosinemia may be present in the first few weeks of life. Onset of clinical symptoms is highly variable. Ocular lesions may occur as early as two weeks, often within 3–6 months or later, followed by skin lesions.

Gene Mapping and Linkage: TAT (tyrosine aminotransferase) has been mapped to 16q22.1.

Prevention: None known. Genetic counseling indicated.

Treatment: Dietary restriction: low phenylalanine - low tyrosine diet appears uniformly successful. Blood levels of tyrosine in treated patients are preferably maintained below 10mg/dl. If the diet is stopped, symptoms recur.

Prognosis: The oculocutaneous lesions respond readily to the dietary restrictions of tyrosine and phenylalanine.

Two young children, less than three years of age at the time of the report, born to an untreated woman with oculocutaneous tyrosinemia, have had normal physical and psychomotor development.

Detection of Carrier: Unknown. Oral tyrosine load tests have not succeeded in differentiating carriers from control.

Special Considerations: An oculocutaneous disorder described by Richner and Hanhart in 1938 appears to be identical to this disorder. Some of the earlier reported patients with *Richner-Hanhart Syndrome* have been studied and the presence of an abnormality in tyrosine metabolism has been confirmed (Balato et al, 1986).

References:
Richner H: Hornhautaffektion bei keratoma palmare et plantare hereditarium. Klin Monatsbl Augenheilkd 1938; 100:580–588.
Bardelli MM, et al.: Familial tyrosinemia with eye and skin lesions. presentation of two cases. Ophthalmologica (Basel) 1977; 175:5–9.
Faull KF, et al.: Metabolic studies on two patients with nonhepatic tyrosinemia using deurated tyrosine loads. Pediatr Res 1977; 11:631–637.
Goldsmith LA, et al.: Hepatic enzymes of tyrosine metabolism in tyrosinemia II. J Invest Dermatol 1979; 73:500–522.
Ney D, et al.: Dietary management of oculocutaneous tyrosinemia in an 11-year-old child. Am J Dis Child 1983; 137:995–1000.
Balato N, et al.: Tyrosinemia type II in two cases previously reported as Richner-Hanhart syndrome. Dermatoloaica 1986; 173:66–74.
Nyhan WL, Sakati NA: Oculocutaneous tyrosinemia. In: Nyhan WL, ed: Diagnostic recognition of genetic disease. Philadelphia: Lea & Febiger, 1987:112–119. *

SH017
NY000

Carol S. Shear
William L. Nyhan

Tyrosinemia III
See TYROSINEMIA I
Tyrosinemia with eye and skin lesions, familial
See TYROSINEMIA II, OREGON TYPE
Tyrosinemia-plantar and palmar keratosis-ocular keratitis
See TYROSINEMIA II, OREGON TYPE
Tyrosinosis, acute and chronic
See TYROSINEMIA I
TYS
See SCLEROTYLOSIS

❖ U ❖

'U'-shaped hearing loss
   See *DEAFNESS (SENSORINEURAL), MIDFREQUENCY*
UDP-galactose-epimerase deficiency
   See *GALACTOSE EPIMERASE DEFICIENCY*
UDP-glucuronosyltransferase deficiency, type I
   See *UDP-GLUCURONOSYLTRANSFERASE, SEVERE DEFICIENCY TYPE I*

UDP-GLUCURONOSYLTRANSFERASE, SEVERE DEFICIENCY TYPE I   0961

Includes:
   Crigler-Najjar syndrome, type I
   Hyperbilirubinemia, Crigler-Najjar type
   Jaundice without bilirubin glucuronide in bile
   UDP-glucuronosyltransferase deficiency, type I

Excludes:
   Hyperbilirubinemia, conjugated (3009)
   Hyperbilirubinemia, conjugated, Rotor type (3237)
   Hyperbilirubinemia, transient familial neonatal (3238)
   Hyperbilirubinemia, unconjugated (0487)

Major Diagnostic Criteria: Persistent physiologic jaundice of newborn in the absence of hemolysis, serum unconjugated bilirubin concentration in excess of 20 mg/dl, and virtual absence of bilirubin glucuronides in bile.

Clinical Findings: Lifelong nonhemolytic unconjugated hyperbilirubinemia with serum bilirubin concentrations of approximately 15–40 mg/dl (mean, approximately 24 mg/dl). Approximately 75% of affected individuals develop kernicterus during the neonatal period and die in infancy. Survivors may show varied clinical signs of bilirubin encephalopathy. Rarely, signs of kernicterus develop for the first time at or after puberty, usually in association with infection.

Hepatic UDP-glucuronosyltransferase activity with bilirubin as a substrate is undetectable. Activity toward some other substrates, including 4-methylumbelliferone and o-aminophenol, is markedly decreased. Urinary excretion of glucuronides after ingestion of menthol, salicylamide, and n-acetyl-p-aminophenol is decreased to 25% of normal. Fecal urobilinogen excretion is 40–50% of normal.

Serum transaminase, alkaline phosphatase, albumin, and bile salt levels are normal. Gallbladder is normally visualized by oral cholecystography. Morphologic examination of the liver reveals no abnormality except occasional canalicular "bile plugs." Bile contains variable amounts of unconjugated bilirubin. Excretion of unconjugated bilirubin is increased during phototherapy.

Complications: Kernicterus occurs in the vast majority of cases and has a variety of neurologic sequelae.

Associated Findings: None known.

Etiology: Autosomal recessive inheritance of an enzyme defect.

Pathogenesis: Severe inherited deficiency of UDP-glucuronosyltransferase activity toward bilirubin. The clinical disorder results from the toxic effect of unconjugated bilirubin, particularly on the central nervous system.

MIM No.: *21880

CDC No.: 277.400

Sex Ratio: M1:F1

Occurrence: About 70 cases have been reported in the literature.

Risk of Recurrence for Patient's Sib:
   See Part I, *Mendelian Inheritance.*

Risk of Recurrence for Patient's Child:
   See Part I, *Mendelian Inheritance.* Patients often do not live to child-bearing age.

Age of Detectability: Second to third week of life.

Gene Mapping and Linkage: Unknown.

Prevention: None known. Genetic counseling indicated.

Treatment: Exchange transfusion or plasmapheresis during the neonatal period may prevent kernicterus. Maintenance therapy includes phototherapy. Exposure to visible light results in geometric or structural isomerization of bilirubin, which permits its biliary excretion without conjugation.

Recently, liver transplantation has been performed in a few patients. This results in a rapid decrease in serum bilirubin levels.

Patients should not receive drugs, such as sulfonamides or warfarin, that compete with bilirubin for binding sites on albumin, thereby possibly precipitating kernicterus. Phenobarbital administration has no long-lasting effect on serum bilirubin levels in this condition.

Prognosis: Approximately 75% of affected individuals die during the first five years of life from kernicterus or infection. Survival during the neonatal period is improving by the efficient use of plasmapheresis and phototherapy. Liver transplantation may markedly improve the prognosis in older children.

Detection of Carrier: Oral menthol tolerance test (1–2 g for young adults) is useful in distinguishing carriers from normal controls. Urinary menthol glucuronide excretion is quantitated in urine collected for 5 hours after menthol ingestion. Control subjects excrete 39 ± 7.2% of ingested menthol as urinary menthol glucuronide during this period. Heterozygous carriers excrete only about 18% of the given dose during the test period.

Special Considerations: Kernicterus is precipitated by coexisting conditions such as hypoxia, acidosis, sepsis, and prematurity, and is therefore not an obligatory or specific manifestation of this disorder. Because of therapeutic implications, UDP-glucuronosyltransferase deficiency type I must be differentiated from **Hyperbilirubinemia, unconjugated.**

The Gunn strain of mutant Wistar rat has the type I defect.

References:
Crigler JF Jr., Najjar VA: Congenital familial nonhemolytic jaundice with kernicterus. Pediatrics 1952; 10:169–179.
Childs B, et al.: Glucuronic acid conjugation by patients with familial nonhemolytic jaundice and their relatives. Pediatrics 1959; 23:903–913.

Arias IM: Chronic unconjugated hyperbilirubinemia without overt signs of hemolysis in adolescents and adults. J Clin Invest 1962; 41:2233–2245.
Wolkoff AW, et al.: Crigler-Najjar syndrome (type I) in an adult male. Gastroenterology 1979; 76:840–848.
Shevell MI, et al.: Crigler-Najjar syndrome I: treatment by home phototherapy followed by orthotopic hepatic transplantation. J Pediatr 1987; 110:429–431.

CH036 **Jayanta Roy Chowdhury**

UDP-glucuronosyltransferase, severe deficiency type II
See HYPERBILIRUBINEMIA, UNCONJUGATED
UDPG-glycogen transferase
See GLYCOGEN SYNTHETASE DEFICIENCY
Uhl anomaly
See VENTRICLE, RIGHT, UHL ANOMALY
Ulcer, duodenal
See PEPTIC ULCER DISEASES, NON-SYNDROMIC
Ulcer, gastric
See PEPTIC ULCER DISEASES, NON-SYNDROMIC
Ulcer, peptic
See PEPTIC ULCER DISEASES, NON-SYNDROMIC
Ulcer, peptic/hiatal hernia-cafe-au-lait-hypertelorism-myopia
See GASTROCUTANEOUS SYNDROME

ULCER-LEUKONYCHIA-GALLSTONES   2234

Includes:
 Duodenal ulcer-leukonychia-gallstones
 Leukonychia totalis
 Leukonychia-ulcer-gallstones
 Renal calculi-ulcer-leukonychia
Excludes:
 Amyloidoses (1502)
 Histamine excess syndrome (mastocytosis associated)
 Knuckle pads-leukonychia-deafness (0558)
 Endocrine neoplasia, multiple type I (0350)
 Nails, leukonychia (0589)
 Tremor-duodenal ulcer syndrome (0963)

Major Diagnostic Criteria: White nails, duodenal ulcer, and/or cholelithiasis.

Clinical Findings: The clinical picture is recognized when the patient has the combination of leukonychia totalis (white nails), and duodenal ulcer or gallstones. One patient might not have all characteristics present, but is considered likely to be affected if he has one of the characteristics and is a first degree relative to a patient with the complete syndrome. The leukonychia is reportedly present from birth and affects all nails in those patients with the abnormality. Leukonychia has often been considered an incidental finding, but has been noted to be familial.

Limited clinical experience, and limited number of cases makes it difficult to describe a distinct clinical course. The cases reported do not appear to be distinct in their presentation from other patients with gallstones and peptic ulcer, in terms of age of onset or complications.

Complications: Gastric cancer has been reported in one relative, occurring after gastrectomy for an ulcer. Since gastric cancer is generally increased secondary to the peptic ulcer surgery, it is unknown at this time if there is a specific increased evidence of gastric cancer in this syndrome. At this time it would be prudent to suggest close follow up in those patients who have undergone gastrectomy for treatment of their duodenal ulcer.

As regards to other complications, perforation has been reported in one case. Pancreatitis has also been reported in two patients in the literature. The complete history is not available and it is not known if this was a complication of cholelithiasis.

Associated Findings: Renal calculi and sebaceous cyst in association with leukonychia have been reported by Bushkell and Gorlin in a father and son with leukonychia, cysts, and renal calculi. In their review of inherited leukonychia they found one family with 16/19 family members (including the proband) with multiple sebaceous cysts as the only additional feature. One other case was

reported to have peptic ulcer disease and leukonychia, but no sebaceous cysts, or renal calculi. In the three cases with leukonychia and renal calculi and sebaceous cysts, one (age 50) had pancreatitis, one (age 58) had gallbladder disease, and the third was 27 years old, and had not manifested peptic ulcer or gallbladder disease. It is entirely possible that all these features, leukonychia, gallstones, peptic ulcer disease, sebaceous cysts, and renal calculi are all related, and are really one syndrome. This is supported by the tentative evidence that suggests a relationship between renal calculi and duodenal ulcer in specific families.

Etiology: Autosomal dominant inheritance with variable penetrance.

Pathogenesis: Unknown.

MIM No.: *15160

Sex Ratio: M1:F1

Occurrence: Undetermined but presumed rare. Several kindreds have been documented.

Risk of Recurrence for Patient's Sib:
 See Part I, *Mendelian Inheritance.*

Risk of Recurrence for Patient's Child:
 See Part I, *Mendelian Inheritance.*

Age of Detectability: Usually in the third or fourth decade when ulcer or cholelithiasis symptoms present. Leukonychia has been reportedly present from birth.

Gene Mapping and Linkage: Unknown.

Prevention: None known. Genetic counseling indicated.

Treatment: Increased surveillance in the offspring with leukonychia for symptoms of peptic ulcer disease and cholelithiasis, and standard medical symptomatic therapy. Post-gastrectomy patients will need appropriate follow up.

Prognosis: There is no evidence that the prognosis differs markedly from the patients with non-syndromic peptic ulcer disease or cholelithiasis.

Detection of Carrier: Possibly by leukonychia (white nails) in first degree relatives.

References:
Albright SD, Wheeler CE: Leukonychia. Arch Dermatol 1964; 90:392–399.
Bushkell LL, Gorlin RJ: Leukonychia totalis, multiple sebaceous cysts, and renal calculi. Arch Dermatol 1975; 111:899–901.
Rotter JI: The genetics of peptic ulcer: more than one gene, genetics of gastrointestinal disease. Philadelphia: W.B. Saunders, 1980:1–58.
Ingegno AP, Yatto RP: Hereditary white nails (leukonychia totalis) duodenal ulcer and gallstones. NY State J of Med 1982; 82:1797–1800.
Rotter JI: Peptic ulcer. In: Emery AE, Rimoin DL, eds: Principles and practice of medical genetics. New York: Churchill Livingstone, 1983:863–878.

ES005 **Theresa J. Escalante**
Jerome I. Rotter

Ulcerative colitis
See INFLAMMATORY BOWEL DISEASE
Ulcerative proctitis
See INFLAMMATORY BOWEL DISEASE
Ullirch-Turner syndrome
See TURNER SYNDROME
Ullrich syndrome
See NOONAN SYNDROME
Ullrich-Noonan syndrome
See NOONAN SYNDROME
Ulna and fibula, hypoplasia of
See MESOMELIC DYSPLASIA, REINHARDT-PFEIFFER TYPE
Ulnar and fibular absence with severe limb deficiency
See LIMB DEFECT WITH ABSENT ULNA/FIBULA
Ulnar deviation of fingers syndrome
See THUMB, CLASPED
Ulnar drift, congenital
See HAND, ULNAR DRIFT
Ulnar polydactyly-Hirschsprung disease
See HIRSCHSPRUNG DISEASE-CARDIAC DEFECT

ULNAR-MAMMARY SYNDROME 0981

Includes:
    Mammary-ulnar syndrome
    Pallister syndrome
    Schinzel syndrome

Excludes:
    Mesomelic dysplasia, Nievergelt type (0647)
    Mesomelic dysplasia, Reinhardt-Pfeiffer type (0648)

Major Diagnostic Criteria: Combination of absent, hypoplastic, or duplicated ulnar ray structures, with hypoplastic and nonfunctional apocrine and mammary glands, and growth and pubertal delay.

Clinical Findings: This is a complex malformation syndrome with variable expression, characteristically involving a combination of upper limb and mammary gland defects. The abnormalities of the upper limbs may be quite asymmetric. They include clinodactyly; camptodactyly; hexadactyly; and shortness/absence of phalanges/metacarpals of the ulnar digits, of carpal bones, and of the ulna. The thumb, radius, humerus and shoulder girdle may also be involved. The apocrine-mammary defects include absence of body odor and axillary sweating, and developmental functional failure of mammary glands and nipples.

Complications: Physical limitations due to upper limb defects, inability to nurse, and delayed adolescence.

Associated Findings: Scoliosis, absence of teeth, bifid uvula, imperforate hymen, bicornate uterus, cryptorchidism, anal stenosis/atresia, and growth retardation (with late catch-up of growth) and pubertal delay.

Etiology: Autosomal dominant inheritance with variability of expression.

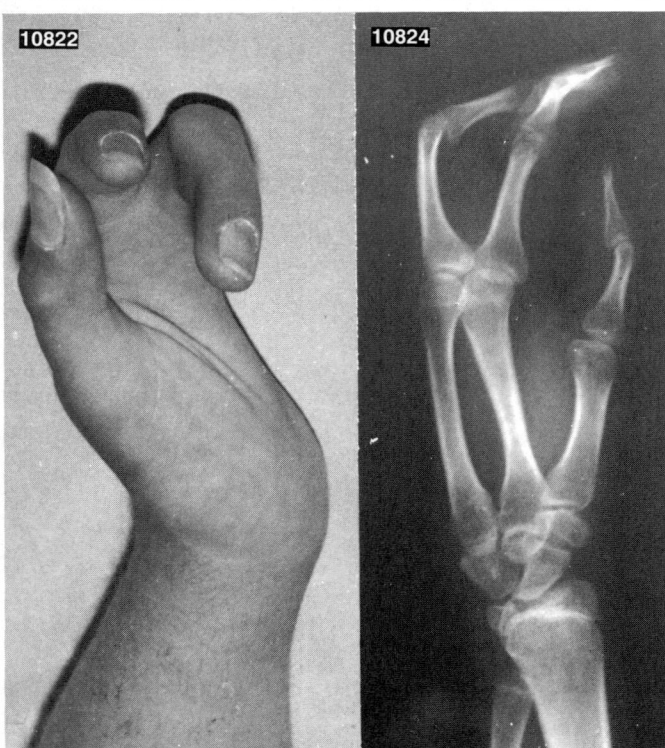

0981A-10822–24: Hypoplasia of distal ulna and absence of ulnar ray derivatives including lateral carpals, 4th and 5th metacarpals, and phalanges.

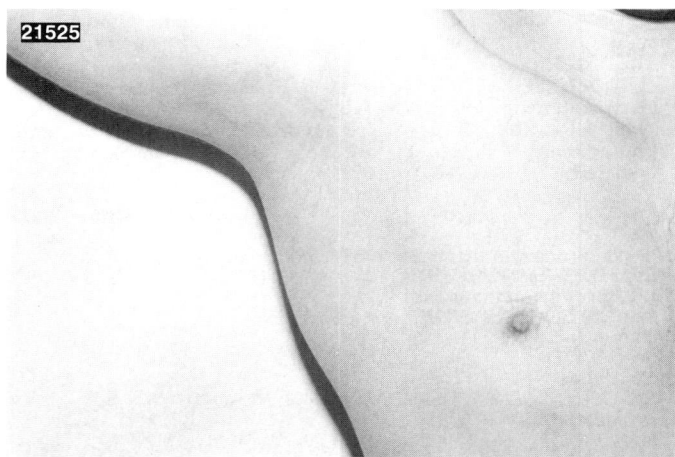

0981B-21525: Total absence of axillary hair, and small nipples.

Pathogenesis: Unknown.

MIM No.: *18145

POS No.: 3420

Sex Ratio: M1:F1

Occurrence: Some 16 cases in four families have been documented.

Risk of Recurrence for Patient's Sib:
    See Part I, *Mendelian Inheritance.*

Risk of Recurrence for Patient's Child:
    See Part I, *Mendelian Inheritance.*

Age of Detectability: At birth.

Gene Mapping and Linkage: Unknown.

Prevention: None known. Genetic counseling indicated.

Treatment: Orthopedic surgery for upper limb malformations; plastic surgery for breast and nipple hypoplasia; hymenotomy; orchiopexy.

Prognosis: Good.

Detection of Carrier: Variability of gene expression may be such that very minimally affected persons may have severely affected offspring. The hand malformation may be totally absent.

References:
Gonzalez CH, et al.: Studies of malformation syndromes of man 42B: mother and son affected with the ulnar-mammary syndrome type Pallister. Eur J Pediatr 1976; 123:225–235.

Pallister PD, et al.: Studies of malformation syndromes in man 42: a pleiotropic dominant mutation affecting skeletal, sexual and apocrine-mammary development. BD:OAS XII(5). New York: Alan R. Liss, for The National Foundation-March of Dimes, 1976:247–254.

Hecht JT, Scott CI, Jr.: The Schinzel syndrome in a mother and daughted. Clin Genet 1984; 25:63–67.

Schinzel A: Ulnar-mammary syndrome. J Med Genet 1987; 24:778–781.

Schinzel A, et al.: The ulnar-mammary syndrome: an autosomal dominant pleiotropic gene. Clin Genet 1987; 32:160–168. (Erratum: Clin Genet 1987; 32:425 only).

HE023
PA010

                    Jürgen Herrmann
                    Philip D. Pallister

Umbilical cord deformation sequence
See UMBILICAL CORD, LONG
Umbilical cord hernia
See OMPHALOCELE
Umbilical cord looping
See UMBILICAL CORD, LONG
Umbilical cord torsion (coarctation)
See UMBILICAL CORD, LONG
Umbilical cord true knot
See UMBILICAL CORD, LONG

UMBILICAL CORD, LONG   2956

Includes:
Umbilical cord deformation sequence
Umbilical cord looping
Umbilical cord torsion (coarctation)
Umbilical cord true knot

Excludes:
Neu-Laxova syndrome (2092)
Umbilical cord, short (2955)
Umbilical cord, short umbilical cord syndrome (2957)

Major Diagnostic Criteria: In abortuses, a long cord measures in excess of 2.5 times the crown-rump length. In preterm infants, the umbilical cord measures 2 SD or more above the mean length as corrected for sex. At term gestation, the cord length exceeds 80 cm; cords measuring more than 300 cm have been detected.

Clinical Findings: During the prenatal period, polyhydramnios is usually, but not always, present. Ultrasonographic visualization is possible (but is usually unreliable) after the first trimester. During parturition, cord prolapse, along with mechanical compression (compromise) of the fetal circulation may occur. The latter condition results in changes in fetal heart rate and ultimately leads to fetal distress (hypoxia). Umbilical vein thromboses and cord entanglements (body loops, knots) are much more common in long cords. True knots are common in long cords and increase the blood pressure required to maintain normal fetal perfusion. Constrictive loops around a fetal part (neck, arm, shoulder, trunk) rarely may impart deep grooves in the underlying fetal tissues and may lead to significant structural deformation.

Complications: Long cords are significantly (p <0.001) prone to accidents (loops, knots, prolapse). The long cord accident rate is 60%. The incidence of anomalies (velamentous insertion, hematoma, vein thrombosis, single umbilical artery, and torsion) is also increased in the fetus with a long cord (19%) compared with normal (14%) and short (17%) cords. Long cords are prone to coiling (looping), true knot formation (0.4–0.5% of deliveries), and cord prolapse at delivery. Following large volume amniocentesis, long cords are at greater risk for knot and loop formations. In each of these conditions, the fetal vascular supply may be compromised. The incidence of frequent variable decelerations of the baseline fetal heart rate is significantly increased in fetuses with long cords (p <0.05) as are FHR patterns, suggesting fetal distress (p <0.05).

Associated Findings: Twinning, polyhydramnios, abdominal pregnancy, fetal hyperkinesia, fetal hypertension (e.g., maternal drugs: amphetamines, cocaine, xanthines), and fetal growth retardation.

Etiology: Undetermined but presumably nongenetic.

Pathogenesis: Current theories include excessive fetal movement (hyperkinesia), excessive stretch during development (e.g., polyhydramnios, abdominal pregnancy), and fetal hypertension.

Sex Ratio: M1:F1

Occurrence: Long cords are seen in 11% of abortus specimens. Long cords occur in 7% of all deliveries. In pregnancies complicated by polyhydramnios, as many as 12% of cords may be classified as long.

Risk of Recurrence for Patient's Sib: Presumably low.

Risk of Recurrence for Patient's Child: Unknown.

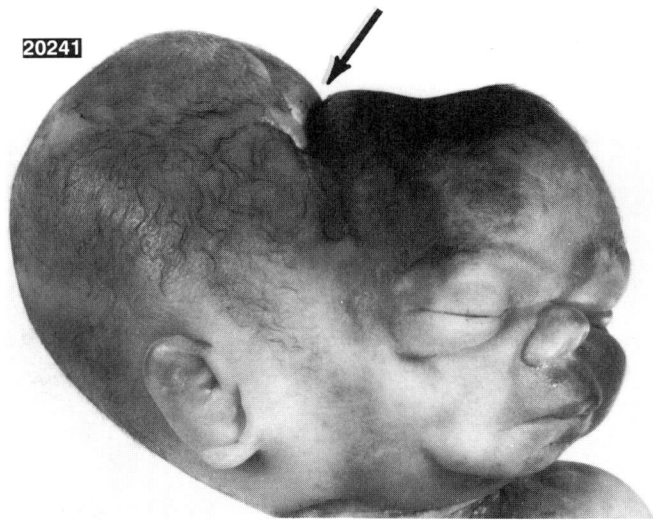

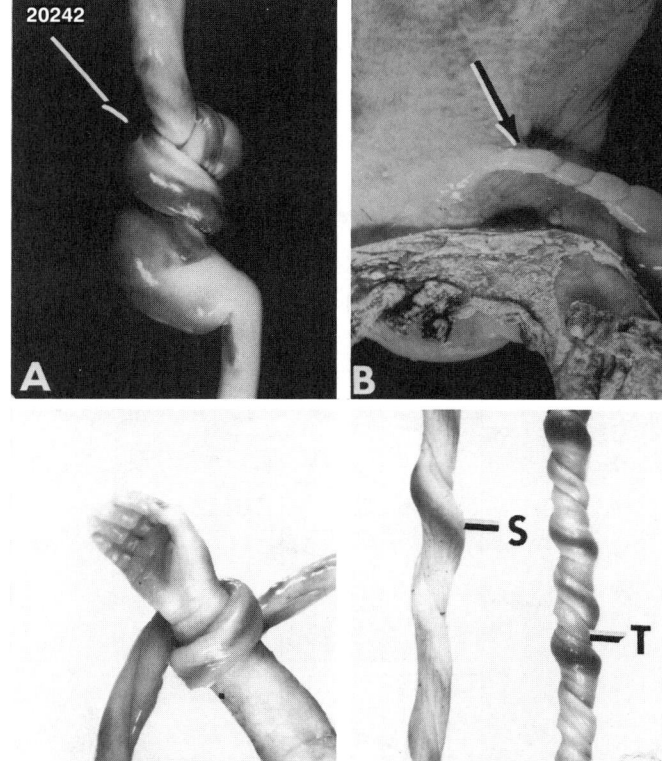

2956A-20241: Newborn with an 80 cm long umbilical cord showing significant deformation of the skull due to an umbilical cord loop (arrow). **20242:** Abnormalities associated with "long umbilical cord": A. True knot with vascular compression; B. Torsion of cord near fetal abdomen (arrow); C. Cord loop around fetal arm; D. Long cords showing normal (left hand) vascular spiral (S) as opposed to cord twists (T).

Age of Detectability: Possibly evident on fetal ultrasound after 12 weeks gestation or shortly thereafter. Most are not detected until delivery.

Gene Mapping and Linkage: Unknown.

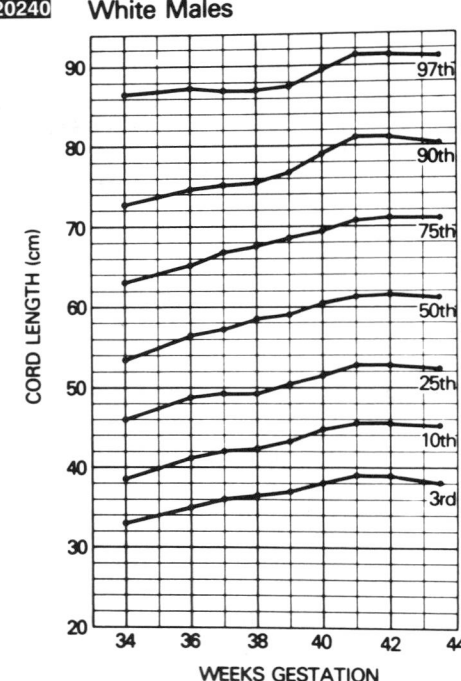

20240 White Males

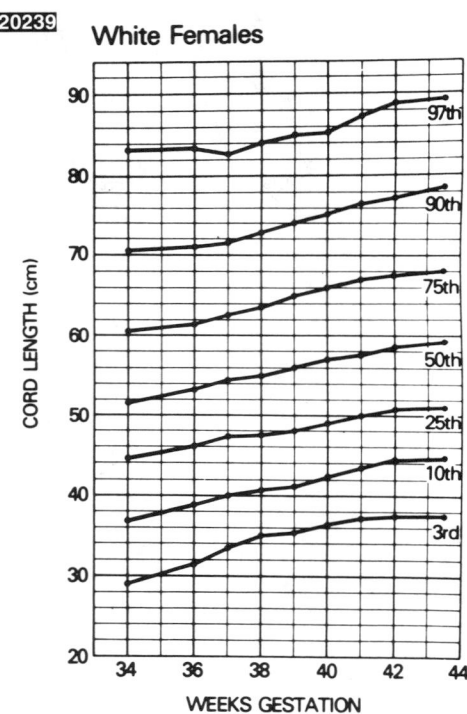

20239 White Females

2956B-20240: Umbilical cord length by gestational age in US white males (Mills et al). **20239:** Umbilical cord length by gestational age in US white females (Mills et al).

Prevention: No known methods currently available except when maternal drugs induce fetal hypertension (e.g., amphetamines, cocaine, xanthines). In the latter cases, drugs should be discontinued.

Treatment: None necessary except that during delivery efforts should be directed toward preventing compromise of the fetal vascular supply; fetal monitoring is indicated.

Prognosis: Excellent if complications of hypoxia are avoided during intrauterine development at delivery.

Detection of Carrier: Unknown.

References:
Javert CT, Barton B: Congenital and acquired lesions of the umbilical cord and spontaneous abortion. Am J Obstet Gynecol 1952; 63:1065–1077.
Rayburn WF, et al.: Umbilical cord length and intrapartum complications. Obstet Gynecol 1981; 57:450–452.
Mossenger AC, et al.: Umbilical cord length as an index of fetal activity: experimental study and clinical implications. Pediatr Res 1982; 16:109–112.
Mills JL, et al.: Standards for measuring umbilical cord length. Placenta 1983; 4:423–426.

BL002   **Will Blackburn**

UMBILICAL CORD, MULTIPLE VESSELS   **2576**

Includes:
    Umbilical arteries, multiple
    Umbilical veins, multiple

Excludes: Umbilical vein, persistent right

Major Diagnostic Criteria: Multiple umbilical arteries and veins.

Clinical Findings: Duplicated umbilical vessels have been reported in both normal infants and infants with major or multiple congenital anomalies.

Complications: None directly from the duplicated vessels, but as in babies with single umbilical artery, the extent of the complications in infants with multiple umbilical cord vessels depends on the severity of the associated congenital malformations.

Associated Findings: None known.

Etiology: Unknown.

Pathogenesis: Abnormal division of the umbilical vessels within the Wharton's jelly portion of the cord at 3–5 weeks gestation.

Sex Ratio: M1:F1

Occurrence: Karchmer et al (1966) examined the umbilical cords of 40 malformed infants. From this population, two were identified with cords containing three umbilical arteries.

Risk of Recurrence for Patient's Sib: Unknown.

Risk of Recurrence for Patient's Child: Unknown.

Age of Detectability: At birth.

Gene Mapping and Linkage: Unknown.

Prevention: None known. Genetic counseling indicated.

Treatment: Unknown.

Prognosis: Unknown.

Detection of Carrier: Unknown.

References:
Karchmer S, et al.: Anomalies del cordon umbilical y coexistencia de malformaciones congenitas. Ginecologia y Obstetricia de Mexico 1966; 21:831–837.
Painter D, Russell P: Four-vessel umbilical cord associated with multiple congenital anomalies. Obstet Gynecol 1977; 50:505–507.
Beck R, Naulty CM: A human umbilical cord with four arteries. Clin Pediatr 1985; 24:118–119.

EL013   **Sami B. Elhassani**

UMBILICAL CORD, SHORT   2955

Includes:
Fetal constraint
Short cord

Excludes:
Cerebroarthrodigital syndrome
Umbilical cord, long (2956)
Umbilical cord, short umbilical cord syndrome (2957)

Major Diagnostic Criteria: Short umbilical cords measure more than 10 cm but less than 35.5 cm at term delivery.

Clinical Findings: The umbilical cord attains most of its growth during the first and second trimesters; a slow rate of growth is attained during the third trimester and postterm periods. Short umbilical cords measure more than 10 cm but less than 35.5 cm at term delivery. Short cords during the fetal period are those with lengths in the lower 6th percentile corrected for sex and gestational age. The cord, although short, is usually structurally normal. The surface amnion may show signs of amnion nodosum and other structural abnormalities. A slight reduction of cord length has been associated with **Chromosome 21, trisomy 21** and infants born to mothers with hypertension. Unfortunately, intrauterine diagnosis is difficult.

Complications: A cord length of 35.5 cm is thought to be necessary for the normal progression of a vaginal delivery. Short cords are susceptible to traumatic traction or avulsion and fetal exsanguination during vaginal delivery. Short cords are at increased risk for failure of fetal descent, uterine inversion, placental abruption, abnormal fetal heart rate (63%), and cord anomalies (17%).

Associated Findings: Short cords are most often associated with conditions that produce intrauterine constraint (e.g., oligohydramnios, uterine anomalies, or deformations), fetal constraint (e.g., amniotic bands-adhesions, skin disease), fetal limb anomalies (e.g., amelia, **Sirenomelia sequence**, arthrogryposis), and fetal hypokinesia (e.g., CNS and neuromuscular diseases). Body wall defects are common (cyllosomus, pleurosomus, omphalocele) as are signs of fetal compression (Potter facies, thoracic and lung hypoplasia, abnormal limb position, and limb deformations). Fetal renal disease (e.g., renal agenesis, dysplasia, or cystic disease) is common. Both genetic and nongenetic syndromes are also encountered.

Table 1   Factors Associated with Short Umbilical Cord

Intrauterine Environmental Constraint
  Oligohydramnios
    Fetal Oliguria-Anuria
    Amnionic Fluid Leakage
  Amniotic bands syndrome
  Uterine Malformations-Deformations
  Multiple Pregnancy
Fetal Cutaneous Constraint
  Restrictive Dermopathy
  Skin, localized absence of
  Congenital **Contractures**
  Epidermolysis bullosum
  Stomach, pyloric atresia
Fetal Cutaneous Constraint + Hypokinesia
  "Cocoon" Fetus
  Neu-Laxova syndrome
  Ectrodactyly
  Pterygium syndrome
Fetal Hypokinesia
  Chromosome Abnormalities
    Chromosome 21, trisomy 21
      (mild degrees of cord shortening)
    Chromosome triploidy
    Prader-Willi syndrome (possibly)
  Lissencephaly-Associated Syndromes
    Neu-Laxova syndrome

  Pena-Shokeir syndrome
  Cerebro-oculo-facio-skeletal syndrome
  Cerebro-hepato-renal syndrome
  Lissencephaly syndrome
  Muscular dystrophy, congenital with mental retardation
  Neuromuscular
    Spinal muscular atrophy (prenatal)
    Muscular dystrophy, congenital with mental retardation
  Limb Anomalies
    Amelia
    Arthrogryposes
    Cranio-carpo-tarsal dysplasia, whistling face type
  Acardiac Fetus
  Maternal Hypertension
    (mild degrees of cord shortening)
Fetal Hypotension
  Maternal Drugs
  Acardiac Fetus

Etiology: Both genetic and nongenetic associations have been reported.

Pathogenesis: A variety of conditions are known to promote umbilical cord growth (fetal blood pressure, fetal movement, and cord stretch or increased tension); hence, most theories embrace the concept that short cords are due to situations leading to reduced stretch (e.g., constraint syndromes), reduced fetal movement, or reduced fetal blood pressure.

Sex Ratio: Variable due to diverse associations.

Occurrence: About 0.8 to 1.2% of all umbilical cords are short.

Risk of Recurrence for Patient's Sib: Variable depending on nature of etiology and pathogenesis.

Risk of Recurrence for Patient's Child: Unknown.

Age of Detectability: Usually evident by the end of the second trimester and by ultrasonography during the third trimester. Most commonly noted in association with reduced fundal height (e.g., oligohydramnios).

Gene Mapping and Linkage: Unknown.

Prevention: In conditions in which oligohydramnios is due to obstruction of the lower urinary tract (posterior urethral bands, urethral stenosis, or agenesis), the placement of an intrauterine catheter to drain urine continuously into the amniotic cavity prevents progressive renal degeneration and enhances lung growth by expanding the amniotic fluid volume.

Treatment: Cesarean section delivery may be indicated because of risk for umbilical cord laceration or avulsion during vaginal delivery.

Prognosis: Variable depending on provoking condition. Short umbilical cord is associated with decreased Apgar scores, the need for resuscitation at delivery, hypotonia, jittery-tremorous newborns, and subsequent psychomotor abnormalities.

Detection of Carrier: Only possible when associated with known genetic conditions.

References:
Purola E: The length and insertion of the umbilical cord. Ann Chir Gynaecol Fenn 1968; 57:621–622.
Punnett HH, et al.: Syndrome of ankylosis, facial anomalies and pulmonary hypoplasia. J Pediatr 1974; 85:375–377.
Miller ME, et al.: Short umbilical cord: its origin and relevance. Pediatrics 1981; 67:618–621.
Moessinger AC, et al.: Umbilical cord length as an index of fetal activity: experimental study and clinical implications. Pediatr Res 1982; 16:109–112.
Mills JL, et al.: Standards for measuring umbilical cord length. Placenta 1983; 4:423–426.
Naeye RL: Umbilical cord length: clinical significance. J Pediatr 1985; 107:278–281.

Will Blackburn

UMBILICAL CORD, SHORT UMBILICAL CORD SYNDROME
2957

Includes:
> Acordia
> Flying fetus syndrome
> SUC syndrome
> Tethered fetus syndrome
> Umbilical cord agenesis
> Umbilical cord aplasia

Excludes:
> Acardiac twin
> Amniotic adhesions
> **Amniotic bands syndrome** (0874)
> Amniotic rupture sequence
> Single umbilical artery
> **Umbilical cord, long** (2956)
> **Umbilical cord, short** (2955)

Major Diagnostic Criteria: The amniotic sac is intact, and amniotic bands (adhesions) are absent; the fetus is almost directly apposed or tethered to the placenta. The umbilical cord and sometimes its structures are extremely short, measuring 10 cm or less at term gestation. A single umbilical artery is usually present. An abdominal wall defect (omphalocele) is present and may lie in direct contact with the amniotic surface of the placental plate. The fetal trunk (spine) is sharply bent in the direction of umbilical cord tethering, which results in pleurosomus- or cyllosoma-like deformations.

Deformations of the extremities are present (e.g., clubfoot, abnormal rotation, or asymmetry). Internal anomalies are always present (e.g., diaphragmatic hernia, gastrointestinal, or genitourinary). SUC syndrome infants look alike; infants with amniotic rupture sequence also have very short umbilical cords but do not look alike.

Clinical Findings: Clinical signs appear by the end of the first trimester and include decreased fundal height, decreased fetal growth, and reduced amniotic fluid volume. Ultrasonography reveals close approximation of fetus and placenta and usually no visible umbilical cord. The fetus is progressively bent (pleurosomus; "flying fetus") in the direction of tethering, and body orientation (position) does not change as pregnancy proceeds. Reduced fetal movement (hypokinesia) is present. Sirenoid malformations have been reported in a few cases.

At birth, the placenta and fetus are delivered together, but occasionally the placenta may be avulsed from the fetus. Inspection reveals undeveloped body stalk elements (short, "naked" umbilical vessels surrounded by little or no Wharton jelly) and close approximation of placenta, fetal membranes, and fetal body wall elements (e.g., omphalocele membrane). X-ray studies reveal skeletal abnormalities (kyphoscoliosis, pleurosomus, pelvic hypoplasia, fused or abnormal ribs), signs of diaphragmatic hernia (persistent pleuroperitoneal canal), and severe, asymmetric, thoracic hypoplasia.

Complications: Due to fetal tethering, fetal descent during parturition does not occur; abnormal fetal presentation is the rule. Abruptio placenta and inversion of the uterus may occur. During vaginal delivery, avulsion of the placenta and funicular hemorrhage are common. Affected infants usually survive to term and are remarkably well developed; respiratory distress due to pulmonary hypoplasia is noted immediately after birth and is a common cause of death.

Associated Findings: Necropsy studies reveal internal anomalies involving the skeletal, gastrointestinal, and genitourinary systems.

Etiology: Unknown. Genetic mechanisms have not been described.

Pathogenesis: Current theories include a generalized failure in body stalk growth with subsequent failure of umbilical artery growth. When sirenoid malformations are present a "vascular steal" mechanism has been considered.

Sex Ratio: M1:F1

Occurrence: Unknown. Necropsy studies reveal an incidence of 1:600 necropsies.

Risk of Recurrence for Patient's Sib: Presumably low.

Risk of Recurrence for Patient's Child: Affected individuals do not survive to reproduce.

Age of Detectability: Usually at 12–14 weeks gestation.

Gene Mapping and Linkage: Unknown.

Prevention: None known. Genetic counseling indicated.

Treatment: Delivery by cesarean section is recommended due to high risk for placental vessel avulsion, fetal exsanguination, and abnormal fetal presentation. No treatment is currently available.

Prognosis: All patients have died shortly after birth due to respiratory insufficiency. A few have died *in utero*.

Detection of Carrier: Unknown.

References:
Gruenwald P, Mayberger HW: Differences in abnormal development of monozygotic twins. Arch Pathol 1960; 70:685–695.
Miller ME, et al.: Short umbilical cord: its origin and relevance. Pediatrics 1981; 67:618–621.
Barr M, Heidelberger KP: Short umbilical cord: cause or effect of fetal anomalies? Proc Greenwood Genet Center 1983; 2:100–101.
Blackburn WR, Cooley NR, Jr.: Short umbilical cord syndrome: an anomaly complex recognizable during the prenatal period. Clin Res 1984; 32:884A.

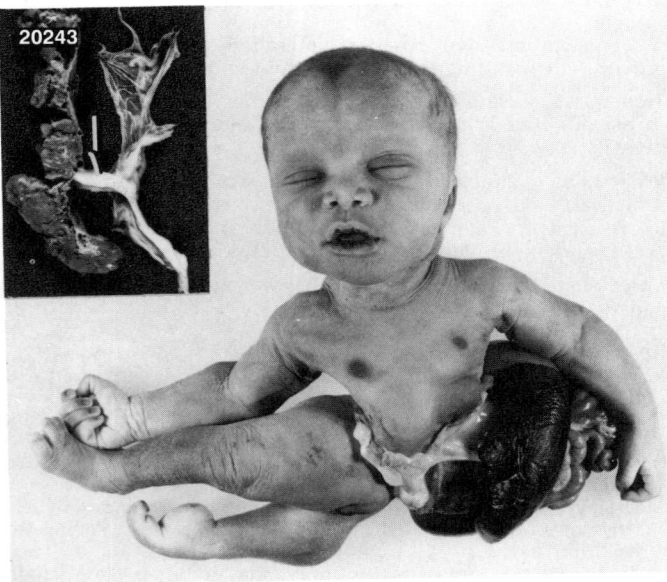

2957-20243: Newborn with short umbilical cord syndrome. Note the short cord (inset, arrow) and the infant's pleurosomus deformation. The omphalocele membrane is in close approximation to the fetal surface of the placenta (inset).

BL002

Will Blackburn

UMBILICAL CORD, SINGLE ARTERY 2500

Includes: Artery, umbilical cord, single

Excludes: Umbilical vessel defects, other

Major Diagnostic Criteria: Absence of one of the two umbilical arteries during routine newborn physical examination. Because 14% of infants with single umbilical artery die perinatally, and the incidence of major anomalies in those who die is 53%, a thorough physical as well as an earlier and a closer than usual follow-up examination should be performed.

Clinical Findings: While the occurrence of single umbilical artery by itself is a benign condition, the pathologic clinical signs are related to associated malformations. Such malformations include those of skeletal, gastrointestinal, cardiovascular and nervous systems. The condition is also frequently found in babies with **Chromosome 13, trisomy 13** and **Chromosome 18, trisomy 18**.

Complications: The extent of the complications is dependent on the severity of the congenital anomalies associated with single umbilical artery.

Associated Findings: None known.

Etiology: Single umbilical artery has been said to be associated with a variety of high-risk pregnancies such as advanced maternal age, high parity, multiple gestation, diabetes, intrauterine growth retardation, and reduced placental weight.

Pathogenesis: It is not known whether absence of the second umbilical artery is due to primary aplasia or atrophy. Monie (1970) reported the presence of single umbilical artery in normal human embryos 3–4 mm in length; therefore, the finding of the condition at birth may be due to the persistence of the normally transient single umbilical artery.

CDC No.: 747.500

Sex Ratio: M1:F1

Occurrence: Single umbilical artery is one of the most common congenital malformations, occurring in about 1% of neonates. Microscopic examination of the umbilical cord of 48 affected infants showed no significant differences in congenital anomalies or neonatal mortality between infants with agenesis of one of their arteries and infants with arterial obliteration.

Risk of Recurrence for Patient's Sib: Unknown.

Risk of Recurrence for Patient's Child: Unknown.

Age of Detectability: At birth, or prenatally by ultrasound imaging.

Gene Mapping and Linkage: Unknown.

Prevention: None known. Genetic counseling indicated.

Treatment: Unknown.

Prognosis: Unknown.

Detection of Carrier: Unknown.

Special Considerations: Because 10.3% of malformed fetuses and 17.1% of chromosomally abnormal fetuses have single umbilical artery, karyotyping of malformed newborns with single umbilical artery is advisable. The following are recommended for babies with single umbilical artery: 1) thorough physical examination, with special attention to intra-abdominal masses, dysmorphic features of the face, and anomalies of the hands and feet. 2) prenatal counseling, emphasizing the expected normal development of the majority of infants with single umbilical artery. 3) earlier and closer than usual follow-up examination, again with special attention to the abdomen, face, hands, and feet. 4) special procedures (invasive or noninvasive) not indicated at the time of the diagnosis should be reserved for the detection of additional anomalies, particularly a suspected intra-abdominal mass.

References:

Monie IW: Genesis of single umbilical artery. Am J Obstet Gynecol 1970; 108:400–405.

Collaborative Perinatal Study of the National Institute of Neurologic Diseases and Stroke: Women and their Pregnancies. DHEW publi-cation No. (NIH) 73–379. Washington, D.C.: U.S. Department of Health, Education, and Welfare, 1972.

Altshuler G, et al.: Single umbilical artery: correlation of clinical status and umbilical cord histology. Am J Dis Child 1975; 129:697 only.

Bjoro K, Jr: Vascular anomalies of the umbilical cord: obstetric impli-cations. Early Human Development 1983; 8:118–127.

Heifetz SA: Single umbilical artery: a statistical analysis of 237 autopsy cases and review of the literature. Perspect Pediatr Pathol 1984; 8:345–377.

Byrne J, Blanc WA: Malformations and chromosome anomalies in spontaneously aborted fetuses with single umbilical artery. Am J Obstet Gynecol 1985; 151:340–342.

EL013 **Sami B. Elhassani**

URACHAL ANOMALIES 2573

Includes:
  Bladder diverticulum, superior
  Patent urachus
  Umbilical cord (giant), associated with patent urachus
  Urachal cyst or sinus

Excludes:
  Omphalomesenteric duct anomalies (2574)
  Umbilical cord, long (2956)
  Umbilical cord tumors

Major Diagnostic Criteria: Urine discharges from the umbilicus. The diagnosis may be confirmed by injecting a radiopaque material into the umbilical orifice, thus outlining the patency of the urachal lumen or by introducing a colored dye into the bladder through a urethral catheter.

Clinical Findings: *Completely patent urachus*: a small or giant umbilical bud which discharges urine. Radiopaque material injected into the umbilical orifice demonstrates the patent urachal tract. Bladder outlet obstruction may be an associated anomaly; a voiding cystourethrogram is advisable.

Urachal cyst: a superficial infraumbilical midline mass with a high susceptibility to infection. The diagnosis is frequently made by physical examination. In addition, a cystogram should be obtained to determine if there is any communication with the bladder.

Urachal sinus: urine discharges from the umbilical stump. Sometimes the urachal sinus can be felt as a thick cord beneath the skin coursing toward the bladder. Contrast studies should be obtained to outline the sinus tract.

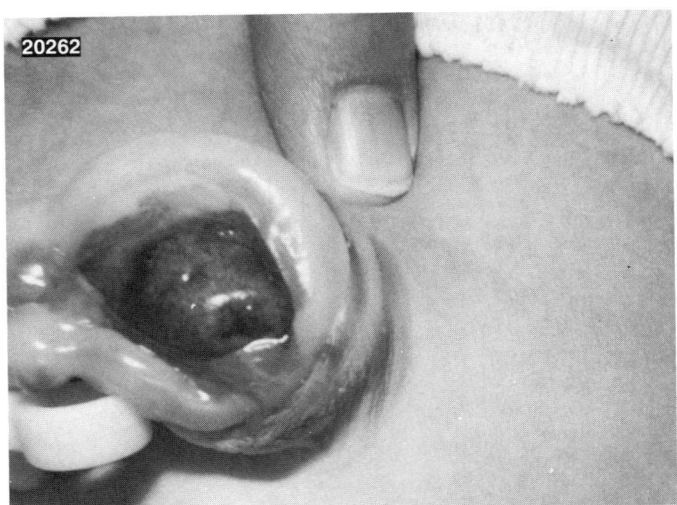

2573-20262: Patent urachus; note the orifice in the umbilical stump.

Urachal diverticulum: usually asymptomatic; it can be demonstrated only by cystogram.

Complications: Recurrent infections are likely in all untreated urachal malformations.

Associated Findings: None known.

Etiology: Persistence of the embryonic luminal communication between the bladder and the umbilicus.

Pathogenesis: Failure of the normal obliteration of the distal allantois may result in any of the four types of urachal anomalies.

Sex Ratio: M2:F1

Occurrence: 1:629 births.

Risk of Recurrence for Patient's Sib: Unknown.

Risk of Recurrence for Patient's Child: Unknown.

Age of Detectability: The majority of urachal anomalies are detected at birth. Occasionally, a patent urachus is not recognized until after the cord has fallen off and urine escapes from the umbilicus. This rare clinical manifestation is usually associated with a giant umbilical cord.

Gene Mapping and Linkage: Unknown.

Prevention: None known. Genetic counseling indicated.

Treatment: Excision of the urachal tract is the treatment of choice to avoid recurrent urinary tract infections.

Prognosis: Unknown.

Detection of Carrier: Unknown.

References:
Ente G, Penzer PH: Giant umbilical cord associated with patent urachus. Am J Dis Child 1970; 120:82–83.

EL013   **Sami B. Elhassani**

URETHRAL VALVES, POSTERIOR   2407

Includes: Prostatic male urethra, obstruction

Excludes:
Urethral diverticula
Urethral polyps
Urethral strictures

Major Diagnostic Criteria: Visualization of posterior valves by voiding cystourethrogram.

Clinical Findings: Congenital obstruction of the prostatic urethra. Presenting findings include decreased urinary stream (25%), distended bladder (67%), urinary infection (50%), abdominal distention (30%), renal failure (33%), papable kidneys (50%), hematuria (10%), failure to thrive (50%), fever of unknown origin (25%), vomiting and diarrhea (33%), and hypertension (5%).

Symptoms may manifest in early infancy, but may go undetected until later in infancy or childhood.

Complications: Urinary infections, hydronephrosis, bladder neck hypertrophy, vesicoureteral reflux, renal failure, hypertension.

Associated Findings: Obstruction of the ureteropelvic or ureterovesicular junction, rectal prolapse, renal dysplasia, renal agenesis, and pulmonary hypoplasia.

Etiology: Unknown.

Pathogenesis: Posterior valves may arise from 1) an embryonic remnant of the urogenital membrane, 2) an anomalous junction of the Wollfian duct and the prostatic utricle, 3) persistence of the Wollfian ducts, or 4) fusion of the epithelial colliculus with the roof of the posterior urethra.

CDC No.: 753.600

Sex Ratio: M1:F0

Occurrence: Undetermined but presumed rare.

Risk of Recurrence for Patient's Sib: Presumably low.

Risk of Recurrence for Patient's Child: Unknown.

Age of Detectability: The majority of patients present during the first year of life, with one-third given medical assistance within the first three months. However, posterior valves may go undetected until later in childhood or even in adulthood. Prenatal ultrasonography may expedite early detection and treatment.

Gene Mapping and Linkage: Unknown.

Prevention: None known. Genetic counseling indicated.

Treatment: The objectives of management include establishing adequate drainage of the urinary tract and removal of the lesion. Surgical strategies vary depending on the severity of the obstruction or the age of the patient. Adequate urinary drainage may be accomplished by inserting an indwelling bladder catheter or may require a suprapubic or upper urinary tract diversion. Removal of valves is usually performed by transurethral endoscopic fuguration.

Prognosis: Unknown.

Detection of Carrier: Unknown.

Special Considerations: Early detection and surgical intervention can greatly improve the prognosis by reducing the morbidity and mortality associated with urinary infections and acute renal failure. Additionally, early intervention can reduce the incidence of chronic renal failure and end-stage kidney disease caused by posterior valves. In recent years, in utero detection of hydronephrosis by prenatal ultrasound may lead to early diagnosis and management in the immediate post natal period. Fetal surgery has been recently attempted, but this procedure still remains experimental.

References:
Mayor G, et al.: Renal function in obstructive uropathy: long-term effect of reconstructive surgery. Pediatrics 1975; 56:740–747.
Harrison MR, et al.: Fetal surgery for congenital hydronephrosis. New Engl J Med 1982; 306:591–593.
Warshaw BL, et al.: Prognostic features in infants with obstructive uropathy due to posterior urethral valves. J Urol 1985; 133:240–242.
Hulbert WC, et al.: Current views on posterior urethral valves. Ped Annal 1988; 17:31–36.

HY001   **Leonard C. Hymes**

Uric acid metabolism-central nervous system disorder
  See LESCH-NYHAN SYNDROME
Uric acid urolithiasis
  See RENAL HYPOURICEMIA
Uridine diphosphate galactose 4'-epimerase deficiency
  See GALACTOSE EPIMERASE DEFICIENCY
Urinary reflux, primary, congenital, or idiopathic
  See VESICO-URETERAL REFLUX
Urinary tract and digital defects-nephrosis-deafness
  See NEPHROSIS-DEAFNESS-URINARY TRACT AND DIGITAL DEFECTS

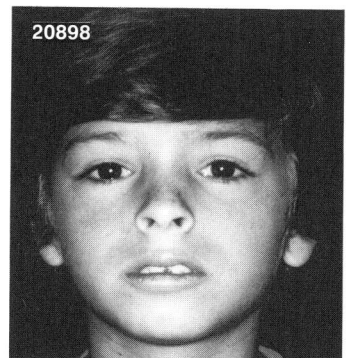 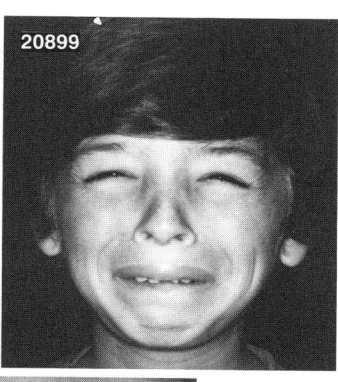

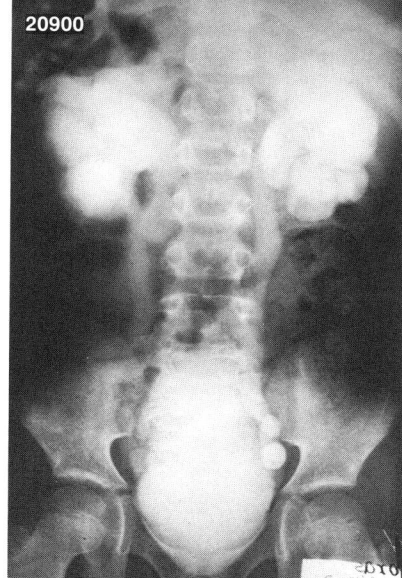

UROFACIAL SYNDROME   2527

Includes:
  Bladder (dysplastic)-hydronephrosis-hydroureter-grimacing facies
  Facial palsy, partial-urinary abnormalities*
  Hydronephrosis-dysmorphic facies, Ochoa type
  Hydronephrosis-hydroureter-dysplastic bladder-grimacing facies
  Ochoa syndrome
  Smile, inverted-occult neuropathic bladder

Excludes:
  Hydronephrosis due to posterior urethral valves
  Hydronephrosis due to ureteral stenosis
  Hydronephrosis without facial abnormalities
  Kidney, polycystic disease, dominant (0859)
  Kidney, polycystic disease, recessive (2003)
  Renal agenesis, bilateral (0856)

2527-20898: Note normal facial expression. **20899:** Grimace or inverted facial expression when laughing. **20900:** IVP shows bilateral hydronephrosis and a trabeculated bladder.

Major Diagnostic Criteria: The condition should be considered in all newborns and children who present with hydronephrosis and pyelonephritis, usually bilateral. There are two characteristics that differentiate this condition from other types of pyelonephritis and hydronephrosis: the peculiar appearance of the face and occult neuropathic bladder, with retention and severe bladder changes in the absence of neurologic or obstructive problems. At first it is difficult to recognize the characteristic facies, but, once known, it becomes diagnostic; and children with it should undergo a complete evaluation of the urinary tract. Most children show hydronephrosis and hydroureter, which vary from mild to severe including trabeculation, diverticula, vesicoureteral reflux, urinary tract infections, and spastic posterior urethra.

Some patient have impaired growth, but others have normal growth and psychomotor development. About 60% have constipation.

Clinical Findings: Appearance of the face is usually diagnostic. Noticeable at birth, it can be easily recognized through life. It is most noticeable when the patient smiles or laughs.

Early signs of the condition are diurnal and nocturnal enuresis (20% have both). Urinary tract infections were found in all patients. Hypertension developed in 13.8% of the patients reported by Ochoa and Gorlin (1987). Six (14%) had severe renal failure with uremia. Urodynamic evaluation of the bladder showed a hypertonic, hyperreflexic bladder, with uninhibited contractions of the detrusor. The bladder is macroscopically abnormal, with diverticulae and trabeculation; some are even congenital. It is suspected that there is a histologic abnormality producing the noted defects and also the hypertrophic neck of the bladder. It is likely that these changes induce ureteral reflux and

retention of urine, with the consequent infections, hydronephrosis, and hydroureter.

Complications: Urinary tract abnormalities, constipation, infections, hydronephrosis, renal failure, enuresis, retention of urine. Renal failure is probably the most concerning of the complications and could be prevented by early diagnosis and surgical treatment of the urinary tract obstruction.

Associated Findings: Neural tube defects, spina bifida occulta, **Meningocele.** Cryptorchidism was found in all affected males and may be causally related to the syndrome. One patient had psychomotor developmental delay, which does not appear to be a major constituent of the condition since all others have normal intellectual performance.

Etiology: Autosomal recessive inheritance, although some researchers believe that dominant inheritance cannot be fully ruled out. The extent of consanguinity is a topic of debate.

Pathogenesis: It is likely that there is a generalized abnormality of the neural tissue of the bladder and perhaps of the ureters and urethra that induces urine retention, ureteral reflux, dilation infection, dilated ureters, hydronephrosis, and pyelonephritis with renal failure. The earliest manifestations that we have seen are in newborns or children, but given the severity of the lesions seen in newborns, it is possible that the condition affects the fetus and produces severe damage to the urinary tract with the consequent oligohydramnios and pulmonary hypoplasia, although there have been no reports of an affected fetus.

About two-thirds of the patients have constipation, which may be a manifestation of the abnormality of the neural tissue of the abdominal viscera.

MIM No.: *23673

POS No.: 4264

Sex Ratio: M1.25:F1

Occurrence: Twenty-three families with 36 affected children (reported by Ochoa and Gorlin, 1987) and 19 probable cases recognized by case histories are known to be affected in Colombia. Reports exist of at least three other families, two in the United States and one in England.

Risk of Recurrence for Patient's Sib:
See Part I, *Mendelian Inheritance.*

Risk of Recurrence for Patient's Child:
See Part I, *Mendelian Inheritance.*

Age of Detectability: At birth, or possibly the condition can be detected in utero by sonography of the GU tract.

Gene Mapping and Linkage: Unknown.

Prevention: None known. Genetic counseling indicated.

Treatment: There is no specific treatment for the tissue and neural defect of this condition. Treatment is geared to correct the urinary tract obstruction and to cure the infection to prevent chronic renal failure. In some cases reconstructive surgery of the ureters and the ureterovesicular junction, ureterostomies, and ileal derivations are necessary depending on the severity of the compromise of the bladder. If severe renal damage has occurred, peritoneal dialysis, hemodialysis, and even kidney transplant are permanent therapeutic approaches, but the limitations imposed by the abnormal bladder need to be kept in mind when planning for these types of procedures.

Prognosis: The prognosis depends greatly on 1) the severity of the lesions at the time of diagnosis, 2) the degree of impairment of the renal function, 3) the success of the surgical correction of the anatomic defects, and 4) the presence of other malformations, such as meningocele, which could make the complications more severe and more difficult to treat. The rate of death in childhood or in the early teen years appears to be high in the severe cases, but long survival of the mild ones is a distinct possibility.

Detection of Carrier: Unknown.

Special Considerations: It is likely that this is a common syndrome, affecting many of those children who have hydronephrosis and hydroureter with an abnormal bladder, but that it is not accurately diagnosed because most physicians dealing with these malformations of the urinary tract are not aware of the association of such malformations with the peculiar facies.

References:
Elajalde BR: Genetic and diagnostic considerations in three families with abnormalities of facial expression and congenital urinary obstruction: "the Ochoa syndrome." Am J Med Genet 1979; 3:97–108.
Ochoa B, Gorlin RJ: Urofacial (Ochoa) syndrome. Am J Med Genet 1987; 27:661–667.

EL002
EL014

B. Rafael Elejalde
Maria Mercedes de Elejalde

Urogenital adysplasia
See RENAL AGENESIS, BILATERAL
Urolithiasis, 2,8-dihydroxyadenine (DHA)
See ADENINE PHOSPHO-RIBOSYL-TRANSFERASE (APRT) DEFICIENCY
Uromelia
See SIRENOMELIA SEQUENCE
Uroporphyrinogen decarboxylase deficiency
See PORPHYRIA CUTANEA TARDA
Uroporphyrinogen III cosynthase deficiency
See PORPHYRIA, ERYTHROPOIETIC

URORECTAL SEPTUM MALFORMATION SEQUENCE 3161

Includes:
    Cloacal dysgenesis with female virilization
    Cloacal membrane, persistence of

Excludes:
    Androgen insensitivity syndrome, incomplete (0050)
    Androgen steroidogenesis, disorders of
    Prune-belly syndrome (2007)
    Sex chromosome abnormalities
    Steroid 21-hydroxylase deficiency (0908)
    Vater association (0987)

Major Diagnostic Criteria: Presence of a phallus-like structure (1.5 to 2 cm long), absent labia, no perineal openings (no anus, urethra, or introitus), vesicovaginorectal fistula, oligohydramnios, normal chromosomes, and normal adrenal gland function.

Clinical Findings: All of the reported cases had normal female karyotype (46,XX) in association with ambiguous genitalia. The abnormalities of the genitalia consisted of a phallus-like perineal structure, no urethral or vaginal openings, imperforate anus, vesicovaginorectal communication, and Mullerian duct defects. Urinary abnormalities, including renal agenesis or dysplasia, hydronephrosis, severe bladder dilation, or absence of the urethra were present in about 70% of the cases. Even with urethral agenesis, abdominal distention was seen in only 29% of the cases; its absence probably owes to absorption of fetal urine in the colon after passage through the vesicovaginorectal fistula. Ninety-four percent of the patients had abnormalities of the uterus and vagina. The ovaries were grossly and histologically normal. A history of oligohydramnios was usually present.

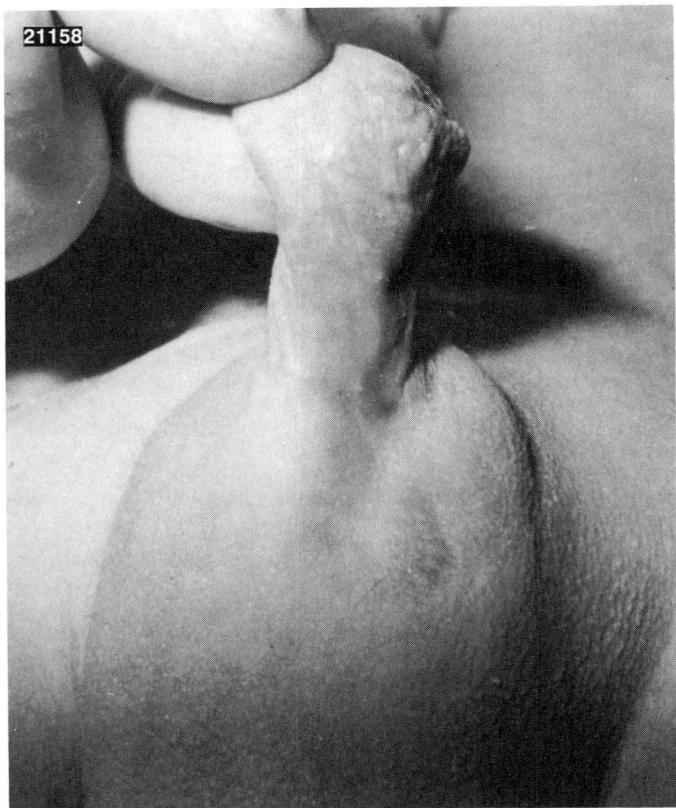

3161-21158: Note the phallus-like structure and a perineum without urethral or vaginal opening.

Complications: Most newborns die within the first 48 hours of life from severe respiratory distress secondary to lung hypoplasia or, rarely, pulmonary edema. The lung hypoplasia probably results from the oligohydramnios. Acute renal failure may be present in those cases in which renal abnormalities have severely compromised kidney function. Chronic renal failure has developed as late as age three years. Abdominal distension also may be caused by GI tract obstruction and may require surgical intervention.

Associated Findings: Persistent urachus, sacral agenesis, clinodactyly of the fifth finger, tracheoesophageal fistula, malrotation of the gut, and absent left radius and sometimes the thumb have been reported.

Etiology: All reported cases have been sporadic.

Pathogenesis: The cloaca is the most distal portion of the embryonic hindgut. By the sixth week of the development of a coronal sheet of mesenchyme, the urorectal septum, proliferates caudally and makes contact with the cloacal membrane, thus dividing the cloaca into an anterior cavity, the urogenital sinus, and a posterior one, the rectum and upper anal canal. The cloacal membrane, as a result of its fusion with the urorectal septum, is divided into the urogenital diaphragm ventrally and the anal membrane dorsally. These two membranes normally break down, leaving the urogenital sinus and anal canal connected to the outside (amniotic cavity). Recently, Escobar et al (1987) hypothesized that this condition is the result of failure of the urorectal septum to divide the cloacal cavity properly or to fuse with the cloacal membrane. These deficiencies lead to persistence of the cloacal cavity and membrane, with abnormal differentiation of both the internal and external genitalia and anal ampulla. The cause of phallic growth is undetermined.

Sex Ratio: M0:F1. This condition has only been recognized in females. In males, persistence of the cloaca may not be recognized, because it is diagnosed either as **Vater association** or urethral obstruction sequence with imperforate anus.

Occurrence: Between 1959 and 1987, nineteen cases were reported in the literature.

Risk of Recurrence for Patient's Sib: Presumably less than one percent.

Risk of Recurrence for Patient's Child: There are no reports of a pregnancy in an affected individual.

Age of Detectability: Prenatal diagnosis has been accomplished by ultrasound detection of a septated cystic structure in the fetal pelvis, no detectable bladder, fetal hydronephrosis, and oligohydramnios. The condition may be detected clinically at, or shortly after birth.

Gene Mapping and Linkage: Unknown.

Prevention: None known. Genetic counseling indicated.

Treatment: Surgery is usually required to alleviate the imperforate anus and urethral obstruction. Later, in surviving children, reconstructive surgery of the genitourinary system is needed. Respiratory distress, if present, may require intensive respiratory support.

Prognosis: Stillborn cases have been reported. Long-term survival of affected individuals is unusual. Seventy-six percent die of respiratory complications or renal failure during the first month of life. Chronic renal failure may lead to premature death in those who survive infancy.

Detection of Carrier: Unknown.

Special Considerations: Although this phenotype is distinctive, chromosomal analysis in the neonatal period should be done to distinguish this condition from males with ambiguous genitalia and from chromosomal aberrations.

References:
Lubinsky M: Female pseudohermaphroditism and associated anomalies. Am J Med Genet 1980; 6:123–136.
Wenstrup R, Pagon R: Female pseudohermaphroditism with anorectal, mullerian duct, and urinary tract malformations: report of four cases. J Pediatr 1985; 107:771–775.

Escobar LF, et al.: Urorectal septum malformation sequence: report of six cases and embryological analysis. Am J Dis Child 1987; 141:1021–1024. *

ES004
WE005
BI017

Luis F. Escobar
David D. Weaver
David Bixler

UROS deficiency
See PORPHYRIA, ERYTHROPOIETIC

URTICARIA PIGMENTOSA (UP) 3263

Includes:
   Mast cell disease
   Mastocytosis
   Telangiectasia macularis eruptiva perstans

Excludes:
   Urticaria
   Xeroderma pigmentosum (1005)

Major Diagnostic Criteria: Hyperpigmented macules or papules on the skin. Dariers sign: erythema and edema of skin lesions in response to trauma. Histology of the skin: mast cell infiltrate in the upper third of the dermis; occasionally nodular aggregates of mast cells extend into the subcutaneous fat and eosinophils are scattered within the infiltration.

Clinical Findings: Four clinical forms of urticaria pigmentosa exist: (1) Localized; mastocytoma. (2) Generalized: (a) maculopapular; (b) telangiectasia macularis eruptiva perstans; (c) erythrodermic, diffuse.

In addition, systemic mastocytosis may occur; organs involved include bone, gastrointestinal tract, lymphatic systems, spleen and liver.

The skin lesions present as multiple red-brown macules and papules distributed on the trunk and occasionally the limbs. Multiple nodular, lichenoid and plaquelike lesions may be seen, and a rare bullous variety exists.

Ten percent of cases are solitary; a mastocytoma is a red-brown, pink or yellow nodule.

Telangiectasia macularis eruptiva perstans, a confluent pattern of telangiectatic and hyperpigmented macules, is a rare variant.

Symptoms of UP are a wheal and flare response to skin trauma, pruritis and flushing. Most patients are asymptomatic. Flushing is precipitated by exercise, hot baths, stress, cold exposure and drugs (especially aspirin and codeine).

Complications: Unknown.

Associated Findings: None known.

Etiology: Autosomal dominant inheritance, possibly with reduced expressivity.

Pathogenesis: The accumulation of mast cells in various organs of the body is the hallmark of mastocytosis. Degranulation of mast cells leads to release of chemical mediators into the skin and other tissues, which results in increased vascular permeability and smooth muscle constriction, and affects leucocyte migration and platelet ulceration.

MIM No.: 15480

Sex Ratio: M1:F1

Occurrence: Some 150 cases were seen at the Mayo clinic between 1917 and 1952 (Klaus, 1962). Most affected persons are Caucasians. Familial cases are rare; approximately 50 cases reported in world literature.

Risk of Recurrence for Patient's Sib:
   See Part I, *Mendelian Inheritance*. Reduced expressivity is possible.

Risk of Recurrence for Patient's Child:
   See Part I, *Mendelian Inheritance*. Reduced expressivity is possible.

Age of Detectability: Urticaria pigmentosa usually presents in childhood.

Gene Mapping and Linkage: Unknown.

Prevention: None known. Genetic counseling indicated.

Treatment: Symptomatic treatment with antihistamines is recomended. Ketotifen may be of use as a mast cell stabiliser.

Prognosis: In the absence of systemic involvement, life span is normal.

Detection of Carrier: Unknown.

Special Considerations: As many as 50 familial cases of urticaria pigmentosa have been recorded. Uniovular twins have been concordant for UP in all but two reported families (Selamonowitz et al, 1970). The inheritance in these families has been autosomal dominant. However, it is important to note that the majority of urticaria pigmentosa or mastocytosis of any type is not familial.

References:
Klaus SN, Winkelmann RK: Course of urticaria pigmentosa in children. Arch Derm 1962; 86:68–71.
Shaw JM: Genetic aspects of urticaria pigmentosa. Arch Derm 1968; 97:137–138.
Selamonowitz VJ, et al.: Uniovular twins discordant for cutaneous mastocytosis. Arch Derm 1970; 102:34–41.
Di Bacco RS, De Leo VA: Mastocytosis and the mast cell. J Am Acad Derm 1982; 7:709–722.
Fowler JF, et al.: Familial urticaria pigmentosa. Arch Derm 1986; 122:80–81.

WI055   **Ingrid M. Winship**

Urticaria syndromes, acquired
See COLD HYPERSENSITIVITY

URTICARIA, DERMO-DISTORTIVE TYPE   3124

Includes:
Dermodistortive urticaria
Vibratory angioedema

Excludes:
Angioedema, hereditary (0054)
Dermographia
Pressure urticaria

Major Diagnostic Criteria: The presence of physical urticaria secondary to stretching or vibration of the skin is sufficient to suggest the diagnosis.

Clinical Findings: The rather sudden (i.e., within a few minutes) appearance of transient, pruritic, erythematous wheals in areas of skin exposed to repetitive vibratory or stretching stimulation characterizes the disorder. These wheals usually disappear within one hour. If extensive stimulation is present, systemic manifestations such as faintness, facial flushing, and headache appear.

Complications: Unknown.

Associated Findings: None known.

Etiology: Probably autosomal dominant inheritance with a high degree of penetrance.

Pathogenesis: Unknown. Histamine may be the mediator of the responses.

MIM No.: 12563

Sex Ratio: Presumably M1:F1.

Occurrence: One family of Christian Lebanese ethnic origin has been reported.

Risk of Recurrence for Patient's Sib:
See Part I, *Mendelian Inheritance.*

Risk of Recurrence for Patient's Child:
See Part I, *Mendelian Inheritance.*

Age of Detectability: Symptoms can occur soon after birth.

Gene Mapping and Linkage: Unknown.

Prevention: None known. Genetic counseling indicated.

Treatment: Unknown. Avoidance of precipitating stimuli is beneficial.

Prognosis: Good. Although annoying, this condition does not affect life span or intelligence.

Detection of Carrier: Unknown.

Special Considerations: Dermodistortive urticaria and vibratory angioedema could be the same condition.

References:
Epstein PA, Kidd KK: Dermo-distortive urticaria: an autosomal dominant dermatologic disorder. Am J Med Genet 1981; 9:307–315.
Epstein PA, et al.: Genetic linkage analysis of dermo-distortive urticaria. Am J Med Genet 1981; 9:317–321.

T0007   **Helga V. Toriello**

URTICARIA-DEAFNESS-AMYLOIDOSIS   0982

Includes:
Amyloidosis-deafness-urticaria
Deafness-urticaria-amyloidosis
Muckle-Wells syndrome

Excludes:
Amyloidoses (other)
Fever, familial mediterranean (FMF) (2161)

Major Diagnostic Criteria: Include "aguey bouts" with characteristic skin rash, progressive perceptive deafness, nephropathy, and typical perireticulin amyloidosis.

Clinical Findings: During adolescence "aguey bouts" (chills, fever, malaise) make their appearance and recur continually thereafter. Over the next two to four decades perceptive deafness appears and progresses; finally nephropathy appears and leads to death. The "aguey bouts" recur every three weeks or so, lasting 24 to 48 hours. They are accompanied by malaise, a geographic urticarial rash, no particular alteration of leukocytes, but with hyperglobulinemia and raised sedimentation rate. Pes cavus, short metacarpals, short stature, and some skin thickening are usually present. Nephropathy is of the sclerotic amyloid variety, combining predominantly azotemic manifestations with substantial proteinuria. Permanganate-sensitive amyloid deposition is also present in other parts of the body in the pattern characteristic of typical (i.e., perireticulin) amyloidosis plus pulmonary parenchymal involvement. Antigenically, the deposits consist of AA protein alone. The changes in the ear include degeneration of the organ of Corti and vestibular sensory epithelium, atrophy of the cochlear nerve, and ossification of the basilar membrane.

Deafness always develops, and the condition is transmitted as an autosomal dominant. It thus differs from **Fever, familial mediterranean (FMF)**, which does not include deafness and is autosomal recessive. It also differs from the deafness in other forms of hereditary but dominantly nephropathic amyloidosis, and all of the other types of hereditary **Amyloidosis**.

Complications: Loss of libido and eventually uremic renal failure (seen in all but one case).

Associated Findings: Glaucoma was reported in two patients.

Etiology: Autosomal dominant inheritance with incomplete penetrance.

Pathogenesis: Unknown.

MIM No.: *19190

POS No.: 3130

Sex Ratio: Presumably M1:F1 (M1.3:F1 observed).

Occurrence: Eight families with this condition have been described, the most recent in 1988 (Messier), as well as six sporadic cases. In addition, three families have been described with what appears to be an incomplete variant, comprising all the features of the clinical syndrome but lacking amyloidosis. Finally, a family with *dominantly* inherited **Fever, familial mediterranean (FMF)**, which included neither deafness nor urticaria, was reported by Bergman and Warmenius (1968).

Risk of Recurrence for Patient's Sib:
See Part I, *Mendelian Inheritance.*

Risk of Recurrence for Patient's Child:
See Part I, *Mendelian Inheritance.*

Age of Detectability: In early adolescence, at clinical appraisal of "aguey bouts" which are an initial manifestations. The full syndrome not established before the third decade of life.

Gene Mapping and Linkage: Unknown.

Prevention: None known. Genetic counseling indicated.

Treatment: From an early age, hearing aids, auditory and speech training, and lip-reading instruction may be helpful. Eventually, the usual supportive therapy or more radical treatment for renal failure will be required.

Prognosis: Usually death from uremia during the fifth or sixth decade.

Detection of Carrier: Possibly by clinical examination of first degree relatives.

References:
Muckle TJ, Wells MV: Urticaria, deafness and amyloidosis: a new heredo-familial syndrome. Q J Med 1962; 31:235–248.
Bergman F, Warmenius S: Familial perireticular amyloidosis in a Swedish family. Am J Med 1968; 45:601–606.
Alexander F, Atkins EL: Familial renal amyloidosis: case reports, literature review and classification. Am J Med 1975; 59:121–128.
Letosa RM, et al.: Sindrome de Muckle-Wells: estudio de una familia. Rev Clin Española 1978; 149:93–96.
Muckle TJ: The Muckle-Wells syndrome: a review. Br J Dermatol 1979; 100:87–92. *
Sweeney PJ, et al.: Muckle-Wells syndrome: first Irish case. J Irish Coll Phys Surg 1979; 9:68 only.
Messier G, et al.: Overt or occult renal amyloidosis in the Muckle-Wells syndrome. Siciety de Nephrologie des Paris, 1988.

MU002   **Thomas J. Muckle**

USHER SYNDROME   0983

Includes:
Deafness (sensorineural)-retinitis pigmentosa
Hallgren syndrome
Retinitis pigmentosa-hearing loss (sensorineural)

Excludes:
Alstrom syndrome (0041)
Cockayne syndrome (0189)
Cockayne syndrome, type II (2787)
Enzyme deficiencies, disorders with multiple peroxisomal
Fetal rubella syndrome (0384)
Nephritis-deafness (sensorineural), hereditary type (0708)
Phytanic acid oxidase deficiency, infantile type (2278)
Phytanic acid storage disease (0810)

Major Diagnostic Criteria: Sensorineural hearing loss and **Retinitis pigmentosa**. May be documented by electrophysiologic methods.

Clinical Findings: The cardinal manifestations of sensorineural hearing loss and retinitis pigmentosa are variable in time of onset and severity, leading most observers to comment on heterogeneity in Usher syndrome. While two separate classification schemes have been devised to group families according to severity (Merin et al., 1974; Gorlin et al., 1979), other studies have found considerable intrafamilial variability for both otic and optic manifestations (Bateman et al., 1980). Over 90% of patients have profound congenital deafness, with onset of retinitis pigmentosa by age 10 years. The minority will have either severe congenital deafness with retinitis manifested in the second decade or progressive hearing loss with retinitis appearing around puberty. The ophthalmologic findings may be characteristic with pallor of the optic nerve, arteriolar narrowing, and "bone spicule" concretions of pigment. Recently, the possibility of biochemical diagnosis has been raised by finding a decreased content of polyunsaturated fatty acids in plasma phospholids from patients with Usher syndrome.

Complications: Several investigators comment on a typical psychosis in Usher syndrome patients; when mental deficiency and psychosis are present, the disorder is termed *Hallgren syndrome.* Labyrinthine ataxia is relatively frequent and necessitates discrimination from Refsum disease (see **Phytanic acid storage disease**) by phytanic acid measurement. Posterior sublenticular cataracts are a later complication. Since Usher syndrome accounts for 6–10% of the congenitally deaf population, all hearing-impaired individuals under age 25 years should be screened for decreasing dark adaptation or peripheral vision. Early recognition of such individuals allows social and vocational preparation for life as a deaf and blind adult.

Associated Findings: Abnormalities of nasal cilia and sperm axonemes have been described.

Etiology: Unsually autosomal recessive inheritance; a rare X-linked form was suggested by two pairs of affected brothers whose mothers were sisters.

Pathogenesis: The abnormalities in nasal cilia, sperm, and photoreceptor axonemes provides one potential route for gene expression; serum fatty acid abnormalities in Usher syndrome, and various peroxisomal disorders having retinitis with deafness, provides another.

MIM No.: *27690, 31265

POS No.: 3421

Sex Ratio: M1:F1

Occurrence: Prevalence has been estimated at 3.6–5:100,000 (Grondahl, 1987). A prevalence of 3:1,000 normal individuals was estimated in Denmark. Clusters of patients have been reported in Berlin (Mainly Jews), Finland, Norway (particularly among Lapps), and Louisiana (French Cajuns).

Risk of Recurrence for Patient's Sib:
See Part I, *Mendelian Inheritance.*

Risk of Recurrence for Patient's Child:
See Part I, *Mendelian Inheritance.*

Age of Detectability: In most patients, profound sensorineural hearing loss is recognized at birth or during infancy. Less than 10% will have progressive hearing loss recognized in the first decade. Retinitis pigmentosa may not be diagnosed until after puberty.

Gene Mapping and Linkage: GC (group-specific component (vitamin D binding protein)) has been mapped to 4q12-q13.

Prevention: None known. Genetic counseling indicated.

Treatment: Special education, cataract removal.

Prognosis: Life span is normal, but severe deafness and blindness are anticipated in most patients. The sensorineural hearing loss is described as stable by most observers, but some reports describe deterioration with age.

Detection of Carrier: One report cites the presence of gyrate atrophy in heterozygotes.

Special Considerations: Usher syndrome is undoubtedly a heterogenous group of autosomal recessive disorders, to be further delineated by clinical, metabolic, and DNA marker studies.

References:
Usher CH: Bowman's lecture: on a few hereditary eye affections. Trans Ophthalmol Soc UK 1935; 55:164–245.
Merin S, et al.: Usher's and Hallgren's syndromes. Acta Genet Med Gemellol 1974; 23:45–55.
Gorlin RJ, et al.: Usher's syndrome type III. Arch Otolaryngol 1979; 105:353–354.
Bateman JB, et al.: Heterogeneity of retinal degeneration and hearing impairment syndromes. Am J Ophthalmol 1980; 90:755–767. †
Boughman JA, et al.: Usher syndrome: definition and estimate of prevalence from two high-risk populations. J Chronic Dis 1983; 36:595–604.
Bazan NG, et al.: Decreased content of docosahexanoate and arachidonate in plasma phospholipids in Usher's syndrome. Biochem Biophys Res Commun 1986; 141:600–604.
Hunter DG, et al.: Abnormal sperm and photoreceptor axonemes in Usher's syndrome. Arch Ophthalmol 1986; 104:385–389.

Shinkawa H, Nadol JB, Jr.: Histopathology of the inner ear in Usher's syndrome as observed by light and electron microscopy. Ann Otol Rhinol Laryng 1986; 95:313–318.

Grondahl J: Estimation of prognosis and prevalence of retinitis pigmentosa and Usher syndrome in Norway. Clin Genet 1987; 31:225–264.

WI024   **Golder N. Wilson**

UVULA, CLEFT   0184

Includes:
    Bifid uvula
    Uvula, split
Excludes:
    Cleft lip (0178)
    Cleft palate (0180)
Major Diagnostic Criteria: Mid-line separation of uvula.

Clinical Findings: Cleft uvula varies from a notching of uvula to complete cleft of uvula extending to the posterior border of the soft palate.

Complications: Hypernasality.

Associated Findings: Submucous cleft palate.

Etiology: Multifactorial inheritance, although an autosomal dominant form may exist.

Pathogenesis: Failure of complete fusion of the uvular portion of the medial halves of the soft palate during embryogenesis.

MIM No.: 19210

CDC No.: 749.080

Sex Ratio: M1.2:F1

Occurrence: One percent among Caucasians, 10% among Mongolians including American Indians.

Risk of Recurrence for Patient's Sib: About ten percent without an affected parent, 30% with an affected parent.

Risk of Recurrence for Patient's Child: About ten percent.

Age of Detectability: At birth.

Gene Mapping and Linkage: Unknown.

Prevention: None known. Genetic counseling indicated.

Treatment: Surgical correction is seldom needed, but available.

Prognosis: Normal life expectancy.

Detection of Carrier: Unknown.

Special Considerations: Some cases of cleft uvula may be microforms of cleft palate. In persons with cleft uvula the complete removal of the adenoid pad during tonsillectomy and adenoidectomy may produce hypernasal speech.

References:
Meskin LH, et al.: Abnormal morphology of the soft palate. I. the prevalence of cleft uvula. Cleft Palate J 1964; 1:342–346. *
Meskin LH, et al.: Abnormal morphology of the soft palate. II. the genetics of cleft uvula. Cleft Palate J 1965; 2:40–45. *
Richardson ER: Cleft uvula: incidence in negroes. Cleft Palate J 1970; 7:669–672.
Chosack A, Eidelman E: Cleft uvula: prevalence and genetics. Cleft Palate J 1987; 5:63–67.

J0027   **Ronald J. Jorgenson**

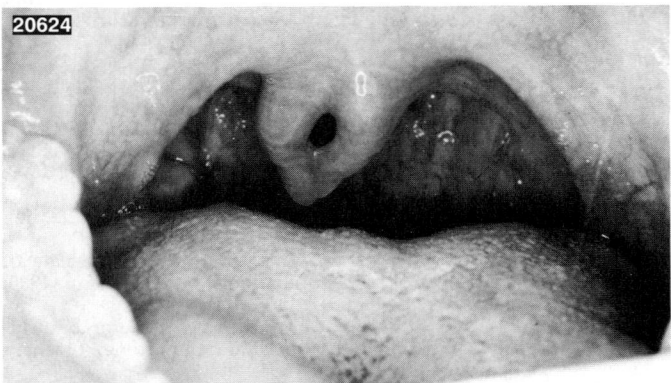

0184-20624:   Cleft uvula.

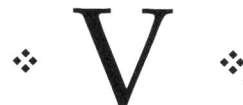

VAGINAL ATRESIA   0984

Includes: Vagina, absence, congenital (one form)

Excludes:
    Hymen, imperforate (0483)
    Mullerian aplasia (0682)
    Pseudohermaphroditism, all forms of male and female
    Renal-genital-middle ear anomalies (0860)
    Vaginal septum, transverse (0985)

Major Diagnostic Criteria: Atresia of the lower vagina in a female (46,XX) with a normal upper vagina, uterus, external genitalia, and ovaries.

Clinical Findings: The lower one-fifth to one-third of the vagina is replaced by 2–3 cm of fibrous tissue. The remaining (superior) portion of the vagina is well differentiated. External genitalia are normal for females. The uterine cervix and corpus, fallopian tubes, and ovaries are likewise normal. Usually somatic anomalies are not present, although renal anomalies have been reported. At puberty female secondary sexual development is normal, except for absence of menses.

Vaginal atresia should be differentiated from **Mullerian aplasia**, a condition in which the cephalad portion of the vagina and the uterus are absent. Some authors group both these conditions under "congenital absence of vagina." In addition, an autosomal recessive trait characterized by vaginal atresia, renal hypoplasia or agenesis, and middle ear anomalies (see **Renal-genital-middle ear anomalies**) has been described.

Complications: Menstrual products cannot pass because of the atretic lower vagina. Hydrometrocolpos may lead to amenorrhea, as well as abdominal pain or palpable masses as the result of accumulation of fluid.

Associated Findings: Renal anomalies have been reported.

Etiology: Undetermined. Familial aggregates are very rare. Limitation of the defect to a single organ system is compatible with polygenic/multifactorial inheritance.

Pathogenesis: The caudal portion of the vagina is formed from invagination of the urogenital sinus, whereas the cephalad portion is of müllerian origin. In vaginal atresia the urogenital sinus presumably fails to contribute the caudal portion of the vagina.

CDC No.: 752.410

Sex Ratio: M0:F1

Occurrence: Occurs in perhaps 5–10% of females said to have "absence of the vagina", as opposed to **Mullerian aplasia** which is more common.

Risk of Recurrence for Patient's Sib: Probably not greater than 1–5% for female sib to be affected, assuming multifactorial etiology.

Risk of Recurrence for Patient's Child: No more than 1–5% for a female child to be affected, assuming multifactorial etiology.

Age of Detectability: Usually at puberty, when hydrometrocolpos causes primary amenorrhea. Occasionally mucocolpos occurs in neonates.

Gene Mapping and Linkage: Unknown.

Prevention: None known. Genetic counseling indicated.

Treatment: Surgical extirpation of the fibrous tissue. The thickness of atretic portion precludes simple incisional drainage.

Prognosis: Normal life span; normal fertility.

Detection of Carrier: Unknown.

References:
Dennison WM, Bacsich P: Imperforate vagina in the newborn: neonatal hydrocolpos. Arch Dis Child 1961; 36:156–160.
Simpson JL: Disorders of sexual differentiation: etiology and clinical delineation. New York: Academic Press, 1976:345–346.
Jones HW Jr, Rock JA: Reparative and constructive surgery of the female generative tract. Baltimore: Williams & Wilkins, 1983:161–164.

SI018   **Joe Leigh Simpson**

VAGINAL SEPTUM, TRANSVERSE   0985

Includes:
    Hydrometrocolpos-postaxial polydactyly-congential heart anomalies
    Kaufman-McKusick syndrome
    McKusick-Kaufman syndrome
    Transverse vaginal septum

Excludes:
    Chondroectodermal dysplasia (0156)
    Hymen, imperforate (0483)
    Mullerian aplasia (0682)
    Mullerian fusion, incomplete (0684)
    Vaginal atresia (0984)
    Vaginal septum, longitudinal

Major Diagnostic Criteria: Transverse vaginal septum, with or without a perforation, in a 46,XX individual with normal ovaries, normal external genitalia, and otherwise normal müllerian derivatives.

Clinical Findings: Transverse septa are usually located near the junction of the upper one-third and lower two-thirds of the vagina; however, septa may be present in the middle or lower one-third. These septa are about 1 cm thick and may or may not have a perforation. A perforation, if present, is usually central in location; however, it may occasionally be eccentric. The external genitalia, uterine cervix, uterine corpus, fallopian tubes, and ovaries are normal. The most frequent presenting symptom is primary amenorrhea. Hydrometrocolpos or hematometrocolpos may be noted on pelvic examination. No somatic abnormalities are present. At puberty normal secondary sexual development occurs.

Longitudinal vaginal septa, sagittal or coronal, have been reported, but these septa represent an entity different from transverse vaginal septa. Longitudinal septa rarely produce clinical problems.

Complications: If no perforation is present, mucus and menstrual fluid cannot be expelled and, hence, hydrometrocolpos may develop. Coital difficulties or abnormalities of the second stage of labor have been reported.

Associated Findings: Polydactyly and cardiac anomalies have been associated with transverse vaginal septum, but usually no associated anomalies are present.

Etiology: Although autosomal recessive inheritance appears to be responsible for transverse vaginal septa in the Amish, heritable tendencies have not been verified in other ethnic groups. Whether the presence of polydactyly and/or heart anomalies indicates a separate condition (*Kaufman-McKusick syndrome*) has not been determined.

Pathogenesis: Vaginal septa probably result from failure of the urogenital sinus derivatives and the müllerian duct derivatives to fuse or canalize properly in order to form a normal vagina. Although this explanation is accepted by most investigators, the situation may be more complex. Some data suggest that abnormal mesodermal proliferation may occur.

MIM No.: *23670

CDC No.: 752.380

Sex Ratio: M0:F1

Occurrence: At least six families, and many individual cases (some associated with consanguinity), have been documented.

Risk of Recurrence for Patient's Sib:
See Part I, *Mendelian Inheritance*. In the Amish 1:4 for 46,XX sibs; 1:8 for all sibs. In other ethnic groups, similar risk figures may or may not be appropriate.

Risk of Recurrence for Patient's Child:
See Part I, *Mendelian Inheritance*. Some forms could be inherited in polygenic/multifactorial fashion, in which case the risk is estimated at less than 5%.

Age of Detectability: Usually at puberty, because of primary amenorrhea with or without hydrometrocolpos, or hematometrocolpos. Occasionally mucocolpos is noted at birth, and Farrell et al (1986) described prenatal diagnosis. Some affected patients have been detected because of coital difficulties or abnormalities during labor.

Gene Mapping and Linkage: Unknown.

Prevention: None known. Genetic counseling indicated.

Treatment: Surgical extirpation or creation of an opening in the septum if no perforation is present; enlargement of the perforation may be necessary if the opening is very small.

Prognosis: Normal life span.

Detection of Carrier: Glandular hypospadias and prominent scrotal raphe are claimed by some to be manifestations in the male.

References:
McKusick VA, et al.: Recessive inheritance of a congenital malformation syndrome. J Am Med Asso 1968; 204:113–116.
Simpson JL: Disorders of sexual differentiation: etiology and clinical delineation. New York: Academic Press, 1976:348–351.
Sarto GE, Simpson JL: Abnormalities of the Müllerian and Wolffian duct systems. BD:OAS XIV(6c). New York: Alan R. Liss, for The National Foundation-March of Dimes, 1978:37–55.
Robinow M, Shaw A: The McKusick/Kaufman syndrome: recessively inherited vaginal atresia, hydrometrocolpos, uterovaginal duplications, anorectal anomalies, postaxial polydactyly, and congenital heart disease. J Pediatr 1979; 94:776–778.
Suidan FG, Azoury RS: The transverse vaginal septum: a clinicopathologic evaluation. Obstet Gynecol 1979; 54:278–283.
Goecke T, et al.: Hydrometrocolpos, postaxial polydactyly, congenital heart disease, and anomalies of the gastrointestinal and genitourinary tracts. Eur J Pediatr 1981; 136:297–305.
Jones HW Jr, Rock JA: Reparative and constructive surgery of the female generative tract. Baltimore: Williams & Wilkins, 1983:158–164.
Pinsky L: Origin of the "associated" anomalies in Kaufman-McKusick syndrome. (Letter) Am J Med Genet 1983; 14:791–792.
Farrell SA, et al.: Abdominal distension in Kaufman-McKusick syndrome. Am J Med Genet 1986; 25:205–210.

SI018   **Joe Leigh Simpson**

Valine transaminase deficiency
See HYPERVALINEMIA
Valinemia
See HYPERVALINEMIA
Valium^, fetal effects
See FETAL BENZODIAZEPINE EFFECTS
Vallecular cyst
See EPIGLOTTIS, VALLECULAR CYST
Valproate sensitivity
See ORNITHINE TRANSCARBAMYLASE DEFICIENCY
Valproic acid and conjoined twins
See TWINS, CONJOINED, TERATOGENICITY
Valproic acid, fetal damage from
See FETAL VALPROATE SYNDROME
Valproic acid, fetal effects
See MENINGOMYELOCELE
Valvar aortic stenosis
See AORTIC VALVE STENOSIS
Van Allen type amyloidosis
See AMYLOIDOSIS, IOWA TYPE
Van Bogaert spongy degeneration of the CNS
See BRAIN, SPONGY DEGENERATION
Van Buchem disease
See ENDOSTEAL HYPEROSTOSIS

VAN DEN BOSCH SYNDROME   0986

Includes: Anhidrosis-mental retardation-eye and skeletal defects

Excludes:
    Choroideremia (0925)
    Ectodermal dysplasia, Christ-Siemens-Touraine type (0333)
    X-linked mental retardation (1509)

Major Diagnostic Criteria: Anhidrosis, mental retardation, choroideremia, acrokeratosis verruciformis, and winged scapulae.

Clinical Findings: Anhidrosis associated with mental deficiency; delayed somatic growth; ophthalmologic abnormalities (horizontal nystagmus, myopia, choroideremia, abnormal retinogram); winged scapulae; acrokeratosis verruciformis; and bronchial and skin infections.

Complications: Hyperthermia, intolerance to heat, and bronchial and skin infections.

Associated Findings: None known.

Etiology: X-linked recessive inheritance.

Pathogenesis: Unknown.

MIM No.: *31450

POS No.: 3424

Sex Ratio: M1:F0

Occurrence: Described in a single Dutch kindred.

Risk of Recurrence for Patient's Sib:
See Part I, *Mendelian Inheritance*.

Risk of Recurrence for Patient's Child:
See Part I, *Mendelian Inheritance*.

Age of Detectability: In neonatal period.

Gene Mapping and Linkage: A small deletion on the long arm of the X-chromosome could explain the concurrence of the different components of this syndrome, which have been described as isolated X-linked traits.

Prevention: None known. Genetic counseling indicated.

Treatment: Avoid high environmental temperature, encourage hydration; special education as needed.

Prognosis: Unknown.

Detection of Carrier: Possibly altered sweat pores in carrier.

References:
Van Den Bosch, J: A new syndrome in three generations of a Dutch family. Ophthalmologica 1959; 137:422–423.

WI021   **R.S. Wilroy, Jr.**

van der Woude syndrome
 See CLEFT LIP/PALATE-LIP PITS OR MOUNDS
Van Gelderen syndrome
 See ALOPECIA-SKELETAL ANOMALIES-SHORT STATURE-MENTAL RETARDATION
Van Lohuizen syndrome
 See CUTIS MARMORATA
Varadi-Papp syndrome
 See ORO-PALATAL-DIGITAL SYNDROME, VARADI TYPE
Varicella embryopathy
 See FETAL EFFECTS FROM VARICELLA-ZOSTER
Varicella-zoster, fetal effects
 See FETAL EFFECTS FROM VARICELLA-ZOSTER
Vascular anomalies-congenital heart defects-distichiasis
 See DISTICHIASIS-HEART DEFECT-PERIPHERAL VASCULAR DISEASE/ANOMALIES
Vascular dysplasia-sternal malformation association
 See STERNAL MALFORMATION-VASCULAR DYSPLASIA ASSOCIATION
Vascular formations, familial
 See RETINA, CAVERNOUS HEMANGIOMA
Vascular malformations of middle ear
 See EAR, OSSICLE AND MIDDLE EAR MALFORMATIONS
Vascular malformations, familial
 See HEMANGIOMAS OF THE HEAD AND NECK
Vascular tumors hemangioid cell derivation-spontaneous hemorrhage
 See HEMANGIOMA-THROMBOCYTOPENIA SYNDROME
Vasolidator, fetal effects
 See FETAL EFFECTS FROM MATERNAL VASODILATOR
Vasopressin-resistant
 See DIABETES INSIPIDUS, VASOPRESSIN RESISTANT TYPES I AND II
Vasotec^, fetal effects
 See FETAL ANGIOTENSIN CONVERTING ENZYME (ACE) INHIBITION RENAL FAILURE
Vasquez syndrome
 See X-LINKED MENTAL RETARDATION-GROWTH-HEARING AND GENITAL DEFECTS

VATER ASSOCIATION   0987

Includes:
 Imperforate anus-polydactyly syndrome
 Polydactyly-imperforate anus
 VACTEL association
 VACTERL association

Excludes:
 Anus-hand-ear syndrome (0072)
 Charge association (2124)
 Heart-hand syndrome (0455)
 MURCS association (2406)
 Renal agenesis, unilateral (0857)
 Tracheal agenesis-multiple anomaly association (2849)

Major Diagnostic Criteria: The VATER association is diagnosed, according to the criteria of Quan and Smith (1973), on the basis of the presence of three of five designated VATER ascertainment abnormalities: Vertebral dysgenesis, Anal atresia, Tracheosophageal fistula with Esophageal atresia, and Renal and Radial limb dysgenesis in the absence of a chromosome aberration.

Clinical Findings: While many additional malformations are observed in VATER patients, and result in a high average number of anomalies (seven to eight) per patient, central system abnormalities are minimally increased and mental retardation is only an occasional problem. The malformations are widely distributed throughout the body, with approximately two-thirds located in the lower body segment, notably those of the distal intestinal and genitourinary tracts, lumbosacrococcygeal vertebrae, pelvis, and lower limbs. Anomalies observed in the upper body segment include esophageal atresia with or without tracheoesophageal fistula, radial limb dysgenesis, heart, proximal intestinal tract, rib, and respiratory tract abnormalities. Hypersegmentation (13–14 ribs and/or thoracic vertebrae; 6–7 lumbar vertebrae) occurs in approximately 10% of VATER patients.

Complications: Respiratory, cardiac, and renal failure can be severe in VATER patients neonatally.

Associated Findings: Monozygotic twinning is increased (6%), while maternal diabetes and situs inversus have low incidences when compared with those of patients with the **Sacrococcygeal dysgenesis syndrome**.

Etiology: Nearly all cases have been sporadic, although a few familial cases have been reported (Auchterlonie and White, 1982).

Pathogenesis: Unknown.

MIM No.: 19235

POS No.: 3425

Sex Ratio: M1:F1

Occurrence: About 250 cases have been documented. Probably underreported, since patients previously identified to have only multiple anomalies can now be diagnosed as having the VATER association.

Risk of Recurrence for Patient's Sib: Minimal, except in familial cases.

Risk of Recurrence for Patient's Child: Unknown.

Age of Detectability: At birth or shortly thereafter.

Gene Mapping and Linkage: Unknown.

Prevention: None known. Genetic counseling indicated.

Treatment: Surgical correction or medical management of spine, limb, cardiovascular, urinary, intestinal, and other malformations as indicated.

Prognosis: The overall survival of 46 VATER patients was 72% (Weaver et al., 1986) but the series did not include fetal deaths or stillbirths. The prognosis of each VATER patient will depend on the particular combination and severity of abnormalities present, and on the availability of surgical and medical correction.

Detection of Carrier: Unknown.

Special Considerations: VATER is an acronym used to identify a sporadic, nonrandom association of specified abnormalities. It is probably best to confine the designation of VATER association to patients who rigidly meet the original criteria of Quan and Smith (1973).

References:
Quan L, Smith DW: The VATER association, vertebral defects, anal atresia, T-E fistula with esophageal atresia, radial and renal dysplasia: a spectrum of associated defects. J Pediatr 1973; 82:104–107.
Smith DW, et al.: Monozygotic twinning and the Duhamel anomalad (imperforate anus to sirenomelia); a non-random association between two aberrations in morphogenesis. BD:OAS XII(5). New York: March of Dimes Birth Defects Foundation, 1976:53–63.
Auchterlonie IA, White MP: Recurrence of the VATER association within a sibship. Clin Genet 1982; 21:122–124.
Khoury MJ, et al.: A population study of the VACTERL association: evidence for its etiologic heterogeneity. Pediatrics 1983; 71:815–820.
Duncan PA, et al.: Distinct caudal regression syndrome identified by associated malformation pattern and demographic features. (Abstract) Proc Greenwood Genet Center 1986; 5:142 only.
Weaver DD, et al.: The VATER association: analysis of 46 patients. Am J Dis Child 1986; 140:225–229.
Duncan PA, Shapiro LR: Seronomelia and VATER association: possi-

ble interrelated disorders with common embryologic pathogenesis. Dysmorphol Clin Genet 1988; 2:96–103.

DU003   Peter A. Duncan
SH009   Lawrence R. Shapiro

Vein of Galen aneurysm
See CNS ARTERIOVENOUS MALFORMATION

VELO-CARDIO-FACIAL SYNDROME   2129

Includes: Shprintzen syndrome

Excludes:
    Arthro-ophthalmopathy, hereditary, progressive, Stickler type (0090)
    Cardio-auditory syndrome (0123)
    Cleft palate-micrognathia-glossoptosis (0182)
    Fetal alcohol syndrome (0379)
    G syndrome (0401)
    Hypertelorism-hypospadias syndrome (0505)
    Immunodeficiency, thymic agenesis (0943)
    Myotonic dystrophy (0702)
    Tricho-rhino-phalangeal syndrome
    Vena cava, persistent left superior joined to coronary sinus (0807)

Major Diagnostic Criteria: Numerous physical, psychological, and behavioral findings have been documented in this common syndrome of clefting. However, with the exception of some of the cardiac anomalies and **Cleft palate**, the majority of anomalies associated with this syndrome are minor and occur with frequency in the general population. However, the following combination of anomalies should lead to a strong suspicion of this syndrome:

1) cleft, submucous cleft, or occult submucous cleft of the secondary palate, or hypernasal speech, 2) **Ventricular septal defect** (VSD) alone or in combination with other cardiac anomalies, including **Aortic arch, right** and **Heart, tetralogy of Fallot**, 3) learning disabilities or mental retardation, hypotonia, and mildly delayed developmental milestones, 4) relatively small stature, 5) relatively small head circumference, often **Microcephaly**, 6) slender, tapered hands and digits, often hyperextensible, 7) retrognathia, 8) characteristic facies, including a prominent nose with a large, squared nasal root and narrow alar base, malar flatness, vertical maxillary excess, long philtrum, and open-mouth posture, bluish suborbital venous congestion (often referred to as "allergic shiners"), occasional mild facial asymmetry, 9) small auricles, often with thickened helical rims, occasionally asymmetrical with one slightly larger than the other, 10) cephalometric X-rays show platybasia (obtuse angulation of the cranial base) with relatively normal mandibular morphology, 11) frequent upper respiratory illness with apparent immunologic deficiency, 12) tortuous retinal vessels and occasionally other eye anomalies, including microphthalmia and ocular coloboma, 13) medial displacement of the internal carotid arteries in the posterior pharyngeal wall, 14) absent or small thymus, tonsils or adenoids, and 15) hypocalcemia and hypotonia in infancy.

Clinical Findings: Birth weight is usually normal. Growth often proceeds normally during infancy and young childhood, though "failure to thrive" has been reported in approximately 25% of affected neonates. This has been associated with obstructive apnea in a number of neonates. Obstructive apnea has been seen in affected neonates and is precipitated by both retrognathia and pharyngeal hypotonia. Hypocalcemia has been reported in approximately 10% of known cases. In several of these cases, hypocalcemia has occurred in association with absent thymus and right sided aortic arch, thus leading to the diagnosis of **Immunodeficiency, thymic agenesis** occurring in association with velo-cardio-facial syndrome. As the children get older, growth is constant though they tend to remain relatively small, usually falling between the second and twenty-fifth percentile.

Developmental milestones are usually mildly delayed, though they may be barely within normal limits. Nearly all of the reported cases have been "floppy babies" remaining relatively hypotonic throughout childhood. However, intellectual impairment is generally not evident in preschool years. Language development is often mildly delayed and speech is almost always characterized by hypernasality, with or without overt clefting of the palate. With advancing age, especially after entering school where more abstract reasoning becomes necessary, learning disabilities and perhaps even mild intellectual impairment become apparent. The majority of the children require some type of special class placement or supplementary educational services, especially in earlier school years, but are eventually "mainstreamed" and graduate from high school. Several affected individuals have also completed college. However, the range of IQ scores in secondary school age children with this syndrome is reported at 69–87 on a performance scale (with mean scores of 79 and 70 respectively).

Hypernasal speech has been observed in nearly all documented cases to date, whether obtained from cleft palate centers or cardiac clinics. Hypernasality has been related to both the frequent occurrence of **Cleft palate** (including submucous and occult submucous cleft palate) and to hypotonia of the pharynx. It is of interest to note that obstructive sleep apnea has been reported following pharyngeal flap surgery, including one reported case of sudden death one month postoperatively. Surgical risk is also increased by the observation of medial displacement of the internal carotid arteries in approximately 25% of cases examined nasopharyngoscopically.

Patients have displayed a very characteristic personality. They have a bland affect, are disinhibited, impulsive, and very affectionate.

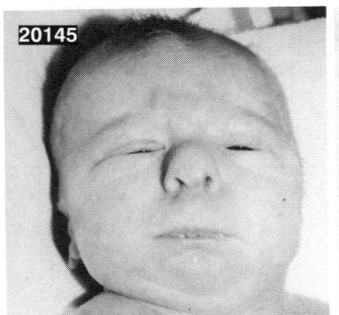
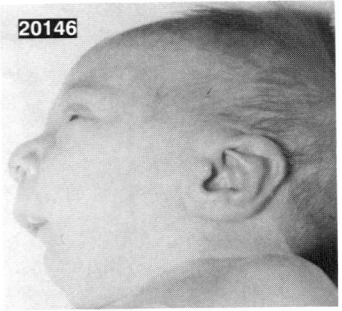
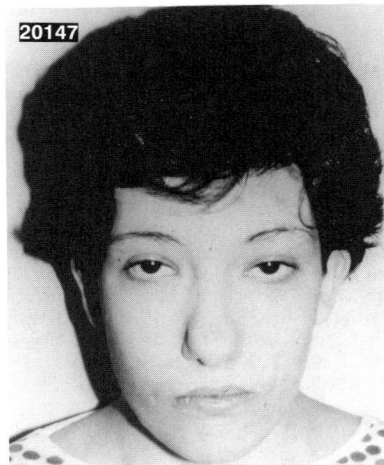

2129-20145: Note prominent nose with squared nasal root, long philtrum and mild facial asymmetry. **20146:** Lateral view of the face; the micrognathia is not characteristic and is an associated finding in this infant. **20147:** Adult subject; note prominent nose with squared root and narrow alar base.

Based upon approximately 150 cases clinical findings can be summarized as learning disabilities (100%); **Cleft palate** including submucous and occult submucous cleft palate (98%); hypernasal speech and high pitched voice (98%); pharyngeal hypotonia (90%); retrognathia (87%); cardiac anomalies (80%), including **Ventricular septal defect** (65%), **Aortic arch, right** (35%), **Heart, tetralogy of Fallot** (21%), aberrant left subclavian artery (20%), and a variety of associated cardiac anomalies which occurred in less than 10% of reported cases.

Characteristic facies, including in any combination: "long face" with vertical maxillary excess (85%), prominent nose with squared nasal root and narrow alar base and resultant compromise of the nasal airway (75%), long philtrum and upper lip (70%), malar flatness (70%), narrow palpebral fissures (65%), blue suborbital venous congestion, or "allergic shiners" (50%), and abundant scalp hair (50%); obtuse angulation of the cranial base, or platybasia (75%); intermittent conductive hearing loss secondary to frequent serous otitis media and cleft palate (75%); small auricles and minor auricular anomalies, including thickened helical folds (60%); slender hands and tapered digits, generally small by measurement (60%); tortuous retinal vessels (50%); small or absent tonsils and adenoids (50%); mental retardation (40%); **Microcephaly** (40%); small stature (30%); medial displacement of the internal carotid arteries (25%); **Hernia, inguinal** (25%); **Hernia, umbilical** (20%); scoliosis (15%); **Cleft palate-micrognathia-glossoptosis** (15%); hypospadias (10% of affected males); absent thymus (approximately 10%); hypocalcemia (approximately 10%);

With the exception of cardiac X-rays (chest films, cardiac catheterizations, echocardiograms, etc.), X-ray findings to date have been limited to cephalometry which has shown anomalies of the basicranium (platybasia) and videofluoroscopic phonation studies of the pharynx which has shown hypotonia of the pharyngeal walls in approximately 80% of the cases examined.

Complications: Obstructive sleep apnea has been frequently observed in nearly half of the cases who were seen as neonates for the first time. There were several factors contributing to this upper airway compromise, including retrognathia, pharyngeal (and generalized) hypotonia, and severe constriction of the nose. Several patients have developed obstructive sleep apnea following pharyngeal flap surgery to relieve hypernasal speech. Palatal and other surgery may be complicated by cardiac anomalies. Medial displacement of the internal carotid arteries may also lead to bleeding complications during pharyngeal surgery. A small number of infants have died because of the severity of their cardiac anomalies.

Associated Findings: **Holoprosencephaly**, diastasis recti, synophrys, sensori-neural hearing loss, and cryptorchidism.

Etiology: Autosomal dominant inheritance.

Pathogenesis: The numerous vascular anomalies may point towards a major effect on the circulatory system. Numerous patients have had karyotypes and no chromosome anomalies have been found. Similarly, numerous biochemical tests have been performed because of early failure to thrive, but no metabolic or immunologic factors have been found with the exception of absent thymic hormone in patients with absent thymus. Cleft palate is clearly a primary feature of the syndrome and is not secondary to retrognathia. Retrognathia is caused by posterior displacement of the temporomandibular joint which is related to the flattening of the cranial base (platybasia). The mandible is morphologically normal. Similarly, the prominence of the nasal root and the malar deficiency which result in the characteristic facies are caused by the abnormal flexion of the cranial base and the abnormal arrangement and orientation of the facial bones.

Neurologic investigations have failed to show any identifiable abnormalities within the brain to account for hypotonia, learning disabilities, or mental retardation. However, it should be noted that nearly all patients have relatively small head circumferences with approximately 40% of the patients being microcephalic. Small stature is a primary feature of the syndrome and is not secondary to cardiac anomalies.

MIM No.: *19243

POS No.: 3132

Sex Ratio: M1:F1

Occurrence: Common syndrome of clefting, comprising as much as 5% of the population of individuals with cleft palate without cleft lip. At least 150 cases have been observed.

Risk of Recurrence for Patient's Sib:
See Part I, *Mendelian Inheritance.*

Risk of Recurrence for Patient's Child:
See Part I, *Mendelian Inheritance.*

Age of Detectability: Can be detected at birth if the association of cleft palate and cardiac anomalies is present, or if **Cleft palate-micrognathia-glossoptosis** or **Immunodeficiency, thymic agenesis** is present. Characteristic facies may not be apparent until later in childhood. Speech disorders, language impairment, and learning disabilities are valuable aids in the diagnosis of this syndrome, but are also not evident until at least 2–3 years of age.

Gene Mapping and Linkage: Unknown.

Prevention: None known. Genetic counseling indicated.

Treatment: Symptomatic treatment for cardiac, palatal, speech, hearing, and learning problems can be very effective. If patient feels it is necessary, aesthetic surgery (rhinoplasty, maxillary and mandibular osteotomies) can remove facial stigmata. Early failure to thrive is most often related to obstructive apnea and is best temporarily relieved by placement of a nasopharyngeal tube. Several patients have required glossopexy which was usually divided by six months of age.

Prognosis: Life span is normal. All documented cases to date have had learning disabilities, especially in the areas of mathematics and reading comprehension. Forty percent of documented cases have been mildly mentally retarded. However, the prognosis for normal social functioning is good.

Detection of Carrier: Unknown.

Special Considerations: This syndrome is one of the most common syndromes of clefting, but because affected children are not severely dysmorphic, diagnosis may be difficult. However, identification is important because of special treatment considerations for speech, language, and learning deficits. Early identification can lead to the interception of anticipated learning disabilities and more effective educational management.

References:
Strong WB: Familial syndrome of right-sided aortic arch, mental deficiency, and facial dysmorphism. J Pediatr 1968; 73:882–888.
Shprintzen RJ, et al.: A new syndrome involving cleft palate, cardiac anomalies, typical facies, and learning disabilities: velo-cardio-facial syndrome. Cleft Palate J 1978; 15:56–62.
Young D, et al.: Cardiac malformations in the velocardiofacial syndrome. Am J Cardiol, 1980; 46:643–648.
Shprintzen RJ, et al.: The velo-cardio-facial syndrome: a clinical and genetic analysis. Pediatrics 1981; 67:167–172.
Aruystas M, Shprintzen RJ: Craniofacial morphology in the velo-cardio-facial syndrome. J Craniofac Genet Dev Biol 1984; 4:39–45.
Golding-Kishner K, Weller G: Velo-cardio-facial syndrome: language and psychological profiles. J Craniofacial Genet Devel Biol 1985; 5:259–266.
Williams MA, et al.: Male-to-male transmission of the velo-cardio-facial syndrome: a case report and review of 60 cases. J Craniofacial Genet Devel Biol, 1985; 5:175–180.
Wraith JE, et al.: Velo-cardio-facial syndrome presenting as holoprosencephaly. Clin Genet 1985; 27:408–410.
Beemer FA, et al.: Additional eye findings in a girl with velo-cardio-facial syndrome. Am J Med Genet 1986; 24:541–542.
Williams MA, et al.: Adenoid hypoplasia in the velo-cardio-facial syndrome. J Craniofac Genet Devel Biol 1987; 7:23–26.

SH040   **Robert J. Shprintzen**

Velopharyngeal incompetence
See PALATOPHARYNGEAL INCOMPETENCE
Velopharyngeal insufficiency
See PALATOPHARYNGEAL INCOMPETENCE
Vena cava connecting to right atrium via coronary sinus
See VENA CAVA, PERSISTENT LEFT SUPERIOR JOINED TO CORONARY SINUS

VENA CAVA, ABSENT HEPATIC SEGMENT 0528

Includes:

    Azygos continuation of inferior vena cava
    Inferior vena cava, absent
    Inferior vena cava, absent hepatic segment
    Infrahepatic interruption of inferior vena cava

Excludes: N/A

Major Diagnostic Criteria: As an isolated defect, absence of the hepatic segment of the inferior vena cava (IVC) gives rise to no symptoms. Associated cardiac defects are frequently present and signs and symptoms are dependent on the specific abnormalities. The condition is frequently present in the polysplenia syndrome.

Clinical Findings: In this condition the IVC is absent between the renal veins and the hepatic veins. The systemic venous drainage from below the interruption is via an enlarged azygos vein to the superior vena cava. Less often, the hemiazygos vein is the alternative venous pathway and empties into a persistent left superior vena cava.

The anomaly by itself does not alter hemodynamics and is not responsible for symptomatology. It may be identified on X-ray by absence of the IVC density at the cardiophrenic angle in the lateral view. The collateral route of flow to the right SVC by the azygos vein creates a large rounded density seen in the right lung field just above the SVC-RA junction. This anomaly is almost invariably present when the radiograph shows the stomach in a malposed position. In other words, if the thoracic contents are in their usual position (situs solitus) and the stomach is right-sided, or if the thoracic contents indicate situs inversus and the stomach is left-sided, absent hepatic segment of the IVC is present until proven otherwise.

This may occur as an isolated anomaly, but usually there are associated cardiovascular defects. It is particularly common as part of the polysplenia syndrome.

Complications: Inadvertent ligation of the azygos vein may lead to death. During cardiopulmonary bypass, the surgeon must recognize and deal with the altered systemic venous drainage.

Associated Findings: Multiple spleens, abnormal cardiac situs, isolated abdominal situs inversus.

Etiology: Unknown.

Pathogenesis: Hypoplasia or aplasia of the anastomosis that normally develops between right subcardinal and proximal vitelline venous systems (renal and posthepatic segments of the IVC).

CDC No.: 747.480

Sex Ratio: Presumably M1:F1

Occurrence: About 1:100 patients with congenital heart disease. Rare in the absence of congenital cardiac disease.

Risk of Recurrence for Patient's Sib: Unknown.

Risk of Recurrence for Patient's Child: Unknown.

Age of Detectability: From birth by selective angiography.

Gene Mapping and Linkage: Unknown.

Prevention: None known. Genetic counseling indicated.

Treatment: Unknown.

Prognosis: In the rare situation where there are no associated cardiac anomalies, longevity is normal. Interruption of the IVC with azygos continuation does not influence the prognosis of other conditions.

Detection of Carrier: Unknown.

References:

Anderson RC, et al.: Anomalous inferior vena cava with azygos continuation (infrahepatic interruption of the inferior vena cava): report of 15 new cases. J Pediatr 1961; 59:370.

Lucas RV Jr.: Anomalous venous connection, pulmonary and systemic. In: Adams FH, Emmanouilides GC, eds: Heart disease in infants, children, and adolescents. Baltimore: Williams & Wilkins, 1983:486–488.

LU003   **Russell V. Lucas, Jr.**

VENA CAVA, PERSISTENT LEFT SUPERIOR JOINED TO CORONARY SINUS 0807

Includes: Vena cava connecting to right atrium via coronary sinus

Excludes:

    Vena cava, persistent left superior connecting to left atrium
    Pulmonary venous connection, total anomalous (0842)

Major Diagnostic Criteria: A persistent left superior vena cava (LSVC) is virtually always an incidental finding. Angiography or catheter passage confirms the diagnosis.

Clinical Findings: In this anomaly, a persistent LSVC connects to the coronary sinus. The physiology is normal. Its importance lies in the frequent coexistence of other congenital cardiac defects and in the technical complications it may engender during cardiac catheterization or cardiac surgery. From the junction of the left subclavian and left internal jugular veins the LSVC descends vertically in front of the aortic arch. A short distance from its origin, it receives the superior left intercostal vein, then passes in front of the left pulmonary hilum. It receives the hemiazygos vein, penetrates the pericardium and crosses the posterior wall of the left atrium obliquely, receives the greater cardiac vein and enters the coronary sinus.

The coronary sinus and its right atrial ostium are larger than normal. As a rule, the persistent LSVC is part of a bilateral superior caval system. Rarely the RSVC may be absent.

X-ray features: The shadow of the LSVC may be seen along the left upper border of the mediastinum. Diagnosis may be confirmed by passage of a cardiac catheter into the LSVC via the left subclavian vein or by way of the coronary sinus from the heart.

0528-12167: Absent hepatic segment of inferior vena cava. Two views.

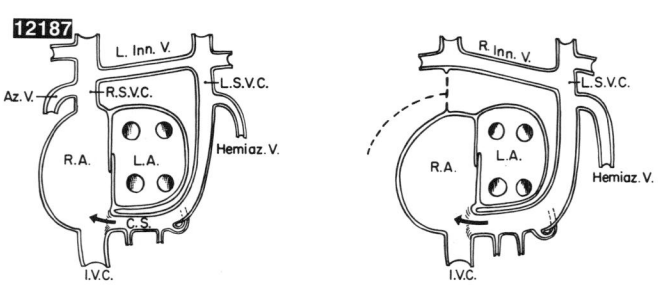

0807-12187: Diagrams illustrating persistent left superior vena cava connected to coronary sinus.

Echocardiographic features: The enlarged coronary sinus may produce an abnormal echo in the left atrium. This echo is similar to the left atrial echoes produced by TAPVC to coronary sinus and cor triatriatum.

Complications: Utilization of the LSVC for catheter passage in a right heart study may interfere with the satisfactory completion of the procedure. At operation, ligation of the LSVC may be fatal when the RSVC is absent. Cannulation of the LSVC via the coronary sinus is necessary during cardiopulmonary bypass.

Associated Findings: Heart, tetralogy of Fallot, Ventricular septal defect, sinus venosus atrial septal defect, cyanotic congenital cardiac defects, particularly those with malposition of the heart or abdominal viscera. A high incidence of leftward P axis is found in patients with persistent LSVC.

Etiology: Unknown.

Pathogenesis: Embryologically, persistence of the LSVC is a consequence of simple failure of obliteration of the left common cardinal vein.

CDC No.: 747.410

Sex Ratio: Presumably M1:F1.

Occurrence: Prevalence 1:330 in the general population. 1:30 in patients with congenital heart disease.

Risk of Recurrence for Patient's Sib: Unknown.

Risk of Recurrence for Patient's Child: Unknown.

Age of Detectability: From birth, by catheterization or angiography.

Gene Mapping and Linkage: Unknown.

Prevention: None known. Genetic counseling indicated.

Treatment: Unknown.

Prognosis: Excellent when occurring as an isolated anomaly.

Detection of Carrier: Unknown.

References:
Winter FS: Persistent left superior cava: survey of the world literature and report of 30 additional cases. Angiology 1954; 5:90. *
Lucas RV Jr., Schmidt R: Anomalous venous connection, pulmonary and systemic. In: Adams FH, Emmanouilides GC, eds: Heart disease in infants, children, and adolescents, 3rd ed. Baltimore: Williams & Wilkins, 1983:482–484. *

LU003   **Russell V. Lucas, Jr.**

Venezuelan equine encephalitis (VEE)
See FETAL VENEZUELAN EQUINE ENCEPHALITIS INFECTION
Venous aneurysm of external ear, pulsating
See EAR, ARTERIOVENOUS FISTULA
Venous return, anomalous (partial)
See PULMONARY VENOUS CONNECTION, PARTIAL ANOMALOUS
Ventricle, anomalous muscle bundle of right
See VENTRICLE, OBSTRUCTION WITHIN RIGHT VENTRICLE OR ITS OUTFLOW TRACT

VENTRICLE, DIVERTICULUM   0988

Includes:
Aneurysm, congenital left ventricular
Diverticular aneurysm of the left ventricle
Diverticulosis of the left ventricle
Diverticulum of left ventricle
Diverticulum of right ventricle

Excludes:
Arrhythmogenic right ventricular dysplasia
Ventricular aneurysm due to Chagas' disease
Ventricular aneurysm due to ischemic cardiac disease
Ventricular aneurysm due to open heart surgical procedures

Major Diagnostic Criteria: Although acceptable resolution for diagnosis could be expected with two-dimensional echocardiography, digital subtraction X-ray with peripheral intravenous injec-

tion, or with nuclear magnetic resonance imaging, the current standard for diagnosis is contrast ventriculography. Angled angiographic views may be required, depending upon the size and location of the diverticulum. Criteria for diagnosis with noninvasive imaging may be established as greater experience with these rare defects is accumulated.

Clinical Findings: Clinical manifestations are related to the size of the diverticulum and to its anatomic location. A subxiphoid, palpable pulsating mass in the epigastrium may be due to an apical left ventricular diverticulum with associated midline defects of the diaphragm or anterior abdominal wall. Usually, however, there are not physical findings specifically suggesting the presence of a ventricular diverticulum and murmurs are uncommon. Congestive cardiac failure, peripheral emboli, ventricular arrhythmias including ventricular tachycardia and ventricular fibrillation, and sudden death due to arrhythmia or aneurysm rupture are among the other presentations of a ventricular diverticulum. A congenital left ventricular diverticular aneurysm may also present as an asymptomatic abnormality on routine chest X-ray or electrocardiography in a healthy, asymptomatic adult. Atypical chest pain syndromes and endocarditis have been attributed to LV diverticulae.

Electrocardiographic findings are frequent but not diagnostic. Left ventricular hypertrophy, left ventricular strain, T wave abnormalities, ST segment elevation, and "pseudoinfarction" patterns have been described.

Symptoms and findings may be present due to associated cardiovascular anomalies.

Complications: Rupture of ventricular diverticulum; arrhythmias, including ventricular tachycardia or ventricular fibrillation; sudden death from rupture or arrhythmias; infective endocarditis; and peripheral embolic and congestive cardiac failure are among the possible complications.

Associated Findings: Congenital coronary anomalies, pericardial defects, midline defects of the diaphragm or anterior abdominal wall, and omphalocele have been reported. Associated congenital cardiac anomalies can include single ventricle, **Atrial septal defects, Ventricular septal defect, Aorta, coarctation, Ductus arteriosus, patent**.

Etiology: Unknown.

Pathogenesis: Possibilities include focal myocarditis occurring during intrauterine development, or a focal ischemic myocardial event occurring during fetal development.

Sex Ratio: Presumably M1:F1.

Occurrence: Less than 1:200,000 births (less than 0.05% of congenital heart disease). The incidence of mild and unrecognized cases, however, is obviously unknown.

Risk of Recurrence for Patient's Sib: Unknown.

Risk of Recurrence for Patient's Child: Unknown.

Age of Detectability: From birth, by ventriculography

Gene Mapping and Linkage: Unknown.

Prevention: None known. Genetic counseling indicated.

Treatment: Resection of a large diverticulum is likely to be required. Surgical repair of associated midline or intracardiac congenital defects may be required. Medical or surgical treatment of a patient with arrhythmias due to a diverticulum may be required.

Prognosis: Without treatment, the presence of a large diverticulum is associated with death in infancy in the majority of cases. The prognosis may be limited by the type of associated anomalies in those cases with other congenital cardiovascular defects in addition to ventricular diverticulum.

Detection of Carrier: Unknown.

References:
Powell SJ: Diverticulum of the left ventricle: case report with special reference to electrocardiographic findings. Am Heart J 1958; 55:518–522.
Edget JW, et al.: Diverticulum of the heart: part of the syndrome of

congenital cardiac and midline thoracic and abdominal defects. Am J Cardiol 1969; 24:580–583.

Norton JB, et al.: Congenital diverticulum of the left ventricle. Am J Dis Child 1973; 126:702–704.

Treistman B, et al.: Diverticular aneurysm of left ventricle. Am J Cardiol 1973; 32:119–123. *

Baltaxe HA, et al.: Diverticulosis of the left ventricle. AJR 1979; 133:257–261. *

Fellows CL, et al.: Ventricular dysrhythmias associated with congenital left ventricular aneurysms. Am J Cardiol 1986; 57:997–999.

JE006   **Larry S. Jefferson**
BR014   **J. Timothy Bricker**

VENTRICLE, DOUBLE CHAMBERED RIGHT   2414

Includes:

Anomalous muscle bundle of the right ventricle
Anomalous right ventricular muscles
Double chambered right ventricle
Obstructing muscular bands of the right ventricle
Obstruction within the right ventricular body
Right ventricular anomalous muscle bundle
Right ventricular obstruction by aberrant muscular bands
Right ventricular subinfundibular obstruction
Two-chambered right ventricle

Excludes:

Combined valvular and infundibular stenosis
Heart, tetralogy of Fallot (0938)
Infundibular stenosis, primary
Pulmonary valve, stenosis (0839)
Subvalvular pulmonary stenosis

Major Diagnostic Criteria: A holosystolic ejection-type murmur usually best localized to the mid-precordial region coupled with the electrocardiographic finding of right ventricular hypertrophy usually isolated to the far right (V_4R–V_3R) precordial leads are indicative of the diagnosis. The vectorcardiogram further supports the electrocardiographic features and the phonocardiogram allows positive identification of the appearance of the murmur. Echocardiographic and Doppler studies allow noninvasive positioning of the obstruction and gradient determination. Cardiac catheterization and angiocardiography confirm the diagnosis invasively but are not positively necessary.

Clinical Findings: The anatomical configuration is generally considered to be of two types. In both the right ventricle is divided by muscular elements into a high pressure inflow and low pressure outflow chamber. A low type of obstruction is produced when the muscular structure arises at or near the apical region of the right ventricle and courses obliquely to approximate a point superior to the tricuspid valve annulus. In the high type the obstruction encircles the right ventricle in a more circumferential fashion just superior to the tricuspid annulus and below the usual position of the supraventricular crest.

The nature of these structures has been debated with earlier reports considering the low type of obstruction to be secondary to hypertrophy of the moderator band. However, electro-physiologic studies following surgical resection of this structure have failed to confirm specific alterations in the right ventricular excitation sequence casting doubt upon this consideration. Nonetheless the appearance with detailed angiographic study as well as at the time of surgery is that of muscular structures at least approximating the expected positions of both the moderator band and the septomarginal band in the respective types, involving hypertrophy of each component to greater or lesser degree to cause the varying appearances.

The age at presentation is highly variable due both to a wide spectrum of severity of obstruction and to the natural history of a tendency for the obstruction to be progressive with time. It has rarely been diagnosed in infancy but with improved non-invasive diagnostic techniques this may change. Additionally, the condition is frequently associated with other cardiac abnormalities

which not infrequently are discovered before the obvious signs of double chambered right ventricle are identified.

Symptoms and clinical findings are dependent upon both the severity of obstruction and associated defects. The patients are usually acyanotic, but extreme obstruction combined with an appropriately positioned large ventricular septal defect may cause sufficient right to left shunt to result in cyanosis. The presence of a systolic murmur with characteristic phonocardiographic appearance and a highly specific electro-vectorcardiographic pattern usually allow inclusion of the diagnosis on clinical grounds. The murmur is of holosystolic duration with ejection appearance. It is therefore unusual for the more common forms of right ventricular outlet obstruction; similarly it is unlike the murmur generated by ventricular septal defect to which it is similar in duration.

The position of the murmur, which is best localized to the midprecordial area, is also unlike that of these more common congenital cardiac malformations. The principal electrocardiographic feature is a displacement of the right ventricular hypertrophy pattern further rightward so that it is usually only seen in the right chest leads V_3R-V_4R; also frequently seen is failure to find evidence for right ventricular hypertrophy both in lead aVR and the left precordial leads. The vectorcardiogram confirms this unusual appearance which has been shown to likely be due to displacement of a segment of hypertrophied myocardium localized to the superomedial aspect of the right ventricle. Of note is the fact that associated abnormalities have not been shown to alter either the auscultatory-phonocardiographic findings or the electro-vectorcardiographic appearance.

The two-dimensional echocardiogram is usually indicative of hypertrophy of the obstructing muscular structures but by itself does not positively diagnose the abnormality. Combining the two-dimensional echocardiogram with Doppler flow mapping will usually allow both positioning of the level of obstruction and calculation of its degree.

Invasive study can be largely eliminated by appropriately combining the non-invasive evaluations but still may be necessary for the delineation of the presence and severity of associated malformations.

Once the anatomy is clearly defined, surgical relief is quite straightforward and is indicated when the lesion is hemodynamically significant.

Complications: The usual problems resulting from congenital cardiac lesions must be considered. Foremost amongst these is endocarditis. Others include progression to higher grades of obstruction with occasional production of cyanosis, brain abscess, and rarely right ventricular failure. Surgical complications include difficulty with tricuspid valvular chordal attachments when the obstructive elements are resected.

Associated Findings: Other forms of congenital cardiac malformations are frequent, occurring in at least 75% of reported cases. The principal association is with **Ventricular septal defect. Chromosome 21, trisomy 21** has also been described.

Etiology: Presumably multifactorial inheritance.

Pathogenesis: Only the trabecular component of the right ventricle is involved with uniform sparing of the outlet zone. There thus appears to be a primary defect in the formation of trabecular components of the right ventricle and may represent malformation of normally occurring structures.

Sex Ratio: M1:F1

Occurrence: Less than 0.5% of all congenital cardiac abnormalities.

Risk of Recurrence for Patient's Sib: Unknown.

Risk of Recurrence for Patient's Child: Unknown.

Age of Detectability: At birth.

Gene Mapping and Linkage: Unknown.

Prevention: None known. Genetic counseling indicated.

Treatment: Primary surgical resection of the obstructing elements, and repair of associated defects. Use of non-invasive methodology should allow earlier detection and enhance management. Echo-Doppler investigation for gradient determination would be expected to reduce need for cardiac catheterization in most instances.

Prognosis: Depends on the severity of obstruction and its progression. Patients with low grade obstruction may not require surgery at any time, but will require non-invasive follow-up to determine progression. Corrective surgery for those hemodynamically significant should result in normal life span.

Detection of Carrier: Unknown.

References:

Fellows KE, et al.: Angiography of obstructing muscular bands of the right ventricle. Am J Roentgenol 1972; 128:249–256.

Byrum CJ, et al.: Excitation of the double chamber right ventricle: electrophysiologic and anatomic correlation. Am J Cardiol 1982; 49:1254–1258.

Folger GM Jr: Electro-vectorcardiographic features of double-chambered right ventricle. Eur Heart J 1984; 5:1043–1053.

Folger GM Jr: Right ventricular outflow pouch associated with double-chambered right ventricle. Am Heart J 1985; 109:1044–1049.

Folger GM Jr: The right ventricular pouch: a proposed explanation for the electro-vectorcardiographic pattern of double chambered right ventricle. Angiology 1986; 37:483–486.

El Tohami ETA, et al.: The murmur of double-chambered right ventricle: phonocardiographic evaluation. Clin Cardiol 1987; 10:309–315.

F0002   **Gordon M. Folger, Jr.**

VENTRICLE, DOUBLE OUTLET LEFT   0581

Includes:

Double outlet l. ventricle-atresia of r. ventricular infundibulum
Double outlet left ventricle-pulmonary stenosis
Double outlet left ventricle-ventricular septal defect
Left ventricle, double outlet

Excludes:

Great vessels arising from a common left or primitive ventricle
Ventricle, double outlet right, with ventricular inversion.

Major Diagnostic Criteria: The origin of both the pulmonary artery and aorta are entirely or predominantly above the left ventricle.

Clinical Findings: This rare anomaly occurs when both the pulmonary artery and the aorta arise entirely or predominantly above the morphological left ventricle. Both semilunar valves may have fibrous continuity with the mitral valve. The right ventricle may be normally formed, but may be hypoplastic with infundibular atresia. The atria and viscera are usually in solitus arrangement, with concordant relation of the atria and ventricles. The semilunar valves may be in the same coronal plane, or the aortic valve level may be anterior or posterior to the pulmonary valve level. The aorta is usually to the right of the pulmonary trunk. The ventricular septal defect (VSD) may be subaortic or subpulmonic in location or confluent with both great vessels.

The presence or absence of pulmonary stenosis largely determines the clinical course. Cyanosis is prominent with significant pulmonary stenosis and VSD, and the clinical picture may be indistinguishable from that of tetralogy of Fallot. Clinical signs in this group include a prominent ejection systolic murmur due to pulmonary stenosis, and an accentuated single second heart sound at the base. EKGs show right axis deviation and right ventricular hypertrophy. Chest X-ray shows slight cardiac enlargement and decreased pulmonary vascular markings.

In contrast, patients with VSD but without pulmonary stenosis are relatively acyanotic initially and present with congestive cardiac failure. Pulmonary artery hypertension with increased pulmonary blood flow is clinically evident. The precordium is hyperactive, and the second heart sound is split with pulmonary closure accentuation. A pansystolic murmur is present at the lower left sternal border, sometimes with a prominent mid-diastolic flow murmur. EKG shows combined ventricular hyper-

trophy. The chest X-ray shows a large heart with increased pulmonary vascularity. These findings may suggest the diagnosis of transposition of the great arteries with VSD.

Hemodynamic data from the published cases showed a systolic pressure gradient at the pulmonary or subpulmonary valve level in 4 cases; right ventricular infundibular atresia was present in 1 patient, and no obstruction was present in the remaining 2. Right ventricular hypertension was present in all patients. In the infant with an intact ventricular septum, the right ventricular peak systolic pressure was greater than the systemic level. The observation of almost identical oxygen saturations in the aorta, pulmonary artery and left ventricle in a cyanotic patient suspected clinically as having tetralogy of Fallot, seems to be an important clue to the diagnosis of double outlet left ventricle with pulmonary stenosis.

Selective biplanar angiography with injections into both the right and left ventricle establishes the diagnosis by demonstrating both vessels arising predominantly to the left of the septum above the morphological left ventricle, and establishes the presence or absence of pulmonary or subpulmonary stenosis, the presence or absence of a VSD, and the status of the atrio-ventricular valves.

At surgery, external inspection of the position of the great arteries has not been helpful in suggesting the diagnosis of double outlet left ventricle, since the great arteries may be similar in appearance to that seen in patients with tetralogy of Fallot, or they may be malposed in a manner similar to that noted in complete transposition of the great arteries or double outlet right ventricle. However, careful analysis of arterioventricular connections during cardiopulmonary bypass can establish the diagnosis.

Complications: Congestive heart failure, pulmonary hypertension, cyanosis.

Associated Findings: VSD, pulmonary stenosis, right ventricular infundibular atresia, tricuspid valve stenosis, atresia or straddling.

Etiology: Unknown.

Pathogenesis: Van Praagh postulated abnormal conal growth resulting in essentially no conal tissue beneath both the great vessels, which leaves them in a side-by-side position above the left ventricle with both semilunar valves in fibrous continuity with the mitral valve. Anderson emphasized rather an absorptive process involving both the right and left ventricular conus.

Sex Ratio: M1.5:F1, based on 111 cases.

Occurrence: Van Praagh and Weinberg (1983) reviewed 111 well-documented cases based upon personal examinations and the literature.

Risk of Recurrence for Patient's Sib: Unknown. Predictably low risk because of the rarity of the lesion.

Risk of Recurrence for Patient's Child: Unknown.

Age of Detectability: From birth.

Gene Mapping and Linkage: Unknown.

Prevention: None known. Genetic counseling indicated.

Treatment: *Palliative surgery:* systemic-pulmonary artery shunt for cyanotic infants with diminished pulmonary blood flow; pulmonary artery banding for acyanotic infants with markedly increased pulmonary blood flow.

Corrective surgery for both groups: intraventricular diversion of blood from right ventricle to pulmonary artery with patch repair of VSD; radical reconstruction with pericardial tunnel or extracardiac valve-bearing conduit from right ventricle to pulmonary artery and patch closure of VSD; Fontan-type procedure when coexistent tricuspid atresia.

Prognosis: Following intracardiac repair, patients reported alive and improved.

Detection of Carrier: Unknown.

References:

Pacifico AD, et al.: Surgical treatment of double-outlet left ventricle. Circulation 1973; III-19, 23, 47–48.

Bharati S, et al.: Morphologic spectrum of double outlet left ventricle and its surgical significance. Circulation 1977; 56:43.

Van Praagh R, Weinberg PM: Double outlet left ventricle. In: Moss AJ, et al., eds: Heart disease in infants, children, and adolescents. 3rd ed. Baltimore: Williams & Wilkins, 1983:370–385. *

N0003   **James J. Nora**

VENTRICLE, DOUBLE-OUTLET RIGHT WITH ANTERIOR SEPTAL DEFECT   0297

Includes:
>   Taussig-Bing syndrome
>   Ventricular septal defect-double outlet right ventricle

Excludes:
>   **Heart, transposition of great vessels** (0962)
>   **Ventricle, double-outlet right with posterior septal defect** (0298)

Major Diagnostic Criteria: Clinical evidence of cyanosis, cardiomegaly, heart failure, increased pulmonary arterial vascularity and biventricular hypertrophy in an infant who also demonstrates, on plain chest roentgenogram, gross enlargement of the relatively normally situated main pulmonary artery is suggestive of DORV with anterior VSD. The exact anatomic diagnosis depends upon 2-D echocardiography and selective angiocardiography.

Clinical Findings: Double outlet right ventricle (DORV) with anterior ventricular septal defect (VSD) is that cardiac malformation in which both the aorta and pulmonary artery arise entirely from the right ventricle. The only outlet from the left ventricle is via a large VSD anterior to or above the crista supraventricularis. This position of the VSD is just inferior to the pulmonary artery. Thus, the pulmonary artery overrides the defect to a varying extent, but arises in otherwise normal fashion from the right ventricular infundibulum. The pulmonary trunk and aorta are normally interrelated externally. However, the aortic valve is displaced to the right and lies higher than normal at about the same level as the pulmonic valve in both the cross-sectional and coronal body planes. Thus, the aortic valve cannot be in continuity with the anterior leaflet of the mitral valve. Right ventricular infundibular obstruction is not seen, but pulmonic valvar stenosis occurs rarely.

Clinical features mimic complete transposition of the great arteries with a VSD. The position of the VSD beneath the pulmonic valve results in selective streaming of left ventricular (oxygenated) blood into the pulmonary artery. The aorta receives primarily right ventricular (desaturated) blood. Thus, the patient is cyanotic from birth, although this may be mild in early infancy. Heart failure, chronic respiratory infections and growth retardation are usually present. A harsh systolic murmur is present at the upper left sternal border but is usually not accompanied by a thrill. The second sound is narrowly split or single and the pulmonic component is accentuated. A diastolic murmur of pulmonic insufficiency is occasionally heard. The EKG shows right axis deviation, right atrial enlargement and biventricular hypertrophy. Plain chest roentgenograms demonstrate markedly increased pulmonary vascularity of a shunt type, a prominent pulmonary artery segment, cardiomegaly involving both ventricles and left atrial enlargement. This is one of the few admixture lesions that is overtly cyanotic with a normally positioned pulmonary artery segment.

Since a great anatomic spectrum exists in this lesion, the echocardiographic differential diagnosis for DORV includes abnormalities in the tetralogy/truncus group as well as those in the transposition group. Identification of septal-aortic override or septal-pulmonic override with mitral semilunar discontinuity is essential for making this diagnosis. It was initially reported that an anterior displacement of the posterior great vessel from the mitral valve was diagnostic of this disorder. However, it has recently been pointed out that great difficulties arise in demonstrating this anterior-posterior displacement. Further, the presence of a subaortic or subpulmonic conus separating this posterior great vessel semilunar valve from the mitral valve is at least as important in delineating these malformations as is the anterior-posterior displacement. Secondary characteristics involving abnormal great

vessel orientation may be of use in defining this group. See also **Heart, tetralogy of Fallot.**

Cardiac catheterization and angiocardiography are necessary to establish the precise anatomy. Significant systemic arterial desaturation is present, and pulmonary artery oxygen saturation exceeds systemic artery saturation. This is in contrast to DORV with a posterior VSD. Catheter position may suggest the abnormal location of the aortic valve. Selective right ventricular angiography will demonstrate denser opacification of the aorta than of the pulmonary artery, while selective left ventricular angiography will demonstrate the VSD and denser opacification of the pulmonary artery than of the aorta. Angiocardiography also demonstrates the abnormal position of the aortic valve and its lack of relation to anterior leaflet of the mitral valve.

Complications: Chronic heart failure, frequent respiratory infection, growth failure, and cyanosis may result in early death. With increasing age, pulmonary vascular disease will occur.

Associated Findings: None known.

Etiology: Presumably multifactorial inheritance.

Pathogenesis: Failure of transfer of the posterior great artery (aorta) to the left ventricle results in DORV. The pathogenesis of the VSD is variable, but apparently is due to faulty development in both the conus septum and the muscular ventricular septum. Recently it has been appreciated that neural crest cells contribute importantly to cardiac morphogenesis. In fact, experimental removal of certain regions of the cranial neural crests causes double outlet right ventricle.

MIM No.: 12100, 14050

Sex Ratio: M1:F1

Occurrence: Less than 1:100 cases of congenital heart disease.

Risk of Recurrence for Patient's Sib: Unknown.

Risk of Recurrence for Patient's Child: Unknown.

Age of Detectability: From birth.

Gene Mapping and Linkage: Unknown.

Prevention: None known. Genetic counseling indicated.

Treatment: In infancy, palliative surgery may be necessary. Creation of an atrial septal defect and pulmonary artery banding will increase the amount of intracardiac mixing and thus increase the supply of oxygenated blood to the aorta. The total complex is now amenable to surgical correction by use of either senning procedure, or the Mustard procedure, originally designed for complete transposition of the great arteries. The atrial portion of the operation is performed as usual. The VSD is closed by a patch in such a way as to transfer the pulmonary artery to the left ventricle. Anatomic correction by use of the vatene procedure can also be considered.

Other therapy as necessary for congestive heart failure and pulmonary infection.

Prognosis: Overall prognosis is poor with pulmonary arteriolar vascular disease being a common early complication. Survival beyond childhood without surgery is unlikely. With successful corrective surgery, prognosis is favorable.

Detection of Carrier: Unknown.

References:

Van Praagh R: What is the Taussig-Bing malformation? Circulation 1968; 38:445–449.

Sridaromont S, et al.: Double-outlet right ventricle: anatomic and angiographic correlations. Mayo Clinic Proceedings 1978; 53:555–577.

Hagler DJ, et al.: Double-outlet right ventricle: wide-angle two-dimensional echocardiograph observations. Circulation 1981; 63:419–428. †

Wilcox BR, et al.: Surgical anatomy of double-outlet right ventricle with situs solitus and atrioventricular concordance. J Thorac Cardiovasc Surg 1981; 82:405–417.

Hagler DJ, et al.: Double-outlet right ventricle. In: Adams FH, Emmanouilledes GC, eds: Moss' heart disease in infants, children and adolescents, 3rd ed. Baltimore: Williiams & Wilkins, 1983:351–369. * †

Pacifico AD, et al.: Intra-ventricular tunnel repair for Taussig-Bing heart and related cardiac anomalies. Circulation 1986; 74:53–66. * †

Kirby ML: Cardiac morphogenesis: recent research advances. Pediatr Res 1987; 21:219–224.

GE013   **Ira H. Gessner**

VENTRICLE, DOUBLE-OUTLET RIGHT WITH POSTERIOR SEPTAL DEFECT   **0298**

Includes: Great vessels from right ventricle-posterior septal defect

Excludes:
  Heart, tetralogy of Fallot (0938)
  Heart, transposition of great vessels (0962)
  Ventricle, double-outlet right with anterior septal defect (0297)
  Ventricular septal defect (0989)

Major Diagnostic Criteria: Clinical evidence of a large left-to-right ventricular level shunt with pulmonary hypertension and a superiorly oriented, counterclockwise frontal plane (QRS) loop should arouse suspicion of double outlet right ventricle (DORV) with posterior ventricular septal defect (VSD) and no pulmonic stenosis. Selective angiography and/or comprehensive 2-D echocardiograph can establish a correct diagnosis. DORV with posterior VSD and pulmonic stenosis simulates tetralogy of Fallot almost exactly. The presence of marked right atrial enlargement and of atrioventricular conduction delay would suggest DORV with pulmonic stenosis, but selective angiocardiography and/or 2-D echocardiograph can establish the exact anatomy.

Clinical Findings: DORV with posterior VSD is that cardiac malformation in which both the aorta and pulmonary artery arise entirely from the right ventricle. The only outlet from the left ventricle is via a large VSD which is posteriorly located, i.e. below the crista supraventricularis. The pulmonary trunk and aorta are normally interrelated externally. However, the aortic valve is displaced to the right and lies higher than normal at about the same level as the pulmonic valve in both the cross-sectional and coronal body planes. The displaced aortic valve causes lack of continuity between the anterior leaflet of the mitral valve and the aortic valve. Obstruction to flow into the pulmonary artery is common due to right ventricular infundibular hypertrophy. Subaortic obstruction is rarely seen.

Clinical features are determined by the degree of pulmonic obstruction. Without pulmonic obstruction, the clinical features closely resemble a large VSD with right ventricular hypertension. Poor growth, frequent respiratory infection and heart failure are present in infancy. A precordial systolic thrill and a grade IV/VI harsh systolic murmur along the lower left sternal border, a narrowly split and accentuated second sound, and an apical diastolic murmur of increased mitral valve flow indicate the presence of a large VSD with elevated right ventricular pressure. Cyanosis is usually minimal or absent because the posterior location of the VSD allows left ventricular output to be directed through the VSD towards the aortic valve; thus significant mixing in the right ventricle may not occur. With time, pulmonary arteriolar disease may develop resulting in increased pulmonary vascular resistance. Cyanosis will then become a prominent feature. The EKG demonstrates left atrial enlargement and biventricular hypertrophy. A distinctive EKG feature commonly seen is marked left axis deviation and superior counterclockwise frontal plane QRS forces, similar to that seen in an endocardial cushion defect. Plain chest X-rays demonstrate a large pulmonary artery segment, increased pulmonary vascularity of the shunt type, left atrial enlargement and cardiomegaly, findings which are not specific for this malformation. In the presence of significant pulmonic obstruction, the clinical features mimic those of tetralogy of Fallot and indeed may be indistinguishable. Cyanosis is present from early infancy. A left lower parasternal systolic thrill and murmur and a single second sound are found. There is no mitral flow murmur.

The EKG frequently demonstrates right atrial enlargement and always shows right ventricular hypertrophy of the type commonly seen in tetralogy of Fallot. In DORV with pulmonary stenosis, right axis deviation is seen and the QRS forces are directed inferiorly. Delayed atrioventricular conduction time and intraventricular conduction delay are commonly seen. Right atrial enlargement and delayed atrioventricular conduction are unusual in tetralogy of Fallot, providing one of the few distinguishing clinical features between these two malformations. Plain chest X-rays demonstrate decreased pulmonary arterial vascularity, a prominent aorta, mild cardiomegaly involving the right heart, a small right ventricular outflow tract with absence of a pulmonary artery segment, and no left atrial enlargement; these features are commonly seen in tetralogy of Fallot as well.

Since a great anatomic spectrum exists in this lesion, the echocardiographic differential diagnosis for DORV includes abnormalities in the tetralogy/truncus group as well as those in the transposition group. Identification of septal-aortic override or septal-pulmonic override with mitral semilunar discontinuity is essential for making this diagnosis. It was initially reported that an anterior displacement of the posterior great vessel from the mitral valve was diagnostic of this disorder. However, it has recently been pointed out that great difficulties arise in demonstrating this anterior-posterior displacement. Further, the presence of a subaortic or subpulmonic conus separating this posterior great vessel semilunar valve from the mitral valve is at least as important in delineating these malformations as is the anterior-posterior displacement. Doppler echocardiograph can be used to quantitate pulmonic stenosis, if present. Secondary characteristics involving abnormal great vessel orientation may be of use in defining this group. See also **Heart, tetralogy of Fallot.**

Cardiac catheterization and selective angiocardiography are necessary to establish the precise anatomic and hemodynamic diagnosis. Without pulmonic obstruction, the catheterization findings are those of a large VSD with equal pressures in the left and right ventricles. Mild systemic arterial desaturation is usually seen, although, as mentioned above, streaming of left ventricular blood into the aorta may be so precise that little systemic arterial desaturation is found. Systemic arterial oxygen saturation is significantly greater than pulmonary oxygen saturation. Position of the catheter in the great vessels may suggest the abnormal location of the aortic valve. Selective right and left ventricular angiography will demonstrate the exact anatomic situation; a lack of continuity of the mitral valve with a semilunar valve, a large posterior VSD and the abnormal location of the aortic valve. In the presence of pulmonic obstruction, the catheterization findings are similar to tetralogy of Fallot. Again, catheter localization of the aortic valve may suggest its abnormal position. However, selective right ventricular angiography is necessary to differentiate between these 2 malformations.

Complications: Without pulmonic stenosis, chronic heart failure, frequent respiratory infections and poor growth occur. Eventual development of pulmonary vascular disease is common. With pulmonic stenosis, hypoxic spells may occur.

Associated Findings: None known.

Etiology: Presumably multifactorial inheritance.

Pathogenesis: Failure of transfer of the posterior great artery (aorta) to the left ventricle results in DORV. The conus septum fails to develop properly and a large VSD results. If the conus septum is displaced anteriorly and becomes hypertrophied, infundibular (pulmonic) obstruction results. Recently, it has been appreciated that neural crest cells contribute importantly to cardiac morphogenesis. Indeed, experimental removal of certain regions of the cranial neural crest causes double outlet right ventricle.

MIM No.: 12100, 14050

Sex Ratio: M1:F1

Occurrence: Less than 1:100 cases of congenital heart defects.

Risk of Recurrence for Patient's Sib: Unknown.

Risk of Recurrence for Patient's Child: Unknown.

Age of Detectability: From birth.

Gene Mapping and Linkage: Unknown.

Prevention: None known. Genetic counseling indicated.

Treatment: Corrective surgery may be accomplished by construction of a tunnel from the VSD to the root of the aorta. If present, infundibular hypertrophy can be resected. When the aorta is too far removed from the VSD for correction, pulmonary artery banding may be performed as a palliative procedure in the absence of infundibular obstruction. Symptomatic therapy for congestive heart failure and pneumonia may be indicated.

Prognosis: Poor; survival is enhanced by a moderate degree of pulmonic obstruction.

Detection of Carrier: Unknown.

Special Considerations: DORV may occur in association with the fundamental ventricular abnormality: ventricular inversion. In that instance, since the anatomic right ventricle is located on the left, both great arteries arise from the left-sided right ventricle.

Complete transposition of the great vessels may occur together with DORV. In that situation, the aorta is located to the left and slightly anteriorly arising from the right ventricular infundibulum. The pulmonary artery arises to the right and posterior of the aorta with lack of continuity between the mitral valve and the pulmonic valve. The physiology is similar to the ordinary case of complete transposition of the great vessels with a VSD.

References:

Sridaromont S, et al.: Double-outlet right ventricle: anatomic and angiographic correlations. Mayo Clinic Proceedings 1978; 53:555–577. * †

Hagler DJ, et al.: Double-outlet right ventricle: wide-angle two-dimensional echocardiograph observations. Circulation 1981; 63:419–428. †

Wilcox BR, et al.: Surgical anatomy of double-outlet right ventricle with situs solitus and atrioventricular concordance. J Thorac Cardiovasc Surg 1981; 82:405–417.

Hagler DJ, et al.: Double-outlet right ventricle. In: Adams FH, Emmanouiledes GC, eds: Moss' heart disease in infants, children and adolescents, 3rd ed. Baltimore: Williiams & Wilkins, 1983:351–369. * †

Kirby ML: Cardiac morphogenesis: recent research advances. Pediatr Res 1987; 21:219–224.

GE013

Ira H. Gessner

VENTRICLE, ENDOCARDIAL FIBROELASTOSIS OF LEFT VENTRICLE
0348

Includes:
Endocardial fibroelastosis (EFE) of left ventricle
Myocardial hypertrophy-endocardial fibroelastosis
Ventricular, left, endocardial fibrosis fibroelastosis
Ventricular, left, endocardial sclerosis
Ventricular, left, subendocardial fibroelastosis

Excludes:
Cardiomyopathy, nonobstructive
Carnitine deficiency, systemic (2121)
Myocarditis
Ventricle, endocardial fibroelastosis of right ventricle (0349)
Ventricle, endomyocardial fibrosis of left (0353)

Major Diagnostic Criteria: EKG evidence of extreme left ventricular hypertrophy and T-wave changes, radiographic findings of cardiomegaly with enlargement of the left ventricle and left atrium and hemodynamic and angiographic evidence of altered left ventricular performance with mitral insufficiency. When the above findings occur in a young infant, this diagnosis must be considered.

Clinical Findings: This is a condition in which the endocardium of the left ventricle is thickened and noncompliant. Symptoms usually occur in the first 12 months of life, infrequently after 1 year of age or before the first month. Evidence of cardiac decompensation with rapid onset in a previously healthy infant is the characteristic finding in all clinically recognized cases. With progression, if untreated, the terminal state is peripheral collapse accompanied by greyish cyanosis and feeble pulses. Auscultation

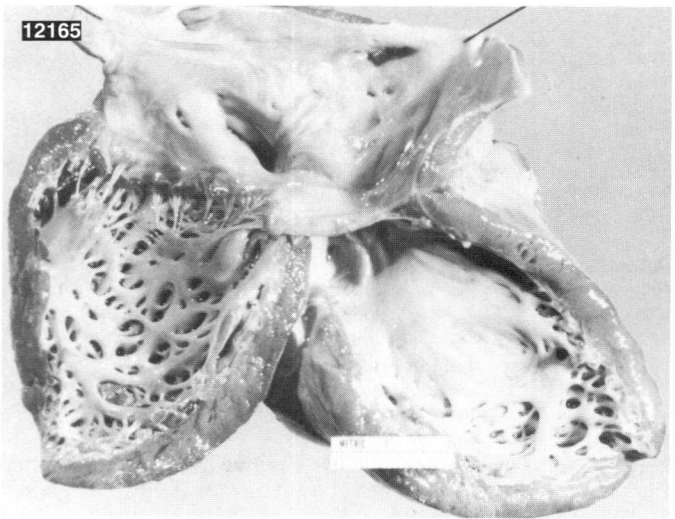

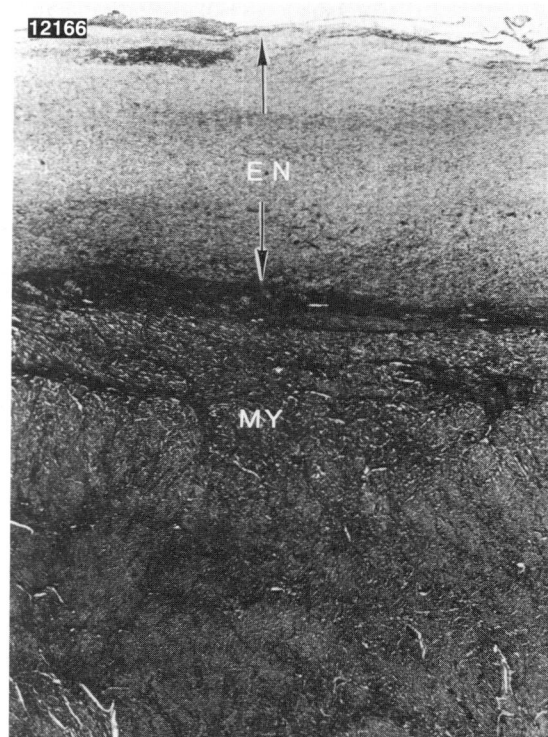

0348-12165: Gross anatomy of endocardial fibroelastosis of the left ventricle. **12166:** Photomicrograph of section of the left ventricle illustrating endocardial fibroelastosis. The endocardium is greatly thickened (between arrows EN) and is comprised principally of fibrous-appearing tissue. The myocardium (MY) is also hypertrophied.

---

of the heart while decompensation is present may reveal only tachycardia and a gallop rhythm. Gross cardiac enlargement is uniformly present. With compensation, a murmur of mitral insufficiency is not uncommonly present and may be clinically obvious in 30–50% of the patients. Most affected infants have accentuated 3rd and 4th heart sounds. The 1st and 2nd sounds may be normal.

Laboratory Findings: The EKG is considered typical and usually forms the basis of the clinical diagnosis. The principal findings are extreme left ventricular hypertrophy with flattening or inversion of the left precordial T waves. These findings occur in 80–90% of patients. X-rays uniformly reveal the heart to be enlarged, particularly the left atrium and ventricle. Evidence of pulmonary venous hypertension or obstruction is invariably present. The functional disorder apparent at cardiac catheterization and angiography is progressive failure of the left ventricle to maintain an adequate contractile state. There is a decrease in left heart output and an increase in left ventricular end systolic, as well as in end diastolic volumes. The result is extreme left ventricular dilatation and failure, although a small number of cases, probably less than 10%, may reveal a nondilated left ventricle. This functional disturbance may be due to the altered endocardium which limits contractility or alters metabolism of the myocardium by reducing the oxygen supply to the subendocardial layer. Valvar regurgitation, principally mitral, due to primary involvement, as well as left ventricular dilatation, demonstrable with left ventricular angiography, further adds to the left ventricular work load. Physiologically, left ventricular end diastolic pressure rises and peak dp/dt falls as myocardial contractility is further embarrassed. Myocardial failure ensues. Left atrial pressure rises as does pulmonary venous pressure.

Echocardiography, at present, cannot routinely differentiate this disease from other forms of congestive cardiomyopathy. The left ventricular and septal walls may be abnormally thickened but the endocardial surface may appear normal. However, it has been demonstrated that dense echoes from thickened endocardium may be identified in certain cases. The wall motion is poor and the left ventricular cavity is usually dilated. The mitral valve motion is attenuated, and the anterior posterior leaflets are seen together. The anterior leaflet is seemingly displaced posteriorly and does not reach the septum in diastole. The left atrium is dilated to a greater or lesser extent, depending upon the degree of left heart failure or mitral insufficiency. Of perhaps greater importance is the ability of the echocardiogram to exclude other abnormalities with similar presentation which may be more amenable to definitive therapy, such as **Artery, coronary, anomalous origin from pulmonary artery**.

Pathologic Anatomy: Grossly, the left ventricle is dilated and thickened. The chordae tendineae of the mitral valve are shortened. The endocardium of the left ventricle and, occasionally of the left atrium, is thickened and presents as a glistening, pearly-white lining of the chamber. The mitral valve usually presents a similar appearance. The aortic valve may also be involved. Microscopically, the fundamental pathologic change is the thickened endocardium composed principally of elastic tissue but with an increased amount of collagenous tissue. However, wide variation in the amounts of these elements has been noted to occur. The condition may thus be less specific and more heterogeneous than previously supposed. Myocardial alterations have also been reported with a decrease in the ratio of capillary to myocardial fiber volume. Electron microscopic studies have indicated the composition of the thickened endocardium to be principally fibrin, but this information lacks confirmation by other investigators.

Complications: Congestive heart failure with coincident failure to thrive and difficult feeding are the principal complications. The decompensation, often amenable initially to therapy with digitalis preparations, frequently becomes intractable with death occurring in 75% by the end of the first year of life. Systemic thromboembolic phenomena represent a serious but little emphasized complication. Emboli from the left ventricle have been reported within all major systemic arterial systems and pulmonary emboli have been reported originating from the right ventricle.

Associated Findings: Associated cardiovascular defects, principally those causing overload of the left ventricle are recognized. Thus, coarctation of the aorta, aortic stenosis and mitral insufficiency are the leading associated abnormalities seen.

Etiology: No specific etiologic agent is known to cause the condition, although a number of agents have been implicated. Originally, the abnormality was thought to be the result of intrauterine infection and was considered a fetal endocarditis. More recently, a number of investigators have reported serologic

and cultural evidence for extrauterine or intrauterine infection with Coxsackie as well as other enteroviruses. A relationship to mumps virus has been suggested because of a reportedly high incidence of positive skin tests to mumps antigen in individuals with endocardial fibroelastosis. However, the initial observation of this relationship has not been confirmed by other investigators.

Evidence of obstruction to the cardiac lymphatics has also been reported, further suggesting an inflammatory etiology. A familial incidence is recognized suggesting a hereditary cause. Secondary EFE, occurring with aortic atresia, mitral valvar disease, usually regurgitation, aortic stenosis and aortic coarctation all suggest overload of the left ventricle as a contributing factor. It is not known, however, whether the EFE in these circumstances is identical to that seen with the isolated lesion.

Pathogenesis: The mode of origin and development of this entity is not known. Whether it develops as a response to one of a number of possible agents over a period of time, or is a basic congenital abnormality of the endocardial surface of the heart, has not been determined. Furthermore, it has not been ascertained whether the lesion is a static one, present as an inherent endocardial defect throughout most of intrauterine and early extrauterine life, or whether if it becomes progressively more severe until it causes left ventricular failure and often death. Thus, if the defect is not progressive, or if progression should be halted, "mild" or subclinical cases might occur. The result would be that the abnormality would be of such a low-grade severity that symptoms might not be produced. Because the lesion is rarely, if ever, accurately diagnosed in an asymptomatic state, and even if entertained in such a state, cannot be definitely proven, the occurrence of sequential structural changes remains conjectural.

MIM No.: *30530, 22600

CDC No.: 425.300

Sex Ratio: M0.6:F1

Occurrence: Approximately 1:6000 live births. Appears to have a higher incidence in colder climates and is less commonly encountered in the tropics. Apparently the incidence has decreased in the past decade in North America.

Risk of Recurrence for Patient's Sib: Empirical risk 3.8%.

Risk of Recurrence for Patient's Child: Unknown.

Age of Detectability: Most commonly within the 1st year of life, infrequent before the 1st month and after the 2nd year. Ventricular enlargement may be detected on ultrasound in the 3rd trimester.

Gene Mapping and Linkage: EFE2 (endocardial fibroelastosis 2) has been provisionally mapped to X.

Prevention: None known. Genetic counseling indicated.

Treatment: Treatment is strictly supportive with efforts to control congestive heart failure. General experience shows that the infant so treated has greater longevity and may survive this disease.

Prognosis: An estimated 50% or greater of diagnosed and treated patients will survive an indefinite period of time. As soon as the disease produces congestive heart failure, the prognosis without treatment is poor and the infant cannot be expected to survive.

Detection of Carrier: Unknown.

References:

Sellers FJ, et al.: The diagnosis of primary endocardial fibroelastosis. Circulation 1964; 29:49–59.

Mitchell SC, et al.: An epidemiologic assessment of primary endocardial fibroelastosis. Am J Cardiol 1966; 18:859–866.

Chen S, et al.: Endocardial fibroelastosis: family studies with special reference to counseling. J Pediatr 1971; 79:385–392–392. *

Westwood M, et al.: Heredity in primary endocardial fibroelastosis. Br Heart J 1975; 37:1077–1084. *

Factor SM: Endocardial fibroelastosis: myocardial and vascular alterations associated with viral-like nuclear particles. Am Heart J 1978; 96:791–801.

Van Der Hauwaert LG, et al.: Long-term echocardiographic assessment of dilated cardiomyopathy in children. Am J Cardiol 1983; 52:1066–1071.

Hodgson S, et al.: Endocardial fibroelastosis: possible X-linked inheritance. J Med Genet 1987; 24:210–214.

F0002   Gordon M. Folger, Jr.

VENTRICLE, ENDOCARDIAL FIBROELASTOSIS OF RIGHT VENTRICLE   0349

Includes:
Endocardial fibroelastosis (EFE) of right ventricle
Right ventricular hypertrophy-endocardial fibroelastosis
Subendocardial fibroelastosis, right ventricular
Ventricular, right, endocardial fibroelastosis

Excludes:
Cardiomyopathy, nonobstructive
Cardiomyopathy, obstructive of right ventricle
Endomyocardial sclerosis
Myocarditis
Ventricle, endocardial fibroelastosis of left ventricle (0348)
Ventricle, endomyocardial fibrosis of right (0354)

Major Diagnostic Criteria: Angiocardiography of the right ventricle demonstrates the small contracted right ventricle. Two-dimensional echocardiograph should suggest the possibility.

Clinical Findings: A rare condition of the right ventricle in which the endocardium is thickened and noncompliant. Although dilation has been observed, the right ventricle is usually contracted and constricted. Most cases have been described as occurring with other right heart malformations, with no more than ten cases of the primary type reported. When EFE of the right ventricle occurs as a primary lesion, it may present findings similar to hypoplasia of the right ventricle with cyanosis, evidence of systemic venous engorgement and reduced pulmonary blood flow.

Laboratory Findings: The EKG pattern is similar to that seen with hypoplasia of the right ventricle in other causes. Radiographically the heart is enlarged, the apex tilted up and the pulmonary conus segment is absent. The pulmonary vasculature is reduced. The findings at cardiac catheterization, as with the other laboratory findings, are similar to those seen in pulmonary atresia or extreme stenosis. The right ventricle is diminutive and there is a massive right-to-left shunt at the atrial level.

Pathology: Isolated primary EFE of the right ventricle such as is seen in the left ventricular form is extremely unusual. In this condition, no obstruction to the otherwise normal right ventricle occurs. The gross appearance, however, is identical to the condition as it occurs as a primary lesion of the left ventricle revealing an opaque white endocardium which is thickened on cut section as well as tough and fibrous. The right ventricle, however, is contracted rather than dilated.

Microscopic: The endocardial layer is increased many times its normal thickness with abundance of elastic fibers and an increase in collagenous tissue. The subendocardial-myocardial junction usually shows a few degenerative muscle fibers.

Complications: Congestive heart failure, right-to-left atrial shunt, hypoxemia and acidosis.

Associated Findings: The condition is nearly always associated with other intracardiac anomalies, principally pulmonary atresia or extreme stenosis with intact ventricular septum.

Etiology: Undetermined. Familial occurrence in 3 generations has been described.

Pathogenesis: Unknown.

MIM No.: *30560, 22600

CDC No.: 425.300

Sex Ratio: Presumably M1:F1

Occurrence: Less than ten cases of the primary type have been substantiated.

Risk of Recurrence for Patient's Sib: Unknown.

Risk of Recurrence for Patient's Child: Unknown.

Age of Detectability: Generally during early infancy, rarely after 2–3 months.

Gene Mapping and Linkage: Unknown.

Prevention: None known. Genetic counseling indicated.

Treatment: Palliative systemic venous to right pulmonary artery anastomosis to improve pulmonary blood flow and reduce right heart work load. Symptomatic therapy for congestive heart failure.

Prognosis: Death in early infancy is nearly inevitable with survival seldom more than a few months unless a palliative procedure is carried out.

Detection of Carrier: Unknown.

References:
Andersen DN, Kelly J: Endocardial fibroelastosis; endocardial fibroelastosis associated with congenital malformations of the heart. Pediatrics 1956; 18:513–521.
Morgan AD, et al.: Endocardial fibroelastosis of the right ventricle in the newborn: presenting the clinical picture of the hypoplastic right heart syndrome. Am J Cardiol 1966; 18:933–937. *
Larson JE, et al.: Isolated endocardial fibroelastosis of the right ventricle associated with pulmonary hypertension. Am Heart J 1984; 107:1286–1290.

F0002   Gordon M. Folger, Jr.

VENTRICLE, ENDOMYOCARDIAL FIBROSIS OF LEFT   0353

Includes:
African cardiopathy
Cardiopathy, constrictive
Davies disease
Endomyocardial fibrosis (EMF) of left ventricle

Excludes:
Endocardial fibroelastosis-primary myocardial hypertrophy
Ventricle, endocardial fibroelastosis of left ventricle (0348)
Ventricle, endomyocardial fibrosis of right (0354)

Major Diagnostic Criteria: Hemodynamic data showing malfunction of the left ventricle and angiocardiography demonstrating reduction of myocardial contractility are the principal features. Angiographic demonstration of apical filling defects in the left ventricle, as well as mitral regurgitation, are usually present. Two-dimensional echocardiograph identifies the findings of left ventricular restrictive disease.

Clinical Findings: Similar to those of endomyocardial fibrosis of the right ventricle. Cardiomegaly is uncommon as this is a restrictive heart disease. Likewise, displacement of the apical impulse is unusual, and it is rarely prominent or heaving. With pulmonary hypertension secondary to mitral regurgitation and advanced left ventricular disease, an accentuated pulmonary component of the second heart sound may be present. A prominent third heart sound is a constant finding and an opening snap may be detected in 1/3 to 1/2 of the cases. A characteristic apical systolic murmur occupying early systole has been reported due to early phase mitral insufficiency with mitral competency occurring in late systole.

Laboratory Findings: Eosinophilia may occur but may be secondary to parasitic infestation. Gamma globulin levels are often elevated. The EKG tracing may be normal and is reportedly rarely helpful. With advanced disease hypertrophy of the left atrium may be seen, and with the development of significant pulmonary hypertension, right atrial hypertrophy and right ventricular hypertrophy develop. Enlargement of the heart is usually present. With pulmonary hypertension, right atrial and ventricular enlargement are usually detectable and left atrial enlargement may be apparent. Pulmonary venous congestion is a frequent finding. Elevation of the left atrial pressure and the left ventricular end diastolic pressure are the usual findings. Pulmonary hypertension is found in nearly 50% of the patients studied but this varies with the degree of left ventricular disease. The left ventricular chamber is frequently small with constant apical filling defects. Contractility is greatly reduced. The left atrium is enlarged and mitral regurgitation is usually present. The echocardiographic findings of small left ventricle and left atrial dilatation indicate the restrictive nature of the abnormality. Apical obliteration of the ventricle by thickened endocardium may be diagnostic of the condition.

Pathologic Anatomy: Grossly, there is a recurring pattern of fibrotic endocardial lesions occurring in two areas - one on the posterior wall of the left ventricle involving the endocardium in the area behind the posterior leaflet of the mitral valve, the chordae of the posterior mitral leaflet and a portion of the endocardium of the outflow tract; and 1 located at the apex of the ventricle tapering toward the endocardium of the septum to terminate at the bases of the posterior papillary muscles. Microscopic findings are the same as endomyocardial fibrosis of right ventricle.

Complications: The development of severe pulmonic hypertension secondary to reduced left ventricular compliance and mitral regurgitation is the principal complication. With pulmonary hypertension, right atrial and ventricular dilatation may occur with the possibility of pulmonary embolic phenomena. Congestive heart failure is a frequent finding and the common cause of death.

Associated Findings: None known.

Etiology: Unknown.

Pathogenesis: Unknown.

Sex Ratio: M1:F1

Occurrence: Unknown.

Risk of Recurrence for Patient's Sib: Unknown.

Risk of Recurrence for Patient's Child: Unknown.

Age of Detectability: Generally early adult life to middle age, rarely in childhood.

Gene Mapping and Linkage: Unknown.

Prevention: None known. Genetic counseling indicated.

Treatment: Anticongestive measures restore compensation for varying periods of time, but the outcome is uniformly fatal, usually in early middle age.

A growing number of cases surgically treated employing endomyocardectomy and replacement of both atrioventricular valves with very satisfactory results has given rise to optimism in the care of some of these patients.

Prognosis: Poor, with death from the condition occurring uniformly.

Detection of Carrier: Unknown.

Special Considerations: For related details, see also **Ventricle, endomyocardial fibrosis of right**.

References:
Cockshott WP: Angiocardiography of endomyocardial fibrosis. Br J Radiol 1965; 38:192–200.
Connor DH, et al.: Endomyocardial fibrosis in Uganda (Davies' disease). I. An epidemiologic, clinical and pathologic study. Am Heart J 1967; 74:687–709.
Connor DH, et al.: Endomyocardial fibrosis in Uganda (Davies' disease). II. An epidemiologic, clinical and pathologic study. Am Heart J 1968; 75:107–124.
Gonzales-Lavin L, et al.: Endomyocardial fibrosis: diagnosis and treatment. Am Heart J 1983; 105:699–705.
Fawzy ME, et al.: Endomyocardial fibrosis: report of eight cases. J Am Coll Cardiol 1985; 5:983–988. *

F0002   **Gordon M. Folger, Jr.**

VENTRICLE, ENDOMYOCARDIAL FIBROSIS OF RIGHT   0354

Includes:
African cardiopathy
Cardiopathy, constrictive
Davies disease
Endomyocardial fibrosis (EMF) of right ventricle

Excludes:
Endocardial fibroelastosis-primary myocardial hypertrophy
Ventricle, endocardial fibroelastosis of right ventricle (0349)
Ventricle, endomyocardial fibrosis of left (0353)

Major Diagnostic Criteria: Hemodynamic changes consist principally of evidence for right ventricular dysfunction with elevation of right atrial pressure and right ventricular end diastolic pressures. Cardiac angiography reveals reduction in right ventricular contractility. Echocardiography reveals the findings of restrictive cardiomyopathy of any cause.

Clinical Findings: A disorder of the cardiac connective tissues characteristically occurring among native of equatorial Africa in which the ventricular endocardium and subendocardial layers, as well as the supportive tissue of the ventricular wall, are thickened and rendered noncompliant. Increased numbers of Caucasians and non-African Blacks are being recognized with the condition around the world.

Characteristically, evidence of right heart failure occurs insidiously. The involved individual is almost invariably a Negro in the early adult years, although children as young as 2 years have been reported to have the condition. Ascites is the most striking feature. Peripheral edema may be present but much less prominent. Hepatosplenomegaly is common with a pulsatile liver frequently present. The cardiac findings consist of enlargement of the heart detectable in 50–60% of patients; a right ventricular lift occurs in approximately half of the patients; an accentuated third heart sound is found in nearly all patients; and the murmur of tricuspid insufficiency is found in 15–25% of cases. Pericardial effusion is common, occurring in nearly 50% of reported cases.

Laboratory Findings: Eosinophilia of significance occurs in some individuals but may be secondary to coexisting parasitic infestation. Elevated gamma globulin levels are commonly encountered. The QRS axis is usually normal. QRS voltages are generally normal or decreased with hypertrophy patterns uncommon. Atrial hypertrophy occurs in approximately 50% of individuals and is more often a P mitral configuration or a pattern suggesting hypertrophy of both atria. Less commonly, right atrial enlargement alone is noted. Characteristic or diagnostic EKG patterns have not been reported. Atrial fibrillation occurs at some time in approximately one-third of cases. Endomyocardial fibrosis is a restrictive heart disease; therefore, gross cardiomegaly is usually due either to enlargement of the right atrium or to the coexistence of a pericardial effusion. Dilatation of the right ventricular infundibular area is, however, a frequent radiographic as well as angiographic finding. Intracardiac calcification may be visualized. Elevation of the right ventricular end diastolic pressure is a constant finding. The right ventricular pressure curve closely resembles that of constrictive pericarditis even though that condition does not coexist. The cardiac output may be normal or reduced. By cardiac angiography, reduced contractility of the right ventricle and a degree of tricuspid insufficiency are common findings. The right ventricular body may appear nearly obliterated with only the dilated infundibular area remaining cavitary. Similarly, the 2-dimensional echocardiograph appearance of apical obliteration of the ventricle by thickened endocardium may be diagnostic.

Pathologic Anatomy: The gross appearance of the heart is that of extreme enlargement of the right atrium, a contracted right ventricle, particularly the apical area with dilatation of the right ventricular outflow area. Significant right ventricular hypertrophy is uncommon. Endocardial fibrosis characteristically is more severe at the apical portion of the right ventricle, usually extending to encase the papillary muscles but sparing the chordae tendineae and the tricuspid valve leaflets. Mural thrombi are often present in the right atrium and may occur in the right ventricle. Calcification in the fibrotic areas occurs occasionally. The microscopic findings are a swollen appearance of the connective tissues of the endocardium and underlying myocardial interstices. The earlier finding that these tissues contain elevated amounts of acid mucopolysaccharide has not been found to be specific for endomyocardial fibrosis. Distinct increase in cardiac muscle fiber size is recognized. Inflammatory changes are not observed.

Complications: Congestive heart failure is a uniform finding and the principal cause of death. Pulmonary emboli secondary to thrombi in the right atrium and ventricle are a major complication.

Associated Findings: None known.

Etiology: No definite etiologic agent has been identified. A number of agents, however, capable of instituting an autoimmune reaction have been considered. Included in these have been infectious agents, toxins and dietary idiosyncracy; none of which have been positively implicated. However, the distribution of the lesion to very specific areas within the heart, and in no other place, and the inability to find immunologically competent cells in areas undergoing change have cast some doubt upon an immunologic origin. Malnutrition has been considered but appears unlikely. Some similarities to rheumatic fever have caused consideration of this disease as the cause of the changes seen but this, too, is unproven.

Pathogenesis: Undetermined, but currently thought to be secondary to an autoimmune mechanism.

Sex Ratio: M1:F1

Occurrence: Undetermined. Found in native African Blacks, much less frequently in Blacks from other world areas. Rare in non-Black populations.

Risk of Recurrence for Patient's Sib: Unknown.

Risk of Recurrence for Patient's Child: Unknown.

Age of Detectability: The disease is seen occasionally in children as young as 2 years, but its clinical onset is more commonly in a young adult.

Gene Mapping and Linkage: Unknown.

Prevention: None known. Genetic counseling indicated.

Treatment: Anticongestive measures restore compensation for varying periods of time, but it appears that the outcome is uniformly fatal. A growing number of cases surgically treated employing endomyocardectomy and replacement of both atrioventricular valves with very satisfactory results has given rise to optimism in the care of some of these patients.

Prognosis: Poor, with death from the condition occurring uniformly, usually in the age range from early adulthood to early middle age.

Detection of Carrier: Unknown.

References:

Cockshott WP: Angiocardiography of endomyocardial fibrosis. Br J Radiol 1965; 38:192–200.
Connor DH, et al.: Endomyocardial fibrosis in Uganda (Davies' disease). I. An epidemiologic, clinical and pathologic study. Am Heart J 1967; 74:687–709.
Connor DH, et al.: Endomyocardial fibrosis in Uganda (Davies' disease). II. An epidemiologic, clinical and pathologic study. Am Heart J 1968; 75:107–124.
Somers K, et al.: Clinical features of endomyocardial fibrosis in the right ventricle. Br Heart J 1968; 30:322–331.
Gonzalez-Lavin L, et al.: Endomyocardial fibrosis: diagnosis and treatment. Am Heart J 1983; 105:699–705. *
Fawzy ME, et al.: Endomyocardial fibrosis: report of eight cases. J Am Coll Cardiol 1985; 5:983–988.

F0002   **Gordon M. Folger, Jr.**

Ventricle, functional obstruction of left
See HEART, SUBAORTIC STENOSIS, MUSCULAR
Ventricle, hypoplasia of right
See TRICUSPID VALVE, ATRESIA

VENTRICLE, OBSTRUCTION WITHIN RIGHT VENTRICLE OR ITS OUTFLOW TRACT   0731

Includes:

Pulmonary stenosis, isolated infundibular
Stenosis of ostium infundibulum
Ventricle, anomalous muscle bundle of right
Ventricle, two-chambered right
Ventricular muscle bands, aberrant right

Excludes:

Heart, tetralogy of Fallot (0938)
Pulmonary valve, stenosis (0839)

Major Diagnostic Criteria: A pulmonary ejection murmur with EKG evidence of right ventricular hypertrophy should suggest the diagnosis. Angiocardiography confirms the diagnosis.

Clinical Findings: Four anatomic types of infundibular pulmonary stenosis have been identified: 1) a fibrous band at the site of the juncture of the infundibulum and right ventricle (stenosis of os infundibulum); 2) diffuse narrowing of the infundibulum by thickened myocardium; 3) anomalous muscle bundles which are proximal to the infundibulum. These bundles are hyperplastic muscle bands passing from the area near the septal leaflet of the tricuspid valve to the anterior ventricular wall. Also, the moderator band may be hyperplastic; and 4) as part of a diffuse idiopathic myocardial hypertrophy in which the hypertrophied ventricular septum obstructs the lumen of the right ventricular outflow tract. Since the location of the right ventricular outflow obstruction varies, differences in the size of the distal or infundibular chamber and the proximal right ventricular cavity result. The right ventricle proximal to the obstruction is hypertrophied, as is the right atrium. Unlike cases with stenosis of pulmonary valve, the pulmonary artery is not dilated.

Infundibular stenosis may also occur secondary to severe stenosis of the pulmonary valve. Here, also, the clinical features vary with the degree of right ventricular outflow obstruction. With mild stenosis, the patients are asymptomatic; in those with severe stenosis, easy fatigability and at times right-sided congestive cardiac failure occur. Cyanosis may be present in the latter group, if a right-to-left shunt occurs through an anatomically patent foramen ovale. A pulmonic systolic ejection murmur is present. It may be located lower along the left sternal border than in valvar stenosis, particularly when the obstruction is located low in the right ventricle. The murmur is longer, and the peak intensity later in severe stenosis. Likewise, the degree of splitting of the second heart sound increases with increasing severity, and the intensity of the pulmonary component is diminished. In contrast to valvar pulmonic stenosis, an ejection click is uncommon.

X-rays of infundibular stenosis are similar to those of valvar pulmonary stenosis, except that poststenotic dilatation of the pulmonary trunk or left pulmonary artery is not usually present.

The EKG demonstrates right ventricular hypertrophy, the severity of which is directly related to the degree of stenosis. Progression of EKG evidence of right ventricular hypertrophy is more frequently observed in this condition than in stenosis of the pulmonary valve.

The outflow tract of the right ventricle is seen by echocardiography, but its precise character is difficult to assess. In this condition, right ventricular and septal hypertrophy occur. In some instances, an abnormal muscle band may be visualized. The pulmonary valve frequently has an early but incomplete closure followed by reopening.

Cardiac catheterization typically reveals a systolic pressure gradient within the right ventricle, although this may be missed if the obstruction is located close to the pulmonary valve. In patients with anomalous muscle bundle, the pressure gradient may be found close to the tricuspid valve. Since the obstruction is generally caused by myocardial tissue, it is dynamic in nature. With exercise or isoproterenol infusion, the degree of obstruction may increase, thereby reducing the effective right ventricular outflow area. The right ventricular end diastolic and right atrial pressures may be elevated, and in severe cases, a right-to-left shunt exists at the atrial level.

Biplane right ventriculography confirms the diagnosis. This demonstrates the muscular narrowing in the infundibular area. Although the obstruction is visualized throughout the cardiac cycle, it is more marked during systole than diastole, again indicating its dynamic nature. Whereas most pulmonary outflow obstructions are best visualized in the lateral projection, an anomalous muscle bundle is best seen in the anteroposterior projection. Since the muscle bundles' course is primarily in an anteroposterior direction, they are seen end on as circular nonopacified areas low in the right ventricle. The pulmonary valve is normal and poststenotic dilatation of the pulmonary artery is usually not present.

Complications: Right-sided cardiac failure, myocardial fibrosis, bacterial endocarditis, **Tricuspid valve, insufficiency**.

Associated Findings: None known.

Etiology: Unknown.

Pathogenesis: Anomalous or hyperplastic muscle bundles may be due to incomplete involution of the embryonic right ventricular trabeculae.

Sex Ratio: M1:F1

Occurrence: Undetermined. Less than 1% of congenital cardiac defects.

Risk of Recurrence for Patient's Sib: Unknown.

Risk of Recurrence for Patient's Child: Unknown.

Age of Detectability: From birth.

Gene Mapping and Linkage: Unknown.

Prevention: None known.

Treatment: If stenosis is severe, surgical excision may be necessary.

Prognosis: Data regarding the natural history of these conditions are scanty. There is, however, one report describing serial cardiac catheterizations. It shows that anomalous muscle bundles become more obstructive with time. The other forms are also believed to be progressive, but there is little evidence to support this.

Detection of Carrier: Unknown.

References:
Lucas RV Jr, et al.: Anomalous muscle bundle of the right ventricle: hemodynamic consequences and surgical considerations. Circulation 1962; 25:443–455.

Hartmann AF Jr, et al.: Development of right ventricular obstruction by aberrant muscular bands. Circulation 1964; 30:679–685.

Rowland TW, et al.: Double-chamber right ventricle: experience with 17 cases. Am Heart J 1975; 89:455–462.

Baumstark A, et al.: Combined double chambered right ventricle and discrete subaortic stenosis. Circulation 1978; 57:299–302.

Emmanouilides GC, Baylen BG: Primary infundibular stenosis. In: Emmanouilides GC, ed: Heart disease in infants, children, and adolescents. Baltimore: Williams & Wilkins, 1983.

M0005   **James H. Moller**

VENTRICLE, RIGHT, UHL ANOMALY   0979

Includes:
> Parchment right ventricle
> Uhl anomaly
> Ventricular myocardium, aplasia of right

Excludes:
> **Tricuspid valve, Ebstein anomaly** (0332)
> **Ventricle, endomyocardial fibrosis of right** (0354)
> Ventricle, hypoplastic right

Major Diagnostic Criteria: The diagnosis may be suspected clinically from the marked cardiomegaly, reduced pulmonary vascular markings, feeble heart tones without significant murmurs and the EKG findings described below. It is established by echocardiography or angiocardiography which demonstrates the enor-

mous but thin-walled and poorly contracting right ventricle devoid of trabeculae, and the normal location of the tricuspid orifice.

Clinical Findings: The pathologic anatomy is characterized by enormous dilatation of the heart, chiefly of the right atrium and right ventricle, and virtual absence of muscle fibers in the wall of the right ventricle. The right atrium is dilated and thick-walled due to hypertrophy and endocardial fibroelastosis. The foramen ovale is often patent; the tricuspid valve is normal. The wall of the grossly dilated right ventricle is thin, translucent and parchment-like, ranging in thickness from 1–2 mm. Its endocardial surface is opaque white due to fibroelastosis. The trabeculae are deficient and flat, the papillary muscles and chordae tendineae are thin and delicate. The crista supraventricularis is likewise flat and hypoplastic. On microscopic examination, the right ventricular wall consists solely of a thickened endocardial layer, showing fibroelastosis, and a subjacent epicardial layer with increased fatty and connective tissue. No intervening muscle fibers are observed between these two layers except, occasionally, a few islands of myocardial cells in areas adjoining the pulmonary ring, tricuspid annulus or diaphragmatic surface. The pulmonary valve is normal but the pulmonary trunk and main branches appear hypoplastic. The left atrium and left ventricle are normal or may reveal hypertrophy with fibroelastosis. The coronary vessels appear normal, as do the systemic and pulmonary veins. The positional relationship of the pulmonary trunk and aorta is normal. The basic physiologic abnormality consists of failure of the right ventricle to function as a pump for the pulmonary circulation. It behaves as a passive reservoir for blood coming from the right atrium, and as such, is a constantly overloaded chamber, which accounts for its enormously dilated state. Pumping is accomplished by right atrial contraction, and cardiac output is accordingly low.

The clinical picture is characterized by heart failure in infancy or early childhood, marked cardiomegaly, feeble heart tones with gallop rhythm and the absence of murmurs. The increased cardiac dullness is unaccompanied by any significant precordial heave or apical impulse. Heart failure is chiefly right-sided, manifested by hepatomegaly, peripheral edema and normal lung findings.

The chest X-rays reveal an enormous cardiac shadow with reduced pulmonary vascular markings. In the frontal projection, there is increased convexity of the right heart border due to right atrial enlargement, and extension of the left heart border to the lateral chest wall caused by the pronounced dilatation of the right ventricle. The pulmonary artery segment is inconspicuous. In the lateral as well as in the right and left anterior oblique projections, there is marked extension of the cardiac borders anteriorly and posteriorly, giving an impression of combined ventricular enlargement. The prominent posterior heart border is, however, mainly due to the posterior displacement of the heart from the right heart dilatation.

The EKG commonly shows broad, peaked and tall P waves due to right atrial enlargement, and small amplitude QRS complexes in the chest lead tracings without a definite ventricular hypertrophy pattern. In addition, the vectorcardiogram reveals counterclockwise posteriorly oriented horizontal QRS loop with the initial forces directed leftwards and anteriorly.

The two-dimensional echocardiogram shows gross enlargement of the right atrium, normal position of the tricuspid valve, and marked dilatation of the right ventricle, with minimum or absent contractions. Doppler flow analysis may reveal normal findings across the tricuspid valve, but normal flow pattern across the pulmonary valve. Unlike **Tricuspid valve, Ebstein anomaly**, an atrial systole-coincident diastolic opening of the pulmonary valve is observed. In Ebstein disease, the septal motion may be paradoxic, whereas in the Uhl anomaly it has been reported to be normal.

At cardiac catheterization, the right atrial presystolic "a" wave is high and of approximately the same magnitude as the right ventricular and pulmonary arterial systolic pressures. Slight systemic arterial oxygen unsaturation may be observed if right-to-left shunting across a patent foramen ovale is present. Angiocardiography is diagnostic. It characteristically reveals gross enlargement of the right ventricle with generalized thinness of its wall, absence of trabeculae, normal location of the tricuspid orifice and prolonged emptying time. Small shunting across a patent foramen ovale may or may not be demonstrated following opacification of the right atrium. The pulmonary trunk and main branches appear hypoplastic.

Complications: Congestive heart failure and death occur in infancy or early childhood.

Associated Findings: An additional abnormality of the left ventricle such as endocardial fibroelastosis or myofibrosis, may be present, and this promotes earlier onset of the intractable heart failure.

Etiology: Unknown.

Pathogenesis: Possibly a congenital defect of the primordium of the right ventricular myocardium.

Sex Ratio: Presumably M1:F1.

Occurrence: Less than 1:100,000 births; under 0.1% of congenital heart disease.

Risk of Recurrence for Patient's Sib: Unknown.

Risk of Recurrence for Patient's Child: Unknown.

Age of Detectability: From birth, by echocardiograph or by cardiac catheterization and angiocardiography.

Gene Mapping and Linkage: Unknown.

Prevention: None known. Genetic counseling indicated.

Treatment: Superior vena cava - right pulmonary artery anastomosis or some other type of right heart bypass surgery, in those with heart failure but without associated left ventricular myocardial disease, to decompress the right heart and improve the pulmonary circulation. Other measures include symptomatic therapy for congestive heart failure.

Prognosis: Poor. In the usual cases where there is almost total absence of the right ventricular myocardium, death from heart failure occurs during infancy. Survival for several years is possible when the myocardial defect is not extensive.

Detection of Carrier: Unknown.

References:

Arcilla RA, Gasul BM: Congenital aplasia or marked hypoplasia of the myocardium of the right ventricle (Uhl's anomaly): clinical angiocardiographic and hemodynamic findings. J Pediatr 1961; 58:381–388. *

Cumming GR, et al.: Congenital aplasia of the myocardium of the right ventricle (Uhl's anomaly). Am Heart J 1965; 70:671–676.

French JW, et al.: Echocardiographic findings in Uhl's anomaly: demonstration of diastolic pulmonary valve opening. Am J Cardiol 1975; 36:349–353.

AR001   **René A. Arcilla**

VENTRICLE, SEPTUM DEXTROPOSITION AND DOUBLE INLET LEFT VENTRICLE   0286

Includes:
  Cor triloculare biatriatum
  Dextroposition of ventricular septum-double inlet left ventricle
  Double inlet left ventricle with ventricular inversion
  Double inlet left ventricle without ventricular inversion
  Holmes heart
  Univentricular heart of the left ventricular type
  Ventricle, single with rudimentary outflow chamber

Excludes:
  Mitral valve atresia (0665)
  Tricuspid valve, atresia (0968)
  Other forms of functional single ventricle

Major Diagnostic Criteria: Clinical evidence of a large left-to-right shunt in a mildly cyanotic infant with electrovectorcardiographic evidence of severe left ventricular hypertrophy should suggest the possibility of double inlet left ventricle with noninversion of the ventricles. Similar clinical findings in the presence of electrovectorcardiographic evidence of right ventricular hypertrophy as evidenced by significant Q waves in lead V_1, plus similar deep Q waves in standard lead III and lead aVF, should suggest the possibility of double inlet left ventricle with inversion of the ventricles. Cardiac catheterization and selective angiocardiography will confirm the exact anatomic situation.

Clinical Findings: Double inlet left ventricle is that cardiac malformation in which both atrioventricular valves open into a large ventricular chamber which morphologically resembles a left ventricle. The left A-V valve communicates exclusively with this large left ventricle. The right A-V valve may also communicate exclusively with the large left ventricle but may override a hypoplastic ventricular septum and open partially into a more or less rudimentary right ventricle. Double inlet left ventricle is usually, but not necessarily, associated with transposition of the great arteries in which case the aorta arises from the rudimentary right ventricle which consists only of a rightward and anteriorly placed infundibular chamber. In the rare instance when the great arteries are normally related (and the ventricles are not inverted), the complex is known as the Holmes heart. The atrial septum is usually intact, although small atrial septal defects may occur. A ventricular septal defect is always present as the route of communication from the large single ventricle to the rudimentary right ventricular infundibular chamber. If the ventricular septal defect is small, there may be functional obstruction to the aorta. Pulmonic or subpulmonic obstruction may also be present, ranging from mild stenosis to complete atresia.

The anatomic complex double inlet left ventricle may also occur in the presence of ventricular inversion. In that condition the large ventricular chamber, which has the internal morphology of a left ventricle and which receives both A-V valves, is located on the right side. The apex of the heart (in situs solitus) usually points to the left, but dextroversion may be present. The pulmonary trunk almost always arises from the main chamber. The left A-V valve may override the ventricular septum in some cases. The hypoplastic right ventricular infundibular chamber is placed leftward, superiorly and anteriorly and gives origin to the aorta. The ventricular septum lies in the sagittal plane. As with noninversion, pulmonic or subpulmonic obstruction may be present.

Clinical features are usually those of a large left-to-right shunt with bidirectional intracardiac mixing and are similar for both inversion and noninversion of the ventricles. In the absence of pulmonary stenosis, cyanosis is initially mild. With increased pulmonary vascular resistance, cyanosis will increase. A harsh systolic murmur and systolic thrill are present along the left sternal border and the second sound is single or narrowly split with accentuation of the pulmonic component. A mitral diastolic flow murmur is common and congestive heart failure is frequently present. When pulmonic or subpulmonic obstruction is present, the clinical findings depend upon the degree of obstruction. When mild, the findings may be unchanged. When severe, cyanosis is prominent, the murmurs may be insignificant, and the second sound is single. When obstruction to aortic outflow is present, the clinical picture frequently mimics aortic atresia or severe coarctation of the aorta and survival beyond a few months of life is unlikely.

The electrovectorcardiographic features depend upon whether inversion or noninversion of the ventricles is present. Regardless of the type of single ventricle, there is almost invariably an alteration of the initial cardiac vectors from the anticipated normal. Additional features suggest noninversion from inversion. With noninversion, the EKG and the vectorcardiogram demonstrate marked left ventricular hypertrophy. The mean frontal QRS axis ranges from $+25°$ to $+75°$ and the initial QRS forces are directed leftward and anteriorly, recording little or no Q wave in any of the usual chest leads (V_3R to V_7). The major QRS forces are shifted leftward and posteriorly resulting in rS complexes in lead V_1 and Rs complexes in lead V_6. Left and right atrial enlargement are frequently present. When pulmonic obstruction is present, the EKG is relatively unchanged except that right atrial enlargement is more marked. In the presence of ventricular inversion, the EKG and vectorcardiogram are quite different. As in ventricular inversion with two ventricles, the initial QRS forces are directed leftward, superiorly and usually posteriorly, resulting in Q waves in standard lead III, lead aVF and lead V_1. However, the major portion of the QRS forces is directed rightward and anteriorly, indicating anterior chamber hypertrophy, and resulting in qRs complexes in lead V_1 and RS complexes in V_6. The QRS axis in the frontal plane is directed somewhat to the right between 100° and 135°. Cardiac arrhythmias, especially varying degrees of atrioventricular block, are more common in the presence of ventricular inversion. As is the case with noninversion, atrial hypertrophy may be present and when pulmonic obstruction is significant, right atrial enlargement is more marked.

The echocardiographic diagnosis of this disorder requires demonstration that two separate atrioventricular valves exist without an intervening ventricular septum. Differential diagnosis of the various forms of single ventricle, as well as some forms of complete atrioventricular canal, is extremely difficult echocardiographically. Nevertheless, the demonstration of the transposed great vessel relationship in the presence of two atrioventricular valves and the absence of an intervening ventricular septal echo may suggest a diagnosis of single ventricle. An additional important feature is the identification of a small outflow tract anteriorly located but unrelated to an atrioventricular valve. It has been reported by some authors that double-inlet left ventricle can be demonstrated reliably with the 2-dimensional echocardiogram, and that this assists in the identification of the type of major ventricular chamber, whether left, right, or undifferentiated.

Chest X-ray findings depend upon the degree of pulmonic obstruction and the position of the right ventricular infundibulum. In the usual case without pulmonic obstruction, there is prominent shunt type vascularity, generalized cardiomegaly, biatrial enlargement and mediastinal findings suggestive of transposition of the great arteries. When pulmonic obstruction is significant, pulmonary arterial vascularity appears normal or decreased, and heart size is normal or slightly enlarged. Chest X-rays may suggest the presence of ventricular inversion by the position of the great arteries and the bulge of the infundibular chamber on the left upper border of the cardiac shadow.

Cardiac catheterization demonstrates a lack of significant shunting at the atrial level, based on fully saturated left atrial blood and no significant oxygen increase in the right atrium. Ventricular and peripheral arterial oxygen values show mild desaturation and are about equal. Selective angiocardiography is necessary to demonstrate the precise anatomy. The presence of ventricular inversion is apparent by the position of the infundibular chamber and the orientation of the ventricular septum. The interrelationship of the great arteries is of little value in distinguishing inversion from noninversion. Angiocardiography will demonstrate the presence of two independent atrioventricular valves entering a large single ventricle, which communicates with a rudimentary right ventricular infundibular chamber.

Complications: Persistent cardiac failure and repeated pulmonary infections frequently prove fatal. When pulmonic obstruction is significant, hypoxic complications may occur. Aortic obstruction may result in low cardiac output, poor systemic perfusion, and death within the first few months of life.

Associated Findings: None known.

Etiology: Probably multifactorial inheritance.

Pathogenesis: Probably due to a failure of alignment of the right portion of the atrioventricular canal with the primitive right ventricle. Thus, the right ventricle does not develop and functions only as an outlet chamber. The reason for the high degree of association of double inlet left ventricle with transposition of the great arteries is unknown.

Sex Ratio: M2:F1

Occurrence: Less than 1:100 cases of congenital heart defects.

Risk of Recurrence for Patient's Sib: Unknown.

Risk of Recurrence for Patient's Child: Unknown.

Age of Detectability: From birth.

Gene Mapping and Linkage: Unknown.

Prevention: None known. Genetic counseling indicated.

Treatment: Palliative procedures such as pulmonary artery banding, or systemic-pulmonary artery shunt in the presence of severe pulmonic stenosis, may prolong life. Other therapy as necessary for congestive heart failure and pneumonia.

Prognosis: Poor; survival into adulthood possible with moderate pulmonic obstruction. Most cases die early in life.

Detection of Carrier: Unknown.

References:
Van Praagh R, et al.: Diagnosis of the anatomic types of single or common ventricle (Review). Am J Cardiol 1965; 15:345.
De la Cruz MV, Miller BL: Double-inlet left ventricle: two pathological specimens with comments on the embryology and on its relation to single ventricle. Circulation 1968; 37:249.
Goldberg SJ, et al.: Pediatric and adolescent echocardiography. Chicago: Year Book Medical Publishers, 1975.
Seward J, et al.: Preoperative and postoperative echocardiographic observations in common ventricle. Circulation 1975; 52 (Suppl II):46.
Gessner IH, et al.: The vectorcardiogram in double inlet left ventricle, with and without ventricular inversion. In: Hoffman I, ed: Vectorcardiography. Amsterdam: North Holland Publishing Co, 1976.
Foale R, et al.: Double-inlet ventricle. Two dimensional echocardiographic findings (abstr). Circulation 1980; 62:III-332.

GE013   **Ira H. Gessner**
EL004   **Larry P. Elliott**
MI020   **B. Lynn Miller**

VENTRICLE, SINGLE LEFT PAPILLARY MUSCLE 0582

Includes:
    Left ventricle, single papillary muscle
    Parachute mitral valve

Excludes: Mitral stenosis, other anatomic forms of congenital

Major Diagnostic Criteria: Short of direct visualization, this parachute deformity is best demonstrated by two-dimensional echocardiograph. Its hemodynamic significance is best assessed by cardiac catheterization.

Clinical Findings: In its pure form, this entity consists of a mitral valve with normal leaflets and commissures. The chordae tendineae, however, are thickened, shortened and converge into a single or nearly single papillary muscle, much as the shrouds of a parachute, hence the descriptive name. While the leaflets and commissures are normal, the short, thickened chordae tendineae with their single point of insertion may severely compromise the effective mitral valve orifice as blood must flow through the interchordal spaces. In addition, the normal mobility of the leaflets is lacking because of the thickened chordae. The clinical manifestations, then, are those of mitral stenosis.

The symptomatology is quite variable and dependent on the presence, or absence, of associated lesions. In general, however, symptoms lead to a diagnosis of congenital heart disease early in life. Dyspnea, congestive heart failure and pulmonary infections are common presenting complaints. Right ventricular hypertrophy can usually be detected during physical examination. A systolic murmur at the apex and accentuated first and second sounds are frequent auscultatory findings. The classic diastolic murmur of mitral stenosis is variable. If a diastolic murmur is present, it may be secondary to increased flow from an associated left-to-right shunt lesion. However, if the murmur has a presystolic accentuation, anatomic mitral valve obstruction should be suspected. Unlike acquired mitral stenosis, the opening snap is an infrequent finding. Either an associated obstructive lesion or congestive heart failure may mask the characteristic murmur.

The chest film may show pulmonary venous obstruction and an enlarged heart with discrete left atrial enlargement. The cardiogram will reflect right-sided enlargement and left atrial enlargement. It cannot be overemphasized, however, that the characteristic physical and laboratory findings may be masked by coexisting lesions.

Coexisting left heart lesions have been stressed in most case reports. These include supravalvar stenosing ring of the mitral valve, aortic stenosis, subaortic stenosis and coarctation of the aorta. Additionally, fibroelastotic changes in the left heart are not uncommon. In at least three cases, however, right ventricular outflow tract obstruction, either at the pulmonic valve or below, has been reported.

Two-dimensional echocardiograph generally delineates the architecture of the mitral valve quite well. Additionally, Doppler interrogation of the transmitral flow will indicate whether there is hemodynamic obstruction.

Cardiac catheterization data usually will show elevated pulmonary artery and pulmonary arterial wedge pressures secondary to obstruction; however, a simultaneous comparison of left atrial pressure with left ventricular diastolic pressure is mandatory to confirm a pressure difference across the valve. As with the clinical findings, catheterization data may be misleading because of associated defects.

Complications: Frequent pulmonary infections, growth failure and death from congestive heart failure.

Associated Findings: None known.

Etiology: Unknown.

Pathogenesis: Unknown.

Sex Ratio: Presumably M1:F1

Occurrence: Undetermined. About eight percent of congenital mitral stenosis is accompanied by this parachute deformity.

Risk of Recurrence for Patient's Sib: Unknown.

Risk of Recurrence for Patient's Child: Unknown.

Age of Detectability: In the neonatal period by clinical evaluations, echocardiography and cardiac catheterizations.

Gene Mapping and Linkage: Unknown.

Prevention: None known. Genetic counseling indicated.

Treatment: Symptomatic therapy for congestive heart failure and respiratory infections, with operative intervention for the severe forms.

Prognosis: Depends on the associated lesions. Most patients are severely symptomatic and die in early childhood. Recently, several successful valve replacements have been reported in children in whom the associated cardiac lesions were not severe. The long-term prognosis for the operative children is not known.

Detection of Carrier: Unknown.

Special Considerations: Congenital mitral stenosis is a very rare lesion. The parachute deformity of the mitral valve is only one form. Undoubtedly there are reported cases of congenital mitral stenosis which include this deformity. Its frequency as a cause of hemodynamic abnormality is not now known. Its significance is related to the inability to correct this lesion with conservative valvotomy. Thus, a decision for the necessity of surgical intervention must include the probability of mitral valve replacement.

References:

Shone JD, et al.: The developmental complex of "parachute mitral valve," supravalvular ring of left atrium, subaortic stenosis and coarctation of aorta. Am J Cardiol 1963; 11:714–725. * †
Terzaki AK, et al.: Successful surgical treatment for "parachute mitral valve" complex: report of 2 cases. J Thorac Cardiovasc Surg 1968; 56:1–10.
Simon AL, et al.: The angiographic features of a case of parachute mitral valve. Am Heart J 1969; 77:809–813.
Glancy DL, et al.: Parachute mitral valve: further observations and associated lesions. Am J Cardiol 1971; 27:309–313.
Ruckman NR, et al.: Anatomic types of congenital mitral stenosis: report of 49 autopsy cases with consideration of diagnosis and surgical implications. Am J Cardiol 1978; 42:592–601. * †
Grenadier E, et al.: Two-dimensional echo Doppler study of congenital disorder of the mitral valve. Am Heart J 1984; 107:319–325.

MI019   **Robert H. Miller**

Ventricle, single with rudimentary outflow chamber
See VENTRICLE, SEPTUM DEXTROPOSITION AND DOUBLE INLET LEFT VENTRICLE
Ventricle, two-chambered right
See VENTRICLE, OBSTRUCTION WITHIN RIGHT VENTRICLE OR ITS OUTFLOW TRACT

VENTRICLES, INVERTED WITH TRANSPOSITION OF GREAT ARTERIES   0540

Includes:
>   Atrioventricular discordance with ventriculoarterial discordance
>   Corrected transposition of great vessels/arteries
>   Inverted transposition of great arteries
>   L-transposition with situs solitus
>   Ventricular inversion with L-transposition (L-TGV)

Excludes:
>   Common ventricle with inversion of infundibular chamber
>   Double inlet left ventricle
>   D-transposition
>   **Heart, transposition of great vessels** (0962)
>   L-transposition with rudimentary ventricle
>   Single ventricle with L-transposition
>   **Ventricles, inverted without transposition of great arteries** (0541)

Major Diagnostic Criteria: Ventricular inversion with L-transposition confirmed by two-dimensional echocardiography or by contrast ventriculography.

Clinical Findings: The hemodynamic findings in ventricular inversion with L-TGV define this malformation. The systemic venous blood enters a normally placed right atrium and then passes to the smooth-walled left ventricle through a bicuspid atrioventricular valve which has fibrous continuity with the pulmonary valve. Blood is ejected into a posterior, medial, and rightward pulmonary trunk before passing into the lungs. The pulmonary venous return empties into a normal left atrium before passage across a tricuspid atrioventricular valve (which is commonly abnormal) to the coarsely trabeculated right ventricle. Finally blood is ejected into the anterior and leftward aorta. The tricuspid atrioventricular valve and aortic valve are separated by the crista supraventricularis and the aortic valve is in a superior position when compared with the pulmonic valve, a reversal of the usual positions. Thus, in this malformation there is atrioventricular discordance and ventriculoarterial discordance. The coronary artery distribution is also abnormal with the right coronary artery arising above the right aortic sinus and giving origin of the anterior descending branch. The left coronary artery arises above the left sinus and traverses posteriorly giving rise to the conal branch and posterior descending artery. Also notable is the malposition of the ventricular conduction system with the AV node, His bundle and bundle branches mirror image in distribution. As a result these patients may have varying degrees of atrioventricular block. Disturbances in conduction/rhythm occur in approximately 60% of patients. Complete heart block occurs in 20–55% of patients while first degree atrioventricular block is seen in 60% of cases. Supraventricular tachycardia, atrial fibrillation, and Wolff-Parkinson-White syndrome may also occur.

The symptoms and physical findings in these patients are generally related to their associated lesions. When no associated malformations are found, these patients may live normal lives with essentially normal life expectancy. In those patients with associated lesions, 75 percent have symptoms in the first month of life. The associated lesions are generally large ventricular septal defects, with or without pulmonary artery obstruction, and the presenting symptoms include those of heart failure with large left-to-right shunts or cyanosis and apnea with pulmonary artery obstruction and right-to-left shunts. Physical examination commonly demonstrates a loud second sound which is frequently palpable at the midleft sternal border and is due to the anatomic position of the semilunar valves. The loudness of this sound is thus due to the proximity of the anterior aortic valve to the chest wall and occurs with aortic valve closure. The pulmonic component is not heard. A soft systolic ejection murmur at the mid-left sternal border from turbulence with ejection into the pulmonary artery is heard in patients without associated defects. Left AV valve (tricuspid) lesions are frequent and generally cause insufficiency, heard as a holosystolic murmur at the lower left sternal border. When pulmonic stenosis is present, a harsh systolic ejection murmur may be auscultated at the mid or lower left sternal border. A ventricular septal defect may cause a harsh murmur at the lower left sternal border.

Commonly associated malformations in this anomaly include: 1) ventricular septal defects in up to 80% of cases. These are generally large, perimembranous defects. Other types of VSDs such as supracristal, muscular, or "swiss-cheese" defects may be seen less commonly; 2) pulmonic stenosis in approximately 70% of patients. The area of stenosis can be either valvar or subvalvar; 3) systemic atrioventricular valve insufficiency in approximately 30% of patients, most of which have Ebstein-like malformation that can also obstruct the right ventricular outflow; 4) rhythm disturbances. Much less commonly associated malformations include: 5) atrial septal defect, 6) patent ductus arteriosus, 7) malpositions of cardiac apex, such as dextroversion, mirror-image dextrocardia, or levoversion; 8) coarctation of the aorta; 9) mitral or tricuspid atresia; 10) situs inversus viscera. Anomalies of pulmonary and systemic venous return are rarely associated.

The chest radiograph of patients with ventricular inversion, L-transposition, and no associated defects may be normal. However, non-diagnostic findings may be noted. A narrow mediastinum with a "straight left heart border" can occur with absence of the pulmonary artery knob or bump, due to the anterior position of the aorta. Occasionally there is hilar prominence of a right pulmonary artery segment which appears elevated with respect to the left. This is the so-called "waterfall" appearance of the right hilus. Cardiomegaly, increased pulmonary vascular markings, and left atrial enlargement may be present. These may be secondary to left-to-right shunt or left AV valve insufficiency. When predominant right-to-left shunting occurs, a prominent left upper heart border bulge may occur due to ascending aorta dilation. If situs solitus and dextroversion are present, the diagnosis of ventricular inversion and L-transposition is correct in approximately 80%.

Electrocardiographic findings include abnormal reversal of the precordial Q wave pattern and clockwise rotation of the frontal plane QRS loops. Left axis deviation is common and both ventricular and atrial enlargement may occur. Rhythm disturbances include first degree AV block, complete AV block, atrial fibrillation, and Wolff-Parkinson-White syndrome.

Echocardiography may be diagnostic with two-dimensional and Doppler examination. The parasternal short axis view can demonstrate the rightward, posterior and medial pulmonary artery and leftward and anterior aorta, as well as right-sided mitral valve. The apical or subxiphoid four-chamber view may show ventricular septal and atrial septal anatomy, respectively, as well as the AV valve anatomy. A trabeculated left-sided ventricle with an infundibular chamber leftward and anteriorly may be demonstrated. Flow patterns of AV valve insufficiency and direction of shunts may be shown by Doppler.

Cardiac catheterization and angiography will show the catheter course from venous ventricle to the posterior, medial pulmonary artery and from systemic ventricle to the anterior aorta. Ventriculography demonstrate the side-by-side position of the ventricles and ventricular septal orientation. The venous ventricle is generally triangular in shape. The systemic trabeculated ventricle is rounded and leftward with an infundibular chamber which is bordered superiorly by the crista supraventricularis. The pulmonary trunk is midline while the aorta is superior and leftward. The shunts and valvar insufficiency may also be ascertained at catheterization. Coronary artery pattern can be outlined by selective aortography.

Complications: Most commonly includes conduction defects, left AV valve insufficiency, and congestive heart failure. Other complications include bacterial endocarditis and recurrent pneumonia.

Associated Findings: Associated cardiovascular anomalies are common. These include: 1) ventricular septal defects; 2) pulmonary stenosis; 3) left atrioventricular valve insufficiency with Ebsteinoid malformation; 4) malposition of the cardiac apex; 5) rhythm disturbances; 6) atrial septal defects; 7) patent ductus arteriosus; 8) coarctation of aorta; 9) mitral atresia; 10) tricuspid

atresia and situs inversus of the viscera. Anomalies of systemic or pulmonary venous return may be encountered rarely.

Etiology: Multifactorial inheritance.

Pathogenesis: Abnormal rotation of the bulboventricular loop during the third to fourth week of gestation. De la Cruz et al. proposed bulboventricular loop twisting leftward instead of rightward with lack of spiral rotation of the conotruncal septum as the major abnormality. Grant proposed this defect to be a disturbance of "polarity" of conotruncal development with the primary defect being the formation of L-loop in situs solitus and D-loop in situs inversus, with secondary loss of truncal septum coiling.

MIM No.: 12100

Sex Ratio: M1.6:F1

Occurrence: About 1:22,000 live births.

Risk of Recurrence for Patient's Sib: Estimated at 1.5%.

Risk of Recurrence for Patient's Child: Unknown.

Age of Detectability: From birth by echocardiography and angiography. Fetal echocardiography is becoming able to diagnose anatomy and rhythm disturbance.

Gene Mapping and Linkage: Unknown.

Prevention: None known. Genetic counseling indicated.

Treatment: Treatment of fetal complete AV block is presently being studied and pacemaker placement shortly after birth is technically feasible if required. Repair of the ventricular septal defect, pulmonic stenosis, and AV valve insufficiency (repair or prosthesis) may be necessary in some cases. Permanent pacemaker implantation may also be required.

Prognosis: This is dependent on associated malformations. Those patients with no associated defects potentially have normal life expectancy. Sudden death due to dysrhythmias may occur. Approximately 60% of patients with associated cardiac anomalies die in the first year of life or in late adolescence due to chronic cardiac failure. Surgical therapy is more difficult technically with the right coronary artery course across the pulmonary outflow tract.

Detection of Carrier: Unknown.

References:

Van Praagh R, Van Praagh S: Isolated ventricular inversion. a consideration of the morphogenesis, definition, and diagnosis of nontransposed and transposed great arteries. Am J Cardiol 1966; 17:395–406.

Allwork SP, et al.: Congenitally corrected transposition of the great arteries. morphologic study of 32 cases. Am J Cardiol 1976; 38:910–923. *

Van Praagh R, et al.: Anatomically corrected malposition of the great arteries (S.D.L.). Circulation 1975; 51:20–31.

Westerman GR, et al.: Corrected transposition and repair of associated intracardiac defects. Circulation 1982; 66(Suppl I):1–197.

BR014   **J. Timothy Bricker**
T0014   **Jeffrey A. Towbin**

VENTRICLES, INVERTED WITHOUT TRANSPOSITION OF GREAT ARTERIES   0541

Includes:

Inversion of ventricles without reversal of arterial trunks
Ventricular inversion, isolated

Excludes: Ventricles, inverted with transposition of great arteries (0540)

Major Diagnostic Criteria: Ventricles inverted without transposition of great arteries. Selective arterial and venous ventriculography are essential to the anatomic confirmation of this entity.

Clinical Findings: The atria, ventricles and their atrioventricular valves are identical to those described for inversion of the ventricles with transposition of the great vessels. Systemic venous blood enters a normally located right atrium and passes through a morphologic mitral valve into a morphologic left ventricle. The aorta, however, arises posteriorly and to the right of the pulmonary artery from the right-sided morphologic left ventricle. The pulmonary veins empty into a normally located left atrium. Blood passes through a morphologic tricuspid valve into a morphologic right ventricle from which the pulmonary trunk arises anteriorly and to the left of the aorta. The right coronary artery arises above the right lateral aortic valve sinus and gives rise to the anterior descending coronary artery. The left coronary artery arises above the left aortic valve sinus and gives rise to the left marginal artery and distal circumflex coronary artery. As in essentially all forms of inversion with 2 ventricles, the coronary artery pattern is inverted. From the side, the great vessels do not appear transposed because the aorta is posterior to the pulmonary trunk. In the frontal view, the aorta lies to the left of the pulmonary trunk, and its ascending portion may be convex to the left. Thus, anatomically, the great vessels are not considered transposed because the anterior leaflet of the mitral valve is in continuity with aortic valve tissue.

As the hemodynamics are the same as in complete transposition of the great arteries, patients having this entity have similar signs and symptoms. In other words, the aorta arises from the venous ventricle and the pulmonary trunk arises from the arterial ventricle. Maintenance of life depends primarily on the associated defects. With only a patent foramen ovale or small atrial septal defect, cyanosis is apparent at birth, and congestive heart failure and poor weight gain occur early in life. A soft systolic murmur, grade 2/6 or less, is heard and the second heart sound is single. If a large ventricular septal defect (VSD) is also present, allowing good mixing of the arterial and venous streams and also an increased pulmonary blood flow, cyanosis is minimal; but congestive heart failure, repeated respiratory infections and poor weight gain are commonly seen. Such patients have a loud systolic murmur and thrill along the lower left sternal border and a diastolic flow murmur over the midprecordium and apex.

The ideal set of associated anomalies is a large VSD and an appropriate degree of pulmonary stenosis. The VSD allows excellent mixing at the ventricular level, and the pulmonary stenosis prevents volume overload of the heart and congestive heart failure. Such patients have a normal sized heart, a single component of S_2 and a harsh systolic murmur along the left sternal border. These patients have mild-to-moderate cyanosis at rest, increasing with activity. With age, cyanosis gradually increases, exercise tolerance decreases and clubbing develops. Besides VSD and various types of right ventricular outflow tract obstruction, patent ductus arteriosus and right aortic arch have been observed.

Analysis of the electrovectorcardiogram shows that the initial QRS forces are directed abnormally to the left and slightly anteriorly. The QRS loop shows slowing of ventricular depolarization, but the pattern of the intraventricular block is not classic right or left heart block. This QRS loop is so inscribed as to record either a QR or R complex in the right precordial leads. This QR pattern, in itself, always suggests inversion of the ventricles. The axis varies from mild right axis deviation to mild left axis deviation.

The echocardiographic demonstration of a right-sided mitral valve and a left-sided tricuspid valve in the presence of ventricular inversion is extremely difficult. Single-crystal findings have appeared unreliable although it has been reported that tricuspid valves can be identified by their lack of semilunar continuity and mitral valves by the presence of semilunar continuity. This is an extremely difficult differential to achieve. High resolution real-time cross-sectional echocardiographic systems can differentiate the morphology of tricuspid and mitral valves as well as their relationship to the atrioventricular septum for the determination of the ventricular situs. The abnormal orientation of ventricles as well as the ventricular septum in this disorder sometimes makes the M-mode differential diagnosis between these disorders and forms of single ventricle extremely difficult.

Chest X-rays are identical to cases with inversion of the ventricles with transposition. With large communications between the 2 circulations, the pulmonary vascularity is prominent and of the shunt type. In the presence of a severe degree of obstruction to pulmonary blood flow, pulmonary vascularity is diminished. There is a relatively higher incidence of right aortic arch.

Cardiac catheterization provides data similar to that obtained in cases of complete transposition of the great arteries. Ventricular angiocardiography is identical to that described for inversion of the ventricles. The diagnosis is based upon the site of origin of the great vessels and the relationship of the right AV valve with aortic valvar tissue. In the AP view, the aorta appears transposed in that it arises to the left of the pulmonary trunk. In the lateral view, however, the great vessels appear normally related. The aorta arises posterior to the pulmonary trunk and there is a fibrous continuity between the anterior leaflet of the right-sided bicuspid AV valve and the aortic valve. The pulmonary trunk arises from the right ventricular infundibulum. The pulmonary valve is superior and anterior to the aortic valve. Associated intracardiac or extracardiac anomalies will be defined in the conventional manner. Another important angiocardiographic finding is the anterior descending coronary artery arising from the right coronary artery as is typical in all cases with the basic ventricular arrangement of inversion of the ventricles with or without transposition of the great arteries.

Complications: Congestive heart failure, recurrent respiratory infections, growth failure are the common complications in infancy. In older individuals, polycythemia and its sequelae are the rule.

Associated Findings: None known.

Etiology: Unknown.

Pathogenesis: Inversion of the ventricles without transposition of the great arteries is due to two embryologic errors: inversion of the bulboventricular loop and that pathologic abnormality which, occurring with a normally developing loop, will result in transposition of the great arteries.

MIM No.: 12100

Sex Ratio: Presumably M1:F1

Occurrence: Undetermined. Less than a dozen cases reported.

Risk of Recurrence for Patient's Sib: Unknown.

Risk of Recurrence for Patient's Child: Unknown.

Age of Detectability: From birth, by selective ventriculography.

Gene Mapping and Linkage: Unknown.

Prevention: None known. Genetic counseling indicated.

Treatment: Palliative surgery in infancy varies with the hemodynamic state. With marked increased pulmonary blood flow, pulmonary artery banding and creation of an atrial septal defect are advised. In those patients with inadequate mixing, a balloon catheter atrial septostomy or Blalock-Hanlon procedure is advisable. With severe right ventricular outflow tract obstruction, a shunt procedure may be indicated. Corrective surgery using the Mustard procedure and correcting the associated defects is feasible.

Therapy for congestive heart failure and upper respiratory infections.

Prognosis: Depends on the associated defects. Best prognosis is when a large VSD and moderate pulmonic stenosis are present. Because of the paucity of cases reported or recognized, no further statements can be made in regard to morbidity, mortality or life expectancy.

Detection of Carrier: Unknown.

References:
Van Praagh R, Van Praagh S: Isolated ventricular inversion: a consideration of the morphogenesis, definition and diagnosis of nontransposed and transposed great arteries. Am J Cardiol 1966; 17:395.
Van Mierop LHS: The heart. In: Netter FH, ed: Ciba collection of medical illustrations. vol. 5. Summit, N.J.: Ciba Publishing, 1969: 118.
Solinger R, et al.: Deductive echocardiographic analysis in infants with congenital heart disease. Circulation 1974; 50:1072.
Henry WL, et al.: Evaluation of atrial ventricular valve morphology in congenital heart disease by real-time cross-sectional echocardiography. Circulation 1975; 50(suppl II):120.
Silverman NH, Snider AR: Two-dimensional echocardiography in

congenital heart disease. Connecticut: Appleton-Century-Crofts, 1982.

EL004
SC013

Larry P. Elliott
Gerold L. Schiebler
L.H.S. Van Mierop

Ventricular cyst of larynx
    See *LARYNGOCELE*
Ventricular fibrillation with prolonged Q-T interval
    See *ARRHYTHMIA, WITH LONG QT INTERVAL WITHOUT DEAFNESS*
Ventricular hypertrophy, hereditary
    See *HEART, SUBAORTIC STENOSIS, MUSCULAR*
Ventricular inversion with L-transposition
    See *VENTRICLES, INVERTED WITH TRANSPOSITION OF GREAT ARTERIES*
Ventricular inversion, isolated
    See *VENTRICLES, INVERTED WITHOUT TRANSPOSITION OF GREAT ARTERIES*
Ventricular muscle bands, aberrant right
    See *VENTRICLE, OBSTRUCTION WITHIN RIGHT VENTRICLE OR ITS OUTFLOW TRACT*
Ventricular myocardium, aplasia of right
    See *VENTRICLE, RIGHT, UHL ANOMALY*
Ventricular preexcitation
    See *ARRHYTHMIA, WOLFF-PARKINSON-WHITE TYPE*

VENTRICULAR SEPTAL DEFECT   0989

Includes:
    Aneurysm of membranous septum with one or more perforations
    Cranioacrofacial syndrome
    Eisenmenger complex
    Membranous septal defect
    Muscular septum, defects in various portions of
    Rabenhorst syndrome
    Ventricular septal defect, supracristal

Excludes:
    Heart, endocardial cushion defects (0347)
    Heart, tetralogy of Fallot (0938)

Major Diagnostic Criteria: For patients with small defects who are asymptomatic and have normal X-ray and EKG, the hallmark of diagnosis is the characteristic VSD murmur. For symptomatic patients and those who have evidence of abnormal hemodynamic overloads, cardiac catheterization can confirm the diagnosis and establish the hemodynamic state. Most defects 3 mm in diameter can be diagnosed with cross section echocardiography.

Clinical Findings: The position of single or multiple defects of the ventricular septum is variable; however, the associated hemodynamic changes are due primarily to the size of the defect. Clinical assessment should be made on the basis of size of the defect, the magnitude of the left-to-right shunt, and the resistance to blood flow through the lungs. The spectrum of clinical findings can be divided into 3 categories: small ventricular septal defects, moderate-to-large defects with large pulmonary blood flow and mild-to-moderate elevation of pulmonary vascular resistance, and large ventricular septal defects with marked elevation of pulmonary vascular resistance and normal-to-diminished pulmonary blood flow.

Small Ventricular Defects have minimal hemodynamic changes and clinical manifestations are inapparent. A harsh systolic murmur along the lower left sternal border is the characteristic finding. Components of the second sound are usually normal. The X-ray findings demonstrate a normal sized heart with normal pulmonary vascularity. The EKG usually is normal or has early biventricular hypertrophy pattern. Some patients, however, demonstrate left axis deviation which possibly is due to an associated anomaly of the left ventricular conduction system. An aneurysm of the membranous septum causes no symptoms unless large enough to obstruct right ventricular outflow.

Moderate-to-Large Ventricular Defect with increased pulmonary blood flow and mild-to-moderate elevation of pulmonary vascular resistance: the clinical manifestations are primarily determined by the magnitude of pulmonary blood flow. Congestive heart failure occurs in approximately one-third of these patients between 1–3 months of age. After 12–16 months of age, large left-to-right shunts are usually tolerated without severe heart failure. The usual systolic murmur is located along the left sternal border and is usually decrescendo in nature. An early faint diastolic blow in the pulmonic area is rarely present as a result of pulmonary insufficiency. There is an apical diastolic murmur of increased mitral flow across the mitral valve. The second sound is loud and usually closely split in those patients with high pulmonary artery pressure. The X-ray demonstrates cardiomegaly and increased pulmonary vascularity commensurate with the magnitude of the left-to-right shunt. In infants, associated pulmonary venous congestion may be evident. Left atrial enlargement usually is present. The EKG demonstrates combined ventricular hypertrophy and left atrial enlargement as a rule.

Large Ventricular Septal Defect with high pulmonary vascular resistance and approximately normal pulmonary blood flow: the major hemodynamic overload is right ventricular hypertension, which is tolerated well throughout early childhood. There are no symptoms throughout infancy and cyanosis is rare until later childhood. Growth proceeds normally. There is no VSD murmur; however, there is frequently a pulmonic ejection murmur in the second left interspace which may be associated with an early diastolic blow of pulmonary insufficiency. The second sound is loud and single. Apical diastolic murmurs are absent. The roentgenographic findings demonstrate a normal to minimally enlarged heart, right ventricular hypertrophy, prominent main pulmonary artery segment and increased hilar markings. There is pronounced contrast between the prominent central pulmonary arterial vessels and the diminished markings in the outer third of the lung field in some cases. The EKG demonstrates right ventricular hypertrophy and right axis deviation. Left atrial and left ventricular hypertrophy are absent. Cardiac catheterization will confirm the presence of a defect, the magnitude of shunting present, the pulmonary vascular resistance and the work load on the left ventricle. Oxygen saturation data and indicator dilution curves are important in assessing systemic and pulmonary blood flow, detection of the site of shunt and evaluating bidirectional shunts.

Echocardiograph is useful to estimate the size of the defect, the degree of left atrial and ventricular enlargement, and to identify any associated defects.

Complications: Death from congestive heart failure and pneumonia; especially in infancy. Bacterial endocarditis. Development of high pulmonary vascular resistance. Aortic insufficiency occasionally occurs.

Associated Findings: An increasingly wide range of associated findings are being reported, including complex syndromes and chromosomal anomalies.

Etiology: Presumably multifactorial inheritance. A high prevalence has been noted in association with chromosomal trisomies.

Pathogenesis: Failure of closure of the subaortic portion of ventricular septum, with anomalous development of any one or several components, i.e. embryonic muscular septum, the endocardial cushions, and conal swellings. Muscular defects may be due to failure of increasing muscle mass to obliterate intratrabecular spaces.

MIM No.: 12285

CDC No.: 745.4

Sex Ratio: M1:F1

Occurrence: Incidence 1:400 full-term live births; slightly higher in prematures.

Risk of Recurrence for Patient's Sib: About 3%.

Risk of Recurrence for Patient's Child: If mother is affected, the empiric risk is about 9.5%. If the father is affected, the empiric risk is about 2%.

Age of Detectability: From birth, by cardiac catheterization or echocardiography. Murmur usually detectable by three weeks of age.

Gene Mapping and Linkage: Unknown.

Prevention: None known. Genetic counseling indicated.

Treatment: Definitive surgery recommended for moderate and large defects with increased pulmonary blood flow. Medical therapy for congestive heart failure and pneumonia prior to surgery.

Prognosis: Patients with small defects have excellent prognosis. Without proper medical or surgical therapy, infants with heart failure have poor prognosis. Those who survive infancy with large defects and high pulmonary pressure have good prognosis during childhood. However, some with high pulmonary artery pressure develop further increases in pulmonary vascular resistance and the Eisenmenge syndrome with increased age.

Detection of Carrier: Unknown.

Special Considerations: The natural history of ventricular defects may involve dynamic changes in the physiologic state of the patient with time. This is also the most common congenital heart defect. Small defects present little physiologic overload, and these patients do well. Also, up to 80% of small ventricular defects may spontaneously close during infancy. Infants with large defects and marked increase in pulmonary blood flow may follow one of several courses between the age of six months to four years: the defect may become smaller and thereby diminish the left-to-right shunt; the size of the defect may remain constant with little change in pulmonary vascular resistance, and thereby the patient may maintain marked increased pulmonary blood flow with associated overload on the left ventricle.

After 12–18 months of age, congestive heart failure may spontaneously improve in the face of an unchanging pulmonary blood flow; in patients with large defects and marked pulmonary blood flow, hypertrophy of the infundibulum may occur with development of pulmonary stenosis; large defects may not change in size and pulmonary vascular resistance may gradually increase with ultimate reduction in pulmonary blood flow. It is this latter group which may progress from the infant picture of large pulmonary blood flow and heart failure, to the childhood state of markedly elevated pulmonary resistance (*Eisenmenger* syndrome). Note: Eisenmenger *syndrome* clinically refers to a physiologic state in which the pulmonary vascular resistance is equal to or exceeds that of the systemic vascular resistance. Eisenmenger *complex* refers specifically to a particular type of large ventricular septal defect; infracristal ventricular septal defect with overriding aorta without infundibular stenosis, which embryologically results from a hypoplasia of the conus septum.

References:
Hoffman JI, Rudolph AM: The natural history of ventricular septal defects in infancy. Am J Cardiol 1965; 16:634–653.
Rudolph AM: The effects of postnatal circulatory adjustments in congenital heart disease. Pediatrics 1965; 36:763–772.
Grosse FR: The Rabenhorst-syndrome: a cardio-acral-facial syndrome. Z Kinderheilk 1974; 117:109–114.
Goldberg SJ, et al.: Pediatric and adolescent echocardiography, 2nd ed. Chicago: Year Book Medical Publishers, 1980:307–328.
Nora JJ, Nora AH: Maternal transmission of congenital heart disease. Am J Cardiol 1987; 59:459–463. *
Graham TP, et al.: Defects of the ventricular septum. In: Adams FH, et al., eds: Heart disease in infants, children, and adolescents, 4th ed. Baltimore: Williams & Wilkins, 1989:189–209. *

GR002
                                           Thomas P. Graham

Ventricular septal defect with absent pulmonary valve
  See PULMONARY VALVE, ABSENT
Ventricular septal defect, endocardial cushion defect type
  See HEART, ENDOCARDIAL CUSHION DEFECTS
Ventricular septal defect, supracristal
  See VENTRICULAR SEPTAL DEFECT
Ventricular septal defect-double outlet right ventricle
  See VENTRICLE, DOUBLE-OUTLET RIGHT WITH ANTERIOR SEPTAL DEFECT
Ventricular septal defect-Hirschsprung disease
  See HIRSCHSPRUNG DISEASE-CARDIAC DEFECT

Ventricular, left, endocardial fibrosis fibroelastosis
  See VENTRICLE, ENDOCARDIAL FIBROELASTOSIS OF LEFT VENTRICLE
Ventricular, left, endocardial sclerosis
  See VENTRICLE, ENDOCARDIAL FIBROELASTOSIS OF LEFT VENTRICLE
Ventricular, left, subendocardial fibroelastosis
  See VENTRICLE, ENDOCARDIAL FIBROELASTOSIS OF LEFT VENTRICLE
Ventricular, right, endocardial fibroelastosis
  See VENTRICLE, ENDOCARDIAL FIBROELASTOSIS OF RIGHT VENTRICLE
Ventriculomegaly
  See HYDROCEPHALY
Verma-Naumoff short rib-polydactyly
  See SHORT RIB-POLYDACTYLY SYNDROME, VERMA-NAUMOFF TYPE

VERMIS AGENESIS   2106

Includes:
    Cerebellar vermis agenesis
    Cerebello-parenchymal disorder IV

Excludes:
    Cerebellar agenesis (2011)
    Hydrocephaly (0481)
    Joubert syndrome (2908)

Major Diagnostic Criteria: Patients with agenesis of the vermis may be asymptomatic or show hypotonia, ataxia and incoordination. Pneumoencephalogram or CT scan show an enlarged IV ventricle.

Clinical Findings: Hypotonia, nystagmus, tremor, and ataxia are present.

Complications: Unknown.

Associated Findings: **Meningocele**, **Encephalocele**, agenesis of corpus callosum, cranioschisis, and heterotopias may be present.

Etiology: Unknown.

Pathogenesis: Failure of fusion of the cerebellar crest is thought to result in agenesis of the vermis. This fusion begins rostrally and the anterior part of the vermis is formed before the posterior portion. Thus, partial agenesis of the anterior vermis does not occur. The insult leading to complete agenesis occurs earlier during development than that resulting in agenesis of the posterior vermis.

MIM No.: *21330

CDC No.: 742.230

Sex Ratio: Unknown.

Occurrence: Unknown.

Risk of Recurrence for Patient's Sib: Unknown.

Risk of Recurrence for Patient's Child: Unknown.

Age of Detectability: In infancy, if symptomatic.

Gene Mapping and Linkage: Unknown.

Prevention: None known. Genetic counseling indicated.

Treatment: Undetermined.

Prognosis: Variable.

Detection of Carrier: Unknown.

References:
Rubinstein HS, Freeman W: Cerebellar agenesis. J Nerv Ment Dis 1940; 92:489–502.
Andermann E, et al.: Three familial midline malformation syndromes of the central nervous system: "agenesis of the corpus callosum and anterior horn cell disease; agenesis of the cerebellar vermis; and atrophy of the cerebellar vermis." BD:OAS XI(2). New York: March of Dimes Birth Defects Foundation, 1975:269.
Macchi G, Bentivoglio M: Agenesis of hypoplasia of cerebellar structures. In: Vinken PJ, Bruyn GW, eds: Congenital malformations of

the brain and skull, part 1: Handbook of clinical neurology. Amsterdam: North Holland, 1977:367–393.

GA018   **Bhuwan P. Garg**

Vertebral anomalies
  See SPONDYLOTHORACIC DYSPLASIA
Vertebral body hypoplasia-lethal short-limbed dwarfism
  See DWARFISM, LETHAL, SHORT-LIMBED PLATYSPONDYLIC TYPE
Vesical exstrophy
  See BLADDER EXSTROPHY
Vesical-ureteral reflux (VUR)
  See VESICO-URETERAL REFLUX

VESICO-URETERAL REFLUX   2408

Includes:
  Ureteral-vesical reflux
  Urinary reflux, primary, congenital, or idiopathic
  Vesical-ureteral reflux (VUR)

Excludes: Reflux secondary to obstructive uropathy

Major Diagnostic Criteria: The presence of vesicoureteral reflux is an objective X-ray sign diagnosed by voiding cystogram, i.e., the retrograde flow of urine into the ureter(s) during micturition. Additional studies may include urine cultures, serum electrolytes, intravenous pyelography, renal sonography, radionuclide techniques, and cystoscopy.

Clinical Findings: Reflux predisposes to infections of the urinary tract. Severe cases may develop pyelonephritis, hydronephrosis, and scarring of renal parenchyma, which may lead to hypertension and sometimes renal failure. The severity of reflux is graded by voiding cystogram and is based on the level of retrograde urine flow within the upper urinary tract, the presence of hydronephrosis, and the degree of ureteral distension and tortuosity.

Complications: Cystitis, pyelonephritis, hydronephrosis, renal scarring, hypertension, and renal failure.

Associated Findings: Reflux may be secondary to obstructive uropathy (**Urethral valves, posterior,** ureteral duplications) or neurogenic bladder, but these entities are excluded from the present discussion of primary vesicoureteral reflux.

Etiology: Reflux may be familial but without a consistent pattern of inheritance.
  On the basis of a family in which three brothers and their maternal grandmother were affected, Middleton et al (1975) concluded that an X-linked form may exist. None of three sisters were affected. Van den Abbeele et al (1987) reported reflux in 27 of 60 (45%) asymptomatic siblings of patients with known reflux.
  Chapman et al (1985) applied complex segregation analysis to data from 88 families with at least one person with this condition. They concluded that a single major locus is the most important causal factor. The mutant allele was estimated to be dominant, with a frequency of about 0.1%. As adults, about 45% of persons with the gene would have vesico-ureteral reflux and/or reflux nephropathy, and 15% develop renal failure, compared to 0.05% and 0.001% respectively, for persons without the gene.

Pathogenesis: Congenital or idiopathic reflux may be a heterogenous entity arising from a shortened intravesicular ureter or, an abnormally positioned ureteral orifice.

MIM No.: 19300, 31455

CDC No.: 753.880

Sex Ratio: M1:F8

Occurrence: Reported in 20–30% of school-aged females with infections of the urinary tract. This disorder is rare in Blacks.

Risk of Recurrence for Patient's Sib:
  See Part I, *Mendelian Inheritance.*

Risk of Recurrence for Patient's Child:
  See Part I, *Mendelian Inheritance.*

Age of Detectability: During infancy or in preschool and school-aged children.

Gene Mapping and Linkage: Unknown.

Prevention: None known. Genetic counseling indicated.

Treatment: Early detection and management is mandatory if recurrent infections and renal injury are to be prevented. Mild reflux is usually managed with prophylactic antibiotics and may resolve later in childhood or adolescence. Surgical reimplantation of the refluxing ureter(s) is recommended for moderate-to-severe degrees of reflux. Surgery may also be required in mildly affected patients who continue to have urinary tract infections despite the use of prophylactic antibiotics.

Prognosis: The prevention of pyelonephritis and scarring of renal parenchyma are the prime objectives of management. Mild cases, with either no or minimal degrees of hydronephrosis, may resolve spontaneously in later childhood. Treatment is directed at preventing infection with prophylactic antibiotics until reflux resolves. In more severe cases, with moderate-to-severe hydronephrosis and tortuous distended ureters, antireflux surgery is usually advocated.

Detection of Carrier: Unknown.

References:
Winberg J, et al.: Epidemiology of symptomatic urinary tract infections in childhood. Acta Paediatr Scand 1974; 252:S1–20. *
Middleton GW, et al.: Sex-linked familial reflux. J Urol 1975; 114:36–39.
Ransley PG, et al.: Vesicoureteral reflux: continuing surgical dilemma. Urology 1978; 12:246–255. *
Lyon RP, et al.: Treatment of vescoureteral reflux. Urology 1980; 16:38–46.
Smellie JM, et al.: Children with urinary tract infection: a comparison of those with and those without vesicoureteral reflux. Kidney Int 1981; 20:717–722. *
Woodard JR: Vesicoureteral reflux: a surgical perspective. Am J Kidney Dis 1983; 3:136–138.
Chapman CJ, et al.: Vesicoureteral reflux: segregation analysis. Am J Med Genet 1985; 20:577–584.
Van den Abbeele AD, et al.: Vesicoureteral reflux in asymptomatic siblings of patients with known reflux: radionuclide cystography. Pediatrics 1987; 79:147–153.

HY001   **Leonard C. Hymes**

Vesiculocephaly
  See COLPOCEPHALY
Viljoen rhizomelic dysplasia
  See OMODYSPLASIA
Vinyl chloride induced scleroderma
  See SCLERODERMA, FAMILIAL PROGRESSIVE
Virilization of the female from maternal extrinsic androgens
  See FETAL EFFECTS FROM MATERNAL EXTRINSIC ANDROGENS

VISCERA, FATTY METAMORPHOSIS   0990

Includes:
  Acyl-CoA dehydrogenase deficiency (some)
  Carnitine deficiency, primary systemic (some)
  Fatty acid oxidation disorders
  Hepatic carnitine palmitoyl transferase deficiency (some)
  Hypoglycemic nonketotic dicarboxylic aciduria (some)
  Liver, steatosis of
  "Reye syndrome-like" manifestations
  Viscera, steatosis of, familial
  White liver disease

Excludes:
  Alpha(1)-antitrypsin deficiency (0039)
  Carnitine deficiency, systemic (2121)
  Cerebro-hepato-renal syndrome (0139)
  Collagen storage disease
  Cystic fibrosis (0237)
  Diabetes mellitus
  Fructose-1-phosphate aldolase deficiency (0395)
  Galactosemia (0403)
  Hepatolenticular degeneration (0469)
  Histiocytosis

Hyperlipoproteinemia, combined (0496)
Jamaican vomiting sickness (hypoglycin A intoxication)
Lipidosis
Phytanic acid oxidase deficiency, infantile type (2278)
Phytanic acid storage disease (0810)
Reye syndrome
Tyrosinemia
Viscera, toxic, nutritional, and inflammatory steatosis of
Wolman disease (1003)

Major Diagnostic Criteria: A group of inborn errors of mitochondrial beta oxidation of fatty acids, most often characterized by acute attacks of vomiting, hypoketotic hypoglycemia, and acidosis, with a variable age of onset and variable degrees of hepatic, CNS, cardiac, and skeletal muscle manifestations. Pathologic findings include various degrees of fatty infiltration of liver parenchymal cells, renal tubular epithelium, myocardium, and skeletal muscle. Gas chromatography mass spectrometry (GCMS) analysis of serum and urine shows excessive accumulation and excretion of secondary metabolites of saturated fatty acids. The diagnosis is confirmed by the demonstration of decreased ability of cultured fibroblasts, mononuclear leukocytes, or liver cells and their mitochondria to oxidize radiolabeled fatty acids or, in the case of **Acidemia, glutaric acidemia II, neonatal onset**, by the detection of deficiency of electron transfer flavoprotein (ETF) or electron transfer flavoprotein: ubiquinone oxidoreductase (ETF:QO) in fibroblasts, using the techniques of enzymatic assay or immunoblotting. In the case **Carnitine deficiency, systemic**, the finding of primary low serum and tissue carnitine levels is diagnostic.

Clinical Findings: A considerable variation exists in the clinical presentation and biochemical picture according to the type and severity of the enzyme defect. The most severe acute cases present in the neonatal period or during infancy with poor feeding, vomiting, "sweaty feet" odor (in **Acidemia, glutaric acidemia II, neonatal onset**), hepatomegaly, hyperbilirubinemia, cardiac arrhythmias, apnea, hypotonia, seizures, and lethargy progressing to coma and death. Less severe cases usually present at a later age with intermittent "Reye syndrome-like" attacks that are provoked by fasting stress and include vomiting, hepatomegaly, elevated liver enzymes, hyperammonemia, and encephalopathy. The episodes usually respond favorably to appropriate treatment, and only negligible symptoms are observed between attacks. The mildest cases are characterized by a chronic course with cardiomyopathy and/or skeletal muscle weakness. Although not the rule, most acute catastrophic cases are caused by **Acyl-CoA dehydrogenase deficiency, long chain type, Acyl-CoA dehydrogenase deficiency, medium chain type, Acidemia, glutaric acidemia II, neonatal onset**, or by **Carnitine deficiency, systemic**. The acute fatal cases are usually characterized by multisystemic fatty infiltration, whereas in milder cases only the liver, myocardium, or skeletal muscle are affected. The fatty changes in liver cells are usually of a macrovesicular type.

Biochemical features that are common to all these disorders during acute attacks include abnormal liver function tests, nonketotic hypoglycemia, metabolic acidosis, carnitine deficiency (primary or secondary), and the overproduction of omega (dicarboxylic acids) and omega-1 oxidation products of fatty acids identified by GCMS analysis of serum and urine. The latter compounds include adipic, suberic, and sebacic acids (C_6-C_{10}-dicarboxylic acids), 5(OH)hexanoic acid, 7(OH)octanoic acid, 9(OH)decanoic acid, hexanoylglycine, and suberylglycine in medium- and long-chain **Acyl-CoA dehydrogenase deficiency** and in **Carnitine deficiency, systemic**; all the above along with ethylmalonic acid, isobutyric acid, 2 methylbutyric acid, isovaleric and glutaric acids and their glycine conjugates, and sometimes sarcosine, are found in **Acidemia, glutaric acidemia II, neonatal onset**. No abnormal organic aciduria has been reported in hepatic carnitine palmitoyl tranferase deficiency.

A family history of death of sibs or clinical episodes suggestive of defective fatty acid oxidation usually exists. The clinical expression and the severity of the specific enzyme defect within a family are consistent, which suggests a complete penetrance.

Complications: Survivors of the acute episodes may develop permanent brain damage, severe hypotonia, and abnormal psychomotor development. The milder cases exhibit cardiomegaly, myopathy, or are free of symptoms.

Associated Findings: Acidemia, glutaric acidemia II, neonatal onset with deficient ETF:QO has been associated with congenital anomalies, including polycystic kidneys, renal dysgenesis, **Kidney, polycystic disease infantile potter type I**, anomalies of the abdominal wall and external genitalia, and cerebral malformations.

Etiology: Autosomal recessive inheritance. Only one family exhibiting an X-linked recessive mode of inheritance has been reported.

Pathogenesis: A defective transport of long-chain fatty acids into the mitochondria is responsible for the derangement in fatty acid oxidation in **Carnitine deficiency, systemic** and hepatic carnitine palmitoyl transferase deficiency. It is not clear whether the primary abnormality in the former is reduced carnitine biosynthesis, abnormal gastrointestinal absorption, a renal tubular defect with loss of carnitine in the urine, or abnormal carnitine transport into tissues.

Seven mitochondrial flavin adenine dinucleotide (FAD) requiring acyl-dehydrogenases, i.e., those specific for dimethylglycine, glutaryl-CoA, isovaleryl CoA, isobutyryl CoA and 2-methylbutyryl CoA, short-chain acyl-CoA, medium-chain acyl-CoA, and long-chain acyl-CoA, appear to be defective in multiple acyl-CoA dehydrogenase deficiency. The primary biochemical abnormality is a deficiency of either ETF or ETF:QO, which are responsible for the transfer of electrons from the flavoprotein acyl-CoA dehydrogenases to the mitochondrial respiratory chain. In some patients the dehydrogenase specific for sarcosine is also involved.

In the isolated medium-chain or long-chain **Acyl-CoA dehydrogenase deficiency**, the defect is at the level of C_6-C_{12} or C_{12}-C_{18} chain mitochondrial beta oxidation, respectively.

MIM No.: *22810

Sex Ratio: M1:F1

Occurrence: Thus far, about 20 kinships have been documented.

Risk of Recurrence for Patient's Sib:
See Part I, *Mendelian Inheritance*.

Risk of Recurrence for Patient's Child:
See Part I, *Mendelian Inheritance*.

Age of Detectability: In neonatal period for severe cases; milder cases can be diagnosed at any age.

Gene Mapping and Linkage: Unknown.

Prevention: None known. Genetic counseling indicated.

Treatment: During acute attacks, intravenous glucose and mannitol, mechanical ventilation, muscle relaxants, and intracranial pressure monitoring. Riboflavin or carnitine administration during acute episodes have only been successful in a few cases. Medical and supportive therapy for chronic cardiomyopathy and skeletal myopathy. Chronic carnitine treatment for **Carnitine deficiency, systemic**.

Prognosis: The acute catastrophic cases, especially those associated with **Acyl-CoA dehydrogenase deficiency, long chain type, Acyl-CoA dehydrogenase deficiency, medium chain type**, and **Acidemia, glutaric acidemia II, neonatal onset**, usually result in rapid deterioration and death, despite aggressive treatment. Survivors may develop permanent brain damage. Milder cases may have acute episodes during fasting, or may suffer from cardiac or skeletal muscle abnormalities, but usually have normal life span and normal intelligence.

Detection of Carrier: Intermediate levels of acyl-CoA dehydrogenase activity or, in the case of **Acidemia, glutaric acidemia II, neonatal onset**, intermediate ETF/ETF:QO activity in cultured fibroblasts or mononuclear leukocytes. No conclusions on the detection of carriers in **Carnitine deficiency, systemic** or hepatic carnitine palmitoyl transferase deficiency have been formulated.

Special Considerations: The fasting-induced nonketotic hypoglycemia observed in this group of disorders is a result of the defective oxidation of fatty acids, which normally produces ketone bodies during fasting and increases gluconeogenesis flux by providing the acetyl-CoA and the reducing equivalents (NADH) necessary for gluconeogenesis. The carnitine deficiency found in all acyl-CoA dehydrogenase deficiency disorders is due to the sequestration of carnitine as acyl-carnitine. The origin of the excessive accumulation of fatty acid metabolites in the beta oxidation disorders is the alternative omega and omega-1 oxidation of fatty acids to dicarboxylic acids and omega-1 hydroxymonocarboxylic acids, respectively, in the microsomes (cytochrome P-450 system), further beta oxidation of these compounds in the peroxisomes, and alternative glycine conjugation. The accumulated fatty acid metabolites are toxic and probably contribute directly to the hepatocerebral toxicity by uncoupling oxidative phosphorylation and by interfering with neuronal membrane function.

In *Mendelian Inheritance in Man* (McKusick, 1988), a heterogenous group of case reports, published in the medical literature between 1964 and 1984, is summarized under the histologic, descriptive heading "Fatty Metamorphosis of Viscera." No detailed biochemical studies, specifically GCMS analysis and enzymatic studies, were performed in any, but one, of those cases. Based on analysis of the cases and the knowledge gathered over the last decade concerning the biochemical lesions and abnormal metabolic blocks in fatty acid degradation, it seems reasonable to conclude that most, if not all, of these case reports belong to the group of inherited inborn errors of mitochondrial fatty acid oxidation described here. Increased awareness of these inherited conditions, especially in patients presenting with "Reye syndrome-like" manifestations, and performance of detailed metabolic investigations will probably result in the detection of many other cases.

References:

Gregersen N, et al.: Suberylglycine excretion in the urine from a patient with dicarboxylic aciduria. Clin Chim Acta 1976; 70:417–425.

Chesney RW, et al.: A three-month-old infant with seizures, hypoglycemia, and apnea. Am J Med Genet 1983; 16:373–388.

Goodman SI, Frerman FE: Glutaric acidaemia type II (multiple acyl-CoA dehydrogenation deficiency). J Inherit Metab Dis 1984; 7:33–37.

Coates PM, et al.: Genetic deficiency of medium-chain acyl coenzyme A dehydrogenase: studies in cultured skin fibroblasts and peripheral mononuclear leukocytes. Pediatr Res 1985; 19:671–676.

Gregersen N: The acyl-CoA dehydrogenation deficiencies. Scand J Clin Lab Invest 1985; (suppl 174):45:1–60.

Rebouche CJ, Paulson DJ: Carnitine metabolism and function in humans. Ann Rev Nutr 1986; 6:41–66.

Moon A, Rhead WJ: Complementation analysis of fatty acid oxidation disorders. J Clin Invest 1987; 79:59–64.

Roe CR, Coates PM: Acyl-CoA dehydrogenase deficiencies. In: Scriver CR, et al, eds: The metabolic basis of inherited disease, 6th ed. New York: McGraw-Hill, 1989:889–914.

ZE004   **Israel Zelikovic**
CH038   **Russell W. Chesney**

VITAMIN B(12) LYSOSOMAL TRANSPORT DEFECT   2994

Includes:
  Cobalamin, defect in lysosomal release of
  Cobalamin F disease
  Methylmalonicaciduria due to B(12) release defect
  Vitamin B(12) lysosomal release defect
  Vitamin B(12) storage disease

Excludes:
  Acidemia, methylmalonic (0658)
  Combined methylmalonic aciduria-homocystinuria diseases
  Methylcobalamin deficiency (2605)
  Transcobalamin II deficiency (2624)

Major Diagnostic Criteria: Methylmalonic aciduria responsive to therapy with vitamin B_{12}; decreased whole cell synthesis of adenosyl-B_{12} and methyl-B_{12} in the presence of elevated unmetabolized vitamin B_{12} in lysosomes. Complementation with cbl C and cbl D fibroblast lines.

Clinical Findings: Stomatitis, glossitis, multifocal seizures, hypotonia, developmental delay, feeding difficulties.

Complications: Unknown.

Associated Findings: In one unpublished case, sudden infant death.

Etiology: Presumably autosomal recessive inheritance.

Pathogenesis: Defect in transfer of free vitamin B_{12} from lysosomes to cytoplasm.

MIM No.: 27738

Sex Ratio: Presumably M1:F1 (M0:F2 observed).

Occurrence: The index case and one additional unrelated patient have been documented since the condition was discovered in 1985.

Risk of Recurrence for Patient's Sib:
  See Part I, *Mendelian Inheritance.*

Risk of Recurrence for Patient's Child:
  See Part I, *Mendelian Inheritance.*

Age of Detectability: During the neonatal period. One unaffected sib of the proband was diagnosed prenatally.

Gene Mapping and Linkage: Unknown.

Prevention: None known. Genetic counseling indicated.

Treatment: The proband was treated with oral and intramuscular vitamin B_{12}.

Prognosis: Unknown.

Detection of Carrier: Unknown.

Special Considerations: Although homocystinuria and megaloblastic anemia was not detected in the original proband, the second patient did have both, as would be expected based on the combined deficiency in methyl-B_{12} and adenosyl-B_{12}.

References:

Rosenblatt DS, et al.: Defect in vitamin B-12 release from lysosomes: newly described inborn error of vitamin B-12 metabolism. Science 1985; 228:1319–1321.

Rosenblatt DS, et al.: New disorder of vitamin B_{12} metabolism (cobalamin F) presenting as methylmalonic aciduria. Pediatrics 1986; 78:51–54.

Watkins D, Rosenblatt DS: Failure of lysosomal release of vitamin B_{12}: a new complementation group causing methylmalonic aciduria (cbl F). Am J Hum Genet 1986; 39:404–408.

Shih VE, et al.: Defective lysosomal release of vitamin B12: hereditary cobalamin metabolic disorder associated with sudden death. Am J Med Genet 1989; 33:555–563.

WA053   **David Watkins**
R0052   **David S. Rosenblatt**

VITAMIN B(12) MALABSORPTION   0992

Includes:

Anemia, pernicous, juvenile
Cobalamin malabsorption
Ileal B(12) transport deficiency
Imerslund-Grasbeck syndrome
Malabsorption of vitamin B(12) (two types)
Pernicious anemia, juvenile-proteinuria

Excludes:

Anemia, pernicious congenital (2656)
Anemia, pernicious, due to deficiency of extrinsic factor
Blind loop syndrome
Diphyllobothrium latum infestation
Folate malabsorption (2166)
Transcobalamin II deficiency (2624)

Major Diagnostic Criteria: Demonstration of vitamin B_{12} deficiency by abnormal Schilling test, reduced serum vitamin B_{12} concentration, and increased excretion of methylmalonic acid and/or homocystine in the urine. Absence of serum antibodies to intrinsic factor and gastric parietal cells. Normal gastric mucosa.

Gastric juice analysis and response to ingested intrinsic factor distinguish three forms of congenital B_{12} malabsorption. Patients with deficiency of intrinsic factor (see **Anemia, pernicious congenital**) will respond clinically and chemically to ingestion of normal gastric juice or to administered intrinsic factor and B_{12}. Patients with functionally impaired intrinsic factor and those with ileal transport defect will have immunologically detectable intrinsic factor in gastric aspirate. Patients with functionally abnormal intrinsic factor will respond to exogenous normal intrinsic factor, while those with the transport defect will not. Patients with B_{12} malabsorption due to specific ilial "receptor site" defect (*Imerslund-Grasbeck syndrome*) will respond only to parenteral administration of physiologic amounts (1 μg/day) of vitamin B_{12}.

Clinical Findings: Megaloblastic anemia noted during the first 1–3 years of life (100%): one group of children lacks gastric intrinsic factor; a second group has an immunologically identifiable, functionally defective intrinsic factor; a third group lacks the ileal transport mechanism for vitamin B_{12}.

Complications: Combined system disease of the central nervous system (CNS).

Associated Findings: Permanent proteinuria is noted in nearly one-half of patients with ileal transport defect. This form of the disorder is also called the *Imerslund-Gräsbeck* syndrome.

Etiology: Autosomal recessive inheritance of a defect affecting either the synthesis of gastric intrinsic factor or the specific vitamin B_{12} transport system in the terminal ileum.

Pathogenesis: Deficiency of vitamin B_{12} leads to megaloblastic anemia, methylmalonic aciduria, and CNS disease.

MIM No.: *26110

Sex Ratio: M1:F1

Occurrence: Over 50 cases have been documented; half in Finland.

Risk of Recurrence for Patient's Sib:
See Part I, *Mendelian Inheritance.*

Risk of Recurrence for Patient's Child:
See Part I, *Mendelian Inheritance.*

Age of Detectability: At one to two years of age.

Gene Mapping and Linkage: Unknown.

Prevention: None known. Genetic counseling indicated.

Treatment: Parenteral administration of vitamin B_{12} (1 μg/day); blood transfusions may be required initially.

Prognosis: Good, if treatment initiated before permanent CNS damage ensues.

Detection of Carrier: Not well defined; both parents of a single patient with ileal transport defect were reported to have moderate impairment of vitamin B_{12} absorption, without anemia.

Special Considerations: The existence of this condition provides strong evidence for single gene control of synthesis of gastric intrinsic factor, and for an ileal "receptor" in the vitamin B_{12} transport process.

References:
McIntyre OR, et al.: Pernicious anemia in childhood. New Engl J Med 1965; 272:981–986.
Mohamed SD, et al.: Juvenile familial megaloblastic anaemia due to selective malabsorption of vitamin B_{12}: a family study and a review of the literature. Q J Med 1966; 35:433–453.
Donaldson RH: Mechanisms of malabsorption of cobalamin. In: Babior BM, ed.: Cobalamin biochemistry and pathophysiology. New York: John Wiley & Sons, 1975:335.
Sennett C, et al.: Transmembrane transport of cobalamin in prokaryotic and eukaryotic cells. Ann Rev Biochem 1981; 50:1053–1086.
Broch H, et al.: Imerslund-Grasbeck anemia: a long-term follow-up study. Acta Paediat Scand 1984; 73:248–253.
Heisel, MA et al.: Congenital pernicious anemia: report of seven patients with studies of the extended family. J Pediatr 1984; 105:564–568.

FL001

David B. Flannery
Leon E. Rosenberg

VOCAL CORD PARALYSIS 2506

Includes:
Gerhardt syndrome
Laryngeal abductor paralysis
Paralysis of vocal cord
Plott syndrome
Vocal cord dysfunction, adductor type

Excludes:
Arytenoid fixation
Glottic scarring, posterior
Laryngeal paralysis (3080)
Vocal cord paralysis, acquired
Vocal cord web

Major Diagnostic Criteria: Flexible laryngoscopy demonstrates abductor paralysis of the vocal cords with paramedian positioning. May be unilateral or bilateral.

Clinical Findings: Symptoms of upper airway obstruction with stridor, abnormal voice or cry, a tendency for aspiration, and recurrent chest infections. Unilateral vocal cord paralysis is often undetected because of the relative paucity of symptoms.

Complications: Airway obstruction may be life threatening with bilateral vocal cord paralysis. Aspiration and recurrent chest infections with unilateral obstruction may also precipitate chronic problems.

Associated Findings: When vocal cord paralysis results from central pathology, such as Arnold-Chiari malformation (see **Anencephaly**), **Hydranencephaly** is a common occurrence. Brainstem abnormalities are also seen frequently.

May be seen with central neurologic defects which commonly affect both vocal cords, including **Meningomyelocele**, anterior horn cell degeneration, or cerebral degeneration or concussion.

Etiology: Congenital forms are associated with birth trauma; forceps delivery or prolonged second stage labor (80% are unilateral, with the left side involved more commonly than the right). Birth anoxia; often with resultant brainstem damage(most commonly bilateral). Idiopathic; involving an equal number of bilateral and unilateral cases. Autosomal dominant and X-linked inheritance have been reported. Holinger et al (1976) reported that paralyses are 55% congenital, 40% acquired, and 5% idiopathic.

Pathogenesis: Central neurologic pathology affects the vagal nuclei contained within the nucleus ambiguus, and results most frequently in bilateral paralysis. Peripheral neurologic trauma most frequently results in unilateral vocal cord paralysis secondary to recurrent laryngeal nerve damage.

Sex Ratio: M1:F:<1 (slight male preponderance).

Occurrence: The third most common congenital laryngeal anomaly, following **Laryngomalacia** and **Subglottic stenosis**.

Risk of Recurrence for Patient's Sib: Varies with etiology.

Risk of Recurrence for Patient's Child: Varies with etiology.

Age of Detectability: Often at birth, but may not be apparent for several weeks or months depending on onset of symptoms.

Gene Mapping and Linkage: Unknown.

Prevention: In cases of surgical trauma, careful dissection with identification of recurrent and superior laryngeal nerves will avoid the problem. Minimizing birth trauma will also decrease the frequency of such lesions.

Treatment: Maintain the airway and treat the precipitating pathology. Careful evaluation of the likelihood of spontaneous recovery should be made.

Unilateral vocal cord paralysis rarely causes major respiratory symptoms. Intermittent stridor, weak cry, and a tendency to chest infections may be seen. Underlying pathology should be treated and paralysis managed expectantly. Vocal cord injection to medialize the cord may be appropriate.

Bilateral vocal cord paralysis nearly always requires a tracheotomy for relief of obstruction. Further management should be based on likelihood of recovery. Many methods of vocal cord

lateralization have been described as methods for improving the airway.

Prognosis: Outlook for spontaneous recovery depends on the etiology. Emery and Fearon (1984) report 100% recovery from birth trauma and acquired idiopathic causes; 60% recovery from peripheral trauma and central neurologic pathology; 20% recovery from congenital idiopathic causes; and 0% from birth anoxia.

Detection of Carrier: Unknown.

References:
Plott D: Congenital laryngeal-abductor paralysis due to nucleus ambiguus dysgenesis in three brothers. New Engl J Med 1964; 271:593–597.
Holinger LD, et al.: Etiology of bilateral abductor vocal cord paralysis. Ann Otol Rhinol Laryngol 1976; 85:428–436.
Cohen SR, et al.: Laryngeal paralysis in children: a long term retrospective study. Ann Otol Rhinol Laryngol 1982; 91:417–424.
Gundfast KM, Milmoe G: Congenital hereditary bilateral abductor vocal cord paralysis. Ann Otol Rhinol Laryngol 1982; 91:564–566.
Emery P, Fearon B: Vocal cord palsy in pediatric practice: a review of 71 cases. Int J Pediatr Otorhinolaryng 1984; 8:147–154.
Cunningham MJ, et al.: Familial vocal cord dysfunction. Pediatrics 1985; 76:750–753.

MY003
OR005

Charles M. Myer III
Peter Orobello

Vogt cephalosyndactyly
See ACROCEPHALOSYNDACTYLY TYPE I
Vohwinkel syndrome
See DEAFNESS-KERATOPACHYDERMIA-DIGITAL CONSTRICTIONS
Volvulus of midgut
See INTESTINAL ROTATION, INCOMPLETE
von Bechterew disease
See ANKYLOSING SPONDYLITIS
von Eulenburg paramyotonia congenita
See PARAMYOTONIA CONGENITA
von Gierke disease
See GLYCOGENOSIS, TYPE Ia

VON HIPPEL-LINDAU SYNDROME 0995

Includes:
Hemangiomatosis, multiple
Lindau disease

Excludes: Cerebellar tumor

Major Diagnostic Criteria: A retinal or cerebellar hemangioblastoma in a patient with a positive family history is indicative of the condition, or the presence of a retinal and central nervous system (CNS) hemangioblastoma in the same patient, is diagnostic.

Clinical Findings: The age of onset varies, but is most common in the fourth decade. There is no age at which individuals at risk can be assumed to be unaffected. The lesions are most frequent in the peripheral retina but may be seen at the disk border or macula, producing complaints of visual disturbance, particularly blurred vision. The lesion is raised, red, and globular. It is fed by a dilated arteriole and drained by a tortuous vein. The retinal lesions are multiple in about one-third of the patients. They may undergo calcification and ossification.

Hemangioblastomas involving the CNS are most common in the posterior fossa. They may be situated in the cerebellar hemispheres, vermis, or the medulla. They may be multiple; most are cystic. An intermittent occipital headache is a frequent early symptom. Vomiting, vertigo, ataxia, nystagmus, dysarthria, and dysmetria are common findings. Mental changes may accompany an increase in intracranial pressure.

The spinal cord is frequently involved, primarily in the cervical and thoracic segments. The hemangioblastoma is usually intramedullary and posterior, producing loss of sensation and proprioception. A spastic paraparesis develops with progressive cord compression.

Approximately 15% of cerebellar hemangioblastomas are associated with polycythemia. A skull X-ray may show signs of

0995-20841: Von Hippel-Lindau syndrome; retina.

increased intracranial pressure. Computed axial tomography (CT) with contrast enhancement is extremely useful in the localization of the tumor. Vertebral angiography is the study of choice to define clearly the extent and vascular supply of a posterior fossa hemangioblastoma. A myelogram and selective segmental angiogram of the spinal cord will identify a spinal cord tumor. Intravenous pyelogram, renal angiography, and CT scan are used to demonstrate renal or adrenal lesions. The CT scan may also show pancreatic lesions.

Complications: The retinal lesions are usually progressive. Exudation occurs at the site of the tumor, causing retinal detachment and eventual blindness. Cataracts and glaucoma may occur as well. The posterior fossa hemangioblastomas produce hydrocephalus by distortion of the aqueduct of Sylvius. Herniation of the cerebellar tonsils can result. Syringomyelia has occasionally been noted in association with a spinal cord hemangioblastoma. Hypertensive crises may complicate an associated pheochromocytoma; renal carcinomas may metastasize. Diabetes mellitus can result from pancreatic involvement.

Associated Findings: Renal, pancreatic, hepatic, and epididymal cysts; renal carcinoma; pheochromocytoma; angiomatosis of liver, ovary, and skin; tumors of epididymis.

Etiology: Autosomal dominant inheritance. Most cases (80–93%) are sporadic.

Pathogenesis: Nervous tissue is secondarily damaged by expanding vascular hamartomatous tumors. One suggestion is that the retinal tumors result from malformation of the mesenchyma in the third month of fetal life, when the retina is vascularized and a mesenchymal plate is formed in the roof of the fourth ventricle.

MIM No.: *19330

POS No.: 3676

CDC No.: 759.620

Sex Ratio: M1:F1

Occurrence: 1:50,000 to 1:60,000

Risk of Recurrence for Patient's Sib:
See Part I, *Mendelian Inheritance.*

Risk of Recurrence for Patient's Child:
See Part I, *Mendelian Inheritance.*

Age of Detectability: Usually by the fourth decade of life, by the presence of retinal and CNS hemangioblastomas.

Gene Mapping and Linkage: VHL (von-Hippel Lindau syndrome) has been mapped to 3p.

Prevention: None known. Genetic counseling indicated.

Treatment: If a retinal tumor is found, photocoagulation or cryocoagulation is the treatment of choice. Diathermy or cryocoagulation may be effective if the lesion is extensive. Follow-up fundus examinations are necessary, as new or recurrent retinal angiomas may occur. Enucleation may be necessary. Treatment of the CNS lesions is surgical, and consideration should be given to surgical removal of a tumor before irreversible CNS damage has occurred.

Once a diagnosis has been made, the patient's entire family should be carefully studied, including annual examination of the retina by indirect ophthalmoscopy from the age of six years, and thorough neurologic examination. Blindness may be prevented if retinal tumors are detected and treated early. CT scanning of the abdomen is the most sensitive screen for renal cysts and carcinoma and pancreatic tumors and cysts, and should occur biennially beginning at 20 years of age. Elevated urinary vanillylmandelic acid (VMA) and serum catecholamine levels suggest a pheochromocytoma. Screening should start at ten years of age. Finally, biennial cranial CT of at risk relatives should begin at 15 years of age.

Prognosis: Usually slowly progressive. Patients tend to die of increased intracranial pressure secondary to the CNS hemangioblastomas.

Detection of Carrier: Unknown.

Special Considerations: The finding of polycythemia in some patients with von Hippel-Lindau disease is of considerable interest. It has been shown that the cyst fluid from some cerebellar hemangioblastomas has a definite erythropoietic stimulator effect, measured by the red cell incorporation of ^{59}Fe in these patients.

The kidney is known to be the principal site of erythropoietin production. Some cystic renal carcinomas produce erythropoietin. Histologically cerebellar hemangioblastomas and renal carcinomas have many similarities. The reappearance of polycythemia following successful removal of a CNS hemangioblastoma might, therefore, suggest a recurrence of the CNS tumor or the development of a renal cell carcinoma.

References:
Melmon KL, Rosen SW: Lindau's disease: a review of the literature and study of a large kindred. Am J Med 1964; 36:595–617.
Horton WA, et al.: Von Hippel-Lindau disease: clinical and pathological manifestations in nine families with 50 affected members. Arch Intern Med 1976; 136:769–777.
Levine E, et al.: CT screening of the abdomen in von Hippel-Lindau disease. Am J Roentgenology (Baltimore) 1982; 139:505–510.
Ionasescu V, Zellweger H: Genetics in neurology. New Yoek: Raven Press, 1983.
Go RCP, et al.: Segregation and linkage analyses of von Hippel-Lindau disease among 220 descendants from one kindred. Am J Hum Genet 1984; 36:131–142.
Huson SM, et al.: Cerebellar haemangioblastoma and von Hippel-Lindau disease. Brain 1986; 109:1297–1310.

HA053   **Robert H.A. Haslam**

Von Mayer-Rokitansky-Kuster anomaly
See MULLERIAN APLASIA
von Recklinghausen disease
See NEUROFIBROMATOSIS

VON WILLEBRAND DISEASE 0996

Includes:
> Pseudohemophilia
> Pseudo (platelet-type) von Willebrand disease
> von Willebrand-like disorders

Excludes: Hemophilia A (0461)

Major Diagnostic Criteria: Prolonged bleeding time (template method) and decreased Factor VIII activity are the most commonly accepted criteria. Ristocetin cofactor activity and von Willebrand protein are often abnormally low. The results of all of these studies may vary in a single individual and among affected members of a family. Particularly in the more common type I and type II von Willebrand disease, the bleeding time may sporadically become normal in a patient who usually has a prolonged bleeding time. Depressed baseline Factor VIII coagulant activity may be elevated into the normal range by stress or pregnancy. The von Willebrand protein normally occurs in multimeric form, and analysis of the protein multamers by SDS-agarose gel electrophoresis or by crossed immunoelectrophoresis is often required to distinguish among the various types and subtypes of von Willebrand disease.

Clinical Findings: Menorrhagia, epistaxis, and excessive bleeding after minor mouth injuries, lacerations, and loss of deciduous teeth, as well as bruising after mild trauma. Patients with the lowest activities of Factor VIII, particularly those with type III von Willebrand disease, have the greatest tendency to easy bruising, periarticular hemorrhages, and other manifestations characteristic of classic hemophilia (see **Hemophilia A**).

A number of distinct types of von Willebrand disease have been characterized. Zimmerman and Ruggeri (1987) list seven: types I, IIA, IIB, IIC, IID, IIE, and III. A large variety of subtypes have also been described (Ruggeri and Zimmerman, 1987).

Complications: Increased risk of bleeding following surgery, dental procedures, and acute trauma. Severe cases may develop permanent joint changes similar to those seen in **Hemophilia A**.

Associated Findings: None known.

Etiology: Autosomal dominant (types I, IIA, IIB, IID, and IIE) and autosomal recessive (types IIC and III) inheritance.

Pathogenesis: *Type I:* This is the most frequent form of von Willebrand disease. A characteristic finding is a proportional decrease in factor VIII coagulant activity (VIII-C) and von Willebrand factor. The multimeric composition of von Willebrand factor, as determined by electrophoresis in agarose gel, is characteristically normal.

Type IIA: As with all of the Type II variants, Type IIA is characterized by an absence of the large von Willebrand factor multimers. Ristocetin cofactor activity is markedly reduced, although the von Willebrand factor protein level may be normal. Factor VIII-C activity is often disproportionately higher than the von Willebrand factor protein level. The bleeding time of affected individuals is consistently prolonged.

Type IIB: The most characteristic finding is an increase over normal of ristocetin-induced platelet aggregation in platelet-rich plasma. Both von Willebrand factor and factor VIII-C levels are decreased or may be normal.

Type IIC: Distinctive findings, demonstrable by agarose gel electrophoresis of plasma, include a marked increase in the smallest multimer component as well as a repeating doublet pattern. The levels of factor VIII-C and von Willebrand factor protein are characteristically normal.

Types IID and IIE: Autosomal dominant forms that differ from types IIA and IIB by the presence of unique structural abnormalities of individual multimers demonstrable by SDS-agar electrophoresis.

Type III: The von Willebrand factor in this rare recessive form is markedly decreased or absent, and affected individuals exhibit severe bleeding manifestations. Factor VIII-C, although also greatly decreased, nevertheless has at least some measurable activity.

MIM No.: *19340, 27748

CDC No.: 286.400

Sex Ratio: M1:F1

Occurrence: Discovered by E.A. von Willebrand on the Aland Islands between Sweden and Finland in 1931, the current incidence is estimated at 30–50:1,000,000.

Risk of Recurrence for Patient's Sib:
See Part I, *Mendelian Inheritance*. Manifestations within a single family can vary markedly.

Risk of Recurrence for Patient's Child:
See Part I, *Mendelian Inheritance*. Manifestations within a single family can vary markedly.

Age of Detectability: Probably at birth, though more often only when accidental injury precipitates bleeding episodes, as in early childhood.

Gene Mapping and Linkage: F8VWF (coagulation factor VIII VWF (von Willebrand factor)) has been mapped to 12pter-p12.

Prevention: None known. Genetic counseling indicated.

Treatment: Cryoprecipitated Factor VIII, fresh plasma, and fresh frozen plasma all will elevate circulating Factor VIII levels (usually more than can be accounted for by the activity of the amount of Factor VIII administered) and reduce the risk of bleeding following surgical and dental procedures. Factor VIII concentrate raises the level of Factor VIII but does not correct the bleeding time because it does not contain von Willebrand factor.

Treatment with any of the agents above may be required to stop persistent bleeding, most frequently epistaxis. If one dose does not suffice, treatment intervals of 24 hours can be employed since severity of bleeding is generally correlated with Factor VIII activity, and the response of the Factor VIII level to therapy is frequently more prolonged than the average T 1/2 of 12 hours observed in classic hemophilia. The correction in bleeding time and platelet function is shorter, with a T 1/2 closer to 6–12 hours. Aspirin should be avoided because it prolongs the bleeding time in these patients.

1-deamino-8-d-arginine vasopressin (desmopressin, DDAVP), a vasopressin analog, may raise the factor VIII and ristocetin cofactor levels, correct the bleeding time, and prevent or treat clinical bleeding in patients with most forms of type I and type IIA von Willebrand disease. Desmopressin is usually not effective in type II or III von Willebrand disease, and is contraindicated in patients with types IIB or platelet-related disease, in whom this treatment may produce thrombocytopenia.

Prognosis: Few patients are substantially handicapped by the defect. However, patients with severe disease may have significant episodes of bleeding throughout their life, and excessive bleeding in female patients is likely with childbirth.

Detection of Carrier: Screening procedures include template bleeding time, level of Factor VIII procoagulant activity, Factor VIII related antigen, and von Willebrand factor, not all of which are consistently abnormal in all patients.

Special Considerations: Because of the risk of transfusion-induced hepatitis B, administration of hepatitis B vaccine is recommended as soon as diagnosis of von Willebrand disease is made.

Acquired forms of von Willebrand-like disorders have also been described in association with **Lupus erythematosis, systemic**; malignancies; and lymphoproliferative disorders. Immunoglobulin inhibitors directed against the factor VIII complex appear to mediate these disorders.

Weiss et al (1982) described a platelet-related form of pseudo-von Willebrand disease in four members, from four generations, of a family whose platelets underwent aggregation by human FVIII/VWF in the absence of ristocetin.

References:
Ruggeri ZM, et al.: Heightened interaction between platelets and factor VIII von Willebrand factor in a new subtype of von Willebrand disease. New Engl J Med 1980; 302:1047–1051.
Weiss HJ, et al.: Pseudo-von Willebrand's disease. New Engl J Med 1982; 306:326–333.
Zimmerman TS, et al.: Factor VIII/von Willebrand factor. Progr in Hemat 1983; 13:279–309.

Ruggeri ZM, Zimmerman TS: Von Willebrand factor and von Willebrand disease. Blood 1987; 70:895–904.
Zimmerman TS, Ruggeri ZM: Von Willebrand disease. Hum Path
1987; 18:140–152.

George R. Honig

H0024

von Willebrand-like disorders
See VON WILLEBRAND DISEASE
Voorhoeve disease
See OSTEOPATHIA STRIATA
Vrolik disease
See OSTEOGENESIS IMPERFECTA
VSR syndrome
*See CONTRACTURES, HERRMANN-OPITZ ARTHROGRYPOSIS
TYPE*

❖ W ❖

W Syndrome
See PALLISTER-W SYNDROME
Waardenburg syndrome variant
*See ALBINISM, WAARDENBURG TYPE-HIRSCHSPRUNG
AGANGLIONOSIS*
Waardenburg syndrome, type I (dystopia canthorum present)
See WAARDENBURG SYNDROMES
Waardenburg syndrome, type II (dystopia canthorum not present)
See WAARDENBURG SYNDROMES
Waardenburg syndrome, type III (Klein-Waardenburg limb anomalies)
See WAARDENBURG SYNDROMES

WAARDENBURG SYNDROMES   0997

Includes:
Hirschsprung disease-pigmentary anomaly
Klein-Waardenburg syndrome
Limb anomalies (upper)-Waardenburg syndrome
Waardenburg-ocular albinism
Waardenburg syndrome, type I (dystopia canthorum
    present)
Waardenburg syndrome, type II (dystopia canthorum not
    present)
Waardenburg syndrome, type III (Klein-Waardenburg limb
    anomalies)

Excludes:
Acrocephalosyndactyly type I (0014)
Albinism, cutaneous (0031)
Albinism, cutaneous-deafness (0030)
Albinism, Waardenburg type-hirschsprung aganglionosis (2823)
Anophthalmia-limb anomalies (3172)
Eye, hypertelorism (0504)
Heterochromia irides, acquired
Oro-facio-digital syndrome

Major Diagnostic Criteria: 1) Dystopia canthorum (lateral displacement of medial canthi, including inferior lacrimal puncta, with normal interpupillary distance), 80–99%; 2) broad nasal bridge usually with lack of frontonasal angle and bulbous nose with hypoplastic alae nasi, 80%; 3) synophrys (confluent eyebrows), 50%; 4) heterochromia irides, 25%; 5) poliosis (white forelock), 20–40%; 6) congenital deafness, 20%.

Clinical Findings: Dystopia canthorum (present in type I, absent in type II); synophrys; heterochromia irides (sometimes restricted to single segment of one eye; if heterochromia is absent, irides are often bright blue in color), may include albinotic fundi, normal-to-subnormal electroretinogram. Deafness may be unilateral or bilateral, sensorineural type, and vestibular function may be impaired; type II has a higher frequency of deafness than type I, and those showing deafness are more likely to demonstrate other stigmata of the syndrome. Poliosis, may be present at birth, then disappear and reappear later; often premature graying of hair, eyelashes, and eyebrows as early as age seven years. Vitiligo in 15% of cases, usually found on arms and face. In type III, there are

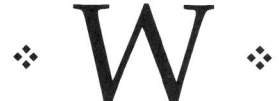
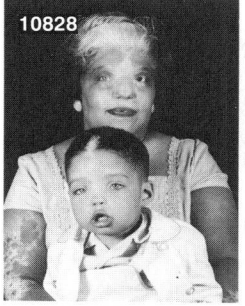
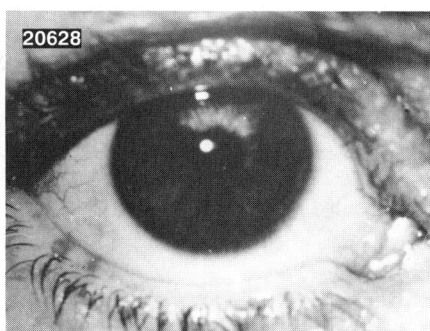
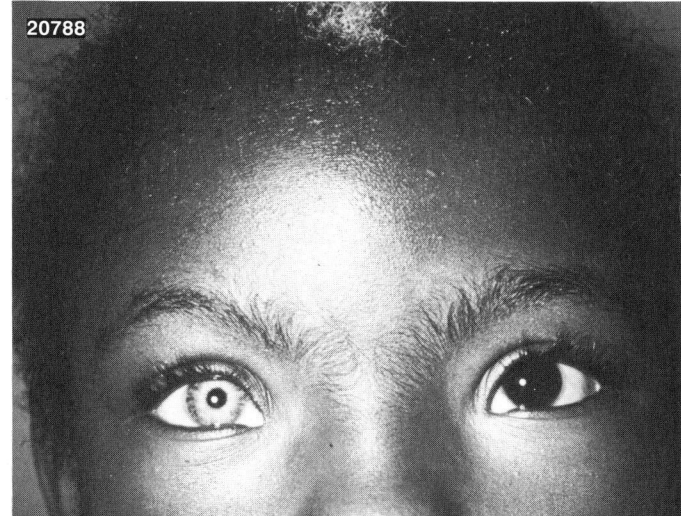

0997-10828: Son has blue irides; mother's right eye is blue; both have dystopia canthorum and patchy depigmentation of skin and limbs. **20628:** Close-up of heterochromia of the iris. **20788:** White forelock, heterochromia of the iris, and lateral displacement of the puncta.

---

bilateral defects of the upper limbs, including hypoplasia, contractures, carpal fusion, and syndactyly.

Complications: Primarily related to deafness, undiagnosed deafness sometimes leading to pseudomental retardation; poor lacrimal conduction; occasional glaucoma.

Associated Findings: Craniosynostosis, high-arched or cleft palate, blepharophimosis (type III), glaucoma, hydrophthalmos, true esotropia (20% of cases), anophthalmia with limb malformations, upper limb-pectoral girdle arthromyodysplasia (type III), Sprengel deformity (winged scapula), Hirschsprung megacolon or atretic disorders of the GI tract (type I and II), unilateral ptosis and the Marcus Gunn phenomenon (type II), congenital heart disease, **Ventricular septal defect, Meningocele,** spina bifida.

Etiology: Autosomal dominant inheritance with variable expression; type I penetrance, 85%; heterogeneity proposed by Hageman and Delleman (1977). A possible recessive variant has been documented in five families (see **Albinism, Waardenburg type-Hirschsprung aganglionosis.**

Pathogenesis: Defect of migration of neural crest cells has been hypothesized.

MIM No.: 14882, *19350, 19351, 27758

POS No.: 3426

CDC No.: 759.800

Sex Ratio: M1:F1

Occurrence: 1:20,000 to 1:40,000; 3% of congenitally deaf children have this syndrome.

Risk of Recurrence for Patient's Sib:
See Part I, *Mendelian Inheritance.*

Risk of Recurrence for Patient's Child:
See Part I, *Mendelian Inheritance.*

Age of Detectability: Unknown.

Gene Mapping and Linkage: WS1 (Waardenburg syndrome, type 1) has been tentatively mapped to 9q34.

Prevention: None known. Genetic counseling indicated.

Treatment: Early recognition and treatment of deafness or ocular complications.

Prognosis: Compatible with normal life span; mental retardation is not a characteristic.

Detection of Carrier: Affected persons often have only subtle signs, and are recognized in retrospect after a more severely affected relative is investigated.

References:
Waardenburg, PJ: A new syndrome combining developmental anomalies of the eyelids, eyebrows, and nose root, with pigmentary defects of the iris and head hair and with congenital deafness. Am J Hum Genet 1951; 3:195–253.
Arias S: Genetic heterogeneity in the Waardenburg syndrome. BD: OAS VII(4). New York: March of Dimes Birth Defects Foundation, 1971:87–101.
Hageman MJ, Delleman JW: Heterogeneity in Waardenburg syndrome. Am J Hum Genet 1977; 29:468–485.
Francois J: Waardenburg's memorial lecture: Waardenburg's syndrome. Int Ophthalmol 1982; 5:3–13.
Goodman RM, et al.: Upper limb involvement in the Klein Waardenburg syndrome. Am J Med Genet 1982; 11:425–433.
Klein D: Historical background and evidence for dominant inheritance of the Klein-Waardenburg syndrome (type III). Am J Med Genet 1983; 14:231–239.
Preus M, et al.: Waardenburg syndrome: penetrance of major signs. Am J Med Genet 1983; 15:383–388.

GA025   **Arthur R. Garrett**

Waardenburg-ocular albinism
See WAARDENBURG SYNDROMES
Waardenburg-Shah syndrome
See ALBINISM, WAARDENBURG TYPE-HIRSCHSPRUNG AGANGLIONOSIS
Waardengurg anophthalmia syndrome
See ANOPHTHALMIA-LIMB ANOMALIES
Wackenheim syndrome
See DYSOSTOSIS, CHEIROLUMBAR
Wagner syndrome
See RETINA, HYALOIDEORETINAL DEGENERATION OF WAGNER
Waisman syndrome
See X-LINKED MENTAL RETARDATION-BASAL GANGLION DISORDER

WALKER-WARBURG SYNDROME   2869

Includes:
Cerebroocular dysgenesis
Cerebroocular dysplasia-muscular dystrophy
Cerebro-oculo-muscular syndrome
Chemke syndrome
HARD syndrome
HARD +/-E syndrome
Hydrocephalus-agyria-retinal dysplasia
Lissencephaly syndrome II
Muscular dystrophy-cerebroocular dysplasia
Pagon syndrome
Warburg syndrome

Excludes:
Craniotelencephalic dysplasia (2791)
Lissencephaly syndrome (0603)
Muscular dystrophy, congenital with mental retardation (2705)
Retinal fold (0867)

Major Diagnostic Criteria: Agyria (or polymicrogyria) with pebbled surface, absent cortical layers, striking glial and vascular proliferation, and white matter edema. Other features include retinal and cerebellar malformations and congenital muscular dystrophy.

Clinical Findings: Among 63 documented patients: type II lissencephaly (61/61); cerebellar malformations (58/58); retinal abnormalities (49/49); congenital muscular dystrophy (25/25); **Hydrocephaly** (60/62); anterior chamber dysgenesis (53/58); vermis hypoplasia (40/40); Dandy-Walker malformation (16/49); posterior encephalocele (19/63); cleft lip/palate (9/63); **Microcephaly** (8/51); and microphthalmia (28/53).

Complications: Seizures.

Associated Findings: Hypoplasia of corpus callosum and/or septum pellucidum. Coloboma (8/36). Elevated serum creatine kinase levels. Congenital contractures.

Etiology: Autosomal recessive inheritance.

Pathogenesis: Unknown.

MIM No.: *23667

POS No.: 3656

CDC No.: 742.240

Sex Ratio: M25:F34 (observed).

Occurrence: About sixty cases have been reported in the literature.

Risk of Recurrence for Patient's Sib:
See Part I, *Mendelian Inheritance.*

Risk of Recurrence for Patient's Child:
See Part I, *Mendelian Inheritance.* Affected individuals are not expected to survive to reproduce.

Age of Detectability: At birth. Has been successfully detected prenatally by high resolution ultrasound based on the presence of fetal hydrocephaly in pregnancies at risk.

Gene Mapping and Linkage: Unknown.

Prevention: None known. Genetic counseling indicated.

Treatment: Supportive.

Prognosis: Most affected infants have decreased life span (median survival nine months), although some patients have been known to survive for several years. Median survival was between 4–9 months. Usually associated with significant mental impairment.

Detection of Carrier: Unknown.

Special Considerations: Walker-Warburg syndrome has also been designated as the HARD -/+E syndrome (Hydrocephaly, Agyria, Retinal Dysplasia, with or without Encephalocele).

References:
Pagon R, et al.: Hydrocephalus, agyria, retinal dysplasia, encephalocele (HARD+/-E) syndrome: an autosomal recessive condition.

BD:OAS XIV(6B). New York: March of Dimes Birth Defects Foundation, 1978:233–241.

Pagon R, et al.: Autosomal recessive eye and brain abnormalities: Warburg syndrome. J Pediatr 1983; 102:542–546. *

Dobyns WB, et al.: Syndromes with lissencephaly II: Walker-Warburg and cerebro-oculo-muscular syndromes and a new syndrome with type II lissencephaly. Am J Med Genet 1985; 22:157–195. * †

Crowe C, et al.: The prenatal diagnosis of the Walker-Warburg Syndrome. Prenat Diagn 1986; 6:177–185.

Dobyns WB, et al.: Diagnostic criteria for Walker-Warburg syndrome. Am J Med Genet 1989; 32:195–210. * †

GR011   **Frank Greenberg**

Walt Disney dwarfism
See *OSTEODYSPLASTICA GERODERMIA, BAMATTER TYPE*

Warburg syndrome
See *WALKER-WARBURG SYNDROME*

Ward-Romano syndrome
See *ARRHYTHMIA, WITH LONG QT INTERVAL WITHOUT DEAFNESS*

Warfarin, fetal effects of
See *FETAL WARFARIN SYNDROME*

Warkany Syndrome
See *CHROMOSOME 8, TRISOMY 8*

Watson syndrome
See *PULMONIC STENOSIS-CAFE-AU-LAIT SPOTS, WATSON TYPE*

WEAVER SYNDROME   2036

Includes: Weaver-Smith syndrome

Excludes:
Beckwith-Wiedemann syndrome (0104)
Cebebral gigantism (0137)
Marshall-Smith syndrome (2193)
Simpson-Golabi-Behmel syndrome (2826)

Major Diagnostic Criteria: Excessive growth of pre- or postnatal onset, characteristic facial features and advanced osseous maturation. The carpal bone development is frequently more advanced than the general skeleton.

Clinical Findings: Based on 27 cases, the pertinent features of this syndrome include:

Major Features of Weaver Syndrome Patients

	Number/Total	Percentage
Excessive Growth		
Postnatally	25/25	100
Prenatally	18/25	72
Performance		
Motor delay	11/11	100
Hoarse and/or low-pitched cry	17/19	90
Developmental delay or mental retardation	20/25	80
Excessive appetite	5/7	71
Hypertonia	15/22	68
Spasticity	4/11	36
Hypotonia	4/22	18
Seizures	3/20	15
Craniofacial		
Micrognathia	21/21	100
Ocular hypertelorism	22/23	96
Large ears	22/23	96
Increased bifrontal diameter	19/20	95
Telecanthus	18/19	95
Long and accentuated philtrum	18/23	78
Macrocephaly	17/22	77
Dysplastic ears	8/15	53
Strabismus	3/6	50
Depressed nasal bridge	9/21	43
Down-slanting palpebral fissures	7/19	37
Flat occiput	5/13	38

	Number/Total	Percentage
Epicanthal folds	2/15	13
Extremities		
Prominent finger pads	11/12	92
Deeply set, narrow or hyperconvexed nails	11/13	85
Limited extension of ankles, wrists, elbows, hips, or knees	10/12	83
Broad thumbs	7/10	70
Hyperextensibility of fingers	4/5	80
Camptodactyly	13/18	72
Talipes equinovarus	6/10	60
Skeleton		
Carpal bone age increased	16/17	94
Flared metaphyses, especially the distal femora and ulnae	18/21	86
Advanced general osseous maturation	16/20	80
Mottled or irregular epiphyses	4/9	44
Scoliosis or kyphosis	4/9	44
Short ribs	2/6	33
Others		
Umbilical hernia	15/15	100
Inguinal hernia	8/8	100
Excessive and loose skin of the neck or extremities	13/14	93
Cryptorchidism	6/10	60
Excessive or prolonged hyper-bilirubinemia	2/4	50
Thin and/or fine scalp hair	2/3	67

The excessive growth is present either at birth or has its onset during infancy. Mental deficiency, when present, is usually mild but ranges from mild to profound. Five individuals are reported to have had normal intellectual function. Most characteristics show considerable variation in the degree of expression. Speech difficulty, particularly dysphasia, may be common. The mean birth lengths for 14 term males and seven term females were 4.94 kg and 3.87 kg, respectively; mean birth lengths for eight term males and five term females were 56.4 cm and 54 cm, respectively, and the mean occipitofrontal circumferences (OFC) of six term males and four term females were 38.7 cm and 35.3 cm, respectively. All values for males are at or above the 97th percentile while length and weight for females is at the 90th percentile and the OFC is at about the 85th percentile.

Complications: Dystocia may occur because of the macrocephaly and/or macrosomia. The megalocephaly is associated with ventriculomegaly which may lead to the impression of hydrocephalus and unnecessary ventricular shunting.

Associated Findings: Features present in two or more of 27 patients with this condition and which are not listed above include spasticity, speech difficulty or no speech, **Eyelid, ptosis, congenital**, prominent lips, maxillary hypoplasia, short neck, inverted nipples, hyperextensibility of fingers, hemangioma, hirsutism, platyspondyly, and anterior wedging of vertebrae. Those found in only one individual are hyperactivity, delayed menarche, amenorrhea, **Myopia, congenital**, **Ear, auditory canal atresia**, widely spaced and irregularly aligned teeth, delayed eruption of permanent teeth, **Ductus arteriosus, patent**, **Ventricular septal defect**, **Hypospadias**, **Pectus excavatum**, hexadactyly, short fourth metatarsals, tapered fingers, large hands and feet, dislocated hips, simian crease, multiple dermal nevi, cervical spinal stenosis, Wormian bones, increased bone density, and hypothyroidism.

Etiology: Unknown.

Pathogenesis: Many features of this syndrome result from excessive growth. The cause of the overgrowth is unknown; no consistent endocrinological disturbance has been found. A pregnancy-related growth factor is unlikely since several infants have

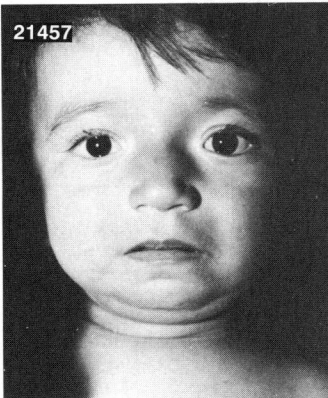

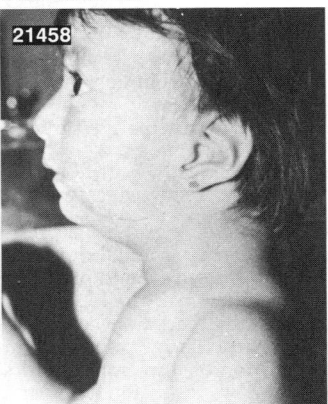

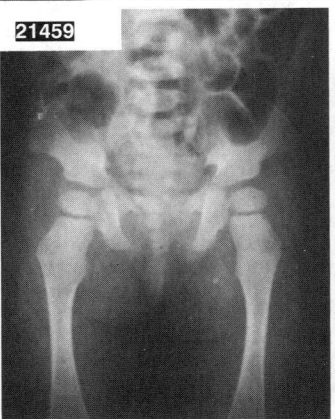

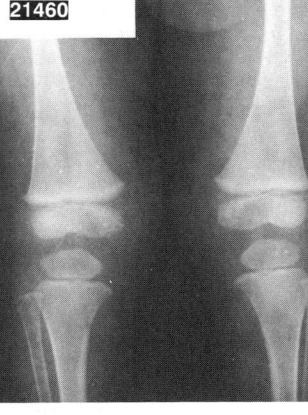

2036-21456: General view shows tall stature. 21457: Close-up shows increased bifrontal diameter, ocular hypertelorism. 21458: Lateral view of the face shows prominent occiput, enlarged ears and micrognathia. 21459–60: X-rays show accelerated maturation and widened femora.

not shown the accelerated growth until after birth and in most the excessive growth rate has continued for years.

POS No.: 3429

Sex Ratio: M17:F7

Occurrence: Twenty-seven cases have been documented in the literature.

Risk of Recurrence for Patient's Sib: All cases have been sporadic.

Risk of Recurrence for Patient's Child: Unknown.

Age of Detectability: At birth.

Gene Mapping and Linkage: Unknown.

Prevention: None known. Genetic counseling indicated.

Treatment: Cesarean section for significant dystocia, appropriate orthopedics.

Prognosis: Functional impairment will depend on degree of mental dysfunction and severity of orthopedic problems. Life span is not known to be altered.

Detection of Carrier: Unknown.

Special Considerations: This condition most likely is separate from the **Marshall-Smith syndrome** that also has accelerated osseous maturation, increased linear growth, and developmental delay. Patients with the latter condition lack the characteristic facial features of Weaver syndrome, usually have a poor weight gain, possess broad middle phalanges of the 3–5 fingers, and often die during infancy.

Roussounis and Crawford (1983) reported siblings whom they believed had Weaver syndrome. However, not enough data are presented to justify this conclusion. A patient reported by Tsukahara et al. is now thought to have **Simpson-Golabi-Behmel syndrome** (Kajii and Tsukahara, 1984).

References:

Weaver DD, et al.: A new overgrowth syndrome with accelerated skeletal maturation, unusual facies, and camptodactyly. J Pediatr 1974; 84:547–552. * †

Fitch N: The syndromes of Marshall and Weaver. J Med Genet 1980; 17:174–178

Majewski F, et al.: The Weaver syndrome: a rare type of primordial overgrowth. Eur J Pediatr 1981; 137:277–282.

Weisswichert PH, et al.: Accelerated bone maturation syndrome of the Weaver type. Eur J Paediatr 1981; 137:329–333.

Roussounis SH, Crawford MJ: Siblings with Weaver syndrome. J Pediatr 1983; 102:595–597

Kajii T, Tsukahara M: The Golabi-Rosen syndrome. Am J Med Genet 1984; 19:819 only.

Ardinger HH, et al.: Further delineation of the Weaver syndrome. J Pediatr 1986; 108:228–235. * †

Greenberg F, et al.: Weaver syndrome: the changing phenotype in an adult. Am J Med Genet 1989; 33:127–129.

WE005
RA023

David D. Weaver
Maria A. Ramos-Arroyo

Weaver-Smith syndrome
See WEAVER SYNDROME

WEAVER-WILLIAMS SYNDROME   2195

Includes:

    Cleft palate-growth/mental retardation-microcephaly-unusual facies

    Growth/mental retardation-microcephaly-unusual facies-cleft palate

    Microcephaly-growth/mental retardation-unusual facies-cleft palate

    Unusual facies-growth/mental retardation-microcephaly-cleft palate

Excludes:

    Cockayne syndrome (0189)

    Marden-Walker syndrome (0629)

    Oro-cranio-digital syndrome (0769)

    Seckel syndrome (0881)

Major Diagnostic Criteria: Based on only two cases, criteria include severe **Microcephaly**, growth and mental retardation, unusual facies, **Cleft palate** and delayed skeletal maturation.

Clinical Findings: The physical characteristics shared by a brother and sister from a nonconsanguineous marriage included severe to profound mental retardation, severe microcephaly (occipitofrontal circumferences were 5 to 6 SDs below the mean), weight deficiency associated with little subcutaneous fat, diminished muscle mass, cupped and hypoplastic ears, orbital hypertelorism, midfacial hypoplasia, malformed and small teeth, cleft palate, down-turned and small mouth, clinodactyly of fingers, generalized hypoplasia of bone and delayed skeletal maturation. Neither had comprehensible speech. Features present only in the brother were moderate hearing deficit, preauricular pit, micrognathia and a long skinny neck. The sister had strabismus, prognathism, a short neck, seizures, spasticity and hemiparesis, findings which were not present in the brother. The adult height of the brother (161 cm) was just below the third percentile. Birth length and weight in both were normal.

Complications: Unknown.

Associated Findings: None known.

Etiology: Possibly autosomal recessive inheritance.

Pathogenesis: Unknown.

POS No.: 4046

Sex Ratio: M1:F1 (observed).

Occurrence: A brother and sister have been reported.

Risk of Recurrence for Patient's Sib:
See Part I, *Mendelian Inheritance.*

Risk of Recurrence for Patient's Child:
See Part I, *Mendelian Inheritance.*

Age of Detectability: At birth.

Gene Mapping and Linkage: Unknown.

Prevention: None known. Genetic counseling indicated.

Treatment: Unknown.

Prognosis: Affected individuals will probably have mental retardation. This condition may be compatible with a normal life span.

Detection of Carrier: Unknown.

References:
Weaver DD, Williams CPS: A syndrome of microcephaly, mental retardation, unusual facies, cleft palate and weight deficiency. BD:OAS XIII(3B). New York: March of Dimes Birth Defects Foundation, 1977:69–84.

WE005   **David D. Weaver**

Webbing, popliteal
  See PTERYGIUM SYNDROME, POPLITEAL
Weemaes chromosome breakage syndrome
  See CHROMOSOME INSTABILITY, NIJMEGEN TYPE
Weill-Marchesani syndrome
  See SPHEROPHAKIA-BRACHYMORPHIA SYNDROME
Weismann-Netter-Stuhl syndrome
  See SKELETAL DYSPLASIA, WEISMANN-NETTER-STUHL TYPE
Weissenbacher-Zweymuller variant of arthro-ophthalmopathy
  See ARTHRO-OPHTHALMOPATHY, WEISSENBACHER-ZWEYMULLER VARIANT
Welander type of muscular dystrophy
  See MUSCULAR DYSTROPHY, DISTAL
Werdnig-Hoffmann disease
  See SPINAL MUSCULAR ATROPHY
Wermer syndrome
  See ENDOCRINE NEOPLASIA, MULTIPLE TYPE I

WERNER SYNDROME   0998

Includes:
  Aging, premature (one form)
  Progeria adultorum
Excludes:
  Mandibuloacral dysplasia (2082)
  Progeria (0825)
  Rothmund-Thomson syndrome (2037)
  Scleroderma, familial progressive (2154)

Major Diagnostic Criteria: Growth arrests at puberty, and cataracts develop in the second or third decade. Premature graying and balding; scleroderma-like involvement of limbs; marked diminution of muscle mass and subcutaneous tissue of limbs; chronic, slowly healing ulcerations over pressure points of feet and ankles; beak-shaped nose; premature development of arteriosclerosis, diabetes mellitus, hypogonadism, and localized soft tissue calcifications.

Clinical Findings: Features first become apparent between ages 15 and 30 years, with habitus of premature aging, shortness of stature, beaked nose, premature graying of hair with alopecia, diabetes mellitus, and cataract formation. There is atrophy with loss of subcutaneous tissue and tightness of the limbs. Circumscribed keratosis and ulcers develop on the skin, persisting over pressure points on the limbs. Poor muscular development and localized soft tissue calcifications are noted in the limbs. Ocular findings, usually noted in the second or third decade, include bilateral juvenile cataracts, macular degeneration, retinitis pigmentosa, and chorioretinitis. Diabetes mellitus and hypogonadism are the two most frequent endocrine abnormalities. Endocrine studies have failed to establish other deficiencies. Sterility, impotence, irregular or absent menses, loss of libido, high-pitched voice, mild gynecomastia, and scant, if any, pubic, axillary, and trunk hair are present. Intelligence was described in 22 cases: Ten of these were noted to be retarded. X-rays reveal osteoporosis, osteomyelitis-type lesions, neurotrophic bone changes in the feet, flat feet and gross foot deformities, osteoarthritis of peripheral

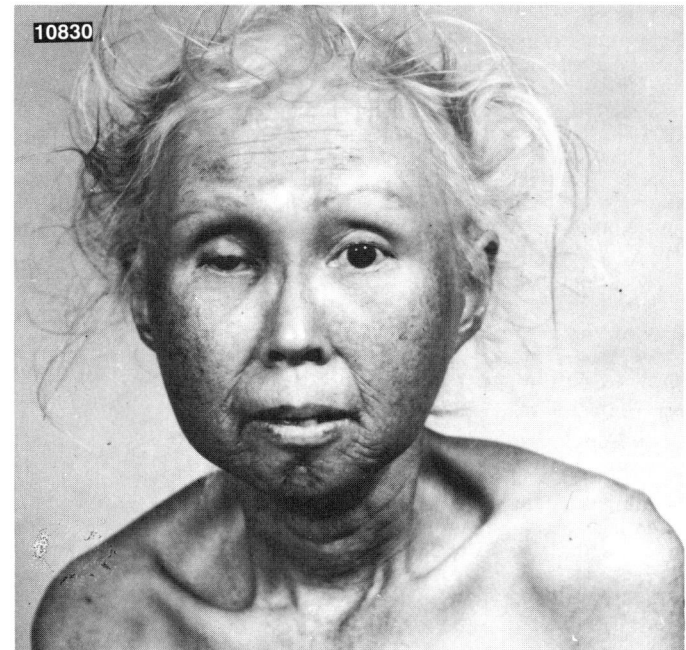

0998-10830: 48-year-old female with prematurely aged appearance.

joints, and spondylotic deformities of the spine. Signs of generalized arteriosclerosis are prominent, with diminished or absent peripheral pulses in the lower limbs, and angina with myocardial infarction is seen. Many cases may go undiagnosed.

Complications: Myocardial infarction, congestive heart failure, ulcerations of limbs, blindness secondary to cataracts; 10% develop neoplasms with a high frequency of sarcomas.

Associated Findings: None known.

Etiology: Autosomal recessive inheritance.

Pathogenesis: Pathologically, patients have shown generalized arteriosclerosis and coronary artery disease. Cardiac findings include calcification of coronary arteries and valves and either typical myocardial infarction or multifocal myocardial fibrosis. Endocrine organs have shown no specific histologic changes except testicular atrophy. Microscopic changes in the skin have included atrophy of the epidermis, thickening of the corium with fibrous tissue, and atrophy or rete pegs. A striking increase in the incidence of neoplasia has been noted and includes melanotic sarcoma, sarcoma of the uterus, fibroliposarcoma, hepatoma, carcinoma of the female breast, and osteogenic sarcoma. Resemblances to progeria in children suggest that the Werner syndrome may represent a later expression of progeria. The scleroderma-type skin lesions, the sclerotic lesions in other organs, and the high incidence of mesenchymal tumors suggest an aberration in connective tissue metabolism. Elevated levels of hyaluronic acid excretion in urine has been reported in many cases from Japan. This suggests that an abnormality in glycosaminoglycan metabolism, a connective tissue component, may be related to the pathogenesis of the disease. Tissue culture studies indicate a striking diminution of the growth potential of fibroblasts in vitro, suggesting that this is a manifestation of senescence at the cellular level. Although there are many resemblances of Werner syndrome to the aging process, important differences exist. In Werner syndrome, there is usually no clinical or pathologic resemblance to senile dementia or to the brain changes noted with aging. Also, while neoplasms are common in old age, the types seen in Werner syndrome (sarcomas, other connective tissue neoplasm, and other unusual tumors) are different from those frequently encountered with advancing age.

MIM No.: *27770

POS No.: 3765

Sex Ratio: M1:F1

Occurrence: Estimated to be 1:50,000 to 1:1,000,000. Many cases may be undiagnosed. Only five to ten living patients are known in the United States.

Over 150 cases have been reported in the world literature since 1904. The condition has been observed in Caucasians, Orientals, and Blacks; it has been reported in North and South America, the Middle East, and Japan, particularly in Caucasians of Jewish ancestry and in Sardinia. As many as 100 cases have been reported in the Japanese literature, probably related to higher consanguinity.

Risk of Recurrence for Patient's Sib:
See Part I, *Mendelian Inheritance.*

Risk of Recurrence for Patient's Child:
See Part I, *Mendelian Inheritance.* Fertility is diminished; 0.4 known children per patient on the average.

Age of Detectability: Detectable clinically by 15 to 30 years of age.

Gene Mapping and Linkage: Unknown.

Prevention: None known. Genetic counseling indicated.

Treatment: Cataracts are surgically resected when mature. **Diabetes mellitus** is usually mild and responds to diet or oral hypoglycemic therapy. Conventional treatments are indicated for arteriosclerotic heart disease, congestive heart failure, cutaneous ulcers, and malignancy.

Prognosis: Many patients survive to the fourth and fifth decades, and a few survive to the sixth and seventh decades. Death is usually caused by malignancy or arteriosclerotic heart disease. Functional impairment from medical complications generally oc-

curs 15–20 years after the onset. Generalized arteriosclerosis and scleroderma-type skin changes are progressive and irreversible.

Detection of Carrier: Increased frequency of premature graying in relatives suggests that heterozygotes may have partial expression.

Special Considerations: There is a striking decrease in the growth potential of fibroblasts in Werner syndrome. Thus, the patient's fibroblasts behave *in vitro* as do those of aged individuals. Cultured skin fibroblasts have a remarkably reduced life span, and there is a slow rate of DNA elongation.

A high frequency of clonally derived chromosomal aberrations termed *verigated translocation mosaicism*, has been seen in cultured fibroblasts. This suggests that Werner syndrome may be considered to be one of several chromosome breakage syndromes, including **Bloom syndrome, Ataxia telangiectasia,** and **Pancytopenia syndrome, Fanconi type.** The elevated excretion of hyaluronic acid could be due to a defect in glycosaminoglycan metabolism, which might explain many of the apparent abnormalities of connective tissue seen in Werner syndrome.

References:

Epstein CJ, et al.: Werner's syndrome: a review of its symptomatology, natural history, pathologic features, genetics and relationship to the natural aging process. Medicine 1966; 45:177–222.

Salk D: Werner's syndrome: a review of recent research with an analysis of connective tissue metabolism, growth control of cultured cells, and chromosomal aberrations. Hum Genet 1982; 62:1–15.

Brown WT: Werner's syndrome. In: German J, ed: Chromosome mutation and neoplasia. New York: Alan R. Liss, 1983:85–93.

Salk D, et al.: Werner's syndrome and human aging. advances in experimental medicine and biology, vol 190. New York: Plenum, 1985.

Bauer EA, et al.: Diminished response of Werner's syndrome fibroblasts to growth factors PDGF and FGF. Science 1986; 234:1240–1243.

BR024   **W. Ted Brown**

Weyers acrofacial dysostosis
*See ACROFACIAL DYSOSTOSIS
also ACROFACIAL SYNDROME, CURRY-HALL TYPE*

Weyers oligodactyly
See HAND, ULNAR AND FIBULAR RAY DEFICIENCY, WEYERS TYPE

Whelan syndrome
See ORO-FACIO-DIGITAL SYNDROME, WHELAN TYPE

Whistling face syndrome
See CRANIO-CARPO-TARSAL 'DYSPLASIA, WHISTLING FACE TYPE

Whitaker Negroes
See ECTODERMAL DYSPLASIA, CHRIST-SIEMENS-TOURAINE TYPE

Whitaker syndrome
See POLYGLANDULAR AUTOIMMUNE SYNDROME

White folded dysplasia of mucosa
See MUCOSA, WHITE FOLDED DYSPLASIA

White liver disease
See VISCERA, FATTY METAMORPHOSIS

White sponge nevus of Cannon
See MUCOSA, WHITE FOLDED DYSPLASIA

Wieacker syndrome
See CONTRACTURES-MUSCLE ATROPHY-OCULOMOTOR APRAXIA

Wieacker-Wolff syndrome
See CONTRACTURES-MUSCLE ATROPHY-OCULOMOTOR APRAXIA

Wiedemann-Rautenstrauch syndrome
See PROGERIA, NEONATAL RAUTENSTRAUCH-WIEDEMANN TYPE

Wiedmann-Beckwith syndrome
See BECKWITH-WIEDEMANN SYNDROME

Wildermuth ear
See EAR, PROMINENT ANTHELIX

Wildervack syndrome
See EYE, DUANE RETRACTION SYNDROME

Wildervanck syndrome
See CERVICO-OCULO-ACOUSTIC SYNDROME

WILLIAMS SYNDROME 0999

Includes:
    Elfin faces-hypercalcemia
    Hypercalcemia-peculiar facies-supravalvular aortic stenosis
    Supravalvar aortic stenosis
    Williams-Beuren syndrome

Excludes:
    Aortic stenosis, supravalvar (0078)
    Hypercalcemia without facial or cardiac anomalies

Major Diagnostic Criteria: Typical facies with full lips, broad nasal bridge, broad nasal tip and anteverted nares; with or without growth and mental deficiency; and supravalvular aortic or pulmonary arterial stenosis. Infantile hypercalcemia may be present.

Clinical Findings: More frequent features include mild short stature, sometimes low birth weight (median of 2.7 kg with range of 1.5–4.0 kg); mild to moderate mental retardation, short attention span with distractibility, hyperverbal speech, loquacious behavior during childhood, with severe behavior problems in one-sixth of patients, IQ most commonly 40–70 (average IQ=56); broad maxilla and mouth with full prominent "cupid's bow" upper lip, anteverted nares with full nasal tip, full pouting cheeks and open mouth with tendency toward inner epicanthic folds, small mandible, prominent ears, and unusual stellate patterning in the iris; and supravalvular aortic stenosis or hypoplasia, peripheral pulmonary artery stenosis, or septal defect in about 75% the patients. There may also be renal artery stenosis with hypertension, hypoplasia of the aorta, and other arterial anomalies. Rarely, may present in infancy with coarse facial features, hepatosplenomegaly, and hernias suggestive of a lysosomal storage disease which resolves with age.

Complications: Renal disease and calcinosis secondary to hypercalcemia. Sudden death has been reported in a few cases.

Associated Findings: Hoarse voice, hyperacusis, strabismus, craniosynostosis, hypodontia, inguinal hernia, kyphosis, kyphoscoliosis, joint contractures and joint limitation, radioulnar synostosis, mitral insufficiency, elevated serum cholesterol and hypercalcemia during infancy (8–18 months), with symptoms and signs such as hypotonia, constipation, anorexia, vomiting, polyuria, polydipsia, renal insufficiency, vicarious calcification, and transient facial palsy. Bladder diverticulae are usually only evident by means of excretory urography. Diverticulitis of the bowel has been

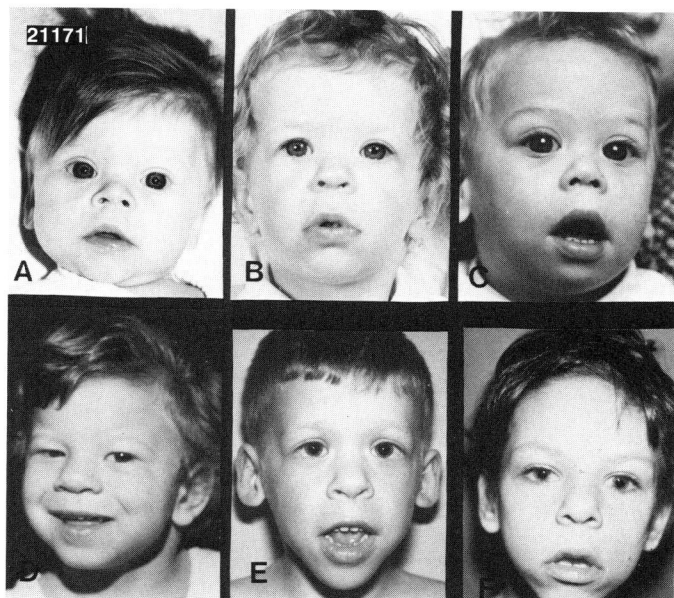

0999B-21171: Note the characteristic facies in these unrelated children.

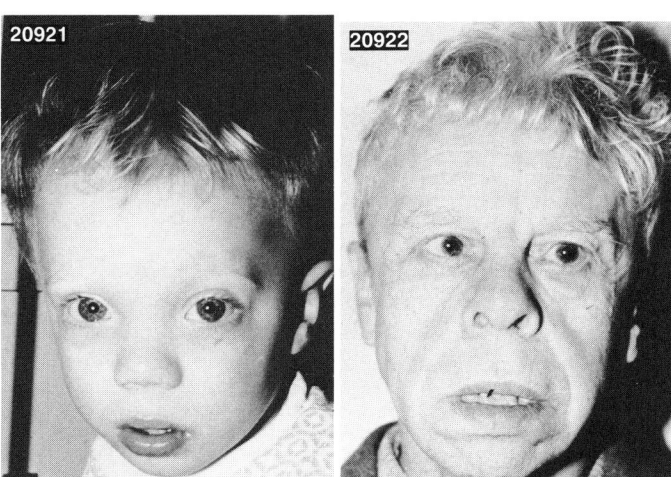

0999A-20921: Williams syndrome in a 2-year-old boy with typical facies; speckled iris, prominent, wide-set eyes, full cheeks, and prominent open mouth. **20922:** The typical facies are still evident in this 65-year-old male with Williams syndrome.

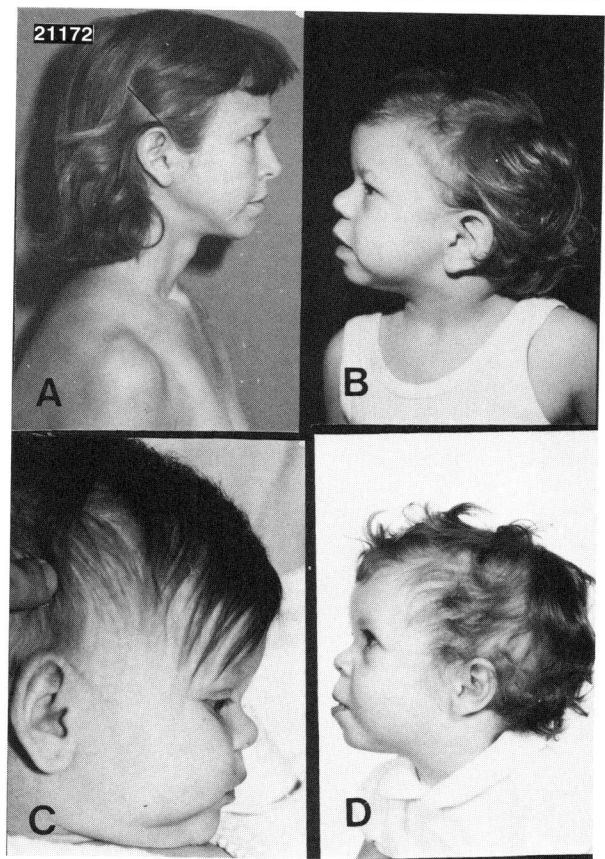

0999C-21172: Lateral view of facies shows full cheeks.

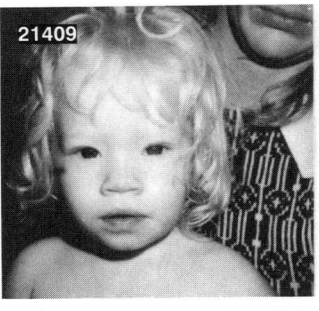
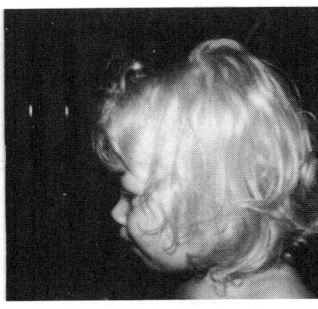

0999D-21409: Note broad forehead, flat nasal bridge and full cheeks.

described in adults. Recurrence of hypercalcemia has been reported in adults. Autism has been reported.

Etiology: Usually a sporadic occurrence, although autosomal dominant inheritance has been suggested, with most cases representing new mutations.

Pathogenesis: Possibly a defect in calcitonin production, release or activity (Culler, 1985). An abnormal synthesis or degradation of 1,25-(OH)2D has been suggested (Burn, 1986).

MIM No.: *19405

POS No.: 3427

Sex Ratio: Presumably M1:F1.

Occurrence: The incidence has been estimated as 1:10,000 (Grimm and Wesselhoeft, 1980).

Risk of Recurrence for Patient's Sib:
See Part I, *Mendelian Inheritance.* Usually sporadic.

Risk of Recurrence for Patient's Child:
See Part I, *Mendelian Inheritance.*

Age of Detectability: From birth to early childhood.

Gene Mapping and Linkage: WMS (William syndrome) has been tentatively mapped to 4q33-qter.

Prevention: None known. Genetic counseling indicated.

Treatment: When hypercalcemia still exists, elimination of vitamin D from the diet and limitation of calcium intake should be considered. Cardiac surgery may be indicated for severe cardiac defects. Individualized educational programs; physical, occupational, and speech therapy may be indicated.

Prognosis: Variable. No average life span can be inferred from existing data.

Detection of Carrier: Unknown.

Support Groups: TX; Klein; Williams Syndrome Association

References:
Williams JCP, et al.: Supravalvular aortic stenosis. Circulation 1961; 24:1311–1318.
Bennett FC, et al.: The Williams elfin facies syndrome. Pediatrics 1978; 61:303–306.
Grimm T, Wesselhoeft H: The genetic aspects of Williams-Beuren syndrome and the isolated form of the supravalvular aortic stenosis; investigation of 128 families. Z Kardiol 1980; 69:168–172.
Preus M: The Williams syndrome: objective definition and diagnosis. Clin Genet 1984; 25:422–428.
Culler FL, et al.: Impaired calcitonin secretion in patients with Williams syndrome. J Pediatr 1985; 107:720–723.
Burn J: Williams syndrome. J Med Genet 1986; 23:389–395.
Biesecker LG, et al.: Renal insufficiency in Williams syndrome. Am J Med Genet 1987; 28:131–135.
Maisuls H, et al.: Cardiovascular finding in the Williams-Beuren syndrome. Am Heart J 1987; 114:897–899.

BU040
GR011

Merlin G. Butler
Frank Greenberg

Williams-Beuren syndrome
See WILLIAMS SYNDROME
Williams-Campbell syndrome
See BRONCHOMALACIA
Wilms tumor
See CANCER, WILMS TUMOR
Wilms tumor-aniridia
See CHROMOSOME 11, PARTIAL MONOSOMY 11p
Wilms tumor-aniridia syndrome
See ANIRIDIA
Wilms tumor-aniridia-gonadoblastoma-mental retardation (WAGR)
See CHROMOSOME 11, PARTIAL MONOSOMY 11p

WILMS TUMOR-PSEUDOHERMAPHRODITISM-GLOMERULOPATHY, DENYS-DRASH TYPE   3139

Includes:
Denys-Drash syndrome
Drash syndrome
Gonadal differentiation (abnormal)-nephropathy-Wilms tumor
Nephropathy-pseudohermaphroditism-Wilms tumor
Pseudohermaphroditism-nephron disorder-Wilms tumor
Wilms tumor-pseudohermaphroditism-nephropathy

Excludes: Colon, atresia or stenosis (0193)

Major Diagnostic Criteria: Gonadal dysfunction usually consisting of male pseudohermaphroditism, glomerulopathy, and **Cancer, Wilms tumor.** According to Habib et al (1985) the syndrome includes patients with either male pseudohermaphroditism or Wilms tumor when associated with the renal histologic lesion of diffuse mesangial sclerosis.

Clinical Findings: The renal disease presents with proteinuria with or without nephrotic syndrome, hypertension, hematuria, and progressive renal insufficiency leading to end-stage renal disease in infancy. The external genitalia are frequently ambiguous, most patients being male pseudohermaphrodites. Wilms tumor occurs in about 55% of cases and may be diagnosed years after the appearance of kidney disease.

Complications: Chronic renal failure. Dysgenetic gonads carry 20–30% risk of malignancy.

Associated Findings: Hydronephrosis, vesicoureteral reflux, urogenital abnormalities.

Etiology: Usually sporadic.

Pathogenesis: May be due to defective embryogenesis of the urogenital ridge.

MIM No.: 19408

POS No.: 4227

Sex Ratio: M1:F>0. The majority of reported patients are male pseudohermaphrodites; however, the syndrome has been also described in females.

Occurrence: About 30 cases have been documented in the literature.

Risk of Recurrence for Patient's Sib: Undetermined, but probably small.

Risk of Recurrence for Patient's Child: Undetermined, but probably small.

Age of Detectability: Usually during early infancy.

Gene Mapping and Linkage: Unknown.

Prevention: None known. Genetic counseling indicated.

Treatment: Since Wilms tumor develops in 55% of patients, bilateral nephrectomy is advised once end-stage renal disease sets in. Removal of gonadal tissue is also advised during the same procedure to avoid malignant transformation. Renal transplantation has been performed successfully.

Prognosis: Untreated patients usually die in infancy.

Detection of Carrier: Unknown.

Special Considerations: This syndrome should be considered in any infant with ambiguous genitalia. Diffuse mesangial sclerosis is the usual histologic lesion in this syndrome, but it may also be a form of infantile nephrotic syndrome, sometimes associated with eye abnormalities (see **Renal mesangial sclerosis-eye defects**).

Support Groups: New York; National Kidney Foundation

References:
Denys P, et al.: Association d'un syndrome anotomopatholgique de psuedohermaphroditisme masculin, d'une tumeur de Wilms, d'une nephropathie parenchymateuse et d'une mosaicisme XX/XY. Arch Fr Pediatr 1967; 24:729–739.
Drash A, et al.: A syndrome of pseudohermaphroditism, Wilms' tumor, hypertension, and degenerative renal disease. J Pediatr 1970; 76:585–593.
Barakat AY, et al.: Pseudohermaphroditism, nephron disorder and Wilms' tumor: a unifying concept. Pediatrics 1974; 54:366–369.
Habib R, et al.: The nephropathy associated with male pseudohermaphroditism and Wilms' tumor (Drash syndrome): a distinctive glomerular lesion-report of 10 cases. Clin Nephrol 1985; 24:269–278.
Barakat AY: Nomenclature of Drash syndrome. (Letter) Clin Nephrol 1988; 29:107 only.

BA065   **Amin Y. Barakat**

Wilms tumor-pseudohermaphroditism-nephropathy
See WILMS TUMOR-PSEUDOHERMAPHRODITISM-GLOMERULOPATHY, DENYS-DRASH TYPE
Wilson disease
See HEPATOLENTICULAR DEGENERATION

WINCHESTER SYNDROME   1000

Includes:
  "Arthritis-like" condition-short stature
  Connective tissue disorder-joint stiffening-short stature
  Winchester-Grossman syndrome

Excludes:
  Arthritis mutilans
  Arthritis, rheumatoid (2517)
  Asymbolia
  Charcot-Marie-Tooth disease
  Gorham disease
  Mucolipidosis
  Mucopolysaccharidosis
  Osteolysis (1521)
  Reticulohistiocytosis, multicentric

Major Diagnostic Criteria: Short stature, joint stiffening with severe flexion contractures, peripheral corneal opacities, skin thickening, X-ray features of progressive carpotarsal osteolysis, and progressive destruction of small joints. Light and electron microscopic evaluation of thickened skin confirms the diagnosis.

Clinical Findings: Winchester syndrome begins before age two years, heralded by symmetric polyarthralgias of large and small joints. Swelling and pain with limitation of motion develop within the first two years of life without associated localized erythema, warmth, or other constitutional symptoms. Intermittent polyarthralgias continue throughout childhood and lead to flexion contractures of the fingers, elbows, hips, knees and ankles. Areas of skin become thickened and leathery, and gradually develop hyperpigmentation and a hypertrophic appearance. Five of seven patients have had coarsened facial features. Peripheral corneal opacities are noted by mid-childhood. Linear growth is retarded from early, childhood leading to dwarfism. Although motor development is retarded, intelligence is normal.

X-rays reveal generalized osteoporosis and progressive osteolysis of carpal and tarsal bones, sometimes with complete resorption by the second decade. Progressive intra- and periarticular erosions of small joints may simulate severe juvenile rheumatoid arthritis; bony anklyosis may develop.

Skin biopsies of affected areas have revealed fibroblastic hyperplasia and, at a later age, abnormal collagen bundle architecture in the deep dermis. Characteristic ultrastructural dilation of mitochondria is observed in fibroblasts. The carpal bones appear to be replaced by dense fibrous tissue, and sections of bone disclose a paucity of trabeculae; growth plates appear normal.

Complications: Severe progressive flexion contractures of major and minor joints lead to immobile "claw hands", and nonambulation that may lead to almost complete disability. Fractures are more common as a result of osteoporosis.

Associated Findings: The lips and gingiva may appear hypertrophic.

Etiology: Autosomal recessive inheritance.

Pathogenesis: Joint contractures, skin thickening, abnormal dermal collagen, and corneal opacities may be due to abnormal fibroblast function. Dwarfism, osteolysis, and osteoporosis appear to be secondary to excessive bone resorption.

MIM No.: *27795

POS No.: 3428

Sex Ratio: Presumably M1:F1 (M3:F4 observed in seven cases).

Occurrence: Undetermined. Recorded cases have occurred in Puerto Rican, Mexican, Indian, and Iranian families.

Risk of Recurrence for Patient's Sib:
  See Part I, *Mendelian Inheritance.*

Risk of Recurrence for Patient's Child:
  See Part I, *Mendelian Inheritance.*

Age of Detectability: Usually by one year of age; before two years of age.

Gene Mapping and Linkage: Unknown.

Prevention: None known. Genetic counseling indicated.

Treatment: Serial casting, continuous passive range of motion machines, or other orthopedic procedures to decrease flexion contractures may be of some benefit.

Prognosis: Normal intelligence, but with significant functional disability.

Detection of Carrier: Possibly by clinical examination of first degree relatives.

Special Considerations: The coarsened facies, thickened skin, corneal clouding, dwarfism, and joint contractures suggest a mucopolysaccharoid storage disease or mucolipidosis. However, the absence of mucopolysacchariduria and presence of rheumatoid-like small joint destruction and carpotarsal osteolysis distinguishe the Winchester syndrome from these latter conditions, as does the absence of lysosomal vacuolization in fibroblasts and chondrocytes. The Winchester syndrome may be differentiated from juvenile **Arthritis, rheumatoid** by the lack of prominent constitutional symptoms, normal erythrocyte sedimentation rate, negative antinuclear antibody and rheumatoid factor, and by extra-skeletal manifestations, particularly the skin changes.

References:
Winchester P, et al.: A new acid mucopolysaccharidosis with skeletal deformities simulating rheumatoid arthritis. Am J Roentgenol Radium Ther Nucl Med 1969; 106:121–128.
Brown SI, Kuwabara T: Peripheral corneal opacification and skeletal deformities: a newly recognized acid mucopolysaccharidosis simulating rheumatoid arthritis. Arch Ophthal 1970; 83:667–677.
Hollister DW, et al.: The Winchester syndrome: a nonlysosomal connective tissue disease. J Pediatr 1974; 84:701–709. *
Cohen AH, et al.: The skin in Winchester syndrome. Arch Dermatol 1975; 111:230–236.
Nabai H, et al.: Winchester syndrome: report of a case from Iran. J Cutan Pathol 1977; 4:281–285.
Irani A, et al.: The Winchester syndrome: a case report. Indian Pediatr 1978; 15:861–863.

G0043   **Donald P. Goldsmith**

Winchester-Grossman syndrome
See WINCHESTER SYNDROME
Wind blown hand
See HAND, ULNAR DRIFT
Wind-mill vain hand
See HAND, ULNAR DRIFT

Windmill vane hand syndrome
 See *CRANIO-CARPO-TARSAL DYSPLASIA, WHISTLING FACE TYPE*
Wing teeth
 See *TEETH, MESIOPALATAL TORSION OF CENTRAL INCISORS*
Winter syndrome
 See *RENAL-GENITAL-MIDDLE EAR ANOMALIES*
Wiskott-Aldrich syndrome
 See *IMMUNODEFICIENCY, WISKOTT-ALDRICH TYPE*
WL symphalangism-brachydactyly syndrome
 See *SYMPHALANGISM*
Wolcott-Rallison syndrome
 See *EPIPHYSEAL DYSPLASIA, MULTIPLE-DIABETES MELLITUS*
Wolf syndrome
 See *CHROMOSOME 4, MONOSOMY 4p*
Wolf teeth
 See *TEETH, LOBODONTIA*
Wolf-Hirschhorn syndrome
 See *CHROMOSOME 4, MONOSOMY 4p*
Wolff syndrome
 See *ALBINISM, CUTANEOUS*
Wolff-Parkinson-White syndrome
 See *ARRHYTHMIA, WOLFF-PARKINSON-WHITE TYPE*
Wolfram syndrome
 See *DIABETES (INSIPIDUS/MELLITUS)-OPTIC ATROPHY-DEAFNESS*

WOLMAN DISEASE   1003

Includes:
 LIPA deficiency
 Lysosomal acid lipase deficiency
 Wolman disease-hypolipoproteinemia-acanthocytosis
 Xanthomatosis, familial-involvement and calcification of
  adrenals

Excludes:
 Analphalipoproteinemia (0048)
 Biliary atresia (0110)
 Cholesteryl ester storage disease (0151)
 Lipogranulomatosis (0598)
 Niemann-Pick disease (0717)

Major Diagnostic Criteria: The diagnosis can be considered certain in a young infant with hepatosplenomegaly, steatorrhea, enlarged and calcified adrenals, foam cells in the marrow, and vacuolization of lymphocytes. Death usually occurs in infancy. Substantiation of the diagnosis depends on demonstration of deficient acid lipase activity in leukocytes and cultured skin fibroblasts.

Clinical Findings: Characteristically, infants present with poor weight gain, vomiting, and loose, frequent stools in the early weeks of life. Symmetrically enlarged, calcified adrenals are seen to have a diffuse punctate pattern of calcification on X-ray examination of the abdomen. Anemia occurs in early infancy. Chronic nutritional failure becomes increasingly severe in spite of all special management efforts (handicapped by foam cell infiltration in the intestinal villi), and the patients die by ages 2–9 months with wasting and infection. Neuromuscular development is retarded, but mostly in a secondary fashion, with neuronal changes of limited distribution when present at all (retina, sympathetic ganglia, myenteric plexus). There is moderate enlargement of the liver and spleen, organs in which the fundamental lipid-laden foam cell diathesis is well visualized: Neutral fat accumulation and cholesterol (80–90% esterified) is marked. Liver cholesterol levels have varied from 3 to 9% of the net weight and spleen; phospholipid levels are normal. Foam cells are found in the bone marrow, and there is prominent vacuolization of the circulating agranulocytes. The possibility has now been raised that some children with this basic syndrome may have a considerably later expression of the GI symptoms, longer survival, and less evident calcification of the adrenals.

Complications: Chronic nutritional failure, and possibly some degree of adrenocortical insufficiency. A positive balance for nutrients and electrolytes, with a margin for support of general development, is extremely difficult to achieve.

Associated Findings: On several occasions, serum alphalipoprotein levels have been found to be very low, although not comparable to those in **Analphalipoproteinemia.**

Wolman disease-hypolipoproteinemia-acanthocytosis, described by Eto and Kitagawa (1970), is a possible variant unique in its hypolipoproteinemia and acanthocytosis.

Etiology: Autosomal recessive inheritance. There is deficient activity of lysosomal acid lipase in cultured fibroblasts, leukocytes, amniocytes, liver, spleen, lymph node, and aortic tissue. With natural substrates the enzyme activity is less than 10% of control. Electrophoresis separates acid lipase into three bands. In Wolman disease there is absence of the least anodal (A) band. This isoenzyme appears to function both as a cholesterol ester hydrolase and triacylglycerol hydrolase, and its deficient activity in Wolman disease leads to lysosomal accumulation of cholesteryl esters and to a lesser extent of triglycerides.

Pathogenesis: The enlargement of liver, spleen, adrenal, and lymph nodes is a consequence of cholesteryl ester and triglyceride accumulation. The adrenal calcification may be a consequence of necrosis and cell infiltrates demonstrated in the fetal adrenal gland of a closely related condition: cholesterol ester storage disease. The degree of cholesteryl ester storage probably is sufficient to lead to cellular malfunction. The lysosomal cholesteryl esterase normally hydrolyzes the cholesteryl esters, which enter the cell via the "Brown and Goldstein" LDL pathway, and the deficient activity of this enzyme in Wolman disease compromises the critical control mechanisms associated with this pathway. These effects probably account for the plasma lipoprotein abnormalities and premature atherosclerosis associated with cholesteryl ester storage disease, in which there is deficiency of the same enzyme. These changes may not be observed in Wolman disease, probably due to their short life span.

MIM No.: *27800, 27810

Sex Ratio: M1:F1

Occurrence: Forty-two cases reported to date. No predilection in any particular group.

Risk of Recurrence for Patient's Sib:
 See Part I, *Mendelian Inheritance.*

Risk of Recurrence for Patient's Child:
 See Part I, *Mendelian Inheritance.* No affected individuals are known to have reproduced.

Age of Detectability: In infancy, clinically. Calcification of the adrenals has been detected within the first few days of life on several occasions, and it should be visible on abdominal X-rays of the mother in later pregnancy. Prenatal diagnosis (lipase studies on cultured fetal cells) has been done.

Gene Mapping and Linkage: LIPA (lipase A, lysosomal acid (Wolman disease)) has been mapped to 10.

Prevention: None known. Genetic counseling indicated.

Treatment: Very unsatisfactory to date. Simplified, high-calorie, high-protein feedings, or low-residue feedings, have not been adequate to allow reasonable weight gain and have been limited by the diarrhea and vomiting. Adrenal corticosteroid supplements have been regularly used. No useful effects have been identified from cholestyramine, d-thyroxine, clofibrate, or medium-chain triglyceride treatments. In the future, enzyme replacement therapy or gene therapy may become feasible. Such approaches are made more hopeful by the absence of significant central nervous system involvement in Wolman disease and by the fact that the acid lipase has been purified and does carry the mannose-6-phosphate ligand, which allows for receptor-mediated targeting to the lysosome.

Prognosis: The usual (infant) patients have expired, in spite of all therapeutic efforts, at ages 1.5 to 9 months, rarely a few months longer. Reports now exist of children with milder symptoms and of later onset who are surviving into middle or late childhood.

Detection of Carrier: Leukocytes or cultured skin fibroblasts of carriers have approximately one-half of the normal activity of acid lipase. This detection is facilitated by a recently developed fluorometric assay.

Special Considerations: **Cholesteryl ester storage disease** is allelic with Wolman disease. Patients with cholesterol ester storage disease are mildly disabled and may live to midadulthood or longer. They have liver disease and premature arteriosclerosis. The relationship between Wolman disease and cholesterol ester storage disease is not clear. Patients with intermediate degrees of severity have been reported. One patient with cholesteryl ester storage disease has shown adrenal calcification, while a patient with Wolman disease lacked it.

References:
Crocker AC, et al.: Wolman's disease: three new patients with a recently described lipidosis. Pediatrics 1965; 35:627–640.
Eto Y, Kitagawa T: Wolman disease with hypolipoproteinemia and acanthocytosis: clinical and biochemical observations. J Pediatr 1970; 77:862–867.
Coates PM, et al.: Prenatal diagnosis of Wolman disease. Am J Med Genet 1978; 2:397–407.
Koch G, et al.: Assignment of LIPA, associated with human lipase deficiency to human chromosome 10 and comparative assignment to mouse chromosome 19. Somatic Cell Genet 1981; 7:345–358.
Nigre A, et al.: New spectrophotometric assays of acid lipase and their use in the diagnosis of Wolman and cholesteryl ester storage disease. Anal Biochem 1985; 145:398–405.
Cagle PT, et al.: Clinicopathological conference: pulmonary hypertension in an 18-year-old girl with cholesteryl ester storage disease (CESD). Am J Med Genet 1986; 24:711–722.
Schmitz G, Assmann G: Acid lipase deficiency: Wolman disease and cholesteryl ester storage disease. In: Scriver CR, et al, eds: The metabolic basis of inherited disease, 6th ed. New York: McGraw-Hill, 1989:1623–1644. *

M0038   **Hugo Moser**

Wolman disease-hypolipoproteinemia-acanthocytosis
 See WOLMAN DISEASE
Word blindness, congenital
 See DYSLEXIA
Wormian bones-blue sclerae-mandibular hypoplasia-campomelia
 See SHORT STATURE-WORMIAN BONES-JOINT DISLOCATIONS

WRINKLY SKIN SYNDROME   2907

Includes: Skin, wrinkly skin syndrome
Excludes:
 Cutis laxa (0233)
 Cutis laxa-growth defect, De Barsy type (2138)
 Ehlers-Danlos syndrome (0338)
 Osteodysplastica gerodermia, Bamatter type (2099)
Major Diagnostic Criteria: Universal features are wrinkly skin of the dorsum of the hands and feet, wrinkly skin of the abdomen, an increased number of palmar and plantar creases, a prominent venous pattern of the skin, and hypoelasticity of the wrinkly skin.

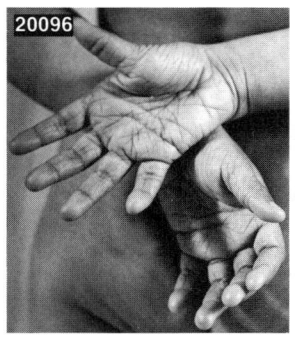 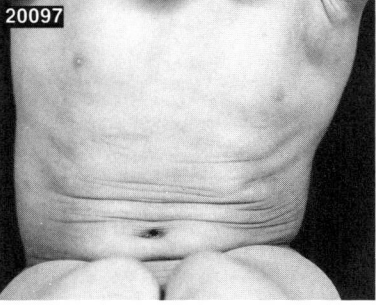

2907-20096: Increased palmar creases and aged appearance of the skin in this 5-year-old. **20097:** Transverse wrinkling of the abdomen in a 5-year-old.

Clinical Findings: The skin findings are present at birth. Progression of the skin findings is unknown; however, described cases do not display the generalized hypoelasticity of **Cutis laxa** or the generalized wrinkling of the skin and aged facial appearance of **Osteodysplastica gerodermia, Bamatter type**. Congenital hip dysplasia (7/7) joint hyperextensibility (5/6), and spinal deformity (6/7) are frequent features. Hypotonia (5/5), **Microcephaly** (4/5), and psychomotor retardation (4/6) occur with sufficient frequency to indicate that this syndrome has significant extracutaneous manifestations. Skin biopsy specimens have been normal in two patients, but one patient showed a decreased number and length of elastic fibers in the wrinkled as opposed to nonwrinkled skin.

Complications: Altered gait due to hip dysplasia and spinal deformities.

Associated Findings: Failure to thrive, short stature, myopia, chorioretinitis, congenital heart disease.

Etiology: Autosomal recessive inheritance, with consanguinity noted in all cases.

Pathogenesis: Some aspects may be due to disordered elastic metabolism.

MIM No.: *27825

POS No.: 3978

Sex Ratio: Presumably M1:F1. M2:F7 observed.

Occurrence: About a dozen cases have been documented in the literature.

Risk of Recurrence for Patient's Sib:
 See Part I, *Mendelian Inheritance.*

Risk of Recurrence for Patient's Child:
 See Part I, *Mendelian Inheritance.*

Age of Detectability: At birth.

Gene Mapping and Linkage: Unknown.

Prevention: None known. Genetic counseling indicated.

Treatment: Orthopedic management of hip dysplasia and spinal deformities.

Prognosis: Life span undetermined. The degree of mental retardation is also undetermined.

Detection of Carrier: Unknown. Carriers are not known to have any clinical manifestations.

References:
Gazit E, et al.: The wrinkly skin syndrome: a new heritable disorder of connective tissue. Clin Genet 1973; 4:186–192. * †
Goodman RM, et al.: The wrinkly skin syndrome and cartilage-hair hypoplasia (a new variant ?) in sibs of the same family. In: Papadatos CJ, Bartsocas CS, eds: Skeletal dysplasias. New York: Alan R. Liss, 1982:205–214.
Karrar ZA, et al.: Cutis laxa, intrauterine growth retardation, and bilateral dislocation of the hips: a report of five cases. In: Papadatos CJ, Bartsocas CS, eds: Skeletal dysplasia. New York: Alan R. Liss, 1982:215–221.
Karrar ZA, et al.: The wrinkly skin syndrome: a report of two siblings from Saudi Arabia. Clin Genet 1983; 23:308–310.
Casamassima AC, et al.: The wrinkly skin syndrome: phenotype and additional manifestations. Am J Med Genet 1987; 27:885–893. * †

CA035   **Anthony C. Casamassima**

Wryneck
 See TORTICOLLIS
WT limb-blood syndrome
 See WT SYNDROME

WT SYNDROME   3145

Includes:
Blood-limb syndrome
Fanconi-like radioulnar hypoplasia-hypoplastic anemia
Limb-blood syndrome
WT limb-blood syndrome

Excludes: Pancytopenia syndrome, Fanconi type (2029)

Major Diagnostic Criteria: Upper limb malformations, especially radial ray defects, in conjunction with hypoplastic anemia, with variable age of onset.

Clinical Findings: Abnormalities of upper extremities, including radioulnar synostosis; digitalized hypoplastic, or absent thumbs; and clinodactyly with or without **Camptodactyly** (usually of the fifth fingers). The anemia is usually chronic megaloblastic anemia with variable intensity and course. Increased mean corpuscular volume (MCV) can precede anemia by years. Bone marrow is usually hypoplastic, with megaloblastic changes in red cell precursors. In some families, pancytopenia is seen. Individuals presenting with severe hypoplastic anemia have decreased life span, often dying within six months to four years of onset of symptoms. Increased chromosome breakage has not been reported.

Complications: Transfusion-dependent treatment for chronic anemia may lead to iron overload, causing organ dysfunction such as congestive heart failure or cirrhosis of the liver. Congestive heart failure is often responsible for death. Affected individuals with pancytopenia may have bleeding and an increased incidence of infection secondary to neutropenia.

Associated Findings: History of easy bruising may precede development of severe hematologic symptoms. In one family reported with WT syndrome, short stature, sensorineural deafness, a characteristic facial appearance (high forehead, midface hypoplasia, upturned nose, and prominant ears) and hyperpigmentation were observed.

Etiology: Autosomal dominant inheritance with variable expression and virtually complete penetrance.

Pathogenesis: Unknown.

MIM No.: 19435

POS No.: 4053

Sex Ratio: Presumably M1:F1; M1.14:F1 (observed).

Occurrence: Three United States families have been documented; two in the Midwest, one in the Rocky Mountains.

Risk of Recurrence for Patient's Sib:
See Part I, *Mendelian Inheritance.*

Risk of Recurrence for Patient's Child:
See Part I, *Mendelian Inheritance.*

Age of Detectability: Limb anomalies are apparent at birth. Hematologic problems are variable in age of onset.

Gene Mapping and Linkage: Unknown.

Prevention: None known. Genetic counseling indicated.

Treatment: Symptomatic treatment of anemia.

Prognosis: Variable, depending on the severity of hematologic symptoms. For severe hypoplastic anemia, death often occurs within six months to 3–4 years of symptom onset.

Detection of Carrier: By physical examination and CBC and red blood cell MCV.

Special Considerations: The condition derives its name from the first two families described; the W. and the T. families. This condition should be distinguished from **Pancytopenia syndrome, Fanconi type** (Fanconi anemia), which is also associated with refractory anemia and radial ray defects. Families reported to have Fanconi anemia and an increased incidence of leukemia and congenital anomalies in nonanemic (or non-Fanconi syndrome) relatives may actually represent the WT syndrome.

References:
Gonzalez CH, et al.: The WT syndrome-a "new" autosomal dominant pleiotropic trait of radial/ulnar hypoplasia with high risk of bone marrow failure and/or leukemia. BD:OAS XIII(3B). New York: March of Dimes Birth Defects Foundation, 1977:31–38.
Smith ACM, et al.: WT syndrome: a third family. Am J Hum Genet 1987; 41:A84.

SM016   **Ann C.M. Smith**

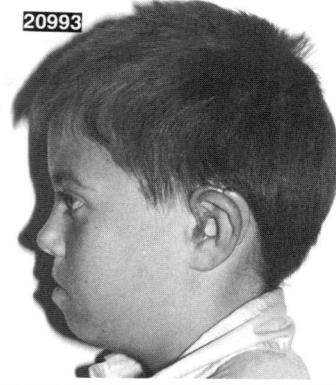

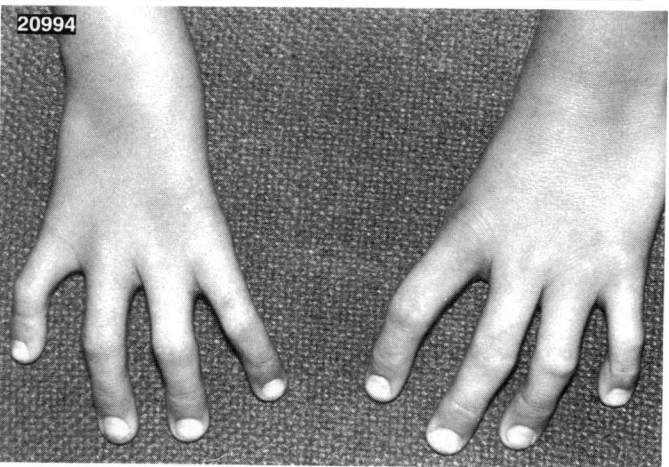

3145-20992: WT syndrome; note high forehead, upturned nose and prominent ears. This 13-year-old male has sensorineural deafness. 20993: Lateral view of the face shows midface hypoplasia. 20994: Bilateral absence of the thumbs.

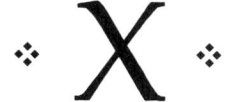

X-linked adult onset spinobulbar muscular atrophy
 See MUSCULAR ATROPHY, SPINAL AND BULBAR, X-LINKED KENNEDY TYPE
X-linked adult spinal muscular atrophy
 See MUSCULAR ATROPHY, SPINAL AND BULBAR, X-LINKED KENNEDY TYPE
X-linked copper malabsorption
 See MENKES SYNDROME
X-linked fragile site
 See X-LINKED MENTAL RETARDATION, FRAGILE X SYNDROME

X-LINKED MENTAL RETARDATION   1509

The concept of X-linked mental retardation has evolved continuously over the last 50 years. (Penrose, 1938) first suggested that the more frequent occurence of mental retardation in males, compared to females, was not due to a number of X-linked genes but to social factors. It now appears that about a third of mental retardation in males may be explainable on the basis of X-linked genes. This concept was later reviewed and confirmed by Morton, et al (1977) and Herbst (1980), and others who suggested that a total of seven to nineteen specific disorders accounted for this sex difference. In the 1960's, Lehrke (1974) also promulgated the idea of the significance of X-linked genes in mental retardation. Progress in understanding X-linked mental retardation was delayed not only by the absence of laboratory diagnosis for these entities, but, at least in retrospect, by the frequent occurence of mildly affected females in many families which obscured the expected pedigree pattern of pure X-linked recessive inheritance. The few publications in this area are generally referenced under the term "non-specific X-linked mental retardation". These included the reports by Martin and Bell (1943) and Renpenning et al (1962). No specific clinical findings within these families were reported in either paper.

In 1969, Lubs reported the marker X, now known as the fragile X, in a family with mental retardation in four males. Giraud et al (1976) and Harvey et al (1977) reported additional cases. At the same time Sutherland (1977) demonstrated the requirements for low folate and low thymidine in culture media for consistent detection of the fragile X. This opened the door to repeatable and planned studies of X-linked mental retardation. The family originally reported by Martin and Bell (1943) was restudied by Richards et al (1981) and proved to have the fragile X. Although *Martin-Bell syndrome* has often been used to describe the fragile X syndrome, it is a confusing reference since neither the clinical features nor the fragile X were observed in the original report and the more descriptive term "fragile X" is preferred.

Most studies have shown that only 30–40% of unselected families with X-linked mental retardation have the fragile X. Nine members of the family reported by Renpenning et al (1962) were restudied by Fox et al (1980). This family proved not to have the fragile X chromosome but did show a moderately consistent pattern of findings, including low mean measurements for height, weight, head circumference and testicular volume, and probably

represents a distinct syndrome. No laboratory tests yet exist for the remaining entities. Very likely, certain of the apparently similar disorders described below will be delineated as clinical entities by linkage and localization studies and others will prove to be overlapping descriptions of a syndrome described under several names by different authors. Only in twelve of the syndromes reported to date have two or more families been reported. The syndromes described by Atkins et al (1985) and by Clark et al (1987), for example, are listed as separate entities although their facial features are quite similar. The "distinguishing features" of hypertelorism and short stature in the Atkins family (compared to hypotelorism and normal stature in the Clark-Baraitser family) may have been familial since other family members had similar findings.

Table 1509–1 presents a working summary of disorders that have been included in the category of non-specific X-linked mental retardation but now have emerging, more specific, features. It does not include all possible entities. X-linked disorders with mental retardation and obvious clinical manifestations, such as hydrocephaly or blindness, are not generally included in this classification. About 80 X-linked disorders may include mental retardation as one manifestation.

References:
Penrose LS: A clinical and genetic study of 1,280 cases of mental defect. Special Rep Ser No. 229, London, Med Res Council, 1938.
Martin JP, Bell J: A pedigree of mental defect showing sex-linkage. J Neurol Psychiatr 1943; 6:154–157.
Renpenning H, et al.: Familial sex-linked mental retardation. Can Med Assoc J 1962; 87:954–956.
Giraud F, et al.: Constitutional chromosomal breakage. Hum Genet 1969; 34:125–136.
Lubs HA: A marker-X chromosome. Am J Hum Genet 1969; 21:231–244.
Lehrke RG: X-linked mental retardation and verbal disability. New York, Intercontinental Medical Book Corporation, 1974. BDOAS X:1–100 (Publication of PhD thesis of the same title, University of Wisconsin, 1968).
Harvey J, et al.: Familial X-linked mental retardation with an X chromosome abnormality. J Med Genet 1977; 14:46–50.
Morton N, et al.: Colchester revisited: a genetic study of mental defect. J Med Genet 1977; 14:1–9.
Sutherland GR: Fragile sites on human chromosomes: demonstration of their dependence on the type of tissue culture medium. Science 1977; 197:265–266.
Fox P, et al.: X-linked mental retardation: Renpenning revisited. Am J Med Genet 1980; 7:491–495.
Herbst DS, Miller JR: Non-specific X-linked mental retardation. II. The frequency in British Columbia. Am J Med Genet 1980; 7:461–469.
Richards BW, et al.: Fragile X-linked mental retardation: the Martin-Bell syndrome. J Ment Defic Res 1981; 25:253–256.
Atkin JF, et al.: A new X-linked mental retardation syndrome. Am J Med Genet 1985; 21:697–705.

Table 1509-1 Selected X-linked Mental Retardation Syndromes

Condition	Distinctive Features	Other Features
TWO OR MORE FAMILIES REPORTED		
X-linked mental retardation, Fragile X syndrome	Fragile X diagnostic Large testes Connective tissue abnormalities with hyperextension, pectus & floppy mitral valve	May have narrow faces, with hypoplastic midface late in childhood with prominent ears. Approximately 1/3 females retarded or dull
X-linked mental retardation, Renpenning type	Small head, short stature Small testes (each 2–25 %ile)	All features are highly variable & may fall in normal range in some family members
X-linked mental retardation, Marfanoid habitus type	Tall (>90 %ile), thin Connective tissue abnormalities with pectus & long, thin hands. Long, narrow face with thin, high nasal bridge, small chin. Large testes (≥90 %ile)	Agenesis corpus callosum in some
Simpson-Golabi-Behmel syndrome	Striking coarse facies Macrostomia Pre + postnatal overgrowth Coccygeal skin tags Midline notching lower lip	Submucous cleft Bone anomalies Cystic kidney Hepatosplenomegaly Early death in some
X-linked mental retardation-growth-hearing and genital defects	Small stature & delayed bone age. Mild-severe deafness. Small scrotum & penis. Cryptorchidism	Severe mental retardation Small palpebral fissures Flat nasal bridge Poor survival
X-linked mental retardation-clasped thumb	Bilateral absence of extensor pollicis brevis tendons with thumb flexion deformity	Usually normal appearance May have growth retardation, lordosis & microcephaly
X-linked mental retardation-Xq duplication	Growth deficiency Short stature (below 3rd %ile) Somatomedin C deficiency Delayed bone age Peculiar face	Small palpebral fissure Bilateral ptosis Tented upper lip Full lower lip Down turned corners of mouth
FG syndrome, Opitz-Kaveggia type	Hypotonia Slow motor development Short stature Abnormal skull/relative macrocephaly High, prominent forehead Frontal cowlick Micrognathia Muscle weakness	Hypertelorism/telecanthus Abnormal (mostly anti-mongoloid) palpebral slant Long philtrum High, arched palate Abnormal dermatoglyphics Striking personality
Coffin-Lowry syndrome	Downslanting palpebral fissures Mild hypertelorism Prominent brow Broad nose Microcephaly Short stature Unusual facial appearance	Thick, soft skin Large hands with tapering fingers
Smith-Fineman-Myers syndrome	Micrognathia Narrow face Patulous lower lip	Minor foot deformities Hyperreflexia Seizures
X-linked mental retardation-choreoathetosis	Choreoathetosis in first year; often constant. Later spasticity, ophthalmoplegia & deafness. Postnatal growth retardation & microcephaly.	Appears normal at birth Later sunken eyes & pinched lower nose
Borjeson-Forssman-Lehmann syndrome	Short stature (<3 %ile) Narrow palpebral fissures Large ears, hypogonadism Seizures	Obesity and swelling of subcutaneous face, hypometabolism, short upturned nose
SINGLE FAMILY REPORTED		
X-linked mental retardation, Atkin type	Short stature Hypertelorism Broad nose and coarse facies Large testes (? familial)	Large, square forehead May have large head & ears. (? familial)

Table 1509-1 (continued) Selected X-linked Mental Retardation Syndromes

Condition	Distinctive Features	Other Features
X-linked mental retardation, Clark-Baraitser type	Normal stature Hypotelorism Broad nose & coarse facies Large testes	Large head (males) & square forehead
X-linked mental retardation, Golabi-Ito-Hall type	Postnatal growth deficiency and micro-cephaly Narrow, triangular face Anteverted ears Upslanted palpebral fissures Laterally displaced inner canthi	Epicanthal folds ASD Brittle, dry hair
X-linked mental retardation-craniofacial abnormalities-club foot	Peculiar facies (coarse) Microcephaly Large anterior fontanel Club foot deformity Early death	Epicanthic folds Flat nasal bridge Anteverted nostrils Abnormal teeth Hypotonia
Seizures, in females, Juberg-Hellman type	Probably X-linked dominant inheritance. Expression limited to females. Seizures with onset 6–18 months. Half also retarded.	
X-linked mental retardation-basal ganglion disorder	Persistent frontal lobe reflexes, cogwheel rigidity, abnormal gait & Parkinsonian tremor. Frontal bossing & large head.	Strabismus Seizures
X-linked mental retardation-skeletal dysplasia	Ridging of metopic suture Fused & hemi-vertebrae Scoliosis & sacral hypoplasia Short mid-phalanges Abducens palsy	Antimongoloid slant & epicanthic folds Broad nasal bridge
Contractures-muscle atrophy-oculo-motor apraxia	Weakness of upper and lower limbs Distal muscle atrophy Dyspraxia of the eye, face and tongue muscles Swallowing difficulties	Overlap of toes Manifestations apparently more restricted to nervous system
X-linked mental retardation-psoriasis	Delayed psychomotor development Normal growth Ataxic gait Seizures	Apparent hypertelorism Large ears, macrostomia Long philtrum
X-linked mental retardation-dystonic movements of hands	Normal growth Dysarthria	No special facial features
X-linked mental retardation-subcortical atrophy-patellar luxation	Facial dysmorphia Clinodactily Ear malformations High nasal bridge Patella luxation Febrile convulsion Abnormalities of fundus of eye	Abnormal teeth Skin dimple of lower back Limb malformation
Hyperkeratosis palmoplantaris-spastic paraplegia-retardation	Pes cavus deformity Abnormal gait	Peculiar face (may be familial)
X-linked mental retardation-muscular weakness-awkward gait	Severe MR Hypotonia Joint contractures Delayed, clumsy walking Awkward, wide-base gait	Hyporeflexia Marked speech defect No special facial features described
Short stature-cerebral atrophy-keratosis follicularis, X-linked	Delayed somatic growth Microcephaly Seizures	Absence of hair and eyelashes Micrognathia Delayed dentition
X-linked mental retardation-short stature-obesity-hypogonadism	Moderate to Severe MR Mild obesity—infancy onset Distinct facial features Short neck	Bitemporal narrowing Almond-shaped palpebral fissures Flat nasal bridge Inverted V-shaped upper lip Short upper lip

Clark RD, Baraitser M: A new X-linked mental retardation syndrome. (Letter) Am J Med Genet 1987; 26:13–15.

LU002
AR011

Herbert A. Lubs
J. Fernando Arena

X-linked mental retardation with fragile X
See X-LINKED MENTAL RETARDATION, FRAGILE X SYNDROME

X-LINKED MENTAL RETARDATION, ATKIN TYPE   2840

Includes: Atkin-Flaitz X-linked mental retardation

Excludes:
  X-linked mental retardation, Clark-Baraitser type (2640)
  X-linked mental retardation (other)

Major Diagnostic Criteria: Expected findings include moderate-to-severe mental retardation in males and normal intelligence or mild mental retardation in females, short stature, **Megalencephaly**, and coarse facial features.

Clinical Findings: Affected individuals have a facial appearance similar to that found in **Coffin-Lowry syndrome**, including large, square forehead; prominent supraorbital ridges; **Eye, hypertelorism**; downslanting palpebral fissure; and broad nasal tip with anteverted nostrils. Other features include **Megalencephaly**, micrognathia, and large ears.

All affected males have moderate-to-severe mental retardation, with developmental delays being noted within the first year of life. Females show mild mental retardation. Twenty-seven percent (3/11) have seizures. Most have a congenial personality, though aggressive behavior has also been exhibited.

Orodental findings include microdontic maxillary lateral inci-

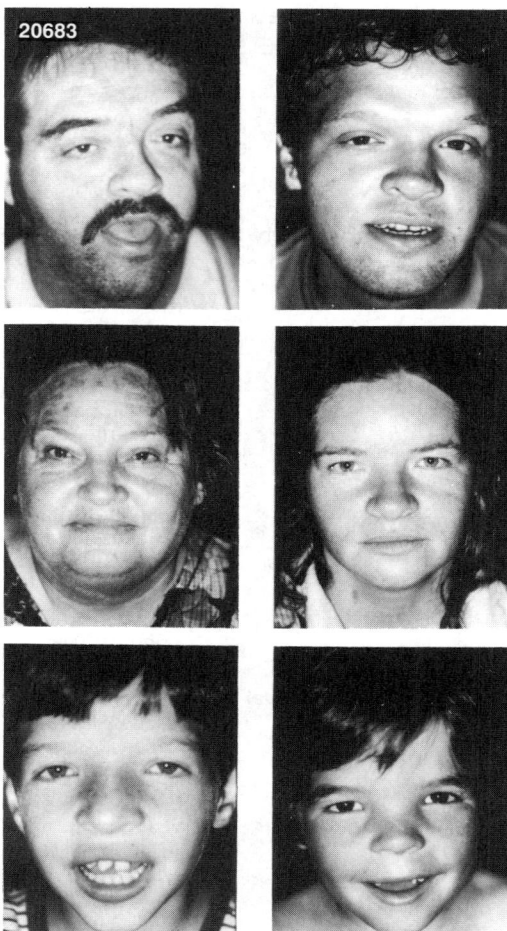

2840B-20683: Faces of representative affected relatives; note Coffin-Lowry-like facies.

---

sors, diastema between maxillary central incisors, palatal torus, and exaggerated median furrow of the tongue.

Other findings include short stature, obesity, and macroorchidism.

Complications: Unknown.

Associated Findings: None known.

Etiology: X-linked inheritance. There is no male-to-male transmission; however, none of the known affected males have reproduced. Women are mildly affected or unaffected.

Pathogenesis: Unknown.

MIM No.: *30953

Sex Ratio: M11:F3 (observed). Limited data suggest that if this is an X-linked condition, females may be affected more often than expected due to lyonization.

Occurrence: One kinship with 14 affected members has been documented.

Risk of Recurrence for Patient's Sib:
  See Part I, *Mendelian Inheritance.*

Risk of Recurrence for Patient's Child:
  See Part I, *Mendelian Inheritance.*

Age of Detectability: Within the first year of life, if family history is positive.

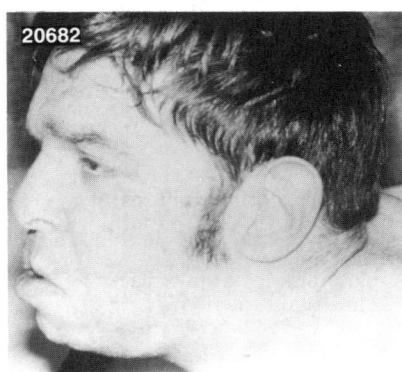

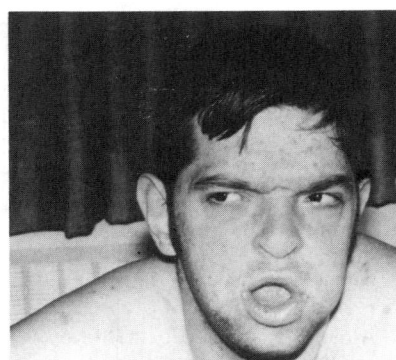

2840A-20682: X-linked mental retardation, Atkin type; note coarse facial features similar to that found in the Coffin-Lowry syndrome with prominent supraorbital ridge, broad nasal tip with anteverted nares and thick lower lip.

Gene Mapping and Linkage: MRX1 (mental retardation, X-linked 1 (non-dysmorphic)) has been mapped to Xp11-q13.

Prevention: None known. Genetic counseling indicated.

Treatment: Treatment of seizures if present, or behavior therapy if needed.

Prognosis: Normal life span.

Detection of Carrier: Unknown.

Special Considerations: Some described features may be familial. The macrocephaly may still be a component of the syndrome as, relatively, the heads are larger than unaffected relatives'. The macroorchidism is likely to be a component of the syndrome, as the average testicular volume in affected individuals is greater than that of unaffected individuals in the same family.

References:
Atkin JF, et al.: A new X-linked mental retardation syndrome. Am J Med Genet 1985; 21:697–705.

AT004   **Joan F. Atkin**

X-linked mental retardation, Chudley-Lowry-Hoar type
  See X-LINKED MENTAL RETARDATION-SHORT STATURE-OBESITY-HYPOGONADISM

X-LINKED MENTAL RETARDATION, CLARK-BARAITSER TYPE   2640

Includes: Clark-Baraitser X-linked mental retardation

Excludes:
  Borjeson-Forssman-Lehmann syndrome (2272)
  Coffin-Lowry syndrome (0190)
  X-linked mental retardation (other)

Major Diagnostic Criteria: **Megalencephaly**, mental retardation of a mild-to-moderate degree, and obesity are present. Affected males have macroorchidism.

Clinical Findings: Affected males are more severely retarded than females; however, both share the facial features of hypotelorism, prominent supraorbital ridges, broad nasal base, thick lower lip, and large ears. Diastema of upper central incisors and small upper lateral incisors are seen. Obesity is moderate, and stature is normal. **Megalencephaly** is present only in males.

Complications: Unknown.

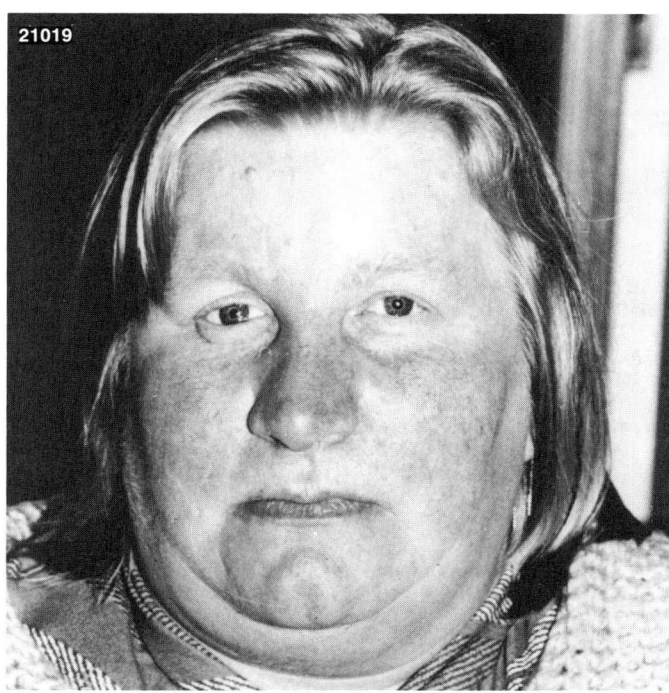

2640B-21019: Mildly retarded and obese mother of sons shown in 21020 & 21021.

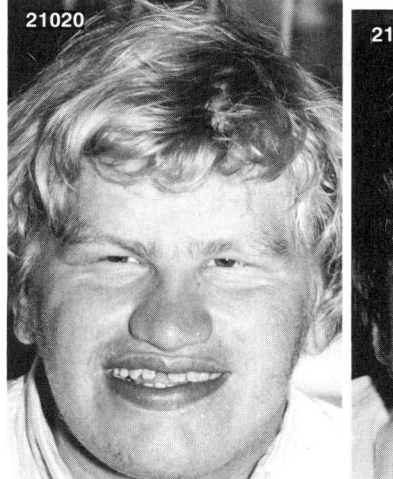 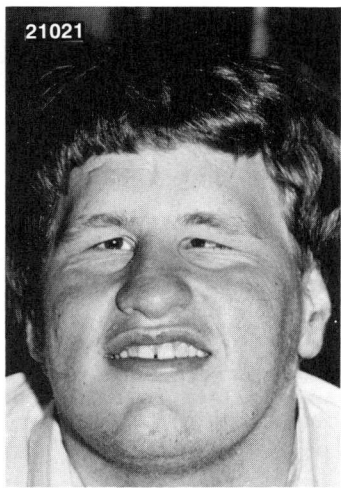

2640A-21020–21: X-linked mental retardation, Clark-Baraitser type; two moderately retarded affected brothers.

Associated Findings: None known.

Etiology: In one family, a mildly affected woman bore two moderately retarded sons and three normal children, including one daughter. This is compatible with X-linked inheritance with decreased expression in the female; however, autosomal dominant inheritance cannot be ruled out.

Pathogenesis: Unknown.

MIM No.: *30953

Sex Ratio: M2:F1 (observed).

Occurrence: One family has been reported in the literature.

Risk of Recurrence for Patient's Sib:
  See Part I, *Mendelian Inheritance.*

Risk of Recurrence for Patient's Child:
  See Part I, *Mendelian Inheritance.*

Age of Detectability: Evident during early childhood by mental retardation and recognizable facies.

Gene Mapping and Linkage: MRX1 (mental retardation, X-linked 1 (non-dysmorphic)) has been mapped to Xp11-q13.

Prevention: None known. Genetic counseling indicated.

Treatment: Unknown.

Prognosis: Apparently normal life span, mild-to-moderate mental retardation.

Detection of Carrier: Clinical examination of females for evidence of the trait is indicated.

Special Considerations: Many similarities exist between this condition and **X-linked mental retardation, Atkin type**. The differences, that those affected who were reported by Atkin were shorter and had **Eye, hypertelorism**, were considered significant by some but not all observers.

References:
Clark RD, Baraitser M: A new X-linked mental retardation syndrome. (Letter) Am J Med Genet 1987; 26:13–15.

CL004
BA058

Robin Dawn Clark
Michael Baraitser

X-linked mental retardation, Fitzsimmons type
*See HYPERKERATOSIS PALMOPLANTARIS-SPASTIC PARAPLEGIA-
RETARDATION*

X-LINKED MENTAL RETARDATION, FRAGILE X SYNDROME   2073

Includes:
> Chromosome, Marker X
> Fragile X chromosome
> Martin-Bell X-linked mental retardation
> Mental retardation, X-linked-marXq28
> X-linked fragile site
> X-linked mental retardation-macroorchidism
> X-linked mental retardation with fragile X

Excludes:
> **X-linked mental retardation, Renpenning type** (2920)
> X-linked mental retardation without the fragile X
> chromosome

Major Diagnostic Criteria: The definitive diagnosis depends upon finding the fragile X chromosome. Males with the fragile X

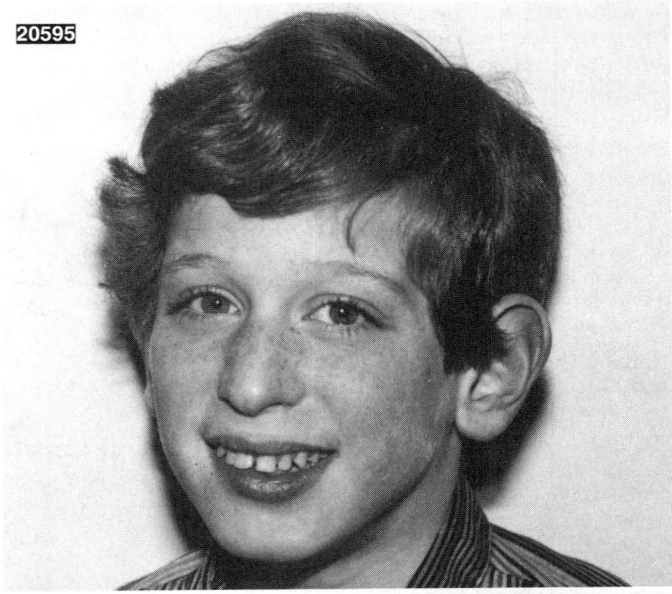

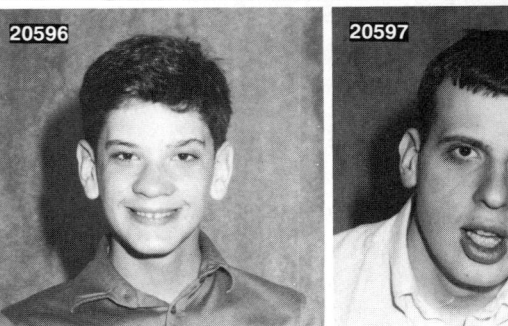

2073B-20595–97: Chromosome X, Fragile X syndrome; note long face with prominent ears and nose, large mouth and thick lips.

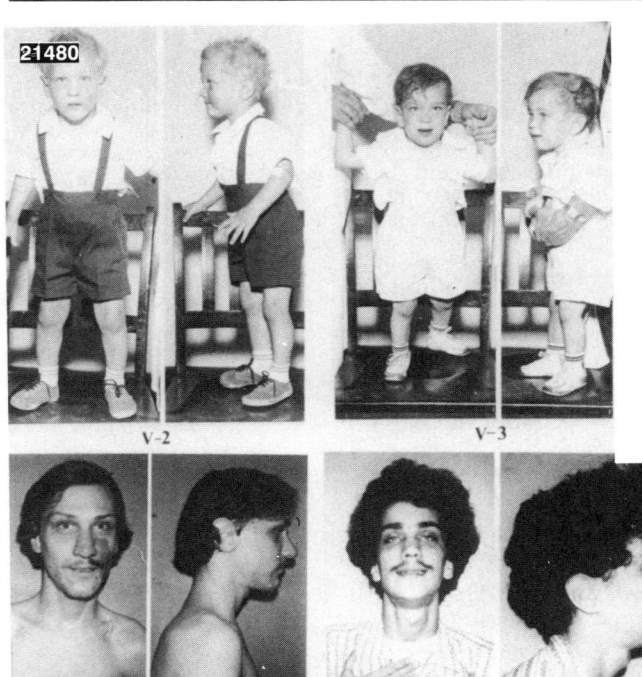

2073A-21480: Original siblings with fragile X described by Lubs (1969). Sib 1 on left at age 3 and 18. Sib 2 at right at 18 mo. and age 17. Both had low set, posteriorly angulated and slightly large ears and broadly based stance. Heads in both at age 17 and 18 are narrower than their normal brother's and father's (not shown). Ears and jaws have changed little in 15 years, although face is longer and more narrow in Sib 2. There is slight pectus and similar size nevus in Sib 1, age 3 and 18.

(abbreviated fra(X)) tend to have mental retardation, large testes and minor connective tissue manifestations. Females are usually of normal intelligence but may be mildly retarded with minor abnormalities. There is often a family history of mental retardation which follows an X-linked pattern of inheritance, but an increasingly large proportion of sporadic cases are now being recognized.

Clinical Findings: The degree of mental retardation in affected males varies from borderline normal to severe.

Unusually large testes (megalotestes or macroorchidism) are found in 80–90% of affected males after puberty. Testicular function is normal. Affected males may have one or both testes of normal size and there is some overlap with normal male testicular size. Prior to puberty, large testes are usually not present but have been described. Large testes (≥30 ml) are sometimes found in retarded males without the fragile X.

Craniofacial features which may be found in affected males are large head, prominent forehead, large ears, and a facies which becomes increasingly long and thin with age. The appearance of a long face is due to a shortening of the interzygomatic distance by about 1 cm. The mandible also becomes particularly prominent in some males after age 20.

Possible connective tissue manifestions include hyperextension of fingers in the majority of children, mild-to-severe pectus excavatum and floppy mitral valve in 80% over age 18 (ordinarily without complications). Occasionally long fingers and hand abnormalities are present. Fine skin and a high-arched palate also have been described.

Behavior is variable. Many are hyperactive, particularly during clinic visits and during the younger years. Management is usually possible at home.

Diagnosis of the fragile X in newborns and young infants on purely clinical criterial is currently difficult. Large, posteriorly rotated ears with minimal folding may be the only physical sign.

Clinical findings in female carriers: Appearance and intelligence are usually normal. A third of carriers have mild mental retardation. A long face has been described in affected carriers and connective tissue manifestations may occur. Increased twinning and fertility have been reported.

Complications: Autistic-like behavior occurs in 5–10% of males. Seizures may occur.

Associated Findings: None known.

Etiology: X-linked inheritance. In affected males, the X chromosome shows a lightstaining gap or fragile site at Xq27.3 in 4–60% cells. The distal portion of Xq may appear bisatellated. A gene at or very closely linked to this fragile site is responsible for the abnormalities in this syndrome. The gene behaves neither as a pure X-linked recessive or dominant gene and may be best described as semi-dominant with decreased penetrance in males.

The fragility of the X, which has not been demonstrated *in vivo*, is probably unrelated to these abnormalities and serves primarily as a marker for the responsible gene. In interspecies somatic cell hybrids, however, crossing-over occurs at the fragile cell hybrids, and may play a role in the pathogenosis of the abnormalities in man.

Males who express neither the clinical nor the cytogenetic manifestations occur and transmit the gene. This may occur in as many as 20% of males with this gene. Nearly all male and female siblings of such transmitting males are normal, as are their obligate carrier daughters. Several mechanisms, including inactivation of the locus during meiosis in certain females, and a stepwise premutation and mutation due to unequal crossing over have been postulated to explain these males. All mothers of sporadic cases are not, as once thought, carriers. Increasingly frequent diagnosis of sporadic cases on clinical grounds will require a new analysis of these data in the future. Isolation of the gene itself will ultimately permit resolution of these uncertainties and an explanation of the unusual genetic mechanisms.

Pathogenesis: Unknown.

MIM No.: *30955

POS No.: 3324

Sex Ratio: M1.0:F0.7

Occurrence: It is estimated that mental retardation due to the fra(X) occurs in at least 1:2,000 male births and is only slightly less frequent in females. The incidence is sufficient to class the fragile X as the most common inherited cause of mental retardation in males.

Risk of Recurrence for Patient's Sib: If mother is a carrier and has a normal intelligence at least 40% and probably 50% of male sibs are affected. One-half of daughters receive the chromosome, and 30–40% will be retarded, for a net risk of 15–20%. The risk of having a retarded female offspring may be higher for retarded heterozygotes.

If fra(X) studies fail to demonstrate any female carriers in the family, current data indicate that a quarter of male siblings and 7–8% of male cousins are affected. It should not be assumed that all mothers of affected, sporadic males are carriers.

Risk of Recurrence for Patient's Child: Few affected males have reproduced. Unaffected carrier males have no risk of affected sons. All daughters are obligate carriers but the risk of retardation is very low. The risks described above for obligate female carriers also hold for their daughters' offspring.

Age of Detectability: An affected male has not yet been diagnosed at birth on clinical grounds alone. During infancy and early childhood, developmental delay and large ears may permit the diagnosis to be suspected. The fragile X chromosome itself in males can be detected cytogenetically at anytime from lymphocytes. Many reports of the prenatal diagnosis of the fragile X in males have been published.

Gene Mapping and Linkage: FRAXA (fragile site, folic acid type, rare, fra(X)(q27.3)) has been mapped to Xq27.3.

Prevention: None known. Genetic counseling indicated.

Treatment: Speech therapy as well as early infant stimulation may be indicated. Psychological consultation in managing hyperactivity and autistic behavior may be helpful. Blind trials with folic acid or folate derivatives have not demonstrated significant improvement in either intelligence or behavior.

Prognosis: Mental retardation is reported in all fragile X expressing males, and in about 30–40% of carrier females.

Detection of Carrier: Blood (lymphocytes) must be cultured in a low-folate and low-thymidine medium such as medium 199 to demonstrate the fragile X. Alternatively, a folate antagonist such as methotrexate or FUdr which blocks thymidylate synthetase can be used. Many obligate carriers show no or a very low, frequency of fragile X positive cells. The demonstration of the fragile X in skin fibroblasts is sometimes difficult. In intelligent female carriers, the fragile X may be hard to detect because the frequency of the fragile X is usually low.

Special Considerations: Chromosome studies to detect the fragile X must be done under special culture medium conditions as described above. Ordinary culture conditions with complete medium obscure the expression of the fragile X. Therefore, if a male is suspected of having the fragile X and has not had special cytogenetic studies designed to screen for the fragile X, chromosome studies must be repeated under correct conditions. These conditions include medium 199 or the addtion of FUdr or methotrexate. The proportion of cells expressing the fragile X varies and 50–100 should be examined. Care should be taken to distinguish the Xq27.3 fragile site from the similar but non-risk bearing fragile site at Xq27.2.

The fragile X can occur in normal males who can transmit it, but not show it cytogenetically. Prenatal diagnosis is still difficult and should only be undertaken in laboratories with significant experience in the detection of the fragile X. Detection of the fragile X from fetal blood from periumbilical blood may be the prenatal diagnostic procedure of choice.

Linkage studies of the fragile X site with DNA markers are available and of use in carrier testing and genetic counseling, but several problems currently limit their usefulness for prenatal diagnosis. The gene order from proximal to distal is DXS51 (a DNA marker), F9 (factor IX), fragile X DXS52 (a DNA marker) and DX515 (still another DNA marker). The recombinational distances currently average about 7% from DXS51 to F9, 22% from F9 to fra(X), 13% from fra(X) to DXS52 and 2% from DXS52 to DXS15. There appears to be genetic heterogeneity with tight linkage (about 18%) between F9 and fra(X) in some families and loose linkage (about 35%) in others. Because of these relatively large recombination distances, the final decision regarding of the fragile X is still best made by its cytogenetic demonstration.

The authors wish to thank Thomas W. Glover and Grant R. Sutherland for their contributions to an earlier version of this article.

Support Groups:
NJ; Bridgeton; National Fragile X Support Group
CO; Denver; The Fragile X Foundation

References:
Lubs HA: A marker X chromosome. Am J Hum Genet 1969; 21:231–244.
Sutherland GR: Heritable fragile sites on human chromosomes. I. Factors affecting expression in lymphocyte culture. Am J Hum Genet 1979; 31:125–135.
Jacobs PA, et al: X-linked mental retardations: a study of 7 families. Am J Med Genet 1980; 7:471–489.
Turner G, et al: Heterozygous expression of X-linked mental retardation and X-chromosome marker fra (X)(q27). New Engl J Med 1980; 303:662–664.
Turner G, et al: X-linked mental retardation, macro-orchidism, and the Xq27 fragile site. J Pediatr 1980; 96:837–841.

Sutherland GR: The fragile X chromosome. Int Rev Cytol 1983; 81:107–141.

Sutherland GR, Hecht F: Fragile sites on human chromosomes. New York: Oxford University Press, 1985.

Brown WT, et al.: Multilocus analysis of the fragile X syndrome. Hum Genet 1988; 78:201–205.

Fryns JP, et al.: A peculiar subphenotype in the fra (X) syndrome: extreme obesity - short stature - stubby hands and feet - diffuse hyperpigmentation. Clin Genet 1988; 32:388–392.

Schwartz CE, et al.: Fragile X monograph. Proc Greenwood Genet Ctr 1988; 7:76–117.

Spano LM, Opitz JM: Bibliography on X-linked mental retardation, the fragile X and related subjects. Am J Med Genet 1988; 30:31–60.

Bridge PJ, Lillicrap DP: Molecular diagnosis of the fragile X [Fra (X)] syndrome: calculation of risks based on flanking DNA markers in small phase-unknown families. Am J Med Genet 1989; 33:92–99.

LU002   **Herbert A. Lubs**
HE007   **Frederick Hecht**

X-LINKED MENTAL RETARDATION, GOLABI-ITO-HALL TYPE   3199

Includes: Golabi-Ito-Hall syndrome

Excludes: X-linked mental retardation (other)

Major Diagnostic Criteria: Mental retardation, postnatal growth deficiency, postnatal **Microcephaly**, narrow triangular face, anteverted ears, upslanted palpebral fissures, epicanthal folds.

Clinical Findings: Mental retardation (one with IQ estimated at 23); postnatal growth deficiency (3/3) noted during the first year of life; postnatal **Microcephaly** (3/3); narrow triangular face (2/3); anteverted ears (3/3); mild hearing loss (1/3); up-slanted palpebral fissures with epicanthal folds (3/3) and laterally displaced inner canthi (2/3). Thin upper lip appeared to be present in (3/3) photographs. Congenital heart defect (**Atrial septal defects** in one case, questionable in the second). Brittle, dry hair (2/3); asymmetric chest (1/3), and chest malformation (1/3). Hypospadias (1/3).

Pertinent normal features include normal testicular size (two prepubertal, one postpubertal), normal results of urine amino acid analysis (two cases reported), and normal chromosomes (one case reported).

Complications: One case developed petit mal seizures.

Associated Findings: Possible congenital heart defect.

Etiology: X-linked recessive inheritance.

Pathogenesis: Unknown.

MIM No.: *30953

POS No.: 3590

Sex Ratio: M3:F0 (observed).

Occurrence: Three individuals in one Caucasian family (two boys, sons of sisters, and their mother's brother) have been clinically evaluated or had their hospital records reviewed.

Risk of Recurrence for Patient's Sib:
See Part I, *Mendelian Inheritance.*

Risk of Recurrence for Patient's Child:
See Part I, *Mendelian Inheritance.*

Age of Detectability: During the first year of life.

Gene Mapping and Linkage: MRX1 (mental retardation, X-linked 1 (non dysmorphic)) has been mapped to Xp11-q13.

Prevention: None known. Genetic counseling indicated.

Treatment: Unknown.

Prognosis: Normal life span is presumed; however, three suspected cases reported in the same family died before ten years of age.

Detection of Carrier: Unknown.

References:
Golabi M, et al: A new X-linked multiple congenital anomalies/mental retardation syndrome. Am J Med Genet 1984; 17:367–374.

AR011   **J. Fernando Arena**
LU002   **Herbert A. Lubs**

X-linked mental retardation, Holmes-Gang type
See X-LINKED MENTAL RETARDATION-CRANIOFACIAL ABNORMALITIES-CLUB FOOT

X-LINKED MENTAL RETARDATION, MARFANOID HABITUS TYPE   2921

Includes: Marfanoid habitus and X-linked mental retardation

Excludes:
  Aicardi syndrome (2320)
  Corpus callosum agenesis (0220)
  Facio-neuro-skeletal syndrome (2339)
  FG syndrome
  X-linked mental retardation (other)

Major Diagnostic Criteria: The combination of psychomotor retardation (usually moderate) with a relatively tall, thin (Marfanoid) habitus; a long, thin face; a high-arched palate; and joint hyperextensibility in one or more persons consistent with X-linked inheritance.

Clinical Findings: The first four males described were from one kindred. All were retarded (IQ range, 40–60) with tall stature (>75th percentile), a large head (>90th percentile), a high-arched palate, small mandible, and hypernasal speech. Three are asthenic (height ≤50th percentile) with long narrow faces and joint hyperextensibility. Despite long fingers, none showed true arachnodactyly or an increased arm span. Other features included **Pectus excavatum** (noted in two) and **Atrial septal defects** (in one case), and large testes (≥ 90th percentile in three).

All test negative for **X-linked mental retardation, Fragile X syndrome**. Complete **Corpus callosum agenesis** was seen in one patient, with partial absence in his brother. One had seizures. Three were poorly coordinated, and all four had attention deficits. Behavior was otherwise variable, showing jocularity, aggressiveness, dependency, and autistic-like mannerisms.

Two further pairs of retarded male siblings (IQ: 56–70), who share similar craniofacial features and the slender, Marfanoid habitus have been reported (Fryns & Buttiens, 1987). These individuals differ, however, in that only one measures below the 75th percentile in height, three show a HC ≤ 50th percentile, and two have short palates with hypernasality. Arm spans exceed height and halluces are short in all, while two have kyphosis and one has kyphoscoliosis. X-rays show an occasional shortening of some metacarpals, metatarsals, and/or proximal phalanges. Testes are normal in two and small in two, with elevated follicle-stimulating hormone levels in one of these. Behavior varies from normal to shy or hyperactive.

All five mothers are of normal intelligence; one has an increased arm span. A female sib from the original kindred had a low-average IQ and was tall and thin with a high-arched palate, retro-micrognathia, and a high-pitched, hypernasal voice. She has had a son who is reported to be "slow," but has not been evaluated.

Complications: Seizures; dental malocclusion and hypernasal speech secondary to craniofacial disproportion and possible velopharyngeal insufficiency; and aggressive or autistic-like behavior.

Associated Findings: It is unclear whether the agenesis of the corpus callosum and the septal defect are an intrinsic part of the syndrome or are associated findings.

Etiology: X-linked recessive inheritance, but one presumed carrier female has mild morphologic changes as well as lower than expected intellectual function.

Pathogenesis: The abnormal gene presumably has a deleterious effect on brain and connective tissue development.

MIM No.: 30952

POS No.: 3705

Sex Ratio: For significant retardation, the ratio is probably M1:F0, but mild manifestations may be seen in an unknown, but probably small, number of female carriers.

Occurrence: Eight males from three kindreds have been documented.

Risk of Recurrence for Patient's Sib:
See Part I, *Mendelian Inheritance.*

Risk of Recurrence for Patient's Child:
See Part I, *Mendelian Inheritance.*

Age of Detectability: Hypotonia and hyperextensibility may be noticeable at birth, especially in a family at risk. Abnormalities of the corpus callosum should likewise be detectable. However, this family was not identified until psychomotor retardation had persisted for several years.

Gene Mapping and Linkage: Unknown.

Prevention: None known. Genetic counseling indicated.

Treatment: Usual intervention for secondary complications, e.g., anticonvulsants, orthodontics, as well as exceptional student education and various therapy modalities as indicated.

Prognosis: Normal life span is presumed. Vocational training has permitted two affected males to be employed under supervision. No progressive cardiovascular symptoms secondary to the apparent connective tissue involvement, except for a questionable prolapsed mitral valve, have been detected.

Detection of Carrier: Female first degree relatives of affected males, who have a Marfanoid habitus, lower than anticipated intelligence, with or without evidence of alterations in the corpus callosum, are probably carriers.

References:
Lujan JE, et al.: A form of X-linked mental retardation with marfanoid habitus. Am J Med Genet 1984; 17:311–322. †
Fryns JP, Buttiens M: X-linked mental retardation with marfanoid habitus. Am J Med Genet 1987; 28:267–274. †

CA016

Mary Esther Carlin

X-LINKED MENTAL RETARDATION, RENPENNING TYPE — 2920

Includes: Renpenning syndrome

Excludes: X-linked mental retardation (other)

Major Diagnostic Criteria: Small head, small testes, and short stature in a pedigree with X-linked mental retardation.

Clinical Findings: All manifestations are variable. Most individuals have severe mental retardation (IQ less than 45 or unmeasurable), a head circumference ranging from the second to the 20th percentile, height less than the 20th percentile, and small testes (usually less than the 25th percentile). One individual with a small head, small testes, and short stature had an IQ of 87. Striking changes occur with age. A relatively normal appearance may be replaced by a marked angulation of the face, loss of facial fat, and development of a somewhat triangular facial appearance. In one kindred, two of four affected individuals showed hyperextensibility of fingers without pectus or other connective tissue signs. Aggressive behavior and repetitive speech are frequently described. The majority have been institutionalized. Laboratory tests for **X-linked mental retardation, Fragile X syndrome** are negative.

Complications: Unknown.

Associated Findings: None known.

Etiology: X-linked recessive inheritance.

Pathogenesis: Unknown.

MIM No.: *30950, 30954

Sex Ratio: M1:F0

Occurrence: At least three kindreds have been reported, including a Dutch Mennonite pedigree from Alberta and Saskatchewan.

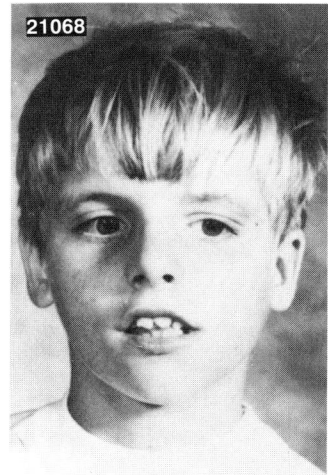
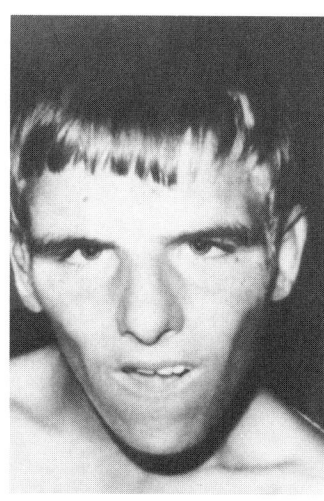
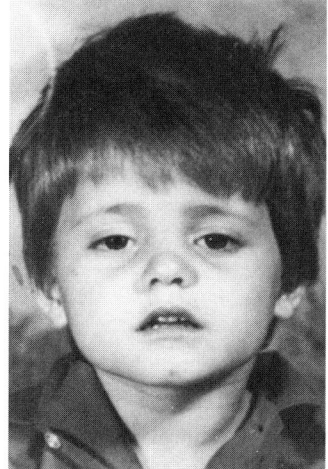
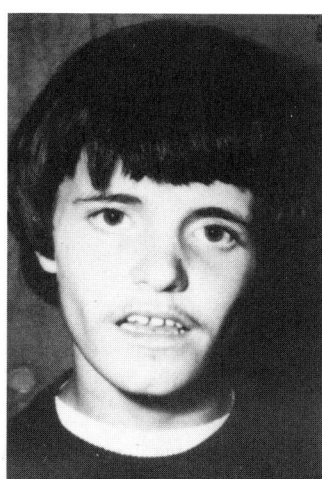

2920-21068: Siblings showing changes in facial appearance with increasing angulation and loss of facial fat with age (sibling 1, aged 12 and 25, upper row, and sibling 2, aged 5 and 20 years, lower row).

Risk of Recurrence for Patient's Sib:
See Part I, *Mendelian Inheritance.*

Risk of Recurrence for Patient's Child:
See Part I, *Mendelian Inheritance.*

Age of Detectability: No data are available for head or testicular size at birth. Since appearance may not become obviously abnormal until the late teens, early diagnosis will probably be difficult unless small head and body size or delayed development are observed in a member of a family with X-linked mental retardation.

Gene Mapping and Linkage: MRX2 (mental retardation, X-linked 2) has been provisionally mapped to Xp22.3-p22.2.

Prevention: None known. Genetic counseling indicated.

Treatment: Unknown.

Prognosis: Normal life span is presumed, with severe retardation most frequent. One individual with a low-normal IQ is known. No major organ complications have been reported.

Detection of Carrier: Only for obligate carriers known from pedigree.

Special Considerations: The original family report by Renpenning et al (1962) demonstrated only nonspecific mental retardation. A restudy by Fox et al in 1980 delineated the major diagnostic criteria and demonstrated the absence of the fragile X. In the interim, the term *Renpenning syndrome* came to be used synonymously with *nonspecific mental retardation*. This practice should be discontinued, and the term *Renpenning syndrome* should be confined to the context of this specific condition.

References:
Renpenning HJ, et al.: Familial sex-linked mental retardation. Can Med Assoc J 1962; 87:954–956.
Fox P, et al.: X-linked mental retardation: Renpenning revisited. Am J Med Genet 1980; 7:491–495.
Sutherland GR, et al.: Linkage studies with the gene for an X-linked syndrome of mental retardation, microcephaly and spastic diplegia (MRX2). Am J Med Genet 1988; 30:493–508.

LU002   **Herbert A. Lubs**

X-linked mental retardation, Schimke type
   See X-LINKED MENTAL RETARDATION-CHOREOATHETOSIS
X-linked mental retardation, Scott type
   See CRANIO-DIGITAL SYNDROME-MENTAL RETARDATION, SCOTT TYPE
X-linked mental retardation, Smith-Fineman-Myers type
   See SMITH-FINEMAN-MYERS SYNDROME
X-linked mental retardation, Urban type (possibly)
   See X-LINKED MENTAL RETARDATION-SHORT STATURE-OBESITY-HYPOGONADISM
X-linked mental retardation, Vasquez type (possibly)
   See X-LINKED MENTAL RETARDATION-SHORT STATURE-OBESITY-HYPOGONADISM

X-LINKED MENTAL RETARDATION-BASAL GANGLION DISORDER   2841

Includes:
   Basal ganglion disorder-mental retardation
   Parkinson disease, early onset-mental retardation
   Waisman syndrome

Excludes:
   Contractures-muscle atrophy-oculomotor apraxia (2832)
   Microcephaly (0659)
   X-linked mental retardation, Atkin type (2840)
   X-linked mental retardation, Fragile X syndrome (2073)
   X-linked mental retardation, Renpenning type (2920)
   X-linked mental retardation (other)

Major Diagnostic Criteria: **Megalencephaly** with increased, nonprogressive, fronto-occipital circumference and frontal bossing; average stature; no macroorchidism. Neurologic symptomatology includes cogwheel rigidity, postural changes, parkinsonian tremors, and shuffling gait. Seizures may be present.

Clinical Findings: Clinical signs manifest in early childhood in the form of psychomotor delays, particularly in areas of speech and language; **Megalencephaly** (on X-ray the calvaria was larger than the facial bones); hyperactivity and seizures in some of the affected boys. There were no signs of dysmorphism, testicular size was normal, and physical appearance resembled that of unaffected family members.

The onset of neurologic symptomatology varied from age two years to later in childhood; all affected males gradually developed tremors, mild choreoathetoid movements, upper and lower limb rigidity of the cogwheel type, and shuffling gait.

In adulthood, persistent frontal lobe reflexes were present, with resting appendicular axial tremors at 3–6 cycles per second. There was paucity of movement, and gait was slow and stooped with poor recovery of balance. Speech was characterized by hypokinetic dysarthria. Affect was appropriate. IQ ranged from 30 to 70 in affected family members.

It is unclear whether the disorder is very slowly progressive or whether differences occurring with age are attributable to neurologic change rather than time progression. The oldest affected male in the family is currently in his late 50s and is not thought to be deteriorating.

Cytogenetic evaluation has been normal in all affected individuals.

Complications: Seizures ranging from grand mal to EEG abnormalities. Affected individuals have difficulty living independently but are able to function with a moderate degree of supervision.

Associated Findings: Two of the affected males had eye abnormalities, consisting of a partial iris coloboma in one and of thinning of the right cornea with a tear in the Descemet membrane in the other.

Etiology: Presumably X-linked recessive inheritance.

Pathogenesis: The neurologic signs are indicative of basal ganglia impairment. No pathologic evaluation has been done on any affected individual.

MIM No.: 31151

Sex Ratio: M13:F:1 (observed). There was one minimally affected female in the described family.

Occurrence: One kindred has been documented in the literature.

Risk of Recurrence for Patient's Sib:
   See Part I, *Mendelian Inheritance*.

Risk of Recurrence for Patient's Child:
   See Part I, *Mendelian Inheritance*. No affected males are known to have reproduced.

Age of Detectability: During early infancy, by developmental delays and macrocephaly.

Gene Mapping and Linkage: The gene has been linked (lod score >5.0) to Xq27-qter markers, DXS52, DXS15, F8, DXS134

Prevention: None known. Genetic counseling indicated.

Treatment: Early childhood special education. L-dopa has been tried experimentally and did not result in measurable improvement.

Prognosis: Life span appears to unaffected, and progression, if present, is extremely slow. The oldest living affected individual is in his 50s.

Detection of Carrier: Unknown.

Support Groups:
   New York; American Parkinson Disease Association
   New York; Parkinson's Disease Foundation
   Chicago; United Parkinson Foundation (UPF)
   CA; Newport Beach; Parkinson's Educational Program (PEP USA)
   FL; Miami; National Parkinson Foundation

References:
Laxova R, et al.: An X-linked recessive basal ganglia disorder with mental retardation. Am J Med Genet 1985; 21:681–689.

LA033   **Renata Laxova**

X-LINKED MENTAL RETARDATION-CHOREOATHETOSIS   2830

Includes:
   Choreoathetosis-mental retardation, X-linked
   Schimke X-linked mental retardation syndrome
   X-linked mental retardation, Schimke type

Excludes:
   Borjeson-Forssman-Lehmann syndrome (2272)
   Lesch-Nyhan syndrome (0588)
   Paraplegia, familial spastic (0295)
   X-linked mental retardation, Fragile X syndrome (2073)
   X-linked mental retardation, Renpenning type (2920)
   X-linked mental retardation-growth-hearing and genital defects (2480)
   X-linked mental retardation (other)

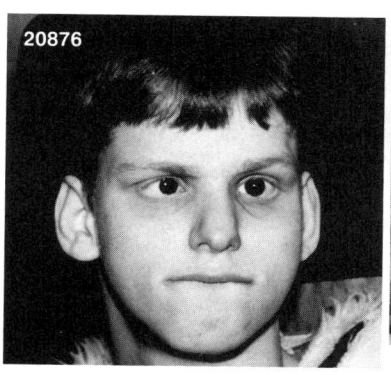
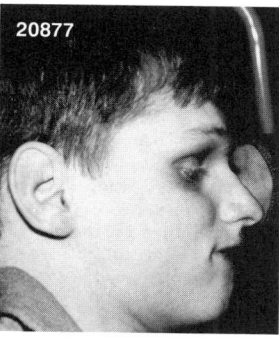

2830-20876–77: X-linked mental retardation-choreoathetosis.

Major Diagnostic Criteria: Childhood onset of choreoathetosis, mental and growth retardation, and postnatal **Microcephaly**.

Clinical Findings: Hypotonia is evident at birth. Choreoathetosis begins in the first year of life; followed later by progressive spasticity. Head circumference is normal at birth, but postnatal **Microcephaly** develops in the first few months. Growth velocity likewise decelerates early. Strabismus is common, and the eyes are sunken. Nerve deafness is present. Feeding difficulties have been noted. Mental retardation is profound.

Complications: Progressive inanition, bronchopneumonia, and contractures.

Associated Findings: None known.

Etiology: Presumably X-linked recessive inheritance.

Pathogenesis: Unknown. One autopsied case showed cystic changes in basal ganglia, spongy degeneration, calcification and gliosis in the thalamus and globus pallidus, and a marked loss of Purkinje cells in the cerebellum.

MIM No.: 31284

Sex Ratio: M1:F0

Occurrence: Four cases from two kinships have been reported in the literature.

Risk of Recurrence for Patient's Sib:
See Part I, *Mendelian Inheritance*.

Risk of Recurrence for Patient's Child:
See Part I, *Mendelian Inheritance*.

Age of Detectability: During the first few months of life.

Gene Mapping and Linkage: Unknown.

Prevention: None known. Genetic counseling indicated.

Treatment: Supportive.

Prognosis: Survival dependent on intensity of supportive care. The oldest male died in his 20s.

Detection of Carrier: Unknown.

References:
Schimke RN, et al.: A new X-linked syndrome comprising progressive basal ganglion dysfunction, mental and growth retardation, external ophthalmoplegia, postnatal microcephaly, and deafness. Am J Med Genet 1984; 17:323–332.

R. Neil Schimke

X-LINKED MENTAL RETARDATION-CLASPED THUMB   **2291**

Includes:
    Adducted thumb-mental retardation
    Bianchine-Lewis syndrome
    Gareis-Mason syndrome
    Mental retardation-aplasia-shuffling gait-adducted thumbs
      (MASA)
    Thumb, congenital clasped-mental retardation
    X-linked mental retardation-clasped-thumb syndrome

Excludes:
    Thumb, adducted thumb syndrome (2075)
    Thumb, clasped (0175)
    X-linked mental retardation, Fragile X syndrome (2073)
    X-linked mental retardation, Renpenning type (2920)
    X-linked mental retardation (other)

Major Diagnostic Criteria: Congenital flexion-adduction contractures of the thumbs with hypoplastic thenar musculature, and mental retardation.

Clinical Findings: *Musculoskeletal abnormalities*: Thumb contractures (13/13) which are variable in severity, and most often symmetric, with hypoplastic thenar eminence. Mild short stature (8/13); lordosis and/or kyphosis (8/13); pes planus (3/13); pes cavus

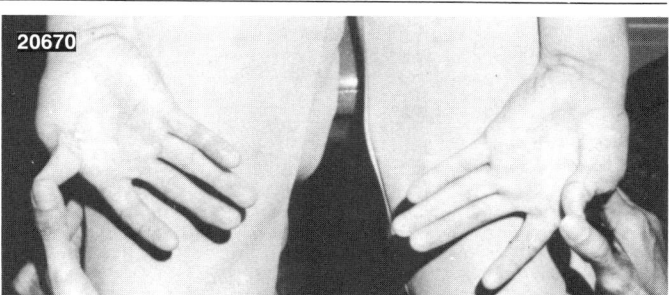
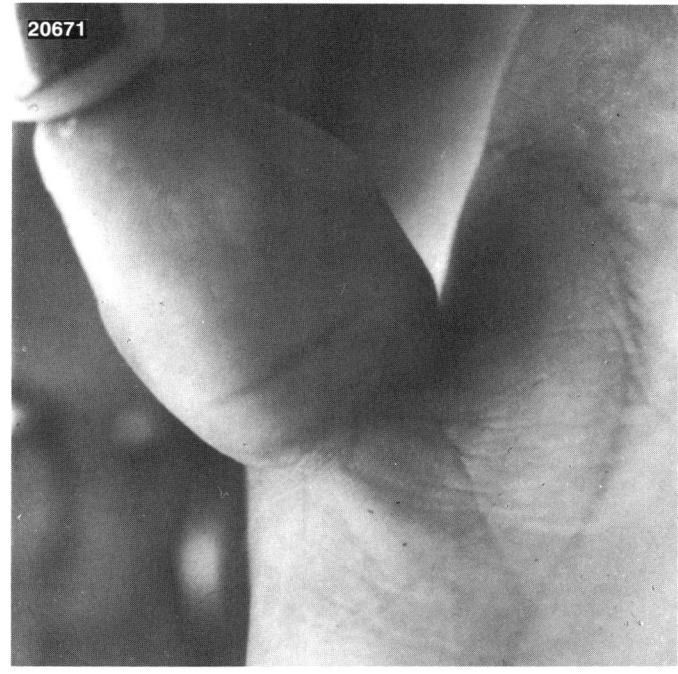

2291-20670–71: Mental retardation-clasped thumb syndrome, Mason-Gareis type; note adducted thumbs with hypoplastic thenar musculature in full view and close up.

(1/13); calcaneovalgus deformity (1/13); and flexion contracture of the second finger (1/13).

CNS abnormalities: Mental retardation (13/13); Lower extremity spasticity (5/13) (an additional two had shuffling gait and hyperactive lower extremity deep tendon reflexes); **Microcephaly** (4/13). Speech abnormalities are variable: All kindreds have individuals with speech abnormalities; the most severely affected was apparently aphasic when examined at eight years of age. Developmental milestones range from severely delayed to normal for the first three years. Developmental history and intelligence of obligate carrier females have not been examined.

Pertinent normal features: Testicular size is normal in postpubertal males. Facial features are normal with no malar or maxillary hypoplasia, enlarged ears, or prominent chin. Chromosomes are normal in all kindreds; one kindred has been evaluated at the sub-band level (maximally "stretched"), and three kindreds tested negative for the presence of **X-linked mental retardation, Fragile X syndrome**.

Unlike the cortical thumbing seen in children with **Cerebral palsy**, and the prenatal contractures seen in the varying **Arthrogryposis**, the contractures associated with this condition are present at birth and are anatomically abnormal, with complete extension impossible.

Complications: Pincer grasp may be compromised.

Associated Findings: **Heart, tetralogy of Fallot** with a double aortic arch, and a peripheral pulmonic stenosis; hairy nevus.

Etiology: X-linked recessive inheritance, with carrier female at risk, presumably from Lyonization. In the four kindreds described, there have been no instances of male-to-male inheritance (in at least three generations), and in three families, four obligate carrier females had affected children with two spouses.

Pathogenesis: Unknown.

MIM No.: 30335, 30925

POS No.: 3432

Sex Ratio: M41:F2 (observed).

Occurrence: Four kindreds have been reported; two Mexican-American, and two Anglo-American. Forty-one affected males and two affected females have been documented, with 20 obligate carriers and 35 females at 50% risk of carrier status.

Risk of Recurrence for Patient's Sib:
See Part I, *Mendelian Inheritance*.

Risk of Recurrence for Patient's Child:
See Part I, *Mendelian Inheritance*.

Age of Detectability: Abduction and extension of the thumb may be seen in the fetus prior to 16 weeks gestation with diagnostic ultrasound. The diagnosis should be approached with great caution, since normal fetuses hold their fingers flexed and thumb flexed and adducted for prolonged periods of time. Mildly affected fetuses with little limitation of extension will not be detectable. The thenar muscle dysplasia is presumed to occur during organogenesis, although this presumption is not proven, and in fact may occur later in pregnancy.

Gene Mapping and Linkage: Unknown.

Prevention: None known. Genetic counseling indicated.

Treatment: Individuals in two families have shown hypoplastic or absent extensor pollicis brevis and longus tendons. Physical therapy alone has not helped mobility and function of affected thumbs. The thumb anomaly may be treatable with orthopedic surgery in some cases.

Prognosis: Normal life span is presumed, with a range of developmental delay from none to severe; mental retardation varies from mild to profound, and some individuals appear to be in the dull normal range. Kyphosis, scoliosis, and lumbar lordosis may develop, as well as spastic lower extremities.

Detection of Carrier: Unknown.

Special Considerations: Clasped thumbs from congenitally hypoplastic extensor muscles have been described as an isolated anomaly, and also as associated with X-linked recessive hydro-

cephalus from aqueductal stenosis (see **Hydrocephaly**). These conditions must be differentiated by appropriate diagnostic tests.

References:
Bianchine JW, Lewis RC: The MASA syndrome: a new heritable mental retardation syndrome. Clin Genet 1974; 5:298–306. *
Gareis FJ, Mason JD: X-linked mental retardation associated with bilateral clasp thumb anomaly. Am J Med Genet 1984; 17:333–338.
Yeatman GW: Mental retardation-clasped thumb syndrome. Am J Med Genet 1984; 17:339–344.
Roberts RM, Lewandowski RC: X-linked mental retardation-clasped thumb syndrome (Gareis-Mason syndrome): further delineation of the phenotype. (Abstract) Dysmorphol Clin Genet 1987; 1:75 only.

R0003   **Richard M. Roberts**

X-linked mental retardation-clasped-thumb syndrome
See X-LINKED MENTAL RETARDATION-CLASPED THUMB

X-LINKED MENTAL RETARDATION-CRANIOFACIAL ABNORMALITIES-CLUB FOOT   3200

Includes:
X   Holmes-Gang syndrome
X   X-linked mental retardation, Holmes-Gang type

Excludes:
FG syndrome
X-linked mental retardation (other)

Major Diagnostic Criteria: Retarded psychomotor development. Peculiar facies with epicanthic folds; flat nasal bridge and anteverted nostrils; low-set ears; and thin upper lip. Club foot deformity and early death.

Clinical Findings: Retarded psychomotor development (3/3); **Microcephaly** (1/3); narrow skull (1/3); large anterior fontanel (3/3); low-set ears (3/3); epicanthal folds (3/3); flat nasal bridge (3/3); short nose with anteverted nostrils (2/3); club foot deformity (3/3); and early death before the second year of life (two at six months; one at 16 months). Autopsy findings in two cases revealed small brain (2/2), kidney hypoplasia and dysplasia (1/2), and hyperplasia and immaturity of pancreatic islet (1/2). The severity of the mental retardation in this disorder is underscored by the fact that none of the three males had any meaningful response to his environment.

Complications: Three cases died before the second year of life from infection.

Associated Findings: Oligohydramnios, abnormal teeth, hypotonia and a harsh, grating cry were present in one patient.

Etiology: Presumably X-linked recessive inheritance.

Pathogenesis: Unknown.

MIM No.: *30953

POS No.: 4082

Sex Ratio: M1:F0

Occurrence: Three individuals in one Caucasian family (one boy and two of his mother's brothers) have been clinically evaluated or had their hospital records reviewed.

Risk of Recurrence for Patient's Sib:
See Part I, *Mendelian Inheritance*.

Risk of Recurrence for Patient's Child:
See Part I, *Mendelian Inheritance*.

Age of Detectability: During the first year of life.

Gene Mapping and Linkage: MRX1 (mental retardation, X-linked 1 (non-dysmorphic)) has been mapped to Xp11-q13.

Prevention: None known. Genetic counseling indicated.

Treatment: Unknown.

Prognosis: The three reported cases died during the first 16 months of life.

Detection of Carrier: The two reported obligate carriers had normal intelligence and appearance.

References:
Holmes LB, Gang DL: An X-linked mental retardation syndrome with craniofacial abnormalities, microcephaly and club foot. Am J Med Genet 1984; 17:375–382.

AR011
LU002

J. Fernando Arena
Herbert A. Lubs

X-LINKED MENTAL RETARDATION-DYSTONIC MOVEMENTS OF THE HANDS   3251

Includes:

Hands, dystonic movements-mental retardation, X-linked
Partington mental retardation

Excludes: X-linked mental retardation (other)

Major Diagnostic Criteria: Mild-to-moderate mental retardation; episodic dystonic movements of the hands; dysarthria; normal height; normal head circumference and facial features.

Clinical Findings: Mild to moderate mental retardation (10/10); dystonic spasms of hands (9/9); dysarthria (7/8); normal height (6/6); normal head circumference (5/6); normal facial features (6/6); postural flexion and abnormal gait (4/6); seizures (2/6); strabismus (1/1); spastic quadriplegia (1/1); death during infancy (2/10).

Complications: Unknown.

Associated Findings: None known.

Etiology: Presumably X-linked recessive inheritance.

Pathogenesis: Unknown.

Sex Ratio: M10:F0 observed.

Occurrence: One family with ten affected males has been reported.

Risk of Recurrence for Patient's Sib:
See Part I, *Mendelian Inheritance.*

Risk of Recurrence for Patient's Child:
See Part I, *Mendelian Inheritance.*

Age of Detectability: During childhood.

Gene Mapping and Linkage: DNA markers DXS41 (p99.6), DXS206 (SJ2.3), DXS84 (p754 and p754–11), DXS (p58.1), DXYS1 (pDP34) and DXS52 (St14) were highly informative. The maximum lod score was 2.11 at O of 0.00 for DXS41. This represents odds in favor of linkage of more than 100:1. These markers are spread between Xp21 and Xcen. The regional localization for the gene for this type of XLMR is likely therefore to be Xpter→Xp21.

Prevention: None known. Genetic counseling indicated.

Treatment: Unknown.

Prognosis: Unknown.

Detection of Carrier: Unknown.

References:
Partington M W, et al.: X-linked mental retardation with dystonic movements of the hands. Am J Med Genet 1988; 30:251–262.

AR011
LU002

J. Fernando Arena
Herbert A. Lubs

X-LINKED MENTAL RETARDATION-GROWTH-HEARING AND GENITAL DEFECTS   2480

Includes:

Juberg-Marsidi mental retardation
Mental retardation-growth/hearing/genital defects, X-linked
Microcephaly, X-linked
Vasquez syndrome

Excludes:
Paraplegia, familial spastic (0295)
X-linked mental retardation, Fragile X syndrome (2073)
X-linked mental retardation (other)

Major Diagnostic Criteria: 1) Mental retardation, severe; 2) growth retardation; 3) delayed bone age; 4) deafness; 5) ocular

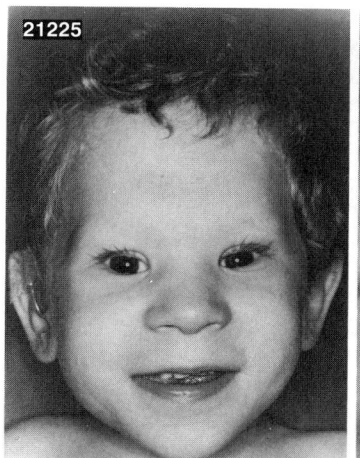
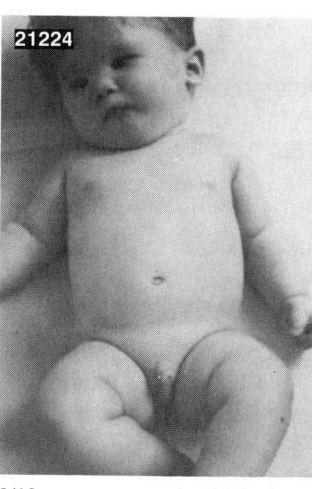

2480A-21225: The proband at 2 8/12 years; note the high forehead, small palpebral fissures, and flat nasal bridge. **21224:** The proband's younger uncle at age 10 months; note the esotropia and microgenitalism.

abnormalities; 6) flat nasal bridge; 7) microgenitalism, small scrotum with cryptorchidism, and small penis; 8) onychodystrophy of fingers and toes.

Clinical Findings: Birth weight <2,500 g (3/3); birth length <50 cm (3/3); growth <3rd percentile (3/3); bone age retarded (3/3); hearing impairment, mild to severe (3/3); narrow palpebral fissures (2/3); strabismus (2/3); epicanthi (1/3); light retinal pigmentation (2/3); flat nasal bridge (3/3); cryptorchidism (3/3); rudimentary scrotum (3/3); small penis (3/3); and severe mental retardation (3/3).

The *Vasquez syndrome* (Vasquez et al, 1979) has additional features of obesity and gynecomastia.

Complications: Those commonly associated with severe mental retardation.

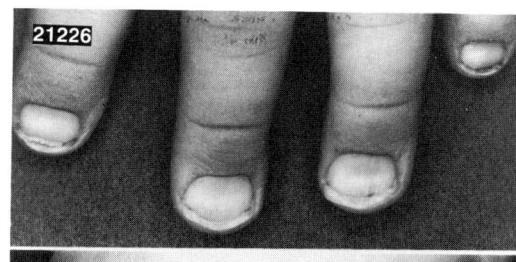
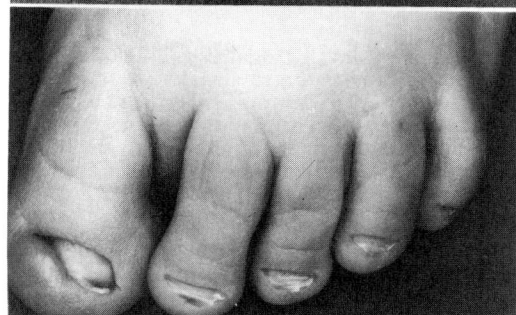

2480B-21226: Note the flat, broad concave fingernails and dysplastic, ingrown toenails.

Associated Findings: High forehead, hemicerebral atrophy, dysplastic ears, highly arched palate.

Etiology: X-linked recessive inheritance.

Pathogenesis: Unknown.

MIM No.: *30959

POS No.: 3584

Sex Ratio: M3:F0 (observed from one kindred).

Occurrence: One kindred each has been reported from Ohio and France.

Risk of Recurrence for Patient's Sib:
See Part I, *Mendelian Inheritance.*

Risk of Recurrence for Patient's Child:
See Part I, *Mendelian Inheritance.*

Age of Detectability: In the neonatal period, by clinical findings.

Gene Mapping and Linkage: Unknown.

Prevention: None known. Genetic counseling indicated.

Treatment: Early childhood educational intervention and special education.

Prognosis: Less than normal life span, perhaps less than 10 years.

Detection of Carrier: Unknown.

References:
Vasquez SB, et al.: X-linked hypogonadism, gynecomastia, mental retardation, short stature, and obesity: a new syndrome. J Pediatr 1979; 94:56–60.
Juberg RC, Marsidi I: A new form of X-linked mental retardation with growth retardation, deafness, and microgenitalism. Am J Hum Genet 1980; 32:714–722. * †
Mattei JF, et al.: X-linked mental retardation, growth retardation, deafness and microgenitalism: a second familial report. Clin Genet 1983; 23:70–74.

JU000   **Richard C. Juberg**

X-linked mental retardation-hypotonia
See X-LINKED MENTAL RETARDATION-MUSCULAR WEAKNESS-AWKWARD GAIT
X-linked mental retardation-macroorchidism
See X-LINKED MENTAL RETARDATION, FRAGILE X SYNDROME
X-linked mental retardation-muscular atrophy
See X-LINKED MENTAL RETARDATION-MUSCULAR WEAKNESS-AWKWARD GAIT

X-LINKED MENTAL RETARDATION-MUSCULAR WEAKNESS-AWKWARD GAIT   3249

Includes:
Allan-Herndon-Dudley (limber neck) mental retardation
Muscular atrophy-mental retardation, X-linked
Neck, limber-mental retardation
X-linked mental retardation-hypotonia
X-linked mental retardation-muscular atrophy

Excludes: X-linked mental retardation (other)

Major Diagnostic Criteria: Severe mental retardation; muscular weakness with moderate atrophy; delayed walking (clumsy attempts at walking between the ages of 3–4 years). Awkward, wide-based, incoordinate gait; marked speech deficit (unintelligible mumbling or gibberish); delayed and poor control of bowel and bladder functions. No evidence of sexual potency. No special facial features described.

Clinical Findings: Based on 24 affected males in the only pedigree described (22 with some clinical information and eight examined in detail): severe mental retardation (21/22); unable to walk or walking with great difficulty (15/22); unable to talk or talked poorly (13/22). Speech ability was not mentioned in nine cases. Muscle atrophy (4/22).

Complications: Moderate contractures of hamstring tendons are frequent, and more severe contractures are present in those patients who do little or no walking.

Associated Findings: None known.

Etiology: Presumably X-linked recessive inheritance.

Pathogenesis: Unknown.

MIM No.: 30960

Sex Ratio: M24:F0

Occurrence: One family with 24 affected males has been reported.

Risk of Recurrence for Patient's Sib:
See Part I, *Mendelian Inheritance.*

Risk of Recurrence for Patient's Child:
See Part I, *Mendelian Inheritance.*

Age of Detectability: After six months of age. At that time, it is noticed that the patients seem weak and are unable to hold up their heads. "Limber neck" is the term used by the affected family to describe the condition at this age.

Gene Mapping and Linkage: Unknown.

Prevention: None known. Genetic counseling indicated.

Treatment: Unknown.

Prognosis: The disease is not progressive. The physical condition of the patients remains the same over a period of years. Affected individuals usually die of intercurrent infections. Age of death in seven cases: one during the first decade; three during the second decade; one during the third decade; and one during the fifth decade.

Detection of Carrier: Unknown.

References:
Allan W, et al.: Some examples of the inheritance of mental deficiency: apparently sex-linked idiocy and microcephaly. Am J Ment Defic 1944; 48:325–334.

AR011   **J. Fernando Arena**
LU002   **Herbert A. Lubs**

X-linked mental retardation-overgrowth syndrome
See SIMPSON-GOLABI-BEHMEL SYNDROME

X-LINKED MENTAL RETARDATION-PSORIASIS   3252

Includes:
Psoriasis-mental retardation, X-linked
Tranebjaerg mental retardation

Excludes: X-linked mental retardation (other)

Major Diagnostic Criteria: Mental retardation; seizures (onset during first five years of life); psoriasis (onset from neonatal period to 11 years of age).

Clinical Findings: Delayed psycomotor development with severe mental retardation (4/4); seizures (4/4); psoriasis (4/4); hypotonia (4/4); long face (4/4); high forehead (4/4); **Eye, hypertelorism** (4/4); broad nasal bridge (4/4); long philtrum (4/4); mouth-breathing facial changes and macrostomia (4/4); prominent lower lips (4/4); mild prognathism (4/4); large, anteverted ears (4/4); ataxic gait (2/4); strabismus (2/4); normal prometaphase chromosomes analysis without fragile X (3/3).

Complications: Unknown.

Associated Findings: Scoliosis (1/4); retarded bone age (1/4).

Etiology: Presumably X-linked recessive inheritance.

Pathogenesis: Unknown.

Sex Ratio: M4:F0 observed.

Occurrence: One family with four affected males has been reported.

Risk of Recurrence for Patient's Sib:
See Part I, *Mendelian Inheritance.*

Risk of Recurrence for Patient's Child:
See Part I, *Mendelian Inheritance.*

Age of Detectability: During infancy.

Gene Mapping and Linkage: Unknown.

Prevention: None known. Genetic counseling indicated.

Treatment: Unknown.

Prognosis: Unknown.

Detection of Carrier: Unknown.

References:
Tranebjaerg, et al.: X-linked mental retardation associated with psoriasis: a new syndrome? Am J Med Genet 1988; 30:263–273.

AR011
LU002

J. Fernando Arena
Herbert A. Lubs

X-LINKED MENTAL RETARDATION-SHORT STATURE-OBESITY-HYPOGONADISM 3147

Includes:
Short stature-mental retardation-obesity-hypogonadism
X-linked mental retardation, Chudley-Lowry-Hoar type
X-linked mental retardation, Urban type (possibly)
X-linked mental retardation, Vasquez type (possibly)
Young-Hughes syndrome

Excludes:
Bardet-Biedl syndrome (2363)
Borjeson-Forssman-Lehmann syndrome (2272)
Dwarfism-dysmorphic facies-retardation, Pitt type (2814)
Prader-Willi syndrome (0823)
X-linked mental retardation (other)

Major Diagnostic Criteria: Mental retardation in a male with moderate short stature, obesity, and hypogonadism.

Clinical Findings: Developmental delay and hypotonia is noted early, usually by 6–9 months of age. Growth parameters show moderate short stature, mild to moderate obesity and hypogonadism beyond puberty. The phallus is normal sized with evidence of small testes. Cryptorchidism has been noted in some affected individuals. The families described by Young & Hughes (1982) and Chudley et al (1988) had hypergonadotropic hypogonadism. The upper extremities may appear shortened distally. **Camptodactyly** was present in some boys, but this is not a consistent feature. Dermatoglyphic analysis in the family reported by Chudley et al (1988) showed a low total finger ridge count with normal palmar creases.

The facial features in affected males were distinct in the cases reported by Chudley et al (1988); consisting of almond-shaped eyes, bitemporal narrowing of the forehead, flat nasal bridge, and a short philtrum with elevated upper lip in the shape of an inverted V. The mouth was large with a high arched palate. The neck was short. The report by Young & Hughes (1982) described a multigeneration family of affected males with a distinctive face with macrostomia, and a thin upper lip and ocular squints; different from the facies in the family reported by Chudley et al (1988). Affected males in the Young & Hughes family had unusual skin diseases, with ichthyosis in one and chronic, atopic and sun-sensitive skin afflictions in the three others.

The diagnosis of **Prader-Willi syndrome** was considered and excluded in all of the affected individuals.

Complications: Unknown.

Associated Findings: Genu valgum and pes planus were seen in the older boys. One boy was born with bilateral dislocated hips. In males who were possibly affected, one died of possible congenital heart disease in infancy and the other died of complications of a seizure disorder. Chronic skin disease in some males.

Etiology: X-linked recessive inheritance.

Pathogenesis: Unknown.

POS No.: 3585

Sex Ratio: M1:F0

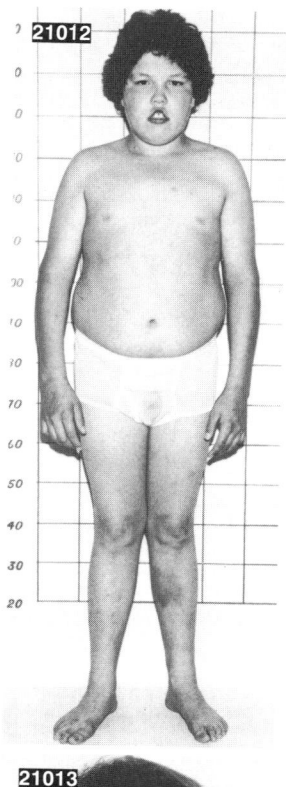

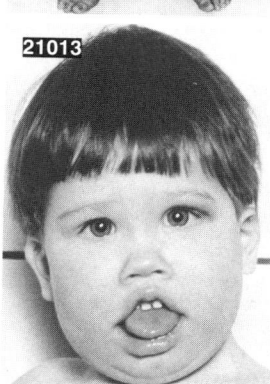

3147-21012: Note relative short stature, obesity, typical facial features, genu valgum and flat feet. 21013: Affected young male; note inverted "V"-shaped upper lip and flat nasal bridge.

Occurrence: Three members of two Canadian families have been reported, and other families with similar conditions have also been documented.

Risk of Recurrence for Patient's Sib:
See Part I, *Mendelian Inheritance.*

Risk of Recurrence for Patient's Child:
See Part I, *Mendelian Inheritance.*

Age of Detectability: Can be suspected in early infancy.

Gene Mapping and Linkage: Based on the family reported by Chudley et al (1988), the gene is possibly located in proximal Xp or Xq region since linkage excluded in distal regions of Xp and Xq. RFLP studies support X chromosome transmission. Since the clinical features in the reported families are not identical, there may be genetic heterogeneity for this disorder with more than one loci on the X chromosome.

Prevention: None known. Genetic counseling indicated.

Treatment: Correction of limb deformities and ocular squints as required. Cryptorchidism by hormonal or surgical intervention.

Prognosis: Unknown. Several of the affected males appear healthy. The oldest described was in his mid-40's. Mental retardation is significant.

Detection of Carrier: Unknown.

References:

Borjeson M, et al.: An X-linked recessively inherited syndrome characterized by grave mental deficiency, epilepsy and endocrine disorder. Acta Med Scand 1962; 171:12–21. †

Urban MD, et al.: Familial syndrome of mental retardation, short stature, contractures of the hands and genital anomalies. J Pediatr 1979; 94:52–55. †

Vasquez SB, et al.: X-linked hypogonadism, gynecomastia, mental retardation, short stature and obesity: a new syndrome. J Pediatr 1979; 94:56–60. †

Young ID, Hughes HE: Sex-linked mental retardation, short stature, obesity and hypogonadism: report of a family. J Ment Defic Res 1982; 26:153–162. * †

Opitz JM, Sutherland GR: Conference report: International Workshop on the Fragile X and X-Linked Mental Retardation. Am J Med Genet 1984; 17:5–94.

Chudley AE, et al.: Mental retardation, distinct facial changes, short stature, obesity and hypogonadism: a new X-linked mental retardation syndrome. Am J Med Genet 1988; 31:741–751. * †

CH030   **Albert E. Chudley**
L0010   **R. Brian Lowry**

X-LINKED MENTAL RETARDATION-SKELETAL DYSPLASIA   2904

Includes:

Abducens palsy-skeletal dysplasia-mental retardation
Christian syndrome
Joint defects with X-linked mental retardation

Excludes:

Aarskog syndrome (0001)
Coffin-Lowry syndrome (0190)
FG syndrome, Opitz-Kaveggia type (0754)
G syndrome (0401)
Hypertelorism-hypospadias syndrome (0505)
X-linked mental retardation, Fragile X syndrome (2073)
X-linked mental retardation, Renpenning type (2920)
X-linked mental retardation (other)

Major Diagnostic Criteria: Moderate mental retardation in males with short stature and skeletal anomalies.

Clinical Findings: Among the skeletal findings are ridging of metopic suture, fusion of cervical vertebrae, thoracic hemivertebrae, scoliosis, sacral hypoplasia, and short middle phalanges. Abducens palsy occurred in 4/4. Carrier females are mentally normal but may (3/5) show fusion of cervical vertebrae, shortened middle phalanges (3/5), or glucose intolerance (3/5).

Complications: Unknown.

Associated Findings: Glucose intolerance (3/4) and imperforate anus (1/4) have been found.

Etiology: X-linked recessive inheritance.

Pathogenesis: Unknown.

MIM No.: 30962

POS No.: 4222

Sex Ratio: M1:F0 (the full syndrome is seen only in males).

Occurrence: Reported in four male first cousins in three sibships connected through females.

Risk of Recurrence for Patient's Sib:
See Part I, *Mendelian Inheritance.*

Risk of Recurrence for Patient's Child:
See Part I, *Mendelian Inheritance.*

Age of Detectability: At birth, or prenatally by linked restriction fragment length polymorphisms.

Gene Mapping and Linkage: MRSD (mental retardation-skeletal dysplasia) has been provisionally mapped to Xq27-q28.

Prevention: None known. Genetic counseling indicated.

Treatment: Special education.

Prognosis: Apparently consistent with a normal life span.

Detection of Carrier: RFLP linkage. Examination of female relatives for skeletal abnormalities.

References:

Christian JC, et al.: X-linked skeletal dysplasia with mental retardation. Clin Genet 1977; 11:128–136.

Dlouhy SR, et al.: Localization of the gene for a syndrome of X-linked skeletal dysplasia and mental retardation to Xq27-qter. Hum Genet 1987; 75:136–139.

H0003   **M.E. Hodes**
CH029   **Joe C. Christian**
DL000   **S.R. Dlouhy**

X-LINKED MENTAL RETARDATION-SUBCORTICAL ATROPHY-PATELLAR LUXATION   3248

Includes: Prieto mental retardation

Excludes: **X-linked mental retardation** (other)

Major Diagnostic Criteria: Mental retardation; facial dysmorphia (low-set malformed ears, prominent nose with high nasal bridge, retrognathia); abnormal growth of teeth (double row of lower incisors in two cases); skin dimple at the lower back; clinodactyly; patella luxation; malformation of lower limbs; abnormal fundus of the eye (partial papillar atrophy); and subcortical atrophy.

Clinical Findings: Based on eight males of the same family: mental retardation (8/8) with subcortical atrophy (6/6); facial dysmorphia (8/8) with prominent nose (5/8), which may have been familial, and retrognathia (4/8); clinodactyly (8/8); ear malformation (7/8); subcortical atrophy (6/8); febrile convulsion (6/8); abnormalities of fundus of eye (5/8); skin dimple at lower back (5/8); patellar luxation (5/8); limb malformation (5/8); abnormal teeth (4/8); bilateral coxa valga (3/8); cranial asymmetry (2/3); and **Eye, hypertelorism** (1/8).

Complications: Unknown.

Associated Findings: None known.

Etiology: Presumably X-linked recessive inheritance.

Pathogenesis: Unknown.

MIM No.: 30961

Sex Ratio: M8:F0

Occurrence: One family with eight affected males has been reported in the literature.

Risk of Recurrence for Patient's Sib:
See Part I, *Mendelian Inheritance.*

Risk of Recurrence for Patient's Child:
See Part I, *Mendelian Inheritance.*

Age of Detectability: During the first year of life.

Gene Mapping and Linkage: Unknown.

Prevention: None known. Genetic counseling indicated.

Treatment: Unknown.

Prognosis: Unknown.

Detection of Carrier: Unknown.

References:

Prieto F, et al.: X-linked dysmorphia syndrome with mental retardation. Clin Genet 1987; 32:326–334.

AR011   **J. Fernando Arena**
LU002   **Herbert A. Lubs**

X-LINKED MENTAL RETARDATION-XQ DUPLICATION 3250

Includes:

Chromosome Xq duplication-mental retardation, X-linked Thode mental retardation

Excludes: X-linked mental retardation (other)

Major Diagnostic Criteria: Severe intellectual handicap; marked short stature; unusual facial appearance characterized by epicanthic folds, ptosis, small palpebral fissures, tented upper lip, and downturned corners of the mouth. Partial duplication of long arm of X (q13.1-q21.1) must be demonstrated.

Clinical Findings: In the report by Thode et al (1988) all three affected males had a characteristic and very similar facial appearance, including small palpebral fissures, bilateral epicanthic folds, ptosis, tented upper lip, and down-turned corners of the mouth. Mid-line depression of the chin was present (2/3), as were bilateral **Hernia, inguinal** (2/3). All had high or impalpable testes, and a 15 degree bent knee posture. Short stature and delayed bone age was present in each. The clinical findings were similar in an earlier report by Vejerslev et al (1985), and in an unpublished report by Leonard.

Complications: Unknown.

Associated Findings: All had low somatomedin C levels. In two, there was a normal growth hormone level, but an elevated growth hormone level was present in the third. The relationship of this duplication and somatomedin C (which has been mapped to chromosome 11p15) is unclear. Gene dosage effect was shown functionally in one affected and two carriers using PKG determinations and a c-DNA probe for this region. In carrier females, the abnormal X was late replicating and their phenotype was normal.

Etiology: Duplication of X (q13.1-q21.1).

Pathogenesis: Unknown.

Sex Ratio: M3:F0 observed.

Occurrence: Three affected families have been reported.

Risk of Recurrence for Patient's Sib:
See Part I, *Mendelian Inheritance.*

Risk of Recurrence for Patient's Child:
See Part I, *Mendelian Inheritance.*

Age of Detectability: Prenatally or at birth.

Gene Mapping and Linkage: Duplication of X (q13.1-q21.1).

Prevention: None known. Genetic counseling indicated.

Treatment: Unknown.

Prognosis: Limited, with severe mental retardation.

Detection of Carrier: By chromosome studies.

References:
Steinbach P, et al.: Tandem duplication dup (dx) (q13q22) in a male proband inherited from the mother showing mosaicism of X-inactivation. Hum Genet 1980; 54:309–313.
Vejerslev LO, et al.: Inherited tandem duplication dup (X) (q131-q212) in a male proband. Clin Genet 1985; 27:276–281.
Thode A, et al.: A new syndrome with mental retardation, short stature and an Xq duplication. Am J Med Genet 1988; 30:239–250.

LU002
AR011

Herbert A. Lubs
J. Fernando Arena

X-linked mixed deafness syndrome
See DEAFNESS WITH PERILYMPHATIC GUSHER
Xanax^, fetal effects
See FETAL BENZODIAZEPINE EFFECTS
Xanthine dehydrogenase/sulfite oxidase/aldehyde oxidase deficiency
See MOLYBDENUM CO-FACTOR DEFICIENCY

XANTHINE OXIDASE DEFICIENCY 2411

Includes: Xanthinuria

Excludes: Molybdenum co-factor deficiency (2412)

Major Diagnostic Criteria: Low serum uric acid (generally < 1 mg/dl, 0.06 mmol/L), low urinary uric acid (generally <50 mg/24 hr, 3 mmol/24 hr) with increased urinary excretion of xanthine and hypoxanthine (oxypurines > 200 mg/24 hr, 12 mmol/24 hr). Some patients develop xanthine stones in the renal tract (40%).

Clinical Findings: No specific clinical findings other than the formation of urinary tract stones in some patients. Low serum uric acid (generally < 1 mg/dl, 0.06 mmol/L), low urinary uric acid (generally <50 mg/24 hr, 3 mmol/24 hr) with increased urinary excretion of xanthine and hypoxanthine (oxypurines > 200 mg/24 hr, 1.2 mmol/24 hr).

Complications: Unknown.

Associated Findings: Pheochromocytoma, hemochromatosis. Xanthinuria has been associated with sulfite oxidase deficiency but this is a different defect associated with **Molybdenum co-factor deficiency**. A myopathy and recurrent polyarthritis has been observed in 6% of cases.

Etiology: Autosomal recessive inheritance.

Pathogenesis: Deficiency of the enzyme xanthine oxidase E.C.1.2.3.2.

MIM No.: *27830

Sex Ratio: M1:F1

Occurrence: At least 58 cases have been documented in the literature, including a Black male.

Risk of Recurrence for Patient's Sib:
See Part I, *Mendelian Inheritance.*

Risk of Recurrence for Patient's Child:
See Part I, *Mendelian Inheritance.*

Age of Detectability: Generally not until adult life.

Gene Mapping and Linkage: Unknown.

Prevention: None known. Genetic counseling indicated.

Treatment: Increased fluid intake to lead to dilution of urine would help in those patients who form renal calculi. Otherwise, none is required.

Prognosis: Normal life span. A few patients may be affected by renal stones.

Detection of Carrier: Unknown.

References:
Dent CE, Philpot GR: Xanthinuria: an inborn error (or deviation) of metabolism. Lancet 1954; I:182–185.
Avazian JH: Xanthinuria and hemochromatosis. New Engl J Med 1964; 270:18–22.
Engelman K, et al.: Clinical, physiological and biochemical studies of a patient with xanthinuria and pheochromocytoma. Am J Med 1964; 37:839–861.
Crawhall JC, et al.: Separation and quantitation of oxypurines by isocratic high pressure liquid chromatography: application to xanthinuria and the Lesch-Nyhan syndrome. Biochem Med 1983; 30:261–270.
Carpenter TO, et al.: Hereditary xanthinuria presenting in infancy with nephrolithiasis. J Pediatr 1986; 109:307–309.
Mateos FA, et al.: Hereditary xanthinuria: evidence for enhanced hypoxanthine salvage. J Clin Invest 1987; 79:847–852.
Holmes EW, Wyngaarden JB: Hereditary xanthinuria. In: Scriver CR, et al, eds: The metabolic basis of inherited disease, 6th ed. New York: McGraw-Hill, 1989:1085–1094.

CR006

John C. Crawhall

Xanthinuria
See XANTHINE OXIDASE DEFICIENCY
Xanthism
See ALBINISM, OCULOCUTANEOUS, RUFOUS TYPE
Xanthoma tuberosum multiplex
See HYPERCHOLESTEREMIA

XANTHOMATOSIS, CEREBROTENDINOUS   2395

Includes:
Cerebral cholesterinosis
Cerebrotendinous xanthomatosis
Cholestanalosis

Excludes: N/A

Major Diagnostic Criteria: Achilles tendon xanthomatosis, progressive neurologic disease (mental retardation, dementia, spinal cord paresis, cerebellar ataxia, and peripheral neuropathy), and cataracts appear most frequently. The diagnosis is confirmed chemically by finding an elevated plasma cholestanol level (>1 mg/dl) in combination with a low or normal plasma cholesterol concentration (<220 mg/dl); increased quantities of C-27 bile alcohol glucuronides are excreted in bile and urine and circulate in plasma.

Clinical Findings: Achilles tendon xanthomas (95%) develop during the second decade. Cataracts (80%) are often present at this time. Neurologic impairment: dementia (90%), spinal cord paresis (95%), and cerebellar ataxia (90%) begin in the second or third decades. Mental retardation (50%) as evidenced by poor school performance is present in one-half of the patients and appears when the affected child enters school. The neurologic diseases progress without remission so that by the fifth decade vital brain functions controlling speech and swallowing become impaired. Because of associated coronary atherosclerosis, fatal myocardial infarctions (10%) have developed. Since the clinical presentation varies among affected family members, it is essential to look for the biochemical abnormalities (plasma cholestanol and plasma, bile, and urine bile alcohol glucuronides) in all sibs. Pulmonary insufficiency (5%) and endocrine hypofunction (3%) have also been noted. Chemically, elevated plasma cholestanol levels in combination with low or normal plasma cholesterol concentrations are diagnostic for cerebrotendinous xanthomatosis (CTX). Increased cholestanol is also present in xanthomas, nerve tissue (brain and peripheral nerve), and bile. Defective hepatic bile acid synthesis is manifested by reduced biliary chenodeoxycholic acid and by the excretion of C-27 bile alcohol glucuronides (bile acid precursors) in bile and urine.

Most subjects with CTX show neurologic dysfunction with dementia, weakness, loss of coordination, and spasticity. As the disease evolves, the neurologic complications worsen. Cataracts affect vision, coronary atherosclerosis leads to angina pectoris and myocardial infarction, pulmonary nodules, shortness of breath, and dyspnea may develop.

Complications: Unknown.

Associated Findings: Hypothyroidism and hypoadrenalism have been detected infrequently. Severe osteoporosis and an increased number of bone fractures have been noted, and urinary calculi appear more frequently.

Etiology: Autosomal recessive inheritance. The basic defect involves incomplete oxidation of the side chain in the conversion of cholesterol to bile acids. The precise enzymatic defect in bile acid synthesis remains controversial, because the mechanism of side chain cleavage in bile acid synthesis has not been defined quantitatively.

Pathogenesis: Reduced synthesis of the two primary bile acids cholic acid and chenodeoxycholic acid leads to deficient enterohepatic bile acid pools. As a result, hepatic cholesterol synthesis is increased. Cholestanol, the 5α-dihydro derivative of cholesterol, is overproduced and is derived from cholesterol directly via the diversion of the bile acid precursor 7α-hydroxycholesterol. Both cholesterol and cholestanol are incorporated into plasma lipoproteins and transported in plasma to various tissues. Because of bile acid synthesis defects, the bile alcohols with 27 carbons and the hydroxyl groups at C-3, C-7, and C-12 resemble cholic acid but contain incompletely oxidized side chains. In addition, hydroxy groups at C-25 accumulate as glucuronides, and these bile alcohol glucuronides are excreted in bile and urine and thus circulate in plasma. It has been hypothesized that the deposition of cholesterol and cholestanol in the central nervous system results from

damage to the blood-brain barrier caused by plasma bile alcohol glucuronides.

Although defective side chain oxidation in cholic acid synthesis exists and large quantities of bile alcohol glucuronides are found, the exact enzymatic defect cannot be defined until the quantitative mechanism of the side chain oxidation in cholic acid synthesis is determined. Two pathways are known (microsomal 25-hydroxylation and mitochondrial 26-hydroxylation), and both may actually produce cholic acid in humans.

MIM No.: *21370

POS No.: 4379

Sex Ratio: Presumably M1:F1, although females have been reported more frequently.

Occurrence: Undetermined, although all populations, including Caucasians, Blacks, and Orientals, have been affected. There is a particularly high occurrence in Sephardic Jews in Israel.

Risk of Recurrence for Patient's Sib:
See Part I, *Mendelian Inheritance*. Although 1:4 is expected, family studies suggest a greater number of affected sibs.

Risk of Recurrence for Patient's Child:
See Part I, *Mendelian Inheritance*.

Age of Detectability: Usually clinically evident by ages 20–30 years, when tendon xanthomas, cataracts, and neurologic disease present.

Gene Mapping and Linkage: Unknown.

Prevention: None known. Genetic counseling indicated.

Treatment: Replacing chenodeoxycholic acid in the enterohepatic circulation of affected persons will inhibit abnormal bile acid synthesis. To date, in 14 of 17 persons treated with chenodeoxycholic acid (750 mg/day), improved neurologic function and lower plasma and cerebrospinal fluid cholestanol levels occurred. However, it is important to emphasize that the earlier the treatment is started (the younger the patient treated), the better the effect. For example, an older patient (aged 74 years) with long-standing neurologic disease is not likely to improve. In contrast, the recognition of the diagnosis before neurologic damage and the institution of treatment will likely prevent the onset of the disease.

Prognosis: In patients with mild neurologic disease, treatment with chenodeoxycholic acid (750 mg/day) has prevented further progression of the disease, and in some cases has reversed it.

Detection of Carrier: Unknown.

References:
Salen G: Cholestanol deposition in cerebrotendinous xanthomatosis: a possible mechanism. Ann Intern Med 1971; 75:843–851.
Berginer VM, et al.: Long-term treatment of cerebrotendinous xanthomatosis with chenodeoxycholic acid. New Engl J Med 1984; 311: 1649–1652.
Berginer VM, et al.: Pregnancy in women with cerebrotendinous xanthomatosis. Am J Med Genet 1988; 31:11–16.
Bjorkhem I, Skrede S: Familial diseases with storage of sterols other than cholesterol: cerebrotendinous xanthomatosis and phytosterolemia. In: Scriver CR, et al, eds: The metabolic basis of inherited disease, 6th ed. New York: McGraw-Hill, 1989:1283–1303.

SA041   **Gerald Salen**

Xanthomatosis, familial-involvement and calcification of adrenals
See WOLMAN DISEASE
Xanthous negros
See ALBINISM, OCULOCUTANEOUS, RUFOUS TYPE
Xerocytosis, hereditary
See ANEMIA, HEMOLYTIC, RED CELL MEMBRANE DEFECTS

XERODERMA PIGMENTOSUM 1005

Includes:
Angioma pigmentosum et atrophicum
Kaposi dermatosis
Photosensitivity with defective DNA synthesis
Pigmented xerodermoid
Trichothiodystrophy-sun sensitivity
Xeroderma pigmentosum with normal DNA repair rates

Excludes:
Cockayne syndrome (0189)
Genodermatoses with defective DNA repair, other
Genodermatoses with malignancy, other
Genodermatoses with ultraviolet hypersensitivity, other
Nevoid basal cell carcinoma syndrome (0101)
Trichothiodystrophy (2559)
Xeroderma pigmentosum-mental retardation (1004)

Major Diagnostic Criteria: Infantile onset of photosensitivity, and/or freckling, and photophobia. Early development of skin and eye cancers. Cellular hypersensitivity to killing by ultraviolet radiation, accompanied by defective DNA repair.

Clinical Findings: *Skin:* Changes are seen almost exclusively on sun exposed skin. Early acute photosensitivity with blistering on minimal sun exposure (seen in about one-half of patients) and/or freckling in response to ultraviolet light (50% by age 18 months); subsequent poikiloderma (increased pigment, decreased pigment, atrophy, and telangiectasia); development of premalignant and benign skin tumors (actinic keratoses, angiomas, and keratoacanthomas); development of malignant skin tumors (2,000-fold in-

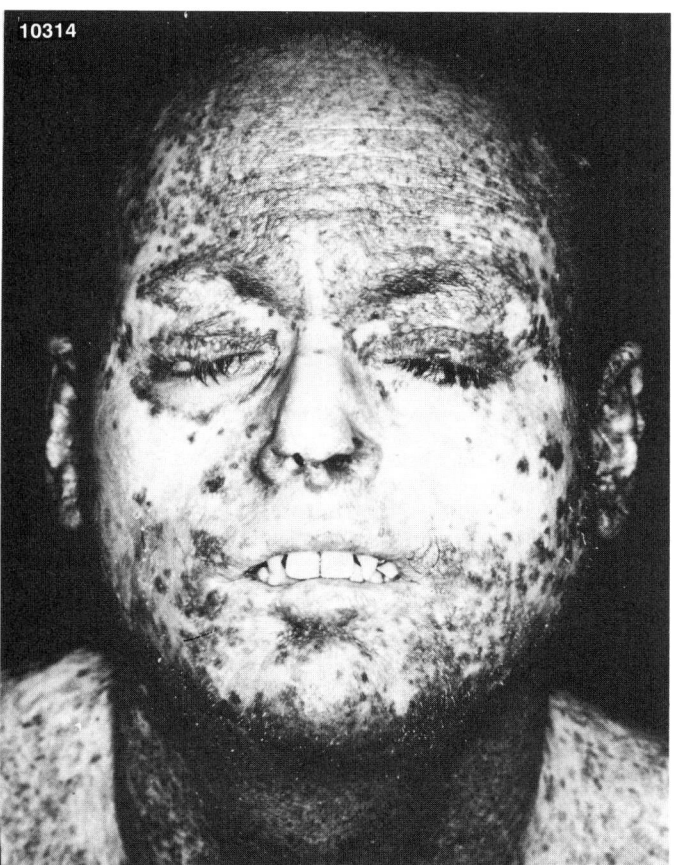
10314

1005-10314: Marked skin changes of xeroderma pigmentosum.

creased frequency by age 20 years). Basal cell and squamous cell carcinomas (50% of tumor patients by age eight years), multiple tumors are common, with >90% on face, head, or neck; malignant melanoma (3–50% of different series); rarely, sarcomas.
Eyes: Symptoms limited to ultraviolet-exposed (anterior) portion of the eye include photophobia (reported for 21% of patients, median age two years); conjunctivitis; keratitis; ectropion, entropion of lids; benign tumors (conjunctival inflammatory masses, papillomas); and malignant neoplasms (2,000-fold increased frequency by age 20 years). Symptoms associated with the anterior eye and lids include epitheliomas, basal cell carcinomas, and melanomas.
Oral: Rarely, squamous cell carcinoma of tip of tongue.
Laboratory findings: Cellular hypersensitivity to killing, and hypermutability to ultraviolet radiation and certain chemical carcinogens such as benzo-a-pyrene (found in cigarette smoke). Defective DNA repair, with a range of residual repair levels observed among patients extending from undetectable to normal. These defects can be demonstrated in cultured fibroblasts, lymphocytes, amniotic fluid cells, and *in vivo* epidermis. Nine excision repair complementation groups have been identified, plus a "variant" form with defective post-replication repair.

Complications: Metastasis of melanoma, squamous cell carcinoma; loss of eyelid; corneal opacification.

Associated Findings: Rarely, internal neoplasms (including four cases of primary brain tumors) have been reported. Two patients have been reported with clinical findings and laboratory tests characteristic of both XP and **Cockayne syndrome**.

Etiology: Autosomal recessive inheritance. Consanguinity reported in 30% of cases. Multiple laboratory forms have been identified, probably with different defects in DNA repair.

Pathogenesis: Failure to repair DNA damage after ultraviolet exposure. Probably defective ultraviolet repair endonuclease(s). Ultraviolet-induced somatic mutations are believed to result in the neoplasms. Eight sub-types have been identified, termed complementation groups A through I.

MIM No.: *27870, *27871, *27872, *27873, *27874, 27875, *27876, *27878, *27879, 27881

CDC No.: 757.360

Sex Ratio: M1:F1

Occurrence: Estimated to be 1:250,000 in the United States, 1:40,000 in Japan, and relatively high in Egypt, Tunisia, and wherever consanguinity is high. Approximately 1,000 English language cases have been reported.

Risk of Recurrence for Patient's Sib:
See Part I, *Mendelian Inheritance.*

Risk of Recurrence for Patient's Child:
See Part I, *Mendelian Inheritance.* Patients have been reported with clinically normal children.

Age of Detectability: *Skin sun sensitivity or freckling:* One-half by 18 months of age, 75% by four years of age, and 95% by 15 years of age. Photophobia can be seen in the neonate. Pigmented xerodermoid with "variant" type repair defects has adult onset of symptoms following extensive sun exposure. All cell types tested, including fetal cells, have a DNA repair defect (excision repair or post-replication repair). Prenatal diagnosis has been reported based on DNA repair studies of cultured amniotic fluid cells.

Gene Mapping and Linkage: XPAC (fast kinetic complementation DNA repair in xeroderma pigmentosum, group A) has been provisionally mapped to 1q.
XPF (xeroderma pigmentosum, complementation group F) has been provisionally mapped to 15.

Prevention: None known. Genetic counseling indicated.

Treatment: Early diagnosis, rigorous protection from ultraviolet radiation and chemical carcinogens such as those present in cigarette smoke, use of physical sunscreens (glasses, long hair, double layers of clothing); use of topical sunscreens (with at least Sun Protection Factor [SPF] 15), baseline photography of skin; regular examination of skin and eyes by parent and physician;

early excision of tumors. For extensive skin disease, prophylactic dermatome shaving, dermabrasion, or excision and grafting of the entire face has been reported. Corneal transplantation may be indicated. Experimental studies with oral retinoids have been demonstrated to prevent new neoplasms, but the dosage required has been toxic.

Prognosis: Survival is generally reduced due to neoplasms, but depends on the form of the disorder and extent of ultraviolet exposure. Five percent of 830 cases reported in the literature were more than 45 years of age, and seven were over 64 years of age. A 70% probability of survival was attained at age 40 years; a 28 year reduction in comparison with the United States general population. However, the few patients who have been diagnosed early in life and rigorously protected from ultraviolet exposure did not develop the severe cutaneous abnormalities.

Detection of Carrier: Most carriers are clinically normal, although there is a suggested increase in skin cancer risk. A few carriers have been reported with abnormal polyADP ribose metabolism, plasminogen activator levels, or increased chromosome breakage following X-ray *in vitro*. At present, there is no laboratory test that will consistently detect XP carriers.

Special Considerations: The Xeroderma Pigmentosum Registry (c/o Dept of Pathology, Room C520, Medical Science Building, CMDNJ-New Jersey Medical School, 100 Bergen St, Newark, NJ 07103) collects information on xeroderma pigmentosum patients and provides educational material to physicians.

Support Groups: NJ; Newark; Xeroderma Pigmentosum Registry

References:

Robbins JH, et al.: Xeroderma pigmentosum: an inherited disease with sun sensitivity, multiple cutaneous neoplasms, and abnormal DNA repair. Ann Intern Med 1974; 80:221–248. †
Kraemer KH, et al.: DNA repair protects against cutaneous and internal neoplasia: evidence from studies of xeroderma pigmentosum. Carcinogenesis 1984; 5:511–514.
Kraemer KH, Slor H: Xeroderma pigmentosum. Clin Dermatol 1985; 3:33–69. †
Kraemer KH: Heritable diseases with increased sensitivity to cellular injury. In: Fitzpatrick TB, et al., eds: Dermatology in general medicine. New York: McGraw Hill, 1987:1791–1796. †
Kraemer KH, et al.: Xeroderma pigmentosum: cutaneous, ocular and neurologic abnormalities in 830 published cases. Arch Dermatol 1987; 123:241–250. *
Kraemer KH, et al.: Prevention of skin cancer in xeroderma pigmentosum with the use of oral isotretinoin. New Engl J Med 1988; 318:1633–1637.
Cleaver J, Kraemer KH: Xeroderma pigmentosum. In: Scriver CR, et al, eds: The metabolic basis of inherited disease, 6th ed. New York: McGraw-Hill, 1989:2949–2973.

KR019   **Kenneth H. Kraemer**

Xeroderma pigmentosum with normal DNA repair rates
See XERODERMA PIGMENTOSUM

XERODERMA PIGMENTOSUM-MENTAL RETARDATION   1004

Includes:
DeSanctis-Cacchione syndrome
Mental retardation-xeroderma pigmentosum
Xeroderma pigmentosum-neurologic abnormalities

Excludes:
Cockayne syndrome (0189)
Photodermatoses with neurologic disease, other
Trichothiodystrophy (2559)
Xeroderma pigmentosum (1005)

Major Diagnostic Criteria: Cutaneous and ocular abnormalities of **Xeroderma pigmentosum** (XP), plus one or more neurologic abnormalities. Cellular hypersensitivity to killing by ultraviolet radiation accompanied by defective DNA repair.

Clinical Findings: Skin and eye abnormalities of **Xeroderma pigmentosum**: photosensitivity, freckling, and photophobia with sub-

sequent neoplasia. Onset may be earlier and more severe than is observed in **Xeroderma pigmentosum** patients without neurologic abnormalities.

In addition, one or more of the following neurologic abnormalities (minimal percentages based on case reports of 154 patients with xeroderma pigmentosum and neurologic abnormalities): progressive mental deterioration, low intelligence (80%); microcephaly (25%); progressive sensorineural deafness (20%); hyporeflexia or areflexia (20%); spasticity, late onset of ataxia and choreoathetoid movements, abnormal electroencephalogram (11%); and neuropathic electromyogram, loss of neurons in cerebral cortex, and demyelination of dorsal columns. Most patients have only a few neurologic abnormalities, such as hyporeflexia and progressive hearing loss. Onset of neurologic symptoms may be in early infancy, or (in 5% or more) delayed until after five to ten years of age.

Some patients may have dwarfism (15%), retarded bone age, and/or immature sexual development (12%).

Complications: Skin and eyes: as in **Xeroderma pigmentosum**. Neurological: in severe cases, loss of ability to walk and talk.

Associated Findings: Rarely, internal neoplasms.

The rare *DeSanctis-Cacchione syndrome* consists of xeroderma pigmentosum and most of the neurologic abnormalities listed above, with the addition of dwarfism and immature sexual development.

Etiology: Probably autosomal recessive inheritance. Consanguinity has been reported in 30%. Multiple molecular forms are likely, probably with different defects in DNA repair.

Pathogenesis: Failure to repair DNA damage after ultraviolet light exposure. The defect is demonstrated in cultured fibroblasts, lymphocytes, and *in vivo* epidermis.

Probably defective ultraviolet repair endonuclease(s). Of nine excision repair complementation groups, five have patients with neurologic abnormalities. Patients in group A may have severe neurologic involvement, or only minimal involvement. Patients in group D generally have later onset of neurologic degeneration, if at all. Two patients have xeroderma pigmentosum plus **Cockayne syndrome** (one in group B and the other in group H). Residual repair rates range from undetectable to 50% of normal in patients with neurologic abnormalities.

MIM No.: 27880
POS No.: 3431
CDC No.: 757.360
Sex Ratio: M1:F1

Occurrence: Prevalence of **Xeroderma pigmentosum** is estimated at 1:250,000 in the United States; 1:40,000 in Japan. Approximately 200 English language cases have been reported with neurological abnormalities, representing about 20% of the total **Xeroderma pigmentosum** cases reported (the proportion is higher in Japan).

Risk of Recurrence for Patient's Sib:
See Part I, *Mendelian Inheritance*. Generally, multiple affected sibs have similar manifestations, however, one kindred was reported with two children with XP, but only the older with neurologic abnormalities.

Risk of Recurrence for Patient's Child:
See Part I, *Mendelian Inheritance*. Of 152 patients reported in a literature survey, none had children.

Age of Detectability: Prenatal diagnosis of xeroderma pigmentosum has been reported based on DNA repair studies of cultured amniotic fluid cells. Skin sun sensitivity or freckling is seen in one-half by six months of age, in 75% by 18 months of age, and in 95% by five years of age. Photophobia is seen in the neonate. Neurological abnormalities usually appear in early childhood, but may have their onset in the second decade of life.

Gene Mapping and Linkage: Unknown.

Prevention: None known. Genetic counseling indicated.

Treatment: *Skin and eyes:* early diagnosis, rigorous protection from ultraviolet radiation and chemical carcinogens such as those present in cigarette smoke, use of physical sunscreens (glasses, long hair, double layers of clothing), use of topical sunscreens (with Sun Protection Factor 15+), baseline photography of skin; regular examination of skin and eyes by parent and physician, and early excision of tumors. For extensive skin disease, prophylactic dermatome shaving, dermabrasion, or excision and grafting of the entire face has been reported. Corneal transplantation may be indicated. Experimental studies with oral retinoids have been shown to prevent new neoplasms, but the doses used have been toxic. *Neurological*: hearing aids may be beneficial.

Prognosis: Survival of patients with xeroderma pigmentosum is generally reduced. Prognosis depends on the form of the disorder and the extent of ultraviolet exposure. Ten percent of 152 cases were less than 30 years old. The survival probability is not significantly different from that of patients with **Xeroderma pigmentosum** without neurological abnormalities.

Detection of Carrier: Carriers of xeroderma pigmentosum are generally clinically normal. There is a possibility of increased skin cancer risk. A few carriers have been reported with abnormal polyADP ribose metabolism, plasminogen activator levels, or *in vitro* hypersensitivity to X-ray-induced chromosome breakage.

Special Considerations: The Xeroderma Pigmentosum Registry (c/o Dept of Pathology, Room C520, Medical Science Building, CMDNJ-New Jersey Medical School, 100 Bergen St, Newark, NJ 07103) is collecting information on xeroderma pigmentosum patients, and provides educational material to physicians.

Support Groups: NJ; Newark; Xeroderma Pigmentosum Registry

References:

Robbins JH, et al.: Xeroderma pigmentosum: an inherited disease with sun sensitivity, multiple cutaneous neoplasms, and abnormal DNA repair. Ann Intern Med 1974; 80:221–248. †

Kraemer KH, Slor H: Xeroderma pigmentosum. Clin Dermatol 1985; 3:33–69. †

Kraemer KH: Heritable diseases with increased sensitivity to cellular injury. In: Fitzpatrick TB, et al., eds: Dermatology in general medicine. New York: McGraw Hill, 1987:1791–1796. †

Kraemer KH, et al.: Xeroderma pigmentosum: cutaneous, ocular and neurologic abnormalities in 830 published cases. Arch Dermatol 1987; 123:241–250. *

Kraemer KH, et al.: Prevention of skin cancer in xeroderma pigmentosum with the use of oral isotretinoin. New Engl J Med 1988; 318:1633–1637.

Cleaver JE, Kraemer KH: Xeroderma pigmentosum. In: Scriver CR, et al, eds: The metabolic basis of inherited disease, 6th ed. New York: McGraw-Hill, 1989:2949–2973.

KR019

Kenneth H. Kraemer

Xeroderma pigmentosum-neurologic abnormalities
See XERODERMA PIGMENTOSUM-MENTAL RETARDATION
Xeroderma-tricho-onychodysplasia
See TRICHO-ONYCHODYSPLASIA-XERODERMA
Xeroderma-trichodysplasia
See TRICHODYSPLASIA-XERODERMA
Xerostomia
See SALIVARY GLAND, AGENESIS
Xk-related chronic granulomatous disease
See GRANULOMATOUS DISEASE, CHRONIC X-LINKED
XX form of pure gonadal dysgenesis
See GONADAL DYSGENESIS, XX TYPE
XX Gonadal dysgenesis
See GONADAL DYSGENESIS, XX TYPE
XX-XY Turner phenotype
See NOONAN SYNDROME
XY form of pure gonadal dysgenesis
See GONADAL DYSGENESIS, XY TYPE
XY gonadal agenesis syndrome
See ANORCHIA
also AGONADIA
XY gonadal dysgenesis
See GONADAL DYSGENESIS, XY TYPE
Xylitol dehydrogenase deficiency
See PENTOSURIA

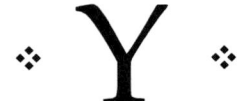

Yellow mutant oculocutaneous albinism
  See ALBINISM, OCULOCUTANEOUS, YELLOW MUTANT
Yellow nail syndrome with familial late-onset lymphedema
  See LYMPHEDEMA II
Yellow teeth
  See TEETH, DEFECTS FROM TETRACYCLINE
Yellow-blue color defect
  See COLOR BLINDNESS, YELLOW-BLUE TRITAN
Young-Hughes syndrome
  *See X-LINKED MENTAL RETARDATION-SHORT STATURE-OBESITY-
  HYPOGONADISM*
Yucheng, congenital
  See FETAL EFFECTS OF POLYCHLORINATED BIPHENYL (PCB)

YUNIS-VARON SYNDROME   2405

Includes:
  Cleidocranial dysplasia-micrognathia-no thumb-distal
    aphalangia
  Cleidocranial dysplasia-micrognathia, Yunis-Varon type
  Micrognathia-cleidocranial dysplasia

Excludes: Cleidocranial dysplasia (0185)

Major Diagnostic Criteria: 1) Craniofacial disproportion; 2) micrognathia; 3) absent or hypoplastic clavicles, thumbs and great toes; 4) aphalangia of fingers or toes with short or absent metacarpals and metatarsal bones; 5) sparse hair; and 6) postnatal short stature.

Clinical Findings: The mean birth weight (2.3 kg) is below average, but body length and head circumference are within normal limits. There is craniofacial disproportion, with marked micrognathia leading to feeding difficulties and failure to thrive. In the one child surviving infancy, growth retardation was progressive and extreme, with relative **Microcephaly**, developmental delay, and moderate mental retardation. The anterior fontanelle is widely open. Hair is sparse, with thin or absent eyebrows and eyelashes. The ears protrude and have a simple pattern. The lips are thin. The clavicles, thumbs, and first toes may be absent or hypoplastic. Fingers and toes may show **Syndactyly** and absent phalanges, and the metacarpals and metatarsals may be short or absent.

The pattern of X-ray findings is distinctive. Cardiac arrhythmia and cardiac enlargement may occur. Routine biochemical tests and chromosomal karyotypes have been normal.

Complications: Death in infancy, presumably from feeding and respiratory difficulties or unrecognized cardiomyopathy.

Associated Findings: None known.

Etiology: Autosomal recessive inheritance.

Pathogenesis: Unknown.

MIM No.: *21634

POS No.: 3485

CDC No.: 755.555

Sex Ratio: M3:F4

Occurrence: Seven patients from five families; one Canadian, one Australian, and three 3 Columbian, have been documented.

Risk of Recurrence for Patient's Sib:
  See Part I, *Mendelian Inheritance.*

Risk of Recurrence for Patient's Child:
  See Part I, *Mendelian Inheritance.*

Age of Detectability: At birth. In theory this condition should be detectable *in utero.*

Gene Mapping and Linkage: Unknown.

Prevention: None known. Genetic counseling indicated.

Treatment: Scrupulous attention to feeding in early infancy; comparable to that in the Pierre Robin sequence. Cardiac arrythmia was controlled by phenytoin in one patient.

Prognosis: Deaths occurred on the first day of life and on days 22, 35, 50, and 65. One survivor spent the first 10 weeks of his life in hospital, but thereafter fed well. He showed progressive growth failure, with a height at 4 1/4 years of age of 84 cm; 19 cm or over four standard deviations below the mean for his age. His head circumference (42 cm) was some six standard deviations below average. Development was slow with a developmental quotient of about 40.

Another survivor has normal intelligence, with growth on the third centile. Cardiomegaly has persisted to age three years.

Detection of Carrier: Unknown.

References:
Yunis E, Varon H: Cleidocranial dysostosis, severe micrognathism, bilateral absence of thumbs and first metatarsal bone and distal aphalangia: a new genetic syndrome. Am J Dis Child 1980; 134:649–653. * †
Hughes HE, Partington MW: The syndrome of Yunis and Varon: report of a further case. Am J Med Genet 1983; 14:539–544. †
Partington MW: Cardiomyopathy added to the Yunis-Varon syndrome. Proc Greenwood Genet Ctr 1988; 7:224–225.

PA026   **M.W. Partington**

Yusho, congenital
  See FETAL EFFECTS OF POLYCHLORINATED BIPHENYL (PCB)

❖ Z ❖

Zayid-Farraj syndrome
See DERMATOARTHRITIS, FAMILIAL HISTIOCYTIC
Zellweger syndrome
See CEREBRO-HEPATO-RENAL SYNDROME
Zestril^, possible fetal effects
*See FETAL ANGIOTENSIN CONVERTING ENZYME (ACE)
INHIBITION RENAL FAILURE*
Zimmermann-Laband syndrome
See GINGIVAL FIBROMATOSIS-DIGITAL ANOMALIES
Zinsser-Cole-Engman syndrome
See DYSKERATOSIS CONGENITA
Zlotogora-Zilberman-Tenenbaum syndrome
See PILI TORTI-CLEFT LIP/PALATE-SYNDACTYLY
Zollinger-Ellison syndrome (some cases)
See ENDOCRINE NEOPLASIA, MULTIPLE TYPE I
Zonana syndrome
See OVERGROWTH, BANNAYAN TYPE
Zonular cataract
See CATARACT, AUTOSOMAL DOMINANT CONGENITAL
Zwerchfell eventration
See DIAPHRAGM, EVENTRATION
Zypokowski-Margolis syndrome
See ALBINISM, CUTANEOUS

GENE MAP TABLE BY SYMBOL NAME

SYMBOL	MARKER NAME	MAP LOCATION	NO	ARTICLE TITLE
AACT	alpha-1-antichymotrypsin	14q32.1	3279	ALPHA-1-ANTICHYMOTRYPSIN DEFICIENCY
ABO	ABO blood group	9q34.1-q34.2	0340	TEETH, ENAMEL AND DENTIN DEFECTS FROM ERYTHROBLASTOSIS FETALIS
ACAD	acyl-Coenzyme A dehydrogenase, multiple	X	2289	ACIDEMIA, GLUTARIC ACIDEMIA II
ACADL	acyl-Coenzyme A dehydrogenase, long chain	unassigned	2228	ACYL-CoA DEHYDROGENASE DEFICIENCY, LONG CHAIN TYPE
ACADM	acyl-Coenzyme A dehydrogenase, C-4 to C-12 straight-chain	1p31	2324	ACYL-CoA DEHYDROGENASE DEFICIENCY, MEDIUM CHAIN TYPE
ACADS	acyl-Coenzyme A dehydrogenase, C-2 to C-3 short chain	12q22-qter	2323	ACYL-CoA DEHYDROGENASE DEFICIENCY, SHORT CHAIN TYPE
AD1	Alzheimer disease 1	21pter-q21	2354	ALZHEIMER DISEASE, FAMILIAL
ADA	adenosine deaminase	20q13.11 or 20q13.2-qter	2196	IMMUNODEFICIENCY, ADENOSINE DEAMINASE DEFICIENCY
ADFN	albinism-deafness syndrome	Xq25-q27	0030	ALBINISM, CUTANEOUS-DEAFNESS
ADH1	alcohol dehydrogenase (class I), alpha polypeptide	4q21-q23	3074	ALCOHOL INTOLERANCE
ADH2	alcohol dehydrogenase (class I), beta polypeptide	4q21-q23	3074	ALCOHOL INTOLERANCE
ADH3	alcohol dehydrogenase (class I), gamma polypeptide	4q21-q23	3074	ALCOHOL INTOLERANCE
ADSL	adenylosuccinate lyase	22	3113	ADENYLOSUCCINATE MONOPHOSPHATE LYASE DEFICIENCY
AGA	aspartylglucosaminidase	4q21-qter	2042	ASPARTYLGLUCOSAMINURIA
AGMX1	agammaglobulinemia, X-linked 1 (Bruton)	Xq21.33-q22	0027	IMMUNODEFICIENCY, AGAMMAGLOBULINEMIA, X-LINKED, INFANTILE
AGS	Alagille syndrome	20p12-p11	2084	ARTERIO-HEPATIC DYSPLASIA
AHC	adrenal hypoplasia, congenital	Xp21.3-p21.2	0024	ADRENAL HYPOPLASIA, CONGENITAL
AHH	aryl hydrocarbon hydroxylase	2pter-q31	2747	CANCER, LUNG, FAMILIAL
AIC	Aicardi syndrome	Xp22	2320	AICARDI SYNDROME
AIED	Aland island eye disease (Forsius-Eriksson ocular albinism	Xp21.3-p21.2	3183	FORSIUS-ERIKSSON SYNDROME
AIH1	amelogenesis imperfecta 1, hypomaturation or hypoplastic (?=AMG & AMGS)	Xp22	0046	TEETH, AMELOGENESIS IMPERFECTA
AIH1	amelogenesis imperfecta 1, hypomaturation or hypoplastic (?=AMG & AMGS)	Xp22	2136	TEETH, SNOW-CAPPED
AIH2	amelogenesis imperfecta 2, hypocalcification (autosomal dominant)	unassigned	0046	TEETH, AMELOGENESIS IMPERFECTA
AK1	adenylate kinase 1	9q34.1-q34.2	2660	ANEMIA, ADENYLATE KINASE DEFICIENCY
AK2	adenylate kinase 2	1p34	2660	ANEMIA, ADENYLATE KINASE DEFICIENCY
AK3	adenylate kinase 3	9p24-p13	2660	ANEMIA, ADENYLATE KINASE DEFICIENCY
ALAD	aminolevulinate, delta-, dehydratase	9q34	3091	DELTA-AMINOLEVULINIC ACID DEHYDRASE DEFICIENCY
ALB	albumin	4q11-q13	0047	ANALBUMINEMIA
ALD	adrenoleukodystrophy	Xq28	2533	ADRENOLEUKODYSTROPHY, X-LINKED
ALDH2	aldehyde dehydrogenase 2, mitochondrial	12q24.2	3074	ALCOHOL INTOLERANCE
ALDOA	aldolase A, fructose-bisphosphate	16q22-q24	2662	ERYTHROCYTE ALDOLASE-A DEFICIENCY
ALDOB	aldolase B, fructose bisphosphate	9q21.3-q22.2	0395	FRUCTOSE-1-PHOSPHATE ALDOLASE DEFICIENCY
ALPL	alkaline phosphatase, liver/bone/kidney	1p36.1-p34	0516	HYPOPHOSPHATASIA
ALS	amyotrophic lateral sclerosis	unassigned	2069	AMYOTROPHIC LATERAL SCLEROSIS, FAMILIAL ADULT AND JUVENILE TYPES
ALS	amyotrophic lateral sclerosis	unassigned	2067	AMYOTROPHIC LATERAL SCLEROSIS
AMG	amelogenin (?=AMGS & AIH)	Xp22.31-p22.1	0046	TEETH, AMELOGENESIS IMPERFECTA
AMH	anti-Mullerian hormone	19p13.3	0683	MULLERIAN DERIVATIVES IN MALES, PERSISTENT
AN1	aniridia 1	2p	0057	ANIRIDIA
AN2	aniridia 2 without Wilms' tumor, GU abnormalities, and M.R.	11p13	0057	ANIRIDIA
AN2	aniridia 2 without Wilms' tumor, GU abnormalities, and M.R.	11p13	2245	CHROMOSOME 11, PARTIAL MONOSOMY 11p
ANCR	Angelman syndrome chromosome region	15q11-q12	2086	ANGELMAN SYNDROME

SYMBOL	MARKER NAME	MAP LOCATION	NO	ARTICLE TITLE
ANK	ankyrin	8p21-p11	0892	SPHEROCYTOSIS
ANK	ankyrin	8p21-p11	2646	ANEMIA, HEMOLYTIC, RED CELL MEMBRANE DEFECTS
AOM	arthroophthalmopathy, progressive (Stickler syndrome)	12q14	2424	ARTHRO-OPHTHALMOPATHY, WEISSENBACHER-ZWEYMULLER VARIANT
AOM	arthroophthalmopathy, progressive (Stickler syndrome)	12q14	0090	ARTHRO-OPHTHALMOPATHY, HEREDITARY, PROGRESSIVE, STICKLER TYPE
APC	adenomatosis polyposis coli	5q21-q22	0536	INTESTINAL POLYPOSIS, TYPE III
APC	adenomatosis polyposis coli	5q21-q22	0535	INTESTINAL POLYPOSIS, TYPE I
APC	adenomatosis polyposis coli	5q21-q22	2739	TURCOT SYNDROME
APOA1	apolipoprotein A-I	11q23-q24	3165	APOLIPOPROTEIN A-I AND C-III DEFICIENCY STATES
APOA1	apolipoprotein A-I	11q23-q24	3096	HYPOALPHALIPOPROTEINEMIA
APOA4	apolipoprotein A-IV	11q23-qter	3096	HYPOALPHALIPOPROTEINEMIA
APOB	apolipoprotein B (including Ag(x) antigen)	2p24-p23	3227	APO B-100, DEFECTIVE, FAMILIAL
APOB	apolipoprotein B (including Ag(x) antigen)	2p24-p23	0002	ABETALIPOPROTEINEMIA
APOB	apolipoprotein B (including Ag(x) antigen)	2p24-p23	2646	ANEMIA, HEMOLYTIC, RED CELL MEMBRANE DEFECTS
APOC1	apolipoprotein C-I	19q13.2	3096	HYPOALPHALIPOPROTEINEMIA
APP	amyloid beta (A4) precursor protein	21q21.2	2354	ALZHEIMER DISEASE, FAMILIAL
APR	apolipoprotein receptor	12q13-q14	3165	APOLIPOPROTEIN A-I AND C-III DEFICIENCY STATES
APR	apolipoprotein receptor	12q13-q14	0048	ANALPHALIPOPROTEINEMIA
APRT	adenine phosphoribosyltransferase	16q24	3104	ADENINE PHOSPHO-RIBOSYL-TRANSFERASE (APRT) DEFICIENCY
APY	atopy (allergic asthma and rhinitis)	11q12-q13	3150	SKIN, ATOPY, FAMILIAL
AR	androgen receptor (dihydrotestosterone receptor; testicular feminization)	Xq12	2954	ANDROGEN INSENSITIVITY (RESISTANCE), MINIMAL
AR	androgen receptor (dihydrotestosterone receptor; testicular feminization)	Xq12	0049	ANDROGEN INSENSITIVITY SYNDROME, COMPLETE
AR	androgen receptor (dihydrotestosterone receptor; testicular feminization)	Xq12	0050	ANDROGEN INSENSITIVITY SYNDROME, INCOMPLETE
ARG1	arginase, liver	6q23	0086	ARGININEMIA
ARSA	arylsulfatase A	22q13.31-qter	0651	METACHROMATIC LEUKODYSTROPHIES
ARSB	arylsulfatase B	5p11-q13	0679	MUCOPOLYSACCHARIDOSIS VI
ARVP	arginine vasopressin (neurophysin II)	20	2611	DIABETES INSIPIDIS, NEUROHYPOPHYSEAL TYPE
ASB	anemia, sideroblastic/hypochromic	X	1518	ANEMIA, SIDEROBLASTIC
ASL	argininosuccinate lyase	7pter-q22	0087	ACIDURIA, ARGININOSUCCINIC
ASMD	anterior segment mesenchymal dysgenesis	4q	0439	EYE, ANTERIOR SEGMENT DYSGENESIS
ASS	argininosuccinate synthetase	9q34-qter	0174	CITRULLINEMIA
AT3	antithrombin III	1q23-q25.1	3066	ANTITHROMBIN III DEFICIENCY
ATA	ataxia telangiectasia (complementation group A)	11q22-q23	0094	ATAXIA-TELANGIECTASIA
ATN	albinism, tyrosinase-negative (?=TYR)	ULG5	0034	ALBINISM, OCULOCUTANEOUS, TYROSINASE NEGATIVE
ATS	Alport syndrome	Xq21.3-q24	0708	NEPHRITIS-DEAFNESS (SENSORINEURAL), HEREDITARY TYPE
B2M	beta-2-microglobulin	15q21-q22.2	3106	AMYLOIDOSIS, HEMODIALYSIS-RELATED
BCEI	breast cancer, estrogen-inducible sequence expressed in	21q22.3	2351	CANCER, BREAST, FAMILIAL
BCH	benign chorea	unassigned	2306	CHOREA, BENIGN FAMILIAL
BCL1	B cell CLL/lymphoma 1	11q13.3	3097	LEUKEMIA/LYMPHOMA, B CELL
BCL2	B cell CLL/lymphoma 2	18q21.3	3097	LEUKEMIA/LYMPHOMA, B CELL
BCL2	B cell CLL/lymphoma 2	18q21.3	3107	LYMPHOMA, NON-HODGKIN
BCP	blue cone pigment	7q22-qter	0199	COLOR BLINDNESS, YELLOW-BLUE TRITAN

SYMBOL	MARKER NAME	MAP LOCATION	NO	ARTICLE TITLE
BCR	breakpoint cluster region	22q11	3092	LEUKEMIA, CHRONIC MYELOID (CML)
BDM	behavior disorder modifier	X	1532	MOOD AND THOUGHT DISORDERS
BFLS	Borjeson-Forssman-Lehmann syndrome	Xq26-q27	2272	BORJESON-FORSSMAN-LEHMANN SYNDROME
BPGM	2,3-bisphosphoglycerate mutase	7q31-q34	2664	ERYTHROCYTE, DIPHOSPHOGLYCERATE MUTASE (2,3) DEFICIENCY
BTS	Batten disease	16	0713	NEURONAL CEROID-LIPOFUSCINOSES (NCL)
BWS	Beckwith-Wiedemann syndrome	11pter-p15.4	0104	BECKWITH-WIEDEMANN SYNDROME
C1NH	complement component 1 inhibitor (angioedema, hereditary)	11q12-q13.1	0054	ANGIOEDEMA, HEREDITARY
C1QA	complement component 1, q subcomponent, alpha polypeptide	1p	3210	COMPLEMENT COMPONENT 1, DEFICIENCY OF
C1QB	complement component 1, q subcomponent, beta polypeptide	1p	3210	COMPLEMENT COMPONENT 1, DEFICIENCY OF
C1R	complement component 1, r subcomponent	12p13	3210	COMPLEMENT COMPONENT 1, DEFICIENCY OF
C1S	complement component 1, s subcomponent	12p13	3210	COMPLEMENT COMPONENT 1, DEFICIENCY OF
C2	complement component 2	6p21.3	2201	COMPLEMENT COMPONENT 2, DEFICIENCY OF
C3	complement component 3	19p13.3-p13.2	2219	COMPLEMENT COMPONENT 3, DEFICIENCY OF
C4A	complement component 4A	6p21.3	2220	COMPLEMENT COMPONENT 4, DEFICIENCY OF
C4B	complement component 4B	6p21.3	2220	COMPLEMENT COMPONENT 4, DEFICIENCY OF
C4BP	complement component 4 binding protein	1q32	2220	COMPLEMENT COMPONENT 4, DEFICIENCY OF
CA2	carbonic anhydrase II	8q22	0863	RENAL TUBULAR ACIDOSIS-SENSORINEURAL DEAFNESS
CA2	carbonic anhydrase II	8q22	3086	RENAL TUBULAR ACIDOSIS-OSTEOPETROSIS SYNDROME
CAE	cataract, zonular pulverulent (FY-linked)	1q21-q25	2342	CATARACT, AUTOSOMAL DOMINANT CONGENITAL
CAE	cataract, zonular pulverulent (FY-linked)	1q21-q25	3174	CATARACT, COPPOCK
CAT	catalase	11p13	0006	ACATALASEMIA
CBBM	color blindness, blue monochromatic	Xq28	0195	COLOR BLINDNESS, BLUE MONOCONE-MONOCHROMATIC
CBS	cystathionine-beta-synthase	21q22.3	0474	HOMOCYSTINURIA
CCA	congenital contractural arachnodactyly	unassigned	0085	ARACHNODACTYLY, CONTRACTURAL BEALS TYPE
CCAT	cataract, congenital	ULG3	3173	CATARACT, HUTTERITE
CCT	cataract, congenital, total	X	0132	CATARACT, CORTICAL AND NUCLEAR
CD11A	antigen CD11A (p180), lymphocyte function-associated antigen 1	16p13.1-p11	2970	GRANULOCYTE GLYCOPROTEIN CD11/CD18 DEFICIENCY
CD13	antigen CD13 (p150)	15q25-qter	2970	GRANULOCYTE GLYCOPROTEIN CD11/CD18 DEFICIENCY
CD18	lymphocyte function-associated antigen 1; macrophage antigen	21q22.3	2970	GRANULOCYTE GLYCOPROTEIN CD11/CD18 DEFICIENCY
CDPX	chondrodysplasia punctata	Xp22.32	2730	CHONDRODYSPLASIA PUNCTATA, X-LINKED DOMINANT TYPE
CECR	cat eye syndrome chromosome region	22pter-q11	0544	CAT EYE SYNDROME
CF	cystic fibrosis	7q31-q32	0237	CYSTIC FIBROSIS
CHE1	cholinesterase (serum) 1	3q26-qter	0152	CHOLINESTERASE, ATYPICAL
CHE2	cholinesterase (serum) 2	2q	0152	CHOLINESTERASE, ATYPICAL
CLG	collagenase, epidermolysis bullosa, dystrophic, (autosomal recessive)	11q21-q22	2562	EPIDERMOLYSIS BULLOSUM, TYPE III
CLS	Coffin-Lowry syndrome	Xp22.2-p22.1	0190	COFFIN-LOWRY SYNDROME
CMM	cutaneous malignant melanoma/dysplastic nevus	1p36	2318	CANCER, MALIGNANT MELANOMA, FAMILIAL
CMM	cutaneous malignant melanoma/dysplastic nevus	1p36	2165	NEVUS, CONGENITAL NEVOMELANOCYTIC
CMT1	Charcot-Marie-Tooth neuropathy 1	1q	2104	NEUROPATHY, HEREDITARY MOTOR AND SENSORY, TYPE I

SYMBOL	MARKER NAME	MAP LOCATION	NO	ARTICLE TITLE
CMT2	Charcot-Marie-Tooth neuropathy 2	17p13.1-q12	2104	NEUROPATHY, HEREDITARY MOTOR AND SENSORY, TYPE I
CMTX	Charcot-Marie-Tooth neuropathy, X-linked	Xq11-q13	2104	NEUROPATHY, HEREDITARY MOTOR AND SENSORY, TYPE I
COD1	cone dystrophy 1 (X-linked)	Xp21.1-p11.3	3228	RETINA, CONE DYSTROPHY, X-LINKED
COL1A1	collagen, type I, alpha 1	17q21.3-q22	0777	OSTEOGENESIS IMPERFECTA
COL1A2	collagen, type I, alpha 2	7q21.3-q22.1	0777	OSTEOGENESIS IMPERFECTA
COL2A1	collagen, type II, alpha 1	12q14.3	0897	SPONDYLOEPIPHYSEAL DYSPLASIA CONGENITA
CORD	cone rod dystrophy (autosomal dominant)	unassigned	0201	RETINA, COMBINED CONE-ROD DEGENERATION
CP	ceruloplasmin	3q23-q25	3077	HYPOCERULOPLASMINEMIA
CPO	coproporphyrinogen oxidase	9	0203	PORPHYRIA, COPROPORPHYRIA
CPP	ceruloplasmin pseudogene	8q21.13-q23.1	3077	HYPOCERULOPLASMINEMIA
CPS1	carbamoyl phosphate synthetase 1, mitochondrial	2p	3022	CARBAMOYL PHOSPHATE SYNTHETASE DEFICIENCY
CRD	choroidoretinal degeneration	X	0869	RETINITIS PIGMENTOSA
CRD	choroidoretinal degeneration	X	0925	CHOROIDEREMIA
CRS	craniosynostosis	7p21	0230	CRANIOSYNOSTOSIS
CSNB1	congenital stationary night blindness 1	Xp21.1-p11.23	0718	NIGHTBLINDNESS, CONGENITAL STATIONARY, X-LINKED RECESSIVE
CTH	cystathionase	16	0236	CYSTATHIONINURIA
CTM	cataract, Marner	16	2342	CATARACT, AUTOSOMAL DOMINANT CONGENITAL
CTM	cataract, Marner	16	0132	CATARACT, CORTICAL AND NUCLEAR
CYBB	cytochrome b-245, beta polypeptide (chronic granulomatous disease)	Xp21.1	0443	GRANULOMATOUS DISEASE, CHRONIC X-LINKED
CYP1	cytochrome P450, subfamily I (aromatic compound-inducible)	15q22-q24	2747	CANCER, LUNG, FAMILIAL
CYP11A	cytochrome P450, subfamily XIA	15	0907	STEROID 20-22 DESMOLASE DEFICIENCY
CYP11B1	cytochrome P450, subfamily XIB, polypeptide 1 (steroid 11-beta-hydroxylase)	8q21-q22	0902	STEROID 11 BETA-HYDROXYLASE DEFICIENCY
CYP11B2	cytochrome P450, subfamily XIB, polypeptide 2 (steroid 11-beta-hydroxylase)	8q21-q22	0902	STEROID 11 BETA-HYDROXYLASE DEFICIENCY
CYP17	cytochrome P450, subfamily XVII (steroid 17-alpha-hydroxylase)	10	0903	STEROID 17 ALPHA-HYDROXYLASE DEFICIENCY
CYP19	cytochrome P450, subfamily XIX (aromatization of androgens)	15q21	2308	GYNECOMASTIA DUE TO INCREASED AROMATASE ACTIVITY, FAMILIAL
CYP21	cytochrome P450, subfamily XXI	6p21.3	0908	STEROID 21-HYDROXYLASE DEFICIENCY
DBH	dopamine beta-hydroxylase (dopamine beta-monooxygenase)	9q34	2883	DOPAMINE BETA-HYDROXYLASE DEFICIENCY, CONGENITAL
DES	desmin	2	3072	MYOPATHY OR CARDIOMYOPATHY DUE TO DESMIN DEFECT
DFN3	deafness, conductive, with fixed stapes	Xq13-q21.2	3116	DEAFNESS WITH PERILYMPHATIC GUSHER
DGCR	DiGeorge syndrome chromosome region	22q11.21-q11.23	0943	IMMUNODEFICIENCY, THYMIC AGENESIS
DGI1	dentinogenesis imperfecta 1	4q12-q23	0279	TEETH, DENTINOGENESIS IMPERFECTA
DHOF	dermal hypoplasia, focal	X	0281	DERMAL HYPOPLASIA, FOCAL
DIA1	diaphorase (NADH) (cytochrome b-5 reductase)	22q13.31-qter	2682	METHEMOGLOBINEMIA, NADH-DEPENDENT DIAPHORASE DEFICIENCY
DIR	diabetes insipidus, renal	Xq28	0287	DIABETES INSIPIDUS, VASOPRESSIN RESISTANT TYPES I AND II
DKC	dyskeratosis congenita	Xq27-q28	2024	DYSKERATOSIS CONGENITA
DM	dystrophia myotonia	19q13.2-q13.3	0702	MYOTONIC DYSTROPHY
DMD	muscular dystrophy, Duchenne and Becker types	Xp21.3-p21.1	0689	MUSCULAR DYSTROPHY, CHILDHOOD PSEUDOHYPERTROPHIC

SYMBOL	MARKER NAME	MAP LOCATION	NO	ARTICLE TITLE
DMD	muscular dystrophy, Duchenne and Becker types	Xp21.3-p21.1	0687	MUSCULAR DYSTROPHY, ADULT PSEUDOHYPERTROPHIC
DTS	diphtheria toxin sensitivity	5q23	3079	DIPHTHERIA, SUSCEPTIBILITY TO
DYT1	dystonia, torsion 1 (autosomal dominant)	9q32-q34	0957	TORSION DYSTONIA
DYT2	dystonia, torsion 2 (autosomal recessive)	unassigned	0957	TORSION DYSTONIA
EBDCT	epidermolysis bullosa dystrophica (Cockayne-Touraine)	unassigned	2560	EPIDERMOLYSIS BULLOSUM, TYPE I
EBN	epilepsy, benign neonatal	20q	3216	CONVULSIONS, BENIGN FAMILIAL NEONATAL
EBR3	epidermolysis bullosa progressiva	ULG4	2562	EPIDERMOLYSIS BULLOSUM, TYPE III
EBS1	epidermolysis bullosa simplex (Ogna)	8	2560	EPIDERMOLYSIS BULLOSUM, TYPE I
EDA	ectodermal dysplasia, anhidrotic (hypohydrotic)	Xq12-q13.1	0333	ECTODERMAL DYSPLASIA, CHRIST-SIEMENS-TOURAINE TYPE
EFE2	endocardial fibroelastosis 2	X	0348	VENTRICLE, ENDOCARDIAL FIBROELASTOSIS OF LEFT VENTRICLE
EJM	epilepsy, juvenile myoclonic	6p	2567	SEIZURES, MYOCLONIC, JUVENILE JANZ TYPE
EKV	erythrokeratodermia variabilis	1	0361	SKIN, ERYTHROKERATODERMIA, VARIABLE
EL1	elliptocytosis 1 (Rh-linked); band 4.1 protein	1pter-p34	2646	ANEMIA, HEMOLYTIC, RED CELL MEMBRANE DEFECTS
EL1	elliptocytosis 1 (Rh-linked); band 4.1 protein	1pter-p34	2665	ELLIPTOCYTOSIS
EMD	Emery-Dreifuss muscular dystrophy	Xq27.3-q28	2491	EMERY-DREIFUSS SYNDROME
EPB3	erythrocyte surface protein band 3	17q21-qter	2646	ANEMIA, HEMOLYTIC, RED CELL MEMBRANE DEFECTS
ETFA	electron transfer flavoprotein, alpha polypeptide (glutaric aciduria II)	15q23-q25	2377	ACIDEMIA, ETHYLMALONIC-ADIPIC
F10	coagulation factor X	13q34	2670	FACTOR X DEFICIENCY
F11	coagulation factor XI	4q35	2671	FACTOR XI DEFICIENCY
F12	coagulation factor XII (Hageman)	5q33-qter	2672	FACTOR XII DEFICIENCY
F13A1	coagulation factor XIII, A1 polypeptide	6p25-p24	2673	FACTOR XIII (FIBRIN STABILIZING FACTOR)
F2	coagulation factor II (prothrombin)	11p11-q12	2679	HYPOPROTHROMBINEMIA
F2L	coagulation factor II (prothrombin)-like	Xpter-q25	2679	HYPOPROTHROMBINEMIA
F2L	coagulation factor II (prothrombin)-like	Xpter-q25	2674	COAGULATION DEFECT, FAMILIAL MULTIPLE FACTORS
F5	coagulation factor V	1q21-q25	2668	FACTOR V DEFICIENCY
F7	coagulation factor VII	13q34	2669	FACTOR VII DEFICIENCY
F8C	coagulation factor VIIIc, procoagulant component (hemophilia A)	Xq28	0461	HEMOPHILIA A
F8VWF	coagulation factor VIII VWF (von Willebrand factor)	12pter-p12	0996	VON WILLEBRAND DISEASE
F9	coagulation factor IX (Christmas disease)	Xq26.3-q27.1	0462	HEMOPHILIA B
FA	Fanconi anemia	unassigned	2029	PANCYTOPENIA SYNDROME, FANCONI TYPE
FAH	fumarylacetoacetate	15q23-q25	0978	TYROSINEMIA I
FGA	fibrinogen, A alpha polypeptide	4q28	2661	AFIBROGINEMIA, CONGENITAL
FGA	fibrinogen, A alpha polypeptide	4q28	0004	FIBRINOGENS, ABNORMAL CONGENITAL
FGB	fibrinogen, B beta polypeptide	4q28	2661	AFIBROGINEMIA, CONGENITAL
FGB	fibrinogen, B beta polypeptide	4q28	0004	FIBRINOGENS, ABNORMAL CONGENITAL
FGDY	faciogenital dysplasia (Aarskog syndrome)	Xq13	0001	AARSKOG SYNDROME
FGG	fibrinogen, gamma polypeptide	4q28	2661	AFIBROGINEMIA, CONGENITAL
FGG	fibrinogen, gamma polypeptide	4q28	0004	FIBRINOGENS, ABNORMAL CONGENITAL
FH	fumarate hydratase	1q42.1	2599	ACIDURIA, FUMARIC
FMD	facioscapulohumeral muscular dystrophy	unassigned	2049	MUSCULAR DYSTROPHY, FACIO-SCAPULO-HUMERAL
FRAXA	fragile site, folic acid type, rare, fra(X)(q27.3)	Xq27.3	2073	X-LINKED MENTAL RETARDATION, FRAGILE X SYNDROME
FRDA	Friedreich ataxia	9q13-q21.1	2714	ATAXIA, FRIEDREICH TYPE
FUCA1	fucosidase, alpha-L- 1, tissue	1p35-p34	0398	FUCOSIDOSIS

SYMBOL	MARKER NAME	MAP LOCATION	NO	ARTICLE TITLE
FY	Duffy blood group	1q21-q25	3065	MALARIA, VIVAX, SUSCEPTIBILITY TO
G6PD	glucose-6-phosphate dehydrogenase	Xq28	0420	GLUCOSE-6-PHOSPHATE DEHYDROGENASE DEFICIENCY
GAA	glucosidase, alpha; acid	17q23	0011	GLYCOGENOSIS, TYPE IIa
GAA	glucosidase, alpha; acid	17q23	2873	GLYCOGENOSIS, TYPE IIb
GAD	glutamate decarboxylase	2	0991	SEIZURES, VITAMIN B(6) DEPENDENCY
GALC	galactosylceramidase	17	0415	LEUKODYSTROPHY, GLOBOID CELL TYPE
GALE	UDP-galactose-4-epimerase	1p36-p35	0357	GALACTOSE EPIMERASE DEFICIENCY
GALK	galactokinase	17q23-q25	0402	GALACTOKINASE DEFICIENCY
GALT	galactose-1-phosphate uridylyltransferase	9p13	0403	GALACTOSEMIA
GBA	glucosidase, beta; acid	1q21	0406	GAUCHER DISEASE
GC	group-specific component (vitamin D binding protein)	4q12-q13	0983	USHER SYNDROME
GC	group-specific component (vitamin D binding protein)	4q12-q13	0446	PLASMA, GROUP-SPECIFIC COMPONENT
GCP	green cone pigment (color blindness, deutan)	Xq28	0196	COLOR BLINDNESS, RED-GREEN DEUTAN SERIES
GCPS	Greig cephalopolysyndactyly syndrome	7p13	2925	POLYSYNDACTYLY-DYSMORPHIC CRANIOFACIES, GREIG TYPE
GGT1	gamma-glutamyltransferase 1	22q11.1-q11.2	0422	GLUTATHIONURIA
GH1	growth hormone 1	17q22-q24	0447	GROWTH HORMONE DEFICIENCY, ISOLATED
GK	glycerol kinase deficiency	Xp21.3-p21.2	2310	GLYCEROL KINASE DEFICIENCY
GLA	galactosidase, alpha	Xq21.3-q22	0373	FABRY DISEASE
GLB1	galactosidase, beta 1	3pter-p21	3215	G(M1)-GANGLIOSIDOSIS, TYPE 3
GLB1	galactosidase, beta 1	3pter-p21	0431	G(M1)-GANGLIOSIDOSIS, TYPE 1
GLI	glioma-associated oncogene homolog (zinc finger protein)	12q13	2839	CANCER, GLIOMA, FAMILIAL
GM2A	GM2 ganglioside activator protein	5	0434	G(M2)-GANGLIOSIDOSIS WITH HEXOSAMINIDASE A DEFICIENCY
GNPTA	UDP-N-acetylgluco.-lysosomal-enzyme N-acetylglucosaminephosphotrans.	4q21-q23	0673	MUCOLIPIDOSIS III
GNPTA	UDP-N-acetylgluco.-lysosomal-enzyme N-acetylglucosaminephosphotrans.	4q21-q23	0672	MUCOLIPIDOSIS II
GNS	N-acetylglucosamine-6-sulfatase (Sanfilippo disease IIID)	12q14	0677	MUCOPOLYSACCHARIDOSIS III
GP2B	glycoprotein IIb (IIb/IIIa complex, platelet, CD41B)	17q21.32	2683	THROMBASTHENIA, GLANZMANN-NAEGELI TYPE
GPI	glucose phosphate isomerase	19q13.1	2750	ANEMIA, GLUCOSE PHOSPHATE ISOMERASE DEFICIENCY
GPX1	glutathione peroxidase 1	3q11-q12	2675	ANEMIA, HEMOLYTIC, GLUTATHIONINE PEROXIDASE DEFICIENCY
GRL	glucocorticoid receptor	5q31-q32	2952	GLUCOCORTICOID RESISTANCE
GSL	galactosialidosis	20	3110	GALACTOSIALIDOSIS
GSR	glutathione reductase	8p21.1	2676	ANEMIA, HEMOLYTIC, GLUTATHIONE REDUCTASE DEFICIENCY
GTS	Gilles de la Tourette syndrome	unassigned	2305	TOURETTE SYNDROME
GUD	genitourinary dysplasia component of WAGR	11p13	2742	CANCER, WILMS TUMOR
GUD	genitourinary dysplasia component of WAGR	11p13	2245	CHROMOSOME 11, PARTIAL MONOSOMY 11p
GUSB	glucuronidase, beta	7q21.2-q22	0680	MUCOPOLYSACCHARIDOSIS VII
HBB	hemoglobin, beta	11p15.5	0886	ANEMIA, SICKLE CELL
HD	Huntington disease	4pter-p16.3	0478	HUNTINGTON DISEASE
HEXA	hexosaminidase A (alpha polypeptide)	15q23-q24	0434	G(M2)-GANGLIOSIDOSIS WITH HEXOSAMINIDASE A DEFICIENCY
HEXB	hexosaminidase B (beta polypeptide)	5q13	0433	G(M2)-GANGLIOSIDOSIS WITH HEXOSAMINIDASE A AND B DEFICIENCY
HFE	hemochromatosis	6p21.3	0460	HEMOCHROMATOSIS, IDIOPATHIC
HHG	hypergonadotropic hypogonadism	ULG5	0556	KLINEFELTER SYNDROME
HHH	hyperornithinemia-hyperammonemia-homocitrullinuria	13q34	3169	HYPERORNITHINEMIA-HYPERAMMONEMIA-HOMOCITRULLINURIA

SYMBOL	MARKER NAME	MAP LOCATION	NO	ARTICLE TITLE
HIGM1	hyper IgM syndrome	Xq24-q27	2524	IMMUNODEFICIENCY, X-LINKED WITH HYPER IgM
HIS	histidase	12	0472	HISTIDINEMIA
HK1	hexokinase 1	10q22	2678	ANEMIA, HEMOLYTIC, ERYTHROCYTE HEXOKINASE DEFICIENCY
HLA-A	major histocompatibility complex, class I	6p21.3	3082	RAGWEED POLLEN SENSITIVITY
HOAC	hypoacusis 2 (autosomal recessive)	ULG4	0271	DEAFNESS (SENSORINEURAL), RECESSIVE PROFOUND
HOMG	hypomagnesemia, secondary hypocalcemia	X	0514	HYPOMAGNESEMIA, PRIMARY
HP	haptoglobin	16q22.1	0452	HAPTOGLOBIN
HPRT	hypoxanthine phosphoribosyltransferase	Xq26	0588	LESCH-NYHAN SYNDROME
HPRT	hypoxanthine phosphoribosyltransferase	Xq26	0441	GOUT
HPT	hypoparathyroidism	Xq26-q27	0515	HYPOPARATHYROIDISM, FAMILIAL
HSAS	hydrocephalus, stenosis of the aqueduct of Sylvius	X	0481	HYDROCEPHALY
HSDB3	hydroxy-delta 5-steroid dehydrogenase, 3 beta- and steroid delta-i somerase	1p13-p11	0909	STEROID 3 BETA-HYDROXYSTEROID DEHYDROGENASE DEFICIENCY
HV1S	herpes simplex virus type 1 sensitivity	3 or 11p11-qter	2988	FETAL HERPES SIMPLEX VIRUS INFECTION
HVBS4	hepatitis B virus integration site 4	2	3008	FETAL EFFECT FROM HEPATITIS B INFECTION
HVBS8	hepatitis B virus integration site 8	17p12-p11.2	3008	FETAL EFFECT FROM HEPATITIS B INFECTION
HYP	hypophosphatemia, vitamin D resistant rickets	Xp22.2-p22.1	0517	HYPOPHOSPHATEMIA, X-LINKED
IC1	ichthyosis 1, (autosomal recessive); congenital ichthyosiform erythroderma	unassigned	2853	ICHTHYOSIS, LAMELLAR RECESSIVE
IC1	ichthyosis 1, (autosomal recessive); congenital ichthyosiform erythroderma	unassigned	2855	ICHTHYOSIS, CONGENITAL ERYTHRODERMIC
IDS	iduronate 2-sulfatase (Hunter syndrome)	Xq27.3-q28	0676	MUCOPOLYSACCHARIDOSIS II
IDUA	iduronidase, alpha-L-	22pter-q11	0675	MUCOPOLYSACCHARIDOSIS I-S
IDUA	iduronidase, alpha-L-	22pter-q11	0674	MUCOPOLYSACCHARIDOSIS I-H
IF	complement component I	4q24-q25	2219	COMPLEMENT COMPONENT 3, DEFICIENCY OF
IFNA	interferon, alpha (leukocyte)	9p22-p13	3090	INTERFERON DEFICIENCY
IFNB1	interferon, beta 1, fibroblast	9p22	3090	INTERFERON DEFICIENCY
IFNB3	interferon, beta 3, fibroblast	2p23-qter	3090	INTERFERON DEFICIENCY
IFNG	interferon, gamma	12q24.1	3090	INTERFERON DEFICIENCY
IFNR	interferon production regulator	16	3090	INTERFERON DEFICIENCY
IGF1	insulin-like growth factor 1	12q23	3100	GROWTH DEFICIENCY, AFRICAN PYGMY TYPE
IGHA1	immunoglobulin alpha 1	14q32.33	0476	SERUM ALLOTYPES, HUMAN
IGHA1	immunoglobulin alpha 1	14q32.33	0521	IMMUNODEFICIENCY, COMMON VARIABLE TYPE
IGHA2	immunoglobulin alpha 2 (A2M marker)	14q32.33	0476	SERUM ALLOTYPES, HUMAN
IGHA2	immunoglobulin alpha 2 (A2M marker)	14q32.33	0521	IMMUNODEFICIENCY, COMMON VARIABLE TYPE
IGHD	immunoglobulin delta	14q32.33	0521	IMMUNODEFICIENCY, COMMON VARIABLE TYPE
IGHD	immunoglobulin delta	14q32.33	0476	SERUM ALLOTYPES, HUMAN
IGHE	immunoglobulin epsilon	14q32.33	0521	IMMUNODEFICIENCY, COMMON VARIABLE TYPE
IGHE	immunoglobulin epsilon	14q32.33	0476	SERUM ALLOTYPES, HUMAN
IGHEP1	immunoglobulin epsilon pseudogene 1	14q32.33	0521	IMMUNODEFICIENCY, COMMON VARIABLE TYPE
IGHEP1	immunoglobulin epsilon pseudogene 1	14q32.33	0476	SERUM ALLOTYPES, HUMAN
IGHG1	immunoglobulin gamma 1 (Gm marker)	14q32.33	0521	IMMUNODEFICIENCY, COMMON VARIABLE TYPE
IGHG1	immunoglobulin gamma 1 (Gm marker)	14q32.33	0476	SERUM ALLOTYPES, HUMAN
IGHG1	immunoglobulin gamma 1 (Gm marker)	14q32.33	2947	IMMUNODEFICIENCY, IgG SUBCLASS DEFICIENCIES
IGHG2	immunoglobulin gamma 2 (Gm marker)	14q32.33	0521	IMMUNODEFICIENCY, COMMON VARIABLE TYPE
IGHG2	immunoglobulin gamma 2 (Gm marker)	14q32.33	0476	SERUM ALLOTYPES, HUMAN
IGHG2	immunoglobulin gamma 2 (Gm marker)	14q32.33	0521	IMMUNODEFICIENCY, COMMON VARIABLE TYPE
IGHG2	immunoglobulin gamma 2 (Gm marker)	14q32.33	2947	IMMUNODEFICIENCY, IgG SUBCLASS DEFICIENCIES

SYMBOL	MARKER NAME	MAP LOCATION	NO	ARTICLE TITLE
IGHG3	immunoglobulin gamma 3 (Gm marker)	14q32.33	2947	IMMUNODEFICIENCY, IgG SUBCLASS DEFICIENCIES
IGHG3	immunoglobulin gamma 3 (Gm marker)	14q32.33	0476	SERUM ALLOTYPES, HUMAN
IGHG3	immunoglobulin gamma 3 (Gm marker)	14q32.33	0521	IMMUNODEFICIENCY, COMMON VARIABLE TYPE
IGHG4	immunoglobulin gamma 4 (Gm marker)	14q32.33	0476	SERUM ALLOTYPES, HUMAN
IGHG4	immunoglobulin gamma 4 (Gm marker)	14q32.33	2947	IMMUNODEFICIENCY, IgG SUBCLASS DEFICIENCIES
IGHG4	immunoglobulin gamma 4 (Gm marker)	14q32.33	0521	IMMUNODEFICIENCY, COMMON VARIABLE TYPE
IGHJ	immunoglobulin heavy polypeptide, joining region	14q32.3	0476	SERUM ALLOTYPES, HUMAN
IGHJ	immunoglobulin heavy polypeptide, joining region	14q32.3	0521	IMMUNODEFICIENCY, COMMON VARIABLE TYPE
IGHM	immunoglobulin mu	14q32.33	0521	IMMUNODEFICIENCY, COMMON VARIABLE TYPE
IGHM	immunoglobulin mu	14q32.33	0476	SERUM ALLOTYPES, HUMAN
IGHV	immunoglobulin heavy polypeptide, variable region (many genes)	14q32.33	0521	IMMUNODEFICIENCY, COMMON VARIABLE TYPE
IGHV	immunoglobulin heavy polypeptide, variable region (many genes)	14q32.33	0476	SERUM ALLOTYPES, HUMAN
IGJ	immunoglobulin J polypeptide	4q21	3073	LEUKEMIA, ACUTE LYMPHOCYTIC, FAMILIAL
IGKC	immunoglobulin kappa constant region	2p12	0476	SERUM ALLOTYPES, HUMAN
IGKC	immunoglobulin kappa constant region	2p12	0521	IMMUNODEFICIENCY, COMMON VARIABLE TYPE
IL6	interleukin 6	7p21-p14	3090	INTERFERON DEFICIENCY
IP1	incontinentia pigmenti 1	Xp11.21-cen	0526	INCONTINENTIA PIGMENTI
IVD	isovaleryl Coenzyme A dehydrogenase	15q14-q15	0547	ACIDEMIA, ISOVALERIC
JPD	juvenile periodontitis	4	0806	TEETH, PERIODONTITIS, JUVENILE
KAL	Kallmann syndrome	Xp22.32	2301	KALLMANN SYNDROME
KMS	Kabuki make-up syndrome	unassigned	2355	KABUKI MAKE-UP SYNDROME
KRT19	keratin 19	17q21-q23	2675	ANEMIA, HEMOLYTIC, GLUTATIONINE PEROXIDASE DEFICIENCY
LCAT	lecithin-cholesterol acyltransferase	16q22.1	2646	ANEMIA, HEMOLYTIC, RED CELL MEMBRANE DEFECTS
LCAT	lecithin-cholesterol acyltransferase	16q22.1	0580	LECITHIN-CHOLESTEROL ACYL TRANSFERASE DEFICIENCY
LCO	liver cancer oncogene	2q14-q21	1505	CANCER, FAMILIAL
LCT	lactase	2	0566	LACTASE DEFICIENCY, CONGENITAL
LDHA	lactate dehydrogenase A	11p15.1-p14	0568	LACTATE DEHYDROGENASE ISOZYMES
LDHB	lactate dehydrogenase B	12p12.2-p12.1	0568	LACTATE DEHYDROGENASE ISOZYMES
LDHC	lactate dehydrogenase C	11	0568	LACTATE DEHYDROGENASE ISOZYMES
LDLR	low density lipoprotein receptor (familial hypercholesterolemia)	19p13.2-p13.1	0488	HYPERCHOLESTEREMIA
LGCR	Langer-Giedion syndrome chromosome region	8q24.11-q24.13	0967	TRICHO-RHINO-PHALANGEAL SYNDROME, TYPE II
LGMD2	limb girdle muscular dystrophy 2 (autosomal recessive)	unassigned	0691	MUSCULAR DYSTROPHY, LIMB-GIRDLE
LIPA	lipase A, lysosomal acid (Wolman disease)	10	0151	CHOLESTERYL ESTER STORAGE DISEASE
LIPA	lipase A, lysosomal acid (Wolman disease)	10	1003	WOLMAN DISEASE
LOX	lysyl oxidase; ?cutis laxa-X; ?Ehlers-Danlos V	X	0338	EHLERS-DANLOS SYNDROME
LOX	lysyl oxidase; ?cutis laxa-X; ?Ehlers-Danlos V	X	3219	OCCIPITAL HORN SYNDROME
LPL	lipoprotein lipase	8p22	0489	HYPERCHYLOMICRONEMIA
LYP	lymphoproliferative syndrome	Xq25-q26	2210	IMMUNODEFICIENCY, X-LINKED LYMPHOPROLIFERATIVE DISEASE
MAA	microphthalmia or anophthalmia and associated anomalies	X	3171	LENZ MICROPHTHALMIA SYNDROME
MAFD1	major affective disorder 1	11p15.5	1532	MOOD AND THOUGHT DISORDERS
MAFD2	major affective disorder 2	Xq27-q28	1532	MOOD AND THOUGHT DISORDERS
MANB	mannosidase, alpha B, lysosomal	19cen-q13.1	2079	MANNOSIDOSIS
MDCR	Miller-Dieker syndrome chromosome region	17p13.3	0603	LISSENCEPHALY SYNDROME

SYMBOL	MARKER NAME	MAP LOCATION	NO	ARTICLE TITLE
MEN1	multiple endocrine neoplasia I	11q12-q13	0350	ENDOCRINE NEOPLASIA, MULTIPLE TYPE I
MEN2A	multiple endocrine neoplasia IIA	10p11.2-q11.2	0351	ENDOCRINE NEOPLASIA, MULTIPLE TYPE II
MEN2B	multiple endocrine neoplasia IIB	10pter-q11.2	0352	ENDOCRINE NEOPLASIA, MULTIPLE TYPE III
MF4	metacarpal 4-5 fusion	X	0923	SYNDACTYLY
MFS	Marfan syndrome	unassigned	0630	MARFAN SYNDROME
MGC1	megalocornea 1 (X-linked)	Xq12-q26	0637	CORNEA, MEGALOCORNEA
MHAM	multiple hamartoma (Cowden syndrome)	unassigned	0412	GINGIVAL MULTIPLE HAMARTOMA SYNDROME
MJD	Machado-Joseph disease	unassigned	2996	MACHADO-JOSEPH DISEASE
MLR	mineralocorticoid receptor (aldosterone receptor)	4q31	0829	ALDOSTERONE RESISTANCE
MNK	Menkes syndrome	Xcen-q13	0643	MENKES SYNDROME
MPO	myeloperoxidase	17q21.3-q23	2214	IMMUNODEFICIENCY, MYELOPEROXIDASE DEFICIENCY TYPE
MRSD	mental retardation-skeletal dysplasia	Xq27-q28	2904	X-LINKED MENTAL RETARDATION-SKELETAL DYSPLASIA
MRX1	mental retardation, X-linked 1 (non dysmorphic)	Xp11-q13	2640	X-LINKED MENTAL RETARDATION, CLARK-BARAITSER TYPE
MRX1	mental retardation, X-linked 1 (non dysmorphic)	Xp11-q13	3199	X-LINKED MENTAL RETARDATION, GOLABI-ITO-HALL TYPE
MRX1	mental retardation, X-linked 1 (non dysmorphic)	Xp11-q13	2840	X-LINKED MENTAL RETARDATION, ATKIN TYPE
MRX1	mental retardation, X-linked 1 (non dysmorphic)	Xp11-q13	3200	X-LINKED MENTAL RETARDATION-CRANIOFACIAL ABNORMALITIES-CLUB FOOT
MRX2	mental retardation, X-linked 2	Xp22.3-p22.2	2920	X-LINKED MENTAL RETARDATION, RENPENNING TYPE
MSS	Marinesco-Sjogren syndrome	ULG5	2031	MARINESCO-SJOGREN SYNDROME
MTM1	myotubular myopathy 1	Xq27-q28	0695	MYOPATHY, MYOTUBULAR
MUT	methylmalonyl Coenzyme A mutase	6p21	0658	ACIDEMIA, METHYLMALONIC
MYC	avian myelocytomatosis viral (v-myc) oncogene homolog	8q24	3089	LYMPHOMA, BURKITT TYPE
NAGA	acetylgalactosaminidase, alpha-N-	22q13-qter	3254	ALPHA-N-ACETYLGALACTOSAMINIDASE DEFICIENCY
NBCCS	nevoid basal cell carcinoma syndrome	1p	0101	NEVOID BASAL CELL CARCINOMA SYNDROME
NCF1	neutrophil cytosolic factor 1	10	0443	GRANULOMATOUS DISEASE, CHRONIC X-LINKED
NDP	Norrie disease (pseudoglioma)	Xp11.4-p11.3	0721	NORRIE DISEASE
NEU	neuraminidase	10pter-q23 or 6	0671	MUCOLIPIDOSIS I
NF1	neurofibromatosis 1 (von Recklinghausen disease, Watson disease)	17q11.2	2776	PULMONIC STENOSIS-CAFE-AU-LAIT SPOTS, WATSON TYPE
NF1	neurofibromatosis 1 (von Recklinghausen disease, Watson disease)	17q11.2	0712	NEUROFIBROMATOSIS
NF2	neurofibromatosis 2 (bilateral acoustic neuroma)	22q11-q13.1	0012	ACOUSTIC NEUROMATA
NHS	Nance-Horan syndrome (congenital cataracts and dental anomalies)	Xp22.3-p21.1	2119	CATARACTS-OTO-DENTAL DEFECTS
NM	neutrophil migration	7q22-qter	2970	GRANULOCYTE GLYCOPROTEIN CD11/CD18 DEFICIENCY
NP	nucleoside phosphorylase	14q11.2	0729	IMMUNODEFICIENCY, NUCLEOSIDE-PHOSPHORYLASE DEFICIENCY
NPS1	nail patella syndrome 1	9q34	0704	NAIL-PATELLA SYNDROME
OA1	ocular albinism 1 (Nettleship-Falls)	Xp22.3	0032	ALBINISM, OCULAR
OAT	ornithine aminotransferase	10q26	0449	GYRATE ATROPHY OF THE CHOROID AND RETINA
OCRL	oculocerebrorenal syndrome of Lowe	Xq25-q26.1	0736	OCULO-CEREBRO-RENAL SYNDROME
OFD1	oral-facial-digital syndrome I	X	0770	ORO-FACIO-DIGITAL SYNDROME I
OI4	osteogenesis imperfecta type IV	7q21.3-q22.1	0777	OSTEOGENESIS IMPERFECTA
OPA1	optic atrophy (autosomal dominant)	unassigned	3069	OPTIC ATROPHY, KJER TYPE

SYMBOL	MARKER NAME	MAP LOCATION	NO	ARTICLE TITLE
OPD	otopalatodigital syndrome	X	2258	OTO-PALATO-DIGITAL SYNDROME, II
OPD	otopalatodigital syndrome	X	0786	OTO-PALATO-DIGITAL SYNDROME, I
OPEM	ophthalmoplegia, external, with myopia	X	0750	OPHTHALMOPLEGIA EXTERNA-MYOPIA
OT	prepro-oxytocin (neurophysin I)	20	2611	DIABETES INSIPIDIS, NEUROHYPOPHYSEAL TYPE
OTC	ornithine carbamoyltransferase	Xp21.1	3023	ORNITHINE TRANSCARBAMYLASE DEFICIENCY
PAH	phenylalanine hydroxylase	12q22-q24.2	0808	PHENYLKETONURIA
PAH	phenylalanine hydroxylase	12q22-q24.2	2236	FETAL EFFECTS FROM MATERNAL PKU
PALB	prealbumin	18q11.2-q12.1	2881	AMYLOIDOSIS, APPALACHIAN TYPE
PALB	prealbumin	18q11.2-q12.1	2141	AMYLOIDOSIS, TRANSTHYRETIN METHIONINE-30 TYPE
PALB	prealbumin	18q11.2-q12.1	2880	AMYLOIDOSIS, ASHKENAZI TYPE
PALB	prealbumin	18q11.2-q12.1	2143	AMYLOIDOSIS, DANISH CARDIAC TYPE
PALB	prealbumin	18q11.2-q12.1	2882	AMYLOIDOSIS, ILLINOIS TYPE
PALB	prealbumin	18q11.2-q12.1	2142	AMYLOIDOSIS, INDIANA TYPE
PBGD	porphobilinogen deaminase	11q23.2-qter	0820	PORPHYRIA, ACUTE INTERMITTENT
PBT	piebald trait	4q12-q21	0031	ALBINISM, CUTANEOUS
PC	pyruvate carboxylase	11q	0850	PYRUVATE CARBOXYLASE DEFICIENCY WITH LACTIC ACIDEMIA
PCCA	propionyl Coenzyme A carboxylase, alpha polypeptide	13q22-q34	0826	ACIDEMIA, PROPIONIC
PEPD	peptidase D	19q12-q13.2	2616	PROLIDASE DEFICIENCY
PFKL	phosphofructokinase, liver type	21q22.3	0428	GLYCOGENOSIS, TYPE VII
PFKM	phosphofructokinase, muscle type	1cen-q32	0428	GLYCOGENOSIS, TYPE VII
PFKM	phosphofructokinase, muscle type	1cen-q32	0429	GLYCOGENOSIS, TYPE VIII
PGK1	phosphoglycerate kinase 1	Xq13	2657	ANEMIA, HEMOLYTIC, ERYTHROCYTE PHOSPHOGLYCERATE KINASE DEFICIENCY
PHK	phosphorylase kinase deficiency, liver (glycogen storage disease type VIII)	X	0430	GLYCOGENOSIS, TYPE IXa
PHK	phosphorylase kinase deficiency, liver (glycogen storage disease type VIII)	X	2303	GLYCOGEN STORAGE DISEASE, X-LINKED WITH NORMAL HEPATIC ENZYMES
PHKA	phosphorylase kinase, alpha	Xq12-q13	0430	GLYCOGENOSIS, TYPE IXa
PHKA	phosphorylase kinase, alpha	Xq12-q13	2303	GLYCOGEN STORAGE DISEASE, X-LINKED WITH NORMAL HEPATIC ENZYMES
PHP	panhypopituitarism	X	0303	DWARFISM, PANHYPOPITUITARY
PI	alpha-1-antitrypsin (protease inhibitor)	14q32.1	0039	ALPHA(1)-ANTITRYPSIN DEFICIENCY
PKD1	polycystic kidney disease 1 (autosomal dominant)	16p13	0859	KIDNEY, POLYCYSTIC DISEASE, DOMINANT
PKLR	pyruvate kinase, liver and RBC	1q21	0852	PYRUVATE KINASE DEFICIENCY
PLG	plasminogen	6q26-q27	3083	PLASMINOGEN DEFECTS
PLP	proteolipid protein (Pelizaeus-Merzbacher disease)	Xq21.3-q22	0803	PELIZAEUS-MERZBACHER SYNDROME
PROC	protein C (inactivator of coagulation factors Va and VIIIa)	2q13-q21	2918	PROTEIN C DEFICIENCY
PROS1	protein S, alpha	3p11-q11.2	2950	PROTEIN S DEFICIENCY
PRPS1	phosphoribosyl pyrophosphate synthetase 1	Xq21-q27	0508	PHOSPHORIBOSYL PYROPHOSPHATE (PRPP) SYNTHETASE ABNORMALITY
PRPS1	phosphoribosyl pyrophosphate synthetase 1	Xq21-q27	0441	GOUT
PTC	phenylthiocarbamide tasting	UlG1	0809	TASTING DEFECT, PHENYLTHIOCARBAMIDE
PTS	6-pyruvyltetrahydropterin synthase	unassigned	2002	BIOPTERIN SYNTHESIS DEFICIENCY
PVS	poliovirus sensitivity	19q12-q13.2	3109	POLIO, SUSCEPTIBILITY TO
PWCR	Prader-Willi syndrome chromosome region	15q11-q12	0823	PRADER-WILLI SYNDROME
PYGL	phosphorylase, glycogen; liver (Hers disease, glycogen storage disease type VI) 14q11.2-q24.3	0427 GLYCO-GENOSIS, TYPE VI		
PYGM	phosphorylase, glycogen (McArdle syndrome)	11q12-q13.2	2877	GLYCOGENOSIS, TYPE V
QDPR	quinoid dihydropteridine reductase	4p15.3	2001	DIHYDROPTERIDINE REDUCTASE DEFICIENCY
RB1	retinoblastoma 1 (including osteosarcoma)	13q14.2	0870	RETINOBLASTOMA

SYMBOL	MARKER NAME	MAP LOCATION	NO	ARTICLE TITLE
RCP	red cone pigment (color blindness, protan)	Xq28	0197	COLOR BLINDNESS, RED-GREEN PROTAN SERIES
RH	Rhesus blood group	1p36.2-p34	3063	ERYTHROBLASTOSIS FETALIS
RP1	retinitis pigmentosa 1	1	0869	RETINITIS PIGMENTOSA
RP2	retinitis pigmentosa 2	Xp11.4-p11.2	0869	RETINITIS PIGMENTOSA
RP3	retinitis pigmentosa 3	Xp21.1-p11.4	0869	RETINITIS PIGMENTOSA
RS	retinoschisis	Xp22.2-p22.1	0871	RETINOSCHISIS
SBMA	spinal and bulbar muscular atrophy (Kennedy disease)	Xq13-q22	0895	SPINAL MUSCULAR ATROPHY
SBMA	spinal and bulbar muscular atrophy (Kennedy disease)	Xq13-q22	2493	MUSCULAR ATROPHY, SPINAL AND BULBAR, X-LINKED KENNEDY TYPE
SCA1	spinal cerebellar ataxia (olivopontocerebellar ataxia)	6p24-p21.3	0742	OLIVOPONTOCEREBELLAR ATROPHY, DOMINANT MENZEL TYPE
SCIDX1	severe combined immunodeficiency, X-linked 1	Xq13-q21.1	0524	IMMUNODEFICIENCY, X-LINKED SEVERE COMBINED
SCZD2	schizophrenia disorder 2	unassigned	1532	MOOD AND THOUGHT DISORDERS
SDYS	Simpson dysmorphia syndrome	X	2826	SIMPSON-GOLABI-BEHMEL SYNDROME
SEDL	spondyloepiphyseal dysplasia, late	Xp22	0898	SPONDYLOEPIPHYSEAL DYSPLASIA, LATE
SI	sucrase-isomaltase	3q25-q26	0920	SUCRASE-ISOMALTASE DEFICIENCY
SMPD1	sphingomyelin phosphodiesterase 1, acid lysosomal	17	0717	NIEMANN-PICK DISEASE
SPG1	spastic paraplegia, complicated	Xq27-q28	0295	PARAPLEGIA, FAMILIAL SPASTIC
SPH1	spherocytosis 1 (clinical type II)	8p21.1-p11.22	0892	SPHEROCYTOSIS
SPH1	spherocytosis 1 (clinical type II)	8p21.1-p11.22	2646	ANEMIA, HEMOLYTIC, RED CELL MEMBRANE DEFECTS
STS	steroid sulfatase (microsomal)	Xp22.32	2532	ICHTHYOSIS, X-LINKED WITH STEROID SULFATASE DEFICIENCY
TAL1	T cell acute lymphoblastic leukemia 1	11p15	3095	LEUKEMIA/LYMPHOMA, T-CELL
TAT	tyrosine aminotransferase	16q22.1	2009	TYROSINEMIA II, OREGON TYPE
TBG	thyroxin binding globulin	Xq21-q22	0950	THYROXINE-BINDING GLOBULIN DEFECTS
TCD	tapeto-choroidal dystrophy, progressive choroidemia	Xq21.1-q21.2	0925	CHOROIDEREMIA
TCN2	transcobalamin II; macrocytic anemia	22q	2624	TRANSCOBALAMIN II DEFICIENCY
TCRA	T cell receptor, alpha (V,D,J,C)	14q11.2	3095	LEUKEMIA/LYMPHOMA, T-CELL
TDD	testicular 17,20-desmolase deficiency	X	0904	STEROID 17,20-DESMOLASE DEFICIENCY
TDF	testis determining factor	Yp11.3	0437	GONADAL DYSGENESIS, XY TYPE
TG	thyroglobulin	8q24	3061	THYROID, THYROGLOBULIN DEFECTS
TKC	torticollis, keloids, cryptorchidism and renal dysplasia	Xq28-qter	2174	CERVICO-DERMO-GU SYNDROME, GOEMINNE TYPE
TPI1	triosephosphate isomerase 1	12p13	2686	ERYTHROCYTE TRIOSEPHOSPHATE ISOMERASE DEFICIENCY
TPO	thyroid peroxidase	2pter-p12	0947	THYROID, PEROXIDASE DEFECT
TRY1	trypsin 1	7q32-qter	0973	TRYPSINOGEN DEFICIENCY
TSC1	tuberous sclerosis 1	9q	0975	TUBEROUS SCLEROSIS
TSHR	thyroid stimulating hormone receptor	22q11-q13	0948	THYROTROPIN UNRESPONSIVENESS
TST1	transforming sequence, thyroid 1	10q11.2	2641	CANCER, THYROID, FAMILIAL PAPILLARY CARCINOMA OF
TYR	tyrosinase	11q14-q21	0034	ALBINISM, OCULOCUTANEOUS, TYROSINASE NEGATIVE
TYS	sclerotylosis	4q	3076	SCLEROTYLOSIS
UMPS	uridine monophosphate synthetase	3cen-q21	0772	ACIDEMIA, OROTIC
UROD	uroporphyrinogen decarboxylase	1p34	3064	PORPHYRIA CUTANEA TARDA
VDD1	vitamin D dependency 1	12q14	0873	RICKETS, VITAMIN D-DEPENDENT, TYPE I
VDR	vitamin D receptor	12	2953	RESISTANCE TO 1,25 DIHYDROXY VITAMIN D
VHL	von-Hippel Lindau syndrome	3p	0995	VON HIPPEL-LINDAU SYNDROME
VMD1	vitelliform macular dystrophy, atypical	8q	0622	RETINA, MACULAR DEGENERATION, VITELLIRUPTIVE

SYMBOL	MARKER NAME	MAP LOCATION	NO	ARTICLE TITLE
VP	variegate porphyria (protoporphyrinogen oxidase)	14q	0822	PORPHYRIA, VARIEGATE
VWS	Van der Woude syndrome	1q32-q41	0177	CLEFT LIP/PALATE-LIP PITS OR MOUNDS
WAGR	Wilms tumor, aniridia, genitourinary abnormalities, and MR	11p13	0057	ANIRIDIA
WAGR	Wilms tumor, aniridia, genitourinary abnormalities, and MR	11p13	2742	CANCER, WILMS TUMOR
WAS	Wiskott-Aldrich syndrome	Xp11.4-p11.21	0523	IMMUNODEFICIENCY, WISKOTT-ALDRICH TYPE
WMS	William syndrome	4q33-qter	0999	WILLIAMS SYNDROME
WND	Wilson disease	13q14.2-q21	0469	HEPATOLENTICULAR DEGENERATION
WS1	Waardenburg syndrome, type 1	9q34	0997	WAARDENBURG SYNDROMES
WT1	Wilms tumor 1	11p13	2742	CANCER, WILMS TUMOR
WT2	Wilms tumor 2	unassigned	2742	CANCER, WILMS TUMOR
XK	Kell blood group precursor (McLeod phenotype)	Xp21.1	2646	ANEMIA, HEMOLYTIC, RED CELL MEMBRANE DEFECTS
XPAC	fast kinetic complementation DNA repair in xeroderma pigmentosum, group A	1q	1005	XERODERMA PIGMENTOSUM
XPF	xeroderma pigmentosum, complementation group F	15	1005	XERODERMA PIGMENTOSUM
ZWS	Zellweger syndrome	7q11	0139	CEREBRO-HEPATO-RENAL SYNDROME

GENE MAP PICTORIALS BY CHROMOSOME

SYMBOL	MARKER NAME	CHROMOSOME	MAP LOCATION	NO	ARTICLE TITLE
EKV	erythrokeratodermia variabilis		1	0361	SKIN, ERYTHROKERATODERMIA, VARIABLE
RP1	retinitis pigmentosa 1		1	0869	RETINITIS PIGMENTOSA
PFKM	phosphofructokinase, muscle type		1cen-q32	0428	GLYCOGENOSIS, TYPE VII
PFKM	phosphofructokinase, muscle type		1cen-q32	0429	GLYCOGENOSIS, TYPE VIII
NBCCS	nevoid basal cell carcinoma syndrome		1p	0101	NEVOID BASAL CELL CARCINOMA SYNDROME
C1QA	complement component 1, q subcomponent, alpha polypeptide		1p	3210	COMPLEMENT COMPONENT 1, DEFICIENCY OF
C1QB	complement component 1, q subcomponent, beta polypeptide		1p	3210	COMPLEMENT COMPONENT 1, DEFICIENCY OF
HSDB3	hydroxy-delta 5-steroid dehydrogenase, 3 beta- and steroid delta-i somerase		1p13-p11	0909	STEROID 3 BETA-HYDROXYSTEROID DEHYDROGENASE DEFICIENCY
ACADM	acyl-Coenzyme A dehydrogenase, C-4 to C-12 straight-chain		1p31	2324	ACYL-CoA DEHYDROGENASE DEFICIENCY, MEDIUM CHAIN TYPE
AK2	adenylate kinase 2		1p34	2660	ANEMIA, ADENYLATE KINASE DEFICIENCY
UROD	uroporphyrinogen decarboxylase		1p34	3064	PORPHYRIA CUTANEA TARDA
FUCA1	fucosidase, alpha-L- 1, tissue		1p35-p34	0398	FUCOSIDOSIS
CMM	cutaneous malignant melanoma/dysplastic nevus		1p36	2165	NEVUS, CONGENITAL NEVOMELANOCYTIC
CMM	cutaneous malignant melanoma/dysplastic nevus		1p36	2318	CANCER, MALIGNANT MELANOMA, FAMILIAL
GALE	UDP-galactose-4-epimerase		1p36-p35	0357	GALACTOSE EPIMERASE DEFICIENCY
ALPL	alkaline phosphatase, liver/bone/kidney		1p36.1-p34	0516	HYPOPHOSPHATASIA
RH	Rhesus blood group		1p36.2-p34	3063	ERYTHROBLASTOSIS FETALIS
EL1	elliptocytosis 1 (Rh-linked); band 4.1 protein		1pter-p34	2646	ANEMIA, HEMOLYTIC, RED CELL MEMBRANE DEFECTS
EL1	elliptocytosis 1 (Rh-linked); band 4.1 protein		1pter-p34	2665	ELLIPTOCYTOSIS
XPAC	fast kinetic complementation DNA repair in xeroderma pigmentosum, group A		1q	1005	XERODERMA PIGMENTOSUM
CMT1	Charcot-Marie-Tooth neuropathy 1		1q	2104	NEUROPATHY, HEREDITARY MOTOR AND SENSORY, TYPE I
GBA	glucosidase, beta; acid		1q21	0406	GAUCHER DISEASE
PKLR	pyruvate kinase, liver and RBC		1q21	0852	PYRUVATE KINASE DEFICIENCY
CAE	cataract, zonular pulverulent (FY-linked)		1q21-q25	2342	CATARACT, AUTOSOMAL DOMINANT CONGENITAL
F5	coagulation factor V		1q21-q25	2668	FACTOR V DEFICIENCY
FY	Duffy blood group		1q21-q25	3065	MALARIA, VIVAX, SUSCEPTIBILITY TO
CAE	cataract, zonular pulverulent (FY-linked)		1q21-q25	3174	CATARACT, COPPOCK
AT3	antithrombin III		1q23-q25.1	3066	ANTITHROMBIN III DEFICIENCY
C4BP	complement component 4 binding protein		1q32	2220	COMPLEMENT COMPONENT 4, DEFICIENCY OF
VWS	Van der Woude syndrome		1q32-q41	0177	CLEFT LIP/PALATE-LIP PITS OR MOUNDS
FH	fumarate hydratase		1q42.1	2599	ACIDURIA, FUMARIC
LCT	lactase		2	0566	LACTASE DEFICIENCY, CONGENITAL
GAD	glutamate decarboxylase		2	0991	SEIZURES, VITAMIN B(6) DEPENDENCY
HVBS4	hepatitis B virus integration site 4		2	3008	FETAL EFFECT FROM HEPATITIS B INFECTION
DES	desmin		2	3072	MYOPATHY OR CARDIOMYOPATHY DUE TO DESMIN DEFECT
AN1	aniridia 1		2p	0057	ANIRIDIA
CPS1	carbamoyl phosphate synthetase 1, mitochondrial		2p	3022	CARBAMOYL PHOSPHATE SYNTHETASE DEFICIENCY
IGKC	immunoglobulin kappa constant region		2p12	0476	SERUM ALLOTYPES, HUMAN
IGKC	immunoglobulin kappa constant region		2p12	0521	IMMUNODEFICIENCY, COMMON VARIABLE TYPE
IFNB3	interferon, beta 3, fibroblast		2p23-qter	3090	INTERFERON DEFICIENCY
APOB	apolipoprotein B (including Ag(x) antigen)		2p24-p23	0002	ABETALIPOPROTEINEMIA
APOB	apolipoprotein B (including Ag(x) antigen)		2p24-p23	2646	ANEMIA, HEMOLYTIC, RED CELL MEMBRANE DEFECTS

1

2

SYMBOL	MARKER NAME	CHROMOSOME	MAP LOCATION	NO	ARTICLE TITLE
APOB	apolipoprotein B (including Ag(x) antigen)		2p24-p23	3227	APO B-100, DEFECTIVE, FAMILIAL
TPO	thyroid peroxidase		2pter-p12	0947	THYROID, PEROXIDASE DEFECT
AHH	aryl hydrocarbon hydroxylase		2pter-q31	2747	CANCER, LUNG, FAMILIAL
CHE2	cholinesterase (serum) 2		2q	0152	CHOLINESTERASE, ATYPICAL
PROC	protein C (inactivator of coagulation factors Va and VIIIa)		2q13-q21	2918	PROTEIN C DEFICIENCY
LCO	liver cancer oncogene		2q14-q21	1505	CANCER, FAMILIAL
HV1S	herpes simplex virus type 1 sensitivity	3	3 or 11p11-qter	2988	FETAL HERPES SIMPLEX VIRUS INFECTION
UMPS	uridine monophosphate synthetase		3cen-q21	0772	ACIDEMIA, OROTIC
VHL	von-Hippel Lindau syndrome		3p	0995	VON HIPPEL-LINDAU SYNDROME
PROS1	protein S, alpha		3p11-q11.2	2950	PROTEIN S DEFICIENCY
GLB1	galactosidase, beta 1		3pter-p21	0431	G(M1)-GANGLIOSIDOSIS, TYPE 1
GLB1	galactosidase, beta 1		3pter-p21	3215	G(M1)-GANCLIOSIDOSIS, TYPE 3
GPX1	glutathione peroxidase 1		3q11-q12	2675	ANEMIA, HEMOLYTIC, GLUTATIONINE PEROXIDASE DEFICIENCY
CP	ceruloplasmin		3q23-q25	3077	HYPOCERULOPLASMINEMIA
SI	sucrase-isomaltase		3q25-q26	0920	SUCRASE-ISOMALTASE DEFICIENCY
CHE1	cholinesterase (serum) 1		3q26-qter	0152	CHOLINESTERASE, ATYPICAL
JPD	juvenile periodontitis	4	4	0806	TEETH, PERIODONTITIS, JUVENILE
QDPR	quinoid dihydropteridine reductase		4p15.3	2001	DIHYDROPTERIDINE REDUCTASE DEFICIENCY
HD	Huntington disease		4pter-p16.3	0478	HUNTINGTON DISEASE
ASMD	anterior segment mesenchymal dysgenesis		4q	0439	EYE, ANTERIOR SEGMENT DYSGENESIS
TYS	sclerotylosis		4q	3076	SCLEROTYLOSIS
ALB	albumin		4q11-q13	0047	ANALBUMINEMIA
GC	group-specific component (vitamin D binding protein)		4q12-q13	0446	PLASMA, GROUP-SPECIFIC COMPONENT
GC	group-specific component (vitamin D binding protein)		4q12-q13	0983	USHER SYNDROME
PBT	piebald trait		4q12-q21	0031	ALBINISM, CUTANEOUS
DGI1	dentinogenesis imperfecta 1		4q12-q23	0279	TEETH, DENTINOGENESIS IMPERFECTA
IGJ	immunoglobulin J polypeptide		4q21	3073	LEUKEMIA, ACUTE LYMPHOCYTIC, FAMILIAL
GNPTA	UDP-N-acetylgluco.-lysosomal-enzyme N-acetylglucosaminephosphotrans.		4q21-q23	0672	MUCOLIPIDOSIS II
GNPTA	UDP-N-acetylgluco.-lysosomal-enzyme N-acetylglucosaminephosphotrans.		4q21-q23	0673	MUCOLIPIDOSIS III
ADH1	alcohol dehydrogenase (class 1), alpha polypeptide		4q21-q23	3074	ALCOHOL INTOLERANCE
ADH2	alcohol dehydrogenase (class 1), beta polypeptide		4q21-q23	3074	ALCOHOL INTOLERANCE
ADH3	alcohol dehydrogenase (class 1), gamma polypeptide		4q21-q23	3074	ALCOHOL INTOLERANCE
AGA	aspartylglucosaminidase		4q21-qter	2042	ASPARTYLGLUCOSAMINURIA
IF	complement component I		4q24-q25	2219	COMPLEMENT COMPONENT 3, DEFICIENCY OF
FGA	fibrinogen, A alpha polypeptide		4q28	0004	FIBRINOGENS, ABNORMAL CONGENITAL
FGB	fibrinogen, B beta polypeptide		4q28	0004	FIBRINOGENS, ABNORMAL CONGENITAL
FGG	fibrinogen, gamma polypeptide		4q28	0004	FIBRINOGENS, ABNORMAL CONGENITAL
FGA	fibrinogen, A alpha polypeptide		4q28	2661	AFIBROGINEMIA, CONGENITAL
FGB	fibrinogen, B beta polypeptide		4q28	2661	AFIBROGINEMIA, CONGENITAL
FGG	fibrinogen, gamma polypeptide		4q28	2661	AFIBROGINEMIA, CONGENITAL
MLR	mineralocorticoid receptor (aldosterone receptor)		4q31	0829	ALDOSTERONE RESISTANCE
WMS	William syndrome		4q33-qter	0999	WILLIAMS SYNDROME

SYMBOL	MARKER NAME	CHROMOSOME	MAP LOCATION	NO	ARTICLE TITLE
F11	coagulation factor XI		4q35	2671	FACTOR XI DEFICIENCY
GM2A	GM2 ganglioside activator protein		5	0434	G(M2)-GANGLIOSIDOSIS WITH HEXOSAMINIDASE A DEFICIENCY
ARSB	arylsulfatase B		5p11-q13	0679	MUCOPOLYSACCHARIDOSIS VI
HEXB	hexosaminidase B (beta polypeptide)		5q13	0433	G(M2)-GANGLIOSIDOSIS WITH HEXOSAMINIDASE A AND B DEFICIENCY
APC	adenomatosis polyposis coli		5q21-q22	0535	INTESTINAL POLYPOSIS, TYPE I
APC	adenomatosis polyposis coli		5q21-q22	0536	INTESTINAL POLYPOSIS, TYPE III
APC	adenomatosis polyposis coli	5	5q21-q22	2739	TURCOT SYNDROME
DTS	diphtheria toxin sensitivity		5q23	3079	DIPHTHERIA, SUSCEPTIBILITY TO
GRL	glucocorticoid receptor		5q31-q32	2952	GLUCOCORTICOID RESISTANCE
F12	coagulation factor XII (Hageman)		5q33-qter	2672	FACTOR XII DEFICIENCY
EJM	epilepsy, juvenile myoclonic		6p	2567	SEIZURES, MYOCLONIC, JUVENILE JANZ TYPE
MUT	methylmalonyl Coenzyme A mutase		6p21	0658	ACIDEMIA, METHYLMALONIC
HFE	hemochromatosis		6p21.3	0460	HEMOCHROMATOSIS, IDIOPATHIC
CYP21	cytochrome P450, subfamily XXI		6p21.3	0908	STEROID 21-HYDROXYLASE DEFICIENCY
C2	complement component 2		6p21.3	2201	COMPLEMENT COMPONENT 2, DEFICIENCY OF
C4A	complement component 4A	6	6p21.3	2220	COMPLEMENT COMPONENT 4, DEFICIENCY OF
C4B	complement component 4B		6p21.3	2220	COMPLEMENT COMPONENT 4, DEFICIENCY OF
HLA-A	major histocompatibility complex, class I		6p21.3	3082	RAGWEED POLLEN SENSITIVITY
SCA1	spinal cerebellar ataxia (olivopontocerebellar ataxia)		6p24-p21.3	0742	OLIVOPONTOCEREBELLAR ATROPHY, DOMINANT MENZEL TYPE
F13A1	coagulation factor XIII, A1 polypeptide		6p25-p24	2673	FACTOR XIII (FIBRIN STABILIZING FACTOR)
ARG1	arginase, liver		6q23	0086	ARGININEMIA
PLG	plasminogen		6q26-q27	3083	PLASMINOGEN DEFECTS
GCPS	Greig cephalopolysyndactyly syndrome		7p13	2925	POLYSYNDACTYLY-DYSMORPHIC CRANIOFACIES, GREIG TYPE
CRS	craniosynostosis		7p21	0230	CRANIOSYNOSTOSIS
IL6	interleukin 6		7p21-p14	3090	INTERFERON DEFICIENCY
ASL	argininosuccinate lyase		7pter-q22	0087	ACIDURIA, ARGININOSUCCINIC
ZWS	Zellweger syndrome		7q11	0139	CEREBRO-HEPATO-RENAL SYNDROME
GUSB	glucuronidase, beta	7	7q21.2-q22	0680	MUCOPOLYSACCHARIDOSIS VII
COL1A2	collagen, type I, alpha 2		7q21.3-q22.1	0777	OSTEOGENESIS IMPERFECTA
OI4	osteogenesis imperfecta type IV		7q21.3-q22.1	0777	OSTEOGENESIS IMPERFECTA
BCP	blue cone pigment		7q22-qter	0199	COLOR BLINDNESS, YELLOW-BLUE TRITAN
NM	neutrophil migration		7q22-qter	2970	GRANULOCYTE GLYCOPROTEIN CD11/CD18 DEFICIENCY
CF	cystic fibrosis		7q31-q32	0237	CYSTIC FIBROSIS
BPGM	2,3-bisphosphoglycerate mutase		7q31-q34	2664	ERYTHROCYTE, DIPHOSPHOGLYCERATE MUTASE (2,3) DEFICIENCY
TRY1	trypsin 1		7q32-qter	0973	TRYPSINOGEN DEFICIENCY
EBS1	epidermolysis bullosa simplex (Ogna)		8	2560	EPIDERMOLYSIS BULLOSUM, TYPE I
ANK	ankyrin		8p21-p11	0892	SPHEROCYTOSIS
ANK	ankyrin		8p21-p11	2646	ANEMIA, HEMOLYTIC, RED CELL MEMBRANE DEFECTS
GSR	glutathione reductase		8p21.1	2676	ANEMIA, HEMOLYTIC, GLUTATHIONE REDUCTASE DEFICIENCY

SYMBOL	MARKER NAME	CHROMOSOME	MAP LOCATION	NO	ARTICLE TITLE
SPH1	spherocytosis 1 (clinical type II)		8p21.1-p11.22	0892	SPHEROCYTOSIS
SPH1	spherocytosis 1 (clinical type II)		8p21.1-p11.22	2646	ANEMIA, HEMOLYTIC, RED CELL MEMBRANE DEFECTS
LPL	lipoprotein lipase		8p22	0489	HYPERCHYLOMICRONEMIA
VMD1	vitelliform macular dystrophy, atypicall		8q	0622	RETINA, MACULAR DEGENERATION, VITELLIRUPTIVE
CYP11B1	cytochrome P450, subfamily XIB, polypeptide 1 (steroid 11-beta-hydroxylase)		8q21-q22	0902	STEROID 11 BETA-HYDROXYLASE DEFICIENCY
CYP11B2	cytochrome P450, subfamily XIB, polypeptide 2 (steroid 11-beta-hydroxylase)		8q21-q22	0902	STEROID 11 BETA-HYDROXYLASE DEFICIENCY
CPP	ceruloplasmin pseudogene		8q21.13-q23.1	3077	HYPOCERULOPLASMINEMIA
CA2	carbonic anhydrase II		8q22	0863	RENAL TUBULAR ACIDOSIS-SENSORINEURAL DEAFNESS
CA2	carbonic anhydrase II		8q22	3086	RENAL TUBULAR ACIDOSIS-OSTEOPETROSIS SYNDROME
TG	thyroglobulin		8q24	3061	THYROID, THYROGLOBULIN DEFECTS
MYC	avian myelocytomatosis viral (v-myc) oncogene homolog		8q24	3089	LYMPHOMA, BURKITT TYPE
LGCR	Langer-Giedion syndrome chromosome region		8q24.11-q24.13	0967	TRICHO-RHINO-PHALANGEAL SYNDROME, TYPE II
CPO	coproporphyrinogen oxidase		9	0203	PORPHYRIA, COPROPORPHYRIA
GALT	galactose-1-phosphate uridylyltransferase		9p13	0403	GALACTOSEMIA
IFNB1	interferon, beta 1, fibroblast		9p22	3090	INTERFERON DEFICIENCY
IFNA	interferon, alpha (leukocyte)		9p22-p13	3090	INTERFERON DEFICIENCY
AK3	adenylate kinase 3		9p24-p13	2660	ANEMIA, ADENYLATE KINASE DEFICIENCY
TSC1	tuberous sclerosis 1		9q	0975	TUBEROUS SCLEROSIS
FRDA	Friedreich ataxia		9q13-q21.1	2714	ATAXIA, FRIEDREICH TYPE
ALDOB	aldolase B, fructose bisphosphate		9q21.3-q22.2	0395	FRUCTOSE-1-PHOSPHATE ALDOLASE DEFICIENCY
DYT1	dystonia, torsion 1 (autosomal dominant)		9q32-q34	0957	TORSION DYSTONIA
NPS1	nail patella syndrome 1		9q34	0704	NAIL-PATELLA SYNDROME
WS1	Waardenburg syndrome, type 1		9q34	0997	WAARDENBURG SYNDROMES
DBH	dopamine beta-hydroxylase (dopamine beta-monooxygenase)		9q34	2883	DOPAMINE BETA-HYDROXYLASE DEFICIENCY, CONGENITAL
ALAD	aminolevulinate, delta-, dehydratase		9q34	3091	DELTA-AMINOLEVULINIC ACID DEHYDRASE DEFICIENCY
ASS	argininosuccinate synthetase		9q34-qter	0174	CITRULLINEMIA
ABO	ABO blood group		9q34.1-q34.2	0340	TEETH, ENAMEL AND DENTIN DEFECTS FROM ERYTHROBLASTOSIS FETALIS
AK1	adenylate kinase 1		9q34.1-q34.2	2660	ANEMIA, ADENYLATE KINASE DEFICIENCY
LIPA	lipase A, lysosomal acid (Wolman disease)		10	0151	CHOLESTERYL ESTER STORAGE DISEASE
NCF1	neutrophil cytosolic factor 1		10	0443	GRANULOMATOUS DISEASE, CHRONIC X-LINKED
CYP17	cytochrome P450, subfamily XVII (steroid 17-alpha-hydroxylase)		10	0903	STEROID 17 ALPHA-HYDROXYLASE DEFICIENCY
LIPA	lipase A, lysosomal acid (Wolman disease)		10p11.2-q11.2	1003	WOLMAN DISEASE
MEN2A	multiple endocrine neoplasia IIA		10pter-q11.2	0351	ENDOCRINE NEOPLASIA, MULTIPLE TYPE II
MEN2B	multiple endocrine neoplasia IIB		10pter-q23	0352	ENDOCRINE NEOPLASIA, MULTIPLE TYPE III
NEU	neuraminidase		10pter-q23 or 6	0671	MUCOLIPIDOSIS I

SYMBOL	MARKER NAME	CHROMOSOME	MAP LOCATION	NO	ARTICLE TITLE
TST1	transforming sequence, thyroid 1		10q11.2	2641	CANCER, THYROID, FAMILIAL PAPILLARY CARCINOMA OF
HK1	hexokinase 1		10q22	2678	ANEMIA, HEMOLYTIC, ERYTHROCYTE HEXOKINASE DEFICIENCY
OAT	ornithine aminotransferase		10q26	0449	GYRATE ATROPHY OF THE CHOROID AND RETINA
LDHC	lactate dehydrogenase C		11	0568	LACTATE DEHYDROGENASE ISOZYMES
F2	coagulation factor II (prothrombin)		11p11-q12	2679	HYPOPROTHROMBINEMIA
CAT	catalase		11p13	0006	ACATALASEMIA
AN2	aniridia 2 without Wilms' tumor, GU abnormalities, and M.R.		11p13	0057	ANIRIDIA
WAGR	Wilms tumor, aniridia, genitourinary abnormalities, and MR		11p13	0057	ANIRIDIA
AN2	aniridia 2 without Wilms' tumor, GU abnormalities, and M.R.		11p13	2245	CHROMOSOME 11, PARTIAL MONOSOMY 11p
GUD	genitourinary dysplasia component of WAGR		11p13	2245	CHROMOSOME 11, PARTIAL MONOSOMY 11p
GUD	genitourinary dysplasia component of WAGR		11p13	2742	CANCER, WILMS TUMOR
WAGR	Wilms tumor, aniridia, genitourinary abnormalities, and MR		11p13	2742	CANCER, WILMS TUMOR
WT1	Wilms tumor 1		11p13	2742	CANCER, WILMS TUMOR
TAL1	T cell acute lymphoblastic leukemia 1		11p15	3095	LEUKEMIA/LYMPHOMA, T-CELL
LDHA	lactate dehydrogenase A		11p15.1-p14	0568	LACTATE DEHYDROGENASE ISOZYMES
HBB	hemoglobin, beta		11p15.5	0886	ANEMIA, SICKLE CELL
MAFD1	major affective disorder 1		11p15.5	1532	MOOD AND THOUGHT DISORDERS
BWS	Beckwith-Wiedemann syndrome		11pter-p15.4	0104	BECKWITH-WIEDEMANN SYNDROME
PC	pyruvate carboxylase		11q	0850	PYRUVATE CARBOXYLASE DEFICIENCY WITH LACTIC ACIDEMIA
MEN1	multiple endocrine neoplasia I		11q12-q13	0350	ENDOCRINE NEOPLASIA, MULTIPLE TYPE I
APY	atopy (allergic asthma and rhinitis)		11q12-q13	3150	SKIN, ATOPY, FAMILIAL
C1NH	complement component 1 inhibitor (angioedema, hereditary)		11q12-q13.1	0054	ANGIOEDEMA, HEREDITARY
PYGM	phosphorylase, glycogen (McArdle syndrome)		11q12-q13.2	2877	GLYCOGENOSIS, TYPE V
BCL1	B cell CLL/lymphoma 1		11q13.3	3097	LEUKEMIA/LYMPHOMA, B CELL
TYR	tyrosinase		11q14-q21	0034	ALBINISM, OCULOCUTANEOUS, TYROSINASE NEGATIVE
CLG	collagenase, epidermolysis bullosa, dystrophic, (autosomal recessive)		11q21-q22	2562	EPIDERMOLYSIS BULLOSUM, TYPE III
ATA	ataxia telangiectasia (complementation group A)		11q22-q23	0094	ATAXIA-TELANGIECTASIA
APOA1	apolipoprotein A-I		11q23-q24	3096	HYPOALPHALIPOPROTEINEMIA
APOA1	apolipoprotein A-I		11q23-q24	3165	APOLIPOPROTEIN A-I AND C-III DEFICIENCY STATES
APOA4	apolipoprotein A-IV		11q23-qter	3096	HYPOALPHALIPOPROTEINEMIA
PBGD	porphobilinogen deaminase		11q23.2-qter	0820	PORPHYRIA, ACUTE INTERMITTENT
HIS	histidase		12	0472	HISTIDINEMIA
VDR	vitamin D receptor		12	2953	RESISTANCE TO 1,25 DIHYDROXY VITAMIN D
LDHB	lactate dehydrogenase B		12p12.2-p12.1	0568	LACTATE DEHYDROGENASE ISOZYMES
TPI1	triosephosphate isomerase 1		12p13	2686	ERYTHROCYTE TRIOSEPHOSPHATE ISOMERASE DEFICIENCY
C1R	complement component 1, r subcomponent		12p13	3210	COMPLEMENT COMPONENT 1, DEFICIENCY OF
C1S	complement component 1, s subcomponent		12p13	3210	COMPLEMENT COMPONENT 1, DEFICIENCY OF

11

SYMBOL	MARKER NAME	CHROMOSOME	MAP LOCATION	NO	ARTICLE TITLE
F8VWF	coagulation factor VIII VWF (von Willebrand factor protein)		12pter-p12	0996	VON WILLEBRAND DISEASE
GLI	glioma-associated oncogene homolog (zinc finger protein)		12q13	2839	CANCER, GLIOMA, FAMILIAL
APR	apolipoprotein receptor		12q13-q14	0048	ANALPHALIPOPROTEINEMIA
APR	apolipoprotein receptor		12q13-q14	3165	APOLIPOPROTEIN A-I AND C-III DEFICIENCY STATES
AOM	arthroophthalmopathy, progressive (Stickler syndrome)		12q14	0090	ARTHRO-OPHTHALMOPATHY, HEREDITARY, PROGRESSIVE, STICKLER TYPE
GNS	N-acetylglucosamine-6-sulfatase (Sanfilippo disease IIID)		12q14	0677	MUCOPOLYSACCHARIDOSIS III
VDD1	vitamin D dependency 1		12q14	0873	RICKETS, VITAMIN D-DEPENDENT, TYPE I
AOM	arthroophthalmopathy, progressive (Stickler syndrome)		12q14	2424	ARTHRO-OPHTHALMOPATHY, WEISSENBACHER-ZWEYMULLER VARIANT
COL2A1	collagen, type II, alpha 1		12q14.3	0897	SPONDYLOEPIPHYSEAL DYSPLASIA CONGENITA
PAH	phenylalanine hydroxylase		12q22-q24.2	0808	PHENYLKETONURIA
PAH	phenylalanine hydroxylase		12q22-q24.2	2236	FETAL EFFECTS FROM MATERNAL PKU
ACADS	acyl-Coenzyme A dehydrogenase, C-2 to C-3 short chain		12q22-qter	2323	ACYL-CoA DEHYDROGENASE DEFICIENCY, SHORT CHAIN TYPE
IGF1	insulin-like growth factor 1		12q23	3100	GROWTH DEFICIENCY, AFRICAN PYGMY TYPE
IFNG	interferon, gamma	**12**	12q24.1	3090	INTERFERON DEFICIENCY
ALDH2	aldehyde dehydrogenase 2, mitochondrial		12q24.2	3074	ALCOHOL INTOLERANCE
RB1	retinoblastoma 1 (including osteosarcoma)		13q14.2	0870	RETINOBLASTOMA
WND	Wilson disease		13q14.2-q21	0469	HEPATOLENTICULAR DEGENERATION
PCCA	propionyl Coenzyme A carboxylase, alpha polypeptide		13q22-q34	0826	ACIDEMIA, PROPIONIC
F7	coagulation factor VII		13q34	2669	FACTOR VII DEFICIENCY
F10	coagulation factor X		13q34	2670	FACTOR X DEFICIENCY
HHH	hyperornithinemia-hyperammonemia-homocitrullinuria	**13**	13q34	3169	HYPERORNITHINEMIA-HYPERAMMONEMIA-HOMOCITRULLINURIA
VP	variegate porphyria (protoporphyrinogen oxidase)		14q	0822	PORPHYRIA, VARIEGATE
NP	nucleoside phosphorylase		14q11.2	0729	IMMUNODEFICIENCY, NUCLEOSIDE-PHOSPHORYLASE DEFICIENCY
TCRA	T cell receptor, alpha (V,D,J,C)		14q11.2	3095	LEUKEMIA/LYMPHOMA, T-CELL
PYGL	phosphorylase, glycogen; liver (Hers disease, glycogen storage disease type VI)		14q11.2-q24.3	0427	GLYCOGENOSIS, TYPE VI
PI	alpha-1-antitrypsin (protease inhibitor)		14q32.1	0039	ALPHA(1)-ANTITRYPSIN DEFICIENCY
AACT	alpha-1-antichymotrypsin		14q32.1	3279	ALPHA-1-ANTICHYMOTRYPSIN DEFICIENCY
IGHJ	immunoglobulin heavy polypeptide, joining region		14q32.3	0476	SERUM ALLOTYPES, HUMAN
IGHJ	immunoglobulin heavy polypeptide, joining region		14q32.3	0521	IMMUNODEFICIENCY, COMMON VARIABLE TYPE
IGHA1	immunoglobulin alpha 1		14q32.33	0476	SERUM ALLOTYPES, HUMAN
IGHA2	immunoglobulin alpha 2 (A2M marker)		14q32.33	0476	SERUM ALLOTYPES, HUMAN
IGHD	immunoglobulin delta		14q32.33	0476	SERUM ALLOTYPES, HUMAN
IGHE	immunoglobulin epsilon		14q32.33	0476	SERUM ALLOTYPES, HUMAN
IGHEP1	immunoglobulin epsilon pseudogene 1		14q32.33	0476	SERUM ALLOTYPES, HUMAN
IGHG1	immunoglobulin gamma 1 (Gm marker)		14q32.33	0476	SERUM ALLOTYPES, HUMAN
IGHG2	immunoglobulin gamma 2 (Gm marker)		14q32.33	0476	SERUM ALLOTYPES, HUMAN
IGHG3	immunoglobulin gamma 3 (Gm marker)		14q32.33	0476	SERUM ALLOTYPES, HUMAN
IGHG4	immunoglobulin gamma 4 (Gm marker)		14q32.33	0476	SERUM ALLOTYPES, HUMAN
IGHM	immunoglobulin mu	**14**	14q32.33	0476	SERUM ALLOTYPES, HUMAN

SYMBOL	MARKER NAME	CHROMOSOME	MAP LOCATION	NO	ARTICLE TITLE
IGHV	immunoglobulin heavy polypeptide, variable region (many genes)		14q32.33	0476	SERUM ALLOTYPES, HUMAN
IGHA1	immunoglobulin alpha 1		14q32.33	0521	IMMUNODEFICIENCY, COMMON VARIABLE TYPE
IGHD	immunoglobulin delta		14q32.33	0521	IMMUNODEFICIENCY, COMMON VARIABLE TYPE
IGHA2	immunoglobulin alpha 2 (A2M marker)		14q32.33	0521	IMMUNODEFICIENCY, COMMON VARIABLE TYPE
IGHE	immunoglobulin epsilon		14q32.33	0521	IMMUNODEFICIENCY, COMMON VARIABLE TYPE
IGHEP1	immunoglobulin epsilon pseudogene 1		14q32.33	0521	IMMUNODEFICIENCY, COMMON VARIABLE TYPE
IGHG1	immunoglobulin gamma 1 (Gm marker)		14q32.33	0521	IMMUNODEFICIENCY, COMMON VARIABLE TYPE
IGHG2	immunoglobulin gamma 2 (Gm marker)		14q32.33	0521	IMMUNODEFICIENCY, COMMON VARIABLE TYPE
IGHG3	immunoglobulin gamma 3 (Gm marker)		14q32.33	0521	IMMUNODEFICIENCY, COMMON VARIABLE TYPE
IGHG4	immunoglobulin gamma 4 (Gm marker)		14q32.33	0521	IMMUNODEFICIENCY, COMMON VARIABLE TYPE
IGHM	immunoglobulin mu		14q32.33	0521	IMMUNODEFICIENCY, COMMON VARIABLE TYPE
IGHV	immunoglobulin heavy polypeptide, variable region (many genes)		14q32.33	0521	IMMUNODEFICIENCY, COMMON VARIABLE TYPE
IGHG1	immunoglobulin gamma 1 (Gm marker)		14q32.33	2947	IMMUNODEFICIENCY, IgG SUBCLASS DEFICIENCIES
IGHG2	immunoglobulin gamma 2 (Gm marker)		14q32.33	2947	IMMUNODEFICIENCY, IgG SUBCLASS DEFICIENCIES
IGHG3	immunoglobulin gamma 3 (Gm marker)		14q32.33	2947	IMMUNODEFICIENCY, IgG SUBCLASS DEFICIENCIES
IGHG4	immunoglobulin gamma 4 (Gm marker)		14q32.33	2947	IMMUNODEFICIENCY, IgG SUBCLASS DEFICIENCIES
CYP11A	cytochrome P450, subfamily XIA	**15**	15	0907	STEROID 20-22 DESMOLASE DEFICIENCY
XPF	xeroderma pigmentosum, complementation group F		15	1005	XERODERMA PIGMENTOSUM
PWCR	Prader-Willi syndrome chromosome region		15q11-q12	0823	PRADER-WILLI SYNDROME
ANCR	Angelman syndrome chromosome region		15q11-q12	2086	ANGELMAN SYNDROME
IVD	isovaleryl Coenzyme A dehydrogenase		15q14-q15	0547	ACIDEMIA, ISOVALERIC
CYP19	cytochrome P450, subfamily XIX (aromatization of androgens)		15q21	2308	GYNECOMASTIA DUE TO INCREASED AROMATASE ACTIVITY, FAMILIAL
B2M	beta-2-microglobulin		15q21-q22.2	3106	AMYLOIDOSIS, HEMODIALYSIS-RELATED
CYP1	cytochrome P450, subfamily I (aromatic compound-inducible)		15q22-q24	2747	CANCER, LUNG, FAMILIAL
HEXA	hexosaminidase A (alpha polypeptide)		15q23-q24	0434	G(M2)-GANGLIOSIDOSIS WITH HEXOSAMINIDASE A DEFICIENCY
FAH	fumarylacetoacetate		15q23-q25	0978	TYROSINEMIA I
ETFA	electron transfer flavoprotein, alpha polypeptide (glutaric aciduria II)		15q23-q25	2377	ACIDEMIA, ETHYLMALONIC-ADIPIC
CD13	antigen CD13 (p150)		15q25-qter	2970	GRANULOCYTE GLYCOPROTEIN CD11/CD18 DEFICIENCY
CTM	cataract, Marner	**16**	16	0132	CATARACT, CORTICAL AND NUCLEAR
CTH	cystathionase		16	0236	CYSTATHIONINURIA
BTS	Batten disease		16	0713	NEURONAL CEROID-LIPOFUSCINOSES (NCL)
CTM	cataract, Marner		16	2342	CATARACT, AUTOSOMAL DOMINANT CONGENITAL
IFNR	interferon production regulator		16	3090	INTERFERON DEFICIENCY
PKD1	polycystic kidney disease 1 (autosomal dominant)		16p13	0859	KIDNEY, POLYCYSTIC DISEASE, DOMINANT
CD11A	antigen CD11A (p180), lymphocyte function-associated antigen 1		16p13.1-p11	2970	GRANULOCYTE GLYCOPROTEIN CD11/CD18 DEFICIENCY
ALDOA	aldolase A, fructose-bisphosphate		16q22-q24	2662	ERYTHROCYTE ALDOLASE-A DEFICIENCY
HP	haptoglobin		16q22.1	0452	HAPTOGLOBIN
LCAT	lecithin-cholesterol acyltransferase		16q22.1	0580	LECITHIN-CHOLESTEROL ACYL TRANSFERASE DEFICIENCY
TAT	tyrosine aminotransferase		16q22.1	2009	TYROSINEMIA II, OREGON TYPE

SYMBOL	MARKER NAME	CHROMOSOME	MAP LOCATION	NO	ARTICLE TITLE
LCAT	lecithin-cholesterol acyltransferase		16q22.1	2646	ANEMIA, HEMOLYTIC, RED CELL MEMBRANE DEFECTS
APRT	adenine phosphoribosyltransferase		16q24	3104	ADENINE PHOSPHO-RIBOSYL-TRANSFERASE (APRT) DEFICIENCY
GALC	galactosylceramidase	17	17	0415	LEUKODYSTROPHY, GLOBOID CELL TYPE
SMPD1	sphingomyelin phosphodiesterase 1, acid lysosomal		17	0717	NIEMANN-PICK DISEASE
HVBS8	hepatitis B virus integration site 8		17p12-p11.2	3008	FETAL EFFECT FROM HEPATITIS B INFECTION
CMT2	Charcot-Marie-Tooth neuropathy 2		17p13.1-q12	2104	NEUROPATHY, HEREDITARY MOTOR AND SENSORY, TYPE I
MDCR	Miller-Dieker syndrome chromosome region		17p13.3	0603	LISSENCEPHALY SYNDROME
NF1	neurofibromatosis 1 (von Recklinghausen disease, Watson disease)		17q11.2	0712	NEUROFIBROMATOSIS
NF1	neurofibromatosis 1 (von Recklinghausen disease, Watson disease)		17q11.2	2776	PULMONIC STENOSIS-CAFE-AU-LAIT SPOTS, WATSON TYPE
KRT19	keratin 19		17q21-q23	2675	ANEMIA, HEMOLYTIC, GLUTATHIONINE PEROXIDASE DEFICIENCY
EPB3	erythrocyte surface protein band 3		17q21-qter	2646	ANEMIA, HEMOLYTIC, RED CELL MEMBRANE DEFECTS
COL1A1	collagen, type I, alpha 1		17q21.3-q22	0777	OSTEOGENESIS IMPERFECTA
MPO	myeloperoxidase		17q21.3-q23	2214	IMMUNODEFICIENCY, MYELOPEROXIDASE DEFICIENCY TYPE
GP2B	glycoprotein IIb (IIb/IIIa complex, platelet, CD41B)	18	17q21.32	2683	THROMBASTHENIA, GLANZMANN-NAEGELI TYPE
GH1	growth hormone 1		17q22-q24	0447	GROWTH HORMONE DEFICIENCY, ISOLATED
GAA	glucosidase, alpha; acid		17q23	0011	GLYCOGENOSIS, TYPE IIa
GAA	glucosidase, alpha; acid		17q23	2873	GLYCOGENOSIS, TYPE IIb
GALK	galactokinase		17q23-q25	0402	GALACTOKINASE DEFICIENCY
PALB	prealbumin		18q11.2-q12.1	2141	AMYLOIDOSIS, TRANSTHYRETIN METHIONINE-30 TYPE
PALB	prealbumin		18q11.2-q12.1	2142	AMYLOIDOSIS, INDIANA TYPE
PALB	prealbumin		18q11.2-q12.1	2143	AMYLOIDOSIS, DANISH CARDIAC TYPE
PALB	prealbumin		18q11.2-q12.1	2880	AMYLOIDOSIS, ASHKENAZI TYPE
PALB	prealbumin		18q11.2-q12.1	2881	AMYLOIDOSIS, APPALACHIAN TYPE
PALB	prealbumin		18q11.2-q12.1	2882	AMYLOIDOSIS, ILLINOIS TYPE
BCL2	B cell CLL/lymphoma 2		18q21.3	3097	LEUKEMIA/LYMPHOMA, B CELL
BCL2	B cell CLL/lymphoma 2		18q21.3	3107	LYMPHOMA, NON-HODGKIN
MANB	mannosidase, alpha B, lysosomal	19	19cen-q13.1	2079	MANNOSIDOSIS
LDLR	low density lipoprotein receptor (familial hypercholesterolemia)		19p13.2-p13.1	0488	HYPERCHOLESTEREMIA
AMH	anti-Mullerian hormone		19p13.3	0683	MULLERIAN DERIVATIVES IN MALES, PERSISTENT
C3	complement component 3		19p13.3-p13.2	2219	COMPLEMENT COMPONENT 3, DEFICIENCY OF
PEPD	peptidase D		19q12-q13.2	2616	PROLIDASE DEFICIENCY
PVS	poliovirus sensitivity		19q12-q13.2	3109	POLIO, SUSCEPTIBILITY TO

SYMBOL	MARKER NAME	CHROMOSOME	MAP LOCATION	NO	ARTICLE TITLE
GPI	glucose phosphate isomerase		19q13.1	2750	ANEMIA, GLUCOSE PHOSPHATE ISOMERASE DEFICIENCY
APOC1	apolipoprotein C-I		19q13.2	3096	HYPOALPHALIPOPROTEINEMIA
DM	dystrophia myotonia		19q13.2-q13.3	0702	MYOTONIC DYSTROPHY
ARVP	arginine vasopressin (neurophysin II)	**20**	20	2611	DIABETES INSIPIDIS, NEUROHYPOPHYSEAL TYPE
OT	prepro-oxytocin (neurophysin I)		20	2611	DIABETES INSIPIDIS, NEUROHYPOPHYSEAL TYPE
GSL	galactosialidosis		20	3110	GALACTOSIALIDOSIS
AGS	Alagille syndrome		20p12-p11	2084	ARTERIO-HEPATIC DYSPLASIA
EBN	epilepsy, benign neonatal		20q	3216	CONVULSIONS, BENIGN FAMILIAL NEONATAL
ADA	adenosine deaminase		20q13.11 or 20q13.2-qter	2196	IMMUNODEFICIENCY, ADENOSINE DEAMINASE DEFICIENCY
AD1	Alzheimer disease 1	**21**	21pter-q21	2354	ALZHEIMER DISEASE, FAMILIAL
APP	amyloid beta (A4) precursor protein		21q21.2	2354	ALZHEIMER DISEASE, FAMILIAL
PFKL	phosphofructokinase, liver type		21q22.3	0428	GLYCOGENOSIS, TYPE VII
CBS	cystathionine-beta-synthase		21q22.3	0474	HOMOCYSTINURIA
BCEI	breast cancer, estrogen-inducible sequence expressed in		21q22.3	2351	CANCER, BREAST, FAMILIAL
CD18	lymphocyte function-associated antigen 1; macrophage antigen		21q22.3	2970	GRANULOCYTE GLYCOPROTEIN CD11/CD18 DEFICIENCY
ADSL	adenylosuccinate lyase		22	3113	ADENYLOSUCCINATE MONOPHOSPHATE LYASE DEFICIENCY
CECR	cat eye syndrome chromosome region	**22**	22pter-q11	0544	CAT EYE SYNDROME
IDUA	iduronidase, alpha-L-		22pter-q11	0674	MUCOPOLYSACCHARIDOSIS I-H
IDUA	iduronidase, alpha-L-		22pter-q11	0675	MUCOPOLYSACCHARIDOSIS I-S
TCN2	transcobalamin II; macrocytic anemia		22q	2624	TRANSCOBALAMIN II DEFICIENCY
BCR	breakpoint cluster region		22q11	3092	LEUKEMIA, CHRONIC MYELOID (CML)
TSHR	thyroid stimulating hormone receptor		22q11-q13	0948	THYROTROPIN UNRESPONSIVENESS
NF2	neurofibromatosis 2 (bilateral acoustic neuroma)		22q11-q13.1	0012	ACOUSTIC NEUROMATA
GGT1	gamma-glutamyltransferase 1		22q11.1-q11.2	0422	GLUTATHIONURIA
DGCR	DiGeorge syndrome chromosome region		22q11.21-q11.23	0943	IMMUNODEFICIENCY, THYMIC AGENESIS
NAGA	acetylgalactosaminidase, alpha-N-		22q13-qter	3254	ALPHA-N-ACETYLGALACTOSAMINIDASE DEFICIENCY
ARSA	arylsulfatase A		22q13.31-qter	0651	METACHROMATIC LEUKODYSTROPHIES
DIA1	diaphorase (NADH) (cytochrome b-5 reductase)		22q13.31-qter	2682	METHEMOGLOBINEMIA, NADH-DEPENDENT DIAPHORASE DEFICIENCY
CCT	cataract, congenital, total		X	0132	CATARACT, CORTICAL AND NUCLEAR
DHOF	dermal hypoplasia, focal		X	0281	DERMAL HYPOPLASIA, FOCAL
PHP	panhypopituitarism		X	0303	DWARFISM, PANHYPOPITUITARY
LOX	lysyl oxidase; ?cutis laxa-X; ?Ehlers-Danlos V		X	0338	EHLERS-DANLOS SYNDROME
EFE2	endocardial fibroelastosis 2		X	0348	VENTRICLE, ENDOCARDIAL FIBROELASTOSIS OF LEFT VENTRICLE

SYMBOL	MARKER NAME	CHROMOSOME	MAP LOCATION	NO	ARTICLE TITLE
PHK	phosphorylase kinase deficiency, liver (glycogen storage disease type VIII)		X	0430	GLYCOGENOSIS, TYPE IXa
HSAS	hydrocephalus, stenosis of the aqueduct of Sylvius		X	0481	HYDROCEPHALY
HOMG	hypomagnesemia, secondary hypocalcemia		X	0514	HYPOMAGNESEMIA, PRIMARY
OPEM	ophthalmoplegia, external, with myopia		X	0750	OPHTHALMOPLEGIA EXTERNA-MYOPIA
OFD1	oral-facial-digital syndrome I		X	0770	ORO-FACIO-DIGITAL SYNDROME I
OPD	otopalatodigital syndrome		X	0786	OTO-PALATO-DIGITAL SYNDROME, I
CRD	choroidoretinal degeneration		X	0869	RETINITIS PIGMENTOSA
TDD	testicular 17,20-desmolase deficiency		X	0904	STEROID 17,20-DESMOLASE DEFICIENCY
MF4	metacarpal 4-5 fusion		X	0923	SYNDACTYLY
CRD	choroidoretinal degeneration		X	0925	CHOROIDEREMIA
ASB	anemia, sideroblastic/hypochromic		X	1518	ANEMIA, SIDEROBLASTIC
BDM	behavior disorder modifier		X	1532	MOOD AND THOUGHT DISORDERS
OPD	otopalatodigital syndrome		X	2258	OTO-PALATO-DIGITAL SYNDROME, II
ACAD	acyl-Coenzyme A dehydrogenase, multiple		X	2289	ACIDEMIA, GLUTARIC ACIDEMIA II
PHK	phosphorylase kinase deficiency, liver (glycogen storage disease type VIII)		X	2303	GLYCOGEN STORAGE DISEASE, X-LINKED WITH NORMAL HEPATIC ENZYMES
SDYS	Simpson dysmorphia syndrome		X	2826	SIMPSON-GOLABI-BEHMEL SYNDROME
MAA	microphthalmia or anophthalmia and associated anomalies		X	3171	LENZ MICROPHTHALMIA SYNDROME
LOX	lysyl oxidase; ?cutis laxa-X; ?Ehlers-Danlos V		X	3219	OCCIPITAL HORN SYNDROME
MNK	Menkes syndrome		Xcen-q13	0643	MENKES SYNDROME
MRX1	mental retardation, X-linked 1 (non dysmorphic)		Xp11-q13	2640	X-LINKED MENTAL RETARDATION, CLARK-BARAITSER TYPE
MRX1	mental retardation, X-linked 1 (non dysmorphic)		Xp11-q13	2840	X-LINKED MENTAL RETARDATION, ATKIN TYPE
MRX1	mental retardation, X-linked 1 (non dysmorphic)		Xp11-q13	3199	X-LINKED MENTAL RETARDATION, GOLABI-ITO-HALL TYPE
MRX1	mental retardation, X-linked 1 (non dysmorphic)		Xp11-q13	3200	X-LINKED MENTAL RETARDATION-CRANIOFACIAL ABNORMALITIES-CLUB FOOT
IP1	incontinentia pigmenti 1		Xp11.21-cen	0526	INCONTINENTIA PIGMENTI
RP2	retinitis pigmentosa 2		Xp11.4-p11.2	0869	RETINITIS PIGMENTOSA
WAS	Wiskott-Aldrich syndrome		Xp11.4-p11.21	0523	IMMUNODEFICIENCY, WISKOTT-ALDRICH TYPE
NDP	Norrie disease (pseudoglioma)		Xp11.4-p11.3	0721	NORRIE DISEASE
CYBB	cytochrome b-245, beta polypeptide (chronic granulomatous disease)		Xp21.1	0443	GRANULOMATOUS DISEASE, CHRONIC X-LINKED
XK	Kell blood group precursor (McLeod phenotype)		Xp21.1	2646	ANEMIA, HEMOLYTIC, RED CELL MEMBRANE DEFECTS
OTC	ornithine carbamoyltransferase		Xp21.1	3023	ORNITHINE TRANSCARBAMYLASE DEFICIENCY
CSNB1	congenital stationary night blindness 1		Xp21.1-p11.23	0718	NIGHTBLINDNESS, CONGENITAL STATIONARY, X-LINKED RECESSIVE
COD1	cone dystrophy 1 (X-linked)		Xp21.1-p11.3	3228	RETINA, CONE DYSTROPHY, X-LINKED
RP3	retinitis pigmentosa 3		Xp21.1-p11.4	0869	RETINITIS PIGMENTOSA
DMD	muscular dystrophy, Duchenne and Becker types		Xp21.3-p21.1	0687	MUSCULAR DYSTROPHY, ADULT PSEUDOHYPERTROPHIC
DMD	muscular dystrophy, Duchenne and Becker types		Xp21.3-p21.1	0689	MUSCULAR DYSTROPHY, CHILDHOOD PSEUDOHYPERTROPHIC
AHC	adrenal hypoplasia, congenital		Xp21.3-p21.2	0024	ADRENAL HYPOPLASIA, CONGENITAL
GK	glycerol kinase deficiency		Xp21.3-p21.2	2310	GLYCEROL KINASE DEFICIENCY
AIED	Aland island eye disease (Forsius-Eriksson ocular albinism)		Xp21.3-p21.2	3183	FORSIUS-ERIKSSON SYNDROME
AIH1	amelogenesis imperfecta 1, hypomaturation or hypoplastic (?=AMG & AMGS)		Xp22	0046	TEETH, AMELOGENESIS IMPERFECTA

X

SYMBOL	MARKER NAME	CHROMOSOME	MAP LOCATION	NO	ARTICLE TITLE
SEDL	spondyloepiphyseal dysplasia, late		Xp22	0898	SPONDYLOEPIPHYSEAL DYSPLASIA, LATE
AIH1	amelogenesis imperfecta 1, hypomaturation or hypoplastic (?=AMG & AMGS)		Xp22	2136	TEETH, SNOW-CAPPED
AIC	Aicardi syndrome		Xp22	2320	AICARDI SYNDROME
CLS	Coffin-Lowry syndrome		Xp22.2-p22.1	0190	COFFIN-LOWRY SYNDROME
HYP	hypophosphatemia, vitamin D resistant rickets		Xp22.2-p22.1	0517	HYPOPHOSPHATEMIA, X-LINKED
RS	retinoschisis		Xp22.2-p22.1	0871	RETINOSCHISIS
OA1	ocular albinism 1 (Nettleship-Falls)		Xp22.3	0032	ALBINISM, OCULAR
NHS	Nance-Horan syndrome (congenital cataracts and dental anomalies)		Xp22.3-p21.1	2119	CATARACTS-OTO-DENTAL DEFECTS
MRX2	mental retardation, X-linked 2		Xp22.3-p22.2	2920	X-LINKED MENTAL RETARDATION, RENPENNING TYPE
AMG	amelogenin (?=AMGS & AIH)		Xp22.31-p22.1	0046	TEETH, AMELOGENESIS IMPERFECTA
KAL	Kallmann syndrome		Xp22.32	2301	KALLMANN SYNDROME
STS	steroid sulfatase (microsomal)		Xp22.32	2532	ICHTHYOSIS, X-LINKED WITH STEROID SULFATASE DEFICIENCY
CDPX	chondrodysplasia punctata		Xp22.32	2730	CHONDRODYSPLASIA PUNCTATA, X-LINKED DOMINANT TYPE
F2L	coagulation factor II (prothrombin)-like		Xpter-q25	2674	COAGULATION DEFECT, FAMILIAL MULTIPLE FACTORS
F2L	coagulation factor II (prothrombin)-like		Xpter-q25	2679	HYPOPROTHROMBINEMIA
CMTX	Charcot-Marie-Tooth neuropathy, X-linked		Xq11-q13	2104	NEUROPATHY, HEREDITARY MOTOR AND SENSORY, TYPE I
AR	androgen receptor (dihydrotestosterone receptor; testicular feminization)		Xq12	0049	ANDROGEN INSENSITIVITY SYNDROME, COMPLETE
AR	androgen receptor (dihydrotestosterone receptor; testicular feminization)		Xq12	0050	ANDROGEN INSENSITIVITY SYNDROME, INCOMPLETE
AR	androgen receptor (dihydrotestosterone receptor; testicular feminization)		Xq12	2954	ANDROGEN INSENSITIVITY (RESISTANCE), MINIMAL
PHKA	phosphorylase kinase, alpha		Xq12-q13	0430	GLYCOGENOSIS, TYPE IXa
PHKA	phosphorylase kinase, alpha		Xq12-q13	2303	GLYCOGEN STORAGE DISEASE, X-LINKED WITH NORMAL HEPATIC ENZYMES
EDA	ectodermal dysplasia, anhidrotic (hypohydrotic)		Xq12-q13.1	0333	ECTODERMAL DYSPLASIA, CHRIST-SIEMENS-TOURAINE TYPE
MGC1	megalocornea 1 (X-linked)		Xq12-q26	0637	CORNEA, MEGALOCORNEA
FGDY	faciogenital dysplasia (Aarskog syndrome)		Xq13	0001	AARSKOG SYNDROME
PGK1	phosphoglycerate kinase 1		Xq13	2657	ANEMIA, HEMOLYTIC, ERYTHROCYTE PHOSPHOGLYCERATE KINASE DEFICIENCY
SCIDX1	severe combined immunodeficiency, X-linked 1		Xq13-q21.1	0524	IMMUNODEFICIENCY, X-LINKED SEVERE COMBINED
DFN3	deafness, conductive, with fixed stapes		Xq13-q21.2	3116	DEAFNESS WITH PERILYMPHATIC GUSHER
SBMA	spinal and bulbar muscular atrophy (Kennedy disease)		Xq13-q22	0895	SPINAL MUSCULAR ATROPHY
SBMA	spinal and bulbar muscular atrophy (Kennedy disease)		Xq13-q22	2493	MUSCULAR ATROPHY, SPINAL AND BULBAR, X-LINKED KENNEDY TYPE
TBG	thyroxin binding globulin		Xq21-q22	0950	THYROXINE-BINDING GLOBULIN DEFECTS
PRPS1	phosphoribosyl pyrophosphate synthetase 1		Xq21-q27	0441	GOUT
PRPS1	phosphoribosyl pyrophosphate synthetase 1		Xq21-q27	0508	PHOSPHORIBOSYL PYROPHOSPHATE (PRPP) SYNTHETASE ABNORMALITY
TCD	tapeto-choroidal dystrophy, progressive choroidemia		Xq21.1-q21.2	0925	CHOROIDEREMIA
GLA	galactosidase, alpha		Xq21.3-q22	0373	FABRY DISEASE
PLP	proteolipid protein (Pelizaeus-Merzbacher disease)		Xq21.3-q22	0803	PELIZAEUS-MERZBACHER SYNDROME

SYMBOL	MARKER NAME	CHROMOSOME	MAP LOCATION	NO	ARTICLE TITLE
ATS	Alport syndrome		Xq21.3-q24	0708	NEPHRITIS-DEAFNESS (SENSORINEURAL), HEREDITARY TYPE
AGMX1	agammaglobulinemia, X-linked 1 (Bruton)		Xq21.33-q22	0027	IMMUNODEFICIENCY, AGAMMAGLOBULINEMIA, X-LINKED, INFANTILE
HIGM1	hyper IgM syndrome		Xq24-q27	2524	IMMUNODEFICIENCY, X-LINKED WITH HYPER IgM
LYP	lymphoproliferative syndrome		Xq25-q26	2210	IMMUNODEFICIENCY, X-LINKED LYMPHOPROLIFERATIVE DISEASE
OCRL	oculocerebrorenal syndrome of Lowe		Xq25-q26.1	0736	OCULO-CEREBRO-RENAL SYNDROME
ADFN	albinism-deafness syndrome		Xq25-q27	0030	ALBINISM, CUTANEOUS-DEAFNESS
HPRT	hypoxanthine phosphoribosyltransferase		Xq26	0441	GOUT
HPRT	hypoxanthine phosphoribosyltransferase		Xq26	0588	LESCH-NYHAN SYNDROME
HPT	hypoparathyroidism		Xq26-q27	0515	HYPOPARATHYROIDISM, FAMILIAL
BFLS	Borjeson-Forssman-Lehmann syndrome		Xq26-q27	2272	BORJESON-FORSSMAN-LEHMANN SYNDROME
F9	coagulation factor IX (Christmas disease)		Xq26.3-q27.1	0462	HEMOPHILIA B
SPG1	spastic paraplegia, complicated		Xq27-q28	0295	PARAPLEGIA, FAMILIAL SPASTIC
MTM1	myotubular myopathy 1		Xq27-q28	0695	MYOPATHY, MYOTUBULAR
MAFD2	major affective disorder 2		Xq27-q28	1532	MOOD AND THOUGHT DISORDERS
DKC	dyskeratosis congenita		Xq27-q28	2024	DYSKERATOSIS CONGENITA
MRSD	mental retardation-skeletal dysplasia		Xq27-q28	2904	X-LINKED MENTAL RETARDATION-SKELETAL DYSPLASIA
FRAXA	fragile site, folic acid type, rare, fra(X)(q27.3)		Xq27.3	2073	X-LINKED MENTAL RETARDATION, FRAGILE X SYNDROME
IDS	iduronate 2-sulfatase (Hunter syndrome)		Xq27.3-q28	0676	MUCOPOLYSACCHARIDOSIS II
EMD	Emery-Dreifuss muscular dystrophy		Xq27.3-q28	2491	EMERY-DREIFUSS SYNDROME
CBBM	color blindness, blue monochromatic		Xq28	0195	COLOR BLINDNESS, BLUE MONOCONE-MONOCHROMATIC
GCP	green cone pigment (color blindness, deutan)		Xq28	0196	COLOR BLINDNESS, RED-GREEN DEUTAN SERIES
RCP	red cone pigment (color blindness, protan)		Xq28	0197	COLOR BLINDNESS, RED-GREEN PROTAN SERIES
DIR	diabetes insipidus, renal		Xq28	0287	DIABETES INSIPIDUS, VASOPRESSIN RESISTANT TYPES I AND II
G6PD	glucose-6-phosphate dehydrogenase		Xq28	0420	GLUCOSE-6-PHOSPHATE DEHYDROGENASE DEFICIENCY
F8C	coagulation factor VIIIc, procoagulant component (hemophilia A)		Xq28	0461	HEMOPHILIA A
ALD	adrenoleukodystrophy		Xq28	2533	ADRENOLEUKODYSTROPHY, X-LINKED
TKC	torticollis, keloids, cryptorchidism and renal dysplasia		Xq28-qter	2174	CERVICO-DERMO-GU SYNDROME, GOEMINNE TYPE
TDF	testis determining factor		Yp11.3	0437	GONADAL DYSGENESIS, XY TYPE

BIRTH DEFECT-NUMBER-TO-PRIME NAME INDEX

0001 AARSKOG SYNDROME
0002 ABETALIPOPROTEINEMIA
0003 EYE, CRYPTOPHTHALMOS WITH OTHER MALFORMATIONS
0004 FIBRINOGENS, ABNORMAL CONGENITAL
0005 SKIN, ACANTHOSIS NIGRICANS
0006 ACATALASEMIA
0007 ACETYLATOR POLYMORPHISM
0008 ACHONDROGENESIS, LANGER-SALDINO TYPE
0009 ACHONDROGENESIS, PARENTI-FRACCARO TYPE
0010 ACHONDROPLASIA
0011 GLYCOGENOSIS, TYPE IIa
0012 ACOUSTIC NEUROMATA
0013 ACROCEPHALOPOLYSYNDACTYLY
0014 ACROCEPHALOSYNDACTYLY TYPE I
0015 ACRODERMATITIS ENTEROPATHICA
0016 ACRODYSOSTOSIS
0017 ACROFACIAL DYSOSTOSIS
0018 ACROMEGALOID PHENOTYPE-CUTIS VERTICIS GYRATA-CORNEAL LEUKOMA
0019 ACROMESOMELIC DYSPLASIA, CAMPAILLA-MARTINELLI TYPE
0020 ACROMESOMELIC DYSPLASIA, MAROTEAUX-MARTINELLI-CAMPAILLA TYPE
0021 ACRO-OSTEOLYSIS, DOMINANT TYPE
0022 ACROPECTOROVERTEBRAL DYSPLASIA
0023 ADRENAL HYPOALDOSTERONISM OF INFANCY, TRANSIENT ISOLATED
0024 ADRENAL HYPOPLASIA, CONGENITAL
0025 ADRENOCORTICAL UNRESPONSIVENESS TO ACTH, HEREDITARY
0026 ADRENOCORTICOTROPIC HORMONE DEFICIENCY, ISOLATED
0027 IMMUNODEFICIENCY, AGAMMAGLOBULINEMIA, X-LINKED, INFANTILE
0028 AGNATHIA-MICROSTOMIA-SYNOTIA
0029 AGONADIA
0030 ALBINISM, CUTANEOUS-DEAFNESS
0031 ALBINISM, CUTANEOUS
0032 ALBINISM, OCULAR
0033 ALBINISM, OCULOCUTANEOUS, HERMANSKY-PUDLAK TYPE
0034 ALBINISM, OCULOCUTANEOUS, TYROSINASE NEGATIVE
0035 ALBINISM, OCULOCUTANEOUS, TYROSINASE POSITIVE
0036 ALBINISM, OCULOCUTANEOUS, YELLOW MUTANT
0037 ALKAPTONURIA
0038 HAIR, ALOPECIA AREATA
0039 ALPHA(1)-ANTITRYPSIN DEFICIENCY
0040 ACIDEMIA, 3-KETOTHIOLASE DEFICIENCY
0041 ALSTROM SYNDROME
0042 BREAST, AMASTIA
0043 RETINA, AMAUROSIS CONGENITA, LEBER TYPE
0044 AMELO-CEREBRO-HYPOHIDROTIC SYNDROME
0045 AMELO-ONYCHO-HYPOHIDROTIC SYNDROME
0046 TEETH, AMELOGENESIS IMPERFECTA
0047 ANALBUMINEMIA
0048 ANALPHALIPOPROTEINEMIA
0049 ANDROGEN INSENSITIVITY SYNDROME, COMPLETE
0050 ANDROGEN INSENSITIVITY SYNDROME, INCOMPLETE
0051 ANEMIA, HYPOPLASTIC CONGENITAL
0052 ANENCEPHALY
0053 AORTIC SINUS OF VALSALVA, ANEURYSM
0054 ANGIOEDEMA, HEREDITARY
0055 ANGIO-OSTEOHYPERTROPHY SYNDROME
0057 ANIRIDIA

0058 PUPIL, ANISOCORIA
0059 EYE, ANISOMETROPIA
0060 EYELID, ANKYLOBLEPHARON
0061 TONGUE, ANKYLOGLOSSIA
0062 PANCREAS, ANNULAR
0063 ARTERY, ANOMALOUS ORIGIN OF CONTRALATERAL SUBCLAVIAN
0064 ARTERY, CORONARY, ANOMALOUS ORIGIN FROM PULMONARY ARTERY
0065 ECTRODACTYLY-ANONYCHIA
0066 NAILS, ANONYCHIA, HEREDITARY
0067 EYE, ANOPHTHALMIA
0068 ANORCHIA
0069 ANORECTAL MALFORMATIONS
0070 ANOSMIA, CONGENITAL
0071 ANTIBODIES TO HUMAN ALLOTYPES
0072 ANUS-HAND-EAR SYNDROME
0073 AORTA, COARCTATION
0074 AORTIC ARCH, CERVICAL
0075 AORTIC ARCH, DOUBLE
0076 AORTIC ARCH INTERRUPTION
0077 AORTIC ARCH, RIGHT
0078 AORTIC STENOSIS, SUPRAVALVAR
0079 AORTIC VALVE ATRESIA
0080 AORTIC VALVE STENOSIS
0081 AORTIC VALVE, TETRACUSPID
0082 AORTICO-LEFT VENTRICULAR TUNNEL
0083 AORTICO-PULMONARY SEPTAL DEFECT
0084 LENS, APHAKIA
0085 ARACHNODACTYLY, CONTRACTURAL BEALS TYPE
0086 ARGININEMIA
0087 ACIDURIA, ARGININOSUCCINIC
0088 ARTHROGRYPOSES
0090 ARTHRO-OPHTHALMOPATHY, HEREDITARY, PROGRESSIVE, STICKLER TYPE
0091 ASPHYXIATING THORACIC DYSPLASIA
0092 ASPLENIA SYNDROME
0093 ATAXIA-HYPOGONADISM SYNDROME
0094 ATAXIA-TELANGIECTASIA
0095 ATRANSFERRINEMIA
0096 ATRIAL SEPTAL DEFECTS
0097 EAR, AUDITORY CANAL ATRESIA
0098 AURICULO-OSTEODYSPLASIA
0099 HAIR, BALDNESS, COMMON
0100 BARTTER SYNDROME
0101 NEVOID BASAL CELL CARCINOMA SYNDROME
0102 ECTODERMAL DYSPLASIA, BASAN TYPE
0103 BASILAR IMPRESSION, PRIMARY
0104 BECKWITH-WIEDEMANN SYNDROME
0105 BERLIN SYNDROME
0106 ACIDURIA, BETA-MERCAPTOLACTATE-CYSTEINE DISULFIDURIA
0107 ACIDURIA, BETA-METHYL-CROTONYL-GLYCINURIA
0108 AORTIC VALVE, BICUSPID
0109 PULMONARY VALVE, BICUSPID
0110 BILIARY ATRESIA
0111 BLEPHAROCHALASIS-DOUBLE LIP-NONTOXIC GOITER
0112 BLOOM SYNDROME
0113 NEVUS, BLUE RUBBER BLEB NEVUS SYNDROME
0114 BRACHYDACTYLY
0115 BRAIN, SPONGY DEGENERATION
0116 GLYCOGENOSIS, TYPE IV
0117 NECK, BRANCHIAL CLEFT, CYSTS OR SINUSES
0118 BRANCHIO-SKELETO-GENITAL SYNDROME
0119 RUBINSTEIN-TAYBI BROAD THUMB-HALLUX SYNDROME
0120 BRONCHIAL ATRESIA

0255 DEAFNESS-DIABETES-PHOTOMYOCLONUS-
     NEPHROPATHY
0256 DEAFNESS, DOMINANT LOW-FREQUENCY
0257 THYROID, HORMONE RESISTANCE
0258 DEAFNESS-HYPERPROLINURIA-ICHTHYOSIS
0259 DEAFNESS-KERATOPACHYDERMIA-DIGITAL
     CONSTRICTIONS
0261 DEAFNESS-MYOPIA-CATARACT-SADDLE NOSE,
     MARSHALL TYPE
0262 DEAFNESS-ONYCHO-OSTEO-DYSTROPHY-
     RETARDATION-SEIZURES (DOORS)
0263 KEUTEL SYNDROME
0265 DEAFNESS-DIVERTICULITIS-NEUROPATHY
0266 DEAFNESS (SENSORINEURAL)-DYSTONIA
0267 DEAFNESS (SENSORINEURAL), MIDFREQUENCY
0268 DEAFNESS-POLYNEUROPATHY-OPTIC ATROPHY
0269 DEAFNESS (SENSORINEURAL), PROGRESSIVE
     HIGH-TONE
0270 DEAFNESS (SENSORINEURAL), RECESSIVE
     EARLY-ONSET
0271 DEAFNESS (SENSORINEURAL), RECESSIVE
     PROFOUND
0272 DEAFNESS, STREPTOMYCIN-SENSITIVITY
0273 DEAFNESS, TUNE
0274 DEAFNESS, UNILATERAL INNER EAR
0275 DEAFNESS-VITILIGO-MUSCLE WASTING
0276 TEETH, DENS INVAGINATUS
0277 TEETH, DENTIN DYSPLASIA, CORONAL
0278 TEETH, DENTIN DYSPLASIA, RADICULAR
0279 TEETH, DENTINOGENESIS IMPERFECTA
0280 DENTINO-OSSEOUS DYSPLASIA
0281 DERMAL HYPOPLASIA, FOCAL
0282 DERMO-CHONDRO-CORNEAL DYSTROPHY,
     FRANCOIS TYPE
0283 NECK/HEAD, DERMOID CYST OR TERATOMA
0284 EYE, DERMOLIPOMA
0285 DEXTROCARDIA-BRONCHIECTASIS-SINUSITIS
     SYNDROME
0286 VENTRICLE, SEPTUM DEXTROPOSITION AND
     DOUBLE INLET LEFT VENTRICLE
0287 DIABETES INSIPIDUS, VASOPRESSIN RESISTANT
     TYPES I AND II
0288 DIAPHRAGM, EVENTRATION
0289 DIAPHRAGMATIC HERNIA
0290 DIAPHYSEAL DYSPLASIA
0291 TEETH, DIASTEMA, MEDIAN INCISAL
0292 DIASTEMATOMYELIA
0293 DIASTROPHIC DYSPLASIA
0294 ACIDURIA, DICARBOXYLIC AMINOACIDURIA
0295 PARAPLEGIA, FAMILIAL SPASTIC
0296 DISTICHIASIS
0297 VENTRICLE, DOUBLE-OUTLET RIGHT WITH
     ANTERIOR SEPTAL DEFECT
0298 VENTRICLE, DOUBLE-OUTLET RIGHT WITH
     POSTERIOR SEPTAL DEFECT
0299 DUBOWITZ SYNDROME
0300 DUODENUM, ATRESIA OR STENOSIS
0301 CONTRACTURE, DUPUYTREN
0302 DWARFISM, LARON
0303 DWARFISM, PANHYPOPITUITARY
0304 DWARFISM, PITUITARY WITH ABNORMAL SELLA
     TURCICA
0306 DYGGVE-MELCHIOR-CLAUSEN SYNDROME
0307 DYSAUTONOMIA I, RILEY-DAY TYPE
0308 DYSCHONDROSTEOSIS
0309 PUPIL, DYSCORIA
0310 DYSOSTEOSCLEROSIS
0311 DYSPLASIA EPIPHYSEALIS HEMIMELICA
0312 EAR, ABSENT TRAGUS
0313 EAR, ARTERIOVENOUS FISTULA
0314 EAR, CUPPED
0315 EAR, INNER DYSPLASIAS
0316 EAR, ECTOPIC PINNA

0317 EAR, EXCHONDROSIS
0318 EAR, EXOSTOSES
0319 EAR, HAIRY
0320 EAR, LOBE, ABSENT
0321 EAR LOBE, CLEFT
0322 EAR LOBE, PIT
0323 EAR LOBE, ATTACHED
0324 EAR LOBE, HYPERTROPHIC THICKENED
0325 EAR, LONG, NARROW, POSTERIORLY ROTATED
0326 EAR, LOP
0327 EAR, LOW-SET
0328 EAR, MOZART TYPE
0329 EAR, PITS
0330 EAR, PROMINENT ANTHELIX
0331 EAR, SMALL WITH FOLDED-DOWN HELIX
0332 TRICUSPID VALVE, EBSTEIN ANOMALY
0333 ECTODERMAL DYSPLASIA, CHRIST-SIEMENS-
     TOURAINE TYPE
0334 ECTODERMAL DYSPLASIA, HIDROTIC
0335 HEART, CORDIS ECTOPIA
0336 ECTRODACTYLY
0337 ECTRODACTYLY-ECTODERMAL DYSPLASIA-
     CLEFTING SYNDROME
0338 EHLERS-DANLOS SYNDROME
0339 SKIN, ELASTOSIS PERFORANS SERPIGINOSA
0340 TEETH, ENAMEL AND DENTIN DEFECTS FROM
     ERYTHROBLASTOSIS FETALIS
0341 TEETH, DEFECTS FROM TETRACYCLINE
0342 TEETH, ENAMEL HYPOPLASIA
0343 ENCEPHALOCELE
0344 ENCEPHALOPATHY, NECROTIZING
0345 ENCHONDROMATOSIS
0346 ENCHONDROMATOSIS AND HEMANGIOMAS
0347 HEART, ENDOCARDIAL CUSHION DEFECTS
0348 VENTRICLE, ENDOCARDIAL FIBROELASTOSIS OF
     LEFT VENTRICLE
0349 VENTRICLE, ENDOCARDIAL FIBROELASTOSIS OF
     RIGHT VENTRICLE
0350 ENDOCRINE NEOPLASIA, MULTIPLE TYPE I
0351 ENDOCRINE NEOPLASIA, MULTIPLE TYPE II
0352 ENDOCRINE NEOPLASIA, MULTIPLE TYPE III
0353 VENTRICLE, ENDOMYOCARDIAL FIBROSIS OF LEFT
0354 VENTRICLE, ENDOMYOCARDIAL FIBROSIS OF RIGHT
0355 EYELID, EPIBLEPHARON
0357 GALACTOSE EPIMERASE DEFICIENCY
0358 EPIPHYSEAL DYSPLASIA, MULTIPLE
0359 EPITHELIOMA, MULTIPLE SELF-HEALING
     SQUAMOUS
0360 TEETH, EPULIS, CONGENITAL
0361 SKIN, ERYTHROKERATODERMIA, VARIABLE
0362 PORPHYRIA, PROTOPORPHYRIA
0363 ESOPHAGUS, ACHALASIA
0364 ESOPHAGUS, ATRESIA
0365 ESOPHAGUS, ATRESIA AND TRACHEOESOPHAGEAL
     FISTULA
0366 ESOPHAGUS, CHALASIA
0367 ESOPHAGUS, DIVERTICULUM
0368 ESOPHAGUS, DUPLICATION
0369 ESOPHAGUS, STENOSIS
0370 EAR, EUSTACHIAN TUBE DEFECTS
0371 EYELID, ECTROPION, CONGENITAL
0372 EYELID, ENTROPION
0373 FABRY DISEASE
0374 FACIAL CLEFT, LATERAL
0375 FACIAL CLEFT, OBLIQUE
0376 DIPLEGIA, CONGENITAL FACIAL
0377 PALSY, CONGENITAL FACIAL
0378 PALSY, LATE-ONSET FACIAL, FAMILIAL
0379 FETAL ALCOHOL SYNDROME
0380 FETAL AMINOPTERIN SYNDROME
0381 FETAL CYTOMEGALOVIRUS SYNDROME
0382 FETAL HYDANTOIN SYNDROME
0383 FETAL RADIATION SYNDROME

0523 IMMUNODEFICIENCY, WISKOTT-ALDRICH TYPE
0524 IMMUNODEFICIENCY, X-LINKED SEVERE COMBINED
0525 IMMUNOGLOBULIN A DEFICIENCY
0526 INCONTINENTIA PIGMENTI
0527 ARTERY, INDEPENDENT ORIGIN OF IPSILATERAL VERTEBRAL
0528 VENA CAVA, ABSENT HEPATIC SEGMENT
0529 HERNIA, INGUINAL
0530 EAR, ANEURYSM OF INTERNAL CAROTID ARTERY
0531 INTESTINAL ATRESIA OR STENOSIS
0532 INTESTINAL DUPLICATION
0533 INTESTINAL ENTEROKINASE DEFICIENCY
0534 INTESTINAL LYMPHANGIECTASIA
0535 INTESTINAL POLYPOSIS, TYPE I
0536 INTESTINAL POLYPOSIS, TYPE III
0537 INTESTINAL ROTATION, INCOMPLETE
0538 MUCOSA (ORAL/EYE), INTRAEPITHELIAL DYSKERATOSIS, BENIGN
0539 CHERUBISM
0540 VENTRICLES, INVERTED WITH TRANSPOSITION OF GREAT ARTERIES
0541 VENTRICLES, INVERTED WITHOUT TRANSPOSITION OF GREAT ARTERIES
0542 THYROID, IODIDE TRANSPORT DEFECT
0543 THYROID, IODOTYROSINE DEIODINASE DEFICIENCY
0544 CAT EYE SYNDROME
0545 INTESTINAL ILEUS, ISOLATED MECONIUM ILEUS
0546 AORTA, ISOLATION OF SUBCLAVIAN ARTERY FROM AORTA
0547 ACIDEMIA, ISOVALERIC
0548 JAW-WINKING SYNDROME
0549 DIABETES MELLITUS, INSULIN DEPENDENT TYPE
0550 DIABETES (INSIPIDUS/MELLITUS)-OPTIC ATROPHY-DEAFNESS
0552 EYE, KERATOCONUS
0553 EYE, KERATOPATHY, BAND-SHAPED
0554 KBG SYNDROME
0555 CRANIOSYNOSTOSIS, KLEEBLATTSCHADEL TYPE
0556 KLINEFELTER SYNDROME
0557 KNIEST DYSPLASIA
0558 KNUCKLE PADS-LEUKONYCHIA-DEAFNESS
0559 NAILS, KOILONYCHIA
0560 KUSKOKWIN SYNDROME
0561 SKIN, KYRLE DISEASE
0562 EAR, LABYRINTH APLASIA
0563 LACRIMAL CANALICULUS ATRESIA
0564 LACRIMAL GLAND, ECTOPIC
0565 LACRIMAL SAC FISTULA
0566 LACTASE DEFICIENCY, CONGENITAL
0567 LACTASE DEFICIENCY, PRIMARY
0568 LACTATE DEHYDROGENASE ISOZYMES
0569 LACTOSE INTOLERANCE
0570 LARSEN SYNDROME
0571 LARYNX, ATRESIA
0572 LARYNX, CYSTS
0573 LARYNX, VENTRICLE PROLAPSE
0574 LARYNX, WEB
0575 LARYNGOCELE
0576 LARYNGOMALACIA
0577 LARYNGO-TRACHEO-ESOPHAGEAL CLEFT
0578 LAURENCE-MOON SYNDROME
0579 OPTIC ATROPHY, LEBER TYPE
0580 LECITHIN-CHOLESTEROL ACYL TRANSFERASE DEFICIENCY
0581 VENTRICLE, DOUBLE OUTLET LEFT
0582 VENTRICLE, SINGLE LEFT PAPILLARY MUSCLE
0583 LENS AND PUPIL, ECTOPIC
0584 LENS, ECTOPIC
0585 LENTICONUS
0586 LENTIGINES SYNDROME, MULTIPLE
0587 LEPRECHAUNISM
0588 LESCH-NYHAN SYNDROME
0589 NAILS, LEUKONYCHIA

0590 LIDDLE SYNDROME
0591 OCULAR DERMOIDS
0592 LIMB-OTO-CARDIAC SYNDROME
0593 NEVUS, EPIDERMAL NEVUS SYNDROME
0594 LIP, DOUBLE
0595 LIP, MEDIAN CLEFT OF UPPER
0596 LIP, PITS OR MOUNDS
0597 LIPASE, CONGENITAL ABSENCE OF PANCREATIC
0598 LIPOGRANULOMATOSIS
0599 SKIN, LIPOID PROTEINOSIS
0600 LIPOMAS, FAMILIAL SYMMETRIC
0601 NECK/FACE, LIPOMATOSIS
0602 LIPOMENINGOCELE
0603 LISSENCEPHALY SYNDROME
0604 LIVER, HAMARTOMA
0605 HEPATIC FIBROSIS, CONGENITAL
0606 LIVER, TRANSPOSITION
0607 TEETH, LOBODONTIA
0608 SKIN, LOCALIZED ABSENCE OF
0610 ARRHYTHMIA, WITH LONG QT INTERVAL WITHOUT DEAFNESS
0611 LUNG, ABERRANT LOBE
0612 LUNG, LOBE SEQUESTRATION
0613 ALVEOLAR RIDGES, LYMPHANGIOMA
0614 LYMPHEDEMA I
0615 LYMPHEDEMA II
0616 HYPERLYSINEMIA
0617 TEETH, MACRODONTIA
0618 MACROGLOSSIA
0619 EAR, MACROTIA
0621 MACULAR COLOBOMA-BRACHYDACTYLY
0622 RETINA, MACULAR DEGENERATION, VITELLIRUPTIVE
0623 EYELID, MADAROSIS
0626 MANDIBULAR PROGNATHISM
0627 MANDIBULOFACIAL DYSOSTOSIS
0628 MAPLE SYRUP URINE DISEASE
0629 MARDEN-WALKER SYNDROME
0630 MARFAN SYNDROME
0631 MAXILLA, MEDIAN ALVEOLAR CLEFT
0632 McDONOUGH SYNDROME
0633 MECKEL DIVERTICULUM
0634 MECKEL SYNDROME
0635 FACE, MEDIAN CLEFT FACE SYNDROME
0636 CLEFTS, LOWER MEDIAN LIP, MANDIBLE AND TONGUE
0637 CORNEA, MEGALOCORNEA
0638 MEGALOCORNEA-MENTAL RETARDATION SYNDROME
0639 OPTIC DISK, MELANOCYTOMA
0640 EYE, MELANOSIS OCULI, CONGENITAL
0641 MELORHEOSTOSIS
0642 MENINGOCELE
0643 MENKES SYNDROME
0645 MESENTERIC CYSTS
0646 MESOMELIC DYSPLASIA, LANGER TYPE
0647 MESOMELIC DYSPLASIA, NIEVERGELT TYPE
0648 MESOMELIC DYSPLASIA, REINHARDT-PFEIFFER TYPE
0649 MESOMELIC DYSPLASIA, WERNER TYPE
0650 METACHONDROMATOSIS
0651 METACHROMATIC LEUKODYSTROPHIES
0652 METAPHYSEAL CHONDRODYSPLASIA, TYPE JANSEN
0653 METAPHYSEAL CHONDRODYSPLASIA, TYPE McKUSICK
0654 METAPHYSEAL CHONDRODYSPLASIA, TYPE SCHMID
0655 METAPHYSEAL CHONDRODYSPLASIA WITH THYMOLYMPHOPENIA
0656 METATROPIC DYSPLASIA
0657 METHIONINE MALABSORPTION
0658 ACIDEMIA, METHYLMALONIC
0659 MICROCEPHALY
0660 TEETH, MICRODONTIA
0661 EYE, MICROPHTHALMIA/COLOBOMA

0663 LENS, MICROSPHEROPHAKIA
0664 EAR, MICROTIA-ATRESIA
0665 MITRAL VALVE ATRESIA
0666 MITRAL VALVE INSUFFICIENCY
0667 MITRAL REGURGITATION-DEAFNESS-SKELETAL DEFECTS
0668 MITRAL VALVE PROLAPSE
0669 MITRAL VALVE STENOSIS
0670 ALOPECIA-EPILEPSY-OLIGOPHRENIA, MOYNAHAN TYPE
0671 MUCOLIPIDOSIS I
0672 MUCOLIPIDOSIS II
0673 MUCOLIPIDOSIS III
0674 MUCOPOLYSACCHARIDOSIS I-H
0675 MUCOPOLYSACCHARIDOSIS I-S
0676 MUCOPOLYSACCHARIDOSIS II
0677 MUCOPOLYSACCHARIDOSIS III
0678 MUCOPOLYSACCHARIDOSIS IV
0679 MUCOPOLYSACCHARIDOSIS VI
0680 MUCOPOLYSACCHARIDOSIS VII
0681 MUCOSA, WHITE FOLDED DYSPLASIA
0682 MULLERIAN APLASIA
0683 MULLERIAN DERIVATIVES IN MALES, PERSISTENT
0684 MULLERIAN FUSION, INCOMPLETE
0685 EXOSTOSES, MULTIPLE CARTILAGINOUS
0687 MUSCULAR DYSTROPHY, ADULT PSEUDOHYPER-TROPHIC
0688 MUSCULAR DYSTROPHY, AUTOSOMAL RECESSIVE PSEUDOHYPERTROPHIC
0689 MUSCULAR DYSTROPHY, CHILDHOOD PSEUDOHYPERTROPHIC
0690 MUSCULAR DYSTROPHY, DISTAL
0691 MUSCULAR DYSTROPHY, LIMB-GIRDLE
0692 MUSCULAR DYSTROPHY, OCULOPHARYNGEAL
0693 MENINGOMYELOCELE
0695 MYOPATHY, MYOTUBULAR
0696 MYOPATHY, NEMALINE
0699 MYOPIA, CONGENITAL
0700 MYOSITIS OSSIFICANS PROGRESSIVA
0701 MYOTONIA CONGENITA
0702 MYOTONIC DYSTROPHY
0703 ECTODERMAL DYSPLASIA, NAEGELI TYPE
0704 NAIL-PATELLA SYNDROME
0705 NASOLACRIMAL DUCT OBSTRUCTION
0706 NASOPHARYNGEAL CYSTS
0707 NOSE, NASOPHARYNGEAL STENOSIS
0708 NEPHRITIS-DEAFNESS (SENSORINEURAL), HEREDITARY TYPE
0709 NEPHROSIS, CONGENITAL
0710 NEPHROSIS, FAMILIAL TYPE
0711 JAW, NEUROECTODERMAL PIGMENTED TUMOR
0712 NEUROFIBROMATOSIS
0713 NEURONAL CEROID-LIPOFUSCINOSES (NCL)
0714 NEUTROPENIA, CYCLIC
0715 NEVUS FLAMMEUS
0716 NEVUS OF OTA
0717 NIEMANN-PICK DISEASE
0718 NIGHTBLINDNESS, CONGENITAL STATIONARY, X-LINKED RECESSIVE
0720 NOONAN SYNDROME
0721 NORRIE DISEASE
0722 NOSE/NASAL SEPTUM DEFECTS
0723 NOSE, ANTERIOR ATRESIA
0724 NOSE, BIFID
0725 NOSE, DUPLICATION
0726 NOSE, GLIOMA
0727 NOSE, POSTERIOR ATRESIA
0728 NOSE, TRANSVERSE GROOVE
0729 IMMUNODEFICIENCY, NUCLEOSIDE-PHOSPHORYLASE DEFICIENCY
0731 VENTRICLE, OBSTRUCTION WITHIN RIGHT VENTRICLE OR ITS OUTFLOW TRACT

0732 FACIO-OCULO-ACOUSTIC-RENAL SYNDROME (FOAR SYNDROME)
0734 OCULAR DRUSEN
0735 OCULO-AURICULO-VERTEBRAL ANOMALY
0736 OCULO-CEREBRO-RENAL SYNDROME
0737 OCULO-DENTO-OSSEOUS DYSPLASIA
0738 OCULO-MANDIBULO-FACIAL SYNDROME
0739 TEETH, ODONTODYSPLASIA
0740 NIGHTBLINDNESS, OGUCHI TYPE
0741 SEIZURES-ICHTHYOSIS-MENTAL RETARDATION
0742 OLIVOPONTOCEREBELLAR ATROPHY, DOMINANT MENZEL TYPE
0743 OLIVOPONTOCEREBELLAR ATROPHY, DOMINANT SCHUT-HAYMAKER TYPE
0744 OLIVOPONTOCEREBELLAR ATROPHY, DOMINANT WITH OPHTHALMOPLEGIA
0745 OLIVOPONTOCEREBELLAR ATROPHY, DOMINANT WITH RETINAL DEGENERATION
0746 OLIVOPONTOCEREBELLAR ATROPHY, LATE-ONSET
0747 OLIVOPONTOCEREBELLAR ATROPHY, RECESSIVE FICKLER-WINKLER TYPE
0748 OMPHALOCELE
0750 OPHTHALMOPLEGIA EXTERNA-MYOPIA
0751 OPHTHALMOPLEGIA, FAMILIAL STATIC
0752 OPHTHALMOPLEGIA, PROGRESSIVE EXTERNAL
0753 OPHTHALMOPLEGIA, TOTAL WITH PTOSIS AND MIOSIS
0754 FG SYNDROME, OPITZ-KAVEGGIA TYPE
0755 OPTIC ATROPHY, INFANTILE HEREDOFAMILIAL
0756 OPTIC DISK PITS
0757 OPTIC DISK, TILTED
0758 OPTIC NERVE HYPOPLASIA
0759 OPTICO-COCHLEO-DENTATE DEGENERATION
0760 ORAL DERMOIDS
0761 ORBITAL AND PERIORBITAL DERMOID CYSTS
0762 ORBITAL CEPHALOCELES
0763 ORBITAL NERVE GLIOMA
0764 ORBITAL HEMANGIOMA
0765 ORBITAL AND PERIORBITAL LYMPHANGIOMA
0766 PULMONARY ARTERY, ORIGIN OF THE LEFT FROM RIGHT PULMONARY ARTERY
0767 PULMONARY ARTERY, ORIGIN FROM ASCENDING AORTA
0768 PULMONARY ARTERY, ORIGIN FROM DUCTUS ARTERIOSUS
0769 ORO-CRANIO-DIGITAL SYNDROME
0770 ORO-FACIO-DIGITAL SYNDROME I
0771 ORO-FACIO-DIGITAL SYNDROME, MOHR TYPE
0772 ACIDEMIA, OROTIC
0773 EAR, OSSICLE AND MIDDLE EAR MALFORMATIONS
0774 JOINTS, OSTEOCHONDRITIS DISSECANS
0775 OSTEODYSPLASTY
0776 OSTEOECTASIA
0777 OSTEOGENESIS IMPERFECTA
0778 OSTEOPATHIA STRIATA
0779 OSTEOPETROSIS, BENIGN DOMINANT
0780 OSTEOPETROSIS, MALIGNANT RECESSIVE
0781 OSTEOPOIKILOSIS
0782 OSTEOPOROSIS, JUVENILE IDIOPATHIC
0783 OSTEOPOROSIS-PSEUDOGLIOMA SYNDROME
0784 OTO-DENTAL DYSPLASIA
0785 OTO-OCULO-MUSCULO-SKELETAL SYNDROME
0786 OTO-PALATO-DIGITAL SYNDROME, I
0787 OTOSCLEROSIS
0788 PACHYDERMOPERIOSTOSIS
0789 NAILS, PACHYONYCHIA CONGENITA
0790 PALATE, FISTULA
0791 PALLISTER-W SYNDROME
0792 SKIN, PALMO-PLANTAR ERYTHEMA
0793 PANCREATITIS, HEREDITARY
0794 PARALYSIS, HYPERKALEMIC PERIODIC
0795 PARALYSIS, HYPOKALEMIC PERIODIC
0796 PARAMYOTONIA CONGENITA

2049 MUSCULAR DYSTROPHY, FACIO-SCAPULO-HUMERAL
2050 PARALYSIS, NORMOKALEMIC PERIODIC
2052 MYOPATHY-CATARACT-GONADAL DYSGENESIS
2054 DEJERINE-SOTTAS DISEASE
2056 MYOPATHY, DISPROPORTIONATE FIBER TYPE I
2058 MYOPATHY, MYOGLOBINURIA-ABNORMAL GLYCOLOSIS, HEREDITARY TYPE
2059 MYOPATHY, FAMILIAL LYSIS OF TYPE I FIBERS
2062 MYOPATHY, REDUCING BODY
2063 MYOPATHY, SARCOTUBULAR
2067 AMYOTROPHIC LATERAL SCLEROSIS
2068 AMYOTROPHIC LATERAL SCLEROSIS, GUAM TYPE
2069 AMYOTROPHIC LATERAL SCLEROSIS, FAMILIAL ADULT AND JUVENILE TYPES
2070 KEARNS-SAYRE DISEASE
2071 NEUROPATHY, HEREDITARY RECURRENT BRACHIAL
2073 X-LINKED MENTAL RETARDATION, FRAGILE X SYNDROME
2075 THUMB, ADDUCTED THUMB SYNDROME
2076 OSTEODYSTROPHY-MENTAL RETARDATION, RUVALCABA TYPE
2078 OCULO-OSTEO-CUTANEOUS SYNDROME, TOUMAALA-HAAPANEN TYPE
2079 MANNOSIDOSIS
2080 PENA-SHOKEIR SYNDROME
2081 DWARFISM, MULIBREY TYPE
2082 MANDIBULOACRAL DYSPLASIA
2083 CHEILITIS GRANULOMATOSA, MELKERSSON-ROSENTHAL TYPE
2084 ARTERIO-HEPATIC DYSPLASIA
2085 NASO-DIGITO-ACOUSTIC SYNDROME, KEIPERT TYPE
2086 ANGELMAN SYNDROME
2087 SINGLETON-MERTEN SYNDROME
2088 BLEPHARO-NASO-FACIAL SYNDROME
2092 NEU-LAXOVA SYNDROME
2093 DENTO-FACIO-SKELETAL DEFECTS, ACKERMAN TYPE
2095 ECTODERMAL DYSPLASIA, CONGENITAL FACIAL, SETLEIS TYPE
2096 SKIN, HYPERKERATOSIS, FOCAL PALMOPLANTAR AND GINGIVAL
2098 SHORT SYNDROME
2099 OSTEODYSPLASTICA GERODERMIA, BAMATTER TYPE
2100 ACROFACIAL DEFECTS, EMERY-NELSON TYPE
2101 SJOGREN SYNDROME
2102 LERI PLEONOSTEOSIS SYNDROME
2103 BLEPHAROPTOSIS-BLEPHAROPHIMOSIS-EPICANTHUS INVERSUS-TELECANTHUS
2104 NEUROPATHY, HEREDITARY MOTOR AND SENSORY, TYPE I
2105 NEUROPATHY, HEREDITARY MOTOR AND SENSORY, TYPE II
2106 VERMIS AGENESIS
2107 HISTIDINURIA
2108 NEUROPATHY, HEREDITARY WITH PRESSURE PALSIES
2109 TEETH, ODONTOBLASTIC DYSPLASIA, FOCAL
2110 RETINA, FLECKED KANDORI TYPE
2112 ARRHYTHMIA, FROM MATERNAL AUTOIMMUNE DISEASE, CONGENITAL
2113 ACIDEMIA, GAMMA-HYDROXYBUTYRIC
2114 ACIDEMIA, 3-HYDROXY-3-METHYLGLUTARIC
2115 RAYNAUD DISEASE
2116 PULMONARY HYPERTENSION, PRIMARY
2117 CANDIDIASIS, FAMILIAL CHRONIC MUCOCUTANEOUS
2118 PALATOPHARYNGEAL INCOMPETENCE
2119 CATARACTS-OTO-DENTAL DEFECTS
2120 OVERGROWTH, RUVALCABA-MYHRE-SMITH TYPE
2122 ARTHRITIS-ARTERITIS SYNDROME
2123 SCHINZEL-GIEDION SYNDROME

2124 CHARGE ASSOCIATION
2125 ANTLEY-BIXLER SYNDROME
2126 ACROFACIAL DYSOSTOSIS, POSTAXIAL TYPE
2127 CRANIO-ECTODERMAL DYSPLASIA
2128 AUTISM, INFANTILE
2129 VELO-CARDIO-FACIAL SYNDROME
2130 CHROMOSOME 12, PARTIAL TRISOMY 12p
2131 CHROMOSOME 15, PARTIAL TRISOMY DISTAL 15q
2132 CHROMOSOME 2, PARTIAL TRISOMY 2p
2133 TEETH, MESIOPALATAL TORSION OF CENTRAL INCISORS
2134 TEETH, ANODONTIA, PARTIAL OR COMPLETE
2135 TEETH, INCISORS, SHOVEL-SHAPED
2136 TEETH, SNOW-CAPPED
2137 TEETH, MOLAR REINCLUSION
2138 CUTIS LAXA-GROWTH DEFECT, DE BARSY TYPE
2139 RIEGER SYNDROME
2140 COLD HYPERSENSITIVITY
2141 AMYLOIDOSIS, TRANSTHYRETIN METHIONINE-30 TYPE
2142 AMYLOIDOSIS, INDIANA TYPE
2143 AMYLOIDOSIS, DANISH CARDIAC TYPE
2144 AMYLOIDOSIS, IOWA TYPE
2145 AMYLOIDOSIS, FINNISH TYPE
2146 AMYLOIDOSIS, ICELANDIC TYPE
2147 AMYLOIDOSIS, CORNEAL
2149 AMYLOIDOSIS, OHIO TYPE
2150 AMYLOIDOSIS, FAMILIAL VISCERAL
2151 DEAFNESS-TRIPHALANGEAL THUMBS-ONYCHODYSTROPHY
2154 SCLERODERMA, FAMILIAL PROGRESSIVE
2155 SYNOVITIS, FAMILIAL HYPERTROPHIC
2157 INFLAMMATORY DISEASE, NEONATAL BATES-LORBER TYPE
2158 DERMATOARTHRITIS, FAMILIAL HISTIOCYTIC
2160 MYXOMA, INTRACARDIAC
2161 FEVER, FAMILIAL MEDITERRANEAN (FMF)
2162 CATARACT-RENAL TUBULAR NECROSIS-ENCEPHALOPATHY, CROME TYPE
2163 HIP, CONGENITAL DISLOCATED
2164 FOOT, TALIPES EQUINOVARUS (TEV)
2165 NEVUS, CONGENITAL NEVOMELANOCYTIC
2166 FOLATE MALABSORPTION
2167 ACROFACIAL DYSOSTOSIS, NAGER TYPE
2168 GLYCOGENOSIS, TYPE Ib
2169 BIEMOND II SYNDROME
2170 CHARLIE M SYNDROME
2172 FACIAL DYSMORPHIA-JOINT HYPEREXTENSIBILITY SYNDROME
2173 NEUROECTODERMAL SYNDROME, FLYNN-AIRD TYPE
2174 CERVICO-DERMO-GU SYNDROME, GOEMINNE TYPE
2175 GROWTH DEFICIENCY-FACIAL DEFECTS-BRACHYDACTYLY
2176 GROWTH-MENTAL DEFICIENCY, MYHRE TYPE
2177 HERRMANN-PALLISTER-OPITZ SYNDROME
2178 HOOFT DISEASE
2179 OCULO-CEREBRO-FACIAL SYNDROME, KAUFMAN TYPE
2180 LACRIMO-AURICULO-DENTO-DIGITAL SYNDROME
2181 LETTERER-SIWE DISEASE
2184 CRANIOSYNOSTOSIS-FIBULAR APLASIA, LOWRY TYPE
2185 CRANIO-FRONTO-NASAL DYSPLASIA
2186 PTERYGIUM SYNDROME, MULTIPLE
2187 NEPHROSIS-HYDROCEPHALUS-THIN SKIN-BLUE SCLERA-GROWTH DEFECT
2188 OCULO-OTO-NASAL MALFORMATIONS WITH OSTEO-ONYCHO DYSPLASIA
2189 PALLISTER-KILLIAN MOSAIC SYNDROME
2191 CAMPTODACTYLY SYNDROME, GUADALAJARA TYPE II

2333 MICROCEPHALY WITH CHORIORETINOPATHY
2334 MICROCEPHALY, ISOLATED AUTOSOMAL
          DOMINANT TYPE
2335 CHROMOSOME 9, TETRASOMY 9p
2336 CHROMOSOME 18, TETRASOMY 18p
2337 DERMO-FACIO-CARDIO-SKELETAL SYNDROME
2338 SHORT STATURE-MENTAL RETARDATION-DELAYED
          SEXUAL MATURITY
2339 FACIO-NEURO-SKELETAL SYNDROME
2340 SHORT STATURE-CEREBRAL ATROPHY-KERATOSIS
          FOLLICULARIS, X-LINKED
2341 ATAXIA-DYSMORPHIC FACIES-TRICHODYSPLASIA
2342 CATARACT, AUTOSOMAL DOMINANT CONGENITAL
2343 CANCER, COLORECTAL
2344 INTESTINAL POLYPOSIS, TYPE II
2345 DEAFNESS-MALFORMED EARS-MENTAL
          RETARDATION
2346 HAIR, ATRICHIA CONGENITA
2348 CHROMOSOME 2, TRISOMY DISTAL 2q
2349 CHROMOSOME 2, MONOSOMY OF MEDIAL 2q
2350 PERRAULT SYNDROME
2351 CANCER, BREAST, FAMILIAL
2352 CANCER, HODGKIN DISEASE, FAMILIAL
2354 ALZHEIMER DISEASE, FAMILIAL
2355 KABUKI MAKE-UP SYNDROME
2356 ALBINISM-BLACK LOCKS-DEAFNESS
2357 ALBINISM, OCULOCUTANEOUS, BROWN TYPE
2358 ALBINISM, OCULOCUTANEOUS, RUFOUS TYPE
2359 ALBINOIDISM
2360 HYPOPIGMENTATION-IMMUNE DEFECT, GRISCELLI
          TYPE
2361 NEUROECTODERMAL MELANOLYSOSOMAL
          SYNDROME
2362 SKIN, HYPERPIGMENTATION, FAMILIAL
2363 BARDET-BIEDL SYNDROME
2364 OCULO-FACIAL SYNDROME, BENCZE TYPE
2365 ABRUZZO-ERICKSON SYNDROME
2366 CHONDRODYSTROPHY-SENSORINEURAL DEAFNESS,
          NANCE-INSLEY TYPE
2368 ORO-PALATAL-DIGITAL SYNDROME, VARADI TYPE
2369 DONLAN SYNDROME
2370 TERATOMA, PRESACRAL-SACRAL DYSGENESIS
2371 JAUNDICE, INTRAHEPATIC CHOLESTATIC, BYLER
          TYPE
2374 CANCER, PANCREAS, FAMILIAL ADENOCARCI-
          NOMA OF
2377 ACIDEMIA, ETHYLMALONIC-ADIPIC
2380 SACROCOCCYGEAL DYSGENESIS SYNDROME
2381 OVERGROWTH, BANNAYAN TYPE
2382 PROTEUS SYNDROME
2385 FETAL EFFECTS FROM MATERNAL HYPERTHERMIA
2386 HYPOBETALIPOPROTEINEMIA
2387 TIBIAL APLASIA/HYPOPLASIA
2388 TIBIAL HYPOPLASIA/APLASIA-ECTRODACTYLY
2390 NEUROPATHY, CONGENITAL SENSORY WITH
          ANHIDROSIS
2392 EPITHELIOMAS, HEREDITARY MULTIPLE CYSTIC
2393 SKIN CREASES, RETICULATE PIGMENTED FLEXURES,
          DOWLING-DEGOS TYPE
2394 HYPERAPOBETALIPOPROTEINEMIA
2395 XANTHOMATOSIS, CEREBROTENDINOUS
2396 CAMPTODACTYLY-CLEFT PALATE-CLUB FOOT,
          GORDON TYPE
2397 HIP, CONGENITAL COXA VARA
2398 ACANTHOCYTOSIS-NEUROLOGIC DEFECTS
2400 HYDATIDIFORM MOLE
2401 ARRHYTHMIA, CARDIAC CONDUCTION DEFECTS,
          NEONATAL
2402 DIGITAL FIBROMA, RECURRING IN INFANTS &
          CHILDREN
2403 APLASIA CUTIS CONGENITA-GASTROINTESTINAL
          ATRESIA

2404 HOMOCYSTINURIA, N(5,10) METHYLENE
          TETRAHYDROFOLATE DEFICIENCY TYPE
2405 YUNIS-VARON SYNDROME
2406 MURCS ASSOCIATION
2407 URETHRAL VALVES, POSTERIOR
2408 VESICO-URETERAL REFLUX
2409 HAND, RADIAL CLUB HAND
2410 HAND, ULNAR DRIFT
2411 XANTHINE OXIDASE DEFICIENCY
2412 MOLYBDENUM CO-FACTOR DEFICIENCY
2414 VENTRICLE, DOUBLE CHAMBERED RIGHT
2415 GALLBLADDER, AGENESIS
2419 CHARCOT MARIE TOOTH DISEASE-DEAFNESS
2421 DYSEQUILIBRIUM SYNDROME
2422 HUTTERITE SYNDROME, BOWEN-CONRADI TYPE
2423 LIPODYSTROPHY-COARSE FACIES-ACANTHOSIS
          NIGRICANS, MIESCHER TYPE
2424 ARTHRO-OPHTHALMOPATHY, WEISSENBACHER-
          ZWEYMULLER VARIANT
2425 TELECANTHUS, HEREDITARY
2426 CHROMOSOME 1, TRISOMY 1q32-qter
2428 CHROMOSOME 1, TRISOMY 1q25-1q32
2429 CHROMOSOME 1, MONOSOMY 1q4
2430 CHROMOSOME 3, TRISOMY 3q2
2431 CHROMOSOME 3, MONOSOMY 3p2
2432 CHROMOSOME 3, TRISOMY 3p2
2433 CHROMOSOME 4, TRISOMY 4p
2434 CHROMOSOME 4, TRISOMY DISTAL 4q
2435 CHROMOSOME 4, MONOSOMY DISTAL 4q
2436 CHROMOSOME 5, TRISOMY 5p
2437 CHROMOSOME 5, TRISOMY 5q3
2438 CHROMOSOME 6, TRISOMY 6p2
2439 CHROMOSOME 6, TRISOMY 6q2
2440 CHROMOSOME 6, RING 6
2442 CHROMOSOME 7, TRISOMY 7q2-3
2443 CHROMOSOME 7, MONOSOMY 7q3
2444 CHROMOSOME 7, MONOSOMY 7q2
2445 CHROMOSOME 7, MONOSOMY 7q1
2446 CHROMOSOME 7, TRISOMY 7p2
2447 CHROMOSOME 7, MONOSOMY 7p2
2449 CHROMOSOME 8, TRISOMY 8p
2450 CHROMOSOME 8, MONOSOMY 8p2
2451 CHROMOSOME 9, TRISOMY 9p
2452 CHROMOSOME 9, TRISOMY 9
2453 CHROMOSOME 9, TRISOMY 9q3
2454 CHROMOSOME 9, RING 9
2455 CHROMOSOME 10, TRISOMY 10q2
2456 CHROMOSOME 10, TRISOMY 10p
2457 CHROMOSOME 10, MONOSOMY 10p
2458 CHROMOSOME 10, MONOSOMY 10q2
2459 CHROMOSOME 11, TRISOMY 11p
2461 CHROMOSOME 12, MONOSOMY 12p
2462 CHROMOSOME 12, TRISOMY 12q2
2463 CHROMOSOME 13, TRISOMY DISTAL 13q
2464 CHROMOSOME 13, TRISOMY 13q1
2465 CHROMOSOME 13, MONOSOMY 13q3
2466 CHROMOSOME 14, TRISOMY 14q
2467 CHROMOSOME 14, RING 14
2468 CHROMOSOME 15, RING 15
2469 CHROMOSOME 16, TRISOMY 16p
2470 CHROMOSOME 16, TRISOMY 16q
2471 CHROMOSOME 17, TRISOMY 17q2
2472 CHROMOSOME 18, TRISOMY 18q2
2473 CHROMOSOME 18, RING 18
2474 CHROMOSOME 19, TRISOMY 19q
2475 CHROMOSOME 20, TRISOMY 20p
2476 CHROMOSOME 21, RING 21
2477 CHROMOSOME 22, RING 22
2478 CHROMOSOME 22, TRISOMY MOSAICISM
2479 SEIZURES, IN FEMALES, JUBERG-HELLMAN TYPE
2480 X-LINKED MENTAL RETARDATION-GROWTH-
          HEARING AND GENITAL DEFECTS
2486 ACHEIROPODY

2638 HAND, LOCKING DIGITS-GROWTH DEFECT
2639 MICROCEPHALY-LYMPHEDEMA
2640 X-LINKED MENTAL RETARDATION, CLARK-BARAITSER TYPE
2641 CANCER, THYROID, FAMILIAL PAPILLARY CARCINOMA OF
2642 MICHELIN TIRE BABY SYNDROME
2643 RADIAL-RENAL-OCULAR SYNDROME
2644 POLYDACTYLY-DISTAL OBSTRUCTIVE UROPATHY
2646 ANEMIA, HEMOLYTIC, RED CELL MEMBRANE DEFECTS
2647 ANEMIA, HEINZ BODY
2650 ANEMIA, DYSERYTHROPOIETIC, TYPE III
2651 ANEMIA, DYSERYTHROPOIETIC, TYPE I
2652 ANEMIA, DYSERYTHROPOIETIC, TYPE II
2656 ANEMIA, PERNICIOUS CONGENITAL
2657 ANEMIA, HEMOLYTIC, ERYTHROCYTE PHOSPHOGLYCERATE KINASE DEFICIENCY
2659 ANEMIA, CONGENITAL SIDEROBLASTIC, NOT B(6) RESPONSIVE
2660 ANEMIA, ADENYLATE KINASE DEFICIENCY
2661 AFIBROGINEMIA, CONGENITAL
2662 ERYTHROCYTE ALDOLASE-A DEFICIENCY
2664 ERYTHROCYTE, DIPHOSPHOGLYCERATE MUTASE (2,3) DEFICIENCY
2665 ELLIPTOCYTOSIS
2666 EOSINOPHILIA, FAMILIAL
2667 ANEMIA, HEMOLYTIC, ERYTHROCYTE PHOSPHOLIPID DEFECT
2668 FACTOR V DEFICIENCY
2669 FACTOR VII DEFICIENCY
2670 FACTOR X DEFICIENCY
2671 FACTOR XI DEFICIENCY
2672 FACTOR XII DEFICIENCY
2673 FACTOR XIII (FIBRIN STABILIZING FACTOR)
2674 COAGULATION DEFECT, FAMILIAL MULTIPLE FACTORS
2675 ANEMIA, HEMOLYTIC, GLUTATIONINE PEROXIDASE DEFICIENCY
2676 ANEMIA, HEMOLYTIC, GLUTATHIONE REDUCTASE DEFICIENCY
2677 ANEMIA, HEMOLYTIC, GLUTATHIONE SYNTHETASE DEFICIENCY
2678 ANEMIA, HEMOLYTIC, ERYTHROCYTE HEXOKINASE DEFICIENCY
2679 HYPOPROTHROMBINEMIA
2681 LEUKOCYTE, MAY-HEGGLIN ANOMALY
2682 METHEMOGLOBINEMIA, NADH-DEPENDENT DIAPHORASE DEFICIENCY
2683 THROMBASTHENIA, GLANZMANN-NAEGELI TYPE
2686 ERYTHROCYTE TRIOSEPHOSPHATE ISOMERASE DEFICIENCY
2687 RENAL DYSPLASIA-RETINAL APLASIA, LOKEN-SENIOR TYPE
2688 IMMUNODEFICIENCY, RETICULOENDOTHELIOSIS WITH EOSINOPHILIA
2689 CANCER, RENAL CELL CARCINOMA
2690 DWARFISM, DYSSEGMENTAL, ROLLAND-DESBUQUOIS TYPE
2691 HYPEROSTOSIS, WORTH TYPE
2692 DYSOSTOSIS, CHEIROLUMBAR
2694 FIBROCHONDROGENESIS
2695 OSTEOMESOPYKNOSIS
2696 SKELETAL DYSPLASIA, FUHRMANN TYPE
2698 DYSOSTOSIS, HUMEROSPINAL
2699 EPIPHYSEAL DYSPLASIA, MULTIPLE RIBBING TYPE
2701 NEUROAXONAL DYSTROPHY, INFANTILE
2702 LUNG, BRONCHOGENIC CYST
2703 LUNG, EMPHYSEMA CONGENITAL LOBAR
2705 MUSCULAR DYSTROPHY, CONGENITAL WITH MENTAL RETARDATION
2706 MUSCULAR DYSTROPHY, CONGENITAL WITH ARTHROGRYPOSIS

2707 MYOPATHY-METABOLIC, MITOCHONDRIAL CYTOCHROME C OXIDASE DEFICIENCY
2709 MYOPATHY-METABOLIC, MYOADENYLATE DEAMINASE DEFICIENCY
2710 MYOPATHY, MALIGNANT HYPERTHERMIA
2711 ALBINISM, OCULOCUTANEOUS, MINIMAL PIGMENT TYPE
2712 ALEXANDER DISEASE
2714 ATAXIA, FRIEDREICH TYPE
2716 ACROMICRIC DYSPLASIA
2718 NOSE, ANTERIOR STENOSIS
2719 NOSE, DISLOCATED NASAL SEPTUM
2720 NOSE, TURBINATE DEFORMITY
2721 SALIVARY GLAND LYMPHANGIOMA
2722 SALIVARY GLAND, AGENESIS
2723 BRANCHIAL CLEFT CYSTS
2724 SALIVARY GLAND, DERMOID CYST
2725 SALIVARY GLAND, DUCTAL CYST
2726 SALIVARY GLAND, HEMANGIOMA
2730 CHONDRODYSPLASIA PUNCTATA, X-LINKED DOMINANT TYPE
2731 FETAL VENEZUELAN EQUINE ENCEPHALITIS INFECTION
2732 FETAL LITHIUM EFFECTS
2733 FETAL EFFECTS OF POLYCHLORINATED BIPHENYL (PCB)
2734 FETAL EFFECTS FROM MATERNAL EXTRINSIC ANDROGENS
2736 CANCER, NEUROBLASTOMA
2739 TURCOT SYNDROME
2742 CANCER, WILMS TUMOR
2743 CANCER, SEBACEOUS GLAND TUMOR-MULTIPLE VISCERAL CARCINOMA
2744 CANCER, MULTIPLE MYELOMA
2745 CANCER, THYMOMA
2746 CANCER, GASTRIC FAMILIAL
2747 CANCER, LUNG, FAMILIAL
2748 CANCER, NEUROEPITHELIAL AND MENINGEAL
2749 CANCER, SOFT TISSUE SARCOMA
2750 ANEMIA, GLUCOSE PHOSPHATE ISOMERASE DEFICIENCY
2752 OCULO-CEREBRO-CUTANEOUS SYNDROME
2754 KYPHOMELIC DYSPLASIA
2755 MICROCEPHALY-HIATUS HERNIA-NEPHROSIS, GALLOWAY TYPE
2756 ACROMEGALOID FACIAL APPEARANCE SYNDROME
2757 RESTRICTIVE DERMATOPATHY
2758 CATARACT-MICROCORNEA SYNDROME
2759 CLEFTING-ECTROPION-CONICAL TEETH
2760 CORNEO-DERMATO-OSSEOUS SYNDROME
2761 CRANIOFACIAL-DEAFNESS-HAND SYNDROME
2762 DEAFNESS-EAR DEFECTS-FACIAL PALSY
2763 DERMO-ODONTODYSPLASIA
2764 EXOSTOSES-ANETODERMIA-BRACHYDACTYLY TYPE E
2765 ALOPECIA-ANOSMIA-DEAFNESS-HYPOGONADISM, JOHNSON TYPE
2766 DWARFISM, LETHAL, SHORT-LIMBED PLATYSPONDYLIC TYPE
2767 FACIAL CLEFTING SYNDROME, GYPSY TYPE
2768 METAPHYSEAL DYSPLASIA-MAXILLARY HYPOPLASIA-BRACHYDACTYLY
2769 PARIETAL FORAMINA-CLAVICULAR HYPOPLASIA
2770 PTERYGIA-DYSMORPHIC FACIES-SHORT STATURE-MENTAL RETARDATION
2771 RADIAL-RENAL SYNDROME
2772 RADIAL HYPOPLASIA-TRIPHALANGEAL THUMBS-HYPOSPADIAS-DIASTEMA
2774 PHARYNX/LARYNX HYPOPLASIA-OMPHALOCELE, SHPRINTZEN-GOLDBERG TYPE
2775 THORACOPELVIC DYSOSTOSIS
2776 PULMONIC STENOSIS-CAFE-AU-LAIT SPOTS, WATSON TYPE

2909 AORTA, COARCTATION, INFANTILE TYPE
2910 DIPHALLIA
2912 MYASTHENIC SYNDROME, CONGENITAL SLOW CHANNEL TYPE
2913 MYASTHENIC SYNDROME, FAMILIAL INFANTILE TYPE
2915 CRANIOSYNOSTOSIS-ARACHNODACTYLY-HERNIA
2918 PROTEIN C DEFICIENCY
2919 TERATOMAS
2920 X-LINKED MENTAL RETARDATION, RENPENNING TYPE
2921 X-LINKED MENTAL RETARDATION, MARFANOID HABITUS TYPE
2922 SCALP DEFECTS-POSTAXIAL POLYDACTYLY
2924 SPONDYLOCOSTAL DYSOSTOSIS-VISCERAL DEFECTS-DANDY WALKER CYST
2925 POLYSYNDACTYLY-DYSMORPHIC CRANIOFACIES, GREIG TYPE
2926 FETAL EFFECTS FROM METHIMAZOLE AND CARBIMAZOLE
2927 FETAL EFFECTS FROM MATERNAL VASODILATOR
2928 TWINS, CONJOINED, TERATOGENICITY
2929 FETAL BENZODIAZEPINE EFFECTS
2930 FETAL BARBITURATE EFFECTS
2931 CEREBRAL PALSY
2932 LIMB, UPPER HYPOPLASIA-MULLERIAN DUCT DEFECTS
2933 INTESTINAL ATRESIAS, MULTIPLE
2934 JEJUNAL ATRESIA
2935 DWARFISM, DYSSEGMENTAL, SILVERMAN-HANDMAKER TYPE
2936 HYDROCEPHALUS-COSTOVERTEBRAL DYSPLASIA-SPRENGEL ANOMALY
2937 SKELETAL BOWING-CORTICAL THICKENING-BONE FRAGILITY-ICTHYOSIS
2938 KNEE, GENU RECURVATUM
2939 PLAGIOCEPHALY
2940 TORTICOLLIS
2941 EYELID, COLOBOMA
2944 BRAIN, ARNOLD-CHIARI MALFORMATION
2945 ERYTHROCYTE, LACTATE TRANSPORTER DEFECT
2946 LYMPHOHISTIOCYTOSIS, FAMILIAL ERYTHROPHAGOCYTIC
2947 IMMUNODEFICIENCY, IgG SUBCLASS DEFICIENCIES
2950 PROTEIN S DEFICIENCY
2952 GLUCOCORTICOID RESISTANCE
2953 RESISTANCE TO 1,25 DIHYDROXY VITAMIN D
2954 ANDROGEN INSENSITIVITY (RESISTANCE), MINIMAL
2955 UMBILICAL CORD, SHORT
2956 UMBILICAL CORD, LONG
2957 UMBILICAL CORD, SHORT UMBILICAL CORD SYNDROME
2958 FETAL MONOZYGOUS MULTIPLE PREGNANCY DYSPLACENTATION EFFECTS
2960 FETAL EFFECTS OF MATERNAL CIGARETTE SMOKING
2961 FETAL DEVELOPMENTAL RETARDATION WITH MATERNAL HYPERTENSION
2962 FETAL ANGIOTENSIN CONVERTING ENZYME (ACE) INHIBITION RENAL FAILURE
2965 PAPILLOMA VIRUS, CONGENITAL INFECTION
2966 SARCOIDOSIS
2967 ACIDURIA, 3-METHYLGLUTACONIC TYPE I
2968 ACIDURIA, 3-METHYLGLUTACONIC TYPE II
2970 GRANULOCYTE GLYCOPROTEIN CD11/CD18 DEFICIENCY
2975 LEUKODYSTROPHY, ADULT-ONSET PROGRESSIVE DOMINANT TYPE
2976 SYNDACTYLY, CENANI TYPE
2977 CUTIS LAXA-DELAYED DEVELOPMENT-LIGAMENTOUS LAXITY
2979 FRONTO-FACIO-NASAL DYSPLASIA
2980 FETAL PARVOVIRUS INFECTION

2981 GASTROCUTANEOUS SYNDROME
2982 FETAL PRIMIDONE EMBRYOPATHY
2984 GAMMA-AMINOBUTYRIC ACID (GABA) TRANSAMINASE DEFICIENCY
2986 FETAL EFFECTS FROM ANGEL DUST (PHENCYCLIDINE OR PCP)
2988 FETAL HERPES SIMPLEX VIRUS INFECTION
2990 HYPERLYSINURIA, ISOLATED
2991 FETAL CARBAMAZEPINE EXPOSURE
2992 FETAL AMINOGLYCOSIDE OTOTOXICITY
2993 OVULATION INDUCTION TRISOMY
2994 VITAMIN B(12) LYSOSOMAL TRANSPORT DEFECT
2995 BRONCHOMALACIA
2996 MACHADO-JOSEPH DISEASE
2998 BRAIN, PORENCEPHALY
2999 BRAIN, MICROPOLYGYRIA
3000 BRAIN, MIDLINE CAVES
3001 BRAIN, SCHIZENCEPHALY
3002 BRAIN, ARACHNOID CYSTS
3003 SPINE, SCOLIOSIS, IDIOPATHIC
3004 SPINE, SPONDYLOLISTHESIS AND SPONDYLOLYSIS
3005 DYSLEXIA
3006 CHROMOSOME X, TRIPLO-X
3007 CHROMOSOME X, POLY-X
3008 FETAL EFFECTS FROM HEPATITIS B INFECTION
3009 HYPERBILIRUBINEMIA, CONJUGATED
3010 ICHTHYOSIS-CHEEK-EYEBROW SYNDROME
3012 PROGEROID SYNDROME WITH EHLERS-DANLOS FEATURES
3013 NEUROPATHY, CONGENITAL MOTOR & SENSORY-SKELETAL-LARYNGEAL DEFECTS
3014 SHORT STATURE-WORMIAN BONES-JOINT DISLOCATIONS
3015 BLADDER EXSTROPHY
3018 KIDNEY, NEPHRONOPHTHISIS-MEDULLARY CYSTIC DISEASE
3019 KIDNEY, MEDULLARY SPONGE KIDNEY
3020 RICKETS, HEREDITARY HYPOPHOSPHATEMIC WITH HYPERCALCIURIA (HHRH)
3022 CARBAMOYL PHOSPHATE SYNTHETASE DEFICIENCY
3023 ORNITHINE TRANSCARBAMYLASE DEFICIENCY
3026 NEPHROSIS-NERVE DEAFNESS-HYPOPARATHY-ROIDISM, BARAKAT TYPE
3028 KIDNEY, RENAL DYSPLASIA, POTTER TYPE II
3029 AASE-SMITH SYNDROME
3030 TRIGONENCEPHALY, AUTOSOMAL DOMINANT TYPE
3031 ALOPECIA-SEIZURES-MENTAL RETARDATION, SHOKEIR TYPE
3032 CORPUS CALLOSUM AGENESIS-SENSORIMOTOR NEUROPATHY, FAMILIAL
3033 ANGIOLIPOMATOSIS
3034 BIEMOND I SYNDROME
3035 BRACHYDACTYLY-LONG THUMB SYNDROME
3036 BRACHYOLMELIA, HOBAEK TYPE
3037 BRANCHIO-OTO-URETERAL SYNDROME
3038 POIKILODERMA, HEREDITARY ACROKERATOTIC, KINDLER-WEARY TYPE
3039 CHANDS
3040 POLYPOSIS-ALOPECIA-PIGMENTATION-NAIL DEFECTS
3041 EDINBURGH MALFORMATION SYNDROME
3042 SYNDACTYLY-POLYDACTYLY-EAR LOBE SYNDROME
3043 IVIC SYNDROME
3044 DERMATO-OSTEOLYSIS, KIRGHIZIAN TYPE
3045 LARYNGEAL ABDUCTOR PARALYSIS-MENTAL RETARDATION
3046 DEAFNESS-NEPHRITIS-MACROTHROMBOPATHIA
3047 MUSCLE-EYE-BRAIN SYNDROME
3048 EPIPHYSEAL DYSPLASIA, MULTIPLE-DIABETES MELLITUS
3049 NASOPALPEBRAL LIPOMA-COLOBOMA SYNDROME
3050 OCULO-RENO-CEREBELLAR SYNDROME

3216 CONVULSIONS, BENIGN FAMILIAL NEONATAL
3217 EPILEPSY, BENIGN CHILDHOOD WITH
CENTROTEMPORAL EEG FOCUS (BEC)
3218 EPILEPSY, BENIGN OCCIPITAL
3219 OCCIPITAL HORN SYNDROME
3220 ARTICULAR HYPERMOBILITY, FAMILIAL
3221 ANEMIA, HEMOLYTIC, GAMMA-GLUTAMYL/
CYSTEINE SYNTHETASE DEFICIENCY
3222 MICROVILLUS INCLUSION DISEASE
3223 MIGRAINE
3224 MYOPATHY, MITOCHONDRIAL-ENCEPHALOPATHY-
LACTIC ACIDOSIS-STROKE
3225 MYOCLONIC EPILEPSY-RAGGED RED FIBERS
3226 LIPID TRANSPORT DEFECT OF INTESTINE
3227 APO B-100, DEFECTIVE, FAMILIAL
3228 RETINA, CONE DYSTROPHY, X-LINKED
3229 ACHOO SYNDROME
3230 THYROTOXICOSIS
3232 TAURODONTISM-SHORT ROOTED TEETH-
MICROCEPHALIC DWARFISM
3233 PTERYGIUM SYNDROME, POPLITEAL, LETHAL
3234 CARDIOMYOPATHY, FAMILIAL DILATED
3235 ANIRIDIA-CEREBELLAR ATAXIA-MENTAL
DEFICIENCY
3236 MUCOSA, ORAL INCLUSION CYSTS OF THE
NEWBORN
3237 HYPERBILIRUBINEMIA, CONJUGATED, ROTOR TYPE
3238 HYPERBILIRUBINEMIA, TRANSIENT FAMILIAL
NEONATAL
3239 EPILEPSY, REFLEX
3240 ATTENTION-DEFICIT HYPERACTIVITY DISORDER
(ADHD)
3241 TRIMETHYLAMINURIA
3242 OCULO-ENCEPHALO-HEPATO-RENAL SYNDROME
3243 PICK DISEASE OF THE BRAIN
3244 CREUTZFELDT-JAKOB DISEASE
3245 GERSTMANN-STRAUSSLER SYNDROME
3246 HAUPTMANN-THANHAUSER SYNDROME
3248 X-LINKED MENTAL RETARDATION-SUBCORTICAL
ATROPHY-PATELLAR LUXATION
3249 X-LINKED MENTAL RETARDATION-MUSCULAR
WEAKNESS-AWKWARD GAIT
3250 X-LINKED MENTAL RETARDATION-Xq DUPLICATION
3251 X-LINKED MENTAL RETARDATION-DYSTONIC
MOVEMENTS OF THE HANDS
3252 X-LINKED MENTAL RETARDATION-PSORIASIS

3254 ALPHA-N-ACETYLGALACTOSAMINIDASE
DEFICIENCY
3255 PEMPHIGUS, BENIGN FAMILIAL
3256 ACROKERATOSIS VERRUCIFORMIS
3257 CRANDALL SYNDROME
3258 SHOVAL-SOFFER SYNDROME
3259 OPHTHALMO-MANDIBULO-MELIC DWARFISM
3260 HYPEREKPLEXIA
3261 ALPERS DISEASE
3262 POIKILODERMA, SCLEROSING, HEREDITARY
3263 URTICARIA PIGMENTOSA (UP)
3264 KERATOSIS PALMARIS ET PLANTARIS OF
UNNA-THOST
3265 HEART-HAND SYNDROME II
3266 HEART-HAND SYNDROME III
3267 SAY-MEYER SYNDROME
3268 HIRSCHPRUNG DISEASE-MICROCEPHALY-
COLOBOMA
3269 HIRSCHSPRUNG DISEASE-POLYDACTYLY-DEAFNESS
3270 JUMPING FRENCHMAN OF MAINE
3271 ISAACS-MERTENS SYNDROME
3272 HEART-HAND SYNDROME IV
3273 NEVO SYNDROME
3274 MUTCHINICK SYNDROME
3275 ACIDEMIA, TRIHYDROXYCOPROSTANIC
3276 CHOLESTASIS, INTRAHEPATIC, RECURRENT BENIGN
3277 BILE DUCTS, INTERLOBULAR, NONSYNDROMIC
PAUCITY
3278 INTRAHEPATIC CHOLESTASIS OF PREGNANCY (ICP)
3279 ALPHA-1-ANTICHYMOTRYPSIN DEFICIENCY
3280 OMODYSPLASIA
3281 FETAL EFFECTS OF NONSTEROIDAL
ANTI-INFLAMMATORY DRUGS (NSAIDS)
3282 EYE, MACULAR DYSTROPHY, NORTH CAROLINA
TYPE
3283 DENTATORUBROPALLIDOLUYSIAN DEGENERATION,
HEREDITARY
3284 CYSTIC HYGROMA
3285 LIMB REDUCTION DEFECTS
3286 HIRSCHSPRUNG DISEASE-CARDIAC DEFECT
3287 NARCOLEPSY
3288 KIDNEY, POLYCYSTIC DISEASE-CATARACT-
BLINDNESS
3289 MAL DE MELEDA
3290 HOWEL-EVANS SYNDROME

MIM-NUMBER-TO-PRIME-NAME INDEX

* 14260 ANEMIA, HEMOLYTIC, ERYTHROCYTE
HEXOKINASE DEFICIENCY
  14267 HIP, DYSPLASIA, NAMAQUALAND TYPE
  14270 HIP, CONGENITAL DISLOCATED
* 14273 DERMATOARTHRITIS, FAMILIAL HISTIOCYTIC
* 14280 RAGWEED POLLEN SENSITIVITY
* 14290 HEART-HAND SYNDROME
* 14300 HORNER SYNDROME
  14305 HUMERO-RADIAL SYNOSTOSIS
  14310 HUNTINGTON DISEASE
* 14320 RETINA, HYALOIDEORETINAL DEGENERATION
OF WAGNER
  14325 HYDROCEPHALUS-COSTOVERTEBRAL
DYSPLASIA-SPRENGEL ANOMALY
* 14350 HYPERBILIRUBINEMIA, UNCONJUGATED
* 14387 HYPERCALCIURIA, FAMILIAL IDIOPATHIC
  14389 HYPERCHOLESTEROLEMIA
  14410 SWEATING, GUSTATORY
* 14425 HYPERLIPOPROTEINEMIA, COMBINED
  14440 HYPERCHOLESTEROLEMIA
  14450 HYPERLIPOPROTEINEMIA, BROAD BETA TYPE
  14460 HYPERTRIGLYCERIDEMIA
  14465 HYPERLIPOPROTEINEMIA V
  14470 CANCER, RENAL CELL CARCINOMA
* 14475 HYPEROSTOSIS, WORTH TYPE
  14480 HYPEROSTOSIS FRONTALIS INTERNA
  14525 SKIN, HYPERPIGMENTATION, FAMILIAL
* 14540 EYE, HYPERTELORISM
* 14541 G SYNDROME
* 14560 KING SYNDROME
* 14560 MYOPATHY, MALIGNANT HYPERTHERMIA
* 14570 HAIR, HYPERTRICHOSIS, LANUGINOSA
* 14575 HYPERTRIGLYCERIDEMIA
* 14590 DEJERINE-SOTTAS DISEASE
  14595 HYPOBETALIPOPROTEINEMIA
  14600 HYPOCHONDROPLASIA
  14615 HYPOMELANOSIS OF ITO
  14616 LIMB, UPPER HYPOPLASIA-MULLERIAN DUCT
DEFECTS
* 14630 HYPOPHOSPHATASIA
  14635 HYPOPHOSPHATEMIA, NON X-LINKED
  14645 HYPOSPADIAS
  14650 DOPAMINE BETA-HYDROXYLASE DEFICIENCY,
CONGENITAL
  14651 HYPOTHALAMIC HAMARTOBLASTOMA
SYNDROME, CONGENITAL
* 14655 HAIR, HYPOTRICHOSIS
* 14659 ICHTHYOSIS HYSTRIX, CURTH-MACKLIN TYPE
* 14660 NEVUS, EPIDERMAL NEVUS SYNDROME
* 14670 ICHTHYOSIS VULGARIS
  14672 ICHTHYOSIS-CHEEK-EYEBROW SYNDROME
  14675 ICHTHYOSIS, LAMELLAR DOMINANT
  14680 ICHTHYOSIFORM HYPERKERATOSIS, BULLOUS
CONGENITAL
  14683 IMMUNODEFICIENCY, COMMON VARIABLE
TYPE
  14683 SERUM ALLOTYPES, HUMAN
* 14690 IMMUNODEFICIENCY, COMMON VARIABLE
TYPE
* 14690 SERUM ALLOTYPES, HUMAN
* 14691 IMMUNODEFICIENCY, COMMON VARIABLE
TYPE
* 14691 SERUM ALLOTYPES, HUMAN
* 14700 IMMUNODEFICIENCY, COMMON VARIABLE
TYPE
* 14700 SERUM ALLOTYPES, HUMAN
* 14701 IMMUNODEFICIENCY, COMMON VARIABLE
TYPE
* 14701 SERUM ALLOTYPES, HUMAN
* 14702 IMMUNODEFICIENCY, COMMON VARIABLE
TYPE
* 14702 SERUM ALLOTYPES, HUMAN
  14706 IMMUNODEFICIENCY, HYPER IgE TYPE

* 14707 IMMUNODEFICIENCY, COMMON VARIABLE
TYPE
* 14707 SERUM ALLOTYPES, HUMAN
* 14710 IMMUNODEFICIENCY, COMMON VARIABLE
TYPE
* 14710 IMMUNODEFICIENCY, IgG SUBCLASS
DEFICIENCIES
* 14710 SERUM ALLOTYPES, HUMAN
* 14711 IMMUNODEFICIENCY, COMMON VARIABLE
TYPE
* 14711 IMMUNODEFICIENCY, IgG SUBCLASS
DEFICIENCIES
* 14711 SERUM ALLOTYPES, HUMAN
* 14712 IMMUNODEFICIENCY, COMMON VARIABLE
TYPE
* 14712 IMMUNODEFICIENCY, IgG SUBCLASS
DEFICIENCIES
* 14712 SERUM ALLOTYPES, HUMAN
* 14713 IMMUNODEFICIENCY, COMMON VARIABLE
TYPE
* 14713 IMMUNODEFICIENCY, IgG SUBCLASS
DEFICIENCIES
* 14713 SERUM ALLOTYPES, HUMAN
* 14716 IMMUNODEFICIENCY, COMMON VARIABLE
TYPE
* 14716 SERUM ALLOTYPES, HUMAN
* 14717 IMMUNODEFICIENCY, COMMON VARIABLE
TYPE
* 14717 SERUM ALLOTYPES, HUMAN
* 14718 IMMUNODEFICIENCY, COMMON VARIABLE
TYPE
* 14718 SERUM ALLOTYPES, HUMAN
  14720 IMMUNODEFICIENCY, COMMON VARIABLE
TYPE
* 14720 SERUM ALLOTYPES, HUMAN
  14725 TEETH, FUSED
  14735 TEETH, MESIOPALATAL TORSION OF CENTRAI
INCISORS
  14740 TEETH, INCISORS, SHOVEL-SHAPED
* 14744 GROWTH DEFICIENCY, AFRICAN PYGMY TYPE
  14748 INTRAHEPATIC CHOLESTASIS OF PREGNANCY
(ICP)
* 14757 INTERFERON DEFICIENCY
* 14762 INTERFERON DEFICIENCY
* 14764 INTERFERON DEFICIENCY
* 14766 INTERFERON DEFICIENCY
* 14775 IVIC SYNDROME
  14777 ALOPECIA-ANOSMIA-DEAFNESS-
HYPOGONADISM, JOHNSON TYPE
* 14779 LEUKEMIA, ACUTE LYMPHOCYTIC, FAMILIAL
* 14780 AASE-SMITH SYNDROME
* 14790 ARTICULAR HYPERMOBILITY, FAMILIAL
* 14790 EHLERS-DANLOS SYNDROME
  14792 KABUKI MAKE-UP SYNDROME
* 14795 KALLMANN SYNDROME
* 14805 KBG SYNDROME
* 14840 KERATOSIS PALMARIS ET PLANTARIS OF
UNNA-THOST
* 14873 SKIN, HYPERKERATOSIS, FOCAL
PALMOPLANTAR AND GINGIVAL
  14880 CRANIOSYNOSTOSIS, KLEEBLATTSCHADEL
TYPE
  14882 WAARDENBURG SYNDROMES
  14886 KLIPPEL-FEIL ANOMALY
  14887 KLIPPEL-FEIL ANOMALY
* 14890 KLIPPEL-FEIL ANOMALY
  14900 ANGIO-OSTEOHYPERTROPHY SYNDROME
* 14920 KNUCKLE PADS-LEUKONYCHIA-DEAFNESS
* 14930 NAILS, KOILONYCHIA
* 14940 HYPEREKPLEXIA
  14950 SKIN, KYRLE DISEASE
* 14970 LACRIMAL CANALICULUS ATRESIA
* 14970 NASOLACRIMAL DUCT OBSTRUCTION

	16282	GRANULOCYTE GLYCOPROTEIN CD11/CD18 DEFICIENCY
	16305	SKIN, VITILIGO
*	16310	NEVUS FLAMMEUS
	16320	NEVUS, EPIDERMAL NEVUS SYNDROME
*	16340	MESOMELIC DYSPLASIA, NIEVERGELT TYPE
*	16350	NIGHTBLINDNESS, CONGENITAL STATIONARY, AUTOSOMAL DOMINANT
*	16370	BREAST, POLYTHELIA
*	16395	NOONAN SYNDROME
	16400	NOSE/NASAL SEPTUM DEFECTS
*	16405	IMMUNODEFICIENCY, NUCLEOSIDE-PHOSPHORYLASE DEFICIENCY
	16418	OCULO-CEREBRO-CUTANEOUS SYNDROME
*	16420	OCULO-DENTO-OSSEOUS DYSPLASIA
	16421	OCULO-AURICULO-VERTEBRAL ANOMALY
*	16430	MUSCULAR DYSTROPHY, OCULOPHARYNGEAL
*	16440	OLIVOPONTOCEREBELLAR ATROPHY, DOMINANT MENZEL TYPE
*	16450	OLIVOPONTOCEREBELLAR ATROPHY, DOMINANT WITH RETINAL DEGENERATION
*	16460	OLIVOPONTOCEREBELLAR ATROPHY, DOMINANT SCHUT-HAYMAKER TYPE
*	16470	OLIVOPONTOCEREBELLAR ATROPHY, DOMINANT WITH OPHTHALMOPLEGIA
	16475	OMPHALOCELE
*	16490	DWARFISM (SHORT LIMBED)-PETERS ANOMALY OF THE EYE
*	16490	OPHTHALMO-MANDIBULO-MELIC DWARFISM
*	16500	OPHTHALMOPLEGIA, FAMILIAL STATIC
	16510	KEARNS-SAYRE DISEASE
	16510	OPHTHALMOPLEGIA, PROGRESSIVE EXTERNAL
	16513	OPHTHALMOPLEGIA, PROGRESSIVE EXTERNAL
*	16550	OPTIC ATROPHY, KJER TYPE
	16555	OPTIC NERVE HYPOPLASIA
*	16580	JOINTS, OSTEOCHONDRITIS DISSECANS
	16600	ENCHONDROMATOSIS
	16600	ENCHONDROMATOSIS AND HEMANGIOMAS
*	16620	OSTEOGENESIS IMPERFECTA
*	16621	OSTEOGENESIS IMPERFECTA
*	16622	OSTEOGENESIS IMPERFECTA
*	16623	OSTEOGENESIS IMPERFECTA
	16624	OSTEOGENESIS IMPERFECTA
	16625	OSTEOGLOPHONIC DYSPLASIA
*	16630	OSTEOLYSIS, CARPAL-TARSAL AND CHRONIC PROGRESSIVE GLOMERULOPATHY
	16645	OSTEOMESOPYKNOSIS
*	16650	OSTEOPATHIA STRIATA-CRANIAL SCLEROSIS-MEGALENCEPHALY
*	16660	OSTEOPETROSIS, BENIGN DOMINANT
*	16670	OSTEOPOIKILOSIS
	16674	SKELETAL BOWING-CORTICAL THICKENING-BONE FRAGILITY-ICTHYOSIS
*	16675	OTO-DENTAL DYSPLASIA
*	16680	OTOSCLEROSIS
*	16690	ELLIPTOCYTOSIS
	16710	PACHYDERMOPERIOSTOSIS
	16720	NAILS, PACHYONYCHIA CONGENITA
	16721	PACHYONYCHIA CONGENITA-STEATOCYSTOMA MULTIPLEX
	16725	BONE, PAGET DISEASE
	16750	PALATOPHARYNGEAL INCOMPETENCE
*	16773	NASOPALPEBRAL LIPOMA-COLOBOMA SYNDROME
	16775	PANCREAS, ANNULAR
*	16780	PANCREATITIS, HEREDITARY
	16787	MOOD AND THOUGHT DISORDERS
	16796	PAPILLOMA VIRUS, CONGENITAL INFECTION
*	16800	CAROTID BODY TUMOR
*	16800	EAR, CHEMODECTOMA OF MIDDLE EAR
*	16830	PARAMYOTONIA CONGENITA
	16840	PARASTREMMATIC DYSPLASIA

	16855	PARIETAL FORAMINA-CLAVICULAR HYPOPLASIA
	16910	DUCTUS ARTERIOSUS, PATENT
	16917	PSEUDOLEPRECHAUNISM, PATTERSON TYPE
	16930	PECTUS EXCAVATUM
*	16950	LEUKODYSTROPHY, ADULT-ONSET PROGRESSIVE DOMINANT TYPE
*	16950	MULTIPLE SCLEROSIS, FAMILIAL
*	16960	PEMPHIGUS, BENIGN FAMILIAL
*	17040	PARALYSIS, HYPOKALEMIC PERIODIC
*	17050	PARALYSIS, HYPERKALEMIC PERIODIC
*	17060	PARALYSIS, NORMOKALEMIC PERIODIC
*	17065	TEETH, PERIODONTITIS, JUVENILE
	17110	IMMUNODEFICIENCY, PLASMA-ASSOCIATED DEFECT OF PHAGOCYTOSIS
*	17120	TASTING DEFECT, PHENYLTHIOCARBAMIDE
*	17140	ENDOCRINE NEOPLASIA, MULTIPLE TYPE II
*	17148	LIMB-OTO-CARDIAC SYNDROME
*	17176	HYPOPHOSPHATASIA
*	17186	GLYCOGENOSIS, TYPE VII
*	17240	ANEMIA, GLUCOSE PHOSPHATE ISOMERASE DEFICIENCY
	17250	DEAFNESS-DIABETES-PHOTOMYOCLONUS-NEPHROPATHY
	17270	PICK DISEASE OF THE BRAIN
*	17280	ALBINISM, CUTANEOUS
*	17310	GROWTH HORMONE DEFICIENCY, ISOLATED
*	17320	SKIN, PITYRIASIS RUBRA PILARIS
*	17335	PLASMINOGEN DEFECTS
*	17365	POIKILODERMA, HEREDITARY ACROKERATOTIC, KINDLER-WEARY TYPE
	17370	POIKILODERMA, SCLEROSING, HEREDITARY
	17375	POLAND SYNDROME
	17380	POLAND SYNDROME
*	17385	POLIO, SUSCEPTIBILITY TO
*	17390	KIDNEY, POLYCYSTIC DISEASE, DOMINANT
*	17400	KIDNEY, NEPHRONOPHTHISIS-MEDULLARY CYSTIC DISEASE
	17405	LIVER, POLYCYSTIC AND MULTICYSTIC DISEASE, ADULT TYPE
*	17420	POLYDACTYLY
	17430	ORO-FACIO-DIGITAL SYNDROME, THURSTON TYPE
	17440	POLYDACTYLY
*	17450	POLYDACTYLY
*	17450	THUMB, TRIPHALANGEAL-DUPLICATED GREAT TOES
*	17460	POLYDACTYLY
*	17470	POLYSYNDACTYLY
	17480	FIBROUS DYSPLASIA, POLYOSTOTIC
*	17490	INTESTINAL POLYPOSIS, JUVENILE TYPE
*	17510	INTESTINAL POLYPOSIS, TYPE I
*	17520	INTESTINAL POLYPOSIS, TYPE II
*	17530	INTESTINAL POLYPOSIS, TYPE III
*	17530	RETINA, CONGENITAL HYPERTROPHY OF RETINAL PIGMENT EPITHELIUM
	17550	POLYPOSIS-ALOPECIA-PIGMENTATION-NAIL DEFECTS
*	17570	POLYSYNDACTYLY-DYSMORPHIC CRANIOFACIES, GREIG TYPE
	17578	BRAIN, PORENCEPHALY
*	17580	SKIN, POROKERATOSIS
	17585	SKIN, POROKERATOSIS
*	17590	·SKIN, POROKERATOSIS
*	17600	PORPHYRIA, ACUTE INTERMITTENT
*	17610	PORPHYRIA CUTANEA TARDA
*	17620	PORPHYRIA, VARIEGATE
*	17627	PRADER-WILLI SYNDROME
	17630	AMYLOIDOSIS, APPALACHIAN TYPE
	17630	AMYLOIDOSIS, ASHKENAZI TYPE
	17630	AMYLOIDOSIS, DANISH CARDIAC TYPE
	17630	AMYLOIDOSIS, ILLINOIS TYPE
	17630	AMYLOIDOSIS, INDIANA TYPE

	18874	MESOMELIC DYSPLASIA, WERNER TYPE
*	18877	MESOMELIC DYSPLASIA, WERNER TYPE
	18930	TONGUE, FOLDING OR ROLLING
*	18950	HYPODONTIA-NAIL DYSGENESIS
	18960	TORTICOLLIS
*	18970	MANDIBLE, TORUS MANDIBULARIS
*	18970	PALATE, TORUS PALATINUS
	18996	ESOPHAGUS, ATRESIA AND TRACHEOESOPH-AGEAL FISTULA
	18996	TRACHEOESOPHAGEAL FISTULA
*	19008	LYMPHOMA, BURKITT TYPE
*	19010	CHIN, TREMBLING
*	19030	TREMOR, HEREDOFAMILIAL
*	19031	TREMOR-DUODENAL ULCER SYNDROME
*	19032	TRICHO-DENTO-OSSEOUS SYNDROME
*	19035	TRICHO-RHINO-PHALANGEAL SYNDROME, TYPE I
	19036	TRICHODYSPLASIA-XERODERMA
	19044	TRIGONENCEPHALY, AUTOSOMAL DOMINANT TYPE
*	19045	ERYTHROCYTE TRIOSEPHOSPHATE ISOMERASE DEFICIENCY
	19060	THUMB, TRIPHALANGEAL
	19068	THUMB, TRIPHALANGEAL-BRACHYECTRODAC-TYLY
*	19090	COLOR BLINDNESS, YELLOW-BLUE TRITAN
*	19110	TUBEROUS SCLEROSIS
	19115	IMMUNODEFICIENCY, TUFTSIN DEFICIENCY TYPE
*	19120	DEAFNESS, TUNE
	19140	MESOMELIC DYSPLASIA, REINHARDT-PFEIFFER TYPE
*	19148	HAIR, UNCOMBABLE-CRYSTALLINE CATARACT
*	19183	RENAL AGENESIS, BILATERAL
*	19183	RENAL AGENESIS, UNILATERAL
*	19190	URTICARIA-DEAFNESS-AMYLOIDOSIS
	19200	MULLERIAN FUSION, INCOMPLETE
	19205	MULLERIAN FUSION, INCOMPLETE
	19210	UVULA, CLEFT
	19235	VATER ASSOCIATION
*	19243	VELO-CARDIO-FACIAL SYNDROME
*	19250	ARRHYTHMIA, WITH LONG QT INTERVAL WITHOUT DEAFNESS
*	19260	HEART, SUBAORTIC STENOSIS, MUSCULAR
	19300	VESICO-URETERAL REFLUX
	19320	SKIN, VITILIGO
*	19325	INTESTINAL ROTATION, INCOMPLETE
*	19330	VON HIPPEL-LINDAU SYNDROME
*	19340	VON WILLEBRAND DISEASE
*	19350	WAARDENBURG SYNDROMES
	19351	WAARDENBURG SYNDROMES
*	19352	PULMONIC STENOSIS-CAFE-AU-LAIT SPOTS, WATSON TYPE
*	19353	ACROFACIAL DYSOSTOSIS
*	19353	ACROFACIAL SYNDROME, CURRY-HALL TYPE
*	19370	CRANIO-CARPO-TARSAL DYSPLASIA, WHISTLING FACE TYPE
*	19390	MUCOSA, WHITE FOLDED DYSPLASIA
*	19405	WILLIAMS SYNDROME
	19407	ANIRIDIA
*	19407	CANCER, WILMS TUMOR
	19408	WILMS TUMOR-PSEUDOHERMAPHRODITISM-GLOMERULOPATHY,DENYS-DRASH TYPE
	19420	ARRHYTHMIA, WOLFF-PARKINSON-WHITE TYPE
	19435	WT SYNDROME
*	19438	ANEMIA, HEMOLYTIC, RED CELL MEMBRANE DEFECTS
*	20010	ABETALIPOPROTEINEMIA
*	20010	ANEMIA, HEMOLYTIC, RED CELL MEMBRANE DEFECTS
	20011	ABLEPHARON-MACROSTOMIA
*	20015	ACANTHOCYTOSIS-NEUROLOGIC DEFECTS
	20017	SKIN, ACANTHOSIS NIGRICANS

*	20040	ESOPHAGUS, ACHALASIA
*	20050	ACHEIROPODY
*	20060	ACHONDROGENESIS, HOUSTON-HARRIS TYPE
*	20060	ACHONDROGENESIS, PARENTI-FRACCARO TYPE
*	20061	ACHONDROGENESIS, HOUSTON-HARRIS TYPE
*	20061	ACHONDROGENESIS, LANGER-SALDINO TYPE
*	20070	GREBE SYNDROME
	20090	METAPHYSEAL CHONDRODYSPLASIA WITH THYMOLYMPHOPENIA
	20097	DENTO-FACIO-SKELETAL DEFECTS, ACKERMAN TYPE
	20098	ACRO-RENAL-MANDIBULAR SYNDROME
	20099	ACROCALLOSAL SYNDROME, SCHINZEL TYPE
*	20100	ACROCEPHALOPOLYSYNDACTYLY
*	20102	ACROCEPHALOPOLYSYNDACTYLY
*	20110	ACRODERMATITIS ENTEROPATHICA
*	20110	NEUROPATHY, MYELO-OPTICO, SUBACUTE TYPE
	20118	ACRO-FRONTO-FACIO-NASAL DYSOSTOSIS
	20120	PROGERIA
*	20125	ACROMESOMELIC DYSPLASIA, CAMPAILLA-MARTINELLI TYPE
*	20125	ACROMESOMELIC DYSPLASIA, MAROTEAUX-MARTINELLI-CAMPAILLA TYPE
*	20130	ACRO-OSTEOLYSIS, NEUROGENIC
	20140	ADRENOCORTICOTROPIC HORMONE DEFICIENCY, ISOLATED
*	20145	ACYL-CoA DEHYDROGENASE DEFICIENCY, MEDIUM CHAIN TYPE
*	20146	ACYL-CoA DEHYDROGENASE DEFICIENCY, LONG CHAIN TYPE
*	20147	ACYL-CoA DEHYDROGENASE DEFICIENCY, SHORT CHAIN TYPE
*	20155	THUMB, ADDUCTED THUMB SYNDROME
*	20171	STEROID 20-22 DESMOLASE DEFICIENCY
*	20181	STEROID 3 BETA-HYDROXYSTEROID DEHYDROGENASE DEFICIENCY
*	20191	STEROID 21-HYDROXYLASE DEFICIENCY
*	20201	STEROID 11 BETA-HYDROXYLASE DEFICIENCY
*	20211	STEROID 17 ALPHA-HYDROXYLASE DEFICIENCY
*	20220	ADRENOCORTICAL UNRESPONSIVENESS TO ACTH, HEREDITARY
	20240	AFIBROGINEMIA, CONGENITAL
*	20250	IMMUNODEFICIENCY, SEVERE COMBINED
	20265	AGNATHIA-HOLOPROSENCEPHALY
*	20270	IMMUNODEFICIENCY, AGRANULOCYTOSIS, INFANTILE KOSTMANN TYPE
*	20292	IMMUNODEFICIENCY, SEVERE COMBINED
*	20310	ALBINISM, OCULOCUTANEOUS, TYROSINASE NEGATIVE
*	20320	ALBINISM, OCULOCUTANEOUS, TYROSINASE POSITIVE
	20328	ALBINISM, OCULOCUTANEOUS, MINIMAL PIGMENT TYPE
*	20329	ALBINISM, OCULOCUTANEOUS, BROWN TYPE
*	20330	ALBINISM, OCULOCUTANEOUS, HERMANSKY-PUDLAK TYPE
*	20331	ALBINISM, OCULAR, AUTOSOMAL RECESSIVE TYPE
	20332	ALBINISM, OCULOCUTANEOUS, YELLOW MUTANT
	20333	PARATHYROID HORMONE RESISTANCE
	20334	ALBINISM-MICROCEPHALY-DIGITAL DEFECTS
*	20340	STEROID 18-HYDROXYLASE DEFICIENCY
*	20341	STEROID 18-HYDROXYSTEROID DEHYDROGENASE DEFICIENCY
	20345	ALEXANDER DISEASE
*	20350	ALKAPTONURIA
	20355	ALOPECIA-SKELETAL ANOMALIES-SHORT STATURE-MENTAL RETARDATION
	20360	ALOPECIA-EPILEPSY-OLIGOPHRENIA, MOYNAHAN TYPE
*	20365	ALOPECIA-MENTAL RETARDATION

* 21490 CHOLESTASIS-LYMPHEDEMA, AAGENAES TYPE
* 21495 ACIDEMIA, TRIHYDROXYCOPROSTANIC
  21500 CHOLESTERYL ESTER STORAGE DISEASE
* 21510 CHONDRODYSPLASIA PUNCTATA, RHIZOMELIC TYPE
* 21515 CHONDRODYSTROPHY-SENSORINEURAL DEAFNESS, NANCE-INSLEY TYPE
* 21515 OTO-SPONDYLO-MEGAEPIPHYSEAL DYSPLASIA
  21555 CIRCUMVALLATE PLACENTA SYNDROME
* 21570 CITRULLINEMIA
  21590 CLEFT LIP
  21610 ORO-CRANIO-DIGITAL SYNDROME
  21630 CLEFT PALATE-STAPES FIXATION-OLIGODONTIA
* 21634 YUNIS-VARON SYNDROME
  21635 RETINA, COATS DISEASE
* 21640 COCKAYNE SYNDROME
  21641 COCKAYNE SYNDROME, TYPE II
* 21650 OCULAR MOTOR APRAXIA, COGAN CONGENITAL TYPE
* 21655 COHEN SYNDROME
  21682 EYE, MICROPHTHALMIA/COLOBOMA
* 21690 COLOR BLINDNESS, TOTAL
* 21695 COMPLEMENT COMPONENT 1, DEFICIENCY OF
* 21700 COMPLEMENT COMPONENT 2, DEFICIENCY OF
* 21703 COMPLEMENT COMPONENT 3, DEFICIENCY OF
  21709 EYE, LIGNEOUS CONJUNCTIVITIS
  21710 AMNIOTIC BANDS SYNDROME
  21710 LIMB AND SCALP DEFECTS, ADAMS-OLIVER TYPE
  21720 EPILEPSY, FAMILIAL
  21720 SEIZURES, FEBRILE
* 21730 CORNEA PLANA
  21740 CORNEAL DYSTROPHY-SENSORINEURAL DEAFNESS
* 21750 EYE, KERATOPATHY, BAND-SHAPED
* 21770 CORNEAL DYSTROPHY, ENDOTHELIAL, CONGENITAL HEREDITARY
* 21780 CORNEAL DYSTROPHY, MACULAR TYPE
* 21800 CORPUS CALLOSUM AGENESIS-SENSORIMOTOR NEUROPATHY, FAMILIAL
  21801 BLINDNESS (CORTICAL)-RETARDATION-POSTAXIAL POLYDACTYLY
* 21830 CRANIO-DIAPHYSEAL DYSPLASIA
* 21833 CRANIO-ECTODERMAL DYSPLASIA
  21835 CRANIOFACIAL DYSSYNOSTOSIS
* 21840 CRANIOMETAPHYSEAL DYSPLASIA
* 21850 CRANIOSYNOSTOSIS
* 21850 CRANIOSYNOSTOSIS-FOOT DEFECTS, JACKSON-WEISS TYPE
  21855 CRANIOSYNOSTOSIS-FIBULAR APLASIA, LOWRY TYPE
* 21860 CRANIOSYNOSTOSIS-RADIAL APLASIA SYNDROME
  21865 CRANIOSYNOSTOSIS-MENTAL RETARDATION-CLEFTING SYNDROME
  21867 CRANIOTELENCEPHALIC DYSPLASIA
* 21870 THYROID, DYSGENESIS
* 21880 UDP-GLUCURONOSYLTRANSFERASE, SEVERE DEFICIENCY TYPE I
* 21890 CATARACT-RENAL TUBULAR NECROSIS-ENCEPHALOPATHY, CROME TYPE
* 21900 EYE, CRYPTOPHTHALMOS WITH OTHER MALFORMATIONS
* 21900 FRASER SYNDROME
* 21910 CUTIS LAXA
* 21915 CUTIS LAXA-GROWTH DEFECT, DE BARSY TYPE
* 21920 CUTIS LAXA-DELAYED DEVELOPMENT-LIGAMENTOUS LAXITY
  21925 CUTIS MARMORATA
  21930 CUTIS VERTICUS GYRATA
* 21950 CYSTATHIONINURIA
* 21970 CYSTIC FIBROSIS

* 21975 CYSTINOSIS
* 21980 CYSTINOSIS
* 21990 CYSTINOSIS
* 22010 CYSTINURIA
* 22011 MYOPATHY-METABOLIC, MITOCHONDRIAL CYTOCHROME C OXIDASE DEFICIENCY
* 22015 RENAL HYPOURICEMIA
  22020 HYDROCEPHALY
* 22040 CARDIO-AUDITORY SYNDROME
* 22050 DEAFNESS-ONYCHO-OSTEO-DYSTROPHY-RETARDATION-SEIZURES (DOORS)
* 22050 DEAFNESS-ONYCHODYSTROPHY
* 22050 DEAFNESS-TRIPHALANGEAL THUMBS-ONYCHODYSTROPHY
* 22070 DEAFNESS (SENSORINEURAL), RECESSIVE PROFOUND
* 22080 DEAFNESS (SENSORINEURAL), RECESSIVE PROFOUND
  22100 DEAFNESS, PFAENDLER TYPE
  22120 DEAFNESS-MYOPIA
* 22130 DEAFNESS-MALFORMED EARS-MENTAL RETARDATION
* 22130 DEAFNESS-MALFORMED, LOW-SET EARS
* 22130 EAR, LOW-SET
* 22135 DEAFNESS-VITILIGO-MUSCLE WASTING
  22140 DEAFNESS-DIVERTICULITIS-NEUROPATHY
  22160 DEAFNESS (SENSORINEURAL), RECESSIVE EARLY-ONSET
  22170 DEAFNESS-ATOPIC DERMATITIS
* 22177 OSTEODYSPLASIA, LIPOMEMBRANOUS POLYCYSTIC-DEMENTIA
* 22180 DERMO-CHONDRO-CORNEAL DYSTROPHY, FRANCOIS TYPE
  22181 DERMATO-OSTEOLYSIS, KIRGHIZIAN TYPE
  22188 LARSEN SYNDROME
* 22190 RETINAL DYSPLASIA
  22210 DIABETES MELLITUS, INSULIN DEPENDENT TYPE
* 22230 DIABETES (INSIPIDUS/MELLITUS)-OPTIC ATROPHY-DEAFNESS
  22250 DIASTEMATOMYELIA
* 22260 DIASTROPHIC DYSPLASIA
* 22269 HYPERDIBASIC AMINOACIDURIA
* 22270 HYPERDIBASIC AMINOACIDURIA
  22273 ACIDURIA, DICARBOXYLIC AMINOACIDURIA
  22276 DIGITO-RENO-CEREBRAL SYNDROME
* 22280 ERYTHROCYTE, DIPHOSPHOGLYCERATE MUTASE (2,3) DEFICIENCY
* 22290 SUCRASE-ISOMALTASE DEFICIENCY
* 22300 LACTASE DEFICIENCY, CONGENITAL
* 22310 LACTASE DEFICIENCY, PRIMARY
* 22336 DOPAMINE BETA-HYDROXYLASE DEFICIENCY, CONGENITAL
* 22337 DUBOWITZ SYNDROME
  22340 DUODENUM, ATRESIA OR STENOSIS
  22340 PYLORODUODENAL ATRESIA, HEREDITARY
* 22380 DYGGVE-MELCHIOR-CLAUSEN SYNDROME
* 22390 DYSAUTONOMIA I, RILEY-DAY TYPE
* 22405 DYSEQUILIBRIUM SYNDROME
* 22410 ANEMIA, DYSERYTHROPOIETIC, TYPE II
* 22412 ANEMIA, DYSERYTHROPOIETIC, TYPE I
  22423. DYSKERATOSIS CONGENITA
* 22430 DYSOSTEOSCLEROSIS
  22440 DWARFISM, DYSSEGMENTAL, ROLLAND-DESBUQUOIS TYPE
  22441 DWARFISM, DYSSEGMENTAL, SILVERMAN-HANDMAKER TYPE
* 22450 TORSION DYSTONIA
  22470 TRICUSPID VALVE, EBSTEIN ANOMALY
* 22490 ECTODERMAL DYSPLASIA, CHRIST-SIEMENS-TOURAINE TYPE
* 22490 ECTODERMAL DYSPLASIA, PASSARGE TYPE

	23575	HIRSCHSPRUNG DISEASE-CARDIAC DEFECT
*	23580	HISTIDINEMIA
*	23583	HISTIDINURIA
	23600	CANCER, HODGKIN DISEASE, FAMILIAL
*	23610	CYCLOPIA
*	23610	HOLOPROSENCEPHALY
*	23620	HOMOCYSTINURIA
*	23625	HOMOCYSTINURIA, N(5,10) METHYLENE TETRAHYDROFOLATE DEFICIENCY TYPE
*	23627	METHYLCOBALAMIN DEFICIENCY
	23630	HOOFT DISEASE
*	23640	HUMERO-RADIAL SYNOSTOSIS
	23645	CEREBRO-NEPHRO-OSTEODYSPLASIA, HUTTERITE TYPE
	23660	HYDROCEPHALY
*	23667	WALKER-WARBURG SYNDROME
*	23668	HYDROLETHALUS SYNDROME
*	23670	VAGINAL SEPTUM, TRANSVERSE
*	23673	UROFACIAL SYNDROME
	23675	HYDROPS FETALIS, NON-IMMUNE
*	23700	HYDROXYPROLINEMIA
	23710	HYMEN, IMPERFORATE
*	23730	CARBAMOYL PHOSPHATE SYNTHETASE DEFICIENCY
	23731	N-ACETYLGLUTAMATE SYNTHETASE DEFICIENCY
	23740	HYPERBETA-ALANINEMIA
*	23745	HYPERBILIRUBINEMIA, CONJUGATED, ROTOR TYPE
*	23750	HYPERBILIRUBINEMIA, CONJUGATED
	23755	HYPERBILIRUBINEMIA, CONJUGATED
*	23780	HYPERBILIRUBINEMIA, CONJUGATED
	23790	HYPERBILIRUBINEMIA, TRANSIENT FAMILIAL NEONATAL
	23820	HYPERCYSTINURIA
*	23830	HYPERGLYCINEMIA, NON-KETOTIC
	23832	KLINEFELTER SYNDROME
*	23860	HYPERCHYLOMICRONEMIA
*	23870	HYPERLYSINEMIA
*	23897	HYPERORNITHINEMIA-HYPERAMMONEMIA-HOMOCITRULLINURIA
*	23900	OSTEOECTASIA
*	23910	ENDOSTEAL HYPEROSTOSIS
	23920	HYPERPARATHYROIDISM, FAMILIAL
*	23950	HYPERPROLINEMIA
*	23951	HYPERPROLINEMIA
*	23980	HYPERTELORISM-MICROTIA-FACIAL CLEFT-CONDUCTIVE DEAFNESS
	23985	OSTEOCHONDRODYSPLASIA WITH HYPERTRICHOSIS
*	24020	ADRENAL HYPOPLASIA, CONGENITAL
*	24030	POLYGLANDULAR AUTOIMMUNE SYNDROME
*	24050	IMMUNODEFICIENCY, COMMON VARIABLE TYPE
*	24050	SERUM ALLOTYPES, HUMAN
*	24060	GLYCOGEN SYNTHETASE DEFICIENCY
*	24080	HYPOGLYCEMIA, FAMILIAL NEONATAL
*	24108	HYPOGONADISM-DIABETES-ALOPECIA-DEAFNESS-RETARDATION-EKG ANOMALIES
	24109	HYPOGONADISM-PARTIAL ALOPECIA
*	24120	BARTTER SYNDROME
*	24150	HYPOPHOSPHATASIA
*	24151	HYPOPHOSPHATASIA
*	24153	RICKETS, HEREDITARY HYPOPHOSPHATEMIC WITH HYPERCALCIURIA (HHRH)
	24175	HYPOSPADIAS
*	24190	HAIR, ATRICHIA CONGENITA
	24205	RENAL HYPOURICEMIA
*	24210	ICHTHYOSIS, CONGENITAL ERYTHRODERMIC
*	24210	ICHTHYOSIS, LAMELLAR RECESSIVE
	24215	ICHTHYOSIFORM ERYTHROKERATODERMA, ATYPICAL WITH DEAFNESS
*	24217	TRICHOTHIODYSTROPHY
*	24230	ICHTHYOSIS, CONGENITAL ERYTHRODERMIC
*	24230	ICHTHYOSIS, LAMELLAR RECESSIVE
*	24250	ICHTHYOSIS, HARLEQUIN FETUS
*	24260	IMINOGLYCINURIA
*	24270	IMMUNODEFICIENCY, NEZELOF TYPE
	24286	IMMUNODEFICIENCY WITH CENTROMERIC INSTABILITY
*	24309	LIPODYSTROPHY-COARSE FACIES-ACANTHOSIS NIGRICANS, MIESCHER TYPE
*	24309	SKIN, ACANTHOSIS NIGRICANS
*	24315	INTESTINAL ATRESIA OR STENOSIS
*	24315	INTESTINAL ATRESIAS, MULTIPLE
*	24318	INTESTINAL PSEUDO-OBSTRUCTION SYNDROMES
	24330	CHOLESTASIS, INTRAHEPATIC, RECURRENT BENIGN
*	24340	ACETYLATOR POLYMORPHISM
*	24340	NEUROPATHY, HERITABLE ISONIAZIDE TYPE (INH)
	24345	ANOSMIA, CONGENITAL
*	24350	ACIDEMIA, ISOVALERIC
*	24360	JEJUNAL ATRESIA
*	24370	IMMUNODEFICIENCY, HYPER IgE TYPE
*	24380	JOHANSON-BLIZZARD SYNDROME
	24410	JUMPING FRENCHMAN OF MAINE
*	24420	KALLMANN SYNDROME
*	24440	DEXTROCARDIA-BRONCHIECTASIS-SINUSITIS SYNDROME
*	24445	OCULO-CEREBRO-FACIAL SYNDROME, KAUFMAN TYPE
	24450	EYE, KERATOCONUS
	24485.	KERATOSIS PALMARIS ET PLANTARIS OF UNNA-THOST
*	24500	HYPERKERATOSIS PALMOPLANTARIS-PERIODONTOCLASIA
*	24515	KEUTEL SYNDROME
	24519	KNIEST-LIKE DYSPLASIA
*	24520	LEUKODYSTROPHY, GLOBOID CELL TYPE
	24521	MENINGOCELE-CONOTRUNCAL HEART DEFECT, KOUSSEFF TYPE
	24534	ERYTHROCYTE, LACTATE TRANSPORTER DEFECT
*	24560	LARSEN SYNDROME
	24565	LARSEN SYNDROME, LETHAL TYPE
	24580	LAURENCE-MOON SYNDROME
	24590	ANEMIA, HEMOLYTIC, RED CELL MEMBRANE DEFECTS
*	24590	LECITHIN-CHOLESTEROL ACYL TRANSFERASE DEFICIENCY
*	24620	LEPRECHAUNISM
*	24640	LETTERER-SIWE DISEASE
*	24645	ACIDEMIA, 3-HYDROXY-3-METHYLGLUTARIC
	24650	BERLIN SYNDROME
*	24660	LIPASE, CONGENITAL ABSENCE OF PANCREATIC
	24670	LIPID TRANSPORT DEFECT OF INTESTINE
*	24710	SKIN, LIPOID PROTEINOSIS
*	24720	LISSENCEPHALY SYNDROME
	24741	LYMPHEDEMA-HYPOPARATHYROIDISM
	24795	HYPERLYSINURIA, ISOLATED
	24800	MEGALENCEPHALY
*	24825	HYPOMAGNESEMIA, PRIMARY
*	24830	MAL DE MELEDA
*	24837	MANDIBULOACRAL DYSPLASIA
	24839	MANDIBULOFACIAL DYSOSTOSIS, TREACHER COLLINS TYPE, RECESSIVE
*	24850	MANNOSIDOSIS
*	24860	MAPLE SYRUP URINE DISEASE
*	24870	MARDEN-WALKER SYNDROME
	24877	FACIO-NEURO-SKELETAL SYNDROME
*	24880	MARINESCO-SJOGREN SYNDROME
	24895	McDONOUGH SYNDROME
*	24900	MECKEL SYNDROME

* 24910   FEVER, FAMILIAL MEDITERRANEAN (FMF)
  24920   COLON, AGANGLIONOSIS
* 24921   INTESTINAL HYPOPERISTALSIS, MEGACYSTIS-MICROCOLON TYPE
* 24931   MEGALOCORNEA-MENTAL RETARDATION SYNDROME
  24940   NEUROCUTANEOUS MELANOSIS
  24942   OSTEODYSPLASTY
  24960   MIETENS-WEBER SYNDROME
  24962   MENTAL RETARDATION-HEART DEFECTS-BLEPHAROPHIMOSIS
  24963   MUTCHINICK SYNDROME
* 24965   ACIDURIA, BETA-MERCAPTOLACTATE-CYSTEINE DISULFIDURIA
  24966   RENAL MESANGIAL SCLEROSIS-EYE DEFECTS
  24967   HEART-HAND SYNDROME IV
  24970   MESOMELIC DYSPLASIA, LANGER TYPE
  25000   METACHROMATIC LEUKODYSTROPHIES
* 25010   METACHROMATIC LEUKODYSTROPHIES
  25020   METACHROMATIC LEUKODYSTROPHIES
* 25025   METAPHYSEAL CHONDRODYSPLASIA, TYPE McKUSICK
  25042   METAPHYSEAL DYSOSTOSIS-DEAFNESS
  25045   EXOSTOSES-ANETODERMIA-BRACHYDACTYLY TYPE E
* 25060   METATROPIC DYSPLASIA
* 25080   METHEMOGLOBINEMIA, NADH-DEPENDENT DIAPHORASE DEFICIENCY
* 25090   METHIONINE MALABSORPTION
* 25095   ACIDURIA, 3-METHYLGLUTACONIC TYPE I
* 25095   ACIDURIA, 3-METHYLGLUTACONIC TYPE II
* 25100   ACIDEMIA, METHYLMALONIC
* 25117   ACIDEMIA, MEVALONIC
* 25120   MICROCEPHALY
  25124   MICROCEPHALY-RETARDATION-SKELETAL AND IMMUNE DEFECTS
* 25126   CHROMOSOME INSTABILITY, NIJMEGEN TYPE
* 25126   MICROCEPHALY, AUTOSOMAL RECESSIVE WITH NORMAL INTELLIGENCE
* 25127   MICROCEPHALY WITH CHORIORETINOPATHY
* 25130   MICROCEPHALY-HIATUS HERNIA-NEPHROSIS, GALLOWAY TYPE
  25175   LENS, MICROSPHEROPHAKIA
* 25180   EAR, MICROTIA-ATRESIA
* 25210   ORO-FACIO-DIGITAL SYNDROME, MOHR TYPE
* 25215   MOLYBDENUM CO-FACTOR DEFICIENCY
  25220   HAIR, MONILETHRIX
* 25240   MUCOLIPIDOSIS I
* 25250   MUCOLIPIDOSIS II
* 25260   MUCOLIPIDOSIS III
* 25265   MUCOLIPIDOSIS IV
* 25280   MUCOPOLYSACCHARIDOSIS I-H
* 25280   MUCOPOLYSACCHARIDOSIS I-S
* 25290   MUCOPOLYSACCHARIDOSIS III
* 25292   MUCOPOLYSACCHARIDOSIS III
* 25293   MUCOPOLYSACCHARIDOSIS III
* 25294   MUCOPOLYSACCHARIDOSIS III
* 25300   MUCOPOLYSACCHARIDOSIS IV
  25301   MUCOPOLYSACCHARIDOSIS IV
* 25320   MUCOPOLYSACCHARIDOSIS VI
* 25322   MUCOPOLYSACCHARIDOSIS VII
* 25325   DWARFISM, MULIBREY TYPE
* 25326   BIOTINIDASE DEFICIENCY
* 25327   CARBOXYLASE DEFICIENCY, HOLOCARBOXY-LASE DEFICIENCY TYPE
* 25328   MUSCLE-EYE-BRAIN SYNDROME
  25329   PTERYGIUM SYNDROME, MULTIPLE LETHAL
* 25330   SPINAL MUSCULAR ATROPHY
  25331   CONTRACTURES, CONGENITAL LETHAL FINNISH TYPE
* 25340   SPINAL MUSCULAR ATROPHY
* 25355   SPINAL MUSCULAR ATROPHY
* 25360   MUSCULAR DYSTROPHY, LIMB-GIRDLE

* 25370   MUSCULAR DYSTROPHY, AUTOSOMAL RECESSIVE PSEUDOHYPERTROPHIC
* 25380   MUSCULAR DYSTROPHY, CONGENITAL WITH MENTAL RETARDATION
* 25390   MUSCULAR DYSTROPHY, CONGENITAL WITH ARTHROGRYPOSIS
  25400   MYOPATHY-CATARACT-GONADAL DYSGENESIS
* 25415   ANOSMIA, CONGENITAL
* 25420   MYASTHENIC SYNDROME, CONGENITAL SLOW CHANNEL TYPE
* 25421   MYASTHENIC SYNDROME, FAMILIAL INFANTILE TYPE
  25450   CANCER, MULTIPLE MYELOMA
* 25460   IMMUNODEFICIENCY, MYELOPEROXIDASE DEFICIENCY TYPE
* 25475   MYOPATHY-METABOLIC, MYOADENYLATE DEAMINASE DEFICIENCY
  25477   SEIZURES, MYOCLONIC, JUVENILE JANZ TYPE
* 25478   SEIZURES, PROGRESSIVE MYOCLONIC, LAFORA TYPE
* 25480   SEIZURES, PROGRESSIVE MYOCLONIC, UNVERRICHT-LUNDBORG TYPE
* 25511   MYOPATHY-METABOLIC, CARNITINE PALMITYL TRANSFERASE DEFICIENCY
* 25512   MYOPATHY-METABOLIC, CARNITINE PALMITYL TRANSFERASE DEFICIENCY
* 25515   MYOPATHY, MYOGLOBINURIA-ABNORMAL GLYCOLOSIS, HEREDITARY TYPE
  25516   MYOPATHY, FAMILIAL LYSIS OF TYPE I FIBERS
  25517   MYOPATHY-CATARACT-GONADAL DYSGENESIS
  25520   MYOPATHY, MYOTUBULAR
* 25531   MYOPATHY, DISPROPORTIONATE FIBER TYPE I
  25550   MYOPIA, CONGENITAL
  25560   MUSCULAR DYSTROPHY, CONGENITAL WITH ARTHROGRYPOSIS
* 25570   MYOTONIA CONGENITA
* 25580   CHONDRODYSTROPHIC MYOTONIA, SCHWARTZ-JAMPEL TYPE
* 25596   MYXOMA, INTRACARDIAC
  25598   NASO-DIGITO-ACOUSTIC SYNDROME, KEIPERT TYPE
  25599   OTO-OCULO-MUSCULO-SKELETAL SYNDROME
* 25600   ENCEPHALOPATHY, NECROTIZING
* 25603   MYOPATHY, NEMALINE
  25604   DIGITAL DEFECTS-NODULAR ERYTHEMA-EMACIATION, NAKAJO TYPE
* 25605   SKELETAL DYSPLASIA, DE LA CHAPELLE TYPE
* 25610   KIDNEY, NEPHRONOPHTHISIS-MEDULLARY CYSTIC DISEASE
  25620   NEPHROSIS-DEAFNESS-URINARY TRACT AND DIGITAL DEFECTS
* 25630   NEPHROSIS, CONGENITAL
  25634   NEPHROSIS-NERVE DEAFNESS-HYPOPARATHYROIDISM, BARAKAT TYPE
  25635   NEPHROSIS, FAMILIAL TYPE
* 25650   ICHTHYOSIS, LINEARIS CIRCUMFLEXA
* 25652   NEU-LAXOVA SYNDROME
* 25654   GALACTOSIALIDOSIS
* 25655   MUCOLIPIDOSIS I
* 25660   NEUROAXONAL DYSTROPHY, INFANTILE
  25669   NEURO-FACIO-DIGITO-RENAL SYNDROME
  25670   CANCER, NEUROBLASTOMA
* 25671   NEUROECTODERMAL MELANOLYSOSOMAL SYNDROME
* 25673   NEURONAL CEROID-LIPOFUSCINOSES (NCL)
* 25680   NEUROPATHY, CONGENITAL SENSORY WITH ANHIDROSIS
* 25685   NEUROPATHY, GIANT AXONAL
* 25720   NIEMANN-PICK DISEASE
* 25722   NIEMANN-PICK DISEASE
* 25725   NIEMANN-PICK DISEASE
* 25727   NIGHTBLINDNESS, CONGENITAL STATIONARY, AUTOSOMAL RECESSIVE

	25730	CHROMOSOME 13, TRISOMY 13
	25730	CHROMOSOME 18, TRISOMY 18
	25730	KLINEFELTER SYNDROME
	25735	NECK, CYSTIC HYGROMA, FETAL TYPE
	25770	OCULO-AURICULO-VERTEBRAL ANOMALY
*	25780	GINGIVAL FIBROMATOSIS-DEPIGMENTATION-MICROPHTHALMIA
	25791	DWARFISM, OCULO-PALATO-CEREBRAL TYPE
*	25797	OCULO-RENO-CEREBELLAR SYNDROME
	25798	ODONTO-ONYCHODERMAL DYSPLASIA
*	25810	NIGHTBLINDNESS, OGUCHI TYPE
*	25830	OLIVOPONTOCEREBELLAR ATROPHY, RECESSIVE FICKLER-WINKLER TYPE
	25832	CLEFT PALATE-OMPHALOCELE
*	25836	ONYCHO-TRICHODYSPLASIA-NEUTROPENIA
*	25840	OPHTHALMOPLEGIA, TOTAL WITH PTOSIS AND MIOSIS
	25845	OPHTHALMOPLEGIA, PROGRESSIVE EXTERNAL
	25848	OPSISMODYSPLASIA
	25865	DEAFNESS-POLYNEUROPATHY-OPTIC ATROPHY
*	25870	OPTICO-COCHLEO-DENTATE DEGENERATION
*	25885	ORO-FACIO-DIGITAL SYNDROME, SUGARMAN TYPE
	25886	ORO-FACIO-DIGITAL SYNDROME, BARAITSER-BURN TYPE
*	25887	GYRATE ATROPHY OF THE CHOROID AND RETINA
*	25890	ACIDEMIA, OROTIC
	25892	ACIDEMIA, OROTIC
	25927	OSTEODYSPLASTY
*	25940	OSTEOGENESIS IMPERFECTA
	25941	OSTEOGENESIS IMPERFECTA
*	25942	OSTEOGENESIS IMPERFECTA
	25950	OSTEOSARCOMA
	25960	OSTEOLYSIS, RECESSIVE CARPAL-TARSAL
	25961	OSTEOLYSIS, ESSENTIAL
*	25970	OSTEOPETROSIS, MALIGNANT RECESSIVE
	25971	OSTEOPETROSIS, MILD RECESSIVE
	25972	OSTEOPETROSIS, MALIGNANT RECESSIVE
*	25973	OSTEOPETROSIS, MALIGNANT RECESSIVE
*	25973	RENAL TUBULAR ACIDOSIS-OSTEOPETROSIS SYNDROME
	25975	OSTEOPOROSIS, JUVENILE IDIOPATHIC
*	25977	OSTEOPOROSIS-PSEUDOGLIOMA SYNDROME
	25978	OTO-ONYCHO-PERONEAL SYNDROME
	26013	NAILS, PACHYONYCHIA CONGENITA
	26035	CANCER, PANCREAS, FAMILIAL ADENOCARCINOMA OF
*	26040	SHWACHMAN SYNDROME
	26050	CNS NEOPLASMS
	26053	SKIN, PARANA HARD SKIN SYNDROME
*	26080	PENTOSURIA
	26095	TEETH, PERIODONTITIS, JUVENILE
*	26100	ANEMIA, PERNICIOUS CONGENITAL
*	26110	VITAMIN B(12) MALABSORPTION
	26154	DWARFISM (SHORT LIMBED)-PETERS ANOMALY OF THE EYE
*	26155	MULLERIAN DERIVATIVES IN MALES, PERSISTENT
*	26160	FETAL EFFECTS FROM MATERNAL PKU
*	26160	PHENYLKETONURIA
*	26163	DIHYDROPTERIDINE REDUCTASE DEFICIENCY
*	26164	BIOPTERIN SYNTHESIS DEFICIENCY
	26170	ANEMIA, HEMOLYTIC, ERYTHROCYTE PHOSPHOGLYCERATE KINASE DEFICIENCY
*	26175	GLYCOGENOSIS, TYPE IXb
	26180	CLEFT PALATE-MICROGNATHIA-GLOSSOPTOSIS
	26200	CRANDALL SYNDROME
	26200	DEAFNESS-PILI TORTI, BJORNSTAD TYPE
	26202	TRICHODENTAL DYSPLASIA WITH REFRACTIVE ERRORS
*	26219	LIPODYSTROPHY-COARSE FACIES-ACANTHOSIS NIGRICANS, MIESCHER TYPE
	26235	DWARFISM-DYSMORPHIC FACIES-RETARDATION, PITT TYPE
*	26240	GROWTH HORMONE DEFICIENCY, ISOLATED
*	26250	DWARFISM, LARON
*	26260	DWARFISM, PANHYPOPITUITARY
	26270	DWARFISM, PITUITARY WITH ABNORMAL SELLA TURCICA
	26310	KIDNEY, POLYCYSTIC DISEASE-CATARACT-BLINDNESS
*	26320	HEPATIC FIBROSIS, CONGENITAL
*	26320	KIDNEY, POLYCYSTIC DISEASE, RECESSIVE
*	26320	LIVER, CONGENITAL CYSTIC DILATATION OF INTRAHEPATIC DUCTS
	26351	SHORT RIB-POLYDACTYLY SYNDROME, VERMA-NAUMOFF TYPE
*	26352	SHORT RIB-POLYDACTYLY SYNDROME, TYPE II
*	26353	SHORT RIB-POLYDACTYLY SYNDROME, TYPE I
	26354	HEART-HAND SYNDROME IV
	26363	POLYSYNDACTYLY-CARDIAC MALFORMATIONS
*	26365	PTERYGIUM SYNDROME, POPLITEAL, LETHAL
*	26370	PORPHYRIA, ERYTHROPOIETIC
	26375	ACROFACIAL DYSOSTOSIS, POSTAXIAL TYPE
*	26409	PROGERIA, NEONATAL RAUTENSTRAUCH-WIEDEMANN TYPE
	26413	PROLIDASE DEFICIENCY
*	26415	PSEUDOACHONDROPLASTIC DYSPLASIA
	26416	PSEUDOACHONDROPLASTIC DYSPLASIA
*	26430	STEROID 17-KETOSTEROID REDUCTASE DEFICIENCY
*	26435	ALDOSTERONE RESISTANCE
*	26460	STEROID 5 ALPHA-REDUCTASE DEFICIENCY
*	26470	RICKETS, VITAMIN D-DEPENDENT, TYPE I
*	26480	PSEUDOXANTHOMA ELASTICUM
*	26490	FACTOR XI DEFICIENCY
*	26500	PTERYGIUM SYNDROME, MULTIPLE
	26550	PULMONARY VALVE, STENOSIS
	26560	NEPHROSIS, CONGENITAL
*	26570	FIBROMATOSIS, JUVENILE HYALINE
*	26580	PYKNODYSOSTOSIS
	26585	GROWTH DEFICIENCY, AFRICAN PYGMY TYPE
*	26590	PYLE DISEASE
*	26595	PYLORODUODENAL ATRESIA, HEREDITARY
*	26610	SEIZURES, VITAMIN B(6) DEPENDENCY
*	26613	ACIDEMIA, PYROGLUTAMIC
	26614	ANEMIA, HEMOLYTIC, RED CELL MEMBRANE DEFECTS
	26614	ELLIPTOCYTOSIS
*	26615	PYRUVATE CARBOXYLASE DEFICIENCY WITH LACTIC ACIDEMIA
*	26620	PYRUVATE KINASE DEFICIENCY
	26627	GINGIVAL FIBROMATOSIS-CHERUBISM-SEIZURES, RAMON TYPE
	26640	RETINAL DYSPLASIA
	26650	PHYTANIC ACID STORAGE DISEASE
*	26690	RENAL DYSPLASIA-RETINAL APLASIA, LOKEN-SENIOR TYPE
*	26700	OVERGROWTH-RENAL HAMARTOMA, PERLMAN TYPE
*	26730	RENAL TUBULAR ACIDOSIS-SENSORINEURAL DEAFNESS
	26740	RENAL-GENITAL-MIDDLE EAR ANOMALIES
*	26743	RENAL TUBULAR DYSGENESIS
*	26750	IMMUNODEFICIENCY, SEVERE COMBINED
*	26770	IMMUNODEFICIENCY, RETICULOENDOTHELIOSIS WITH EOSINOPHILIA
*	26770	LYMPHOHISTIOCYTOSIS, FAMILIAL ERYTHROPHAGOCYTIC
*	26800	RETINITIS PIGMENTOSA
	26801	RETINITIS PIGMENTOSA
	26802	RETINITIS PIGMENTOSA
	26803	RETINITIS PIGMENTOSA
	26805	RETINOPATHY-MICROCEPHALY-MENTAL RETARDATION

	27758	WAARDENBURG SYNDROMES
*	27760	SPHEROPHAKIA-BRACHYMORPHIA SYNDROME
*	27770	WERNER SYNDROME
	27772	CRANIO-CARPO-TARSAL DYSPLASIA, WHISTLING FACE TYPE
*	27790	HEPATOLENTICULAR DEGENERATION
*	27795	WINCHESTER SYNDROME
*	27800	WOLMAN DISEASE
	27810	WOLMAN DISEASE
*	27825	WRINKLY SKIN SYNDROME
*	27830	XANTHINE OXIDASE DEFICIENCY
	27840	ALBINISM, OCULOCUTANEOUS, RUFOUS TYPE
*	27870	XERODERMA PIGMENTOSUM
*	27871	XERODERMA PIGMENTOSUM
*	27872	XERODERMA PIGMENTOSUM
*	27873	XERODERMA PIGMENTOSUM
*	27874	XERODERMA PIGMENTOSUM
	27875	XERODERMA PIGMENTOSUM
*	27876	XERODERMA PIGMENTOSUM
*	27878	XERODERMA PIGMENTOSUM
*	27879	XERODERMA PIGMENTOSUM
	27880	XERODERMA PIGMENTOSUM-MENTAL RETARDATION
	27881	XERODERMA PIGMENTOSUM
*	30010	ADRENOLEUKODYSTROPHY, X-LINKED
*	30020	ADRENAL HYPOPLASIA, CONGENITAL
*	30025	ADRENOCORTICAL UNRESPONSIVENESS TO ACTH, HEREDITARY
*	30030	IMMUNODEFICIENCY, AGAMMAGLOBULINE-MIA, X-LINKED, INFANTILE
*	30040	IMMUNODEFICIENCY, X-LINKED SEVERE COMBINED
*	30050	ALBINISM, OCULAR
*	30060	FORSIUS-ERIKSSON SYNDROME
	30065	ALBINISM, OCULAR-LATE-ONSET-SENSORINEURAL DEAFNESS, X-LINKED
*	30070	ALBINISM, CUTANEOUS-DEAFNESS
	30080	PARATHYROID HORMONE RESISTANCE
*	30100	IMMUNODEFICIENCY, WISKOTT-ALDRICH TYPE
*	30105	NEPHRITIS-DEAFNESS (SENSORINEURAL), HEREDITARY TYPE
*	30110	TEETH, AMELOGENESIS IMPERFECTA
*	30110	TEETH, SNOW-CAPPED
*	30120	TEETH, AMELOGENESIS IMPERFECTA
*	30122	AMYLOIDOSIS, FAMILIAL CUTANEOUS
*	30130	ANEMIA, SIDEROBLASTIC
	30131	ANEMIA, SIDEROBLASTIC
	30141	ANENCEPHALY
*	30150	FABRY DISEASE
	30170	ANOSMIA, CONGENITAL
	30180	ANORECTAL MALFORMATIONS
	30190	BORJESON-FORSSMAN-LEHMANN SYNDROME
	30195	BRANCHIAL ARCH SYNDROME, X-LINKED
*	30220	CATARACT, CORTICAL AND NUCLEAR
	30230	CATARACT, CORTICAL AND NUCLEAR
*	30235	CATARACTS-OTO-DENTAL DEFECTS
	30238	DIGITO-PALATAL SYNDROME, STEVENSON TYPE
	30270	METACHROMATIC LEUKODYSTROPHIES
*	30280	NEUROPATHY, HEREDITARY MOTOR AND SENSORY, TYPE I
	30290	CHARCOT MARIE TOOTH DISEASE-DEAFNESS
*	30295	CHONDRODYSPLASIA PUNCTATA, X-LINKED DOMINANT TYPE
	30296	CHONDRODYSPLASIA PUNCTATA, X-LINKED DOMINANT TYPE
*	30310	CHOROIDEREMIA
	30311	CHOROIDEREMIA
	30320	CHOROIDEREMIA
	30320	RETINITIS PIGMENTOSA
	30335	X-LINKED MENTAL RETARDATION-CLASPED THUMB
*	30360	COFFIN-LOWRY SYNDROME

	30365	COLON, ATRESIA OR STENOSIS
	30370	COLOR BLINDNESS, BLUE MONOCONE-MONOCHROMATIC
*	30380	COLOR BLINDNESS, RED-GREEN DEUTAN SERIES
*	30390	COLOR BLINDNESS, RED-GREEN PROTAN SERIES
	30400	COLOR BLINDNESS, YELLOW-BLUE TRITAN
	30402	RETINA, CONE DYSTROPHY, X-LINKED
	30403	RETINA, CONE DYSTROPHY, X-LINKED
	30405	AICARDI SYNDROME
*	30410	CORPUS CALLOSUM AGENESIS
	30411	CRANIO-FRONTO-NASAL DYSPLASIA
	30412	OTO-PALATO-DIGITAL SYNDROME, II
*	30415	EHLERS-DANLOS SYNDROME
*	30415	OCCIPITAL HORN SYNDROME
	30420	CUTIS VERTICUS GYRATA
	30430	ANOSMIA, CONGENITAL
	30435	DEAFNESS-HYPOGONADISM
*	30440	DEAFNESS WITH PERILYMPHATIC GUSHER
*	30480	DIABETES INSIPIDUS, VASOPRESSIN RESISTANT TYPES I AND II
*	30490	DIABETES INSIPIDIS, NEUROHYPOPHYSEAL TYPE
*	30500	DYSKERATOSIS CONGENITA
	30505	DEAFNESS (SENSORINEURAL)-DYSTONIA
*	30510	ECTODERMAL DYSPLASIA, CHRIST-SIEMENS-TOURAINE TYPE
*	30520	EHLERS-DANLOS SYNDROME
*	30530	VENTRICLE, ENDOCARDIAL FIBROELASTOSIS OF LEFT VENTRICLE
*	30540	AARSKOG SYNDROME
*	30545	FG SYNDROME, OPITZ-KAVEGGIA TYPE
*	30560	DERMAL HYPOPLASIA, FOCAL
*	30560	VENTRICLE, ENDOCARDIAL FIBROELASTOSIS OF RIGHT VENTRICLE
*	30562	FRONTOMETAPHYSEAL DYSPLASIA
	30570	GERM CELL APLASIA
*	30590	GLUCOSE-6-PHOSPHATE DEHYDROGENASE DEFICIENCY
*	30595	ACIDEMIA, GLUTARIC ACIDEMIA II
*	30600	GLYCOGEN STORAGE DISEASE, X-LINKED WITH NORMAL HEPATIC ENZYMES
*	30600	GLYCOGENOSIS, TYPE IXa
	30605	SIMPSON-GOLABI-BEHMEL SYNDROME
*	30610	GONADAL DYSGENESIS, XY TYPE
*	30640	GRANULOMATOUS DISEASE, CHRONIC X-LINKED
*	30670	HEMOPHILIA A
	30680	HEMOPHILIA A
*	30690	HEMOPHILIA B
*	30700	HYDROCEPHALY
*	30703	GLYCEROL KINASE DEFICIENCY
	30715	HAIR, HYPERTRICHOSIS, X-LINKED
	30740	ATAXIA-HYPOGONADISM SYNDROME
	30750	SHOVAL-SOFFER SYNDROME
*	30760	HYPOMAGNESEMIA, PRIMARY
*	30770	HYPOPARATHYROIDISM, FAMILIAL
*	30780	HYPOPHOSPHATEMIA, X-LINKED
	30781	HYPOPHOSPHATEMIA, X-LINKED
*	30800	GOUT
*	30800	LESCH-NYHAN SYNDROME
	30805	LIMB REDUCTION-ICHTHYOSIS
*	30810	ICHTHYOSIS, X-LINKED WITH STEROID SULFATASE DEFICIENCY
*	30823	IMMUNODEFICIENCY, X-LINKED WITH HYPER IgM
*	30824	IMMUNODEFICIENCY, X-LINKED LYMPHOPROLIFERATIVE DISEASE
	30828	TEETH, IMPACTED
*	30830	INCONTINENTIA PIGMENTI
*	30870	KALLMANN SYNDROME

POSSUM-NUMBER-TO-PRIME-NAME INDEX

3001 AARSKOG SYNDROME
3003 PRUNE-BELLY SYNDROME
3004 ACHONDROGENESIS, LANGER-SALDINO TYPE
3004 ACHONDROGENESIS, PARENTI-FRACCARO TYPE
3006 ACHONDROPLASIA
3007 ACROCEPHALOSYNDACTYLY TYPE I
3008 ACROCEPHALOPOLYSYNDACTYLY
3008 ACROCEPHALOSYNDACTYLY TYPE V
3010 ACROCEPHALOPOLYSYNDACTYLY
3010 ACROCEPHALOSYNDACTYLY TYPE III
3011 ACRODYSOSTOSIS
3012 ACROFACIAL DYSOSTOSIS
3013 ACRO-OSTEOLYSIS, DOMINANT TYPE
3013 HAJDU-CHENEY SYNDROME
3014 ACROMESOMELIC DYSPLASIA, CAMPAILLA-MARTINELLI TYPE
3015 ACROMESOMELIC DYSPLASIA, MAROTEAUX-MARTINELLI-CAMPAILLA TYPE
3016 ACROPECTOROVERTEBRAL DYSPLASIA
3017 CAMPTODACTYLY-TRISMUS SYNDROME
3018 AICARDI SYNDROME
3019 ARTERIO-HEPATIC DYSPLASIA
3020 ALSTROM SYNDROME
3021 AMELO-CEREBRO-HYPOHIDROTIC SYNDROME
3022 AMELO-ONYCHO-HYPOHIDROTIC SYNDROME
3023 FABRY DISEASE
3025 SCHINZEL-GIEDION SYNDROME
3026 ANUS-HAND-EAR SYNDROME
3027 ARACHNODACTYLY, CONTRACTURAL BEALS TYPE
3028 ACIDURIA, ARGININOSUCCINIC
3029 OCULO-CEREBRO-FACIAL SYNDROME, KAUFMAN TYPE
3030 ARTHRO-OPHTHALMOPATHY, HEREDITARY, PROGRESSIVE, STICKLER TYPE
3030 ARTHRO-OPHTHALMOPATHY, WEISSENBACHER-ZWEYMULLER VARIANT
3031 BLEPHAROCHALASIS-DOUBLE LIP-NONTOXIC GOITER
3032 ASPHYXIATING THORACIC DYSPLASIA
3033 ATAXIA-TELANGIECTASIA
3035 AURICULO-OSTEODYSPLASIA
3036 BECKWITH-WIEDEMANN SYNDROME
3038 DEAFNESS-PILI TORTI, BJORNSTAD TYPE
3039 BLEPHARO-NASO-FACIAL SYNDROME
3040 BLOOM SYNDROME
3041 HYPERHIDROSIS-PREMATURE GREYING-PREMOLAR APLASIA
3042 BRACHYDACTYLY
3043 SPHEROPHAKIA-BRACHYMORPHIA SYNDROME
3044 OCULO-OSTEO-CUTANEOUS SYNDROME, TOUMAALA-HAAPANEN TYPE
3045 CRANIODIAPHYSEAL DYSPLASIA, LENZ-MAJEWSKI TYPE
3046 BRANCHIO-SKELETO-GENITAL SYNDROME
3047 NASO-DIGITO-ACOUSTIC SYNDROME, KEIPERT TYPE
3048 C SYNDROME
3049 CAMPOMELIC DYSPLASIA
3051 CAMPTODACTYLY SYNDROME, TEL HASHOMER TYPE
3053 OSTEOLYSIS, CARPAL-TARSAL AND CHRONIC PROGRESSIVE GLOMERULOPATHY
3054 ACROCEPHALOPOLYSYNDACTYLY
3055 CEBEBRAL GIGANTISM
3056 CEREBRO-COSTO-MANDIBULAR SYNDROME
3057 CEREBRO-HEPATO-RENAL SYNDROME
3059 CERVICO-OCULO-ACOUSTIC SYNDROME
3060 CHEDIAK-HIGASHI SYNDROME

3061 METAPHYSEAL CHONDRODYSPLASIA, TYPE McKUSICK
3062 CHONDRODYSTROPHY-SENSORINEURAL DEAFNESS, NANCE-INSLEY TYPE
3064 CHONDRODYSPLASIA PUNCTATA, RHIZOMELIC TYPE
3064 RHIZOMELIC SYNDROME, URBACH TYPE
3065 CHONDRODYSPLASIA PUNCTATA, MILD SYMMETRIC TYPE
3066 CHONDROECTODERMAL DYSPLASIA
3067 CHROMOSOME 3, TRISOMY 3p2
3069 CHROMOSOME 4, MONOSOMY 4p
3070 CHROMOSOME 4, TRISOMY 4p
3071 CHROMOSOME 4, TRISOMY DISTAL 4q
3072 CHROMOSOME 4, MONOSOMY DISTAL 4q
3073 CHROMOSOME 5, MONOSOMY 5p
3075 CHROMOSOME 6, TRISOMY 6p2
3077 CHROMOSOME 8, TRISOMY 8
3078 CHROMOSOME 8, TRISOMY 8p
3079 CHROMOSOME 9, TRISOMY 9p
3080 CHROMOSOME 9, TRISOMY 9
3081 CHROMOSOME 9, PARTIAL MONOSOMY 9p
3083 CHROMOSOME 10, TRISOMY 10q2
3084 CHROMOSOME 10, TRISOMY 10p
3085 CHROMOSOME 10, MONOSOMY 10p
3086 TUBULAR STENOSIS
3087 CHROMOSOME 11, MONOSOMY 11q
3088 CHROMOSOME 12, PARTIAL TRISOMY 12p
3090 CHROMOSOME 13, TRISOMY 13
3091 CHROMOSOME 13, MONOSOMY 13q3
3094 CHROMOSOME 18, TRISOMY 18
3095 CHROMOSOME 18, MONOSOMY 18p
3096 CHROMOSOME 18, MONOSOMY 18q
3098 ORO-FACIO-DIGITAL SYNDROME, SUGARMAN TYPE
3099 CHROMOSOME 20, TRISOMY 20p
3100 CHROMOSOME 21, TRISOMY 21
3101 DWARFISM, PANHYPOPITUITARY
3104 TURNER SYNDROME
3105 CHROMOSOME X, POLY-X
3106 CHROMOSOME X, POLY-X
3107 KLINEFELTER SYNDROME
3112 CHROMOSOME 1, MONOSOMY 1q
3113 LAURENCE-MOON SYNDROME
3114 CHROMOSOME TRIPLOIDY
3115 CHROMOSOME TETRAPLOIDY
3118 CHROMOSOME 1, MONOSOMY 1q4
3121 ENCHONDROMATOSIS
3122 CHROMOSOME 7, MONOSOMY 7q1
3124 CHROMOSOME 12, TRISOMY 12q2
3125 CHROMOSOME 13, MONOSOMY 13q
3126 CHROMOSOME 1, TRISOMY 1q32-qter
3130 URTICARIA-DEAFNESS-AMYLOIDOSIS
3131 OSTEODYSTROPHY-MENTAL RETARDATION, RUVALCABA TYPE
3132 VELO-CARDIO-FACIAL SYNDROME
3133 BRANCHIO-OTO-RENAL DYSPLASIA
3134 LISSENCEPHALY SYNDROME
3135 PENA-SHOKEIR SYNDROME
3136 CEREBRO-OCULO-FACIO-SKELETAL SYNDROME
3137 ECTODERMAL DYSPLASIA, RAPP-HODGKIN TYPE
3138 ORO-CRANIO-DIGITAL SYNDROME
3139 CLEFT LIP/PALATE-FILIFORM FUSION OF EYELIDS
3140 CLEFT LIP/PALATE-LIP PITS OR MOUNDS
3141 CLEFT LIP/PALATE-ECTODERMAL DYSPLASIA-SYNDACTYLY
3143 ACROFACIAL DYSOSTOSIS
3143 ACROFACIAL DYSOSTOSIS, NAGER TYPE
3145 CLEFT PALATE-STAPES FIXATION-OLIGODONTIA

CDC-NUMBER-TO-PRIME-NAME INDEX

090.000	FETAL SYPHILIS SYNDROME
171.800	CANCER, EWING SARCOMA
189.000	CANCER, WILMS TUMOR
190.500	RETINOBLASTOMA
191.000	CANCER, GLIOMA, FAMILIAL
191.000	CNS NEOPLASMS
194.000	CANCER, NEUROBLASTOMA
214.800	LIPOMAS, FAMILIAL SYMMETRIC
237.700	NEUROFIBROMATOSIS
238.000	TERATOMAS
238.040	TERATOMA, SACROCOCCYGEAL TERATOMA
239.200	CYSTIC HYGROMA
239.200	NECK, BRANCHIAL CLEFT, CYSTS OR SINUSES
239.200	NECK, CYSTIC HYGROMA, FETAL TYPE
239.200	NECK/HEAD, DERMOID CYST OR TERATOMA
251.200	HYPOGLYCEMIA, FAMILIAL NEONATAL
255.200	STEROID 3 BETA-HYDROXYSTEROID DEHYDROGENASE DEFICIENCY
255.200	STEROID 11 BETA-HYDROXYLASE DEFICIENCY
255.200	STEROID 17 ALPHA-HYDROXYLASE DEFICIENCY
255.200	STEROID 17,20-DESMOLASE DEFICIENCY
255.200	STEROID 17-KETOSTEROID REDUCTASE DEFICIENCY
255.200	STEROID 18-HYDROXYLASE DEFICIENCY
255.200	STEROID 18-HYDROXYSTEROID DEHYDROGENASE DEFICIENCY
255.200	STEROID 20-22 DESMOLASE DEFICIENCY
255.200	STEROID 21-HYDROXYLASE DEFICIENCY
257.800	ANDROGEN INSENSITIVITY SYNDROME, COMPLETE
270.100	PHENYLKETONURIA
270.200	ALBINISM, CUTANEOUS
270.200	ALBINISM, OCULAR
270.200	ALBINISM, OCULAR, AUTOSOMAL RECESSIVE TYPE
270.200	ALBINISM, OCULOCUTANEOUS, BROWN TYPE
270.200	ALBINISM, OCULOCUTANEOUS, HERMANSKY-PUDLAK TYPE
270.200	ALBINISM, OCULOCUTANEOUS, MINIMAL PIGMENT TYPE
270.200	ALBINISM, OCULOCUTANEOUS, RUFOUS TYPE
270.200	ALBINISM, OCULOCUTANEOUS, TYROSINASE NEGATIVE
270.200	ALBINISM, OCULOCUTANEOUS, TYROSINASE POSITIVE
270.200	ALBINISM, OCULOCUTANEOUS, YELLOW MUTANT
270.200	ALBINISM-BLACK LOCKS-DEAFNESS
270.200	TRICHOMEGALY-RETARDATION-DWARFISM-RETINAL PIGMENTARY DEGENERATION
270.300	MAPLE SYRUP URINE DISEASE
270.600	ACIDURIA, ARGININOSUCCINIC
270.700	HYPERGLYCINEMIA, NON-KETOTIC
271.000	GLYCOGEN STORAGE DISEASE, X-LINKED WITH NORMAL HEPATIC ENZYMES
271.000	GLYCOGEN SYNTHETASE DEFICIENCY
271.000	GLYCOGENOSIS, TYPE Ia
271.000	GLYCOGENOSIS, TYPE Ib
271.000	GLYCOGENOSIS, TYPE Ic
271.000	GLYCOGENOSIS, TYPE IIa
271.000	GLYCOGENOSIS, TYPE IIb
271.000	GLYCOGENOSIS, TYPE IId
271.000	GLYCOGENOSIS, TYPE III
271.000	GLYCOGENOSIS, TYPE IV
271.000	GLYCOGENOSIS, TYPE V
271.000	GLYCOGENOSIS, TYPE VI
271.000	GLYCOGENOSIS, TYPE VII
271.000	GLYCOGENOSIS, TYPE VIII
271.000	GLYCOGENOSIS, TYPE IXa
271.000	GLYCOGENOSIS, TYPE IXb
271.000	GLYCOGENOSIS, TYPE IXc
277.000	CYSTIC FIBROSIS
277.010	CYSTIC FIBROSIS
277.400	HYPERBILIRUBINEMIA, CONJUGATED
277.400	HYPERBILIRUBINEMIA, CONJUGATED, ROTOR TYPE
277.400	HYPERBILIRUBINEMIA, TRANSIENT FAMILIAL NEONATAL
277.400	HYPERBILIRUBINEMIA, UNCONJUGATED
277.400	UDP-GLUCURONOSYLTRANSFERASE, SEVERE DEFICIENCY TYPE I
277.510	MUCOPOLYSACCHARIDOSIS I-H
277.620	ALPHA(1)-ANTITRYPSIN DEFICIENCY
277.630	CHOLINESTERASE, ATYPICAL
279.200	IMMUNODEFICIENCY, SEVERE COMBINED
279.200	IMMUNODEFICIENCY, X-LINKED SEVERE COMBINED
282.000	SPHEROCYTOSIS
282.000	TEETH, ENAMEL AND DENTIN DEFECTS FROM ERYTHROBLASTOSIS FETALIS
282.100	ELLIPTOCYTOSIS
282.200	GLUCOSE-6-PHOSPHATE DEHYDROGENASE DEFICIENCY
282.600	ANEMIA, SICKLE CELL
286.000	HEMOPHILIA A
286.000	HEMOPHILIA B
286.400	VON WILLEBRAND DISEASE
330.100	G(M1)-GANGLIOSIDOSIS, TYPE 1
330.100	G(M1)-GANGLIOSIDOSIS, TYPE 2
330.100	G(M2)-GANGLIOSIDOSIS WITH HEXOSAMINIDASE A AND B DEFICIENCY
330.100	G(M2)-GANGLIOSIDOSIS WITH HEXOSAMINIDASE A DEFICIENCY
335.000	SPINAL MUSCULAR ATROPHY
336.000	SYRINGOMYELIA
352.600	DIPLEGIA, CONGENITAL FACIAL
362.700	RETINITIS PIGMENTOSA
425.300	VENTRICLE, ENDOCARDIAL FIBROELASTOSIS OF LEFT VENTRICLE
425.300	VENTRICLE, ENDOCARDIAL FIBROELASTOSIS OF RIGHT VENTRICLE
426.705	ARRHYTHMIA, WOLFF-PARKINSON-WHITE TYPE
427.900	ARRHYTHMIA, SUPRAVENTRICULAR TACHYCARDIAS, CONGENITAL
427.900	ARRHYTHMIA, WITH LONG QT INTERVAL WITHOUT DEAFNESS
520.600	TEETH, NATAL OR NEONATAL
524.080	CLEFT PALATE-MICROGNATHIA-GLOSSOPTOSIS
550.000	HERNIA, INGUINAL
550.100	HERNIA, INGUINAL
550.900	HERNIA, INGUINAL
553.100	HERNIA, UMBILICAL
658.800	AMNIOTIC BANDS SYNDROME
740.0	ANENCEPHALY
741	MENINGOMYELOCELE
742.0	ENCEPHALOCELE
742.100	MICROCEPHALY
742.230	VERMIS AGENESIS
742.240	LISSENCEPHALY SYNDROME
742.240	WALKER-WARBURG SYNDROME
742.260	HOLOPROSENCEPHALY
742.280	BRAIN, MICROPOLYGYRIA
742.280	BRAIN, MIDLINE CAVES
742.280	BRAIN, SCHIZENCEPHALY
742.3	HYDROCEPHALY
742.320	HYDRANENCEPHALY

742.400	MEGALENCEPHALY
742.410	BRAIN, PORENCEPHALY
742.420	BRAIN, ARACHNOID CYSTS
742.480	BRAIN, ARNOLD-CHIARI MALFORMATION
742.520	DIASTEMATOMYELIA
742.580	SPINAL CORD, NEURENTERIC CYST
742.800	JAW-WINKING SYNDROME
742.810	DYSAUTONOMIA I, RILEY-DAY TYPE
743.000	EYE, ANOPHTHALMIA
743.100	EYE, MICROPHTHALMIA/COLOBOMA
743.200	GLAUCOMA, CONGENITAL
743.220	CORNEA, MEGALOCORNEA
743.300	LENS, APHAKIA
743.310	LENS, MICROSPHEROPHAKIA
743.310	SPHEROPHAKIA-BRACHYMORPHIA SYNDROME
743.325	CATARACT, POLAR AND CAPSULAR
743.326	CATARACT, AUTOSOMAL DOMINANT CONGENITAL
743.326	CATARACT, CORTICAL AND NUCLEAR
743.330	LENS, ECTOPIC
743.380	LENTICONUS
743.420	ANIRIDIA
743.430	EYE, MICROPHTHALMIA/COLOBOMA
743.440	LENS AND PUPIL, ECTOPIC
743.480	EYE, ANTERIOR SEGMENT DYSGENESIS
743.520	OPTIC DISK PITS
743.520	OPTIC DISK, MELANOCYTOMA
743.520	OPTIC DISK, MORNING GLORY ANOMALY
743.520	OPTIC DISK, TILTED
743.520	OPTIC NERVE HYPOPLASIA
743.580	EYE, VITREOUS, PERSISTENT HYPERPLASTIC PRIMARY
743.600	BLEPHAROPTOSIS-BLEPHAROPHIMOSIS-EPICANTHUS INVERSUS-TELECANTHUS
743.600	EYELID, PTOSIS, CONGENITAL
743.610	EYELID, ECTROPION, CONGENITAL
743.620	EYELID, ENTROPION
743.630	DISTICHIASIS
743.630	EYE, CRYPTOPHTHALMOS WITH OTHER MALFORMATIONS
743.630	EYELID, EPIBLEPHARON
743.635	BLEPHAROPTOSIS-BLEPHAROPHIMOSIS-EPICANTHUS INVERSUS-TELECANTHUS
743.635	EYELID, ANKYLOBLEPHARON
743.636	EYELID, COLOBOMA
743.640	LACRIMAL CANALICULUS ATRESIA
743.660	LACRIMAL GLAND, ECTOPIC
743.660	LACRIMAL SAC FISTULA
744.010	EAR, MICROTIA-ATRESIA
744.020	EAR, OSSICLE AND MIDDLE EAR MALFORMATIONS
744.030	EAR, INNER DYSPLASIAS
744.030	EAR, LABYRINTH APLASIA
744.090	DEAFNESS-EAR PITS
744.200	EAR, MACROTIA
744.230	EAR, ECTOPIC PINNA
744.230	EAR, EXCHONDROSIS
744.230	EAR, EXOSTOSES
744.230	EAR, LOBE, ABSENT
744.230	EAR, LOP
744.230	EAR, MOZART TYPE
744.230	EAR, PROMINENT ANTHELIX
744.245	EAR, LOW-SET
744.246	EAR, LONG, NARROW, POSTERIORLY ROTATED
744.250	EAR, EUSTACHIAN TUBE DEFECTS
744.280	EAR, CRYPTOTIA
744.280	EAR, DARWIN TUBERCLE
744.280	EAR, SMALL WITH FOLDED-DOWN HELIX
744.400	BRANCHIAL CLEFT CYSTS
744.900	CYSTIC HYGROMA
744.900	NECK, CYSTIC HYGROMA, FETAL TYPE
745.000	HEART, TRUNCUS ARTERIOSUS
745.010	AORTICO-PULMONARY SEPTAL DEFECT
745.1	HEART, TRANSPOSITION OF GREAT VESSELS
745.2	HEART, TETRALOGY OF FALLOT
745.4	VENTRICULAR SEPTAL DEFECT
745.5	ATRIAL SEPTAL DEFECTS
745.6	HEART, ENDOCARDIAL CUSHION DEFECTS
746.000	PULMONARY VALVE, ATRESIA
746.010	PULMONARY VALVE, STENOSIS
746.020	PULMONARY VALVE, INCOMPETENCE
746.080	PULMONARY VALVE, BICUSPID
746.080	PULMONARY VALVE, TETRACUSPID
746.100	TRICUSPID VALVE, ATRESIA
746.100	TRICUSPID VALVE, STENOSIS
746.105	TRICUSPID VALVE, INSUFFICIENCY
746.200	TRICUSPID VALVE, EBSTEIN ANOMALY
746.300	AORTIC VALVE STENOSIS
746.400	AORTIC VALVE, BICUSPID
746.480	AORTIC VALVE ATRESIA
746.500	MITRAL VALVE STENOSIS
746.505	MITRAL VALVE ATRESIA
746.600	MITRAL VALVE INSUFFICIENCY
746.800	DEXTROCARDIA-BRONCHIECTASIS-SINUSITIS SYNDROME
746.820	HEART, COR TRIATRIATUM
746.850	HEART, PERICARDIUM AGENESIS
746.870	ARRHYTHMIA, HEART BLOCK, CONGENITAL COMPLETE
746.880	ARRHYTHMIA, CARDIAC CONDUCTION DEFECTS, NEONATAL
746.880	ARRHYTHMIA, FROM MATERNAL AUTOIMMUNE DISEASE, CONGENITAL
746.880	HEART, CORDIS ECTOPIA
746.885	ARTERY, CORONARY, ARTERIOVENOUS FISTULA
747.000	DUCTUS ARTERIOSUS, PATENT
747.1	AORTA, COARCTATION
747.1	AORTA, COARCTATION, INFANTILE TYPE
747.215	AORTIC ARCH INTERRUPTION
747.220	AORTIC STENOSIS, SUPRAVALVAR
747.230	AORTIC ARCH, RIGHT
747.240	AORTIC SINUS OF VALSALVA, ANEURYSM
747.250	AORTIC ARCH, DOUBLE
747.290	AORTICO-LEFT VENTRICULAR TUNNEL
747.380	PULMONARY ARTERY, COARCTATION
747.380	PULMONARY ARTERY, ORIGIN FROM ASCENDING AORTA
747.380	PULMONARY ARTERY, ORIGIN FROM DUCTUS ARTERIOSUS
747.380	PULMONARY ARTERY, ORIGIN OF THE LEFT FROM RIGHT PULMONARY ARTERY
747.410	VENA CAVA, PERSISTENT LEFT SUPERIOR JOINED TO CORONARY SINUS
747.420	PULMONARY VENOUS CONNECTION, TOTAL ANOMALOUS
747.480	LIVER, VENOUS ANOMALIES
747.480	VENA CAVA, ABSENT HEPATIC SEGMENT
747.500	UMBILICAL CORD, SINGLE ARTERY
747.610	ARTERY, RENAL FIBROMUSCULAR DYSPLASIA
747.680	PULMONARY HYPERTENSION, PRIMARY
747.800	CNS ARTERIOVENOUS MALFORMATION
748.000	NOSE, ANTERIOR ATRESIA
748.000	NOSE, ANTERIOR STENOSIS
748.000	NOSE, POSTERIOR ATRESIA
748.110	NOSE, DUPLICATION
748.120	NOSE, BIFID
748.180	NOSE, GLIOMA
748.180	NOSE, GRANULOSIS RUBRA NASI
748.180	NOSE, NASOPHARYNGEAL STENOSIS
748.180	NOSE, TRANSVERSE GROOVE
748.180	NOSE, TURBINATE DEFORMITY
748.185	NOSE, PROBOSCIS LATERALIS
748.2	LARYNX, WEB
748.300	LARYNGOCELE
748.300	LARYNGOMALACIA
748.300	LARYNX, ATRESIA

748.300	LARYNX, VENTRICLE PROLAPSE
748.320	TRACHEOMALACIA
748.350	BRONCHIAL ATRESIA
748.380	LARYNX, CYSTS
748.385	LARYNGO-TRACHEO-ESOPHAGEAL CLEFT
748.390	LARYNGO-TRACHEO-ESOPHAGEAL CLEFT
748.480	LUNG, BRONCHOGENIC CYST
748.520	LUNG, LOBE SEQUESTRATION
748.580	LUNG, CONGENITAL LOBAR ADENOMATOSIS
748.580	LUNG, EMPHYSEMA CONGENITAL LOBAR
748.690	LUNG, ABERRANT LOBE
749.0	CLEFT PALATE
749.080	UVULA, CLEFT
749.1	CLEFT LIP
749.190	CLEFTS, LOWER MEDIAN LIP, MANDIBLE AND TONGUE
749.2	CLEFT LIP
750.000	TONGUE, ANKYLOGLOSSIA
750.110	HYPOGLOSSIA-HYPODACTYLIA
750.120	MACROGLOSSIA
750.140	CLEFTS, LOWER MEDIAN LIP, MANDIBLE AND TONGUE
750.140	TONGUE, CLEFT
750.180	TONGUE, FISSURED
750.180	TONGUE, FOLDING OR ROLLING
750.180	TONGUE, GEOGRAPHIC
750.180	TONGUE, PIGMENTED PAPILLAE
750.180	TONGUE, PLICATED
750.210	PALATOPHARYNGEAL INCOMPETENCE
750.230	SALIVARY GLAND, AGENESIS
750.260	LIP, PITS OR MOUNDS
750.270	LIP, CHEILITIS GLANDULARIS
750.270	LIP, DOUBLE
750.280	MANDIBLE, TORUS MANDIBULARIS
750.3	TRACHEOESOPHAGEAL FISTULA
750.300	ESOPHAGUS, ATRESIA
750.310	ESOPHAGUS, ATRESIA AND TRACHEOESOPH-AGEAL FISTULA
750.340	ESOPHAGUS, STENOSIS
750.420	ESOPHAGUS, DIVERTICULUM
750.430	ESOPHAGUS, DUPLICATION
750.480	ESOPHAGUS, ACHALASIA
750.480	ESOPHAGUS, CHALASIA
750.510	PYLORIC STENOSIS
750.600	HERNIA, HIATAL
750.740	STOMACH, DIVERTICULUM
750.750	STOMACH, DUPLICATION
750.780	STOMACH, HYPOPLASIA
750.780	STOMACH, PYLORIC ATRESIA
750.780	STOMACH, TERATOMA
751.000	OMPHALOMESENTERIC DUCT ANOMALIES
751.010	MECKEL DIVERTICULUM
751.1	INTESTINAL ATRESIA OR STENOSIS
751.100	INTESTINAL ATRESIAS, MULTIPLE
751.100	PYLORODUODENAL ATRESIA, HEREDITARY
751.190	JEJUNAL ATRESIA
751.230	ANORECTAL MALFORMATIONS
751.240	ANORECTAL MALFORMATIONS
751.3	COLON, AGANGLIONOSIS
751.490	INTESTINAL ROTATION, INCOMPLETE
751.600	LIVER, AGENESIS
751.610	HEPATIC FIBROSIS, CONGENITAL
751.610	LIVER, CYST, SOLITARY
751.610	LIVER, POLYCYSTIC AND MULTICYSTIC DISEASE, ADULT TYPE
751.620	LIVER, ACCESSORY LOBE
751.620	LIVER, ARTERIAL ANOMALIES
751.620	LIVER, HAMARTOMA
751.620	LIVER, HEMANGIOMATOSIS
751.620	LIVER, TRANSPOSITION
751.630	GALLBLADDER, AGENESIS
751.640	GALLBLADDER, ANOMALIES
751.650	BILIARY ATRESIA

751.660	BILE DUCT CHOLEDOCHAL CYST
751.720	PANCREAS, ANNULAR
751.780	PANCREATITIS, HEREDITARY
751.810	INTESTINAL DUPLICATION
751.880	INFLAMMATORY BOWEL DISEASE
751.880	INTESTINAL ENTEROKINASE DEFICIENCY
751.880	INTESTINAL HYPOPERISTALSIS, MEGACYSTIS-MICROCOLON TYPE
751.880	INTESTINAL LYMPHANGIECTASIA
751.880	INTESTINAL POLYPOSIS, JUVENILE TYPE
751.880	INTESTINAL PSEUDO-OBSTRUCTION SYNDROMES
751.880	JAUNDICE, INTRAHEPATIC CHOLESTATIC, BYLER TYPE
752.380	VAGINAL SEPTUM, TRANSVERSE
752.410	VAGINAL ATRESIA
752.430	HYMEN, IMPERFORATE
752.600	HYPERTELORISM-HYPOSPADIAS SYNDROME
752.600	HYPOSPADIAS
752.610	EPISPADIAS
752.700	HERMAPHRODITISM, TRUE
752.710	GONADAL DYSGENESIS, XY TYPE
752.720	GONADAL DYSGENESIS, XX TYPE
752.800	ANORCHIA
752.860	DIPHALLIA
753.000	RENAL AGENESIS, BILATERAL
753.010	RENAL AGENESIS, UNILATERAL
753.110	KIDNEY, POLYCYSTIC DISEASE, RECESSIVE
753.120	KIDNEY, POLYCYSTIC DISEASE, DOMINANT
753.140	KIDNEY, NEPHRONOPHTHISIS-MEDULLARY CYSTIC DISEASE
753.150	KIDNEY, MEDULLARY SPONGE KIDNEY
753.150	KIDNEY, NEPHRONOPHTHISIS-MEDULLARY CYSTIC DISEASE
753.320	KIDNEY, HORSESHOE
753.500	BLADDER EXSTROPHY
753.600	URETHRAL VALVES, POSTERIOR
753.880	VESICO-URETERAL REFLUX
754.020	NOSE, DISLOCATED NASAL SEPTUM
754.050	PLAGIOCEPHALY
754.070	TRIGONENCEPHALY, AUTOSOMAL DOMINANT TYPE
754.200	SPINE, SCOLIOSIS, IDIOPATHIC
754.300	HIP, CONGENITAL DISLOCATED
754.430	KNEE, GENU RECURVATUM
754.500	FOOT, TALIPES EQUINOVARUS (TEV)
754.520	FOOT, METATARSUS VARUS
754.735	FOOT, VERTICAL TALUS
754.800	PECTUS CARINATUM
754.810	PECTUS EXCAVATUM
754.820	PENTALOGY OF CANTRELL
754.840	HAND, RADIAL CLUB HAND
754.880	HAND, LOCKING DIGITS-GROWTH DEFECT
754.880	HAND, ULNAR DRIFT
755.0	ECTRODACTYLY-POLYDACTYLY
755.0	POLYDACTYLY
755.1	SYNDACTYLY
755.2	LIMB REDUCTION-ICHTHYOSIS
755.2	LIMB, UPPER HYPOPLASIA-MULLERIAN DUCT DEFECTS
755.250	ECTRODACTYLY
755.250	ECTRODACTYLY-POLYDACTYLY
755.250	TIBIAL HYPOPLASIA/APLASIA-ECTRODACTYLY
755.280	RADIAL DEFECTS
755.350	ECTRODACTYLY
755.350	TIBIAL HYPOPLASIA/APLASIA-ECTRODACTYLY
755.365	TIBIAL APLASIA/HYPOPLASIA
755.365	TIBIAL HYPOPLASIA/APLASIA-ECTRODACTYLY
755.380	FEMORAL HYPOPLASIA-UNUSUAL FACIES SYNDROME
755.440	HAND, ULNAR AND FIBULAR RAY DEFICIENCY, WEYERS TYPE
755.500	CAMPTODACTYLY
755.500	THUMB, ADDUCTED THUMB SYNDROME

755.500 THUMB, CLASPED
755.500 THUMB, TRIPHALANGEAL
755.500 THUMB, TRIPHALANGEAL-DUPLICATED GREAT
        TOES
755.510 DIGITO-TALAR DYSMORPHISM
755.510 HAND, ULNAR AND FIBULAR RAY DEFICIENCY,
        WEYERS TYPE
755.536 RADIAL-ULNAR SYNOSTOSIS
755.555 CLEIDOCRANIAL DYSPLASIA
755.555 PARIETAL FORAMINA-CLAVICULAR HYPOPLASIA
755.555 YUNIS-VARON SYNDROME
755.556 SPRENGEL DEFORMITY
755.616 FOOT, VERTICAL TALUS
755.660 HIP, CONGENITAL COXA VARA
755.660 HIP, DYSPLASIA, NAMAQUALAND TYPE
755.800 ARTHROGRYPOSES
755.800 ARTHROGRYPOSIS, AMYOPLASIA TYPE
755.800 ARTHROGRYPOSIS, DISTAL TYPES
755.810 LARSEN SYNDROME
755.810 LARSEN SYNDROME, LETHAL TYPE
756.000 CRANIOSYNOSTOSIS
756.030 CRANIOSYNOSTOSIS, KLEEBLATTSCHADEL TYPE
756.040 CRANIOFACIAL DYSOSTOSIS
756.040 CRANIOFACIAL DYSOSTOSIS-DIAPHYSEAL
        HYPERPLASIA
756.045 MANDIBULOFACIAL DYSOSTOSIS
756.045 MANDIBULOFACIAL DYSOSTOSIS, TREACHER
        COLLINS TYPE, RECESSIVE
756.046 OCULO-MANDIBULO-FACIAL SYNDROME
756.055 ACROCEPHALOSYNDACTYLY TYPE I
756.056 ACROCEPHALOSYNDACTYLY TYPE III
756.057 ACROCEPHALOSYNDACTYLY TYPE V
756.057 CRANIOSYNOSTOSIS-FOOT DEFECTS,
        JACKSON-WEISS TYPE
756.060 OCULO-AURICULO-VERTEBRAL ANOMALY
756.080 LIMB AND SCALP DEFECTS, ADAMS-OLIVER TYPE
756.085 EYE, HYPERTELORISM
756.085 HYPERTELORISM-HYPOSPADIAS SYNDROME
756.110 KLIPPEL-FEIL ANOMALY
756.130 SPINE, SPONDYLOLISTHESIS AND
        SPONDYLOLYSIS
756.170 SACROCOCCYGEAL DYSGENESIS SYNDROME
756.400 ASPHYXIATING THORACIC DYSPLASIA
756.410 ENCHONDROMATOSIS
756.420 ENCHONDROMATOSIS AND HEMANGIOMAS
756.430 ACHONDROPLASIA
756.445 DIASTROPHIC DYSPLASIA
756.446 METATROPIC DYSPLASIA
756.447 THANATOPHORIC DYSPLASIA
756.450 METAPHYSEAL CHONDRODYSPLASIA WITH
        THYMOLYMPHOPENIA
756.450 METAPHYSEAL CHONDRODYSPLASIA, TYPE
        JANSEN
756.450 METAPHYSEAL CHONDRODYSPLASIA, TYPE
        McKUSICK
756.450 METAPHYSEAL CHONDRODYSPLASIA, TYPE
        SCHMID
756.450 METAPHYSEAL DYSPLASIA-MAXILLARY
        HYPOPLASIA-BRACHYDACTYLY
756.460 SPONDYLOEPIPHYSEAL DYSPLASIA CONGENITA
756.460 SPONDYLOEPIPHYSEAL DYSPLASIA, LATE
756.470 EXOSTOSES, MULTIPLE CARTILAGINOUS
756.470 EXOSTOSES-ANETODERMIA-BRACHYDACTYLY
        TYPE E
756.480 CRANIODIAPHYSEAL DYSPLASIA,
        LENZ-MAJEWSKI TYPE
756.480 SKELETAL BOWING-CORTICAL THICKENING-
        BONE FRAGILITY-ICTHYOSIS
756.480 SKELETAL DYSPLASIA, 3-M TYPE
756.480 SKELETAL DYSPLASIA, DE LA CHAPELLE TYPE
756.480 SKELETAL DYSPLASIA, FUHRMANN TYPE
756.480 SKELETAL DYSPLASIA, SCHNECKENBECKEN TYPE

756.480 SKELETAL DYSPLASIA, WEISMANN-NETTER-
        STUHL TYPE
756.500 OSTEOGENESIS IMPERFECTA
756.510 FIBROUS DYSPLASIA, POLYOSTOTIC
756.520 CHONDROECTODERMAL DYSPLASIA
756.525 CHONDROECTODERMAL DYSPLASIA
756.530 CORTICAL HYPEROSTOSIS, INFANTILE
756.540 OSTEOPETROSIS, BENIGN DOMINANT
756.540 OSTEOPETROSIS, MALIGNANT RECESSIVE
756.540 OSTEOPETROSIS, MILD RECESSIVE
756.550 DIAPHYSEAL DYSPLASIA
756.560 OSTEOPOIKILOSIS
756.570 EPIPHYSEAL DYSPLASIA, MULTIPLE
756.570 EPIPHYSEAL DYSPLASIA, MULTIPLE RIBBING TYPE
756.570 EPIPHYSEAL DYSPLASIA, MULTIPLE, RECESSIVE
        TARDA TYPE
756.575 CHONDRODYSPLASIA PUNCTATA, MILD
        SYMMETRIC TYPE
756.575 CHONDRODYSPLASIA PUNCTATA, RHIZOMELIC
        TYPE
756.580 OSTEOCHONDRODYSPLASIA WITH
        HYPERTRICHOSIS
756.580 OSTEODYSPLASTY
756.580 OSTEOECTASIA
756.580 OSTEOFIBROUS DYSPLASIA OF TIBIA AND FIBULA
756.580 OSTEOGLOPHONIC DYSPLASIA
756.580 OSTEOLYSIS, CARPAL-TARSAL AND CHRONIC
        PROGRESSIVE GLOMERULOPATHY
756.580 OSTEOLYSIS, ESSENTIAL
756.580 OSTEOLYSIS, RECESSIVE CARPAL-TARSAL
756.580 OSTEOMESOPYKNOSIS
756.580 OSTEOPATHIA STRIATA
756.580 OSTEOPATHIA STRIATA-CRANIAL
        SCLEROSIS-MEGALENCEPHALY
756.580 OSTEOPOROSIS, JUVENILE IDIOPATHIC
756.580 OSTEOPOROSIS-PSEUDOGLIOMA SYNDROME
756.610 DIAPHRAGMATIC HERNIA
756.620 DIAPHRAGM, EVENTRATION
756.700 OMPHALOCELE
756.710 GASTROSCHISIS
756.720 PRUNE-BELLY SYNDROME
756.800 POLAND SYNDROME
756.830 NAIL-PATELLA SYNDROME
756.850 EHLERS-DANLOS SYNDROME
756.860 TORTICOLLIS
756.880 MYOPATHY OR CARDIOMYOPATHY DUE TO
        DESMIN DEFECT
756.880 MYOPATHY, CENTRAL CORE DISEASE TYPE
756.880 MYOPATHY, DISPROPORTIONATE FIBER TYPE I
756.880 MYOPATHY, FAMILIAL LYSIS OF TYPE I FIBERS
756.880 MYOPATHY, MALIGNANT HYPERTHERMIA
756.880 MYOPATHY, MITOCHONDRIAL-
        ENCEPHALOPATHY-LACTIC ACIDOSIS-STROKE
756.880 MYOPATHY, MYOGLOBINURIA-ABNORMAL
        GLYCOLOSIS, HEREDITARY TYPE
756.880 MYOPATHY, MYOTUBULAR
756.880 MYOPATHY, NEMALINE
756.880 MYOPATHY, SARCOTUBULAR
756.880 MYOPATHY-CATARACT-GONADAL DYSGENESIS
756.880 MYOPATHY-METABOLIC, CARNITINE
        DEFICIENCY, PRIMARY AND SECONDARY
756.880 MYOPATHY-METABOLIC, CARNITINE PALMITYL
        TRANSFERASE DEFICIENCY
756.880 MYOPATHY-METABOLIC, GLYCOPROTEIN-
        GLYCOSAMINOGLYCANS STORAGE TYPE
756.880 MYOPATHY-METABOLIC, MITOCHONDRIAL
        CYTOCHROME C OXIDASE DEFICIENCY
756.880 MYOPATHY-METABOLIC, MYOADENYLATE
        DEAMINASE DEFICIENCY
757.000 LYMPHEDEMA I
757.000 LYMPHEDEMA II
757.100 ICHTHYOSIS, HARLEQUIN FETUS
757.120 SJOGREN-LARSSON SYNDROME

757.190   GIROUX-BARBEAU SYNDROME
757.190   ICHTHYOSIFORM HYPERKERATOSIS, BULLOUS
          CONGENITAL
757.190   ICHTHYOSIS HYSTRIX, CURTH-MACKLIN TYPE
757.190   ICHTHYOSIS, CONGENITAL ERYTHRODERMIC
757.190   ICHTHYOSIS, LAMELLAR DOMINANT
757.190   ICHTHYOSIS, LAMELLAR RECESSIVE
757.190   ICHTHYOSIS, LINEARIS CIRCUMFLEXA
757.190   SKIN, ERYTHROKERATODERMIA, PROGRESSIVA
          SYMMETRICA
757.190   SKIN, ERYTHROKERATODERMIA, VARIABLE
757.190   SKIN, ERYTHROKERATOLYSIS HIEMALIS
757.195   ICHTHYOSIS VULGARIS
757.197   ICHTHYOSIFORM ERYTHROKERATODERMA,
          ATYPICAL WITH DEAFNESS
757.330   EPIDERMOLYSIS BULLOSUM, TYPE I
757.330   EPIDERMOLYSIS BULLOSUM, TYPE II
757.330   EPIDERMOLYSIS BULLOSUM, TYPE III
757.340   BERLIN SYNDROME
757.340   ECTODERMAL DYSPLASIA, BASAN TYPE
757.340   ECTODERMAL DYSPLASIA, CHRIST-SIEMENS-
          TOURAINE TYPE
757.340   ECTODERMAL DYSPLASIA, HIDROTIC
757.346   ECTODERMAL DYSPLASIA, CONGENITAL FACIAL,
          SETLEIS TYPE
757.346   ECTODERMAL DYSPLASIA, HAY-WELLS TYPE
757.346   ECTODERMAL DYSPLASIA-ADRENAL CYST
757.350   INCONTINENTIA PIGMENTI
757.360   XERODERMA PIGMENTOSUM
757.360   XERODERMA PIGMENTOSUM-MENTAL
          RETARDATION
757.370   CUTIS LAXA
757.380   NEVUS FLAMMEUS
757.380   NEVUS OF OTA
757.380   NEVUS, BLUE RUBBER BLEB NEVUS SYNDROME
757.380   NEVUS, CONGENITAL NEVOMELANOCYTIC
757.380   NEVUS, EPIDERMAL NEVUS SYNDROME
757.390   CUTIS MARMORATA
757.395   SKIN, LOCALIZED ABSENCE OF
757.400   HAIR, ALOPECIA AREATA
757.400   HAIR, ATRICHIA CONGENITA
757.410   HAIR, MONILETHRIX
757.450   HAIR, HYPERTRICHOSIS, LANUGINOSA
757.450   HAIR, HYPERTRICHOSIS, X-LINKED
757.480   HAIR, BALDNESS, COMMON
757.500   NAILS, ANONYCHIA, HEREDITARY
757.516   NAILS, PACHYONYCHIA CONGENITA
757.520   NAILS, KOILONYCHIA
757.530   NAILS, LEUKONYCHIA
757.600   BREAST, AMASTIA
757.650   BREAST, POLYTHELIA
757.680   GYNECOMASTIA DUE TO INCREASED
          AROMATASE ACTIVITY, FAMILIAL
757.900   DARIER DISEASE
757.900   ECTODERMAL DYSPLASIA, NAEGELI TYPE
757.900   SKIN PEELING SYNDROME
757.900   SKIN TUMORS, MULTIPLE GLOMUS
757.900   SKIN, ACANTHOSIS NIGRICANS
757.900   SKIN, CUTANEOUS MELANOSIS, DIFFUSE
757.900   SKIN, ELASTOSIS PERFORANS SERPIGINOSA
757.900   SKIN, HYPERKERATOSIS, FOCAL PALMOPLANTAR
          AND GINGIVAL
757.900   SKIN, HYPERPIGMENTATION, FAMILIAL
757.900   SKIN, KERATOSIS FOLLICULARIS SPINULOSA
          DECALVANS
757.900   SKIN, KYRLE DISEASE
757.900   SKIN, LEIOMYOMAS, MULTIPLE
757.900   SKIN, LIPOID PROTEINOSIS
757.900   SKIN, PAINFUL PLANTAR CALLOSITIES
757.900   SKIN, PALMO-PLANTAR ERYTHEMA
757.900   SKIN, PITYRIASIS RUBRA PILARIS
757.900   SKIN, POROKERATOSIS
757.900   SKIN, PSORIASIS VULGARIS

757.900   SKIN, VITILIGO
758.0   CHROMOSOME 21, TRISOMY 21
758.1   CHROMOSOME 13, TRISOMY 13
758.2   CHROMOSOME 18, TRISOMY 18
758.300   CHROMOSOME 21, MONOSOMY 21
758.310   CHROMOSOME 5, MONOSOMY 5p
758.320   CHROMOSOME 4, MONOSOMY 4p
758.330   CHROMOSOME 13, MONOSOMY 13q
758.340   CHROMOSOME 18, MONOSOMY 18q
758.350   CHROMOSOME 18, MONOSOMY 18p
758.500   CHROMOSOME 8, TRISOMY 8
758.520   CHROMOSOME 22, TRISOMY MOSAICISM
758.585   CHROMOSOME TETRAPLOIDY
758.586   CHROMOSOME TRIPLOIDY
758.600   TURNER SYNDROME
758.610   TURNER SYNDROME
758.7   KLINEFELTER SYNDROME
758.800   CHROMOSOME MOSAICISM, 45,X/46,XY TYPE
758.990   BRANCHIO-OCULO-FACIAL SYNDROME
758.990   CHROMOSOME 1, MONOSOMY 1q
758.990   CHROMOSOME 1, MONOSOMY 1q4
758.990   CHROMOSOME 1, TRISOMY 1q25-1q32
758.990   CHROMOSOME 1, TRISOMY 1q32-qter
758.990   CHROMOSOME 2, MONOSOMY OF MEDIAL 2q
758.990   CHROMOSOME 2, PARTIAL TRISOMY 2p
758.990   CHROMOSOME 2, TRISOMY DISTAL 2q
758.990   CHROMOSOME 3, MONOSOMY 3p2
758.990   CHROMOSOME 3, TRISOMY 3p2
758.990   CHROMOSOME 3, TRISOMY 3q2
758.990   CHROMOSOME 4, MONOSOMY DISTAL 4q
758.990   CHROMOSOME 4, RING 4
758.990   CHROMOSOME 4, TRISOMY 4p
758.990   CHROMOSOME 4, TRISOMY DISTAL 4q
758.990   CHROMOSOME 5, MONOSOMY 5q INTERSTITIAL
758.990   CHROMOSOME 5, TRISOMY 5p
758.990   CHROMOSOME 5, TRISOMY 5q3
758.990   CHROMOSOME 6, MONOSOMY DISTAL 6q
758.990   CHROMOSOME 6, MONOSOMY PROXIMAL 6q
758.990   CHROMOSOME 6, RING 6
758.990   CHROMOSOME 6, TRISOMY 6p2
758.990   CHROMOSOME 6, TRISOMY 6q2
758.990   CHROMOSOME 7, MONOSOMY 7p2
758.990   CHROMOSOME 7, MONOSOMY 7q1
758.990   CHROMOSOME 7, MONOSOMY 7q2
758.990   CHROMOSOME 7, MONOSOMY 7q3
758.990   CHROMOSOME 7, MOSAIC TRISOMY 7
758.990   CHROMOSOME 7, TRISOMY 7p2
758.990   CHROMOSOME 7, TRISOMY 7q2-3
758.990   CHROMOSOME 8, MONOSOMY 8p2
758.990   CHROMOSOME 8, TRISOMY 8p
758.990   CHROMOSOME 9, PARTIAL MONOSOMY 9p
758.990   CHROMOSOME 9, RING 9
758.990   CHROMOSOME 9, TETRASOMY 9p
758.990   CHROMOSOME 9, TRISOMY 9
758.990   CHROMOSOME 9, TRISOMY 9p
758.990   CHROMOSOME 9, TRISOMY 9q3
758.990   CHROMOSOME 10, MONOSOMY 10p
758.990   CHROMOSOME 10, MONOSOMY 10q2
758.990   CHROMOSOME 10, TRISOMY 10p
758.990   CHROMOSOME 10, TRISOMY 10q2
758.990   CHROMOSOME 11, MONOSOMY 11q
758.990   CHROMOSOME 11, PARTIAL MONOSOMY 11p
758.990   CHROMOSOME 11, PARTIAL TRISOMY 11q
758.990   CHROMOSOME 11, TRISOMY 11p
758.990   CHROMOSOME 12, MONOSOMY 12p
758.990   CHROMOSOME 12, PARTIAL TRISOMY 12p
758.990   CHROMOSOME 12, TRISOMY 12q2
758.990   CHROMOSOME 13, MONOSOMY 13q3
758.990   CHROMOSOME 13, TRISOMY 13q1
758.990   CHROMOSOME 13, TRISOMY DISTAL 13q
758.990   CHROMOSOME 14, MONOSOMY 14q (q24.3-q32.1)
758.990   CHROMOSOME 14, PARTIAL TRISOMY 14q
758.990   CHROMOSOME 14, RING 14

758.990 CHROMOSOME 14, TRISOMY 14 MOSAIC
758.990 CHROMOSOME 14, TRISOMY 14q
758.990 CHROMOSOME 15, PARTIAL TRISOMY DISTAL 15q
758.990 CHROMOSOME 15, RING 15
758.990 CHROMOSOME 15, TRISOMY 15q1
758.990 CHROMOSOME 16, MONOSOMY 16q
758.990 CHROMOSOME 16, TRISOMY 16p
758.990 CHROMOSOME 16, TRISOMY 16q
758.990 CHROMOSOME 17, INTERSTITIAL DELETION 17p
758.990 CHROMOSOME 17, TRISOMY 17q2
758.990 CHROMOSOME 18, RING 18
758.990 CHROMOSOME 18, TETRASOMY 18p
758.990 CHROMOSOME 18, TRISOMY 18p AND q11
758.990 CHROMOSOME 18, TRISOMY 18q2
758.990 CHROMOSOME 19, TRISOMY 19q
758.990 CHROMOSOME 20, PERICENTRIC INVERSION
758.990 CHROMOSOME 20, TRISOMY 20p
758.990 CHROMOSOME 21, RING 21
758.990 CHROMOSOME 22, MONOSOMY 22
758.990 CHROMOSOME 22, MONOSOMY 22q
758.990 CHROMOSOME 22, RING 22
758.990 CHROMOSOME 22, SUPERNUMERARY DER 22, T(11:22)
758.990 CHROMOSOME INSTABILITY, NIJMEGEN TYPE
758.990 CHROMOSOME X, POLY-X
758.990 CHROMOSOME X, TRIPLO-X
758.990 CHROMOSOME XYY
758.990 CHROMOSOME, NUCLEOLAR ORGANIZER REGION, TRANSLOCATION
758.990 CHROMOSOMES, COMPLEX REARRANGEMENTS
759.000 ASPLENIA SYNDROME
759.010 SPLEEN, CONGENITAL ISOLATED HYPOSPLENIA
759.080 SPLEEN, CYSTS
759.110 ADRENAL HYPOPLASIA, CONGENITAL
759.210 THYROID, DYSGENESIS
759.220 THYROGLOSSAL DUCT REMNANT
759.3   SITUS INVERSUS VISCERUM
759.4   TWINS, CONJOINED
759.500 TUBEROUS SCLEROSIS
759.600 INTESTINAL POLYPOSIS, TYPE II
759.610 STURGE-WEBER SYNDROME
759.620 VON HIPPEL-LINDAU SYNDROME
759.630 INTESTINAL POLYPOSIS, TYPE III
759.800 CRANIO-CARPO-TARSAL DYSPLASIA, WHISTLING FACE TYPE

759.800 NOONAN SYNDROME
759.800 ORO-FACIO-DIGITAL SYNDROME I
759.800 ORO-FACIO-DIGITAL SYNDROME, BARAITSER-BURN TYPE
759.800 ORO-FACIO-DIGITAL SYNDROME, MOHR TYPE
759.800 ORO-FACIO-DIGITAL SYNDROME, THURSTON TYPE
759.800 ORO-FACIO-DIGITAL SYNDROME, WHELAN TYPE
759.800 WAARDENBURG SYNDROMES
759.820 BARDET-BIEDL SYNDROME
759.820 COCKAYNE SYNDROME
759.820 COCKAYNE SYNDROME, TYPE II
759.820 DE LANGE SYNDROME
759.820 LAURENCE-MOON SYNDROME
759.820 SECKEL SYNDROME
759.820 SILVER SYNDROME
759.820 SILVER SYNDROME, X-LINKED
759.820 SMITH-LEMLI-OPITZ SYNDROME
759.820 SMITH-LEMLI-OPITZ SYNDROME, TYPE II
759.840 ANGIO-OSTEOHYPERTROPHY SYNDROME
759.840 HEART-HAND SYNDROME
759.840 RUBINSTEIN-TAYBI BROAD THUMB-HALLUX SYNDROME
759.840 THROMBOCYTOPENIA-ABSENT RADIUS
759.860 ARTHRO-OPHTHALMOPATHY, HEREDITARY, PROGRESSIVE, STICKLER TYPE
759.860 MARFAN SYNDROME
759.870 BECKWITH-WIEDEMANN SYNDROME
759.870 CEREBRO-COSTO-MANDIBULAR SYNDROME
759.870 CEREBRO-HEPATO-RENAL SYNDROME
759.870 INTESTINAL ILEUS, ISOLATED MECONIUM ILEUS
759.870 LEPRECHAUNISM
759.870 MENKES SYNDROME
759.870 NEPHRITIS-DEAFNESS (SENSORINEURAL), HEREDITARY TYPE
759.870 PRADER-WILLI SYNDROME
759.890 HEMIHYPERTROPHY
759.890 MECKEL SYNDROME
760.710 FETAL ALCOHOL SYNDROME
760.750 FETAL HYDANTOIN SYNDROME
771.090 FETAL RUBELLA SYNDROME
771.210 FETAL CYTOMEGALOVIRUS SYNDROME
771.210 FETAL TOXOPLASMOSIS SYNDROME

ILLUSTRATION CREDITS BY PUBLISHER₁

Academic Press
New chromosome syndromes, 1977:245-272, 21498

Acta Geneticae Medical et Gemellologiae
1970:19:421-424, 20475

American Journal of Diseases of Children
1976, 10715
1966:112:79-81, 10758
1972:123:254-258, 11008
1972:123:254-258, 11009
1964:107:49, 12236
1964:107:49, 12237
1964:107:49, 12249
1964:107:49, 12250
1964:107:49, 12254
1964:107:49, 12257
1984:138:821, 20175
1984:138:821, 20176
1984:138:821, 20177
1984:138:821, 20178
1984:138:821, 20179
1984:138:821, 20180
1974:127:408-409, 20577
1974:127:408-409, 20578
1976:130:1244, 21499
1974:127:408-409, 20579
1975:129:360-362, 21123
1987:141:1021-1024, 21158
1981:135:729-731, 21161
1970:120:255-257, 21165
1970:120:255-257, 21166
1970:120:255-257, 21167
1980:134:285-289, 21174
1971:122:443, 21328

American Journal of Human Genetics
1972:24:189-213, 21507
1975:27:521-527, 20419
1980:32:714-722, 21224
1980:32:714-722, 21225
1981:33:455, 21416
1981:33:455, 21417
1981:33:455, 21418
1972:24:189-213, 21497
1972:24:189-213, 21501
1972:24:189-213, 21502
1972:24:189-213, 21506

American Journal of Medical Genetics
1987:27:943-952, 20050
1987:27:943-952, 20051
1983:14:335-346, 20066
1983:14:335-346, 20067
1983:14:335-346, 20068
1983:14:335-346, 20069
1983:14:335-346, 20070
1987:26:207-215, 20298
1987:26:207-215, 20299
1987:26:207-215, 20300
1987:26:207-215, 20301
1984:18:781-788, 20305
1984:18:781-788, 20306
1982:11:329-336, 20363
1982:11:329-336, 20364
1978:1:291-299, 20391
1978:1:291-299, 20392
1978:1:291-299, 20393
1978:1:291-299, 20394
1978:1:291-299, 20395
1986:25:29-39, 20406
1986:25:29-39, 20407
1986:25:29-39, 20408
1986:25:29-39, 20409
1983:15:29-38, 20418
1984:18:671, 20458

1984:18:671, 20459
1984:18:671, 20460
1984:18:671, 20461
1985:21:137-142, 20462
1985:21:137-142, 20463
1986:25:1-8, 20464
1986:25:1-8, 20465
1985:22:311-314, 20466
1985:22:311-314, 20467
1985:431-439, 20477
1985:431-439, 20478
1985:431-439, 20479
1980:5:179-188, 20508
1985:22:243-253, 20515
1985:22:243-253, 20516
1984:19:653-664, 20519
1984:19:653-664, 20520
1985:20:597-606, 20539
1984:19:487-499, 20554
1984:19:487-499, 20555
1987:26:217-220, 20559
1986:25:537-541, 20562
1986:25:537-541, 20563
1983:16:213-224, 20584
1984:17:809-826, 20585
1980:7:75-83, 20588
1985:22:685, 20593
1985:22:685, 20594
1982:12:327-331, 20626
1986:25:467-471, 20680
1986:25:467-471, 20681
1985:21:697-705, 20682
1985:21:697-705, 20683
1983:14:225-229, 20685
1983:14:225-229, 20686
1983:14:225-229, 20688
1983:14:225-229, 20689
1985:20:283-294, 20866
1985:20:283-294, 20867
1985:20:283-294, 20870
1985:20:283-294, 20872
1987:27:661-667, 20898
1987:27:661-667, 20899
1987:27:661-667, 20900
1985:21:669-680, 20938
1985:21:669-680, 20939
1985:21:669-680, 20940
1985:21:669-680, 20941
1985:21:669-680, 20942
1984:19:307, 20970
1984:19:307, 20971
1987:28:297-302, 20990
1982:11:185-239, 22125
1987:28:297-302, 20991
1980:7:91-102, 21000
1980:7:91-102, 21001
1987:26:13-15, 21019
1987:26:13-15, 21020
1987:26:13-15, 21021
1985:22:501-512, 21040
1985:22:531-543, 21042
1985:22:531-543, 21043
1985:22:531-543, 21044
1985:22:531-543, 21045
1986:SUP2:53-63, 21050
1986:SUP2:53-63, 21051
1985:21:569-574, 21066
1984:19:161-169, 21073
1982:11:185-239, 21124
1982:11:383-395, 21280
1982:11:383-395, 21281
1982:11:383-395, 21282
1982:11:383-395, 21283
1983:14:335-346, 21314
1983:14:335-346, 21316

1. The illustration number, in numeric order, as it appears in the text, follows the Publisher citation.

1983:14:335-346, 21317
1983:14:335-346, 21318
1983:14:335-346, 21323
1985:20:325-339, 21329
1985:20:325-339, 21330
1986:2:53-63, 21369
1986:2:53-63, 21370
1987:28:303-309, 21373
1987:28:303-309, 21374
1979:3:269-279, 21375
1979:3:65-80, 21386
1979:3:65-80, 21387
1979:3:65-80, 21388
1979:3:65-80, 21389
1979:3:65-80, 21390
1979:3:65-80, 21391
1985:21:417-432, 21393
1985:21:417-432, 21394
1985:21:417-432, 21396
1985:21:417-432, 21397
1983:14:501-511, 21411
1983:14:501-511, 21412
1983:14:501-511, 21413
1983:14:501-511, 21414
1987:26:207-215, 21421
1987:26:207-215, 21422
1985:20:159-163, 21423
1985:20:159-163, 21424
1985:20:159-163, 21425
1984:19:487, 21426
1984:19:369-377, 21431
1984:19:369-377, 21432
1981:9:139-146, 21445
1981:9:139-146, 21446
1981:9:139-146, 21447
1981:9:139-146, 21448
1988:29:573-579, 21450
1988:29:573-579, 21451
1984:17:133-144, 21480
1989:32:461-467, 21481
1989:32:461-467, 21482
1989:32:461-467, 21483

American Journal of Medicine
1973:54:793-800, 21234
1973:54:793-800, 21235
1973:54:793-800, 21236

American Journal of Ophthalmology
1988:105:40-45, 21272

American Journal of Physical Anthropology
1976:45:109-116, 20266

Annales de Genetique
1978:21:247-251, 21340
1979:22:165-167, 20514

Annals of Internal Medicine
1987:106:538-545, 20405
1976:84:393-397, 11311
1976:84:393-397, 11313
1976:84:393-397, 11315
1976:84:393, 11317
1976:84:393, 11319
1976:84:393, 11321
1987:106:538-545, 20404

Annals of Otology, Rhinology & Laryngology
1979:88:100-104, 21067

Applied Neurophysiology
1963:23:1, 10218

Archives of Dermatology
1966:93:194-201, 21263
1970:101:699, 10295

Archives of Ophthalmology
1986:104:61-64, 21159
1986:104:61-64, 21160

Archives of Otolaryngology
1973:98:124-128, 21011

Birth Defects Original Article Series
1974:10:41-50, 10675
1974:10:41-50, 10676
1974:10:41-50, 10677
1974:10:167-170, 10709
1974:10:22, 10902
1974:10:22, 10903
1974:10:22, 10904
1974:10:23, 10905
1974:10:23, 10906
1974:10:23, 10907
1976:12:309, 10908
1974:10:337, 10910
1974:10:25, 10911
1974:10:25, 10912
1974:10:25, 10913
1974:10:337, 10914
1974:10:337, 10915
1974:10:216, 10922
1974:10:216, 10923
1977:13:53-67, 20547
1977:13:53-67, 20548
1977:13:53-67, 20549
1977:13:53-67, 20552
1977:13:53-67, 20553
1976:12:275-278, 20571
1977:13:167, 21454
1976:12:275-278, 20572
1978:14:287-78, 21187
1978:14:287-78, 21188
1978:14:287-78, 21189
1969:5:79-95, 21194
1969:5:79-95, 21195
1969:5:79-95, 21196
1969:5:79-95, 21197
1969:5:79-95, 21198
1969:5:79-95, 21199
1975:11:30-33, 21294
1975:11:30-33, 21295
1975:11:30-33, 21296
1975:11:30-33, 21297
1975:11:30-33, 21298
1975:11:30-33, 21299
1977:13:167, 21452
1977:13:167, 21453

Bulletin of the Johns Hopkins Hospital
1964:114:402-411, 10711

Charles C. Thomas
10108

Clinical Genetics
1974:5:294, 10714
1976:16:1-18, 21368
1974:5:1, 10798
1984:25:68-72, 20154
1983:24:140-146, 20272
1983:24:140-146, 20273
1983:24:140-146, 20274
1985:27:414, 20346
1985:27:414, 20347
1981:19:321-330, 20480
1981:19:321-330, 20481
1981:19:321-330, 20482
1981:19:321-330, 20483
1981:19:321-330, 20484
1980:17:209-212, 20509
1985:28:251-254, 20513
1984:26:308-317, 20526
1984:26:308-317, 20527
1984:26:308-317, 20528
1987:32:28-34, 21076
1987:32:28-34, 21077
1987:32:28-34, 21078
1981:19:23-25, 21079
1981:19:23-25, 21080
1978:14:251-256, 21081
1978:14:251-256, 21082
1974:5:363-367, 21089
1974:5:363-367, 21090
1980:18:413-416, 21149
1980:18:413-416, 21150

1981:20:1-5, 21153
1981:20:1-5, 21154
1974:5:127-132, 21155
1974:5:127-132, 21156
1976:10:319-324, 21164
1976:10:319-324, 21168
1976:10:319-324, 21169
1976:10:319-324, 21170
1984:25:422-448, 21171
1984:25:422-448, 21172
1983:23:376-379, 21218
1986:29:83-87, 21237
1981:19:202-206, 21334
1981:19:202-206, 21335
1976:16:1-18, 21362
1976:16:1-18, 21363
1976:16:1-18, 21364
1976:16:1-18, 21365
1976:16:1-18, 21366
1976:16:1-18, 21367

Dental Clinics of North America
1975:19:1-27, 10613
1975:19:1-27, 10610
1975:19:1-27, 10611
1975:19:1-27, 10612

Dermatologica
1982:164:293-304, 20064
1982:164:293-304, 20065

Dysmorphology and Clinical Genetics
1987:1:17-20, 20188
1987:1:17-20, 20189
1987:1:17-20, 20190
1987:1:142-144, 20586
1987:1:142-144, 20587
1988:2:104-108, 20601
1988:2:104-108, 20602
1988:2:104-108, 20603
1984:2(4):29-30, 20794
1984:2(4):29-30, 20795
1989:3, 21456
1989:3, 21457
21458
21459
21460
1989:3:103-107, 21461
1989:3:103-107, 21462
1989:3:103-107, 21463
1989:3:103-107, 21464
1989:3:103-107, 21465
1989:3:103-107, 21466
1989:3:28-32, 21471
1989:3:28-32, 21474
1989:3:28-32, 21475
1989:3:28-32, 21478
1989:3:28-32, 21479
1989:4:97-102, 21515
1989:4:97-102, 21516
1989:4:97-102, 21517
1990:4, 21518
1990:4, 21519
1989:3:61-64, 21525

Editions Medecine et Hygiene
1969:17:45-52, 21064
1969:17:45-52, 21063

European Journal of Pediatrics
1982:138:301-303, 20072
1979:130:65, 20582
1979:130:65, 20583

Helvetica Paediatrica Acta
1980:35:243-251, 21293
1980:35:243-251, 21289
1980:35:243-251, 21290
1980:35:243-251, 21291
1980:35:243-251, 21292

Human Genetics
1985:69:243-245, 20161
1985:69:243-245, 20162
1976:31:219-225, 20403

1980:56:231-234, 20510
1978:40:231-234, 20511
1977:36:243-247, 20512
1981:57:210-213, 21157
1978:40:311-324, 21240
1978:40:311-324, 21241
1978:40:311-324, 21243
1978:40:311-324, 21244
1978:40:311-324, 21247
1979:50:241-246, 21249
1979:47:233-237, 21338
1979:47:233-237, 21339
1979:48:151-156, 21384
1979:48:151-156, 21385

Humangenetik
1975:29:233-241, 21343
1973:19:341-343, 21173
1975:29:233-241, 21341
1975:29:233-241, 21342

Internationale Stiftung Mozarteum
21442

Journal of Bone and Joint Surgery
1975:57:542, 10716
1972:54:509, 21217
1975:57:542, 10717
1976:58B:343-346, 21083
1976:58B:343-346, 21084
1976:58B:343-346, 21085
1976:58B:343-346, 21086

Journal of Clinical Dysmorphology
1985:3:2-9, 20252

Journal of Medical Genetics
1970:7:11-19, 10345
1985:22:46-53, 20311
1985:22:46-53, 20313
1985:22:46-53, 20315
1985:22:46-53, 20316
1986:32:355-359, 20675
1986:32:355-359, 20676
1974:11:287-291, 20873
1974:11:287-291, 20874
1983:20:277, 20959
1983:20:277, 20960
1973:42:428-434, 21288
1983:20:277, 20961
1985:22:36-38, 21054
1987:24:204-206, 21069
1987:24:204-206, 21070
1987:24:204-206, 21071
1987:24:9-13, 21091
1987:24:9-13, 21092
1987:24:9-13, 21093
1988:25:157-163, 21175
1988:25:157-163, 21176
1981:18:129-133, 21250
1981:18:129-133, 21251
1981:18:129-133, 21252
1985:22:78-80, 21253
1985:22:78-80, 21254
1977:14:144-147, 21255
1977:14:144-147, 21256

Journal of Neurosurgical Sciences
1983:59:215-228, 20308
1983:59:215-228, 20309
1983:58:89-102, 21126
1983:59:215-228, 20310

Journal of Pediatric Ophthalmology and Strabismus
1988:25:93-98, 20591

Journal of Pediatrics
1960:56:778, 10737
1960:56:778, 10738
1960:56:778, 10739
1960:56:778, 10740
1960:56:778, 10741
1975:86:388, 21470
1960:56:778, 10742
1970:77:856, 20977

1975:87:280-284, 20999
1987:110:747-750, 21145
1987:110:747-750, 21146
1981:98:92-95, 21148
1971:79:450-455, 21151
1971:79:450-455, 21152
1969:74:755-762, 21158
1969:74:755-762, 21159
1969:74:755-762, 21160
1969:74:755-762, 21164
1986:109:469-475, 21344
1986:109:469-475, 21345
1986:109:469-475, 21346
1986:109:469-475, 21347
1986:109:469-475, 21348
1986:109:469-475, 21349
1986:109:469-475, 21350
1986:109:469-475, 21355
1986:109:469-475, 21356

Klinische Paediatrie
1973:185:181-186, 21062
1973:185:181-186, 21061

Lea & Febiger
Nyhan, WL: Diagnostic recognition, 1987:126, 20183
Nyhan, WL: Diagnostic recognition, 1987:142, 20184
Diagnosis and treatment 2nd ed., 1984, 21127

Minerva Pediatrica
1967:19:2187, 10444

Neurology
1967:17:961, 12228
1967:17:961, 12229
1967:17:961, 12230
1967:17:961, 12231
1967:17:961, 12232
1967:17:961, 12233

Neuropediatrics
1980:11:291-297, 20350

New England Journal of Medicine
1986:314:1542-1546, 21131
1986:314:1542-1546, 21130

Oral Surgery
1964:17:683-690, 10592
1964:18:409-418, 10603
1964:18:409-418, 10604

Pediatric Clinics of North America
1986:33:1277-1297, 21143
1986:33:1277-1297, 21144

Pediatric Dentistry
1985:7:326-328, 20281
1985:7:326-328, 20282

Pediatric Radiology
1981:10:155-160, 20580
1981:10:155-160, 20581
1980:10:46-50, 21219
1980:10:46-50, 21220
1980:10:46-50, 21221

Pediatrics
1971:48:756-765, 10340
1971:48:756-765, 10341
1971:48:756-765, 10342
1971:47:610-612, 21142
1971:48:756-765, 10343
1978:61:12-15, 21136
1978:61:12-15, 21139
1978:61:12-15, 21140

Pergamon Press
1961, 10123

Plastic and Reconstructive Surgery
1971:48:542-500, 10543
1971:48:542-500, 10544
1971:48:542-500, 10545

Postgraduate Medical Journal
1977:53:507-515, 21222

Radiology
1970:95:129-134, 20862
1970:95:129-134, 20863
1970:95:129-134, 20864
1970:95:129-134, 20865

South African Medical Journal
1979:21:659-665, 21087
1979:21:659-665, 21088
1979:21:659-665, 21223

Springer-Verlag
Wackenheim, A: Cheirolumbar dysostosis, 1980, 20331
Wackenheim, A: Cheirolumbar dysostosis, 1980, 20332
Wackenheim, A: Cheirolumbar dysostosis, 1980, 20333
Wackenheim, A: Cheirolumbar dysostosis, 1980, 20334
Wackenheim, A: Cheirolumbar dysostosis, 1980, 20335
Wackenheim, A: Cheirolumbar dysostosis, 1980, 20336
Wackenheim, A: Cheirolumbar dysostosis, 1980, 20337
Wackenheim, A: Cheirolumbar dysostosis, 1980, 20338
Wackenheim, A: Cheirolumbar dysostosis, 1980, 20339
Wackenheim, A: Cheirolumbar dysostosis, 1980, 20340
Wackenheim, A: Cheirolumbar dysostosis, 1980, 20341
Wackenheim, A: Cheirolumbar dysostosis, 1980, 20342
Wackenheim, A: Cheirolumbar dysostosis, 1980, 20343

St. Justine Clinic of Medical Genetics
10374

Surgery in Gynecology and Obstetrics
1958:107:602-614, 20677
1958:107:602-614, 20678
1958:107:602-614, 20679

Syndrome Identification
1977:5:14-18, 20052
1977:5:14-18, 20053
1977:5:14-18, 20054
1977:5:14-18, 20055
1977:5:14-18, 20056
1987:26:551-556, 20564
1987:26:551-556, 20565

University of Minnesota Dermatology
10307

W.B. Saunders
Smith, DW: Recognizable patterns of human malformation, 1982:228., 20279
Smith, DW: Recognizable patterns of human malformation, 1982:228, 20280
Smith, DW: Recognizable patterns of human malformation, 3rd Ed., 1982:439, 20518
Smith, DW: Recognizable patterns of human malformation, 3rd ed., 1982:439, 20521
Smith, DW: Recognizable patterns of human malformation, 4th ed., 1988:605, 20573
Smith, DW: Recognizable patterns of human malformation, 4th ed., 1988:605, 20574

Year Book Medical Publishers
Current Problems in Surgery, 1966, 10370
Current Problems in Surgery, 1966, 10371

Z Kinderheilkd
1975:120:1, 20558
1968:102:1-4, 20448
1968:102:1-4, 20449
1968:102:1-4, 20450
1968:102:1-4, 20451
1968:102:1-4, 20452
1968:102:1-4, 20453
1975:120:231, 20556

ILLUSTRATION CREDITS BY CONTRIBUTOR

Dagfinn Aarskog
20350, 20418, 20977, 20978, 20979

Louise C. Abbott
10613

Albert M. Abrams
10610, 10611, 10612

Kirk Aleck
20445, 20447

Judith Allanson
21091, 21092, 21093

Rudolph Angermuller
21442

Holly Hutchison Ardinger
20518, 20519, 20520, 20521

Joan F. Atkin
20682, 20683

Gerald D. Aurbach
11269, 11271, 11272

Biagio Azzarelli
20929

Michael Baraitser
21002, 21003, 21006, 21007, 21009, 21010

Amin Y. Barakat
20700

Bruce J. Bart
10239, 10240, 10314, 11386, 11421

Christos S. Bartsocas
10479

Harold N. Bass
21398, 21400, 21401

J. Bronwyn Bateman
20016, 20842, 21273, 21274, 21275, 21276, 21277

Arthur L. Beaudet
10718, 10719, 21470

Frits A. Beemer
20344, 20345

Peter Beighton
10716, 10717, 11311, 11313, 11315, 11317, 11319, 11321, 11640, 11646, 20522, 20523, 20526, 20527, 20528, 21073, 21079, 21080, 21081, 21082, 21083, 21084, 21085, 21086, 21087, 21088, 21089, 21090, 21201, 21207, 21210, 21211, 21214, 21215, 21217, 21218, 21219, 21220, 21221, 21222, 21223

Renee Bernstein
20311, 20313, 20315, 20316

Diana W. Bianchi
20222, 21313

Josette W. Bianchine
10649, 10995

David Bixler
10160, 10162, 10163, 10636, 21014

F. Owen Black
21011

Will Blackburn
20235, 20236, 20237, 20238, 20239, 20240, 20241, 20242, 20243

E.M. Bleeker-Wagemakers
20156, 20157, 20158, 20159

Zvi Borochowitz
20001, 20002, 20003, 20071, 20082, 20468, 20604, 21402, 21403, 21443

Sylvia S. Bottomley
20614, 20615, 20616

Jack Brown
21263

Kenneth S. Brown
20628

W. Ted Brown
20595, 20596, 20597

Merlin G. Butler
20601, 20602, 20603

Mary Louise Buyse
10383, 10573

Jose-Maria Cantu
20161, 20162, 20163, 20508, 20510, 20513, 20514, 21031, 21032, 21033

J. Aidan Carney
20225

Nancy J. Carpenter
20215, 20216

Anthony C. Casamassima
20096, 20097

Florence Char
20701, 20702, 20704, 20705, 20706, 20707, 20710, 20711, 20712, 20713, 20715, 20716, 20717, 20719, 20720, 20721, 20722, 20723, 20724, 20725, 20726, 20729, 20730, 20731, 20734, 20735, 20737, 20738, 20739, 20740, 20741, 20742, 20744, 20745, 20746, 20747, 20748, 20749, 20750, 20752, 20755, 20756, 20757, 20759, 20763, 20764, 20765, 20766, 20768, 20769, 20770, 20771, 20772, 20773, 20774, 20775, 20776, 20779, 20780, 20783, 20784, 20786, 20788, 20790, 20791, 20792, 20793, 20794, 20795

Harold Chen
20195, 20196, 20584, 20585, 21000, 21001, 21038, 21039, 21405, 21406, 21407, 21408, 21409, 21410, 21411, 21412, 21413, 21414

Albert E. Chudley
21013

Robin Dawn Clark
21019, 21020, 21021

Sterling K. Clarren
20588, 21143, 21144, 21147, 21148

David Cogan
10220

M. Michael Cohen
10008, 10032, 10044, 10045, 10046, 10047, 10048, 10093, 10094, 10095, 10096, 10097, 10098, 10143, 10144, 10145, 10216, 10229, 10242, 10243, 10251, 10253, 10254, 10435, 10436, 10437, 10438, 10439, 10440, 10441, 10528, 10529, 10530, 10531, 10532, 10582, 10583, 10614, 10673, 10674, 10793, 10794, 10795, 10796, 10797, 10916, 10917, 10928, 10930, 10931, 10932, 10949, 10951, 11131, 11132, 11149, 11150, 11151, 11307, 11309, 12204, 12205

David E.C. Cole
20014, 20015

J. Michael Connor
20515, 20516

Kenneth L. Garver
21162, 21163, 21164, 21168, 21169, 21170

Mark C. Gebhardt
20569

Ekkart Genee
21063, 21064

James German
21116

Ronald E. Gier
10120, 10121, 10122

Enid F. Gilbert-Barness
20485, 20486, 20487

Mitchell S. Golbus
21288

Morton F. Goldberg
10402, 10403, 10627, 10640, 10646

Donald Goldsmith
20488, 20489

Stanley Goldstein
20866, 20867, 20870, 20872

Thomaz Rafael Gollop
20685, 20686, 20688, 20689, 20692, 20693, 20694, 20695

Richard M. Goodman
10868, 10869, 10873, 10874, 20328, 20329, 20476

Hymie Gordon
10302, 10304, 10306

Robert J. Gorlin
10119, 10133, 10135, 10136, 10148, 10149, 10321, 10322, 10323, 10324, 10325, 10326, 10358, 10427, 10430, 10737, 10738, 10739, 10740, 10741, 10742, 12271, 20898, 20899, 20900, 20975, 20976, 21194, 21195, 21196, 21197, 21198, 21199

John M. Graham
21050, 21051, 21369, 21370

Frank Greenberg
20293, 20294, 20295, 20296, 20297

Fahed Halal
20100, 20101, 20102, 20103, 20104, 20106, 20107, 20108, 20109, 20122, 20123, 20124, 20128

Bryan D. Hall
10099, 10101, 10102, 10150, 10659, 21174, 21187, 21188, 21189

Judith G. Hall
11360, 11361, 11362, 21123, 21124, 21126, 22125

Carol Haynes
20517

Jurgen Herrmann
10009, 10675, 10676, 10677, 10709, 10744, 10746, 10747, 10748, 10749, 10822, 10824, 10839, 10840

Riitta Herva
20477, 20478, 20479, 20480, 20481, 20482, 20483, 20484

Reba Michels Hill
20599, 20600

Richard Hoefnagel
10408, 10620, 10787, 11200, 11202, 11204

Georg Hoffmann
20181, 20182

Thomas M. Holder
10370, 10371

Lewis B. Holmes
10726

George R. Honig
20164

H. Eugene Hoyme
20980, 20981, 20982

Alasdair G.W. Hunter
21240, 21241, 21243, 21244, 21247, 21278, 21279, 21280, 21281, 21282, 21283, 21375

Victor Ionasescu
20013, 20305, 20306, 20308, 20309, 20310

Harry Israel
20173, 20174

Elizabeth J. Ives
12270

Ian Jeffries
20875

Jan E. Jirasek
10382

John P. Johnson
20083, 20613

Virginia P. Johnson
20593, 20594, 20607, 20608, 20609, 20610, 20611, 20612

Ronald J. Jorgenson
10030, 10155, 10245, 10247, 10274, 10276, 10514, 10572, 10593, 10597, 10598, 10609, 10617, 10920, 10967, 11057, 11089, 11103, 11104

Ronald J. Jorgenson
20396, 20397, 20399, 20401, 20402

Ronald J. Jorgenson
20540, 20541, 20542

Richard C. Juberg
10130, 21155, 21156, 21157, 21158, 21159, 21160, 21164, 21224, 21225, 21226, 21416, 21417, 21418

Stephen G. Kahler
20667, 20668, 20669

Stephen G. Kaler
20244, 20245, 20246, 21518, 21519

Raymond S. Kandt
20351

James R. Kasser
20884, 20885, 20886

Donald Kaufman
21097

Robert L. Kaufman
10257, 10259, 10260, 10979, 10980, 10982

Harris J. Keene
10592

Thaddeus E. Kelly
10922, 10923

Nancy G. Kennaway
20201

Kenneth R. Kenyon
11073

Yukio Kitano
20698, 20699

Jane Kivlin
20589, 21159, 21160

Steven E. Kopits
11257, 11261

Boris G. Kousseff
20017, 20018, 20026, 20030, 20042, 20043, 20044, 20045, 20046, 20047, 20048, 20049, 20197, 20198, 20199, 20200, 20410, 20411, 20412, 20413, 20416, 21255, 21256, 21303, 21304, 21305, 21306, 21307, 21308, 21309

K.S. Kozlowski
20577, 20578, 20579, 20580, 20581

Celeste M. Krauss
20210, 20211, 20212, 21423, 21424, 21425

Dhavendra Kumar
20154

Jurgen Kunze
20072, 20996, 20997, 20998

A. Kurtz
20627

Michael Edison Labhard
20169, 20170, 20171, 20172

Roger L. Ladda
21132, 21133, 21134, 21136, 21139, 21140, 21185, 21186

Charlotte Z. Lafer
20490, 20491, 20492

Leonard O. Langer
21113, 21114, 21115

Lawrence G. Leichtman
20188, 20189, 20190

Richard Alan Lewis
20637, 20638, 20639, 20640, 20896

Raymond M. Lewkonia
21072

Richard Lindenberg
20930, 20931, 20932

R.B. Lowry
11026, 11027, 21012, 21040, 21042, 21043, 21044, 21045

Herbert A. Lubs
21068, 21480

Russell V. Lucas
12156, 12167, 12187, 12191, 12192, 12193, 12194, 12195

Philip M. Marden
10758

Pierre Maroteaux
20284, 20285, 20286, 20287, 20647, 20648, 20649, 20650, 20651, 20652, 20653, 20654, 21022, 21023, 21024, 21025, 21026, 21027

John T. Martsolf
20052, 20053, 20054, 20055, 20056, 20391, 20392, 20393, 20394, 20395

Victor A. McKusick
10123, 10207, 10238, 10261, 10262, 10292, 10296, 10297, 10298, 10308, 10320, 10344, 10359, 10389, 10390, 10411, 10452, 10480, 10481, 10489, 10490, 10492, 10493, 10498, 10505, 10506, 10507, 10508, 10509, 10515, 10650, 10651, 10656, 10657, 10722, 10724, 10752, 10806, 10809, 10810, 10828, 10844, 10845, 10846, 10851, 10852, 10864, 10865, 10881, 10886, 10887, 10888, 10889, 10890, 10891, 10892, 10893, 10894, 10895, 10897, 10908, 10918, 10936, 10953, 10954, 10955, 10956, 10957, 10978, 11003, 11013, 11028, 11029, 11031, 11032, 11038, 11040, 11041, 11044, 11045, 11046, 11047, 11049, 11052, 11053, 11054, 11070, 11071, 11085, 11086, 11087, 11088, 11090, 11153, 11154, 11155, 11181, 11250, 11251, 11253, 11255, 11267, 11268, 11278, 11281, 11326, 21270

Peter Meinecke
21065, 21300, 21301, 21302, 21433, 21434, 21435, 21461, 21462, 21463, 21464, 21465, 21466, 21525

Heirie M.M. Mendez
20220, 20221

Paul Merlob
21253, 21254

David F. Merten
20213, 20214

Lawrence H. Meskin
10546

Louise Brearley Messer
10605, 10606

Virginia V. Michels
20110, 20252

Joyce A. Mitchell
21268

Cynthia A. Moore
21035

Merle E. Morris
12158, 12159

Gabriel Mortimer
20493, 20494

John E. Murphy
20403

Charles M. Myer
20943, 20945, 20948, 20949, 20950, 20951, 20953, 20954, 20955, 20956, 20958

George Nager
10131, 10132

Samir S. Najjar
20207

Giovanni Neri
20057, 20058, 20529, 20530, 21373, 21374

Richard Neu
21142

Gerhard Neuhauser
20556, 20558

Buford L. Nichols
10725, 11082

Pat Nichols
20111, 20112, 20117, 20119

Norio Niikawa
20217, 20531

Sirkka-Liisa Noponen
20477, 20478, 20479, 20480, 20481, 20482, 20483, 20484

James J. Nora
12139

Fiorella Nuzzo
20665, 20666

William L. Nyhan
12169, 20183, 20184

John M. Opitz
10763, 10764, 10765, 10814, 11331, 12211, 12224, 12225, 21431, 21432

B.A. Paes
21471, 21474, 21475, 21478, 21479

Philip D. Pallister
10782, 10783, 10784, 20881, 20882, 20883

Michael W. Partington
20454

Sharon G. Paryani
21130, 21131

Eberhard Passarge
10626, 11352

Michael A. Patton
20298, 20299, 20300, 20301, 21421, 21422

Sergio D.J. Pena
20902

Rudolf A. Pfeiffer
21177, 21178, 21182

Marta Pinheiro
20359, 20360, 20361, 20362, 20367, 20368, 20369, 20375, 20376, 20377, 20378, 20379, 20380, 20381, 20386, 20387, 20388

Leonard Pinsky
21098, 21099, 21100

Andrew E. Poole
20247, 20248, 20250, 20251

Andrew K. Poznanski
10151, 10152, 10153, 20862, 20863, 20864, 20865

Marilyn Preus
10705, 10706, 10714, 10715, 21171, 21172

Zvonimir Puretic
20008, 20009, 20010

David T. Purtilo
20404, 20405

Qutub H. Qazi
20061, 21165, 21166, 21167

Mark M. Ravitch
20677, 20678, 20679

Salomon H. Reisner
10134

J. Marc Rhoads
21484

Arthur R. Rhodes
20205, 20206

David L. Rimoin
10316, 10319, 10332, 10333, 10334, 10348, 10350, 10351, 10472, 10473, 10474, 10939, 10940, 10941, 10942, 10988, 10989, 10990, 10991, 10992, 10993, 11266

Richard M. Roberts
20670, 20671, 20672, 20673, 20674

Meinhard Robinow
10467, 10477, 10478, 10801, 10803, 11058, 11060, 11762, 20175, 20176, 20177, 20178, 20179, 20180, 20228, 20590, 21104, 21105, 21106, 21266, 21267, 21445, 21446, 21447, 21448, 21450, 21451

Luther K. Robinson
20455, 20456

Karol Rondou
20031, 20032, 20033, 20038, 20039, 20040, 20041, 20078, 20079, 20080, 20081, 20091, 20092, 20093, 20094, 20095, 20470, 20471, 20472, 20473, 20562, 20563, 20564, 20565, 20566, 20567, 20850, 20851, 20852, 20853, 20854, 20855, 20907, 20908, 20909, 20910, 20911, 20912, 20913, 20914, 20915, 20917, 20918, 20919, 20920, 20921, 20922, 20923, 20924, 20925, 20926, 20928, 21046, 21047, 21048, 21049

Allen Root
20253, 20254, 20255, 20256

Jack H. Rubinstein
11107, 11108, 11109, 11110

Carlos Ruiz
20330

R.H.A. Ruvalcaba
21149, 21150, 21151, 21152, 21153, 21154

George H. Sack
20938, 20939, 20940, 20941, 20942

Carlos F. Salinas
21521, 21522, 21523, 21524

Riitta Salonen
20458, 20459, 20460, 20461

Jose Sanchez-Corona
20509

Burhan Say
20675, 20676, 21173

R. Neil Schimke
10625, 10750, 10757, 11221, 20876, 20877

Albert A.G.L. Schinzel
20132, 20133, 20134, 20135, 21286, 21287, 21289, 21290, 21291, 21292, 21293

Jerry A. Schneider
20532

C. Ronald Scott
21018

Charles I. Scott
10157, 10158, 10159, 11010, 11012, 11093, 11094, 11098, 11350, 11351

John H. Seashore
21527

Robert E. Sharkey
10118, 10365, 10366, 10381, 11296, 12311

L.J. Sheffield
20168

Robert J. Shprintzen
20139, 20140, 20141, 20142, 20143, 20144, 20145, 20146, 20147, 20148, 20149, 20150, 20151, 20152, 20153

M. Cirillo Silengo
20321, 20322, 20323

Henry K. Silver
12236, 12237, 12249, 12250, 12254, 12257

Dharmdeo N. Singh
20664

William S. Sly
11099, 11100

Ann C.M. Smith
20992, 20993, 20994

Morton E. Smith
20887, 20888

John Stuart Soeldner
21249

Lawrence Solomon
20223, 20224

Annemarie Sommer
21075

Mark A. Sperling
10337, 10338, 10339, 10340, 10341, 10342, 10343, 21392

Jurgen W. Spranger
10455, 10457, 10458, 10459, 10902, 10903, 10904, 10905, 10906, 10907, 10911, 10912, 10913, 11023, 11024, 11025, 11340, 11341, 11342, 21426

Roger E. Stevenson
20191, 20192, 20985, 20986, 20987, 21102, 21103, 21109, 21110, 21111, 21262

Hartmut Stoess
20661, 20662, 20663

Claude Stoll
20165, 20166, 20167, 20431, 20433, 20434, 20435, 20438, 20439, 20440, 20598

Charles Strom
20559

Gerald I. Sugarman
10910, 10914, 10915

Robert Suskind
10295

Kutay Taysi
20086, 20087

A.S. Teebi
21054, 21056, 21057, 21058, 21059

Helga Toriello
20462, 20463, 20464, 20465, 20466, 20467

Robert J. Touloukian
10367, 10368, 10369, 10377, 10380

Philip L. Townes
10963

Elias Traboulsi
20533, 20591, 20592, 21272, 21361

Catherine Turleau
20901, 21334, 21335, 21336, 21337, 21338, 21339, 21340, 21341, 21342, 21343

L. H. S. Van Mierop
10235, 10236

Denis Viljoen
20004, 20005, 20006, 20007, 20011, 20023, 20024, 20025, 20074, 20075, 20076, 20077, 20605

Auguste Wackenheim
20331, 20332, 20333, 20334, 20335, 20336, 20337, 20338, 20339, 20340, 20341, 20342, 20343

Thomas A. Waldmann
10745

Colin E. Wallis
20586, 20587

Mette Warburg
10644, 10648

John Waterson
20535, 20536

David D. Weaver
20226, 20227, 21035, 21052

Avery Weiss
21118, 21119, 21120, 21121, 21122

Chester B. Whitley
20406, 20407, 20408, 20409

Peter Wieacker
20539

Hans-Rudolph Wiedemann
20448, 20449, 20450, 20451, 20452, 20453, 20582, 20583, 21061, 21062

Charles A. Williams
20495, 20990, 20991

R.S. Wilroy
12163, 12164, 21420

Golder N. Wilson
21175, 21176

Miriam G. Wilson
11354, 11355

A.M. Winchester
10345, 10355

Ingrid Winship
20641, 20642, 20643, 20644, 20645, 20646

Robin M. Winter
21066, 21069, 21070, 21071, 21250, 21251, 21252

Carl J. Witkop
10128, 10542, 10557, 10558, 10559, 10590, 10594, 10595, 10596, 10603, 10604, 10616, 10618, 11605, 11620, 11644, 11924, 20617, 20618, 20620, 20622, 20623, 20624, 20625, 21028, 21029, 21030, 21257, 21258, 21259, 21260, 21261

Beverly Phyllis Wood
11034, 11036, 11037

Yoshifumi Yamamoto
20680, 20681

Elaine H. Zackai
20999

Ismail Zayid
21234, 21235, 21236

Hans Zellweger
10788

Janice Zunich
21419